The Difficult Diagnosis in

Surgical Pathology

The Difficult Diagnosis in

Surgical Pathology

Noel Weidner, M.D.
Professor of Pathology
Chief, Surgical Pathology
University of California, San Francisco
San Francisco, California

W.B. SAUNDERS COMPANY
A Division of Harcourt Brace & Company
Philadelphia   London   Toronto   Montreal   Sydney   Tokyo

W.B. SAUNDERS COMPANY
A Division of
Harcourt Brace & Company

The Curtis Center
Independence Square West
Philadelphia, Pennsylvania 19106

Library of Congress Cataloging-in-Publication Data

The difficult diagnosis in surgical pathology   /   [edited by] Noel
Weidner.

        p.   cm.

    ISBN 0-7216-6464-4
    1. Pathology, Surgical.   I. Weidner, Noel.
    [DNLM: 1. Pathology, Surgical.   WO 142 D569 1996]

RD57.D54   1996   617'.075—dc20

DNLM/DLC   95–19481

The Difficult Diagnosis in Surgical Pathology   ISBN 0–7216–6464–4

Copyright © 1996 by W. B. Saunders Company

All rights reserved. No part of this publication may be reproduced or transmitted in any form or by any means, elec-
tronic or mechanical, including photocopy, recording, or any information storage and retrieval system, without permission in writing from the publisher.

Printed in the United States of America

Last digit is the print number: 9   8   7   6   5   4   3   2

Contributors

Daniel A. Arber, M.D.
  Staff Pathologist, City of Hope National Medical Center,
  Duarte, California
  Lymph Node

Kenneth W. Barwick, M.D.
  Chief of Anatomic Pathology, Baptist Medical Center,
  Jacksonville, Florida
  The Esophagus and Stomach

Kenneth P. Batts, M.D.
  Assistant Professor of Pathology, Mayo Medical School;
  Consultant, Department of Pathology and Laboratory
  Medicine, Mayo Clinic, Rochester, Minnesota
  The Esophagus and Stomach

John K. C. Chan, M.B.B.S., M.R.C.Path., F.R.C.P.A.
  Consultant Pathologist, Queen Elizabeth Hospital,
  Kowloon, Hong Kong
  Uterus and Fallopian Tubes

Karen L. Chang, M.D.
  Staff Pathologist, City of Hope National Medical Center,
  Duarte, California
  Lymph Node

Cheryl M. Coffin, M.D.
  Associate Professor, University of Utah School of
  Medicine; Chief, Department of Pathology, Primary
  Children's Medical Center, Salt Lake City, Utah
  *Diagnostic Challenges in Soft Tissue Pathology: A
  Clinicopathologic Review of Selected Lesions*

Carolyn C. Compton, M.D., Ph.D.
  Associate Professor of Pathology, Harvard Medical
  School; Associate Pathologist, Director of
  Gastrointestinal Pathology, Massachusetts General
  Hospital, Boston, Massachusetts
  Diseases of the Pancreas

P. Anthony di Sant'Agnese, M.D.
  Professor of Pathology and Laboratory Medicine,
  Director of Surgical Pathology, University of Rochester
  Medical Center, Rochester, New York
  The Genitourinary Tract

Diane C. Farhi, M.D.
  Associate Professor of Pathology, Emory University
  School of Medicine; Director of Hematopathology,
  Emory University Hospital, Atlanta, Georgia
  Bone Marrow; The Spleen

Linda D. Ferrell, M.D.
  Professor of Pathology, University of California, San
  Francisco, San Francisco, California
  *Colon, Appendix, and Anorectum; Liver and Gallbladder
  Pathology*

Elliott Foucar, M.D.
  Clinical Associate Professor of Pathology and
  Dermatology, University of New Mexico School of
  Medicine; Director of Surgical Pathology, Presbyterian
  Hospital, Albuquerque, New Mexico
  Diagnostic Decision-Making in Surgical Pathology

Ronald L. Goldman, M.D.*
  Clinical Associate Professor, Department of Pathology,
  University of California, San Francisco, San Francisco,
  California
  Diseases of the Ovary and Pelvic Peritoneum; Triviomas

Samuel Hensley, M.D.
  Neuropathologist, Mississippi Baptist Medical Center,
  Jackson, Mississippi
  The Central Nervous System

James K. Kelly, M.B., B.Ch., B.A.O., F.R.C.Path.
  Vice Chief, Department of Laboratories, Chief of
  Anatomical Pathology, Greater Victoria Hospital Society,
  Victoria, British Columbia, Canada
  Colon, Appendix, and Anorectum

---

* Deceased

Michael Kyriakos, M.D.
Professor of Pathology, Washington University School of Medicine; Pathologist, Barnes Hospital, St. Louis, Missouri
Diagnostic Challenges in Soft Tissue Pathology: A Clinicopathologic Review of Selected Lesions

Janice M. Lage, M.D.
Professor of Pathology, Director of Surgical Pathology, Georgetown University Medical Center, Washington, D.C.
Placenta and Gestational Trophoblastic Disease

Philip E. LeBoit, M.D.
Associate Professor of Clinical Pathology and Dermatology, University of California, San Francisco, San Francisco, California
Dermatopathology

L. Jeffrey Medeiros, M.D.
Associate Professor of Pathology, Brown University School of Medicine; Director, Hematopathology, Rhode Island Hospital, Providence, Rhode Island
Adrenal Gland: Tumors and Tumor-Like Lesions

Clara E. Mesonero, M.D.
Assistant Professor of Pathology and Laboratory Medicine, University of Rochester Medical Center, Rochester, New York
The Genitourinary Tract

Cesar A. Moran, M.D.
Chief, Mediastinal Pathology, Department of Pulmonary and Mediastinal Pathology, Armed Forces Institute of Pathology, Washington, D.C.
Pulmonary System

Shirin Nash, M.D.
Associate Professor, Tufts University School of Medicine, Boston, Massachusetts; Associate Pathologist, Baystate Medical Center, Springfield, Massachusetts
Small Intestine

Joseph A. Regezi, D.D.S., M.S.
Professor, Oral Pathology and Pathology, University of California, San Francisco, San Francisco, California
Head and Neck

James G. Smirniotopoulos, M.D.
Associate Professor of Radiology and Nuclear Medicine, Uniformed Services University of the Health Services; Senior Scientist and Chief of Neuroradiology, Armed Forces Institute of Pathology, Washington, D.C.
The Central Nervous System

Saul Suster, M.D.
Associate Clinical Professor of Pathology, University of Miami School of Medicine, Miami, Florida; Director of Surgical Pathology, Arkadi M. Rywlin Department of Pathology and Laboratory Medicine, Mount Sinai Medical Center of Greater Miami, Miami Beach, Florida
Mediastinal Pathology

Paul E. Swanson, M.D.
Assistant Professor of Pathology, Washington University School of Medicine, St. Louis, Missouri
Diagnostic Challenges in Soft Tissue Pathology: A Clinicopathologic Review of Selected Lesions

William Y. W. Tsang, M.B.B.S., F.R.C.P.A.
Senior Pathologist, Department of Pathology, Queen Elizabeth Hospital, Kowloon, Hong Kong
Uterus and Fallopian Tubes

Noel Weidner, M.D.
Professor of Pathology, Chief, Surgical Pathology, University of California, San Francisco, San Francisco, California
Head and Neck; Diseases of the Ovary and Pelvic Peritoneum; Breast Diseases; Triviomas

Lawrence M. Weiss, M.D.
Director, Surgical Pathology, City of Hope National Medical Center, Duarte, California
Adrenal Gland: Tumors and Tumor-Like Lesions; Lymph Node

Barbara C. Wolf, M.D.
Associate Professor of Pathology and Laboratory Medicine, Albany Medical College; Director of Anatomic Pathology and Hematopathology, Albany Medical Center, Albany, New York
The Spleen

Charles Zaloudek, M.D.
Professor of Clinical Pathology, University of California, San Francisco, San Francisco, California
The Vulva, Vagina, and Cervix

Preface

Arriving at a correct diagnosis is generally a routine matter in the majority of cases presented to the surgical pathologist. Usually the major requirement of the pathologist is that he or she pay close attention to detail, as when assessing specimen margins or in determining the presence or absence of lymph node metastases. Nevertheless, as many as 5% to 10% of cases (depending on your practice situation) pose difficult diagnostic problems for which the pathologist will have to seek assistance, either by reviewing the existing literature related to the case or by consulting with colleagues. Although a number of first-rate surgical pathology textbooks provide general information on a vast array of common lesions, because of space limitations, most do not provide in-depth discussions on uncommon lesions or difficult diagnostic situations.

This book, *The Difficult Diagnosis in Surgical Pathology,* fills that gap. It was conceived as an extension of the more general textbooks of surgical pathology. When the information in the general texts regarding a particular diagnostic situation has been exhausted, *The Difficult Diagnosis in Surgical Pathology* will provide added insight. In this multi-authored textbook, pathologists with special expertise in various organ systems focus on many diagnostic problems that they have confronted in their own practices and expand the current fund of knowledge available on them. Among the many kinds of diagnostic problems discussed are atypical presentations of common lesions (e.g., morphologic variants or presentation in unusual sites); uncommon and/or obscure lesions that may not be well known to general pathologists; and different lesions with similar clinicopathologic features that can arise in an organ but that, for therapeutic and prognostic reasons, must be clearly differentiated from each other. Virtually all organ systems are covered except bone; however, by virtue of the rarity of bone lesions in general, they are best covered in textbooks devoted exclusively to bone pathology. Pertinent endocrine lesions are covered within the appropriate organ systems.

Even a large text such as this, exclusively devoted to diagnostic problems in surgical pathology, cannot be all-inclusive because of space limitations. Thus, the authors have described diagnostic settings that they have encountered with some degree of relative frequency. Extensive reference lists are also included to provide sources for information on many other rare lesions not extensively discussed here.

Finally, this is our first edition, and the editor welcomes your comments for improving the text in the future. In the interim, please enjoy *The Difficult Diagnosis in Surgical Pathology.*

NOEL WEIDNER, M.D.
Professor of Pathology
Chief, Surgical Pathology
University of California, San Francisco
505 Parnassus Avenue
San Francisco, California 94143-0102

Contents

CHAPTER 1

Diagnostic Decision-Making in Surgical Pathology

Elliott Foucar, M.D.

The ability to translate findings on a glass slide into clinically useful information is referred to in surgical pathology as having an "eye" for tissue evaluation. The diagnostic "eye" encompasses both the factual foundation and the problem-solving skills of surgical pathology and therefore symbolizes the domain of expertise that provides the justification for the clinical specialty of surgical pathology.

It is self-evident that pathologists have wide variation in their factual knowledge base. However, data collection and manipulation skills, which represent the "art" of surgical pathology, also are quite variable from one individual to another. Some internists and some radiologists[1-3] have made efforts to establish an intellectual foundation for the study of problem-solving in their specialty areas, but surgical pathologists share with the majority of their clinical colleagues a lack of interest in the *methods* used to apply facts to diagnostic problems. In part, this lack of interest results because there is no comprehensive description of diagnostic decision-making in an area of this complexity, and in fact, there is no generally accepted theory of complex problem-solving.

Can the art of surgical pathology be taught, i.e., is there a scientific basis for obvious differences in diagnostic skills, or is diagnostic decision-making just a semi-mystical combination of intuition, speculation, and anecdotes that some residents "get" after a period of exposure, and some do not? It is certainly possible that even routine diagnosis is essentially an art form that cannot be productively studied except by evaluating the final product of the process, i.e., the diagnosis. However, this concept of the diagnostic process as highly individual, idiosyncratic behavior is in conflict with the expectations of our clinical colleagues, who strongly feel that like findings should receive like diagnoses. It is also in conflict with the self-image of many surgical pathologists, who are justifiably proud of their rigorous, scientific approach to diagnosis.

The underlying premise of this chapter is that the successful approach to diagnostic decisions in surgical pathology should be pursued as a science, in spite of our current inadequate ability to offer precise definitions and explanations. This study of diagnosis requires a reductionist approach, in which a complex system is broken down into its parts and their interactions with each other. Those pathologists reluctant to accept this seemingly simplistic approach should offer an alternative. The development of a viable diagnostic science is an important goal that heretofore has received far too little attention.

TYPES OF DIAGNOSTIC PROBLEMS

In order to attempt a discussion of the nuts and bolts of diagnosis, it must be recognized at the start that the intellectual processes used to approach routine and complex cases are quite different.[4] For routine cases, the surgical pathologist uses straightforward techniques that are sometimes referred to as "deterministic." Although each case in medicine is unique in some way, in fact, in all relevant details, the experienced surgical pathologist has seen most cases many times before. The problem solver makes use of standard solutions that have already proved their value in previous cases and applies these solutions to new, apparently similar cases. Features of these routine cases become part of a well-structured knowledge base that can be accessed rapidly and efficiently. These typical situations, sometimes referred to as "prototypes of the profession,"[5] are stored in memory as "chunks" of information, i.e., combinations of familiar stimuli that after repeated exposure become recognizable as units or patterns.[6] Individuals with similar training can be expected to apply the same facts and decision-making methods to these deterministic cases, resulting in a very high rate of diagnostic agreement.

In every practice, in addition to these deterministic cases there are randomly admixed cases that do not allow the surgical pathologist, no matter what his or her level of expertise, to treat the case as routine. For these latter cases, the surgical pathologist does not have a solution available in memory or in readily available texts or papers. Making a diagnosis calls for a novel action, a new application of available information, or simply a best guess. Some of these difficult cases masquerade as just another case to approach with deterministic diagnostic methods, whereas others are recognized from the outset as something new and different. In one major subtype of difficult case, there is an ill-defined threshold for establishing a clinically significant diagnosis. The differential diagnostic considerations are obvious, but the threshold is not clear-cut.[7] The second major subtype of difficult case is one in which distinctive findings are identified, but the pathologist does not have a personal experience with such findings and is not aware of pertinent literature. For these latter cases, the pathologist must locate the pertinent literature, or determine that no literature presently exists that will directly assist in diagnosis. Variation in diagnosis is a not unexpected outcome of the evaluation of these difficult cases.

Interestingly, the major educational goal of the surgical pathologist is to master easily applied rules that move problems out of the realm of complex decision-making and into the realm of deterministic reasoning. For example, on the first day of the residency, virtually every case requires complex decision-making skills, and the resident often spends a great deal of time examining even straightforward slides in an exhaustive effort to obtain all information possible.[8] As training progresses, the resident is able to use "chunks" of diagnostically useful information to rapidly solve routine diagnostic problems. The subspecialist with a large referral practice provides an extreme example of the conversion of cases from difficult to deterministic. Certain "once in a decade" cases for most of us may be the daily contents of the "in" basket, and these cases are approached by the consultant not as problems requiring complex decision-making but rather as routine. Because the consultant may go through the differential diagnostic possibilities for a certain type of "once in a decade" case several times a week, he or she can avoid the treacherous waters of complex decision-making and simply handle the case in a deterministic fashion—seemingly having turbocharged the decision-making process. Deterministic reasoning does not guarantee a "correct" result, but does considerably narrow the diagnostic variation that is an inherent consequence of complex decision-making.

OVERVIEW OF TOOLS OF DIAGNOSTIC DECISION-MAKING

Although each case, whether difficult or routine, has unique features, the diagnostician has standard tools that are applied to case evaluation. The major tools are the following: (1) diagnostic rules of thumb, (2) data collection and valuation, and (3) hypothesis manipulation skills, i.e., activation, evaluation, and verification.

For routine cases, at the very simplest level, the process condenses to "If I see A, the diagnosis is B." Such deterministic cases have been described as instant pattern recognition or glance diagnosis cases, and the diagnostic steps are rapid and inapparent. In contrast, for the difficult case, the use of diagnostic tools is readily apparent, and because of variation in case features, successful diagnosis emphasizes different diagnostic tools. For example, if the clinical or morphologic findings of the disease are quite subtle, the case may require finely honed data collection skills. In contrast, a diagnosis may hinge on a morphologic abnormality that is quite prominent but of obscure significance, placing emphasis on hypothesis activation skills. Some difficult cases will be solved when a diagnostic heuristic leads in the correct direction.

Complex decision-making uses poorly defined factors such as "luck," "intuition," "flair," or "imaginative insight." However, as Peter Medawar pointed out when discussing the role of such factors in basic research, a lottery winner has actively become eligible for luck by purchasing a ticket.[9] In surgical pathology, eligibility for diagnostic luck generally derives from years of effort to improve the application of the basic diagnostic tools.

Heuristics

Problem-solving heuristics, or judgment heuristics, are the thousands of rules of thumb arising directly out of thoughtful experience.[10, 11] These rules are used to organize the diagnostic process. "If I see squamous metaplasia of prostatic glandular epithelium, I should think of infarction and begin looking for other supportive findings." Heuristics have been learned through trial and error in similar cases, or through exposure to journals, teachers, textbooks, or other sources. Tested rules allow data gathering (e.g., looking at slides, talking to clinicians, reviewing laboratory data), hypothesis activation, and hypothesis testing to proceed with an efficient, often parallel attack on a diagnostic problem, rather than as separate sequential steps. During the diagnostic process, heuristics organize rapid switches between information acquisition, hypothesis activation, and hypothesis verification, enabling the specific pursuit of appropriate additional information by branching the diagnostic process in fruitful directions. Heuristics are constantly tested and modified in the course of diagnostic work, with failed heuristics discarded, and successful heuristics modified to include new information and techniques that prove to be valuable. For example, there are published lists of routine histologic heuristics that are currently used to aid in the distinction between melanoma and Spitz nevus.[12, 13] In the past, similar lists of light microscopic heuristics were used to distinguish between large cell lymphoma and undifferentiated carcinoma.[14] Since the 1980s, these latter heuristics have been largely replaced by the heuristics that guide the immunoperoxidase evaluation of large cell malignancies.

Data Collection

When examining a glass slide, the surgical pathologist must first detect an abnormality before this feature can be identified and then used to support or refute diagnostic possibilities.[15] Clearly, the diagnostic process is largely driven by the data that are collected, and marked differences in the native ability to collect data are readily apparent (Table 1–1). Information-gathering skills vary from the almost purely visual (e.g., detecting on a glass slide a specific feature with diagnostic usefulness) to complex techniques of abnormality identification. Heuristics guide the process of data collection by directing the surgical pathologist's attention to the diagnostically useful features of the slide.[16] Without a heuristic that says "Look for X in Y situation," a finding on the glass slide will often become part of "background." The pathologists of my generation who for years looked at sections of stomach without ever noting *Helicobacter* will agree with this opinion, as will those who never noted koilocytosis in cervical biopsies or never noted nuclear grooves or nuclear inclusions in papillary carcinoma of the thyroid.

In general, successful diagnosticians divide the useful surgical pathology observations into mini-tests. The simplest tests involve evaluation of discrete variables—those that can take on only a limited number of values, and the simplest of these are binary (i.e., they have two possible results labeled "positive" and "negative").[1, 17] An example is evaluation of a lymph node for the presence of metastatic disease. However, most histologic observations are continuous variables (e.g., glandular architecture) that must be arbitrarily transformed

Table 1–1. **Variation in Routine Slide Data Collection Skills**

Level of Ability	Definition	Example
I	Consistently discovers clinically unexpected subtle findings	Discovers a rare small granuloma in the myometrium of a routine hysterectomy specimen
II	Lacks Level I ability, but consistently discovers clinically expected subtle findings	Discovers a rare granuloma in a liver biopsy submitted to rule out primary biliary cirrhosis
III	Lacks Level II ability, but discovers subtle findings when told that the findings are present	Finds a granuloma in a colon biopsy when told that the biopsy contains a granuloma
IV	Lacks Level III ability, and has difficulty detecting subtle findings when told that they are present	Cannot find a granuloma in an appendiceal germinal center when told that a slide shows this finding

into discrete variables (e.g., normal, atypical, highly atypical, malignant) in order to have an associated useful diagnostic value. If "prominent" nucleoli are to be used to distinguish between well-differentiated prostatic adenocarcinoma and adenosis, one must devise a threshold measurement on the continuum of nucleolar size by which a nucleolus will become "prominent."[18] Successful data collection requires **technical sensitivity** (finding or detecting important things that are hard to find), **technical specificity** (ignoring look-alikes), and **precision** (consistency in the interpretation of identical findings).

In addition to the enormous amount of visual information on surgical pathology slides, the surgical pathologist often has available numerous separate and distinct additional sources of information—the clinical laboratory, the clinician, radiology findings, and so on—and the experienced diagnostician uses all of these data together with the histopathologic findings in the diagnostic process. Data are collected in a seemingly disorganized fashion from these various sources and is used to modify the strength of belief in existing hypotheses. The skipping around in data acquisition is legitimate and rational, and is generally organized by heuristics that have worked for the surgical pathologist in the past. In fact, when data from diverse sources support a certain hypothesis, there often is a much higher diagnostic certainty. For example, the likelihood of defining the specific significance of a histopathologic abnormality such as lymphocyte epidermotropism is greatly improved by knowing such information as patient age, duration and clinical appearance of the skin lesions, and the presence or absence of circulating Sézary cells. With complete clinical information, a difficult histopathologic diagnosis can sometimes become quite straightforward.

Assignment of Value to Data

The differing value of individual data elements prompts different responses during the data-gathering process. Often

a new piece of data becomes available that activates the heuristic "If you see A, then look for B." For example, a prostate biopsy specimen with an area of small, crowded glands immediately prompts a search for large nucleoli. Other data may have such a high diagnostic value to the experienced diagnostician that they either end the process by "clinching" the diagnosis or, alternatively, lead to a completely new approach to data-gathering by decreasing the likelihood of or even excluding previously plausible hypotheses. A positive HMB-45 stain obtained in the course of evaluating what had been thought to be an atypical histiocytic proliferation within a lymph node is an example. The value of diagnostic data is largely dependent on their ability to distinguish among the diagnostic alternatives. Ideally a finding would always be present in patients with the disease in question and would never be present in patients who do not have this disease. In practice, very few histopathologic observations have this high diagnostic value.

Before a finding can be useful in the diagnostic process, the surgical pathologist must know the probability that this finding will be present in the proposed disease and, conversely, must know the probability that this finding may incorrectly identify an individual who does not have the disease. Is the positive HMB-45 in and of itself such a valuable finding that it is diagnostic of melanoma in an atypical nodal sinus proliferation? What if the patient is a 12-year-old with no evident atypical cutaneous pigmented lesion? Without a reproducible system to attribute diagnostic value to data, the diagnostic process founders. How is this value assignment accomplished?

Even though, except in the very simplest of settings, clinical diagnosis cannot be reduced to specific probabilities or numbers, skilled diagnosticians have the ability to develop useful probability estimates. Most discussions of this topic focus on sensitivity and specificity, but predictive value can also be used to value data. Successful diagnosis is largely based on an intuitive understanding of how application of these statistical concepts allows the surgical pathologist to determine how each new piece of data collected during the diagnostic process increases or decreases the probability of each diagnostic consideration. Table 1–2 illustrates the definitions of these basic statistical terms with an example from the current literature in which the authors investigated the value of Leu-M1 in distinguishing primary adenocarcinoma of the lung from mesothelioma.[19]

Instead of looking at diagnostic data in terms of their sensitivity, specificity, or predictive value, some authors prefer to estimate the likelihood of a certain finding in the disease of interest, and then to compare this likelihood to the likelihood of the same finding in patients without the disease in question, resulting in a likelihood ratio.[20, 21] For example, it is potentially of diagnostic interest that papillary carcinoma of the thyroid has "Orphan Annie" nuclei as a "constant" finding.[22] However, clinical studies have shown that physicians differ markedly in their interpretation of such terms as *rarely*, *often*, and so on, and presumably pathologists have the same problem.[23] Until it is known how likely clear nuclei are to be present in both papillary carcinoma and lesions that may be confused with papillary carcinoma, the information is difficult to use diagnostically. One study found clear nuclei in 83% of cases of papillary carcinoma, and such nuclear changes were also present in approximately 5% of a group of 62 other lesions

Table 1–2. **Statistical Definitions, Using Leu-M1 in Adenocarcinoma of Lung vs. Mesothelioma as an Example**

Item	Group Studied	Descriptive Definition	Definition
Sensitivity* or "true-positive rate"	Individuals with the target disorder	Frequency of a positive test result among those patients with the disease of interest, expressed as a percentage	TP/(TP + FN) × 100‡
Example§	Individuals with primary adenocarcinoma of the lung	Percentage of lung cancer patients tested who had a positive Leu-M1	79/(79 + 24) × 100 = 77%
Specificity† or "true-negative rate"	Individuals without the target disorder	Frequency of a negative test result in those patients without the disease of interest, expressed as a percentage	TN/(TN + FP) × 100‡
Example§	Individuals with mesothelioma	Percentage of mesothelioma patients tested who had a negative Leu-M1	32/(32 + 2) × 100 = 94%
Predictive value positive	Individuals with a positive result in the test of interest	Frequency of disease of interest among those patients with a positive test result, expressed as a percentage	TP/(TP + FP) × 100‡
Example§	Individuals with a positive Leu-M1 and either adenocarcinoma of the lung or mesothelioma	Percentage of total positive results that are attributed to patients with adenocarcinoma	79/(79 + 2) × 100 = 97%
Predictive value negative	Individuals with a negative result in the test of interest	Frequency of lack of the disease of interest among those patients with a negative test result, expressed as a percentage	TN/(TN + FN) × 100‡
Example§	Individuals with a negative Leu-M1 and either adenocarcinoma of the lung or mesothelioma	Percentage of total negative results that are attributed to patients with adenocarcinoma	32/(32 + 24) × 100 = 57%

* Sensitivity should not be confused with analytical sensitivity, which is the ability to detect a small amount of substance (or cells).
† Specificity should not be confused with analytical specificity, which is the ability of an analytical method to detect a single target substance and no other.
‡ TP, true-positive; TN, true-negative; FP, false-positive; FN, false-negative.
§ Example of the usefulness of Leu-M1 to identify adenocarcinoma of the lung when the differential diagnosis is restricted to mesothelioma and when patients with adenocarcinoma are approximately three times as common as are patients with mesothelioma.
Data from Brown RW, Clark GM, Tandon AK, et al: Multiple-marker immunohistochemical phenotypes distinguish malignant pleural mesothelioma from pulmonary adenocarcinoma. Hum Pathol 24:347–354, 1993.

(follicular adenomas, follicular carcinoma, diffuse hyperplasia).[24] The presence of the "Orphan Annie" nuclei feature by itself, when used in the diagnostic setting described in the paper, would then have a likelihood ratio (true-positive rate/false-positive rate) of 16.6, favoring a diagnosis of papillary thyroid carcinoma. If, based on information gathered prior to looking for clear nuclei, the pathologist felt that the odds of the patient having papillary carcinoma were 1:1, then the finding of clear nuclei would modify these odds in the following manner:[25]

Pretest odds for papillary carcinoma		Likelihood ratio		Post-test odds for papillary carcinoma
1:1	×	16.6	=	16.6:1

The post-test odds or probability for one observation becomes the pretest odds for a second, independent diagnostic observation.

If a finding is just as likely in persons without the target disease as it is in those with the target disease, the finding has no effect on the probability that the patient has the target disease. When a finding is more common in people who do not have the disease in question than it is in patients who do have this disease, the likelihood ratio is less than one. The ratio rises toward infinity as a finding becomes progressively more likely in a certain disease and progressively less likely in patients who do not have that disease. This likelihood ratio model for assigning value to data is quite intuitive, and in fact closely resembles the thought processes of experienced diagnosticians.

Hypothesis Activation, Evaluation, and Verification

The process of hypothesis activation, also known as diagnostic triggering, begins at the very earliest stages of the diagnostic process, when perhaps only scant clinical information and/or initial morphologic findings are available.[26] These provisional hypotheses serve as organizers for data collection, resulting in a manageable number of categories under which findings are "filed."[27] Once a diagnostic hypothesis has been activated, there is established an expectation of what things should be present and what things should not be present if the patient in fact has the disease in question.

Rather than functioning as a "factual vacuum cleaner" to deal with the flood of diagnostic data, the morphologist engages in organized and meaningful observations that are designed to evaluate these preliminary hypotheses.[28] A blank mind ritualistically collecting information about a "tumor" of the ovary will be unlikely to notice nuclear grooves of tumor cells, but this finding may be quite obvious if the diagnosis of adult granulosa cell tumor is activated as a possibility.[29] It is a common experience that features suddenly become visible once the expectation of their presence has been established by a hypothesis.

Only a limited number of hypotheses (approximately 4 ± 2 in clinical decision-making studies) can be entertained at any one time, and information is gathered to build a case for (corroborative) or against (refutative) the most likely candidates.[27, 29] The diagnostician searches for high-value data among an essentially infinite number of clinical and pathologic signals, attempting to shorten the list of hypotheses, and to follow the shortest diagnostic pathway to a single diagnostic threshold. While following this shortest diagnostic pathway, the diagnostician must keep active the hypothesis "some other disease"—maintaining an open mind to subtle morphologic or clinical information that would suggest a new working hypothesis. The use of reliable heuristics to activate new hypotheses and to quickly change the direction of the morphologic investigation is one distinguishing characteristic of the experienced morphologist. Heuristics activated by the hypothesis then assist the surgical pathologist in selecting the smallest subset of variables that contains all of the discriminating information necessary to confirm the hypothesis—or at least to establish a best-guess diagnosis.

Just as it is critical that "value" be assigned to data collected during the diagnostic process, it is also critical that some reproducible system be developed to assign value or "probability of correctness" to hypotheses, and to modify this probability as data are collected. In statistical terms, the probability that a hypothesis is correct lies somewhere on a scale of 0 (certain not to be correct) to 1.0 (certain to be correct),[30] but in practice, the results are often qualitative, ranging from "very unlikely to be the diagnosis" through various shades of "maybe" to an "established" diagnosis. If you know nothing about the patient, the prior probability of a target disease is simply the prevalence of the disease in the population from which the patient was drawn. You modify this basic prevalence (probability) when, for example, you reason even before looking at node biopsy sections that a large lymph node in the left axilla of a 59-year-old woman may contain tumor from a clinically occult breast cancer. An informal value or prior probability that the patient has metastatic breast cancer is assigned to this hypothesis. Each important new piece of clinical or morphologic information alters this prior probability that the patient has breast cancer, producing a new posterior probability. For example, the probability of breast cancer as an explanation for this patient's nodal disease becomes relatively lower if you learn that 3 years ago she had a deep nodular melanoma of the left arm. In contrast, the probability of breast carcinoma would have been modified upward if it were found that the patient had a mammographically suspicious lesion in the left breast. The mathematical model that describes the degree of change of diagnostic probabilities as incremental data are collected and evaluated is usually referred to as Bayes' theorem.[31] Simplistically, the theorem allows calculation of the probability that a patient belongs to a given clinical class, given the presence of a certain finding or test result.[32] Even though no one uses the exact formulas in diagnostic work, because neither exact prior probabilities for hypotheses nor exact sensitivities and specificities for most clinical observations are available, the *underlying* principles are generally used. As additional clinical, laboratory, and morphologic data are accumulated, diagnostic success is dependent on knowing how each of the additional pieces of information, individually and as a group, modify the likelihood of each of the diagnostic possibilities.

In a simple case, the diagnostician can quickly follow available data (clinical algorithm or mapping approach) to an established diagnosis, or the sequential, iterative process can occur over hours, days, or even weeks.[33, 34] However, simultaneous assessment of multiple variables (pattern recognition approach) is also an important component of hypothesis evaluation. In the pattern recognition approach, multiple facts (often from various sources in addition to the glass slides) are collected within a short period of time, and these facts fit a diagnostic heuristic, resulting in rapid diagnosis, seemingly in a single step of deterministic logic. In Bayesian terms, deterministic diagnoses are characterized by a rapid leap from prior probability to a confirmatory posterior probability. The skilled diagnostician rapidly changes diagnostic approaches to deal with the evolving data base, moving back and forth between the sequential assessment of data and the simultaneous, often deterministic assessment of data. Usually these changes in diagnostic approach are made without conscious recognition that different methods are being used.

A diagnosis can be considered to be confirmed when it is the simplest explanation that accounts for all the patient's major normal and abnormal findings. Because diagnosis is probabilistic, diagnoses are made with more or less confidence.[35] Achieving a diagnostic threshold usually means combining or synthesizing the diagnostic value of multiple variables to satisfy the requirements of a hypothesis-confirming heuristic. Making a positive diagnosis requires selecting a threshold along the scale of evidence, with values above the threshold level leading to a positive diagnosis, and those below being negative. Thresholds become a problem for the surgical pathologist when significant numbers of cases have features in the region of but not clearly beyond the threshold, and yet crossing the threshold significantly changes the clinical approach to the patient, perhaps initiating a cascade of intervention. Breast and prostate[36] biopsies provide everyday examples of the phenomenon in which a meaningful threshold is difficult to establish for some cases. Unfortunately, the patient and the clinician can be confused when lesions on either side of a threshold have very similar histopathologic features but very different names (e.g., atypical hyperplasia or carcinoma).

USING DIAGNOSTIC LABELS FOR PREDICTION

One of the major benefits of the "scientific" approach to problems is the ability to make useful predictions, and it is clear that one of the major expectations of both patients and their physicians is that the surgical pathology report will provide some foreknowledge or at least a reasonable expectation of the future. However, the entire area of prediction is fraught with confusion.[37] How is it possible that in 1705, the English astronomer Edmond Halley successfully predicted that the comet that now bears his name would return in 1758, but in modern America patients who have been told that they have 6 months to live sometimes attend their physicians' funerals years later?

It must first be recognized that Halley's problem was of an entirely different magnitude of complexity than the one facing individuals attempting to make predictions in such fields as economics, the weather, or biology, where large numbers of variables often make problems intractable.[38] Additionally, there is an important distinction between predictions for a group, and predictions for an individual within that group. This distinction is well understood by the soothsayers whose predictions line the supermarket checkout lines.[39] For example, these soothsayers know that predicting a calamity will befall a certain politician during the coming year is quite a long shot, even given specific knowledge of the individual's propensity for self-destructive behavior. In contrast, predicting that calamity will befall an as yet unnamed individual who is part of the risk group "famous persons" during the same year is essentially a sure thing.

At the same time that we recognize that making specific predictions in complex systems is a truly daunting task, we know that selected types of predictions in such systems are in fact quite easy. For example, I predict that most January nights in Minneapolis in the year 2000 will be very cold. I predict that the stock market is not going to do well in the short term if inflation is running at 20% and unemployment is 30%. I predict that a patient with lung cancer associated with positive mediastinal lymph nodes and bone and lung metastases will not survive for very long. Exceptions are possible, especially in a biologic system, but such predictions are "Halley predictions," i.e., I have in hand all the variables necessary to make a correct statement.

Some of the problems in using surgical pathology reports to make predictions derive from a misunderstanding of the characteristics of the group that the diagnosis identifies. When a surgical pathology report notes the presence in a patient's liver of multiple metastases from colon cancer, the information can be used to make very specific predictions about the future of that individual patient. What predictive value does my report have for a specific patient when it notes focal non-necrotizing intraductal carcinoma of the female breast? Will psychological harm be done to the patient when she is labeled as a cancer victim?[40] If we accept as externally valid the papers stating that this patient is now a member of a group known to be at an increased risk for the development of invasive carcinoma, which of the currently therapeutic options available to that patient can be applied with confidence that this therapy will lead to a better clinical outcome for the patient than will no therapy at all? When the surgical pathology report on a prostate needle biopsy notes the presence of focal well-differentiated adenocarcinoma of the prostate in a 70-year-old man, what are the implications for the patient's future? An extreme and unworkable view is that if everyone in a diagnostic category (e.g., measured level of melanoma invasion) does not have the same clinical outcome, then why even use this technique to divide patients into prognostic groups?[41] Just as dysfunctional is the view that if a diagnosis places the patient in a group with elevated risk, then the patient should be approached therapeutically as if it is known that the patient will experience the negative outcome that the group is at risk for. In order to play the prediction game, the surgical pathologist must have some knowledge about whether a diagnosis makes a Halley prediction about the patient or simply puts the patient in a risk category with a significant "p" value—but insignificant "c" (clinical) value.

METHODS FOR DIAGNOSTIC IMPROVEMENT

Diagnosis in clinical medicine has been described as the process of making adequate diagnoses with inadequate information.[42] While those of us who practice morphologic diagnosis may feel our decisions are better founded on hard data than those of our clinical colleagues, our diagnostic process

is certainly a long way from the world of the basic scientist. Nevertheless, the decision-making of successful surgical pathologists shows organized patterns of behavior that are continually being refined by the daily successes and failures of the diagnostic experience. For the most skillful diagnosticians, the diagnostic experience is used to improve diagnostic tools through an informal program of continuous diagnostic improvement. This activity is analogous to the process of continuous quality improvement that industry has pioneered to produce "quality" products.[43] In surgical pathology, this quality product is the diagnostic "label" that best serves the needs of our patients. Key to the development of a successful program of continuous diagnostic improvement is an understanding of the limitations and pitfalls of each of our diagnostic tools. At the simplest level, diagnostic improvement is achieved by moving cases out of the realm of complex decision-making and into the routine. Yesterday's difficult case that was solved using complex decision-making becomes part of the deterministic repertoire of the surgical pathologist. The failure of the diagnostic improvement process is marked by the permanent division of cases into (1) cases that I can diagnose with repeatedly proven deterministic techniques, and (2) cases that someone else should tell me the answer to.

Heuristics

The best defense against diagnostic errors is a continuous evaluation of diagnostic heuristics through diagnostic experience and literature review. The process of modifying existing heuristics, discarding failed heuristics, and adding new ones is central to continuous diagnostic improvement. Biases that damage the value of heuristics and consequently lead to diagnostic dysfunction have been well described.[44, 45] A few of the major biases are described below:

1. *Availability.* Heuristics can be inappropriately applied because of their availability in memory rather than their appropriateness for the case under consideration. Slightly pink vessels or stroma may reliably bring to mind the possibility of amyloid, but further pursuit of that heuristic may be appropriate only occasionally. An easily remembered diagnostic heuristic can be mistakenly thought to have a higher probability of being appropriate to the diagnostic problem than a heuristic that is difficult to recall. However, availability in memory is often affected by factors other than likelihood of disease. For example, if the consequences of past failure to apply the heuristic were great, the heuristic may be applied in many circumstances where it is inappropriate—"just in case." Similarly, it is true that physicians are heavily influenced by the characteristics of their own easily remembered recent cases, in spite of the danger that these recent cases (because of sampling error) may have misleading features.

2. *Representativeness.* A patient is considered to be highly likely to have a certain disease when the features of the disease closely resemble the surgical pathologist's previous experience with that disease. In psychological terms, if a new instance is sufficiently similar to category members, then this new instance is itself likely to be a category member.[46] However, inaccurate heuristics can result when the diagnostician has had only a limited experience with a disease category, and this biased view results in biased heuristics and diagnostic dysfunction. A diagnostician who sees only five or six brain biopsies a year, most of which are straightforward primary or metastatic neoplasms, may be completely unaware that the clinical and pathologic presenting features of multiple sclerosis can overlap closely with those of glial neoplasms.[47] In order to acquire a realistic

view of the total spectrum of all but the most common diseases, personal experience must be supplemented by information from the literature, and diagnostic heuristics must be appropriately modified using this published information. It follows that acquiring the skills to interpret and apply the research done by others is a necessary skill for the practice of surgical pathology.

3. *Hindsight Bias.* This is a form of diagnostic overconfidence that occurs when a case is reviewed following the collection of additional relevant information. For example, knowledge that an event such as a metastasis has occurred can give the surgical pathologist the feeling that the event was inevitable, and the heuristics that would be used to evaluate the primary lesion if it were 1 of 50 cases in a day's work are sometimes abandoned. It is surprising how often a truly difficult case is judged to have been bungled at the time of original diagnosis, based not on the facts and findings available at the time but on the view through the "retrospectoscope."

Data Collection

Technical errors in tissue processing cause errors in both the detection and the identification of abnormalities and are the most basic cause of diagnostic difficulty in surgical pathology interpretation. If the information needed to establish a diagnosis simply is not on the slide because the specimen is small, crushed, poorly sectioned, or overstained, the surgical pathologist cannot contribute to an understanding of the patient's problem. Clumsy processing of a specimen sometimes creates so much "noise" that data "signals" are difficult to identify. If slides of poor technical quality are accompanied by misleading clinical clues that create inaccurate prior probabilities, the likelihood of a diagnostic error increases substantially.

In addition to technical preparation problems, the diagnostician should be aware that failures in data-gathering and therefore in hypothesis activation and verification often result directly from the characteristics of the data that we work with.

1. Our data are characterized by thresholds that are superficially similar to those of our clinical pathology colleagues. A bilirubin level can be normal or abnormal, and endometrial architecture can be benign or malignant. However, our data are more analogous to panels of clinical laboratory data, where there is often considerable information between major thresholds, and complex interactions between variables. Bilirubin level below a threshold is just "normal," while endometrial architecture below the malignant threshold may be proliferative, secretory, or atrophic, and multiple histologic features contribute to the assignment of an endometrial biopsy specimen to one of these categories.

2. Most data are continuous, and the distinction between normal and various stages of abnormal is often subjective both for quantitative data (e.g., number of mitoses per 10 high-power fields) and for descriptive data (e.g., atypia). Even when continuous morphologic data can be measured directly on the glass slide (e.g., the depth of invasion of melanoma), there can be significant technical problems in achieving a reproducible measurement. Critical points or break points are by definition arbitrary, and no rational person expects the individuals within prognostic groups to have a uniform outcome.[41, 48] Extreme examples on the spectrum of continuous data are usually easily identified, and interpretation is relatively easy because reliable estimates of the sensitivity/specificity of the observation can be culled from personal experience or from the literature. In contrast, the interpretation of morphologic or clinical abnormalities that are not extreme can be frustrating, with no clear guidelines available for determining what combination of abnormalities reaches a diagnostic threshold.

3. Some findings, such as stromal invasion, are always important, and must be explained by the final diagnosis. Other findings, such

as lymphocytes within a tumor, are conditionally important; i.e., in some settings the finding is critical, whereas in other settings it is of marginal importance or even trivial. Often the "setting" that modifies the value of variables, such as patient age, is itself on a continuous scale that does not have clear-cut thresholds.

4. Establishing a diagnosis generally requires multiple data elements, each of which often has the characteristics of (1), (2), and (3) above. This situation of multiple data elements is particularly troublesome when major clinical decisions depend on the subjective evaluation of multiple data continuums. It is well known that increasing the number of variables in a problem increases the likelihood that the problem will be intractable.[38]

5. A final problem in data collection seems to result from a built-in level of human error that is an expected part of all complex activity. Over the last year, I saw three fairly straightforward cutaneous melanomas that were all originally identified as nevi by three different pathologists, two of whom are dermatopathology subspecialty board–certified. Reading through the reports, it is apparent that in each case, it never crossed the pathologist's mind that the case was atypical, much less malignant. Because the atypical features were never noted, the hypothesis "Could this lesion be malignant?" was never activated. With regard to the problem of human error in the blood bank setting, Dr. Howard Taswell of the Mayo Clinic has stated: "No matter how much you reprimand or retrain a person, they are not going to improve over this low error rate. You now need to design a better system for technologists to work in."[49] Technology to alter the blood bank work environment, such as automated crossmatching and bar coding, is now being introduced, but no clear vision of how human error can be significantly reduced in surgical pathology has emerged. Some institutions have experimented with having multiple pathologists review selected cases, but as the melanoma example points out, problem cases are often those not thought initially to be a problem. Can we afford to have two pathologists review every case? If two is good, would five be better?

Diagnostic Value of Data

It is of critical importance in the interpretation of diagnostic data to understand that "specificity rules." High or low sensitivity is a secondary feature that makes a highly specific feature more or less valuable. Knowledge that a finding is present in a high percentage or even all of the examples of a certain disease (high sensitivity) becomes useful only when it is known that this finding is not present or is present only very infrequently in other disease states that could be confused with the diagnosis under consideration (high specificity or low false-positive rate). Unfortunately, whereas specificity data are the most valuable to the diagnostic process, sensitivity data are much easier to gather from the literature or from personal experience. Information about diagnostic sensitivity is sometimes presented in the literature in the following format: Of 100 cases of disease X, 89 had the finding Y. Unfortunately, without specificity data, this information is almost worthless.

EXAMPLE 1. A paper on Merkel cell tumor would reasonably tell us what percentage of Merkel cell tumors have a globular paranuclear keratin pattern (sensitivity of this finding) and would consider small cell carcinoma of the lung and lymphoma in the differential diagnosis (specificity).[50] But what if the patient has medullary carcinoma of the thyroid or some other "neuroendocrine" primary, and skin biopsy shows a small cell carcinoma with globular keratin? Knowing that globular keratin is a highly sensitive and specific feature of Merkel cell tumor when the differential diagnosis includes lymphoma and small cell carcinoma of the lung is not helpful. A new question concerning the specificity of globular paranuclear keratin has been raised, and must be answered before a diagnosis can be made.

EXAMPLE 2. A beginner evaluating a large, fast-growing soft tissue mass might attempt to support the diagnosis of nodular fasciitis by pointing to the lesion's numerous mitotic figures. Literature could easily be produced to show that mitoses are characteristic and to be expected, and therefore are highly sensitive for the identification of nodular fasciitis.[51] However, when malignancy is a consideration in the differential diagnosis, the finding of mitoses completely lacks specificity, and the variable "numerous mitoses present" is worthless for establishing the diagnosis of nodular fasciitis. In contrast, if the differential diagnosis is changed (e.g., "Is this nodular fasciitis or a scar?"), the mitotic variable does acquire some specificity and could be diagnostically useful.

EXAMPLE 3. Roses et al. base the histologic diagnosis of melanoma on a total of 20 architectural, cytologic, and adjunctive features found to be present in cases that they judged to be melanoma.[52] Unfortunately, one simply cannot make a diagnosis with sensitivity data, which is all that these authors are presenting. For example, 100% of melanomas will be characterized by the presence of cells and collagen, but this information is useless because all benign melanocytic lesions have these same findings. Each of these 20 features recorded by Roses et al. will be present in some (many?) melanomas. The specificity side of the issue is left to the reader, who must determine how often and to what degree some, many, or all of these features will be found in benign lesions that could be confused with melanoma.

Working with Hypotheses

HYPOTHESIS ACTIVATION. Routine hypothesis activation begins almost immediately in the diagnostic process and is data-driven. Activation can be improved both through improving data-gathering skills and through improving the heuristics that link specific data to specific diagnostic possibilities. It follows that common reasons for "I never thought of that diagnosis" include "I never saw that subtle finding" and "I didn't know to link that finding with that hypothesis." Hypothesis activation in difficult cases may require skills of creativity or intuition that perhaps cannot be acquired as a specific set of skills, but as Medawar has suggested, hypothesis activation can be encouraged by "acquiring the habit of reflection."[53] Clinical studies of the diagnostic process have found that the best predictor of arriving at a correct diagnosis is including the correct diagnosis among the initial ones considered.[54]

HYPOTHESIS EVALUATION. An accurate estimate of the prior probability of a certain disease greatly decreases the likelihood of diagnostic error, and an inaccurate initial estimate can poison the diagnostic process. It cannot be overemphasized that the interpretation of new information depends on beliefs held before the new information became available, in part because there is a tendency to "anchor" or become inflexible about estimated disease probability very early in the diagnostic process.[26] For example, if a 25-year-old woman with a breast mass is considered to have a very low clinical probability of having malignant disease, then the findings on needle biopsy may be considered difficult to interpret in spite of overt malignant features. An extreme example of low anchoring is seen in the individual who avoids rare diagnoses, with a logic pattern that goes something like "I've been in practice 20 years and have never seen one so this couldn't be one." Although it certainly is appropriate to be cautious about making low-probability diagnoses, there is an important distinction between caution and diagnostic paralysis. In contrast, some diagnosticians tend to give rare events excessively high probability assessments (so-called zebra hunting). If a diagnosis is inappropriately considered to be highly likely because the diagnostician has anchored on a high prior probability, much effort and money can be wasted before this diagnosis is determined to be incorrect. For example, a few lymphocytes in the epidermis of a patient with dermatitis may set off an effort to establish the diagnosis of cutaneous T-cell lymphoma, including lymph node biopsy and immunohistochemical and clinical studies.

HYPOTHESIS CONFIRMATION. For those diseases in which the criteria for diagnosis are well accepted and unambiguous, the task of hypothesis confirmation is mainly one of data acquisition. In contrast, when the published criteria are controversial, or the clinical data gathered are conflicting, the task is much more complicated, and diagnosticians will vary in their final diagnosis. As hypothesis confirmation becomes more and more subjective, it becomes progressively more important for the surgical pathologist to be well versed in the clinical implications of both overdiagnosis and underdiagnosis. If the response of your clinical colleagues to a positive diagnosis will be innocuous and possibly even beneficial, it is best to overdiagnose. If the clinicians' response to a positive diagnosis will be toxic and of questionable value, err on the side of underdiagnosis.

The most important attribute of a confirmed hypothesis is **accuracy**, which can be described as the closeness that a diagnostic label describes the true clinical significance of an abnormality. Often in surgical pathology there are lesions (e.g., superficial highly atypical melanocytic lesions) for which there is no biologic gold standard, so we are left with **consistency** (internal and external) as the best available standard. If I cannot consistently attach similar labels to similar lesions, I have an internal consistency problem. If the labels that other observers attach to my cases are different from my labels, I have an external consistency problem. Sometimes an expert outside observer simply "doesn't know that he/she doesn't know" the accurate answer, but in the absence of a gold standard for accuracy, we all have to take seriously any lack of consistency.

CONCLUSION

Central to the acceptance of surgical pathology diagnosis in the arena of patient care is the assumption that the field has a scientific basis that results in acceptably low levels of diagnostic variation when cases are later reviewed by the original pathologist or a different pathologist. Recording of diagnoses in a standard format is a good first step,[55] but even more important would be an effort to optimize and standardize the steps that lead to filling in the diagnostic form. If surgical pathology is to remain a respected subspecialty of clinical medicine, we must continue our progress toward evidence-based medicine, as exemplified by the use of immunoperoxidase techniques, and away from the cult of personality that was so important to the field in the past. As Peter Huber has pointed out in his book *Galileo's Revenge: Junk Science in the Courtroom*, an observation such as the effects of ''N rays'' that is visible to only a select few can often best be explained by imagination.[56]

It is not impossible that in the near future, we will begin to look at variations in the diagnostic decision-making process of surgical pathologists with the idea of codifying behavior that leads to improved outcomes. Traditionally, the specialty has attempted to tap the best diagnosticians for educational leadership roles, and no doubt, much can be learned from studying the decision-making of the ''greats,'' the ''naturals,'' the people who virtually always ''get it right.'' Interestingly, the process may also be studied by looking at the behavior of the people who more than occasionally ''get it wrong.'' Perhaps a useful analogy is in the study of the coagulation system, which yielded its mysteries through careful studies of patients whose serum was missing key factors. Diagnostic decision-making, which is also a complex multistep process, may be better understood by systematically studying diagnostic malfunction. For example, some pathologists have great difficulty at the level of detecting abnormalities on a glass slide. Others have major problems in the ''guts'' of diagnostic decision-making, often failing in the transition from detection to identification. A few pathologists share with some of our clinical colleagues[57] an inability to summarize facts into a specific decision, even when all the necessary diagnostic information has been skillfully gathered.

Acknowledgments

Some of the concepts in this chapter were originally developed for the following chapter: Foucar E, Foucar K: Diagnostic decision making in bone marrow pathology. In Foucar K (ed): Bone Marrow Pathology. Chicago, ASCP Press (In press).

The author is grateful for the review of this chapter by Drs. Peter Banks, Kathy Foucar, and James Linder.

References

1. Doubilet PM: Statistical techniques for medical decision making: Applications to diagnostic radiology. AJR 150:745–750, 1988.
2. O'Connor GT, Sox HC: Bayesian reasoning in medicine: The contributions of Lee B. Lusted. Med Decis Making 11:107–111, 1991.
3. Kassirer JP: Clinical problem-solving—a new feature in the Journal. N Engl J Med 326:60–61, 1992.
4. Ridderikhoff J: Medical problem-solving: An exploration of strategies. Med Educ 25:196–207, 1991.
5. Heller RF, Saltzstein HD: Heuristics in medical and non-medical decision-making. Q J Med Psychol 44:211–235, 1992.
6. Kassirer JP, Sonnenberg FA: Diagnostic reasoning. In Kelley WN (ed): Textbook of Internal Medicine, 2nd ed, Vol I. Philadelphia, JB Lippincott, 1992, p 12.
7. Foucar E: Noncomedo ductal carcinoma in situ [letter]. Am J Clin Pathol 101:788–790, 1994.
8. McGuire CH: Medical problem-solving: A critique of the literature. J Med Educ 60:587-595, 1985.
9. Medawar PB: Induction and intuition in scientific thought. Jane Lectures for 1968. Memoirs of the American Philosophical Society 75:33–34, 1969.
10. Sox HC, Blatt MA, Higgins MC, et al: Probability: Quantifying uncertainty. In Sox HC, Blatt MA, Higgins MC, et al: Medical Decision Making. Boston, Butterworth-Heinemann, 1988, pp 27–64.
11. Schwartz S, Griffin T: Evaluating medical information. In Schwartz S, Griffin T: Medical Thinking. The Psychology of Medical Judgement and Decision Making. New York, Springer-Verlag, 1986, p 62.
12. Paniago-Pereira C, Maize JC, Ackerman AB: Nevus of large spindle and/or epithelioid cells (Spitz's nevus). Arch Dermatol 114:1811–1823, 1978.
13. Casso EM, Grin-Jorgensen CM, Grant-Kels JM: Spitz nevi. J Am Acad Dermatol 27:901–913, 1992.
14. Morgan TW, Banks PM: Large cell neoplasia: An evaluation of criteria for the distinction of lymphoid from epithelial malignancies [abstract]. Lab Invest 40:273, 1979.
15. Thomas JP: Detection and identification: How are they related? J Opt Soc Am A 2:1457–1467, 1985.
16. Kinchla RA: Attention. Annu Rev Psychol 43:711–742, 1993.
17. Statland BE, Winkel P, Burke MD: Quantitative approaches used in evaluating laboratory measurements and other clinical data. In Henry JB (ed): Clinical Diagnosis and Management by Laboratory Methods, 16th ed, Vol I. Philadelphia, WB Saunders, 1979, p 526.
18. Kramer CE, Epstein JI: Nucleoli in low-grade prostate adenocarcinoma and adenosis. Hum Pathol 24:618–623, 1993.
19. Brown RW, Clark GM, Tandon AK, et al: Multiple-marker immunohistochemical phenotypes distinguish malignant pleural mesothelioma from pulmonary adenocarcinoma. Hum Pathol 24:347–354, 1993.
20. Sox HC, Blatt MA, Higgins MC, et al: Understanding new information: Bayes' theorem. In Sox HC, Blatt MA, Higgins MC, et al: Medical Decision Making. Boston, Butterworth-Heinemann, 1988, p 75.
21. Jaeschke R, Guyatt GH, Sackett DL: Users guide to the medical literature. III. How to use an article about a diagnostic test. B. What are the results and will they help me in caring for my patients? JAMA 271:703–707, 1994.
22. Rosai J, Carcangui ML, DeLellis RA: Papillary carcinoma. In Rosai J, Sobin LH (eds): Tumors of the Thyroid Gland. Atlas of Tumor Pathology, Third Series, Fascicle 5. Washington, DC, Armed Forces Institute of Pathology, 1992, p 72.
23. Bryant GD, Norman GR: Expressions of probability. Words and numbers [letter]. N Engl J Med 302:411, 1980.
24. Hapke MR, Dehner LP: The optically clear nucleus. A reliable sign of papillary carcinoma of the thyroid? Am J Surg Pathol 3:31–38, 1979.
25. Sackett DL, Haynes RB, Guyatt GH, et al: The interpretation of diagnostic data. In Sackett DL, Haynes RB, Guyatt GH, et al: Clinical Epidemiology. A Basic Science for Clinical Medicine, 2nd ed. Boston, Little, Brown, 1991, p 123.
26. Kassirer JP: Diagnostic reasoning. Ann Intern Med 110:893–900, 1989.
27. Elstein AS, Kagan N, Shulman LS, et al: Methods and theory in the study of medical inquiry. J Med Educ 47:85–92, 1972.
28. Dudley HAF: The clinical task. Lancet 2:1353–1354, 1970.
29. Campbell EJM: The diagnosing mind. Lancet 1:849–851, 1987.
30. Sox HC, Blatt MA, Higgins MC, et al: Introduction. In Sox HC, Blatt MA, Higgins MC, et al: Medical Decision Making. Boston, Butterworth-Heinemann, 1988, pp 3–4.
31. Edwards W: Conservatism in human information processing. In Kahneman D, Slovic P, Tversky A (eds): Judgement Under Uncertainty: Heuristics and Biases. New York, Cambridge University Press, 1982, pp 359–369.
32. Statland BE, Winkel P, Burke MD, Galen RS: Quantitative approaches used in evaluating laboratory measurements and other clinical data. In Henry JB (ed): Clinical Diagnosis and Management by Laboratory Methods, 16th ed, Vol I. Philadelphia, WB Saunders, 1979, p 527.
33. Sox HC, Blatt MA, Higgins MC, et al: Understanding new information: Bayes' theorem. In Sox HC, Blatt MA, Higgins MC, et al: Medical Decision Making. Boston, Butterworth-Heinemann, 1988, p 93.
34. Elstein AS: Clinical judgement: Psychological research and medical practice. Science 194:696–700, 1976.
35. Swets JA: The science of choosing the right decision threshold in high-stakes diagnostics. Am Psychol 47:522–532, 1992.
36. Koss LG, Suhrland MJ: Atypical hyperplasia and other abnormalities of prostatic epithelium. Hum Pathol 24:817–818, 1993.
37. Medawar P: Expectation and prediction. In Medawar P: Pluto's Republic. Oxford, Oxford University Press, 1982, p 298.
38. Traub JF, Wozniakowski H: Breaking intractability. Sci Am 270:102–107, 1994.
39. Paulos JA: Probability and coincidence. In Paulos JA: Innumeracy. Mathematical Illiteracy and Its Consequences. New York, Vintage Books, 1988, p 38.
40. Sackett DL, Haynes RB, Guyatt GH, et al: The interpretation of diagnostic data. In Sackett DL, Haynes RB, Guyatt GH, et al: Clinical Epidemiology. A Basic Science for Clinical Medicine, 2nd ed. Boston, Little, Brown, 1991, pp 166–167.
41. Green MS, Ackerman AB: Thickness is not an accurate gauge of prognosis of primary cutaneous melanoma. Am J Dermatopathol 15:461–473, 1993
42. Elstein AS, Shulman LS, Sprafka SA: Foreword. In Elstein AS, Shulman LS, Sprafka SA: Medical Problem Solving: An Analysis of Clinical Reasoning. Cambridge, Harvard University Press, 1978, p vii.
43. Blumenthal D: Total quality management and physicians' clinical decisions. JAMA 269:2775–2778, 1993.
44. Schwartz S, Griffin T: Judgment heuristics and biasis. In Schwartz S, Griffin T: Medical Thinking. The Psychology of Medical Judgement and Decision Making. New York, Springer-Verlag, 1986, pp 63–73.
45. Dawson NV, Arkes HR: Systematic errors in medical decision making: Judgement limitations. J Gen Intern Med 2:183–187, 1987.
46. Rips LJ, Collins A: Categories and resemblance. J Exp Psychol [Gen] 122:468–486, 1993.

47. Zagzag D, Miller DC, Kleinman GM, et al: Demyelinating disease versus tumor in surgical neuropathology. Clues to correct pathological diagnosis. Am J Surg Pathol 17:537–545, 1993.

48. Vollmer RT: Do not abandon the Breslow thickness. Am J Dermatopathol 15:478–479, 1993.

49. Check WA: Keeping up with transfusion QA. CAP Today 7:15–18, 1993.

50. Battifora H, Silva EG: The use of antikeratin antibodies in the immunohistochemical distinction between neuroendocrine (Merkel cell) carcinoma of the skin, lymphoma, and oat cell carcinoma. Cancer 58:1040–1046, 1986.

51. Bernstein KE, Lattes R: Nodular (pseudosarcomatous) fasciitis, a nonrecurrent lesion: Clinicopathologic study of 134 cases. Cancer 49:1668–1678, 1982.

52. Roses DF, Harris MN, Ackerman AB: Clinical and histologic features of malignant melanomas. In Ebert PA (consulting editor): Diagnosis and Management of Cutaneous Malignant Melanoma. Major Problems in Clinical Surgery, Vol XXVII. Philadelphia, WB Saunders, 1983, pp 35–37.

53. Medawar PB: Induction and intuition in scientific thought. Jane Lectures for 1968. Memoirs of the American Philosophical Society 75:57, 1969.

54. Weinstein MC, Fineberg HV: Sources of probability. In Weinstein MC, Fineberg HV: Clinical Decision Analysis. Philadelphia, WB Saunders, 1980, pp 176–177.

55. Kempson RL: The time is now. Checklists for surgical pathology reports. Arch Pathol Lab Med 116:1107–1108, 1992.

56. Huber PW: Galileo's Revenge: Junk Science in the Courtroom. New York, Basic Books (a division of HarperCollins Publishers), 1991, pp 28–31.

57. Hurst JW: The Bench and Me: Teaching and Learning Medicine. New York, Igaku-Shoin, 1992, p 17.

CHAPTER 2

Head and Neck

Noel Weidner, M.D., and Joseph A. Regezi, D.D.S., M.S.

This chapter is divided into three sections: (1) lesions that mimic other benign or malignant neoplasms, (2) uncommon presentations of common lesions, and (3) uncommon lesions worth knowing about but not covered in the previous sections.

LESIONS THAT MIMIC OTHER BENIGN OR MALIGNANT PROCESSES

Benign Head and Neck Lesions

Fibrous Dysplasia

The benign fibro-osseous diseases of the jaws represent a diverse group of conditions that vary widely in their clinical-radiographic presentations and biologic behaviors (Table 2–1). Fibro-osseous lesions share the common characteristic of replacement of resident bone with a benign fibroblastic matrix in which new bone is formed. Because of this histologic overlap, diagnosis on microscopic grounds alone can be difficult. It cannot be overemphasized that diagnosis should be made only in the context of knowledge of clinical and radiographic features. This is a clinical-pathologic determination in which the clinician and pathologist may have to work closely together to arrive at a definitive diagnosis.

Fibrous dysplasia is a condition of unknown cause that results in the replacement of normal bone with fibrous connective tissue and structurally weak fibrillar bone.[1] It may be limited to one bone (monostotic type), or it may involve several bones (polyostotic type). When the polyostotic type occurs in association with endocrine abnormalities, particularly precocious puberty, and pigmented skin macules, it is referred to as **Albright's syndrome.** Fibrous dysplasia is a self-limiting process that starts in childhood, but because of its slow growth, it may go unnoticed until adulthood. The process usually stabilizes during puberty, persisting in a quiescent state indefinitely. As the name indicates, it is generally regarded as a dysplastic process rather than a neoplastic one.

CLINICOPATHOLOGIC FEATURES. Patients with fibrous dysplasia experience gradual (usually asymptomatic and unilateral) swelling of the bone(s) affected. In the craniofacial complex, this most commonly occurs in the maxilla and calvaria, whereas in the remainder of the skeleton, it is most frequently seen in the rib, femur, and tibia. Jaw lesions may result in severe facial deformity. Involvement of the orbits, sinuses, and/or cranial ostia can result in nasal obstruction, sinusitis, headaches, and hearing and visual disturbances. Outside the craniofacial complex, pain is the most common pre-senting symptom. Radiographically, fibrous dysplasia has ill-defined margins that blend into surrounding bone. They typically are diffusely radiopaque lesions ranging from the characteristic ground-glass appearance to sclerotic. Although the tumor bone may surround teeth, looseness or exfoliation is not seen. Serum laboratory values are usually within normal limits, unless the patient has extensive disease, resulting in an elevation of serum alkaline phosphatase level.

When treatment is necessary to alleviate unacceptable facial deformity, surgical "remodeling" rather than complete excision is often an acceptable procedure because of the lesion's size and benign behavior.[2] The lesion recurs in approximately 25% of these cases. Complete or partial excision with bone grafting has recently been used with some success. An increased risk of malignant transformation of fibrous dysplasia to sarcoma has been observed, often following therapeutic radiation of the involved bone.

Microscopically, fibrous dysplasia consists of a relatively vascular benign fibrous connective tissue stroma surrounding immature, fibrillar, or woven bony trabeculae (Figs. 2–1 and 2–2). The stroma is usually only slightly to moderately cellular. The incompletely calcified bony trabeculae are somewhat regular in size and are uniformly distributed throughout, gradually blending into normal surrounding bone.[3] Osteoclasts are typically inconspicuous, and osteoblasts are scant, providing an appearance to the tumor bone that has been referred to as "osseous metaplasia." Occasional stromal giant cells are seen. Lack of haphazard cellularity and nuclear atypia help separate fibrous dysplasia from **low-grade osteosarcoma.** Lack of inflammatory cells helps separate it from **osteomyelitis.** If the affected bone has been previously biopsied or treated, the classic histologic features described here may be lost, leaving a non-specific picture. Also, as patients with fibrous dysplasia age, tumor bone may show some maturation in the form of lamellar bone.[4] In these cases, the clinical-radiographic features will likely dictate the final diagnosis. Other than polarization microscopy to verify the immature nature of the new bone, there are no adjunctive procedures that can be used to establish the diagnosis of fibrous dysplasia.

DIFFERENTIAL DIAGNOSIS. In the craniofacial complex, this condition is most often confused with **ossifying fibroma.** Distinguishing these two lesions is important because they have differing prognoses and are treated differently. Ossifying fibroma is a neoplasm that, if left untreated, may grow considerably and destroy bone; however, ossifying fibroma is well circumscribed and usually easily excised when small. Microscopically, the new bone in ossifying fibroma is well demar-

Table 2–1. **Clinicopathologic Features of Fibro-osseous Lesions of the Jaws**

	Fibrous Dysplasia	Ossifying Fibroma	Chronic Osteomyelitis	Periapical Cemental Dysplasia
Age:	1–2 decades	3–4 decades	Any decade	4–5 decades
Site:	Max > mand	Mand > max	Mand > max	Anterior mand
S&S:	None	None	Low-grade pain	None
X-ray:	Diffusely opague, ill-defined margins	Opaque foci or relatively opaque, well-defined margins	Mottled lucent-opaque, indistinct margins	Lucent to opaque
Cause:	Unknown	Unknown	Pulpitis, trauma, periodontitis	Unknown
LM:	New bone is fibrous and immature, uniform trabeculae, few osteoblasts and osteoclasts, low to moderate cellularity, no inflammation, no atypia, blends into adjacent bone.	Bone in uniform islands or trabeculae, few osteoclasts, moderate to high cellularity, no inflammation, no atypia, separated from adjacent bone.	Irregular bony trabeculae, mature bone, osteoblasts and osteoclasts, reversal lines, few inflammatory cells, no atypia, blends into adjacent bone.	Irregular bony islands and trabeculae in benign fibrous matrix, osteoblastic rimming and some osteoclasts, moderate cellularity, blends into adjacent bone.

Max, maxilla; Mand, mandible; S&S, signs and symptoms; LM, light microscopy.

cated from surrounding resident bone and is seen as uniform trabeculae or oval (spherical) islands (Figs. 2–3 and 2–4). Osteoblasts are usually prominent, typically rimming the new bone. Lamellar bone in some cases may be a prominent feature.[5] Stromal cellularity of ossifying fibroma may be relatively high compared with that of fibrous dysplasia, and it may vary from one area to another. Lesions composed predominantly of the oval (spherical) hard tissue islands have been referred to as **cementifying fibromas.** This distinction is essentially academic, since the behaviors of the so-called cementifying fibroma and ossifying fibroma are the same (**suggesting that as a group these two lesions and intermediate forms be called cemento-ossifying fibromas**). An incompletely defined (and not universally accepted) variant

of ossifying fibroma has been designated as **juvenile ossifying fibroma.**[4, 6] It has been claimed that this variant exhibits greater tumor cellularity, appears in a younger age group, and may have the potential for considerable growth. Sometimes cemento-ossifying fibromas may extend into the meninges and show aneurysmal bone cyst–like changes. In the latter setting, these may be misdiagnosed as meningiomas.

Another lesion with microscopic features that may occasionally overlap with fibrous dysplasia is **low-grade or mild chronic osteomyelitis** of the jaws. The latter may have only scant inflammatory cells, and there can be much new bone formation. However, the new bony trabeculae are of irregular size and distribution, and reversal lines are likely to be evident. Both osteoblasts and osteoclasts may be seen. Clinical-

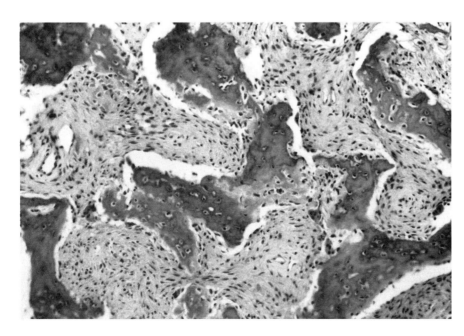

FIGURE 2–1. Fibrous dysplasia showing immature trabeculae in relatively hypocellular fibrovascular stroma. Osteoblasts and osteoclasts are inconspicuous. (H&E, ×40)

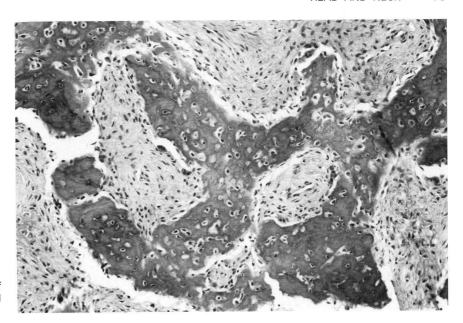

FIGURE 2–2. Immature bony trabeculae of fibrous dysplasia. Few osteoblasts and osteoclasts are evident. (H&E, ×100)

pathologic correlation may be critical. **Chronic osteomyelitis usually occurs in the mandible, typically related to a devital tooth or extension of periodontal disease.**

Periapical cemental dysplasia and its close relative **florid osseous dysplasia** exhibit features that approximate fibrous dysplasia (see Table 2–1). These lesions, believed to originate from periodontal ligament, appear more like ossifying fibroma but tend to blend into surrounding hard tissue. Their association with vital anterior mandibular teeth in middle-aged women, particularly in African-Americans, can often be a discriminating factor. Although so-called **familial fibrous dysplasia, or cherubism,** has clinical features that are shared by fibrous dysplasia, it is microscopically dissimilar.

Ameloblastoma

Recognized and studied for over a century, the clinical characteristics and behavior of **ameloblastoma** are well known. It is generally believed that this tumor arises from the neoplastic transformation of cyst epithelium or from epithelium involved in the formation of teeth. Specifically, the epithelial origin may be from the epithelial lining of an **odontogenic cyst (especially the dentigerous cyst); the enamel organ; remnants of the enamel organ (reduced enamel epithelium)** found overlying the crown of an unerupted tooth; **remnants of Hertwig's epithelial root sheath (rests of Malassez),** which are found throughout the periodontal ligament; or **epithelial remnants of the dental lamina (rests of Serres)** found in the bones of the jaw or the connective tissue of the gingiva. The stimulus for this neoplastic transformation, however, is unknown.

Ameloblastoma may be confused with other jaw lesions and occasionally with infiltrating neoplasms of the maxillary sinus. New information about this lesion and other odontogenic tumors has been slow in coming over the past decades.

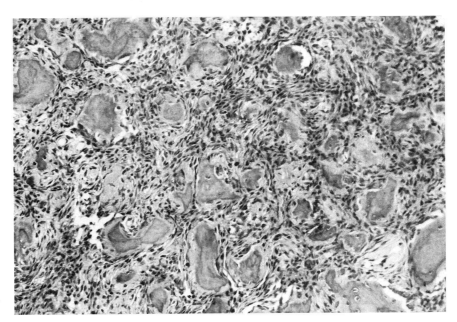

FIGURE 2–3. Ossifying fibroma with evenly distributed islands of bone in benign cellular matrix. (H&E, ×100)

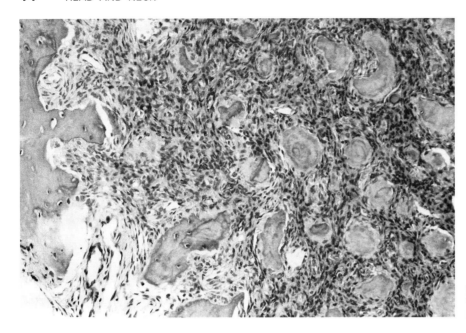

FIGURE 2–4. Ossifying fibroma with uniform trabeculae in a cellular stroma. Note prominent osteoblasts. (H&E, ×100)

Of greatest significance has been the recognition of subtypes and variants that exhibit different biologic behaviors.

CLINICOPATHOLOGIC FEATURES. Ameloblastoma typically occurs around the age of 40 years; however, children are also rarely affected. Odontogenic tumors that are more likely to appear in children are **adenomatoid odontogenic tumor** and **ameloblastic fibroma (both of which have decidedly different biologic behaviors).** Ameloblastoma may appear anywhere in the jaws, although the molar-ramus of the mandible is the favored location. Affected patients are asymptomatic, and lesions are usually discovered during routine radiographic examination or because of jaw swelling. Extraosseous gingival tumors are rarely seen.

Radiographically, ameloblastomas usually appear as well-defined lucencies. These lesions may be unilocular or multi-locular. When unilocular tumors exhibit microscopic intramural or intraluminal tumor growth, the designation of **unicystic ameloblastoma** has been used.

Ameloblastomas characteristically exhibit a slow but unrelenting and destructive growth pattern that has been likened to that seen with basal cell carcinomas. Microscopically, ameloblastomas exhibit a remarkable similarity to **basal cell carcinoma** as well. These shared features are likely related to shared histogenic origins.

Ameloblastomas can exhibit numerous histologic patterns, but these microscopic variants do not differ in their biologic behaviors.[7] Some lesions may exhibit only one histologic pattern, whereas others, especially large lesions, may exhibit several. The common denominator to all ameloblastomas is the presence of well-differentiated palisaded cells

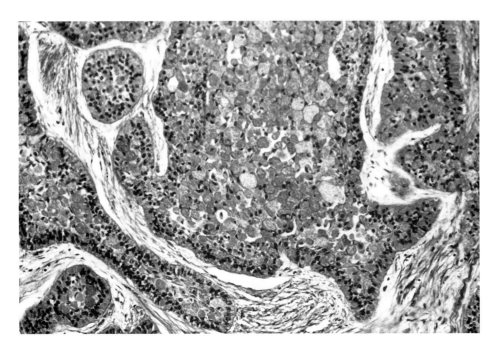

FIGURE 2–5. Granular cell ameloblastoma. (H&E, ×100)

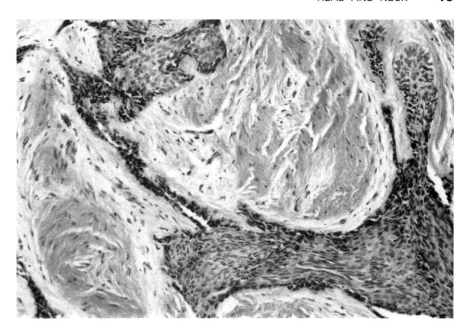

FIGURE 2–6. Desmoplastic ameloblastoma. (H&E, ×40)

around the periphery of nests, strands, and networks of epithelium. The nuclei of these palisaded cells are typically polarized away from the basement membrane. Budding of epithelium from these proliferative nests and strands is also characteristic of this lesion. These features result in a microscopic picture that roughly mimics the appearance of the enamel organ. Palisading cells and budding epithelium are found in all the **microscopic subtypes (follicular, cystic, plexiform, acanthomatous, and granular cell** [Fig. 2–5]). A recently recognized variant with a predilection for the anterior jaws and that features spindled epithelial cells and a desmoplastic stroma is known as **desmoplastic ameloblastoma** (Fig. 2–6). Keratinization in the form of ghost cells can be seen in ameloblastomas as well as in other odontogenic tumors and cysts (particularly the **calcifying odontogenic cyst**) (Fig. 2–7).

Recently there has been a trend to divide ameloblastomas into two clinical-pathologic subtypes: **small unicystic lesions and large multicystic (or solid) lesions.**[8] The unicystic ameloblastoma is a cyst with intraluminal or mural ameloblastomatous change (Fig. 2–8). Occasionally, the lining exhibits a plexiform pattern, prompting the designation of **plexiform unicystic ameloblastoma** (Fig. 2–9). Unicystic lesions, which are believed to represent early small ameloblastomas in a preexisting cyst, are treated conservatively (curettage) and have a low recurrence rate (<10%). The multicystic (or solid) ameloblastomas require more extensive treatment and have a higher recurrence rate (50% to 90%).

Two rare malignant variants of ameloblastoma have been described.[9] One lesion, known as **malignant or metastatic ameloblastoma,** exhibits microscopic features of well-

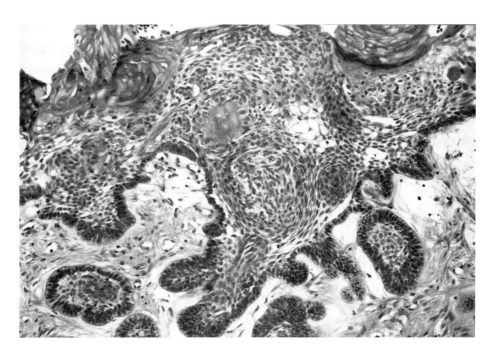

FIGURE 2–7. Ameloblastoma showing "ghost cell" keratinization (*top right and left*). (H&E, ×100)

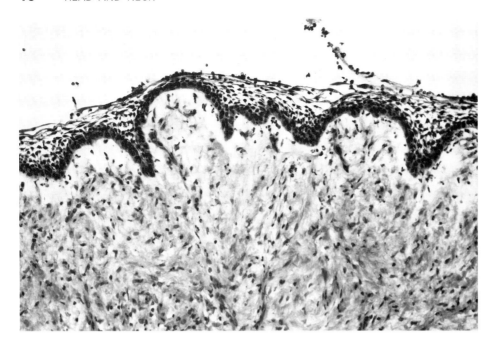

FIGURE 2–8. Unicystic ameloblastoma. Note palisaded basal layer, loose keratinocytes, pointed rete ridges, and paucity of inflammatory cells. (H&E, ×100)

differentiated ameloblastoma, which are found in both primary and metastatic sites (Fig. 2–10). The second lesion, designated as **ameloblastic carcinoma,** microscopically resembles ameloblastoma but exhibits microscopic signs of malignancy (i.e., squamous cell carcinoma) in its primary and metastatic sites. In either case, metastasis from an ameloblastoma is rare. The lung is the most common metastatic site, presumably owing to aspiration at the time of surgery; local lymph nodes are very rarely affected.

DIFFERENTIAL DIAGNOSIS. Distinguishing ameloblastoma from hyperplastic cyst wall is the usual problem associated with making a definitive diagnosis. **Hyperplastic cystic epithelium** may appear as a reticulum similar to ameloblastoma, but peripherally palisaded cells with polarized nulcei are

absent. The cyst wall is also more likely to contain an inflammatory cell infiltrate than ameloblastoma.

Another benign lesion that mimics ameloblastoma (acanthomatous type) is **squamous odontogenic tumor** (Fig. 2–11).[10] This lesion, which usually involves the alveolar process, is well circumscribed and is usually associated with the roots of teeth. It is typically small and seems to have limited growth potential. Microscopically, it appears as islands of bland squamous epithelium without an inflammatory infiltrate. Peripheral palisades are not seen.

Malignancies seen in the jaws that may occasionally resemble ameloblastoma include **primary intraosseous carcinoma or mucoepidermoid carcinoma of the jaws**[11] and **adenocarcinoma and squamous cell carcinoma of maxillary sinus**

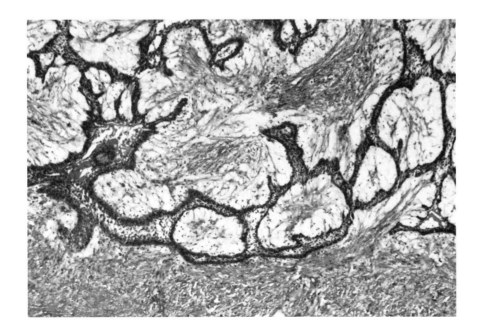

FIGURE 2–9. Plexiform unicystic ameloblastoma showing network of odontogenic epithelium lining a cystic space (lumen at top) in absence of inflammatory cell infiltrate. (H&E, ×100)

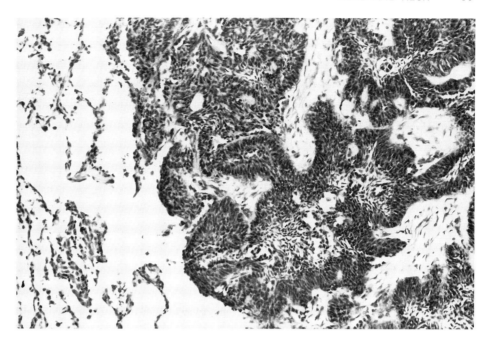

FIGURE 2–10. Metastatic ameloblastoma to lung. (H&E, ×100)

origin. These malignancies have atypical nuclei and mitotic figures, features not seen in ameloblastomas.

Hairy Leukoplakia

Oral hairy leukoplakia (HL), originally described in 1984 in human immunodeficiency virus (HIV)–positive men, is an expression of Epstein-Barr virus (EBV) that has served as a sign before acquired immunodeficiency syndrome (AIDS). Subsequently, HL has been found in patients immunosuppressed for other reasons, such as organ transplantation. EBV proteins and DNA have been identified in the keratinocytes of HL and in the normal mucosa of AIDS patients. EBV assembly has also been detailed in HL keratinocytes.[12]

CLINICOPATHOLOGIC FEATURES. HL presents as a white patch, which may be flat, corrugated, or papillated (hairy). It has a strong predilection for the lateral margin of the anterior half of the tongue. It is often bilateral and may extend onto the dorsum or floor of the mouth. It is rarely seen on the buccal mucosa and palate. Patients are asymptomatic, although secondary infection by *Candida albicans* may cause discomfort. Lesions are usually discovered on routine oral examination and occasionally on self-examination. Clinically, HL appears similar to frictional **hyperkeratosis and idiopathic leukoplakia.**

HL has a distinctive and often diagnostic microscopic appearance in hematoxylin and eosin (H&E) sections. The surface is hyperparakeratotic and may exhibit numerous

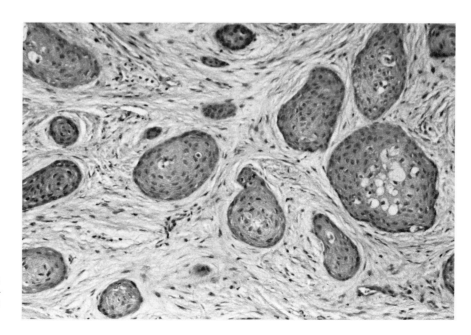

FIGURE 2–11. Squamous odontogenic tumor of mandible. Bland islands of epithelium are found in non-inflamed fibrous stroma. (H&E, ×100)

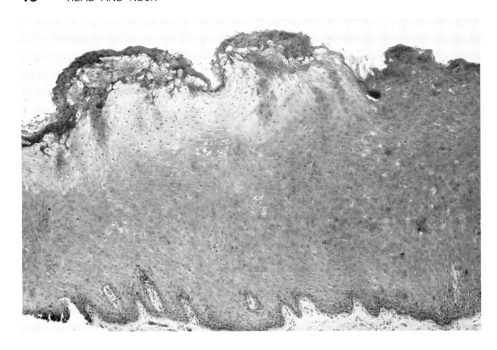

FIGURE 2–12. Hairy leukoplakia. Note pale-staining keratinocytes below keratotic surface projections. There is no inflammatory cell infiltrate. (H&E, ×40)

bacteria-covered filamentous projections (Fig. 2–12), and *Candida* hyphae are frequently found penetrating the parakeratin. Supporting the keratin are spinous cells that exhibit ballooning degeneration and perinuclear halos (Fig. 2–13). The nuclei of these cells show the features that are exclusive to HL, as all the other features may occasionally be seen in other conditions. **Pale red to blue intranuclear inclusions, and homogeneous "smudgy" nuclei are indicative of Epstein-Barr virus infection** (Fig. 2–14). The homogeneous nuclei are usually "peppered" or marginated with deep basophilic dots of residual nuclear chromatin.[13, 14] *In situ* hybridization with Epstein-Barr virus probes can be used to confirm the presence of virus in these cells for the very occasional equivocal case. Only a limited inflammatory cell infiltrate is seen in the supporting connective tissue.

DIFFERENTIAL DIAGNOSIS. The lesion from which HL must be differentiated is **simple hyperkeratosis.** Hyperkeratosis may show any or all of the cytoplasmic features described earlier (Fig. 2–15). Intracellular edema is common in oral mucosa and should not be confused with the virally infected balloon cells of HL. The nuclear changes seen in the context of the cytoplasmic changes noted previously are not seen in any other oral condition, including **herpes simplex, herpes zoster,** and **cytomegalovirus infections.** The virally induced nuclear changes can be used to confirm the clinical diagnosis of HL. However, because of the subjective nature of H&E section interpretation, some diagnostic caution might be exercised when the clinical setting is inconsistent with HIV infection. In these cases, it would be prudent to defer definitive diagnosis until there is confirmatory *in situ* hybridization testing of the biopsy specimen.

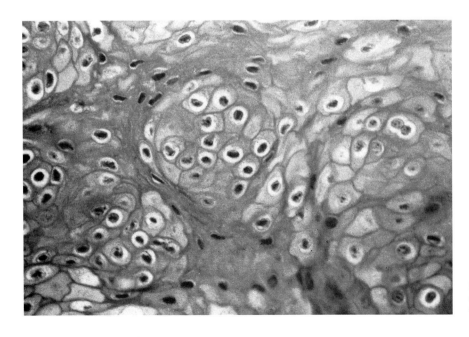

FIGURE 2–13. Hairy leukoplakia showing characteristic pale-staining "balloon cells" with intranuclear inclusions. (H&E, ×250)

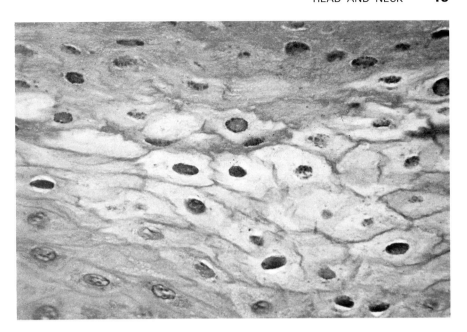

FIGURE 2-14. Hairy leukoplakia showing characteristic nuclear homogenization with clumps of chromatin. (H&E, ×250)

Lymphocytic or Epimyoepithelial Sialadenitis (LESA): Salivary Gland Component of Sjogren's Syndrome

Sjogren's syndrome by definition includes xerostomia, keratoconjunctivitis sicca, and rheumatoid arthritis or other "collagen vascular disease." It has become common practice to classify patients into either primary or secondary types. In primary Sjogren's syndrome, the patients have both eye (keratoconjunctivitis sicca) and oral (lymphocytic sialadenitis) components but no collagen vascular disease. In secondary Sjogren's syndrome, patients have eye and/or oral components plus a systemic collagen vascular disease, usually rheumatoid arthritis.[15]

The xerostomia is associated with salivary gland changes, which are reflected in all major and minor salivary tissues. The basic tissue process is a T- and B-lymphocyte infiltration resulting in replacement of salivary parenchyma. More T cells than B cells are seen in the infiltrate, and in the T-cell population, more CD4 lymphocytes than CD8 lymphocytes are seen.[16] The morphologic lesions in the salivary glands have been referred to as **lymphocytic or epimyoepithelial sialadenitis (LESA)** or, alternatively, **benign lymphoepithelial lesions.** LESA shows a spectrum of morphologic features ranging from focal and non-specific lymphoid infiltration through dense, extensive, and confluent lymphoid infiltration associated with epimyoepithelial island formation. B-cell lymphomas can eventually evolve from LESA, and they may have clinicopathologic features in common with other lymphomas arising from **mucosa-associated lymphoid tissue (MALT).** Like other MALT lymphomas, salivary gland lymphomas arising in association with LESA are indolent, low-grade, B-cell lymphomas that often remain localized to the salivary gland or other MALT sites. Because MALT

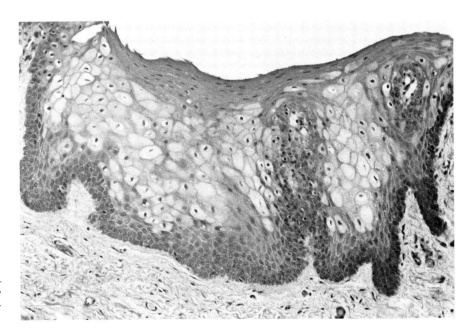

FIGURE 2-15. Normal mucosa with "balloon cells" that are similar to those in hairy leukoplakia. Note normal-appearing nuclei. (H&E, ×250)

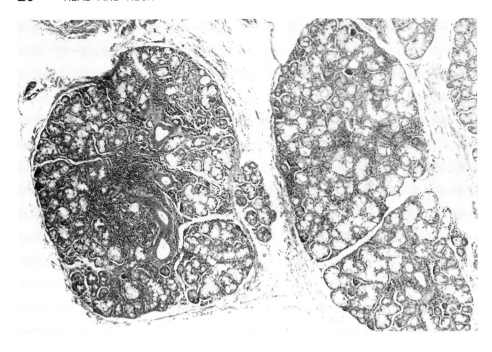

FIGURE 2–16. Lobules from labial salivary gland biopsy showing lymphoid foci consistent with the salivary component of Sjogren's syndrome. (H&E, ×40)

lymphomas tend to be low-grade and remain localized, they are very amenable to regional therapies such as surgery and radiation. Nonetheless, some low-grade MALT lymphomas can become systemic and dedifferentiate to higher-grade, large-cell lymphomas.[17-19]

CLINICOPATHOLOGIC FEATURES. Currently, the diagnosis of Sjogren's syndrome is based on (1) evidence of keratoconjunctivitis sicca using established clinical tests, (2) demonstration of lymphocytic infiltration in salivary gland biopsy, and (3) medical confirmation of rheumatoid arthritis or other collagen vascular disease. The salivary component can be best evaluated by **labial salivary gland biopsy,** because morbidity is low compared with parotid gland biopsy, and sensitivity appears to be as good or possibly better. The determination of the salivary involvement in Sjogren's syndrome has also

been done using salivary flow measurements, contrast radiography, and scintigraphy. However, none of these measures is as specific and reliable as salivary gland biopsy.

Labial salivary gland biopsies should include several glands, preferably five or more, which should all show some evidence of characteristic pathologic change (Fig. 2–16). The infiltrate associated with Sjogren's syndrome is predominantly lymphocytic, although significant numbers of plasma cells can be seen. The cells are typically found in focal aggregates in the gland parenchyma, often involving small ducts and vessels (Figs. 2–17 and 2–18). Ducts may also exhibit concomitant epithelial hyperplasia. As the disease progresses, the focal aggregates become confluent, replacing glandular parenchyma as they increase in size. The distinctive epimyoepithelial islands seen in Sjogren's syndrome of major glands

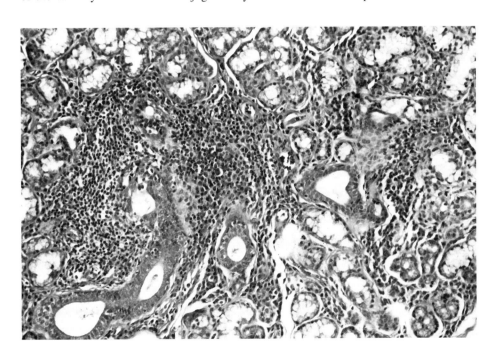

FIGURE 2–17. Lymphocytic sialadenitis seen in association with Sjogren's syndrome. Note persistence of salivary acini. (H&E, ×100)

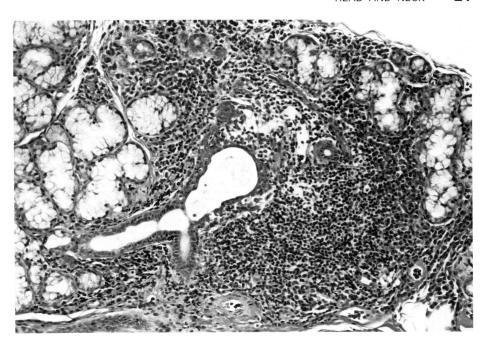

FIGURE 2–18. Lymphocytic sialadenitis seen in association with Sjogren's syndrome. Note ductal inflammation and hyperplasia (*center*). (H&E, ×100)

(**benign lymphoepithelial lesion**) are infrequently seen in labial salivary gland biopsies. Of particular importance is the finding of intact acini adjacent to lymphocytic foci in the absence of non-specific or obstructive changes that are frequently noted in salivary tissue (Fig. 2–19).[20, 21]

DIFFERENTIAL DIAGNOSIS. Diagnosis of **Sjogren's-associated lymphocytic or epimyoepithelial sialadenitis** requires separation from normal gland (which may contain scattered mononuclear cells) and non-specific sialadenitis. The following inflammatory changes would *not* support the diagnosis: (1) parenchymal scarring, (2) ductal dilatation, (3) neutrophilic infiltrate, and (4) acinar atrophy with ductal persistence.

An objective, reliable scheme has been devised for the microscopic diagnosis of **Sjogren's-associated lymphocytic** sialadenitis.[21, 22] In this scheme, **a search is made for aggregates of lymphocytes (plasma cells) in labial salivary glands; 50 or more cells is defined as a focus, and if two or more foci are found in 4 mm² of glandular tissue (assisted with an ocular graticule), the infiltrate is regarded as significant.** In making this assessment it is necessary to consider the non-specific inflammatory changes described previously. Also, all glands should show foci of lymphoid cells, although the severity of infiltration can vary among glands. The biopsy, then, that meets these criteria would be interpreted as lymphocytic sialadenitis (consistent with the salivary component of Sjogren's syndrome). Definitive diagnosis would be based on combined oral (salivary), eye, and systemic findings.

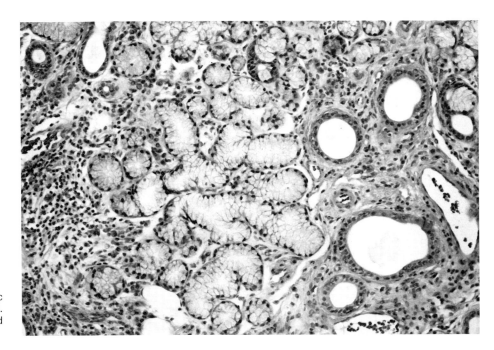

FIGURE 2–19. Chronic non-specific sialadenitis of labial salivary gland. Note ductal dilatation and associated scar (*right*). (H&E, ×100)

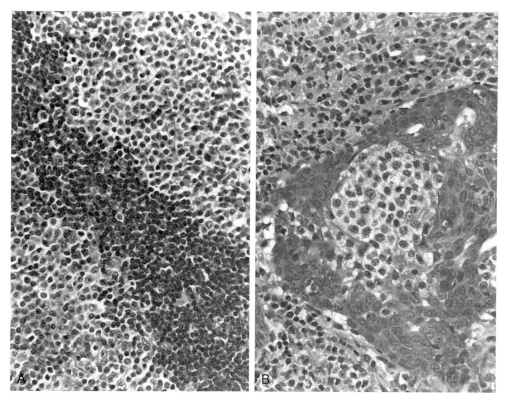

FIGURE 2–20. *A,* Low-grade B-cell lymphoma, MALT-type, in salivary gland. Shown are two pale-staining clusters of "centrocyte-like" lymphoma cells with monocytoid B-cell features separated by a band of benign small lymphocytes. (H&E, original magnification [OM] ×50) *B,* Shown is a lymphoepithelial lesion (LEL) characterized as a pale-staining cluster of "centrocyte-like" cells with monocytoid B-cell features within an epimyoepithelial island, features characteristic of low-grade, B-cell lymphomas of MALT type. (H&E, OM ×100)

Finally, LESA must be distinguished from malignant lymphoma; indeed, the increased risk of developing lymphoma in patients with lymphocytic sialadenitis is well known.[23] The lymphomas arising in LESA are characterized by the development of an expanded population of so-called centrocyte-like cells showing light-chain restriction.[18] These cells stand out as an expanded population centered around and sometimes infiltrating the epimyoepithelial islands (Fig. 2–20). Although "benign" lymphocytes may infiltrate the epimyoepithelial islands in LESA, when the intraepithelial

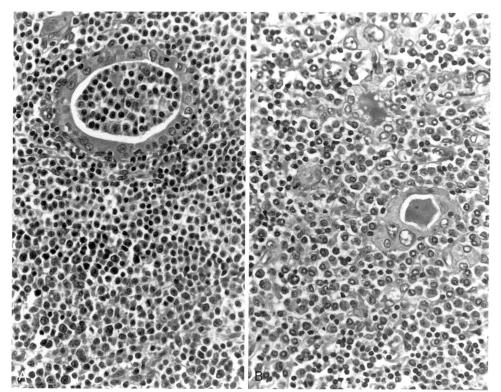

FIGURE 2–21. *A,* Note the lymphoepithelial lesion (LEL) characterized as a pale-staining cluster of "centrocyte-like" lymphoma cells within a follicle of a thyroid containing a MALT-type, low-grade B-cell lymphoma. (H&E, OM ×10) *B,* Shown is thyroid with Hashimoto's thyroiditis. Note the Hurthle cell changes and the absence of LEL lesions, which are better developed in thyroids containing low-grade B-cell lymphomas of MALT type. (H&E, OM ×100)

lymphocytes form well-defined clusters or aggregates (**lymphoepithelial lesions, or LELs**), the findings are more suggestive of lymphoma (Fig. 2–20). A similar process occurs in thyroids containing lymphoma, wherein thyroid follicles become filled by a monomorphous population of lymphoma cells and form LELs (Fig. 2–21). These centrocyte-like cells vary from pale-staining, medium-sized, rounded cells with well-defined cytoplasmic borders and clear cytoplasm (clear-cell or ''monocytoid'' variant) (see Fig. 2–20) to more typical centrocytes (resembling intermediate to small cleaved lymphocytes), to blast-like centrocytes having larger and more prominent nucleoli. Hyjek et al.[18] and Falzon and Isaacson[24] proposed that the presence of an expanded population of these centrocyte-like cells combined with the immunohistochemical (or molecular biologic) demonstration of light-chain restriction pointed toward a diagnosis of lymphoma. However, Fishleder et al.[25] detected clonal immunoglobulin (Ig) gene rearrangements in five ''histologically'' benign examples of LESA, suggesting that clonal populations of B cells did not indicate malignancy, but rather a prelymphomatous state. Also, similar monotypic populations of plasma cells have been detected in labial salivary glands of patients with Sjogren's syndrome, a finding which predicted the development of a systemic monoclonal lymphoproliferative disease.[26] Additional clinicopathologic studies with more cases, long follow-up, and detailed histologic, immunohistochemical, and molecular biologic studies are needed to understand further these atypical cases of LESA.

Wegener's Granulomatosis

Wegener's granulomatosis (WG) commonly involves the mucosa of the head-and-neck region (>90% of cases), and, because of its accessibility, a nasal mucosal biopsy is often used to establish the diagnosis. WG is one of many different diseases known to cause the **lethal or non-healing midline granuloma (LMG) syndrome.**[27–29] The major disorders causing this LMG syndrome include destructive **foreign-body, granulomatous reactions, infections** (bacterial, fungal, spirochetal, and parasitic), **malignant tumors** (sarcoma, carcinoma, and lymphoma), **vasculitides** (especially WG), **angiocentric immunoproliferative lesions** (also known as malignant midline reticulosis [MMR], polymorphous reticulosis [PMR], or lymphomatoid granulomatosis [LYG]), and a variety of **idiopathic diseases,** including **sarcoid** and **idiopathic midline destructive disease (IDMM).**[28, 30] Accurate diagnosis is critical, because therapy and prognosis vary with each disorder causing LMG.

CLINICOPATHOLOGIC FEATURES. WG typically involves the lungs, kidneys, skin, and/or upper aerodigestive tract; however, atpyical presentations of disease clinically isolated to only one of these locations can occur. Also, peculiar initial presentations of WG in the conjunctivae or middle ear can occur and cause considerable diagnostic confusion. Colby et al.[31] reviewed this area (including 52 biopsies from 36 of their own patients) and found that certain pathologic features were useful in diagnosing WG in biopsies from the nose, sinuses, mouth, pharynx, larynx, ear, eye, orbit, and salivary glands. These features include: **(1) mucosal ulceration; (2) acute and chronic (chronic-active) inflammation; (3) active vasculitis of small arteries, veins, and capillaries (granulomatous or non-granulomatous and with or without fibrinoid**

necrosis); **(4) necrosis (especially extravascular foci); and (5) granulomatous changes** (Fig. 2–22). Also, a distinctive microvasculitis with inflammatory cell cuffing of small vessels is sometimes observed, and neutrophils often aggregate into small clusters, eventually forming small microabscesses. In some cases, eosinophils can be prominent. Sinus biopsies are better for diagnosis than nasal biopsies; tissue samples should be more than 0.5 cm in aggregate size; and special stains and cultures for infectious organisms should be negative.

Colby et al.[31] and Devaney et al.[32] have summarized the diagnostic criteria and terminology for WG in head and neck biospy specimens. When **granulomatous inflammation, necrosis, and vasculitis** all are present and there is evidence of head and neck, lung, and/or kidney involvement, the diagnosis of WG should be made. When two of these histologic findings are present, the diagnosis of WG should be made only if the head and neck, lung, and kidney are involved; otherwise a ''probable'' diagnosis of WG should be made and further biopsies suggested. When only one of these histologic features is present, the biopsy should be considered ''suggestive'' of WG if head and neck and lung or head and neck and kidney involvement is present. Further biopsies in doubtful cases may lead to a definitive diagnosis.

A useful serologic test for WG was reported by van der Woude et al.[33] involving the detection of circulating autoantibodies against the cytoplasm of neutrophils and monocytes (**antineutrophilic cytoplasmic antibody [ANCA]**). These antibodies produce a diffuse granular cytoplasmic fluorescence pattern on ethanol-fixed neutrophil preparations (cANCA), and they immunoreact against proteinase-3 present in neutrophilic granules. The vast majority of patients with generalized WG (96%) and most with limited disease (67%) show cANCA immunoreactivity.[34] Also, occasional patients with WG exhibit perinuclear staining of ANCA (pANCA). The latter autoantibodies, which are directed against myeloperoxidase, elastase, and other lysosomal enzymes, are not specific for WG. They can more frequently be found in so-called pauci-immune crescent glomerulonephritis and other systemic vasculitides such as hypersensitivity vasculitis. Although cANCA is most frequent in WG, non-WG patients with hypersensitivity vasculitis, pulmonary hemorrhage (secondary to capillaritis, which can be life threatening), and/or crescentic glomerulonephritis can have either cANCA or pANCA, or immune-complex–mediated, or anti–glomerular basement membrane (GBM) antibody-mediated disease.[35] Finally, some investigators believe that ANCA may produce vascular injury by activating neutrophils and monocytes, whereas others believe ANCA is an epiphenomenon in these disorders.

DIFFERENTIAL DIAGNOSIS. Before making a diagnosis of WG, it is first most important to **rule out infection** with special stains and/or culture when available. **Sarcoma, carcinoma, or lymphoma** is recognized when the malignant cells are adequately represented in the biopsy material. Appropriate immunohistochemistry and/or electron microscopy should distinguish the different tumor types. Ferry et al.[36] reported on a series of 13 nasal lymphomas and found a high proportion of **angioinvasive, diffuse, large-cell lymphomas** with a predominance of T-cell type and a relatively good prognosis when treated with radiation therapy. Occasional cases of B-cell lymphomas also occur in this site, most often associated with systemic disease. **Angiocentric immunoprolifer-**

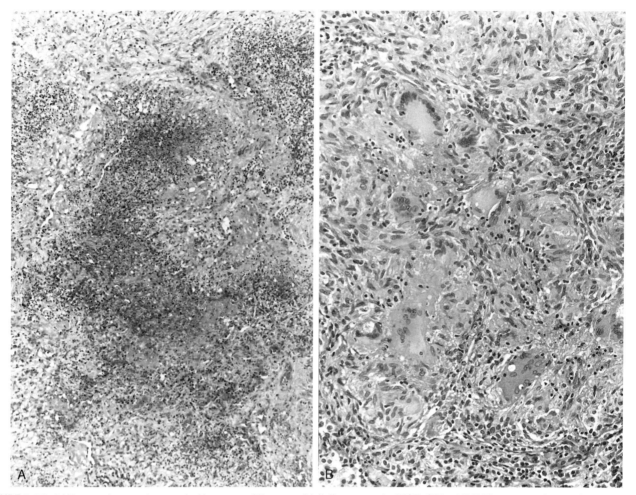

FIGURE 2–22. *A,* Wegener's granulomatosis. Note central "geographic" dirty necrosis. (H&E, OM ×10) *B,* Tissue contains a polymorphous mixture of inflammatory cells with clusters of multinucleated giant cells. (H&E, OM ×100)

ative lesions (AILs) can present more diagnostic problems (Fig. 2–23).[37] AILs represent a spectrum of lesions from benign lymphocytic vasculitis to angiocentric lymphomas. They have a polymorphous and sometimes pleomorphic cellular composition and a behavioral spectrum ranging from benign to frankly malignant. AILs can involve the lung, skin, kidneys, gastrointestinal (GI) tract, hematolymphoid system, central nervous system, and upper aerodigestive tract (especially the nasopharynx, palate, and paranasal sinuses). AILs contain angiocentric, angioinvasive, and sometimes angiodestructive infiltrates of mixed lymphoid cells, plasma cells, and histiocytes. Ischemic tissue necrosis may be present and (although much less commonly) is sometimes seen as fibrinoid necrosis of vessel walls. AILs may be associated with a reactive hemophagocytic syndrome caused by the activation of benign histiocytes throughout the body. When this occurs, the patient may have pancytopenia, fever, and hepatosplenomegaly.

The term **benign lymphocytic vasculitis (BLV)** may be appropriate for those very low grade AILs that lack cytologic atypia and are composed predominantly of small lymphocytes (corresponding to grade 1, with no large or bizarre lymphoid cells). These BLVs often respond to conservative management, but some low-grade AILs may progress to lymphoma. Like Jaffe,[38] we favor the term AIL (usually grade 2, with a polymorphous inflammation, some cytologic atypia in small lymphoid cells, and occasional large, bizarre lymphoid cells) for the more polymorphous and atypical AILs previously reported as polymorphous reticulosis, malignant midline reticulosis, and/or lymphomatoid granulomatosis. The term high-grade AIL (usually grade 3 or monotonous and highly atypical) or angiocentric lymphoma is appropriate for AILs that are clearly malignant lymphomas on cytologic grounds. AILs can cause death, sometimes after conversion to overt malignant lymphoma. Medeiros et al.[39] studied eight cases of AIL and found gene rearrangements (T-cell) in only one, and EBV gene sequences were found in one of four cases using the highly sensitive, polymerase chain reaction technique. The relative rarity of "clonality" by these measures may help to rule out "true" angiocentric lymphoma, but this distinction becomes vague in grades 2 and 3 AIL lesions. High-grade AILs frequently show an abnormal T-cell phenotype characterized by the loss of CD3, CD5, and/or CD7.

Distinction of WG from AIL is usually not difficult. Giant cells, neutrophils, and abscess-like necrosis are usually not present in AIL, whereas coagulation necrosis and lymphoid cells (especially with atypia) are features noted in AIL but not in WG. Also, AIL should not be confused with **angiotropic or intravascular large-cell lymphoma (so-called angioendotheliomatosis),** a disease process that can present in the nose

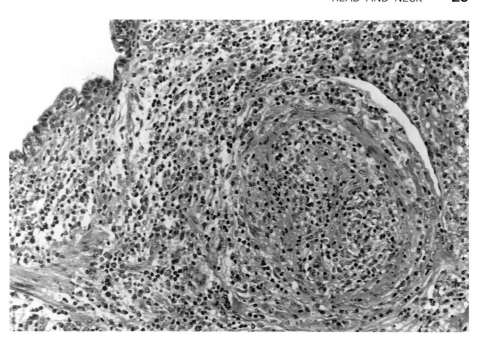

FIGURE 2–23. Angiocentric immuno-proliferative lesion of the nasopharynx showing the polymorphous inflammatory infiltrate associated with an angiocentric and angioinfiltrative pattern (right side of photomicrograph). (H&E, OM ×50)

but is more commonly found as a systemic disease, especially with central nervous system (CNS) symptomatology.[40, 41]

Sarcoid and foreign-body granulomas can be confused with WG, but the non-caseating, "hard" granulomas of sarcoid and the finding of foreign bodies by polarization microscopy combined with the absence of abscess-like necrosis and vasculitis should lead to the correct diagnosis of these two disorders. **Allergic angiitis and granulomatosis (Churg-Strauss vasculitis)** can cause a lethal midline granuloma syndrome but is extraordinarily rare and associated with asthma and peripheral eosinophila. Although more common on the tongue, **traumatic ulcerative granuloma with stromal eosinophilia (TUGSE, or Riga-Fede's disease)**[42] can occur on the palate and produce non-healing ulcers and associated non-specific mixed inflammatory infiltrates mimicking WG. Some TUGSE-like lesions have been described as **atypical histiocytic granuloma** because of their cytologic resemblance to a hematolymphoid malignancy.[43] Although usually causing lip swelling, **cheilitis granulomatosa (CG)** may also involve the buccal, palatal, sublingual, and gingival mucosa. Histologically, CG is characterized by peri- and paravascular mononuclear inflammatory infiltrates with edema, non-caseating granulomas, and multinucleated Langhans'-type giant cells. Patients may also present with other components of the **Melkersson-Rosenthal syndrome** (orofacial swelling, facial nerve paralysis, and plicated tongue).[44] **Oral Crohn's disease** and **recurrent aphthous ulceration (RAU)** with or without Behçet's syndrome (BS) should be included in this differential diagnosis.[45, 46] Oral Crohn's disease as a diagnostic problem is rare, but RAU probably affects 20% of the population and is usually clinically diagnostic. BS may include uveitis, aphthous ulcers, skin ulcers, genital ulcers, and gastrointestinal ulcers, as well as vascular and neurologic features. RAUs can manifest as crops of herpetiform tiny ulcers or as single or multiple ulcers from a few millimeters to several centimeters in diameter. Effective treatment of RAU may depend on finding and treating an underlying systemic disease, such as Crohn's disease, celiac disease, and folate, iron, and/or vita-

min B_{12} deficiency. RAUs, which are usually not associated with systemic disease, are treated with topical steroids, antibiotics, and immunomodulators.

If, after all these entities have been eliminated by careful clinicopathologic studies, the findings remain non-specific and the patient has destructive lesions of the upper aerodigestive tract, then **idiopathic midline destructive disease (IMDD)** should be considered. Tsokos et al.[30] have outlined the **criteria for diagnosing IMDD: (1) presence of locally destructive lesions restricted to the upper aerodigestive tract; (2) absence of systemic disease; (3) presence of acute and chronic inflammation with variable necrosis; and (4) absence of atypical cells, frank vasculitis, and demonstrable infection.** IMDD appears very responsive to radiation therapy.[30, 47]

Basal Cell Tumors of Salivary Glands

The 1972 World Health Organization (WHO) classification divided salivary gland adenomas into two basic categories, **pleomorphic adenoma (mixed tumor) and monomorphic adenomas,** the latter including **adenolymphoma (Warthin's tumor), oxyphil adenoma,** and other types. Thus, **monomorphic adenomas** consisted of a diverse and confusing group of tumors, which were not always monomorphic or monocellular. The much improved and modified 1989 WHO classification included not only pleomorphic adenoma but also **myoepithelioma, basal cell adenoma, Warthin's tumor (adenolymphoma), oncocytoma, canalicular adenoma, sebaceous adenoma, sebaceous lymphadenoma, inverted ductal papilloma, intraductal papilloma, sialadenoma papilliferum, papillary cystadenoma, and mucinous cystadenoma.**[48, 49] "Monomorphic" adenoma as a diagnostic term is now in disfavor, but it is still used to describe the occasional salivary gland adenoma with features not characteristic of any clear-cut category. This section focuses on basal cell tumors, which include **basal cell adenoma, basal cell adenocarcinoma, and the solid type of adenoid cystic carcinoma.**

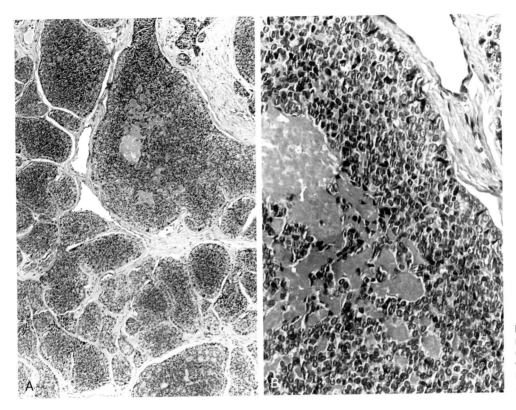

FIGURE 2–24. *A,* Basal cell adenoma, membranous pattern. (H&E, OM ×2.5) *B,* Note deposition of intercellular, hyaline, basal lamina–like material. (H&E, OM ×100)

Distinguishing these tumors is important because each has a different prognosis.

CLINICOPATHOLOGIC FEATURES. Basal cell adenomas are composed of isomorphic cells that form a prominent palisaded basal cell layer. They have a distinct basement membrane architecture and sometimes develop basosquamous whorls. The basaloid cells grow in four distinct patterns: solid, trabecular, tubular, and membranous (Figs. 2–24 to 2–28). Although one pattern usually predominates, basal cell adenomas can show mixed patterns. By definition, there is no mucoid stromal

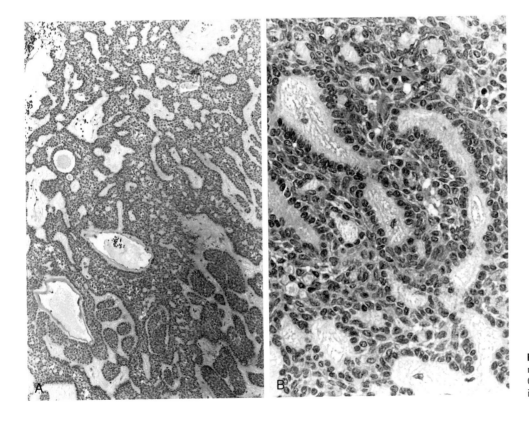

FIGURE 2–25. *A,* Basal cell adenoma, membranous type. (H&E, OM ×2.5) *B,* Note peripheral palisading. (H&E, OM ×100)

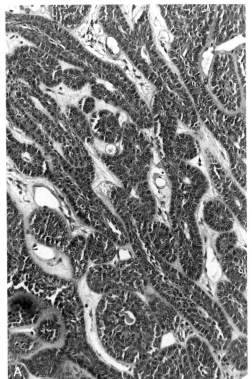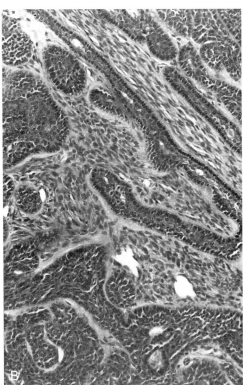

FIGURE 2–26. *A,* Basal cell adenoma, trabecular variant without cellular stroma. (H&E, OM ×50) *B,* Basal cell adenoma, trabecular variant with cellular spindled myoepithelial stroma. (H&E, OM ×50)

component as found in pleomorphic adenomas, but Dardick et al.[50] have proposed a subtype of **basal cell adenoma with a very cellular, spindled myoepithelial-cell stroma,** which is located between the anastomosing or trabecular cords of epithelial tumor cells (see Fig. 2–26).

Basal cell adenomas are rare (1% to 2% of all salivary gland adenomas) and tend to occur in late adulthood (mean age, 60 years; range, 0.1–93), with 70% occurring in the parotid and the remainder arising from submandibular or minor salivary glands.[51] Congenital tumors of the salivary

glands often resemble basal cell adenomas.[52] The solid variant is characterized by tumor cells arranged in small, rounded to large irregular islands and masses (see Fig. 2–28). Although basement membrane material is present, it is less well developed than in the membranous type (see Figs. 2–24 and 2–25). The trabecular pattern shows tumor cells arranged in anastomosing cords and bands (see Fig. 2–26). The tubular pattern is characterized by prominent duct-like lumen formation within the anastomosing cords (also known as salivary duct adenoma, tubular adenoma variant) (see Fig. 2–27), and

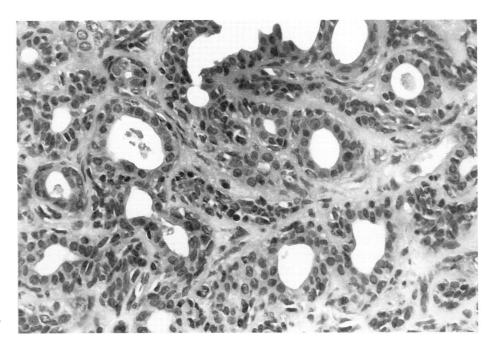

FIGURE 2–27. Basal cell adenoma, tubular variant. (H&E, OM ×50)

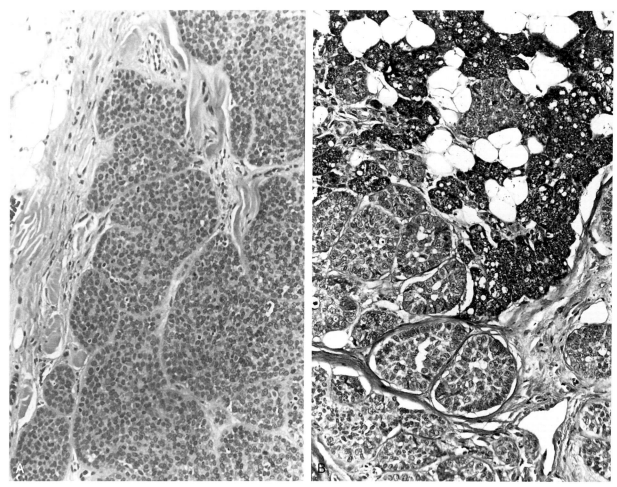

FIGURE 2–28. *A,* Basal cell adenomatous tumor (solid pattern) with invasive cell clusters at the periphery, consistent with so-called basal cell adenocarcinoma. (H&E, OM ×10) *B,* Note the "solid" nests of invasive basal cell adenocarcinoma cells extending into adjacent salivary gland tissues. Cytologic atypia greater than that encountered in non-invasive basal cell adenomas is not needed for a diagnosis of basal cell adenocarcinoma, but in addition they show invasion of surrounding tissues. (H&E, OM ×100)

the membranous variant shows a prominent palisading pattern of peripheral cell layers, excessive hyaline basal membrane material (PAS positive), sometimes focal squamous metaplasia, and focal prominent intercellular hyaline deposits (see Figs. 2–24 and 2–25). Basal cell adenomas are non-infiltrating tumors, but they are often multifocal and multinodular and sometimes associated with ductal hyperplasia-microadenomas and/or **concomitant dermal cylindromas-trichoepitheliomas.**[53, 55] Because these patterns closely resemble dermal cylindromas (especially the membranous pattern), Batsakis and Brannon[56] have proposed that they be termed **dermal analogue tumors** of major salivary glands. Finally, Nagao et al.[57] studied 40 basal cell adenomas and, in addition to the patterns described here, found areas that they characterized as "papillary," cystic, and/or adenoid cystic–like.

Ellis and Wiscovitch[53] were among the first to describe **basal cell adenocarcinomas ("malignant basal cell tumor")** of the salivary glands (see Fig. 2–28). These tumors grew in all the multifocal and multinodular patterns of benign basal cell adenoma, but by definition they were also infiltrative into adjacent tissues as strands and nests of tumor cells extending into normal acini, muscle, fat, and/or dermis. Some showed perineural and/or intravascular invasion; they often

had more frequent mitoses (mean, 2 per 10 HPF; range, 0–9) and sometimes more cytologic atypia and tumor-cell necrosis. The most common growth pattern was that of solid cell nests, smaller hyaline membrane structures, and less frequent trabecular-tubular structures. The recurrence rate was about 25%, the metastasis rate was about 10%, concomitant occurrence with dermal cylindromas was about 10%, and the predominant site was the parotid gland. Basal cell adenocarcinoma is considered the malignant counterpart of basal cell adenoma, and malignant transformation of the latter to adenocarcinoma has been described.[58]

The **solid type of adenoid cystic carcinoma (ACC)** constitutes about 10% of ACC tumors and is often confused with basal cell adenocarcinoma or other tumors, such as poorly differentiated squamous carcinoma, basaloid-squamous carcinoma, or small-cell undifferentiated carcinoma. The solid type of ACC grows as chromatin-dark epithelial islands composed of polygonal to oval cells with hyperchromatic nuclei and high nucleocytoplasmic ratios (Fig. 2–29). The solid cell nests may have sporadic glandular structures or cribriform patterns and/or central necrosis. Mitoses are stated to be fewer than those found in basal cell adenocarcinomas,[51] yet Batsakis et al.[59] and Chomette et al.,[60] respectively, state that in the solid (or basaloid) variant of ACC "mitoses are easily found" and

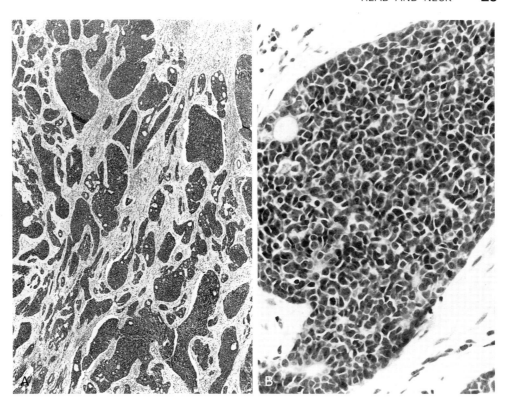

FIGURE 2–29. *A,* Solid type of adenoid cystic carcinoma associated with poorest prognosis. (H&E, OM ×25) *B,* Note high nucleocytoplasmic ratios and occasional gland within an otherwise solid nest of adenoid cystic carcinoma. (H&E, OM ×100)

"are fairly numerous." Greater sampling may show more "classic" areas of ACC growing as the glandular-cribriform and/or trabecular-tubular type (Fig. 2–30A). Some suggest that at least 30% of the tumor should be solid to be considered the solid variant; however, any measure of solid pattern may portend a worse prognosis.[55]

The **glandular-cribriform type of ACC,** which constitutes about 50% of all ACCs, has cribriform ("Swiss cheese") spaces, sieve-like configurations, pseudocysts with mucoid and/or hyaline material, small glands with mucinous secretion, fibrous (hyalinized) stroma, and minimal cellular stromal reaction (Fig. 2–30B). The trabecular-tubular type of ACC accounts for about 30% of all ACCs and grows as epithelial strands or cords with well-developed tubules (see Fig. 2–30). Between the tumor cells there is a hyaline/desmoplastic stromal reaction. The glandular-cribriform and **trabecular-tubular types** are often admixed and usually show prominent perineural invasion. The trabecular-tubular type has the best prognosis, whereas the solid type has the worst prognosis, with numerous early recurrences and metastases associated with high mortality. The classic glandular-cribriform type of ACC is stated to have an intermediate prognosis.[61] Because ACCs frequently show mixed patterns, the predominant pattern (usually but not always >50%) should be used to place each tumor into an appropriate group of trabecular-tubular, glandular-cribriform, or solid.[57] Other investigators have suggested that the numbers of gland-like spaces per square millimeter of tumor, excluding supporting stroma and small areas with the tubular pattern, appeared to be a better measure of aggressiveness of the cribriform and solid patterns.[62] Mitotic activity, perineural invasion, vascular invasion, and necrosis remain controversial as predictors of prognosis, yet they are most frequently seen in the solid pattern of ACCs.[63] Nascimento et al.[63] reported that ACCs located in minor salivary

glands, whose symptoms lasted less than 1 year, and those with advanced clinical stage were associated with a poorer prognosis than those without these features.

DIFFERENTIAL DIAGNOSIS. The differential diagnosis of basal cell tumors primarily includes **pleomorphic adenoma, myoepithelioma, canalicular adenoma, low-grade polymorphous adenocarcinoma, basaloid-squamous carcinoma, undifferentiated carcinoma, and neuroendocrine carcinoma.** Pleomorphic adenomas exhibit a myoepithelium-derived myxochondroid matrix in addition to duct epithelial differentiation (Fig. 2–31). Yet, Dardick et al.[50] recognized a subtype of basal cell adenoma with myoepithelial cell–derived "stroma" (see Fig. 2–26). Also, some salivary gland tumors are overwhelmingly composed of myoepithelial elements, which may be spindle-shaped (Fig. 2–32A), plasmacytoid-hyaline (Fig. 2–32B), oncocytic, and/or a combination of these patterns admixed with minor components of ductular differentiation. Whether the latter salivary gland tumors are best considered separately as myoepitheliomas or as variants of pleomorphic adenomas with a predominant myoepithelial component is controversial and of little clinical importance because both behave biologically the same and are treated with conservative yet complete excision. **Canalicular adenomas** (Fig. 2–33B) are benign tumors that occur predominantly in the upper lip (90%) and the buccal mucosa (10%).[51] They consist of columnar epithelial cells arranged in anastomosing bilayered strands separated by a loose, vascular stroma. They resemble trabecular-type basal cell adenomas (Fig. 2–33A). Low-grade, polymorphous adenocarcinomas have a bland, uniform, cytologic presentation (see later discussion).

Basaloid-squamous carcinomas (BSCs) can be easily mistaken for solid variants of ACC, especially those with central necrosis (Fig. 2–34). BSCs arise from the pyriform

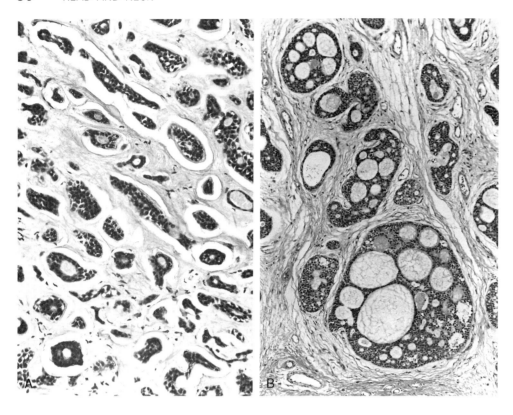

FIGURE 2–30. *A,* Trabecular-tubular type of adenoid cystic carcinoma associated with best prognosis. (H&E, OM ×25) *B,* Glandular-cribriform type of adenoid cystic carcinoma associated with intermediate prognosis. (H&E, OM ×25)

sinus, hypopharynx, base of tongue, tonsil, and larynx.[64–68] BSCs are rare but distinctive tumors associated with a grave prognosis. They occur most commonly in elderly males and do not become apparent until they reach an advanced stage. Cytologically, BSCs present as lobules of moderately pleomorphic basaloid cells forming solid tumor growths often closely apposed to the surface mucosa (see Fig. 2–34). The lobulated, sometimes anastomosing nests of tumor frequently have central, comedo-like necrosis and are admixed with intercellular deposits of globular and ribbon-like stromal hyalin material (Figs. 2–34 and 2–35). Foci of ducts and/or cribriform foci may also be present, and there may be associated

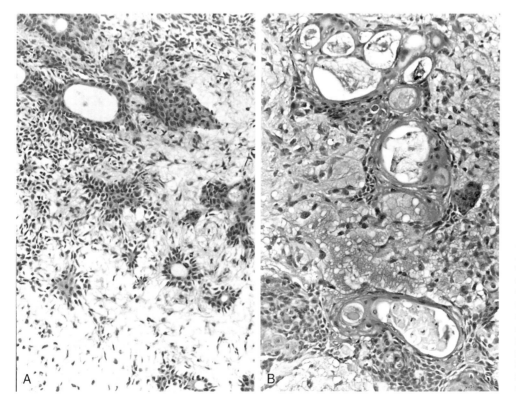

FIGURE 2–31. *A,* Pleomorphic adenoma. Note the mixed ductal and myxochondroid elements with transitional myoepithelial cells spindling off epithelial clusters. (H&E, OM ×10) *B,* Pleomorphic adenoma with myxochondroid and ductal epithelial clusters showing squamous and mucinous differentiation. This pattern of pleomorphic adenoma can be mistaken for mucoepidermoid carcinoma. (H&E, OM ×100)

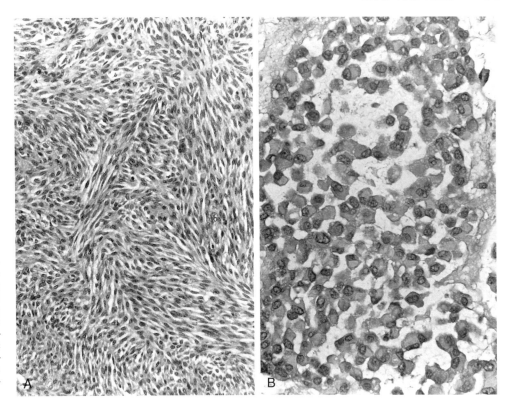

FIGURE 2–32. *A,* Spindled myoepithelial cells from a pleomorphic adenoma showing overwhelming myoepithelial differentiation (so-called spindle cell myoepithelioma). (H&E, OM ×100) *B,* Plasmacytoid myoepithelial cells from a pleomorphic adenoma showing overwhelming myoepithelial differentiation (so-called plasmacytoid myoepithelioma). (H&E, OM ×100)

squamous dysplasia of surface mucosa, focal squamous differentiation within the tumor, and/or foci of conventional squamous carcinoma present. **Undifferentiated and neuroendocrine carcinomas** are covered in the section on undifferentiated carcinoma.

Oncocytoma

Oncocytomas are rare salivary gland tumors, accounting for less than 1% of all salivary gland neoplasms. Most oncocytomas occur in the major salivary glands, but some cases have arisen in the minor salivary glands.[69] Importantly, other

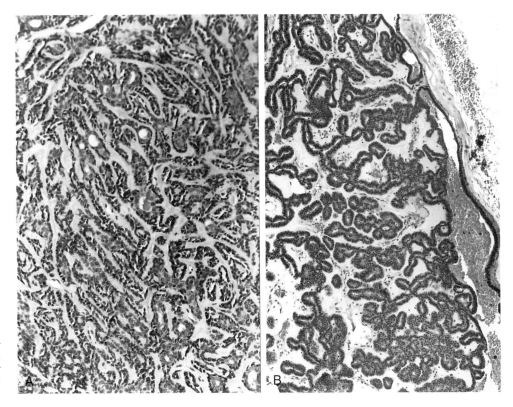

FIGURE 2–33. *A,* Basal cell adenoma, trabecular variant. (H&E, OM ×10) *B,* Canalicular adenoma from upper lip. (H&E, OM ×10)

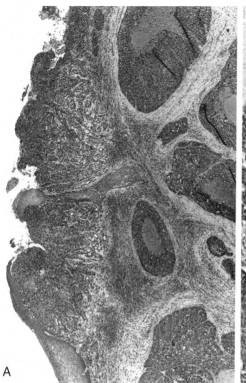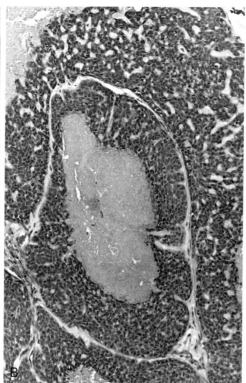

FIGURE 2-34. *A,* Basaloid-squamous cell carcinoma of larynx. Note typical invasive squamous carcinoma at the surface, with rounded nests of basaloid-squamous cell carcinoma below. (H&E, OM ×2.5) *B,* Invasive nests and sheets of basaloid-squamous cell carcinoma show central comedo-like necrosis and adenoid cystic-like pattern. (H&E, OM ×50)

salivary gland tumors can show "oncocytic changes," such as pleomorphic and monomorphic adenomas.[70] Rare examples of "oncocytoma" have also been reported in the ovary, stomach, liver, pituitary, lacrimal sac or caruncle, lower respiratory tract, pancreas, breast, esophagus, thymus, and kidney.[71] Thus, it is this rarity of occurrence and their histologic overlap with other tumors that make their diagnosis difficult. Also, secondary salivary gland tumors such as pleomorphic adenoma and mucoepidermoid carcinoma can also occur in these patients, sometimes in association with a history of radiation

exposure. Finally, oncocytic carcinoma is even rarer, constituting an estimated 0.0005% of all salivary gland tumors.[72]

CLINICOPATHOLOGIC FEATURES. Brandwein and Huvos[73] studied 44 patients with 68 tumors of major salivary glands; 84% occurred in the parotid gland, 11% were in the submandibular gland, and 5% were incidentally found in upper cervical lymph nodes (apparently arising from salivary gland rests). The mean patient age was 58 years (range, 23–89), the incidence in males and females was about equal, and 20% had a history of prior radiation exposure. Bilateral tumors occurred

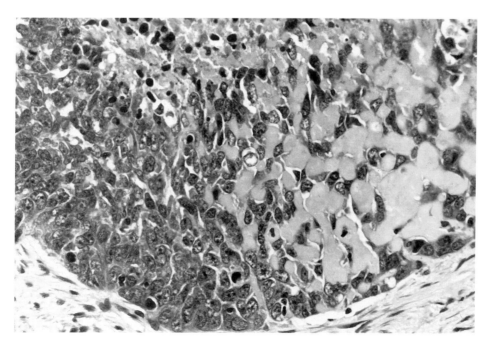

FIGURE 2-35. Abundant basal lamina material is often deposited between tumor cells in basaloid-squamous cell carcinoma. Mitotic figures and cytologic atypia are prominent. (H&E, OM ×100)

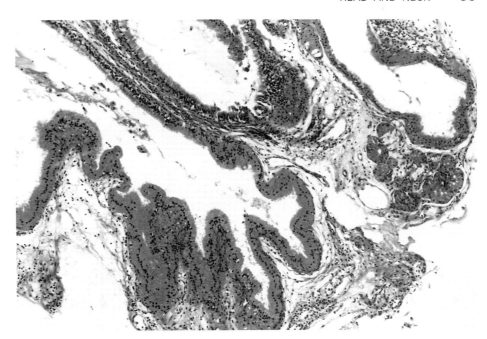

FIGURE 2–36. Oncocytic papillary cystadenomatosis with multifocal oncocytic hyperplasia of the duct epithelium of the seromucinous glands, producing simple oncocytic cysts to small oncocytomas. (H&E, OM ×25)

in four patients, which correlated with extensive clear-cell changes and greater recurrences.

Brandwein and Huvos[73] defined oncocytoma as a single neoplasm in contrast to **nodular hyperplasia or nodular oncocytosis,** which referred to two or more distinct tumor nodules. These nodules may become so numerous and enlarged as to replace the entire parotid gland with a multinodular or lobulated oncocytic tumor. **Oncocytosis** referred to formation of micronodules as a result of oncocytic metaplasia and hyperplasia of small and large ducts; however, this change

was so common around oncocytic lesions that the distinction between an oncocytoma and nodular oncocytic hyperplasia may be very arbitrary. Oncocytic papillary cystadenomatosis refers to multifocal oncocytic hyperplasia of the duct epithelium of the seromucinous glands, producing simple oncocytic cysts to small oncocytomas (Fig. 2–36).[74]

Grossly, oncocytic tumors appear as single or multiple soft, tan-brown nodules, but cystic change can occur. The classic oncocyte has a uniform round, centrally located nucleus within abundant pink and uniformly granular cytoplasm (Fig. 2–37).

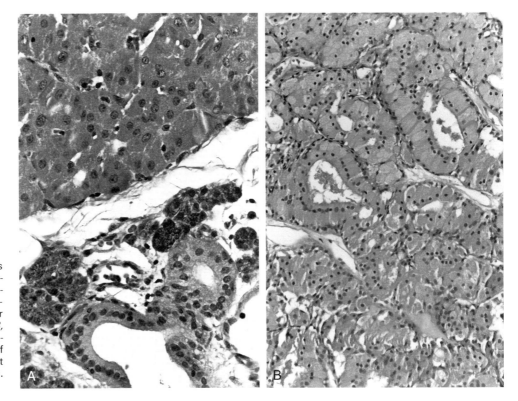

FIGURE 2–37. *A,* Oncocytoma is shown in upper left-hand portions of the photograph. Immediately adjacent, some oncocytic intercalated ductal cells for comparison. (H&E, OM ×50) *B,* Some oncocytomas have cytologic features like those of Warthin's tumor but without the lymphoid cell–rich stroma. (H&E, OM ×25)

After 48 hours of incubation, phosphotungstic acid hematoxylin (PTAH) stain will demonstrate mitochondria as blue granules. Nucleoli can be single and prominent or multiple (Fig. 2–38). It is important that the intensity of the oxyphilia can vary, and interspersed or transitions to clear cells are not unusual. Indeed Ellis[75] has described a **"clear-cell"** variant of **oncocytoma** of salivary gland (see Fig. 2–38). These benign clear-cell oncocytomas can be confused with other clear-cell tumors of salivary glands, which are for the most part of low-grade malignant potential but occasionally frankly malignant. Salivary gland oncocytomas have rare mitotic figures (0–1 per 20 HPF). Lesions are nodular and grow in acinar, trabecular, and/or follicular patterns (see Fig. 2–37). Areas resembling Warthin's tumor may be present, with tall oncocytes forming cysts and papillae, but they lack the lymphoid stroma. Other unusual features include focal sebaceous, goblet-cell, and/or squamous differentiation as well as myxoid, hyaline, and even cartilagenous stroma.

Taxy[76] has recently re-emphasized that **oncocytic salivary gland tumors can sometimes show tumor necrosis associated with squamous metaplasia, mucinous metaplasia, and/or a desmoplastic stromal reaction, which can be associated with enough cytologic atypia to simulate carcinoma** (Fig. 2–39). These changes are most commonly encountered in Warthin's tumors; a finding also referred to as metaplastic or infarcted ("infected") Warthin's tumor (see Fig. 2–39).[77, 78] The tumor necrosis and metaplasia are reminiscent of necrotizing sialometaplasia, thought to be ischemic in origin.[76] But care must be exercised before true malignant change is totally ruled out, because **"oncocytic" adenocarcinomas and malignant lymphomas can rarely arise within Warthin's tumors.**[79, 80]

The recurrence rate of benign oncocytomas is roughly 10%. Brandwein and Huvos[73] found that so-called aggressive features such as capsular invasion, pseudopod-like infiltration, perineural spread, oncocytes "hugging" vascular spaces, cellular pleomorphism, adjacent oncocytosis, and mitotic rate were not significant for predicting recurrence. Stromal hyalinization and marked vascularity may give the false impression of invasion as well. However, very rarely, **oncocytic carcinomas** do occur, and Seifert et al.[78] discussed two "criteria" necessary to establish this diagnosis. First, the tumor cells must be clearly identified as oncocytes, and second, the tumor must be malignant. But, as outlined by Brandwein and Huvos,[73] benign oncocytomas may have "aggressive" cytoarchitectural features, which are not necessarily predictive of a poor outcome. Thus, like some neuroendocrine tumors, it may be that lymph node and/or distant metastases are the only absolute indicators of malignancy. However, large tumor size, tumor necrosis, and numerous mitoses (especially if atypical) should be considered ominous findings.

DIFFERENTIAL DIAGNOSIS. The differential diagnosis of oncocytoma includes **other salivary gland tumors showing oncocytic changes.** These include pleomorphic and monomorphic adenomas. Close attention to other areas of these tumors should disclose their true identity. Moreover, certain oncocytes are distinctive for oncocytic tumors: cells with shrunken pyknotic nuclei (pyknocytes), tall oncocytes with tapered or blunt ends, and occasional binucleated oncocytes. Also, a variety of low- and high-grade clear-cell tumors need to be distinguished from the so-called "clear-cell" variant of oncocytoma. These include some pleomorphic adenomas, sebaceous adenoma and sebaceous adenocarcinoma, some mucoepidermoid carcinomas, acinic cell carcinoma, epithelial-myoepithelial carcinoma, and metastatic renal cell carcinoma or clear-cell thyroid carcinoma. Again, close attention to other areas of these clear-cell lesions should disclose their true identity; hence, extensive tumor sampling is indi-

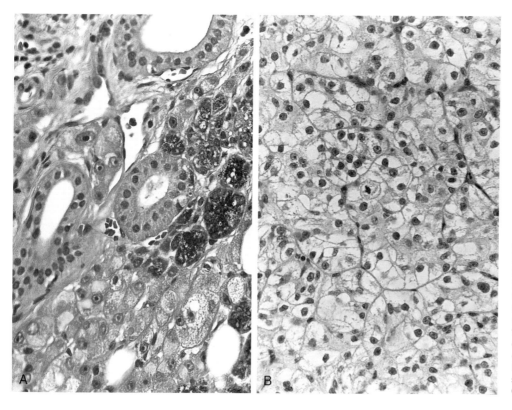

FIGURE 2–38. A, Atypical cytologic features are apparent in this infiltrating oncocytic tumor, but these aggressive cytoarchitectural features are not necessarily predictive of malignant oncocytoma, an extremely rare tumor. (H&E, OM ×100) B, Glycogen-rich, clear-cell variant of oncocytoma, a pattern that can be easily confused with metastatic renal carcinoma. (H&E, OM ×100)

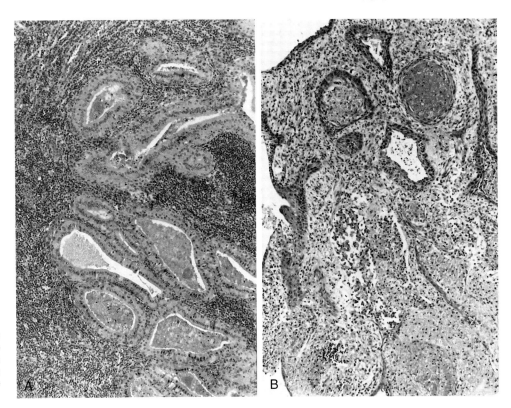

FIGURE 2–39. *A,* Warthin's tumor. (H&E, OM ×25) *B,* Warthin's tumor with focal necrosis and squamous metaplasia. This pattern can be mistaken for carcinoma. (H&E, OM ×25)

cated in these difficult cases. Salivary duct carcinomas are typically "apocrinoid," and thus mimic oncocytic carcinoma. Indeed, some cases of reported oncocytic carcinoma may now be considered examples of salivary duct carcinoma.

Squamous Cell Papilloma

Squamous papillary lesions of the head-and-neck region include both malignant and benign proliferations. This review focuses on the benign lesions, especially those with epithelial atypia/dysplasia. Many of these papillary lesions are associated with **human papillomavirus (HPV)** infection. Benign squamous papillomas have been associated with HPV 6 or 11, whereas some malignant papillomas have either shown no association with HPV or been associated with HPV 6, 11, 16, and/or 18, sometimes in combination with types 31, 33, and 35.[81–83] Distinguishing benign from malignant squamous papillomas is complicated by the finding of **epithelial atypia/ dysplasia in otherwise benign squamous papillomas, especially in rapidly growing, recurrent lesions** (Fig. 2–40). Because the outcome for these two lesions is quite different, their distinction is critical.[84]

CLINICOPATHOLOGIC FEATURES. Squamous papillomas (exophytic papillary growths of the squamous and/or admixed respiratory mucosa) have been divided into the **solitary** (usually non-recurring) and **multiple** (often recurring) forms. Although both forms can involve any head and neck mucosal site in both children and adults (including the trachea [2% to 26% of cases] and lung [<1% of cases]), the solitary form is most common in the oral mucosa of adults, whereas the multiple recurring form is most common in the larynx and tracheobronchial mucosa of children. Malignant transformation rarely occurs in multiple recurring lesions, usually in adult-onset disease and when there is a previous history of

irradiation, smoking, and/or cytotoxic drug exposure.[83] However, invasive papillomatosis can occur without cytologic atypia or metastases.[85]

Although classified as benign lesions, squamous papillomas commonly show epithelial atypia/dysplasia, which can be severe enough to cause a misdiagnosis of **carcinoma in situ** or **papillary carcinoma** (see Fig. 2–40).[81, 84] Quick et al.[84] reviewed 32 cases of laryngeal papillomatosis and found that in those papillomas with a high rate of recurrence and growth, the epithelial atypia/dysplasia tended to be most pronounced. Although in some the atypia/dysplasia was "quite disturbing," there was no evidence of development of invasive carcinoma. Crissman et al.[81] reported seven adult patients with recurrent papillomas with a mean age of 42.7 years at the time of study (range, 25–76) and a mean age of 13.3 years at initial diagnosis (range, 4–40). All had various degrees of epithelial atypia, and their lesions contained either HPV 6 or 11; six cases revealed abnormal DNA. The most common diagnosis in the biopsies from these patients was dysplastic papilloma, and a diagnosis of either severe dysplasia/carcinoma in situ or papillary carcinoma had been rendered for all seven patients. None of the patients were treated for malignancy, and none developed carcinoma. Illustrations of the atypia/dysplasia from this study of recurrent papillomatosis showed little or no epithelial maturation; there was, however, increased cellularity, giant hyperchromatic nuclei with variable epithelial maturation, and pronounced nuclear atypia with "attempts at surface keratinization" and a "hint of koilocytotic change."[81] These investigators described six patients with papillary carcinoma (mean age at onset of disease, 63.3 years; range, 46–79); three had invasion. No HPV was detected in these carcinomatous lesions, and all showed abnormal DNA content.

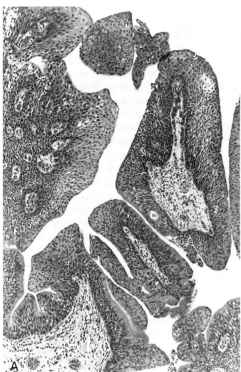
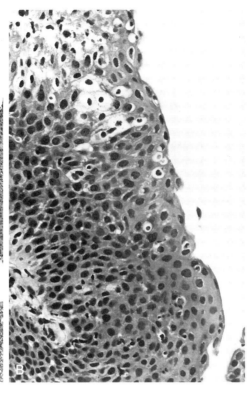

FIGURE 2–40. *A*, Laryngeal papillomatosis, recurrent. (H&E, OM ×10) *B*, Recurrent laryngeal papillomatosis showing mild atypia. Care should be taken not to over-diagnose atypia as carcinoma in recurrent, rapidly growing laryngeal papillomatosis. (H&E, OM ×100)

DIFFERENTIAL DIAGNOSIS. Epithelial atypia/dysplasia in squamous papillomas in the adolescent are well described and should not be a diagnostic problem (in fact, in the vast majority, the findings can be ignored); however, when squamous papillomas persist into adulthood or develop in adulthood, the differential diagnosis must include papillary squamous carcinoma in situ and/or invasive carcinoma.[81] As Crissman et al.[81] indicate, "this problem is compounded when a history of recurrent papillomatosis is not available or if the pathologist is not cognizant of the range of histologic and cytologic cellular atypia, which can be observed in recurrent papillomatosis." This can cause the overdiagnosis of carcinoma in this setting. Although uncommon, true squamous carcinomas occur in the larynx of children and young adults.[86, 87] True papillary carcinomas tend to occur in older patients, are not associated with a history of previous recurrent papillomatosis, and show more diffuse full-thickness malignant epithelium. In doubtful cases, a biopsy of the underlying stroma should be performed to rule out invasive squamous carcinoma, and consideration should be given to HPV typing. In contrast to recurring laryngeal papillomatosis, true papillary carcinomas are much less likely to be associated with HPV infection.

The differential diagnosis of benign squamous papilloma also includes verrucous carcinoma, verrucous-squamous carcinoma, well-differentiated (verruciform) squamous carcinoma, superficial extending carcinoma, verrucous hyperplasia, pseudoepitheliomatous hyperplasia (PEH), verruca vulgaris, and verruciform xanthoma. **Verrucous carcinomas**[88] are exophytic, sessile and papillary, hyperkeratotic, and acanthotic squamous lesions that infiltrate subepithelial connective tissue as broad invaginating folds of highly differentiated, minimally atypical squamous epithelium,

often with adjacent chronic inflammation (Fig. 2–41). Verrucous carcinomas are warty lesions that look malignant clinically, but paradoxically are histologically benign. Treatment is surgery, but neck dissection is not necessary because lymph nodal and/or distant metastases do not occur. Verrucous carcinomas should be sampled widely, because less well differentiated areas of conventional invasive squamous carcinoma can be found in as many as 20% of cases. These lesions are best considered **verrucous-squamous carcinomas**[89] and are more likely to recur locally. Well-differentiated (verruciform) squamous carcinomas show greater cytologic atypia than verrucous carcinoma (Fig. 2–42). The term **superficial extending carcinoma (SEC)** is used for a superficially yet diffusely invasive squamous carcinoma, which is usually moderately to poorly differentiated and is invasive only into the mucosa or limited to a few underlying glandular and/or muscular structures, but may show lymph nodal and/or lymphatic vessel invasion.[90] Although SEC is like other head and neck squamous carcinomas, it is especially prone to be associated with other synchronous and/or metachronous squamous lesions, and its extent of invasion is frequently underestimated by clinicians. **Verrucous hyperplasia** is the term for a verrucous epithelial proliferation that clinically mimics verrucous carcinoma and histologically shows exuberant acanthosis and keratosis. **Verrucous hyperplasia, however, is purely exophytic and extends no deeper than the level of the adjacent normal epithelial basement membrane.**[91] Yet, verrucous hyperplasias may be associated with verrucous carcinoma, intraepithelial dysplasia, and/or conventional squamous carcinoma. Thus, verrucous hyperplasia should be regarded as potentially precancerous, often eventually becoming verrucous carcinoma and/or squamous carcinoma.

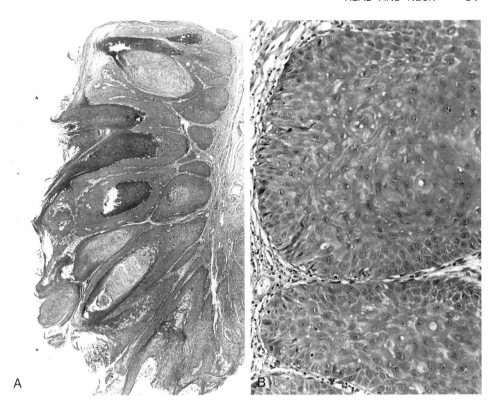

FIGURE 2–41. *A,* Verrucous carcinoma. Note the invagination of blunt epithelial "tongues" into adjacent stroma. Hyperparakeratosis is prominent. (H&E, OM ×2.5) *B,* Invaginating tongues of squamous cells show only mild cytologic atypia. (H&E, OM ×100)

Pseudoepitheliomatous hyperplasia often occurs in benign squamous epithelium adjacent to chronic-active ulcers or overlying granular cell tumors (Fig. 2–43).

Recently, Krutchkoff et al.[92] have outlined the more subtle morphologic features of *in situ* squamous dysplasia in head and neck squamous mucosa. This reference is worth reviewing. Cytologically bland verruciform and keratotic squamous lesions with numerous foamy histiocytes in the upper laminal propria are known as **verruciform xanthoma.**[93] They are of unknown cause and not associated

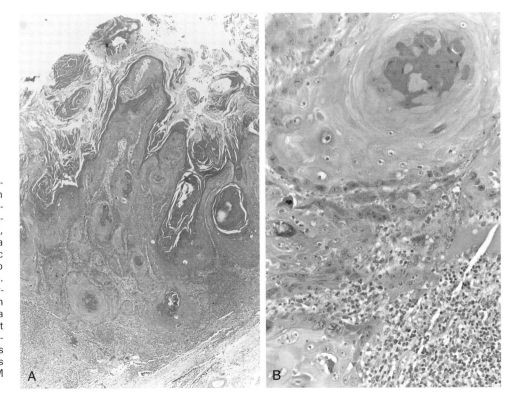

FIGURE 2–42. *A,* Well-differentiated squamous carcinoma with verrucous carcinoma-like features. (H&E, OM ×10) *B,* In contrast to verrucous carcinoma, invasive squamous carcinoma cells show greater cytologic atypia and the tendency to invade as small clusters of cells. So-called hybrid squamous carcinomas show features of both invasive squamous carcinoma and verrucous carcinoma, and it is likely that a continuum of well-differentiated squamous tumors occurs among tumors of this general category. (H&E, OM ×100)

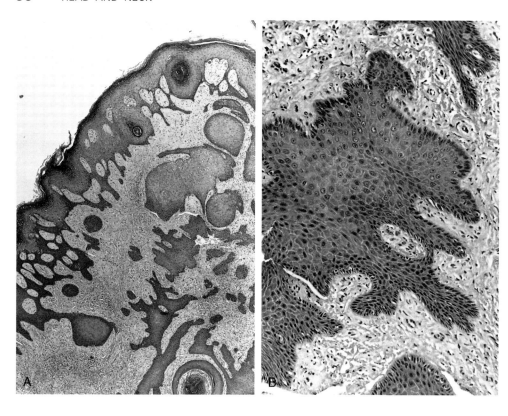

FIGURE 2–43. *A,* Pseudoepitheliomatous hyperplasia (PEH). Note irregular-sized and -shaped nests of squamous epithelium separated by abundant fibroblastic stroma. (H&E, OM ×2.5) *B,* Note benign cytologic features of PEH; but such bland squamous islands can grow down fistula tracts into bone. (H&E, OM ×100)

with any systemic illness. HPV lesions mimicking verruca vulgaris of the skin have been described in the larynx, and they may be confused with verrucous carcinoma.[94] Thus, when viewing any verruciform, hyperplastic, and/or epitheliomatous squamous lesion, take care to examine the tips of the connective tissue papillae close to the squamous epithe-

lium for foamy histiocytes, and if present, consider verruciform xanthoma.

Granular Cell Tumor

Granular cell tumors are uncommon tumors of probable neural origin. Although the vast majority are benign, occa-

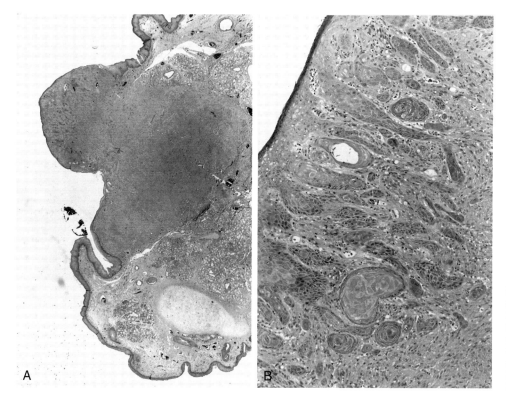

FIGURE 2–44. *A,* Granular cell tumor of the larynx. (H&E, OM ×2.5) *B,* Note prominent pseudoepitheliomatous hyperplasia of overlying squamous epithelium with "detached" clusters of squamous epithelial cells simulating invasive carcinoma. (H&E, OM ×50)

sional malignant examples occur.[95] They are important because they are frequently associated with overlying benign PEH of the squamous mucosa (Figs. 2–44 and 2–45), which can cause the **overdiagnosis of invasive squamous carcinoma.** The consequences of overtreatment can be catastrophic to the patient.

The histogenesis of granular cell tumors remains controversial, but most examples are strongly positive for S-100 protein, suggesting Schwann cell differentiation.[96] This is also supported by the identification of axons in some lesions, finding similar-appearing granular cells in degenerating nerve, and focal findings of granular cells in occasional schwannomas. Yet, this theory does not explain all examples, because granular cells occur in basal cell carcinomas, ameloblastomas, ameloblastic fibromas, and rarely, in close association with smooth muscle.[97, 98]

CLINICOPATHOLOGIC FEATURES. Granular cell tumors are usually asymptomatic, unless they impinge on a vital structure. They occur anywhere on the skin or mucous membranes and are found in any age group. About one third to one half occur in the tongue, about one third occur in the skin, and the remainder involve other mucosal covered structures, especially the larynx or tracheobronchial tree. About one half have associated PEH, which can closely mimic invasive, well-differentiated squamous carcinoma (see Fig. 2–44). **Congenital epulis** occurs exclusively on the gingiva of newborn infants, and it is microscopically identical to other granular cell tumors, except there is no PEH and they may be S-100 negative. Granular cells are usually polygonal or spindled cells with abundant granular cytoplasm (see Fig. 2–45). The granules are pink periodic acid-Schiff (PAS) positive, and irregular in size and shape (this last feature helps separate granular cell tumor from oncocytic granules, which are uniform). The granules are lysosomal structures thought to be autophagic vacuoles. Granular cells, although commonly positive for S-100 protein, are also CD68 positive and may be S-100 negative,[99] and they show desmin and actin immunoreactivity in those cases associated with smooth muscle.[97]

Malignant granular cell tumors have been broken down into two groups by Gamboa.[100] One group was clinically malignant without histologic evidence of malignancy, and the other was both clinically and histologically malignant. Cellular and nuclear pleomorphism, prominent nucleoli, and mitotic figures are now regarded as highly suggestive of malignancy in a granular cell tumor.[101]

DIFFERENTIAL DIAGNOSIS. The purpose of including granular cell tumors within this chapter was to emphasize the concomitant PEH, which can be overdiagnosed as invasive well-differentiated squamous carcinoma. To avoid this mistake, always consider the possibility of an underlying granular cell tumor before making a final diagnosis of invasive well-differentiated squamous carcinoma. Look for polygonal to spindled cells with granular cytoplasm. If suspicious cells are present, perform PAS and S-100 staining and/or electron microscopy until a clear diagnosis is reached. Separating granular cell tumors from oncocytomas is aided by the observation that the granules of granular cell tumors are irregular in size and shape, whereas the granules of oncocytic lesions are small, regular, and uniform in size and shape. PAS stain, PTAH stain, and/or electron microscopy should resolve problematic cases.

Malignant Head and Neck Lesions

Osteosarcoma and Juxtacortical Osteosarcoma

Jaw osteosarcomas are more commonly seen in the mandible than the maxilla and constitute approximately 5% of all

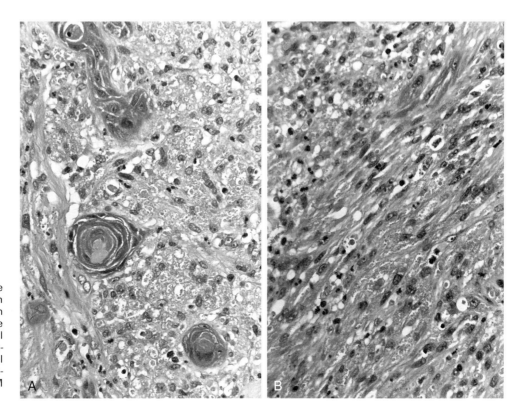

FIGURE 2–45. *A,* Shown are the epithelioid granular cells with irregularly granular cytoplasm admixed with pseudoinvasive clusters of squamous epithelial cells. (H&E, OM ×100) *B,* Granular cells can form polygonal shapes but also spindle cell configurations as well. (H&E, OM ×100)

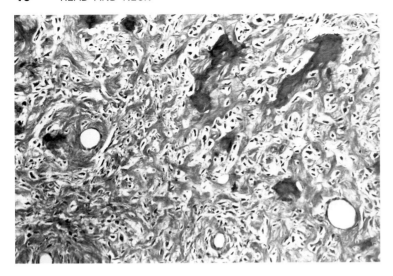

FIGURE 2–46. Osteoblastic osteosarcoma of the mandible. Note irregular trabeculae and calcification. (H&E, ×100)

osteosarcomas. They may originate from the medullary cavity or the periosteum of the jaws (**juxtacortical osteosarcomas**). Lesions originating from the periosteum are separated from central lesions because of differences in clinical features, microscopy, and biologic behavior. Although osteosarcomas and juxtacortical osteosarcomas are not commonly seen by surgical pathologists, they may cause diagnostic problems because most of these jaw lesions are relatively well differentiated. Separation from fibro-osseous and chondroid lesions, and occasionally giant cell lesions, may be difficult.

CLINICOPATHOLOGIC FEATURES. Osteosarcomas of the jaws exhibit some behavioral features that distinguish them from lesions of the rest of the skeleton. Jaw lesions tend to occur at an older mean age (fourth decade versus second decade for non-jaw lesions). Swelling, pain, and paresthesia are more typical of jaw lesions. A uniformly widened periodontal membrane space is often seen when the lesion involves the alveolus,[102–104] and there is a wide range of radiographic presentations, from radiolucent to radiopaque with classic "sunburst" pattern.

As a group, jaw osteosarcomas have been generally described as being better differentiated than lesions of the remainder of the skeleton. In well-differentiated osteosarcoma, the nuclei are usually dark and angular. Mitotic figures may or may not be seen. New bone tends to be more haphazard in size and distribution. The histologic subtypes of jaw osteosarcomas include (in order of descending frequency) osteoblastic (Figs. 2–46 and 2–47), chondroblastic (Fig. 2–48), fibroblastic (Fig. 2–49), and telangiectatic, depending on the predominant type of stroma. The importance of recognition of histologic subtypes relates to accurate classification of these lesions as osteosarcomas, rather than as **chondrosarcomas, fibrosarcomas,** or **benign connective tissue lesions.** The histologic subtypes do not exhibit different clinical behaviors. Definitive diagnosis is based upon H&E microscopy taken in an appropriate clinical context. Immunohistochemistry using

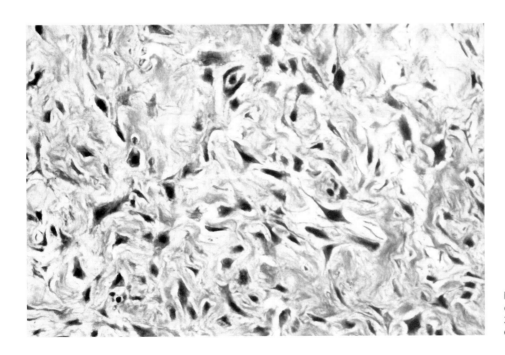

FIGURE 2–47. High magnification of osteosarcoma illustrated in Figure 2–46 showing angular and hyperchromatic cells. (H&E, ×250)

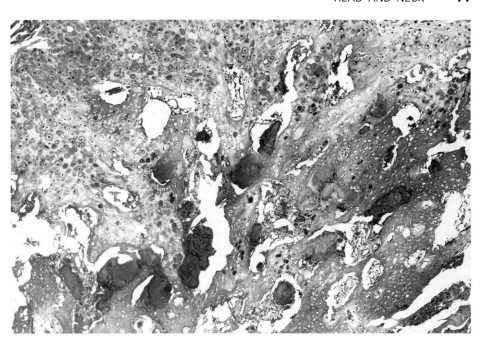

FIGURE 2–48. Chondroblastic osteosarcoma with a predominantly cartilaginous field. (H&E, ×100)

currently available antibodies appears to offer no particular advantage in tumor classification.[105]

Metastases from a jaw lesion are very uncommon compared with those from similar lesions in other bones; thus, the prognosis is correspondingly more favorable for jaw lesions. The 5-year survival rate for non-jaw lesions is approximately 20% (30% to 40% for jaw tumors) when treated with surgery alone. When surgery is combined with chemotherapy, survival rates have been significantly increased (50% to 60%).[106] Patients with jaw lesions would be expected to fare better than patients with osteosarcomas in other bones.

Juxtacortical osteosarcomas have been subdivided into **parosteal** and **periosteal** types because of clinicopathologic differences.[107] The parosteal subtype, the more common of the two, affects patients at an average age of 40 years, as opposed to 20 years for those with periosteal osteosarcoma.[108] Radiographically, the parosteal subtype is relatively dense, particularly at its base, and the periosteal subtype is relatively lucent; both are discontinuous with the underlying marrow.

The prognosis for juxtacortical osteosarcoma is better than for marrow-derived osteosarcoma, and parosteal has a better prognosis than periosteal osteosarcoma. Although recurrence of juxtacortical lesions is not uncommon, metastasis is apparently vary rare.

Histologically, parosteal sarcomas are well-differentiated lesions showing new calcified bone at the base and a cellular fibrous and/or cartilaginous cap (Figs. 2–50 and 2–51). Periosteal osteosarcomas are poorly differentiated and are composed predominantly of lobules of malignant cartilage admixed with lesser amounts of tumor osteoid.[109]

DIFFERENTIAL DIAGNOSIS. Diagnosis of central osteosarcoma requires the finding of malignant cells in association with osteoid. Because most lesions are relatively well differentiated, osteosarcomas, particularly the fibroblastic type, may be confused with benign fibro-osseous lesions. Atypical cytologic features and haphazard microscopic patterns would be expected in osteosarcomas. In benign lesions, maturation of bony trabeculae is seen, and the periphery is well defined, as

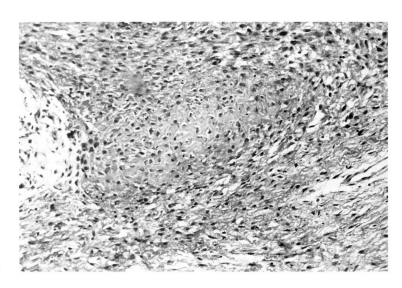

FIGURE 2–49. Fibroblastic osteosarcoma. (H&E, ×100)

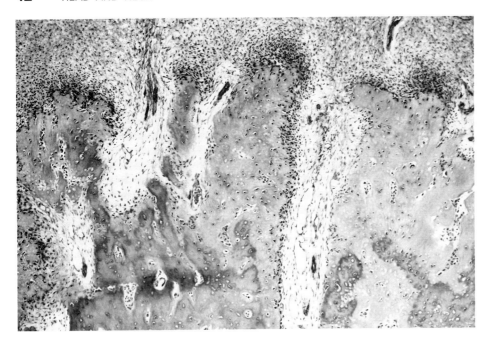

FIGURE 2–50. Parosteal osteosarcoma. Upper cellular zone represents the expanding outer surface. (H&E, ×40)

in ossifying fibroma and osteoblastoma.[110] Ossifying fibroma may be particularly cellular, but nuclei are uniform. Clinical and radiographic features may also provide valuable diagnostic information that would help sort out lesions in which microscopic features overlap.

Chondroblastic osteosarcoma, the most common subtype in the jaws, may be confused with chondrosarcoma. By definition, any chondroblastic malignancy that exhibits *any* tumor bone formation is classified as an osteosarcoma. This definition seems to have effectively made chondrosarcoma a very rare tumor in the jaws. The telangiectatic type may be confused with **aneurysmal bone cyst** or **central giant cell granuloma.** Cellular atypia is not seen in the latter lesions. Because they are well differentiated, parosteal osteosarcomas may be

underdiagnosed as **osteoma** or **osteochondroma.** This diagnosis should be considered for any recurring cellular "exostosis" or "torus." Clinicopathologic correlation may help in the diagnosis of parosteal sarcomas.

Early Oral Kaposi's Sarcoma

HIV-associated Kaposi's sarcoma (KS) is a well-known component of the acquired immunodeficiency syndrome (AIDS). Much evidence points to this lesion as a neoplastic proliferation of blood vascular endothelial cells (i.e., CD31 and CD34 positive), although there is support for the opinion that it represents a reactive process that is sustained by virus or virus products. Oral lesions may occur in the company of

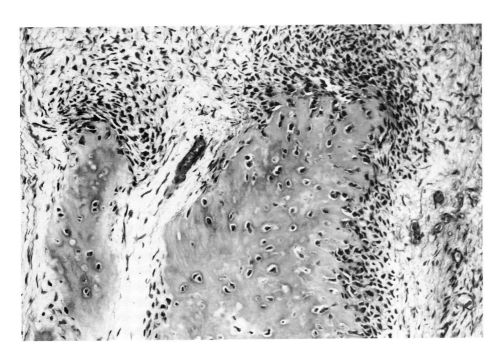

FIGURE 2–51. High magnification of tissue illustrated in Figure 2–50. (H&E, ×100)

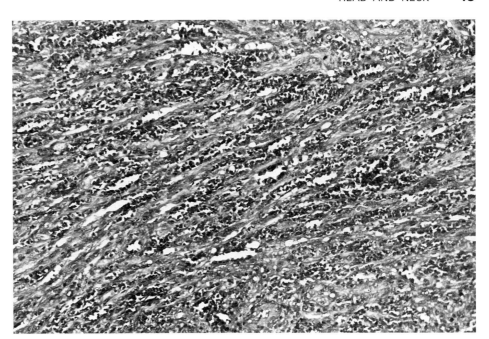

FIGURE 2–52. Advanced oral Kaposi's sarcoma exhibiting spindle-shaped cells and slit-like vascular spaces. (H&E, ×100)

cutaneous lesions, or they may be the first sign of the disease. Histologic diagnosis is relatively straightforward when the lesions are advanced; however, when small or early, oral KS may be a considerable challenge to the surgical pathologist.[111]

CLINICOPATHOLOGIC FEATURES. HIV-associated oral KSs present clinically as flat or nodular lesions that are characteristically red to purple in color. Rarely, a nodular lesion may be the same color as the surrounding tissue. The flat or macular lesions are believed to represent an early stage in the development of KS. Oral lesions are frequently multiple and may occur simultaneously with cutaneous lesions. The most frequent sites of occurrence are the palate and gingiva. Pain and ulceration are usually absent.[112]

Histologically, oral KS can be divided into two subtypes: small well-delineated lesions, and larger infiltrative lesions.

The larger advanced lesions have distinct microscopic features (Figs. 2–52 and 2–53). Among the most important microscopic changes noted in large lesions are well-differentiated spindle cells, slit-like and bizarre (angular, branching, open) vascular channels, high cellularity, extravasation of red blood cells, hemosiderin, and hyaline globules. Nuclear atypia and mitotic figures may be present, but they tend to be minimal and may vary from one lesion to another.

Small (early) lesions often challenge the interpretive skills of the surgical pathologist. Clinical correlation can be of considerable importance in making diagnostic decisions, because clinical appearance is usually suggestive of the diagnosis even when the histology is subtle or equivocal. A history of AIDS or HIV infection would obviously be of help, although oral KS may be the first recognized sign of AIDS.

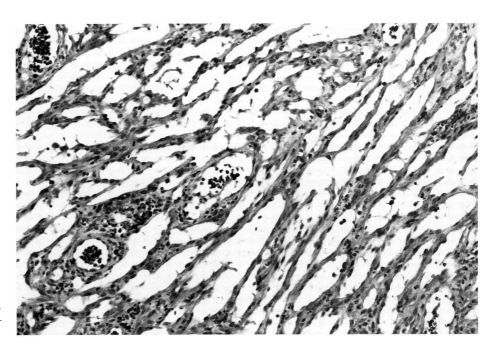

FIGURE 2–53. Advanced oral Kaposi's sarcoma showing bizarre vascular spaces. (H&E, ×100)

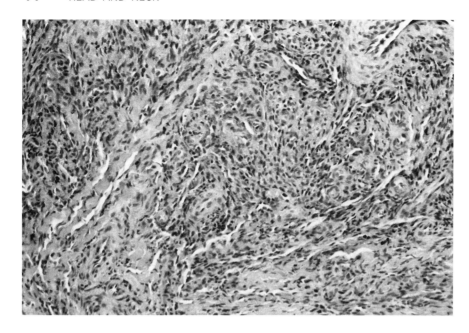

FIGURE 2–54. Small (early) oral Kaposi's sarcoma found as multiple small spindle cell nodules in submucosa. (H&E, ×40)

Small lesions characteristically contain inconspicuous proliferations of spindle to oval cells, often forming ill-defined vascular spaces (Figs. 2–54 and 2–55). These incipient or poorly developed vascular spaces are usually lined by spindle cells, although oval or polygonal cells are also noted (Figs. 2–56 and 2–57). Lymphocytes are usually found in small numbers and appear to be scattered in and around the lesions. Occasionally, rounded capillaries are noted toward the periphery of these lesions. The spindle and oval cells are usually seen in patches, but occasionally they form solitary nodules. Red blood cell extravasation is almost always seen, and hemosiderin and hyaline globules are frequently seen. Nuclear atypia is not evident, and mitotic figures are infrequent. Most spindle cells strongly express CD34 antigen when stained immunohistochemically, a feature that can be used to confirm histologic impressions if necessary (Fig. 2–58).

DIFFERENTIAL DIAGNOSIS. A combination of several microscopic features can be used to separate small KS lesions from **pyogenic granulomas.** In KS, vascular spaces are inconspicuous, overlying epithelium is intact, and the lesion is separated from the overlying epithelium by a connective tissue band. In pyogenic granuloma, vascular spaces are prominent and round, there is often surface ulceration, and granulation tissue making up the lesion is found directly beneath the surface epithelium or ulcer. Extravasated red blood cells and hemosiderin are much more commonly found in KS than in pyogenic granuloma. A high mitotic index would favor pyogenic granuloma over small KS. Although hyaline globules are relatively specific for KS, they can also occasionally be seen in pyogenic granulomas.

Bacillary angiomatosis, a recently recognized cutaneous infection caused by *Bartonella henselae* that mimics KS both

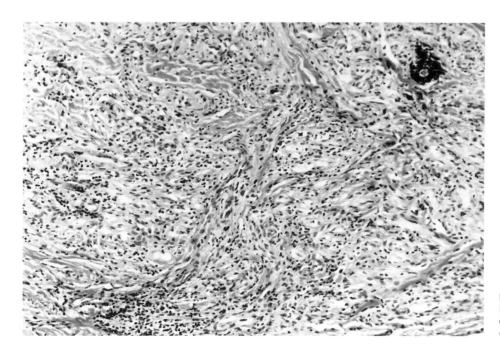

FIGURE 2–55. Small (early) oral Kaposi's sarcoma with lymphoid cells. Note spindle cells without obvious vascular channels. (H&E, ×40)

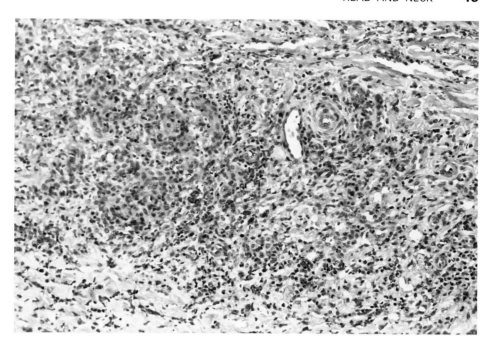

FIGURE 2–56. Nodule of small (early) Kaposi's sarcoma. (H&E, ×100)

clinically and microscopically, might be considered in a differential diagnosis because it has been seen intraorally, although rarely.[113–115] Features that would suggest bacillary angiomatosis include a circumscribed lobular tumor with round blood vessels, polygonal endothelial cells, and clusters of neutrophils with basophilic granules of bacteria.

Acinic Cell Carcinoma

Acinic cell carcinomas (ACCs) are low-grade carcinomas that constitute about 1% of all salivary gland tumors and 10% to 15% of malignant salivary gland tumors.[116] Ellis and Corio[117] followed 244 cases of ACCs and found a recurrence rate of 12%, a metastatic rate of 7.8%, and a death rate of 6.1%. ACCs exhibit a number of cytoarchitectural patterns, which may cause diagnostic difficulty.

CLINICOPATHOLOGIC FEATURES. The overwhelming majority of ACCs arise in the parotid gland, but examples have occurred in the submaxillary, sublingual, and minor salivary glands, including the nasal cavity.[116] There is a slight male predominance and a peak incidence in the third decade of life (mean age, 38 years; range, 5–84).[117] ACCs are slow growing (mean tumor duration, 3.0 years; range, 0.1–30 years), sometimes painful, and usually less than 3 cm in diameter at presentation (mean size, 2.3 cm; range, 0.2–13 cm).[117] Ellis and Corio[117] identified four growth patterns and five cell types. The growth patterns were (1) solid, characterized by sheets or nodules of uniform basophilic cells (Fig. 2–59A); (2) micro-

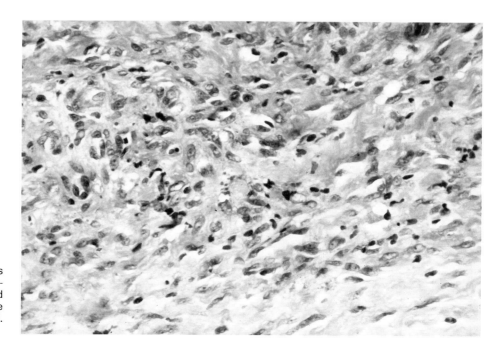

FIGURE 2–57. Small (early) Kaposi's sarcoma showing spindle cells, ill-defined capillaries, and extravasated red blood cells. Hyaline globules are evident in the center of the field. (H&E, ×250)

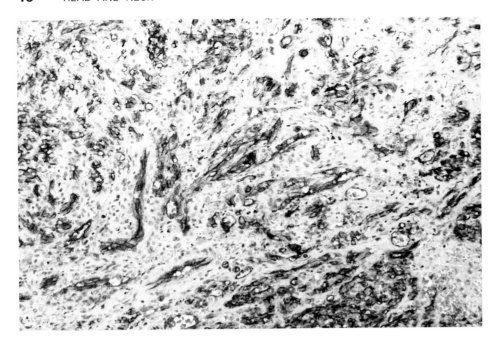

FIGURE 2–58. Small (early) Kaposi's sarcoma stained with anti-CD34 antibody. Most cells are immunoreactive. (H&E, ×100)

cystic, tumor cell masses with variable sizes and numbers of intercellular spaces owing to cell breakdown and accumulation of fluids (Fig. 2–59*B*); (3) papillary-cystic, characterized by larger cystic spaces into which extend papillary growths of epithelial cells; and (4) follicular, characterized by cell masses forming septa of epithelial cells and surrounding spaces containing colloid-like material that mimics thyroid follicles. The five cell types included (1) acinous, characterized by round to polyhedral basophilic cells, which resembled normal serous acinar cells (see Fig. 2–59*A*); (2) intercalated-

duct, composed of cuboidal or low columnar cells with eosinophilic cytoplasm mimicking intercalated duct cells; (3) vacuolated, characterized by rounded cells with intracytoplasmic vacuoles, which may produce cell membrane distention (see Fig. 2–59*B*); (4) non-specific glandular, characterized by lightly eosinophilic or amophilic cells with indistinct cell borders; and (5) clear cells, characterized by absent or poorly staining cytoplasm. According to Ellis and Corio,[117] mitotic figures and cytologic atypia are rare. Furthermore, the stroma is often sparse, but may be abundant, and it can contain a

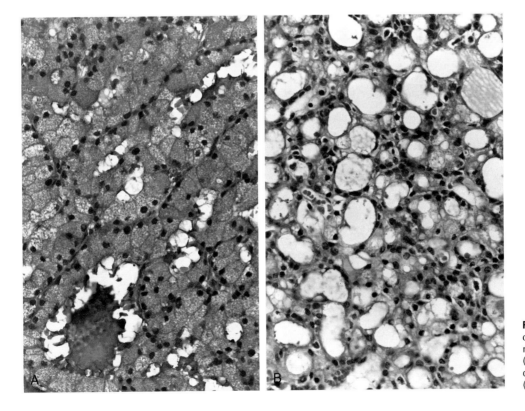

FIGURE 2–59. *A,* Acinic cell carcinoma, solid pattern simulating normal salivary gland acini. (H&E, OM ×100) *B,* Acinic cell carcinoma, microcystic pattern. (H&E, OM ×100)

marked lymphoid reaction with germinal centers. Calcification can occur. Mixed cytoarchitectural patterns are commonly found in the same tumor.

Some authors have attempted to subclassify ACCs into low- and high-grade variants,[118] based on the relative peripheral demarcation of the tumors, cellular differentiation, and growth pattern. Indeed, some consider the papillary-cystic and/or abundant fibrous stroma growth patterns to be more aggressive, in contrast to the lymphocyte-rich stroma, which is considered to have a favorable prognosis.[118] Perzin and LiVolsi[119] reported that increased mitotic activity, marked cellular atypia, and infiltrative growth correlated with aggressive behavior. Ellis and Corio[117] did not include tumors with increased mitotic activity and marked cytologic atypia in their study of ACCs, preferring to classify such pleomorphic tumors in different categories. Among these relatively cytologically bland ACCs, Ellis and Corio[117] found a high incidence of infiltrative growth, multinodularity and stromal hyalinization in ACCs that recurred and/or metastasized. Also, they found all four cytoarchitectural growth patterns and five cell types in tumors that recurred, metastasized, and/or caused death of the patient. Thus, there seems to be no clear consensus that histologic subtyping of ACCs is useful prognostically; but most agree that the gravity of the prognosis depends on the extent of local invasion and completeness of surgical removal.[118] DNA content has thus far not proved useful because the vast majority of ACCs are "diploid."[120]

DIFFERENTIAL DIAGNOSIS. Given the cytoarchitectural diversity of ACCs, the differential diagnosis is quite broad and includes virtually any salivary gland tumor capable of showing glandular, papillary, microcystic, and/or clear-cell morphology. The key to diagnosing ACC lies in the fact that more than 50% of ACCs exhibit one or more of the cytoarchitectural patterns outlined previously, most often the classic solid and/or microcystic pattern combined with the well-differentiated acinic-cell cytology. Therefore, in difficult cases, extensive tumor sampling should yield material with the classic cytoarchitectural features, thus distinguishing it from ACC look-alikes. However, predominantly papillary-cystic or follicular variants can occur and cause confusion; becoming proficient in recognizing these patterns of ACC is encouraged.[117–119, 121] In fact, pure cystic ACCs occur with intracystic papillary growth.[121] The intracystic papillary components can be easily confused with **papillary cystadenocarcinoma** of salivary gland.[122] Fortunately, both are low-grade carcinomas, making their distinction less clinically important. ACCs have also been reported in unusual instances such as in ectopic salivary gland tissues of the neck[123] and in the laryngotracheal junction 46 years after thyroid irradiation.[124] A benign lesion potentially confused with ACC is **sialadenosis.**[125] Sialadenosis is characterized by enlargement of the serous acinar cells and slight compression of the duct system by the swollen acini. The nuclei of the acinar cells are displaced toward the basal part of the cell. There is no inflammatory infiltrate. Patients present with recurrent painless, bilateral swelling of the parotid glands. This lesion is associated with endocrine disorders, malnutrition, alcoholism, cirrhosis, and dysfunction of the autonomic nervous system.

Polymorphous Low-grade Adenocarcinoma

Polymorphous low-grade adenocarcinoma (PLAC) was initially popularized by Batsakis et al.[126] as **terminal duct**

carcinoma, but this tumor has also been reported as **lobular carcinoma of salivary glands.**[127] These tumors are now most frequently called PLAC, which is a better term because it emphasizes the diverse morphologic features of the tumor.[128] It is very likely that most surgical pathologists will encounter examples of PLAC during their careers, and they must guard against underdiagnosing them as **pleomorphic adenoma** or overdiagnosing them as **adenoid cystic carcinoma.** PLACs are indolent tumors, which are locally invasive but slow to metastasize. About 12% recur, 10% develop cervical nodal metastases, and less than 1% of patients eventually die of local disease. Usually many years are required for metastasis and/or local recurrences to develop.

CLINICOPATHOLOGIC FEATURES. PLACs occur almost exclusively in the intraoral minor salivary glands, especially those located at the junction of the hard and soft palate. Yet, very rare examples of PLAC occur wherever salivary gland tissue occurs, including in the nose and major salivary glands (the latter may be associated with PLAC ex pleomorphic adenoma).[129] There is a 2 : 1 female predominance and the ages vary widely, but the peak incidence is in the fifth and sixth decades (mean age, 49 years; range, 23–79).[130] Swelling has been the most frequent symptom. Histologically, PLACs are characterized by cytologic uniformity and architectural diversity (Figs. 2–60 to 2–62). The cells are uniform, cytologically bland cells with oval to spindle nuclei with fine chromatin and inconspicuous nucleoli; tumor cell cytoplasm is scant to moderate, and eosinophilic or clear; cell borders are indistinct. Mitotic figures are uncommon and necrosis is rare. PLAC tumors, although circumscribed, invade adjacent tissues such as bone, muscle, fat, salivary glands, and nerves (the last quite extensively) (see Fig. 2–61). A polymorphous growth pattern can be observed within the same tumor. These patterns include tubular, cribriform, papillary, solid, and fascicular (see Figs. 2–60 to 2–62). Combinations and transitions between these patterns are common, and the stroma may be mucoid, hyaline, and/or mucohyaline. At the periphery, infiltration of tumor as duct-like structures and/or elongated cords forming a single-file pattern (lobular) is common.

DIFFERENTIAL DIAGNOSIS. The polymorphous growth patterns encountered in PLAC overlap with a number of other salivary gland tumors, including pleomorphic adenoma, monomorphic adenoma, and adenoid cystic carcinoma. Pleomorphic adenomas are usually well circumscribed and show the characteristic biphasic epithelial and myxochondroid matrix differentiation. Monomorphic adenomas are likewise well circumscribed and are not polymorphous as the name implies. PLACs are invasive tumors, and careful attention to the periphery of the lesion and its infiltrative nature will allow its recognition if the other uniform cytologic and polymorphous architectural features are also present. Adenoid cystic carcinoma can be clearly distinguished from PLAC by the presence of hyperchromatic basaloid cells with scant cytoplasm in adenoid cystic carcinoma, and cuboid, columnar, and/or spindled cells in PLACs, which have vesicular to oval nuclei, fine chromatin, inconspicuous nucleoli as well as conspicuous eosinophilic cytoplasm.[130]

Epithelial-Myoepithelial Carcinoma

Epithelial-myoepithelial carcinoma (EMC) is a rare carcinoma of salivary glands initially described in 1972.[131] It is

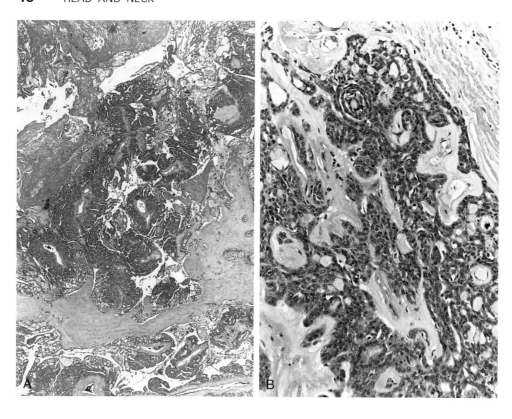

FIGURE 2–60. *A,* Polymorphous low-grade adenocarcinoma. (H&E, OM ×2.5) *B,* Infiltrating trabeculae of polymorphous low-grade adenocarcinoma cells admixed with hyalinized and vascular stroma. (H&E, OM ×100)

a biphasic tumor composed of duct luminal epithelial cells and clear myoepithelial cells. Most tumors are low-grade in behavior, but about 50% recur locally. Fonseca and Soares[132] studied 22 cases and found death due to neoplastic disease in 40% of their cases. Other series have reported distant metastases in 5% to 10% of cases and death from neoplastic disease in less than 5%.[132] Recognition of this tumor requires understanding its pathologic features and the pathologic features of other lesions with clear-cell morphology.

CLINICOPATHOLOGIC FEATURES. Most EMCs originate in the parotid gland, but minor salivary gland examples occur with a major to minor salivary gland ratio of from 8:1 to

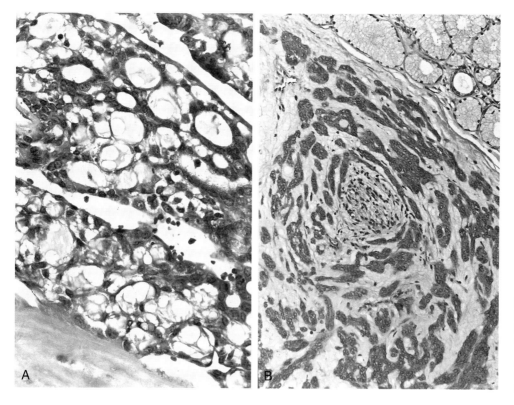

FIGURE 2–61. *A,* Polymorphous low-grade adenocarcinoma having an area with a microcystic or cribriform pattern. (H&E, OM ×100) *B,* Perineural invasion is often a prominent finding in polymorphous low-grade adenocarcinoma. (H&E, OM ×50)

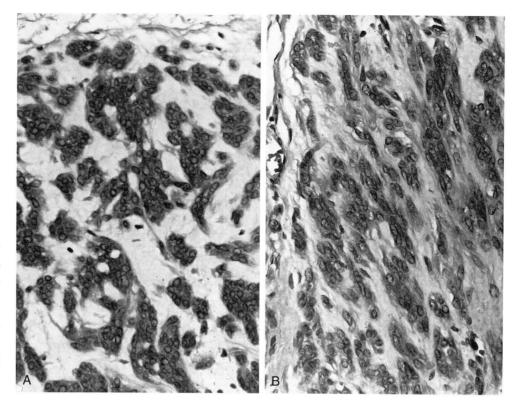

FIGURE 2–62. *A,* Polymorphous low-grade adenocarcinoma with an invasive area composed of small nests of tumor cells separated by myxomatous stroma. Note the bland uniform nuclei and homogeneous chromatin pattern, which have an optically clear quality. (H&E, OM ×100) *B,* Invasive tumor cells of polymorphous low-grade adenocarcinoma may show spindle cell morphology. (H&E, OM ×100)

1.4 : 1.[132] There is a slight female predominance, and most patients are in the fifth to eighth decades of life (mean reported ages of presentation vary from 59 to 76 years).[132] EMCs present as indolent single, firm, lobulated tumor masses, usually 2 to 8 cm in greatest diameter. Some may have cystic spaces, and although grossly "circumscribed," EMCs infiltrate adjacent tissues; indeed, facial paralysis and bone invasion may occur. EMCs form islands and clusters of tumor cells separated by dense bands of connective tissue.

Two cell types predominate in EMCs. The first type is a centrally disposed, cuboidal, often eosinophilic, duct epithelial cell with central or basal nuclei. These cells form duct lumina and are surrounded by the second cell type, a clear, glycogen-containing, vacuolated myoepithelial cell (Fig. 2–63). The tumors closely resemble the so-called adenomyoepithelioma of breast. The duct luminal epithelial cells are strongly positive for keratin, whereas the myoepithelial cells are positive for S-100 protein, vimentin, smooth muscle actin, muscle-specific actin (HHF-35), and keratin (especially the high-molecular-weight types). Fonseca and Soares[132] identified four distinct architectural types, almost always occurring in various combinations within the same tumor. The types included (1) a solid type that forms multiple nodules composed predominantly of clear cells; (2) a tubular type wherein tubules regularly formed by an inner layer of duct-like cells and an outer layer of clear, myoepithelial cells resemble the usual organization of normal intercalated ducts; (3) a cribriform type mimicking adenoid cystic carcinoma; and (4) a papillary type that forms thin papillae lined by the typical double-layered structure. Fonseca and Soares[132] also noted that, in addition to the clear, vacuolated myoepithelial cells, myoepithelial cells in some tumor areas were spindle-shaped, and that hyaline basement membrane material often surrounded solid, clear-cell groups or

tubular double-layered structures. Some examples are dominated by solid, variably hyalinized, multinodal masses composed of spindled and polygonal cells with variable cytoplasmic clearing (Fig. 2–64). Ductular differentiation can be inconspicuous, as in some cases of benign myoepithelioma of salivary glands. Possibly, these cases may be better labeled malignant myoepithelioma.

DIFFERENTIAL DIAGNOSIS. Although EMC is a fairly distinctive tumor, other salivary gland tumors may show clear-cell areas and, thus, should be considered in the differential diagnosis. These lesions include **pleomorphic adenoma, acinic cell carcinoma, adenoid cystic carcinoma, mucoepidermoid carcinoma, sebaceous carcinoma, clear-cell variant of oncocytoma, metastatic renal carcinoma, "true" clear-cell carcinoma of minor salivary glands, and clear-cell rhabdomyosarcoma.** Pleomorphic adenomas are not as infiltrative and contain myxochondroid stroma. Acinic carcinomas, adenoid cystic carcinomas, oncocytomas, and sebaceous carcinomas are not biphasic, and with complete sampling should show areas characteristic of each of these tumors. Low-grade mucoepidermoid carcinomas contain mucin; are composed of mixtures of mucin-secreting goblet cells, intermediate cells, and well-differentiated squamous cells; and form variably sized cystic spaces filled with mucin (Fig. 2–65). The mucin-secreting and intermediate cells usually predominate, and they should not be a diagnostic problem if the tumor is well sampled. Examples of high-grade mucoepidermoid carcinoma closely resemble moderate to poorly differentiated squamous carcinoma, but the squamous carcinoma cells also contain scattered intracytoplasmic mucin vacuoles, which become apparent with mucicarmine stain. The clinical relevance of separating high-grade mucoepidermoid carcinoma from invasive moderate to poorly differentiated squamous carcinoma has never been clear to us.

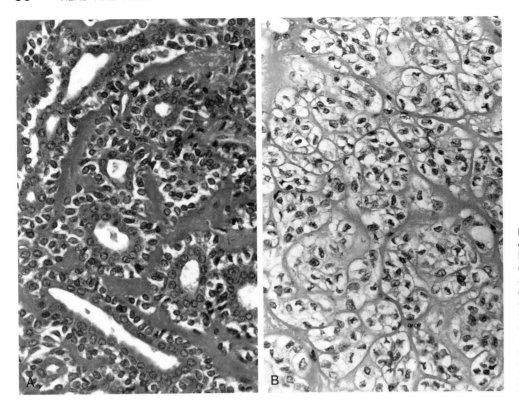

FIGURE 2–63. *A,* Epithelial-myo-epithelial carcinoma. Note the biphasic morphology: central duct luminal epithelial differentiation surrounded by a rim of clear myoepithelial cells. (H&E, OM ×100) *B,* Some epithelial-myoepithelial carcinomas are dominated by the clear-cell myoepithelial component, and multiple sections may be necessary to find the more classic biphasic differentiation shown in *A.* (H&E, OM ×100)

Unfortunately, we have encountered salivary gland tumors that show mixed patterns. For example, we have seen adenoid cystic carcinomas containing areas identical to EMC, and carcinomas ex pleomorphic adenoma may take on features of EMC. For therapeutic decision-making, we classify such combined tumors by the most aggressive pattern and detail the microscopic findings in an accompanying note. Rare examples of hyalinizing, glycogen-rich, clear-cell carcinomas, which are non-myoepithelial and monomorphic, have been described in the salivary glands.[133] These are low-grade tumors

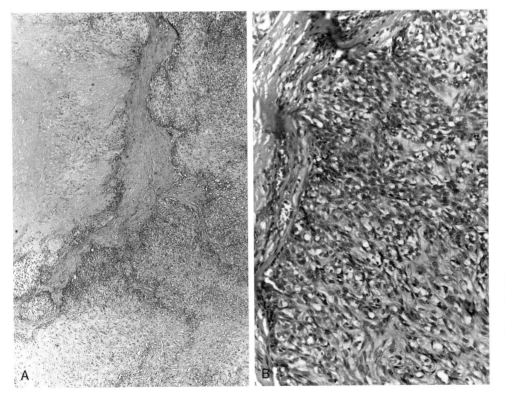

FIGURE 2–64. *A,* A less well differentiated example of epithelial-myoepithelial carcinoma is shown and characterized by spindle and clear-cell myoepithelial differentiation. (H&E, OM ×2.5) *B,* Spindle-cell and clear-cell myoepithelial component is more apparent at higher magnification. (H&E, OM ×50)

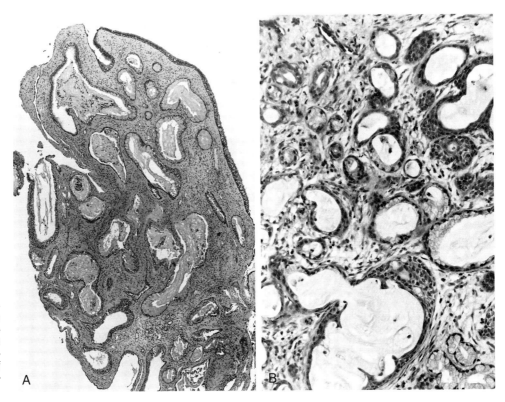

FIGURE 2–65. *A,* Mucinous microcysts are clearly shown in this low-grade mucoepidermoid carcinoma. (H&E, OM ×2.5) *B,* Note the numerous goblet cells and intermediate cells characteristic of low-grade mucoepidermoid carcinomas. (H&E, OM ×100)

and must be separated from metastatic renal carcinoma, which is best ruled out with appropriate imaging studies. Finally, rarely, rhabdomyosarcoma can present with clear cells.[134]

Salivary Duct Carcinoma

Some malignant adenocarcinomas of the salivary glands display a **striking histologic resemblance to intermediate or high-grade *in situ* and infiltrating ductal carcinomas of the breast.** Indeed, such tumors in the salivary glands have been called **salivary duct carcinoma (SDC).** These tumors have a dismal prognosis, with about 66% of reported cases developing recurrences, 66% developing lymph node metastases, 66% developing distant metastases, and 70% of patients dying of tumor.[130] It is important that they be distinguished from less aggressive variants of salivary gland malignancy.

CLINICOPATHOLOGIC FEATURES. SDCs occur primarily in the parotid gland with occasional examples in the submandibular gland. Yet, we have seen a case apparently arising from the minor salivary glands of the nasal cavity. There is a 3:1 male predominance, and most patients are in their seventh and eighth decades (mean age, 64 years; range, 27–83). Tumors are rapidly growing masses (usually 2–6 cm) and are often associated with pain and/or enlarged cervical lymph nodes. Grossly, SDCs are firm masses, but they may have foci of necrosis and cellularity. Comedo-type necrosis is often prominent, but solid, papillary, and/or cribriform patterns can be seen, sometimes with a desmoplastic stroma simulating infiltrating "ductal" carcinoma of the breast (Fig. 2–66). SDC cells are relatively large and have abundant eosinophilic apocrine-like cytoplasm, pleomorphic-hyperchromatic nuclei, and frequent mitotic figures. Comedonecrosis is not always present, and mucin production is not a striking feature,

although luminal mucin is present in some cases. The infiltrating components frequently invade nerves, salivary gland, lymphatics, and adjacent structures.

DIFFERENTIAL DIAGNOSIS. The differential diagnosis of SDC includes **carcinoma in (ex) pleomorphic adenoma (CEPA), high-grade mucoepidermoid carcinoma, oncocytic carcinoma, mucus-producing adenopapillary carcinoma (also known as papillary cystadenocarcinoma), and PLAC.** CEPAs usually show features of salivary duct carcinoma arising in close association with or from within an "old" hyalinized pleomorphic adenoma,[135] whereas the remainder show carcinomas of various types, including undifferentiated carcinoma, PLAC, adenoid cystic carcinoma, and myoepithelial carcinoma. Tortoledo et al.[135] further reported that only those CEPA patients having carcinomas invasive at least 8 mm beyond the capsule of the benign pleomorphic adenoma died of disease.

PLAC and papillary cystadenocarcinoma are separated from SDC by their low-grade (relatively bland) cytologic features. Intracytoplasmic mucous production and squamous differentiation are features of mucoepidermoid carcinoma, not SDC. Oncocytic carcinomas are extremely rare, and oncocytes contain numerous mitochondria, which are not found in SDC. Also, comedonecrosis and papillary-cribiform growth are not features of oncocytic carcinomas.

Undifferentiated Carcinomas of the Head and Neck

Many **undifferentiated carcinomas** of the head and neck can be divided into **sinonasal undifferentiated carcinoma (SNUC), large-cell undifferentiated carcinoma, small-cell carcinomas (neuroendocrine and non-neuroendocrine**

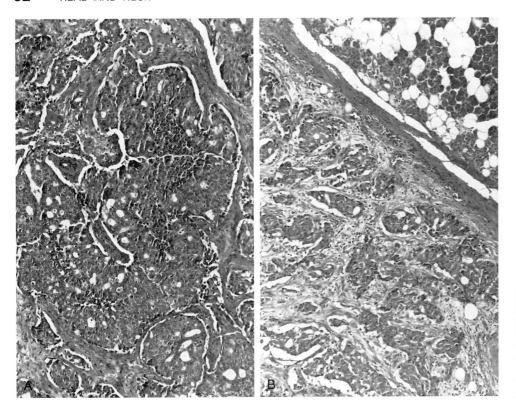

FIGURE 2–66. *A,* High-grade salivary duct carcinoma. Note the close resemblance to infiltrating ductal carcinoma of the breast with *in situ* cribriform and comedo necrosis patterns. (H&E, OM ×25) *B,* Salivary duct carcinoma showing invasive ductal elements. (H&E, OM ×25)

types), and undifferentiated carcinoma with lymphoid stroma or of the nasopharyngeal type.[136–138] By definition, undifferentiated carcinomas are devoid of any phenotypic expression that would allow them to be otherwise classified by light microscopy. A discussion of these types of undifferentiated carcinomas is included here because they are highly aggressive tumors that can be confused with benign lesions such as benign lymphoepithelial lesions, as well as other malignant tumors with quite different therapies and prognoses, such as **neuroepithelioma** and **olfactory neuroblastoma.**

CLINICOPATHOLOGIC FEATURES. **SNUC** is a highly aggressive and often lethal undifferentiated carcinoma that occurs

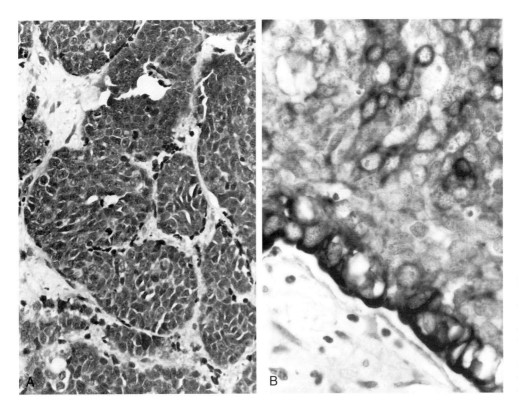

FIGURE 2–67. *A,* Sinonasal undifferentiated carcinoma (SNUC) is shown forming organoid clusters or nests of tumor cells, a pattern simulating olfactory neuroblastoma. (H&E, OM ×25) *B,* The tumor cells were strongly reactive for cytokeratin, especially in the periphery of the cell nests. (H&E, OM ×100)

in the nasal cavity and paranasal sinuses.[136] Patients may be current or former smokers, and they range in age from 30 to 77 years, present with multiple symptoms, and have tumors that usually extend into the orbital bones and/or invade the cranial cavity. SNUCs are composed of medium-sized cells with small amounts of cytoplasm, which grow in nests, trabeculae, and/or sheets (Fig. 2–67). Nuclei are round or oval and contain prominent nucleoli. Mitoses, tumor necrosis, and vascular invasion are characteristic findings. SNUCs are frequently positive for keratin, epithelial membrane antigen, and/or ''neuron-specific'' enolase. Tumor cells can have small desmosomes and rare neurosecretory-like granules. Cytoplasmic processes are not present.

Undifferentiated carcinomas of the salivary glands usually fall into the categories of small-cell carcinoma, large-cell undifferentiated carcinoma, or undifferentiated carcinoma with lymphoid stroma. The small-cell carcinomas may resemble their lung tumor (oat cell) and/or cutaneous (Merkel cell) counterparts (Fig. 2–68). Small-cell carcinomas grow in sheets of uniform, densely hematoxyphilic cells with scanty cytoplasm. Necrosis is common, and focal duct differentiation may be present. Hui et al.[138] studied 16 cases of undifferentiated carcinomas forming masses of the major salivary glands (15 parotid, 1 submandibular) in patients ranging from 48 to 80 years (mean, 67). The male:female ratio was 3:1, and seven had cervical metastases at presentation. Twelve were small-cell carcinomas (cells < 30 μm in diameter), and four were designated large-cell undifferentiated carcinomas. The latter were composed of tumor cells two to three times the size of small-cell carcinoma cells, showing abundant cytoplasm and having vesicular nuclei with up to three nucleoli (Fig. 2–69). Both tumor types grew as solid clusters and/or organoid nests. Electron microscopy in 12 tumors disclosed six with neurosecretory granules; five of these were small-

cell carcinomas, and one was a large-cell undifferentiated carcinoma. Four tumors (three small-cell carcinomas and one large-cell undifferentiated carcinoma) were simply undifferentiated carcinomas, whereas others showed some ductal and/ or myoepithelial features. All the undifferentiated carcinomas immunoreacted for keratin, and two reacted for vimentin. Ten of the 16 patients were dead of disease within 4.5 years of diagnosis, and only tumor size (>4.0 cm) correlated with outcome. In this study, cell size and/or neuroendocrine differentiation had little bearing on prognosis.[138]

The term undifferentiated carcinoma with lymphoid stroma of salivary glands has been adopted by the WHO over **malignant lymphoepithelial lesion** or **lymphoepithelial carcinoma** (Fig. 2–70).[139] Although whites and blacks can have the disease, undifferentiated carcinoma with lymphoid stroma occurs mostly in Mongolian races (North American Eskimos [**''Eskimoma''**], native Greenlanders, and Southern Chinese). Undifferentiated carcinomas with lymphoid stromata occur in the parotid or submandibular glands; patient ages range from 20 to 60 years; cases in females outnumber those in males; EBV is likely causally related; 40% of patients have metastases to cervical nodes at presentation; and local recurrence and/or systemic spread have been recorded in 20% to 50%. Tumor cells may form anastomosing, syncytium-like, epithelial masses surrounded by variably fibrotic lymphoplasmacytoid stroma, which closely resembles the epimyoepithelial islands of BLELs (Fig. 2–70B). Yet, undifferentiated carcinoma with lymphoid stroma may be indistinguishable from undifferentiated carcinoma of the nasopharyngeal type (Fig. 2–71) (either of the Regaud's or Schmincke's patterns) by light, ultrastructural, and/or immunohistochemical studies. Foci of squamous differentiation may occur, but the usual tumor cells are large, with vesicular or spindled nuclei and prominent nucleoli. A high mitotic rate, marked anaplasia,

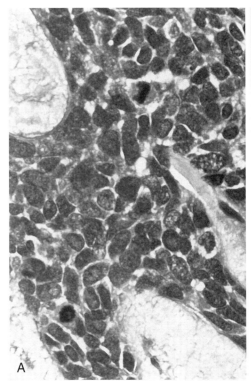
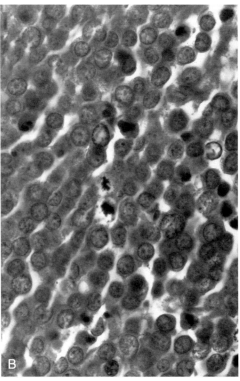

FIGURE 2–68. *A,* Small-cell undifferentiated carcinoma (SCUC) of the salivary gland, showing nuclear molding, frequent mitotic figures, and focal gland formation in the upper left-hand corner. No neuroendocrine differentiation was present by ultrastructural and chromogranin ipox studies. (H&E, OM ×250) *B,* A second pattern of small-cell carcinoma of salivary gland, showing features similar to primary cutaneous neuroendocrine carcinomas (so-called Merkel cell carcinoma). Note the round uniform cells with ''optically clear'' nuclei. This tumor showed prominent neuroendocrine features by both ultrastructural and chromogranin ipox studies; hence, this is a case of small-cell neuroendocrine carcinoma (SCNC) or poorly differentiated neuroendocrine carcinoma. In cases like these, metastatic disease should always be ruled out. (H&E, OM ×250)

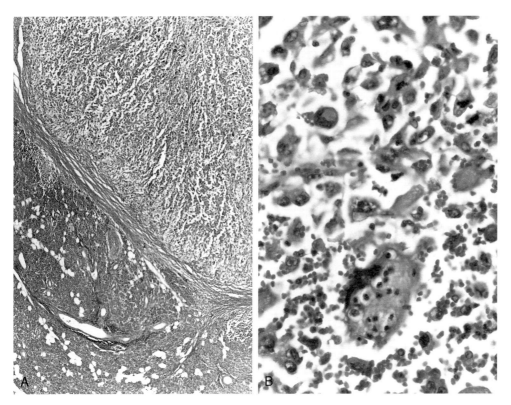

FIGURE 2–69. *A,* Salivary gland carcinoma is shown pushing into adjacent salivary gland tissues. (H&E, OM ×25) *B,* This tumor showed no differentiation features by light microscopy, and ultrastructure and ipox studies confirmed the epithelial nature of the tumor. Thus, this tumor, which contained many neutrophils (some within tumor cells), was classified as large-cell undifferentiated carcinoma of salivary gland. (H&E, OM ×100)

necrosis, and areas simulating lymphoma are thought to be adverse findings, whereas spindling of tumor cells and BLEL-like growth are considered favorable findings. Because undifferentiated carcinoma with lymphoid stroma may appear as a malignant caricature of BLEL, some have considered them to arise from BLEL, but this has not been shown conclusively.

Nasopharyngeal carcinomas have been classified by the WHO into squamous cell carcinomas, non-keratinizing carcinoma, and undifferentiated carcinoma.[140] These tumors can occur in children younger than 10 years and adults older than 90 years (bimodal peaks between 15–25 and 60–69), with many patients of Mongolian origin (especially

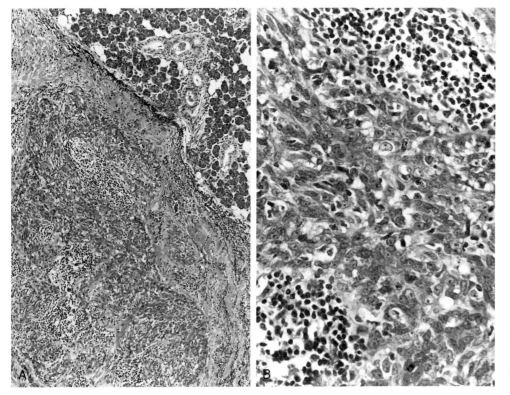

FIGURE 2–70. *A,* Undifferentiated carcinoma with lymphoid stroma (UCLS) arising from parotid gland. These tumors have been referred to as malignant lymphoepithelial lesions or "Eskimomas." (H&E, OM ×25) *B,* In this setting, note the close resemblance of UCLS to benign lymphoepithelial lesions, although UCLS shows more cytologic atypia. (H&E, OM ×100)

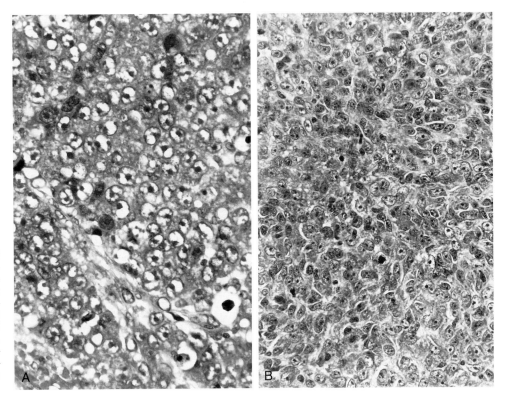

FIGURE 2–71. *A,* Undifferentiated nasopharyngeal carcinoma composed of poorly differentiated carcinoma cells having vesicular nuclei and prominent, often central, nucleoli. This pattern may be misdiagnosed as large-cell lymphoma, immunoblastic type. (H&E, OM ×100) *B,* A second pattern of undifferentiated carcinoma, showing less conspicuous nucleoli. (H&E, OM ×100)

Southern Chinese men) and with a well-documented association with EBV infection. Importantly, nasopharyngeal carcinomas present with metastases to upper cervical lymph nodes, with an occult primary in more than 50% of cases. The nonkeratinizing type forms a plexiform growth pattern resembling transitional cell carcinomas of the bladder and with variable anaplasia. Undifferentiated carcinomas of the nasopharyngeal type (**"lymphoepithelioma"**) grow as diffuse sheets of tumor cells with clear vesicular nuclei, often containing a single prominent nucleolus (round cells) (see Fig. 2–71). But spindled cells, clear cells, and anaplastic cells can occur separately or admixed with the other forms. Keratinizing examples have

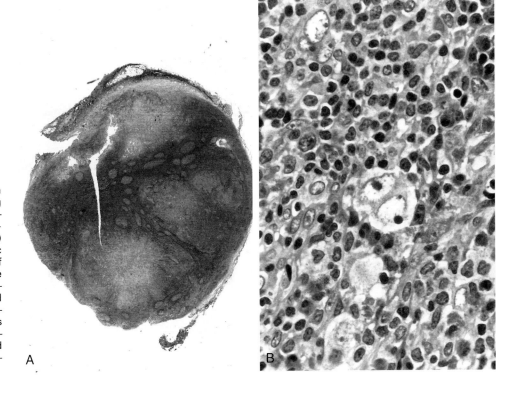

FIGURE 2–72. *A,* A cervical lymph node, containing pale-staining islands of metastatic undifferentiated carcinoma (a.k.a. "lymphoepithelioma"). (H&E, OM ×2.5) *B,* Some examples of metastatic undifferentiated carcinoma of nasopharyngeal origin simulate primary Hodgkin's disease, complete with RS-like cells and admixed polymorphous inflammatory infiltrate with numerous eosinophils. Note the RS-like carcinoma cells, which showed strong cytokeratin immunoreactivity. (H&E, OM ×100)

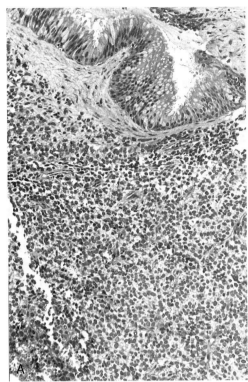
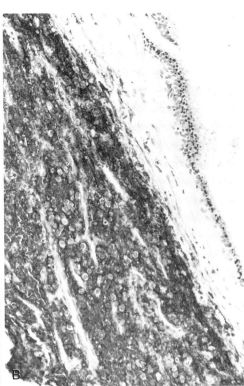

FIGURE 2–73. *A,* Immediately adjacent to respiratory mucosa (*top*) are sheets of small round cells, which contain abundant glycogen by special stains. (H&E, OM ×10) *B,* The small round cells were strongly positive for the monoclonal antibody O13, which is immunoreactive for the MIC2 gene product. The latter is frequently and strongly expressed on Ewing's sarcomas or peripheral neuroepitheliomas. (H&E, OM ×10)

a worse prognosis than the non-keratinizing and undifferentiated variants; the latter are further subdivided into prognostic groups based on the degree of anaplasia and pleomorphism.[141] Nonetheless, cure rates of higher than 50% can be achieved with radiation therapy. Reactive lympho-plasmacytoid stroma is common, imparting a resemblance to lymphoma.

DIFFERENTIAL DIAGNOSIS. Undifferentiated carcinoma can be confused with a variety of benign and malignant lesions. These lesions include **lymphoma, plasmacytoma,**

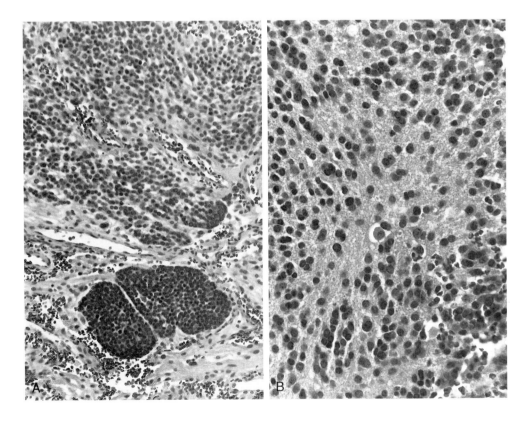

FIGURE 2–74. *A,* Olfactory neuroblastoma showing an island of tumor cells as well as sheet-like growth patterns. (H&E, OM ×25) *B,* Note the small round tumor cells separated by abundant fibrillary matrix. (H&E, OM ×100)

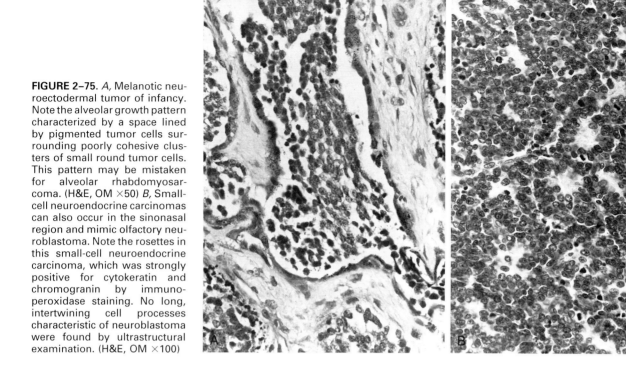

FIGURE 2–75. *A,* Melanotic neuroectodermal tumor of infancy. Note the alveolar growth pattern characterized by a space lined by pigmented tumor cells surrounding poorly cohesive clusters of small round tumor cells. This pattern may be mistaken for alveolar rhabdomyosarcoma. (H&E, OM ×50) *B,* Small-cell neuroendocrine carcinomas can also occur in the sinonasal region and mimic olfactory neuroblastoma. Note the rosettes in this small-cell neuroendocrine carcinoma, which was strongly positive for cytokeratin and chromogranin by immunoperoxidase staining. No long, intertwining cell processes characteristic of neuroblastoma were found by ultrastructural examination. (H&E, OM ×100)

chordoma, malignant melanoma, rhabdomyosarcoma, post-radiation polyphenotypic small-cell tumor, neuroendocrine carcinoma, paraganglioma, olfactory neuroblastoma, small-cell osteosarcoma, and Ewing's sarcoma/ peripheral neuroepithelioma (ES/PN). Metastatic undifferentiated carcinoma, nasopharyngeal type, to major salivary glands should be ruled out before making a diagnosis of undifferentiated carcinoma with lymphoid stroma. Metastatic undifferentiated carcinoma with lymphoid stroma or undifferentiated carcinoma, nasopharyngeal type, to cervical lymph nodes can very closely mimic Hodgkin's disease or immunoblastic lymphoma[142, 143] (Fig. 2–72). Immunohistochemical and ultrastructural studies will separate these lesions if carefully applied and interpreted. Yet, difficulties in distinguishing these various lesions could become problematic with small biopsies, crushed specimens, and/or poorly fixed specimens. It is important to keep in mind that small-cell osteosarcoma should show foci of osteoid, react with vimentin, and not stain for keratin.[144] ES/PN should react strongly with anti-MIC2 antibodies such as O13 (Fig. 2–73),[145] although exam-

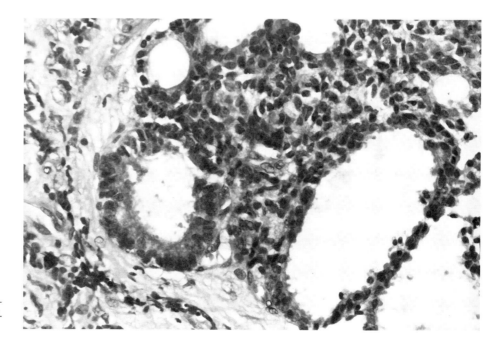

FIGURE 2–76. Olfactory neuroblastoma with glandular component. (H&E, OM ×100)

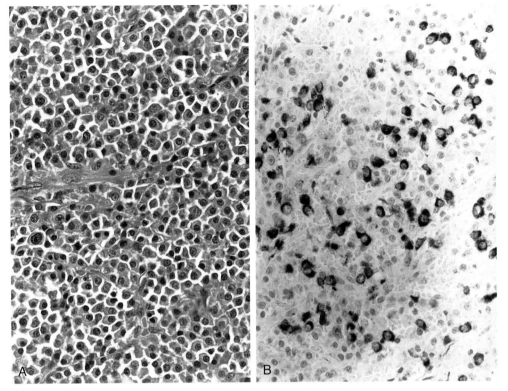

FIGURE 2–77. *A,* Plasmacytoma of the head and neck. Note the sheets of monomorphous cells, which on close inspection show some plasmacytic features. The latter may be quite subtle in small biopsy specimens. (H&E, OM ×25) *B,* Cytokeratin stain (CAM 5.2 + AE1/3) on the same plasmacytoma. Strong cytokeratin immunoreactivity is obvious and potentially misleading. Plasma cells are also frequently epithelial membrane antigen positive and negative for antibodies to leukocyte common antigen. Demonstration of kappa and lambda light-chain restriction and/or electron microscopy would be very helpful in making the correct diagnosis in a small biopsy specimen. (H&E, OM ×100)

ples of these lesions will show keratin and neurofilament immunoreactivity. Olfactory neuroblastomas usually show the characteristic neurofibrillary matrix (sometimes forming Homer Wright rosettes) and neurosecretory granules, but they may react with keratin (Fig. 2–74).[146] **Melanotic neuroectodermal tumor of infancy** (Fig. 2–75A)[147] and **heterotopic glial nodules**[148] may show neural processes, the latter sometimes associated with markedly sclerotic stroma. Some examples of small-cell neuroendocrine carcinoma may show rosettes, which can mimic Homer Wright rosettes found in

olfactory neuroblastoma, and some examples of olfactory neuroblastoma may show glandular differentiation (mixed olfactory neuroblastoma and carcinoma) (Fig. 2–76). Olfactory neuroblastomas do not react with epithelial membrane antigen, in contrast to undifferentiated, small-cell carcinomas.[149] Keratin immunoreactivity can also be seen in plamacytomas (Fig. 2–77), chordomas (Fig. 2–78), smooth-muscle tumors, and rhabdomyosarcomas; but desmin, muscle-specific actin, and myoglobin immunostains combined with electron microscopy should lead to a clear diagnosis in most cases. Lymphomas

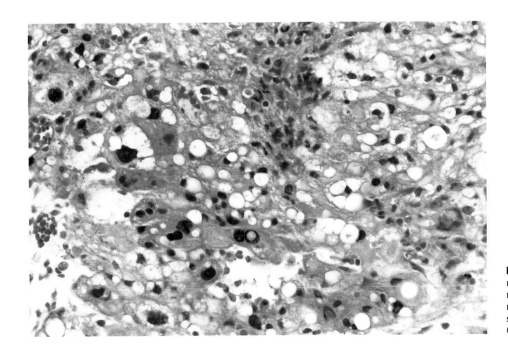

FIGURE 2–78. Chordoma showing multivacuolated physaliferous cells, many with atypical nuclei. Nuclei may also show cytoplasmic inclusions simulating melanoma. (H&E, OM ×100)

but not plasmacytomas are positive for leukocyte common antigen. Chordomas are strongly positive for cytokeratin and S-100 protein and show the characteristic vacuolated physaliphorous cells. Vimentin is also usually well expressed in rhabdomyosarcoma, but much less commonly so in olfactory neuroblastoma and undifferentiated carcinomas. Also to be considered in the differential diagnosis are rare small blue-cell tumors of the head and neck, which have occurred after radiation therapy for retinoblastoma and resemble peripheral neuroepithelioma (with or without myogenous and/or epithelial features).[150] Paragangliomas, which might also be considered, are keratin and calcitonin negative and usually show slender S-100–positive sustentacular cells around the periphery of the organoid nests of cells.[151–153]

Neuroendocrine carcinomas of the sinonasal area as defined by Silva et al.[154] appear to have a much better prognosis than undifferentiated carcinomas in this region (100% 5-year and 77% 10-year survival). These neuroendocrine tumors are composed of polygonal to spindled cells with little anaplasia, a low mitotic rate (<3/10 HPF), no vascular invasion, minimal focal necrosis, and numerous neurosecretory granules (see Fig. 2–75). SNUC lesions are much more anaplastic.

Wenig et al.[155,156] have proposed that the spectrum of neuroendocrine tumors in the larynx starts with a lesion analogous to a classic carcinoid tumor, which they designated well-differentiated neuroendocrine carcinoma, and extends to tumors analogous to classic small-cell neuroendocrine carcinomas, including both the oat cell and intermediate types, which they designated poorly differentiated neuroendocrine carcinoma. However, the most common form of laryngeal neuroendocrine tumor has features between these two extremes and is analogous to atypical carcinoid, well-differentiated neuroendocrine carcinoma, and/or malignant carcinoid of the lung, which Wenig et al.[156] designated moderately differentiated neuroendocrine carcinoma (Fig. 2–79).

These moderately differentiated laryngeal neuroendocrine carcinomas have many features in common with thyroid medullary carcinoma (both can present as neck masses with cervical metastases and have very similar histologic features including argyrophilia, mucicarminophilia, hyaline stroma, abundant neurosecretory granules, and positive staining for amyloid, calcitonin, and carcinoembryonic antigen. The only clear distinctions are site of origin and the usual absence of elevated serum calcitonin, which is present in thyroid medullary carcinoma but not in laryngeal neuroendocrine carcinoma.[157]

Like others, we have noted the rather confusing and inconsistent nomenclature applied to the spectrum of neuroendocrine carcinomas encountered at many different body sites. Just like in other carcinoma types, we believe there are well, moderately, and poorly differentiated forms of neuroendocrine carcinoma. However, we believe that the term *carcinoid* should be retained for those tumors arising in the appropriate sites that have well-characterized features (carcinoid cytoarchitecture, no necrosis, no or only rare mitoses, and a very favorable prognosis). Referring to classic carcinoids as well-differentiated neuroendocrine carcinomas is confusing, because this term is used for a higher grade neuroendocrine carcinoma of the lung. Also, the term small-cell neuroendocrine carcinoma should be retained for both the oat cell and intermediate types, because these tumors are well characterized, and literature describing their clinicopathologic features is well established. But, calling small-cell neuroendocrine carcinomas poorly differentiated neuroendocrine carcinomas (small-cell type) is an acceptable alternative. Greater controversy about nomenclature develops with those neuroendocrine carcinomas with clinicopathologic features intermediate to classic carcinoid and small-cell or poorly differentiated neuroendocrine carcinoma. Using terms like **atypical carcinoid** or **malignant carcinoid** is confusing because these tumors look

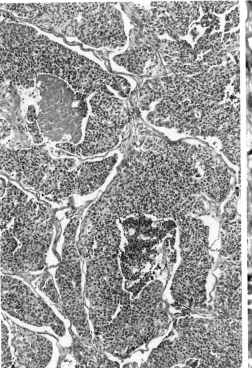
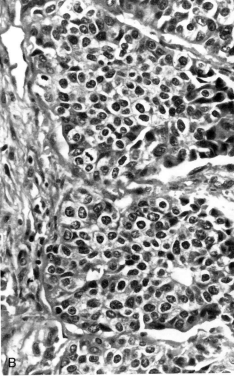

FIGURE 2–79. *A,* Moderately differentiated neuroendocrine carcinoma of the larynx. Note the organoid growth pattern and patchy central necrosis. (H&E, OM ×5) *B,* Same tumor showing relatively uniform population of cells with abundant cytoplasm, organoid growth pattern, and occasional mitotic figure (less than 5 mitotic figures per 10 HPF in this tumor). (H&E, OM ×100)

and behave like overt carcinomas. In this setting, the terms **well-differentiated or moderately differentiated neuroendocrine** are more appropriate. For example, we have observed well-differentiated, carcinoid-like, neuroendocrine carcinomas that have more necrosis and/or greater mitotic activity and cytologic atypia than that found in classic carcinoid but less than that found in the higher grade, moderately differentiated examples of neuroendocrine carcinoma. Mark and Ramirez[158] have suggested that the finding of five or more mitotic figures per 10 high-power fields could be used to distinguish lower from higher grade examples of these carcinoid-like, neuroendocrine carcinomas. Travis et al.[159] have also suggested that mitotic figure content is important in grading or subclassifying neuroendocrine tumors of the lung.

Therefore, we would suggest that the following scheme be considered for classifying the spectrum of neuroendocrine tumors (Table 2–2). Proceeding from the least to the most aggressive tumors: first, there is **classic carcinoid tumor** with no necrosis and one or fewer mitotic figures per 10 HPF; next, **well-differentiated neuroendocrine carcinoma** showing carcinoid-like cytoarchitecture, mild necrosis, and/or one to five mitotic figures per 10 HPF; next, **moderately differentiated neuroendocrine carcinoma** showing carcinoid-like cytoarchitecture, moderate necrosis, and/or 6 to 10 mitotic figures per 10 HPF; and finally, **poorly differentiated neuroendocrine carcinoma** with carcinoid-like and/or classic small-cell, diffuse cytoarchitecture, severe necrosis, and/or very frequent mitotic figures (>10 mitotic figures per 10 HPF). Neuroendocrine carcinomas partially or completely composed of large cells but sometimes showing extensive necrosis and/or very frequent mitotic figures could be considered a form of poorly differentiated neuroendocrine carcinoma (large-cell, or mixed small-cell and large-cell type). Poorly differentiated large-cell carcinomas, which do not appear carcinoid-like at low magnification but show neuroendocrine differentiation by electron microscopy and/or immunoperoxidase studies, would be considered large-cell undifferentiated carcinomas with neuroendocrine features. Using criteria like these, we believe most pathologists would more reliably and reproducibly grade and/or stratify neuroen-

docrine carcinomas along this spectrum, rather than struggle to place these neuroendocrine tumors into a variety of confusing and variably defined "pigeonholes." This problem is compounded by the fact that occasional neuroendocrine carcinomas show mixed differentiation such as squamous, glandular, exocrine, neuroendocrine, chondrosarcomatous, and rhabdomyosarcomatous features.[160]

Sarcomatoid Carcinoma

Sarcomatoid carcinomas are usually biphasic tumors composed of both carcinomatous and sarcomatous elements.[161–214] Although uncommon, they occur in numerous sites, especially in the upper aerodigestive tract,[161–181] including the esophagus.[182–185] Other locations for sarcomatoid carcinomas include the lower respiratory tract,[161, 186, 187] urogenital tract,[161, 188–190] stomach,[161, 190, 191] small intestine,[192] pancreas,[193] colon,[194] anus,[195] liver,[161] gallbladder,[161] breast,[161, 196] skin,[161, 197, 198] thyroid,[161] conjunctiva,[200] and salivary glands.[161, 201] Traditionally, sarcomatoid carcinomas have been controversial lesions.[161–181] The controversy has centered around not only their presumed histogenesis but also their biologic behavior and appropriate therapy.[161–181]

Authors have variably referred to these tumors as carcinosarcoma,[161, 162, 181] pseudosarcoma,[164, 168, 172, 175] spindle cell carcinoma,[166, 169, 173, 176] pleomorphic carcinoma,[165] polypoid carcinoma,[182, 183] and metaplastic carcinoma.[161, 168] Anonsen et al.[163] have nicely reviewed the controversy of this tumor's histogenesis. Three theories have evolved:[161] that the tumor represents a "collision" tumor or a dual growth of sarcoma and carcinoma (i.e., arising from two distinct but adjacent malignant clones);[162] that the tumor is a squamous carcinoma with an atypical but benign connective-tissue reaction (so-called pseudosarcoma); and that the tumor is a squamous carcinoma that has developed a spindle-cell component (i.e., sarcomatous metaplasia).[163] Very few favor the unlikely event of two independent malignant clones arising separately and growing adjacent to each other.[161–165, 168] Some authors have reserved the term **carcinosarcoma** for these presumed collision tumors,[161–163, 168] but this does not have to be the case. Diamandopoulos and Meissner[202] define carcinosarcoma as

Table 2–2. **Proposed Scheme for Classifying the Spectrum of Neuroendocrine Tumors**

	Classic Carcinoid	Spectrum of Neuroendocrine Carcinoma by Differentiation		
		Well	*Moderate*	*Poor*
Incidence (Relative):	Common	Rare	Uncommon	Common
LM Pattern (Low-magnification):	Classic carcinoid	Carcinoid-like	Carcinoid-like	Classic small-cell with or without carcinoid-like areas* or large-cell with carcinoid-like areas
Necrosis:	None	None to mild (spotty or small clusters of cells)	None to moderate (patchy or focally comedo-like)	None to extensive and confluent
Mitotic Activity:	Very rare or ≤ 1 mf per 10 HPF	> 1 but ≤ 5 mfs per 10 HPF	> 5 but ≤ 10 mfs per 10 HPF	> 10 mfs per 10 HPF

* Includes classic small-cell neuroendocrine carcinoma of the oat cell, polygonal, or intermediate morphology. Neuroendocrine carcinomas partially or completely composed of large cells but showing a carcinoid-like pattern at low magnification and frequent mitotic figures (with or without extensive necrosis) could be considered a form of poorly differentiated neuroendocrine carcinoma (large-cell or mixed small- and large-cell type). However, poorly differentiated large-cell carcinomas, which do not resemble carcinoid at low magnification but show neuroendocrine differentiation by electron microscopy and/or immunoperoxidase studies, would be classified as large-cell undifferentiated carcinomas with neuroendocrine features.

LM, light microscopic; mf, mitotic figure; HPF, high-power field.

"a cancer containing a mixture of carcinomatous and sarcomatous elements." Moreover, Gould[203] suggests that it is better to classify tumors based on what they are, as defined by phenotypic-differentiation markers, rather than on the basis of questionable assumptions about their origins. Sharing this belief, we feel the term *carcinosarcoma* nicely describes tumors showing both carcinomatous and sarcomatous differentiation, especially when the latter shows malignant bone, cartilage, and/or muscle. When used in this descriptive sense, *carcinosarcoma* need not imply that these mixed tumors are of carcinomatous or sarcomatous origin, nor does it necessarily imply that the tumor arose from one or two malignant cell clones.[194]

The most popular theory is that the pleomorphic spindle cells derive from sarcomatous metaplasia of the malignant epithelial cells.[161–181, 209] Although Krompecher[161, 169] in the early 1900s proposed sarcomatous transformation of carcinoma cells, Battifora[169] reported convincing ultrastructural evidence of this process. That carcinoma cells can undergo sarcomatous metaplasia is based on the following observations: (1) frequent observation of transitional areas between the biphasic components; (2) demonstration of immunoreactive keratin in spindle cells; (3) retained ultrastructural features of epithelial cells in spindle cells (desmosomes and tonofibrils); (4) shared features of both epithelium and mesenchyme in some spindle cells; and (5) the numerical predominance of carcinomas in locations where sarcomatoid carcinomas occur.[161–181] In a study of sarcomatoid carcinomas of the upper aerodigestive tract, Zarbo et al.[166] demonstrated immunoreactive keratin in the spindle cell components in 44% of 18 biphasic tumors and in 57% of seven monophasic spindle cell tumors devoid of demonstrable squamous carcinoma. Most spindle cells were also positive for vimentin (sometimes co-expressed with cytokeratin), thus confirming mesenchymal metaplasia. At the same time, 41% of 13 tumors studied by electron microscopy retained ultrastructural features of epithelial differentiation. When electron microscopic and immunohistochemical techniques were combined, epithelial differentiation could be demonstrated in the spindle cells in 60% of cases.

Just as the histogenesis of sarcomatoid carcinoma has generated controversy, so has the prognosis and treatment of these tumors. Appleman and Oberman[210] considered polypoid lesions to have a good prognosis regardless of histologic findings, whereas tumors of any other configuration had a poor prognosis. Himalstein and Humphrey[211] found the best predictor of prognosis to be the histologic grade of the associated squamous carcinoma. Still others[212, 213] have emphasized size and location as correlating best with outcome. Leventon and Evans[167] reported 20 cases and found that 9 of 10 patients died whose tumors invaded muscle, bone, salivary glands, or accessory respiratory glands, whereas all 10 patients survived whose tumors were superficial and did not extend into any of these structures. A history of ionizing irradiation to the tumor site and tumor location in the oral cavity correlated with invasiveness and thus a poor outcome. Other than invasiveness, histologic features and gross configuration were not found to be of significant prognostic importance. In contrast, after studying 59 cases from the oral cavity, Ellis and Corio[176] found that no clinical or histomorphologic characteristic other than distant metastasis was a reliable prognostic indicator. In their series, the most common metastatic site was cervical lymph nodes (11 cases) followed by lung (6 cases); there was one case each of metastases to heart, skin, and bone.

Batsakis et al.[162] have reviewed the natural history of sarcomatoid carcinoma in the head and neck and correlated their findings by anatomic site. When considering all tumor sites, he and his coworkers found that 42% of 154 reported patients had died of or with disease. Sixty percent of 53 patients with oral cavity lesions had died within 1 to 72 months, 77% of 13 patients with sinonasal tract lesions had died within 6 to 30 months, and 33% of 65 patients with laryngeal lesions had died within 4 to 24 months. Polypoid glottic tumors appeared to have the most favorable prognosis (estimated 90% 3-year survival), whereas sarcomatoid carcinomas at all other locations did poorly regardless of their gross appearance.[162, 164] Batsakis et al.[162] concluded that, although accurately predicting biologic behavior of individual cases may be difficult, sarcomatoid carcinomas, as a group, manifest biologic behavior that is more aggressive than that of most conventional carcinomas. In addition, he and his coworkers believed that management of the individual patient should be based on experience derived from the whole group of sarcomatoid carcinomas. Unlike those cases occurring in the head and neck, in sarcomatoid carcinoma of the esophagus, patients have shown approximately 50% survival.[182–185] This contrasts sharply with the 4% 5-year survival for patients with the usual esophageal carcinoma.[182–185]

CLINICOPATHOLOGIC FEATURES. Sarcomatoid carcinomas present as rapidly growing, usually polypoid or exophytic masses, although endophytic nodular or sessile examples occur. Exophytic lesions outnumber endophytic lesions by roughly 2 to 1.[166, 167] In two series combined,[166, 167] 43% of 35 cases occurred in the larynx, 40% in the oral cavity, 20% in the hypopharynx and pyriform sinuses, 14% in the sinonasal tract, and 11% in the oropharynx. Numerous cases have also been described in the esophagus,[182–184] where polypoid lesions are most common. Males predominate in most series; male to female ratios have ranged from 4:1 to 2:1.[162–181] Patient ages have been reported to range from 14 to 93 years, with median ages from 55 to 65 years.[162–181] Depending on tumor location, patients complain of pain, burning, dyspnea, dysphagia, hoarseness, hemorrhage, otalgia, loose teeth, swelling, and/or persistent ulcer.[162–181] In the series of Leventon and Evans,[167] 95% of 19 patients indulged in snuff, smoked, or chewed tobacco; 81% of 16 patients had evidence of longstanding oral neglect; 24% of 17 patients admitted to alcohol abuse; and 32% of 19 patients had undergone ionizing irradiation to the tumor site. Macroscopically, most sarcomatoid carcinomas are exophytic polypoid masses attached to the mucosa by a stalk; however, endophytic fungating or ulcerating infiltrative masses occur.[162–181] The tumor surfaces are frequently ulcerated and capped by a friable pseudomembrane. The tumor substance is firm, gray-white to tan-white, and usually without central necrosis (a feature attributed to well-developed vascularity).[176]

Microscopically, most sarcomatoid carcinomas are predominantly composed of pleomorphic spindle cells and lesser portions of carcinoma.[161–185] With the exception of examples in the esophagus, where adenosquamous carcinomas occasionally occur,[185] the carcinomatous component is almost always squamous (Fig. 2–80). It is usually present at the base or stalk of the tumor, and numerous histologic sections may be necessary to find it. Carcinoma may not be demonstrable

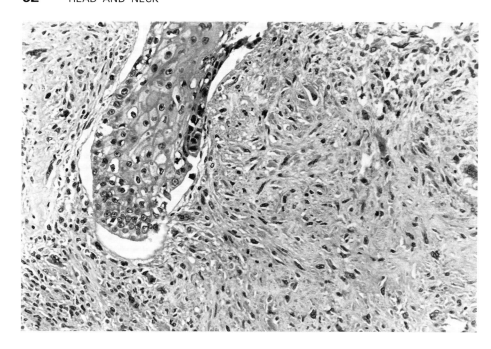

FIGURE 2–80. Sarcomatoid carcinoma showing malignant spindle cell stroma adjacent to an island of atypical squamous epithelium. (H&E, OM ×100)

in all cases; in fact, 28% of cases in the series of Zarbo et al.[166] were totally devoid of demonstrable squamous carcinoma. The squamous component can be invasive, *in situ,* verrucous, or "transitional";[162–181] sometimes it has been described as dysplastic rather than overtly malignant.[176] The sarcomatous elements contain plump spindle cells showing variable but usually marked pleomorphism (see Fig. 2–80). Nuclei demonstrate malignant features of clumped dense chromatin, prominent nucleoli, irregular nuclear profiles, and numerous

(frequently atypical) mitotic figures. A diffuse ill-defined streaming pattern predominates in most cases, but storiform, myxoid, microcystic, xanthomatous, hemangiopericytomatous, tumor giant cell, and/or malignant osteocartilaginous areas may be present in variable combinations.[161–185] Tumors showing malignant osteocartilaginous areas are frequently associated with a history of previous ionizing irradiation to the site of the tumor.[162–185] Osteoclast-like giant cells, which are likely benign cells derived from bone marrow monocytes,

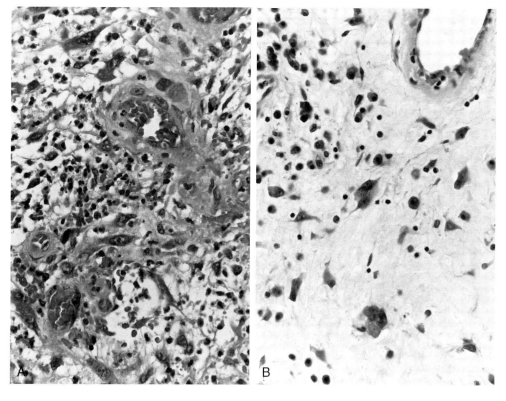

FIGURE 2–81. *A,* Atypical stromal and endothelial cells sometimes encountered in atypical granulation-tissue reactions following radiation therapy. These lesions can be overdiagnosed as recurrent malignancy. (H&E, OM ×100) *B,* Atypical stromal cells, sometimes encountered in inflammatory polyps of the sinonasal area. Care should be taken not to misdiagnose these lesions as malignant. (H&E, OM ×100)

are present within the sarcomatous stroma in many cases. Rarely, rhabdomyosarcomatous differentiation has been described.[181]

DIFFERENTIAL DIAGNOSIS. Malignant tumors that might simulate sarcomatoid carcinoma of the upper aerodigestive tract include **soft-tissue sarcomas, mucosal melanoma, true malignant mixed tumors of salivary glands, malignant spindle cell myoepithelioma, mucoepidermoid carcinoma with spindle cell stroma, teratocarcinosarcoma of the sinonasal tract, and laryngeal blastoma.** Benign lesions that need to be separated from sarcomatoid carcinoma include sinonasal polyps with stromal atypia (Fig. 2–81B), bizarre (pseudomalignant) granulation-tissue reactions after ionizing radiation exposure (Fig. 2–81A), nodular (''pseudosarcomatous'') fasciitis, and benign spindle cell myoepithelioma. Soft-tissue sarcomas are rare in the upper-aerodigestive tract; in fact, in a review of malignant laryngeal lesions by Batsakis et al.,[162] only 0.3% were classified as sarcomas.[162] They emphasized that this low frequency demands that sarcomatoid carcinoma be ruled out before a diagnosis of soft-tissue sarcoma is made. Nevertheless, among the soft-tissue sarcomas, synovial sarcoma might prove occasionally difficult to separate from sarcomatoid carcinoma (Figs. 2–82 and 2–83). **Synovial sarcomas** occur in the upper aerodigestive tract, can present as polypoid or sessile mucosal masses, and occasionally demonstrate squamous metaplasia.[215, 216] However, they usually display nests of plump epithelioid cells interspersed throughout a monotonous cellular fibrosarcomatous stroma (see Fig. 2–82). Cellular pleomorphism is less than that found in most sarcomatoid carcinomas, and, unlike the latter, synovial sarcomas may demonstrate slit-like and/or frond-like papillary structures lined by cuboidal epithelioid cells (see Fig. 2–83). To complicate matters, synovial sarcoma cells may immunoreact with keratin and/or vimentin antibodies and have ultrastructural features of epithelial cells.[215–217] **Monophasic variants** lack morphologic features of epithelial differentiation and appear similar to fibrosarcoma or neurosarcoma, two additional soft-tissue sarcomas that can occur within the upper aerodigestive tract and mimic sarcomatoid carcinoma.[162, 218] **Malignant fibrous histiocytomas** have also been described in this region as mucosal masses.[219, 220] The gross and microscopic presentations can exactly mimic those of sarcomatoid carcinoma; indeed, some of the reported cases may have been sarcomatoid carcinomas wherein the original squamous carcinoma had been destroyed and the spindle cells had lost immunologic and ultrastructural features of epithelial cells. Such a tumor is a malignant fibrous histiocytoma; if one chooses to name tumors strictly by the types of differentiation they show, such tumors may behave more as sarcomas than as carcinomas. In either event, both tumors show similar aggressive behavior and should be treated accordingly.

In the pediatric age group, sarcomatoid carcinoma is very rare; nevertheless, a polypoid tumor involving the left maxillary ridge has been described in a 14-year-old boy.[180] Because the tumor was devoid of squamous carcinoma, its differentiation from **rhabdomyosarcoma** was especially difficult. Electron microscopy revealed desmosomes in the spindle cells and confirmed the diagnosis of sarcomatoid carcinoma. This distinction is important, because sarcomatoid carcinoma is best treated with surgery, whereas rhabdomyosarcoma is best treated with ionizing radiation and chemotherapy.[180] Only very rare examples of sarcomatoid carcinoma have shown rhabdomyosarcomatous differentiation.[181] **Mucosal melanoma** forming spindle cells could produce an ulcerated exophytic mass, and they need not contain pigment either grossly or microscopically.[221] In the nasal cavity, about one third of cases are

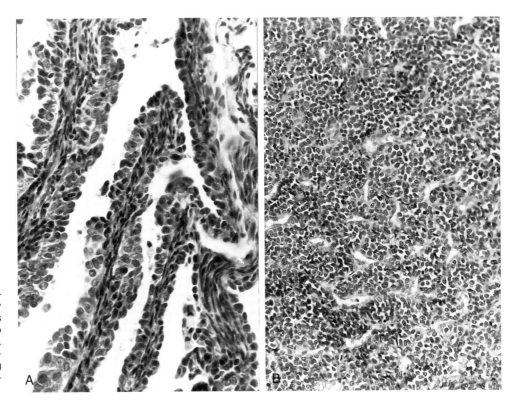

FIGURE 2–82. *A,* Biphasic synovial sarcoma showing papillary pattern with epithelial cells lining the papillae, which also have dense spindle cell cores. (H&E, OM ×100) *B,* Monophasic synovial sarcoma showing a hemangiopericytoma-like vascular pattern. (H&E, OM ×50)

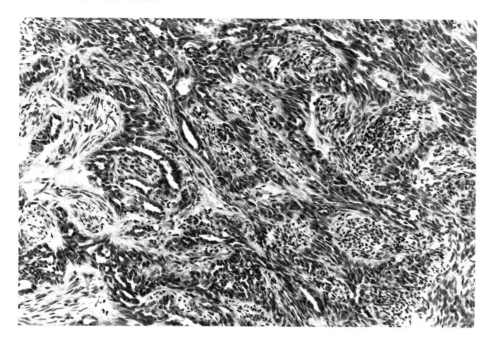

FIGURE 2–83. Biphasic synovial sarcoma showing more common biphasic pattern of trabeculae of epithelial cells forming gland-like spaces surrounded by spindle cells. (H&E, OM ×50)

amelanotic.[221] Ultrastructural study for premelanosomes and/or immunohistochemical stains for S-100 should resolve diagnostic problems in most cases. Sarcomatoid carcinoma of the lip needs to be differentiated from **neurotropic melanoma,**[222] a form of **spindle cell (desmoplastic) melanoma.** Recognition of neurotropic melanoma depends on finding a dysplastic melanocytic lesion within adjacent epidermis (although absent in about 20% of cases), endoneurial invasion (so-called neurotropism), poorly defined margins, and atypical neuroma-like growth patterns. Melanin pigment is usually not present,

and in difficult cases, S-100 immunoreactivity should help resolve diagnostic problems. Salivary gland tumors can mimic sarcomatoid carcinoma. The most likely is so-called **true malignant mixed tumor (carcinosarcoma).**[223] In contrast to **carcinoma ex pleomorphic adenoma,** true malignant mixed tumors show both carcinoma and sarcoma (Fig. 2–84). Within the sarcomatous component, chondrosarcoma usually predominates and is present in greater amounts than is usually seen in sarcomatoid carcinoma, in which chondrosarcomatous metaplasia is usually absent or only focal. Less common sali-

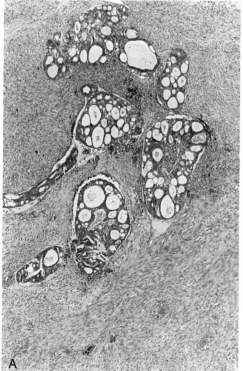

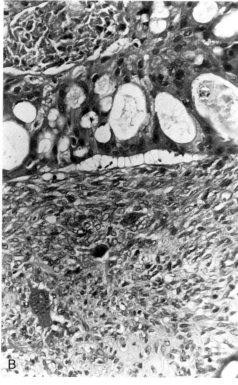

FIGURE 2–84. *A,* Carcinosarcoma of salivary gland. Note central salivary duct–like carcinoma surrounded by invasive spindle cell elements. Some might consider this case a true malignant mixed tumor. (H&E, OM ×10) *B,* Cytologic features of the carcinosarcoma become more apparent at higher magnification. (H&E, OM ×100)

vary gland lesions to consider are **malignant myoepithelioma,**[224] and **spindle cell mucoepidermoid carcinoma.**[225] A spindle cell malignancy containing cells showing mixed epithelial and smooth muscle features by electron microscopy and immunoreactivity for S-100, keratin, and actin favors myoepithelial differentiation, whereas mucin-producing carcinoma cells suggest mucoepidermoid carcinoma. Within the sinonasal tract, a unique mixed tumor, **teratocarcinosarcoma,** has been described by Shanmugaratnam et al.[226] and Heffner and Hyams.[227] This tumor shows combined histologic features of carcinosarcoma and teratoma. A similar-appearing tumor has been described by Eble et al.[228] in the larynx and is referred to as **laryngeal blastoma.** Both deserve consideration in the differential diagnosis of sarcomatoid carcinoma.

Although one could argue the usefulness of separating some of these lesions from sarcomatoid carcinoma, it is important to distinguish benign from malignant lesions. First, **sinonasal polyps with stromal atypia** have been described by Compagno et al.[229] (see Fig. 2–81B). These atypical lesions neither display associated carcinoma nor have the mitotic index frequently found in sarcomatoid carcinoma. Similar polyps have been described in the bladder and lower female genital tract.[230, 231] Next, **bizarre (pseudomalignant) granulation tissue reactions following ionizing radiation** exposure can occur and simulate sarcomatoid carcinoma[231] (see Fig. 2–81A). These lesions are especially treacherous because they have occurred in the upper aerodigestive tract in patients known to have had carcinoma. In addition, they showed marked cytologic atypia and numerous (sometimes atypical) mitotic figures. Central to their recognition as benign are their granulation tissue growth pattern and the roughly equivalent cytologic atypia found in both stromal and endothelial cells. Similar pseudomalignant lesions have been described following trauma in the bladder and cervix.[232–234] Third, **nodular**

(pseudosarcomatous) fasciitis can occur in the upper aerodigestive tract and present as a rapidly growing polypoid mass.[235] They tend to be myxoid, contain extravasated red blood cells, and show numerous normal-appearing mitotic figures. The benign cytologic features and tissue culture–like appearance of the spindle cells are central to their recognition as benign. Finally, the **spindle cell variant of benign myoepithelioma** arising from salivary glands could be confused with a sarcomatoid carcinoma (see Fig. 2–32A).[235] However, the benign cytologic features, mixed ultrastructural features of epithelium and smooth muscle, and immunoreactivity for S-100, cytokeratin, and actin should lead to the correct diagnosis.[224]

Variants of Papillary Thyroid Carcinoma

Although it is not the purpose of this discussion to review all the clinical pathologic features of **typical papillary thyroid carcinoma (PTC),** it is worth describing some of the PTC variants, because they can be mistaken for benign disorders. These variants include **diffuse sclerosing (DS) variant of PTC,**[236, 237] **PTC with exuberant nodular fasciitis-like stroma,**[238] **macrofollicular variant of PTC, encapsulated follicular variant of PTC, papillary oxyphil and clear-cell variant,** and **papillary microcarcinoma.**

DS-PTC should be recognized, because it can be confused with a **diffuse lymphocytic thyroiditis or early phases of subacute (granulomatous) thyroiditis,** and it may have a worse prognosis than the usual forms of PTC. DS-PTC can diffusely involve one or both thyroid lobes. It can be recognized by the presence of numerous tumor islands within lymphatic spaces, tumor nests with papillae and/or squamous metaplasia (resembling endometrial morula), large numbers of psammoma bodies, marked lymphocytic infiltration, and prominent fibrosis (Fig. 2–85). In contrast to typical PTC,

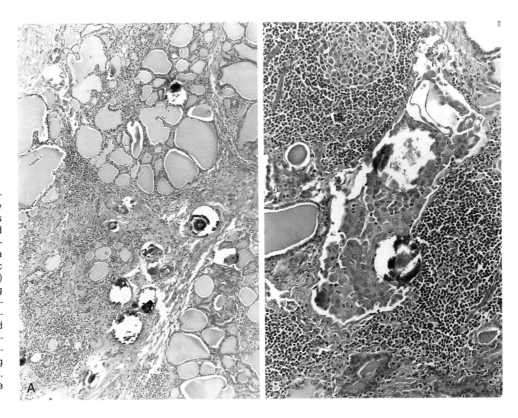

FIGURE 2–85. *A,* Diffuse sclerosing variant of invasive papillary carcinoma. Note numerous psammoma bodies distributed between normal thyroid follicles. The thyroid parenchyma shows fibrosis and chronic inflammation. (H&E, OM ×2.5) *B,* In the diffuse sclerosing variant of invasive papillary carcinoma, invasive nests of papillary carcinoma are found scattered throughout the thyroid parenchyma within lymphatic spaces and showing squamous morule-like features. Note the numerous psammoma bodies. (H&E, OM ×100)

DS-PTC has a greater incidence of cervical lymph node and lung metastases, and it occurs in a younger age group. The more frequent presence of diffuse thyroid gland involvement and reduced disease-free survival suggest that total and near-total thyroidectomy is justified, followed by the administration of radioactive iodine to attempt elimination of metastases.[237] Overall survival may still be quite favorable.[239, 240] Of interest, Chan et al.[241] have described a form of **sclerosing mucoepidermoid carcinoma of the thyroid with prominent eosinophilia** and arising from a background of Hashimoto's thyroiditis. These tumors formed masses composed of infiltrating tumor cells that had mild to moderate nuclear pleomorphism, distinct nucleoli, squamous differentiation, mucin pools, and abundant dense fibrohyaline stroma, which was infiltrated by numerous eosinophils in all cases. The tumors were negative for thyroglobulin and calcitonin.

Although the well-developed granulomatous (multinucleated giant cell containing) stage of **subacute thyroiditis** is easily recognized, occasional cases presenting early may show no or few multinucleated giant cells and/or neutrophilic microabscesses. Instead, early examples of subacute thyroiditis may show focal or patchy thyroid involvement characterized by a desmoplastic stroma-like reaction surrounding clusters of colloid-poor follicles. Some of the affected follicles contain a "follicle-centered" discohesive lymphocytic and epithelioid histiocytic infiltrate, sometimes with apparent loss of and/or columnar alteration of the follicular epithelium. The epithelioid histiocytes predominate, and focal nuclear atypia may be present. Overall, this pattern may closely mimic an infiltrating, multifocal and/or diffuse sclerosing thyroid malignancy. In subacute thyroiditis, multiple sections performed to look for the more characteristic "follicle-centered" multinucleated giant cells and/or neutrophilic microabscesses should lead to the correct diagnosis.

Additional cases of **primary mucinous or mucoepider-moid carcinomas of the thyroid** have been reported.[242–244] Their histogenesis is unclear, yet their natural history is like that of PTC. Furthermore, Mlynek et al.[245] studied 142 cases of thyroid cancer and found mucicarmine-positive tumor cells in 50% of papillary, 50% of medullary, 35% of follicular, and 21% of anaplastic cancers. Chan and Tse[244] found 17% of metastatic PTCs had intracytoplasmic mucicarmine-positive material. Thus, mucin production by follicular and parafollicular thyroid tumors is more common than usually thought, and that mucin positivity does not rule out a thyroid primary. Moreover, PTCs with significant areas of **trabecular growth** (>50%), **tall cell** (>30% of the tumor cells are twice as tall as they are wide and have oxyphilic cytoplasm), and/or **columnar cell** features (pseudostratified hyperchromatic nuclei imparting an endometroid look) may follow a more aggressive course.

PTC with exuberant nodular fasciitis-like stroma (NFS) was reported by Chan et al.[238] as representative of a variant form of PTC with a prominent stromal component, which at low magnification resembled fibroadenoma, phyllodes tumor, and/or fibrocytic changes of the breast. The abundant stroma was like nodular fasciitis, because it was composed of fascicles of spindled cells separated by mucoid matrix, collagen, and extravasated red blood cells. The carcinoma cells exhibited cytologic features of PTC (overlapping and relatively large nuclei, optically clear nucleoplasm, occasional cytoplasmic nuclear inclusions, and prominent numbers of tumor nuclei with nuclear grooves), but grew in anastomosing narrow tubules, cluster glands, solid sheets (sometimes with squamous metaplasia), and/or papillae. It is important not to confuse PTC-NFS with a benign fibroproliferative thyroid lesion and with dedifferentiated or anaplastic thyroid carcinomas.

There are pitfalls in the diagnosis of PTC that should be emphasized.[246] First, not all papillae in thyroid lesions indicate PTC. Papillae, which have central fibrovascular stalks lined

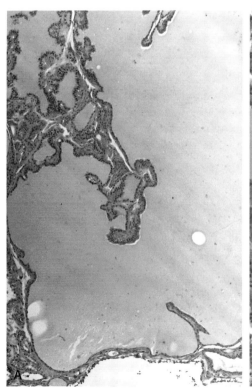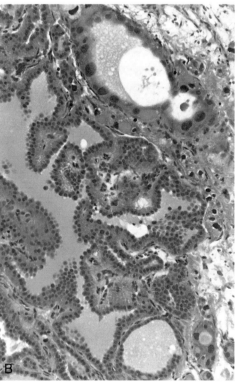

FIGURE 2–86. *A*, Nodular hyperplasia (nodular goiter) showing so-called pseudopapillae. Note that the pseudopapillae point toward the center of the large dilated cystic follicle and contain follicles within their cores. (H&E, OM ×2.5) *B*, Patient with Graves' disease, previously treated with ^{131}I, showing blunt pseudopapillae and focal cytologic atypia. Such patients can develop recurrent hyperplasia as well as benign and malignant thyroid tumors. (H&E, OM ×100)

by a row of epithelial cells, can occur in Graves' disease, Hashimoto's disease, nodular hyperplasia, and follicular adenoma. These **"pseudopapillae"** are relatively short and stubby; they often have edematous stalks with small follicles within them, lack branching, orient with their tips toward the center of large follicular cysts, and are lined by columnar cells with normochromatic nuclei arranged in a regular basilar-oriented row (Fig. 2–86A). Also, in patients with Graves' disease previously treated with radioactive iodine, recurrent lesions may be nodular, associated with fibrosis, marked cytologic atypia, and intranuclear cytoplasmic inclusions (Fig. 2–86B). Psammoma bodies within the fibrovascular stalks of the papillae are highly suggestive of PTC; however, when they are found within the colloid of follicles, they are indicative of benign follicular neoplasms, especially those showing Hurthle cell changes.[247] It should be emphasized that the diagnosis of PTC is based on a set of cytologic and architectural features. The papillae of PTC are "complex" and arborizing; they are lined by one or more cell layers having centrally located and overlapping nuclei, which are optically clear, contain cytoplasmic nuclear inclusions, and reveal numerous nuclear grooves. PTC cells also react with antibodies to S-100 and high-molecular-weight keratins, and in contrast to benign lesions, their luminal surface is coated by alcian blue and anti-EMA–positive material. The tumor cells of PTC also tend to be larger than the benign follicle lining cells found in the adjacent thyroid parenchyma. PTCs can have follicular, solid, and squamous areas without being considered some other tumor or a more aggressive variant. The presence of increased nuclear hyperchromasia or anaplasia, increased mitotic activity, necrosis (sometimes in a peritheliomatous pattern), and/or a nested insular growth pattern (sometimes with microfollicles, artifactual retraction from fibrohyaline stroma, and/or central necrosis) should suggest dedifferentiation of low-grade PTC to a **poorly differentiated ("insular")**

(Fig. 2–87) **or anaplastic carcinoma.**[248] Additional sections of the tumor in these cases should clarify the diagnosis.

Further variants of PTC have been described, and they are reviewed by LiVolsi,[240] Vickery et al.,[236] and Rosai et al.[249] We have recently encountered the **papillary oxyphil and clear-cell variant** described by Dickersin et al.[250] (Fig. 2–88A), which has a quite aggressive behavior. It should be emphasized that clear-cell changes in primary thyroid tumors can occur in both benign and malignant lesions and should not be taken to indicate that all thyroid tumors containing clear cells are malignant or so-called clear-cell carcinomas.[251] When clear-cell changes are prominent, metastatic renal carcinoma should be considered (Fig. 2–89).

In addition to predominantly "follicular" examples of PTC, we have encountered cases of the so-called **macrofollicular variant of PTC,** which closely mimics benign macrofollicular adenoma or nodular goiter.[252] Key to the diagnosis is the presence of epithelial cells with cytologic features characteristic of PTC lining the macro- and microfollicles (Fig. 2–90). These lesions have a very good prognosis. Another variant of PTC known as the **diffuse follicular variant of PTC** is probably more aggressive than classic PTC, occurs in young patients, mimics diffuse goiter, diffusely involves the thyroid without nodules, and has a predominant follicular pattern without fibrosis and a high frequency of lymph nodal and distant metastases, but responds well to radioactive iodine.[252] **The encapsulated PTC** variant can be mistaken for benign adenoma, because invasion is not required to make the diagnosis. The diagnosis depends on finding the classic and well-developed cytologic features of PTC, which are discussed in more detail in the next section. The WHO committee has defined **papillary microcarcinoma** as a papillary carcinoma measuring 1.0 cm or less in diameter—a term that replaces occult sclerosing carcinoma, non-encapsulated sclerosing tumor, and occult papillary carcinoma. Although papil-

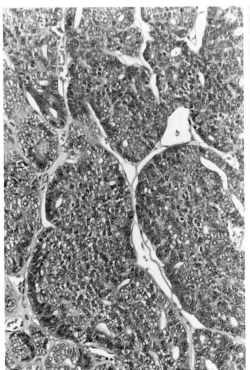
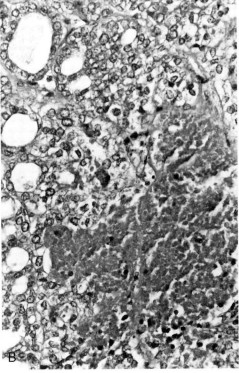

FIGURE 2–87. *A,* Poorly differentiated or insular carcinoma of the thyroid. Note the insular arrangement of the tumor cells and focal thyroid follicle differentiation. (H&E, OM ×25) *B,* An island of poorly differentiated carcinoma is shown with central necrosis and focal thyroid follicular differentiation. (H&E, OM ×100)

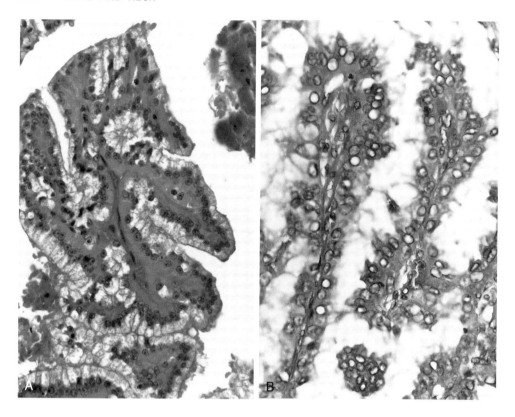

FIGURE 2–88. *A,* Papillary carcinoma variant characterized by biphasic cells showing oncocytic granular cytoplasm subnuclearly and clear, vacuolated cytoplasm supranuclearly. (H&E, OM ×100) *B,* Classic cytoarchitectural features of well-differentiated papillary carcinoma of thyroid type. Note the numerous optically clear nuclei. (H&E, OM ×100)

lary microcarcinomas have a very good prognosis, cervical nodal metastasis can be present, and rare examples have been reported to cause death.

Differential Diagnosis of Follicular Thyroid Tumors

Follicular carcinomas have been subdivided into two broad categories based on the extent of invasion: **encapsulated, minimally invasive (MIFC), and widely invasive (WIFC) types.**[253, 254] Although the prognosis of encapsulated MIFC is very good (70% to 95% 10-year survival) compared with WIFC (30% to 45% 10-year survival), the distinction of **follicular adenoma** from follicular carcinoma is important, given differences in the therapies and psychosocial impact on the patient.

Because the prognosis for MIFC is very good and close to that of follicular adenoma, there is no need for overdiagnosing MIFC.[254] Thus, strict criteria must be maintained in making the diagnosis of MIFC. Rosai et al.[249] and Franssila et al.[253] indicate that follicular neoplasms with clear-cut, obvious, and/or unquestionable evidence of tumor thrombi in blood vessels or equally clear-cut evidence of invasive tumor beyond the capsule should be considered MIFC. In contrast, WIFC includes those extensively (often grossly evident) invasive follicular carcinomas that are not encapsulated or those that are encapsulated yet show abundant or marked tissue and/or vascular invasion (greater than four blood vessels invaded, according to Lang et al.[254]). Rosai et al.[249] state that vessel invasion should involve medium-sized veins, located within the capsule or beyond, and have lumina partially or totally occluded by a tumor thrombus, which should be attached to the wall (often polypoid plugs) and which may or may not have an endothelial covering (Fig. 2–91*A*). Yet, a tumor

thrombus can have a free-floating tail and, depending on the plane of section, the attachment point may not be present.[253] Tumor cell nests slightly bulging into thin-walled vessels should not be regarded as vascular invasion (Fig. 2–91*B*), especially if the latter formations are within the tumor substance or even at the inner margins of the capsule. It is also important not to mistake tissue retraction around a cluster of thyroid cells or a "floater" (no endothelial lining) artifactually forced into a vessel during tissue processing as vessel invasion. Furthermore, the criteria for capsular invasion should be even more strict: the tumor should spread in an invasive fashion well beyond the capsule into the surrounding benign thyroid tissues or extrathyroid tissues. Capsular irregularities and/or clusters of follicular cells embedded in the capsule are not evidence of invasion; however, if suspicious tumor islands within the capsule are present, additional sections and/or tissue should be examined. Although follicular carcinomas tend to show fibrous capsules, more cellularity, increased mitotic figures, and greater nuclear atypia as compared with follicular adenoma (Fig. 2–92), these features (including Hurthle cell changes) cannot be used as criteria for the diagnosis of MIFC.[253] The capsule of follicular tumors should be widely sampled (at least 10 generous blocks), but if atypical features are noted, further extensive sampling and deeper cuts should be performed.

Vascular invasion is clearly the most important morphologic predictor of aggressive behavior in encapsulated follicular neoplasms. This observation is underscored by a recent study by van Heerden et al.,[255] in which 20 patients with "follicular carcinomas" diagnosed by capsular invasion were followed up for a median of 11 years and experienced no recurrences, but 12 of 45 patients (27%) with follicular carcinomas diagnosed by vascular invasion with or without capsular invasion died of disease within the same time.

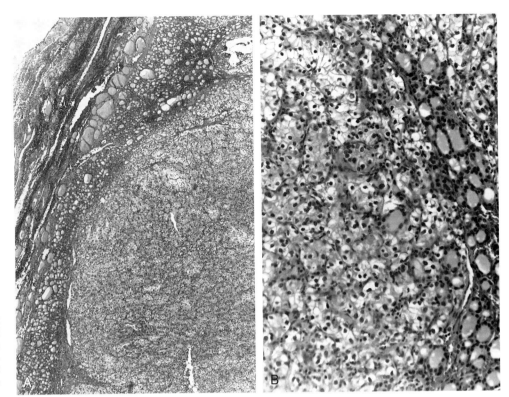

FIGURE 2–89. *A*, Metastatic clear-cell carcinoma from the kidney, simulating a primary clear-cell tumor of the thyroid. (H&E, OM ×2.5) *B,* The clear-cell features of the metastatic renal carcinoma are more apparent at higher magnification. Admixed are thyroid follicles from an adenomatous nodule (goiter), which made distinction from a primary thyroid tumor difficult. (H&E, OM ×50)

Evans,[256] however, defined encapsulated follicular carcinomas as tumors that did not invade surrounding thyroid but had capsular invasion that was characterized by nests, cords, or nodules of tumor cells located within the capsule (Fig. 2–93). The capsules of the latter were at least moderately thick (and often very thick) over most of their extent. The substantial majority of follicular adenomas had capsules that were entirely or in large part very thin (<0.1 mm thick) or even imperceptible. ''Thus, a circumscribed follicular tumor was considered an encapsulated follicular carcinoma if it had a

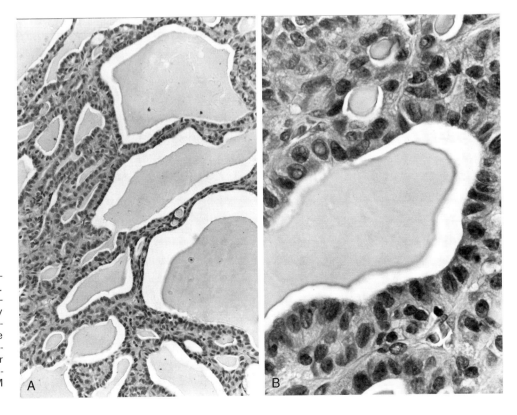

FIGURE 2–90. *A*, Papillary carcinoma, macrofollicular variant. (H&E, OM ×10) *B,* In the macrofollicular variant of papillary carcinoma, the follicular architecture is maintained and the cytology is that of classic papillary carcinoma. Note the nuclear grooves and intranuclear cytoplasmic inclusions. (H&E, OM ×100)

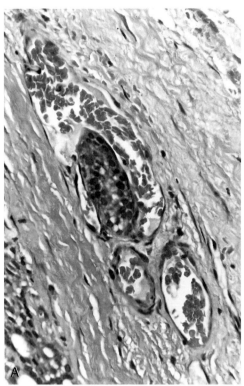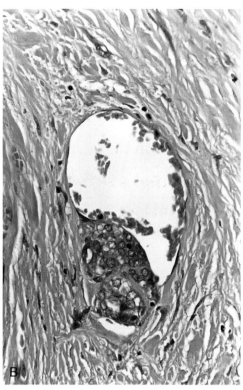

FIGURE 2–91. *A,* A clear-cut example of angioinvasion in follicular carcinoma of the thyroid. The vascular tumor embolus is covered by an endothelial-cell layer. (H&E, OM ×100) *B,* Follicular neoplastic cells pushing along the endothelialized wall of a thin-walled blood vessel. This is not sufficient to be considered angioinvasion. (H&E, OM ×100)

capsule that was entirely or predominantly at least moderately thick *and* it demonstrated invasion of that capsule (but not further), and was considered a follicular adenoma if it had a capsule that was entirely or predominantly thin or imperceptible or it had a thicker capsule with no invasion.''[256] Invasive follicular carcinomas had invasion into adjacent benign thyroid tissues. Importantly, none of 19 follicular adenomas metastasized, three of seven encapsulated follicular carcinomas metastasized (40%), and 9 of 11 invasive follicular carcinomas metastasized (80%). Vascular invasion was not present

in any of the ''encapsulated follicular carcinomas.'' Indeed, we have seen two **encapsulated follicular carcinomas as defined by Evans**[256] metastasize to bones. Nevertheless, because these lesions remain controversial, at present, we call Evans' ''encapsulated follicular carcinomas''[256] atypical follicular adenomas and provide an accompanying comment describing the various criteria and controversies.

Psammoma bodies within the fibrovascular stalks of the papillae are highly suggestive of PTC; however, when they are found within the colloid of follicles, they are also consis-

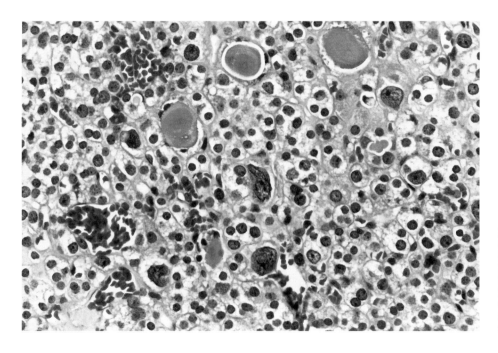

FIGURE 2–92. Shown is a follicular adenoma with focal cytologic atypia. Cytologic atypia within thyroid follicular neoplasms is not indicative of follicular carcinoma; yet, atypical features within a follicular neoplasm should trigger a hunt for angioinvasion and/or clear-cut capsular invasion. (H&E, OM ×100)

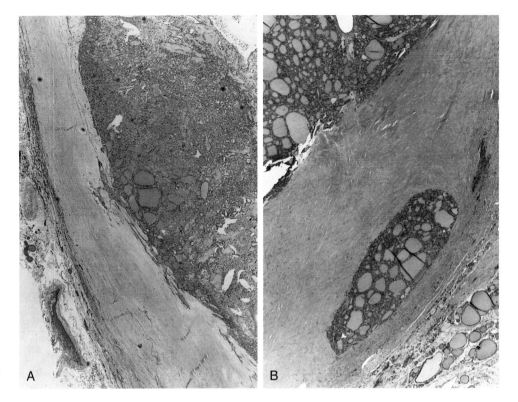

FIGURE 2-93. *A,* Follicular neoplasm of the thyroid, which is surrounded by a broadly thickened fibrous capsule. Although no clear-cut angioinvasion was detected, this lesion produced a bone metastasis. (H&E, OM ×10) *B,* Within the thick capsule, islands of isolated thyroid tissue were present. Although classification is controversial, some authors would consider this capsular invasion as evidence of follicular carcinoma. Others insist on full-thickness penetration of the capsule, such that follicular carcinoma cells penetrate into adjacent benign thyroid parenchyma. (H&E, OM ×25)

tent with benign follicular neoplasms, especially those showing Hurthle cell changes (Fig. 2–94*A*).[247] The diagnosis of PTC is based on a set of cytologic and architectural features. PTCs can have follicular, solid, and squamous areas without being considered some other tumor or a more aggressive variant. In fact, some encapsulated thyroid tumors have cyto-

logic features identical to papillary thyroid carcinoma, and some are entirely follicular. Such tumors should be considered **well-differentiated carcinomas of the papillary type (encapsulated follicular variant).**[257] In these, capsular and/or angioinvasion may or may not be present. Other follicular neoplasms may show well-developed cytologic features

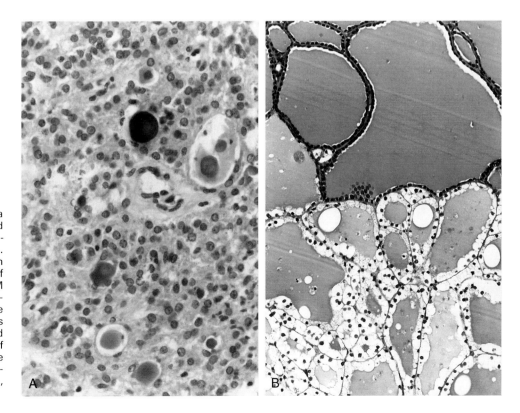

FIGURE 2-94. *A,* Psammoma bodies may form within colloid of follicular adenomas, especially Hurthle cell variants. Psammoma bodies formed in this manner are not indicative of papillary carcinoma. (H&E, OM ×50) *B,* Peculiar area of clear-cell change within an otherwise benign thyroid. This area was thyroglobulin positive and apparently representative of some form of degenerative change and of no clear-cut clinicopathologic significance. (H&E, OM ×2.5)

of papillary carcinoma only focally, and they should be considered **benign follicular adenoma with focal well-differentiated papillary carcinoma (follicular variant)** (Fig. 2–95). Follicular neoplasms with capsular and/or vascular invasion and imperfectly developed cytologic features of papillary carcinoma should be considered **well-differentiated (minimally invasive, encapsulated) carcinomas, not otherwise specified.** Follicular neoplasms without invasion and imperfectly developed features of papillary carcinoma should be considered **follicular adenoma.** Also, the **hyalinizing-trabecular variant of follicular adenoma** may show well-developed nuclear cytoplasmic inclusions and nuclear grooves (Fig. 2–96).[258]

Unfortunately, the newer techniques of immunohistochemistry, flow ploidy analysis, histomorphometrics, and molecular biology have as yet been unable to solve all the diagnostic problems outlined in the last two sections. With these special techniques, much overlap exists between the benign and malignant follicular thyroid lesions. Thus, resolution of these problems currently relies on the strict application of time-honored criteria, which are based on careful gross and light microscopic examinations of the specimens.

As a final note to this section, rarely **parathyroid carcinoma** can present in the thyroid as an invasive lesion and mimic a follicular carcinoma. Parathyroid carcinoma can be difficult to recognize, and a number of criteria have been proposed for identifying malignancy in parathyroid lesions. These criteria include increased mitotic activity, a thick capsule with capsular invasion, thick fibrous bands within the lesion, a trabecular growth pattern, spindle cells, large nuclei, and vascular invasion. However, all these features can be found in benign parathyroid lesions. Although most would agree that the diagnosis of parathyroid carcinoma is secure when the parathyroid lesion produces a metastasis and/or invades adjacent tissues (such as thyroid and/or skeletal muscle), some morphologic findings can be strongly suggestive of parathyroid carcinoma. These include high mitotic counts (i.e., >5–8/10 HPF) together with a thick fibrous capsule demonstrating capsular invasion or an invasive contour with lack of encapsulation, but occasional parathyroid carcinomas do not show these features and behave in a malignant fashion.

Variants of Medullary Thyroid Carcinoma

Medullary thyroid carcinomas (MTCs) constitute 5% to 10% of all thyroid carcinomas.[259, 260] The classic histologic pattern is present in most MTCs and includes nests and/or sheets of uniform spindle to rounded cells separated by a variably fibrovascular stroma with amyloid and containing ''neuroendocrinoid'' nuclei, which are surrounded by moderate amounts of eosinophilic to amphophilic granular cytoplasm (Fig. 2–97). With the exception of an occasional ''higher grade'' lesion, classic MTCs have few mitoses, and necrosis is uncommon. A suspected diagnosis of classic MTC is easily confirmed by showing that the tumor cells are argyrophilic, contain neurosecretory granules, and/or are immunoreactive with antibodies to chromogranin, calcitonin, and/or carcinoembryonic antigen.[261, 262] But variant patterns of MTC occur, which complicates the easy recognition of MTC. These **variant patterns include predominantly epithelial, oxyphil, squamous, insular, amyloid-rich, amyloid-poor, true papillary, pseudopapillary, glandular (tubular and/or follicular), anaplastic (giant-cell, small-cell, neuroblastoma-like), encapsulated, mucin-producing, melanin-producing, clear-cell, calcitonin-free, multihormone-producing, and MTC admixed with other thyroid carcinomas (follicular carcinoma or papillary carcinoma).**[263, 264]

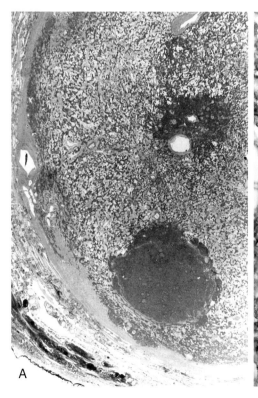
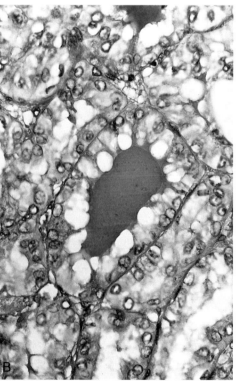

FIGURE 2–95. *A,* Shown is a follicular adenoma of the thyroid, within which are two discrete nodules of papillary carcinoma, follicular variant. (H&E, OM ×2.5) *B,* The cytoarchitectural features of the nodules of papillary carcinoma are shown at left. Note the follicular architecture, optically clear nuclei, and scalloped dark-staining colloid. (H&E, OM ×100)

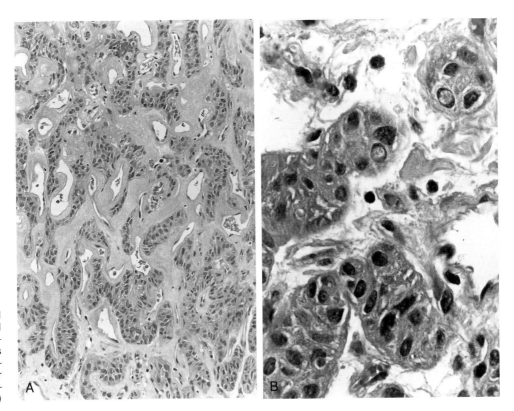

FIGURE 2–96. *A,* Hyalinized and trabecular adenoma. (H&E, OM ×10) *B,* Tumor cells of hyalinized and trabecular adenomas often show intranuclear cytoplasmic inclusions and nuclear grooves, thus simulating papillary carcinoma. (H&E, OM ×100)

The predominantly epithelial variant resembles carcinoma composed of oval to polygonal tumor cells with eosinophilic granular cytoplasm and little intervening stroma.[264] The oxyphil variant is composed of large eosinophilic cells indistinguishable at the light microscopic level from Hurthle cells,[265] and rare MTCs may exhibit focal squamous differentiation.[265]

Nuclei of the oxyphils may contain cytoplasmic inclusions like those described in classic papillary thyroid carcinomas.[266] The "insular" variant has a carcinoid-like appearance but may show central necrosis.[264] The amyloid-rich variant is composed of compact groups of small round or spindled cells, with extremely hyperchromatic nuclei and scanty clear cytoplasm

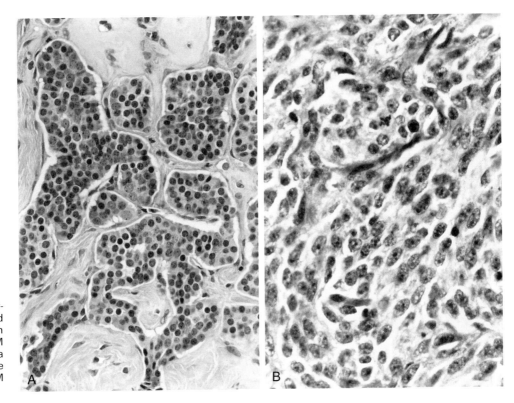

FIGURE 2–97. *A,* Medullary carcinoma showing trabecular and nested growth pattern with amyloid-rich stroma. (H&E, OM ×50) *B,* Medullary carcinoma showing polygonal to spindle cell morphology. (H&E, OM ×100)

separated by large septa of hyalinized, glassy amyloid.[264] As many as 10% to 25% of MTCs show no amyloid at the light microscopic level; the absence of such is apparently more common in the small infiltrating types of MTC.[267] Although artifactual "falling apart" of central portions of an MTC cause the pseudopapillary pattern, true papillae with fibrovascular cores of MTC can occur (Fig. 2–98).[267] Glandular variants of MTC with tubules and/or follicles occur and mimic follicular neoplasms (Fig. 2–99), but they are negative for thyroglobulin even though some follicles are filled with colloid-like material.[268] Both anaplastic giant-cell and small-cell variants of MTC have been reported.[269, 270] The small-cell variant may have abundant mitotic activity, and some have shown neuroblastoma-like features.[271] Occasional examples of MTC are encapsulated and resemble follicular thyroid tumors. Some have been called C-cell adenomas, but because metastasis can occur, they should be considered MTC.[272] Also, peculiar variants of MTC have been well documented to produce melanin pigment, sometimes enough to blacken the tumor.[273] Multihormone production in MTC is well known and sometimes causes Cushing's syndrome.[259, 274]

Mucin production within MTC has been reported in about 40% of cases,[264] but this is also a finding in about 10% of other types of thyroid carcinomas. The mucin production can be intracellular, extracellular, or both.[264] MTC can metastasize to cervical lymph nodes, and mucin production by the tumor cells does not rule out metastatic MTC. This problem is confounded by the concomitant presence of prominent follicular and mucin-producing components in some examples of MTC.[275] Also, some cases of MTC (5% to 20%) may show no or borderline immunoreactivity for calcitonin (calcitonin-free variant).[262] In these cases, ultrastructural studies coupled with anti–carcinoembryonic antigen (CEA) (positive in 88% to 100%), anti-chromogranin (nearly 100% positive), anti-

CGRP (calcitonin gene-related–peptide-positive in 80% to 95%), and/or calcitonin mRNA *in situ* hybridization should demonstrate the true differentiation of the tumor.[276] Some authors have suggested that MTC with prominent CEA immunoreactivity and reduced calcitonin immunoreactivity may follow a more aggressive course.[277] The number of MTC tumor cells in DNA synthesis phase as shown by increased mitotic activity and/or increased proliferating cell nuclear antigen staining (PCNA) may also correlate with a poorer prognosis.[278] Necrosis, tumor size, and increased cellular pleomorphism, as shown by small cells or focal giant anaplastic cells, may also indicate a poorer outcome; but stage (lymph node status) remains the best predictor of outcome.

Although still controversial,[279, 280] we believe very good evidence exists that **mixed medullary-follicular (follicular-parafollicular) carcinomas of the thyroid** occur (see Fig. 2–99).[281–284] When sensitive techniques are applied, there appears to be a continuum of mixed follicular-neuroendocrine tumors occurring within the thyroid. For example, the presence of cells demonstrating neuroendocrine markers in carcinomas staining mainly for thyroglobulin (follicular carcinomas) is frequent among the more poorly differentiated examples of mucoepidermoid and mucinous carcinomas of the thyroid. Furthermore, Holm et al.[284] found thyroglobulin immunoreactivity in 5 of 27 MTCs, suggesting that the co-expression of follicular and medullary differentiation is more frequent than generally thought. Yet, it is best to use the WHO criteria for applying this terminology (mixed medullary-follicular carcinoma) to those tumors showing both the morphologic features of medullary carcinoma together with immunoreactivity for calcitonin, and the morphologic features of follicular carcinoma together with immunoreactivity for thyroglobulin.[285] Because mixed medullary-follicular carcinomas of the thyroid concentrate radioactive iodine, whenever

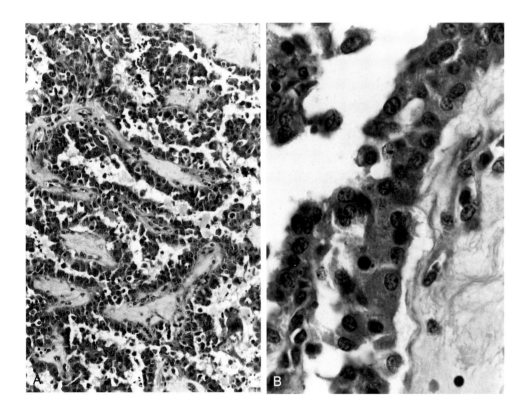

FIGURE 2–98. *A,* Medullary carcinoma, papillary variant. (H&E, OM ×10) *B,* Higher magnification shows the cytologic features, with tumor cells showing abundant eosinophilic, granular cytoplasm. (H&E, OM ×100)

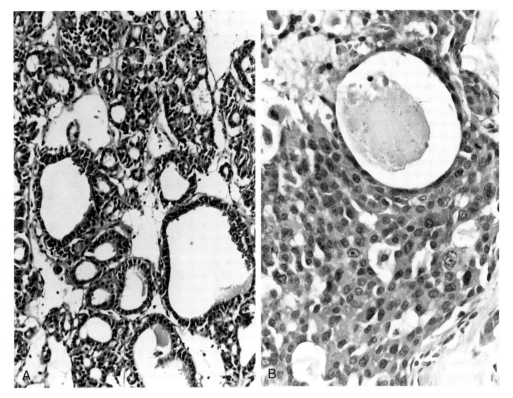

FIGURE 2–99. *A,* Some medullary carcinomas may show a prominent follicular growth pattern, but these follicular cells were thyroglobulin negative. (H&E, OM ×25) *B,* Mixed follicular-parafollicular carcinoma (mixed follicular-medullary carcinoma) is shown. Polygonal cells were calcitonin and chromogranin positive, whereas the polygonal cells lining the colloid containing follicles were positive for thyroglobulin and some were also positive for calcitonin and chromogranin. (H&E, OM ×100)

there is doubt, it is worthwhile to consider treating MTCs showing thyroglobulin immunoreactivity with this modality, especially because there are no efficient alternatives for treating MTC.[283] Finally, **mixed medullary-papillary carcinomas of the thyroid** have been described,[286] and, very rarely, separate and distinctly different primaries can occur (collision tumors), such as the concurrence of follicular carcinoma, papillary carcinoma, and medullary carcinoma.[287]

MTC can occur in sporadic and familial settings.[280, 288] The sporadic type of MTC occurs in one lobe, whereas the familial variant (10% to 25% of cases) is usually bilateral and multicentric, in which the tumor is preceded by C-cell hyperplasia. Familial MTC is associated with **multiple endocrine neoplasia** (MEN) type II syndrome, which has been divided into types IIA and IIB (or III). Pheochromocytoma and hyperparathyroidism occur in both variants, although hyperparathyroidism is only occasionally seen in MEN IIB. The MEN IIB syndrome is additionally characterized by neurogangliomatosis, mucosal neuromas, marfanoid habitus, and skeletal abnormalities. Sporadic and symptomatic familial cases of MTC frequently present with larger tumors, cervical lymph nodal metastases (40% of cases), and distant metastases (20%), whereas familial patients with C-cell disease picked up by screening (abnormal serum serotonin levels) have smaller tumors and fewer positive cervical lymph nodes (14%) and distant metastases (0%).[266] Therefore, it is important to recognize familial disease so that proper serum screening can be initiated in relatives. Unfortunately, sporadic and index familial cases are generally detected only by clinical symptoms. When MTC is detected in a thyroid, a search for C cells should be undertaken, and if they are present, the clinician alerted to the possibility of familial disease.

Unfortunately, the diagnosis of **C-cell hyperplasia** is not easy, and criteria remain disputed. When present, the C-cell hyperplasia occurs predominantly in the lateral portions of the middle third and upper third of the thyroid lobes, also the most common location of MTC (Fig. 2–100).[286] In the normal thyroid, C cells are rare, constituting less than 0.1% of the epithelial cell mass.[289] Normally, C cells are located among the follicles between the basal lamina and follicular epithelial cells, and a finding of C-cell groups in sites other than those of their normal location could represent C-cell hyperplasia, especially if the groups are microscopic clusters (>20 C cells) and nodules of enlarged cells. Nevertheless, an increase in C cells in their usual site, or the presence of follicular clusters composed of more than three calcitonin-positive cells, has been considered C-cell hyperplasia by some authors. Tomita and Millard[290] have carefully counted C cells in the human thyroid. They stated that more than 72 C cells per 271.3 mm^2 was consistent with C-cell hyperplasia, a calculation equivalent to the mean value plus twice the standard deviation. It is important not to confuse squamous metaplasia, palpation thyroiditis, and tangentially cut follicles with C-cell hyperplasia.

This all seems straightforward, but what makes the diagnosis of C-cell hyperplasia difficult is the observation that C-cell hyperplasia can occur with hypercalcemia of various causes, hyperparathyroidism (primary or secondary), hypergastrinemia, in partially thyroidectomized patients, Hashimoto's thyroiditis patients, and rarely in patients with other thyroid tumors or apparently even sporadic MTC.[275, 291, 292] Also, peculiar ''solid cell nests'' of C cells can be found in up to 14% of autopsy thyroids,[291] a finding of uncertain significance and cause but apparently not representative of a form of C-cell hyperplasia associated with increased risk of MTC. Nonetheless, if increased numbers of C cells are present in a patient with MTC (especially when there are multifocal and bilateral MTCs), and when the previously described other causes are

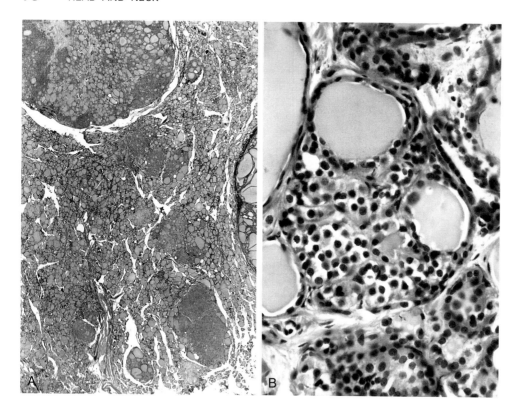

FIGURE 2–100. *A*, Patient with multiple endocrine neoplasia syndrome. Note the foci of C-cell hyperplasia and micromedullary carcinoma (*upper left*). (H&E, OM ×2.5) *B*, Microscopic focus of C-cell hyperplasia. (H&E, OM ×100)

excluded, the clinician should be alerted to the possibility of familial C-cell disease. Additional history should be taken, and screening instituted for the family members at risk. When detected early in these familial patients, MTC can be treated early and cured with total thyroidectomy. Also important is at what size does a focus of nodular C-cell hyperplasia become MTC? One series of MTCs, occurring in MEN IIA syndrome, reported the MTCs to range from 1 mm to greater than 4.0 cm in diameter, and 4 of 27 patients with MTCs smaller than 0.7 cm had lymph node metastases, although none of the MTC patients with tumors up to 1.5 cm in diameter had died of disease. Also, Aldabagh et al.[275] reported a sporadic case of MTC measuring 2 mm that presented with cervical node metastasis that also showed C-cell hyperplasia in the immediate vicinity of the primary. Carney et al.[293] have suggested that the term "*in situ* MTC" may be superior to C-cell hyperplasia, because of the propensity of early development of metastatic MTC in patients with the MEN IIB syndrome.

Anaplastic Thyroid Carcinoma

Anaplastic thyroid carcinoma constitutes about 15% of all thyroid malignancies.[294] Also known as **undifferentiated, sarcomatoid, and dedifferentiated carcinomas,** they are highly malignant, rapidly growing tumors composed of variable combinations of spindle cells and giant cells, with or without a squamoid component.[294–306] At one time, a group of "small-cell" undifferentiated carcinomas were included in the anaplastic category; however, by using electron microscopic and immunohistochemical techniques, most of these small-cell tumors have now been subclassified as either malignant lymphomas, poorly differentiated ("insular") carcinomas, or small-cell variants of medullary or follicular

carcinoma.[294–299] **Pure squamous carcinomas of the thyroid** (0.3% to 1% of all thyroid tumors) are best regarded as separate from anaplastic carcinoma, although they have a natural history like that of anaplastic carcinoma.[294–300] It is also important to separate **mucoepidermoid carcinoma of the thyroid** from anaplastic carcinoma, because the mucoepidermoid tumors resemble papillary carcinoma in their natural history.[301]

Anaplastic carcinomas are generally considered to be the result of dedifferentiation of a preexisting well-differentiated tumor.[294, 295, 302] The reported coexistence of well-differentiated and anaplastic tumors varies in the literature from 10% to 89%.[302] The better-differentiated components have most commonly been papillary or follicular carcinomas; however, Hurthle cell, poorly differentiated, or medullary carcinomas have also been reported.[201, 294, 295] Some authors have suggested a role for prior irradiation in stimulating anaplastic transformation,[303] whereas others have postulated that dedifferentiation represents the natural course of well-differentiated thyroid tumors (possibly the consequence of chronic stimulation by thyroid-stimulating hormone).[295, 304] We emphasize that well-differentiated thyroid tumors dedifferentiate very infrequently, and the fear of this occurrence should not influence the therapy.[294] The incidence of anaplastic thyroid carcinoma appears to be dropping, apparently because of increased thyroid surgery to remove these low-grade precursor lesions.[305]

Anaplastic carcinomas are one of the most aggressive tumors of the human body. Most are fatal within 6 months to 1 year from the time of diagnosis.[294, 295, 302] The cause of death is usually extensive local recurrence with invasion of vital regional structures. A few long-term survivors have been reported; however, these patients tend to have focal (intrathyroid) disease or tumors showing "small-cell" histology. After re-evaluation, most cases of so-called small-cell anaplastic carcinomas have been found to be lymphoma or medullary carcinoma.[294, 302]

CLINICOPATHOLOGIC FEATURES. Patients with anaplastic thyroid carcinoma are usually elderly women. In one series of 82 cases,[302] the mean age of patients at presentation was 65 years. Although the ages of the patients in this series ranged from 18 to 87 years, only seven patients (8.5%) were younger than 50 years. In most series, male:female ratios were reported to be from 1:1.4 to 1:4.3.[295, 302] Anaplastic carcinoma usually presents as a rapidly growing thyroid mass (approximately 80%), but slow-growing examples also occur.[302] Evidence of recent growth is frequently superimposed on a preexisting goiter.[302] These tumors are usually hard and fixed, and patients describe various combinations of dyspnea, hoarseness, dysphagia, cough, cervical pain, and weight loss.[302] Although there is a single case report of anaplastic thyroid carcinoma (''small-cell type'') causing hyperthyroidism, the vast majority of patients are usually euthyroid.[307]

Gross specimens have usually shown gray-white tumor tissue extensively infiltrating thyroid and extrathyroid structures.[295] Tumors often contain foci of necrosis and hemorrhage, and occasional examples are cystic.[295] Microscopically, anaplastic carcinomas display various patterns that usually mimic sarcomas, especially malignant fibrous histiocytoma (all subtypes), malignant hemangiopericytoma, angiosarcoma, and fibrosarcoma.[294] In addition, osseous and cartilagenous metaplasia occasionally occur, producing areas simulating osteosarcoma or chondrosarcoma.[294] Some examples contain numerous osteoclast-like giant cells (Fig. 2–101).

Generally, three major growth patterns occur in various combinations of spindle-cell, giant-cell, and squamoid patterns.[294-296] Undifferentiated spindle-cell and giant-cell patterns predominate, whereas squamoid areas are found in a minority of cases and always in association with undifferentiated areas.[294, 295] Pleomorphic cells, high mitotic rates (with many atypical forms), necrotic foci, and marked tissue invasiveness are common to all anaplastic carcinomas, although

it must be emphasized that occasional anaplastic thyroid carcinomas occur that are deceptively benign appearing and mimic **Riedel's struma** (Fig. 2–102). Close attention to complete tumor sampling, more subtle and focal cytologic atypia, and increased mitotic activity should lead to the correct diagnosis of carcinoma. Tumor cells of anaplastic thyroid carcinomas invade not only vascular spaces but also large-vessel walls (so-called angiotropism).[294, 295]

Although occasional tumors are encountered that ultrastructurally are indistinguishable from sarcoma, epithelial features are usually suggested following electron microscopic study.[294, 295] These include cell-to-cell junctions, microvilli, tonofibrils, and gland-like lumina. Immunohistochemical studies of anaplastic carcinoma have shown that from 50% to 100% have immunoreactivity for a low-molecular-weight keratin,[294-296] a reaction that can be observed in formalin-fixed, paraffin-embedded material. CEA immunoreactivity can be found in tumors with squamoid differentiation, but assays for thyroglobulin immunoreactivity have been negative in most tumors.[294-296] Anaplastic variants of medullary carcinoma have been reported that have argyrophilia and immunoreactivity for calcitonin.[296, 308, 309] Although reported by some authors to account for 64% of anaplastic carcinomas, medullary tumors more likely represent only a small fraction of the anaplastic group.[296, 309] We emphasize that entrapped non-neoplastic thyroid follicles, non-specific absorption of thyroglobulin by tumor cells, and non-specificity of reagents (e.g., to calcitonin) may lead to spurious interpretations of immunohistochemical preparations.[294, 295]

DIFFERENTIAL DIAGNOSIS. Anaplastic thyroid carcinomas can be difficult, if not impossible, to differentiate from sarcomas, especially **fibrosarcoma, malignant fibrous histiocytoma, malignant hemangiopericytoma, osteogenic sarcoma, and angiosarcoma.**[294] Rosai et al. believe that the vast majority of thyroid tumors having a sarcoma-like appearance are of epithelial derivation. This is a near certainty for those tumors that are associated with a well-differentiated component, have clear-cut epithelial (squamoid) foci, have ultra-

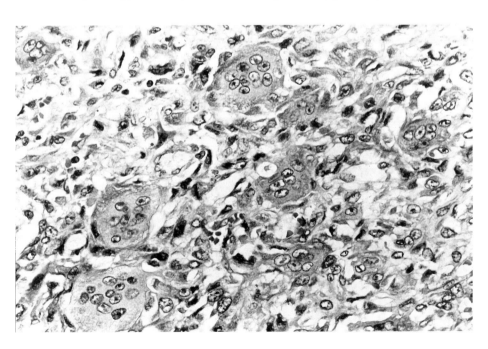

FIGURE 2–101. Anaplastic thyroid carcinoma with admixed osteoclast-like giant cells. (H&E, OM ×100)

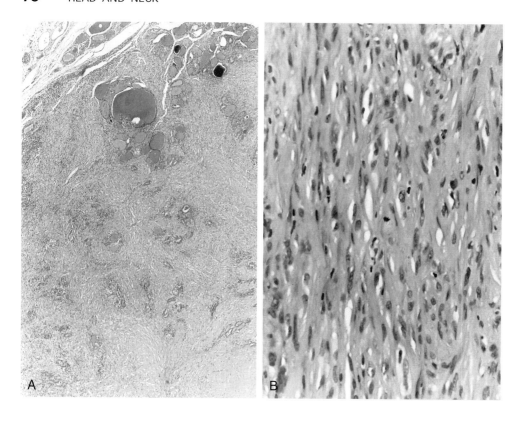

FIGURE 2–102. *A,* Anaplastic thyroid carcinoma simulating Riedel's struma. (H&E, OM ×2.5) *B,* The spindled cells were quite bland, but close inspection of multiple sections revealed increased cytologic atypia and mitotic activity. (H&E, OM ×100)

structural markers of epithelial differentiation, and/or are immunoreactive for cytokeratin and/or epithelial membrane antigen.[294, 295] This does not eliminate the possibility that true sarcomas occur as primary thyroid tumors, and (although controversial) malignant hemangioendotheliomas of the thyroid have been reported, especially in Europe.[310] The "carcinoma versus sarcoma" issue is further complicated by the observation of vimentin immunoreactivity (a presumed mesenchymal marker) in some otherwise typical anaplastic thyroid carcinomas.[294, 311]

How should those highly malignant thyroid tumors that lack epithelial features be classified? If one presumes that these anaplastic tumors are all of epithelial derivation, they should be called anaplastic carcinoma. However, if one favors a classification of tumors based strictly on cellular differentiation, certainly some of these anaplastic tumors would be classified as sarcomas. In either event, all anaplastic tumors within this group manifest highly malignant behavior and, for the time being, require a uniform therapeutic approach.

As found in the illustrated case, osteoclast-like, multinucleated giant cells are dispersed among the anaplastic tumor cells in approximately 10% of cases (see Fig. 2–101).[294] Although Silverberg and DeGiorgi reported a peculiar case with 6-year survival, most authors believe that the **osteoclastoma-like thyroid tumors** are variants of anaplastic carcinoma.[294, 295, 312, 313] As in typical anaplastic carcinoma, death usually occurs within 1 year of diagnosis; peak incidence is in late adulthood; there is a predilection for women; there is frequently a preexisting goiter; special studies frequently reveal epithelial features in stromal cells; and as in the current case, co-existing well-differentiated thyroid tumors are well documented.[313]

Similar appearing but not necessarily identical osteoclastoma-like tumors have been reported in a variety of organ systems, including liver,[314] salivary glands,[315, 316] pancreas,[317] breast,[318] lung,[319] renal pelvis,[320] skin,[321] orbit,[322] heart,[323] colon,[324] kidney,[325] bladder,[326] ovary,[327] and soft tissues.[328] Tumors within this group have displayed different biologic behaviors and have been variably interpreted to be of either epithelial, mesenchymal, or indeterminate origin.[315] As a result, prognostication and therapy need to be individualized for extraskeletal osteoclastoma-like tumors—with due consideration given to the organ system involved.

The origin of the osteoclast-like giant cells remains an enigma. They are not malignant cells, and current data suggest that they are analogous to normal bone osteoclasts and likely derived from bone marrow (i.e., probably monocytes).[294, 295] It has been suggested that they are attracted to the tumor, perhaps in response to a secretion that is either neoplastic or inflammatory in origin.[294, 295, 327] Of interest in the current case is the fact that similar-appearing multinucleated giant cells were found within adjacent benign thyroid follicles. These appeared to be foreign body–type multinucleated giant cells, apparently reacting to thyroid colloid.

Finally, and as previously mentioned, anaplastic thyroid carcinoma must be differentiated from **Riedel's struma.** Clearly, occasional cases of anaplastic carcinoma mimic this inflammatory fibrosclerotic process (see Fig. 2–102). The clinicopathologic features of Riedel's struma are outlined in the section following on tumefactive fibroinflammatory lesions of the head and neck. Also to be considered in the differential diagnosis of anaplastic thyroid carcinoma are **ectopic thymoma, spindle-cell epithelial tumor with thymus-like elements (SETTLE), solitary fibrous tumor, and carcinoma showing thymus-like elements (CASTLE),** although these lesions are extremely rare.[329] **Keratin-positive, epithelioid angiosarcomas** can occur in the thyroid and in deep soft-tissue sites, indicating that keratin positivity does not rule out sarcoma (Fig. 2–103);[330] and, not all epithelioid angiosarcomas (a.k.a. **malignant hemangioendothelioma of the thyroid**) are keratin positive.[331] The distinction of carcinoma from angiosarcoma is compounded by the fact that **carcinomas can show considerable ''pseudoangiosarcomatous'' changes.**[332]

UNCOMMON PRESENTATIONS OF COMMON LESIONS IN THE HEAD AND NECK

Benign Lesions

Tumefactive Fibroinflammatory Lesions and Inflammatory Pseudotumors

The term **tumefactive fibroinflammatory lesion (TFL)** is used to describe mixed inflammatory and fibrotic masses of the head and neck that clinically appear malignant but are actually benign yet locally destructive and invasive lesions.[333, 334] TFLs are closely related to and can occur concomitantly with other fibrosclerotic disorders of soft tissue, which can also clinically simulate malignancy but are histologically benign. These lesions include **retroperitoneal fibrosis, sclerosing cholangitis, mediastinal fibrosis, Riedel's thyroiditis, and pseudotumor of the orbit.** Any possible combination of these fibrosclerotic disorders can occur, and, when present, the combination is referred to as **multifocal fibrosclerosis.**[335] Steroid therapy is suggested as the first line of management; surgery and/or radiation

is reserved for persistent disease. The cause of TFL is unknown, but it appears most likely to be a form of hypersensitivity and/or autoimmune reaction.

Closely related to, but somewhat distinctive from, TFL is **inflammatory (myofibroblastic) pseudotumor (IPT),** which represents a homogeneous group of inflammatory myofibroblastic and histiocytic proliferations occurring throughout the body, including lung, liver, spleen, skin, lymph nodes, salivary glands, pancreas, and deep soft tissues.[336] Synonyms for IPT include **plasma cell granuloma, plasma cell/histiocytoma complex, histiocytoma, xanthomatous pseudotumor, postinflammatory pseudotumor, fibrous xanthoma, inflammatory myofibroblastic tumor, and inflammatory myofibrohistiocytic proliferation.**[336] IPT differs from TFL in both clinical presentation and histopathologic features. Both lesions are presented here because they can be confused both clinically and pathologically with other benign and malignant processes. IPT rarely recurs after surgical therapy. The cause of IPT remains unknown.

CLINICOPATHOLOGIC FEATURES. TFLs present as masses of the head and neck in adult men and women (mean, 47 years; range, 33–71), but cases of TFL in children (10 years) have been reported.[337] TFLs usually involve the neck or parotid gland, but the antrum, nasal cavity, tongue, nasopharynx, and buccal space may be involved. In about one third of patients, mutiple fibrosclerotic lesions may occur at any of these head and neck sites in a synchronous or dysynchronous pattern and with sclerosing cholangitis, mediastinal fibrosis, retroperitoneal fibrosis, or pseudotumors of the orbit.[334] Grossly, TFLs are firm and gray-tan, and although circumscribed, they are not encapsulated and can invade into surrounding structures, including veins and arteries.[334] The histologic appearance of TFL is identical to that of the other inflammatory fibrosclerotic lesions in this group, such as mediastinal and retroperitoneal

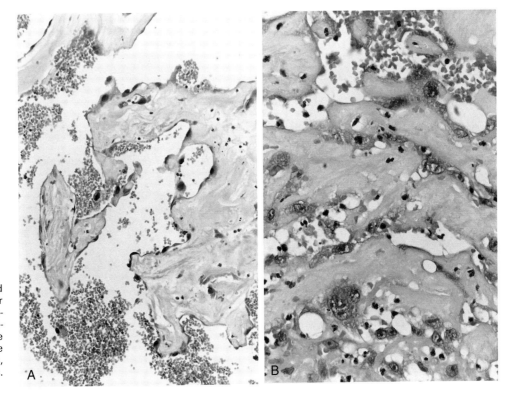

FIGURE 2–103. *A,* Epithelioid angiosarcoma of thyroid. Tumor cells were positive for both keratin and Factor VIII–related antigen. (H&E, OM ×10) *B,* Note marked cytologic atypia of the epithelioid angiosarcoma cells, which line vascular spaces. (H&E, OM ×100)

fibrosis. TFLs are composed of prominent fibrotic tissue (sometimes hyalinized) with prominent numbers of admixed lymphocytes, plasma cells, and scattered polys (including eosinophils) (Fig. 2–104A). Germinal centers and fat necrosis can be present.

Like TFLs, IPTs of the head and neck tend to occur in adult men and women (mean, 70 years; range, 46–87), frequently as a mass or swelling in the parotid gland.[336] They are lobulated, yellow-gray firm nodules that are circumscribed but not encapsulated. Histologically, IPTs are composed of haphazardly arranged sweeping fascicles of ovoid to spindle cells, sometimes forming a vague storiform pattern (Fig. 2–105). Lesion cells may be positive for CD68, muscle-specific actin (HHF-35), and even cytokeratin. Some tumors contain foci of xanthoma cells and Touton-like giant cells. A uniformly distributed, but variably dense, lymphoplasmacytic infiltrate containing many plasma cells is present throughout IPTs (Fig. 2–105B). Germinal centers and/or a lymphoid cuff may be present. Overall, IPTs tend to be more cellular and "active" appearing than TFLs, which are more densely collagenized.

DIFFERENTIAL DIAGNOSIS. TFLs and IPTs are different from the other fibroproliferative lesions found in the head-and-neck region. These other entities include fibromatosis (see Fig. 2–104B), which lacks the inflammatory components of TFL and IPT; various soft-tissue sarcomas; and sarcomatoid carcinoma. The latter two show malignant cytology. Nodular fasciitis, which is very similar to IPTs and a form of inflammatory (myofibroblastic) tumor, often shows a more edematous "tissue culture-like" appearance to the lesional cells. In immunosuppressed patients, atypical mycobacteria may produce spindle-cell lesions very similar to IPT.[338]

Malignant Lesions

Intestinal-Type Adenocarcinoma of the Nasopharynx

In addition to the better known minor salivary gland tumors that can occur in the nasal cavity, occasionally a patient will present with an **adenocarcinoma that closely mimics a colon carcinoma.**[339] At least 80% of these patients eventually die of the tumor as a result of uncontrolled local growth, but systemic metastases can occur. These tumors have been called **sinonasal enteric-type adenocarcinomas (ETACs).** Some of these patients have a history of long exposure to dusts, especially hardwood dust encountered by sanders in furniture manufacturing or workers in the shoe industry exposed to leather dust.[340–344]

CLINICOPATHOLOGIC FEATURES. ETAC occurs predominantly in middle-aged men, who present with nasal obstruction and/or epistaxis. They often provide the pertinent occupational exposure listed previously. ETACs closely resemble the variably differentiated adenocarcinomas that arise within the gastrointestinal tract, especially the colon. Usually they are composed of papillae covered by enteric-type columnar cells and goblet cells, but argentaffin-positive neuroendocrine and/or Paneth cells may be present (Fig. 2–106). "Dirty" necrosis may be present, as it often is with colonic adenocarcinomas.

DIFFERENTIAL DIAGNOSIS. ETAC must be differentiated from **low-grade, nasopharyngeal papillary adenocarcinoma (LGNPPA),**[345] **papillary-cystic acinic-cell carcinoma,**[117] and **metastatic adenocarcinomas** to the sinonasal region. **Papillary-cystic acinic-cell carcinoma** and LGNPPA

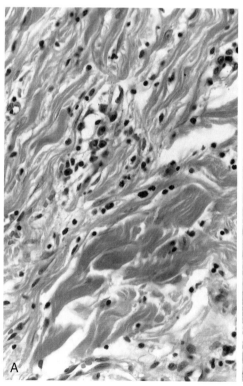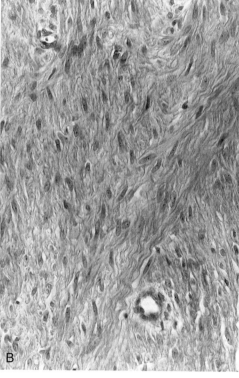

FIGURE 2–104. *A,* Tumefactive fibroinflammatory lesion. Note dense focally hyalinized collagen admixed with chronic inflammatory cells. (H&E, OM ×100) *B,* Aggressive fibromatosis. Note mature, scar-like fibrous tissue with bland fibroblasts, mature collagen, and scarcity of inflammatory cells. (H&E, OM ×100)

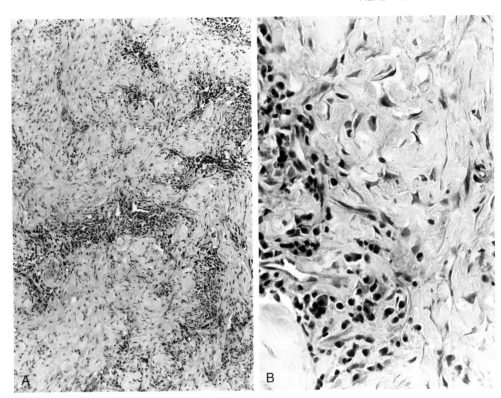

FIGURE 2–105. *A,* Inflammatory pseudotumor or inflammatory myofibroblastic proliferation. Note the admixture of fibrous tissue and chronic inflammatory cells, especially around blood vessels. (H&E, OM ×2.5) *B,* Plasma cells and reactive-appearing myofibroblasts predominate. (H&E, OM ×100)

show modestly atypical cells growing in papillary and glandular patterns with uncommon mitoses. The cells do not have the colon carcinoma–like character of ETAC. Most importantly, a metastatic bowel carcinoma should be ruled out by obtaining pertinent history.

UNCOMMON LESIONS WORTH KNOWING ABOUT, BUT NOT OTHERWISE COVERED

Benign Lesions

Necrotizing Sialometaplasia

Necrotizing sialometaplasia (NSM) is a non-neoplastic, nodular or ulcerated, self-healing lesion of salivary glands, which can be confused clinically and histologically with **squamous or mucoepidermoid carcinoma.**[346] In fact, President Grover Cleveland's maxillectomy for a palatal ''malignancy'' (called epithelioma or sarcoma) may be the most famous case of misdiagnosis of NSM, especially because he survived 15 years without radiation and/or chemotherapy.[346] Light microscopic diagnosis eliminates the need for further therapy, because all reported patients have healed completely within 1 to 3 months.[347] Most authors favor an ischemic cause, and there is no known association with a systemic disease. Walker et al.[348] documented a case in the larynx secondary to atheromatous embolization after manipulation of an atherosclerotic aneurysm.

CLINICOPATHOLOGIC FEATURES. NSM presents in adults (mean age, 48 years; range, 17–80) as an asymptomatic nodule or deep ulcer usually on the hard palate, but NSM has been reported on the mucobuccal fold, retromolar trigone, tongue, incisive canal, lip, maxillary sinus, nose, nasopharynx, larynx, and major salivary glands.[346] Some patients have a history of prolonged smoking and/or ethanol abuse, and extrapalatal lesions most often arise after surgery, trauma, and/or radiation. Because the palatal lesions arise spontaneously, the cause of palatal and extrapalatal lesions may be different. The microscopic features include mucosal ulceration with **pseudoepitheliomatous hyperplasia (PEH),** lobular necrosis of the salivary glands, dissolution of acinar walls, release of mucus, mucus escape reaction with neutrophils and foamy histiocytes, granulation-tissue response, and prominent squamous metaplasia of salivary acini and ducts (Fig. 2–107). These findings variably involve multiple lobules, and importantly the normal lobular architecture of the salivary gland is preserved. The metaplastic nests have bland cytologic features.[349]

DIFFERENTIAL DIAGNOSIS. The differential diagnosis primarily includes **squamous cell carcinoma** and **mucoepidermoid carcinoma.** The PEH, squamous metaplasia of ducts and acini, and necrosis associated with prominent stromal repair reaction mimic both *in situ* and invasive, well-differentiated squamous carcinoma. Also, residual mucus cells in ducts adjacent to squamous metaplasia simulate mucoepidermoid carcinoma. To avoid a mistake, look closely for preservation of lobular architecture of underlying salivary gland, infarct pattern of necrosis adjacent to viable salivary gland, absence of cystic spaces, intense mixed inflammation, and the bland appearance of the squamous metaplastic cells. The invasive carcinomas are much more haphazard.

Benign Lymphoepithelial Cysts

Bernier and Bhaskar[350] defined **benign lymphoepithelial cysts (BLCs)** as solitary or multiple cysts within lymph nodes

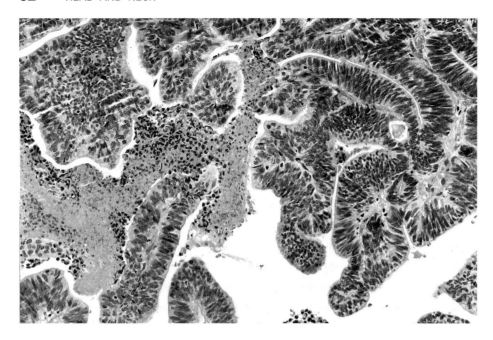

FIGURE 2–106. Intestinal-type adeno-carcinoma of the sinonasal region. Note the close resemblance to primary adenocarcinomas of the gastrointestinal tract. (H&E, OM ×50)

associated with salivary glands. These authors believed that BLCs result from the cystic degeneration of salivary gland inclusions within lymph nodes.[350, 351] Other authors favor remnants of the branchial arch as the origin of BLCs, and, many cases have been reported as ''branchial cyst.''[352–358]

Although uncommon, they have been reported in the periodic literature[350, 352–361] and are mentioned in a variety of textbooks.[362–366] Yet, their histopathologic characteristics are often incompletely described; hence, pathologists are not always familiar with them. So far as we know, ultrastructural features of BLCs and the cytologic findings in specimens obtained by fine-needle aspiration have not been reported. We have reviewed the features of five intraparotid BLCs studied by light microscopy. Also, in three of these cases, we were able to carry out cytologic studies, and in one case, electron microscopic studies. The results have

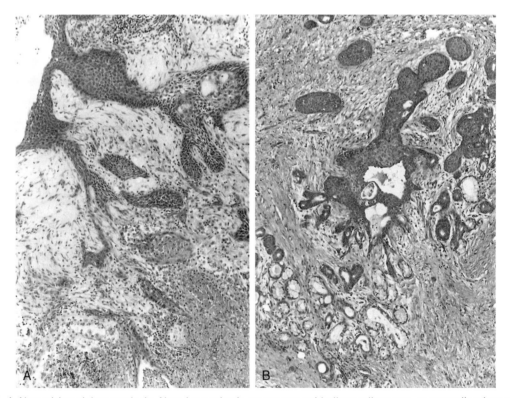

FIGURE 2–107. *A,* Necrotizing sialometaplasia. Note hyperplastic squamous epithelium adjacent to or extending into area of necrotic minor salivary glands. (H&E, OM ×25) *B,* Note squamous metaplasia conforming to distribution of minor salivary gland ducts. (H&E, OM ×25)

been previously discussed, but they are reviewed again here.[366]

Clinicopathologic Features

The patients ranged in age from 29 to 78 years (average, 58 years) and had consulted their physicians because of parotid nodules that had been present for from 1 to 6 months (average, 3 months). Three of the patients were women. The nodules were estimated to range from 1 to 2 cm in diameter. Four caused no pain; one was slightly tender. In none of these cases was there clinical evidence of facial nerve involvement. Fine-needle aspiration in three cases yielded specimens that suggested several entities, including **mucocele, Warthin's tumor,** and **mucoepidermoid carcinoma.** All five patients were treated with superficial parotidectomy, and there have been no recurrences 2, 3, 6, 8, and 96 months later. None of the patients manifested features of Sjogren's syndrome or other autoimmune disease.

All of the lesions were cystic, well circumscribed, and confined to the parotid gland (Fig. 2–108). The cyst contents were white and mucoid in three cases, and caseous and yellow in two. In all cases the cyst walls were firm and white to tan. All five lesions contained epithelium-lined, multiloculated cystic spaces encased by dense lymphoid tissue composed of small lymphocytes, plasma cells, and germinal centers. A variably thick band of collagen surrounded much of the lymphoid stroma; the remaining periphery was composed of sharply defined, dense lymphoid tissue minimally intermixed with adjacent parotid-gland tissue. No subcapsular or medullary lymphatic sinusoids were apparent. All the lesions had areas of subepithelial fibrosis. The epithelial nuclei were homogeneous and contained pale, evenly distributed chromatin and inconspicuous nucleoli. Mitotic figures were rare; those that were present had a normal configuration.

In three cases, the epithelium appeared "mucoepidermoid," composed of variable mixtures of cuboidal cells and mucin-producing columnar cells. In these cases, the epithelium was either stratified or composed of a single layer of cuboidal cells. Histologic examination by light microscopy showed no keratin or intercellular bridges. In a few areas, invagination of the epithelium into adjacent lymphoid or fibrous stroma formed small epithelial nests that were both solid and microcystic. In other areas, the epithelium was papillary. In two lesions, the epithelial component was entirely squamous and contained well-defined intracellular bridges. In one of these cases, a granulomatous (foreign-body) response to keratinous debris was focally prominent.

DIFFERENTIAL DIAGNOSIS. Within the category of BLCs, various types of epithelium have been reported. The most frequent has been squamous,[350, 353–362] but variable combinations of cuboidal,[350, 360–362] columnar,[353, 359, 361, 362] ciliated columnar,[353, 354] and mucin-producing[359] epithelia also have been reported. In addition, rare examples of squamous epithelium containing sebaceous differentiation have been documented.[352]

Thus far, BLCs have not been known to recur or metastasize. Thus, they should be differentiated from more aggressive lesions, especially cystic low-grade mucoepidermoid carcinoma. This problem in differential diagnosis is underscored by the recent report of a **low-grade mucoepidermoid carcinoma arising within an intraparotid lymph node.**[367]

Three of our cases contained mucoepidermoid epithelium resembling that found in cystic **low-grade mucoepidermoid carcinomas.** The distinction between these two lesions is admittedly difficult in some cases; indeed, it may be that the mucoepidermoid subtype of BLC should be classified at the benign end of the spectrum of cystic low-grade mucoepidermoid carcinoma. However, given the well-documented, benign behavior of the mucoepidermoid subtype of BLC, it hardly seems justified to consider these cysts as carcinomas.

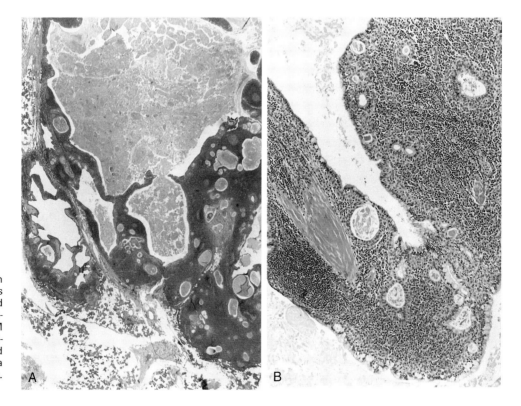

FIGURE 2–108. *A,* A benign lymphoepithelial cyst (BLC) is shown centrally and surrounded by lymphoid cell stroma containing smaller cysts. (H&E, OM ×2.5) *B,* Note the columnar epithelial cells, focal hyalinized stroma, and lymphoid stroma containing small lymphoid cells. (H&E, OM ×50)

Features favoring the diagnosis of cystic low-grade mucoepidermoid carcinoma are a high proportion of mucin-producing cells relative to squamous-like intermediate cells, the presence of macrocysts combined with a major component of microcysts and solid-cell nests, and the absence of intimately associated lymphoid stroma containing germinal centers,[367-370] although mucoepidermoid carcinomas with prominent lymphoid stroma occasionally occur.

The presence of malignant cytologic features, of course, strongly supports a diagnosis of cancer. It should be recognized, however, that aspiration cytology of low-grade mucoepidermoid carcinoma may at times yield only mucoid material and benign-appearing, mucin-producing cells.[371] In such cases, a false-negative diagnosis may be unavoidable. Conversely, reactive epithelial atypia in the cells lining a BLC could conceivably result in a false-positive diagnosis. Where small lymphocytes are a prominant feature, BLC is a more likely diagnosis than is low-grade mucoepidermoid carcinoma.

BLCs have not been associated with **Sjogren's syndrome and/or benign lymphoepithelial lesion (so-called Milkulicz's disease).**[350, 362] However, it may be difficult to differentiate between BLCs and cystic examples of **benign lymphoepithelial lesions (BLLs)** (Fig. 2–109). BLLS are lined by epithelium identical to that found in epimyoepithelial islands. BLL epithelium resembles squamous epithelium, lacks epithelial mucin, is often permeated by lymphocytes, and contains abundant pericellular hyaline material, suggesting basement membrane. Usually lacking the features of lymph nodes, the associated lymphoid cells tend to infiltrate adjacent salivary gland tissues in an irregular fashion. Involved salivary gland tissues frequently display areas of acinar atrophy and periacinar fibrosis and contain satellite lesions composed of epimyoepithelial islands and lymphoid cells. **Cystic lymphoid hyperplasia in AIDS** is characterized by grossly visible cystic spaces lined by squamous epithelium surrounded by lymphoid tissue showing follicular or diffuse lymphoid hyperplasia, reactive vascularity, and neoplastic epimyoepithelial islands.[125] The lesions resemble markedly cystic examples of BLL with associated follicular hyperplasia.

Dermoid and keratinous cysts resemble squamous examples of BLCs, except that they are not surrounded by a mass of dense lymphoid tissue containing germinal centers. Although BLCs are similar to Warthin's tumor, they do not have the oncocytic and double-layered columnar epithelium characteristic of the latter.[372] Fine-needle aspirates from Warthin's tumors, however, may yield only inflammatory cells and mucoid material that may also contain metaplastic squamous cells and mucin-producing cells.[373] In the absence of the characteristic oncocytes, such specimens could not be distinguished cytologically from BLCs. Foreign-body granulomatous inflammation (in response to keratin debris) may be found in all these benign cystic tumors. Other cystic disorders occurring in the salivary glands include **mucoceles** (extravasation and retention types), **salivary duct cysts, ranula,** and **cystic parotid disease** (dysgenetic polycystic disease).[125]

Middle-Ear Adenomatous Tumors

The majority of surgical specimens removed from the middle ear result from inflammatory diseases, with diverse histologic features, including acute and chronic inflammation, granulation tissue, necrosis, fibrosis, cholesterol granuloma, and xanthogranulomatous inflammations. Yet, neoplasms occur and must be considered in the differential diagnosis of middle-ear lesion. **Adenomatous tumors of the middle ear** are unusual and morphologically heterogeneous tumors, which may recur locally and invade bone. Rarely, if ever, do

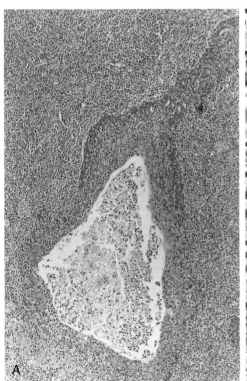 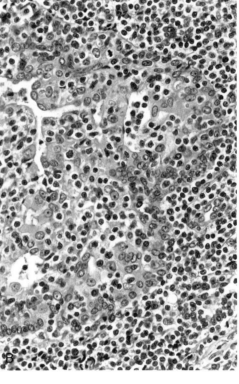

FIGURE 2–109. *A*, Cystic benign lymphoepithelial lesion (BLL) or epimyoepithelial island. (H&E, OM ×10) *B*, Small lymphocytes infiltrate the epimyoepithelial cells as single cells or in small 2- to 3-cell clusters in benign epimyoepithelial sialadenitis. (H&E, OM ×100)

they metastasize to distant sites. Difficulties in classification exist as evidenced by the varied names given to them (**middle-ear adenoma, adenomatous tumor, adenomatous neoplasm, monomorphic adenoma, carcinoma, mixed carcinoid, low-grade adenocarcinoma, aggressive papillary middle-ear tumor, ceruminoma, and amphicrine tumor**).[374–380] Clinically, these tumors are often mistakenly considered **glomus tumors (paragangliomas), acoustic neuromas, ceruminomas, cholesteatomas, vascular tumor, or metastasis.**

CLINICOPATHOLOGIC FEATURES. Most middle-ear adenomatous tumors present as middle-ear masses (usually 0.5–2 cm) in adults (mean age, 38 years; range, 16–69) with the expected regional symptomatology (hearing loss, tinnitus, vertigo, discharge pain, headaches, perforated tympanic membrane, and/or chronic otitis) and destruction of middle-ear structures such as the ossicles and regional bone. Mills and Fechner[377] have suggested there are two distinct types of **middle-ear adenomatous tumors:** those that have a predominantly **solid** growth pattern and those that are clearly **papillary.** The solid variant (middle-ear adenomas) is composed of broad sheets of tightly packed, cytologically uniform round, ovoid, or carcinoid-like cells, but areas of trabeculae, ribbons, duct-like structures, and/or cribriform areas are also commonly present. Both mucin production and neuroendocrine differentiation are well documented, leading some authors to suggest amphicrine differentiation (combined endocrine and exocrine differentiation in the same cells) for these tumors.[377] These tumors are frequently positive for keratin, chromogranin, and/or vimentin. Indeed, three cell types can be demonstrated. Type A cells are slender, darkly staining cells that line the glandular lumina, show exocrine differentiation, and stain strongly for keratin. Type B cells have abundant, pale cytoplasm, contain neurosecretory granules, and stain for chromogranin, keratin, vimen-

tin, and multiple neuroendocrine polypeptides. The third cell is an amphicrine cell with features of both A and B cells. Invasion is limited, and the recurrence rate is less than 5%; all recurrences have been resectable by subsequent surgeries.[377]

In contrast, the papillary variant is a more locally aggressive tumor.[375, 378] In fact, Heffner[375] has suggested that these **papillary tumors are more likely of endolymphatic sac origin,** secondarily involving the middle ear (Fig. 2–110). Although the papillary variants are likewise slow growing and do not metastasize, they are usually associated with extensive local invasion, destruction of the temporal bone, and/or extension into the posterior fossa. As a consequence, Heffner considers these **aggressive papillary tumors a form of low-grade adenocarcinoma.** They occur in patients of wide age range (mean age, 41; range, 15–71 years) without gender preference. They are papillary-cystic glandular tumors composed of low columnar cells, often with clear cytoplasm, bland cytologic features, and rare mitotic figures (see Fig. 2–110). Some crowded glands are filled with colloid-like material causing a resemblance to thyroid, and many of these tumors can have areas of hypocellular fibrosis, hemorrhage, cholesterol clefts, and other reactive-reparative changes. Tumor cells are positive for keratin, and some cells may stain for S-100, GFAP, Leu-7, and synaptophysin. Electron micrographic studies have shown epithelial features with glycogen and some secretion granules. Recurrences are frequent and death can rarely occur, especially if these locally aggressive papillary tumors are not totally resected.

DIFFERENTIAL DIAGNOSIS. The differential diagnosis of middle-ear adenomatous tumors includes **paraganglioma (glomus tumor), ceruminomatous tumors, plasmacytoma, cholesteatoma, adenoid cystic carcinoma, choroid plexus tumors, meningioma, acoustic neuroma, salivary gland choristoma,**[381] and **metastatic carcinoma (especially thy-**

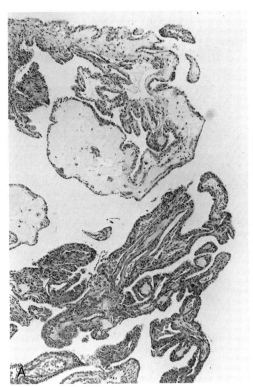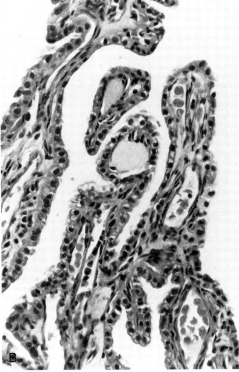

FIGURE 2–110. *A,* Papillary middle-ear adenomatous tumor of probable endolymphatic sac origin. (H&E, OM ×25) *B,* Note the papillary architecture and bland cytologic features. (H&E, OM ×100)

roid or renal). Paragangliomas tend to be more vascular tumors whose cells (often with more abundant granular cytoplasm) grow in organoid nests surrounded by numerous vessels. Although both middle-ear adenomatous tumors and paragangliomas stain for chromogranin, paragangliomas are negative for keratin and calcitonin. Plasmacytomas can present as polygonal cell tumors; and, although the nuclei with the characteristic peripherally clumped chromatin are usually eccentric and adjacent to a pale Golgi complex, nuclei of neoplastic plasma cells may be more centrally disposed and contain less clumped chromatin and more prominent nucleoli. Also, plasma cells may be positive for keratin and epithelial membrane antigen and negative for leukocyte common antigen. Kappa and lambda stains could be a tremendous help, if the plasmacytoma is secreting these paraproteins. Recently, *in situ* hybridization with kappa and lambda mRNA probes has become commercially available and practical. If all else fails, electron microscopy should clearly demonstrate the characteristic features of plasma cells versus the neuroendocrine and/or epithelial features of middle-ear adenomatous tumors. When numerous plasma cells are admixed with large, polygonal histiocytes with vesicular nuclei and prominent nucleoli, consider **Rosai-Dorfman disease (sinus histiocytosis with massive lymphadenopathy [SHML]).**[382] The histiocytes should be strongly positive for S-100 protein, as well as other macrophage markers. Emperipolesis is not as well developed in extranodal sites as in nodal SHML. Ceruminomatous tumors (benign or malignant) and adenoid cystic carcinoma are geographically centered in the external auditory canal rather than the middle ear, whereas meningiomas and choroid plexus tumors are geographically centered within the dura and CNS, although there may be overlap in the extension of both. Thoughtful search for the characteristic features of each should lead to the correct diagnosis. Acoustic neuromas are spindle-cell tumors with characteristic strong S-100 positivity, keratin negativity, and Schwann-cell ultrastructural features. Salivary gland choristomas resemble normal salivary gland tissue, and metastatic renal and thyroid carcinoma can be ruled out by careful history, appropriate examinations of the thyroid and kidneys, and thyroglobulin immunostain. Cholesteatoma does not show the characteristic cytology of middle-ear adenomatous tumors, although both may show concomitant mixed inflammation and fibrosis. Finally, it should be remembered that rarely both rhabdomyosarcoma and Langerhans' granulomatosis can present as middle-ear masses.[383]

Phosphaturic Mesenchymal Tumors

Oncogenic or tumor-induced osteomalacia-rickets is a syndrome characterized by hypophosphatemia, renal phosphate wasting, and decreased serum 1,25-dihydroxyvitamin D$_3$ levels.[384-386] The tumors secrete a phosphaturic substance that causes total-body phosphate depletion leading to osteomalacia or rickets.

Obviously, once a suspicious mass in bone, skin, or soft tissue is found, it should be surgically removed with a clear margin and examined by a pathologist. The morphologic features of the tumor may help confirm the diagnosis of oncogenic osteomalacia-rickets, especially if it has the unique morphologic features of a phosphaturic mesenchymal tumor (mixed connective tissue variant). Postoperatively, serum phosphate and 1,25-dihydroxyvitamin D$_3$ should be measured, because

biochemical abnormalities may begin to resolve within hours. In other cases, it may take days to weeks for these chemicals to return to normal levels.

If the abnormal chemistries resolve, the patient's symptoms disappear, and the tumor appears totally resected and benign, then the diagnosis is confirmed and the prognosis is excellent. But if this does not occur and the tumor shows features not typical for phosphaturic mesenchymal tumors, then one should continue the search for the "right" tumor or consider an alternative diagnosis. If the patient's serum chemistries and symptoms only partially improve, there may be residual or multifocal tumor, especially if the tumor appears only partially resected or shows malignant cytologic features. In the latter event, additional surgery, chemotherapy, and/or radiation therapy may be necessary to effect the cure. If it is not possible to find or eradicate the tumor causing the osteomalacia or rickets, then supplemental phosphorus and vitamin D therapy is indicated.

CLINICOPATHOLOGIC FEATURES. Most patients present with severe debilitating bone pain (sometimes with fractures), osteopenia, hypophosphatemia, hyperphosphaturia, normocalcemia, and decreased serum 1,25-dihydroxyvitamin D$_3$. The tumors can occur in bone, skin, or soft tissue, and they may be small and difficult to find. Although these tumors are histologically polymorphous, personal review of 16 tumors documented to cause this syndrome revealed four groups. The first contained 10 unique-appearing, mixed connective tissue tumors having variably prominent vessels, osteoclast-like giant cells, focal microcystic changes, dystrophic calcification, osseous metaplasia, and/or poorly developed cartilage-like areas. With one exception, all tumors of this group occurred in soft tissue and were benign (Fig. 2–111). The single malignant tumor originated in bone, recurred locally, and metastasized to lung.

The remaining tumors occurred in bone and showed benign clinical behavior. They resembled tumors known to occur in bone, that is, osteoblastoma-like (three tumors), non-ossifying fibroma–like (two tumors), and ossifying fibroma–like (one tumor).

DIFFERENTIAL DIAGNOSIS. Before diagnostic evaluation, it is important to consider the differential diagnostic possibilities. The common clinical causes of osteomalacia include renal failure, intestinal malabsorption, chronic acidosis, and unusual dietary habits. In renal failure, the serum phosphorus level is high. Although severe hypophosphatemia can occur in diabetic ketoacidosis, acute alcoholism, and severe dietary restriction of phosphorus, serum phosphorus levels in these conditions are usually only slightly low. In these conditions, and in sharp contrast to oncogenic osteomalacia-rickets, the urine is almost phosphate free. Finally, it is important to separate oncogenic osteomalacia-rickets from other tumor-associated osteomalacia or hypophosphatemic syndrome, such as tumor-induced malabsorption or diarrhea, ectopic parathyroid hormone production, and phosphorus uptake by leukemia/lymphoma cells.

Oncogenic osteomalacia-rickets should be suspected in any patient who presents with hypophosphatemia and inappropriate phosphaturia.[358, 386] The serum 1,25-dihydroxyvitamin D$_3$ level is low always, and the serum alkaline phosphatase level should be elevated. Because clinical osteomalacia or rickets may not be present when the biochemical abnormalities first develop, a bone biopsy might be helpful

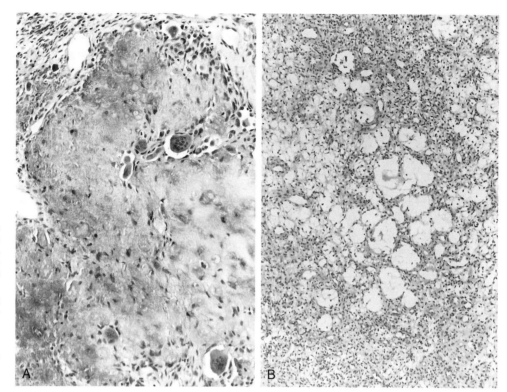

FIGURE 2–111. *A,* Phosphaturic mesenchymal tumor, mixed connective tissue variant. Note the cartilage-like stroma and peripherally located clusters of small mesenchymal cells with admixed osteoclast-like giant cells. (H&E, OM ×50) *B,* Phosphaturic mesenchymal tumor, mixed connective tissue variant, showing a microcystic pattern within a stroma composed of numerous small mesenchymal cells. (H&E, OM ×25)

in securing a diagnosis. Tetracycline labeling should precede biopsy.

If there is no clinical evidence to suggest another cause for osteomalacia, a vigorous and meticulous search for a small, inconspicuous tumor should be initiated. The mesenchymal tumors can occur in almost any location. Approximately 53%

have occurred in bone, 45% in soft tissues, and 3% in skin. About 44% have involved the lower extremities, 27% the head and neck area, and 17% the upper extremities. The patient should be asked about the presence of a tumor and given a whole-body clinical examination. In addition, computed tomography, regional tomograms, and bone scans

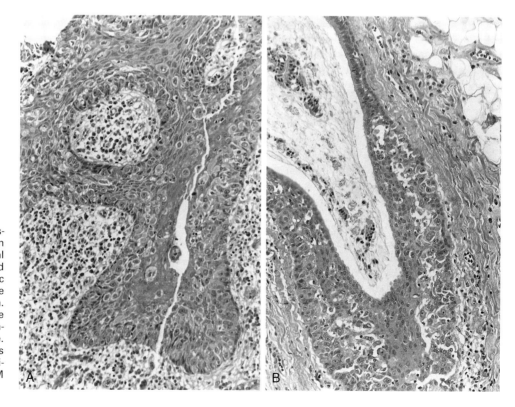

FIGURE 2–112. *A,* Paget's disease of the oral mucosa. Shown is a segment of superficial oral mucosa containing scattered single and clusters of neoplastic cells located mainly within the lower parts of the mucosa. These neoplastic cells were CAM 5.2 positive and occasionally mucicarmine positive. (H&E, OM ×100). *B,* The Paget's cells extended down minor salivary gland ducts. (H&E, OM ×100)

should be administered until a tumor is either found or ruled out. One phosphaturic mesenchymal tumor (mixed connective tissue variant) showed marked uptake of technetium 99m methylene diphosphonate, a property that, if present, can hasten tumor discovery. Finally, if a phosphaturic mesenchymal tumor is not found, one should consider other tumors that cause oncogenic osteomalacia-rickets. These tumors include prostate cancer, breast cancer, oat cell carcinoma, fibrous dysplasia, and soft-tissue tumors occurring in neurofibromatosis.

Malignant Lesions

Metastatic Tumors to the Major Salivary Glands

Separating metastatic from primary salivary gland tumors is very important for therapeutic and prognostic reasons. In this regard, there are two general types of metastasis to salivary glands: metastatic tumors originating from the head and neck region and metastatic tumors from distant sites.[387] About **two thirds of such metastatic tumors are from the head and neck region,** with most being metastatic squamous carcinomas of the face (70%) and malignant melanoma of the face (27%) and the remainder divided among undifferentiated carcinoma nasopharyngeal type, oral squamous carcinoma, and meibomian gland carcinoma. Clearly, undifferentiated carcinoma nasopharyngeal type can metastasize to the parotid and be confused with undifferentiated carcinoma with lymphoid stroma. The remaining metastases to the major salivary glands are from **distant sites** and most commonly include **lung carcinomas** (to be differentiated from primary undifferentiated carcinomas), **renal carcinomas** (to be differentiated from various clear-cell primary carcinomas and clear-cell oncocytoma), **breast carcinomas** (to be differentiated from salivary duct carcinoma), **colonic carcinoma, thyroid carcinoma,** and **uterine carcinomas** (the last three to be separated from papillary cystadenocarcinoma). It is fortunate that prostate carcinoma only very rarely metastasizes to salivary glands, because pleomorphic adenomas, mucoepidermoid carcinomas, adenoid cystic carcinomas, and adenocarcinomas (not otherwise specified) primary to salivary glands can immunoreact with antibodies to prostate-specific antigen and prostatic acid phosphatase.[388]

Extramammary Paget's Disease of the Oral Mucosa

On very rare occasions, Paget's disease can present in the oral cavity (Fig. 2–112), and it may be associated with carcinoma *in situ* and/or invasive poorly differentiated carcinoma of the underlying minor salivary glands.[389] Clinically, oral Paget's disease can cause extensive, multifocal, and rapidly spreading erythroplakia of the oral mucosa, accompanied by a relatively small invasive salivary gland carcinoma. The *in situ* components may be recurrent and very difficult to control. The invasive component can metastasize to distant sites, resulting in the patient's death.

References

1. Stompro B, Wolf P, Haghighi P: Fibrous dysplasia of bone. Am Fam Physician 39:179–184, 1989.
2. Camilleri AE: Craniofacial dysplasia. J Laryngol Otol 105:662–666, 1991.
3. Slootweg PJ, Muller H: Differential diagnosis of fibro-osseous jaw lesions. J Craniomaxillofac Surg 18:210–214, 1990.
4. Waldron CA: Fibro-osseous lesions of the jaws. J Oral Maxillofac Surg 43:249–262, 1985.
5. Eversole LR, Leider AS, Nelson K: Ossifying fibroma: A clinicopathologic study of sixty-four cases. Oral Surg Oral Med Oral Pathol 60:505–511, 1985.
6. Slootweg PJ, Muller H: Juvenile ossifying fibroma. Report of four cases. J Craniomaxillofac Surg 18:125–129, 1990.
7. Waldron C, El-Mofty S: A histopathologic study of 116 ameloblastomas with special reference to the desmoplastic variant. Oral Surg Oral Med Oral Pathol 63:441–451, 1987.
8. Leider A, Eversole LR, Barkin M: Cystic ameloblastoma. Oral Surg Oral Med Oral Pathol 60:624–630, 1985.
9. Slootweg P, Muller H: Malignant ameloblastoma or ameloblastic carcinoma. Oral Surg 57:168–176, 1984.
10. Leider A, Jonker A, Cook H: Multicentric familial squamous ondontogenic tumor. Oral Surg Oral Med Oral Pathol 68:175–181, 1989.
11. Ruskin J, Cohen D, Davis L: Primary intraosseous carcinoma: Report of two cases. J Oral Maxillofac Surg 46:425–432, 1988.
12. Rabanus JP, Greenspan D, Peterson V, et al: Subcellular distribution and life cycle of Epstein-Barr virus in keratinocytes of oral hairy leukoplakia. Am J Pathol 139:185–197, 1991.
13. Fernandez JF, Benito MAC, Lizaldez EB, Montanes MA: Oral hairy leukoplakia: A histopathologic study of 32 cases. Am J Dermatol 12:571–578, 1990.
14. Fowler CB, Reed KD, Brannon RB: Intranuclear inclusions correlate with the ultrastructural detection of herpes-type virions in oral hairy leukoplakia. Am J Surg Pathol 13:114–119, 1989.
15. Daniels TE: Clinical assessment and diagnosis of immunologically mediated salivary gland diseases in Sjogren's syndrome. J Autoimmun 2:529–541, 1989.
16. Fox RI, Carstens SA, Fong S, et al: Use of monoclonal antibodies to analyze peripheral blood and salivary gland lymphocyte subsets in Sjogren's syndrome. Arthritis Rheum 25:419–426, 1982.
17. Isaacson PG, Wright DH: Extranodal malignant lymphoma arising from mucosa-associated lymphoid tissue. Cancer 53:2515–2524, 1984.
18. Hyjek E, Smith WJ, Isaacson PG: Primary B-cell lymphoma of salivary glands and its relationship to myoepithelial sialadenitis. Hum Pathol 19:766–776, 1988.
19. Pelstring RJ, Essell JH, Kurtin PJ, et al: Diversity of organ site involvement among malignant lymphomas of mucosa-associated tissues. Am J Clin Pathol 96:738–745, 1991.
20. Daniels TE: Salivary histopathology in diagnosis of Sjogren's syndrome. Scand J Rheumatol Suppl 61:36–43, 1986.
21. Greenspan JS, Daniels TE, Talal N, Sylvester RA: The histopathology of Sjogren's syndrome in labial salivary gland biopsies. Oral Surg 37:217–229, 1974.
22. Chisholm DM, Mason DK: Labial salivary gland biopsy in Sjogren's syndrome. J Clin Pathol 21:656–660, 1968.
23. Hyman GA, Wolff M: Malignant lymphoma of the salivary glands. Review of the literature and report of 33 new cases, including four cases associated with the lymphoepithelial lesion. Am J Clin Pathol 65:421–429, 1976.
24. Falzon M, Isaacson PG: The natural history of benign lymphoepithelial lesion of the salivary gland in which there is a monoclonal population of B cells. A report of two cases. Am J Surg Pathol 15:59–65, 1991.
25. Fishleder A, Tubbs R, Hesse B, Levine H: Uniform detection of immunoglobulin-gene rearrangement in benign lymphoepithelial lesions. N Engl J Med 316:1118–1121, 1987.
26. Bodeutsch C, de Wilde PCM, Kater L, et al: Monotypic plasma cells in labial salivary glands of patients with Sjogren's syndrome: Prognosticator for systemic lymphoproliferative disease. J Clin Pathol 46:123–128, 1993.
27. Crissman JD, Weiss MA, Gluckman J: Midline granuloma syndrome. A clinicopathologic study of 13 patients. Am J Surg Pathol 6:335–346, 1982.
28. Batsakis JG, Luna MA: Midfacial necrotizing lesions. Semin Diagn Pathol 4:90–116, 1987.
29. Grange C, Cabane J, DuBois A, et al: Centrofacial malignant granulomas. Clinicopathologic study of 40 cases and review of the literature. Medicine 71:179–196, 1992.
30. Tsokos M, Fauci AS, Costa J: Idiopathic midline destructive disease (IDMM). A subgroup of patients with the "midline granuloma" syndrome. Am J Clin Pathol 77:162–168, 1982.
31. Colby TV, Tazelaar HD, Specks U, DeRemee RA: Nasal biopsy in Wegener's granulomatosis. Hum Pathol 22:101–104, 1991.
32. Devaney KO, Travis WD, Hoffman T, et al: Interpretation of head-and-neck biopsies in Wegener's granulomatosis. A pathologic study of 126 biopsies in 70 patients. Am J Surg Pathol 14:555–564, 1990.
33. van der Woude FJ, Rasmussen N, Lobato S, et al: Autoantibodies against neutrophils and monocytes: Tool for diagnosis and marker of disease activity in Wegener's granulomatosis. Lancet 1:425–429, 1985.
34. Nolle B, Specks U, Ludemann J, et al: Anticytoplasmic autoantibodies: Their immunodiagnostic value in WG. Ann Intern Med 149:2461–2465, 1989.
35. Falk RJ, Jennette JC: Wegener's granulomatosis, systemic vasculitis, and antineutrophil cytoplasmic autoantibodies. Annu Rev Med 42:459–469, 1991.
36. Ferry JA, Sklar J, Zukerberg LR, Harris NL: Nasal lymphoma. A clinicopathologic study with immunophenotypic and genotypic analysis. Am J Surg Pathol 15:268–279, 1991.

37. Lipford EH, Margolick JB, Longo DL, et al: Angiocentric immunoproliferative lesions: A clincopathologic spectrum of post thymic T-cell proliferations. Blood 72:1674–1681, 1988.

38. Jaffe ES: Post-thymic lymphoid neoplasia. In Jaffe ES (ed), Bennington JL (consulting ed): Surgical Pathology of the Lymph Nodes and Related Organs. Vol. 16 in the series Major Problems in Pathology. Philadelphia, WB Saunders, 1985, pp 218–246.

39. Medeiros LJ, Peiper SC, Elwood L, et al: Angiocentric immunoproliferative lesions: A molecular analysis of eight cases. Hum Pathol 22:1150–1157, 1991.

40. Stroup RM, Sheibani K, Moncada A, et al: Angiotropic (intravascular) large cell lymphoma. Cancer 66:1781–1788, 1990.

41. Wick MR, Banks PM, McDonald TJ: Angioendotheliomatosis of the nose with fatal systemic dissemination. Cancer 48:2510–2517, 1981.

42. Elzay RP: Traumatic ulcerative granuloma with stromal eosinophilia (Riga-Fede's disease and traumatic eosinophilic granuloma). Oral Surg Oral Med Oral Pathol 55:497–506, 1983.

43. Eversole LR, Leider AS, Jacobsen PL, Kidd PM: Atypical histiocytic granuloma. Cancer 55:1722–1729, 1985.

44. Worsaae N, Hristensen KC, Schiodt M, Reibel J: Melkersson-Rosenthal syndrome and cheilitis granulomatosa. Oral Surg Oral Med Oral Pathol 54:404–413, 1982.

45. Tyldesley WR: Oral Crohn's disease and related conditions. Br J Oral Surg 17:1–9, 1979.

46. Greenspan JS: Infections and non-neoplastic diseases of the oral mucosa. J Oral Pathol 12:139–166, 1983.

47. Friedmann I, Sando I, Balkany T: Idiopathic pleomorphic midfacial granuloma (Stewart's type). J Laryngol Otol 92:601–611, 1978.

48. Seifert G, Brocheriou C, Cardesa A, Eveson JW: WHO international histological classification of tumors. Tentative histological classification of salivary gland tumors. Pathol Res Pract 186:555–581, 1990.

49. Seifert G, Sobin LH: The WHO's histological classification of salivary gland tumors. A commentary on the second edition. Cancer 70:379–385, 1992.

50. Dardick I, Daley TD, van Nostrand AWP: Basal-cell adenoma with myoepithelial cell-derived "stroma": A new major salivary gland entity. Head Neck Surg 8:257–267, 1986.

51. Seifert G, Kratochvil F, Auclair P, Ellis G: Clinical features of 160 cases of basal cell adenoma and 121 cases of canalicular adenoma. Oral Surg Oral Med Oral Pathol 70:605, 1990.

52. Harris MD, McKeever P, Robertson JM: Congenital tumors of the salivary gland: A case report and review. Histopathology 17:155–157, 1990.

53. Ellis GL, Wiscovitch JG: Basal-cell adenocarcinomas of the major salivary glands. Oral Surg Oral Med Oral Pathol 69:461–469, 1990.

54. Gardner DG, Daley TD: The use of the terms monomorphic adenoma, basal cell adenoma, and canalicular adenoma as applied to salivary gland tumors. Oral Surg Oral Med Oral Pathol 56:608–615, 1983.

55. Herbst EW, Utz W: Multifocal dermal-type basal cell adenomas of parotid glands with co-existing dermal cylindromas. Virchows Arch [A] 403:95–102, 1984.

56. Batsakis JG, Brannon RB: Dermal analogue tumours of major salivary glands. J Laryngol Otol 95:155–164, 1981.

57. Nagao K, Matsuzaki O, Saiga H, et al: Histopathologic studies of basal cell adenoma of the parotid gland. Cancer 50:736–745, 1982.

58. Hyma BA, Scheithauer BW, Weiland LH, Irons GB: Membranous basal cell adenoma of the parotid gland. Malignant transformation in a patient with multiple dermal cylindromas. Arch Pathol Lab Med 112:209–211, 1988.

59. Batsakis JG, Luna MA, el-Naggar A: Histopathologic grading of salivary gland neoplasms. III. Adenoid cystic carcinomas. Ann Otol Rhinol 99:1007–1009, 1990.

60. Chomette G, Auriol M, Tranbaloc P, Vaillant JM: Adenoid cystic carcinoma of minor salivary glands. Analysis of 86 cases. Virchows Arch [Pathol Anat] 395:289–301, 1982.

61. Matsuba HM, Spector GJ, Thawley SE, et al: Adenoid cystic salivary gland carcinoma. A histopathologic review of treatment failure patterns. Cancer 57:519–524, 1986.

62. Santucci M, Bondi R: New prognostic criterion in adenoid cystic carcinoma of salivary gland origin. Am J Clin Pathol 91:132–136, 1989.

63. Nascimento AG, Amaral ALP, Prado LAF, et al: Adenoid cystic carcinoma of salivary glands. A study of 61 cases with clinicopathologic correlation. Cancer 57:312–319, 1986.

64. Bands ER, Frierson HF, Mills SE, et al: Basaloid squamous cell carcinoma of the head and neck. A clinicopathologic and immunohistochemical study of 40 cases. Am J Surg Pathol 16:939–946, 1992.

65. Wain SL, Kier R, Vollmer RT, Bossen EH: Basaloid-squamous carcinoma of the tongue, hypopharynx, and larynx. Report of 10 cases. Hum Pathol 17:1158–1166, 1986.

66. Luna MA, el-Naggar A, Parichatikanond P, et al: Basaloid squamous carcinoma of the upper aerodigestive tract. Cancer 66:537–542, 1990.

67. McKay MJ, Bilous AM: Basaloid-squamous carcinoma of the hypopharynx. Cancer 63:2528–2531, 1989.

68. Tsan WYW, Chan JKC, Lee KC, et al: Basaloid-squamous carcinoma of the upper aerodigestive tract and so-called adenoid cystic carcinoma of the oesophagus: The same tumor? Histopathology 19:35–46, 1991.

69. Yaku Y, Mori Y, Kanda T, et al: Ultrastructural study of glycogen-rich oxyphilic adenoma of the nasopharyngeal minor salivary gland. Virchows Arch [A] 407:151–158, 1985.

70. Palmer TJ, Gleeson MJ, Eveson JW, Cawson RA: Oncocytic adenomas and oncocytic hyperplasia of salivary glands. A clinico-pathologic study of 26 cases. Histopathology 16:487–495, 1990.

71. Cotton DWK: Oncocytomas. Histopathology 16:507–509, 1990.

72. Hamperl H: Benign and malignant oncocytoma. Cancer 15:1019–1027, 1962.

73. Brandwein MS, Huvos AG: Oncocytic tumors of major salivary glands. A study of 68 cases with follow-up of 44 patients. Am J Surg Pathol 15:514–528, 1991.

74. Yamase HT, Putman HC: Oncocytic papillary cystadenomatosis of the larynx. Cancer 44:2306–2311, 1979.

75. Ellis GL: "Clear-cell" oncocytoma of salivary gland. Hum Pathol 19:862–867, 1988.

76. Taxy JB: Necrotizing squamous/mucinous metaplasia in oncocytic salivary gland tumors. A potential diagnostic problem. Am J Clin Pathol 97:40–45, 1992.

77. Eveson JW, Cawson RA: Infarcted ("infected") adenolymphomas. A clinicopathologic study of 20 cases. Clin Otolaryngol 14:205–210, 1989.

78. Seifert G, Bull HG, Donath K: Histologic subclassification of the cystadenolymphoma of the parotid gland. Virchows Arch A Pathol Anat Histopathol 388:13–38, 1980.

79. Therkildsen MH, Christensen N, Andersen LJ, et al: Malignant Warthin's tumor: A case study. Histopathology 21:167–171, 1992.

80. Griesser GH, Hansmann M-L, Bogman MJJT, et al: Germinal center derived malignant lymphoma in cystadenolymphoma. Virchows Arch [Pathol Anat] 408:491–496, 1986.

81. Crissman JD, Kessis T, Shah KV, et al: Squamous papillary neoplasia of the adult upper aerodigestive tract. Hum Pathol 19:1387–1396, 1988.

82. Popper HH, Wirnsberger G, Juttner-Smolle FM, et al: The predictive value of human papilloma virus (HPV) typing in the prognosis of bronchial squamous cell papillomas. Histopathology 21:323–330, 1992.

83. Guillou L, Sahli R, Chauber P, et al: Squamous cell carcinoma of the lung in a nonsmoking, nonirradiated patient with juvenile laryngotracheal papillomatosis. Evidence of human papillomavirus-11 DNA in both carcinoma and papillomas. Am J Surg Pathol 15:891–898, 1991.

84. Quick CA, Foucar E, Dehner LP: Frequency and significance of epithelial atypia in laryngeal papillomatosis. Laryngoscope 89:550–560, 1979.

85. Fechner RE, Fitz-Hugh GS: Invasive tracheal papillomatosis. Am J Surg Pathol 4:79–86, 1980.

86. Gindhart TD, Johnston WH, Chism SE, Dedo HH: Carcinoma of the larynx in childhood. Cancer 46:1683–1687, 1980.

87. Lee SS, Ro JY, Luna MA, Batsakis JG: Squamous cell carcinoma of the larynx in young adults. Semin Diagn Pathol 4:150–152, 1987.

88. Ferlto A, Recher G: Ackerman's tumor (verrucous carcinoma) of the larynx. Cancer 46:1617–1630, 1980.

89. Medina JE, Dichtel W, Luna MA: Verrucous-squamous carcinomas of the oral cavity. Arch Otolaryngol 110:437–440, 1984.

90. Carbone A, Volpe R: Superficial extending carcinoma (SEC) of the larynx and hypopharynx. Pathol Res Pract 188:729–738, 1992.

91. Shear M, Pindborg JJ: Verrucous hyperplasia of the oral mucosa. Cancer 46:1855–1862, 1980.

92. Krutchkoff DJ, Eisenberg E, Anderson C: Dysplasia of oral mucosa: A unified approach to proper evaluation. Mod Pathol 4:113–119, 1991.

93. Buchner A, Hansen LS, Merrell PW: Verruciform xanthoma of the oral mucosa. Report of five cases and review of the literature. Arch Dermatol 117:563–565, 1981.

94. Fechner RE, Mills SE: Verruca vulgaris of the larynx: A distinctive lesion of probable viral origin confused with verrucous carcinoma. Am J Surg Pathol 6:357–362, 1982.

95. Uzoaru I, Firfer B, Ray V, et al: Malignant granular cell tumor. Arch Pathol Lab Med 116:206–208, 1992.

96. Stefansson K, Wollmann RL: S100 protein in granular cell tumors (granular cell myoblastomas). Cancer 49:1834–1838, 1982.

97. Shimokama T, Watanabe T: Leiomyoma exhibiting a marked granular change: Granular cell leiomyoma versus granular cell schwannoma. Hum Pathol 23:327–331, 1992.

98. Sobel HJ, Marquet E, Schwarz R: Granular degeneration of appendiceal smooth muscle. Arch Pathol Lab Med 92:427–432, 1971.

99. LeBoit PE, Barr RJ, Burall S, et al: Primitive polypoid granular-cell tumor and other cutaneous granular-cell neoplasms of apparent nonneural origin. Am J Surg Pathol 15:48–58, 1991.

100. Gamboa LG: Malignant granular cell myoblastoma. Arch Pathol Lab Med 60:663–668, 1955.

101. Klima M, Peters J: Malignant granular cell tumor. Arch Pathol Lab Med 111:1070–1073, 1987.

102. Bertoni F, Dallera P, Bacchini P, et al: The Istituto Rizzoli-Beretta experience with osteosarcoma of the jaws. Cancer 68:1555–1563, 1991.

103. Tanzawa H, Uchiyama S, Sato K: Statistical observation of osteosarcoma of the maxillofacial region in Japan. Oral Surg Oral Med Oral Pathol 72:444–448, 1991.

104. Vege D, Borges A, Aggrawal K, et al: Osteosarcoma of the craniofacial bones. J Craniomaxillofac Surg 19:90–93, 1991.

105. Regezi J, Zarbo R, McClatchey K, Courtney R: Osteosarcomas and chondrosarcomas of the jaws: Immunohistochemical correlations. Oral Surg Oral Med Oral Pathol 64:302–307, 1987.

106. Goorin A, Abelson H, Frei E: Osteosarcoma: Fifteen years later. N Engl J Med 313:1637–1643, 1985.

107. Unni K, Dahlin D, Beabout J: Periosteal osteogenic sarcoma. Cancer 37:2476–2485, 1976.

108. Millar B, Browne R, Flood T: Juxtacortical osteosarcoma of the jaws. Br J Oral Maxillofac Surg 28:73–79, 1990.

109. Zarbo R, Regezi J, Baker S: Periosteal osteogenic sarcoma of the mandible. Oral Surg Oral Med Oral Pathol 57:643–647, 1984.

110. Bertoni F, Unni K, McLeod R, Dahlin D: Osteosarcoma resembling osteoblastoma. Cancer 55:416–426, 1985.

111. Lummerman H, Freedman PD, Kerpel SM, Phelan JA: Oral Kaposi's sarcoma: A clinicopathologic study of 23 homosexual and bisexual men from the New York metropolitan area. Oral Surg Oral Med Oral Pathol 65:711–716, 1988.

112. Lozada F, Silverman S, Migliorati CA, et al: Oral manifestations of tumor and opportunistic infections in the acquired immunodeficiency syndrome (AIDS): Findings in 53 homosexual men with Kaposi's sarcoma. Oral Surg Oral Med Oral Pathol 56:491–494, 1983.

113. Cockerell CJ, LeBoit PE: Bacillary angiomatosis: A newly characterized, pseudoneoplastic, infectious cutaneous vascular disorder. J Am Acad Dermatol 22:501–512, 1990.

114. Welch DF, Pickett DA, Slater LN, et al: *Rochalimaea* sp. nov., a cause of septicemia, bacillary angiomatosis, and parenchymal bacillary peliosis. J Clin Microbiol 30:275–280, 1992.

115. Speight PM, Zakrzewska J, Fletcher CDM: Epithelioid angiomatosis affecting the oral cavity as a first sign of HIV infection. Br Dent J 171:367–370, 1990.

116. Perzin KH, Cantor JO, Johannsen JV: Acinic cell carcinoma arising in nasal cavity. Cancer 47:1818–1822, 1981.

117. Ellis GL, Corio RL: Acinic cell adenocarcinoma. A clinicopathologic analysis of 294 cases. Cancer 52:542–549, 1983.

118. Spiro RH, Huvos AG, Strong EW: Acinic cell carcinoma of salivary gland origin. A clinicopathologic study of 67 cases. Cancer 41:924–935, 1978.

119. Perzin KH, LiVolsi VA: Acinic cell carcinomas arising in salivary glands: A clinicopathologic study. Cancer 44:1434–1457, 1979.

120. Hamer K, Mausch H-E, Caselitz J, et al: Acinic cell carcinoma of the salivary glands: The prognostic relevance of DNA cytophotometry in a retrospective study of long duration (1965–1987). Oral Surg Oral Med Oral Pathol 69:68–75, 1990.

121. Hanson TA: Acinic cell carcinoma of the parotid salivary gland presenting as a cyst. Cancer 36:570–575, 1975.

122. Allen MS, Fitz-Hugh GS, Marsh WL: Low-grade papillary adenocarcinoma of the palate. Cancer 33:153–158, 1974.

123. Perzin KH, LiVolsi VA: Acinic cell carcinoma arising in ectopic salivary gland tissue. Cancer 45:967–972, 1980.

124. Spires JE, Mills SE, Cooper PH, et al: Acinic cell carcinoma. Its occurrence in the laryngotracheal junction after thyroid radiation. Arch Pathol Lab Med 105:266–268, 1981.

125. Seifert G: Tumor-like lesions of the salivary glands. The new WHO classification. Pathol Res Pract 188:836–846, 1992.

126. Batsakis JG, Pinkston GR, Luna MA, et al: Adenocarcinoma of the oral cavity: A clinicopathologic study of terminal duct carcinomas. J Laryngol Otol 97:825–835, 1983.

127. Freedman PD, Lumerman H: Lobular carcinoma of intraoral minor salivary gland origin. Report of twelve cases. Oral Surg 56:157–165, 1983.

128. Evans HL, Batsakis JG: Polymorphous low-grade adenocarcinomas of minor salivary glands: A study of 14 cases of a distinctive neoplasm. Cancer 53:935–942, 1984.

129. Ritland F, Lubensky I, LiVolsi A: Polymorphous low-grade adenocarcinoma of the salivary gland. Arch Pathol Lab Med 117:1261–1263, 1993.

130. Luna MA, Batsakis JG, Ordonez NG, et al: Salivary gland adenocarcinomas: A clinicopathologic analysis of three distinctive types. Semin Diagn Pathol 4:117–135, 1987.

131. Donath K, Seifert G, Schmutz R: Zur diagnose und ultrastruktur des tubularen speichelgangkarzinomas. Epithelial-myoepitheliales schaltstuckkarzinom. Virchows Arch (A) 356:16–31, 1972.

132. Fonseca I, Soares J: Epithelial-myoepithelial carcinoma of the salivary glands. A study of 22 cases. Virchows Arch A Pathol Anat Histopathol 422:389–396, 1993.

133. Milchgrub S, Gnepp DR, Vuitch F, et al: Hyalinizing clear-cell carcinoma of salivary gland. Am J Surg Pathol 18:74–82, 1994.

134. Chan JKC, Ng H-K, Wan KY, et al: Clear cell rhabdomyosarcoma of the nasal cavity and paranasal sinuses. Histopathology 14:391–399, 1989.

135. Tortoledo ME, Luna MA, Batsakis JG: Carcinomas ex pleomorphic adenoma and malignant mixed tumors. Arch Otolaryngol 110:172–176, 1984.

136. Frierson HF, Mills SE, Fechner RE, et al: Sinonasal undifferentiated carcinoma. An aggressive neoplasm derived from schneiderian epithelium and distinct from olfactory neuroblastoma. Am J Surg Pathol 10:771–779, 1986.

137. Mills SE, Fechner RE: ''Undifferentiated'' neoplasms of the sinonasal region: Differential diagnosis based on clinical, light microscopic, immunohistochemical, and ultrastructural features. Semin Diagn Pathol 6:316–328, 1989.

138. Hui KK, Luna MA, Batsakis JG, et al: Undifferentiated carcinomas of the major salivary glands. Oral Surg Oral Med Oral Pathol 69:76–83, 1990.

139. Cleary KR, Batsakis JG: Undifferentiated carcinoma with lymphoid stroma of the major salivary glands. Ann Otol Rhinol Laryngol 99:236–238, 1990.

140. Shanmugaratnam K, Sobin L: Histologic typing of upper respiratory tract tumors. No. 19. Geneva, World Health Organization, 1978.

141. Hsu H-C, Chen C-L, Hsu M-M, et al: Pathology of nasopharyngeal carcinoma. Proposal of a new histologic classification correlated with prognosis. Cancer 59:945–951, 1987.

142. Carbone A, Micheau C: Pitfalls in microscopic diagnosis of undifferentiated carcinoma of nasopharyngeal type (lymphoepithelioma). Cancer 50:1344–1351, 1982.

143. Zarate-Osorno A, Jaffe ES, Medeiros J: Metastatic nasopharyngeal carcinoma initially presenting as cervical lymphadenopathy. A report of two cases that resembled Hodgkin's disease. Arch Pathol Lab Med 116:862–865, 1992.

144. Frierson HF, Ross GW, Stewart FM, et al: Unusual sinonasal small-cell neoplasms following radiotherapy for bilateral retinoblastomas. Am J Surg Pathol 13:947–954, 1989.

145. Weidner N, Tjoe J: Immunohistochemical profile of monoclonal antibody O13: An antibody that recognizes glycoprotein p30/32^{MIC2} and is useful in diagnosing Ewing's sarcoma and peripheral neuroepithelioma. Am J Surg Pathol 18:486–494, 1994.

146. Taxy JB, Bharani NK, Mills SE, et al: The spectrum of olfactory neural tumors: A light-microscopic immunohistochemical and ultrastructural analysis. Am J Surg Pathol 10:687–695, 1986.

147. Johnson RE, Scheithauer BW, Dahlin DC: Melanotic neuroectodermal tumor of infancy. A review of seven cases. Cancer 52:661–666, 1983.

148. Theaker JM, Fletcher CDM: Heterotopic glial nodules: A light microscopic and immunohistochemical study. Histopathology 18:255–260, 1991.

149. Frierson HF, Ross GW, Mills SE, Frankfurter A: Olfactory neuroblastoma. Additional immunohistochemical characterization. Am J Clin Pathol 94:547–553, 1990.

150. Saw D, Chan JKC, Jagirdar J, et al: Sinonasal small cell neoplasm developing after radiation therapy for retinoblastoma. Hum Pathol 23:896–899, 1992.

151. Kliewer KE, Cochran AJ: A review of the histology, ultrastructure, immunohistology, and molecular biology of extra-adrenal paragangliomas. Arch Pathol Lab Med 113:1209–1218, 1989.

152. Milroy CM, Rode J, Moss E: Laryngeal paragangliomas and neuroendocrine carcinomas. Histopathology 18:201–209, 1991.

153. Googe PB, Ferry JA, Bhan AK, et al: A comparison of paraganglioma, carcinoid tumor, and small-cell carcinoma of the larynx. Arch Pathol Lab Med 112:809–815, 1988.

154. Silva EG, Butler JJ, Mackay B, Goepfert H: Neuroblastomas and neuroendocrine carcinomas of the nasal cavity. A proposed new classification. Cancer 50:2388–2405, 1982.

155. Wenig BM, Gnepp DR: The spectrum of neuroendocrine carcinomas of the larynx. Semin Diagn Pathol 6:329–350, 1989.

156. Wenig BM, Hyams VJ, Heffner DK: Moderately differentiated neuroendocrine carcinoma of the larynx. A clinicopathologic study of 54 cases. Cancer 62:2658–2676, 1988.

157. Woodruff JM, Huvos AG, Erlandson RA, et al: Neuroendocrine carcinomas of the larynx. A study of two types, one of which mimics thyroid medullary carcinoma. Am J Surg Pathol 9:771–790, 1985.

158. Mark EJ, Ramirez JF: Peripheral small-cell carcinoma of the lung resembling carcinoid tumor. Arch Pathol Lab Med 109:263–269, 1985.

159. Travis WD, Linnoila I, Tsokos MG, et al: Neuroendocrine tumors of the lung with proposed criteria for large-cell neuroendocrine carcinoma. Am J Surg Pathol 15:529–553, 1991.

160. Doglioni C, Ferlito A, Chiamenti C, et al: Laryngeal carcinoma showing multidirectional epithelial neuroendocrine and sarcomatous differentiation. ORL J Otorhinolaryngol Relat Spec 52:316–326, 1990.

161. Saphir O, Vass A: Carcinosarcoma. Am J Cancer 33:331–361, 1938.

162. Batsakis JG, Rice DH, Howard DR: The pathology of head and neck tumors: Spindle-cell lesions (sarcomatoid carcinomas, nodular fasciitis, and fibrosarcoma) of the aerodigestive tracts, part 14. Head Neck Surg 4:499–513, 1982.

163. Anonsen C, Dobie RA, Hoekema D, et al: Carcinosarcoma of the floor of mouth. J Otolaryngol 14:215–220, 1985.

164. Lambert PR, Ward PH, Berci G: Pseudosarcoma of the larynx: A comprehensive analysis. Arch Otolaryngol 106:700–708, 1980.

165. Someren A, Karacioglu Z, Clairmont AA: Polypoid spindle-cell carcinoma (pleomorphic carcinoma). Oral Surg 42:474–489, 1976.

166. Zarbo RJ, Crissman JD, Benkat H, et al: Spindle-cell carcinoma of the upper aerodigestive tract mucosa: An immunohistologic and ultrastructural study of 18 biphasic tumors and comparison with seven monophasic spindle-cell tumors. Am J Surg Pathol 10:741–753, 1986.

167. Leventon GS, Evans HL: Sarcomatoid squamous cell carcinoma of the mucous membranes of the head and neck: A clinicopathologic study of 20 cases. Cancer 48:994–1003, 1981.

168. Lane N: Pseudosarcoma (polypoid sarcoma-like masses) associated with squamous-cell carcinoma of the mouth, fauces, and larynx: Report of ten cases. Cancer 10:19–41, 1957.

169. Battifora H: Spindle-cell carcinoma: Ultrastructural evidence of squamous origin and collagen production by the tumor cells. Cancer 37:2275–2282, 1976.

170. Alguacil-Garcia A, Alonso A, Pettigrew NM: Sarcomatoid carcinoma (so-called pseudosarcoma) of the larynx simulating malignant giant cell tumor of soft parts: A case report. Am J Clin Pathol 82:340–343, 1984.

171. Minckler DS, Meligro CH, Norris HT: Carcinosarcoma of the larynx: Case report with metastases of epidermoid and sarcomatous elements. Cancer 26:195–200, 1970.

172. Lasser KH, Naeim F, Higgins J, et al: ''Pseudosarcoma'' of the larynx. Am J Surg Pathol 3:397–404, 1979.

173. Katholm M, Krogdahl A, Hainau B, et al: Spindle-cell carcinoma of the larynx. Acta Otolaryngol (Stockh) 98:163–166, 1984.

174. Randall G, Alonso WA, Ogura JH: Spindle-cell carcinoma (pseudosarcoma) of the larynx. Arch Otolaryngol 101:63–66, 1974.

175. Eisenbud L, Selub L, Sciubba J: Radiation-induced pseudosarcoma of the tongue. Oral Surg 53:64–68, 1982.

176. Ellis GL, Corio RL: Spindle-cell carcinoma of the oral cavity: A clinicopathologic assessment of fifty-nine cases. Oral Surg 50:523–534, 1980.

177. Leifer C, Miller AS, Putony PB, et al: Spindle-cell carcinoma of the oral mucosa: A light and electron microscopic study of apparent sarcomatous metastasis to cervical lymph nodes. Cancer 34:597–605, 1974.

178. Willis GW: Metastatic metaplastic carcinoma from a pseudosarcoma (Lane tumor) of the mouth. South Med J 70:1467–1468, 1977.

179. Deshotels SJ, Sarma D, Fazio F, et al: Squamous cell carcinoma with sarcomatoid stroma. J Surg Oncol 19:201–207, 1982.

180. Potsic WP, Raney RB, Buck BE, et al: Juvenile spindle cell carcinoma. Otolaryngol Head Neck Surg 87:573–577, 1979.

181. Srinivasan U, Talvalkar GV: True carcinosarcoma of the larynx: A case report. J Laryngol Otol 93:1031–1035, 1979.

182. Osamura RY, Shimamura K, Hata J, et al: Polypoid carcinoma of the esophagus. A unifying term for ''carcinosarcoma'' and ''pseudosarcoma.'' Am J Surg Pathol 2:201–208, 1978.

183. Kuhajda FP, Sun TT, Mendelsohn G: Polypoid squamous carcinoma of the esophagus. A case report with immunostaining for keratin. Am J Surg Pathol 7:495–499, 1983.

184. Takubo K, Tsuchiya S, Nakagawa H, et al: Pseudosarcoma of the oesophagus. Hum Pathol 13:503–505, 1982.

185. Boulay CEH, Isaacson P: Carcinoma of the oesophagus with spindle cell features. Histopathology 5:403–414, 1981.

186. Addis BJ, Corrin B: Pulmonary blastoma, carcinosarcoma and spindle-cell carcinoma: An immunohistochemical study of keratin intermediate filaments. J Pathol 147:291–301, 1985.

187. Zimmerman KG, Sobonya RE, Payne CM: Histochemical and ultrastructural features of an unusual pulmonary carcinosarcoma. Hum Pathol 12:1046–1051, 1981.

188. Wick MR, Perrone TL, Burke BA: Sarcomatoid transitional cell carcinomas of the renal pelvis. An ultrastructural and immunohistochemical study. Arch Pathol Lab Med 109:55–58, 1985.

189. Czernohilsky B, Rotenstreich L, Lancet M: Ovarian dermoid with squamous carcinoma-pseudosarcoma. Arch Pathol 93:141–144, 1972.

190. Steeper TA, Piscioli F, Rosai J: Squamous cell carcinoma with sarcoma-like stroma of the female genital tract. Cancer 52:890–898, 1983.

191. Bansal M, Kaneko M, Gordon RE: Carcinosarcoma and separate carcinoid tumor of the stomach. Cancer 50:1876–1881, 1982.

192. Radi MF, Gray GF, Scott WH: Carcinosarcoma of ileum in regional enteritis. Hum Pathol 15:385–387, 1984.

193. Leman BI, Walker PD: Sarcomatoid carcinoma of the pancreas [abstract]. Am J Clin Pathol 76:351, 1981.

194. Weidner N, Zekan P: Carcinosarcoma of the colon. Report of a unique case with light and immunohistochemical studies. Cancer 58:1126–1130, 1986.

195. Kuwano H, Iwashita A, Enjoji M: Pseudosarcomatous carcinoma of the anal canal. Dis Colon Rectum 26:123–128, 1983.

196. Azzopardi JG, Chepick OF, Hartman WH, et al: The WHO histological typing of breast tumors (second edition). Am J Clin Pathol 78:806–816, 1982.

197. Evans HL, Smith JL: Spindle cell squamous carcinomas and sarcoma-like tumors of the skin. Cancer 45:2687–2697, 1980.

198. Kuwano H, Hashimoto H, Enjoji M: Atypical fibroxanthoma distinguishable from spindle cell carcinoma in sarcomalike lesions. Cancer 55:172–180, 1985.

199. Carcangiu ML, Streeper T, Zampi G, et al: Anaplastic thyroid carcinoma. Am J Clin Pathol 83:135–158, 1985.

200. Cohen B, Green R, Iliff NT, et al: Spindle cell carcinoma of the conjunctiva. Arch Ophthalmol 98:1809–1813, 1980.

201. Auclair PL, Langloss JM, Weiss SW, et al: Sarcomas and sarcomatoid neoplasms of the major salivary gland regions. Cancer 58:1305–1315, 1986.

202. Diamandopoulos GT, Meissner WA: Neoplasia. In Kissane JM (ed): Anderson's Pathology, 8th ed. St. Louis, Mosby, 1985, pp 514–559.

203. Gould VE: Histogenesis and differentiation. A re-evaluation of these concepts as criteria for the classification of tumors. Hum Pathol 17:212–215, 1986.

204. Goellner JR, Devine KD, Weiland LH: Pseudosarcoma of the larynx. Am J Clin Pathol 59:312–326, 1973.

205. Miller D: Pseudosarcoma of the larynx. Can J Otolaryngol 4:314–318, 1975.

206. Stout AP, Lattes R: Tumors of the esophagus. In Atlas of Tumor Pathology, Section V, Fascicle 20. Washington, DC, Armed Forces Institute of Pathology, 1957, p 47.

207. Weidner N: Sarcomatoid carcinoma of the upper aerodigestive tract. Semin Diagn Pathol 4:157–168, 1987.

208. Nappi O, Wick MR: Sarcomatoid neoplasms of the respiratory tract. Semin Diagn Pathol 10:137–147, 1993.

209. Goldman RL, Weidner N: Pure squamous cell carcinoma of the larynx with cervical nodal metastasis showing rhabdomyosarcomatous differentiation. Clinical, pathologic, and immunohistochemical study of a unique example of divergent differentiation. Am J Surg Pathol 2:781–790, 1993.

210. Appelman HD, Oberman HA: Squamous cell carcinoma of the larynx with sarcoma-like stroma. Am J Clin Pathol 44:135–145, 1965.

211. Himalstein MR, Humphrey TR: Pleomorphic carcinoma of the larynx. Arch Otolaryngol 87:389–395, 1968.

212. Sherwin RP, Strong MS, Vaughn CW: Polypoid and junctional squamous cell carcinoma of the tongue and larynx with spindle cell carcinoma (''pseudosarcoma''). Cancer 16:51–60, 1963.

213. Grigg JW, Rachmaninoff N, Robb JM: Pseudosarcoma associated with squamous cell carcinoma of the larynx. Report of a case. Laryngoscope 71:555–561, 1961.

214. Ampil FL: The controversial role of radiotherapy in spindle cell carcinoma (pseudosarcoma) of the head and neck. Radiat Med 3:225–229, 1985.

215. Schmookler BM, Enzinger FM, Brannon RB: Orofacial synovial sarcoma. Cancer 50:269–276, 1982.

216. Mirra JM, Wang S, Bhuta S: Synovial sarcoma with squamous differentiation of its mesenchymal glandular elements. Am J Surg Pathol 8:791–796, 1984.

217. Fisher C: Synovial sarcoma: Ultrastructural and immunohistochemical features of epithelial differentiation in monophasic and biphasic tumors. Hum Pathol 17:996–1008, 1986.

218. Perzin KH, Panyu H, Wechter S: Nonepithelial tumors of the nasal cavity, paranasal sinuses and nasopharynx. A clinicopathologic study XII. Schwann cell tumors (neurilemoma, neurofibroma, malignant schwannoma). Cancer 50:2193–2202, 1982.

219. Perzin KH, Fu Y: Non-epithelial tumors of the nasal cavity, paranasal sinuses and nasopharynx. A clinicopathologic study XI. Fibrous histiocytomas. Cancer 45:2616–2626, 1980.

220. Godoy J, Jacobs JR, Crissman J: Malignant fibrous histiocytoma of the larynx. J Surg Oncol 31:62–65, 1986.

221. Blatchford SJ, Koopmann CF, Coulthard SW: Mucosal melanoma of the head and neck. Laryngoscope 96:929–934, 1986.

222. Reed RJ, Leonard DD: Neurotropic melanoma. Am J Surg Pathol 3:301–311, 1979.

223. Batsakis JG: Tumors of the major salivary glands. In Batsakis JG: Tumors of the Head and Neck. Clinical and Pathological Considerations, 2nd ed. Baltimore, Williams & Wilkins, 1979, pp 1–76.

224. Dardick I: Malignant myoepithelioma of parotid salivary gland. Ultrastruct Pathol 9:163–168, 1985.

225. Love GL, Sarma DP: Spindle cell mucoepidermoid carcinoma of submandibular gland. J Surg Oncol 31:66–68, 1986.

226. Shanmugaratnam K, Kunaratnam N, Chia KB, et al: Teratoid carcinosarcoma of the paranasal sinuses. Pathology 15:413–419, 1983.

227. Heffner DK, Hyams VJ: Teratocarcinosarcoma (malignant teratoma?) of the nasal cavity and paranasal sinuses. Cancer 53:2140–2154, 1984.

228. Eble JN, Hull MT, Bojrab D: Laryngeal blastoma. Am J Clin Pathol 84:378–385, 1985.

229. Compagno J, Hyams VJ, Lepore ML: Nasal polyposis with stromal atypia: Review and follow-up study of 14 cases. Arch Pathol Lab Med 100:224–226, 1976.

230. Young RH: Fibroepithelial polyp of the bladder with atypical stromal cells. Arch Pathol Lab Med 110:241–242, 1986.

231. Norris HJ, Taylor HB: Polyps of the vagina: A benign lesion resembling sarcoma botryoides. Cancer 19:227–232, 1966.

232. Weidner N, Askin FB, Berthrong M, et al: Bizarre (pseudomalignant) granulation-tissue reactions following ionizing-radiation exposure. Cancer 59:1509–1514, 1987.

233. Ro JY, Ayala AG, Ordonez NG, et al: Pseudosarcomatous fibromyxoid tumor of the urinary bladder. Am J Clin Pathol 86:583–590, 1986.

234. Kay S, Schneider V: Reactive spindle cell nodule of the endocervix simulating uterine sarcoma. Int J Gynecol Pathol 4:255–257, 1985.

235. Dahl I, Jarlstedt J: Nodular fasciitis in the head and neck. Acta Otolaryngol 90:152–159, 1980.

236. Vickery AL, Carcangiu ML, Johannessen JV, Sobrinho-Simoes M: Papillary carcinoma. Semin Diagn Pathol 2:90–100, 1985.

237. Carcangiu ML, Bianchi S: Diffuse sclerosing variant of papillary thyroid carcinoma. Clinicopathologic study of 15 cases. Am J Surg Pathol 13:1041–1049, 1989.

238. Chan JKC, Carcangiu ML, Rosai J: Papillary carcinoma of thyroid with exuberant nodular fasciitis-like stroma. Am J Clin Pathol 95:309–314, 1991.

239. Fujimoto Y, Obara T, Ito Y, et al: Diffuse sclerosing variant of papillary carcinoma of the thyroid. Cancer 66:2306–2312, 1990.

240. LiVolsi VA: Papillary neoplasms of the thyroid. Pathologic and prognostic features. Am J Clin Pathol 97:426–434, 1992.

241. Chan JKC, Albores-Saaedra J, Battifora H, et al: Sclerosing mucoepidermoid thyroid carcinoma with eosinophilia. A distinctive low-grade malignancy arising from the metaplastic follicles of Hashimoto's thyroiditis. Am J Surg Pathol 15:438–448, 1991.

242. Franssila KO, Harach HR, Wasenius V-M: Mucoepidermoid carcinoma of the thyroid. Histopathology 8:847–860, 1984.

243. LiVolsi VA: Critical commentary to mucin-producing poorly differentiated carcinoma of thyroid. Pathol Res Pract 189:613–615, 1993.

244. Chan JKC, Tse CCH: Mucin production in metastatic papillary carcinoma of the thyroid. Hum Pathol 19:195–200, 1988.

245. Mlynek M-L, Richter HJ, Leder L-D: Mucin in carcinomas of the thyroid. Cancer 56:2647–2650, 1985.

246. Rosai J, Carcangiu ML: Pitfalls in the diagnosis of thyroid neoplasms. Pathol Res Pract 182:169–179, 1987.

247. Johannessen JV, Sobrinho-Simoes M: The origin and significance of thyroid psammoma bodies. Lab Invest 43:287–296, 1980.

248. Rosai J, Saxen EA, Woolner L: Undifferentiated and poorly differentiated carcinoma. Semin Diagn Pathol 2:123–136, 1985.

249. Rosai J, Zampi G, Carcangiu ML: Papillary carcinoma of the thyroid. A discussion of its several morphologic expressions, with particular emphasis on the follicular variant. Am J Surg Pathol 7:809–817, 1983.

250. Dickersin GR, Vickery AL, Smith SB: Papillary carcinoma of the thyroid, oxyphil cell type, ''clear cell'' variant. Am J Surg Pathol 4:501–509, 1980.

251. Carcangiu ML, Shibley RK, Rosai J: Clear cell change in primary thyroid tumors. Am J Surg Pathol 9:705–722, 1985.

252. Albores-Saavedra J, Gould E, Vardaman C, Vuitch F: The macrofollicular variant of papillary thyroid carcinoma: A study of 17 cases. Hum Pathol 22:1195–1205, 1991.

253. Franssila KO, Ackerman LV, Brown CL, Hedinger CD: Follicular carcinoma. Semin Diagn Pathol 2:101–122, 1985.

254. Lang W, Choritz H, Hundeshagen H: Risk factors in follicular thyroid carcinomas. A retrospective follow-up study covering a 14 year period with emphasis on morphologic findings. Am J Surg Pathol 10:246–255, 1986.

255. van Heerden JA, Hay ID, Goellner JR, et al: Follicular thyroid carcinoma with capsular invasion alone: A nonthreatening malignancy. Surgery 112:1130–1136, 1992.

256. Evans HL: Follicular neoplasms of the thyroid. A study of 44 cases followed for a minimum of 10 years with emphasis on differential diagnosis. Cancer 54:535–540, 1984.

257. Rosai J, Carcangiu ML, DeLillis RA: Tumors of the thyroid. In Atlas of Tumor Pathology, 3rd Series. Washington, DC, Armed Forces Institute of Pathology, 1993.

258. Carney JA, Ryan J, Goellner JR: Hyalinizing trabecular adenoma of the thyroid gland. Am J Surg Pathol 11:583–591, 1987.

259. Holm R, Sobrinho-Simoes M, Nesland JM, et al: Medullary carcinoma of the thyroid gland: An immunohistochemical study. Ultrastruct Pathol 8:25–41, 1985.

260. LiVolsi VA: Medullary carcinoma. In Bennington JL (consulting ed): Surgical Pathology of the Thyroid. Vol. 22 in the Major Problems in Pathology Series. Philadelphia, WB Saunders, 1990, pp 213–252.

261. Harach HR, Wilander E, Grimelius L, et al: Chromogranin A immunoreactivity compared with argyrophilia, calcitonin immunoreactivity, and amyloid as tumour markers in the histopathologic diagnosis of medullary (C-cell) thyroid carcinoma. Pathol Res Pract 188:123–130, 1992.

262. Krisch K, Krisch I, Horvat G, et al: The value of immunohistochemistry in medullary thyroid carcinoma: A systematic study of 30 cases. Histopathology 9:1077–1089, 1985.

263. Albores-Saavedra J, LiVolsi VA, Williams ED: Medullary carcinoma. Semin Diagn Pathol 2:137–146, 1985.

264. Zaatari GS, Saigo PE, Huvos AG: Mucin production in medullary carcinoma of the thyroid. Arch Pathol Lab Med 107:70–74, 1983.

265. Dominguez-Malagon H, Delgado-Chavez R, Torres-Najera M, et al: Oxyphil and squamous variants of medullary thyroid carcinoma. Cancer 63:1183–1188, 1989.

266. Harach HR, Bergholm U: Medullary (C-cell) carcinoma of the thyroid with features of follicular oxyphilic cell tumors. Histopathology 13:645–656, 1988.

267. Bigner SH, Cox EB, Mendelsohn G, et al: Medullary carcinoma of the thyroid in the multiple endocrine neoplasia IIA syndrome. Am J Surg Pathol 5:459–472, 1981.

268. de Micco C, Chapel F, Dor AM, et al: Thyroglobulin in medullary thyroid carcinoma: Immunohistochemical study with polyclonal and monoclonal antibodies. Hum Pathol 24:256–262, 1993.

269. Kadudo K, Miyauchi A, Ogihara T, et al: Medullary carcinoma of the thyroid. Giant cell type. Arch Pathol Lab Med 102:445–447, 1987.

270. Mendelsohn G, Bigner SH, Eggleston JC, et al: Anaplastic variants of medullary thyroid carcinoma. A light-microscopic and immunohistochemical study. Am J Surg Pathol 4:333–341, 1980.

271. Harach HR, Bergholm U: Small cell variant of medullary carcinoma of the thyroid with neuroblastoma-like features. Histopathology 21:378–380, 1992.

272. Driman D, Murray D, Kovacs K, et al: Encapsulated medullary carcinoma of the thyroid. Am J Surg Pathol 15:1089–1095, 1991.

273. Beeran H, Rigaud C, Bogomoletz WV, et al: Melanin production in black medullary thyroid carcinoma (MTC). Histopathology 16:227–233, 1990.

274. Hijazi YM, Nieman LK, Medeiros J: Medullary carcinoma of the thyroid as a cause of Cushing's syndrome: A case with ectopic adrenocorticotropin secretion characterized by double enzyme immunostaining. Hum Pathol 23:592–596, 1992.

275. Aldabagh SM, Trujillo YP, Taxy JB: Occult medullary thyroid carcinoma. Unusual histologic variant presenting with metastatic disease. Am J Clin Pathol 85:247–250, 1986.

276. Sikri KL, Varndell IM, Hamid QA, et al: Medullary carcinoma of the thyroid. An immunocytochemical and histochemical study of 25 cases using eight separate markers. Cancer 56:2481–2491, 1985.

277. Mendelshohn G, Wells SA, Baylin SB: Relationship of tissue carcinoembryonic antigen and calcitonin to tumor virulence in MTC. An immunohistochemical study in early, localized, and virulent disseminated stages of disease. Cancer 54:657–662, 1984.

278. Korkolopoulou P, Papanikolaou A, Hadjiyannakis M: Proliferating cell nuclear antigen (PCNA) in medullary thyroid carcinoma. J Cancer Res Clin Oncol 119:379–381, 1993.

279. Sobrinho-Simoes M: Mixed medullary and follicular carcinoma of the thyroid. Histopathology 23:287–289, 1993.

280. LiVolsi VA: Mixed thyroid carcinoma: A real entity. Lab Invest 57:237–239, 1987.

281. Ljungberg O, Ericsson UB, Bondeson L, Thorell J: A compound follicular-parafollicular cell carcinoma of the thyroid: A new tumor entity. Cancer 52:1053–1061, 1983.

282. Hales M, Rosenau W, Okerlund MD, Galante M: Carcinoma of the thyroid with a mixed medullary and follicular pattern. Cancer 50:1352–1359, 1982.

283. Sobrinho-Simoes M, Nesland JM, Johannessen JV: Farewell to the dual histogenesis of thyroid tumors. Ultrastruct Pathol 8:iii–v, 1985.

284. Holm R, Sobrinho-Simoes M, Nesland JM, et al: Medullary thyroid carcinoma with thyroglobulin immunoreactivity. A special entity? Lab Invest 57:258–268, 1987.

285. Hedinger C, Williams E, Sobin L: Histological typing of thyroid tumours. In World Health Organization International Histological Classification of Tumours, 2nd ed. Berlin, Springer-Verlag, 1988, p 13.

286. Albores-Saavedra J, Gorraez de la Mora T, de la Torre-Rendon F, Gould E: Mixed medullary-papillary carcinoma of the thyroid: A previously unrecognized variant of thyroid carcinoma. Hum Pathol 21:1151–1155, 1990.

287. Gonzalez-Campora R, Lopez-Garrio J, Martin-Lacave I, et al: Concurrence of a symptomatic encapsulated follicular carcinoma, an occult papillary carcinoma and a medullary carcinoma in the same patient. Histopathology 21:380–382, 1992.

288. Mizukammi Y, Michigishi T, Nonomura A, et al: Mixed medullary-follicular carcinoma of the thyroid occurring in familial form. Histopathology 22:284–287, 1993.

289. Autelitano F, Santeusanio G, Tondo UD, et al: Immunohistochemical study of solid cell nests of the thyroid gland found from an autopsy study. Cancer 59:477–483, 1987.

290. Tomita T, Millard DM: C-cell hyperplasia in secondary hyperparathyroidism. Histopathology 21:469–474, 1992.

291. Libbey NP, Nowakowski KJ, Tucci JR: C-cell hyperplasia of the thyroid in a patient with goitrous hypothyroidism and Hashimoto's thyroiditis. Am J Surg Pathol 13:71–77, 1989.

292. Ulbright TM, Kraus FT, O'Neal LW: C-cell hyperplasia developing in residual thyroid following resection for sporadic medullary carcinoma. Cancer 48:2076–2079, 1981.

293. Carney JA, Sizemore GW, Hayles AB: C-cell disease of the thyroid gland in multiple endocrine neoplasia type 2b. Cancer 44:2173–2183, 1979.

294. Rosai J, Saxen EA, Woolneer L: Undifferentiated and poorly differentiated carcinoma. Semin Diagn Pathol 2:123–136, 1985.

295. Carcangiu ML, Steeper T, Zampi G, et al: Anaplastic thyroid carcinoma: A study of 70 cases. Am J Clin Pathol 83:135–158, 1985.

296. Rosai J, Carcangiu ML: Pathology of thyroid tumors: Some recent and old questions. Hum Pathol 15:1008–1012, 1984.

297. Mambo NC, Irwin SM: Anaplastic small cell neoplasms of the thyroid: An immunoperoxidase study. Hum Pathol 15:55–60, 1984.

298. Mendelsohn G, Bigner SH, Eggleston JC, et al: Anaplastic variants of medullary thyroid carcinoma: A light-microscopic and immunohistochemical study. Am J Surg Pathol 4:333–341, 1980.

299. Carcangiu ML, Zampi G, Rosai J: Poorly differentiated (''insular'') thyroid carcinoma: A reinterpretation of Langhans' ''werchernde Struma.'' Am J Surg Pathol 8:655–668, 1984.

300. Shimaoka K, Tsukada Y: Squamous cell carcinomas and adenosquamous carcinomas originating from the thyroid gland. Cancer 46:1833–1842, 1980.

301. Franssila KO, Harach HR, Wasenius V-M: Mucoepidermoid carcinoma of the thyroid. Histopathology 8:847–860, 1984.

302. Nel CJC, van Heerden JA, Goellner JR, et al: Anaplastic carcinoma of the thyroid: A clinicopathologic study of 82 cases. Mayo Clin Proc 60:51–58, 1985.

303. Getaz EP, Shimaoka K, Rao U: Anaplastic carcinoma of the thyroid following external irradiation. Cancer 43:2248–2253, 1979.

304. Kapp DS, LiVolsi VA, Sanders MM: Anaplastic carcinoma following well-differentiated thyroid cancer: Etiological considerations. Yale J Biol Med 55:521–528, 1982.

305. Lampertico P: Anaplastic (sarcomatoid) carcinoma of the thyroid gland. Semin Diagn Pathol 10:159–168, 1993.

306. Casterline PF, Jaques DA, Blom H, et al: Anaplastic giant and spindle-cell carcinoma of the thyroid: A different therapeutic approach. Cancer 45:1689–1692, 1980.

307. Oppenheim A, Miller M, Anderson GH, et al: Anaplastic thyroid cancer presenting with hyperthyroidism. Am J Med 75:702–704, 1983.

308. Martinelli G, Bazzocchi F, Gonvoni E, et al: Anaplastic type of medullary thyroid carcinoma: An ultrastructural and immunohistochemical study. Virchows Arch A 400:61–67, 1983.

309. Kriseman ACN, Bosman FT, Henegouw JCV, et al: Medullary differentiation of anaplastic thyroid carcinoma. Am J Clin Pathol 77:541–547, 1982.

310. Egloff B: The hemangioendothelioma of the thyroid. Virchows Arch A 400:119–142, 1983.

311. Miettinen M, Franssila K, Lehto V-P, et al: Expression of intermediate filament proteins in thyroid gland and thyroid tumors. Lab Invest 50:262–270, 1984.

312. Silverberg SB, DeGiorgi LS: Osteoclastoma-like giant cell tumor of the thyroid: Report of a case with prolonged survival following partial excision and radiotherapy. Cancer 31:621–625, 1973.

313. Esmaili JH, Hafez GR, Warner TFCS: Anaplastic carcinoma of the thyroid with osteoclast-like giant cells. Cancer 52:2122–2128, 1983.

314. Munoz PA, Sambasiva M, Janardan RK: Osteoclastoma-like giant cell tumor of the liver. Cancer 46:771–779, 1980.

315. Balogh K, Wolbarsht RL, Federman M, et al: Carcinoma of the parotid gland with osteoclast-like giant cells: Immunohistochemical and ultrastructural observations. Arch Pathol Lab Med 109:756–761, 1985.

316. Eusebi V, Martin SA, Govoni E, et al: Giant cell tumor of major salivary gland: Report of three cases, one occurring in association with malignant mixed tumor. Am J Clin Pathol 81:666–675, 1984.

317. Rosai J: Carcinoma of pancreas simulating giant cell tumor of bone: Electron microscopic evidence of its acinar origin. Cancer 22:333–344, 1968.

318. Sugano J, Nagao K, Kondo Y, et al: Cytologic and ultrastructural studies of a rare breast cancer with osteoclastlike giant cells. Cancer 52:74–78, 1983.
319. Oyasu R, Battifora HA, Buckingham WB, et al: Metaplastic squamous cell carcinoma of bronchus simulating giant cell tumor of bone. Cancer 39:1119–1128, 1977.
320. Kimura K, Ohnishi Y, Morishita H, et al: Giant cell tumor of the kidney. Virchows Arch A 398:357–365, 1983.
321. Andrew VC, Raitchev R, Nikolova D: Osteoclastoma of the skin. Br J Dermatol 76:40–44, 1964.
322. Abdalla MI, Hosni F: Osteoclastoma of the orbit: Case report. Br J Ophthalmol 50:95–98, 1966.
323. Dorney P: Osteoclastoma of the heart. Br Heart J 29:276–278, 1967.
324. Eshun-Wilson K: Malignant giant-cell tumour of the colon. Acta Pathol Microbiol Immunol Scand A 81:137–144, 1973.
325. Hon LT, Willis RA: Renal carcino-sarcoma, true and false. J Pathol Bacteriol 85:139–144, 1963.
326. Holz F, Fox JE, Abell MR: Carcinosarcoma of the urinary bladder. Cancer 29:294–304, 1972.
327. Bettinger HF: A giant cell tumour of bone in a pseudomucinous cystadenoma of the ovary. Br J Obstet Gynaecol 60:230–232, 1953.
328. Salon R, Sisson HA: Giant-cell tumours of soft tissues. J Pathol 107:27–39, 1972.
329. Chan JK, Rosai J: Tumors of the neck showing thymic or related branchial pouch differentiation: A unifying concept. Hum Pathol 22:349–367, 1991.
330. Eusebi V, Carcangiu ML, Dina R, Rosai J: Keratin-positive epithelioid angiosarcoma of thyroid. A report of four cases. Am J Surg Pathol 14:737–747, 1990.
331. Totsch M, Dobler G, Feichtinger H, et al: Malignant hemangioendothelioma of the thyroid. Its immunohistochemical discrimination from undifferentiated thyroid carcinoma. Am J Surg Pathol 14:69–74, 1990.
332. Banerjee SS, Eyden BP, Wells S, et al: Pseudoangiosarcomatous carcinoma: A clinicopathologic study of seven cases. Histopathology 21:13–23, 1992.
333. Wold LE, Weiland LH: Tumefactive fibroinflammatory lesions of the head and neck. Am J Surg Pathol 7:477–482, 1983.
334. Olsen KD, DeSanto LW, Wold LE, Weiland LH: Tumefactive fibroinflammatory lesions of the head and neck. Laryngoscope 96:940–944, 1986.
335. Comings DE, Skubi KB, van Eyes J, Motulsky AG: Familial multifocal fibrosclerosis. Findings suggestive that retroperitoneal fibrosis, sclerosing cholangitis, Riedel's thyroiditis, and pseudotumor of the orbit may be different manifestations of a single disease. Ann Intern Med 66:884–892, 1967.
336. Williams SB, Foss RD, Ellis GL: Inflammatory pseudotumors of the major salivary glands. Clinicopathologic and immunohistochemical analysis of six cases. Am J Surg Pathol 16:896–902, 1992.
337. Said H, Hadi AR, Akmal SN, Lokman S: Tumefactive fibroinflammatory lesions of the head and neck. J Laryngol Otol 102:1064–1067, 1988.
338. Umlas J, Federman M, Crawford C, et al: Spindle cell pseudotumors due to Mycobacterium avium-intracellulare in patients with acquired immunodeficiency syndrome (AIDS): Positive staining of mycobacteria for cytoskeleton filaments. Am J Surg Pathol 15:1181–1187, 1991.
339. Barnes L: Intestinal-type adenocarcinoma of the nasal cavity and paranasal sinuses. Am J Surg Pathol 10:192–202, 1986.
340. Batsakis JG, Mackay B, Ordonez NG: Enteric-type adenocarcinoma of the nasal cavity. Cancer 54:855–860, 1984.
341. Brinton LA, Blot WJ, Stone BJ, Fraumeni FJ: A death certificate analysis of nasal cancer among furniture workers in North Carolina. Cancer Res 37:3473–3474, 1977.
342. Klintenberg C, Olofsson J, Hellquist H, Sokjer H: Adenocarcinoma of the ethmoid sinuses. A review of 28 cases with special reference to wood dust exposure. Cancer 54:482–488, 1984.
343. Mills SE, Fechner RE, Cantrell RW: Aggressive sinonasal lesion resembling normal intestinal mucosa. Am J Surg Pathol 6:803–809, 1982.
344. Rousch GC: Epidemiology of cancer of the nose and paranasal sinuses. Currrent concepts. Head Neck Surg 2:3–11, 1979.
345. Wenig BM, Hyams VJ, Heffner DK: Nasopharyngeal papillary adenocarcinoma. A clinicopathologic study of a low-grade carcinoma. Am J Surg Pathol 12:946–953, 1988.
346. Lynch DP, Crago CA, Martinez MG: Necrotizing sialometaplasia. A review of the literature and report of two additional cases. Oral Surg 47:63–69, 1979.
347. Jensen JL: Idiopathic diseases. In Ellis GL, Auclair PL, Gnepp DR (eds): Surgical Pathology of the Salivary Glands. Philadelphia, WB Saunders, 1991, pp 60–82.
348. Walker GK, Fechner RE, Johns ME, Kuldeep T: Necrotizing sialometaplasia of the larynx secondary to atheromatous embolization. Am J Clin Pathol 77:221–223, 1982.
349. Batsakis JG, Regezi JA: Selected controversial lesions of salivary tissues. Otolaryngol Clin North Am 10:309–328, 1977.
350. Bernier JL, Bhaskar SN: Lymphoepithelial lesions of salivary glands. Histogenesis and classification based on 186 cases. Cancer 11:1165–1179, 1958.
351. Bhaskar SN, Bernier JL: Histogenesis of branchial cysts. A report of 468 cases. Am J Pathol 35:407–423, 1959.
352. Gnepp DR, Sporck FT: Benign lymphoepithelial parotid cyst with sebaceous differentiation—cystic sebaceous lymphadenoma. Am J Clin Pathol 74:683–687, 1980.
353. Gaisford JC, Anderson VS: First branchial cleft cysts and sinuses. Plast Reconstr Surg 55:299–304, 1975.
354. Olsen KD, Maragos NE, Weiland LH: First branchial cleft anomalies. Laryngoscope 90:423–436, 1980.
355. Richardson GS, Clairmont AA, Erickson ER: Cystic lesions of the parotid gland. Plast Reconstr Surg 61:364–370, 1978.
356. Shaheen NA, Harboyan GT, Nassif RI: Cysts of the parotid gland. Review and report of two unusual cases. J Laryngol Otol 89:435–444, 1975.
357. Weitzner S: Lymphoepithelial (branchial) cyst of parotid gland. Oral Surg 35:85–88, 1973.
358. Work WP: Cysts and congenital lesions of the parotid gland. Otolaryngol Clin North Am 10:339–343, 1977.
359. Buchner A, Hansen LS: Lymphoepithelial cysts of the oral cavity. A clinicopathologic study of thirty-eight cases. Oral Surg 50:441–449, 1980.
360. Hooper R, Saxon R, Tropp A: Cysts of the parotid gland. J Laryngol Otol 89:429–433, 1975.
361. Pieterse AS, Seymour AE: Parotid cysts. An analysis of 16 cases and suggested classification. Pathology 13:225–234, 1981.
362. Batsakis JG: Tumors of the Head and Neck: Clinical and Pathological Considerations. Baltimore, Williams & Wilkins, 1979, p 116.
363. Luna MA: Major salivary glands. In Karcioglu ZA, Someren A (eds): Practical Surgical Pathology. Lexington, MA, Collamore Press, 1985, p 203.
364. Rosai J: Ackerman's Surgical Pathology. St. Louis, CV Mosby, 1981, p 579.
365. Thackray AC, Lucas RB: Tumors of the major salivary glands. Washington, DC, Armed Forces Institute of Pathology, 1974, p 135.
366. Weidner N, Geisinger KR, Sterling RT, et al: Benign lymphoepithelial cysts of the parotid gland: A histologic, cytologic, and ultrastructural study. Am J Clin Pathol 85:395–401, 1986.
367. Smith A, Winkler B, Perzin KH, et al: Mucoepidermoid carcinoma arising in an intraparotid lymph node. Cancer 55:400–403, 1985.
368. Evans HL: Mucoepidermoid carcinoma of salivary glands: A study of 69 cases with special attention to histologic grading. Am J Clin Pathol 81:696–701, 1984.
369. Foote FW, Frazel EL: Tumors of the major salivary glands. Cancer 6:1065–1133, 1953.
370. Stewart FW, Foote FW, Becker WF: Muco-epidermoid tumors of salivary glands. Ann Surg 122:820–844, 1945.
371. Zajicek J, Eneroth CM, Jakobsson P: Aspiration biopsy of salivary gland tumors. VI. Morphologic studies on smears and histologic sections from mucoepidermoid carcinoma. Acta Cytol 20:35–41, 1976.
372. Seifert G, Bull HG, Donath K: Histologic subclassification of the cystadenolymphoma of the parotid gland. Analysis of 275 cases. Virchows Arch A 388:13–38, 1980.
373. Eneroth CM, Zajicek J: Aspiration biopsy of salivary gland tumors. II. Morphologic studies on smears and histologic sections from oncocytic tumors. Acta Cytol 9:355–361, 1965.
374. Faverly DR, Manni JJ, Smedts AAJ, et al: Adeno-carcinoid or amphicrine tumors of the middle ear a new entity? Pathol Res Pract 188:162–171, 1992.
375. Heffner DK: Low-grade adenocarcinoma of probable endolymphatic sac origin. A clinicopathologic study of 20 cases. Cancer 64:2292–2302, 1989.
376. Hosoda S, Tateno H, Inoue HK, et al: Carcinoid tumor of the middle ear containing serotonin and multiple peptide hormones. A case report and review of the pathology literature. Acta Pathol Jpn 42:614–620, 1992.
377. Mills SE, Fechner RE: Middle ear adenoma. A cytologically uniform neoplasm displaying a variety of architectural patterns. Am J Surg Pathol 8:677–685, 1984.
378. Gaffey MJ, Mills SE, Fechner RE, et al: Aggressive papillary middle-ear tumor. A clinicopathologic entity distinct from middle-ear adenoma. Am J Surg Pathol 12:790–797, 1988.
379. Stanley MW, Horwitz CA, Levinson RM, Sibley RK: Carcinoid tumors of the middle-ear. Am J Clin Pathol 87:592–600, 1987.
380. Murphy GF, Pilch BZ, Dickersin GR, et al: Carcinoid tumor of the middle-ear. Am J Clin Pathol 73:816–823, 1980.
381. Kartush JM, Graham MD: Salivary gland choristoma of the middle ear: A case report and review of the literature. Laryngoscope 94:228–230, 1984.
382. Wenig BM, Abbondanzo SL, Childers EL, et al: Extranodal sinus histiocytosis with massive lymphadenopathy (Rosai-Dorfman disease) on the head and neck. Hum Pathol 24:483–492, 1993.
383. Brugler G: Tumors presenting as aural polyps: A report of four cases. Pathology 24:315–319, 1992.
384. Weidner N, Bar RS, Weiss D, Strottmann P: Neoplastic pathology of oncogenic osteomalacia-rickets. Cancer 55:1691–1695, 1985.
385. Weidner N, Santa Cruz D: Phosphaturic mesenchymal tumors, a polymorphous group causing osteomalacia-rickets. Cancer 59:1442–1454, 1987.
386. Weidner N: Review and update: Oncogenic osteomalacia-rickets. Ultrastruct Pathol 15:317–333, 1991.
387. Seifert G, Hennings K, Caselitz J: Metastatic tumors to the parotid and submandibular glands: Analysis and differential diagnosis of 108 cases. Pathol Res Pract 181:684–692, 1986.
388. van Krieken JH: Prostate marker immunoreactivity in salivary gland neoplasms. A rare pitfall in immunohistochemistry. Am J Surg Pathol 17:410–414, 1993.
389. Theaker JM: Extramammary Paget's disease of the oral mucosa with in situ carcinoma of minor salivary gland ducts. Am J Surg Pathol 12:890–895, 1988.

CHAPTER 3

Pulmonary System*

Cesar A. Moran, M.D.

It is common knowledge that lung cancer is one of the leading causes of death in the United States. Even though we are familiar with the most common types of tumors that occur primarily in the lung (i.e., adenocarcinoma, squamous cell carcinoma, undifferentiated large-cell carcinoma, and small-cell carcinoma), there is an extensive array of other tumors, both benign and malignant, that can appear as primary in the lung. These tumors include epithelial, mesenchymal, mixed epithelial/mesenchymal, and other rare entities that, in any given situation, may give rise to problems in diagnosis. It is important to mention the great limitations in diagnosing when a small lung biopsy is obtained. In most circumstances a patient undergoes a lung biopsy as a result of a pulmonary nodule or mass, and the pathologist usually is compelled to provide a diagnosis even though the material obtained is far from ideal for a definitive diagnosis.

In this chapter, several conditions are reviewed that deserve attention in order to properly confront a lung biopsy. Needless to say, in a number of cases, one can only suggest the diagnosis, and a more definitive approach such as complete resection will need to be undertaken before a final diagnosis is rendered. Although in most instances a good hematoxylin-eosin–stained section will suffice, immunohistochemical studies are recommended when one is in doubt about the nature of the neoplasm. Performing further studies such as electron microscopy, flow cytometry, or other more sophisticated analyses should be weighed against the contribution that they may bring in the solution of the problem, which is essentially one of diagnosis for specific treatment. Therefore, many sophisticated studies will play a minor role in the diagnosis.

The emphasis in this chapter, therefore, is on a morphologic approach correlated with the clinical presentation and, in some instances, supported by the use of immunohistochemical studies and electron microscopy.

EPITHELIAL NEOPLASMS

Mucinous (So-Called Colloid) Carcinoma

The existence of primary tumors of the lung characterized by abundant mucus deposition is rare. Terms such as **muci-** **nous carcinoma** or **colloid carcinoma** have not been incorporated in previous classifications of the World Health Organization (WHO).[1] However, a few reports dealing with these tumors have been presented in the literature.[2–4] It has been postulated that these tumors represent a **variant of bronchioloalveolar carcinoma.** Whether these tumors constitute a specific entity or part of the spectrum of differentiation of tumors reported as cystadenomas or cystic tumors of borderline malignancy is still controversial. Nonetheless, it is important to mention that when these tumors are discovered in early stages, their behavior appears to be less aggressive than that of late lesions.

CLINICAL FEATURES. In our study of 24 cases, the patients varied in age from 33 to 81 years. However, more than 80% of patients were older than 40 years.[2] No sex predilection and no specific anatomic site were observed. The tumor was found on a routine physical examination in all patients. Radiographic studies revealed a peripheral lung nodule in 50% of the cases. Nonetheless, the tumor may not be limited to one lobe and, in a few instances, may involve more than one lobe.

GROSS FEATURES. The tumors are usually ill-defined, soft, mucoid, tan-to-brown neoplasms. Their size may vary from less than 1 cm to 1 cm. No cystic structures were described grossly in any of our cases, yet this feature may be an important characteristic in order to separate these tumors from others described as cystadenomas or cystic tumors of borderline malignancy.[3, 4]

HISTOLOGIC FEATURES. The most important characteristic of these tumors is the presence of an overwhelming production of mucus. In some instances, this feature obscures the neoplastic nature of this lesion. The presence of abundant mucin generally obliterates the normal architecture of the lung parenchyma (Fig. 3–1); however, clusters of malignant cells or single malignant cells with large nuclei, prominent nucleoli, and increased nucleocytoplasmic (N/C) ratio are seen floating in the mucus. Some of the single cells may have the appearance of signet ring cells; in other areas, it is possible to note foci of columnar, mucin-secreting epithelium lining the lung alveoli (Figs. 3–2 and 3–3). In a minority of cases, more solid areas with the typical characteristics of adenocarcinoma merging with the "colloid" areas are seen. The mucin deposition is strongly positive with predigested periodic acid-Schiff (PAS)–stained sections. Immunohistochemical studies are noncontributory in these cases, because once the neoplastic areas are found, there is little doubt as to the true nature of the lesion.

The outcome of these tumors depends largely on the stage at which they are found. Even though we could not reach a

---

* The opinions herein expressed are the private views of the author and do not reflect the views of the U.S. Department of the Air Force or the Department of Defense.

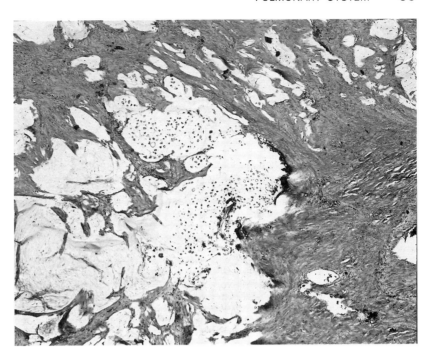

FIGURE 3-1. Colloid carcinoma showing destruction of the pulmonary parenchyma. Note the abundant mucus deposition.

firm correlation between size of the tumor and prognosis in our cases, it is logical to believe that smaller tumors without lymph node metastases will do better. This was supported by the follow-up obtained in some of the cases in our study.

DIFFERENTIAL DIAGNOSIS. The most important diagnosis for these tumors is a **metastasis from a mucin-secreting carcinoma** arising in a location at which these tumors are far more common, i.e., breast, gastrointestinal tract, or ovary.[5, 6] Therefore, a close clinical evaluation is important before rendering the diagnosis of primary lung neoplasm. On the other hand, for those who consider these tumors part of the spectrum of mucinous lesions, cystadenomas and cystic tumors of bor-

derline malignancy may be important differential diagnoses. These last two conditions may prove to be very difficult to differentiate on histopathologic grounds. It is our view that all these tumors should be seen as a variant of bronchioloalveolar carcinoma with the potential to metastasize, as has been proved by our study.

Basaloid Carcinoma

This is a relatively uncommon neoplasm in its pure form (pure basaloid). In a review of 115 lung carcinomas over a

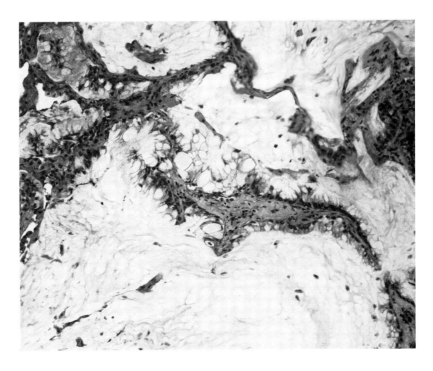

FIGURE 3-2. Colloid carcinoma showing mucin-secreting epithelium lining the alveolar wall.

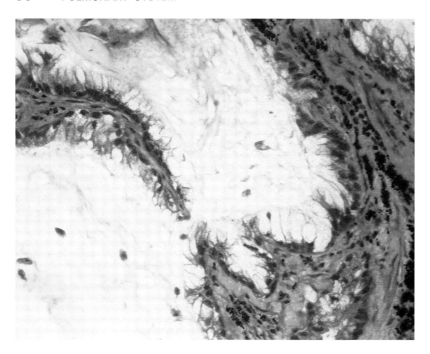

FIGURE 3–3. Mucin-secreting epithelium lining the alveolar wall with abundant mucus deposition.

7-year period, Brambilla et al.[7] described 38 cases of basaloid carcinoma, of which 19 were pure basaloid carcinoma. The authors noted that this histologic feature may also be seen in association with other more conventional tumors such as squamous cell carcinoma or large-cell carcinoma. The latter observation has also been shared by us. In a large number of non–small-cell carcinomas, careful examination may lead to the finding of focal areas of "basaloid" carcinoma. Nonetheless, Brambilla et al.[7] believe that this type of lung carcinoma deserves to be separated from other types in view of the poor prognosis that it conveys.

CLINICAL FEATURES. There appears to be a predominance for males and for the lobar or segmental bronchi in these tumors. The age of presentation varies from 36 to 79 years,

with a median age of 60 years. Most of the patients are in stage I of the disease, whereas fewer cases are in stage III.

GROSS FEATURES. The tumor may present as an exophytic endobronchial lesion and may vary from 1 to 6 cm in greatest diameter.

HISTOLOGIC FEATURES. The hallmark for the diagnosis of this tumor is the presence of islands of tumor composed of medium-sized cells with an oval or spindle appearance, scant cytoplasm, and prominent nucleoli with **peripheral palisading** (Figs. 3–4 and 3–5). These islands are separated by fibro-connective tissue, which imparts a rather lobular pattern to the tumor on scanning magnification. The mitotic rate may be high. Immunohistochemical studies for keratin demonstrate the epithelial nature of this neoplasm, and the presence of

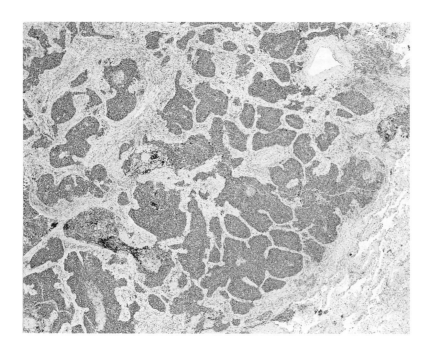

FIGURE 3–4. Numerous islands of malignant cells in a basaloid carcinoma.

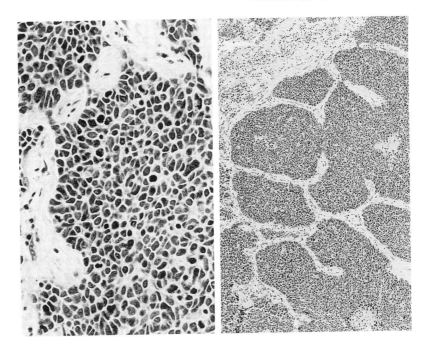

FIGURE 3–5. *Right,* Islands of epithelial cells separated by fibroconnective tissue. *Left,* A closer view of the cellular detail of a basaloid carcinoma composed of relatively larger cells with round to oval nuclei and some cells with prominent nucleoli.

desmosomes and/or tonofilaments with electron microscopy supports such an interpretation.

The outcome for patients with this type of tumor seems to be rather poor, because they metastasize in approximately 80% of the cases.[7]

DIFFERENTIAL DIAGNOSIS. An important differential diagnosis is that of a **metastatic basal-cell carcinoma** from the head-and-neck area or a **cloacogenic carcinoma.**[8–11] These two conditions can be excluded by a careful clinical evaluation of the patient. Another tumor that may be confused with this entity is a **large-cell neuroendocrine carcinoma.** In the latter case, immunohistochemical studies using neuroendocrine markers for chromogranin, synaptophysin, and Leu-7 are of most value in arriving at a correct diagnosis.

Small-Cell Carcinoma

This type of tumor accounts for approximately 20% of primary lung malignancies.[12, 13] They carry a poor prognosis, mainly owing to their rapid growth and widespread metastases. Small-cell carcinomas have been linked to cigarette smoking.[14, 15] Even though immunohistochemical and ultrastructural studies may be used as an aid in diagnosis, in the ultimate analysis, the diagnosis is made by conventional light microscopy.

CLINICAL FEATURES. Small-cell carcinomas occur essentially in adult individuals in the fifth or sixth decade of life. Although at one time the ratio of men to women showed a male predominance, it is now being narrowed to about 2:1. This increase in the incidence in the female population may be due to increased smoking in this group. Small-cell carcinomas are central lesions in about 90% of cases. They are usually found in lobar or mainstem bronchi growing in the submucosa or along the peribronchial connective tissue. Peripheral tumors may be seen, and they are usually accompanied by lymph node or mediastinal involvement. Cough, dyspnea, hemoptysis, or other symptoms related to obstruction may be seen in patients with small-cell carcinoma. When the tumor is in an advanced stage (namely when it is invading mediastinal structures), the symptomatology may become more dramatic, exhibiting superior vena cava syndrome among others. Other symptoms that have been associated with small-cell carcinoma include inappropriate secretion of antidiuretic hormone and Cushing's syndrome. Radiographically, the most common presentation is that of a hilar or perihilar mass often associated with mediastinal widening.[16, 17]

GROSS FEATURES. It is difficult to truly assess the gross features of this tumor, because theoretically no tumor resection is performed in view of the treatment used for these tumors. Therefore, most of the gross characteristics are usually found in autopsy material and after the patient has been treated with radiation and/or chemotherapy.

HISTOLOGIC FEATURES. At low power, the most striking feature is the **crush artifact** that is consistently seen in transbronchial biopsies. When the biopsy is more extensive, areas of necrosis may be seen in association with the tumor cells. The tumors are composed of a **homogeneous cell population forming sheaths of cells with scant cytoplasm, finely dispersed chromatin (so-called salt and pepper), round to oval nuclei, and rather inconspicuous nucleoli. Mitoses are very common.** Rarely does the tumor show a nesting pattern, ductules, or ribbons.

By immunohistochemistry, the tumor cells may show positive reaction for keratin, neuron-specific enolase (NSE), chromogranin, synaptophysin, and Leu-7. Nonetheless, these neuroendocrine markers show only focal and weakly positive reaction. In a number of cases, all immunohistochemical markers may turn out to be negative (including keratin).

UNUSUAL VARIANTS. Mixed small-cell and large-cell carcinoma (SC/LC) is a rare presentation for either small-cell carcinomas or large-cell carcinomas. However, it has been estimated that approximately less than 5% of tumors may have this distinct combination.[18] Histologically, these tumors show areas of conventional small-cell carcinoma with areas of rather larger cells with or without an organoid pattern. The large-cell component may at times be difficult to distinguish from the small-cell component. Nonetheless, the presence of rather larger cells with moderate amounts of cytoplasm, round nuclei, and prominent nucleoli is diagnostic for this component. The prognosis of this tumor probably does not differ significantly from that of the small-cell carcinoma.

Another combination of small-cell carcinoma is with a conventional non–small-cell tumor such as squamous cell carcinoma, adenocarcinoma, or spindle cell carcinoma.[18, 19] However, this association is rather infrequent. The histologic features are those of combined conventional carcinomas.

DIFFERENTIAL DIAGNOSIS. The tumors that may be confused with a small-cell carcinoma are, in essence, **lymphocytic lymphoma** and **primitive neuroectodermal tumor.** These entities may also occur primarily as lung tumors. In lymphocytic lymphoma, the presence of crush artifact, nuclear molding, and high mitotic activity are useful discriminants. In addition, the negative keratin and positive leukocyte common antigen (LCA) reaction are more in keeping with the diagnosis of lymphoma. In primitive neuroectodermal tumor, the morphologic features may not be so obvious. The presence of rosettes and more extensive areas of hemorrhage are useful features. In addition, the presence of abundant quantities of glycogen by PAS histochemical stain and negative results for epithelial and neuroendocrine markers also help differentiate these tumors. In addition, a **carcinoid** may be confused with small-cell carcinoma. However, the presence of cellular atypia, high mitotic index, crush artifact, necrosis, and hemorrhage are features more often seen in small-cell carcinoma. In addition, immunohistochemical stains using neuroendocrine markers (chromogranin, synaptophysin, and Leu-7) show a much stronger positive reaction in carcinoids.

Large-Cell Neuroendocrine Carcinoma

This tumor in essence **represents a poorly differentiated carcinoma with a characteristic organoid pattern under light microscopy.** The tumor is uncommon and probably represents what used to be called in previous reports **"intermediate-cell carcinoma."**[20, 21] However, it is currently recognized as a separate category in the spectrum of neuroendocrine neoplasms.[22]

CLINICAL FEATURES. The tumor does not have sex predilection and is common in adult individuals in the sixth decade of life. Its presence appears to correlate with cigarette smoking, and unlike with other neuroendocrine neoplasms, ectopic hormone production has not been reported thus far.

GROSS FEATURES. There are no gross pathologic features that allow distinction of this tumor from other neoplasms. The tumors may vary in size from a few centimeters to up to 8 to 10 cm in greatest dimension. As with other high-grade neoplasms, areas of hemorrhage and/or necrosis may be seen. The tumor is unencapsulated but may be well circumscribed. Central location is more often seen; however, peripheral tumors may be encountered.

HISTOLOGIC FEATURES. The low-power appearance of this tumor is that of an organoid tumor with a trabecular growth pattern (Fig. 3–6). The tumor cells are a little larger than in regular small-cell carcinoma and often show more cytoplasm and prominent nucleoli (Fig. 3–7). The mitotic rate is high, and areas of necrosis and/or hemorrhage are often seen. Areas showing rosette-like structures are also frequently observed.

Immunohistochemical studies using neuroendocrine markers including chromogranin, synaptophysin, adrenocorticotropic hormone (ACTH), and calcitonin are useful in arriving at a correct interpretation. Dense core granules may be seen using ultrastructural studies.[22]

Regarding the behavior of these tumors, **it is logical to believe that they carry a prognosis similar to that of small-cell carcinomas.** However, a more comprehensive study in a large number of cases is necessary to evaluate the natural course of these neoplasms.

DIFFERENTIAL DIAGNOSIS. The differential diagnosis of these tumors may be a wide one, because they can be confused with tumors such as a **poorly differentiated adenocarcinoma, large-cell carcinoma with neuroendocrine features, small-cell carcinoma, or basaloid carcinoma.** In this con-

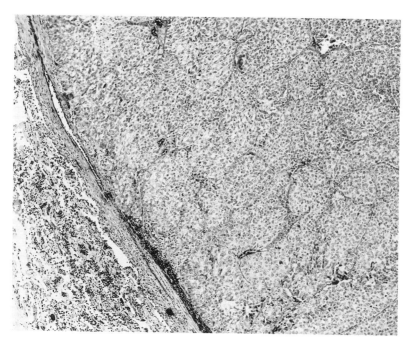

FIGURE 3–6. Low-power view of a large-cell neuroendocrine carcinoma showing nesting pattern.

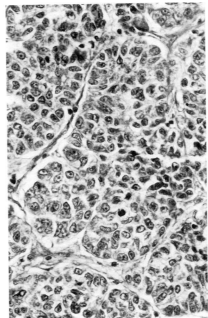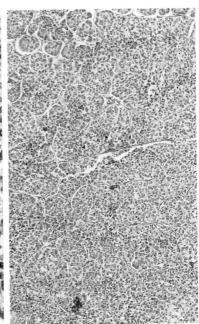

FIGURE 3–7. *Right,* The characteristic nesting pattern of a large-cell neuroendocrine carcinoma. *Left,* Closer view of the cellular detail composed of rather larger cells with moderate amount of cytoplasm, round to oval nuclei, and prominent nucleoli.

text, the careful evaluation of the histologic features of the neoplasm coupled with positive staining for neuroendocrine markers will lead to the correct diagnosis.

Atypical Carcinoid

Carcinoid tumors are generally believed to represent a low-grade malignant neoplasm. However, cases of atypical carcinoid are considered to have a more aggressive behavior.[23] Therefore, it is important to separate atypical carcinoids from the conventional **carcinoid tumor.**

CLINICAL FEATURES. The symptomatology in these tumors is not different from that of other endobronchial lesions and may present with symptoms of obstructive pneumonia, hemoptysis, and/or dyspnea.[24] As with other neuroendocrine neoplasms, ectopic production of hormones may be seen, leading to conditions such as Cushing's syndrome or carcinoid syndrome.[25, 26]

GROSS FEATURES. Carcinoid tumors can be found either centrally or peripherally. In their central location, they are usually endobronchial, polypoid lesions. The presence of a large tumor with hemorrhage or necrosis should alert one to the possibility of an atypical carcinoid. These latter features probably represent the most important gross features to differentiate typical from atypical carcinoids.

HISTOLOGIC FEATURES. The hallmark of these tumors is their organoid pattern (Fig. 3–8). The cell population appears to be homogeneous and composed of rather small cells with eosinophilic cytoplasm and round nuclei with finely dispersed chromatin. However, a closer view of these tumors shows areas of cellular pleomorphism, mitotic activity (5–10 mitoses × 10 HPF) (Fig. 3–9), necrosis, and/or hemorrhage. Morphologically, these features alone are the most important to separate atypical from conventional carcinoid tumors. Other histologic growth patterns that may occur in these tumors include the **oncocytic variant,** which is composed of cells with abundant eosinophilic cytoplasm, thus the term oncocytic. Another variant of carcinoids is the one termed **melano-**

cytic carcinoids, characterized by a conventional growth pattern with areas of pigment deposition, mimicking a malignant melanoma. However, immunohistochemical stains prove the neuroendocrine nature of these tumors.

The behavior of atypical carcinoids is more aggressive than that of the conventional carcinoid tumor. Therefore, correct diagnosis is clinically relevant. The mortality reported in some studies varies but is higher than in conventional carcinoid.[24, 27]

Immunohistochemical studies using neuroendocrine markers including chromogranin, synaptophysin, and calcitonin are useful in arriving at a correct diagnosis. Ultrastructural studies can also be helpful. The presence of dense core granules confirms the neuroendocrine nature of these tumors.

DIFFERENTIAL DIAGNOSIS. The most important differential diagnosis is from a conventional **carcinoid** and from **small-cell carcinoma.** The distinction from the former should be based on the presence of cellular pleomorphism, high mitotic count, hemorrhage, and/or necrosis. The distinction from a small-cell carcinoma may be more subtle. In small-cell carcinoma, there is marked cellular anaplasia and cellular pleomorphism with a high mitotic count, often as high as 20 or more mitoses per 10 HPF. Immunohistochemical studies using neuroendocrine markers may help in the distinction from small-cell carcinoma. Whereas small-cell carcinomas usually show only a focal and weak positive reaction for these markers, atypical carcinoids show more marked and diffuse positivity. Immunohistochemical studies to differentiate atypical carcinoid from the conventional carcinoid are of no help, because both tumors may show a strong positive reaction for neuroendocrine markers.

Pleomorphic Carcinoma

This subset of tumors **encompasses a mixture of histologic growth patterns, including the spindle cell carcinoma and giant cell carcinoma.** However, the term **pleomorphic carcinoma** attempts to further categorize those tumors that would

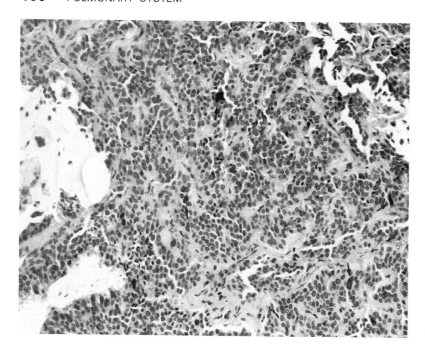

FIGURE 3–8. Atypical carcinoid showing areas of more conventional carcinoid; however, there is focal cellular atypia *(arrows).*

otherwise be labeled as **sarcomatoid carcinoma, giant cell carcinoma with sarcomatous stroma, or large-cell carcinoma with giant cell features and sarcomatous components.**[28–34]

CLINICAL FEATURES. The tumor is seen in adults and more often in the sixth decade of life, with slight male predilection of approximately 2:1. Chest pain, cough, or hemoptysis may be the presenting symptoms. However, asymptomatic patients may also be seen. In more than 25% of cases, the tumor is of a high clinical stage at presentation.

GROSS FEATURES. The majority of these tumors present as solitary masses that may vary from a few centimeters to more than 10 cm in greatest dimension. The tumors are white or yellow-tan, with or without hemorrhage or necrosis. In more

than 60% of cases, they may have a peripheral location. However, endobronchial tumors may also be found.

HISTOLOGIC FEATURES. The hallmark of these tumors is the presence of a **mixture of spindle cell and giant cells** (Fig. 3–10). The spindle cell component shows elongated cells with moderate amounts of eosinophilic cytoplasm, which are arranged in fascicles or storiform pattern giving the impression of a sarcoma. The giant cell component contains multinucleated cells showing different degrees of anaplasia and often showing bizarre forms. These giant cells may be seen in clusters or distributed haphazardly, admixed with the undifferentiated large-cell carcinoma or the spindle cell component. **In some cases, one can observe conventional areas of adenocarcinoma or squamous cell**

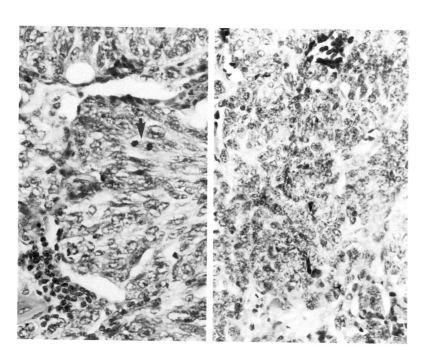

FIGURE 3–9. *Right,* Atypical carcinoid showing marked cellular atypia. *Left,* Mitoses are present *(arrow).*

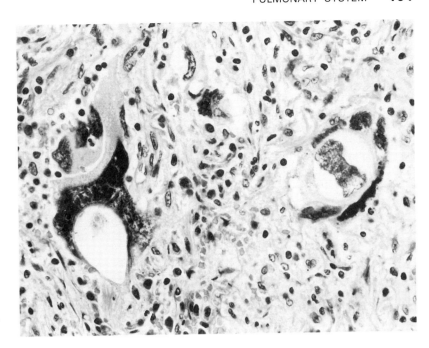

FIGURE 3–10. Numerous giant cells are present in this pleomorphic carcinoma.

carcinoma. **In rare cases, it is possible to see a small-cell carcinomatous component.** Nonetheless, the predominant features are those of a mixed spindle cell and giant cell carcinoma. Areas of necrosis and/or hemorrhage may be seen in these tumors.

Immunohistochemically, the presence of positive reaction for epithelial markers, including keratin and epithelial membrane antigen (EMA), is helpful in arriving at a correct interpretation. Vimentin antibodies may also be positive in these tumors.

The survival of patients with pleomorphic carcinoma is in essence linked to staging. In our study, the prognosis of the patients with this tumor was rather poor, with a median survival of 10 months and only 10% surviving 5 years.

DIFFERENTIAL DIAGNOSIS. The most important differential diagnosis is that of a sarcomatous lesion, namely **malignant fibrous histiocytoma** or a **high-grade leiomyosarcoma.** These two sarcomatous tumors may be easily ruled out by the presence of a positive reaction of tumor cells for epithelial markers (keratin-EMA) and negative results for desmin and/or smooth muscle actin. In cases of malignant fibrous histiocytoma (MFH), one should expect to find a more prominent storiform pattern with numerous giant cells of the Touton type and negative results for keratin and EMA.

Adenosquamous Carcinoma

As its name implies, this tumor is composed of an admixture of adenocarcinoma and a squamous cell carcinoma. However, no definitive criteria exist as to the amount of each component in order to make this diagnosis. This tumor is rare and probably represents fewer than 5% of all tumors of the lung.[35–40]

CLINICAL FEATURES. This tumor is more common in adults in their fifth or sixth decade of life. There appears to be a male predominance for this tumor. In a large series of cases, more than 70% of the tumors were found in male patients.[38] A history of smoking is obtained in more than 90% of the patients. Clinically, the patients may present with symptoms of hemoptysis, dyspnea, weight loss, anorexia, etc. There appears not to be a predilection for any particular lobe or lung.

GROSS FEATURES. These tumors have no special characteristics that allow gross distinction from other non–small-cell carcinomas. Nonetheless, they are more often peripheral in location.[36]

HISTOLOGIC FEATURES. The hallmark of this tumor is the **presence of a bona fide squamous cell carcinoma with its characteristic histology (i.e., intercellular bridges, keratinization, and so forth) and the presence of an adenocarcinoma with its typical features (i.e., glandular, acinar, or papillary proliferation with presence of intracellular and extracellular mucin).** These two components may be intermixed or may be separated. On rare occasions, this tumor may show an amyloid-like stroma.[41]

Immunohistochemical studies are rarely used in the diagnosis of this tumor, because the diagnosis of this lesion is essentially a morphologic one. However, in the cases reported with amyloid stroma, the cells may show positivity for antibodies against keratin, EMA, vimentin, and S-100 protein. In view of these latter results, it is possible that this particular variant of adenosquamous carcinoma may be more closely related to salivary gland–like tumors.

Although survival may be related to stage, it has been claimed that these tumors have a worse prognosis than conventional adenocarcinomas or squamous cell carcinomas.[37]

DIFFERENTIAL DIAGNOSIS. The most important differential diagnosis of these tumors is that of **high-grade mucoepidermoid carcinoma.** However, the finding of a peripheral lesion and absence of low-grade areas of mucoepidermoid carcinoma leads to the correct interpretation.

MIXED EPITHELIAL AND MESENCHYMAL TUMORS

The presence of intrapulmonary tumors showing a mixture of epithelial and mesenchymal elements is rare, but when encountered, may pose a problem in diagnosis. Among the most common tumors of this type are **pulmonary blastoma** and **carcinosarcoma.**

Pulmonary Blastoma

This tumor is **also known as a well-differentiated fetal adenocarcinoma, pulmonary endodermal tumor resembling fetal lung, well-differentiated adenocarcinoma simulating fetal lung tubules, and pulmonary adenocarcinoma of fetal type.**[42-44] Pulmonary blastomas account for fewer than 1% of all primary intrapulmonary tumors.[45, 46]

CLINICAL FEATURES. There is no sex predilection for this tumor, and it usually occurs in adults. In more than 75% of patients, a history of smoking is obtained.[43, 47] Clinically, the patients may present with cough, chest pain, and/or hemoptysis. However, about 25% of the patients may be asymptomatic.[43]

GROSS FEATURES. Blastomas typically present as solitary tumors. They are white to tan soft tissue masses that may vary in size from a few centimeters to over 20 cm in greatest dimension. They are not encapsulated and may show cystic structures and hemorrhagic areas. On rare occasions, the tumor may present as a bronchial lesion.

HISTOLOGIC FEATURES. On scanning magnification, the typical pattern is that of a proliferation of glandular elements obliterating the normal lung parenchyma (Fig. 3–11). These glandular elements are distributed in a back-to-back or cribriform pattern. The gland-like structures are composed of a non-ciliated, pseudostratified epithelium with cells showing round nuclei and clear cytoplasm, often with subnuclear vacuolization resembling fetal lung epithelium in weeks 9 to 11 of gestation (Fig. 3–12). Rosette-like structures may occasionally be seen. The stromal background where these glandular structures are embedded may show a distinct cellular proliferation. A sarcomatous component containing predominantly

atypical spindle cells is often seen. **"Morules" (small balls of epithelial-looking cells) are commonly seen in blastomas,** and their presence is an important feature for diagnosis. Less often one can see numerous multinucleated syncytiotrophoblast-like giant cells distributed haphazardly in the stroma. Necrosis and mitoses are commonly encountered in the epithelial component of the tumor. However, the presence of mitoses does not appear to correlate with the prognosis of the tumor. **One important histologic feature of blastomas is the so-called hepatoid growth pattern, which resembles a yolk sac tumor of the gonads, i.e., small tubules embedded in a myxoid stroma composed of rather small cells with vacuolated cytoplasm.** However, in very rare instances, actual liver tissue may be seen. It is also important to mention that in a small number of cases, one can find immature cartilage and muscle. Nonetheless, the presence of these features should not be interpreted as evidence of **carcinosarcoma** or other mesenchymal tumor.

Histochemically, PAS stain shows abundant glycogen. However, mucin stains (mucicarmine and periodic acid–Schiff after diastase [DPAS]) are usually negative at the intracellular level. Immunohistochemically, blastomas may show positive reaction against antibodies for chromogranin and neuron specific enolase in the glandular (epithelial) component of the tumor and in the morules.[43] Other immunohistochemical stains used include keratin, carcinoembryonic antigen (CEA), EMA, and alpha-fetoprotein. In biphasic blastomas with a sarcomatous component, desmin, muscle-specific actin, myoglobin, and/or S-100 protein may be used to further delineate the sarcomatous component.

The treatment of choice for pulmonary blastomas appears to be surgical resection. However, when metastases are present, co-adjuvant therapy in the form of chemotherapy may be used. The prognosis for these tumors depends largely on the stage at which they are diagnosed. However, tumors showing a biphasic component with sarcomatous elements seem to have a poor prognosis.[43, 45]

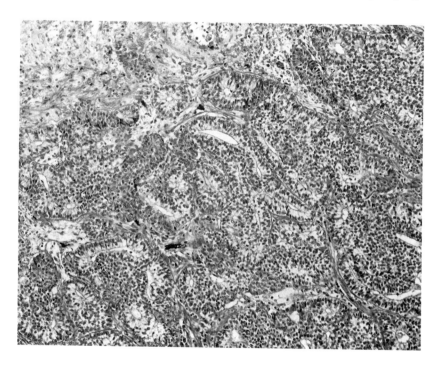

FIGURE 3–11. Pulmonary blastoma showing a glandular proliferation resembling fetal lung.

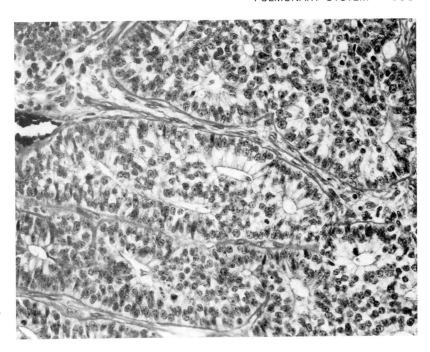

FIGURE 3–12. Closer view of the glandular proliferation in a pulmonary blastoma showing a non-ciliated, pseudostratified epithelium.

DIFFERENTIAL DIAGNOSIS. Pulmonary blastomas may be confused with primary as well as with metastatic neoplasms of the lung. A **well-differentiated adenocarcinoma with clear-cell features** may be confused with a pulmonary blastoma. However, the presence of an endometrioid-like appearance and the presence of morules, cartilage, or muscle should lead to a correct interpretation. **Carcinosarcoma** is another tumor that may be mistaken for pulmonary blastoma. In carcinosarcomas of the lung, however, one should expect to see malignant cartilage, bone, or muscle in association with typical areas of adenocarcinoma or squamous cell carcinoma with absence of fetal or embryonic type of proliferation. Lastly, the occurrence of a metastasis from a possible female genital tract source should be investigated by careful clinical evaluation.

Carcinosarcoma

As the name implies, **carcinosarcomas are neoplasms composed of two different cell lines: one, a well-defined carcinoma (i.e., squamous cell carcinoma or adenocarcinoma), and the other, a mesenchymal neoplasm (i.e., rhabdomyosarcoma, leiomyosarcoma, osteosarcoma, and/or chondrosarcoma).** These are rare neoplasms that may represent less than 0.5% of lung malignancies.[48] More recently, the term **biphasic sarcomatoid carcinoma** has been proposed for these tumors.[49]

CLINICAL FEATURES. Although much of what has been reported in the literature may include a variety of tumors that by today's standards would not fit into the category of carcinosarcomas, it is believed that carcinosarcoma affects more often adult men than women who are middle-aged and smokers.[50–54] Clinically, the symptoms depend on the anatomic site of the tumor. When the tumor is in an endobronchial location, symptoms related to obstruction such as cough, dyspnea, and hemoptysis may be encountered.

GROSS FEATURES. The tumor may present as a solitary, well-circumscribed, peripheral mass or as an endobronchial tumor. When peripheral, the tendency of the tumor is to invade pleura and chest wall. The tumor is often a white-gray mass with areas of necrosis and hemorrhage. The size of the tumor may vary from a couple of centimeters to more than 6 cm in greatest dimension.

HISTOLOGIC FEATURES. The combination of a well-defined squamous cell carcinoma or an adenocarcinoma with a well-defined osteosarcoma, chondrosarcoma, leiomyosarcoma or rhabdomyosarcoma is the hallmark of these tumors (Figs. 3–13 and 3–14). Once these two components are identified, the diagnosis of carcinosarcoma is confirmed. Immunohistochemically, the use of antibodies to distinguish muscle, such as smooth muscle actin, desmin, and myoglobin, may be used. However, the diagnosis of carcinosarcoma is more often confirmed by light microscopy.

Surgical resection appears to be the treatment of choice. In some instances, postoperative chemotherapy has been used, but the usefulness of this treatment is still not well defined. The prognosis for this tumor is rather poor, with approximately 75% of patients dying after 2 years following diagnosis.

DIFFERENTIAL DIAGNOSIS. The most important differential diagnosis of this tumor is **pleomorphic carcinoma** and **pulmonary blastoma.** In the former, the absence of a clear mesenchymal component such as osteosarcoma, chondrosarcoma, etc., and the presence of keratin expression in the spindle cell component help establish the correct diagnosis. In the latter, the presence of a fetal-like glandular proliferation with presence of morules, giving the appearance of an endometrioid carcinoma, or with areas resembling an endodermal sinus tumor is more in keeping with pulmonary blastoma.

SALIVARY GLAND–LIKE TUMORS OF THE LUNG

The occurrence of primary tumors in the lung bearing resemblance to salivary gland tumors has been known for

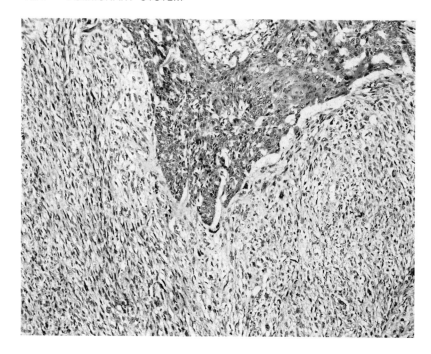

FIGURE 3-13. Pulmonary carcinosarcoma showing a biphasic cell population. A squamous cell carcinoma with areas of a spindle cell sarcoma.

some time. However, it was not until recently that reports on a series of cases of this type of tumor have become available. Nonetheless, these tumors are quite unusual in the lung, and their diagnosis has to be weighed against a possible metastatic tumor from a more common site such as the parotid gland.

Mucoepidermoid Carcinoma

This tumor seems to be the most common salivary gland–like tumor of the lung and represents the counterpart of the salivary gland neoplasms.[55-62] It may account for fewer than 5% of all lung tumors but constitutes about 50% of the tumors

of this kind. As in the salivary gland, these tumors in the lung have also been divided into high- and low-grade tumors.

CLINICAL FEATURES. The tumor seems to be more often encountered in women than in men in the second and third decades of life. However, cases of mucoepidermoid tumors in children have also been reported. Because of the endobronchial nature of this neoplasm, the symptoms are related to obstruction of the airway, giving rise to related symptoms such as cough, dyspnea, and/or hemoptysis. Tobacco use, although not clearly identified as a factor in the development of this tumor, has been observed in some cases.[62]

GROSS FEATURES. The tumor presents as an exophytic, polypoid, endobronchial growth. They are single, well-

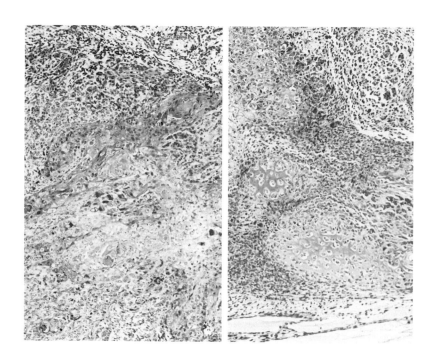

FIGURE 3-14. *Right,* A pulmonary carcinosarcoma showing malignant osteoid areas. *Left,* Sarcomatous areas admixed with squamous cell carcinoma.

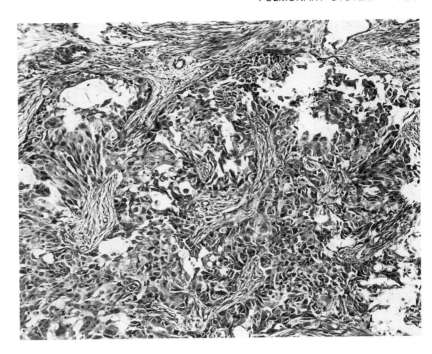

FIGURE 3–15. Mucoepidermoid carcinoma showing solid neoplastic areas in a lobular pattern separated by fibrous connective tissue.

circumscribed tumors ranging in size from less than 1 cm to more than 5 cm in greatest diameter. On cut surface, the tumors may show solid and cystic areas with hemorrhage and necrosis. No predilection for a particular side or lobe has been identified.

HISTOLOGIC FEATURES. Low-grade tumors are characterized by a mixture of solid and cystic components. The solid component is distributed in sheets of epithelial cells composed of round to oval cells with clear or eosinophilic cytoplasm, round nuclei, and inconspicuous nucleoli (Figs. 3–15 and 3–16). In some areas, this solid component shows features more like a squamous cell carcinoma, whereas in other areas, the solid component may appear basaloid. The cystic component is composed of glands lined by mucin-secreting epithe-lium, which may have fair amounts of mucin within their lumen. Both components may be embedded in a myxoid stroma or separated by thick bands of collagenous stroma. Mild cellular atypia and scattered mitoses are the usual findings in cases of low-grade tumors. **In cases of high-grade tumors, one can expect to find classic areas of low-grade tumor; however, areas of necrosis, hemorrhage, marked cellular atypia, and mitoses are the features that separate these two categories.**

Histochemical stains for mucin are useful in defining the mucus component in the glandular or cystic areas lined by mucin-secreting epithelium. Immunohistochemical studies using epithelial markers (keratin, EMA) are positive in these tumors.

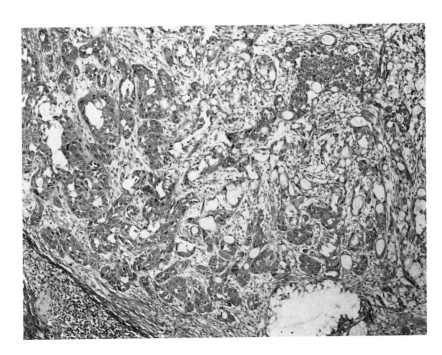

FIGURE 3–16. Both glandular and solid areas are admixed in this mucoepidermoid carcinoma.

The clinical course of these tumors depends on the grade and stage at which they are diagnosed. Nonetheless, it has been stated that tumors belonging to the low-grade category should be treated by surgical resection alone, whereas those of high grade should be treated very much the same as conventional squamous cell carcinoma or adenocarcinoma.[62]

DIFFERENTIAL DIAGNOSIS. The most important differential diagnosis is that of an **adenosquamous carcinoma** for the high-grade tumors. However, the presence of an endobronchial tumor and the finding of areas of **low-grade mucoepidermoid** tumor are in favor of **mucoepidermoid carcinoma.** In cases of low-grade tumor, the possibility of a **metastasis from salivary gland origin** should be carefully ruled out by a detailed clinical history and physical evaluation.

Adenoid Cystic Carcinoma

This neoplasm, as well as other salivary gland–like tumors of the lung, shares the same morphologic features as its counterpart in the salivary glands. It is generally believed that adenoid cystic carcinomas are slow-growing tumors of low malignant potential.[63-70] However, staging of the tumor may play a more important prognostic role for these tumors.

CLINICAL FEATURES. There does not appear to be any lung or lobe predilection for these tumors. The tumor appears to be more common in adults in the fifth decade of life. Because these tumors in the majority of cases present as an endobronchial lesion, the symptoms are those related to obstruction. These symptoms include cough, wheezing, dyspnea, and hemoptysis.

GROSS FEATURES. As previously mentioned, these tumors most often present as endobronchial tumors. They may be soft, tan, and well circumscribed. However, in a few cases, the lesion may be ill-defined and locally infiltrative. They may be small lesions, less than 1 cm in greatest dimension to well over 3 cm.

HISTOLOGIC FEATURES. The morphologic features of adenoid cystic carcinoma in the lung are the same as those seen in their more common location such as the salivary gland. The most common histologic growth pattern is the cribriform pattern (cylindromatous), which typically displays nests of tumor cells containing numerous well-defined luminal spaces filled with mucinous material (Figs. 3–17 to 3–19). The cells are small, with a round nuclei and moderate amounts of eosinophilic cytoplasm. In some areas a basaloid appearance may be seen. However, typical cylindromatous areas are the predominant feature. These glandular areas are often separated by a hyalinized fibroconnective stroma with myxoid features. The two other histologic features, tubular and solid growth pattern, are less frequent. In the tubular pattern, one often sees a proliferation of gland-like spaces with open lumina lined by two or three layers of small cells. In the solid pattern, one typically sees a cellular proliferation without the more usual organoid or cylindromatous pattern. Mitotic activity in either growth pattern is inconspicuous. Peripheral invasion is often seen. However, lymphatic or vascular invasion is not a common finding.

Immunohistochemically, adenoid cystic carcinomas are usually stained with antibodies for keratin, actin, and vimentin. Antibodies against S-100 protein also may be positive in a minority of cases.

The behavior of these tumors in the lung, although largely regarded as of low malignant potential, may be more directly affected by the stage at which the tumor is diagnosed. Cases exhibiting more aggressive behavior, with metastases to different organs, have been documented.[70] The treatment of choice for these tumors appears to be surgical resection with clear margins.

DIFFERENTIAL DIAGNOSIS. The most important issue is separating a primary from a **metastatic tumor.** This can be solved by obtaining a careful clinical history and physical examination. Other tumors that may be confused with adenoid cystic carcinoma include a **well-differentiated adenocarcinoma** and

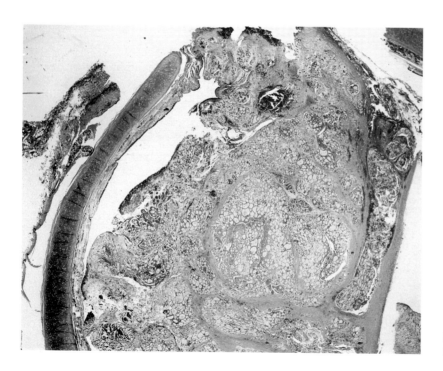

FIGURE 3–17. Endobronchial growth of an adenoid cystic carcinoma.

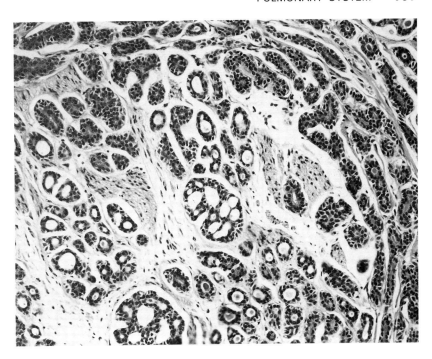

FIGURE 3–18. The classic cylindromatous pattern of an adenoid cystic carcinoma.

a **mixed tumor (pleomorphic adenoma)** of the lung. In the former, the presence of a cribriform or cylindromatous growth pattern separated in islands by fibroconnective tissue indicates the correct diagnosis. In addition, immunohistochemical stains for keratin and actin are helpful in clarifying the issue. In the latter, the diagnosis is more difficult and one that relies on morphology alone. The presence of a cylindromatous pattern, mucin in the lumen of the glandular structures, and absence of other mesenchymal components leads to the correct diagnosis.

Mixed Tumor (Pleomorphic Adenoma)

The occurrence of mixed tumors (pleomorphic adenoma) primary in the lung is a rare event. However, mixed tumors

of the lung bearing similar features to their counterpart in the salivary glands have been reported in a few instances. As expected, these tumors in the lung, just as in the salivary gland, may be benign or malignant.[71-76]

CLINICAL FEATURES. The tumor appears in adults without any gender preference or specific portion of the lung. Most of the cases present as endobronchial lesions. However, cases of peripheral tumors have been reported. Because of the nature of the neoplasm, namely its endobronchial presentation, symptoms are related to airway obstruction, including cough, dyspnea, and hemoptysis. The tumors present as a single pulmonary neoplasm that may vary from 1 cm to more than 4 cm in greatest dimension. On rare occasions, the tumor may reach more than 10 cm in greatest dimension.[76] At resection,

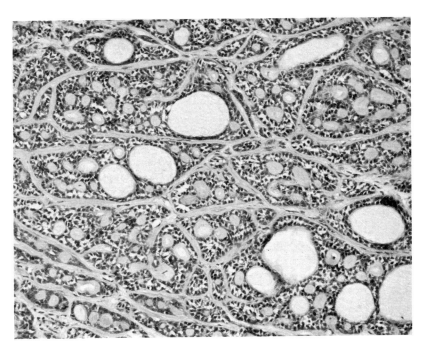

FIGURE 3–19. The cylindromatous pattern showing islands of tumor cell separated by areas of fibroconnective tissue.

the tumors are gray-to-white, soft, and rubbery, with a myxoid cut surface.

HISTOLOGIC FEATURES. The hallmark of these tumors is the presence of a **myoepithelial cell proliferation embedded in a myxoid or chondroid stroma** (Figs. 3–20 to 3–22). The myoepithelial cell proliferation is characterized by a cellular component arranged in ducts, glands, or solid sheets of rather small cells with a moderate amount of cytoplasm, round to oval nuclei, and inconspicuous nucleoli. The ductal or glandular structures may be lined by two distinct layers of cells, one composed of columnar cells with basally oriented nuclei with abundant eosinophilic cytoplasm and an outer layer composed of flattened or round cells with clear cytoplasm. The stroma in which this myoepithelial cell proliferation is embedded may vary from a myxoid background to chondroid stroma to frank areas of well-defined cartilage. It is important to note that the formation of cartilage in cases of mixed tumors of the lung is not as prominent as it is in the salivary gland counterparts. In the benign cases, mitoses, necrosis, and/or hemorrhage are absent. However, in cases of malignant mixed tumors, these latter features are part of the histologic features of the tumor.

Immunohistochemically, the myoepithelial component shows positive reaction for antibodies against CAM 5.2, keratin, muscle-specific actin, and vimentin. Other immunostains using S-100 protein and glial fibrillary acidic protein (GFAP) may also be positive in these tumors.

The benign variants of mixed tumor have favorable prognosis, whereas those showing malignant features tend to do poorly. The treatment of choice for these tumors appears to be surgical resection.

DIFFERENTIAL DIAGNOSIS. The most important distinction should be with similar **metastatic tumors of salivary gland origin** or arising at other sites where these tumors occur. In our experience,[76] we noted that mixed tumors in the lung do not form well-defined cartilage and duct-like structures as often as their salivary gland counterparts. In addition, the clinical history plays a very important role in arriving at a more correct interpretation. Other tumors that may pose a problem include **carcinosarcoma, hamartoma,** and **pulmonary blastoma.** In carcinosarcomas, one expects to identify malignant epithelial areas as well as mesenchymal areas (chondrosarcoma, osteosarcoma). The latter findings are not seen in mixed tumors of the lung. In pulmonary hamartoma, the lesion is expected to show mature cartilaginous areas mixed with mature fatty tissue and invagination of respiratory epithelium. Lastly, pulmonary blastoma shows the typical embryonic epithelium that is the hallmark of this tumor.

Acinic Cell Carcinoma (Fechner's Tumor)

Acinic cell carcinoma primary in the lung represents one of the rarest salivary gland–like tumors of the lung. Only a few reports of these tumors are encountered in the literature.[77–81] The term *Fechner's tumor* was coined honoring the first original description of this tumor in the lung.

CLINICAL FEATURES. The tumors can occur essentially at any age; however, it is more common in adults. No sex or lung predilection has been observed in any of the previous reports. Although the lesion may occur as an endobronchial polypoid tumor, cases of intraparenchymal tumors have also been described. When these tumors are in an endobronchial location, one expects to see symptoms of airway obstruction, such as dyspnea, cough, hemoptysis, and the like, as the presenting signs. However, in our experience, patients may be completely asymptomatic. The tumors tend to be single and well circumscribed.

HISTOLOGIC FEATURES. The morphologic features of these tumors in the lung may be as varied as their counterparts in the salivary gland. The tumors are composed of a cellular proliferation of relatively large cohesive cells replacing the normal lung parenchyma. In some areas, the sheets of cells may be separated by thick fibrous connective tissue bands.

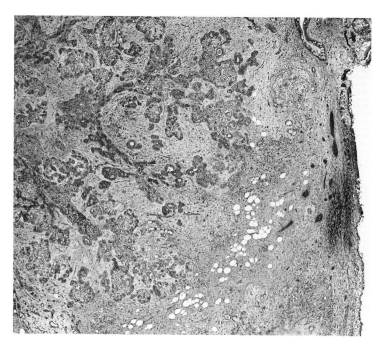

FIGURE 3–20. Mixed tumor (pleomorphic adenoma) in an endobronchial location.

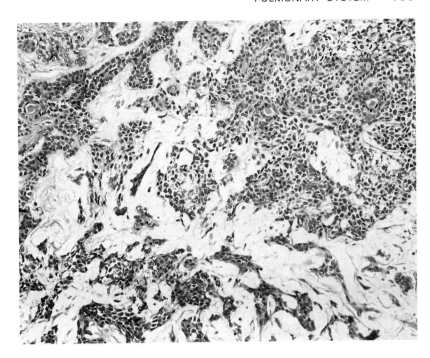

FIGURE 3–21. Mixed tumor with areas of myoepithelial proliferation embedded in a loose myxoid background.

An inflammatory infiltrate may be present in these areas. The tumor may show different growth patterns, including areas showing acinar and microcystic structures composed of an acinar type of cell with eccentric nuclei (Fig. 3–23), a solid variant composed of a proliferation of acinar cells with central nuclei and moderate amounts of eosinophilic cytoplasm (Fig. 3–24), and areas showing microcystic and papillocystic structures. In some cases, the cellular proliferation is composed of polygonal cells with central nuclei and moderate amounts of eosinophilic cytoplasm, whereas in other cases, the cells have a clear granular cytoplasm with an eccentric nuclei.

Histochemical stains for mucin, such as PAS, DPAS, and mucicarmine, are useful. Usually the tumor shows strong positive reaction for PAS and is negative for DPAS and mucicarmine. However, in our experience, DPAS and mucicarmine may show focal positive reaction. The former may even show a strong positive reaction in tumor cells. Immunohistochemically, the tumor may also show a positive reaction for antibodies against keratin and/or EMA. Ultrastructurally, the presence of granules of varying electron density are diagnostic in cases of acinic cell carcinoma.

The prognosis of these tumors appears to be quite good, and surgical resection alone is the treatment of choice.

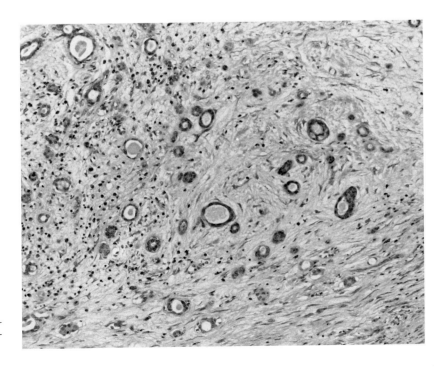

FIGURE 3–22. Mixed tumor showing loose connective tissue with ductal and glandular structures.

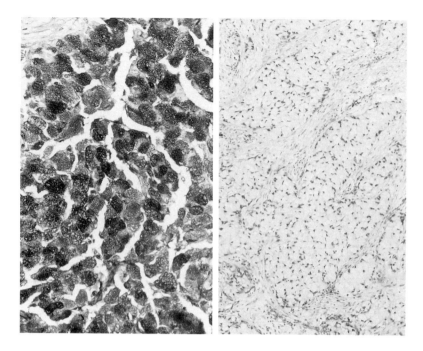

FIGURE 3–23. *Right,* An acinic cell carcinoma showing an acinar proliferation of clear cells with nuclei displaced toward the periphery. *Left,* PAS stain showing the prominent granular features of this tumor.

DIFFERENTIAL DIAGNOSIS. The most important differential diagnosis is a **metastasis from a salivary gland origin.** In this case, a careful clinical history and physical examination will lead to the correct interpretation. Acinic cell carcinoma may also be confused with a **carcinoid tumor.** In this setting, the presence of areas showing papillocystic and microcystic structures would be unusual for a carcinoid tumor. In addition, the use of neuroendocrine markers such as chromogranin and/or synaptophysin would be most helpful in separating a carcinoid tumor from an acinic cell carcinoma of the lung.

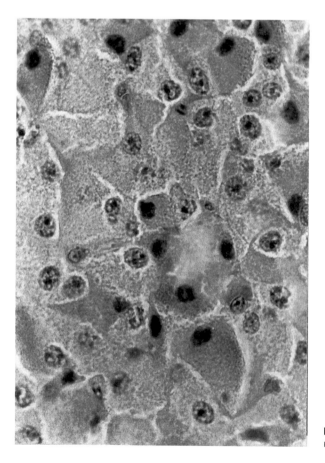

FIGURE 3–24. Acinic cell carcinoma showing a cellular proliferation with more oncocytic features.

Oncocytoma

This tumor in the lung represents the rarest of all salivary gland–like tumors. Only a few case reports have been described.[82-84]

The tumors may also present in an endobronchial location and may vary in size from less than 1 cm to more than 2.5 cm. Histologically, the tumors share similar features with oncocytomas described elsewhere, namely the presence of a cellular proliferation composed of relatively larger cells with abundant eosinophilic cytoplasm and an eccentrically placed nuclei. Mitoses, necrosis, and cellular atypia are inconspicuous. The presence of numerous mitochondria in ultrastructural studies is diagnostic for this tumor.

Because of the similarities with other tumors that may show oncocytic features, **oncocytomas should not be confused with acinic cell carcinoma or oncocytic carcinoid.** In the former, the presence of electron dense granules and absence of mitochondria in ultrastructural studies lead to the correct diagnosis. In the latter, the presence of positive results for neuroendocrine markers and absence of abundant mitochondria in ultrastructural studies are more in keeping with an oncocytic carcinoid.

MESENCHYMAL TUMORS OF THE LUNG

The lung may be the primary site of a number of tumors that bear the same histologic features as those of sarcomas in the soft tissues. Because of the similar features exhibited by these tumors, it is of crucial importance to establish that the lesion in the lung is a primary tumor. This can be accomplished only by a good clinical history and a physical examination. Otherwise, one must assume that the lesion in the lung is a metastasis until proven otherwise. Because essentially any type of sarcoma can potentially present as a primary lung tumor, we deal here with those that are relatively more common and those that may pose a problem in diagnosis.

Malignant Fibrous Histiocytoma (MFH)

This tumor represents the most common soft tissue sarcoma. The presence of this type of tumor in the lung has been well documented in the literature.[85-89] Its histogenesis has been the subject of much debate and remains unclear.

CLINICAL FEATURES. MFH occurs in adult individuals without predilection for gender or specific site in the lung. The tumor may appear as a central or peripheral mass that may vary in size from a few centimeters to more than 10 cm in greatest dimension. The patients may present with symptoms of cough, chest pain, hemoptysis, and/or shortness of breath. In a few instances, the tumor has been described as an endobronchial tumor.[86]

HISTOLOGIC FEATURES. The tumor in the lung, the same as its counterpart in the soft tissue, shows a distinctive growth pattern. Typically, there is a spindle cell proliferation arranged in a storiform or cartwheel pattern composed of spindle cells with light eosinophilic cytoplasm, elongated nuclei, and inconspicuous nucleoli (Figs. 3–25 and 3–26). Marked pleomorphism is seen with the presence of larger cells with large nuclei, prominent nucleoli, and abundant eosinophilic and often vacuolated cytoplasm. Scattered giant cells of the Touton type are seen in most instances. Mitoses, necrosis, and hemorrhage are commonly seen in these tumors. Occasionally, the tumors may show a prominent myxoid background separating the neoplastic cell proliferation. Inflammatory mononuclear cells are often seen in the stroma of the tumor. Occasionally, areas of hemangiopericytic-like appearance are seen admixed with more conventional areas of MFH.

Immunohistochemically, there is not a single stain that is specific for MFH. Even though immunostains using antibodies for vimentin, alpha-1-antitrypsin, and chymotrypsin may be

FIGURE 3–25. MFH showing the classic storiform pattern.

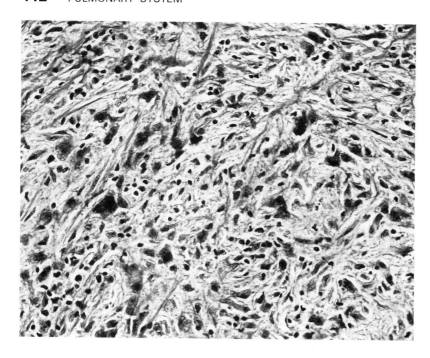

FIGURE 3–26. Closer view of areas with marked cellular pleomorphism. Note the scattered bizarre forms.

positive, these positive results are not necessarily diagnostic of MFH.

Different treatments have been used in these tumors, including surgery, chemotherapy, and/or radiation therapy, yet the prognosis remains poor. However, staging at the time of diagnosis is important, because tumors that are more extensive at the time of diagnosis have a worse prognosis than those that are limited to the lung.

DIFFERENTIAL DIAGNOSIS. Tumors that may be confused with MFH include **leiomyosarcoma, hemangiopericytoma,** and **fibrosarcoma.** In the case of leiomyosarcoma, the use of immunohistochemical stains with positive results using antibodies for muscle, actin, and desmin leads to the correct diagnosis. MFH can be distinguished from fibrosarcoma or hemangiopericytoma by the presence of a distinctive storiform pattern with numerous giant cells and marked pleomorphism. Immunohistochemistry does not play a significant role for diagnosis with the latter. In small biopsies, an important differential diagnosis is that of **inflammatory pseudotumor.** In such instances, the presence or absence of cellular pleomorphism, mitoses, necrosis, or hemorrhage leads to the correct diagnosis.

Fibrosarcoma

Fibrosarcomas are unusual primary malignant mesenchymal neoplasms.[90–92] Most of what has been published on this condition is the result of studies done before the advent of immunohistochemistry; therefore, cases that in the past were labeled as fibrosarcomas, by today's standards with more modern techniques may not necessarily meet the criteria for that diagnosis. An example of this is seen in some cases that in the past were categorized as childhood fibrosarcoma and now are coined under the category of congenital myofibroblastic tumors.[93]

CLINICAL FEATURES. Fibrosarcomas in adults may occur essentially at any age (young adults and older individuals) but probably are more common in the fifth decade of life. The tumors may occur as an intraparenchymal lesion or as an endobronchial lesion. Therefore, symptoms may vary according to the location of the neoplasm. Those tumors found in endobronchial location present with symptoms of airway obstruction such as cough, hemoptysis, and dyspnea. In a number of cases, the patients are asymptomatic.

GROSS FEATURES. The tumors presenting as an endobronchial lesion have a tendency to be smaller than those in an intraparenchymal location, probably because symptoms are more common and diagnosis becomes more rapid. Whatever the cause, they may vary from 1 to 3 cm in greatest dimension, whereas those in intraparenchymal location can be larger than 10 cm in greatest dimension. The tumors are firm, white to gray, and non-encapsulated. Areas of necrosis and/or hemorrhage may be seen mainly in larger tumors.

HISTOLOGIC FEATURES. At low power, there is evidence of a spindle cell proliferation obliterating the normal architecture of the lung parenchyma. This spindle cell proliferation is arranged in a "**herringbone pattern**" of fusiform cells with scant cytoplasm and oval nuclei intermixed with abundant collagen (Figs. 3–27 and 3–28). Mitoses are easily found and are numerous. Necrosis and/or hemorrhage may be seen, especially in larger tumors.

Immunohistochemical studies for vimentin are positive. However, stains for muscle, neurogenic, or epithelial markers are negative. Therefore, the diagnosis by immunohistochemical standards becomes one of exclusion.

The treatment for these tumors is surgical resection. The use of radiation therapy and chemotherapy is raised for those tumors that are unresectable. The prognosis in these tumors is essentially based on the stage, size of the tumor, and number of mitoses (>10 HPF). It appears to be that tumors larger than 5 cm with numerous mitoses have a worse prognosis than those under 5 cm with fewer mitoses.

DIFFERENTIAL DIAGNOSIS. The most difficult condition to distinguish it from is the **intrapulmonary fibrous tumors**

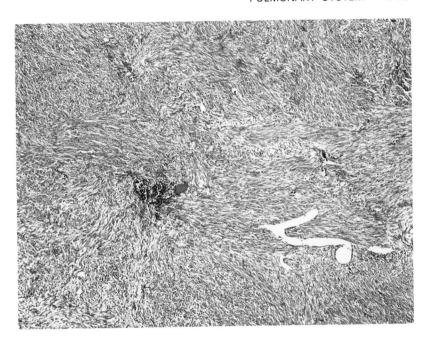

FIGURE 3–27. Fibrosarcoma showing a prominent atypical spindle cell proliferation.

(intrapulmonary localized fibrous mesothelioma).[94] Whether fibrosarcomas and intrapulmonary fibrous tumors represent the same entity is debatable. However, so far, no malignant counterparts of the fibrous tumors in intrapulmonary location have been described. That may be a clue to the similarities that they share with bona fide cases of fibrosarcoma. Therefore, a separation of these two conditions may be arbitrary. Other sarcomas that could be mistaken for fibrosarcomas include **leiomyosarcoma** and **neurogenic sarcoma.** However, positive results using muscle antibodies or S-100 protein lead to the correct interpretation. If inflammatory pseudotumor is a consideration, the presence of cellular atypia and mitoses and absence of an inflammatory background with foamy macrophages lead to the correct interpretation.

Leiomyosarcoma

Malignant smooth muscle tumors arising primarily in the lung are rare but paradoxically probably more common than benign smooth muscle tumors.[90, 95–101]

CLINICAL FEATURES. The tumors may occur at any age from childhood to adult. However, they present more often in adults in the fifth decade of life, with a slight predilection for men. Essentially, the tumor may occur in three different forms: intraparenchymal, endobronchial, or arising from the pulmonary artery. Depending on the location of the tumor, symptoms may appear; the endobronchial tumors have symptoms related to airway obstruction, whereas intraparenchymal tumors are more often asymptomatic.

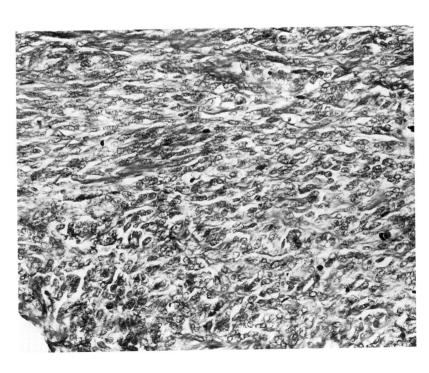

FIGURE 3–28. Fibrosarcoma with scattered mitoses and prominent cellular pleomorphism.

GROSS FEATURES. The tumors may show a polypoid configuration when in endobronchial location, whereas those in intraparenchymal location may be larger. They usually present as well-defined tumor masses, firm, white to gray. Necrosis and/or hemorrhage may be seen more often in larger lesions.

HISTOLOGIC FEATURES. At low power, there is a spindle cell proliferation replacing the lung parenchyma, frequently arranged in a storiform pattern. The cellular proliferation is composed of elongated cells with cigar-shaped nuclei, prominent nucleoli, and finely fibrillary cytoplasm (Fig. 3–29). Areas showing large, bizarre cells are seen. Mitoses are common and often numerous. Areas showing more discohesive malignant cells may be observed. Areas of necrosis and/or hemorrhage are often seen mainly in larger tumors. Results of immunohistochemical studies using muscle markers such as muscle-specific actin and desmin are usually positive. Rare cases of leiomyosarcomas showing keratin positivity have been reported; therefore, the positive result for an epithelial marker in a spindle cell proliferation should not deter one from the diagnosis of smooth muscle tumor.

The treatment of choice for these tumors is surgical resection, and the prognosis of the tumor appears to be determined by the size and mitotic activity. Tumors showing a mitotic count of more than 10 mitoses/10 HPF and a size greater than 10 cm in greatest dimension appear to have a poor prognosis.

DIFFERENTIAL DIAGNOSIS. An important consideration is the possibility of **metastatic leiomyosarcoma.** In such cases, a careful clinical history and physical examination play an important role. Ample sampling should be obtained in larger tumors to rule out the possibility of a **carcinosarcoma.** In the latter instance, the finding of an epithelial component is diagnostic.

Epithelioid Hemangioendothelioma

This tumor is of ubiquitous distribution and may present in the lung as a primary neoplasm. Originally this tumor was described as an **intravascular, bronchiolar,** and **alveolar tumor (IVBAT)** of the lung.[102–104] However, it is now recognized as a tumor of vascular origin.

CLINICAL FEATURES. The majority of patients are young women who may present with symptoms of cough, dyspnea, chest pain, and so on. Radiologically, it is common to see numerous bilateral intrapulmonary nodules that raise the clinical suspicion of a metastatic tumor. On the other hand, the patients may be asymptomatic, and the finding of pulmonary nodules is made after a routine chest radiograph.

GROSS FEATURES. The pulmonary nodules may vary in size from a few millimeters to about 1 cm in greatest dimension. They are soft-rubbery, tan lesions with occasional areas of calcification.

HISTOLOGIC FEATURES. At low power, one observes discrete pulmonary nodules destroying the normal lung architecture. The nodules show an acellular and often sclerotic center surrounded by a rim containing more cellular areas exhibiting intra-alveolar growth. The acellular areas are composed of a myxoid or hyalinized matrix, whereas the cellular areas are composed of rather smaller cells with a plump appearance, round-to-oval nuclei, finely dispersed chromatin, and inconspicuous nucleoli (Figs. 3–30 and 3–31). Mitoses are rare. Immunohistochemical studies using factor VIII and *Ulex europaeus* are positive in these tumors. Ultrastructurally, Weibel-Palade bodies, microfilaments, cytoplasmic vacuoles, and microtubules are observed.

The behavior of these neoplasms is variable. In some cases there is slow progress, and patients may survive for over a decade; in other cases, the course is more aggressive, leading to respiratory insufficiency and death. The treatment of choice for these tumors is still unknown.

DIFFERENTIAL DIAGNOSIS. Because of the multinodular presentation, a metastasis is usually one of the first considerations. **Chondrosarcoma or chordoma** may be often confused with this tumor. However, in chondrosarcoma, one often sees a malignant cartilage that is not seen in epithelioid hemangioendothelioma. In addition, the presence of factor VIII and

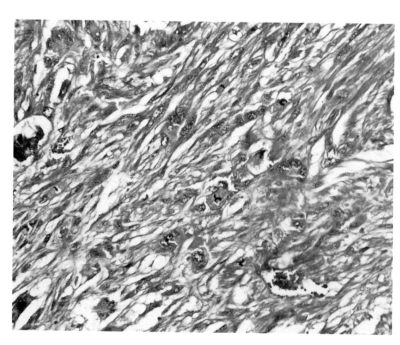

FIGURE 3–29. Pulmonary leiomyosarcoma showing cellular pleomorphism.

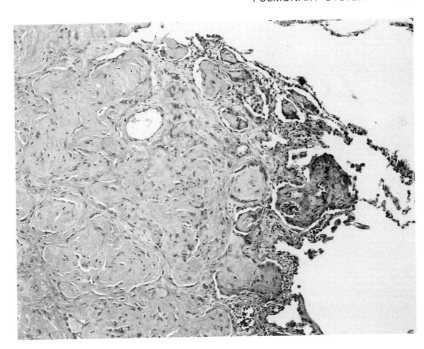

FIGURE 3-30. Epithelioid hemangioendothelioma showing a myxoid nodule replacing pulmonary parenchyma.

Ulex europaeus positivity in tumor cells should lead to the correct interpretation. In cases of chordoma, the absence of a more myxoid background with positive results for vascular markers and negative results for epithelial markers and S-100 protein are also more in keeping with the diagnosis of epithelioid hemangioendothelioma.

Mesenchymal Cystic Hamartoma

This term was designated for a group of cystic lesions occurring in patients with a wide range of ages. These tumors are exceptionally rare, and only a few cases have been reported.[105]

CLINICAL FEATURES. In the initial description of the five cases of this particular entity,[105] the patients varied in age from 1 to 53 years. Although patients can be asymptomatic, they may also present with symptoms of dyspnea, hemothorax, pneumothorax, and hemoptysis.

GROSS FEATURES. The lesions are typically cystic and of about 1 cm in greatest dimension. They can present as single cystic tumors or as numerous cystic nodules in the lung parenchyma. No site of predilection in the lung has been observed.

HISTOLOGIC FEATURES. The tumor is characterized by a primitive mesenchymal-looking cellular proliferation. Papillary areas may be seen as well as small airways lined with respiratory epithelium. Cystic structures are evident, and some are lined by normal-looking respiratory epithelium. A cam-

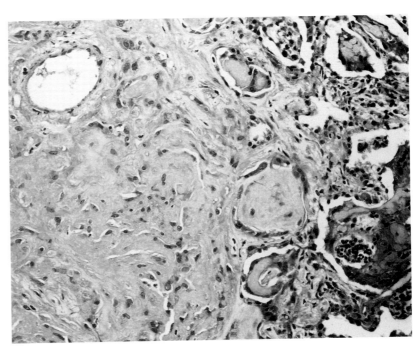

FIGURE 3-31. Hyalinized relatively acellular areas extending into alveolar spaces.

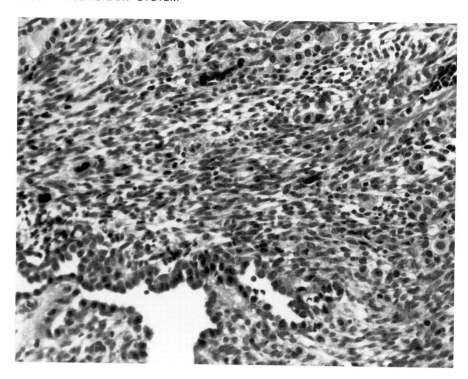

FIGURE 3–32. Mesenchymal cystic hamartoma showing a cystic area. Note the spindle cell proliferation at the margin of the cyst.

bium layer of primitive spindle mesenchymal cells is also seen (Figs. 3–32 and 3–33). Underneath the cysts, within the cambium layer, small cystic structures are often seen mimicking a vascular neoplasia. Adjacent areas show inflammatory changes.

Even though this tumor was initially thought to be a benign neoplasm, reports of malignancy arising in these tumors have been presented.[106, 107] Therefore, it is wise not only to completely resect the tumor but also to closely follow up these patients. On the other hand, it is possible that the tumor represents a **variant of another low-grade malignant mesen-** **chymal neoplasm.** However, further studies of this entity are needed to properly assess the malignant potential of these tumors.

DIFFERENTIAL DIAGNOSIS. The lesions that can be confused with this tumor are numerous and are essentially those representing sarcomatous lesions of the lung. **Rhabdomyosarcoma** may look like these tumors. However, the cystic nature of the tumor and special studies using muscle antibodies lead to the correct diagnosis. Other sarcomatous lesions of the lung have to be carefully ruled out by detailed histologic characteristics and by the use of immunohistochemical studies. Also,

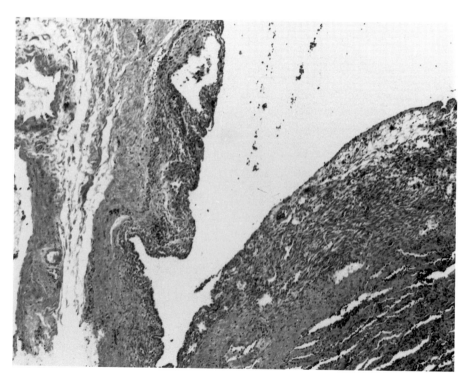

FIGURE 3–33. Closer view of the spindle cell proliferation showing focal areas of cellular atypia. Note the normal epithelial lining.

it is important to rule out metastatic sarcoma with a "cystic" growth component, especially **metastatic endometrial stromal sarcoma or dematofibrosarcoma protuberans.**

Primitive Neuroectodermal Tumor

This term encompasses several other entities, including **extraskeletal Ewing's sarcoma, malignant small-cell tumor of the thoracopulmonary region, paravertebral round cell tumor,** and **neuroepithelioma.**[108–112]

We have observed a few cases in intrapulmonary location (unpublished data). The cases that we have observed have been in young adults who clinically may present with history of hemoptysis, cough, chest pain, and dyspnea.

Histologically, these tumors are characterized by sheets of malignant cells, in some areas arranged in small nests. The cellular proliferation is rather discohesive and composed of rather small cells with scant cytoplasm, round nuclei, and inconspicuous nucleoli. Rosettes of the Homer-Wright type are seen scattered in the tumor. Areas of necrosis and/or hemorrhage are commonly seen in these cases. Histochemical stains for PAS show moderate amounts of glycogen in the tumor cells. Immunohistochemical stains for NSE are probably the most common marker found positive in these tumors.

DIFFERENTIAL DIAGNOSIS. These tumors must be distinguished from other most common small-cell tumors in intrapulmonary location. Essentially, **small-cell carcinomas** and **other neuroendocrine tumors** as well as **malignant lymphoma** are considerations when dealing with primitive neuroectodermal tumor. In this setting, the presence of positive markers using epithelial, neuroendocrine, and lymphoid markers is helpful in arriving at the correct diagnosis.

Rhabdomyosarcoma

CLINICAL FEATURES. Primary rhabdomyosarcomas of the lung are rare.[113–116] Rhabdomyosarcomas can present as an intraparenchymal mass or as an endobronchial tumor. The symptoms depend on the location of the tumor.

GROSS FEATURES. The tumor may appear cystic or solid, gray to white, and of soft consistency. Areas of hemorrhage and necrosis are common.

HISTOLOGIC FEATURES. The alveolar and embryonal growth patterns can be seen. As with rhabdomyosarcomas in other locations, the tumor is characterized by the presence of a malignant cellular proliferation with strap-like rhabdomyoblasts with cross-striations (Figs. 3–34 and 3–35). This latter feature is more easily seen with phosphotungstic acid hematoxylin (PTAH) histochemical stain. Immunohistochemically, rhabdomyosarcomas show positive reaction using muscle markers, namely desmin and myoglobin. Ultrastructurally, the presence of sarcomeres with Z-bands is diagnostic of rhabdomyosarcoma.

DIFFERENTIAL DIAGNOSIS. Other sarcomatous lesions, such as **peripheral neuroepithelioma,** or **metastatic tumors with rhabdoid features** should be considered in the differential diagnosis. However, the use of muscle markers helps arrive at a correct diagnosis.

Kaposi's Sarcoma

CLINICAL FEATURES. Currently, with the **acquired immunodeficiency syndrome (AIDS)** epidemic, the presence of this tumor in the lung should be considered a metastases until proved otherwise. Nonetheless, the tumor can occur primarily in intrapulmonary location.[117]

HISTOLOGIC FEATURES. Kaposi's sarcoma in the lung shows a perivascular or peribronchial distribution, extending along the vascular channels. The tumor is characterized by the presence of a spindle cell proliferation with vascular spaces interspersing the cellular proliferation. The spindle cells do not show striking atypia, and mitoses are rare. Within the cellular proliferation, there are numerous **eosinophilic globules that are PAS positive.** Adjacent areas of hemorrhage or necrosis may be seen in association with this tumor.

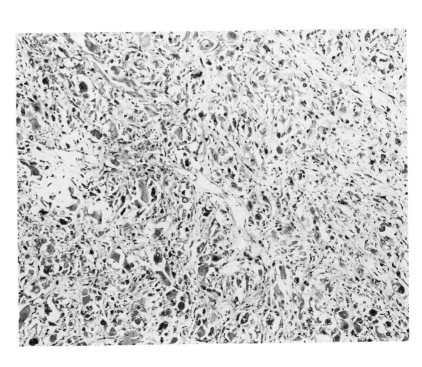

FIGURE 3–34. Pulmonary rhabdomyosarcoma showing marked cellular pleomorphism and numerous rhabdomyoblasts.

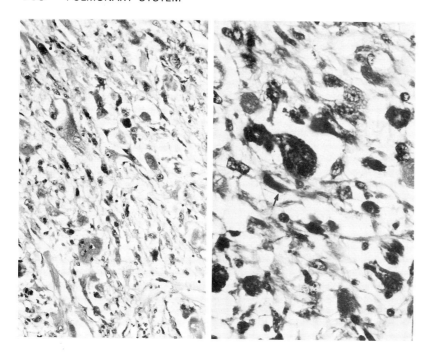

FIGURE 3–35. *Right,* PTAH stain showing cross striations *(arrow)*. *Left,* Closer view of a rhabdomyosarcoma with numerous rhabdomyoblasts present. (H&E)

DIFFERENTIAL DIAGNOSIS. The most important differential diagnosis is with other sarcomas, namely **leiomyosarcoma** or **angiosarcoma.** In the former, the presence of interlacing fascicles with numerous mitoses and cellular atypia, in addition to positive results with muscle markers, leads to the correct diagnosis. In the latter, the presence of cellular atypia with occasional areas of more solid pattern in combination with positive results for endothelial markers (*Ulex europaeus* and factor VIII) in tumor cells leads to a correct diagnosis.

Angiosarcoma

CLINICAL FEATURES. This tumor as primary intrapulmonary tumor is rare. However, a few cases have been reported in the literature.[118–120] Because **angiosarcoma in the lung is often a metastasis from other more common sites** such as heart or skin, careful clinical history is important. Clinically, patients may present with symptoms of cough and/or hemoptysis.

HISTOLOGIC FEATURES. The tumor is characterized by the presence of numerous anastomosing vascular spaces filled with red blood cells and lined by atypical endothelial cells. In some areas, the tumor shows more solid areas formed with polygonal or spindle cells with round or elongated nuclei. Cellular atypia and mitoses are easily found. Occasionally the tumor extends into alveolar spaces, vascular channels, and bronchi. Immunohistochemically, *Ulex europaeus* and factor VIII show positive reaction in tumor cells.

DIFFERENTIAL DIAGNOSIS. The most important differential diagnosis is to separate angiosarcoma from **Kaposi's sarcoma.** The presence of areas with more solid growth pattern and cellular atypia, in addition to positive reaction of tumor cells for vascular markers, leads to the correct diagnosis.

Hemangiopericytoma

CLINICAL FEATURES. This tumor is relatively uncommon in intrapulmonary location. However, several reports dealing with this entity have been published.[121–123] The tumors appear to affect adults, and the patients often are asymptomatic. The tumor is frequently found on a routine physical examination. When symptoms are present, cough, hemoptysis, and chest pain are more common. The tumor appears to be well circumscribed and encapsulated. Necrosis and/or hemorrhage may be seen on gross examination.

HISTOLOGIC FEATURES. The tumor is characterized by a spindle cell proliferation with numerous vascular spaces. An important characteristic of hemangiopericytomas is the presence of "staghorn" blood vessels lined with flattened endothelium. The spindle cells have an oval nuclei and inconspicuous nucleoli. Mitoses are seen occasionally. Necrosis and/or hemorrhage are often present, especially in larger tumors. Although all hemangiopericytomas should be considered potentially malignant tumor, there have been proposed criteria for malignancy that include large size (>8 cm), pleural and bronchial wall involvement, cellular pleomorphism, and high mitotic activity (>10 HPF).

DIFFERENTIAL DIAGNOSIS. One important differential diagnosis is **intrapulmonary thymoma, spindle cell variant.** In this case the presence of foamy histiocytes in vascular spaces, focal areas of mononuclear cell (namely lymphocytes), and positive reaction against epithelial markers lead to the correct diagnosis. One other important differential diagnosis is the **intrapulmonary localized fibrous tumor of the pleura (intrapulmonary fibrous mesothelioma).** This latter entity can be indistinguishable from hemangiopericytoma. However, acellular areas with abundant collagen deposition alternating with more cellular areas and the presence of the so-called patternless pattern should lead to a correct interpretation. It is possible that cases reported or diagnosed as hemangiopericytomas may fall in the category of what today is called intrapulmonary localized fibrous tumors.

Chondrosarcoma

CLINICAL FEATURES. This is a rare slow-growing cartilaginous tumor in the lung.[124, 125] Two possibilities have been mentioned about its presence as a lung neoplasm: that the tumor arises *de novo,* and that the tumor arises from a preexisting hamartomatous chondroma.

Clinically, the patients may present with symptoms of airway obstruction when the tumor is in endobronchial location.

HISTOLOGIC FEATURES. At low power, the tumor appears formed by large lobules of malignant cartilage with nests of pleomorphic and hyperchromatic chondrocytes in lacunae. Occasional bizarre cells may be seen. The tumor may be seen extending into vascular spaces. Necrosis and/or hemorrhage are not common.

DIFFERENTIAL DIAGNOSIS. The most important differential consideration is to separate this tumor from a **metastasis from an osseous site.** In this regard, the presence of numerous lesions in the lung parenchyma and a good clinical history may be of help.

Osteosarcoma

This is a very rare neoplasm in intrapulmonary location.[126] Of the cases described, the tumor has been an intraparenchymal, lobulate, firm, white tumor mass without association with bronchi.

Microscopically, the tumor shows a spindle cell proliferation with prominent areas of osteoid and immature bone. Because this tumor is rare in lung, the presence of osteosarcoma-like features in a lung neoplasm should alert the pathologist to properly sample the specimen and to rule out the possibility of a carcinosarcoma. The diagnosis of primary osteosarcoma of the lung should be used with care after an ample sampling of the tumor in question.

Lipomas

CLINICAL FEATURES. Primary benign fatty tumors of the lung are rare.[127–129] In four cases that we have the opportunity to review, the patients were adult males. No predilection for specific site was noted. The lesions were endobronchial, and the symptoms of the patients were related to airway obstruction. The tumors were described as well circumscribed, soft, yellow tumors ranging from 1 to 3 cm in greatest dimension.

HISTOLOGIC FEATURES. The hallmark of these tumors is the presence of mature fat tissue. However, the tumors may show myxoid areas and spindle cell features similar to lipomas in soft tissues. No necrosis, hemorrhage, or cellular atypia is seen in these cases (Fig. 3–36). However, rarely a lipoma may show atypical features.[127]

DIFFERENTIAL DIAGNOSIS. Conditions that should be considered in the differential diagnosis include a **hamartomatous chondroma** and a **liposarcoma.** In hamartomatous chondroma, the fat tissue is admixed with cartilaginous areas with invagination of the respiratory epithelium. In cases of liposarcoma, it is expected to see evidence of cellular atypia and lipoblasts.

Liposarcoma

CLINICAL FEATURES. These are exceedingly rare neoplasms.[130] Because the tumor may present as an endobronchial lesion, symptoms related to airway obstruction may be present.

HISTOLOGIC FEATURES. As with other similar tumors in soft tissue, liposarcomas in lung are characterized by the presence

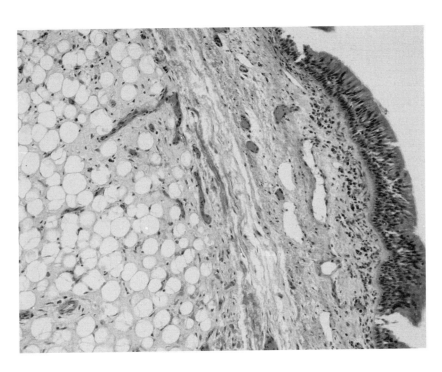

FIGURE 3–36. Endobronchial lipoma showing a proliferation of mature fat cells underneath a normal bronchial epithelium.

of fat tissue with lipoblast and cellular atypia. The tumor shows a fine but prominent vascular network. High mitotic activity is not common.

DIFFERENTIAL DIAGNOSIS. The most important is to separate benign from malignant fat tissue tumors. In this regard, **lipoma** becomes the most important entity to rule out. The presence of cellular atypia and lipoblasts is in keeping with the diagnosis of liposarcoma.

TUMORS ARISING FROM ECTOPIC OR EMBRYONICALLY DISPLACED TISSUES

Intrapulmonary Thymoma

Thymomas are the most **common tumors in the anterior mediastinum.** However, they **can occur in the lung or growing along the pleural surface.**[131-139] Nonetheless, before rendering the diagnosis of ectopic primary thymoma, an anterior mediastinal location must be ruled out by radiographic means or by exploratory surgery.

CLINICAL FEATURES. The tumor usually occurs in an adult, although younger patients have been reported.[131] No gender or racial predilection has been observed. Clinically, the patients may have a history of myasthenia gravis or pulmonary obstruction, or they may be asymptomatic. Radiographically, intrapulmonary thymomas may present as a hilar mass or intralobar mass. In cases of pleural thymomas, the radiographic features may mimic a mesothelioma with encasement of the lung.

GROSS FEATURES. There are no specific gross features that allow differentiation from other more common intrapulmonary tumors. The size of the tumor may vary. However, in the cases reported, it seems that the tumors are rarely more than 5 cm in greatest diameter. The tumor may show cystic structures or may have a more solid or fleshy appearance.

HISTOLOGIC FEATURES. The morphologic features of intrapulmonary or pleural thymomas are not different from those of conventional mediastinal thymomas. They are characterized by a biphasic cell population consisting of epithelial cells and lymphocytes with the characteristic fibrous septa separating large areas into lobules. In rare occasions, the tumor may be predominantly spindle cell type.

Immunohistochemically, the use of epithelial markers, including keratin or EMA, may prove useful in arriving at a correct diagnosis. Ultrastructural studies provide useful information by showing the presence of tonofilaments or desmosomes, thus supporting an epithelial origin.

DIFFERENTIAL DIAGNOSIS. Clinically, the tumor may be confused with other more common intrapulmonary tumors. However, on morphologic grounds, the characteristic features of thymomas allow easy recognition. Nonetheless, when the tumor is a predominantly spindle cell thymoma, it can be confused with other neoplasms including **hemangiopericytoma.** In this context, immunohistochemical or ultrastructural studies are most helpful in leading to a correct diagnosis.

Meningioma

Primary meningiomas of the lung are exceedingly rare. Only a few reports of this unusual neoplasm have appeared as a primary intrapulmonary tumor.[140-145]

CLINICAL FEATURES. The cases reported have been in adults, more often women. No particular site in the lung seems to be affected. The lesion may appear as a subpleural lung neoplasm or as an intraparenchymal tumor. It is usually a single tumor mass, and reports of the lesion having been present for at least 3 years prior to removal of the tumor have been documented. This latter characteristic would speak in favor of this being a slow-growing tumor with low aggressive potential.

GROSS FEATURES. The lesion appears as a single mass that can vary in size from a few centimeters to more than 5 cm

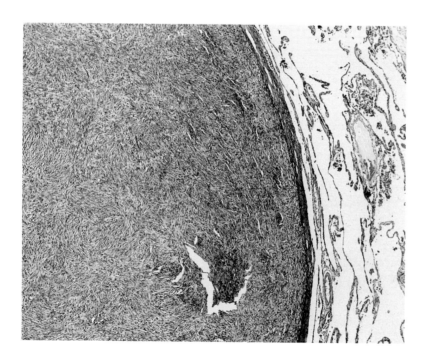

FIGURE 3–37. Pulmonary meningioma showing a well-circumscribed pulmonary tumor.

in greatest dimension. This tumor may show similar gross features to those seen in its more common intracranial location.

HISTOLOGIC FEATURES. At low power, it is possible to see a well-demarcated tumor mass replacing the normal pulmonary parenchyma. The tumor is composed of a spindle cell proliferation with a distinctive whorled pattern (Fig. 3–37). The cells are elongated with oval nuclei and fibrillary eosinophilic cytoplasm (Fig. 3–38). Lamellar calcified bodies may or may not be seen distributed within the tumor. Mitoses and cellular pleomorphism are not common. Immunohistochemical studies that may be of help in corroborating this diagnosis include EMA, keratin, and vimentin positivity.

The treatment of choice appears to be surgical resection, and the prognosis for these tumors appears good.

DIFFERENTIAL DIAGNOSIS. The most important consideration is to make sure that one is not dealing with a **metastatic meningioma.** Therefore, a good clinical history and physical examination are very important. On the other hand, meningiomas may be confused with other sarcomas or benign neurogenic tumors. In this context, the characteristic whorled pattern and the immunohistochemical findings should lead to the correct interpretation.

Glomus Tumor

This tumor is exceedingly rare in the lung. Only two cases of this entity have been reported.[146, 147]

CLINICAL FEATURES. It is difficult to assess the predominant clinical features of this tumor in view of the scarcity of reported cases. The cases in the literature occurred in adults.

HISTOLOGIC FEATURES. At low power, well-demarcated tumor is seen that shows a prominent vascular component admixed with areas of more solid growth. The areas of solid growth are composed of round to oval cells with distinct cell borders, round nuclei, inconspicuous nucleoli, and eosinophilic cytoplasm (Fig. 3–39). The cellular proliferation surrounds vascular structures that are scattered throughout the tumor. In other areas, the cellular proliferation is arranged in strands or ribbons of cells embedded in a myxomatous stroma (Fig. 3–40). Mitoses, necrosis, and cellular atypia are uncommon.

Immunohistochemically, the tumors show positive reaction for antibodies against actin. Ultrastructurally, glomus tumors show smooth muscle differentiation with the presence of pinocytotic vesicles, basement membrane, and intracytoplasmic filaments with focal condensations. The treatment of choice is surgical resection of the tumor, and the prognosis seems to be good.

DIFFERENTIAL DIAGNOSIS. The most difficult diagnosis is probably to separate this tumor from a smooth muscle tumor such as **leiomyoblastoma** or **epithelioid leiomyosarcoma.** A possible clue to differentiate them is the very prominent vascularity in cases of glomus tumors. In addition, the presence of more conventional areas of benign glomus tumor may also help in arriving at a more accurate diagnosis. Ultrastructurally and immunohistochemically, both tumors show similar features. In addition, both tumors are rare as primary or as metastatic tumors.

Granular Cell Tumor

These tumors are also rare as primary lung neoplasms.[148–150] Their histogenesis continues to be a matter of debate.

CLINICAL FEATURES. These tumors have been reported in adults and probably occur more often in the fifth decade of life. Because of the endobronchial location of most of the cases, symptoms related to airway obstruction may be seen, including cough, dyspnea, and hemoptysis. However, they can present as intraparenchymal lesions, in which case the lesion is probably asymptomatic and discovered on routine physical examination.

GROSS FEATURES. In the vast majority of cases, these tumors present as well-circumscribed endobronchial lesions,

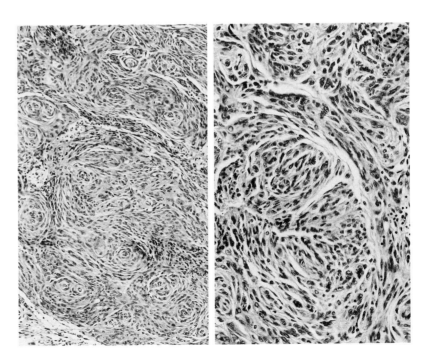

FIGURE 3–38. *Right,* Meningioma showing spindle cell proliferation formed by elongated cells with fibrillary cytoplasm. *Left,* The characteristic whorled pattern.

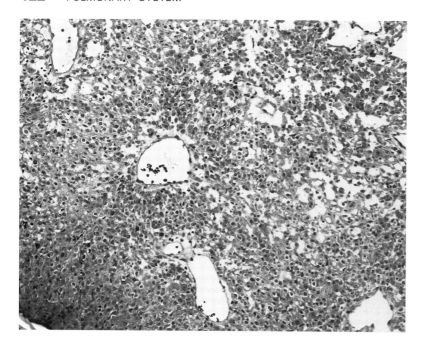

FIGURE 3–39. Solid areas of a glomus tumor composed of elongated cells with oval nuclei with prominent vascular features.

without any lung site predilection. The lesions can be less than 1 cm to more than 5 cm.

HISTOLOGIC FEATURES. Typically the tumor shows a homogeneous cellular proliferation composed of relatively large cells with distinct cell borders, round nuclei, and abundant granular eosinophilic cytoplasm (Figs. 3–41 and 3–42). The cellular proliferation appears to be uniform throughout the tumor. Mitoses, cellular atypia, and necrosis are uncommon. Immunohistochemically, the tumor may show positive reaction with antibodies for S-100 protein and neuron-specific enolase. Ultrastructurally, the presence of lysosomes is diagnostic of granular cell tumors.

Surgical resection appears to be the treatment of choice, and the prognosis for these tumors is good.

DIFFERENTIAL DIAGNOSIS. Tumors showing histiocytic or oncocytic changes may be confused with granular cell tumor. However, the presence of relatively larger cells with prominent granular eosinophilic cytoplasm is diagnostic of granular cell tumor. In cases in which one suspects another tumor with oncocytic features (such as **oncocytic carcinoid,** which can also present as an endobronchial lesion), the use of immunohistochemical stains for neuroendocrine markers leads to the correct diagnosis.

Malignant Melanoma

Malignant melanoma is a tumor of ubiquitous distribution that can present as a primary lung neoplasm.[151–153] Distinction

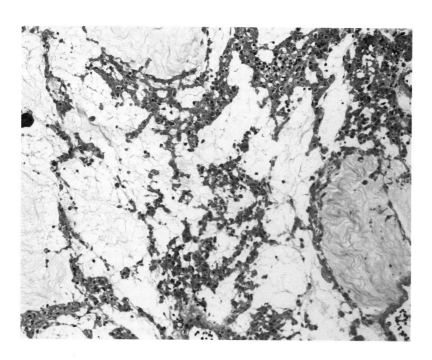

FIGURE 3–40. Strands and ribbons of cells embedded in a myxoid stroma can be seen in glomus tumor.

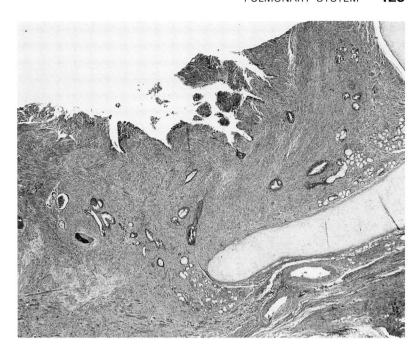

FIGURE 3-41. Granular cell tumor showing an endobronchial growth with a homogeneous cellular proliferation.

from metastatic melanoma can be made only by clinical means.

CLINICAL FEATURES. The tumor seems to occur in adults, without gender or lung predilection. In the cases described, no previous history of melanoma has been obtained. Because these tumors may present as an endobronchial lesion, symptoms related to airway obstruction may be seen.

GROSS FEATURES. Most reported cases of primary melanoma of the lung are described as an endobronchial lesion. However, flat melanomas have also been described.

HISTOLOGIC FEATURES. The most important feature suggesting lung primary is the transition between relatively normal bronchial epithelium and an atypical melanocytic proliferation (melanoma *in situ*) in a patient without evidence of a tumor elsewhere. As with melanomas elsewhere, these tumors may

show different growth patterns, including the common nesting pattern composed of large cells with round nuclei, prominent nucleoli, and eosinophilic cytoplasm. Bizarre cells may be observed in the tumor. Pigment may or may not be evident. In addition, other histologic features such as spindle cells may be observed in cases of melanoma. Immunohistochemically, S-100 protein and HMB-45 show diffuse positive staining of tumor cells. Premelanosomes may be identified on ultrastructural studies.

The behavior of the tumor is unpredictable. Either it will behave aggressively or it may follow a protracted course. Survival of more than a decade has been observed in some cases.

DIFFERENTIAL DIAGNOSIS. The most important problem in differential diagnosis is to determine whether the tumor repre-

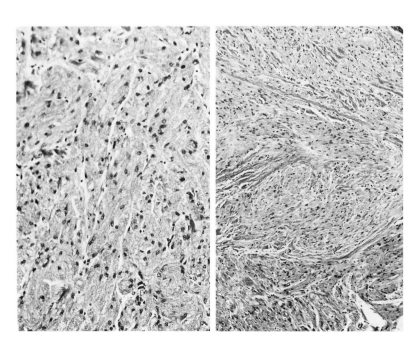

FIGURE 3-42. *Right,* Rather large cells with abundant eosinophilic cytoplasm. *Left,* Closer view showing prominent granular cytoplasm with round to oval nuclei toward the periphery of the cells.

sents a **metastasis from another source.** Careful clinical history is essential in this context.

LYMPHOPROLIFERATIVE DISORDERS

A variety of lymphoproliferative disorders may present with lung involvement. Herein we will include those entities that may pose a difficulty for the diagnosis and that may rarely be encountered in the lung.

Pseudolymphoma

Pulmonary pseudolymphomas are relatively rare primary lymphoid lesions,[154] even though there are some authors who doubt the existence of such a condition.[155] **In the past, a good number of cases coded as pseudolymphomas of the lung would today be reclassified as malignant lymphomas.** However, the existence of pseudolymphoma as an entity has been recognized in the literature. Whether these lesions are premalignant lesions or part of a spectrum of low-grade lymphoproliferative lesions is still controversial.

CLINICAL FEATURES. Pulmonary pseudolymphomas have been more often reported in adults. In a good number of cases, the patients present with a history of an autoimmune process such as systemic lupus erythematosus. The majority of patients, however, are usually asymptomatic, and the pulmonary mass is discovered on a routine physical examination. In rare occasions, numerous intrapulmonary nodules can be seen radiographically.

HISTOLOGIC FEATURES. Low-power magnification shows areas of lung parenchyma replaced by a lymphoid infiltrate showing numerous germinal centers (Fig. 3–43). Closer view of the infiltrate demonstrates the presence of a polymorphous cellular infiltrate composed of mature lymphocytes and plasma cells with numerous Russell bodies (Fig. 3–44). Giant

cells and granulomas are often seen. Necrosis is rare in cases of pseudolymphoma.

Immunohistochemically, the infiltrate shows a polyclonal population of B lymphocytes. Even though the prognosis for cases of pseudolymphoma is good, these patients deserve a close follow up for the eventuality of a recurrence or the progression to malignant lymphoma.

DIFFERENTIAL DIAGNOSIS. The most important problem in differential diagnosis is to separate these lesions from a **low-grade malignant lymphoma.** Histologically, the presence of a polymorphous infiltrate with numerous plasma cells and germinal centers, in addition to the evidence of polyclonality, leads to the correct diagnosis.

Pulmonary Plasmacytoma

Plasmacytomas occurring as primary lung neoplasms are exceedingly rare. Nonetheless, they have been reported in the literature.[156–161]

CLINICAL FEATURES. In a review of this unusual neoplasm, Geetha et al.[156] found 19 patients with this condition. Men and women were affected equally, and the median age was 42 years. Reports of this tumor in children have also been documented. It appears that in many instances, the pulmonary mass is found on a routine physical examination.

HISTOLOGIC FEATURES. The growth pattern of pulmonary plasmacytomas is similar to those found elsewhere. At low power there is a diffuse, homogeneous cellular proliferation at times separated by thin fibrous septa. Closer view of the cellular infiltrate shows the presence of the characteristic plasma cell proliferation (Figs. 3–45 and 3–46). Focal cellular atypia is seen, but this feature is not common. Immunohistochemically, the use of kappa and lamda stains should help in arriving at a correct diagnosis because the tumor shows a monoclonal staining pattern.

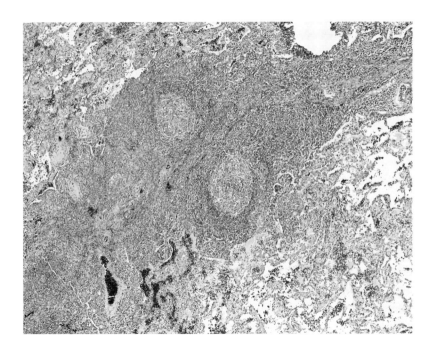

FIGURE 3–43. Pulmonary pseudolymphoma showing a lymphoid proliferation with presence of germinal centers.

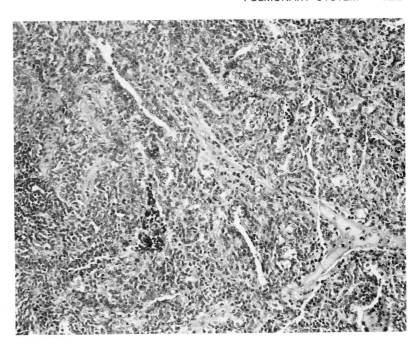

FIGURE 3–44. Pulmonary pseudolymphoma showing a polymorphous cellular infiltrate with numerous plasma cells.

The treatment for patients with pulmonary plasmacytoma may vary from individual to individual. However, surgical resection seems to be the most often used treatment. In some instances, radiation therapy and chemotherapy have been used after surgical resection. The prognosis for these patients is also variable. The tumor may follow an indolent course, or the patient may develop multiple myeloma.

DIFFERENTIAL DIAGNOSIS. It is most important not to confuse pulmonary plasmacytoma with a **plasmacytoid malignant lymphoma.** The presence of a virtually homogeneous cell population composed of plasma cells without significant atypia leads to the correct diagnosis. Another possible entity to be considered is a plasma cell granuloma. However, in the latter case, the presence of collections of foamy macrophages and spindle cells in addition to the presence of a polyclonal infiltrate would be against the diagnosis of pulmonary plasmacytoma.

Malignant Lymphoma (Low-Grade Malignant Lymphoma of Balt)

CLINICAL FEATURES. Adults are more often affected by this condition. However, younger individuals may also be affected. There appears to be no gender predilection for this tumor, and a significant portion of the patients are discovered to have this tumor on a routine chest radiograph.[162–165]

The tumor may present a solitary mass or pulmonary infiltrates. Grossly, the tumor may show its characteristic appear-

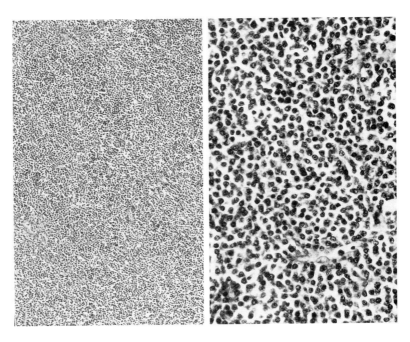

FIGURE 3–45. *Left,* Diffuse infiltrate replacing normal lung parenchyma. *Right,* The infiltrate is exclusively of plasma cells.

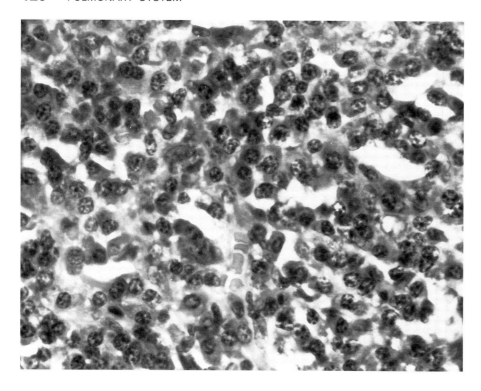

FIGURE 3–46. Closer view of the plasma cell infiltrate in a pulmonary plasmacytoma.

ance of "fish flesh." Necrosis and/or hemorrhage are uncommon.

HISTOLOGIC FEATURES. At low power, there is a diffuse homogeneous cellular proliferation obliterating the normal lung architecture (Fig. 3–47). At higher power, the tumor is composed almost exclusively of atypical lymphocytes (Fig. 3–48). In some areas, a plasmacytoid appearance may be observed. The neoplastic cellular proliferation usually extends into vascular structures. In addition, the tumor cells have predilection to spread into lymphatic routes, pleura, and bronchial cartilage. The presence of numerous multinucleated giant cells or a striking granulomatous reac-

tion may be seen in these cases. Germinal center may also be seen.

Even though the diagnosis can confidently be made on morphologic grounds, immunohistochemical studies using lymphoid markers can be used to further classify the immunophenotype of the tumor. Most of these cases are B-cell lymphomas; therefore, immunohistochemical stain for L-26 (B-cell marker) is expected to be positive. However, a small group of lymphomas sharing the histologic features previously described show a predominance for T cells (positive UCHL-1 marker).[164] These tumors are very uncommon, and their clinical significance is still unknown.

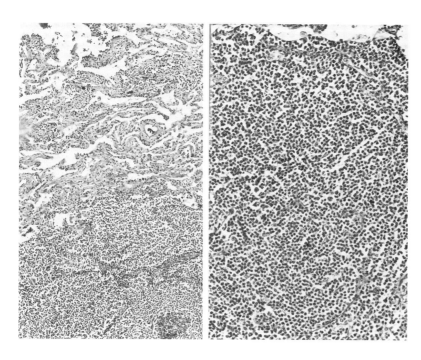

FIGURE 3–47. *Left,* Lymphoid proliferation infiltrating the lung parenchyma. *Right,* A homogeneous lymphoid infiltrate of a malignant lymphoma.

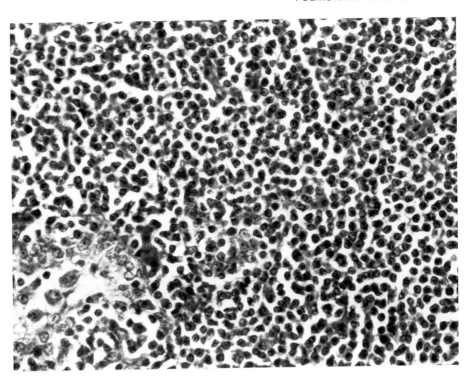

FIGURE 3–48. Closer view of the lymphoid infiltrate in a malignant lymphoma of lung.

DIFFERENTIAL DIAGNOSIS. Possible entities that may be considered include **lymphocytic interstitial pneumonitis** and **pseudolymphoma.** However, the presence of an atypical infiltrate invading bronchial cartilage, vascular structures, and pleura, in addition to monoclonal reactivity with lymphoid markers, is more in keeping with the diagnosis of lymphoma.

Angiocentric Immunoproliferative Processes

This term encompasses several lesions that have been coded under different names, including **lymphomatoid granulomatosis (LYG), polymorphic reticulosis, benign and malignant angiitis** and **granulomatosis,** and **angiocentric immunoproliferative lesions (AIL).**[166–170] Current universal terminology for these lesions is still controversial. However, it is possible that all these terms represent a spectrum of differentiation for these lesions. We will concentrate our description on LYG/AIL as an encompassing term.

CLINICAL FEATURES. This condition appears to affect adults more often. However, younger patients have been described. Common symptomatology observed in these patients includes chest pain and dyspnea. In some patients, besides the pulmonary manifestations, skin involvement may also co-exist. The lesion in the lung may appear as a multinodular tumor that can be bilateral.

HISTOLOGIC FEATURES. At low-power magnification, there may be the presence of discrete nodular areas composed predominantly of lymphocytes. In some areas, the lymphoid infiltrate may expand into the interstitium. However, the **infiltrate especially follows vascular tracts and often infiltrates vascular structures.** The atypical cellular proliferation shows a more polymorphous cell population with presence of lymphocytes with twisted nuclei. Areas of necrosis are commonly seen. In addition, large cells with bilobate nuclei (Reed-Sternberg–like cells) are often seen. Granulomas are not part of the morphologic picture of LYG/AIL. Depending on the cytologic appearance of the infiltrate, a grading system has been proposed. Lesions that show marked cytologic atypia of the lymphoid cells, a more monomorphous appearance, extensive necrosis, and increased proportion of large cells have been designated as high-grade. The opposite conditions would indicate low-grade lesions. Even though an intermediate group may also be possible, for practical terms, it is easier to relate those lesions as high- or low-grade. Most of the cases of this condition are in the high grade category. Immunohistochemically, most cases show a T-cell positivity (UCHL-1 positive).

DIFFERENTIAL DIAGNOSIS. It can include other lymphoproliferative lesions such as **Hodgkin's disease, small lymphocytic lymphoma of bronchus-associated lymphoid tissue (BALT), or large-cell lymphoma.** In this regard, immunohistochemical markers coupled with careful evaluation of the histologic features of the angiocentric lesion would be of help in arriving at a correct interpretation.

Hodgkin's Disease

CLINICAL FEATURES. Primary Hodgkin's disease of the lung is extremely rare.[171, 172] When present, an extension from another source such as mediastinum should be excluded. In a study of 15 patients[172] in whom Hodgkin's disease was found in the lung, the patients appear to be older than the patients affected by nodal Hodgkin's disease. In addition, the number of women seems to be higher than the number of men.

The histologic features of Hodgkin's disease in the lung are similar to those described in other locations such as mediastinum or lymph node.

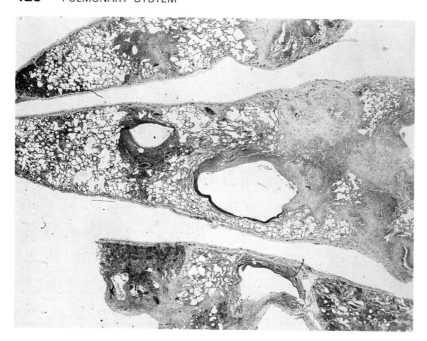

FIGURE 3–49. Eosinophilic granuloma of lung showing numerous nodules in the lung parenchyma.

Eosinophilic Granuloma of Lung (Histiocytosis X)

CLINICAL FEATURES. Men and women are affected around the fourth decade of life. A number of the patients provide a history of smoking. However, this association has not been clearly defined. The symptomatology may be variable, including pneumothorax, dyspnea, cough, and chest pain.[173–175]

HISTOLOGIC FEATURES. The classic presentation of pulmonary eosinophilic granuloma is that of numerous nodules replacing portions of the normal lung parenchyma (Fig. 3–49). These nodules may or may not contain a variable amount of eosinophils; however, their absence does not preclude the diagnosis of eosinophilic granuloma. These nodules may also show a variable degree of cellularity. In some nodules, areas of fibrosis are often seen. The latter feature may relate to the various stages of development of these nodules. At high-power magnification, the cellular proliferation consists of mixed infiltrate of lymphocytes with or without eosinophils and histiocytes with grooving of the nuclei (Fig. 3–50). Adjacent lung parenchyma may show collections of macrophages filling the alveolar spaces.

Immunohistochemical stains for S-100 protein are useful to identify Langerhans cells, and the presence of Birbeck granules under electron microscopy is diagnostic of eosinophilic granuloma.

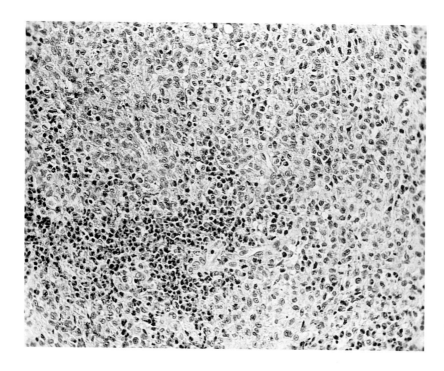

FIGURE 3–50. Eosinophilic granuloma of lung showing small accumulation of eosinophils admixed with a histiocytic cellular process.

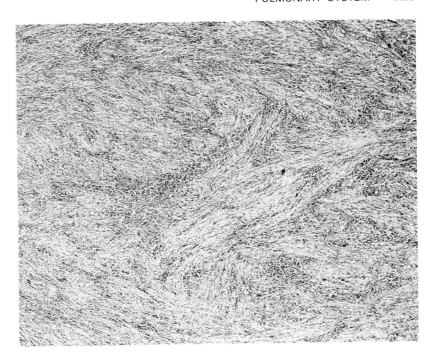

FIGURE 3–51. Inflammatory pseudotumor showing a spindle cell proliferation replacing normal lung parenchyma.

Once the diagnosis is established, treatment with steroids may be indicated. Progression to pulmonary fibrosis may occur.

DIFFERENTIAL DIAGNOSIS. Reactive eosinophilic pleuritis may show some of the histologic features of eosinophilic granuloma of the lung. However, in reactive eosinophilic pleuritis, even though the patient may present with history of spontaneous pneumothorax, the infiltrate seems to be along the pleural surface and not in the nodular intraparenchymal location as with eosinophilic granuloma. Another consideration may be **Hodgkin's disease;** however, the absence of Reed-Sternberg cells and positive reaction using S-100 protein antibodies are more in keeping with the diagnosis of eosinophilic granuloma.

TUMORS OF UNKNOWN HISTOGENESIS

Inflammatory Pseudotumor (Plasma Cell Granuloma)

This is a benign condition that, as its name implies, mimics a pulmonary neoplasm and must be distinguished from other malignant neoplasms. In the past, this lesion has been known by several names, including **fibroxanthoma, histiocytoma, xanthofibroma, xanthoma,** and **xanthogranuloma.** More recently, the term **inflammatory myofibroblastic tumor** was introduced as a synonym for **plasma cell granuloma.**[176–182]

CLINICAL FEATURES. This condition can be seen at any age and possibly represents the majority of benign intrapulmonary lung tumors in children.[177] There is no gender or lung predilection. When symptoms are present, they include cough, fever, dyspnea, and the like. In many cases, a history of respiratory infection is obtained. However, in a good number of cases, there are no clinical symptoms, and the lesion is found in a routine chest radiograph. In most instances, the lesion appears as a single, well-defined tumor. On a few occasions, the tumor may appear as multiple nodules distributed throughout the lung parenchyma, affecting both lungs or affecting the mediastinum.

HISTOLOGIC FEATURES. At low magnification, there is obliteration of the normal lung parenchyma by a spindle cell proliferation (Fig. 3–51) with scattered Masson bodies mainly at the periphery of the lesion. However, at higher magnification, one can see a mixture of inflammatory cells including plasma cells, lymphocytes, macrophages, and eosinophils admixed with a marked fibroblastic proliferation (Fig. 3–52). Because of the presence of a mixture of components, inflammatory pseudotumors have been categorized in different subtypes. Nonetheless, an overlap of morphologic features may be seen in those subtypes. The plasma cell granuloma type is characterized by a mixture of spindle cells, probably representing fibroblasts or myofibroblasts, and collagen admixed with a heavy plasma cell component. Areas showing collections of macrophages with other inflammatory cells may be seen distributed haphazardly throughout. No granulomas are seen in this lesion. The fibrohistiocytic variant of inflammatory pseudotumor is characterized by the presence of a spindle cell proliferation probably representing fibroblasts or myofibroblast admixed with macrophages (xanthoma cells). This spindle cell proliferation is arranged in a storiform pattern with scattered areas of inflammatory cells. Touton giant cells may be observed in this lesion. Even though mitotic figures may be seen, they are rare. Necrosis and anaplasia are unusual.

Immunohistochemical positivity for vimentin and muscle-specific actin may be seen in the spindle cell component. Lysozyme and alpha-1-antichymotrypsin positivity may be seen in macrophages. The plasma cell component, as expected, shows a polyclonal reaction.

The treatment of choice for this lesion appears to be surgical excision. Although this condition is considered benign, reports

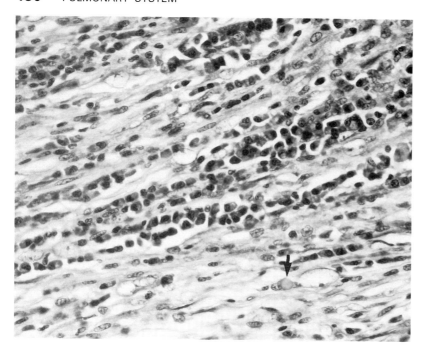

FIGURE 3–52. Inflammatory pseudotumor showing spindle cells admixed with numerous plasma cells. A Russell body is seen *(arrow)*.

of infiltration outside the lung parenchyma have been documented.[180]

DIFFERENTIAL DIAGNOSIS. Because of the presence of a spindle cell proliferation, this lesion may be confused with a **sarcoma.** In the cases with more fibrohistiocytic features and presence of Touton giant cells, the most important consideration is a **malignant fibrous histiocytoma.** However, the presence of an inflammatory background with numerous plasma cells and collections of macrophages with absence of anaplasia are more in keeping with the diagnosis of inflammatory pseudotumor. If another sarcoma is considered, one may have to rely on the use of immunohistochemical studies. In cases in which invasion of adjacent organs is present, one

may have to carefully sample and review the lesion before a diagnosis of pseudotumor is made.

Sclerosing Hemangioma

This tumor represents an unusual benign neoplasm of uncertain histogenesis. The tumor has been coded in the past as **papillary pneumocytoma** and **fibroxanthoma** among others. Several theories have been proposed to explain its origin in the lung. However, its histogenesis remains uncertain.[183–188]

CLINICAL FEATURES. The tumor can occur at any age, and patients vary from young adults to middle-aged individuals.

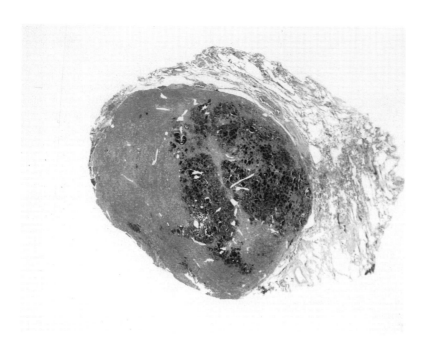

FIGURE 3–53. Low-power view of a sclerosing hemangioma showing a well-demarcated pulmonary nodule.

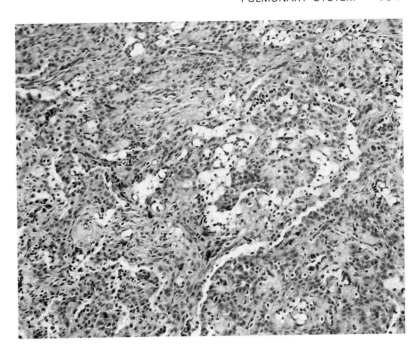

FIGURE 3–54. Sclerosing hemangioma showing solid areas separated by collagenous tissue and presence of scattered macrophages.

It is more common in women, and a great number of patients are asymptomatic. Radiologically, there is generally a single tumor mass that may show central calcifications.

GROSS FEATURES. The tumor size may vary from smaller than 1 cm to more than 5 cm. Usually, the tumor is a single intraparenchymal reddish mass. However, multiple lesions as well as metastasis to regional lymph nodes have been described.

HISTOLOGIC FEATURES. The tumors may show different growth patterns admixed with one another (Fig. 3–53). Areas of papillary features admixed with more solid areas or areas of sclerosis and/or hemorrhage may be observed in the same tumor. In addition, collections of foamy macrophages and inflammatory infiltrate may be seen. The cellular proliferation may be composed of round cells with oval nuclei and inconspicuous nucleoli (Figs. 3–54 and 3–55). In the areas of papillary growth, the lining cells appear cuboidal with eosinophilic cytoplasm. More recently, we described a case of sclerosing hemangioma admixed with numerous multinucleated giant cells that represents the granulomatous variant of this entity.[189]

Immunohistochemical studies for keratin, EMA, CEA, vimentin, and surfactant apoprotein have been reported to stain the round interstitial cellular proliferation.

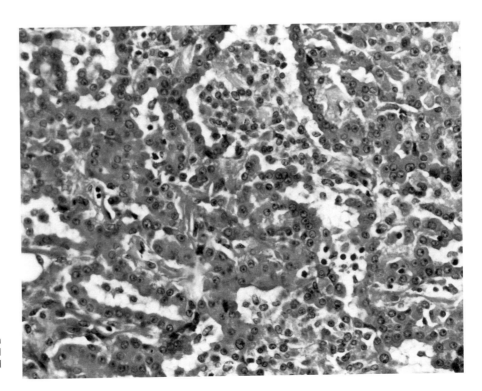

FIGURE 3–55. Closer view of a solid area of a sclerosing hemangioma composed of polygonal cells with round to oval nuclei and eosinophilic cytoplasm.

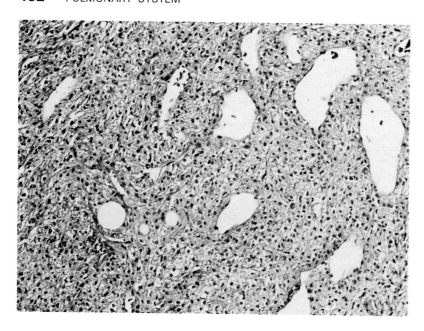

FIGURE 3–56. "Sugar tumor" showing the characteristic clear cellular proliferation admixed with numerous vascular spaces.

The treatment of choice is surgical excision, and the prognosis is good.

DIFFERENTIAL DIAGNOSIS. Sclerosing hemangioma may be confused with an **inflammatory pseudotumor** because of the presence of foamy macrophages and inflammatory infiltrate. However, the presence of papillary and solid areas admixed with sclerosis are more in keeping with a sclerosing hemangioma. In addition, sclerosing hemangioma may be confused with **carcinoid tumors.** In this setting, the use of neuroendocrine markers leads to the correct diagnosis.

Clear-Cell Tumor (Sugar Tumor) of Lung

This represents an unusual neoplasm of the lung.[190-192] Because of its close similarity to tumors in other organs, the diagnosis is not easily made, and in many cases, it is confused with other more common tumors. Its histogenesis is still controversial.

CLINICAL FEATURES. The tumor affects both sexes and is more common in adults. Most of the patients are asymptomatic, and the pulmonary mass is found on a routine physical examination.

GROSS FEATURES. The tumors are well-circumscribed intrapulmonary masses with no direct association with airways. At resection, the tumors appear well demarcated, with no hemorrhage or necrosis.

HISTOLOGIC FEATURES. At low power there is a homogeneous cellular proliferation with numerous dilated vascular spaces (Fig. 3–56). Closer view of the cellular proliferation shows cells characterized by clear cytoplasm (Fig. 3–57); in some areas the cytoplasm can be slightly eosinophilic or granular. However, the most striking feature is the large cells with eccentric nuclei and clear cytoplasm. The dilated vascular structures are often hyalinized or fibrotic. No necrosis or mitotic activity is seen.

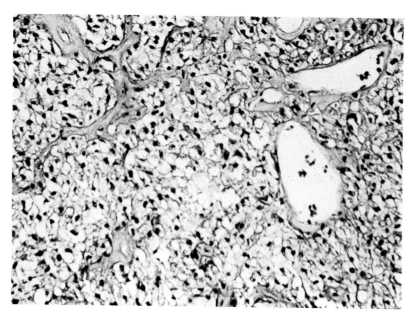

FIGURE 3–57. Closer view of the clear cellular proliferation of a "sugar tumor." Hyalinization of the adjacent vessels is common in these tumors.

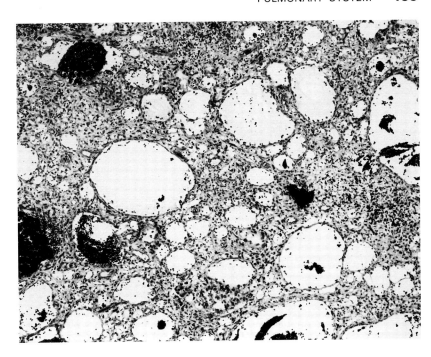

FIGURE 3-58. Alveolar adenoma showing dilated structures admixed with more solid areas.

Histochemical stains for PAS are useful to demonstrate the presence of glycogen. Immunohistochemically, numerous antibodies have been shown to produce a positive reaction in the clear cells. However, characteristically and probably more practical and useful is the presence of positive reaction for HMB-45.

This tumor is benign and surgical resection alone is curative.

DIFFERENTIAL DIAGNOSIS. Essentially **any tumor showing clear-cell features** should be considered in the differential diagnosis. Among the most common, **renal cell carcinoma** and **clear-cell carcinoma of the thyroid** are at the top of the list. However, the absence of tumors in these areas plus the presence of positive staining for HMB-45 should lead to the correct diagnosis.

Alveolar Adenoma

This term was coined by Yousem and Hochholzer[193] for a benign pulmonary neoplasm that can occur only sparingly as a primary lung tumor.

CLINICAL FEATURES. In the original description of six cases,[193] the patients were adults with a mean age of 59 years. The tumor is usually found on routine physical examination.

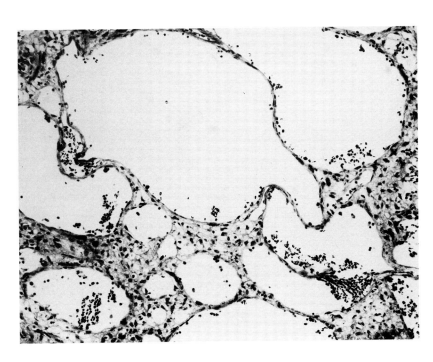

FIGURE 3-59. Alveolar adenoma showing dilated spaces mimicking a lymphangioma.

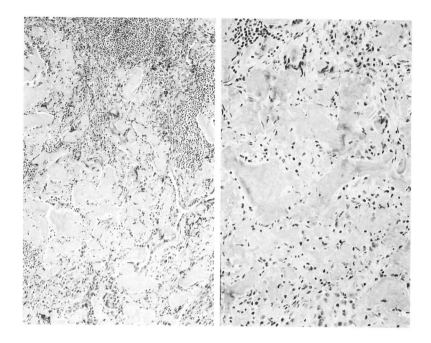

FIGURE 3–60. Two different fields of a pulmonary mass composed of an amorphous acellular material admixed with inflammatory cells and occasional giant cells, typical of pulmonary amyloidosis.

GROSS FEATURES. The tumor is well circumscribed with hemorrhagic and cystic areas and can vary in size from 1 to 2.5 cm. No predilection for a particular lung or lobe has been appreciated.

HISTOLOGIC FEATURES. At low power, the tumor appears well circumscribed and cystic (Fig. 3–58). At higher power, the cystic structures are lined by alveolar pneumocytes, some showing a hobnail-shaped appearance. Within these cystic structures, collections of foamy macrophages are found. At times the tumors give the impression of a vascular neoplasm, and many cases were interpreted as pulmonary **lymphangiomas** in the past (Fig. 3–59). An inflammatory background can be seen as well as the formation of more fibrotic areas. Immunohistochemical stains for keratin and CEA may show positive reaction in the alveolar lining.

The treatment for these tumors is surgical excision, and the prognosis is good.

DIFFERENTIAL DIAGNOSIS. Vascular tumors, namely **lymphangiomas,** are the most important in the differential diagnosis. In this regard the use of negative staining for factor VIII and positive staining for keratin and CEA helps clarify the issue. From the histologic point of view, even though the tumor may look vascular, the cystic spaces are lined by alveolar cells and not endothelial cells.

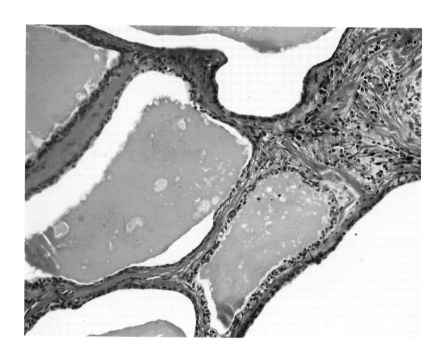

FIGURE 3–61. Mucous gland adenoma composed of dilated mucous glands filled with mucus.

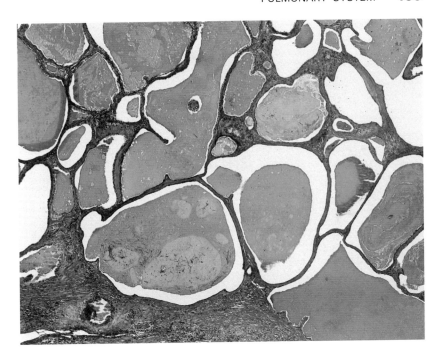

FIGURE 3–62. Dilated mucous glands filled with mucus without cellular atypia.

MISCELLANEOUS TUMORS

Pulmonary Amyloidosis (Amyloidoma)

CLINICAL FEATURES. It is a rare condition that can present as one or multiple pulmonary nodules. If the condition presents as a solitary nodular mass, it is likely that the patient is asymptomatic; the opposite occurs with multiple pulmonary nodules. Pulmonary amyloidosis may be associated with other medical conditions, including Sjogren's syndrome and other lymphoproliferative lesions.[194, 195]

GROSS FEATURES. The nodule or nodules may vary in size from 0.5 cm to more than 10 cm and have a waxy or hard consistency. Calcifications may be present.

MICROSCOPIC FINDINGS. The pulmonary parenchyma is replaced by a dense, homogeneous, eosinophilic amorphous material. An inflammatory infiltrate consisting of lymphocytes or plasma cells may be present, usually at the periphery of the nodule. Multinucleated giant cells at the periphery of the nodule are often seen (Fig. 3–60). Congo Red histochemical stain with an apple-green birefringency confirms the diagnosis.

Surgical resection of the nodules is the treatment of choice. The prognosis is good.

Lymphangiomyomatosis (LAM)

CLINICAL FEATURES. This condition is seen exclusively in women.[196–198] The clinical presentation may be related to the

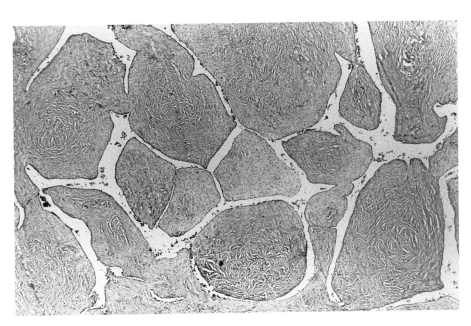

FIGURE 3–63. Adenofibroma showing spindle cell proliferation in a papillary-like pattern and lined by cuboidal epithelium.

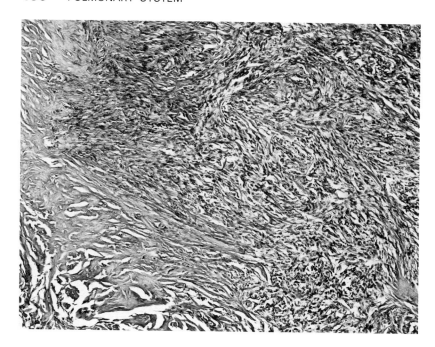

FIGURE 3–64. Localized fibrous tumor showing merging of rather acellular areas with more solid areas of spindle cell proliferation.

extent of the disease and may include respiratory symptoms such as cough, dyspnea, and other symptoms of obstruction.

HISTOLOGIC FEATURES. At low power, the lung parenchyma appears cystic. Higher power shows the presence of smooth muscle proliferation in the interstitium. In some areas, the smooth muscle proliferation appears more immature with some cytologic atypia. Adjacent lung parenchyma may show hemosiderin-laden macrophages. **Recently, it was shown that the cells in LAM stain positively for HMB-45.**

This condition can progress to pulmonary insufficiency followed by death.

DIFFERENTIAL DIAGNOSIS. The most important is a **leiomyoma.** However, the cystic nature of the process with smooth muscle proliferation along cysts without forming a mass is in keeping with LAM.

Mucous Gland Adenoma

CLINICAL FEATURES. It is a rare benign epithelial lesion that can occur in children and adults. Because of the bronchial location of the lesion, airway obstructive symptoms may be present. The lesions can be as large as 2 cm in greatest dimension.[199–201]

HISTOLOGIC FEATURES. The lesion is **essentially an exaggerated dilation of the mucous glands, which are usually filled with mucus** (Figs. 3–61 and 3–62). Focal papillary protrusions may be seen. In some occasions, the lesion is composed of glands lined by goblet cells. The dilation of the glands imparts a cystic appearance to these lesions. No cytologic atypia is seen in these lesions. Surgical excision is curative.

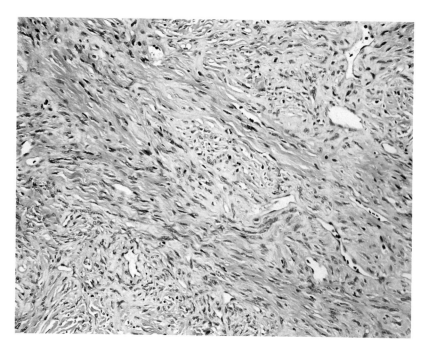

FIGURE 3–65. Localized fibrous tumor showing spindle cell proliferation with a wavy pattern reminiscent of a neural tumor.

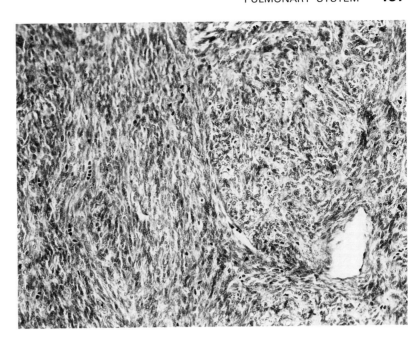

FIGURE 3–66. Localized fibrous tumor showing a more sarcomatous pattern similar to the one observed in monophasic synovial sarcoma.

DIFFERENTIAL DIAGNOSIS. Because of the mucus deposition in the glands, the lesion may be confused with a colloid carcinoma or mucoepidermoid carcinoma. However, the absence of atypia, solid growth pattern of a carcinomatous process, and mucin-secreting epithelium lining the alveoli is in keeping with the diagnosis of mucous gland adenoma.

Pulmonary Adenofibroma

It is an unusual benign tumoral condition in the lung. The cases described have occurred in adults.[202] The patients are asymptomatic, and the lesion is discovered on incidental chest radiographs. The lesion presents as a solitary coin lesion that can range in size from 1 to 2 cm in greatest diameter. Histologically, the tumors are characterized by a hyalinized spindle cell proliferation that in low power appears as papillary projections. These papillary-like structures are lined by a simple cuboidal epithelium (Fig. 3–63). Immunohistochemically, vimentin antibodies strongly stain the spindle cell proliferation, whereas the epithelial lining is strongly positive for keratin and EMA.

Although the tumor is benign, it should be separated from the conventional **chondromatous hamartoma.** Nonetheless, we consider that pulmonary adenofibroma represents an unusual type of hamartoma.

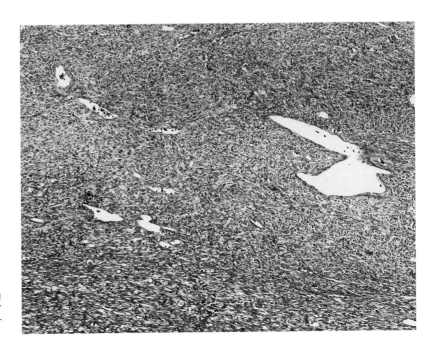

FIGURE 3–67. Localized fibrous tumor showing spindle cell proliferation with numerous vascular structures similar to the one observed in hemangiopericytoma.

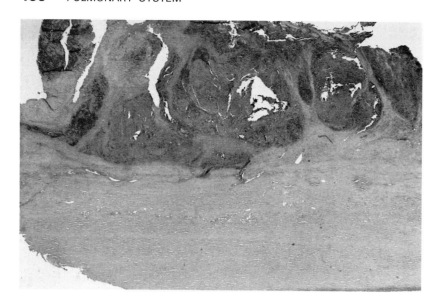

FIGURE 3-68. Thymoma growing along the pleural surface. Note the thickened pleura.

PLEURAL CONDITIONS

Localized Fibrous Tumor (Fibrous Mesothelioma)

These tumors are rather uncommon and have been also known by other names such as **fibroma, submesothelial fibroma,** or **fibrous mesothelioma.** Although originally described as a pleural tumor, intrapulmonary tumors have been described.[94, 204-206]

CLINICAL FEATURES. The tumors seem to affect men and women in equal proportions and usually occur in the sixth decade of life. The patients may present with symptoms of chest pain, pleural effusion, dyspnea, or hypoglycemia. Radiologically, the tumor presents as a well- or ill-defined tumor in any portion of the pleura. The tumor, as its name implies, is localized, and diffuse pleural thickening is not a feature of this tumor.

GROSS FEATURES. The tumor may vary in size from a few centimeters to well over 25 cm in greatest dimension. It is firm, white, and may be surrounded by a glistening membrane. In some cases, a pedicle may be identified.

HISTOLOGIC FEATURES. The growth pattern of solitary fibrous tumors of the pleura is diverse.[211] Although it is possible that the short storiform pattern (so-called patternless pattern) may be the most commonly identified (Fig. 3–64), the tumors may show features mimicking a neurogenic tumor (Fig. 3–65) or a monophasic synovial sarcoma (Fig. 3–66). Often the tumor shows a striking hemangiopericytic pattern (Fig. 3–67). Therefore, one must be familiar with the histologic growth patterns that this tumor may show. In addition, the clinical presentation of the tumor (pleural based) along with the histologic features is most helpful in arriving at a correct interpretation. Increased mitotic activity, hypercellularity, cellular atypia, necrosis, and hemorrhage have been interpreted as features associated with malignant tumors.

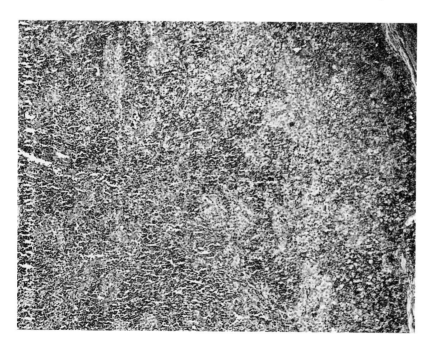

FIGURE 3–69. Pleural thymoma showing a biphasic cell population composed of epithelial cells and lymphocytes.

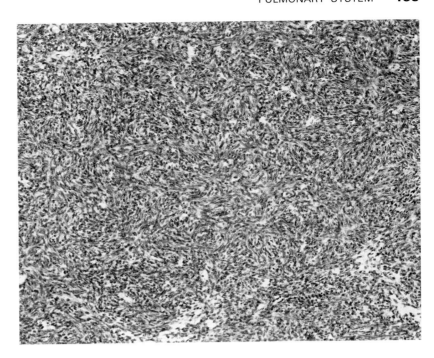

FIGURE 3-70. Pleural thymoma showing the spindle cell pattern.

However, one of the most important factors for prognosis is the gross features of the neoplasm. Even though the histologic features of a localized tumor of the pleura may be interpreted as atypical, if a tumor is attached to the pleura by a pedicle and is completely resected, the prognosis is good. On the other hand, even though the morphologic features of the tumor are benign, if a tumor is not resectable, the possibility of recurrence is high.

Immunohistochemically, vimentin is the most consistent antibody that shows positive reaction. However, focal positivity using actin and desmin has been reported. Keratin and S-100 protein are negative.

Pleural Thymomas

Thymomas are tumors more commonly seen in anterior mediastinum. However, in rare instances the tumor may be seen arising in the pleura in a manner clinically indistinguishable from mesothelioma.[139, 207]

CLINICAL FEATURES. In our study of eight cases, we did not identify any preference for gender or pleural site. All the patients were adults who presented with symptoms of chest pain, fever, and shortness of breath. However, the patients may also be asymptomatic. Radiographically, pleural thickening with encasement of the lung may occur without the presence of an anterior mediastinal mass.

GROSS FEATURES. In the cases that we reviewed, the tumor appeared to grow along the pleural border in a fashion similar to pleural mesothelioma.

HISTOLOGIC FEATURES. The tumor exhibits similar features as those of thymomas described in the anterior mediastinum, essentially a biphasic cell population composed of lymphocytes and epithelial cells separated in a typical lobular pattern (Figs. 3-68 and 3-69). It is also possible to find a spindle cell thymoma with the characteristic cellular proliferation of fusiform cells and numerous vascular spaces mimicking a vascular neoplasm, namely hemangiopericytoma (Fig. 3-70).

In this context, immunohistochemical studies may be of help in arriving at a proper diagnosis. Epithelial markers such as EMA or keratin show positive staining.

References

1. WHO: Histological Typing of Lung Tumors, 2nd ed. Geneva, Switzerland, World Health Organization, 1981.
2. Moran CA, Hochholzer L, Fishback N, et al: Mucinous (so-called colloid) carcinomas of lung. Mod Pathol 5(6):634, 1992.
3. Graeme-Cook F, Mark EJ: Pulmonary mucinous cystic tumors of borderline malignancy. Hum Pathol 22:185, 1991.
4. Kragel PJ, Devaney KO, Meth BM, et al: Mucinous cystadenoma of the lung. Arch Pathol Lab Med 114:1053, 1990.
5. Young RH, Gilks CB, Scully RE: Mucinous tumors of the appendix associated with mucinous tumors of the ovary and pseudomyxoma peritonei. Am J Surg Pathol 15:415, 1991.
6. McDivitt RW, Stewart FW, Berg JW: Tumors of the Breast Fasc #2, 2nd series. Washington, D.C., Armed Forces Institute of Pathology, 1968.
7. Brambilla E, Moro D, Veale D, et al: Basal cell (basaloid) carcinoma of the lung. A new morphologic and phenotypic entity with separate prognostic significance. Hum Pathol 23:993, 1992.
8. Wain SL, Kier R, Vollmer RT, et al: Basaloid squamous carcinoma of the tongue, hypopharynx, and larynx: Report of 10 cases. Hum Pathol 17:1158, 1986.
9. McKay MJ, Bilous AM: Basaloid squamous carcinoma of the hypopharynx. Cancer 63:2528, 1989.
10. Kheir S, Hickey RC, Martin RG, et al: Cloacogenic carcinoma of the anal canal. Arch Surg 104:407, 1972.
11. Klotz RG, Pamukcoglu T, Souilliard DH: Transitional cloacogenic carcinoma of the anal canal. Clinicopathologic study of 373 cases. Cancer 20:1727, 1967.
12. Haque AK: Pathology of carcinoma of the lung: An update on current concepts. J Thorac Imaging 7(1):9, 1991.
13. Pietra GC: The pathology of carcinoma of the lung. Semin Roentgenol 25(1):25, 1990.
14. Yesner R, Carter D: Pathology of carcinoma of the lung. Changing patterns. Clin Chest Med 3(2):257, 1982.
15. Yesner R: Histopathology of lung cancer. Semin Ultrasound CT MR 9(1):4, 1988.
16. Rosado-de-Christenson ML, Moran CA: Primary Lung Cancer: Pathology and Presenting Features. (Categorical course on imaging of cancers.) Reston, VA, American College of Radiology, 1992, pp 1–8.
17. Rosado-de-Christenson ML, Templeton P, Moran CA: Bronchogenic carcinoma: Radiologic-pathologic correlation. Radiographics 14:429–446, 1994.
18. Fraire AE, Johnson EH, Yesner R, et al: Prognostic significance of histopathologic subtype and stage in small cell lung cancer. Hum Pathol 23:520, 1992.
19. Sehested M, Hirsch FR, Osterlind K, Olsen JE: Morphologic variations of small cell lung cancer. A histopathologic study of pretreatment and posttreatment specimens in 104 patients. Cancer 11:1592, 1993.
20. Gould VE, Linnoila RI, Memoli VA, Warren WH: Neuroendocrine cells and neuroendocrine neoplasms of the lung. Pathol Annu 18:287, 1983.

21. Mooi WJ, Dewar A, Springall D, et al: Non-small cell lung carcinomas with neuroendocrine features. A light microscopic, immunohistochemical and ultrastructural study of 11 cases. Histopathology 13:329, 1988.

22. Travis WD, Linnoila RI, Tsokos MG, et al: Neuroendocrine tumors of the lung with proposed criteria for large-cell neuroendocrine carcinoma. An ultrastructural, immunohistochemical, and flow cytometric study of 35 cases. Am J Surg Pathol 15(6):529, 1991.

23. Arrigoni MG, Woolner LB, Bernatz PE: Atypical carcinoid tumors of the lung. J Thorac Cardiovasc Surg 64:413, 1972.

24. McCaughan BC, Martini N, Bains MS: Bronchial carcinoids. Review of 124 cases. J Thorac Cardiovasc Surg 89:8, 1985.

25. Pass HI, Doppman JL, Nieman L, et al: Management of the ectopic ACTH syndrome due to thoracic carcinoids. Ann Thorac Surg 50:52, 1990.

26. Ricci C, Patrassi N, Massa R, et al: Carcinoid syndrome in bronchial adenoma. Am J Surg 126:671, 1973.

27. Paladugu RR, Benfield JR, Pak HY, et al: Bronchopulmonary Kulchitzky cell carcinomas. A new classification scheme for typical and atypical carcinoids. Cancer 64:1304, 1989.

28. Ginsberg SS, Buzaid AC, Stern H, Carter D: Giant cell carcinoma of the lung. Cancer 70:606, 1992.

29. Herman DL, Bullok WK, Waken JK: Giant cell carcinoma of the lung. Cancer 19:1337, 1966.

30. Humphrey PA, Scroggs MW, Roggli VL, Shelburne JD: Pulmonary carcinomas with a sarcomatoid element: An immunohistochemical and ultrastructural analysis. Hum Pathol 19:155, 1989.

31. Matsui K, Kitagawa M: Spindle cell carcinoma of the lung. A clinicopathologic study of three cases. Cancer 67:2361, 1991.

32. Matsui K, Kitagawa M, Miwa A: Lung carcinoma with spindle cell components: Sixteen cases examined by immunohistochemistry. Hum Pathol 23:1289, 1992.

33. Ro JY, Chen JL, Lee JS, et al: Sarcomatoid carcinoma of the lung: Immunohistochemical and ultrastructural study of 14 cases. Cancer 69:376, 1992.

34. Fishback NF, Travis WD, Moran CA, et al: Pleomorphic (spindle/giant cell) carcinoma of the lung: A clinicopathologic study of 78 cases. Cancer 73:2936–2945, 1994.

35. Sridhar KS, Raub WA, Duncan RC, et al: The increasing recognition of adenosquamous lung carcinoma (1977–1986). Am J Clin Oncol 15:356, 1992.

36. Ishida T, Kaneko S, Yokoyama H, et al: Adenosquamous carcinoma of the lung. Clinicopathologic and immunohistochemical features. Am J Clin Pathol 97:678, 1992.

37. Takamori S, Noguchi M, Morinaga S, et al: Clinicopathologic characteristics of adenosquamous carcinoma of the lung. Cancer 67:649, 1991.

38. Sridhar KS, Bounassi MJ, Raub W, et al: Clinical features of adenosquamous lung carcinoma in 127 patients. Am Rev Respir Dis 142:19, 1990.

39. Naunheim KS, Taylor JR, Skosey C, et al: Adenosquamous lung carcinoma: Clinical characteristics, treatment and prognosis. Ann Thorac Surg 44:462, 1987.

40. Fitzgibbons PL, Kern WH: Adenosquamous carcinoma of the lung: A clinical and pathologic study of seven cases. Hum Pathol 16:463, 1985.

41. Yousem SA: Pulmonary adenosquamous carcinomas with amyloid-like stroma. Mod Pathol 2:420, 1989.

42. Kodama T, Shimosato Y, Watanabe S, et al: Six cases of well differentiated adenocarcinoma simulating fetal lung tissues in pseudoglandular stage: Comparison with pulmonary blastoma. Am J Surg Pathol 8:725, 1984.

43. Koss M, Hochholzer L, O'Leary T: Pulmonary blastomas. Cancer 67:2368, 1991.

44. Kradin R, Young R, Dickersin G, et al: Pulmonary blastoma with argyrophil cells lacking sarcomatous features (pulmonary endodermal tumor resembling fetal lung). Am J Surg Pathol 6:165, 1982.

45. Francis D, Jacobsen M: Pulmonary blastoma. Curr Top Pathol 73:265, 1983.

46. Jacobsen M, Francis D: Pulmonary blastoma. A clinicopathologic study of eleven cases. Acta Pathol Microbiol Scand (A) 88:151, 1980.

47. Nakatani Y, Dickersin G, Mark E: Pulmonary endodermal tumor resembling fetal lung: A clinicopathologic study of five cases with immunohistochemical and ultrastructural characterization. Hum Pathol 21:1097, 1990.

48. Davis MP, Eagan RT, Weiland LH, Pairolero PC: Carcinosarcoma of the lung: Mayo Clinic experience and response to chemotherapy. Mayo Clin Proc 59:598, 1984.

49. Nappi O, Wick MR: Sarcomatoid neoplasms of the respiratory tract. Semin Diagn Pathol 137, 1993.

50. Addis B, Corrin B: Pulmonary blastoma, carcinosarcoma, and spindle-cell carcinoma: An immunohistochemical study of keratin intermediate filaments. J Pathol 147:291, 1985.

51. Ishida T, Tateishi M, Kaneko S, et al: Carcinosarcoma and spindle cell sarcoma of the lung. Clinicopathologic and immunohistochemical studies. J Thorac Cardiovasc Surg 100:844, 1990.

52. Ludwigsen E: Endobronchial carcinosarcoma: A case with osteosarcoma of pulmonary invasive part, and a review with respect to prognosis. Virchows Arch A 373:293, 1977.

53. Prive L, Tellem M, Meranze D, Chodoff R: Carcinosarcoma of the lung: Immunohistochemical and ultrastructural studies of 14 cases. Cancer 69:376, 1992.

54. Stackhouse E, Harrison E, Ellis F: Primary mixed malignancies of lung: Carcinosarcoma and blastoma. J Thorac Cardiovasc Surg 57:385, 1969.

55. Dowling EA, Miller RE, Johnson IM, Collier FCD: Mucoepidermoid tumors of the bronchi. Surgery 52:600, 1962.

56. Turnbull AD, Huvos AG, Goodner JT, Foote FW: Mucoepidermoid tumors of the bronchial glands. Cancer 28:539, 1971.

57. Ozlu C, Christopherson WM, Allen JD: Muco-epidermoid tumors of the bronchus. J Thorac Cardiovasc Surg 42:24, 1961.

58. Axelsson C, Burcharth F, Johansen A: Mucoepidermoid lung tumors. J Thorac Cardiovasc Surg 65:902, 1973.

59. Klacsmann PG, Olson JL, Eggleston JC: Mucoepidermoid carcinoma of the bronchus. Cancer 43:1720, 1979.

60. Barsky SH, Martin SE, Matthews M, et al: "Low grade" mucoepidermoid carcinoma of the bronchus with "high grade" biologic behavior. Cancer 51:1505, 1983.

61. Mullins JD, Barnes RP: Childhood bronchial mucoepidermoid tumors. Cancer 44:315, 1979.

62. Yousem SA, Hochholzer L: Mucoepidermoid tumors of the lung. Cancer 60:1346, 1987.

63. Enterline HT, Schoenberg HW: Carcinoma (cylindromatous type) of trachea and bronchi and bronchial adenoma: A comparative study. Cancer 7:663, 1954.

64. Inoue H, Iwashita A, Kanegae H, et al: Peripheral pulmonary adenoid cystic carcinoma with substantial submucosal extension to the proximal bronchus. Thorax 46:147, 1991.

65. Conlan AA, Payne WS, Woolner LB, Sanderson DR: Adenoid cystic carcinoma (cylindroma) and mucoepidermoid carcinoma of the bronchus. J Thorac Surg 76:369, 1978.

66. Markel SF, Abell MR, Haight L, French AJ: Neoplasms of the bronchus commonly designated as adenomas. Cancer 17:590, 1964.

67. Payne WS, Ellis FH, Woolner LB, Moersch HJ: The surgical treatment of cylindroma (adenoid cystic carcinoma) and mucoepidermoid tumors of the bronchus. J Thorac Cardiovasc Sug 38:709, 1959.

68. Nomori H, Kaseda S, Kobayashi T, et al: Adenoid cystic carcinoma of the trachea and main-stem bronchus. A clinical, histopathologic and immunohistochemical study. J Thorac Cardiovasc Surg 96:271, 1988.

69. Heilbrunn A, Crosby IK: Adenoid cystic carcinoma and mucoepidermoid carcinoma of the tracheobronchial tree. Chest 61:145, 1972.

70. Moran CA, Suster S, Koss MN: Primary adenoid cystic carcinoma of the lung. A clinicopathologic and immunohistochemical study of 16 cases. Cancer 73: 1390–1397, 1994.

71. Hayes MMM, Van der Westhuizen NG, Forgie R: Malignant mixed tumor of the bronchus: A biphasic neoplasm of epithelial and myoepithelial cells. Mod Pathol 6:85, 1993.

72. Payne WS, Scier J, Woolner LB: Mixed tumors of the bronchus (salivary gland type). J Thorac Cardiovasc Surg 49:663, 1965.

73. Sakamoto H, Uda H, Tanaka T, et al: Pleomorphic adenoma in the periphery of the lung. Report of a case and review of the literature. Arch Pathol Lab Med 115:393, 1991.

74. Spencer H: Bronchial mucous gland tumors. Virchows Arch A [Pathol Anat] 383:101, 1979.

75. Wright ES, Pike E, Couves CM: Unusual tumors of the lung. J Surg Oncol 24:23, 1983.

76. Moran CA, Suster S, Askin FB, Koss MN: Benign and malignant salivary gland-like mixed tumors of the lung. Clinicopathologic and immunohistochemical study of 8 cases. Cancer 74:2251–2260, 1994.

77. Fechner RE, Bentinck BR, Askew JB: Acinic cell tumor of the lung. A histologic and structural study. Cancer 29:501, 1972.

78. Gharpure KJ, Deshpande RK, Vishweshvara RN, et al: Acinic cell tumor of the bronchus (a case report). Indian J Cancer 22:152, 1985.

79. Katz DR, Bubis JJ: Acinic cell tumor of the bronchus. Cancer 38:830, 1976.

80. Yoshida K, Koyama J, Matsui T: Acinic cell tumor of the bronchial gland. Nippon Geka Gakkai Zasshi 90:1810, 1989.

81. Moran CA, Suster S, Koss MN: Acinic cell carcinoma of the lung ("Fechner tumor"). A clinicopathologic, immunohistochemical, and ultrastructural study of five cases. Am J Surg Pathol 16:1039, 1992.

82. Fechner RE, Bentinck BR: Ultrastructure of bronchial oncocytoma. Cancer 31:1451, 1973.

83. Black WC: Pulmonary oncocytoma. Cancer 23:1347, 1969.

84. Santos-Briz A, Terron J, Sastre R, et al: Oncocytoma of the lung. Cancer 40:1330, 1977.

85. Bedrossian CWM, Verani R, Unger KM, Salman J: Pulmonary malignant fibrous histiocytoma: Light and electron microscopic studies of one case. Chest 75:186, 1979.

86. Yousem SA, Hochholzer L: Malignant fibrous histiocytoma of the lung. Cancer 60:2532, 1987.

87. McDonnell T, Kyriakos M, Roper C, Mzoujian G: Malignant fibrous histiocytoma of the lung. Cancer 61:137, 1988.

88. Sajjad SM, Begin LR, Dail DH, Lukeman JM: Fibrous histiocytoma of lung—a clinicopathologic study of two cases. Histopathology 5:325, 1981.

89. Lee TJ, Shelburne JD, Linder J: Primary malignant fibrous histiocytoma of the lung. A clinicopathologic and ultrastructural study of five cases. Cancer 53:1124, 1984.

90. Guccion J, Rosen S: Bronchopulmonary leiomyosarcoma and fibrosarcoma. Cancer 30:836, 1972.

91. Gebauer C: The postoperative prognosis of primary pulmonary sarcomas: A review with a comparison between the histological forms and the other primary endothoracal sarcomas based on 474 cases. Scand J Thorac Cardiovasc Surg 16:91, 1982.

92. Nascimento A, Unni K, Bernatz P: Sarcomas of the lung. Mayo Clin Proc 57:355, 1982.

93. Pettinato G, Manivel JC, Saldana MJ, et al: Primary bronchopulmonary fibrosarcoma of childhood and adolescence: Reassessment of a low-grade malignancy.

Clinicopathologic study of five cases and review of the literature. Hum Pathol 20:463, 1989.

94. Yousem S, Flynn S: Intrapulmonary localized fibrous tumor: Intraparenchymal so-called localized fibrous mesothelioma. Am J Clin Pathol 89:365, 1988.

95. Yellin A, Rosenman Y, Lieberman Y: Review of smooth muscle tumours of the lower respiratory tract. Br J Dis Chest 78:337, 1984.

96. Wick MR, Scheithauer BW, Piehler JM, Pairolero PC: Primary pulmonary leiomyosarcomas. Arch Pathol Lab Med 106:510, 1982.

97. Jimenez JF, Uthman EO, Townsend JW, et al: Primary brnchopulmonary leiomyosarcoma in childhood. Arch Pathol Lab Med 110:348, 1986.

98. Gal AA, Brooks JSJ, Pietra GG: Leiomyomatous neoplasms of the lung: A clinical, histologic, and immunohistochemical study. Mod Pathol 2:209, 1989.

99. Beluffi G, Bertolotti P, Mietta A, et al: Primary leiomyosarcoma of the lung in a girl. Pediatr Radiol 16:240, 1986.

100. Ramanathan T: Primary leiomyosarcoma of the lung. Thorax 29:482, 1974.

101. Morgan PGM, Ball J: Pulmonary leiomyosarcomas. Br J Dis Chest 74:245, 1980.

102. Dail DH, Liebow AA: Intravascular bronchioloalveolar tumor [abstract]. Am J Pathol 78:6, 1975.

103. Dail DH, Liebow AA, Gmelich JT, et al: Intravascular, bronchiolar, and alveolar tumor of the lung (IVBAT): An analysis of 20 cases of a peculiar sclerosing endothelial tumor. Cancer 51:452, 1983.

104. Azumi N, Churg A: Intravascular and sclerosing bronchioloalveolar tumor: A pulmonary sarcoma of probable vascular origin. Am J Surg Pathol 5:587, 1981.

105. Mark EJ: Mesenchymal cystic hamartoma of the lung. N Engl J Med 315:1255, 1986.

106. Hedlund GL, Bisset GS, Bove KE: Malignant neoplasms arising in cystic hamartomas of the lung in childhood. Radiology 173:77, 1989.

107. Bove KE: Sarcoma arising in pulmonary mesenchymal cystic hamartoma (Case 6). Pediatr Pathol 9:785, 1989.

108. Angerval L, Enzinger FM: Extraskeletal neoplasms resembling Ewing's sarcoma. Cancer 101:446, 1977.

109. Askin FB, Rosai J, Sibly R, et al: Malignant small cell tumor of the thoracopulmonary region in children. Cancer 43:2438, 1979.

110. Gould V, Jannson D, Warren W: Primitive neuroectodermal tumors (PNET) of the chest wall in adults [abstract] Mod Pathol 4:115A 1991.

111. Hashimoto H, Enjoji M, Nakajima T, et al: Malignant neuroepithelioma (peripheral neuroblastoma). Am J Surg Pathol 7:309, 1983.

112. Tefft M, Vawter GF, Metus A: Paravertebral ''round cell'' tumors in children. Radiology 92:1501, 1969.

113. Avagnina A, Elsner B, DeMarco L, et al: Pulmonary rhabdomyosarcoma with isolated small bowel metastasis. Cancer 53:1948, 1984.

114. Allan BT, Day DL, Dehner LP: Primary pulmonary rhabdomyosarcoma of the lung in children: Report of two cases presenting with spontaneous pneumothorax. Cancer 59:1005, 1987.

115. Lee SH, Rengaciary SS, Paramesh J: Primary pulmonary rhabdomyosarcoma: A case report and review of the literature. Hum Pathol 12:92, 1981.

116. Erikson A, Thunell M, Lundquist G: Pedunculated endobronchial rhabdomyosarcoma with fatal asphyxia. Thorax 37:390, 1982.

117. Nash G, Fliegiel S: Kaposi's sarcoma presenting as pulmonary disease in the acquired immunodeficiency syndrome: Diagnosis by lung biopsy. Hum Pathol 10:999, 1984.

118. Spragg RG, Wolf PL, Haghigi P, et al: Angiosarcoma of the lung with fatal pulmonary hemorrhage. Am J Med 74:1072, 1983.

119. Tralka GA, Katz S: Hemangioendothelioma of the lung. Am Rev Respir Dis 87:107, 1963.

120. Yousem SA: Angiosarcoma presenting in the lung. Arch Pathol Lab Med 110:112, 1986.

121. Yousem SA, Hochholzer L: Primary pulmonary hemangiopericytoma. Cancer 59:549, 1987.

122. Shin MS, Ho KJ: Primary pulmonary hemangiopericytoma of lung: Radiology and pathology. AJR 133:1077, 1979.

123. Meade JB, Whitwell F, Bickford BJ, Waddington JKB: Primary hemangipericytoma of lung. Thorax 29:1, 1974.

124. Morgan AD, Salama FD: Primary chondrosarcoma of the lung: Case report and review of the literature. J Thorac Cardiovasc Surg 64:460, 1972.

125. Sun CCJ, Kroll M, Miller JE: Primary chondrosarcoma of the lung. Cancer 50:1864, 1982.

126. Reingold IM, Amromin GD: Extraosseous osteosarcoma of the lung. Cancer 28:491, 1971.

127. Matsuba K, Saito T, Ando K, Shirakusa T: Atypical lipoma of the lung. Thorax 4:865, 1991.

128. Iannicello CM, Shoenut JP, Sharma GP, McGoey JS: Endobronchial lipoma. Can J Surg 30:430, 1987.

129. Moran CA, Suster S, Koss MN: Endobronchial lipomas: A clinicopathologic correlation of four cases. Mod Pathol 7:212–214, 1994.

130. Sawamura K, Hashimoto T, Nanjo S, et al: Primary liposarcoma of the lung: Report of a case. J Surg Oncol 19:243, 1982.

131. Crane AR, Carrigan PT: Primary subpleural intrapulmonic thymoma. J Thorac Surg 25:600, 1953.

132. Fukayama M, Maeda Y, Funata N, et al: Pulmonary and pleural thymoma. Diagnostic application of lymphocyte markers to the thymoma of unusual site. Am J Clin Pathol 89:617, 1988.

133. Green WR, Pressoir R, Gumb RV, et al: Intrapulmonary thymoma. Arch Pathol Lab Med 111:1074, 1987.

134. Kalish PE: Primary intrapulmonary thymoma. N Y State J Med 63:1705, 1963.

135. Kung IT, Loke SL, So SY, et al: Intrapulmonary thymoma: Report of two cases. Thorax 40:471, 1985.

136. McBurney RP, Claggett OT, McDonald JR: Primary intrapulmonary neoplasm (thymoma ?) associated with myasthenia gravis: Report of a case. Proc Staff Meetings Mayo Clin 26:345, 1951.

137. Thorburn JD, Stephens HB, Grimes OF: Benign thymoma in the hilus of the lung. J Thorac Surg 24:540, 1952.

138. Yeoh CB, Ford JM, Lattes R, et al: Intrapulmonary thymoma. J Thorac Cardiovasc Surg 51:131, 1966.

139. Moran CA, Travis WD, Rosado-de-Christenson M, et al: Thymomas presenting as pleural tumors. Report of eight cases. Am J Surg Pathol 16:138, 1992.

140. Strimlan CV, Golembiewski RS, Celko DA, Fino GJ: Primary pulmonary meningioma. Surg Neurol 29:410, 1988.

141. Chumas JC, Lorelle CA: Pulmonary meningioma: A light and electron microscopic study. Am J Surg Pathol 6:795, 1982.

142. Kemnitz P, Spormann H, Heinrich P: Meningioma of lung: First report with light and electron microscopic findings. Ultrastruct Pathol 3:359, 1982.

143. Drlicek M, Grisold W, Lorber J, et al: Pulmonary meningioma. Immunohistochemical and ultrastructural features. Am J Surg Pathol 15:455, 1991.

144. Flynn SD, Yousem SA: Pulmonary meningiomas: A report of two cases. Hum Pathol 22:469, 1991.

145. Robinson PG: Pulmonary meningioma. Am J Clin Pathol 97:814, 1992.

146. Tang CK, Toker C, Foris NP, Trump BF: Glomangioma of the lung. Am J Surg Pathol 2:103, 1978.

147. Garcia-Prats MD, Sotelo-Rodriguez MT, Ballestin C, et al: Glomus tumour of the trachea: Report of a case with microscopic, ultrastructural and immunohistochemical examination and review of the literature. Histopathology 19:459, 1991.

148. Deavers M, Guinee D, Koss MN, Travis WD: Granular cell tumors of the lung: Clinicopathologic study of 15 cases [abstract]. Mod Pathol 6:129A, 1993.

149. McSwain GR, Colpitts R, Kreutner A, et al: Granular cell myoblastoma. Surg Gynecol Obstet 150:703, 1980.

150. Oparah SS, Subramanian VA: Granular cell myoblastoma of the bronchus: Report of 2 cases and review of the literature. Ann Thorac Surg 22:199, 1976.

151. Allen MS, Drash EC: Primary melanoma of lung. Cancer 21:154, 1968.

152. Jensen OA, Egedorf J: Primary malignant melanoma of the lung. Scand J Respir Dis 48:127, 1967.

153. Jennings TA, Axiotis CA, Kress Y, Carter D: Primary malignant melanoma of the lower respiratory tract. Report of a case and literature review. Am J Clin Pathol 94:649, 1990.

154. Koss MN, Hochholzer L, Nichols PW, et al: Primary non-Hodgkin's lymphoma and pseudolymphoma of lung: A study of 161 patients. Hum Pathol 14:1024, 1983.

155. Addis BJ, Hyjek E, Isaacson PG: Primary pulmonary lymphoma: A re-appraisal of its histogenesis and its relationship to pseudolymphoma and lymphoid interstitial pneumonia. Histopathology 13:1, 1988.

156. Geetha J, Pandit M, Korfhage L: Primary pulmonary plasmacytoma. Cancer 71: 721, 1993.

157. Amin R: Extramedullary plasmacytoma of lung. Cancer 56:152, 1985.

158. Morinaga S, Gemma A, Nakajima T, et al: Plamacytoma of the lung associated with nodular deposits of immunoglobulin. Am J Surg Pathol 11:989, 1987.

159. Baroni CD, Mineo TC, Ricci C, et al: Solitary secretory plasmacytoma of the lung in a 14-year-old boy. Cancer 40:2329, 1977.

160. Roikjaer O, Thompsen JK: Plasmacytoma of the lung. Cancer 58:2671, 1986.

161. Wile A, Olinger G, Peter JB, Dornfeld L: Pulmonary plasmacytoma with M-protein. Cancer 37:2338, 1976.

162. Kennedy JL, Nathwani BN, Burke JS, et al: Pulmonary lymphomas and other pulmonary lymphoid lesions. A clinicopathologic and immunologic study of 64 patients. Cancer 56:539, 1985.

163. L'Hoste RJ, Filippa DA, Lieberman PH, Bretsky S: Primary pulmonary lymphomas. A clinicopathologic analysis of 36 cases. Cancer 54:1397, 1984.

164. Li G, Hansmann ML: Primary lymphomas of the lung: Morphological, immunohistochemical, and clinical features. Histopathology 16:519, 1990.

165. Turner RR, Colby TV, Doggett RS: Well-differentiated lymphocytic lymphoma. A study of 47 patients with primary manifestations in the lung. Cancer 54:2088, 1984.

166. Katzenstein AL, Carrington CB, Liebow AA: Lymphomatoid granulomatosis. A clinicopathologic study of 152 cases. Cancer 43:360, 1979.

167. Koss MN, Hochholzer L, Langloss JM, et al: Lymphomatoid granulomatosis: A clinicopathologic study of 42 patients. Pathology 18:283, 1986.

168. DeRemee RA, Weiland LH, McDonald TJ: Polymorphic reticulosis, lymphomatoid granulomatosis. Two diseases or one? Mayo Clin Proc 53:634, 1978.

169. Saldana MJ, Patchefsky AS, Israel HI, et al: Pulmonary angiitis and granulomatosis. Hum Pathol 8:391, 1977.

170. Jaffe ES, Lipford EH, Margolick JB, et al: Lymphomatoid granulomatosis and angiocentric lymphoma: Spectrum of post thymic T-cell proliferations. Semin Respir Med 10:167, 1989.

171. Harper PG, Fischer C, McLennan K, Souhammi RL: Presentation of Hodgkin's disease as an endobronchial lesion. Cancer 53:147, 1984.

172. Yousem SA, Weiss LM, Colby TV: Primary pulmonary Hodgkin's disease: A clinicopathologic study of 15 cases. Cancer 57:1217, 1986.

173. Travis WD, Borok Z, Roum JH, et al: Pulmonary Langerhans cell granulomatosis (histiocytosis X): A clinicopathologic study of 48 cases. Am J Surg Pathol 17(10):971, 1993.

174. Soler P, Chollet S, Jacque C, et al: Immunocytochemical characterization of pulmonary histiocytosis X cells in lung biopsies. Am J Pathol 118:439, 1985.

175. Colby TV, Lombard C: Histiocytosis X in the lung. Hum Pathol 14:847, 1983.

176. Pettinato G, Manivel J, De Rosa N, Dehner L: Inflammatory myofibroblastic tumor (plasma cell granuloma). Clinicopathologic study of 20 cases with immunohistochemical and ultrastructural observations. Am J Clin Pathol 94:538, 1990.

177. Hartman GE, Shochat SJ: Primary pulmonary neoplasms of childhood: A review. Ann Thorac Surg 36:108, 1983.

178. Berardi R, Lee S, Chen H, Stines G: Inflammatory pseudotumor of the lung. Surg Gynecol Obstet 156:89, 1983.

179. Buell R, Wang NS, Seemayer TA, Ahmed MN: Endobronchial plasma cell granuloma (xanthomatous pseudotumor): A light and electron microscopic study. Hum Pathol 7:411, 1976.

180. Hong HY, Castelli MJ, Walloch JL: Pulmonary plasma cell granuloma (inflammatory pseudotumor) with invasion of thoracic vertebra. Mt Sinai J Med 57:117, 1990.

181. Monzon C, Gilchrist G, Burgert E, et al: Plasma cell granuloma of the lung in children. Pediatrics 70:268, 1982.

182. Spencer H: The pulmonary plasma cell/histiocytoma complex. Histopathology 8:903, 1984.

183. Liebow AA, Hubbell DS: Sclerosing hemangioma (histiocytoma, xanthoma) of the lung. Cancer 9:53, 1956.

184. Nagata N, Dairaku M, Ishida T, et al: Sclerosing hemangioma of the lung: Immunohistochemical characterization of its origin as related to surfactant apoprotein. Cancer 55:116, 1985.

185. Spencer H, Nambu S: Sclerosing hemangioma of lung. Histopathology 10:477, 1986.

186. Yousem SA, Wick MR, Singh G, et al: So-called sclerosing hemangioma of lung: An immunohistochemical study supporting a respiratory epithelial origin. Am J Surg Pathol 12:582, 1988.

187. Katzenstein AL, Weise DL, Fulling K, Battifora H: So-called sclerosing hemangioma of the lung. Evidence for mesothelial origin. Am J Surg Pathol 7:3, 1983.

188. Huszar M, Suster S, Herczeg E, Geiger B: Sclerosing hemangioma of the lung. Immunohistochemical demonstration of mesenchymal origin using antibodies to tissue-specific intermediate filaments. Cancer 58:2422, 1986.

189. Moran CA, Zeren H, Koss MN: The granulomatous variant of sclerosing hemangioma of the lung. Arch Pathol Lab Med 118:1028–1030, 1994.

190. Gal AA, Koss MN, Hochholzer L, Chejfec G: An immunohistochemical study of benign clear cell (sugar) tumor of the lung. Arch Pathol Lab Med 115:1034, 1991.

191. Gaffey MJ, Mills SE, Zarbo RJ, et al: Clear cell tumor of the lung. Immunohistochemical and ultrastructural evidence of melanogenesis. Am J Surg Pathol 15:644, 1991.

192. Liebow AA, Castleman B: Benign clear cell (sugar) tumor of the lung. Yale J Biol Med 43:213, 1971.

193. Yousem SA, Hochholzer L: Alveolar adenoma. Hum Pathol 17:1066, 1986.

194. Chen KTK: Amyloidosis presenting in the respiratory tract. Pathol Annu 24:253, 1989.

195. Hui AN, Koss MN, Hochholzer L, Wehunt WD: Amyloidosis presenting in the lower respiratory tract. Clinicopathologic, radiologic, immunohistochemical, and histochemical studies on 48 cases. Arch Pathol Lab Med 110:212, 1986.

196. Corrin B, Liebow A, Friedman PJ: Pulmonary lymphangiomyomatosis: A review. Am J Pathol 79:347, 1975.

197. Carrington CB, Cugell DW, Gaensler EA, et al: Lymphangioleiomyomatosis: Physiologic, pathologic, radiologic correlations. Am Rev Respir Dis 116:977, 1977.

198. Bonin M, Myers J, Roche P, Colby T: Pulmonary lymphangiomyomatosis (LAM): An immunohistochemical analysis of 22 cases. Mod Pathol 5:112A, 1992.

199. Key BM, Oritchett PS: Mucous gland adenoma of the bronchus. South Med J 72:83, 1979.

200. Edwards CW, Matthews HR: Mucous gland adenoma of the bronchus. Thorax 36:147, 1981.

201. Emory WB, Mitchel WT, Hatch HG: Mucous gland adenoma of the bronchus. Am Rev Resp Dis 108:1407, 1973.

202. Suster S, Moran CA: Pulmonary adenofibroma: Report of two cases of an unusual type of hamartomatous lesion of the lung. Histopathology 23:547–551, 1993.

203. England DM, Hochholzer L, McCarthy MJ: Localized benign and malignant fibrous tumors of the pleura. A clinicopathologic review of 223 cases. Am J Surg Pathol 13:640, 1989.

204. Scharifker D, Kaneko M: Localized fibrous ''mesothelioma'' of pleura (submesothelial fibroma): A clinicopathologic study of 18 cases. Cancer 43:627, 1979.

205. Said JW, Nash G, Banks-Schlegel S, et al: Localized fibrous mesothelioma: An immunohistochemical and electron microscopy study. Hum Pathol 15:440, 1984.

206. Moran CA, Suster S, Koss MN: The spectrum of histologic growth patterns in benign and malignant fibrous tumors of the pleura. Semin Diagn Pathol 9:169, 1992.

207. Honma K, Shimada K: Metastasizing ectopic thymoma arising in the right thoracic cavity and mimicking diffuse pleural mesothelioma. An autopsy study of a case with review of the literature. Wien Klin Wochenschr 98:14, 1986.

CHAPTER 4

Mediastinal Pathology

Saul Suster, M.D.

Although tissues from the mediastinum represent a relatively infrequent source of biopsy and surgical resection material for the average practicing pathologist, they may pose a considerable challenge for diagnosis because of the large variety of structures contained within this anatomic compartment that may be involved in pathologic processes. Virtually all types of tumors may arise as a primary in this location, in addition to this being a frequent site of metastases from distant or adjacent organs. For the most part, the diagnosis of lesions in the mediastinum is still dependent on a thorough familiarity by the pathologist with the hematoxylin and eosin (H&E) appearance of such lesions. Close correlation of the H&E morphology with the clinical circumstances will guide the pathologist in the choice of further specialized diagnostic techniques. The major emphasis in this chapter thus rests on the light microscopic appearances of the different processes that may pose difficulties for diagnosis in the mediastinum, with mention of the role and applications of special techniques when appropriate within the context of differential diagnosis.

ATYPICAL PRESENTATION OF COMMON LESIONS

Epithelial Neoplasms

Thymoma

The term *thymoma* in a generic sense refers to a neoplasm composed of thymic epithelial cells.[1] The morphologic hallmark of thymomas is their characteristic biphasic composition, displaying a variable admixture of epithelial cells and thymic lymphocytes. Other distinctive features of thymomas include coarse lobulation, thick fibrous bands separating the lobules at sharp angles, perivascular spaces, and the so-called areas of medullary differentiation. Traditionally, thymomas have been classified histologically according to the relative amounts of lymphocytes/epithelial cells and by the shape of their cells, namely, into lymphocyte-rich, epithelial-rich, mixed, and spindle cell thymomas.[1, 2] Unusual patterns, however, are not infrequently encountered.

Thymoma with Hemangiopericytic Growth Pattern

These tumors are characterized by numerous dilated, branching vascular spaces scattered among the neoplastic epithelial cells. The vascular spaces often show an ''antler-like'' configuration characteristic of hemangiopericytomas (Fig. 4–1). Exaggeration of the hemangiopericytic pattern may result in a trabecular growth pattern, with the creation of slender parallel cords of epithelial cells separated from one another by gaping vascular channels. Rarely, the epithelial cords may adopt a serpiginous disposition resembling the adenoid pattern of some skin adnexal tumors (Fig. 4–2). The hemangiopericytic pattern is more often observed as a focal phenomenon in thymoma, and attention to the features in the surrounding areas should permit a correct diagnosis. In rare instances, however, this pattern may predominate, raising the possibility of **hemangiopericytoma** or other tumors with a hemangiopericytic growth pattern (i.e., **solitary fibrous tumor, synovial sarcoma, leiomyosarcoma,** and so on). Immunostains for keratin antibodies are of value in demonstrating the epithelial nature of the cells surrounding the vascular spaces.

Thymoma with Epithelial Rosette-like Structures

Such structures may be present as a focal event, or may be widespread and overshadow the other components of the tumor, in which case the lesions closely resemble thymic carcinoid or other neuroendocrine neoplasm. The epithelial pseudorosettes are in most instances composed of small clusters of plump epithelial cells disposed radially about a center without a lumen (Fig. 4–3). Unlike neural rosettes or the microacinar structures found in carcinoid tumors, the rosette-like structures in thymomas stain strongly positive for keratin antibodies and fail to immunoreact with neuroendocrine or neural markers.

Thymoma with Unusual Spindle Cell Patterns

In addition to the conventional solid spindle pattern of growth seen in spindle cell thymoma, a few unusual variations on the theme may also occur. The spindle cells in spindle cell thymoma may occasionally adopt a prominent cartwheel or storiform configuration simulating a fibrohistiocytic tumor (Fig. 4–4); absence of mitotic activity and the coarsely lobular growth pattern of the tumor on low magnification serve to identify the lesion as a thymoma. Spindle cell thymoma may also grow in anastomosing cords of spindle epithelial cells separated by a very cellular fibrovascular stroma rich in spindled fibroblasts, imparting the lesion with a striking biphasic

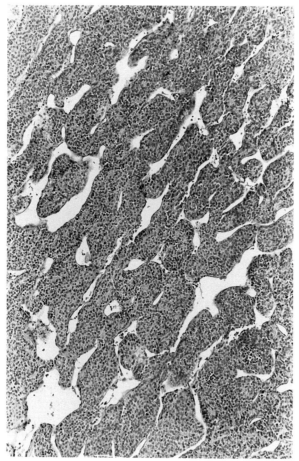

FIGURE 4–1. Thymoma with prominent hemangiopericytic growth pattern.

appearance (Fig. 4–5); the spindled fibroblasts in such cases, however, are not part of the neoplastic proliferation. Occasionally, spindle cell thymoma may undergo extensive xanthomatous degeneration that may closely resemble that seen in **schwannian neoplasms** (Fig. 4–6).

Thymoma with Cystic Changes

Cystic changes in thymoma have been thought to represent an exaggeration of the mechanism of formation of perivascular spaces, with the larger cysts being formed as a result of progressive enlargement and coalescence of such structures.[3] Infrequently, the cystic changes may reach such magnitude as to make identification of the underlying neoplasm very difficult. Unusual variations of this pattern include a fine, microcystic pattern, or larger, coalescent and more diffusely scattered cystic spaces with a marked cribriform appearance simulating **adenoid cystic carcinoma** (Fig. 4–7).

Other Unusual Features in Thymoma

Germinal centers have been observed in thymomas of patients with myasthenia gravis in up to 10% of cases; Hassall's corpuscles and epithelial-lined cysts are rare in thymomas but may be observed in a small number of cases. An unusual thymoma with a prominent rhabdomyomatous stro-

mal component has been described (Fig. 4–8); this tumor should be distinguished from other tumors with a "rhabdoid" morphology.[4] A **plasma cell–rich variant of thymoma** also exists that is characterized by a prominent background polyclonal population of plasma cells.[5] Benign thymomas may also undergo spontaneous infarction and necrosis; in some instances, the areas of necrosis may be traced to cystically dilated Hassall's corpuscles displaying severe inflammatory changes. The necrotic areas are most likely related to the cystic/inflammatory changes of the organ and should not be misconstrued as evidence of malignancy.

Thymic Carcinoma

Thymic carcinoma is defined as a primary thymic epithelial neoplasm displaying obvious cytologic evidence of malignancy.[2,6] Because of their rarity and their numerous histologic variants and growth patterns, these tumors have remained very poorly categorized. Suster and Rosai[7] presented a study of 60 patients with thymic carcinoma. They were able to divide these lesions into two groups according to their prognostic features: (1) low-grade thymic carcinoma were tumors characterized by a relatively favorable prognosis, with a 5-year survival rate approaching 90%; (2) high-grade thymic carcinomas were characterized clinically by a highly aggressive behavior, with most cases proving rapidly fatal within 15 months. The tumors in the low-grade group included well-differentiated squamous cell carcinoma, mucoepidermoid car-

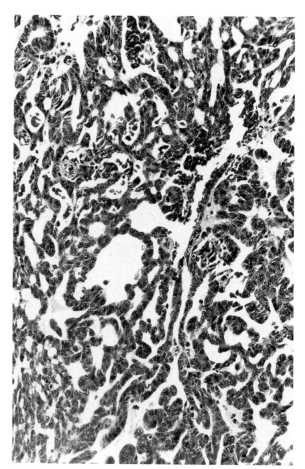

FIGURE 4–2. Thymoma with adenoid growth pattern.

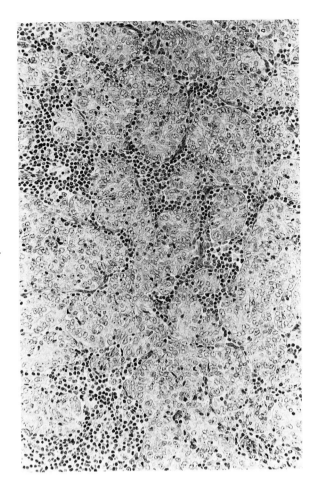

FIGURE 4–3. Epithelial pseudorosettes in thymoma.

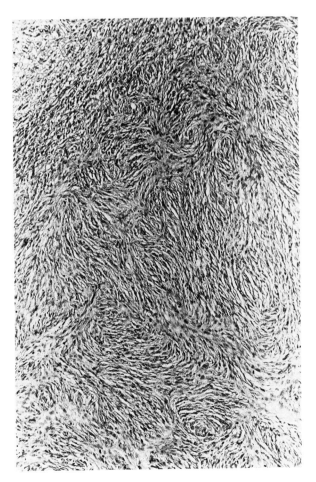

FIGURE 4–4. Thymoma with prominent storiform pattern resembling fibrohistiocytic tumor.

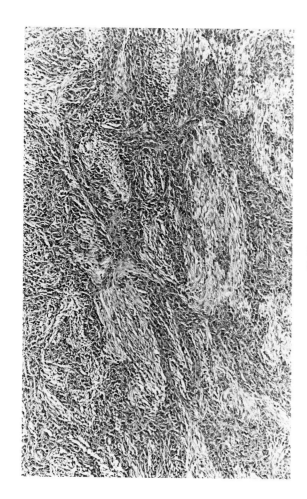

FIGURE 4–5. Spindle cell thymoma with prominent fibroblastic stromal component.

FIGURE 4–6. Spindle cell thymoma with xanthomatous degeneration.

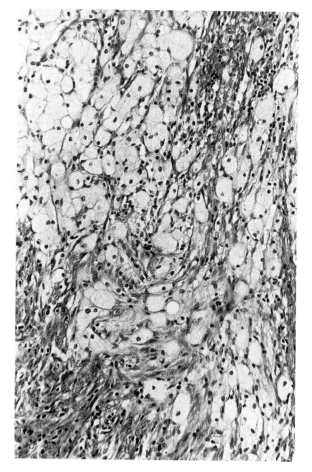

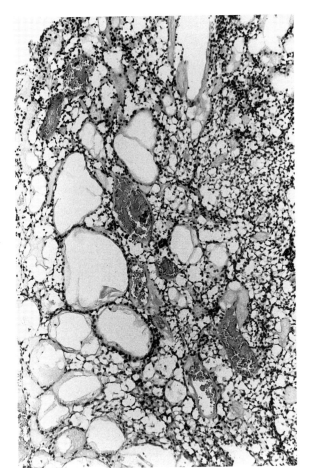

FIGURE 4–7. Cribriform spaces in cystic thymoma simulating adenoid cystic carcinoma.

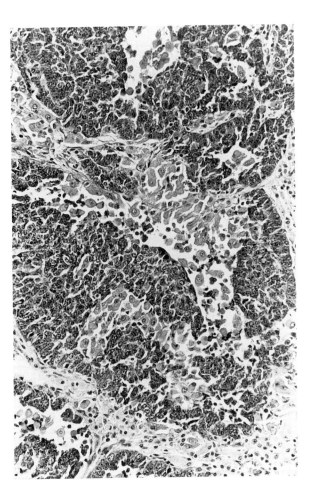

FIGURE 4–8. Benign thymoma with prominent rhabdomyomatous component (rhabdomyomatous thymoma).

147

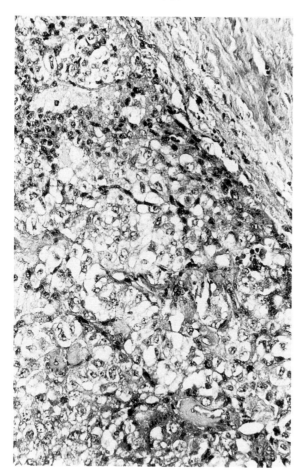

FIGURE 4–9. Well-differentiated squamous cell carcinoma of the thymus with focal clear-cell changes.

cinoma, and basaloid carcinoma; the tumors in the high-grade group included poorly differentiated (lymphoepithelioma-like) squamous cell carcinoma, small-cell/neuroendocrine, clear-cell, sarcomatoid, and anaplastic/undifferentiated carcinoma. The morphologic features of the various histologic variants of thymic carcinoma have been adequately illustrated in previous publications;[6–10] however, certain unusual variations on the theme deserve further mention.

Low-grade Thymic Carcinoma

Well-differentiated squamous cell carcinoma of the thymus may show focally areas with prominent clear-cell change (Fig. 4–9), a phenomenon that has been previously described for squamous cell carcinoma at other sites.[11, 12] **Basaloid carcinoma of the thymus** may show focally the formation of papillary structures (Fig. 4–10); this should not be mistaken for **metastatic papillary carcinoma.** Identification of the more conventional features of basaloid carcinoma of the thymus helps establish the correct diagnosis. Basaloid carcinoma of the thymus is often associated with prominent cystic changes and may also occasionally harbor a prominent myoid cell component (Fig. 4–11); this should not be misinterpreted as **carcinosarcoma** with rhabdomyosarcomatous differentiation, as the rhabdomyomatous cell component does not appear to influence the favorable prognosis of this tumor.[7]

High-grade Thymic Carcinoma

Small-cell/neuroendocrine carcinoma of the thymus may occasionally show a focally trabecular pattern of growth that vaguely resembles that of carcinoid tumors (Fig. 4–12); however, the predominantly confluent growth pattern, extensive areas of necrosis, and high mitotic activity that characterize these tumors generally betray the high-grade malignant potential of these lesions. Small-cell/neuroendocrine carcinoma of the thymus may also show prominent areas of squamous differentiation (Fig. 4–13); a phenomenon that has been previously observed in primary small-cell/neuroendocrine carcinomas at other locations.[13] Small-cell/neuroendocrine carcinoma may also occasionally show areas of transition with **poorly differentiated (lymphoepithelioma-like) squamous cell carcinoma of the thymus,** demonstrating the continuum that exists among these different cell lines (Fig. 4–14). **Clear-cell carcinoma** is characterized by sheets of large cells with abundant clear cytoplasm with sharply outlined cell borders (Fig. 4–15). The differential diagnosis includes **large-cell lymphoma (clear-cell type), seminoma, and metastatic carcinoma,** particularly from kidney, adrenal, or thyroid. The first two diagnostic dilemmas can be resolved with the aid of special stains; the last one, however, requires strict clinicopathologic correlation to rule out the possibility of an occult primary in one of those organs. The **sarcomatoid variant of thymic carcinoma** is characterized by a biphasic composition,

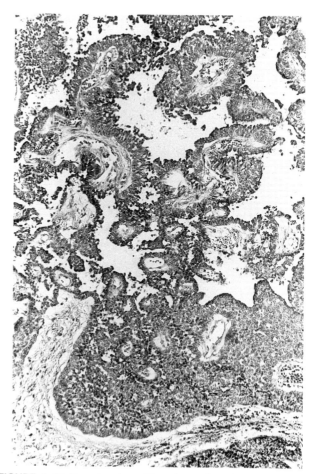

FIGURE 4–10. Prominent papillary formations in basaloid carcinoma of the thymus.

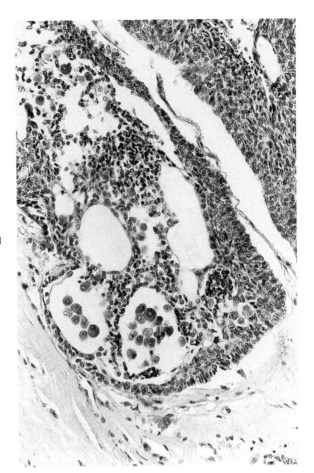

FIGURE 4–11. Basaloid carcinoma of the thymus with focal myoid cell component.

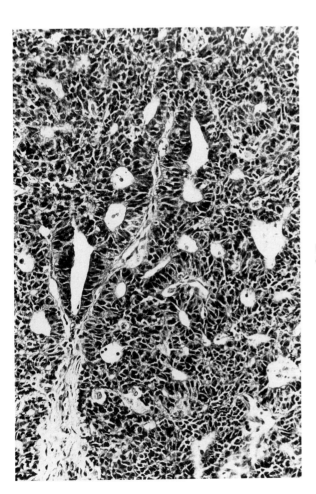

FIGURE 4–12. Trabecular growth pattern in small-cell/neuroendocrine carcinoma of the thymus.

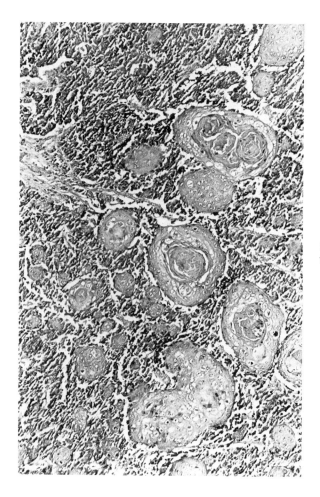

FIGURE 4–13. Foci of squamous differentiation in small-cell carcinoma of the thymus.

FIGURE 4–14. Focal areas of poorly differentiated (lymphoepithelioma-like) carcinoma of the thymus arising in association with small-cell carcinoma.

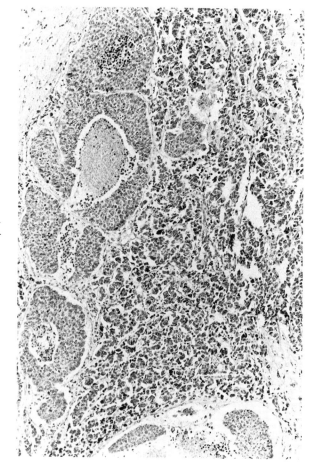

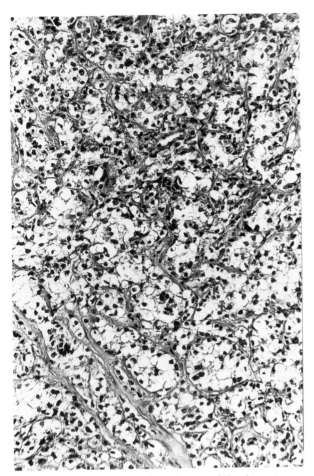

FIGURE 4–15. Clear-cell carcinoma of the thymus.

introduce features that may obscure the diagnosis. It is well known that HD in the thymus often induces cystic changes in the epithelial component of this organ.[16] Occasionally, the cystic changes may overshadow the underlying neoplastic process, with only small scattered islands of atypical lymphoreticular infiltrates remaining among the cystic structures (Fig. 4–17). In other instances, the predominant stimulus to the gland takes the form of thymic epithelial hyperplasia without cystic change, raising the alternative diagnosis of thymoma. Unlike thymomas, in which the cells form tumor lobules separated by broad bands of fibrous tissue, the epithelial hyperplasia in such instances is characterized by long, slender, often branching strands of benign thymic epithelium. Identification of small foci containing an atypical lymphoreticular infiltrate with RS cells establishes the diagnosis. The lymphocyte-depleted variant of HD may also create difficulties for diagnosis because of its close resemblance to large-cell lymphoma with sclerosis. Identification of RS cells scattered among the infiltrate and the application of immunohistochemical stains may be of aid in diagnosis. RS cells and its variants characteristically react with CD15 (Leu-M1), but are negative for CD45 (leukocyte common antigen [LCA]) in formalin-fixed paraffin-embedded sections. In contrast, the neoplastic cells of most non-Hodgkin's lymphomas are CD45+ and CD15−.[17, 18] Great difficulties may arise, however, in separating **anaplastic large-cell lymphoma ("Ki-1 lymphoma")** from HD. Both entities may share a similar morphology, particu-

with clusters and strands of atypical epithelial cells admixed with a background of atypical spindle cells. It is not certain whether the spindle cell component represents spindle cell carcinoma or whether it constitutes a separate mesenchymal element of the tumor (i.e., carcinosarcoma). Finally, an interesting feature that may be observed in **undifferentiated/anaplastic carcinomas of the thymus** is the presence of focal areas containing **syncytial trophoblastic-type giant cells,** raising the possibility of **choriocarcinomatous differentiation** in a primitive germ cell tumor (Fig. 4–16). Immunohistochemical determination of human chorionic gonadotropin (HCG) and other oncofetal peptides is of help in defining the diagnosis in such instances.

Lymphoid Proliferations

Hodgkin's Disease

Mediastinal Hodgkin's disease (HD) may arise primarily in the thymus, or may involve mediastinal lymph nodes as part of systemic disease.[14, 15] Although it has been claimed that the majority of cases of mediastinal HD are of the nodular sclerosing type, all histologic variants of HD may be seen in this location. Traditionally, the diagnosis of HD rests on the identification of Reed-Sternberg (RS) cells and its variants against the appropriate background. When primary in the thymus, however, certain characteristics intrinsic to this organ

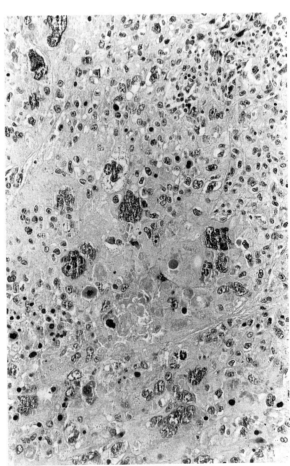

FIGURE 4–16. Undifferentiated carcinoma of the thymus with focus of trophoblast-like giant cells.

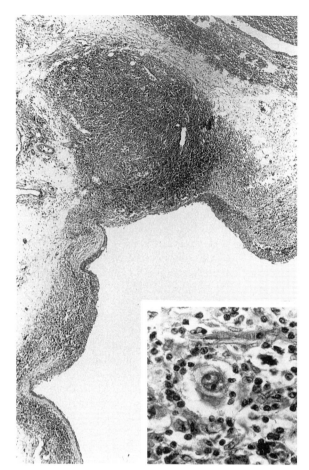

FIGURE 4–17. Cystic Hodgkin's disease. Notice atypical lymphoreticular infiltrate with Reed-Sternberg cells in wall of the cyst (*inset*).

larly the lymphocyte-depleted variant of HD, and both are immunoreactive with the CD30 (Ki-1/BerH2) antigen.[19, 20] Application of additional markers such as EMA, Leu-M1, LCA, and L26 (pan-B cell marker) may be of aid in defining the diagnosis although, admittedly, there are cases in which this distinction is not possible.[21] Another potential source of confusion is with the **syncytial variant of HD,**[22] which is characterized by clustering of RS cells and its variants around areas of necrosis (Fig. 4–18). Examination of adjacent areas for more typical features of HD may be necessary in such cases to arrive at the correct diagnosis. Another unusual phenomenon that was first described by Toker[23] and later documented in mediastinal Hodgkin's is the **sarcomatous transformation of HD.**[24] Such cases are characterized by the emergence of areas composed of atypical spindle cells adopting a prominent storiform pattern virtually indistinguishable from that seen in malignant fibrous histiocytoma (Fig. 4–19). Identification of residual lymphoreticular elements displaying the characteristic features of HD serves to establish the diagnosis. Several types of altered histologic appearances may also be induced as a result of radiation therapy of Hodgkin's disease, including **massive fibrosis and cystic hyperplasia,** which may simulate a recurrent neoplasm.[25] Finally, transitions and combinations between HD and B-cell non-Hodgkin's lymphoma may occasionally occur in the region of the mediastinum, creating many difficulties for classification (Fig. 4–20).

Non-Hodgkin's Lymphomas

Non-Hodgkin's malignant lymphoma may present in the mediastinum as a manifestation of disseminated disease or as a primary mediastinal neoplasm.[26, 27] The majority of non-Hodgkin's lymphomas of the mediastinum correspond to **diffuse large-cell lymphomas,** followed in frequency by **lymphoblastic lymphoma.**[26–28]

Large-cell lymphomas of the mediastinum are often extranodal and extensively involve the thymus; in fact, some authors regard them as primary B-cell neoplasms of the thymus.[29] The majority of those tumors that have been studied by cell markers have been of B-cell type, although lymphomas with a T-cell phenotype have also been described.[30] Most large-cell lymphomas are of large non-cleaved cell type, characterized by large cells with vesicular nuclei and multiple small nucleoli. B-immunoblastic lymphomas characterized by large cells with prominent eosinophilic nucleoli and abundant cytoplasm may also involve the mediastinum. One of the hallmarks of large-cell lymphomas in the mediastinum is their tendency to undergo extensive sclerosis.[31, 32] The sclerotic bands frequently separate the cells into small compartments, creating a histologic appearance that may simulate an epithelial, germ cell, or endocrine neoplasm (Fig. 4–21). In other instances, the fibrotic stroma induces artifactual compression of the cells, creating a spindled appearance reminiscent of a sarcoma. In more advanced cases, the sclerosis takes the form

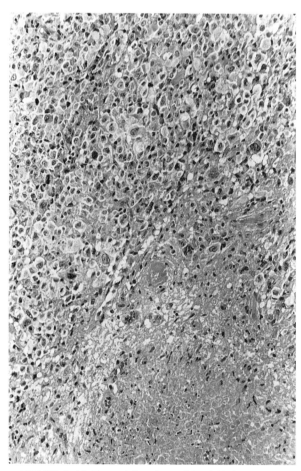

FIGURE 4–18. Syncytial variant of Hodgkin's disease.

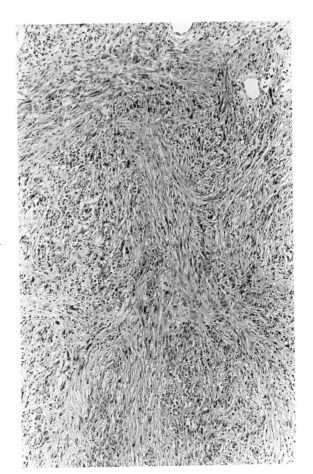

FIGURE 4–19. Sarcomatous transformation of Hodgkin's disease in the thymus. Notice prominent storiform pattern.

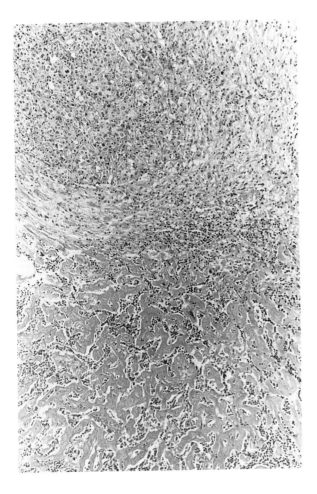

FIGURE 4–20. Composite Hodgkin's/non-Hodgkin's lymphoma of the mediastinum. Notice variegated nature of lymphoid infiltrate in HD component (*top half*).

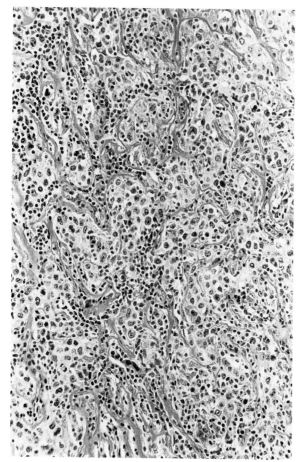

FIGURE 4–21. Large-cell lymphoma of the mediastinum with sclerosis. Notice prominent compartmentalization of tumor cells by thin fibrous bands.

of a fine network that entraps individual cells. The final stages of this process result in an almost acellular picture that may resemble sclerosing mediastinitis. Prominent cytoplasmic clearing is another feature that may be encountered in mediastinal large-cell lymphoma;[33] such cases are characterized by large cells surrounded by abundant amphophilic cytoplasm with clearly defined cell borders, raising the possibility of seminoma or clear-cell carcinoma in the differential diagnosis (Fig. 4–22).

Another source of confusion arises from the presence of prominent multinucleated and RS-like tumor cells in pleomorphic large-cell lymphomas of the mediastinum, suggesting the diagnosis of Hodgkin's disease. Immunohistochemical studies demonstrate a B-cell phenotype in such cells (LCA[+], L26[+], kappa/lambda light chain restriction), thus establishing the diagnosis of non-Hodgkin's lymphoma. An unusual variant of large-cell lymphoma of the mediastinum exhibiting marked tropism for germinal centers has also been described.[34] Such cases are characterized by a proliferation of large atypical cells arranged in clusters that encroach upon mantle zones and invade germinal centers (Fig. 4–23). Their unusual growth pattern may be easily confused for primary or metastatic carcinoma, seminoma, or metastatic melanoma. Immunohistochemical stains are necessary in such instances to demonstrate a lymphoid cell lineage and rule out alternative diagnostic possibilities. As with HD of the thymus, large-cell

lymphoma of the mediastinum is also capable of inducing hyperplastic changes of thymic epithelium that result in either cystic dilatation of Hassall's corpuscles or the formation of solid cords of hyperplastic thymic epithelial cells (Fig. 4–24). In the latter instance, distinction between lymphoma and lymphocyte-rich thymoma may pose a problem; in thymoma, however, the epithelial cells are usually scattered singly and evenly throughout the lesion, whereas in lymphoma, the hyperplastic thymic epithelium usually takes the form of elongated, often branching, solid strands of epithelial cells resulting from compression and displacement of the residual thymic epithelial elements by the neoplastic proliferation. Immunoperoxidase stains for keratin bring out this distinction nicely (Fig. 4–25). Large-cell lymphomas of the mediastinum may also rarely show marked angiotropism. This feature may be manifested as solid clusters of atypical lymphoid cells lying within dilated lymphatic and vascular spaces, thus simulating a metastatic epithelial malignancy (Fig. 4–26A), or as frank invasion of vessel walls (Fig. 4–26B). Although the latter feature has been described as being distinctive for T-cell lymphomas, we have also observed this phenomenon in large-cell lymphomas of the mediastinum of B-cell type. Other unusual variants of malignant lymphoma that may present as primary in the mediastinum include **large-cell lymphoma with high content of epithelioid histiocytes (Lennert's phenomenon, lymphoepithelioid lymphoma), monocytoid B-cell lymphoma, small-cell lymphoma/CLL, and low-grade**

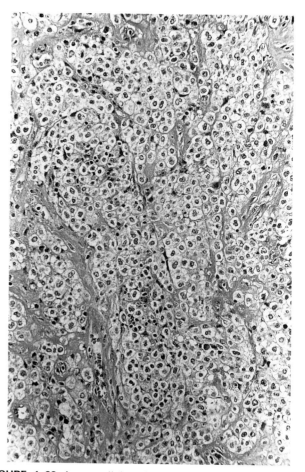

FIGURE 4–22. Large-cell lymphoma of the mediastinum with prominent cytoplasmic clearing of the cells.

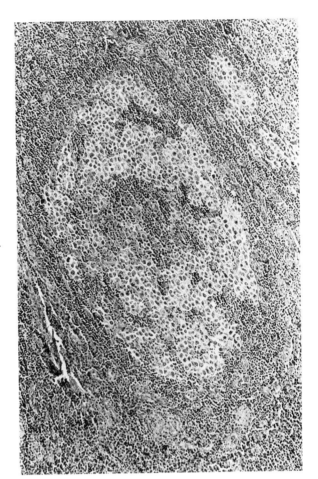

FIGURE 4–23. Large-cell lymphoma of the mediastinum with marked tropism for germinal centers.

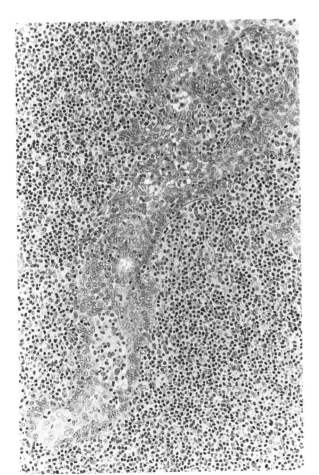

FIGURE 4–24. Elongated strands of hyperplastic thymic epithelium are seen in a patient with mediastinal lymphoma.

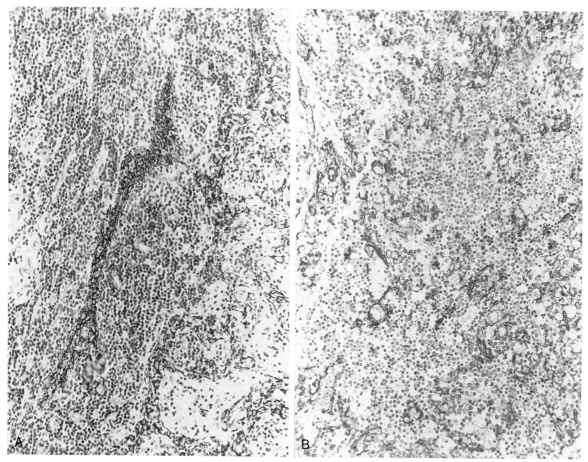

FIGURE 4–25. *A,* Keratin immunostain in large-cell lymphoma of the mediastinum highlights elongated, branching structures formed by hyperplastic thymic epithelium. *B,* For comparison, pattern of keratin immunostain in lymphocyte-rich thymoma shows even distribution of keratin-positive epithelial cells that are scattered singly among the lymphoid cells.

B-cell lymphoma of mucosa-associated lymphoid tissue (MALT) involving the thymus.[35, 36]

Lymphoblastic lymphoma represents the most common mediastinal lymphoma in children, although it may also occur in adults.[28, 37] It is characterized by diffuse sheets of lymphoblasts with convoluted nuclear membranes, small inconspicuous nucleoli, and frequent mitotic figures and is often associated with extensive areas of necrosis. Tingible body macrophages are usually present in fair numbers, creating the typical "starry-sky" appearance. A feature that is often seen in lymphoblastic lymphoma, particularly at the periphery of the tumor, is the arrangement of the neoplastic cells in a linear or single-file pattern. Lymphoblastic lymphoma may also occasionally show prominent incrustation of DNA material around vessel walls, resulting in a picture that closely simulates small-cell carcinoma (Fig. 4–27). The diagnosis of lymphoblastic lymphoma is confirmed by demonstrating the presence of intranuclear terminal deoxynucleotidyl transferase (TdT), along with CD1, CD4, CD8, CD14, and CD38 positivity, indicative of an immature cortical thymocyte phenotype.[38]

Other Lymphoproliferative and Myeloproliferative Conditions

Granulocytic Sarcoma

This condition may rarely present as a mediastinal mass and can be mistaken for large-cell lymphoma.[39] Eosinophilic myelocytes, when present, suggest this diagnosis. Helpful aids for diagnosis on paraffin sections include a positive chloroacetate esterase stain (Leder stain) and immunochemical stains for lysozyme.[40]

Extramedullary Plasmacytoma

Extramedullary plasmacytoma has also been described in the mediastinum.[41] Such cases are characterized by a monotonous proliferation of monotypic plasma cells with immunohistochemical demonstration of light chain restriction.

Castleman's Disease

Castleman's disease (angiofollicular lymphoid hyperplasia) is a benign disorder with a special predilection for the mediastinum. It usually involves mediastinal lymph nodes but may also be found arising within the thymus.[42] Two histologic variants have been described: the **hyaline vascular and plasma cell types.** Characteristic morphologic features of this condition include follicular lymphoid hyperplasia with prominent vessels within germinal centers containing hyaline material, and concentric, "onion-skin" layering of mantle-zone lymphocytes around germinal centers. Penetration of germinal centers by elongated vessels creates the distinctive "lollipop" appearance (Fig. 4–28). In the plasma cell variant, the interfollicular areas show marked plasmocytosis with

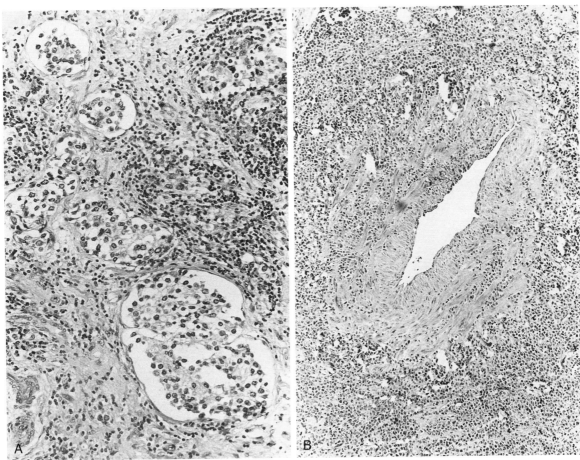

FIGURE 4–26. *A,* Invasion of vascular lumina by lymphoma cells in large-cell lymphoma of the mediastinum. *B,* Invasion of vessel wall by lymphoma cells in B-cell lymphoma of the mediastinum.

varying amounts of vascularity and sclerosis. In advanced stages, the germinal centers show a tendency to undergo massive hyalinization resulting in structures that resemble Hassall's corpuscles, a feature that may lead to confusion with thymoma. Confluence of hyalinized germinal centers may also lead to extensive areas of hyalinization with metaplastic ossification (Fig. 4–29), which may obscure the underlying process and lead to confusion with other fibrosing processes. Another feature of Castleman's disease is the tendency to induce florid hyperplastic changes of thymic epithelium that may lead to a mistaken diagnosis of thymoma on small mediastinoscopic biopsies. The prominent plasmacytosis and elongated, branching appearance of the epithelial elements are helpful clues for arriving at the correct diagnosis.

Thymic Lymphoid Hyperplasia

It is important to distinguish this condition from true thymic hyperplasia. The latter is defined as an enlargement of the gland beyond that considered to be the upper limit of normal for a particular age group, but with conservation of the normal ratio of lymphocytes and epithelial cells of the normal thymus.[2] In thymic lymphoid hyperplasia, the thymus is usually not enlarged; the term **hyperplasia** in such instances refers to the presence of an increased number of lymphoid follicles with prominent germinal centers in the medullary region of the gland. Lymphoid hyperplasia of the thymus is most frequently

associated with myasthenia gravis,[43] although it can also be observed in a number of other immune-mediated disorders such as lupus erythematosus, scleroderma, rheumatoid arthritis, and thyrotoxicosis.[44, 45] Thymic lymphoid hyperplasia may also infrequently be accompanied by florid epithelial hyperplasia. The diffuse and haphazard distribution of the latter in such instances helps avoid a misdiagnosis of thymoma.

Extramedullary Hematopoiesis

This condition may present as large solitary mediastinal masses, usually located in the posterior mediastinum along the paravertebral column.[46] The lesions are histologically characterized by immature myeloid precursors admixed with atypical magakaryocytes against a fibrous background.

Neuroendocrine Neoplasms

Carcinoid Tumors

It is now well established that neoplastic neuroendocrine proliferations may arise in the thymus.[47, 48] The most frequent form of primary mediastinal neuroendocrine neoplasm is thymic carcinoid. Histologically, the typical thymic carcinoid is characterized by a proliferation of monotonous round cells with large, round or oval nuclei containing finely dispersed

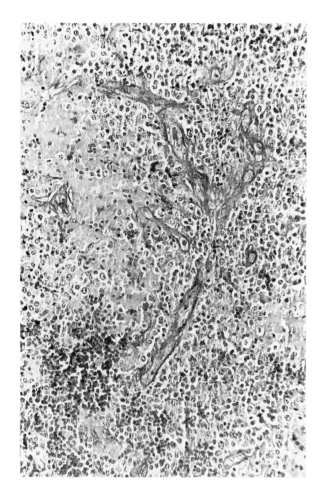

FIGURE 4–27. Prominent incrustation of vessel walls by DNA material is seen in this lymphoblastic lymphoma.

FIGURE 4–28. Vessel wall penetrating germinal center in Castleman's disease creating distinctive "lollipop" appearance.

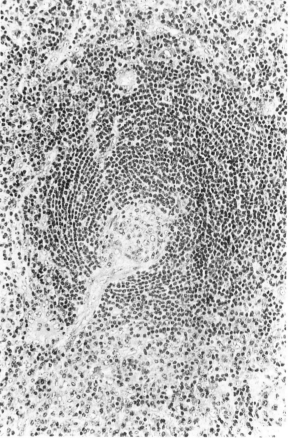

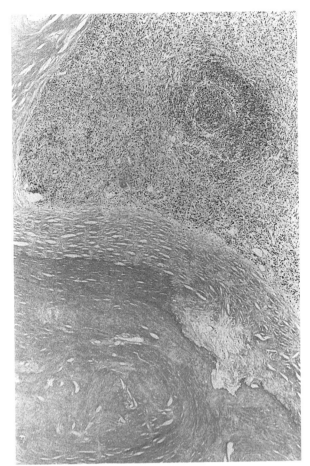

FIGURE 4–29. Massive hyalinization with ossification in an example of Castleman's disease of the posterior mediastinum.

chromatin ("salt and pepper" nuclei) and inconspicuous nucleoli. The tumor cells are arranged in cords and ribbons and separated by a delicate fibrovascular stroma. The formation of rosettes or microacinar-like structures is particularly prominent in these tumors. Another distinctive feature of thymic carcinoids is their tendency to show foci of dystrophic calcification, which accounts for their often gritty texture of the cut section on gross inspection.

Several **histologic variants** of thymic carcinoid have now been recognized, including a **spindle cell type,**[49] **pigmented carcinoid,**[50] a variant closely **resembling medullary thyroid carcinoma with amyloid stroma,**[51] and **sclerotic and diffuse variants.**[52] Carcinoids resembling medullary carcinoma of the thymus are characterized by the presence of stromal amyloid (Fig. 4–30), which is best identified by the use of Congo red stains. These must be distinguished from extension of medullary carcinoma of the thyroid into the superior mediastinum. A **desmoplastic variant of thymic carcinoid** has also been described that is characterized by a prominent sclerotic stroma containing small islands and scattered tumor cells adopting a single-file configuration (Fig. 4–31); such lesions are often mistaken for metastatic carcinoma. Some thymic carcinoids may assume a diffuse growth pattern, with sheets of monotonous tumor cells without intervening stroma; these cases may be readily mistaken for lymphoid proliferations or thymoma on cursory examination. Identification of areas in the periphery showing the more conventional features of thymic

carcinoid helps direct the pathologist toward the correct diagnosis. Other unusual variants of thymic carcinoid include **tumors composed exclusively of cells featuring abundant oncocytic cytoplasm (oncocytic carcinoid)** (Fig. 4–32) and a variant of **thymic carcinoid characterized by the production of abundant stromal mucin** (Fig. 4–33).

Regardless of the histologic variant, thymic carcinoids exhibit a consistent histochemical staining pattern characterized by argyrophilia with the Grimelius, Sevier-Munger, or Churukian-Schenk techniques and negative staining with argentaffin stains.[52] The most helpful aid in diagnosis for these tumors is demonstration of chromogranin immunoreactivity by immunohistochemical methods.[53] Other neuroendocrine markers such as neuron-specific enolase (NSE), Leu-7, and synaptophysin may yield inconsistent results and may not all be present in a given lesion. Thymic carcinoids may additionally secrete a variety of neuropeptide hormones and amines such as met-enkephalin, endorphins, serotonin, adrenocorticotropic hormone (ACTH), somatostatin, and so on.[54] Demonstration of dense-core neurosecretory granules in the cytoplasm of the cells by electron microscopy provides additional supportive evidence of neuroendocrine differentiation in equivocal cases.

Mediastinal Paraganglioma

Most **mediastinal paragangliomas** occur in association with aorticopulmonary chemoreceptors located in the antero-

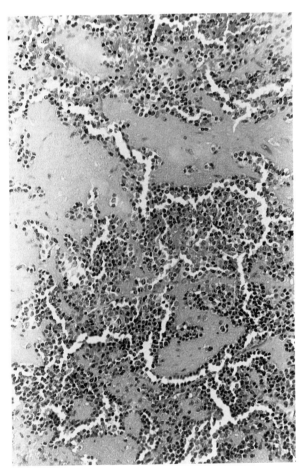

FIGURE 4–30. Thymic carcinoid simulating medullary carcinoma of the thyroid.

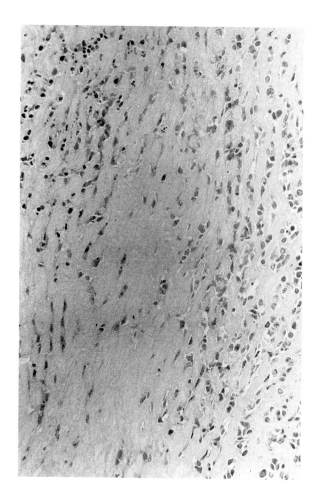

FIGURE 4–31. Desmoplastic variant of thymic carcinoid simulating metastatic breast carcinoma.

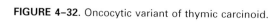

FIGURE 4–32. Oncocytic variant of thymic carcinoid.

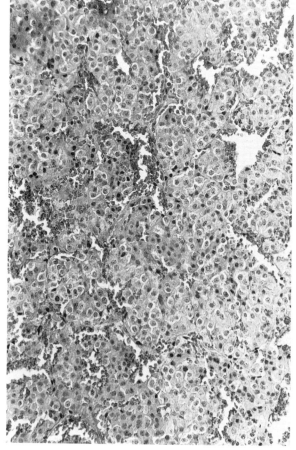

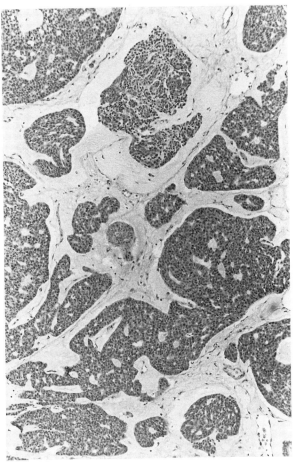

FIGURE 4–33. Thymic carcinoid with abundant mucin production simulating metastatic mucin-secreting carcinoma.

superior mediastinum; others arise from mediastinal aortico-sympathetic paraganglia and occur posteriorly, along the costovertebral sulcus.[55] Their morphologic appearances are identical to paragangliomas in other locations, i.e., the tumors are composed of a uniform population of large, polygonal cells arranged in tight nests (''Zellballen'') separated by dense fibrovascular septa. Cytologic features include round or oval nuclei with dispersed chromatin and rare mitotic figures. Nuclear pleomorphism can be striking in these neoplasms and does not correlate with biologic behavior. A few morphologic variants have been described, including spindle cell paraganglioma, granular cell paraganglioma, and a hyalinizing, angiectatic variant (Fig. 4–34).[56] Other unusual features in mediastinal paraganglioma include the formation of gland-like lumen in the Zellballen, and areas displaying a solid pattern of growth. The most important differential diagnosis for these lesions, particularly when located in the anterior mediastinum, is that of thymic carcinoid. Although carcinoids share many morphologic features with paraganglioma, paragangliomas never display ribbons, cords, or festoons, nor do they contain rosettes or microacinar structures. Additionally, cytomegaly, a prominent and almost constant feature in paragangliomas, is rarely a feature of carcinoids. From the immunohistochemical point of view, both share immunoreactivity for chromagranin and other neuroendocrine markers. **Paragangliomas, however, are usually negative for keratin intermediate fila-**

ments, unlike carcinoids, which stain positive with this marker.[56] S-100 protein–positive sustentacular cells are usually a prominent feature in paragangliomas, although such cells have also been described in carcinoid tumors.[57] Ultrastructural examination is of limited help in distinguishing these two conditions; however, the presence of whorled aggregates of intermediate filaments in perinuclear location favors thymic carcinoid over paraganglioma.

Germ Cell Neoplasms

Seminoma

Seminomas of the mediastinum arise almost exclusively from the thymus; they have been described only in males. Their microscopic appearance in general is similar to that of their gonadal counterpart. The tumors are characterized by sheets or clusters of large, atypical cells surrounded by abundant clear cytoplasm and containing round to oval nuclei with prominent, irregular nucleoli. The tumor cells are separated by fibrous septa infiltrated by lymphocytes and plasma cells. A florid granulomatous stromal reaction is a frequent component. Occasional tumors exhibit a more pronounced degree of nuclear pleomorphism and high mitotic activity, thus qualifying for the designation of anaplastic seminoma. Features of these tumors that are specific for their thymic location include prominent cystic changes, reactive follicular hyperplasia, and fibrosis.[16] Cystic change in seminoma is a frequent feature of these tumors; occasionally, the cystic changes can be of such magnitude that the seminomatous components may be reduced to a minimal expression and the process may be mistakenly diagnosed as a benign thymic cyst (Fig. 4–35).[58] Careful search for discrete foci containing the characteristic large cells with prominent nucleoli is therefore mandatory when evaluating cystic lesions of the mediastinum. Another common feature of mediastinal seminomas is the frequent presence of reactive lymphoid follicular hyperplasia. Small clusters of seminoma cells characteristically are distributed along the periphery of the mantle zones in the lymphoid follicles (Fig. 4–36). Mediastinal seminoma may also be accompanied by extensive fibrosis; in some instances, thick fibrous bands may separate the thymic parenchyma into discrete nodules that resemble HD or thymoma on scanning magnification. Identification of the seminoma cells and absence of RS cells on careful search help reach a correct diagnosis. Another unusual feature of seminoma is the occurrence of thymic epithelial hyperplasia, which may lead to the incorrect diagnosis of thymoma (Fig. 4–37). As with Hodgkin's and non-Hodgkin's lymphomas, attention to the growth pattern of the epithelial cell islands is important for diagnosis: reactive epithelial hyperplasia generally manifests as slender, elongated, often branching strands and cords of normal-appearing epithelial cells surrounded by lymphocytes and other stromal elements, in contrast with the epithelial component in thymoma, which is evenly scattered (lymphocyte-rich variant) or forms solid, angulated lobules (epithelial-rich thymoma).

The differential diagnosis for mediastinal seminoma includes large-cell lymphoma, Hodgkin's disease, thymoma, and clear-cell thymic carcinoma. Application of immunostains may be helpful in this setting; seminomas are negative for lymphoid markers and generally show negative or very focal

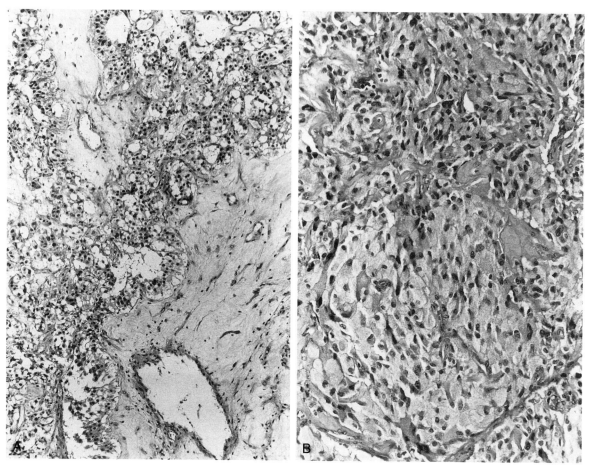

FIGURE 4–34. *A,* Posterior mediastinal paraganglioma with prominent angiectatic areas and stromal hyalinization. *B,* Mediastinal paraganglioma with granular cell change.

weak positivity with keratin antibodies. Placental alkaline phosphatase has been described as a good marker for testicular seminomas; however, it may show only weak or variable reactivity on paraffin-embedded tissues.[59] Electron microscopy may help establish the diagnosis in equivocal cases by demonstrating the characteristically dispersed filamentous nucleolonema. Other ultrastructural features of seminoma include cytoplasmic glycogen and rare desmosomes.[60]

Non-seminomatous Germ Cell Tumors

Non-seminomatous germ cell tumors of the mediastinum include embryonal carcinoma, endodermal sinus tumor, and choriocarcinoma. Histologically they are indistinguishable from their gonadal counterparts. **Embryonal carcinomas** are characterized by primitive-appearing cells growing in sheets with focal primitive glandular or papillary formations. Mitoses are numerous, and there are often large areas of necrosis. Focally these tumors may sometimes adopt a pseudoangiosarcomatous growth pattern, with highly atypical cells lining apparent vascular spaces containing extravasated red blood cells (Fig. 4–38). **Endodermal sinus tumor** is characterized by a variety of growth patterns, including microcystic, solid, alveolar, glandular, and papillary. Schiller-Duval bodies are distinctive for this type of tumor but may often be hard to find. Hyaline globules are also characteristic, but not specific. The most common diagnostic pitfall is mistaking a predomi-

nantly papillary yolk sac tumor for metastatic carcinoma (Fig. 4–39). **Choriocarcinomas** are characterized by the admixture of cytotrophoblastic and syncytiotrophoblastic elements against a highly hemorrhagic background. As in other extragonadal locations and in the gonads, admixtures of various types of germ cell tumors are common. Such tumors are referred to as **mixed germ cell tumors.** One of the most frequent combinations is between seminomatous and nonseminomatous elements.[61] An unusual occurrence in mediastinal germ cell tumors is the development of sarcomatous components such as angiosarcoma or rhabdomyosarcoma (Fig. 4–40).[62] Immunohistochemistry may play an important role in the diagnosis of germ cell tumors of the mediastinum. Embryonal carcinoma strongly immunoreacts in most instances with antibodies against placental alkaline phosphatase (PLAP), and to a lesser degree with alpha-fetoprotein (AFP), human chorionic gonadotropin (HCG), and widespectrum keratin. Endodermal sinus tumors are characterized by strong immunoreactivity for AFP; they may also be positive for PLAP, carcinoembryonic antigen (CEA), and keratin. Choriocarcinomas are strongly positive for HCG and may also stain with PLAP, CEA, and keratin. There is, however, a certain degree of overlap between the staining specificities for these markers, and a sharp distinction between the different types of germ cell tumors may not be possible in many instances owing to their propensity for containing admixtures of the different cell types.

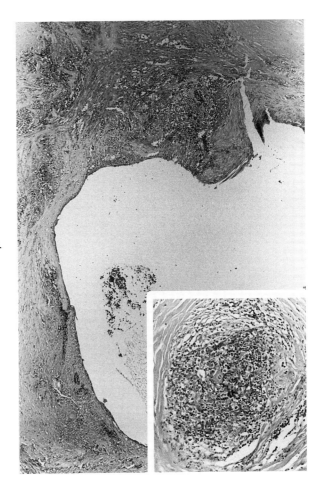

FIGURE 4–35. Mediastinal seminoma with prominent cystic changes. Notice atypical cellular infiltrate in the wall of the cyst (*inset*).

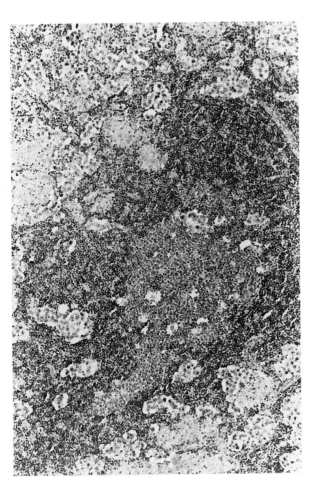

FIGURE 4–36. Lymphoid follicular hyperplasia in mediastinal seminoma. Note large, clear seminoma cells arranged in clusters around mantle zones of germinal centers.

163

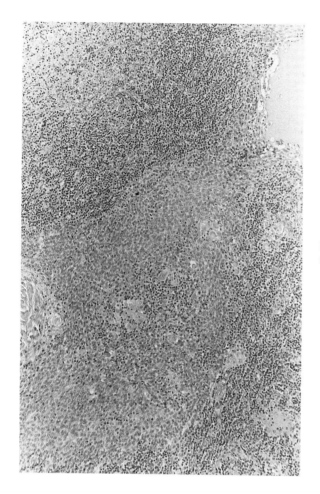

FIGURE 4–37. Areas of reactive thymic epithelial hyperplasia in thymic seminoma.

FIGURE 4–38. Embryonal carcinoma of the mediastinum with pseudo-angiosarcomatous pattern.

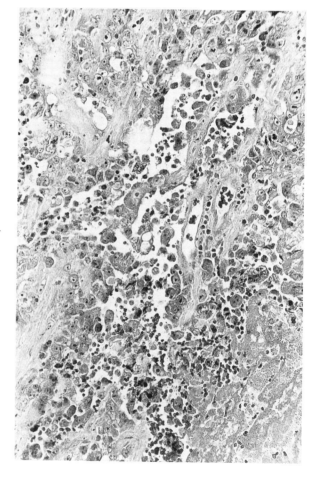

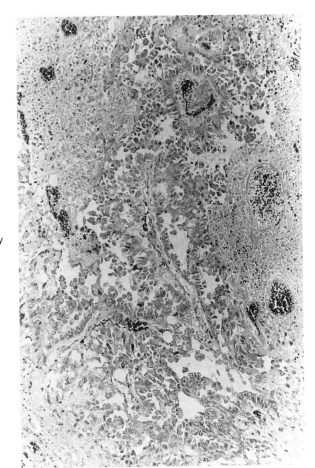

FIGURE 4–39. Yolk sac tumor of mediastinum with predominant papillary growth pattern.

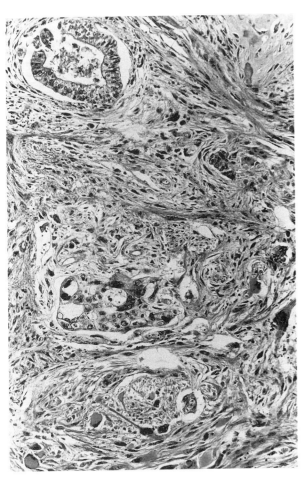

FIGURE 4–40. Foci of rhabdomyosarcomatous differentiation in embryonal carcinoma of the mediastinum.

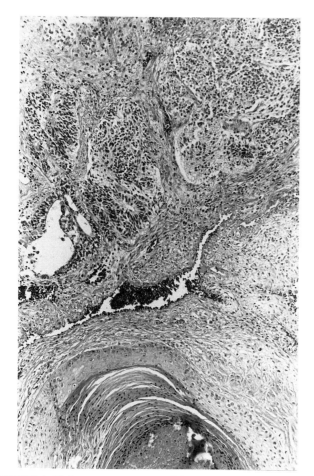

FIGURE 4–41. Immature teratoma of the mediastinum with primitive neural elements (*top*).

Teratomas

Mature cystic teratomas represent the most common type of mediastinal germ cell neoplasms. Their microscopic appearance resembles that of the more common mature cystic teratoma of ovary (dermoid cyst). **Immature teratomas** are characterized by the presence of immature epithelial, mesodermal, or neural elements without a component of embryonal carcinoma (Fig. 4–41). **Malignant teratoma** refers to the combination of embryonal carcinoma and mature teratoma; it may also contain elements of immature teratoma. As with other types of germ cell tumors, malignant teratoma may also show the development of a sarcomatous component, such as angiosarcoma or rhabdomyosarcoma.[63]

Neural Neoplasms

Peripheral Nerve Sheath Tumors

Benign peripheral nerve sheath tumors include schwannoma and neurofibroma. The majority of such cases present in the posterior mediastinum, although they can also arise in the anterior and superior compartments of the mediastinum.[64] **Schwannomas** are the most common benign peripheral nerve sheath tumors of the posterior mediastinum and are characterized by cellular foci of spindle cells with prominent palisading

(Antoni A) admixed with paucicellular, often myxoid areas (Antoni B). As with schwannomas elsewhere, they exhibit a wide range of degenerative changes, including perivascular hyalinization, cystic changes, and xanthomatous degeneration. Marked pleomorphism and cellular atypia may be present occasionally in some of these tumors (ancient schwannoma); however, in the absence of necrosis and mitotic activity, these features are of no biologic significance. Rare variants of schwannoma that may be occasionally encountered in the mediastinum include the melanotic schwannoma, characterized by deposition of melanin pigment, and the so-called glandular schwannoma, characterized by the presence of glandular structures scattered among the spindle cell elements. An unusual finding in schwannomas is the presence of palisaded areas of collagen deposition that may often adopt a stellate configuration (so-called amianthoid fibers) (Fig. 4–42). **Neurofibromas** are the second most common benign neural tumors in the mediastinum and most often arise in the setting of neurofibromatosis.[65] Histologically they are composed of a uniform spindle cell population without obvious palisading. Degenerative changes such as those associated with schwannomas (i.e., foci of myxoid degeneration, cystic changes, and so forth) are lacking. Nuclear pleomorphism is not a feature in the benign forms, and mitotic activity is generally absent. Mast cells may be a prominent component and can be easily highlighted by the use of metachromatic stains. Neurofibromas are often the site of malignant degenera-

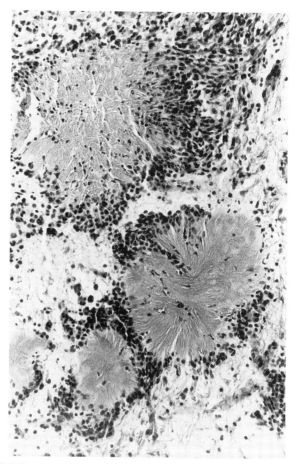

FIGURE 4–42. Posterior mediastinal schwannoma with palisaded areas of abnormal collagenization (so-called amianthoid fibers).

tion, particularly when multiple or plexiform. Areas of atypia or mitoses should warrant careful examination for malignant degeneration. Finally, a highly unusual variant of schwannoma has been described by Carney and designated "psammomatous melanotic schwannoma," in which melanotic epithelioid and spindle cell elements of intramediastinal spinal roots are found admixed with psammoma bodies (Fig. 4–43).[66] Over half of the patients with these tumors present with a familial complex of myxomas, spotty pigmentation, and endocrine overactivity; about 10% of these tumors are capable of metastases.

Malignant peripheral nerve sheath tumors (malignant schwannoma, neurofibrosarcoma, neurogenic sarcoma) are more common in the posterior mediastinum but may also arise in the anterior compartment.[67] Although some may occur sporadically or secondary to prior radiation, the majority of cases arise in the setting of neurofibromatosis. Histologically they may show two predominant patterns of growth: a fascicular growth pattern characterized by elongated fascicles of spindle cells adopting a prominent "herringbone" pattern, and an epithelioid variant characterized by large, round to oval cells with abundant cytoplasm arranged in a diffuse or lobular configuration (Fig. 4–44). Mitoses are numerous in these tumors, and areas of hemorrhage and necrosis may be frequently present. In a small percentage of cases, malignant schwannomas may show areas featuring alternate lines of differentiation, such as rhabdomyosarcomatous (malignant

"triton" tumor), angiosarcomatous, and chondrosarcomatous or osteosarcomatous.[68, 69] Another rare variant is the malignant counterpart of glandular schwannoma, characterized by the presence of benign-appearing glandular structures set against a background of atypical spindle elements. The diagnosis of peripheral nerve sheath tumors is facilitated by immunohistochemical demonstration of S-100 protein immunoreactivity in the neoplastic cells. Absence of staining for this marker, however, may occur in as many as 50% of cases, making a negative result unreliable for definitive determination.[70, 71] Electron microscopy may be a valuable aid for diagnosis in equivocal cases by demonstrating slender, interdigitating cell processes with cell junctions and basal lamina material, as well as mesoaxon formation and other neural features distinctive for tumors of peripheral nerve sheath.[70, 72]

Ganglion Cell Tumors

Tumors derived from the sympathetic nervous system in the chest cavity arise almost exclusively in the posterior mediastinum. They differ from their retroperitoneal counterparts in that those in the mediastinum tend to exhibit a higher degree of differentiation. **Ganglioneuroma** is the most common tumor in this group, and is composed histologically of an admixture of mature ganglion cells with spindle cells that may be either fibroblastic or schwannian in nature. **Ganglioneuroblastoma** represents an intermediate stage of differentiation, similar to differentiating neuroblastoma in the retroperitoneum, and is composed of an admixture of immature neuroblastic elements with an abundant neurofibrillary matrix. Clusters of ganglion cells may be present scattered throughout the lesion. Neuroblastoma is predominantly composed of immature neuroblastic elements supported by a fibrillary matrix. These tumors may display foci of necrosis; areas of calcification are a frequent finding (Fig. 4–45). Homer-Wright pseudorosettes are rarely seen in these tumors in the mediastinum. The more cellular variants may mimic blastic lymphoma, Ewing's sarcoma, or metastatic small-cell carcinoma.[73]

COMMON LESIONS THAT SHARE FEATURES WITH OTHER LESIONS WITH WHICH THEY MAY BE CONFUSED

Benign Lesions

Encapsulated Thymoma

Benign thymomas may occasionally exhibit morphologic features that can lead to confusion with other neoplastic and reactive conditions of that organ. Lymphocyte-rich thymomas may contain numerous scattered tingible-body macrophages, imparting them with a distinctive "starry-sky" appearance (Fig. 4–46). Care should be taken not to mistake such cases for malignant lymphoma; careful identification of the epithelial cells of thymoma and attention to the lobular growth pattern and good circumscription of the lesion are essential for correct diagnosis. In equivocal cases, application of keratin stains highlights thymic epithelial cells scattered throughout the lesion. Prominent formation of germinal centers may occa-

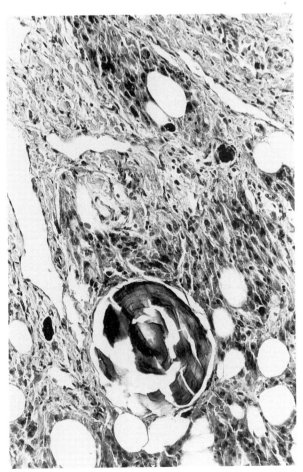

FIGURE 4–43. Psammomatous melanotic schwannoma arising in posterior mediastinum.

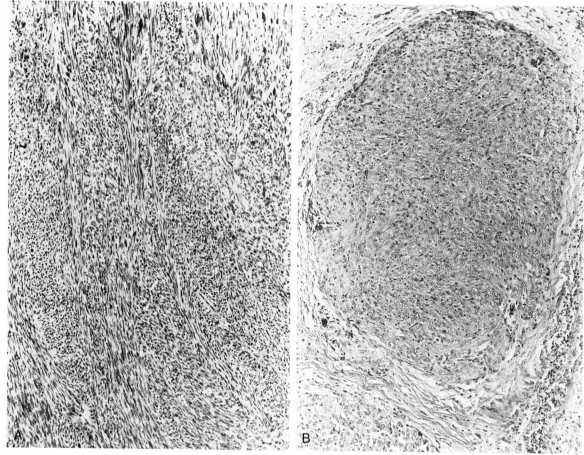

FIGURE 4–44. *A,* Malignant schwannoma with fascicular growth pattern. *B,* Epithelioid malignant schwannoma composed of large round cells with abundant cytoplasm and prominent lobulation.

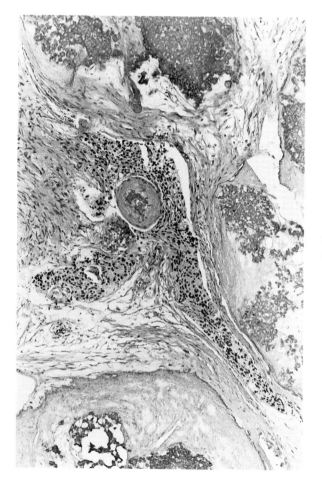

FIGURE 4–45. Neuroblastoma of the posterior mediastinum with extensive calcification.

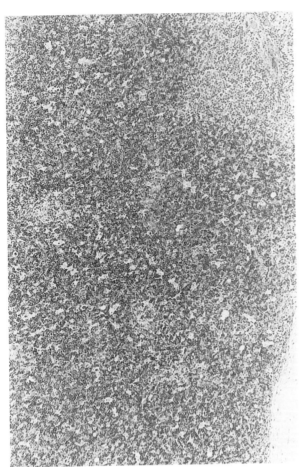

FIGURE 4–46. Lymphocyte-rich thymoma with prominent tingible-body macrophages resulting in a "starry-sky" appearance.

sionally be encountered in encapsulated thymomas of patients with myasthenia gravis; the presence of such structures should not lead to confusion with thymic follicular hyperplasia of myasthenia gravis. Other patterns of thymoma that may be confused with other neoplasms have been discussed in the section dealing with atypical presentation of common lesions.

Hyperplastic and Regressive Changes of the Thymus

A variety of hyperplastic and regressive changes may take place in the thymus. **True thymic hyperplasia** is a rare condition characterized by global enlargement of the thymus with preservation of the normal ratio of lymphocytes and epithelial cells.[74] Such lesions may be mistaken both clinically and histologically for thymoma or other neoplasm. Thymic hyperplasia has been recognized as a complication of chemotherapy for Hodgkin's disease in children[75] and germ cell tumors in adults[76] and has been interpreted under such circumstances to represent an immunologic "rebound" phenomenon. A similar enlargement of the thymus has also been observed in children recovering from thermal burns[77] and after cessation of administration of corticosteroids in infants.[78] Histologically, the lesions show the features of a normal thymus without formation of the distinctive angulated lobules, perivascular spaces, or other features associated with thymoma.

Thymic involution may be either physiologic or secondary to stress. In physiologic involution of the thymus, the gland experiences gradual and progressive atrophic changes, which in its late stages results in a picture consisting of atrophic lobules of thymic epithelium depleted of lymphocytes, with partly cystic, closely aggregated Hassall's corpuscles and abundant intervening adipose tissue.[79] In stress involution, a condition related to episodes of severe stress in which there is sudden release of corticosteroids from the adrenal cortex, the gland is characterized by prominent karyorrhexis of lymphocytes with active phagocytosis by macrophages, resulting in a striking "starry sky" appearance confined to the cortex.[80] Such changes may be easily confused on small biopsy specimens for lymphoblastic lymphoma. An analogous process has been observed in patients with acquired immunodeficiency syndrome (AIDS), in which the involuting process is accompanied by effacement of the corticomedullary junction, marked lymphocytic depletion, fibrosis, and lack or paucity of Hassall's corpuscles.[81, 82]

Mediastinal Cysts

Congenital cysts account for approximately 20% of primary mediastinal mass lesions.[83] Included in this group are cysts arising from pericardial, bronchogenic, enteric, and thymic epithelium. For the most part, congenital cysts of the mediastinum are asymptomatic and usually discovered incidentally on routine chest x-ray examinations, or may be discovered because of compression symptoms depending on their size and location. Malignant changes may exceptionally take place in them.[84] **Thymic cysts** may be of developmental origin or the result of an acquired, reactive process. The former are usually unilocular, translucent, and lined by a single layer of simple cuboidal to columnar ciliated epithelium. **Multilocular thymic cysts** are more often the result of hyperplastic proliferation and cystic transformation of thymic epithelium induced by an acquired inflammatory process.[85] Histologically they are characterized by cystic cavities lined by squamous, columnar, or cuboidal epithelium (with some having features of dilated Hassall's corpuscles) and by scattered nests or islands of normal thymic tissue within the cyst walls, often in continuity with the cyst lining epithelium (Fig. 4–47). Additional features that are a constant component of these lesions include severe acute and chronic inflammation, fibrovascular proliferation, necrosis, hemorrhage, cholesterol granulomas, and reactive lymphoid hyperplasia with prominent germinal centers. These cysts may often create diagnostic problems because of their apparent invasive character on gross inspection, their variegated microscopic features, and the fact that a great number of primary thymic neoplasms may be accompanied by similar profuse cystic changes. In view of this last feature, extensive sampling is mandatory in all multilocular cysts of the mediastinum to exclude the possibility of other processes, including Hodgkin's disease, seminoma, and non-Hodgkin's lymphoma. Another feature that may be seen in multilocular thymic cysts is the development of pseudoepitheliomatous hyperplasia in the cyst lining epithelium.[86] Such phenomenon should not be mistaken for the development of a malignancy arising from the cyst wall.

Localized Fibrous Tumor and Other Benign Mesenchymal Neoplasms

Fibrous tumors arising from serosal surfaces (**solitary fibrous tumor,** submesothelial fibroma, fibrous mesotheli-

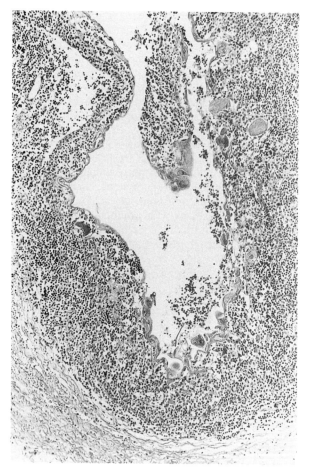

FIGURE 4–47. Multilocular thymic cyst showing cystic dilatation of Hassall's corpuscles.

oma) most often present as polypoid, pedunculated lesions attached to the parietal or visceral pleura of the lung; however, they have also been described presenting as mediastinal masses.[87] Histologically, they are characterized by their variegated appearance, with a combination of areas exhibiting a cellular spindle cell population and areas displaying diffuse fibrosis evident in the majority of cases. In a study by Moran et al.,[88] these tumors were found to exhibit a variety of histologic patterns, including angiofibroma and hemangiopericytoma-like, fibrosarcoma-like, monophasic synovial sarcoma–like, and malignant schwannoma-like appearances (Fig. 4–48). Fibrous tumors of the mediastinum may thus be easily mistaken for a variety of soft tissue sarcomas, including fibrosarcoma, malignant fibrous histiocytoma, malignant schwannoma, and monophasic synovial sarcoma. The tumor cells are immunoreactive only with vimentin antibodies, thus, immunohistochemistry may play a limited role in their diagnosis. Close attention to the gross features of the lesion is critical for diagnosis, namely, that of a well-circumscribed, encapsulated, polypoid mass attached to a serosal surface by a pedicle.

Other types of benign mesenchymal neoplasms originating in the mediastinum include **lymphangioma, lymphangiomyoma, hemangioma, lipoma, rhabdomyoma, leiomyoma,** and **extraskeletal chondroma.**[89] Lipomas, lymphangiomas, and hemangiomas represent the most common ones in this group. Lymphangioma and lymphangiomyoma most often

arise in the anterosuperior mediastinum in children, often in continuity with a cervical component. Hemangiomas in adults are usually of the cavernous type. In children, they may have a very cellular appearance and appear infiltrative, similar to cutaneous juvenile hemangioendotheliomas of infancy; however, they display a benign behavior.[90]

Malignant Tumors

Malignant Lymphoma

Malignant lymphomas of the mediastinum may share features with many other lymphoid and non-lymphoid conditions. The various morphologic patterns of Hodgkin's and non-Hodgkin's lymphomas have already been detailed in a previous section. Some points, however, deserve emphasis. The most common source of confusion in diagnosis for malignant lymphoma of the mediastinum has traditionally been with epithelial-rich thymoma and metastatic carcinoma. Prior to the advent of immunohistochemistry, such lesions would often be misdiagnosed as epithelial neoplasms. The propensity for large-cell lymphoma in this location to undergo sclerosis with "packaging" and compartmentalization of small groups of cells by thin fibrous bands often creates the impression of an epithelial malignancy. Additionally, lymphomas often elicit a hyperplastic response in the thymus that takes the form of thin, elongated, often branching strands of thymic epithelium composed of a single- or double-cell layer, surrounded by or circumscribing dense connective tissue in a fibroepitheliomatous fashion. Similar formations are commonly seen at the periphery of multilocular thymic cysts, in Castleman's disease, and in seminomas, teratomas, and other neoplasms of the thymus. In malignant lymphomas, however, these strands of thymic epithelial cells are seen not only around but also within the tumor, where they may be surrounded and infiltrated by the neoplastic elements. Because of this latter feature, ultrastructural examination from the lesions can often lead to misinterpretation of the process as epithelial in nature, owing to the presence of cells with intercellular junctions and other epithelial characteristics. Immunohistochemical stains for keratin may be extremely useful for diagnosis in this setting by delineating these structures and highlighting their distinctive net-like pattern. Additionally, application of lymphoid markers demonstrates the lymphoid nature of the atypical cells circumscribing these structures. Hodgkin's disease in the mediastinum may also pose several difficulties of its own for diagnosis and may share features with a variety of other conditions affecting this region. The tendency of HD to undergo extensive sclerosis may yield areas displaying only a sparse chronic inflammatory infiltrate and massive fibrosis in small biopsies taken from the periphery of the lesions, leading to confusion with sclerosing mediastinitis. For this reason, definitive diagnosis may not be possible on small mediastinoscopic biopsies, and complete resection of the lesion may offer the only possibility for adequate evaluation of the lesion. The propensity of HD and non-Hodgkin's lymphoma to undergo extensive cystic degeneration has already been mentioned. Another feature of HD that deserves mention is the development of large epithelial-lined thymic cysts after the administration of radia-

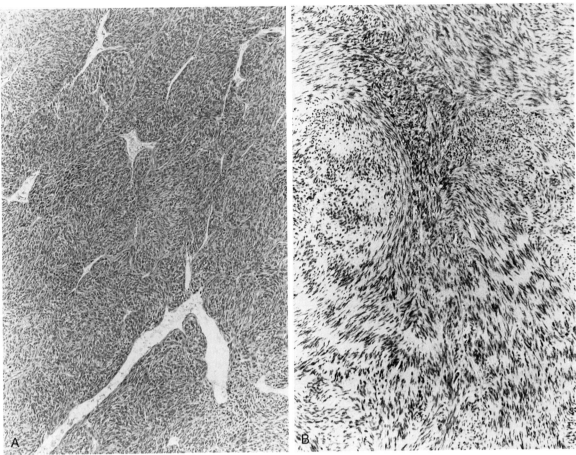

FIGURE 4–48. *A,* Solitary fibrous tumor of the mediastinum with hemangiopericytic growth pattern. *B,* Solitary fibrous tumor with neural-type palisading.

tion therapy, which may simulate radiographically tumor relapse.[91, 92]

Sarcomas

Virtually every type of soft tissue sarcoma may occur in the mediastinum. In addition to neural tumors (which have been reviewed in a previous section), tumors of vasoformative tissues, adipose tissue, chondro-osseous tissues, and smooth and skeletal muscle and fibroblastic and fibrohistiocytic tumors have been described.

Malignant Vascular Neoplasms

These fall into two general categories: **epithelioid hemangioendothelioma** and **angiosarcoma.** Epithelioid hemangioendotheliomas are low-grade vascular malignancies that are characterized by a proliferation of round to oval cells with abundant, often vacuolated cytoplasm lacking overt features of malignancy, such as atypia or mitotic activity (Fig. 4–49). The epithelioid appearance of the cells often leads to confusion with carcinoma. The endothelial nature of the epithelioid cells can be demonstrated by positive staining for factor VIII–related antigen.[93] Occasional examples may display abundant osteoclast-type giant cells and metaplastic bone admixed with the endothelial cells,[94, 95] as well as intravascular papillary

tufting.[93] Conventional angiosarcomas are extremely rare but may arise in the posterior mediastinum.

Liposarcomas

Liposarcoma is one of the most common sarcomas of the mediastinum. Most of the cases described in the literature have been located in the posterior mediastinum. Only two cases have been described of a **sarcoma of thymic stroma with features of liposarcoma** originating from the anterior mediastinum.[96] Histologically, **mediastinal liposarcomas** show the same features as liposarcomas in other locations, including well-differentiating, sclerosing, myxoid, round cell, and pleomorphic variants.

Myogenic Sarcomas

Leiomyosarcomas in the mediastinum most often represent secondary extension from tumors arising in thoracic viscera or from the walls of major vessels,[97, 98] although primary tumors arising from the soft tissue in both mediastinal compartments unassociated with vascular or other structures can also occur.[99] **Rhabdomyosarcomas** occur most often in children and are mostly located in the posterior mediastinum or arise as a component of malignant teratomas.[100] Histologically, embryonal rhabdomyosarcomas are the most frequent, although the alveolar variant may also be encountered. Immunohistochem-

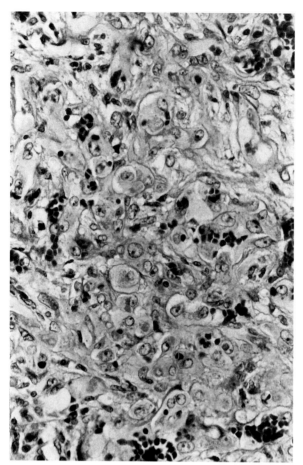

FIGURE 4–49. Epithelioid hemangioendothelioma of the anterior mediastinum. Notice vacuolation and abundant cytoplasm of the neoplastic cells.

istry is of value for diagnosis by demonstrating expression of desmin and muscle-specific actin within the tumor cells.[101] Primary rhabdomyosarcoma arising in pure form in the mediastinum has also been described.[102] These tumors must be distinguished from other small blue-cell tumors originating at these sites or from distant metastases.

Chondrosarcoma and Osteosarcoma

Primary osteosarcoma and chondrosarcoma of the mediastinum are extremely rare; only a handful of cases are reported in the literature. The majority of chondrosarcomas described have been associated with the tracheobronchial tree or thoracic vertebrae. An unusual case of extraskeletal mesenchymal chondrosarcoma of the posterior mediastinum unassociated with bony structures has also been documented.[103] Extraosseous osteosarcomas have been described in the posterior mediastinum unassociated to regional bony structures,[104] and a rare case of extraskeletal osteosarcoma involving the anterior mediastinum arising from an ectopic hamartomatous thymus has been reported.[105]

Malignant Fibroblastic and Fibrohistiocytic Neoplasms

Fibrosarcomas of the mediastinum, although once thought to be quite common, are now vanishingly rare. The majority of the cases classified under this diagnosis in the past would probably be reclassified today under a variety of other designations. The most important diagnostic pitfall for these tumors is confusing them with benign solitary fibrous tumor of the mediastinum. It is likely that cases of mediastinal fibrosarcoma previously reported in association with hypoglycemia correspond to solitary fibrous tumors.[106, 107] Separation between the two may be impossible on a histological basis; attention to the gross features of the lesion are mandatory for adequate interpretation. The same caveat applies to tumors previously designated as **hemangiopericytomas** in mediastinal location. Some authors have regarded the term *fibrosarcoma* as synonymous with the malignant counterpart of solitary fibrous tumors.[108] Although the benign and malignant variants of the latter entity have been variously separated on the basis of cellularity, atypia, and increased mitotic activity, these may not represent reliable predictive criteria. Lesions exhibiting increased cellularity, atypia, and brisk mitotic activity but that are otherwise well-circumscribed, encapsulated, and attached by a pedicle may behave in a benign fashion.[88] Cases of **malignant fibrous histiocytoma (MFH)** have also been described in both anterior and posterior mediastinum.[109, 110] As with fibrosarcoma, the main differential diagnosis for these lesions is with solitary fibrous tumors, which may also exhibit focally a prominent storiform pattern with nuclear pleomorphism, atypia, and mitoses creating a picture that is virtually indistinguishable from MFH. Extensive sampling in search of some of the other features and growth patterns of solitary fibrous tumors and careful attention to the gross features of the lesion are necessary for correct diagnosis.

Other Sarcomas

Synovial sarcoma may also involve mediastinal tissues adjacent to the aorta or pulmonary hila.[111] These tumors grow as biphasic neoplasms similar to their soft tissue counterparts, with sheets of monotonous spindle cells admixed with glandular epithelial structures. We have seen two examples of **alveolar soft part sarcoma** arising as a primary in the mediastinum.

Metastatic Tumors

The mediastinum can be the repository of metastases from intrathoracic and extrathoracic primaries. Quite frequently, metastases to the mediastinum simulate clinically and radiographically a primary tumor. Lung cancer, for example (small-cell carcinoma in particular), often presents as a huge mediastinal mass owing to hilar lymph node metastasis from a small bronchial primary. Direct extension simulating clinically a mediastinal primary can also occur with tumors of the esophagus, pleura, chest wall, vertebra, or trachea. Other tumors that may metastasize to the mediastinum include carcinomas of the breast, thyroid, stomach, kidney, prostate, and testis; soft tissue sarcomas; and melanomas (Fig. 4–50).[112, 113] The main differential diagnosis for these lesions is with primary thymic carcinoma. Because of the great number of histologic variants of thymic carcinoma described, all such tumors presenting in the mediastinum must be tentatively regarded as metastatic until proved otherwise. A helpful hint for diagnosis is the type of lymphoid infiltrate surrounding the metastatic epithelial elements. Identification of a peripheral rim of lymph nodal tissue would favor a metastasis to hilar lymph nodes over a

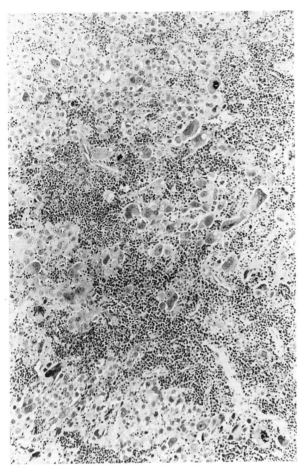

FIGURE 4–50. Metastatic large-cell undifferentiated carcinoma of the lung to mediastinal lymph nodes.

thymic primary. When normal lymph node landmarks are not available, immunohistochemical stains for lymphoid markers may help clarify the issue; predominant staining with B-cell markers identifies the tissue as lymph node over thymus, which is mainly composed of T lymphocytes.

UNCOMMON LESIONS OF THE MEDIASTINUM WORTH KNOWING ABOUT

Ectopias

Alterations of the normal embryologic development of the thymus may give rise to a series of congenital abnormalities. One of the anomalies most frequently encountered is the presence of **parathyroid gland** tissue within the thymus; such ectopic rests most often are found within the capsule of the thymus or in close proximity to it.[114] **Ectopic sebaceous glands** have also been reported in the thymus;[115] these are believed to be related to the contribution of the ectodermically derived cervical sinus to the developing thymus. Another developmental malformation that has been documented in the thymus is the presence of **ectopic salivary gland tissue.** It has been reported as a component of an intrathoracic cyst that contained within its walls normal thymus and parathyroid

tissue,[116] or incidentally found within the capsule of the normal thymus.[114]

Sclerosing Mediastinitis

Fibrosing inflammation of the mediastinum is often the sequela of infections by fungal organisms such as *Histoplasma, Aspergillus, Cryptococcus,* and *Mucor.*[117] In a large number of cases, a specific etiologic infectious agent cannot be identified in patients with chronic fibrosing mediastinitis. Such cases have been generally designated as idiopathic sclerosing mediastinitis. Histologically, the lesion consists of bundles of relatively acellular, hyalinized connective tissue admixed with inflammatory cells that often form lymphoid follicles and entrap nerve bundles at the periphery of the lesions. Special stains for organisms are invariably negative. The fibrous process usually extends beyond the confines of the mediastinal compartment and infiltrates adjacent structures, invading and encasing the walls of veins and bronchi. Sclerosing mediastinitis must be distinguished from several other fibrosing conditions affecting the mediastinum, such as Hodgkin's disease, large-cell lymphoma, thymic seminoma, and fibrosarcoma. Appropriate sampling in search of more distinctive features is indicated in such cases to rule out these alternative diagnoses.

Histiocytosis X

Langerhans cell granulomatosis may involve the mediastinum, especially in children.[118] The lesions show identical features to those of the same condition in other locations, i.e., a proliferation of cells with elongated, vesicular nuclei, prominent nuclear membrane convolutions, nuclear grooves, and small nucleoli, admixed with eosinophils. Positive stains for S-100 protein are useful in identifying the cells as Langerhans cells; demonstration of racquet- or zipper-shaped structures in the cytoplasm by electron microscopy may be confirmatory in equivocal cases.

Thymolipoma

It is not yet clear whether thymolipoma represents a true neoplasm, a hamartoma, or simply fatty replacement of a previously hyperplastic thymus. In any event, the term describes a large, well-circumscribed mass composed of mature fat admixed with normal thymic tissue.[119] These lesions are usually asymptomatic; however, a small percentage of patients may present with symptoms as a result of compression of regional structures or in association with Graves' disease, myasthenia gravis, red cell aplasia, and hypogammaglobulinemia. An unusual variant of this condition has been recently described by Moran et al.[120] that is characterized by a prominent fibrous component; such lesions have been designated **thymofibrolipoma.**

Thyroid Lesions Involving the Mediastinum

Thyroid tumors and tumor-like conditions can present as superior mediastinal masses. The most common of these is the so-called **substernal goiter,** in which a thyroid gland afflicted by nodular follicular hyperplasia grows down into the mediastinum and causes compression symptoms.[121] Rarely, **malignant thyroid neoplasms** may show the same phenomenon and present as apparent anterior superior mediastinal masses. Diagnostic problems may arise when invasion of superior mediastinal structures takes place by **poorly differentiated ("insular") carcinoma of the thyroid,** raising the possibility of thymic carcinoid or neuroendocrine carcinoma in the differential diagnosis (Fig. 4–51).

Parathyroid Tumors Involving the Mediastinum

Because of the common embryologic derivation of the thymus and the parathyroid glands, parathyroid rests often may be encountered in the region of the thymus. Such rests may occasionally give rise to neoplasms that recapitulate hyperplastic and neoplastic conditions of these glands in cervical locations. Because such lesions are usually relatively small, they generally come to the attention of the physician as a result of signs and symptoms of hyperparathyroidism. **Hyperplasia and adenomas** of parathyroid in the mediastinum present as well-circumscribed masses usually contained within the confines of the thymus. Parathyroid hyperplasia and adenoma may be indistinguishable morphologically and are generally

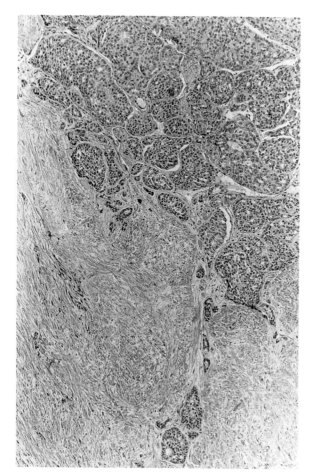

FIGURE 4–51. Poorly differentiated ("insular") carcinoma of the thyroid infiltrating anterosuperior mediastinum.

characterized by sheets, trabeculae, or islands of round to polygonal cells with bland nuclear features and evenly dispersed chromatin. Mitotic figures are generally scarce. Occasional examples may show bizarre nuclear features; however, this is of no prognostic significance in the absence of mitotic activity. Lesions having a higher content of intratumoral adipose tissue have been designated as lipoadenomas.[122] **Parathyroid carcinoma** may also rarely arise in the mediastinum.[123] Such lesions are generally characterized by more pronounced cellular pleomorphism, increased mitotic activity, trabecular growth pattern, and vascular and capsular infiltration. The differential diagnosis of mediastinal parathyroid lesions includes thymic carcinoid, paraganglioma, clear-cell thymic carcinoma, and seminoma. The most important discriminatory parameter for diagnosis is immunoreactivity for parathyroid hormone or demonstration of elevated serum levels of parathyroid hormone and hypercalcemia.

Other Unusual Conditions

Sinus histiocytosis with massive lymphadenopathy (SHML) has been shown to involve the mediastinum and may be accompanied by transient immunologic defects.[124] Attention to the distinctive features of this condition in extranodal sites, namely, a proliferation of S-100–positive histiocytes with striking emperiopolesis admixed with a prominent lymphoplasmactyic infiltrate, helps define the diagnosis. Mediastinal lymphadenopathy due to **infectious mononucleosis** has also been described.[125] Such cases could be mistakenly diagnosed as Hodgkin's disease or non-Hodgkin's lymphoma on small mediastinoscopic biopsies. A variety of unusual benign and malignant neoplasms have been occasionally reported as arising in the mediastinum, including **mediastinal myxoma,**[126] **oncocytoma,**[127] **meningioma,**[128] **salivary gland–type mixed tumor,**[129] **granular cell tumor,**[130] **melanotic progonoma of infancy,**[131] and **ependymoma.**[132]

References

1. Rosai J, Levine GD: Tumors of the thymus (Fascicle 13, 2nd Series). In Atlas of Tumor Pathology. Washington, DC, Armed Forces Institute of Pathology, 1976, pp 34–166.
2. Levine GD, Rosai J: Thymic hyperplasia and neoplasia: A review of current concepts. Hum Pathol 9:495–515, 1978.
3. Suster S, Rosai J: Cystic thymomas. A clinicopathologic study of 10 cases. Cancer 69:92–97, 1992.
4. Moran CA, Koss MN: Rhabdomyomatous thymoma. Am J Surg Pathol 17:633–636, 1993.
5. Moran CA, Suster S, Koss MN: Plasma cell-rich thymoma. Am J Clin Pathol 102:199–201, 1994.
6. Wick MR, Scheithauer BW, Weiland LH, Barnaz PE: Primary thymic carcinomas. Am J Surg Pathol 6:613–630, 1982.
7. Suster S, Rosai J: Thymic carcinoma. A clinicopathologic study of 60 cases. Cancer 67:1025–1032, 1991.
8. Snover DC, Levine GD, Rosai J: Thymic carcinoma: Five distinctive histologic variants. Am J Surg Pathol 6:451–470, 1982.
9. Kuo T-T, Chang J-P, Lin F-J, et al: Thymic carcinomas: Histopathologic varieties and immunohistochemical study. Am J Surg Pathol 14:24–34, 1990.
10. Shimosato Y, Kameya T, Nagai K, Suemasu K: Squamous cell carcinoma of the thymus: An analysis of eight cases. Am J Surg Pathol 1:109–121, 1977.
11. Kuo T-T: Clear cell carcinoma of the skin. A variant of squamous cell carcinoma that simulates sebaceous carcinoma. Am J Surg Pathol 4:573–583, 1980.
12. Katzenstein AL-L, Prioleau PG, Askin FB: The histologic spectrum and significance of clear cell change in lung carcinoma. Cancer 45:943–947, 1980.
13. Gould E, Albores-Saavedra J, Dubner B, et al: Eccrine and squamous differentiation in Merkel cell carcinoma. Am J Surg Pathol 12:768–772, 1988.
14. Burke WA, Burford TH, Dorfman RF: Hodgkin's disease in the mediastinum. J Thorac Cardiovasc Surg 3:287–296, 1967.

15. Keller AR, Castleman B: Hodgkin's disease of the thymus gland. Cancer 33:1615–1623, 1974.

16. Rosai J: The pathology of thymic neoplasia. In Berard CW, Dorfman RF, Kaufman N (eds): Malignant Lymphoma (Monograph No. 29). Baltimore, Williams & Wilkins, 1987, pp 161–183.

17. Chittal SM, Cavariviere P, Schwarting R, et al: Monoclonal antibodies in the diagnosis of Hodgkin's disease. The search for a rational panel. Am J Surg Pathol 12:9–21, 1988.

18. Dorfman RF, Gatter KC, Pulford KAF, Mason DY: An evaluation of the utility of anti-granulocyte and anti-leukocyte monoclonal antibodies in the diagnosis of Hodgkin's disease. Am J Pathol 123:508–509, 1986.

19. Agnarsson BA, Kadin ME: Ki-1 positive large cell lymphoma. A morphologic and immunologic study of 19 cases. Am J Surg Pathol 12:264–274, 1988.

20. Miettinen M: CD30 distribution. Immunohistochemical study on formaldehyde-fixed, paraffin-embedded Hodgkin's and non-Hodgkin's lymphomas. Arch Pathol Lab Med 116:1197–1201, 1992.

21. Frizzera G: The distinction of Hodgkin's disease from anaplastic large cell lymphoma. Semin Diagn Pathol 9:291–296, 1992.

22. Strickler JG, Michie SA, Warnke RA, Dorfman RF: The ''syncytial variant'' of nodular sclerosing Hodgkin's disease. Am J Surg Pathol 10:470–477, 1986.

23. Toker C: Tumors: An Atlas of Differential Diagnosis. Baltimore, University Park Press, 1983, pp 278–279.

24. Suster S: Transformation of Hodgkin's disease into malignant fibrous histiocytoma. Cancer 57:264–268, 1986,

25. Kin HC, Nosher J, Haas A, et al: Cystic degeneration of thymic Hodgkin's disease following radiation therapy. Cancer 55:354–356, 1985.

26. Lichtenstein AK, Levine A, Taylor CT, et al: Primary mediastinal lymphoma in adults. Am J Med 68:509–514, 1980.

27. Levitt LJ, Aisenberg AC, Harris NH, et al: Primary non-Hodgkin's lymphoma of the mediastinum. Cancer 50:2486–2492, 1982.

28. Nathwani BN, Kim H, Rappaport H: Malignant lymphoma, lymphoblastic. Cancer 38:964–983, 1976.

29. Lamarre L, Jacobson JO, Aisenberg AC, Harris NL: Primary large cell lymphoma of the mediastinum. A histologic and immunophenotypic study of 29 cases. Am J Surg Pathol 13:730–739, 1989.

30. Waldron JA Jr, Dohring EJ, Farber LR: Primary large cell lymphoma of the mediastinum. An analysis of 20 cases. Semin Diagn Pathol 2:281–295, 1985.

31. Perrone T, Frizerra G, Rosai J: Mediastinal diffuse large cell lymphoma with sclerosis. A clinicopathologic study of 60 cases. Am J Surg Pathol 10:176–191, 1986.

32. Menestrina F, Chilosi M, Bonnetti F, et al: Mediastinal large cell lymphoma of B-type, with sclerosis. Histopathological and immunohistochemical study of eight cases. Histopathology 10:589–600, 1986.

33. Moller P, Lammler B, Eberlein-Gonska M, et al: Primary mediastinal clear cell lymphoma of B-cell type. Virchows Arch A [Anat Pathol] 409:79–92, 1986.

34. Suster S: Large cell lymphoma of the mediastinum with marked tropism for germinal centers. Cancer 69:2910–2916, 1992.

35. Jenkins PF, Ward MJ, Davies P, et al: Non-Hodgkin's lymphoma, chronic lymphatic leukemia and the lung. Br J Dis Chest 75:22–30, 1981.

36. Isaacson PG, Chan JKC, Tang C, Addis BJ: Low-grade B-cell lymphoma of mucosa-associated lymphoid tissue arising in the thymus. A thymic lymphoma mimicking myoepithelial sialadenitis. Am J Surg Pathol 14:342–351, 1990.

37. Streuli RA, Kaneko Y, Variakojis D, et al: Lymphoblastic lymphoma in adults. Cancer 47:2510–2516, 1981.

38. Braziel, RM, Keneklis T, Donlon JA, et al: Terminal deoxynucleotidyl transferase in non-Hodgkin's lymphomas. Am J Clin Pathol 80:655–659, 1983.

39. Toback A, Hasbrouck DJ, Blaustein J, Ershier WB: Granulocytic sarcoma of the anterior mediastinum. Am J Med Sci 290:206–208, 1985.

40. Neiman RS, Barcos M, Berard C, et al: Granulocytic sarcoma. A clinicopathologic study of 61 biopsied cases. Cancer 48:1426–1437, 1981.

41. Niwa K, Tanaka T, Mori H, et al: Extramedullary plasmacytoma of the mediastinum. Jpn J Clin Oncol 17:95–100, 1987.

42. Keller AR, Hochholzer L, Castleman B: Hyaline-vascular and plasma-cell types of giant lymph node hyperplasia of mediastinum and other locations. Cancer 29:670–683, 1972.

43. Castleman B: The pathology of the thymus gland in myasthenia gravis. Ann N Y Acad Sci 135:496–503, 1966.

44. Trotter JL, Ferguson TP, Garvey WF: Studies on the thymus from patients with multiple sclerosis and myasthenia gravis. J Neuroimmunol 3:99–111, 1982.

45. Goldstein G, Mackey IR: Contrasting abnormalities in the thymus in systemic lupus erythematosus and myasthenia gravis: A quantitative histologic study. Aust J Exp Biol Med Sci 43:381–390, 1965.

46. Verani R, Olson J, Moake JL: Intrathoracic extramedullary hematopoiesis. Report of a case in a patient with sickle-cell disease–beta-thalassemia. Am J Clin Pathol 73:133–138, 1980.

47. Rosai J, Higa E: Mediastinal endocrine neoplasms of probable thymic origin, related to carcinoid tumor: Clinicopathologic study of eight cases. Cancer 29:1061–1074, 1972.

48. Wick MR, Rosai J: Neuroendocrine neoplasms of the mediastinum. Semin Diagn Pathol 8:35–51, 1991.

49. Wick MR, Carney JA, Bernatz PE, Brown LR: Primary mediastinal carcinoid tumors. Am J Surg Pathol 6:195–205, 1982.

50. Levine GD, Rosai J: A spindle cell variant of thymic carcinoid tumor. A clinical, histologic, and fine structural study with emphasis on its distinction from spindle cell thymoma. Arch Pathol 100:293–300, 1976.

51. Ho FCS, Ho JCI: Pigmented carcinoid tumor of the thymus. Histopathology 1:363–369, 1977.

52. Rosai J, Levine G, Weber WR, Higa E: Carcinoid tumors and oat-cell carcinomas of the thymus. Pathol Annu 2:201–226, 1976.

53. Wick MR, Simpson RW, Niehans GA, et al: Anterior mediastinal tumors: A clinicopathologic study of 100 cases, with emphasis on immunohistochemical analysis. Prog Surg Pathol 11:79–119, 1990.

54. Herbst WM, Kummer W, Hofmann W, et al: Carcinoid tumors of the thymus: An immunohistochemical study. Cancer 60:2465–2470, 1987.

55. Olson JL, Salyer WR: Mediastinal paraganglioma (aortic body tumor): A report of four cases and a review of the literature. Cancer 41:2405–2412, 1978.

56. Moran CA, Suster S, Fishback N, Koss MN: Mediastinal paragangliomas. A clinicopathologic and immunohistochemical study of 16 cases. Cancer 72:2358–2364, 1993.

57. Achilles E, Padberg BC, Holl K, et al: Immunohistochemistry of paragangliomas—value of staining for S-100 protein and glial fibrillary acidic protein in diagnosis and prognosis. Histopathology 18:453–458, 1991.

58. Burns BF, McCaughey WTE: Unusual thymic seminomas. Arch Pathol Lab Med 110:539–541, 1986.

59. Beckstead JH: Alkaline phosphatase histochemistry in human germ cell neoplasms. Am J Surg Pathol 7:341–349, 1983.

60. Levine GD: Primary thymic seminoma. A neoplasm ultrastructurally similar to testicular seminoma and distinct from epithelial thymoma. Cancer 31:729–741, 1973.

61. Hurt RD, Bruckman JE, Farrow GM, et al: Primary anterior mediastinal seminoma. Cancer 49:1658–1663, 1982.

62. Manivel C, Wick MR, Abenoza P, Rosai J: The occurrence of sarcomatous components in primary mediastinal germ cell tumors. Am J Surg Pathol 10:711–717, 1986.

63. Ulbright TM, Loehrer PJ, Roth LM, et al: The development of non-germ cell malignancies within germ cell tumors. A clinicopathologic study of 11 cases. Cancer 54:1824–1833, 1984.

64. Davidson KG, Walbaum PR, McKormack RJM: Intrathoracic neural tumors. Thorax 33:359–367, 1978.

65. Oberman HA, Abell MR: Neurogenous neoplasms of the mediastinum. Cancer 13:882–898, 1960.

66. Carney JA: Psammomatous melanotic schwannoma. A distinctive, heritable tumor with special associations, including cardiac myxoma and the Cushing syndrome. Am J Surg Pathol 14:206–222, 1990.

67. Ducataman BS, Scheithauer BW, Piepgras DG, et al: Malignant peripheral nerve sheath tumors. A clinicopathologic study of 120 cases. Cancer 57:2006–2021, 1986.

68. Woodruff JM, Chernick NL, Smith NC, et al: Peripheral nerve tumors with rhabdomyosarcomatous differentiation (malignant ''triton'' tumors). Cancer 32:426–439, 1973.

69. Ducataman BS, Scheithauer BW: Malignant peripheral nerve sheath tumors with divergent differentiation. Cancer 54:1049–1057, 1984.

70. Fisher C: The value of electronmicroscopy and immunohistochemistry in the diagnosis of soft tissue sarcomas: A study of 200 cases. Histopathology 16:441–454, 1990.

71. Weiss SW, Langloss JM, Enzinger FM: The role of S-100 protein in the diagnosis of soft tissue tumors with particular reference to benign and malignant Schwann cell tumors. Lab Invest 49:299–305, 1983.

72. Erlandson RA, Woodruff JM: Peripheral nerve sheath tumors: An electron microscopic study of 43 cases. Cancer 49:273–287, 1982.

73. de Lorimier AA, Bragg KU, Linden G: Neuroblastoma in childhood. Am J Dis Child 118:441–450, 1969.

74. Ricci C, Pescamona E, Rendina EA, et al: True thymic hyperplasia: A clinicopathological study. Ann Thorac Surg 47:741–745, 1989.

75. Shin MS, Ho KT: Diffuse thymic hyperplasia following chemotherapy for nodular sclerosis Hodgkin's disease. Cancer 57:30–33, 1983.

76. Due W, Dieckman K-P, Stein H: Thymic hyperplasia following chemotherapy for a testicular germ cell tumor. Immunohistochemical evidence for a simple rebound phenomenon. Cancer 63:446–449, 1989.

77. Gelfland DW, Goldman AS, Law AJ: Thymic hyperplasia in children recovering from thermal burns. J Trauma 12:813–817, 1972.

78. Caffey J, Sibley R: Regrowth and overgrowth of the thymus after atrophy induced by oral administration of corticosteroids to human infants. Pediatrics 26:762–770, 1960.

79. Smith SM, Ossa-Gomez LJ: A quantitative histologic comparison of the thymus in 100 healthy and diseased adults. Am J Clin Pathol 76:657–665, 1981.

80. Selye H: Thymus and adrenals in the response of the organism to injuries and intoxication. Br J Exp Pathol 17:234–248, 1936.

81. Seemayer TA, Laroche AC, Russo P, et al: Precocious thymic involution manifest by epithelial injury in the acquired immune deficiency syndrome. Hum Pathol 15:469–474, 1984.

82. Grody VW, Fligliel S, Naeim F: Thymus involution in the acquired immune deficiency syndrome. Am J Clin Pathol 84:85–96, 1985.

83. Silverman NA, Sabiston DC Jr: Primary tumors and cysts of the mediastinum. Curr Probl Cancer 2:1–55, 1977.

84. Chuang MT, Barba FA, Kaneko M, Teirstein AS: Adenocarcinoma arising in an intrathoracic duplication cyst of foregut origin. A case report with review of the literature. Cancer 47:1887–1890, 1981.

85. Suster S, Rosai J: Multilocular thymic cyst: An acquired reactive process. Study of 18 cases. Am J Surg Pathol 15:388–398, 1991.

86. Suster S, Barbuto D, Carlson D, Rosai J: Multilocular thymic cysts with pseudoepitheliomatous hyperplasia. Hum Pathol 22:455–460, 1991.

87. Witkin GB, Rosai J: Solitary fibrous tumor of the mediastinum. A report of 14 cases. Am J Surg Pathol 13:547–557, 1989.

88. Moran CA, Suster S, Koss MN: The spectrum of histologic growth patterns in benign and malignant fibrous tumors of the pleura. Semin Diagn Pathol 9:169–180, 1992.

89. Swanson PE: Soft tissue neoplasms of the mediastinum. Semin Diagn Pathol 8:14–34, 1991.

90. Awotwi JD, Zusman J, Waring WW, Beckerman RC: Benign hemangioendothelioma—a rare type of posterior mediastinal mass in children. J Pediatr Surg 18:581–584, 1983.

91. Baron RL, Sagel SS, Baglan RJ: Thymic cysts following radiation therapy for Hodgkin's disease. Radiology 141:593–597, 1981.

92. Kim HC, Nosher J, Haas A, et al: Cystic degeneration of thymic Hodgkin's disease following radiation therapy. Cancer 55:354–356, 1985.

93. Suster S, Moran CA, Koss MN: Epithelioid hemangioendothelioma of the anterior mediastinum. Clinicopathologic, immunohistochemical and ultrastructural study of 12 cases. Am J Surg Pathol 18:871–881, 1994.

94. Lamovec J, Sobel HJ, Zidar A, Jermon J: Epithelioid hemangioendothelioma of the anterior mediastinum with osteoclast-like giant cells. Light microscopic, immunohistochemical, and electron microscopic study. Am J Clin Pathol 93:813–817, 1990.

95. Weidner N: Atypical tumor of the mediastinum: Epithelioid hemangioendothelioma containing metaplastic bone and osteoclast-type giant cells. Ultrastruct Pathol 15:481–488, 1991.

96. Havlicek F, Rosai J: A sarcoma of thymic stroma with features of liposarcoma. Am J Clin Pathol 82:217–224, 1984.

97. Griff LE, Cooper J: Leiomyosarcoma of the esophagus presenting as a mediastinal mass. AJR 101:472–481, 1967.

98. Davis GL, Bergmann M, O'Jane H: Leiomyosarcoma of the superior vena cava. A first case with resection. J Thorac Cardiovasc Surg 72:408–412, 1976.

99. Moran CA, Suster S, Perino G, et al: Malignant smooth muscle neoplasms presenting as mediastinal soft tissue masses. A clinicopathologic study of 10 cases. Cancer 74:2251–2260, 1994.

100. Crist WM, Raney RB, Newton W, et al: Intrathoracic soft tissue sarcomas in children. Cancer 50:598–604, 1982.

101. Wick MR, Swanson PE, Manivel JC: Immunohistochemical analysis of soft tissue sarcomas. Comparison with electron microscopy. Appl Pathol 6:169–196, 1980.

102. Suster S, Moran CA, Koss MN: Primary rhabdomyosarcomas of the anterior mediastinum. Report of 4 cases unassociated with germ cell, teratomatous or thymic carcinomatous components. Hum Pathol 25:349–356, 1994.

103. Chelty R: Extraskeletal mesenchymal chondrosarcoma of the mediastinum. Histopathology 17:261–278, 1990.

104. Greenwood SM, Meschter SC: Extraskeletal osteogenic sarcoma of the mediastinum. Arch Pathol Lab Med 113:430–433, 1989.

105. Valderrama E, Kahn LB, Wind E: Extraskeletal osteosarcoma arising in an ectopic hamartomatous thymus. Report of a case and review of the literature. Cancer 51:1132–1137, 1983.

106. Baldwyn RS: Hypoglycemia associated with fibrosarcoma of the mediastinum. Ann Surg 160:975–977, 1964.

107. Walsh CH, Wright AD, Coore HG: Hypoglycemia associated with an intrathoracic fibrosarcoma. Clin Endocrinol 4:393–398, 1975.

108. Carter D, Otis CN: Three types of spindle cell tumor of the pleura: Fibroma, sarcoma and sarcomatoid mesothelioma. Am J Surg Pathol 12:747–753, 1988.

109. Mills SA, Breyer RH, Johnston FR, et al: Malignant fibrous histiocytoma of the mediastinum and lung. A report of three cases. J Thorac Cardiovasc Surg 84:367–372, 1982.

110. Morshius WJ, Cox AL, Lacquet LK, et al: Primary malignant fibrous histiocytoma of the mediastinum. Thorax 45:154–155, 1990.

111. Witkin GB, Miettinen M, Rosai J: A biphasic tumor of the mediastinum with features of synovial sarcoma. A report of four cases. Am J Surg Pathol 13:490–499, 1989.

112. Lindell MM, Doubleday LC, Von Eschenbach AC, Libshitz HI: Mediastinal metastases from prostatic carcinoma. J Urol 128:331–334, 1982.

113. McCloud TC, Kalisher L, Stark P, Green R: Intrathoracic lymph node metastases from extrathoracic neoplasms. AJR 131:403–407, 1978.

114. Suster S, Rosai J: Histology of the normal thymus. Am J Surg Pathol 14:284–303, 1990.

115. Woolf M, Rosai J, Wright DH: Sebaceous glands within the thymus: Report of three cases. Hum Pathol 15:341–343, 1984.

116. Becklet IA, Johnston DG: Choristoma of the thymus. Am J Dis Child 92:175–178, 1956.

117. Schowengerdt CG, Suyemoto R, Main FB: Granulomatous and fibrous mediastinitis. A review and analysis of 180 cases. J Thorac Cardiovasc Surg 57:365–379, 1969.

118. Siegal GP, Dehner LP, Rosai J: Histiocytosis X (Langerhans' cell granulomatosis) of the thymus. A clinicopathologic study of four childhood cases. Am J Surg Pathol 9:117–124, 1985.

119. Otto HF, Loning TH, Lachenmayer L, et al: Thymolipoma in association with myasthenia gravis. Cancer 50:1623–1628, 1982.

120. Moran CA, Zeren H, Koss MN: Thymofibrolipoma. A histologic variant of thymolipoma. Arch Pathol Lab Med 118:281–282, 1994.

121. Katlic MR, Wang C, Grillo HC: Substernal goiter. Ann Thorac Surg 39:391–399, 1985.

122. Woolf M, Goodman EN: Functioning lipoadenoma of a supernumerary parathyroid gland in the mediastinum. Head Neck Surg 2:302–307, 1980.

123. Murphy MN, Glennon PG, Diocee MS, et al: Nonsecretory parathyroid carcinoma of the mediastinum. Cancer 58:2468–2476, 1986.

124. Becroft DMO, Dix MR, Gillman JC, et al: Benign sinus histiocytosis with massive lymphadenopathy. Transient immunological defects in a child with mediastinal involvement. J Clin Pathol 26:463–469, 1973.

125. Rosenthal T, Hertz M: Mediastinal lymphadenopathy in infectious mononucleosis. Report of two cases. JAMA 233:1300–1301, 1975.

126. Jaituni S, Arkee MSK, Caterine JM: Mediastinal myxoma. A case report. J Iowa Med Soc 64:107–110, 1974.

127. Meijer S, Hoitsma HFW: Malignant intrathoracic oncocytoma. Cancer 49:97–100, 1982.

128. Wilson AJ, Ratliff JL, Lagios MD, Agullar MJ: Mediastinal meningioma. Am J Surg Pathol 3:557–562, 1979.

129. Feigin GA, Robinson B, Marchevsky A: Mixed tumor of the mediastinum. Arch Pathol Lab Med 110:80–81, 1984.

130. Robinson JM, Knoll R, Henry DA: Intrathoracic granular cell myoblastoma of the posterior mediastinum. South Med J 81:1453–1457, 1988.

131. Misugi K, Okajima H, Newton WA, et al: Mediastinal origin of a melanotic progonoma or retinal anlage tumor. Ultrastructural evidence for neural crest origin. Cancer 18:477–484, 1965.

132. Doglioni C, Bontempini L, Iuzzolino P, et al: Ependymoma of the mediastinum. Arch Pathol Lab Med 112:194–196, 1988.

CHAPTER 5

The Esophagus and Stomach

Kenneth P. Batts, M.D., and Kenneth W. Barwick, M.D.

ESOPHAGUS

Most clinically significant tumors of the esophagus are malignant, with **squamous cell carcinomas** being the most common; however, the frequency of adenocarcinomas, most of which are associated with Barrett's esophagus, appears to be increasing. When compared with the rest of the gastrointestinal tract, benign neoplasms of the esophagus are relatively unusual. They also tend to be small and rarely cause symptoms.[1] This discussion of uncommon esophageal neoplasms excludes "usual" squamous cell carcinomas and adenocarcinomas. Epithelial neoplasia is discussed first, followed by mesenchymal and melanocytic neoplasia.

Epithelial Neoplasia

Benign Epithelial Neoplasms (Squamous Papilloma)

The only benign squamous neoplasm is the rare **squamous papilloma.** A literature review in 1980 noted only 17 cases; the authors reported an additional three cases found in 6157 endoscopic procedures.[2] Nearly all squamous papillomas of the esophagus have been incidental findings at autopsy or during endoscopy. Grossly, papillomas are sessile lesions with papillary projections above the mucosal surface that typically range in size from several millimeters to 2 cm,[3, 4] although polyps as large as 5 to 6 cm have been reported.[5] The lesions are usually single, although approximately 30% have been multiple, and usually occur in the distal third of the esophagus.[2] Microscopically, the lesions are composed of variably hyperplastic, benign-appearing, digitiform squamous epithelial structures with relatively thin central fibrovascular stalks that connect with the lamina propria (Fig. 5–1).

Most squamous papillomas in adults are likely the result of chronic irritation, given the usual distal location and frequency of hiatal hernias and other conditions that favor reflux.[2–4] Papillomas of the distal esophagus have not been associated with malignant change.[3, 6] There are very rare case reports of viral-associated esophageal papillomas. Multiple esophageal papillomas have occurred in a girl with **hypopharyngeal papillomatosis**[7] and in a boy whose mother had vulvar condylomata at the time of his birth.[8] Furthermore, **human papillomavirus** (HPV) has been demonstrated in rare cases.[9] Thus, there is a theoretical basis for distinguishing between distal papillomas in a reflux-prone adult and those occurring in the setting of HPV ("squamous papillomas with viral features").

Adenomas

Benign gastric epithelium in the esophagus is best classified as heterotopic if present in the proximal esophagus and discontinuous from the stomach and as metaplastic (Barrett's) if present in contiguity with the stomach mucosa. The only examples of "true" adenomas have occurred in the background of Barrett's esophagus[10] and are thus better designated as "polypoid dysplasia" in Barrett's esophagus.

Malignant Epithelial Neoplasms

Spindling Squamous Cell Carcinoma

A rare, typically polypoid malignancy of the esophagus composed of a mixture of squamous cell carcinoma and a spindle cell component has gone by a confusing variety of names such as **sarcomatoid carcinoma,**[11] **carcinosarcoma,**[12, 13] **esophageal carcinoma with prominent spindle cells,**[14] **spindle cell squamous carcinoma of the esophagus,**[15] **and polypoid squamous carcinoma.**[16, 17] The majority of reports of this entity consist of single case reports or very small series and nearly all address the concept of pathogenesis. The major issue concerns whether the spindling component is truly a sarcoma (justifying "carcinosarcoma"), a spindling "metaplastic" form of squamous carcinoma ("sarcomatoid" or "spindling squamous cell carcinoma"), or atypical reactive stromal metaplasia ("pseudosarcoma").[18] Because these neoplasms are usually polypoid, the unifying term **polypoid carcinoma** has been proposed.[17]

We prefer the use of the term **spindling squamous cell carcinoma or carcinoma with stromal (spindle cell) metaplasia,** which would seem to be more appropriate than "carcinosarcoma" for most lesions. A number of immunohistochemical[14, 16, 19] and ultrastructural[20, 21] studies have shown that the spindled, sarcomatoid component likely represents mesenchymal metaplasia of squamous carcinoma. Certainly, the metaplasia may be so complete that no vestiges of carcinoma remain, and malignant bone and cartilage may be present.[19] Polypoid carcinoma is a less desirable term because most but not all polypoid squamous carcinomas have spindling elements and only 75% of carcinosarcomas are elevated.[97]

Patients with spindling squamous cell carcinomas usually present with dysphagia.[12] Lesions are frequently polypoid

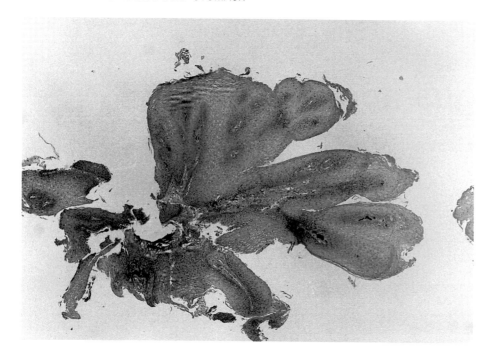

FIGURE 5–1. Squamous papilloma of the esophagus, biopsy specimen. Cytologically bland squamous epithelium with central connective tissue cores form finger-like extensions that appear warty grossly. (H&E, ×45)

(75%) but may be ulcerated. They range in size from 2 to 15 cm, and most (70%) occur in the middle third of the esophagus.[12] Microscopically, the stromal component frequently predominates, being characterized by variably anaplastic spindled cells that may contain areas of bizarre anaplasia. The squamous cell carcinoma is usually typical in appearance and may contain an extensive *in situ* component; adenocarcinoma elements may be seen in some cases (Fig. 5–2). Metastases may reflect either the squamous cell or "sarcomatoid" component.

Survival appears to be dependent on depth of invasion. Appelman noted that only one of nine lesions limited to the mucosa had metastasized, versus 17 of 20 cases with submucosal or deeper invasion.[22] Size is likely also important as tumors 8 cm or larger always metastasized, versus about 40% of those less than 8 cm.[23] Although the early prognosis for spindle cell carcinoma seems to be somewhat better than squamous cell carcinoma (63% versus 28% 3-year survival), by 5 years survival rates are similar for the two groups (27% versus 22%).[12] It has been suggested that this may reflect the tendency for spindle cell carcinoma to show a lesser degree of invasion, leading to high resectability rate, but later tendency for hematogenous metastasis.

It remains debatable whether **"pseudosarcoma"** should be distinguished from spindling squamous cell carcinoma. Although both are polypoid, it has been suggested that "pseudosarcoma" can be distinguished from spindling squamous cell carcinoma by virtue of the fact that the former contains a "reactive," bland-appearing stroma that does not metastasize.[1] In practice, this seems to be difficult,[17, 24] and we agree with others that the term *pseudosarcoma* of the esophagus should be avoided.[1]

Verrucous Squamous Cell Carcinoma

In the original description of esophageal verrucous squamous cell carcinoma by Minielly et al., the authors were able to identify only five cases among Mayo Clinic patients from 1906 through 1967.[25] In a 1991 review by Biemond et al., only an additional seven cases have been reported.[26] Clinically, long delays from the time of first symptoms to final diagnosis are common, the median age is 61 (range, 36–76), and males outnumber females 7 to 4.[26] Risk factors for verrucous squamous cell carcinoma are similar to those of "usual" squamous cancer, namely smoking, heavy alcohol use, achalasia, and strictures associated with acid or lye ingestion.

Verrucous squamous cell carcinomas of the esophagus are grossly and microscopically similar to those seen in other organs. Grossly, they form large, soft warty growths that may deeply infiltrate adjacent tissues but rarely show metastases. Microscopically, the surface is deceptively bland and well differentiated; hyperkeratotic squamous epithelium is present in a papillary growth pattern. Invasion occurs by means of broad, pushing fronts rather than slender tongues or single cells (Fig. 5–3). Thus, the diagnosis of malignancy may be difficult to establish histologically, particularly with small, superficial biopsies.

Similar to verrucous carcinoma in other organ sites, nodal metastases are exceptional and deaths were due to local strictures, fistulae, aspiration pneumonia, and anastomotic dehiscence. Only 3 of 11 patients were felt to be cured of disease, all by surgical resection.[26]

Paget's Disease

Rare case reports of squamous cell carcinoma of esophagus with features of Paget's disease have been reported.[27, 28] Lateral "pagetoid" spread may be noted at some distance from the primary neoplasm. One study failed to demonstrate convincing Paget's disease in 100 control esophageal adenocarcinomas.[27]

Small-Cell Carcinoma

Small-cell carcinoma of the esophagus is a rare neoplasm that constitutes approximately 0.8% to 2.4% of all esophageal

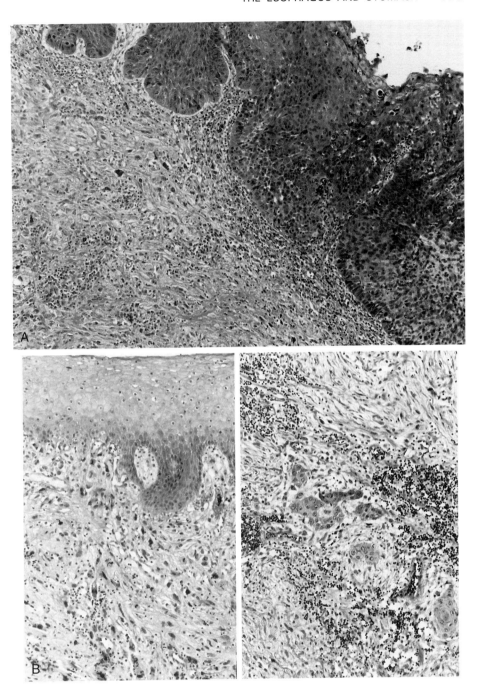

FIGURE 5–2. Spindle cell carcinoma, resection. *A,* Squamous cell carcinoma *in situ* overlies a malignant spindle cell process. *B,* Additional sampling shows areas where only the sarcomatous elements are evident *(left),* whereas in other sections an invasive squamous cell carcinoma can be seen admixed with the spindling elements *(right).* (H&E, ×125)

malignancies.[29, 30] As of 1991, a total of 134 cases have been reported;[29] the topic remains popular, as a number of other reports have also reviewed the existing literature.[31–35] Most small-cell carcinomas resemble **oat cell carcinoma of the lung** morphologically, ultrastructurally, and immunohistochemically; however, approximately 25% are "mixed," showing squamous (19%) or, less likely, adenocarcinoma elements or carcinoid tumor elements.[29] Thus, it would appear that the majority of small-cell carcinomas arise from normal argyrophil cells that have been identified in the basal layer of the esophageal mucosa in 28% of normal necropsies,[36] whereas a minority represent "small-cell" squamous cell carcinomas or adenocarcinomas. The term *non–oat cell small-cell carcinoma* has been used for oat cell–like carcinomas in which neurosecretory granules cannot be identified.[37]

One can distinguish "pure" oat cell carcinoma from mixed forms through careful sampling to exclude squamous or adenocarcinoma elements, presence of nuclear molding, the absence of prominent nucleoli, and (ideally) positive histochemical, immunohistochemical, or ultrastructural evidence of neuroendocrine derivation. Clinically, however, there appears to be no clinical difference between oat cell and non–oat cell types,[1] and the two are discussed together here.

Clinically, patients with esophageal small-cell carcinoma range in age from 29 to 88 years, with a mean of 64 years; males outnumber females 2 : 1.[29] Dysphagia is the most common presenting symptom (78%), although anorexia and weight loss are also commonly noted (42%).[29] **Ectopic hormone production** is present in 10% of cases; adrenocorticotropic hormone is the most common, but calcitonin, somato-

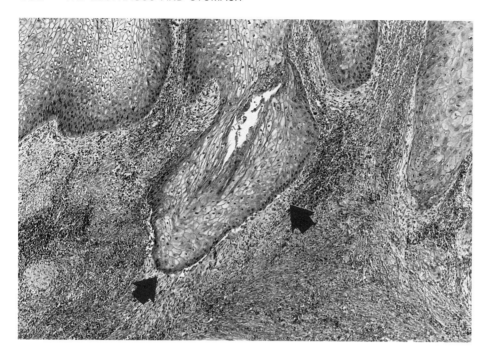

FIGURE 5-3. Verrucous squamous cell carcinoma. Cytologically bland squamous epithelium infiltrates the underlying stroma by a broad, pushing front *(arrows)*. This invasion may be extremely difficult to appreciate in a biopsy specimen. (H&E, ×80)

statin, antidiuretic hormone, and vasoactive intestinal peptide also have been reported.

Most tumors are located in the middle and lower esophagus and present as friable exophytic masses with frequent ulceration; they are rarely pedunculated. Tumors range from 1 to 14 cm, with a mean of 5.8 cm. Metastases are present in 70% at the time of initial diagnosis; paraesophageal and mediastinal nodes are most commonly involved (85%), with supraclavicular (28%) and abdominal nodes (26%) less common.[29] Visceral and musculoskeletal metastases are not uncommon, the liver being the most common extranodal site of metastasis (48% of cases).[29]

Survival is very poor, with a mean of 5.3 months and 6-month and 1-year survival rates of 37% and 10%, respectively.[29] There have been some partial responses[23, 38] and occasionally long-term remission[39] with chemotherapy and radiotherapy. Interestingly, serum neuron-specific enolase has been used as a serum marker for remission or relapse in small-cell carcinoma of the esophagus.[40]

Carcinoid Tumors

Very few case reports of esophageal carcinoid tumors exist. Inasmuch as some oat cell carcinomas have been shown to have areas resembling carcinoid tumors and atypical carcinoid tumors, it would seem reasonable that these tumors represent a spectrum of **neuroendocrine neoplasia.** It is not clear why reports of esophageal oat cell carcinomas outnumber those of carcinoids at least 20 to 1, although some carcinoid tumors may be included in series of ''oat cell'' tumors. Tumors have ranged in size from 2 to 12 cm,[41, 42] and aggressive behavior with nodal[42,43] and widespread[43] metastases has been noted. An interesting variant is a mucin-producing carcinoid of the proximal esophagus that resembles glandular carcinoids of the midgut.[41]

Choriocarcinoma

Choriocarcinoma of the esophagus is a very rare neoplasm; we are aware of only five case reports in the English literature.[44–48] There have been three males and two females, their ages being 40, 42, 44, 49, and 74. The tumors were generally large and friable and located in the mid[49] and low[50] esophagus and associated with widespread metastases. The tumors were uniformly fatal. These tumors all morphologically resemble typical choriocarcinoma with cytotrophoblastic and syncytiotrophoblastic elements. The two cases in which serum and/or urine studies were performed showed elevated human chorionic gonadotropin (hCG),[45, 48] and the single case analyzed immunohistochemically showed positivity with anti-hCG and anti-human placental lactogen (HPL).[44] One case also contained an adenocarcinoma component.[45] The diagnosis of esophageal choriocarcinoma requires the presence of cyto- and syncytiotrophoblastic elements, because hCG immunoreactive cells have been found in 21% of esophageal squamous cell carcinomas, a frequency comparable to that seen in gastric and colonic adenocarcinomas.[51] Furthermore, the presence of serum hCG is not diagnostic of choriocarcinoma, as one study showed that 44% of gastrointestinal carcinoma patients have elevated serum hCG levels.[52]

Adenoid Cystic Carcinoma

Adenoid cystic carcinoma is an uncommon esophageal tumor, at least 54 cases having been reported in the English literature as of 1992.[53–55] In a 1986 review of 44 cases, it was noted that the mean age of patients was 65 years and the male:female ratio was 3.4 : 1.[56] Among well-documented cases, 19 of 25 had metastasized at the time of diagnosis, and only 8 of 44 patients (23%) survived more than 1 year.[56] Most tumors are present in the middle and lower esophagus, and fungating lesions are very common, followed by ulcerative and infiltrative type of growth.[57] Small, asymptomatic tumors are uncommon.[53]

Histologically, the tumors resemble their salivary gland counterparts, with a mixture of epithelial cells, myoepithelial cells, and basement membrane.[58] There seems to be a greater tendency for esophageal tumors to have solid or basaloid areas, greater pleomorphism, necrosis, and higher mitotic activity.[3, 59] Some neoplasms are associated with adjacent squamous cell carcinoma *in situ*.[57] The preponderance of evidence suggests that esophageal adenoid cystic carcinomas arise from the intercalated ducts of the submucosal esophageal glands.

It is generally acknowledged that adenoid cystic carcinomas of the esophagus are much more aggressive than their salivary gland counterparts and associated with grim prognosis. As Enterline and Thompson have pointed out, however, this is based on scanty facts because many cases have limited follow-up.[3] It would appear (not unreasonably) that small, superficial tumors and those without metastases have a better prognosis.

Mucoepidermoid and Adenosquamous Carcinoma

Esophageal neoplasms composed of a mixture of glandular and squamous elements have gone by a confusing array of terms such as **mucoepidermoid carcinoma, adenosquamous carcinoma, adenoacanthoma,** and **squamous cell carcinoma with pseudoglandular features.**[3, 60] The term *mucoepidermoid carcinoma* should be restricted to neoplasms, with three cell types generally recognized in salivary mucoepidermoid carcinoma: mucin-secreting, squamous cells, and intermediate cells.[3, 61] In contrast, the term **adenosquamous carcinoma** is probably best reserved for primarily squamous cell carcinomas in which there are glandular elements[141] or marked mucin production[3] (Fig. 5–4). Finally, *adenoacan-*

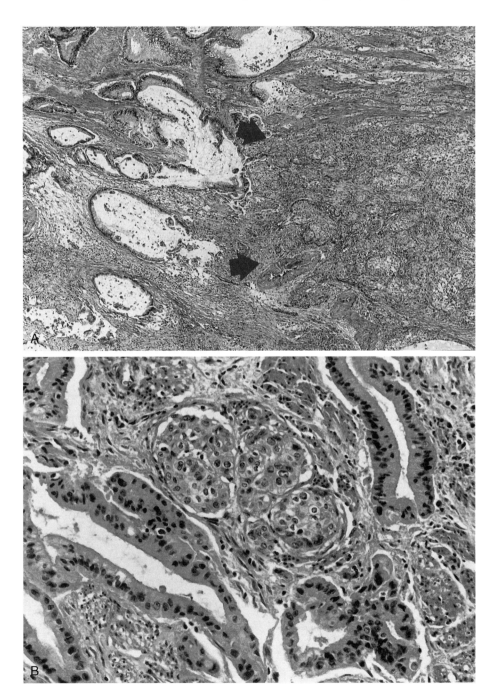

FIGURE 5–4. Adenosquamous carcinoma. *A,* The tumor comprises both glandular elements with abundant mucin *(left)* as well as nests of squamous cell carcinoma *(right, arrows).* (H&E, ×73) *B,* At higher power, both the glandular and squamous elements appear malignant, justifying the diagnostic term *adenosquamous carcinoma.* (H&E, ×233)

thoma should be restricted to primarily glandular tumors with focal areas of bland squamous differentiation.[3, 62]

Although a 1990 review noted a total of 20 cases of esophageal "mucoepidermoid" carcinoma, the presence of signet cells in some and origin from Barrett's esophagus in others make the "purity" of this series suspect.[63] This study reports that the majority of mucoepidermoid carcinomas occur in the sixth decade (mean, 60 years; range, 47–81) and the male : female ratio is 3 : 1. The tumors are almost uniformly ulcerated or indurated; they always involve at least the muscularis propria, 82% involve adventitia, and 80% have nodal involvement.[63] One year survival is only 65%, and only one patient has survived more than 40 months.[63] It is likely that true mucoepidermoid carcinoma of the esophagus, analogous to that seen arising from salivary glands, is less common than would appear from the literature. The prognosis is difficult to assess owing to "contamination" of review series by adenosquamous carcinoma, but does not seem to be different from that for patients with squamous cell carcinoma.[64]

Mesenchymal Neoplasms

Leiomyoma

As opposed to the rest of the gut, the common stromal tumors of the esophagus tend to resemble typical extraintestinal leiomyomas both microscopically and grossly. If careful serial histologic sectioning is performed, the most common leiomyomas are tiny (<7 mm) subclinical lesions that can be found in close to 10% of cases and may be multiple.[65] These lesions have been referred to as "seedling" leiomyomas and are usually found in the gastroesophageal junction region. Most arise from the inner circular portion of the muscularis propria, although they may arise from the outer longitudinal muscle or muscularis mucosae.

In contrast, most symptomatic cases of leiomyomas are 2 to 5 cm in diameter, with leiomyomas up to 5000 g having

been reported.[66] Esophageal leiomyomas are present in about twice as many men as women.[65, 66] Grossly evident leiomyomas are seen in only approximately 1 in 1100 autopsies.[66] More than half are found in the distal third, 30% in the middle, and the remainder are in the proximal esophagus.[66] The gross appearance is typically round to oval, and intramural masses are the rule. Calcification is uncommon.[66] An unusual variant has been referred to as "diffuse leiomyomatosis of the esophagus." This condition generally affects younger women, is associated with dysphagia, and is characterized by circumferential, confluent smooth muscle lesions of the muscularis propria of variable size.[67, 68] Very rare associations with esophageal leiomyoma include familial congenital esophageal stenosis with leiomyoma and leiomyosarcoma,[69] esophagogastric and vulvar leiomyomatosis,[70] and familial esophageal leiomyomatosis and an Alport-like nephropathy,[71] and hypertrophic osteoarthropathy.[72]

Hemangioma

Vascular neoplasms of the esophagus are very rare. In an exhaustive review of 1,400,000 case records of the Mayo Clinic in 1949, a total of 106 vascular tumors of the gastrointestinal tract were noted, and only 10 (nine benign, one malignant) arose from the esophagus.[73] An incidence of 1 per 1862 autopsies was noted in one series.[74] Hemangiomas are usually asymptomatic. Among reported cases, however, approximately 40% of patients suffered hemorrhage, and 33% dysphagia.[75] Larger lesions may be pedunculated and cause obstructive symptoms; the largest reported lesion has been 12 cm.[76] Although the majority of hemangiomas are cavernous,[75] capillary types exist as well (Fig. 5–5).

Granular Cell Tumor

Granular cell tumor (GCT) is a not uncommon, readily recognized mesenchymal neoplasm that may occur in virtually

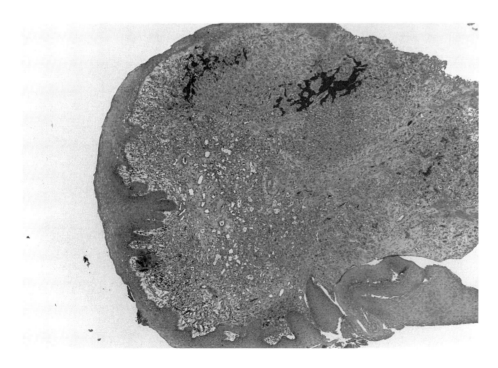

FIGURE 5–5. Esophageal hemangioma, capillary type. This polypoid lesion was an incidental finding at endoscopy. (H&E, ×73)

any body site.[77] Originally felt to be of striated muscle origin (granular cell ''myoblastoma''), they are now known to be of schwannian origin.[77] Most GCTs are benign lesions that rarely cause significant symptoms and are frequently incidental findings. Multicentricity, noted in 10% to 15% of cases, may make the distinction between benign and the rare (2%) malignant granular cell tumor difficult.[77]

Esophageal GCTs are relatively uncommon, constituting approximately 1% of all GCTs[78] and 30% of all gastrointestinal tract GCTs.[79] A 1985 literature review noted 119 cases of esophageal GCT.[80] As with GCTs in general, most patients are in the fourth, fifth, or sixth decade of life.[79] The majority of esophageal GCTs are asymptomatic and found incidentally, typically consisting of small (<2 cm), poorly circumscribed yellowish submucosal nodules; they are occasionally present in muscle or adventitia.[79] When the patient is symptomatic, dysphagia is the predominant complaint;[81] in one case, an associated dysmotility disorder was documented.[82] Multiple esophageal lesions occur occasionally, and ''miliary'' esophageal GCTs consisting of large numbers of 2- to 4-mm lesions have been described.[83] The presence of synchronous GCTs in other organs is not uncommon.[81, 84]

Microscopically, esophageal GCTs are identical to those seen elsewhere, being composed of uniform polygonal cells, the small centrally placed nuclei, and abundant coarsely granular cytoplasm.[77] Although about half show some acanthosis and pseudoepitheliomatous hyperplasia (Fig. 5–6), the degree seems to be less than that seen in the tongue and anorectal region.[79] Nonetheless, at least one resected tumor was initially diagnosed as ''squamous cell carcinoma'' on biopsy.[85] Ultra-

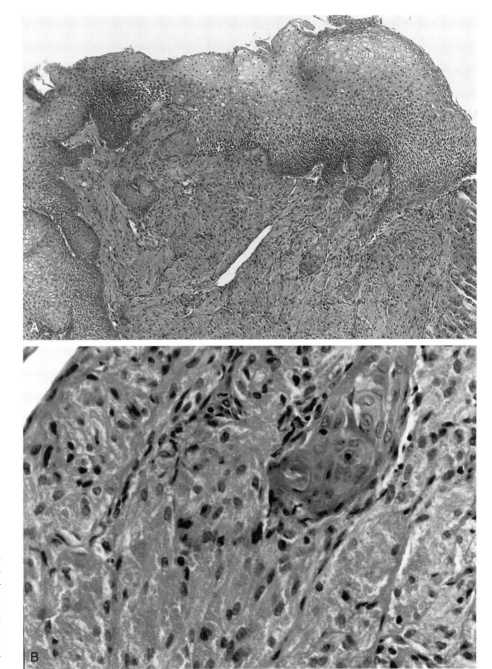

FIGURE 5–6. Esophageal granular cell tumor. *A,* The squamous epithelium shows mild epithelial hyperplasia but no dysplasia. A submucosal neoplasm is evident. (H&E, ×90) *B,* On higher power, the characteristic features of a granular cell tumor are evident: spindled to oval cells with uniform nuclei and abundant granular cytoplasm. (H&E, ×250)

structurally, the granular cytoplasm in GCT is a result of autophagic granules (lysosomes). The reaction of GCTs with KP-1, a putative histiocytic marker, has led to the conclusion that this antibody is actually directed against lysosomes.[51] The natural history of esophageal GCTs seems to be very indolent, and thus small tumors can probably be followed by endoscopy.[86] The distinction between benign and malignant GCT may be difficult at times, although size, pleomorphism, mitotic activity, and most importantly the presence of metastases are useful.[77] A few reports of "malignant" granular cell tumor exist,[85, 87, 88] although only one has demonstrated metastatic capability.[87]

Fibrovascular Polyp

An uncommon lesion with a sometimes spectacular clinical presentation is the fibrovascular polyp. This lesion has gone by a variety of monikers, including **pedunculated fibroma, fibrolipoma, lipoma, myxofibroma, and hamartomatous polyp.**[89] Approximately 60 esophageal fibrovascular polyps had been reported by 1989.[89] These lesions tend to be large, polypoid, smooth-surfaced intraluminal masses that may have long stalks, measure up to 18 cm in maximum dimension, and commonly insert just below the attachment of the cricopharyngeal muscle. The most common symptom is dysphagia, although large lesions may cause tracheal compression and respiratory difficulties, may be regurgitated, and in rare cases may cause asphyxiation due to regurgitation and aspiration.[90]

Histologically, fibrovascular polyps are composed of variably cellular spindle cell stroma with focal myxoid change, prominent blood vessels, occasional lymphoid aggregates, and adipose tissue in varying amounts. These lesions are benign, do not recur following excision, and should be removed because of the risk of asphyxiation.

Inflammatory Pseudotumor (Inflammatory Fibroid Polyp)

Rare inflammatory pseudotumors of the esophagus have been reported.[91, 92] These tumors are also known as "inflammatory fibroid polyps" and are likely analogous to their more common counterparts in the stomach and intestines. Inflammatory pseudotumors are commonly polypoid but occasionally may be largely intramural. They are composed of a mixture of spindled cells and a mixed inflammatory infiltrative that may contain numerous plasma cells and eosinophils. The spindled cells may mimic a sarcoma or carcinosarcoma; however, these are benign lesions that may represent an exuberant response to injury.

Miscellaneous Benign Mesenchymal Lesions

Very rare benign mesenchymal lesions include **osteochondroma (tracheobronchial choristoma)**[93] and a tumor initially termed **melanocytic tumor of the esophagus,**[94] which appears to represent an example of what is now known as **"psammomatous melanotic Schwannoma."**[95]

Malignant Mesenchymal Neoplasms

Leiomyosarcoma

Leiomyosarcoma is the most common esophagus sarcoma. Although they have been said to account for 0.5% to 1% of all esophageal malignancies,[96] the actual incidence may be even lower. A 1988 review noted fewer than 60 cases in the published literature; however, 10% were associated with squamous cell carcinoma.[97] Thus, as Appelman has pointed out, the actual number of esophageal leiomyosarcomas is likely even less than the literature would suggest, because leiomyosarcoma may mimic **spindle cell carcinoma** clinically, grossly, and histologically.[22] There seem to be fewer recent reports of leiomyosarcoma, possibly reflecting better recognition of the distinction between leiomyosarcoma and spindled carcinomas. Clinically, there appears to be a slight male predominance, and the age range has been 27 to 78 years, with most occurring in the sixth decade of life.[97] The most common complaints are dysphagia (75%), weight loss (50%), and substernal pain (45%), with gastrointestinal bleeding being uncommon.[3] The tumors may be present throughout the esophagus and may be polypoid, infiltrating, or a combination.[97] Most (60% to 70%) have been described as polypoid.

Leiomyosarcomas resemble those found in extra-intestinal sites histologically; however, "organ-specific" criteria for distinguishing "atypical" esophageal leiomyomas from leiomyosarcoma (size, mitotic activity, and so on) have not been proposed. In keeping with characteristics in other organ sites, leiomyosarcomas would be expected to show increased size and mitotic activity, variable pleomorphism, and a tendency toward local invasion, necrosis, and of course metastasis. Furthermore, smooth muscle differentiation should be apparent either by light microscopy, immunohistochemistry, or ultrastructural analysis. An associated squamous cell cancer should make the diagnosis of leiomyosarcoma very suspect.

The prognosis for esophageal leiomyosarcoma is fairly poor; only one third with resectable lesions survive 5 years. Surgical treatment appears to be the most promising therapeutic approach.[97]

Rhabdomyosarcoma

Except for leiomyosarcoma, other esophageal sarcomas are extremely rare. Although 12 cases of esophageal rhabdomyosarcoma had been reported as of 1980, Vartio et al. accepted only five cases (including their own) as being undisputed.[98] Attesting to the rarity of the tumor, a search of the English literature from 1980 to 1991 revealed only one reported case.[99] Rhabdomyosarcomas tend to occur most frequently in the sixth through eighth decades, the most common symptom is dysphagia, and about 80% of those affected are males.[99] Polypoid tumors are slightly more common than ulcerated lesions, and nearly all occur in the middle and lower esophagus. As striated muscle is confined to the upper and middle esophagus, presumably esophageal rhabdomyosarcomas arise from either "totipotential" stem cells or primitive mesenchymal cells displaced to the esophagus during embryogenesis.

Kaposi's Sarcoma

Gastrointestinal involvement by Kaposi's sarcoma is much more common in forms related to transplantation and **acquired immunodeficiency syndrome (AIDS)** than in chronic or lymphadenopathic forms.[77, 100] Although it is generally silent clinically, at autopsy the majority of patients with cutaneous Kaposi's sarcoma have visceral involvement.[100, 101] Esophageal involvement by Kaposi's sarcoma has been documented in the post-transplant setting[102] and is likely frequent in disseminated visceral Kaposi's sarcoma. The gross and histologic features are similar to those in other visceral organs.

Other Sarcomas

We are aware of three reported cases of esophageal **synovial sarcoma**.[103, 104] These lesions tend to be polypoid or pedunculated lesions in the proximal esophagus that may be amenable to local surgical excision.[104]

At least four cases of esophageal **liposarcoma** have been reported.[105-108] Similar to many other esophageal sarcomas, these tend to be polypoid and have a broad pedicle and may infiltrate the esophageal wall. Myxoid liposarcoma is the most common type.[105, 106, 108] Although follow-up is limited in most reports, in one case, clinical recurrence took more than 6 years even after incomplete excision.

Isolated case reports of esophageal **osteogenic sarcoma**[109] and **chondrosarcoma**[110] exist. A "**malignant mesenchymoma**" of the esophagus, containing rhabdomyosarcomatous, osteosarcomatous, and malignant fibrous histiocytoma-like areas, has been reported; however, because the lesion also contained probable squamous cell carcinoma *in situ,* the possibility of a "metaplastic" squamous cell carcinoma exists.[111]

Malignant Melanoma

Primary malignant melanoma of the gastrointestinal tract has been convincingly demonstrated only as arising from the esophagus, gallbladder, and anus.[112] As of 1989, 139 cases of primary esophageal melanoma (EM) had been reported.[113] It has been estimated that 0.5% of all non-cutaneous melanomas arise in the esophagus, resulting in an incidence of 0.0036/100,000, or approximately eight new cases per year.[114] Although the concept of primary EM was in doubt at one point, the demonstration of benign melanocytes in 8% of consecutive necropsies[115] and the frequent observation of a junctional melanocytic component to the tumor have solidified the concept of melanomas arising from the esophagus.

Clinically, EM tends to occur in the sixth and seventh decades (range, 7–86 years; mean, 60.5), and has a male:female ratio of 2:1.[113] The most common symptom is dysphagia (80%), although weight loss (38%) and post-swallowing substernal discomfort (33%) were also common; melena is uncommon (7%).

Grossly, most tumors are polypoid, range in size from 2 to 17 cm (average, 5.7 cm), and are usually pigmented.[113] The distal esophagus is the most common site for EM (43%); 18% are present at the junction of the middle and lower thirds, 29% in the middle third, and 10% in the proximal third. The surrounding mucosa may show satellite nodules (12%) or melanosis that may be focal (18%) or diffuse (5%).

Microscopically, they resemble melanomas of other sites and thus on occasion may mimic other malignant tumors, particularly when non-pigmented (10%). Junctional activity is seen in 40% of cases and is helpful in proving the esophagus as being the primary site (Fig. 5–7). Distinction between metastatic melanoma and primary EM may be difficult and is ultimately a diagnosis of exclusion. A reasonable set of criteria is listed by Sabanathan et al., the tumor being considered primary when (1) it has the characteristic light microscopic, immunohistochemical, and/or ultrastructural features; (2) the adjacent epithelium contains melanocytes; (3) the

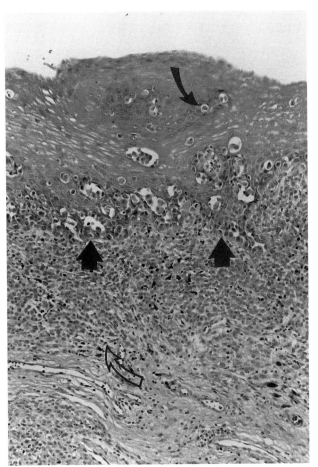

FIGURE 5–7. Primary esophageal malignant melanoma. Analogous to cutaneous melanoma, the neoplastic cells can be seen in a "pagetoid" intraepithelial pattern *(closed curved arrow),* as single cells and nests along the "dermal-epidermal" junction *(broad arrows),* and in the "dermis" *(open curved arrow).* The intraepithelial pattern allows one to identify this tumor as primary rather than metastatic. (H&E, ×133)

tumor is polypoid; (4) junctional changes are present in the adjacent epithelium; and (5) no other likely primary sites are evident.[113] Application of these criteria is important because 4% of patients dying with metastatic cutaneous melanoma have esophageal involvement at autopsy.[116] Metastases are present in 41% at the time of discovery, the most common sites being mediastinal lymph nodes, liver, lungs, pleura, and supraclavicular lymph nodes. Prognosis is dismal, with overall survival of 9.8 months and 5-year survival of 1.7%.[113] Surgical excision yields a bit more hope than non-surgical treatment (4.25% versus 0% 5-year survival). Rare long-term survivors have been reported after surgical excisions, even in the presence of local metastases.[117]

Malignant Lymphoma

Although the gastrointestinal tract is involved in approximately 10% to 20% of all lymphomas,[15] esophageal involvement is seen in only 1.5%.[118] The esophageal involvement is usually due to extension of the tumor from the stomach or mediastinal lymph nodes, primary malignant lymphoma of the esophagus being exceedingly rare. To be regarded as primary in the esophagus, a lymphoma should have a predominant esophageal mass, nodal involvement should be restricted to "draining" lymph nodes with no evidence of mediastinal or peripheral adenopathy, and the liver, spleen, marrow, and peripheral blood should be uninvolved.[119]

Relatively few cases meet these criteria. A literature review of 1989 accepted only seven cases of primary non-Hodgkin's lymphoma, three of which were associated with **AIDS;**[120] at least two subsequent reports exist.[89, 121] We have recently seen an anaplastic large-cell lymphoma ("Ki-1 lymphoma") that appears to be a primary esophageal lymphoma (Fig. 5–8). A case of primary Hodgkin's disease of the esophagus has been reported,[122] as have two cases of plasmacytic neoplasms.[32, 123]

THE STOMACH

The Normal Gastric Biopsy: General Commentary

Perhaps the most difficult task in examining gastric mucosal biopsies (and gastrointestinal tract biopsies in general) is recognition of normal tissue and its histophysiologic range within the population. The designation "mild chronic inflammation" is probably the most commonly rendered and undoubtedly the most abused diagnosis in interpretation of gastrointestinal

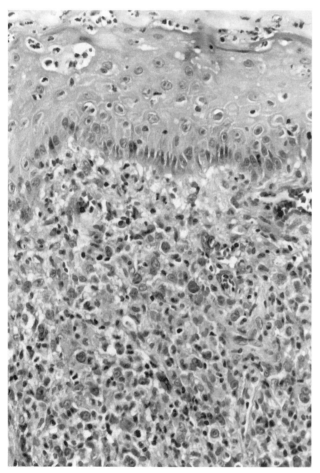

FIGURE 5–8. Primary esophageal lymphoma, anaplastic large-cell type, Ki-1 (CD30 positive) phenotype. At resection, the process was limited to the mucosa, forming multiple (three) ulcerated masses up to 5 cm in diameter. There was no evidence of extraesophageal disease at the time of resection. (H&E, ×240)

biopsies. There is no absolute remedy for this because appreciation for the range of normal comes only after a large, non-passive clinical experience that has been integrated with clinical opinions and patient outcomes. Certain observations and guidelines, however, may be worthy of consideration. First, an increase in density of round cells within the lamina propria independent of any other structural or acute epithelial changes (such as mucin depletion or polarization of epithelial nuclei) is likely to be of no clinical significance. Second, mild to moderate edema of the lamina propria and extravasation of red blood cells beneath the surface epithelium are likely to be artifacts or related to the procedure if there are no accompanying abnormal histologic changes. This is especially true in the lower gastrointestinal tract. Third, in the absence of clinical symptoms, "mild chronic inflammation" may be physiologic and not pathologic and should be offered only cautiously as a pathologic diagnosis. Fourth, acute cellular injury patterns such as marked mucin depletion and proliferative changes such as stratification of nuclei in the absence of cellular inflammation may have as much or more clinical significance as cellular infiltrates. These changes should be described in the diagnostic note in appropriate clinical settings (e.g., in the question of drug-associated gastritis or of acute mucosal injury of uncertain derivation). Finally, with non-neoplastic gastrointestinal biopsies, it is often wise to resist the urge to "make a diagnosis" and to be prepared to offer observation and opinion instead. The diagnostic statement "minor histologic changes of uncertain (or improbable) clinical significance" followed by a consultation note describing their possible relevance (or lack thereof) to the patient in question may provide a far more useful commentary than a terse diagnosis such as "mild chronic inflammation." This is most possible and most useful in the clinical setting where endoscopists and surgeons provide relevant history and ask specific questions and where pathologists examine the tissues in view of that information, taking great care to answer the specific questions. It is the obligation of clinicians and pathologists alike to create this environment in spite of current restrictions of time and resource to the practice of medicine.

Endocrine Cell Hyperplasia

The gastrointestinal tract is home for several types of endocrine cells that secrete hormones and interact with autonomic nerves and ganglia of the gut. These cells are interspersed between the epithelial cells and are located throughout the entire gastrointestinal tract. Their distribution is not uniform, however, in that certain types of cells tend to be distributed within specific locations.[124, 125] Gastrin cells, for example, are located primarily within the gastric antrum and the upper duodenum. At least 16 different types of endocrine cells are now recognized and are categorized primarily by their secretory products and by morphologic parameters (Table 5–1). A number of reviews have addressed current classification of this endocrine population within the gut.[124–126] Pathologic alterations of these cells ranging from simple hyperplasia to dysplasia and neoplasia have been defined, especially within the clinicopathologic spectrum of chronic gastritis.[127–129] This section focuses on hyperplasia and neoplasia of gastrin-producing cells and enterochromaffin-like cells.

Table 5–1. **Gastrointestinal Endocrine Cells and Their Location**

Cell	Secretory Product	Stomach Corpus	Stomach Antrum	Small Bowel Proximal	Small Bowel Distal	Colon
D	Somatostatin	++	+	+	+	+
ECL	Histamine (?)	+	−	−	−	−
EC1	Serotonin, substance P	+/−	+	+	+	+
EC2	Serotonin, motilin	+/−	+	+	+/−	+/−
G	Gastrin	−	++	+	−	−
I	Cholecystokinin	−	−	+	+	−
K	Gastrin inhibitory protein	−	−	+	+	−
L	Enteroglucagon	−	−	+	+	+
M	Motilin	−	−	+	+/−	−
N	Neurotensin	−	−	+/−	+	−
P	Bombesin-like	+/−	+	+	+/−	+/−
PP	Pancreatic polypeptide	−	−	−	−	+
S	Secretin	−	−	+	+	−
X	Unknown	+	−	−	−	−

ECL, enterochromaffin-like; EC, enterochromaffin.

Recognition and characterization of endocrine cell hyperplasia have become possible in large part as a result of immunohistochemical techniques that allow better definition of the presence and number of these cells. Both primary and secondary forms of hyperplasia affecting many of the different types of endocrine cells within the gut are now recognized. At the current time, however, the clinical significance of these hyperplasias is incompletely understood and appears to be limited, with the exceptions of primary gastrin cell hyperplasia and enterochromaffin-like cell proliferation. Endocrine cell hyperplasia is defined as an increased number or cell mass of a particular type of cell. Clinical application of this definition is difficult, however, in that there is limited knowledge regarding normal ranges of most of these cell types.

Primary Antral G-Cell Hyperplasia

Primary G-cell hyperplasia is a clinical entity of unknown cause associated with persistent or recurrent peptic ulcer disease.[126, 130] This cannot be clinically distinguished from **Zollinger-Ellison syndrome** and previously has been labeled **pseudo–Zollinger-Ellison syndrome.** Pathologists are on occasion asked to document primary gastrin cell hyperplasia after unsuccessful localization of a presumed gastrinoma. This differential can be approached by clinical laboratory tests including the secretin stimulation test and calcium stimulation test and by immunohistochemical analysis of tissue, but quantitation of the G-cell population on biopsy or resection specimen is especially useful for differentiating primary G-cell hyperplasia from the Zollinger-Ellison syndrome. Antral-based G cells are diffusely hyperplastic in the former condition and normal in the latter. Argyrophilic stains, such as the Grimelius and Sevier-Munger stains, can be used to provide a rough estimate of the number of G cells within the gastric antrum, but the unpredictability of the silver stain for G cells prevents accurate quantitation. G-cell quantitation is much more reliably provided by immunohistochemical analysis using primary antibodies against gastrin. In primary G-cell hyperplasia, gastrin-producing cells are diffusely distributed in increased numbers, allowing quantitation by endoscopic biopsies that are full thickness and of sufficient size.[130] Lewin et al. studied five cases of primary gastrin cell hyperplasia and defined normal numbers to be 20 ± 10 per 0.1 mm length of mucosa and hyperplasia to be greater than 50 per 0.1 mm length of mucosa.[130] They noted that in normal control cases G cells were largely confined to the lower third of the middle portion of the mucosa, whereas in G-cell hyperplasia the endocrine cells were closely clustered and occupied areas above and below the usual zone where these cells reside (Fig. 5–9).

Secondary Antral G-Cell Hyperplasia

Hyperplasia of G cells within the antrum and pyloric region occurs secondary to a number of clinical conditions, including chronic atrophic gastritis, pernicious anemia, gastric outload obstruction, chronic hypercalcemic states, post-vagotomy state, and duodenal ulcer disease.[130–132] The distribution of G cells is identical in secondary and primary G-cell hyperplasia, thus these conditions must be differentiated on clinical grounds. In both variants, overgrowth of G cells can be seen in virtually all the antral glands, occupying both the lower and intermediate portions of the glands. In their normal state, these cells are confined to the lower third to the lower half of the glands. The hyperplastic pattern is usually a diffuse distribution of individual cells and small groups of cells, but occasionally clusters of G cells occur within the glands and adjacent lamina propria, creating micronodules that rarely may progress to functioning G-cell carcinoid tumors or gastrinomas. This progression from hyperplasia to G-cell carcinoid tumor is analogous to that of enterochromaffin-like cells in patients with chronic atrophic gastritis as described in greater detail in the following section.

Enterochromaffin-like Cell Hyperplasia

One of the more common questions in the area of gastric endocrine cell hyperplasia that confronts the surgical pathologist is definition and diagnosis of abnormalities affecting the enterochromaffin-like (ECL) cells in fundic **chronic atrophic gastritis** with or without **pernicious anemia** (type A gastritis). In the normal gastric fundus, ECL cells are primarily located in the lower third of the mucosa and constitute about 45% of

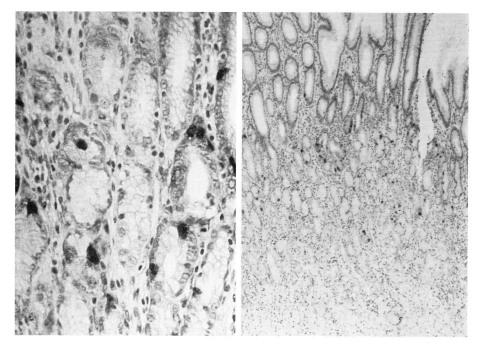

FIGURE 5–9. Minimal hyperplasia of gastrin-producing cells as detected by immunohistochemistry with anti-gastrin antibodies. The left field illustrates G cells located individually without clustering within gastric glands. The right field shows that the cells are not retained in the base of the mucosa but are located up within the gastric pits as well. In spite of this abnormal distribution, the number of cells was 28 per 0.1 mm mucosa, below the level of G-cell hyperplasia as defined by Lewin et al.[130] (Immunoperoxidase, ×250 & ×90)

the endocrine population. In chronic type A gastritis, proliferative ECL cells may reach the foveolar regions and may constitute as much as 70% of the endocrine cell population.[133] In type A gastritis, a pathophysiologic sequence has been defined that is initiated by atrophic gastritis involving the fundus, with its attendant loss of parietal cells and consequent hypochlorhydria.[129, 134, 135] This in turn evokes hypergastrinemia. The ECL cell is sensitive to serum gastrin levels and may be induced to progress through simple hyperplasia into dysplasia and carcinoid tumor formation. Solcia et al. have classified nonantral gastric endocrine cell proliferation into hyperplasia, dysplasia, and neoplasia.[129] They have further divided hyperplastic states into three patterns: linear or diffuse, micronodular, and adenomatoid. Linear hyperplasia is overgrowth of ECL cells inside the basement membranes of glands leading to a relatively uniform line of such proliferating cells just above the muscularis mucosae. Micronodular hyperplasia consists of clusters of these cells either within the glands or within the lamina propria measuring less than 150 microns (Fig. 5–10). Adenomatoid hyperplasia is defined as aggregates of micronodules, usually five or more, situated deep within the mucosa above the muscularis mucosae.

Endocrine cell dysplasia results from continued enlargement and fusion of micronodules. Nuclear features of these enlarging clusters may be the same as those in simple hyperplasia or may show enlargement, variation in size, and hyper-

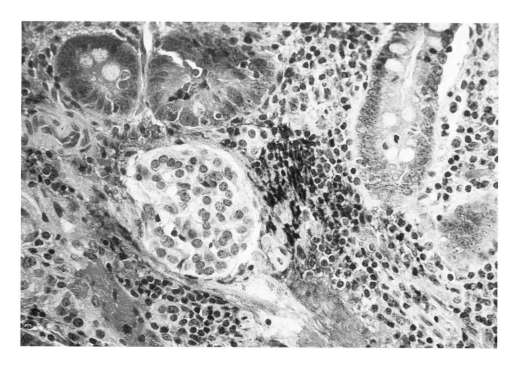

FIGURE 5–10. A micronodule of ECL cells in a surveillance biopsy from a patient with chronic gastritis and history of a small gastric carcinoid tumor treated earlier by endoscopic piecemeal removal. The patient refused further therapy. (H&E, ×250)

chromasia. These dysplastic foci often exhibit less affinity for silver stains, making them difficult to define by this histochemical technique.

The clinical significance of ECL hyperplasia in patients with atrophic gastritis is an increased risk of developing gastric carcinoid tumor.[12, 134, 136, 137] Although it is now clear that such a risk does exist, it is small (about 5%), and most patients with endocrine cell hyperplasia show no obvious progression into neoplasia.[128, 138, 139] Those who do usually progress slowly over a period of years. The question of whether to clinically monitor these patients by endoscopic biopsy and quantitation of endocrine cells remains unresolved.[140] It is likely, however, that the surgical pathologist will be asked from time to time to assess and perhaps quantitate endocrine cell hyperplasia in atrophic gastritis patients. Immunohistochemical analysis of biopsies using antibodies to such markers as chromagranin A or neuron-specific enolase allows such assessment.[126] The nomenclature of early carcinoid tumor formation is confusing because of the various terminologies that have been used in the descriptive literature. In an attempt to resolve this, Itsuno et al. meticulously studied six resected gastric specimens from patients with type A gastritis carcinoids by histologic mapping.[133] They observed that **endocrine cell micronests** (ECMs) measuring less than 0.1 mm often did not display invasive characteristics, whereas larger ECMs frequently did. From their observations they offered the following definitions of **microcarcinoids** (neoplastic ECMs): (1) ECMs measuring more than 0.1 mm in largest diameter, (2) ECMs that infiltrate into muscularis mucosae or submucosa even if smaller than 0.1 mm, (3) ECMs that show carcinoid-like structures such as trabecular or ribbon-like features even if smaller than 0.1 mm, and (4) ECMs that show large atypical cells regardless of size (Fig. 5–11). Tumors that reach 0.5 cm have reached the carcinoid stage.[124]

Patients with chronic atrophic gastritis do have a small but definable increased risk of developing gastric carcinoids.

Such patients may develop multiple carcinoids that have a distinctly less aggressive pathobiology than the solitary carcinoid that characteristically occurs independent of atrophic gastritis.[140, 141] Bordi et al. recently studied 23 examples of gastric carcinoid, including 19 associated with chronic atrophic gastritis A and four without this association.[136] The latter tumors, which were all single, were more aggressive and were not associated with endocrine cell proliferation or signs of gastrin hypersecretion. Larger series of solitary carcinoids occurring independent of atrophic gastritis demonstrate metastasis in as many as 55%.[141a] In contrast, only 9% of the 133 cases of multiple carcinoids associated with hypergastrinemia studied by Solcia et al. metastasized.[129]

Therapy for patients with multiple carcinoid tumors in the setting of atrophic gastritis is controversial.[87, 99, 142] Earlier literature recommended total gastrectomy for these patients to remove the entire mucosa at risk for development of carcinoids. A number of more recent reports, however, have demonstrated that antrectomy alone is successful in reducing serum levels of gastrin and resulting in regression of mucosal carcinoid tumors within the gastric fundus.[140, 143] This lesser form of surgery appears to be a viable option for nonmetastatic multiple carcinoid tumors.

Eosinophilic Infiltrates of the Stomach

Eosinophilic infiltration of the stomach or any other portion of the gastrointestinal tract may occur as either diffuse or localized forms and in neither case can be regarded as a distinct diagnostic entity.[144] The eosinophil is a resident cell within the lamina propria of the bowel but may also be a component of inflammation. Although its presence in increased numbers often signifies an allergic response, the broad differential of lesions that are associated with eosinophilic infiltration makes its histologic presence alone essen-

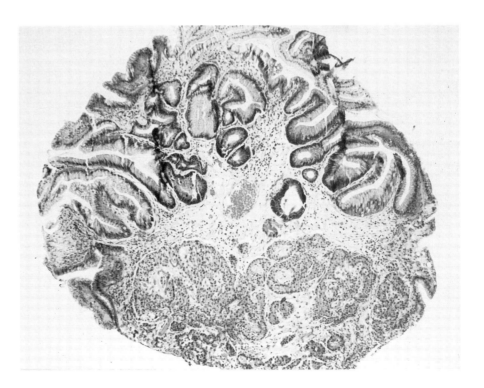

FIGURE 5–11. A microcarcinoid by the definition of Itsuno et al.[133] (see text) because of size greater than 0.1 mm. This patient had areas of endocrine cell hyperplasia demonstrated in several random gastric biopsies. (H&E, ×90)

tially non-specific. Similar to the problem with lymphocytic and plasmacytic infiltrates within gastrointestinal mucosa, there are no well-defined guidelines as to what number and density of eosinophils are abnormal. Within the normal gastric lamina propria, eosinophils are rare, never clustered, and without epithelial infiltration.[145]

Clinical and laboratory investigation has generated much new knowledge regarding the nature and function of the eosinophil.[146–148] This cell was first identified by Ehrlich in 1879 and has since been recognized by its familiar cytoplasmic granules. These membrane-bound granules consist of an electron-dense crystalloid core with an electron-lucent matrix. They are made up primarily of several cationic proteins, which include eosinophil peroxidase, major basic protein, eosinophilic cationic protein, and eosinophil-derived neurotoxin. In addition, eosinophils produce a variety of inflammatory mediators such as platelet activating factors and leukotriene C4. These various proteins and mediators have been shown to be responsible for killing parasites but are also recognized to be toxic to host tissue.[146] Within the gut, they may be induced to release reactive oxygen metabolites that have a more prolonged and more cytotoxic effect than neutrophils.

Much of the literature examining eosinophilic infiltration within the stomach has focused on the differentiation of eosinophilic gastroenteritis and inflammatory fibroid polyp, one from the other, and from other less-specific types of eosinophilic infiltration.[144, 148]

Inflammatory Fibroid Polyp

This rare lesion owes much of the confusion regarding its nature to the several terms that have been employed to describe it. These include **eosinophilic granuloma, inflammatory pseudotumor, hemangiopericytoma, fibrous inflammatory polyp, inflammatory polyp, neurofibroma, submucosal granuloma, and gastric fibroma with eosinophilic infiltration.**[144, 149, 150] The term *inflammatory fibroid polyp* is now generally accepted, however. This lesion can occur anywhere within the gastrointestinal tract, but approximately 70% of cases occur in the gastric antrum.[144, 149–151] An additional 15% to 20% occur within the small bowel.[152, 153]

Clinical symptoms vary depending on location and size of the lesion within the gastrointestinal tract. In general, symptoms are obstructive: gastric outlet obstruction for antral lesions, dysphasia for esophageal lesions, and intussusception for small intestinal lesions. Asymptomatic cases found incidentally during surgery for other lesions or at autopsy are also well described.

The macroscopic appearance of inflammatory fibroid polyp is generally that of a solitary sessile or pedunculated lesion usually measuring 2 to 6 cm, although examples as large as 19 cm have been described. The overlying mucosal surfaces are usually smooth, but they may be ulcerated, especially over the apex of larger lesions. In those cases without mucosal ulceration, an underlying smooth muscle tumor or carcinoid tumor may be simulated.

Histologically, inflammatory fibroid polyps are characterized by two predominant features: (1) loose mesenchymal stroma with characteristic concentric arrangement of fibroblasts around capillaries and arterioles, and (2) modest to marked eosinophilic infiltration.[144, 154] The loose proliferation of fibroblasts, capillaries, and inflammatory infiltrates often simulates granulation tissue. The characteristic concentric pattern of fibroblasts around arterioles led to the earlier impression that this lesion was a variant of hemangiopericytoma, a conjecture that has since been discarded. Although the eosinophil is usually the predominant inflammatory cell, this is variable, and some lesions show a predominance of plasma cells. The stroma is typically loose or even myxoid, although regions of more dense arrangements of fibroblasts and fibrocytes led to earlier speculation that this lesion represented a true fibroma, again a conjecture that has been discarded.

The etiology and pathogenesis of inflammatory fibroid polyp are undefined. It is generally accepted that the lesion is not associated with systemic manifestations or peripheral eosinophilia, and it is generally regarded as a localized proliferation of vascular granulation tissue, perhaps responding to an undefined local stimulus.[155] Inflammatory fibroid polyp is not neoplastic, but it can be mistaken for a malignant neoplasm, making its recognition essential before radical therapy.[50, 156] Small examples of this lesion can be successfully removed endoscopically.[157]

Eosinophilic Gastroenteritis

This lesion is also rare, and its diagnosis can be established only by clinical and pathologic exclusion of other causes of eosinophilic infiltration.[158–161] The term *eosinophilic gastroenteritis* is actually a misnomer in that the entire gastrointestinal tract can be involved and often does show histologic disease even in those patients with prominent upper gastrointestinal symptomatology. Unlike inflammatory fibroid polyp, eosinophilic gastroenteritis is often associated with systemic manifestations. One half to three quarters of patients have a personal or family history of allergic conditions such as asthma, hypersensitivity to drugs, or food intolerance. Peripheral eosinophilia usually has been observed in more than 90% of patients. The erythrocyte sedimentation rate has typically been reported to be normal or only slightly elevated, although one study observed moderate elevation in 10 of 40 patients.[161] A 3 : 2 predominance of men, with a bimodal age distribution peaking in the third and sixth decades, has been observed in eosinophilic gastroenteritis.[144]

After the observations of Klein et al. in 1970, three principal clinical and pathologic variances of eosinophilic gastroenteritis had been defined.[162] The first of these is predominant eosinophilic infiltration into the mucosa in which patients present with abdominal pain, nausea, and vomiting. Diarrhea and malabsorption are observed in those patients with more distal disease in the colon and small bowel. The second pattern is that of predominant muscular involvement resulting in rigidity and thickening of the bowel wall. These patients give signs and symptoms of obstruction usually presenting either as gastric outlet obstruction or small intestinal obstruction. The third pattern is that of serosal and subserosal infiltration that results in eosinophilic ascites. Subsequent clinical studies have demonstrated much overlap of these three subtypes, however, and one recent study of 40 patients found no significant demographic, symptomatic, or laboratory parameter differences among the three groups, with the exception that the subserosal group manifested ascites and higher peripheral eosinophilic counts.[161] This study also observed that peripheral eosinophilia was absent in 9 of the 40 patients and suggested that the diagnosis of eosinophilic gastroenteritis should be entertained even in the absence of peripheral eosinophilia in the setting of unexplained gastrointestinal symptoms and eosinophilic infiltration of the bowel.

Endoscopic and gross features of eosinophilic gastroenteritis obviously vary depending on localized versus more diffuse involvement and predominantly mucosal versus predominantly deeper level infiltration. In the more common situation of diffuse mucosal disease, the gastric mucosa often shows thickening with prominent folds and a cobblestone appearance. Endoscopically, nodular polypoid intraluminal masses can be observed, and polypoid filling defects can be seen by upper gastrointestinal imaging studies. In resection specimens in which there is predominant muscular involvement, the wall may be thickened and rigid and give a pale non-specific fibrous appearance on cut surface.

The histology of eosinophilic gastroenteritis is essentially that of dense and eosinophilic infiltration and is otherwise not specific. Various definitions of inclusion into studies ranging from eosinophil counts of 50 to 100/HPF have been employed, although there is no consensus as to what defines the borderline between upper normal and abnormal.[144, 161] Talley et al. defined eosinophilic gastroenteritis using three criteria:[161] (1) presence of gastrointestinal symptoms, (2) biopsies showing eosinophilic infiltration of one or more areas of the gastrointestinal tract from esophagus to colon, and (3) no evidence of paracytic or extraintestinal disease. In their study, abnormal eosinophilic infiltration was defined as at least 20 eosinophils per HPF, but no further attempt at exact quantification was undertaken. Mucosal involvement may be patchy, and multiple biopsies are indicated in patients for whom there is clinical suspicion. Mucosal biopsies overlying deep muscular or subserosal involvement may be normal. In fully characteristic biopsies, the eosinophilic infiltration is striking, constituting the majority of cells within the lamina propria with or without epithelial infiltration.

Differential Diagnosis

As previously indicated, the optimal interpretation of eosinophils within the stomach and remainder of the gastrointestinal tract is contingent on clinical and pathologic exclusion of more specific disorders. Differential diagnosis must include **intestinal vasculitis,** especially **polyarteritis nodosa, inflammatory bowel disease** (especially **Crohn's disease**), **parasitic infestation, peptic ulcer disease, gastric carcinoma, intestinal lymphoma,** and **hypereosinophilic syndrome.** Rarely **histiocytosis X** and **granulomatous gastritis** can present with conspicuous eosinophilic infiltration of the gastric mucosa.

Crohn's disease affects the upper gastrointestinal tract in a surprisingly high percentage of patients with this disorder, but in most this is a microscopic disease only. Such involvement occurs in one quarter to one half of adults with Crohn's disease, but involvement is even more frequent in children and adolescents in whom the stomach and duodenum may show microscopic disease in up to almost three quarters of patients.[163, 164] Rarely the stomach may be involved by Crohn's disease without other gastrointestinal manifestations.[165] A small percentage of patients with Crohn's colitis develop cologastric fistulas; an incidence of 0.6% was reported in one large series.[166] The histology of Crohn's disease is not different from elsewhere in the gastrointestinal tract. A wide array of non-specific and relatively specific histologic patterns may occur. In the absence of highly suggestive histology with granulomas, the diagnosis of Crohn's disease in the stomach should depend on a combination of clinical and histologic features because there is much overlap with the histologic patterns of peptic disease and gastritis. A brisk infiltrate of eosinophils may be seen in any of these injury patterns.

Ischemic Gastritis, Erosive Gastritis, and Stress Ulceration

Ischemic injury to the stomach is considered to be very rare owing to the rich blood supply and extensive collateral circulation. It has become apparent, however, that there is a spectrum of lesions that occurs within the stomach in which ischemia appears to play either a primary or an important contributing role. This spectrum includes **erosive gastritis, stress ulceration, drug-associated injury, chemical injury,** and **atherosclerotic (cholesterol) embolism.** These conditions have varied etiologic factors but are linked by a common histologic expression that underscores the role of cellular ischemia as a final pathway of injury.[167, 168]

Gastric Ischemia

Overt ischemic compromise to the stomach is unusual. Five arteries serve the stomach: (1) the left gastric arising from the celiac artery, (2) the right gastric arising from the hepatic artery, (3) the right gastroepiploic arising from the hepatic artery, (4) the left gastroepiploic arising from the splenic artery, and (5) the short gastric arteries arising from the splenic artery. All these vessels interanastomose at the level of the mucosa, making overt occlusive ischemic injury unusual. Nonetheless, lesser forms of ischemic injury to the gastric mucosa are more common, especially in elderly patients with cardiovascular compromise and in patients undergoing intense physiologic or psychological stress.[169] In our aging population, we will see an increased incidence of such ischemia-mediated episodes of gastric mucosa in hospitalized critically ill elderly patients.[42, 170] Although most such episodes are diagnosed by endoscopic appearance, the increasing clinical complexity of these patients will undoubtedly increase the number of biopsies seeking clarification of the clinical condition.

One source of both upper and lower gastrointestinal bleeding that follows local mucosal ischemia is **cholesterol embolism,** usually as a part of the cholesterol embolism syndrome.[171, 172] Multiple organ cholesterol showers can occur after angiography, vascular surgery, or anticoagulative therapy or as a spontaneous event.[171, 173] Gastric biopsies or resection specimens may show characteristic cholesterol clefts wedged within the lumina of small submucosal arteries. There may be intimal proliferation and ultimately obliterative sclerosis (Fig. 5–12). In older cases, a prominent giant-cell reaction can be seen within the vascular wall and adventitia.[174]

Erosive Gastritis

The pathogenesis of acute erosive and hemorrhagic forms of gastritis is multifactorial and complex and is betrayed by the relatively uniform histologic expression resulting from final common pathophysiologic modes of injury at a cell

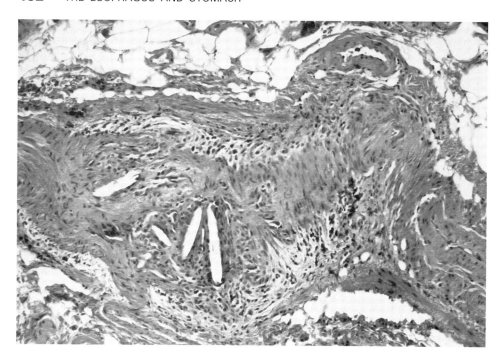

FIGURE 5–12. This submucosal artery was within a partial gastrectomy specimen removed for uncontrolled upper gastrointestinal bleeding. The patient had no definable risks for cholesterol embolism except generalized atherosclerosis. Note the intimal proliferation response to the embolism. (H&E, ×200)

level.[167, 175] The last few years have borne forth much new knowledge of mediators and mechanisms of gastric and duodenal mucosal injury.[168, 176] Recognition of the important role of prostaglandins and sulfhydryls as mediators of cytoprotection as well as a fuller understanding of mechanisms to cell injury rendered by hypoxia, chemical injury, and inflammatory/immune injury has led to recognition that a given pathologic injury expressed within the gastric mucosa usually follows a complex war between injurious and protective pathophysiologic mechanism.[167, 177] The degree to which these various factors impact on each other can result in a spectrum of outcomes ranging from minimal, clinically silent lesions to diffuse or massive necrotizing lesions resulting in necrosis, hemorrhage, and death. Mucosal biopsies may be received from patients virtually anywhere within this spectrum. Erosive gastritis is common in patients receiving aspirin and other non-steroidal anti-inflammatory drugs (NSAIDs) or in the setting of stress lesions in seriously ill patients.[42, 178, 179] In an autopsy study of 249 patients receiving NSAIDs, premortem non-specific ulcerations of the stomach and duodenum were observed in 22%.[178] Drug-associated gastric injury secondary to these agents is also on the rise in children.[180] The antrum is most sensitive to injury mediated by NSAIDs.[181] The endoscopist may see areas of diffuse erythema or mucosal hemorrhage or alternatively may see scattered erosions over the mucosal surface coated by white yellow exudate. These lesions either can occur within the fundus or the antrum or may be randomly located throughout the stomach.

The histology of erosive gastritis shares some similarities with early ischemic colitis. In very early lesions, which are seldom biopsied, there may be ectasia of mucosal capillaries, especially within the foveolar region and superficial glandular region of the mucosa. Coagulative necrosis of the luminalmost areas of the lamina propria associated with necrosis and sloughing of surface foveolar epithelial cells is characteristic of slightly more severe lesions. This process may be coated by a thin mucosanguineous pseudomembrane, all of which

may overlie a relatively intact lower mucosal compartment (Fig. 5–13). Again, similar to what occurs in the colon, viable epithelial cells at the interface between necrotic and nonnecrotic regions may show intense regenerative changes to the point of mimicking dysplasia or even *in situ* carcinoma. As the lesion evolves, there may be a brisk infiltrate of neutrophils ultimately accompanied by lymphocytes and plasma cells resulting in a histologic picture of gastritis that may not be distinguishable from non-erosive, non-specific forms of chronic gastritis. Interpretation of these biopsies is aided by knowledge of clinical history but may still be unresolvable in elderly patients owing to the high prevalence of chronic non-specific forms of gastritis, upon which may be superimposed more acute erosive forms of injury. In such cases, monitoring clinical progression may be the only means of determining appropriate interpretation. It is important, however, for the surgical pathologist to be mindful that both of these injury mechanisms can be co-expressed, especially in critically ill elderly patients.

Stress Ulceration of the Upper Gastrointestinal Tract

Many stress ulcers within the gastroduodenal mucosa are the more severe end of a spectrum that includes gastric hyperemia and erosive gastritis in compromised patients. Stress ulceration has a rich history in the surgical literature, including its recognition as a **Curling's ulcer** in burn patients, as a **Cushing's ulcer** in patients with cranial damage, and as sources of exsanguinating hemorrhage in patients who have suffered injuries from trauma, burns, sepsis, or intracranial events.[170] Again, there is evidence that mucosal ischemia is a common pathogenic factor.[167, 175, 182] Experimentation with animal models, confirmed in biopsy tissues of human patients, has shown that much of the cellular injury actually occurs during reperfusion.[168, 177] During this interval, reactive oxygen metabolites including superoxide, hydroxyl radical, and hydrogen peroxide are generated. These agents alter vascular

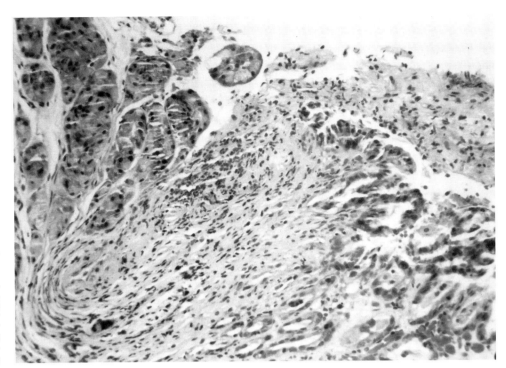

FIGURE 5–13. Superficial gastric ulceration of probable ischemic derivation in an elderly woman with severe postprandial pain (abdominal angina). At upper endoscopy the stomach showed diffuse areas of erythema and erosion. Here an area of coagulative necrosis of the gastric pit region is overlain by a thin fibrinoid membrane. (H&E, ×150)

permeability by directly injuring cell membranes of endothelial cells.

Stress ulcerations are usually confined to the mucosa and typically occur in the body and fundus of the stomach. They may be single or multiple and are usually small, measuring 1 cm or less. Histologically, their acute appearance is superficial coagulative necrosis and hemorrhage with minimal associated inflammation (Fig. 5–14). As the lesions evolve, however, a brisk neutrophilic infiltrate and ultimately a lymphoplasmacytic infiltrate complicates the acute appearance. In the patient who recovers, there is usually no structural after-math of the superficial stress ulcer in that minimal granulation tissue and fibrin deposition are precipitated. In those lesions, however, that involve the muscularis mucosae or penetrate into the submucosa, mucosal fibrosis may ensue.

Precancerous Lesions

Precursors of gastric carcinoma may be separated into two major categories: precancerous conditions and precancerous lesions.[19, 120] Precancerous conditions are clinical conditions

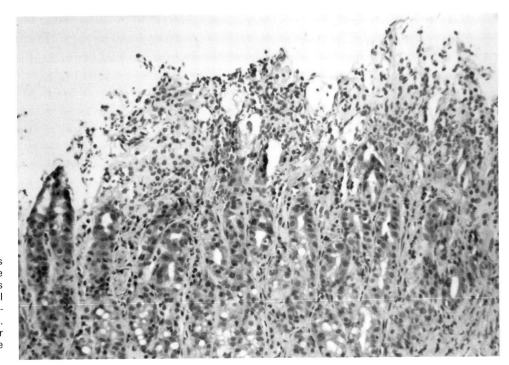

FIGURE 5–14. Superficial stress ulcer in a patient post-operative for common duct stones. In this illustration, there is superficial coagulative necrosis with no significant inflammatory response. Epithelial cells below the ulcer show vacuolar degenerative injury. (H&E, ×150)

associated with an increased risk of carcinoma and include severe chronic atrophic gastritis with intestinal metaplasia, post-gastrectomy state, immunodeficiency disorders, Menetrier's disease, and perhaps chronic gastric ulcer. Precancerous lesions, in contrast, are pathologic lesions and are essentially limited to two entities: epithelial dysplasia and adenomas. There is some overlap between these two lesions, as the epithelium that forms the gastric adenoma may be, and often is, described as dysplastic. In the following discussion, we first consider epithelial dysplasia as a discrete entity and then examine its presence and implication in the larger context of gastric adenomas.

Gastric Dysplasia

Gastric epithelial dysplasia lacks a uniformly accepted definition. In its broadest sense, dysplasia implies abnormal growth. Relative to the stomach, the Pathology Panel of the International Study Group on Gastric Cancer has defined dysplastic gastric epithelium as "one showing prominent cellular and structural abnormalities and believed to have high propensity to malignant transformation, irrespective of the presence or absence of metaplastic changes."[183] At least two factors, however, have complicated this understanding of dysplasia: (1) difficulty in recognition and grading of epithelial dysplasia, especially regarding its separation from regenerative changes, and (2) the clinical observation that dysplasia, especially mild to moderate grades, often spontaneously regresses.[184, 185] Thus, there are difficulties both in histologic recognition of gastric dysplasia and in defining the clinical implication for the patient in whom it is demonstrated.

The first hurdle facing the surgical pathologist confronted with an abnormal gastric biopsy that raises the question of dysplasia is triage into a hyperplastic versus a dysplastic category. The Pathology Panel of the International Study Group on Gastric Cancer has recognized and defined two categories of **hyperplasia:** simple and atypical.[186] Simple hyperplasia is distinguished from dysplasia in that the hyperplastic cells are uniform in size and shape with basally or centrally located nuclei (Fig. 5–15). Pseudostratification is absent or minimal. This process typically demonstrates maturation and differentiation toward the luminal surface. Atypical (or severe) hyperplasia describes a similar process of immature epithelium but one in which there is more pseudostratification and less luminal maturation (Fig. 5–16). Although this process may demonstrate minimal loss of polarity even in the surface region, the cells lack pleomorphism and abnormal mitoses, which would indicate dysplasia or carcinoma. This category of histologic change has, however, been recognized by other investigators as mild dysplasia or indefinite for dysplasia. Still others have used the term *severe hyperplasia* for this change. Ming, who uses the term *severe hyperplasia,* has observed that others classify these changes as mild dysplasia, but indicates that there is no evidence that it is premalignant.[187] We agree and concur with the Pathology Panel of the International Study Group on Gastric Cancer that these changes should be retained in a regenerative category and not considered precancerous.

Histologic features that distinguish dysplasia can be divided into architectural changes and cytologic changes (Table 5–2). Architectural changes of dysplasia include glandular crowding with back-to-back glands and irregular proliferation of glands with loss of luminal orientation. Cribriform pattern and cystic dilatation may also occur. Cytologic changes are manifested primarily in the nucleus and include hyperchromasia, enlarged nuclei with variation in size, prominent irregular nucleoli, and pseudostratification (Fig. 5–17). Frequent mitoses are usual, and atypical mitoses may be present. These changes occur throughout the length of the abnormal gland and are manifested on the luminal surface as well as deep within the glands. In contrast, features of regenerative hyperplasia not characteristic of dysplasia include relative maturation of the epithelium at the surface, immature cells concentrated at the base of the foveolae, hyperchromatic but basal nuclei, and enlarged but regular nucleoli.

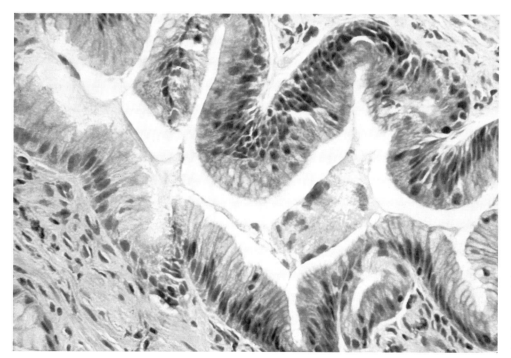

FIGURE 5–15. Simple hyperplasia within the foveolar type epithelium of a regenerative polyp. The nuclei are hyperchromatic but remain regular, basally located, and without nucleoli. Also, there is maturation toward the luminal surface (to the left in this field). (H&E, ×250)

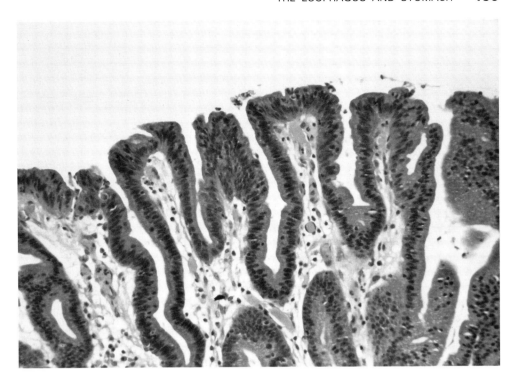

FIGURE 5–16. Severe hyperplasia of gastric foveolar epithelium showing incomplete maturation at the luminal surface and minimal stratification of nuclei. The nuclei are regular, however, and lack significant nuclear abnormalities of size and shape. (H&E, ×200)

Numerous grading systems exist for gastric dysplasia, including a commonly employed one that recognizes mild, moderate, and severe grades.[188] Other classifications recognize hyperplastic versus adenomatous type, whereas others recognize types according to the relationship to metaplastic lesions versus non-metaplastic epithelium. In the United States, where gastric dysplasia is uncommonly encountered, it seems reasonable to recognize high-grade and low-grade categories, as is done in the colon. In this schema, high-grade dysplasia would have histologic features similar to carcinoma *in situ*. This appears to be justified, in that prospective studies implicate only severely dysplastic epithelium as precancerous.[186, 189]

The significance of gastric dysplasia was the topic of an international symposium held in 1988.[186] Combined data from the several participating centers showed a strong association of carcinoma with severe dysplasia (54%) and a weak association with moderate dysplasia (9%). It was noted that the vast majority of carcinomas that were discovered by surveillance were found within 2 years of the diagnosis of dysplasia, and many were found immediately upon repeat endoscopic procedures. Because of this, a major conclusion of that symposium was that high-grade gastric dysplasia should be considered *para*cancerous rather than *pre*cancerous. This would indicate a need for immediate repeat endoscopy procuring numerous biopsies after demonstration of severe dysplasia.

Recommendations for management of patients in whom gastric dysplasia is demonstrated very significantly include on the aggressive side proposals for partial gastrectomy after the demonstration of severe dysplasia. The broader consensus, however, indicates that a more conservative approach with follow-up examination is indicated for low-grade dysplasia.[186] Some investigators have recommended follow-up intervals of 6 to 12 months for low-grade dysplasia and immediate reexamination with multiple biopsies for high-grade dysplasia. The existing data indicate that it is of paramount importance to search for a co-existing carcinoma for high-grade dysplasia patients. Until such carcinoma is found, frequent follow-up endoscopy with biopsy is indicated.[190–194]

Gastric Polyps

The primary challenge for the surgical pathologist who encounters a gastric polyp is to place it into one of two broad and general categories: neoplastic and non-neoplastic. Although this can usually be readily accomplished by recognition of the dysplastic or neoplastic epithelium that by definition is present in adenomas, separation from atypical regenerative changes within non-neoplastic polyps can be very difficult, especially on endoscopic biopsies. When available, study of multiple biopsies and of biopsies of adjacent mucosa to determine the presence or absence of gastritis can be useful to determine the nature of the overall pathologic process.[195] Adenomas tend to express their most

Table 5–2. **Histology of Regeneration versus Dysplasia**

Regeneration	Dysplasia
Maturation usually occurs at mucosal surface.	Maturation is lacking at the mucosal surface.
Mitoses are usually restricted to base of glands or pits.	Mitoses may occur at surface.
Nuclei are usually uniform in size and shape.	Nuclei are often irregular in size and shape.
Nuclei tend to be basal.	Nuclei are often stratified.
Nucleoli are usually modest and regular.	Irregular macronucleoli may be present.
Chromatin may appear increased, but is uniform.	Chromatin is often irregular and clumped.
Architectural pattern generally preserved; foveolar hyperplasia evident.	Cribriform and back-to-back glandular patterns may occur.
Regenerative changes non-uniform, accentuated near inflammation.	Dysplastic changes tend to be regionally uniform.

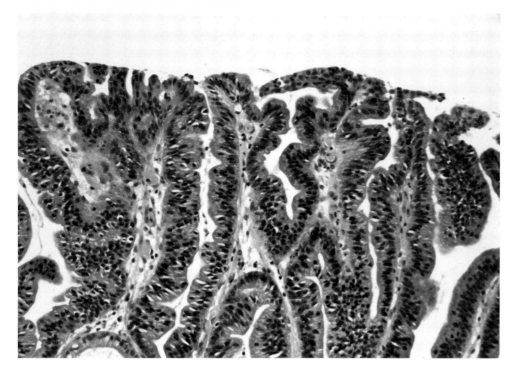

FIGURE 5-17. High-grade dysplasia of gastric mucosa adjacent to an invasive carcinoma in a gastrectomy specimen. Comparison with Figure 5-16 highlights irregular architectural features, including nuclear stratification and lack of surface maturation. Also, even at this low power, nucleoli and chromatin irregularities can be appreciated. (H&E, ×200)

severe dysplastic changes superficially, whereas regenerative atypia often occurs below an ulcerated surface or more toward the center of a lesion. This and the other criteria described previously and listed in Table 5-2 are applicable for recognizing hyperplasia versus dysplasia in both polypoid and flat mucosal lesions.

INCIDENCE. Gastric polyps are relatively uncommon but are encountered in approximately 3% to 5% of endoscopies. The majority of these lesions are non-neoplastic, with about three quarters of them being hyperplastic polyps. In most series, adenomas account for approximately 8% to 10% of lesions.

CLASSIFICATION. Classification of epithelial gastric polyps is confusing because of the numerous competing systems that have been published.[196-199] Most systems emphasize two general categories, with one being non-neoplastic and the second being neoplastic.[196] Table 5-3 provides a histologic classification of gastric polyps using this general approach.

Hyperplastic Polyps

Hyperplastic polyps typically occur in a background of chronic gastritis or other chronic injury process (such as post–partial gastrectomy). They are part of a spectrum ranging from inflammation and granulation tissue within the foveolar region of the mucosa to hyperplasia of foveolar epithelium through redundant overgrowth of this epithelium forming a nodule or polyp. This proposed mechanism maintains that hyperplastic polyps result from exuberant regenerative growth of the normal proliferative zone of the gastric epithelium located in the neck region of the gastric gland at the base of the foveolae as a consequence of chronic inflammation.[197] The foveolar overgrowth that forms the primary constituent of hyperplastic polyps may also occur diffusely, leading to prominent gastric folds.

The most common histology underlying **prominent gastric folds** is, in fact, hyperplastic foveolar epithelium,[197] a finding

that may induce both pathologist and endoscopist to surmise that they have not defined the lesion. In an analysis of 31 patients with hyperplastic gastropathy using full-thickness biopsies, 58% were found to have peptic ulcer disease with the prominent folds due to foveolar hyperplasia, edema, and inflammation.[200] The remainder of patients had **Zollinger-Ellison syndrome, Menetrier's disease,** or **hyperplastic hypersecretory gastropathy.**

Hyperplastic polyps are characterized histologically by dilated and elongated foveolae often with cystic formation. Usually the epithelial cells lining the cystic and elongated glands have the appearance of normal foveolar cells, but they may show proliferative change, including hyperchromatic nuclei, nucleoli, and abundant mucinous cytoplasm. Various degrees of inflammation may be evident within the lamina propria, and the surface may be eroded or ulcerated.

The most common diagnostic challenge occurring during examination of endoscopic biopsies of regenerative polyps is distinguishing between regenerative changes and dysplasia. In the setting of moderate to severe acute inflammation, the foveolar cells tend to extrude their mucus and undergo reparative regeneration, thereby creating a high nuclear to cytoplasmic ratio. Although prominent nucleoli may be present within the proliferating nuclei, they are typically uniform and lack the patchy hyperchromatism seen in truly dysplastic nucleus. Regenerative changes are also regionally non-uniform within the biopsy and tend to be most manifest near the inflammation, gradually undergoing transition to more normal-appearing epithelium even within the same gastric pit (Fig. 5-18). In those cases in which a determination of regenerative atypia versus low-level dysplasia cannot be made, it is prudent to establish absence of carcinoma deeper by cuts into the biopsy, but in its absence there is probably no further clinical significance of this distinction.

Historically it has been debated whether there is true malignant potential of hyperplastic polyps, with the vast abundance

Table 5–3. **Gastric Epithelial Polyps**

Non-neoplastic
Hyperplastic polyp
    Localized and diffuse
       foveolar hyperplasia
Inflammatory polyps
Hamartomas
    Fundic gland polyp
    Peutz-Jeghers polyp

Neoplastic
Adenomas
    Tubular
    Tubulovillous
    Villous
Polypoid carcinomas

of data indicating that this risk is exceedingly low. Nonetheless, there are well-documented case reports of carcinoma present within a regenerative polyp.[201] Because hyperplastic polyps have their genesis in atrophic gastritis, which also give rise to a higher likelihood of gastric carcinoma, some of these cases probably represent secondary invasion of a hyperplastic polyp by an otherwise unrelated carcinoma. Rare examples of mixed hyperplastic adenomatous polyps are encountered, and these are best classified as neoplastic polyps. These lesions typically have two histologic domains, with one clearly being adenoma and the other being hyperplastic. This is far less common than foci of marked regenerative atypia that occur within the inflamed hyperplastic polyp, and in general there appears to have been a tendency to overdiagnose regenerative and reparative changes within inflamed and ulcerated hyperplastic polyps as dysplasia.

Fundic Gland Polyps

A gastric polyp that is often underdiagnosed despite its relative frequency is the fundic gland polyp.[202–205] Fundic gland polyps are usually multiple, have a female predominance (about 4:1), and occur within the fundic (parietal/chief cell-bearing) region of the stomach. Unlike hyperplastic polyps, fundic gland polyps do not have an association with chronic gastritis, hypochlorhydria, or hypergastrinemia.[206] Their cystic dilatation within the lower portion and just deep to the foveolar region contributes to the speculation that the fundic gland polyp is a hamartoma of the gastric mucosa. The small cysts are lined by native gastric mucosal cells (mucous neck, parietal, and chief), which become atrophic as the cysts dilate (Fig. 5–19).

Fundic gland polyposis is linked to familial polyposis and is the most frequent gastric abnormality in this genetic syndrome.[203, 207] The lesions more commonly occur sporadically, however,[204, 205] and in neither case show intrinsic risk of malignant change.[208] Many appear, in fact, to regress spontaneously.[203, 209] The two most significant contributions to be made by a pathologist encountering a fundic gland polyp are to recognize it as a non-neoplastic lesion and to alert the endoscopist to the possible association with familial polyposis.

Adenomas

The histogenesis of gastric adenoma is incompletely understood, although its frequent relationship with atrophic gastritis and its histologic similarity to intestinal metaplasia suggest a relationship with chronic gastritis and intestinal metaplasia. In general, gastric adenomas resemble colonic adenomas, and they may be histologically indistinguishable. Intestinal features such as goblet cells, Paneth cells, argentaffin cells, acidic mucin, and occasionally a striated surface border help define the similarity to colonic lesions.

The World Health Organization's classification of gastric adenomas again reflects the similarities to those in the colon.[199] In this schema, gastric adenomas are divided into tubular, tubulovillous, and villous types. Microscopically flat and exo-

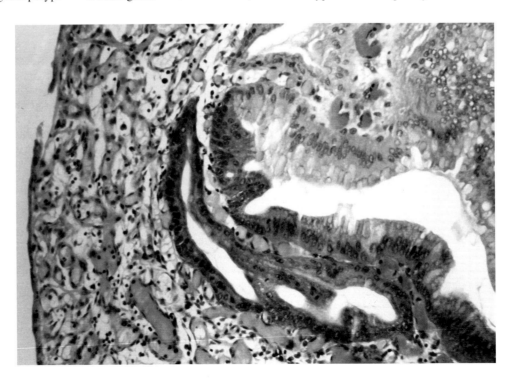

FIGURE 5–18. Atypical regenerative changes near the eroded surface of a hyperplastic gastric polyp. These nuclei show some features of true dyplasia, including stratification, variation in size and shape, and nucleoli. These changes are not striking, however, and, more importantly, were not uniform within regions of the polyp. They were most evident near areas of erosion or inflammation. These changes do not constitute "adenomatous foci." (H&E, ×200)

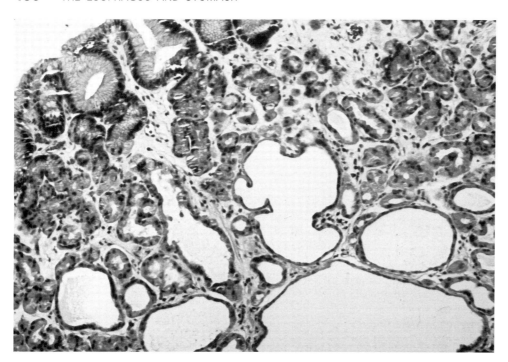

FIGURE 5–19. Fundic gland polyp. These presumedly hamartomatous lesions contain normal gastric mucosal elements. Characteristically cystic dilatation of gastric glands occurs immediately beneath the foveolae, as is illustrated in this biopsy. (H&E, ×150)

phytic (papillary) forms are recognized. Unlike hyperplastic polyps, adenomas are typically solitary, and when multiple, usually are no more than two or three.

DEPRESSED AND FLAT ADENOMAS. These morphologic variants of gastric adenoma deserve mention because of their potential unique biology and their potential gross and endoscopic confusion with variants of early gastric carcinoma. Depressed adenomas present as shallow depressions of the mucosa often along the lesser curvature and may not be recognized until after resection for another lesion.[210] When they are recognized by the endoscopist, the initial impression is often a depressed variant of early gastric carcinoma,[210–212] although they may also simulate a re-epithelialized peptic ulcer.[213] The adenomatous epithelium of the depressed adenoma occupies the entire thickness of the mucosa and is histologically and histochemically identical to non-depressed gastric adenomas.[211, 212] In spite of this, the depressed adenoma appears to have a higher malignant potential.[210, 212]

The flat adenoma presents to the endoscopist as a slightly raised or plaque-like lesion often having a central depression. Similar to adenomas in general, the adenomatous epithelium of this lesion is present without maturation at the surface. Dissimilar to other types, however, the neoplastic epithelium frequently occupies only the upper third to one half of the gastric mucosa. Deeper beneath the neoplastic epithelium, histologically normal mucosa is found lining glands that are often cystically dilated (Fig. 5–20). Characteristically, the level of dysplasia within this flat adenoma is only minimal to moderate. Mitoses are few, and follow-up studies have demonstrated that these lesions tend to be relatively stable without progression in size and may even regress.[214] In spite of this, however, these lesions are clearly neoplastic and have a relatively high incidence of malignant change. Similar to the depressed adenoma, the flat adenoma is typically small (less than 2 cm) and may be confused with a variant of early gastric carcinoma.

Papillary adenomas of the stomach are most common within the antrum and may grow as large as 10 cm or more, although the average size is 2 to 4 cm. Histologically, these lesions comprise neoplastic columnar cells often with pseudostratified nuclei located either basally or centrally within the cell. Unlike flat adenomas, papillary adenomas frequently show pleomorphism and abundant mitoses. A difficult task for the pathologist can be to distinguish high-grade dysplasia within an endoscopic biopsy from early carcinoma in these polypoid lesions. This challenge is ameliorated to some extent by the recognition that a neoplastic polyp within the stomach should be removed once its neoplastic nature is demonstrated independent of whether malignant transformation has occurred.

MALIGNANT TRANSFORMATION. Malignant change in gastric adenoma increases with the size of the lesion and grade of dysplasia. A wide range of malignant transformation has been reported—from 6% to 75%. Tsujitani et al. observed an 83% likelihood of associated carcinoma in adenomas larger than 4 cm, but this was much less likely in adenomas less than 2 cm.[215] Although flat adenomas have a lower incidence of malignant change than papillary adenomas, again, the degree of risk of change correlates with size and level of dysplasia. With the recognized risk of malignant transformation of the neoplastic epithelial polyp within the stomach, there is consensus that larger lesions (2 cm or above) should be endoscopically or surgically removed whenever possible.[215] For lesions smaller than 2 cm, a more conservative approach may be possible, in that these lesions seem to progress at a relatively slow rate.[210]

Gastrointestinal Stromal Tumors

The two major difficulties in diagnosis of gastrointestinal stromal tumors are division of benign from malignant and determination of cell of origin.

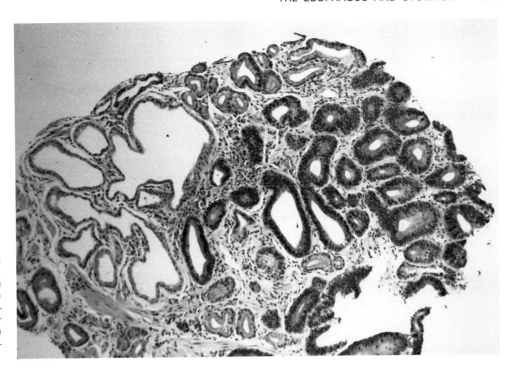

FIGURE 5–20. Small endoscopic biopsy of a gastric flat adenoma. The luminal epithelium (visible here in the right side of the field) shows relatively bland adenomatous epithelium. Deeper within the mucosa (to the left) are dilated non-neoplastic gastric glands. (H&E, ×150)

Criteria for dividing benign versus malignant smooth tumors of the gastrointestinal tract are not absolute. This division is best accomplished by using a constellation of gross and histologic parameters (Table 5–4).[22] Those most commonly employed are numbers of mitoses, cellularity, pleomorphism, necrosis, size of tumor, and location.[216–219]

The single most useful criterion for dividing benign versus malignant tumors has been number of mitoses, with most studies recognizing tumors containing at least 5 mitoses/10 HPF as being malignant.[216, 218] It is clear, however, that some tumors containing fewer mitoses or even no mitoses can behave aggressively.[218] In general, it has been observed that lesions with many mitoses (>10/50 HPF) probably behave aggressively and that tumors with fewer (<5/50 HPF) are less likely to do so. One study of 131 gastrointestinal stromal tumors found that all lesions with less than 2 mitoses/50 HPF were clinically benign provided they did not present as symptomatic lesions.[217]

Dense cellularity, particularly when combined with nuclear pleomorphism, predicts a tendency toward more aggressive behavior. Reproducible criteria that quantitate degree of cellularity with clinical correlation are not available, however. Lesions made up of cells containing uniform small round dense nuclei tend to behave aggressively.[22]

Pleomorphism has been recognized as predictive of malignant behavior in some gastric leiomyosarcomas.[218] This criterion must be used cautiously, however, as ischemic and degenerative changes can induce nuclear pleomorphism similar to that which occurs in uterine leiomyomas. Pleomorphism is also not invariable in malignant gastrointestinal smooth muscle tumors that metastasize, notably those with small uniform cells.

Tumor necrosis can be used as another indicator of malignant status, but necrosis may be seen occasionally in smooth muscle tumors that do not display malignant behavior. Necrosis is best assessed in conjunction with other histologic features in an overall determination of tumor grade.[220]

Size of tumor also correlates with biologic behavior in gastrointestinal smooth muscle tumors, although there is considerable variation in the literature as to which size should be employed to separate likely benign from likely malignant.[22] Five to 6 cm seems to be the criterion most commonly used for this purpose.[218–220]

Location of gastrointestinal stromal tumors may aid in prognostic assessment. Almost all smooth muscle tumors of the esophagus are benign. The stomach is a comparatively favorable location relative to the intestine and colon.[221] Within the stomach, gastrointestinal stromal tumors showing epithelioid

Table 5–4. **Guidelines for Grading Gastrointestinal Stromal Tumors**

Feature	Benign	Sarcoma, Low Grade	Sarcoma, High Grade
Mitoses	None	<5/10 HPF	5–10 or more/10 HPF
Cellularity	Sparse to moderate	Moderate	Dense
Pleomorphism	Absent to mild	Absent to mild	Moderate to marked
Necrosis	Usually absent	Absent to minimal	Minimal to marked
Location	May occur anywhere	Uncommon in esophagus	Uncommon in esophagus
DNA index	Diploid	Usually diploid	Usually aneuploid
Immunochemistry	Usually positive for multiple markers	Usually positive for multiple markers	Usually positive for few markers

histology are likely to be malignant when arising in the cardia or fundus, whereas they may be benign or malignant when occurring in the body or antrum.[22] Obviously invasion of the tumor either grossly or microscopically into adjacent structures or adjacent tissue indicates malignancy,[219, 222] but this is not commonly seen.

More recent analysis has suggested that DNA analysis and immunohistochemical characterization of gastrointestinal stromal tumors provide prognostic information. One study of 41 lesions observed that aneuploid status predicted adverse behavior.[223, 224] Lesions that express multiple markers of differentiation (smooth muscle actin, muscle specific actin, vimentin, and desmin) may have less aggressive biology than those that express vimentin alone.[225]

The large, histologically high-grade, mitotically active gastric smooth muscle tumor is easily recognized as sarcoma. Similarly a small circumscribed lesion with bland cells and no mitoses can be designated as at least probably benign. Those tumors with intermediate characteristics remain problematic, but by analyzing number of mitoses, cellularity, pleomorphism, necrosis, and size of tumor most lesions can be placed within a benign, borderline–probably benign, borderline–probably malignant, or malignant category.

A second topic that has received much recent attention relative to gastrointestinal stromal tumors has been consideration of cell of origin. It has long been assumed that most spindle cell neoplasms that arise within the gastrointestinal tract are in fact smooth muscle tumors; ultrastructural and immunohistochemical studies have indicated that a variable percentage of these lesions have apparent fibroblastic or schwannoid or even histocytic derivation.[142, 226] The ability of the cells making up these lesions to express more than one intermediate filament subtype, including keratin proteins,[36] complicates this issue and suggests that the cells are relatively immature and undifferentiated. Using a panel of antibodies, including four that indicated myoid differentiation, Franquemont and Frierson recently demonstrated at least one muscle marker in 85% of 46 tumors. Still, with the lack of overall consensus regarding histogenesis, the term *gastrointestinal stromal tumor* is often employed.[225]

Epithelioid stromal tumors of the gastrointestinal tract were first described in the English literature in detail in 1962 by Stout, having been described in the French literature 2 years earlier.[22] Since that time, there has been much speculation about the natural history, cell of origin, and appropriate name for these lesions. The terms **bizarre smooth muscle tumors** and **leiomyoblastoma** are still used, but **epithelioid smooth muscle tumor** appears to have gained widest usage and is endorsed by the World Health Organization. The most characteristic histologic feature of these neoplasms is cytoplasmic clearing around the nuclei, a feature that is a fixation artifact not present in cryostat-prepared sections (Fig. 5–21). Following the early description by Stout, epithelioid smooth muscle tumors tended to be described as neoplasms of intermediate biologic aggressiveness between benign and malignant smooth muscle tumors of routine histology. This impression undoubtedly is generated in part by the facts that (1) the vast majority of gastrointestinal epithelioid stromal tumors occur in the stomach, and (2) gastric stromal tumors in general have less aggressive biology than their intestinal counterparts.[22] Nonetheless, the assumption of intermediate aggressiveness has not held up under scrutiny.[22]

In their analysis of 127 gastric epithelioid leiomyomatous lesions, Appelman found no single criterion capable of dividing benign from malignant.[22] Features that in constellation predicted malignant behavior were (1) location in the cardia, fundus, or posterior wall, (2) clinical history of weight loss, (3) size of tumor, (4) microscopic evidence of infiltration, (5) size of tumor, (6) presence of small compact tumor cells, and (7) number of mitoses. Similar observations have been made relative to the overall spectrum of gastrointestinal stromal tumors by others. In his analysis of 56 gastrointestinal smooth muscle tumors, Evans found mitoses to be the strongest predictor of clinical behavior and observed no biologic significance for epithelioid histology.[216] He recommended that criteria for analysis of behavior be applied uniformly to all gastrointestinal smooth muscle cell tumors and that the term *leiomyoblastoma* be dropped. Apart from its strong tendency to occur in the stomach, epithelioid histology of gastrointestinal stromal tumors has no independent prognostic significance.

Gastric Lymphoma

In the 1990s, there is no area of gastric pathology in greater flux than gastric lymphoma. Great advances have been gained in understanding these lesions relative to their histogenesis, classification, and therapy. Nonetheless, more information will be required before unanswered questions in each of these areas can be resolved.[227] This section cannot provide a comprehensive review of the histogenesis and classification of gastrointestinal lymphomas, and the reader is referred to current reviews that detail these topics.[228–230] This section provides a brief overview of these issues and concentrates on methods of gastric biopsy interpretation of lymphoid infiltrates in the stomach.

The current understanding of malignant lymphomas affecting the gastric mucosa owes much to advances in understanding of the normal **mucosa-associated lymphoid tissue (MALT)**.[228, 231] Similar to the lungs, salivary glands, and other mucosal organs, the gastrointestinal tract has an intrinsic organized lymphoid tissue that is associated with the mucosa. These lymphoid tissues are most concentrated in Waldeyer's ring, Peyer's patches, and the appendix but are widely dispersed throughout most of the gut. Of interest for this discussion, lymphoid tissue is absent in the normal stomach but is acquired in response to various inciting agents such as *Helicobacter pylori* infection.[228, 232] MALT demonstrates several relatively specific features, including reactive follicles, prominent marginal zones, infiltration of the overlying epithelium by lymphocytes, and plasma cells located immediately beneath the surface epithelium.[228, 233] In normal and reactive MALT, there is a capacity and a tendency of mature lymphocytes to infiltrate glandular epithelium. These cells play a functional role in antigen recognition and processing within the gastrointestinal tract.

The major advance in understanding gastrointestinal lymphomas came with the recognition that there is a group of lymphomas that recapitulate the structure of native and aquired mucosa-associated lymphoid tissue (**MALT lymphomas).** This concept has been largely defined by Isaacson et al., who proposed the concept of low-grade B-cell lymphoma of mucosa-associated tissue.[229] Similar to the lymphoid tissue

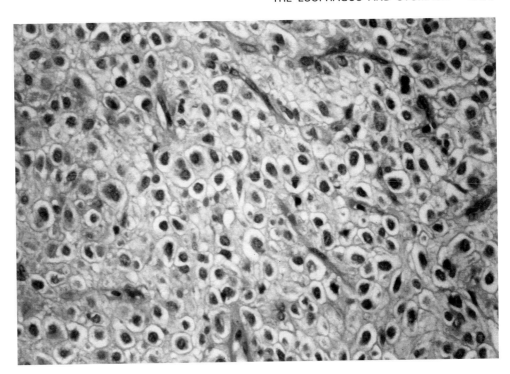

FIGURE 5–21. Epithelioid smooth muscle tumor of stomach demonstrating the characteristic perinuclear cytoplasmic clearing. These lesions usually have bland nuclear features, but are assessed for malignant potential in the same fashion as other gastrointestinal smooth muscle tumors (see text and Table 5–4). (H&E, ×250)

of Waldeyer's ring and Peyer's patches, the structure of low-grade MALT lymphomas is that of a lymphoid follicle surrounded by a diffuse infiltration of B cells that infiltrate glandular epithelium, resulting in characteristic lymphoepithelial complexes. The neoplastic cells of the perifollicular infiltrate are slightly larger than small lymphocytes and have more abundant cytoplasm and irregular nuclear outlines. These features cause them to resemble small cleaved cells or centrocytes, resulting in designation of the term *centrocyte-like cells (CLCs)*. These relatively innocuous appearing CLCs are now known to be the lesional cells of conditions formerly called **pseudolymphoma** and **benign lymphoepithelial lesion.**[231, 234]

Histologically, there are two broad categories of lymphomas that occur primarily within the gastric mucosa: low grade and intermediate to high grade. The general principles for biopsy recognition of these two types differ somewhat. Most gastric lymphomas (about 75%) are intermediate to high grade. Here the diagnostic difficulty is not so much recognizing the presence of a malignant neoplasm but distinguishing poorly differentiated carcinoma from large-cell lymphoma. The two primary diagnostic tools beyond morphology are mucin histochemistry and immunohistochemistry. Mucin stains demonstrate acid mucin in many poorly differentiated carcinomas and allow their division from malignant lymphoma. Beyond this, immunohistochemical analysis with markers for epithelial cells versus lymphoid cells resolves most cases. A standard diagnostic approach uses keratin antibodies for recognition of carcinomas and leukocyte common antigen antibodies for recognition of lymphomas.

Low-grade lymphomas of the stomach are diagnostically more challenging.[235] The clinical questions are also broader, in that separation from benign inflammatory conditions such as chronic gastritis and lymphoid reaction about benign ulcers is often a major question raised by endoscopic biopsies. Reliable morphologic criteria are now defined that allow recognition of these low-grade lymphomas by morphology alone in

many cases.[110, 236] As mentioned previously, these low-grade MALT lymphomas have histologic features that are reminiscent of native or acquired MALT. These features include prominent reactive-appearing follicles with neoplastic cells occupying marginal zones, a mixture of small lymphocytes and small atypical cells that resemble cleaved follicular center cells or centrocytes, monocytoid cells with more abundant cytoplasm, and neoplastic plasma cells usually distributed in distinct subepithelial or interfollicular zones. Occasional follicles contain an excess of cleaved or monocytoid cells. Finally the CLCs tend to infiltrate glandular epithelium, resulting in the characteristic lymphoepithelial complex. Zukerberg et al. defined the **lymphoepithelial complex** of MALT lymphomas as infiltration of mucosal epithelium by small aggregates (three to six cells) of lymphoid cells located inside the glandular basement membrane[110] (Fig. 5–22). Clusters of plasma cells tend to be located in superficial subepithelial locations and may be either reactive or part of neoplasm. When they are neoplastic, they often display intranuclear Dutcher bodies. Recognition of these features in endoscopic biopsies of low-grade gastric lymphomas can allow diagnosis or a high level of suspicion.[110, 236] In a comparison of 25 low-grade gastric lymphomas with 58 benign inflammatory infiltrates in the stomach, Zukerberg et al. recognized the following features to be associated with lymphomas: prominent (2–3 or more) lymphoepithelial complexes, Dutcher bodies, and moderate cytologic atypia.[110] One or more of these three features was present in 18 of 25 gastric lymphomas. Features less specific for low-grade lymphoma included dense lymphoid aggregates, rare or questionable lymphoepithelial lesions, muscularis mucosae invasion by lymphoid tissue, ulceration, and mild cytologic atypia. Finally, germinal centers, crypt abscesses, and reactive epithelial atypia were seen with equal frequency in both neoplastic and non-neoplastic categories.

In a study of endoscopic biopsies from 29 patients with gastric lymphoma, Arista-Nasr et al. noted that diagnostic

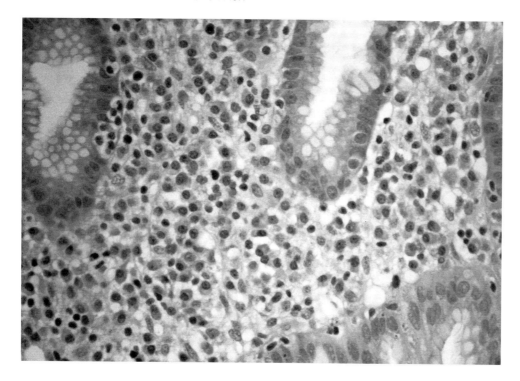

FIGURE 5–22. Low-grade mucosa-associated lymphoid tissue B-cell lymphoma showing a characteristic lymphoepithelial complex within the gland in the left side of the field. (H&E, ×250)

errors can occur because of morphologic similarity of lymphoid infiltration in chronic gastritis and/or peptic ulcer disease with low-grade lymphoma.[236] They indicated, however, that careful morphologic study using the following criteria usually allows diagnosis or a high level of suspicion: (1) marked increase in density of the lymphoid infiltrate in the gastric mucosa, (2) massive substitution of gastric glands by lymphoid infiltration, and (3) lymphocytes infiltrating and partially destroying glandular epithelium (the lymphoepithelial complex) (Fig. 5–23).

Although histologic criteria of low-grade mucosa-based lymphomas are now well defined, it is nonetheless true that endoscopic biopsies are often insufficient to conclusively discriminate lymphoma from reactive lymphoid processes.[237] In these cases, the diagnostic pathologist should be prepared to employ phenotypic and genotypic methods of analysis.[233, 237–239] Immunohistochemical stains for kappa or lamda light chain can be used on paraffin sections and may identify a monoclonal plasmacytic component. Utilization of these antibodies in paraffin-embedded tissue may be difficult,

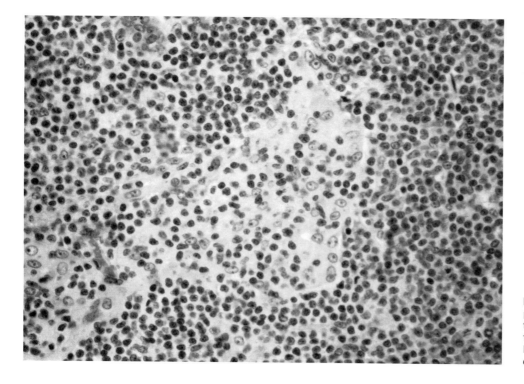

FIGURE 5–23. Advanced lymphoepithelial complex wherein the gland in the center of the field is heavily infiltrated and largely destroyed by neoplastic centrocyte-like cells. (H&E, ×250)

however, even in the hands of highly experienced histotechnicians and pathologists. It is therefore preferable to have mucosal biopsies that have been quick frozen to $-70°C$ for more reliable analysis. Utilizing such tissues, immunochemical stains for kappa and lamda light chain may show light chain restriction in the surface immunoglobulins of the CLCs. In addition, these neoplastic cells are usually reactive for pan-B cell markers such as CD19, CD20, or CD22 (alternatively B-4, B-1, or Leu-14). Whether these assays are immediately available or obtainable by consultation, the diagnostic pathologist must be prepared to handle and triage endoscopic biopsies for complete analysis. Specific recommendations for the gastric biopsy containing a lymphoid infiltrate are offered in the following paragraph.

In any gastric biopsy demonstrating a poorly differentiated malignant neoplasm, mucin stains may be employed to facilitate recognition of poorly differentiated carcinomas. If this fails, a panel of immunostains with epithelial markers (keratin) and lymphoid markers (leukocyte common antigen) may be employed to differentiate high-grade lymphoma from poorly differentiated carcinoma. In the biopsy containing a mature-appearing lymphoid infiltrate, careful histologic study using the criteria outlined previously often allows segregation of reactive processes from low-grade lymphoma. In equivocal cases, however, it is advisable to employ further studies. In cases in which there is well-preserved paraffin-embedded tissue, immunohistochemical analysis for kappa and lamda chains might be employed to document monoclonality. This failing, additional biopsies should be requested and quickly frozen for phenotypic and genotypic analysis. In any case, if there is a pre-endoscopic suspicion of lymphoma, delay can be avoided by rapidly freezing some of the biopsies procured before fixation. Cryosections can be examined to determine whether there is indication for additional studies and the tissue triaged appropriately without the necessity of returning for additional biopsies.[237]

Early recognition of mucosa-based malignant lymphomas appears to be important prognostically.[240] One recent study of 240 gastric lymphomas concluded that the major prognostic factors for survival were low stage, low-grade histology, and surgical resectability.[241] A similar study of 145 primary gastric lymphomas reached very similar conclusions, with low stage, low grade, and resectability being favorable features.[242] Although the prognosis for early-stage, low-grade lymphomas is good, late recurrence is not uncommon, likely caused in part by the recognized multifocality of these lymphomas within the gastric mucosa.[232] This demonstrated multifocality and recognized propensity for recurrence indicate that these patients should be followed up with regular endoscopy and gastric biopsy.

Finally, the lesion of **gastric pseudolymphoma** should be specifically addressed. Sufficient clinical, immunophenotypic, and genetic data now exist to conclude that this lesion represents low-grade B-cell lymphoma in an early indolent form.[243-245] Current recommendations for therapy for this lesion differ and range from frequent endoscopic surveillance with biopsies[244] to immediate treatment by surgical excision.[243, 246] In general, once the diagnosis of gastric lymphoma is established, most patients are counseled to receive therapy.[247] Whether this is indicated in all patients with the indolent form of low-grade lymphoma formerly called pseudolymphoma is a question awaiting further clinical data.

References

1. Ming S-C: Tumors of the esophagus and stomach. In Ming S-C: Atlas of Tumor Pathology 7, second series. Bethesda, MD, Armed Forces Institute of Pathology, 1973, p 16.
2. Colina F, Solis JA, Munoz MT: Squamous papilloma of the esophagus. A report of three cases and review of the literature. Am J Gastroenterol 74:410–414, 1980.
3. Enterline H, Thompson J: Benign epithelial tumors and plaques. In Enterline H, Thompson J (eds): Pathology of the Esophagus. New York, Springer-Verlag, 1984, pp 128–144.
4. Orlowska J, Jarosz D, Gugulski A, et al: Squamous cell papillomas of the esophagus: Report of 20 cases and literature review. Am J Gastroenterol 89:434–437, 1994.
5. Walker JH: Giant papilloma of the thoracic esophagus. Am J Roentgenol 131:519–520, 1978.
6. Carr NJ, Monihan JM, Sobin LH: Squamous cell papilloma of the esophagus: A clinicopathologic and follow-up study of 25 cases. Am J Gastroenterol 89:245–248, 1994.
7. Frootko NJ, Rogers JH: Oesophageal papillomata in the child. J Laryngol Otol 92:823–827, 1978.
8. Nuwayhid NR, Ballard ET, Cotto R: Esophageal papillomatosis. Ann Otol Rhinol Laryngol 86:623–625, 1977.
9. Winkler B, Capo V, Rwumann W, et al: Human papillomavirus infection of the esophagus. A clinicopathological study with demonstration of papillomavirus antigen by the immunoperoxidase technique. Cancer 55:149–155, 1985.
10. Lee RG: Adenomas arising in Barrett's esophagus. Am J Clin Pathol 85:629–632, 1986.
11. Weidner N: Sarcomatoid carcinoma of the upper aerodigestive tract. Semin Diagn Pathol 4:157–168, 1987.
12. Iyomasa S, Kato H, Tachimori Y, et al: Carcinosarcoma of the esophagus: A twenty case study. Jpn J Clin Oncol 20:99–106, 1990.
13. Xu L, Sun C, Wu LH, et al: Clinical and pathological characteristics of carcinosarcoma of the esophagus: Report of four cases. Ann Thorac Surg 37:197–203, 1984.
14. Gal AA, Martin SE, Kernen JA, Patterson MJ: Esophageal carcinoma with prominent spindle cells. Cancer 60:2244–2250, 1987.
15. Agha FP, Keren DF: Spindle-cell squamous carcinoma of the esophagus: A tumor with biphasic morphology. AJR 145:541–545, 1985.
16. Kuhajda FP, Sun TT, Mendelsohn G: Polypoid squamous carcinoma of the esophagus. A case report with immunostaining for keratin. Am J Surg Pathol 7:495–499, 1983.
17. Osamura RY, Shimamura K, Hata J, et al: Polypoid carcinoma of the esophagus. A unifying term for "carcinosarcoma" and "pseudosarcoma." Am J Surg Pathol 2:201–208, 1978.
18. Iezzoni JC, Mills SE: Sarcomatoid carcinomas (carcinosarcomas) of the gastrointestinal tract: A review. Semin Diagn Pathol 10:176–187, 1993.
19. Hanada M, Nakano K, Yamashita H: Carcinosarcoma of the esophagus with osseous and cartilaginous production. A combined study of keratin immunochemistry and electron microscopy. Acta Pathol Jpn 34:669–678, 1984.
20. Battifora H: Spindle cell carcinoma. Ultrastructural evidence of squamous origin and collagen production by the tumor cells. Cancer 37:2275–2282, 1976.
21. DuBoulay CEH, Isaacson P: Carcinoma of the esophagus with spindle cell features. Histopathology 5:403–414, 1981.
22. Appelman HD: Mesenchymal tumors of the gut: Historical perspectives, new approaches, new results, and does it make any difference? In Goldman H, Appelman HD, Kaufman N (eds): Gastrointestinal Pathology. Baltimore, Williams & Wilkins, 1990, pp 220–246.
23. Isolauri J, Mattila J, Kallioniemi OP: Primary undifferentiated small cell carcinoma of the esophagus: Clinicopathological and flow cytometric evaluation of eight cases. J Surg Oncol 46:174–177, 1991.
24. Martin MR, Kahn LB: So-called pseudosarcoma of the esophagus. Nodal metastases of the spindle cell element. Arch Pathol Lab Med 101:604–609, 1977.
25. Minielly JA, Harrison EG, Fontana FS, et al: Verrucous squamous cell carcinoma of the esophagus. Cancer 20:2078–2087, 1967.
26. Biemond P, ten Kate FJW, van Blankenstein M: Esophageal verrucous carcinoma: Histologically a low-grade malignancy but clinically a fatal disease. J Clin Gastroenterol 13:102–107, 1991.
27. Yates DR, Koss LS: Paget's disease of the esophageal epithelium. Report of first case. Arch Pathol 86:447–452, 1968.
28. Nonomura A, Kimura A, Mizukami Y, et al: Paget's disease of the esophagus. J Clin Gastroenterol 16:130–135, 1993.
29. Beyer KL, Marshall JB, Diaz-Arias AA, et al: Primary small-cell carcinoma of the esophagus. Report of 11 cases and review of the literature. J Clin Gastroenterol 13:135–141, 1991.
30. Nichols GL, Kelsen DP: Small cell carcinoma of the esophagus. The Memorial Hospital experience 1970–1987. Cancer 64:1531–1533, 1989.
31. Attar BM, Levendoglu H, Rhee H: Small cell carcinoma of the esophagus. Report of three cases and review of the literature. Dig Dis Sci 35:145–152, 1990.
32. Mulder LD, Gardiner GA, Weeks DA: Primary small cell carcinoma of the esophagus: Case presentation and review of the literature. Gastrointest Radiol 16:5–10, 1991.
33. Tennvall J, Johansson L, Albertsson M: Small cell carcinoma of the esophagus: A clinical and immunohistopathological review. Eur J Surg Oncol 16:109–115, 1990.

34. McCullen M, Vyas SK, Winwood PJ, et al: Long-term survival associated with metastatic small cell carcinoma of the esophagus treated by chemotherapy, autologous bone marrow transplantation, and adjuvant radiation therapy. Cancer 73:1–4, 1994.

35. Nishimaki T, Suzuki T, Fukuda T, et al: Primary small cell carcinoma of the esophagus with ectopic gastrin production. Report of a case and review of the literature. Dig Dis Sci 38:767–771, 1993.

36. Tauchi K, Tsutsumi Y, Yoshimura S, et al: Immunohistochemical and immunoblotting detection of cytokeratin in smooth muscle tumors. Acta Pathol Jpn 40:574–580, 1990.

37. Kishida H, Sodemoto Y, Ushigome S, et al: Non-oat cell small cell carcinoma of the esophagus. Report of a case with ultrastructural observation. Acta Pathol Jpn 33:403–413, 1983.

38. Kelsen DP, Weston E, Kurtz R, et al: Small cell carcinoma of the esophagus. Treatment by chemotherapy alone. Cancer 45:1558–1561, 1980.

39. Hussein AM: Combination chemotherapy and radiotherapy for small-cell carcinoma of the esophagus. Am J Clin Oncol 13:369–373, 1990.

40. Sasajima K, Watanabe M, Ando T, et al: Serum neuron-specific enolase as a marker of small-cell carcinoma of the esophagus. J Clin Gastroenterol 12:384–388, 1990.

41. Chong FK, Graham JH, Madoff IM: Mucin-producing carcinoid (''composite tumor'') of upper third of esophagus. A variant of carcinoid tumor. Cancer 44:1853–1859, 1979.

42. Reusser P, Gyr K, Scheidegger D, et al: Prospective endoscopic study of stress erosions and ulcer in critically ill neurosurgical patients. Crit Care Med 18:270–274, 1990.

43. Brenner S, Heimlich H, Widman M: Carcinoid of esophagus. N Y State J Med 69:1337–1339, 1969.

44. Kikuchi Y, Tsuneto Y, Kawai T, et al: Choriocarcinoma of the esophagus producing chorionic gonadotropin. Acta Pathol Jpn 38:489–499, 1988.

45. McKechnie JC, Fechner RE: Choriocarcinoma and adenocarcinoma of the esophagus with gonadotropin secretion. Cancer 27:694–702, 1971.

46. Trillo A, Accettullo LM, Yeiter TL: Choriocarcinoma of the esophagus: Histologic and cytologic findings—a case report. Acta Cytol 23:69–74, 1979.

47. Wasan HS, Schofield JB, Krausz T, et al: Combined choriocarcinoma and yolk sac tumor arising in Barrett's esophagus. Cancer 73:514–517, 1994.

48. Sasano N, Abe S, Satake O, et al: Choriocarcinoma mimicry of an esophageal carcinoma with urinary gonadotrophic activities. Tohoku J Exp Med 100:153–163, 1970.

49. Agha FP, Schnitzer B: Esophageal involvement in lymphoma. Am J Gastroenterol 80:412–416, 1985.

50. Adachi Y, Mori M, Iida M, et al: Inflammatory fibroids polyp of the stomach. Report of three unusual cases. J Clin Gastroenterol 15:154–158, 1992.

51. Tsang WYW, Chan JKC: KP-1 staining for granular cell neoplasms: Is KP-1 a marker for lysosomes rather than histiocytic lineage? Histopathology 21:84–86, 1992.

52. Birkenfeld S, Noiman G, Krispin M, et al: The incidence and significance of serum hCG and CEA in patients with gastrointestinal malignant tumors. Eur J Surg Oncol 15:103–108, 1989.

53. Blaauwgeers JLG, Allema JH, Bosma A, et al: Early adenoid cystic carcinoma of the upper esophagus. Eur J Surg Oncol 16:77–81, 1990.

54. Cerar A, Jutersek A, Vidmar S: Adenoid cystic carcinoma of the esophagus. A clinicopathologic study of three cases. Cancer 67:2159–2164, 1991.

55. Kim JH, Lee MS, Cho SW, et al: Primary adenoid cystic carcinomas of the esophagus: A case report. Endoscopy 23:38–41, 1991.

56. Petursson SR: Adenoid cystic carcinoma of the esophagus: Complete response to chemotherapy. Cancer 57:1464–1467, 1986.

57. Fenoglio-Preiser CM, Lantz PE, Listrom MB, et al: Gastrointestinal Pathology. An Atlas and Text. New York, Raven Press, 1989, p 101.

58. Sweeney EC, Cooney T: Adenoid cystic carcinoma of the esophagus: A light and electron microscopic study. Cancer 45:1516–1525, 1980.

59. Epstein JI, Sears DL, Tucker RA, et al: Carcinoma of the esophagus with adenoid cystic differentiation. Cancer 53:1131–1136, 1984.

60. Lam KY, Dickens P, Loke SL, et al: Squamous cell carcinoma of the oesophagus with mucin-secreting component (muco-epidermoid carcinoma and adenosquamous carcinoma): A clinicopathologic study and a review of literature. Eur J Surg Oncol 20:25–31, 1994.

61. Kay S: Mucoepidermoid carcinoma of the esophagus. Report of two cases. Cancer 22:1053–1059, 1968.

62. Bell-Thompson J, Haggitt RC, Ellis FH: Mucoepidermoid and adenoid cystic carcinomas of the esophagus. J Thorac Cardiovasc Surg 79:438–446, 1980.

63. Sasajima K, Watanabe M, Takubo K, et al: Mucoepidermoid carcinoma of the esophagus: Report of two cases and review of the literature. Endoscopy 22:140–143, 1990.

64. Fegelman E, Law SY, Fok M, et al: Squamous cell carcinoma of the esophagus with mucin-secreting component. Mucoepidermoid carcinoma. J Thorac Cardiovasc Surg 107:62–67, 1994.

65. Takubo K, Nakagawa H, Tsuchiya S, et al: Seedling leiomyoma of the esophagus and esophagogastric junction zone. Hum Pathol 12:1006–1010, 1981.

66. Serametis MG, Lyons WS, deBuzman VC, et al: Leiomyomata of the esophagus—an analysis of 838 cases. Cancer 38:2166–2177, 1976.

67. Hendel RC, Cuenoud HF, Giansiracusa DF, et al: Multiple cholesterol emboli syndrome. Bowel infarction after retrograde angiography. Arch Intern Med 149:2371–2374, 1989.

68. Kabuto T, Taniguchi K, Iwanaga T, et al: Diffuse leiomyomatosis of the esophagus. Dig Dis Sci 25:388–391, 1980.

69. Cohen SR, Thompson JW, Sherman NJ: Congenital stenosis of the lower esophagus associated with leiomyoma and leiomyosarcoma of the gastrointestinal tract. Ann Otol Rhinol Laryngol 97:454–459, 1988.

70. Schapiro RL, Sandrock AR: Esophagogastric and vulvar leiomyomatosis: A new radiologic syndrome. J Can Assoc Radiol 24:184–187, 1973.

71. Lonsdale RN, Roberts PF, Vaughn R, et al: Familial oesophageal leiomyomatosis and nephropathy. Histopathology 20:127–133, 1992.

72. Kaymakcalan H, Sequeria W, Baretta R, et al: Hypertrophic osteoarthropathy with myogenic tumors of the esophagus. Am J Gastroenterol 74:17–20, 1980.

73. Gentry RW, Dockerty MB, Clagett OT: Vascular malformations and vascular tumors of the gastrointestinal tract. Int Abstr Surg 88:281–323, 1949.

74. Schmidt HW, Clagett OT, Harrison EG Jr: Benign tumors and cysts of the esophagus. J Thorac Cardiovasc Surg 41:717–732, 1961.

75. Hanel JH, Talley NA, Hunt DR: Hemangioma of the esophagus: An unusual case of upper gastrointestinal bleeding. Dig Dis Sci 26:257–263, 1981.

76. Feist JH, Siconolfi EP, Gilman E: Giant cavernous hemangioma of the esophagus. JAMA 235:1146–1147, 1976.

77. Enzinger FM, Weiss SW: Soft Tissue Tumors. St. Louis, CV Mosby, 1983, pp 745–753.

78. Paskin DL, Hull JD, Cookson PS: Granular cell myoblastomas: A comprehensive review of 15 years experience. Ann Surg 175:501–504, 1972.

79. Johnson J, Helwig EB: Granular cell tumors of the gastrointestinal tract and perianal region. A study of 74 cases. Dig Dis Sci 26:807–816, 1981.

80. Coutinho DS, Soga J, Yoshikawa T, et al: Symptomatic granular cell tumors of esophagus. A report of two cases and review of the literature. Am J Gastroenterol 80:758–762, 1985.

81. Sarma DP, Rodriquez FH, Deiparine EM, et al: Symptomatic granular cell tumor of the esophagus. J Surg Oncol 33:246–249, 1986.

82. Cappell MS, Lebwohl O: Esophageal dysmotility from a small granular cell tumor. J Clin Gastroenterol 13:432–435, 1991.

83. Meroni E, Spinelli P, Cerrai F: Esophageal miliary granular cell tumor [letter]. Gastrointest Endosc 35:274, 1984.

84. Rubesin S, Herlinger H, Sigal H: Granular cell tumors of the esophagus. Gastrointest Radiol 10:11–15, 1985.

85. Ohmori T, Arita N, Uraga N, et al: Malignant granular cell tumor of the esophagus. A case report. Acta Pathol Jpn 37:775–783, 1987.

86. Brady PG, Nord HJ, Connar RG: Granular cell tumors of the esophagus: Natural history, diagnosis and therapy. Dig Dis Sci 33:1329–1333, 1988.

87. Obiditsch-Mayer I, Salzer-Kuntschik M: Malignant ''granular cell neuroma,'' so-called ''myoblastoma'' of the esophagus. Beitr Pathol Anat 125:357–373, 1961.

88. Wyatt MG, O'Donoghue DS, Clarke TJ, et al: Malignant granular cell tumor of the esophagus. J Surg Oncol 17:388–391, 1991.

89. Penagini R, Ranzi T, Velio P, et al: Giant fibrovascular polyp of the oesophagus: Report of a case and effects on oesophageal function. Gut 30:1624–1629, 1989.

90. Jang GC, Clouse ME, Fleischner FG: Fibrovascular polyp—a benign intraluminal tumor of the esophagus. Radiology 30:1624–1629, 1969.

91. Li Volsi VA, Perzin KH: Inflammatory pseudotumors (inflammatory fibrous polyps) of the esophagus: A clinicopathologic study. Am J Dig Dis 20:475–481, 1975.

92. Wolf BC, Khettry U, Leonardi HK, et al: Benign lesions mimicking malignant tumors of the esophagus. Hum Pathol 19:148–154, 1988.

93. Mahour GH, Harrison EG Jr: Osteochondroma (tracheobronchial choristoma) of the esophagus. Report of a case. Cancer 20:1489–1493, 1967.

94. Assor D: A melanocytic tumor of the esophagus. Cancer 35:1438–1443, 1975.

95. Carney JA: Psammomatous melanocytic schwannoma—a distinctive, heritable tumor with special associations including cardiac myxoma and Cushing's syndrome. Am J Surg 14:206–222, 1990.

96. Lee YTN: Leiomyosarcoma of the gastrointestinal tract: General pattern of metastasis and recurrence. Cancer Treat Rev 10:91–101, 1983.

97. Weinstein EC, Kim YS: Leiomyosarcoma of the esophagus. Mil Med 153:206–209, 1988.

98. Vario T, Nickels J, Hockerstedt K, et al: Rhabdomyosarcoma of the esophagus. Light and electron microscopic study of a rare tumor. Virchows Arch A Pathol Anat Histopathol 386:357–361, 1980.

99. Willen R, Lillo-Gil R, Willen H, et al: Embryonal rhabdomyosarcoma of the esophagus—case report. Acta Chir Scand 155:59–64, 1989.

100. Danzig JB, Brandt LJ, Reinus JF, et al: Gastrointestinal malignancy in patients with AIDS. Am J Gastroenterol 86:715–718, 1991.

101. Sobhani I, Rene E: Kaposi's sarcoma of the gut in acquired immune deficiency syndrome. Eur J Gastroenterol Hepatol 4:404–408, 1992.

102. Siegel JH, Janis R, Alper JC, et al: Disseminated visceral Kaposi's sarcoma. Appearance after human renal allograft homograph operation. JAMA 207:1493–1496, 1969.

103. Amr SS: Synovial sarcoma of the esophagus. Am J Otolaryngol 5:266–269, 1984.

104. Bloch MJ, Iozzo RV, Edmunds LH, et al: Polypoid synovial sarcoma of the esophagus. Gastroenterology 92:229–233, 1987.

105. Baca I, Klempa I, Weber JT: Liposarcoma of the esophagus. Eur J Surg Oncol 17:313–315, 1991.

106. Cooper GJ, Boucher NR, Smith JHF, et al: Liposarcoma of the esophagus. Ann Thorac Surg 51:1012–1013, 1991.

107. Mansour KA, Fritz RC, Jacobs DM, et al: Pedunculated liposarcoma of the esophagus: A first case report. J Thorac Cardiovasc Surg 86:447–450, 1983.

108. Yates SP, Collins MC: Case report: Recurrent liposarcoma of the esophagus. Clin Radiol 42:356–358, 1990.
109. McIntyre M, Webb JN, Browning CGP: Osteosarcoma of the esophagus. Hum Pathol 13:680–682, 1982.
110. Zukerman LR, Ferry JA, Southern JF, et al: Lymphoid infiltrates of the stomach. Evaluation of histologic criteria for the diagnosis of low-grade gastric lymphoma on endoscopic biopsy specimens. Am J Surg Pathol 14:1087–1099, 1990.
111. Haratake J, Jimi A, Horie A, et al: Malignant mesenchymoma of the esophagus. Acta Pathol Jpn 34:925–933, 1984.
112. Mills SE, Cooper PH: Malignant melanoma of the digestive system. In Sommers S, Rosen P (eds): Pathology Annual, Part 2, Vol 18. Norwalk, CT, Appleton-Century-Crofts, 1983, pp 1–26.
113. Sabanathan S, Eng J, Pradhan GN, et al: Primary malignant melanoma of the esophagus. Am J Gastroenterol 84:1475–1481, 1989.
114. Scotto J, Fraumeni JF, Lee JAH: Melanoma of the eye and other non-cutaneous sites: Epidemiologic aspects. J Natl Cancer Inst 56:489–491, 1976.
115. Tateishi R, Taniguchi H, Wada A, et al: Argyrophil cells and melanocytes in esophageal mucosa. Arch Pathol 8:87–89, 1974.
116. DasGupta TK, Brasfield RD: Malignant melanoma of the gastrointestinal tract. Arch Surg 88:969–973, 1964.
117. Hamdy FC, Smith FHF, Kennedy A, et al: Long term survival after excision of a primary malignant melanoma of the oesophagus. Thorax 46:397–398, 1991.
118. Rosenberg SA, Diamond HD, Jaslowicz B, Craver LF: Lymphosarcoma: A review of 1269 cases. Medicine 40:31–84, 1961.
119. Dawson IMP, Cornes JS, Morson BC: Primary malignant lymphoid tumors of the intestinal tract. Br J Surg 49:80–89, 1961.
120. Nagani M, Lavigne BC, Siskind BN, et al: Primary non-Hodgkin's lymphoma of the esophagus. Arch Intern Med 149:193–195, 1989.
121. Mengoli M, Marchi M, Rota E, et al: Primary non-Hodgkin's lymphoma of the esophagus. Scand J Gastroenterol 85:737–741, 1990.
122. Stein HA, Murray D, Warner HA: Primary Hodgkin's lymphoma of the esophagus. Dig Dis Sci 26:457–461, 1981.
123. Ahmed N, Ramos S, Sika J, et al: Primary extramedullary esophageal plasmacytoma. First case report. Cancer 38:943–947, 1976.
124. Dayal Y: Neuroendocrine cells and their proliferative lesions. In Norris HT (ed): Pathology of the Colon, Small Intestine and Anus, 2nd ed. New York, Churchill Livingstone, 1991, pp 305–366.
125. Solcia E, Sessa F, Rindi, et al: Classification and histogenesis of gastroenteropancreatic endocrine tumors. Eur J Clin Invest 20(suppl 1):S72–S81, 1990.
126. Lewin KJ: The endocrine cells of the gastrointestinal tract. The normal endocrine cells and their hyperplasias. In Sommer SC, Rosen PP, Fechner RE (eds): Pathology Annual, Vol 21. Norwalk, CT, Appleton-Century-Crofts, 1986, pp 1–27.
127. Borch K: Atrophic gastritis and gastric carcinoid tumors. Ann Med 21:291–297, 1989.
128. Borch K, Renvall H, Liedberg G: Gastric endocrine cell hyperplasia and carcinoid tumors in pernicious anemia. Gastroenterology 88:638–648, 1985.
129. Solcia E, Fiocca R, Villani L, et al: Morphology and pathogenesis of endocrine hyperplasias, precarcinoid lesions, and carcinoids arising in chronic atrophic gastritis. Scand J Gastroenterol 26(suppl 180):146–159, 1991.
130. Lewin KJ, Yang K, Ulcich T, et al: Primary gastrin cell hyperplasia: Report of five cases and a review of the literature. Am J Surg Pathol 8:821–832, 1984.
131. Keuppens F, Willems G, Degraef J, et al: Antral gastrin cell hyperplasia in patients with peptic ulcer. Ann Surg 191:276–281, 1980.
132. Graham DY, Lew GM, Lechago J: Antral G-cell and D-cell numbers in Helicobacter pylori infection: Effect of H. pylori eradication. Gastroenterology 104:1655–1660, 1993.
133. Itsuno M, Watanabe H, Iwafuchi M, et al: Multiple carcinoids and endocrine cell micronests in type A gastritis. Their morphology, histogenesis and natural history. Cancer 63:881–890, 1989.
134. Berendt RC, Jewell LD, Shnitka TK, et al: Multicentric gastric carcinoid complicating pernicious anemia. Origin from the metaplastic endocrine cell population. Arch Pathol Lab Med 113:399–403, 1989.
135. Sjoblom SM, Sipponen P, Karonen SL: Mucosal argyrophil endocrine cells in pernicious anemia and upper gastrointestinal carcinoid tumors. J Clin Pathol 42:371–377, 1989.
136. Bordi C, Yu J-Y, Baggi MT, et al: Gastric carcinoids and their precursor lesions. A histologic and immunohistochemical study of 23 cases. Cancer 67:663–672, 1991.
137. Nosaka T, Habu H, Endo M, et al: Multiple carcinoid tumors of the stomach with hypergastrinemia. Am J Gastroenterol 87:766–770, 1992.
138. Solcia E, Rindi G, Silini E, Villani L: Enterochromaffin-like (ECL) cells and their growths: Relationships to gastrin, reduced acid secretion and gastritis. Baillieres Clin Gastroenterol 7:149–165, 1993.
139. Stockbrugger RW, Menon GG, Beilby JO, et al: Gastroscopic screening in 80 patients with pernicious anemia. Gut 24:1141–1147, 1983.
140. Hirshcowitz BI, Griffin J, Pellegrin D, et al: Rapid progression of enterochromaffinlike cell gastric carcinoids in pernicious anemia after antrectomy. Cancer 102:1409–1418, 1992.
141. Solcia E, Capella C, Fiocca R, et al: The gastroenteropancreatic endocrine system and related tumors. Gastroenterol Clin North Am 18:671–693, 1989.
141a. Godwin JD: Carcinoid tumors: An analysis of 2,837 cases. Cancer 36:560–569, 1975.
142. Hurlimann J, Gardiol D: Gastrointestinal stromal tumours: An immunohistochemical study of 165 cases. Histopathology 19:311–320, 1991.

143. Kern SE, Yardley JH, Lazenby AJ, et al: Reversal by antrectomy of endocrine cell hyperplasia in the gastric body in pernicious anemia, a morphometric study. Mod Pathol 3:561–566, 1990.
144. Blackshaw AJ, Levison DA: Eosinophilic infiltrates of the gastrointestinal tract. J Clin Pathol 39:1–7, 1986.
145. Goldman H, Proujansky R: Allergic proctitis and gastroenteritis in children. Clinical and mucosal biopsy features in 53 cases. Am J Surg Pathol 10:75–86, 1986.
146. Gleich GJ, Ottesen EA, Leiferman KM, et al: Eosinophils and human disease. Int Arch Allergy Appl Immunol 88:59–62, 1989.
147. Spry CJF: Eosinophil Structure, Constituents, and Metabolism in Eosinophils, a Comprehensive Review and Guide to the Scientific and Medical Literature. Oxford University Press, 1988, pp 48–65.
148. Walsh RE, Gaginella TS: The eosinophil in inflammatory bowel disease. Scand J Gastroenterol 26:1217–1224, 1991.
149. Johnstone JM, Morson BC: Inflammatory fibroid polyp of the gastrointestinal tract. Histopathology 2:349–361, 1978.
150. Shimer GR, Helwig EB: Inflammatory fibroid polyps of the intestine. Am J Clin Pathol 81:708–714, 1984.
151. Harned RK, Buck JL, Shekitka KM: Inflammatory fibroid polyps of the gastrointestinal tract: Radiologic evaluation. Radiology 182:863–866, 1992.
152. Assarian GS, Sundareson A: Inflammatory fibroid polyp of the ileum. Hum Pathol 16:488–493, 1985.
153. Dawson PM, Shousha S, Burn JI: Inflammatory fibroid polyp of the small intestine presenting as intussusception. Br J Clin Pract 44:495–497, 1990.
154. Kolodziejczyk P, Yao T, Tsuneyoshi M: Inflammatory fibroid polyp of the stomach. A special reference to an immunohistochemical profile of 42 cases. Am J Surg Pathol 17:1159–1168, 1993.
155. Trillo AA, Rowden G: The histogenesis of inflammatory fibroid polyps of the gastrointestinal tract. Histopathology 19:431–436, 1991.
156. Ali J, Qi W, Hanna SS, Huang SN: Clinical presentations of gastrointestinal inflammatory fibroid polyps. Can J Surg 35:194–198, 1992.
157. Tada S, Iida M, Yao T, et al: Endoscopic removal of inflammatory fibroid polyps of the stomach. Am J Gastroenterol 86:1247–1250, 1991.
158. Case records of the Massachusetts General Hospital. Weekly clinicopathological exercises. Case 20–1992. N Engl J Med 326:1342–1349, 1992.
159. Cello JP: Eosinophilic gastroenteritis—a complex disease entity. Am J Med 67:1097–1114, 1979.
160. Lee CM, Changchien CS, Chen PC, et al: Eosinophilic gastroenteritis: 10 years experience. Am J Gastroenterol 88:70–74, 1993.
161. Talley NJ, Shorter RG, Phillips SF, et al: Eosinophilic gastroenteritis: A clinicopathologic study of patients with disease of the mucosa, muscle layer and subserosal layers. Gut 31:34–38, 1990.
162. Klein NC, Hargrove MD, Sleisenger MH, et al: Eosinophilic gastroenteritis. Medicine 49:299–311, 1970.
163. Cameron DJ: Upper and lower gastrointestinal endoscopy in children and adolescents with Crohn's disease: A prospective study. J Gastroenterol Hepatol 6:355–358, 1991.
164. Lenaerts C, Roy CC, Vaillancourt M, et al: High incidence of upper gastrointestinal tract involvement in children with Crohn disease. Pediatrics 83:777–781, 1989.
165. Cary ER, Tremaine WJ, Banks PM, et al: Isolated Crohn's disease of the stomach. Mayo Clin Proc 64:776–779, 1989.
166. Greenstein AJ, Present DH, Sachar DB, et al: Gastric fistulas in Crohn's disease. Report of cases. Dis Colon Rectum 32:888–892, 1989.
167. Cho CH, Koo MW, Garg GP, et al: Stress-induced gastric ulceration: Its aetiology and clinical implications. Scand J Gastroenterol 27:257–262, 1992.
168. Szabo S: Gastroduodenal mucosal injury—acute and chronic: Pathways, mediators and mechanisms. J Clin Gastroenterol 13(suppl 1):S1–S8, 1991.
169. Johnston G, Vitikainen K, Knight R, et al: Changing perspective on gastrointestinal complications in patients undergoing cardiac surgery. Am J Surg 163:525–529, 1992.
170. Chueng LY: Thomas G Orr Memorial Lecture. Pathogenesis, prophylaxis and treatment of stress gastritis. Am J Surg 156:437–440, 1988.
171. Lie JT: Cholesterol atheromatous embolism. The great masquerader revisited. Pathol Ann 27(Pt 2):17–50, 1992.
172. Moolenaar W, Lamers CB: Cholesterol crystal embolization and the digestive system. Scand J Gastroenterol 188(Suppl):69–72, 1991.
173. Fine MJ, Kapoor W, Falanga V: Cholesterol crystal embolization: A review of 221 cases in the English literature. Angiology 38:769–784, 1987.
174. Kennedy A, Cumberland D, Gaines P: The pathology of cholesterol embolism arising as a complication of intra-aortic catheterization. Histopathology 15:515–521, 1989.
175. Pilchman J, Lefton HB, Braden GL: Cytoprotection and stress ulceration. Med Clin North Am 75:853–863, 1991.
176. Silen W: What is cytoprotection of the gastric mucosa? Gastroenterology 94:232–235, 1988.
177. Schiessel R, Feil W, Wenzl E: Mechanism of stress ulceration and implications for treatment. Gastroenterol Clin North Am 19:101–120, 1990.
178. Allison MC, Howatson AG, Torrance CV, et al: Gastrointestinal damage associated with the use of nonsteroidal antiinflammatory drugs. N Engl J Med 327:749–754, 1992.
179. Soll AH: Non-steroidal anti-inflammatory drugs and peptic ulcer. Ann Intern Med 114:307–319, 1991.
180. Gryboski JD: Peptic ulcer disease in children. Med Clin North Am 75:889–902, 1991.

181. Hoftiezer JM, O'Laughlin JC, Ivey KJ: Effects of 24 hours of aspirin, Bufferin, paracetamol and placebo on human gastrointestinal mucosa. Gut 23:692–697, 1982.
182. Martin LF: Stress ulcers are common after aortic surgery. Endoscopic evaluation of prophylactic therapy. Am Surg 60:169–174, 1994.
183. Ming S-C, Bajtai A, Correa P, et al: Gastric dysplasia: Significance and pathological criteria. Cancer 54:1794–1801, 1984.
184. Armbrecht U, Stockbrugger RW, Rode J, et al: Development of gastric dysplasia in pernicious anaemia: A clinical and endoscopic follow up study of 80 patients. Gut 31:1105–1109, 1990.
185. Coma del Corral MJ, Pardo-Mindla FJ, Razquin S: Risk of cancer in patients with gastric dysplasia. Follow up study of 67 patients. Cancer 65:2078–2085, 1990.
186. Ming S-C: Significance of epithelial dysplasia in the esophagus and stomach. Endoscopy 21:38–45(S), 1989.
187. Ming S-C: Adenocarcinoma and other malignant tumors of the stomach. In Ming S-C, Goldman H (eds): Pathology of the Gastrointestinal Tract. Philadelphia, WB Saunders, 1992, pp 584–618.
188. Morson BC, Sobin LH, Grundmann E, et al: Precancerous conditions and epithelial dysplasia in the stomach. J Clin Pathol 72:711–721, 1980.
189. Saraga EP, Gardiol D, Costa J: Gastric dysplasia: A histologic follow up study. Am J Surg Pathol 11:788–796, 1987.
190. de Dombal FT, Price AB, Thompson H, et al: The British Society of Gastroenterology early gastric cancer/dysplasia survey: An interim report. Gut 31:115–120, 1990.
191. Di Gregorio C, Morandi P, Fante R, et al: Gastric dysplasia. A follow-up study. Am J Gastroenterol 88:1714–1719, 1993.
192. Lansdown M, Quirke P, Dixon MF, et al: High grade dysplasia of the gastric mucosa: A marker for gastric carcinoma. Gut 31:977–983, 1990.
193. Rugge M, Baffa R, Farinata F, et al: Epithelial dysplasia in atrophic gastritis. Bioptical follow up study. Ital J Gastroenterol 23:70–73, 1991.
194. Sipponen P: Gastric dysplasia. Curr Top Pathol 81:61–76, 1990.
195. Nakano H, Persson B, Slezak P: Study of the gastric mucosal background in patients with gastric polyps. Gastrointest Endosc 36:39–42, 1990.
196. Elster K: Histologic classification of gastric polyps. Curr Top Pathol 63:77–93, 1976.
197. Koch HK, Lesch R, Cremer M, Oehlert W: Polyps and polypoid foveolar hyperplasia in gastric biopsy specimens and their precancerous prevalence. Front Gastrointest Res 4:183–191, 1979.
198. Nakamura T, Nakano G: Histologic classification and malignant change in gastric polyps. J Clin Pathol 38:754–764, 1985.
199. Oota K, Sobin LH: Histologic typing of gastric and esophageal tumors. In International Classification of Tumours. Geneva, 18:37, 1977.
200. Komorowski RA, Caya JG: Hyperplastic gastropathy. Clinicopathologic correlation. Am J Surg Pathol 15:577–585, 1991.
201. Orlowska J, Pietrow D: Multifocal gastric carcinoma arising from hyperplastic and adenomatous polyps. Am J Gastroenterol 85:1629–1634, 1990.
202. Deppisch LM, Rona VT: Gastric epithelial polyps. A 10 year study. J Clin Gastroenterol 11:110–115, 1989.
203. Iida M, Tsuneyoshi Y, Itoh H, et al: Natural history of fundic gland polyposis in patients with familial adenomatous coli/Gardner's syndrome. Gastroenterology 89:1021–1025, 1985.
204. Kinoshita Y, Tojo M, Yano T, et al: Incidence of fundic gland polyps in patients without familial adenomatous polyposis. Gastrointest Endosc 39:161–163, 1993.
205. Lee RS, Burt RW: The histopathology of fundic gland polyposis. Am J Clin Pathol 86:498–503, 1986.
206. Haruma K, Sumii K, Yoshihara M, et al: Gastric mucosa in female patients with fundic glandular polyps. J Clin Gastroenterol 13:565–569, 1991.
207. Domizio P, Talbot IC, Spigelman AD, et al: Upper gastrointestinal pathology in familial adenomatous polyposis: Results from a prospective study of 102 patients. J Clin Pathol 43:738–743, 1990.
208. Hizawa K, Iida M, Matsumoto T, et al: Natural history of fundic gland polyposis without familial adenomatosis coli: Follow-up observations in 31 patients. Radiology 189:429–432, 1993.
209. Iida M, Tsuneyoshi Y, Hidenobu W, et al: Spontaneous disappearance of fundic gland polyposis: Report of three cases. Gastroenterology 79:725–728, 1980.
210. Nakamura K, Sakaguchi H, Enjoji M: Depressed adenoma of the stomach. Cancer 62:2197–2202, 1988.
211. Ito H, Yasui W, Yoshida K, et al: Depressed tubular adenoma of the stomach: Pathological and immunohistochemical features. Histopathology 17:419–426, 1990.
212. Xuan ZX, Ambe K, Enjoji M: Depressed adenoma of the stomach, revisited. Histologic, histochemical and immunohistochemical profiles. Cancer 67:2382–2389, 1991.
213. Coma-del-Corral MJ, Carretero-Albinana L, Ojeda-Gimenez C: Depressed adenoma of the stomach. Conceptual review of five cases. J Clin Gastroenterol 13:353–357, 1991.
214. Kamiya T, Morishita T, Asakura H, et al: Long term follow-up study on gastric adenoma and its relationship to gastric protruded carcinoma. Cancer 50:2496–2503, 1982.
215. Tsujitani S, Furusawa M, Hayashi I: Morphological factors aid in therapeutic decisions concerning gastric adenomas. Hepatogastroenterology 39:56–58, 1992.
216. Evans HL: Smooth muscle tumors of the gastrointestinal tract: A study of 56 cases followed for a minimum of 10 years. Cancer 56:2242–2250, 1985.
217. Morgan BK, Compton C, Talbert M, et al: Benign smooth muscle tumors of the gastrointestinal tract. A 24-year experience. Ann Surg 211:63–66, 1990.
218. Ranchod M, Kempson RL: Smooth muscle tumors of the gastrointestinal tract and retroperitoneum: A pathologic analysis of 100 cases. Cancer 39:255–262, 1977.
219. Shiu MH, Farr GH, Papchristou DN, et al: Myosarcoma of the stomach: Natural history, prognostic factors and management. Cancer 49:177–187, 1982.
220. Grant CS, Kim CH, Farrugia G, et al: Gastric leiomyosarcoma. Prognostic factors and surgical management. Arch Surg 126:985–990, 1991.
221. Ueyama T, Guo KJ, Hashimoto H, et al: A clinicopathologic and immunohistochemical study of gastrointestinal stromal tumors. Cancer 69:947–955, 1992.
222. Ng EH, Pollock RE, Munsell MF, et al: Prognostic factors influencing survival in gastrointestinal leiomyosarcomas. Implications for surgical management and staging. Ann Surg 215:68–77, 1992.
223. Kiyabu MT, Bishop PC, Parker JW, et al: Smooth muscle tumors of the gastrointestinal tract. Flow cytometric quantitation of DNA and nuclear antigen content and correlation with histologic grade. Am J Surg Pathol 12:954–960, 1988.
224. Suzuki H, Sugihira N: Prognostic value of DNA ploidy in primary gastric leiomyosarcoma. Br J Surg 80:1549–1550, 1993.
225. Franquemont DW, Frierson HF: Muscle differentiation and clinicopathologic features of gastrointestinal stromal tumors. Am J Surg Pathol 16:947–954, 1992.
226. Pike AM, Lloyd RV, Appelman HD: Cell markers in gastrointestinal stromal tumors. Hum Pathol 19:830–834, 1988.
227. Thomas CR: Update on gastric lymphoma. J Natl Med Assoc 83:713–718, 1991.
228. Harris NL: Extranodal lymphoid infiltrates and mucosa-associated lymphoid tissue (MALT). A unifying concept. Am J Surg Pathol 15:879–884, 1991.
229. Isaacson P, Spenser J: Malignant lymphoma of mucosal associated lymphoid tissue. Histopathology 11:445–462, 1987.
230. Levison DA, Hall PA, Blackshaw AJ: The gut associated lymphoid tissue and its tumors. Curr Top Pathol 81:133–175, 1990.
231. Isaacson PG: Lymphomas of mucosa associated lymphoid tissue (MALT) [abstract]. Am J Surg Pathol 16:201–202, 1992.
232. Wotherspoon AC, Doglioni C, Isaacson PG: Low grade gastric B-cell lymphoma of the mucosa-associated lymphoid tissue (MALT): A multifocal disease. Histopathology 20:29–34, 1992.
233. Spenser J, Finn T, Pulford K, et al: The human gut contains a novel population of B lymphocytes which resemble marginal zone cells. Clin Exp Immunol 62:607–612, 1985.
234. Nizze H, Cogliatti SB, von Schilling C, et al: Monocytoid B cell lymphoma: Morphologic variants and relationship to low-grade lymphoma of the mucosa-associated lymphoid tissue. Histopathology 18:403–414, 1991.
235. Seifert E, Schulte F, Weismuller J, et al: Endoscopic and bioptic diagnosis of malignant non-Hodgkin's lymphoma of the stomach. Endoscopy 25:497–501, 1993.
236. Arista-Nasr J, Jimenez A, Keirns C, et al: The role of endoscopic biopsy in the diagnosis of gastric lymphoma: A morphologic and immunohistochemical reappraisal. Hum Pathol 22:339–348, 1991.
237. Osborne BM, Pugh WC: Practicality of molecular studies to evaluate small lymphocytic proliferations in endoscopic gastric biopsies. Am J Surg Pathol 16:838–844, 1992.
238. Fend F, Schwaiger A, Weyrer K, et al: Early diagnosis of gastric lymphoma: Gene rearrangement analysis of endoscopic biopsy samples. Leukemia 8:35–39, 1994.
239. van Krieken JH, Raffeld M, Raghoebier S, et al: Molecular genetics of gastrointestinal non-Hodgkin's lymphomas: Unusual prevalence and pattern of c-myc rearrangements in aggressive lymphoma. Blood 76:797–800, 1990.
240. Aozasa K, Ueda T, Kurata A, et al: Prognostic value of histologic and clinical factors in 56 patients with gastrointestinal lymphoma. Cancer 61:309–315, 1988.
241. Radaszkiewicz T, Dragosics B, Bauer P: Gastrointestinal malignant lymphomas of the mucosa-associated lymphoid tissue. Gastroenterology 102:1628–1638, 1992.
242. Cogliatti SB, Schmid U, Schmacher U, et al: Primary B-cell lymphoma: A clinicopathological study of 145 patients. Gastroenterology 101:1159–1170, 1991.
243. Schulman H, Sickel J, Klienman MS, et al: Gastric "pseudolymphoma" with restricted light chain expression in a patient with obscure gastrointestinal blood loss. Dig Dis Sci 36:1495–1499, 1991.
244. Schwartz MS, Sherman H, Smith T, et al: Gastric pseudolymphoma and its relationship to gastric lymphoma. Am J Gastroenterol 84:1555–1559, 1989.
245. Szabo S, Spill WF, Rainsford KD: Non-steroidal anti-inflammatory drug-induced gastropathy. Mechanisms and management. Med Toxicol Adverse Drug Exp 4:77–94, 1989.
246. Sweeny JF, Muus C, McKeown PP, et al: Gastric pseudolymphoma. Not necessarily a benign lesion. Dig Dis Sci 37:939–945, 1992.
247. Frazee RC, Roberts J: Gastric lymphoma treatment. Medical versus surgical. Surg Clin North Am 72:423–431, 1992.

CHAPTER 6

Small Intestine

Shirin Nash, M.D.

DIFFERENTIAL DIAGNOSIS OF ULCERS/STRICTURES IN SMALL INTESTINAL RESECTIONS

Segmental resections of small intestine are submitted for pathologic examination most often as a result of surgery for acute abdominal emergencies. When not related to trauma, neoplasm, or congenital anomalies, the etiology of intestinal ulcers/strictures is often unclear, and the final pathologic diagnosis requires knowledge of specific pathologic features as well as accurate historical data. A correct diagnosis is important not only for prognosis and therapy in any individual case but also for epidemiologic reasons.

The major non-neoplastic causes of small intestinal ulcers/strictures in the adult population are ischemia, iatrogenic causes, and inflammation/infection.

Ischemia

Ischemic ulcers in the small intestine can result from multiple causes, but the majority are due to thromboembolic occlusion of mesenteric arteries or veins and non-occlusive ischemia resulting from a combination of low blood flow or vascular spasm superimposed on moderate to severe atherosclerotic vascular disease. The clinical and pathologic features of each of these are quite well defined.

Arterial Ischemia

Acute mesenteric ischemia is caused by **thromboembolic occlusion of the superior mesenteric artery** (SMA) in 40% to 50% of cases.[1] The patients are elderly, with severe poorly localized visceral pain with or without occult or gross upper or lower gastrointestinal bleeding and with peritoneal signs present in the most severe cases. When all three major gastrointestinal arteries are involved, patients may suffer from chronic ischemia with "abdominal angina," which includes postprandial pain, weight loss, flatulence, constipation, and diarrhea.[1,2] Chronic low flow can progress to acute infarction. Both occlusive and non-occlusive causes result in the easily recognized infarcted intestine with hemorrhagic mucosal necrosis and submucosal and mural edema combined with transmural necrosis in the most severe cases. Less severe injury can result in stricture formation 2 to 8 weeks after the original injury. If this segment is resected because of luminal stenosis and obstruction, the appearances are those of a chronic active ulcer with loss of villous morphology and a flat re-epithelialized surface on a fibrotic submucosa and muscularis propria. Evidence of earlier hemorrhage may be apparent as hemosiderin deposits in the submucosa, and any reactive serosal changes may have converted to serosal adhesions. Examination of the vessels in the resected specimen must be performed but may be unrewarding because the occluded vessels are usually proximal to the mesenteric resection. The differential diagnosis includes ulcers/strictures caused by drugs or radiation and Crohn's disease. Occasionally small intestinal ischemic ulcers may be caused by **atheroemboli** in small distal arteries in the submucosa, and identification of this feature can clinch the etiologic diagnosis of an ischemic ulcer[3] (Fig. 6–1).

Gastrointestinal involvement has been reported in approximately 28% of patients with **systemic vasculitis,** with most cases occurring in patients with polyarteritis nodosa and less often in patients with Wegener's granulomatosis and Churg-Strauss syndrome.[4] Clinical features are similar to those in patients with other causes of ischemia, with occasional fatal outcome related to intestinal vasculitis. Biopsy may show only non-specific inflammation and ulceration with mucosal hemorrhage. Vasculitis is rarely detected even in resected specimens, and diagnosis is often based on clinical signs of associated renal disease and skin rash. Ischemic ulcers due to **arteritis** have also been reported in patients with rheumatoid arthritis.[5] Intestinal infarction may occur without any other systemic manifestations of rheumatoid vasculitis. The pathologic features include a necrotizing vasculitis and a proliferative endarteritis without necrosis of the vessel wall, which can segmentally involve the distal mesenteric arteries.[5] Infarcts in these cases are characteristically multiple and segmental, and lesions may be of varying ages. Buerger's disease has also been reported to involve intestinal arteries and veins, with distal mesenteric vessels occluded by organized and recent thrombi containing microabscesses associated with mild inflammation in the vessel walls.[6] Diagnosis is based on the presence of disease in peripheral extremity vessels presenting before or after the intestinal manifestations in a patient who is a heavy smoker.[7] Intestinal infarction with perforation and peritonitis is reported to be the most common cause of death in Degos' syndrome, which is another unusual form of vasculitis/coagulopathy with intestinal and classic dermal manifestations.[8] Intestinal ulcers in the terminal ileum/jejunum are reported in a large series of Japanese patients with Behçet's disease. The pathology of these perforating and multiple ulcers is not specific, and diagnosis is based on the concurrent pres-

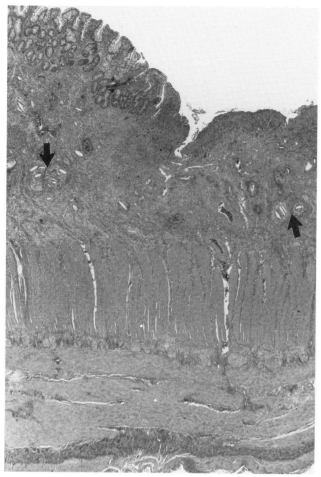

FIGURE 6–1. Chronic active small intestinal ischemic ulcer secondary to atheroemboli (*arrows*). (Elastic stain ×50)

strate decreased arterial flow and the absence of a venous phase.

The bowel received in pathology is hemorrhagic, edematous, and dark, with fan-like thrombi identified in draining veins in a thick hemorrhagic mesentery. Microscopy shows mucosal and mural hemorrhage and necrosis with thrombosed mesenteric veins (even in areas of unaffected bowel) and normal arteries. Recognition of this entity as the cause of infarction by the pathologist is important so that appropriate investigation and therapy can be instituted. The pathologist should also try to identify any fibrous adhesions in an infarcted bowel, because these may be responsible for simple or strangulation obstruction in as many as 50% of cases of small bowel obstruction in adults.[14]

Intestinal venulitis/phlebitis without arteritis has been reported in a patient with systemic lupus erythematosus.[15] A new entity, **idiopathic enterocolic lymphocytic phlebitis,** with thrombi but without arterial lesions as a cause of hemorrhagic mucosal necrosis has been reported in a small series of patients without systemic vasculitis. Although these cases were considered to be idiopathic, all three patients had been treated with hydroxyethyl rutoside for varicose veins.[16] Intestinal infarction secondary to massive amyloid deposits (possibly β_2-microglobulin) in the muscularis propria of the intestinal wall and in the walls of intra- and extramural vessels can occur in patients on long-term hemodialysis.[17] Gastrointestinal involvement is also common in primary (AL) amyloidosis and has been reported in 70% to 80% of patients with systemic disease. It can account for a variety of symptoms and signs, including gastrointestinal hemorrhage and pseudo-obstruction.[18]

Iatrogenic

Intestinal ulcers/strictures with non-specific pathologic appearances are often related to iatrogenic causes, and in these cases, a correct diagnosis is possible only when an accurate history is obtained. It is particularly important for the surgical pathologist to communicate with the primary care physician, because trauma surgeons may or may not be familiar with the history in any given case, especially when operating on an unknown patient on an emergent basis. The most common causes of iatrogenic small intestinal ulcers/strictures after postoperative adhesions are drugs, radiation, and graft-versus-host disease.

Drug-induced Ulcers

Drug-induced ulcers are becoming more common as the armamentarium of therapeutic agents increases. Most reports focus on the actions of oral contraceptives, non-steroidal anti-inflammatory drugs (NSAIDs), and chemotherapeutic agents.

Since their introduction, **oral contraceptives** have been associated with an increased risk of thromboembolic complications. Intra-abdominal vascular compromise with ischemia/infarction of the small intestine and colon has been reported. Patients present with either ''reversible'' enterocolitis showing non-specific pathologic changes on biopsy or small and large bowel infarction most often secondary to thrombosis of the superior mesenteric vein or artery. Resected segments of

ence of ocular inflammation, stomatitis, and genital ulcers.[9] Intestinal involvement may also occur in systemic vasculitis related to drug therapy. The vascular lesions are seen in small vessels with inflammatory infiltrates of mononuclear cells and eosinophils and few neutrophils with occasional granulomas. Necrosis of vessels is not seen. Generalized symptoms of fever, rash, and eosinophilia are often present.[10, 11]

Venous Ischemia

Mesenteric vein thrombosis (MVT) is an uncommon but important cause of intestinal ischemia that should be recognized pathologically. MVT has been recognized as a distinct entity since 1935 and is responsible for approximately 5% to 15% of all cases of intestinal infarction, with the superior mesenteric vein being involved in 95% of cases.[12, 13] MVT can be associated with predisposing factors such as trauma, surgery, estrogens, pancreatitis, renal disease, thrombotic syndromes due to inherited protein deficiencies, sepsis, cirrhosis, and hepatic, colonic, and pancreatic tumors or parasites in as many as one half of cases.[12, 13] The clinical presentation is that of periodic diffuse abdominal pain disproportionate to the abdominal findings, accompanied by fever, nausea, vomiting, and possibly diarrhea. The diagnosis is best made by computed tomography (CT), which shows diffuse thickening of the bowel wall, and by angiography, which may demon-

intestine are gangrenous, dusky or pale, and edematous with occlusive thrombi in mesenteric veins or arteries.[19]

Enteropathy related to the long-term ingestion of NSAIDs has been recognized for almost 20 years. Most patients are apparently symptom free and may have subclinical intestinal inflammation; however, approximately 1% of patients develop ulcers and strictures of the small intestine.[20] Multiple ileal ulcers with perforation have been shown to occur experimentally in rats administered even small doses of NSAIDs. Small intestinal pathology in patients on long-term NSAID therapy has been recently well described in a large English series.[21, 22] These authors reviewed their entire experience with small intestinal resections over 16 years and found an unclassified group of 26 cases in a total of 576 resections. Seven of these showed a distinctive pathology. When correlated with historical data, these patients were found to be on long-term NSAID therapy. In these patients, resected segments of small intestine showed the luminal aspect divided into multiple compartments by thin mucosal diaphragms with orifices ranging from a few millimeters to a few centimeters. These mucosal diaphragms/membranes were unevenly spaced throughout the resected length and were variable in number. Microscopy revealed that these diaphragms resemble exaggerations of normal plicae circularis, with submucosal fibrosis and occasional mucosal erosions and villous irregularity confined to the apex of each diaphragm.[21] It should be emphasized that unlike the transmural inflammation with lymphoid aggregates of Crohn's disease, the pattern in these cases is that of bland fibrosis of greater or lesser degree, confined to the submucosa, with only secondary mild mucosal inflammation and ulceration. These authors have shown that NSAIDs can also cause a less specific and subclinical form of small intestinal inflammation in almost two thirds of patients on long-term therapy, and the effects of these drugs may last as long as 16 months after discontinuation of therapy. This inflammation may progress to ulceration and strictures in an occasional patient.[23] It is obvious that the diagnosis in these cases is entirely dependent on an accurate clinical history.

The association between ingestion of **potassium chloride** and small intestinal ulceration has been known for the past 30 years. A comprehensive series was reported in 1970 on 12 patients with small intestinal ulcers/strictures, most of which appeared to be associated with ingestion of enteric-coated potassium. The pathology in all cases was non-specific, with transverse mucosal ulcers overlying areas of congestion and edema or submucosal fibrosis and involvement of the muscularis propria only in deep ulcers with perforation.[24] The diagnosis can only be supported by a careful drug history, all other cases being reported as "idiopathic" ulceration.

The rapidly proliferating epithelium of the intestine can be readily affected by the action of **chemotherapeutic agents,** including nitrogen mustard, cyclophosphamide, methotrexate, 5-fluorouracil, cytosine arabinoside, and adriamycin.[25-27] Morphologic and functional changes have been described in experimental animals and patients. Nausea, vomiting, hemorrhage, diarrhea, and malabsorption all have been reported in patients while on chemotherapy. It is believed that multiple drug regimens that include cytosine arabinoside are most likely to cause recognizable morphologic changes in the intestinal mucosa.[26] The morphologic changes are predominantly mucosal, with cessation of mitosis and its consequences almost immediately after start of therapy, and return to normal after cessation of medication. Crypt epithelium shows damage, with swollen cells replaced by apoptotic bodies, loss of differentiated epithelial cells, mucin depletion, and conversion of crypts to distended sacs of mucus and cellular debris. Regenerative changes include crypts replaced by large bizarre cuboidal epithelial cells and renewed mitotic activity. Villous loss, with increased vascularity of the lamina propria, can result in ulcerations and hemorrhage that may heal in 14 days but may take as long as 3 to 4 weeks.[27]

Radiation Enteropathy

This is a well-known complication of abdominal radiation therapy for carcinoma of the female genital tract as well as carcinoma of the prostate.[28] Post-radiation injury may occur in anywhere from 5% to 50% of patients and depends on various technical and patient-related factors. The small intestine is particularly susceptible to injury because loops of bowel may be trapped in the pelvis as a result of adhesions.[28-32]

Acute radiation enteritis occurs as early as 2 weeks and results in reversible destruction of the mucosa, which may be associated with bleeding and diarrhea. The more chronic effects are delayed and may last for many years, with injury related to mesenchymal tissues and blood vessels leading to ulcers/strictures and fistulas. Obstruction, malabsorption, and perforation may necessitate early surgery, with mortality often due to the complications of the radiation rather than the original malignancy. Acute mucosal changes can occur within 12 to 24 hours after moderate daily radiation doses, with nuclear pyknosis and karyorrhexis and cell necrosis in the crypts. Decreased numbers of proliferating crypt cells and mitoses finally lead to villous atrophy and cystic crypts within 1 to 2 weeks, with return to normal architecture in 14 days after cessation of therapy. There may be a variable increase in numbers of different types of inflammatory cells in the lamina propria and crypt epithelium. These early effects are rarely significant, and most small intestinal pathology is due to the delayed effects of radiation therapy.[28-32]

The pathologic features of chronic radiation injury have been very well described. The small intestine exhibits long narrow strictures with serosal fibrosis, adhesions, and telangiectasias. The mucosa shows active or healed ulceration with relatively acellular coagulative necrosis (Fig. 6–2A). Submucosal fibrosis with thickened vessels, edema, and hyalinized collagen with atypical fibroblasts all are well-known features. Vessels with atypical endothelium, intimal hyperplasia and foamy macrophages, fibrin thrombi, and fibrinoid necrosis may also be present. The muscularis propria may show focal degeneration and focal hypertrophy with hypertrophied nerves and ganglia. The differential diagnosis includes ischemic and inflammatory ulcers, and an accurate past history of radiation (preferably obtained from the radiation therapist) is very useful for the correct diagnosis. An occasional case of Crohn's disease may occur in a patient with a well-documented history of radiation. In such instances, the presence of fissuring ulceration and aphthous ulcers and the identification of granulomas after extensive specimen sampling enable the pathologist to render the correct diagnosis despite a "misleading" clinical history (Fig. 6–2B).

Graft-Versus-Host Disease (GVHD)

GVHD is an important form of small intestinal injury seen primarily in large medical centers that perform bone marrow

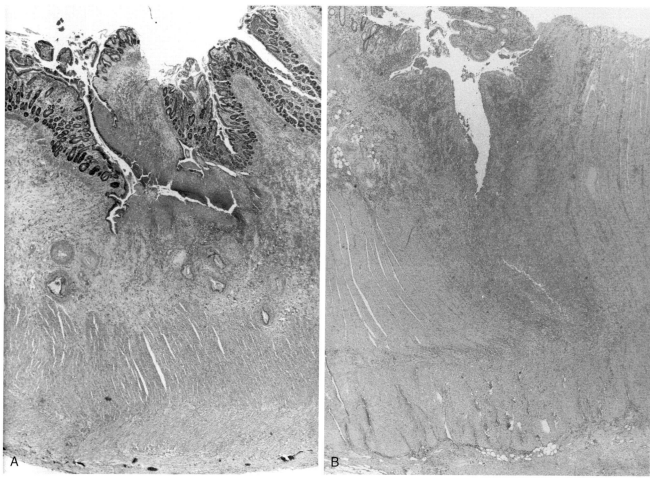

FIGURE 6–2. *A,* Small intestinal ulcer related to radiation therapy. (H&E ×50) *B,* Small intestinal ulcer in patient with Crohn's disease, previously radiated for endometrial carcinoma (compare *A*). (H&E × 50)

transplants for hematologic and solid neoplasms. Severe enteritis following bone marrow transplantation may be treated by resection for perforation, hemorrhage, and ulcer/strictures.[33] Intestinal symptoms usually include nausea, vomiting, and profound watery diarrhea with abdominal cramps and sheets of mucosa sloughed in the stools. Radiologic studies show a diffuse loss of mucosal folds, with a thick bowel and rapid transit of contrast.[34] The disease may be self-limited or life-threatening.

Resected intestinal specimens with severe GVHD show an edematous bowel with diffuse ulceration of the mucosa with "pseudomembranes." Submucosal and mural edema and transmural necrosis are present in very severe cases. Narrowed ulcerated segments alternate with dilated segments lined by more normal mucosa. Microscopically, there is almost complete denudation of the mucosa, with only remnants of lamina propria without epithelium on an edematous and fibrotic submucosa and muscularis (Fig. 6–3). The pathologic hallmark of early GVHD is the presence of single crypt cell necrosis, which is an early and may be an extremely focal finding. Membrane-bound debris from necrotic cells accumulates at the base or sides of crypts and has been referred to as "exploding crypt," or "apoptotic bodies." Initially, there is no increase in numbers of inflammatory cells in the lamina propria. This is followed by crypt dilatation, abscesses, and later

by crypt dropout, which finally results in epithelial denudation. Based on these findings, GVHD has been graded from I to IV, with only the grade I lesion considered to be diagnostic.[35] The differential diagnosis includes chemoradiation toxicity, which is seen within the first 20 days after induction, and viral infections developing in immunosuppressed patients. The latter must be identified using immunohistochemistry and *in situ* hybridization with the appropriate probes. Chronic GVHD usually spares the intestines.

Inflammation/Infection

Strictures with resulting obstruction are a common feature of Crohn's disease and require surgery for the relief of symptoms. The clinical and pathologic features of Crohn's disease are very well known. Ulceration with fissuring and mucosal metaplasias, submucosal fibrosis with neuromatous hyperplasia and arteritis, transmural inflammation with lymphoid aggregates, and fibrosis with fistulas and granulomas (50% of cases) are diagnostic.[36] Intestinal strictures in Crohn's disease are reported to result from a combination of proliferating smooth muscle cells in the muscularis mucosa and propria and an increase in type V collagen produced by these cells.[37]

Yersinia enterocolitica and *pseudotuberculosis* can cause an ileocolitis with mesenteric adenitis for which resections are

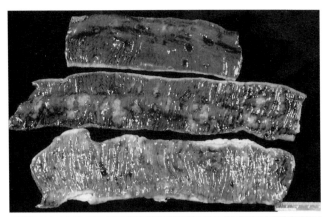

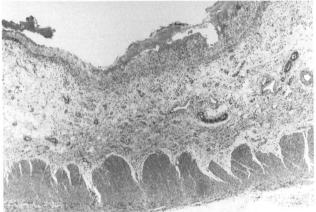

FIGURE 6–3. Small intestinal ulcers identified postmortem in patient with severe GVHD 59 days after bone marrow transplant. (H&E ×50)

occasionally performed. The well-known pathologic features include aphthous mucosal ulcers with granulomatous microabscesses also characteristically noted in the appendix and mesenteric lymph nodes.[38] Cytomegalovirus (CMV) enteritis and enterocolitis have been reported in immunosuppressed organ transplant patients as well as in patients with acquired immunodeficiency syndrome (AIDS), in whom it is the most common reason for emergent ileocolectomy. Symptoms are non-specific and include abdominal pain, diarrhea, and bleeding. Resected specimens show single or multiple ulcers with occasional transmural necrosis and perforation. Diagnosis is based on the recognition of characteristic intranuclear and intracytoplasmic inclusions in all cells, but particularly in endothelial cells, resulting in CMV vasculitis and ischemic ulcers. Diagnosis is important so that appropriate antiviral therapy can be instituted.[39]

Strongyloides stercoralis is the most important helminthic infection causing ulcers/strictures in the small intestine. It is seen in immigrants and Vietnam War veterans but is also endemic in rural areas of the southeastern United States. There is a renewed interest in this infection in the setting of chemotherapy-induced immunosuppression and AIDS.[40, 41] This is the only major helminthic parasite that can complete its life cycle in the human host. Uncomplicated infection is usually asymptomatic and mild, but hyperinfection in immunosuppressed patients can be fatal. In the gastrointestinal tract, most adult female parasites are confined to the superficial mucus layer and the intervillous spaces of the proximal jeju-

num, with the eggs and larvae in the crypts. Ova are produced during the intestinal phase and develop into rhabditiform larvae that are shed in stools (diagnostic of the infection) or occasionally metamorphose into filariform larvae in the bowel wall or in perianal skin, causing autoinfection. Most filariform larvae were found in the lymphatics of the intestinal wall (primarily mucosa and submucosa) and in the mesentery; in one study, the authors have suggested that the major route of larval dissemination in humans is lymphohematogenous.[41] Intestinal pathology can range from active hemorrhagic ulcers with "pseudomembranes," in which both types of larval forms as well as adult worms and ova are present, to chronic changes with fibrotic strictures and eosinophil-rich granulomas.[40–43]

SMALL INTESTINAL BIOPSY

Eosinophilic (Allergic) Gastroenteritis

Eosinophilic infiltrates in the gastrointestinal tract can be associated with parasites, drugs, and inflammatory bowel diseases. However, a specific form of eosinophilic gastroenteritis exists that can involve the mucosa or the gut wall or serosal tissues. This "condition" was originally described in 1937 and has been referred to by a variety of inappropriate terms. In the past two decades it has been recognized as "eosinophilic gastroenteritis," the mucosal form of which most often has an allergic etiology and, as suggested by Goldman, may be quite unrelated to the mural and serosal forms that are probably reaction patterns rather than single disease entities.[44]

Allergic gastroenteritis as defined by Goldman is identified most often in children but is also reported in older patients. Patients may present with colicky abdominal pain, nausea, vomiting, diarrhea, malabsorption with protein-losing enteropathy, and gastrointestinal bleeding with anemia. Asthma, allergy, and peripheral eosinophilia with elevated serum IgE levels are reported in approximately 50% of patients or their families. Endoscopic examination may reveal prominent gastric and/or intestinal folds.[44]

Small intestinal biopsies from patients with allergic gastroenteritis can be highly variable. The characteristic feature is that of **clusters or aggregates of eosinophils** in the lamina propria and submucosa with a focal or diffuse distribution, invading the epithelium and associated with epithelial damage and variable loss of villous architecture (Fig. 6–4*A*). Edema and ulceration of the mucosa are rare. Mononuclear cells and neutrophils are not usually present in increased numbers. Problems with diagnosis arise often because small intestinal biopsies may show only focal infiltrates of few eosinophils associated with minor degrees of epithelial damage. Eosinophils are normally present in the lamina propria of the small intestine, and there is no consensus on what number is considered pathologic.[45] The pathologic features have been best described in pediatric patients in whom morphologic criteria on biopsy are better established. In glandular tissue, lamina propria eosinophils are considered to be increased if they constitute 25% or more of the inflammatory cell population in a single high-power field with 20 or more inflammatory cells. The presence of more than a rare eosinophil in surface or crypt epithelium associated with epithelial damage is also considered abnormal.[46] In difficult cases, additional findings

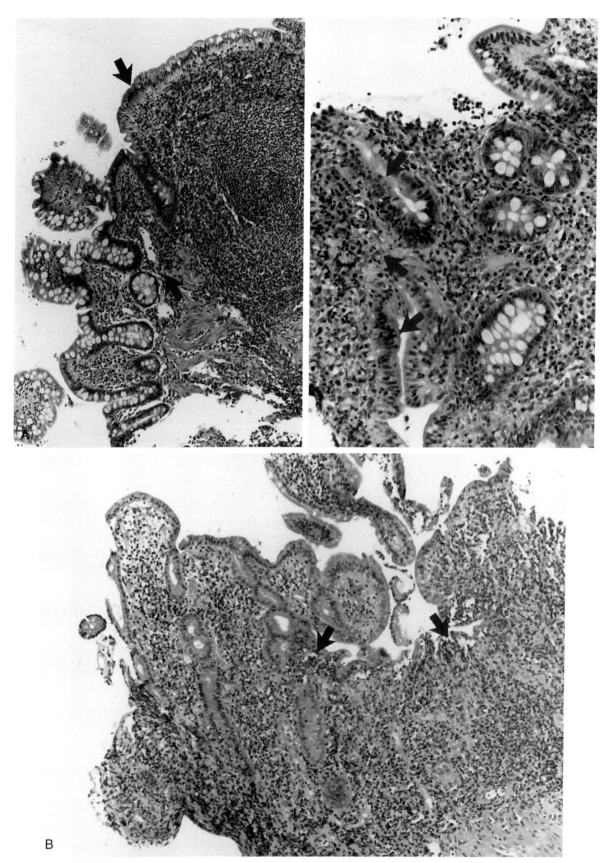

FIGURE 6–4. *A,* Small intestinal biopsy of "granular and erythematous" terminal ileum in 29-year-old male patient with asthma, peripheral eosinophilia, and allergic gastroenteritis. (*Left,* H&E ×250; *right,* H&E ×500) (*Note:* Eosinophils present in lamina propria and epithelium [*arrows*] are not readily seen in black and white photomicrographs.) *B,* Small intestinal biopsy of terminal ileal ulcer in 47-year-old female patient with Crohn's disease. (H&E ×250) (*Note:* Ulcer is associated with mixed inflammatory infiltrate, containing eosinophils [*arrows*].)

in gastric antral biopsies have been shown to be helpful, especially in distinguishing between allergic gastroenteritis, Crohn's disease, and peptic duodenitis.[45] Crohn's disease may show an increase in eosinophils, but these are usually part of a mixed inflammatory infiltrate with numerous neutrophils and mononuclear cells (Fig. 6–4B). Biopsies of Crohn's disease may also show ulcers and edema with glandular metaplasia and occasional granulomas. Peptic duodenitis is another important differential diagnosis that shows mild to moderate loss of villous architecture associated with a mixed inflammatory infiltrate with eosinophils, focal gastric antral-type surface epithelium, and possibly *Helicobacter pylori*. Another entity has been added to the differential diagnosis of increased eosinophils in small intestinal biopsies. Band-like infiltrates of eosinophils associated with mast cells in the deep mucosa with damaged muscle fibers in the muscularis mucosa are special histologic features reported in small intestinal biopsies from patients with connective tissue diseases.[47] In summary, the diagnosis of allergic gastroenteritis should be made only after exclusion of other conditions with increased eosinophils and in association with compatible clinical, radiologic, and laboratory data.[44]

The role of the eosinophil in allergic gastroenteritis is not completely understood; however, it is possible that products of activated eosinophil granules (major basic protein and eosinophil cationic protein) that have been identified in biopsies of patients may be directly toxic to tissues.[48, 49]

Systemic Mast Cell Disease

Systemic mast cell disease (SMCD) occurs in approximately 1 in 8000 to 10,000 persons, with an equal distribution in males and females in all age groups. In 90% of patients, there is only dermatologic involvement (i.e., urticaria pigmentosa). Patients with systemic involvement usually have an indolent course, except for a small subset of patients with mast cell proliferation in bone, spleen, lymph nodes, liver, bowel, and lung who may present with splenomegaly, myeloid hyperplasia/metaplasia, and myelogenous or mast cell leukemia.[50] As many as 80% of patients with SMCD have gastrointestinal symptoms, which include abdominal pain (dyspeptic or crampy) and diarrhea, most likely due to secreted mast cell products, including histamine and prostaglandin D_2.[51, 52] A third of patients may also have signs and symptoms of malabsorption, but this is rarely severe. Endoscopy can confirm the presence of gastritis, duodenitis, or peptic ulcer.[52]

Duodenal biopsies in patients with dyspeptic pain are reported to show duodenal ulcers or severe duodenitis.[51] The few available reports of small intestinal biopsies claim a wide range of pathologic features, from normal architecture to a flat mucosa with total loss of villi and a diffuse infiltrate of mast cells in mucosa and submucosa.[52] The diagnosis of SMCD in small intestinal biopsy can be extremely difficult and the following guidelines may be helpful.

1. In formalin-fixed paraffin-embedded tissues, helpful morphologic features include small intestinal villi with varying degrees of villous atrophy, including a totally flat mucosa. The inflammatory infiltrate (if dense) can consist of increased numbers of mononuclear cells with eosinophils and neutrophils. These mononuclear cells may be small oval or spindle cells with slightly irregular basophilic nuclei

and amphophilic cytoplasm characteristic of mast cells with or without a perivascular distribution.

2. To prove the presence of mast cells, granules should be demonstrated. This can be difficult in formalin-fixed hematoxylin and eosin (H&E)–stained sections. Special stains must be performed and can be very helpful in demonstrating granules even in formalin-fixed tissues. These include Giemsa and toluidine blue stains (metachromatic [purple] granules) and the alphanaphthol chloroacetate esterase stain, which can reveal coarse red granules in mast cells. Mast cells can be distinguished from fibroblasts and histiocytes by immunoperoxidase studies. Mast cells are positive for leukocyte common antigen (LCA) and negative for lysozyme.[50, 52]

3. One-micron sections of tissue fixed in glutaraldehyde and stained with toluidine blue should always be available to better visualize mast cells that may be immature or degranulated. Ultrastructural studies can also be used to identify both mucosal and submucosal mast cells with their characteristic differences in "scroll" morphology.[53]

4. The major problem with the diagnosis of SMCD on gastrointestinal biopsies is the absence of criteria for increased numbers of mast cells in biopsies. Reports and estimates range from 3 to 4 mast cells per high-power field (HPF) to 7 to 10 and 50 to 100 per HPF in patients with SMCD.[54] Numbers of mucosal mast cells detected also vary with the fixative used, being highest in Carnoy's fixative and lowest in formalin-based fixatives.[54] Scott et al. in an older study of jejunal biopsies from 11 patients with untreated celiac disease and 10 control subjects without small intestinal disease showed that the average number of mast cells in both groups was 2 per HPF and suggested that, as reported in skin biopsies, more than 6 mast cells per HPF may represent SMCD. The fixative used was not identified by these authors, although the stain was probably toluidine blue.[55] Other authors have reported an inability to demonstrate mast cells in formalin-fixed tissues stained with toluidine blue and Giemsa stains, but a markedly increased number were demonstrated in Bouin's-fixed tissue stained with astra blue in disease as well as control specimens.[56] For practical purposes, the presence of 6 or more mast cells per HPF identified by special stains in formalin-fixed tissues and supported by toluidine blue–stained 1-micron sections in the appropriate clinical context may suggest a diagnosis of SMCD.

5. The important morphologic differential diagnosis of SMCD in small intestinal biopsies is celiac sprue, which can show similar appearances, with abnormal villi, damaged enterocytes, and an increased mononuclear infiltrate in the mucosa. Subtle differences such as a diffusely flat mucosa in celiac sprue with increased lymphocytes in the lamina propria and surface epithelium versus variable villous alteration and a mixed inflammatory infiltrate in SMCD may be present and helpful in diagnosis. If necessary, a clinical trial on a gluten-free diet may be indicated.

6. Clinical data with symptoms such as flushing, headaches, pruritus, and wheezing are most helpful when present but unfortunately are noted in only 20% of patients, and assays for urinary histamine and its metabolites are not always contributory.[50] Plasma histamine levels have been reported to be elevated in the majority of patients.[51] Finally, because gastrointestinal biopsies may be non-diagnostic even in patients with severe gastrointestinal symptomatology, bone marrow biopsies should be performed and carefully evaluated to establish a final diagnosis.

HIV Infection/Idiopathic AIDS Enteropathy

Enteropathy associated with AIDS was first described by Kotler et al. in 1984 in patients with diarrhea and weight loss in whom pathogens were not identified by routine stool cultures and tissue examination.[57] It is still a confusing term, variably used by some authors to describe pathogen-negative chronic diarrhea in AIDS and by others to describe the morphologic and inflammatory changes seen in gastrointestinal biopsies of patients with human immunodeficiency virus (HIV) infection.[58] Currently, this enteropathy is thought to represent the intermediate phase of HIV infection, with a multifactorial etiology including possibly undiscovered/occult pathogens, the effects of HIV infection, and low-grade bacterial overgrowth secondary to loss of non-immune and immune intestinal defense mechanisms.[59, 60] When diagnostic evaluation includes multiple modalities including electron microscopy, one or more infectious pathogens can be identified in as many as 85% of patients with AIDS; hence, AIDS enteropathy or idiopathic diarrhea in AIDS is seen in only a minority of patients.[59–61]

Small intestinal biopsies in these patients have been described to show a variable morphology similar to that originally described by Kotler in 1984.[57] Specifically these biopsies show partial villous atrophy with crypt hyperplasia, increased intraepithelial lymphocytes, and hyporegenerative features as noted by inappropriately low mitoses per crypt.[57, 58, 61] These appearances are similar to those described in celiac disease, malnutrition, and chemoradiation therapy.[61] HIV proteins, RNA and DNA, in mononuclear cells in the intestinal lamina propria and rare intestinal epithelial cells and a marked decrease in IgA plasma cells have also been described in biopsies of patients with AIDS.[62, 63] The presence of the virus also appears to be associated with decreased or absent mucosal enzymes.[64]

There is increased interest in chronic bacterial enteropathy in patients with AIDS. Several studies have detected increased aerobes and anaerobes in small intestinal luminal fluid in patients with AIDS and diarrhea.[65] Enteroadherent gram-negative coccobacilli have been visualized by light and electron microscopy adherent to enterocytes in mucosal biopsies of 16% to 19% of patients with AIDS and chronic diarrhea from Zambia as well as the United States.[66, 67] It appears likely that some cases of AIDS enteropathy may be bacterial in origin. Severe diffuse small intestinal injury with ulceration is unusual in AIDS enteropathy and has been described only in association with heavy infestation with *Cryptosporidium*.[68, 69] No infectious cause could be identified in an unusual biopsy with an ulcerated intestinal lesion from a terminally ill AIDS patient with starvation and severe malnutrition (Fig. 6–5).

DIFFERENTIAL DIAGNOSIS OF MALIGNANT SMALL INTESTINAL NEOPLASMS

Primary malignant neoplasms are rare in the small intestine and account for less than 1% to 2% of gastrointestinal malignancies. Recent large population–based studies have shown that the most common neoplasms in the small intestine are adenocarcinomas and carcinoids, followed by sarcomas and lymphomas.[70–72] The majority (50%) of adenocarcinomas occur in the second part of the duodenum around the ampulla of Vater, the majority of carcinoids and lymphomas occur in the ileum, and the majority of sarcomas in the jejunum.[70] Metastatic neoplasms in the small intestine are most often from the lung, breast, melanomas, and female genital tract. Contiguous spread may also occur from adjacent gastrointestinal locations.[72] The pathologic diagnosis of malignant small intestinal neoplasms requires an accurate clinical history as well as the appropriate use of special pathologic studies. The majority of primary small intestinal carcinomas have the well-known histologic features of moderately differentiated intestinal/colonic adenocarcinoma and may even be associated with an adenoma. Poorly differentiated mucinous adenocarcinomas with signet cells similar to gastric carcinomas constitute as much as one third of primary periampullary and duodenal neoplasms and should be recognized as such.[72, 73] Risk factors for primary adenocarcinomas include Crohn's

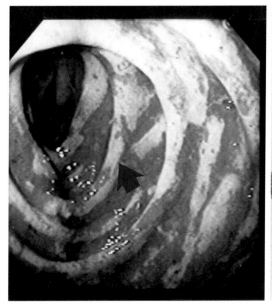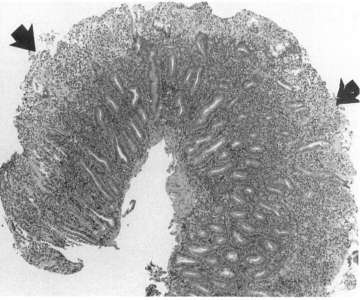

FIGURE 6–5. Duodenal biopsy of severe small intestinal lesion with ulcers (*arrows*) in 30-year-old terminally ill patient with AIDS, diarrhea, and severe malnutrition. No organisms identified. Electron microscopy not performed. (H&E ×100) (Endoscopic photograph courtesy of Dr. Joel Bessoff, Baystate Medical Center, Springfield, MA.)

disease, celiac sprue, and hereditary polyposis syndromes, including Lynch syndrome II.[72, 74]

The usual ileal carcinoid tumor does not present any difficulty in diagnosis. However, some carcinoid tumors may display atypial features such as spindle cell patterns, metaplastic changes, and pleomorphism with rare poorly differentiated features.[75] If hormonal and other immunohistochemical studies are negative, electron microscopy may demonstrate neurosecretory granules. Risk factors include von Recklinghausen's neurofibromatosis, multiple endocrine neoplasia syndrome type 1, and occasionally inflammatory bowel disease and celiac sprue.[72, 76]

Much has been written on gastrointestinal stromal tumors (GISTs) and gastrointestinal autonomic nerve tumors (GANTs, or plexosarcomas).[77, 78] The histogenesis as determined by immunoperoxidase studies appears to be unimportant as a prognostic factor, and diagnosis of malignancy is best made using well-known light microscopic criteria. Risk factors for sarcomas include von Recklinghausen's disease and AIDS.[72, 79]

The gastrointestinal tract is the most common site of extranodal non-Hodgkin's lymphomas, 20% to 40% of which occur in the small intestine.[72, 80] These are a heterogeneous group of neoplasms, and their classification has been difficult. A report on primary lymphomas of the small intestine classified 119 cases using the Kiel European Association for Hematopathology Geneva Workshop scheme on paraffin sections and showed that 66% were B-cell lymphomas and 34% were T-cell lymphomas. The B-cell lymphomas were predominantly high grade (62%), with 20% being low-grade lymphomas of mucosa-associated lymphoid tissue. The T-cell lymphomas were predominantly of the high-grade variety.[80] Immunoperoxidase and possibly cytogenetic and molecular studies are essential for the diagnosis of lymphomas. Risk factors for lymphomas include celiac sprue (T-cell neoplasms), immunoproliferative small intestinal disease (Mediterranean lymphomas), AIDS, and other states of natural and iatrogenic immunodeficiency/immunosuppression (high-grade B-cell lymphomas).[72]

References

1. Ottinger LW: Mesenteric ischemia. N Engl J Med 307:535–537, 1982.
2. Williams LF: Mesenteric ischemia. Surg Clin North Am 68:331–353, 1988.
3. Socinski MA, Frankel JP, Morrow PL, et al: Painless diarrhea secondary to intestinal ischemia. Diagnosis of atheromatous emboli by jejunal biopsy. Dig Dis Sci 29:674–677, 1984.
4. Camilleri M, Pusey CD, Chadwick VS, et al: Gastrointestinal manifestations of systemic vasculitis. Q J Med 206:141–149, 1983.
5. McCurley TL, Collins RD: Intestinal infarction in rheumatoid arthritis. Three cases due to unusual obliterative vascular lesions. Arch Pathol Lab Med 108:125–128, 1984.
6. Rosen N, Sommer I, Knobel B: Intestinal Buerger's disease. Arch Pathol Lab Med 109:962–963, 1985.
7. Broide E, Scapa E, Peer A, et al: Buerger's disease presenting as acute small bowel ischemia. Gastroenterology 104:1192–1195, 1993.
8. Magrinat G, Kerwin KS, Gabriel DA: The clinical manifestations of Degos' syndrome. Arch Pathol Lab Med 113:354–362, 1989.
9. Kasahara Y, Tanaka S, Nishino M, et al: Intestinal involvement in Behcet's disease: Review of 136 surgical cases in the Japanese literature. Dis Colon Rectum 24:103–106, 1981.
10. Mullick EG, McAllister HA, Wagner BM, et al: Drug related vasculitis. Clinicopathologic correlations in 30 patients. Hum Pathol 10:313–325, 1979.
11. Churg J, Churg A: Idiopathic and secondary vasculitis: A review. Mod Pathol 2:144–160, 1989.
12. Case Records of the Massachusetts General Hospital (Case 9-1991). N Engl J Med 324:613–623, 1991.
13. Grendell JH, Ockner RK: Mesenteric venous thrombosis. Gastroenterology 82:358–372, 1982.
14. Case Records of the Massachusetts General Hospital (Case 7-1987). N Engl J Med 316:394–403, 1987.
15. Weiser MM, Andres GA, Brentjens JR, et al: Systemic lupus erythematosus and intestinal venulitis. Gastroenterology 81:570–579, 1981.
16. Saraga EP, Costa J: Idiopathic entero-colic lymphocytic phlebitis. A cause of ischemic intestinal necrosis. Am J Surg Pathol 13:303–308, 1989.
17. Choi HSH, Heller D, Picken MM, et al: Infarction of intestine with massive amyloid deposition in two patients on long-term hemodialysis. Gastroenterology 96:230–234, 1989.
18. Case Records of the Massachusetts General Hospital (Case 43-1985). N Engl J Med 313:1070–1079, 1985.
19. Schneiderman DJ, Cello JP: Intestinal ischemia and infarction associated with oral contraceptives. West J Med 145:350–355, 1986.
20. Banerjee AK: Enteropathy induced by non-steroidal anti-inflammatory drugs. Often subclinical but may mimic Crohn's disease. BMJ 298: 1539–1540, 1989.
21. Lang J, Price AB, Levi AJ, et al: Diaphragm disease: Pathology of disease of the small intestine induced by non-steroidal anti-inflammatory drugs. J Clin Pathol 41:516–526, 1988.
22. Bjarnason I, Price AB, Zanelli G, et al: Clinicopathological features of nonsteroidal antiinflammatory drug-induced small intestinal strictures. Gastroenterology 94:1070–1074, 1988.
23. Bjarnason I, Zanelli G, Smith T, et al: Nonsteroidal antiinflammatory drug-induced intestinal inflammation in humans. Gastroenterology 93:480–489, 1987.
24. Davies DR, Brightmore T: Idiopathic and drug-induced ulceration of the small intestine. Br J Surg 57:134–139, 1970.
25. Shaw MT, Spector MH, Ladman AJ: Effects of cancer, radiotherapy and cytotoxic drugs on intestinal structure and function. Cancer Treat Rev 6:141–151, 1979.
26. Slavin RE, Dias MA, Saral R: Cytosine arabinoside induced gastrointestinal toxic alterations in sequential chemotherapeutic protocols. A clinical-pathologic study of 33 patients. Cancer 42:1747–1759, 1978.
27. Riddell RH: The gastrointestinal tract. In Riddell RH (ed): Pathology of Drug-Induced and Toxic Diseases. New York, Churchill Livingstone, 1982, p 515.
28. Churnratanakul S, Wirzba B, Lam T, et al: Radiation and the small intestine. Future perspectives for preventive therapy. Dig Dis 8:45–60, 1990.
29. Kwitko AO, Pieterse AS, Hecker R, et al: Chronic radiation injury to the intestine: A clinico-pathological study. Aust N Z J Med 12:272–277, 1982.
30. Case Records of the Massachusetts General Hospital (Case 9-1994). N Engl J Med 330:627–632, 1994.
31. Novak JM, Collins JT, Donowitz M, et al: Effects of radiation on the human gastrointestinal tract. J Clin Gastroenterol 1:9–37, 1979.
32. Berthrong M, Fajardo LF: Radiation injury in surgical pathology. Part II. Alimentary tract. Am J Surg Pathol 5:153–177, 1981.
33. Spencer GD, Shulman HM, Myerson D, et al: Diffuse intestinal ulceration after marrow transplantation: A clinicopathologic study of 13 patients. Hum Pathol 17:621–633, 1986.
34. Beschorner WE: Destruction of the intestinal mucosa after bone marrow transplantation and graft-versus-host disease. Surv Synth Pathol Res 3:264–374, 1984.
35. McDonald GB, Shulman HM, Sullivan KN, et al: Intestinal and hepatic complications of human bone marrow transplantation. Part 1. Gastroenterology 90:460–477, 1986.
36. Goldman H: Crohn's disease. In Ming S-C, Goldman H (eds): Pathology of the Gastrointestinal Tract. Philadelphia, WB Saunders, 1992, p 665.
37. Graham MF, Diegelmann RF, Elson CO: Collagen content and types in the intestinal strictures of Crohn's disease. Gastroenterology 94:257–265, 1988.
38. Sheahan DG, Rotterdam H: Small intestine. In Rotterdam H, Sheahan DG, Sommers SC, et al (eds): Biopsy Diagnosis of the Digestive Tract, Vol. 2. New York, Raven Press, 1993, p 381.
39. Nash S: Gastrointestinal and hepatobiliary disease. In Nash G, Said JW (eds): Pathology of AIDS and HIV infection. Philadelphia, WB Saunders, 1992, p 103.
40. Walzer PD, Milder JE, Banwell JG, et al: Epidemiologic features of strongyloides stercoralis infection in an endemic area of the United States. Am J Trop Med 31:313–319, 1982.
41. Haque AK, Schnadig V, Rubin SA, Smith JH: Pathogenesis of human strongyloidiasis: Autopsy and quantitative parasitological analysis. Mod Pathol 7(3):276–288, 1994.
42. Boyd WP, Bachman BA: Gastrointestinal infections in the compromised host. Med Clin North Am 66:743–753, 1982.
43. Case Records of the Massachusetts General Hospital (Case 13-1986). N Engl J Med 314:903–913, 1986.
44. Goldman H: Allergic disorders. In Ming S-C, Goldman H (eds): Pathology of the Gastrointestinal Tract. Philadelphia, W.B. Saunders, 1992, p 180.
45. Blackshaw A, Levison DA: Eosinophilic infiltrates of the gastrointestinal tract. J Clin Pathol 39:1–7, 1986.
46. Goldman H, Proujansky R: Allergic proctitis and gastroenteritis in children. Clinical and mucosal biopsy features in 53 cases. Am J Surg Pathol 10:75–86, 1986.
47. DeSchryver-Kecskemeti K, Clouse RE: A previously unrecognized subgroup of "eosinophilic gastroenteritis." Association with connective tissue diseases. Am J Surg Pathol 8:171–180, 1984.
48. Keshavarzian A, Sayerymuttu SH, Tai PC, et al: Activated eosinophils in familial eosinophilic gastroenteritis. Gastroenterology 88:1041–1049, 1985.
49. Talley NJ, Kephart GM, McGovern TW, et al: Deposition of eosinophil granule major basic protein in eosinophilic gastroenteritis and celiac disease. Gastroenterology 103:137–145, 1992.
50. Case Records of the Massachusetts General Hospital (Case 38-1986). N Engl J Med 315:816–824, 1986.

51. Cherner JA, Jensen RT, Dubois A, et al: Gastrointestinal dysfunction in systemic mastocytosis. A prospective study. Gastroenterology 95:657–667, 1988.
52. Freedman SD, Drews RE, Glotzer DJ, et al: Recurrent gastrointestinal bleeding associated with myelofibrosis and diffuse intestinal telangiectasis. Gastroenterology 101:1432–1439, 1991.
53. Weidner N, Austen KF: Ultrastructural and immunohistochemical characterization of normal mast cells at multiple body sites. J Invest Dermatol 96:26S–31S, 1991.
54. Yardley JH: Malabsorptive disorders. In Ming S-C, Goldman H (eds): Pathology of the Gastrointestinal Tract. Philadelphia, WB Saunders, 1992, p 756.
55. Scott BB, Hardy GJ, Losowsky MS: Involvement of the small intestine in systemic mast cell disease. Gut 16:918–924, 1975.
56. Braverman DZ, Dollberg L, Shiner M: Clinical, histological, and electron microscopic study of mast cell disease of the small bowel. Am J Gastroenterol 80:30–37, 1985.
57. Kotler DP, Gaetz HP, Lange M, et al: Enteropathy associated with the acquired immunodeficiency syndrome. Ann Intern Med 101:421–428, 1984.
58. Greenson JK, Belitsos PC, Yardley JH, Bartlett JG: AIDS enteropathy: Occult enteric infections and duodenal mucosal alterations in chronic diarrhea. Ann Intern Med 114:366–372, 1991.
59. Smith PD, Mai UEH: Immunopathology of gastrointestinal disease in HIV infection. Gastroenterol Clin North Am 21(2):331–345, 1992.
60. Simon D, Brandt LJ: Diarrhea in patients with acquired immunodeficiency syndrome. Gastroenterology 105:1238–1242, 1993.
61. Bartlett JG, Belitsos PC, Sears CL: AIDS enteropathy. Clin Infect Dis 15:726–735, 1992.
62. Kotler DP, Reka S, Borcich A, Cronin WJ: Detection, localization, and quantitation of HIV-associated antigens in intestinal biopsies from patients with HIV. Am J Pathol 139:823–830, 1991.
63. Kotler DP, Scholes JV, Tierney AR: Intestinal plasma cell alterations in acquired immunodeficiency syndrome. Dig Dis Sci 32(2):129–138, 1987.
64. Ulrich R, Zeitz M, Heise W, et al: Small intestinal structure and function in patients affected with human immunodeficiency virus (HIV): Evidence for HIV-induced enteropathy. Ann Intern Med 111:15–21, 1989.
65. Smith P, Quinn TC, Strober W, et al: Gastrointestinal infections in AIDS. Ann Intern Med 116:63–77, 1992.
66. Calamari S, Mathewson J, Stephens A, et al: Microscopic and microbiologic demonstration of enteroadherent bacteria in the colonic mucosa of Zambian patients with the acquired immunodeficiency syndrome. US-CAP Annual Meeting Abstracts, Lab Invest 726:125A, 1994.
67. Kotler DP, Giang TT, Orenstein JM: Chronic bacterial enteropathy in patients with AIDS. Gastroenterology 106(4):A714, 1994.
68. Genta RM, Chappell CL, White AC, et al: Duodenal morphology and intensity of infection in AIDS-related intestinal cryptosporidiosis. Gastroenterology 105: 1769–1775, 1993.
69. Godwin TA: Cryptosporidiosis in the acquired immunodeficiency syndrome: A study of 15 autopsy cases. Hum Pathol 22(12):1215–1225, 1991.
70. Ross RK, Hartnett NM, Bernstein L, et al: Epidemiology of adenocarcinomas of the small intestine: Is bile a small bowel carcinogen? Br J Cancer 63:143–145, 1991.
71. Ashley SW, Wells SA: Tumors of the small intestine. Semin Oncol 15:116–128, 1988.
72. Rotterdam H, Sheahan DG: Malignant tumors of the small intestine. In Rotterdam H, Sheahen DG, Sommers SC, et al (eds): Biopsy Diagnosis of the Digestive Tract, 2nd ed. New York, Raven Press, 1993, pp 484–521.
73. Blackman E, Nash SV: Diagnosis of duodenal and ampullary epithelial neoplasms by endoscopic biopsy: A clinicopathologic and immunohistochemical study. Hum Pathol 16:901–910, 1985.
74. Lynch HT, Smyrk TC, Lynch PM, et al: Adenocarcinoma of the small bowel in Lynch syndrome II. Cancer 64:2178–2183, 1989.
75. Lewin K: Carcinoid tumors and the mixed (composite) glandular—endocrine cell carcinomas. Am J Surg Pathol 11(Suppl 1):71–86, 1987.
76. Burke AP, Sobin LH, Shekitka KM, et al: Somatostatin-producing duodenal carcinoids in patients with von Recklinghausen's neurofibromatosis. Cancer 65:1591–1595, 1990.
77. Ranchod M, Kempson RL: Smooth muscle tumors of the gastrointestinal tract and retroperitoneum. A pathologic analysis of 100 cases. Cancer 39:255–262, 1977.
78. Case Records of the Massachusetts General Hospital (Case 15-1993). N Engl J Med 328:1107–1114, 1993.
79. Chadwick EG, Connor EJ, Hanson ICG, et al: Tumors of smooth-muscle origin in HIV-infected children. JAMA 263:3182–3184, 1990.
80. Domizio P, Owen RA, Shepherd NA, et al: Primary lymphoma of the small intestine. A clinicopathological study of 119 cases. Am J Surg Pathol 17:429–442, 1993.

CHAPTER 7

Colon, Appendix, and Anorectum

James K. Kelly, M.B., B.Ch., B.A.O., F.R.C.Path., and Linda D. Ferrell, M.D.

In the colon, diagnoses of many of the most common neoplastic or inflammatory lesions are straightforward and pose no significant problem to the pathologist. At times, however, rare neoplastic processes or different inflammatory lesions that share some pathologic features can pose diagnostic challenges. In this chapter, we delineate and describe many of these latter clinicopathologic situations.

BENIGN/INFLAMMATORY LESIONS

Acute Self-Limited (Acute Infectious) Colitis

Clinicopathologic features of acute self-limited colitis (ASLC) include acute bloody or non-bloody diarrhea, abdominal cramps, vomiting, tenesmus, fever, leukocytosis, and malaise. Bacterial pathogens such as *Salmonella* spp., *Shigella* spp., *Campylobacter jejuni,* pathogenic *Escherichia coli,* and *Clostridium difficile* are found in 50% of the cases. The histologic diagnosis is based on the following findings: normal crypt architecture, a neutrophil leukocytic infiltrate in the upper half of the mucosa, edema and capillary congestion, normal or minimally increased numbers of plasma cells, absence of basal plasmacytosis, and goblet cell depletion.[1-10] Neutrophilic cryptitis is usually more prominent than crypt abscesses (Fig. 7–1). Look for specific organisms such as *Entamoeba histolytica* or *Cryptosporidium.* It helps if the pathologist knows the length of time from the onset of diarrhea to biopsy. Edema of the lamina propria is an early feature that regresses after several days. Prolonged infections, particularly shigellosis,[9] amebiasis, or chlamydial proctitis, may show crypt regenerative changes and increased numbers of plasma cells resembling inflammatory bowel disease (IBD), and the distinction depends on culture and follow-up.[11, 12]

DIFFERENTIAL DIAGNOSIS. Histologic features identical to ASLC may be seen in **antibiotic colitis, drug-induced colitis,** and **pseudomembranous colitis** at sites without the pseudomembranes. Mild infection may evoke a neutrophilic infiltrate in the lymphoid-glandular complexes and must not be mistaken for focal inflammation of Crohn's disease. In **idiopathic inflammatory bowel disease (IIBD),** the cellular infiltrate involves the lower half of the mucosa as well as the upper. Features that favor a diagnosis of IIBD are crypt architectural distortion and atrophy, villous change, increased chronic inflammatory cells in the lower part of the lamina propria, and Paneth cell or antral metaplasia.[4, 10, 13] When crypts are lost, new crypts are formed by division (fission) of existing crypts. The crypt base becomes bifid and the split moves upward, giving the crypt a branched appearance. Innominate grooves, normal indentations of the mucosa into which several crypts open, should not be mistaken for fission. Crypts in IIBD may also show other forms of architectural distortion, such as shortening, failure to extend to the muscularis mucosae, dilatation, or atrophy. Epithelioid granulomas are highly suggestive of Crohn's disease but can also be found in chlamydiosis,[11, 12] yersiniosis,[7, 8] tuberculosis, schistosomiasis, strongyloidiasis, and syphilis (see later). Inflammation or ulceration lasting 3 months or more is a useful criterion of chronicity. Patients with IIBD may acquire infection by any of the common bacterial or viral agents that cause colitis, and thus, the neutrophilic infiltrate, which is traditionally regarded as evidence of "activity" of IIBD, may be due to superimposed infection. There are no reliable histologic features that would allow this distinction; it can be made only by culture.

Both **cytomegalovirus (CMV) and herpes simplex** have characteristic inclusions and can be identified by immunostaining. CMV colitis complicates immunosuppression due to acquired immunodeficiency syndrome (AIDS), cytotoxic chemotherapy, organ transplantation, renal failure, or severe ulcerative colitis that has been treated with corticosteroids.[14] Rarely, self-limited CMV proctitis follows anal intercourse in immunocompetent patients.[15] Focal deep neutrophil infiltrates and crypt cell apoptosis suggest CMV and demand a search for inclusion bodies. Herpes simplex colitis is extremely uncommon and occurs only in immunocompromised individuals,[16, 17] but proctitis may occur concomitantly with anal infection as multiple and/or diffuse ulcers of the distal rectum. The histologic features include multinucleate giant cells, intranuclear inclusions, and lymphocytic infiltration around submucosal vessels.[17]

Ulcerative Colitis (UC) versus Crohn's Disease

Separation of UC and Crohn's colitis remains important because patients with Crohn's disease are not considered for ileorectal pouch procedures. The endoscopic and clinical features of UC and Crohn's are listed on Table 7–1 (Fig. 7–2).

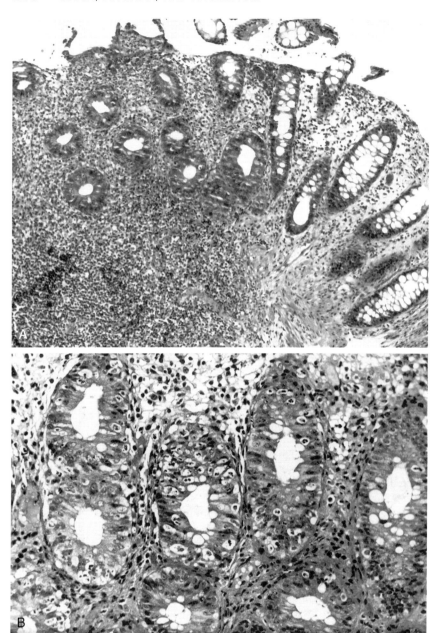

FIGURE 7–1. *A,* Acute infectious colitis. Edema and normal crypt architecture on right; neutrophil infiltration over a lymphoid-glandular complex on the left. *B,* Cryptitis of severe infectious colitis.

Endoscopic biopsy histology is hardly ever pathognomonic of either entity, and even clinically there are rare cases wherein the two diseases seem to overlap (Table 7–2). Inflammation in continuity from the rectum (UC) and discontinuous inflammation (Crohn's) are best documented by multiple biopsies that are labeled according to distance from the anal verge. Sigmoidoscopy alone must not be relied on to diagnose a normal rectum—even if the rectum looks normal, it should be biopsied. If serial sections are cut from endoscopically normal rectal mucosal biopsies from patients with proximal Crohn's disease, granulomas are found in 20% of cases. Granulomas are not found in submucosa or deeper in the bowel wall in ulcerative colitis, but granulomas are occasionally found around ruptured crypts (''mucin granulomas'') in the mucosa. Previous biopsies should be reviewed if there is any disparity clinically or pathologically.

In UC, the rectum may be less diseased than the colon in three circumstances: after steroid enemas, in fulminant colitis,

Table 7–1. **Gross Differences Between Ulcerative Colitis and Crohn's Disease**

Ulcerative Colitis	Crohn's Disease
Disease in continuity from rectum.	Discontinuous disease.
Congested, hemorrhagic or flat, granular mucosa. Large or extensive ulcers in severe disease only.	Distinct ulcers and patchy disease, separated by normal mucosa; or flat mucosal scars of healed ulcers. Mucosa not congested or hemorrhagic; aphthous ulcers.
Strictures rare.	Strictures and sinuses common, especially late in course.
Inflammatory polyps commonly present and numerous.	Inflammatory polyps less common.
Anal lesions uncommon, mainly fissures.	Anal lesions common, mainly fistulas.

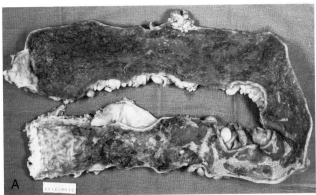
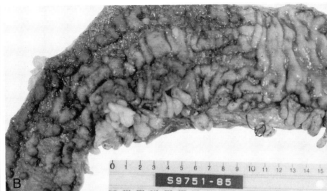
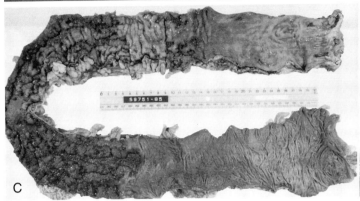

FIGURE 7–2. *A,* Ulcerative colitis. The ulcers are separated by congested and hemorrhagic mucosa. *B,* Crohn's colitis. Ulcers separated by normal-looking mucosa. *C,* Colitis indeterminate. Rectum is spared. Ulcerated area resembles ulcerative colitis in hemorrhagic areas and Crohn's disease in other areas.

and when the disease is entering remission. On the other hand, histologically confirmed segmental disease with normal rectal mucosa is never UC; it may be Crohn's disease, infection, ischemia, or an effect of diverticular disease. Both diseases can be exacerbated or complicated by antibiotic-induced colitis, infection, amebic colitis, or pseudomembranous colitis.

Fulminant Colitis and Colitis Indeterminate

Fulminant colitis presents clinically with fever, blood loss, electrolyte imbalance, and prostration. It may occur at first presentation of IIBD or complicate chronic disease. Approximately 10% of patients with UC develop a fulminant phase at some time, and it may be precipitated by intercurrent infection, antibiotic colitis, pseudomembranous colitis, or combined anticholinergic and narcotic drug treatment.[18] It may be complicated by toxic dilation, which is defined as a flaccid, gas-filled colon measuring 5.5 cm or more in diameter on plain radiograph. The risk of perforation is high as a result of thinning of the wall, ulcers penetrating the muscularis propria, and acute fissures in the floors of ulcers.[18] If a diagnosis of IIBD has not been previously made, differentiation from acute infectious or other forms of colitis may be difficult. Infectious, pseudomembranous, amebic, ischemic, and other forms of colitis may also present as fulminant disease. A specific diagnosis of UC or Crohn's disease is often not possible on the resected colon, and such cases are designated "indeterminate colitis" (see Fig. 7–2*C*).

Differential Diagnosis of Focal Inflammation in a Colorectal Biopsy

Focal inflammation is a hallmark of Crohn's disease but has a wide range of causes, including bacterial infection, CMV infection, graft-versus-host disease, resolving bouts of ulcerative colitis, diversion colitis, non-steroidal anti-inflammatory drug (NSAID) effect, segmental colitis due to infection or diverticular disease, and local trauma by enema tube or endoscope[13] (Fig. 7–3). The edge of a normal solitary lymphoid follicle (lymphoid glandular complex) may resemble focal inflammation, but the foci of inflammation in Crohn's disease contain a mixture of cell types, not just lymphoid cells. The minimal lesion of infectious or antibiotic-associated colitis may appear endoscopically as "red spots" that show

Table 7–2. **Microscopic Differences Between Ulcerative Colitis and Crohn's Disease**

Features Favoring Ulcerative Colitis	Features Favoring Crohn's Disease
Diffuse, evenly distributed mucosal inflammation in continuity from the anus.	Focal chronic inflammation with increased plasma cells, eosinophils, lymphocytes.
Mucosal regeneration, crypts in fission, villous surface, Paneth cells.	Granulomas.
Reactive epithelial hyperplasia/ hyperchromatism.	Sinuses/fissures.
Crypt abscesses.	Normal goblet cells in some foci.
Mucosal lymphoid hyperplasia.	Submucosal lymphoid hyperplasia, transmural inflammation.

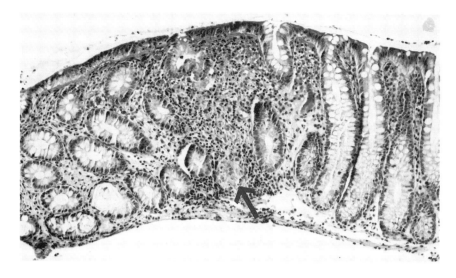

FIGURE 7-3. Crohn's disease in colonic biopsy shows focal inflammation and granuloma *(arrow)*.

focal neutrophilic infiltration confined to the region of a solitary lymphoid follicle. In the early stages of indeterminate colitis, the inflammation may be patchy rather than generalized. Colitis due to enterohemorrhagic *E. coli* may be focal or segmental, but the endoscopically normal mucosa may also show acute inflammation.[6]

Colonic and Appendiceal Granulomas

Colonic granulomas may be caused by Crohn's disease, tuberculosis, schistosomiasis, histoplasmosis, yersiniosis, strongyloidiasis, syphilis, *Chlamydia trachomatis,*[12] chronic granulomatous disease, barium sulfate crystals, sarcoidosis,[19] pneumatosis,[20] diversion colitis,[21] and segmental colitis associated with diverticular disease.[22] In the last two conditions, granulomas are probably a response to leakage of mucin from ruptured crypts. The granulomas of **Crohn's disease** are mainly sarcoid-like, but vary in morphology from pericryptal histiocytic aggregates, through suppurating granulomas with central clusters of neutrophils or eosinophils, to microgranulomas comprised of small aggregates of epithelioid histiocytes without giant cells. Isolated giant cells, when located in the basal portion of the mucosa, are as significant diagnostically as granulomas.[10] Granulomas combined with foci of mixed inflammatory all infiltration of the basal mucosa are highly suggestive of Crohn's disease. **Chronic granulomatous disease, glycogen storage disease type Ib, congenital neutropenia, agammaglobulinemia,** or the **Hermansky-Pudlak syndrome** can show Crohn's-like inflammation of the gut[23-27] (Fig. 7–4). Caseation is the hallmark of **tuberculous** granulomas, but the diagnosis can be established only by the identification of acid-fast bacilli. **Schistosomiasis** is diagnosed by the morphology of the ova, which are typically deposited in the submucosa and induce an eosinophilic inflammatory response and concentric fibrosis. In hyperinfection with ***Strongyloides stercoralis,*** larvae invade the colon and granulomas form in response to dead larvae. The diagnosis is established by identifying the larvae. **Yersinia** colitis displays ulceration over lymphoid follicles, microscopic abscesses, and suppurating granulomas in germinal centers and in the draining lymph nodes.

DIFFERENTIAL DIAGNOSIS. Isolated **Crohn's disease** of the appendix is rare. The majority of cases in which the appendix alone shows a greatly thickened wall, transmural inflammation with lymphoid follicular aggregates, and granulomas do not proceed to develop Crohn's disease of the ileum or colon.[28, 29] These cases represent resolving appendicitis with foreign body granulomatous reaction or inflammatory pseudotumor. Subacute or retrocecal appendicitis may also cause a tumor-like inflammatory reaction and has been referred to as

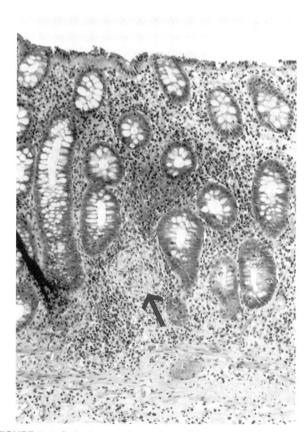

FIGURE 7-4. Colonic granuloma *(arrow)* in a 12-year-old boy with chronic granulomatous disease. The endoscopic findings also resembled Crohn's disease.

appendicular granuloma or ligneous cecitis.[30, 31] **Obliquely cut crypts, submucosal ganglia, nerve trunks,** or **nodules of muscularis mucosae** may simulate granulomas but are easily distinguished on serial or deeper sections.

Colitis of Behçet's Disease

Behçet's disease is an idiopathic relapsing condition characterized by aphthous stomatitis, genital ulcers, and uveitis. Gastrointestinal involvement presents with attacks of vomiting, abdominal pain, flatulence, and diarrhea or constipation. The colon can be involved locally or diffusely, and the ileocecal region is primarily affected. Colonic ulcers are typically large and discrete, but aphthoid, linear, and serpiginous ulcers separated by edematous and friable intervening mucosa also occur. Pseudopolyps have also been described.[32–34] Microscopically, the ulcers penetrate through the muscularis mucosae into the submucosa and sometimes into the muscularis propria. They occasionally spread laterally in ''collar button'' fashion. Deep ulceration predisposes to perforation and bleeding, which are the main complications.[33] Granulomatous inflammation and isolated giant cells occasionally line the ulcers. Anal ulcers or fissures may be present.

The intact mucosa displays areas of patchy inflammation with occasional crypt abscesses.[32] The small veins and venules in the submucosa are frequently inflamed, and all layers of the vessel wall are infiltrated by mononuclear cells, predominantly lymphocytes, with rare neutrophils, but there is no necrosis or fibrinoid change. Leukocytoclastic vasculitis may also occur. The location of vasculitis near small ulcers suggests that it may cause the ulcers. Lymphangiectasia is often present, occasionally with mild lymphangitis.[32]

DIFFERENTIAL DIAGNOSIS. It is not always possible to distinguish Behçet's colitis from Crohn's disease if granulomas are present; some authors describe concurrent Crohn's disease and Behçet's disease. Colitis in Behçet's disease lacks the transmural lymphoid aggregates of Crohn's disease. Venulitis typifies Behçet's disease but is unusual in Crohn's disease.

Collagenous Colitis

Collagenous colitis (CC) is an idiopathic chronic clinicopathologic syndrome characterized by chronic watery diarrhea, occurrence mainly in middle-aged women (male : female ratio, 1 : 4), normal large-bowel endoscopic findings, subepithelial collagen deposition, and preserved crypt architecture.[33–40] CC may be associated with gluten sensitivity, thyroid abnormalities, rheumatoid or seronegative arthritis, and NSAID therapy.

Histologically, the surface epithelium is often lost by the trauma of biopsy, suggesting increased friability. Epithelial lymphocytes are increased in number. The lamina propria contains moderately increased numbers of plasma cells, lymphocytes, and granulocytes. The collagen band beneath the intercrypt surface epithelium is thickened to greater than 10 μm at least focally (Fig. 7–5). Trichrome stain helps emphasize this lesion. The thickness of the band varies from case to case and from biopsy to biopsy. The rectum may not show collagenization, and biopsies should be obtained proximal to the rectum if the diagnosis is suspected.

DIFFERENTIAL DIAGNOSIS. CC presents as watery diarrhea, and the colorectal mucosa looks normal, whereas **IIBD** manifests hematochezia and endoscopic inflammation and ulceration. IIBD does not show collagenization, marked increase in the number of epithelial lymphocytes, or predominance of the inflammation in the upper part of the mucosa. Crypt architectural distortion seen with IIBD is not present in CC. **Ischemia** or **radiation colitis** may include diffuse collagenization of the lamina propria, but this is not limited to the subepithelial zone. When **amyloidosis** involves the mucosa, it is sometimes deposited beneath the surface epithelium forms multiple clumps rather than a uniform band. Trichrome and Congo red stains can differentiate the lesions.

Lymphocytic Colitis

Lymphocytic colitis displays greatly increased numbers of epithelial lymphocytes, increased mononuclear cells in the lamina propria, flattening of surface epithelial cells, and preservation of crypt architecture[41–43] (Fig. 7–6). The normal number of epithelial lymphocytes is less than 1 per 20 epithelial nuclei, and in lymphocytic colitis the number increases to about one per five epithelial nuclei. Thirty percent of patients with celiac disease have this lesion, but the proportion of cases of lymphocytic colitis that are due to gluten sensitivity is unknown. Lymphocytic colitis was originally called microscopic colitis, and it is unclear whether a form of microscopic colitis exists that is distinct from lymphocytic colitis.

DIFFERENTIAL DIAGNOSIS. This lesion differs from CC in that it lacks a collagenous band and does not have a predilection for women.[41] Other differential diagnostic considerations are the same as for collagenous colitis.

Diversion Proctocolitis

Diversion (or bypass) colitis arises in a portion of bowel excluded from the fecal stream[44] and resolves after reanastomosis.[44, 45] It was originally described in patients without prior inflammatory bowel disease who had undergone colostomy or ileostomy with rectal bypass, but it can also arise in patients who have had IIBD formerly. It has also occurred in a sigmoid neovagina. An etiologic factor is the lack of short-chain fatty acids, which are produced by bacterial metabolism and are an important metabolic substrate of colonic epithelial cells. Local application of these fatty acids can result in dramatic clinical improvement.[46]

Most cases of diversion colitis are clinically silent, but symptoms may include tenesmus, passage of blood and mucus, abdominal pain, and watery diarrhea.[45] The lesion may occur as early as 1 month after diversion or not until years later.[44] The bypassed segment shrinks, the lumen is narrowed, and the mucosa shows longitudinal ridges, diffuse nodularity, erythema, friability, petechiae, granularity, and inflammatory polyps. The distal segment is most severely affected, reminiscent of ulcerative colitis.[47, 48]

Microscopic appearances include surface epithelial degeneration, aphthoid ulcers over lymphoid follicles, lymphoid follicular hyperplasia, patchy inflammation of the lamina propria, focal crypt abscesses, preserved crypt architecture, mucin granulomas, and goblet cell depletion or excess.[21, 47–51]

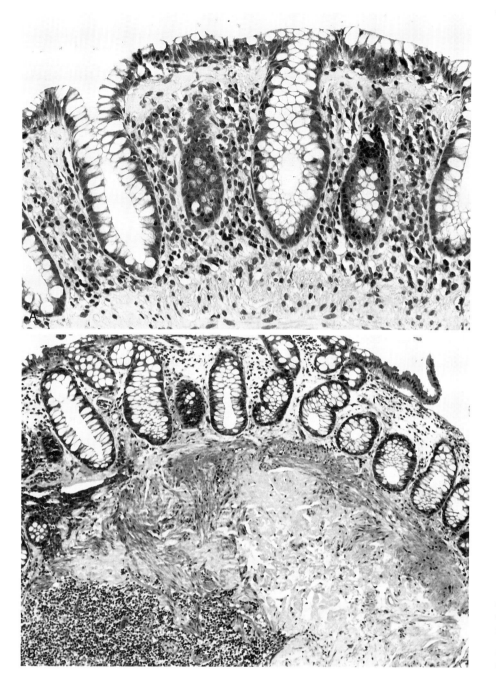

FIGURE 7–5. *A,* Collagenous colitis. Features include the subepithelial collagenous band, mild plasmacytosis, increased epithelial lymphocytes, and mucosal thinning. *B,* Amyloidosis can sometimes mimic collagenous colitis but is more often in the submucosa as here.

DIFFERENTIAL DIAGNOSIS. The main lesions to distinguish from bypass colitis are **ulcerative colitis** and **Crohn's disease.** In patients bypassed for conditions other than IIBD, appearances reminiscent of IIBD, including aphthoid ulcers and focal inflammation, can be confidently attributed to diversion. Granulomas in a bypassed segment of a patient with previous Crohn's disease do not confirm recurrence but would have to be regarded as suggestive of it. It may be impossible to distinguish recurrent Crohn's disease from diversion colitis, and when there is doubt, restoration of bowel continuity should be considered.[49, 50] After subtotal colectomy for UC, the rectal stump may show **florid lymphoid hyperplasia,** changes resembling **pseudomembranous colitis** or **ischemia,** or changes that resemble Crohn's disease, including granulomas near ruptured crypts, transmural inflammation, and fis-

sures. The pathologist should be aware of this spectrum of disease so as not to deny the patient the advantage of a pelvic ileal reservoir.

Segmental Colitis Associated with Diverticular Disease

Segmental colitis associated with diverticular disease is still poorly characterized. Grossly, the mucosa in the vicinity of the diverticular disease displays erythema and friability (independent of polypoid prolapsing mucosal folds). Biopsies show a focal or diffuse increase in laminal chronic inflammatory cells together with neutrophil cryptitis, crypt abscesses, crypt

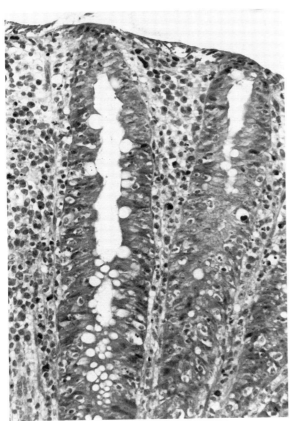

FIGURE 7–6. Lymphocytic colitis. Vast increase in epithelial lymphocytes but no subepithelial collagenization.

regeneration, and sometimes granulomas, resembling idiopathic ulcerative colitis or Crohn's disease.[22, 52-55]

DIFFERENTIAL DIAGNOSIS. If a diffuse chronic proctitis is present, the diagnosis is likely to be **ulcerative colitis;** but if biopsies of the rectum are not inflamed, then segmental colitis is more likely. **Crohn's disease** may affect the sigmoid concomitantly with diverticular disease. **Infectious colitis** can produce a segmental pattern of inflammation.

Cecal Diverticulosis

The spectrum of acquired right-sided diverticulosis includes total colonic diverticulosis, diverticulosis confined to the right colon, and solitary right-sided diverticula. Cecal involvement occurs in only 5% of cases of diverticulosis in the Western Hemisphere and is more common in men.[56, 57] The average age of involvement of cecum is 45 years, as opposed to 60 years for left-sided diverticulosis. **Solitary cecal diverticulum** may ulcerate, mimic appendicitis, perforate, bleed, fistulize into the bladder,[58] or occasionally reach enormous dimensions, up to 10 cm in diameter. An ulcerated solitary diverticulum can be distinguished from a deeply penetrating ulcer by the presence of mucosa at the base of the lesion. Diverticula penetrate alongside blood vessels into the mesocolon, and an inordinate number of cases of massive colonic hemorrhage arise from right-sided diverticula.[59] The proposed mechanism is that fecaliths form a solid surface against which the relentless pounding of the artery causes pressure necrosis and ultimately erosion of the arterial wall. Right-sided colonic

diverticulosis is the most common form of colonic diverticulosis in Asia.[60, 61]

Benign Idiopathic Non-specific Ulcer of the Large Bowel

This is a solitary lesion that is most often found in the cecum of a middle-aged person; however, there is a wide reported age range, including cases in children.[62-66] It presents mainly as perforation, pericolic abscess, or bleeding. Grossly, it varies in size from millimeters to 3 cm and is well circumscribed. Histologically, it is non-specific. The etiology is uncertain. Repeated radiologic examination or endoscopy and biopsy may be necessary to distinguish it from carcinoma.[64]

DIFFERENTIAL DIAGNOSIS. NSAIDs should be considered as possible causes of any idiopathic ulcer. Cecal ulceration as a component of **neutropenic enterocolitis** or **obstructive colitis** is distinguished by the clinical context. Previous removal of polyp and **cauterization** can cause ulceration that is slow to heal and is associated with reparative changes and fibrosis extending into the muscle coat.

Stercoral Ulcers

Stercoral ulcers of the rectum or colon are due to the pressure of impacted feces in bedridden and elderly patients and in patients with dysmotility of the bowel.[67, 68] The ulcers are single or multiple, with irregular outlines, slightly depressed below the mucosal surface, and conform to the shape of the distending mass of feces.[67] The muscle coat may be stretched and thinned, predisposing to free perforation or perirectal abscess. Histologically, the ulcers are non-specific and the inflammatory response is mild. If the ulcer penetrates through the muscle coat, extrarectal suppuration and fat necrosis may occur.[67] Fecal impaction may also be complicated by **obstructive colitis** with perforation of the cecum or of a proximal diverticulum.[69]

DIFFERENTIAL DIAGNOSIS. Chronic ischemia may cause localized stricture with fibrosis and hemosiderin deposition, and typically the splenic flexure is affected. Stercoral ulcers can occur in patients with **systemic sclerosis or other collagen-vascular diseases** when dysmotility leads to chronic constipation, but vasculitis and ischemia may also occur in these patients. Stercoral ulcers are not associated with significant blood vessel pathology other than age-related changes. The ulcers associated with **NSAIDs** are bland, non-specific ulcers that have a predilection for the cecum and for the crests of mucosal folds.

Solitary Rectal Ulcer Syndrome (Rectal Prolapse Syndrome) and Inflammatory Cloacogenic Polyp

Solitary rectal ulcer syndrome (SRUS)[70-76] presents as a single indurated ulcer in the anterior wall of the rectum in 80% of cases, and as multiple ulcers or non-ulcerated, nodular, diffusely erythematous plaques in others. SRUS is due to mucosal prolapse and is an indolent benign condition, refractory to most forms of therapy.[73] Patients present with anorectal pain, passage of blood and mucus, and a feeling of rectal obstruction. The peak incidence is in the third and fourth decades, with equal sex distribution.

Histologic features are tubulovillous architecture with crypt dilatation, ulceration of the superficial epithelium with a pseudomembranous exudate, vascular congestion and fibromuscular obliteration of the lamina propria, thickening of the muscularis mucosae, regenerative proliferation of the epithelium with loss of cytoplasmic mucus, hyperchromatism, nuclear crowding, increased mitotic activity, and a villiform surface configuration, and displacement of glands into the submucosa with mucous cysts due to glandular occlusion (colitis cystica profunda) (Fig. 7–7A).

Inflammatory cloacogenic polyp occurs at the anorectal transitional zone and is similar to solitary ulcer of the rectum. One in four cases protrudes from the anus;[77, 78] others present with rectal bleeding. Patients range in age from 43 to 81 years (median, 66). Most lesions are firm and rubbery, measuring between 1 and 3 cm in diameter, occasionally up to 5 cm. Histologic features are similar to those in SRUS except that the lesions are partially covered by anal squamous mucosa

(Fig. 7–7B). Typical hemorrhoidal dilation of veins and venules in the submucosal plexus can be found in some cases. Others may be variants of solitary ulcer of rectum syndrome.

DIFFERENTIAL DIAGNOSIS. The crypt hyperplastic and regenerative features of both SRUS and inflammatory cloacogenic polyp can be misinterpreted as **dysplasia** or **adenoma.** Displaced glands in the submucosa can be confused with **well-differentiated mucinous adenocarcinoma** but do not show desmoplasia. Small biopsies of the surface ulcer and exudate may resemble **pseudomembranous colitis,** but there is no history of antibiotic therapy.

Colitis Cystica Profunda

In this condition, colonic mucosal glands are displaced into the submucosa and become cystically dilated. The rare generalized form follows a bout of dysentery, and the glands are believed to penetrate into the submucosa through defects left by ulceration of lymphoid-glandular complexes.[79] In the localized form, the displaced glands are a component of a condition such as solitary ulcer of the rectum syndrome,

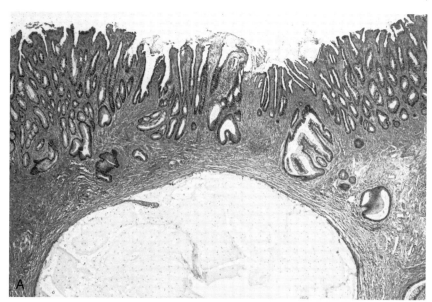

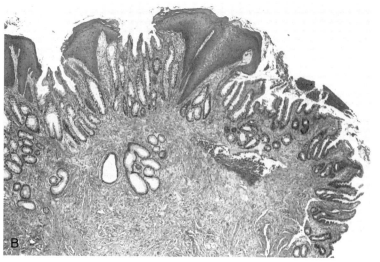

FIGURE 7–7. *A,* Solitary ulcer of the rectum syndrome with localized colitis cystica profunda. Note villiform surface, surface ulceration, epithelial hyperchromatism, and displaced glands in the submucosa forming a cyst. *B,* Inflammatory cloacogenic polyp shows features similar to solitary ulcer syndrome at the squamocolumnar junction.

polyp, chronic inflammatory bowel disease, ischemia, radiation effect, or idiopathic.[79–85] The age range of patients is from 4 to 68 years.[83] Most cases are clinically silent, but large cysts have caused obstruction. Grossly, colitis cystica appears as single or multiple nodular elevations of the mucosa, and on cut surface the nodules are submucosal mucinous cysts. In chronic colitis, the cysts are usually an incidental finding, but, in association with inflammatory polyps, they may create a mass lesion that can simulate a neoplasm.[82] Multiple discrete lesions or segments of affected bowel may be present synchronously or metachronously.[79]

On microscopic examination, the displaced crypts are cystically dilated, and mucinous lakes devoid of an epithelial lining may be present (see Fig. 7–7A). The epithelial lining of the cysts may be columnar or cuboidal and includes absorptive, goblet, endocrine, and metaplastic Paneth cells. Dysplasia is not a feature. There is usually mild reparative fibrosis around the cysts and infiltration by lymphocytes, plasma cells, and eosinophils. The adjacent bowel mucosa can show ulcerative colitis or Crohn's disease. The muscularis mucosae is focally deficient, but in some areas it can appear thickened and fibrotic.

DIFFERENTIAL DIAGNOSIS. Colitis cystica profunda can be distinguished from **mucinous adenocarcinoma** by the presence of epithelial dysplasia, desmoplasia, and invasion in the latter lesion.[84] A case of adenocarcinoma *in situ* in association with colitis cystica profunda has been reported.[85] The cysts of **pneumatosis coli** are lined by connective tissue or histiocytic giant cells, not by epithelium. **Endometriosis** or **endosalpingiosis** can also form tumor-like masses and contain cystic spaces but are distinguished by the morphology of the epithelium, the absence of goblet cells, the presence of endometrial stroma, hemosiderosis, and the marked muscle coat hypertrophy that accompanies endometriosis. Colitis cystica does not usually penetrate the muscularis propria, whereas endometriosis and endosalpingiosis are primarily located in the muscularis propria and serosa. **Colitis cystica superficialis** is cystic dilation of mucosal crypts after bacillary dysentery or pellagra.[86]

Colonic Ischemia

Ischemia is deprivation of blood flow resulting in hypoxia and infarction. The diagnosis is most secure when infarction and vascular occlusion are present, features that are more easily appreciated on a resection specimen than on mucosal biopsies. The main morphologic forms of ischemia are superficial ischemia affecting mucosa alone, acute infarction due to arterial or venous occlusion, ischemic strictures, and multifocal ischemia due to multiple vessel occlusions by vasculitis or emboli.[87, 88]

Acute ischemia results in a spectrum of mucosal changes, from rapid epithelial turnover to infarction. In the mildest ischemic injury, surface epithelial cells are lost and immature crypt cells migrate upward and stretch out to maintain mucosal integrity. The crypt epithelium becomes thinned and the crypts become dilated. With increasing ischemia, ulceration occurs, and fibrin and neutrophils exude to form a diffuse thin pseudomembrane. The inflammatory cell infiltrate in the viable tissue is often scanty. Intact mucosa at the margin of an ischemic ulcer typically shows hyalinization of the lamina propria and

mucosal atrophy (Fig. 7–8A). Biopsies of a mild acute ischemic lesion show a thin mucosa, loss of surface epithelium, loss of mucus, attenuated crypt epithelium, and few neutrophils. Extreme congestion and hemorrhage of mucosa and submucosa typify venous obstruction and may also follow reperfusion after arterial occlusion or hypotensive episodes.

Non-occlusive or transient colonic ischemia is due to arterial spasm, prolonged hypotension (low-flow), dehydration, or combined hypotension and arterial stenosis, and presents with hemorrhagic diarrhea and thumbprinting on barium enema. The ischemic lesions can be unisegmental or multifocal[89, 90] (Fig. 7–8B). An **ischemic stricture** may follow such an episode of acute ischemia that causes circumferential mucosal necrosis. It has a thickened wall, ulcerated mucosa, and congested serosa. Inflammation can range from minimal to heavy and chronic, resembling Crohn's disease. Hemosiderin deposits are often present. The proximal and distal mucosa is normal. **Venous occlusion** occurs by mechanical obstruction, thrombosis, local inflammation, or vasculitis.[91] Vasculitis and emboli are the main causes of **multifocal ischemic lesions,** in addition to non-occlusive or hypoperfusion ischemia.[92–95] Atheromatous emboli have occasionally been diagnosed on colorectal biopsy.[93] Colonic ischemia can also complicate pancreatitis, with resultant strictures and obstruction.[96]

DIFFERENTIAL DIAGNOSIS. Acute lesions of ischemia may be histologically indistinguishable from **enterohemorrhagic E. coli (EHEC)** infection, and this infection probably accounts for cases formerly labeled transient ischemic colitis in young healthy adults.[97] Acute necrosis of the colon rarely follows enemas of **sodium polystyrene sulfonate in sorbitol.**[98] Histology resembles autolysis, except for neutrophilic infiltrates and hemorrhage. **CMV** infects endothelium and may cause secondary ischemia, but the intranuclear inclusions and focal neutrophilic infiltrates should be present. **Segmental colitis** due to infection or associated with diverticular disease is a purely inflammatory condition. Ischemic strictures differ from **Crohn's disease** by lacking multiple foci of inflammation and ulceration, mucosal scars, and granulomas. Ischemic circumferential ulcers often extend for several centimeters, whereas long segmental ulcers are exceptional in Crohn's disease. Submucosal lymphoid aggregates, transmural inflammation, and fissures can be present in both chronic ischemia and Crohn's disease. Organizing arterial thrombi, cholesterol emboli, or vasculitis establishes the diagnosis of ischemia, and it may be necessary to take multiple blocks of mesocolic vessels to identify the vascular pathology. **Chronic radiation enteritis** includes an element of chronic ischemia due to arterial hyalinization and thus can also result in fibrosis and strictures. **Clostridial infection** can simulate ischemia or be triggered by ischemia.

Iatrogenic Colitides

Side effects of medication must be considered when any of the following appearances are found: abundant apoptoses, non-specific ulcers, infectious colitis, ischemia, eosinophilic colitis, collagenous colitis, lymphocytic colitis, pseudo-obstruction, or melanosis coli.[99–122] Examples of colitides facilitated by medications include pseudomembranous colitis by antibiotics; *Yersinia* enterocolitis by deferoxamine; neutropenic enterocolitis by anticancer chemotherapy; neonatal

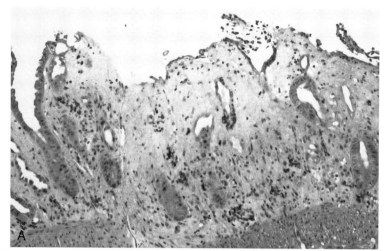

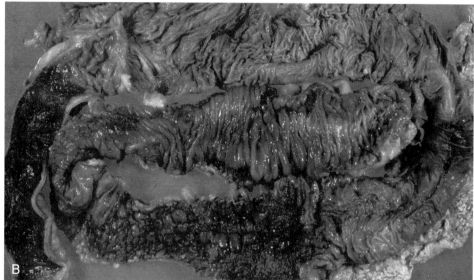

FIGURE 7-8. *A,* Colonic ischemia shows hyalinized lamina propria, focal loss of the surface epithelium, regenerating crypts, and minimal inflammation. Identical features can be seen in enterohemorrhagic *E. coli* infection. *B,* Colonic ischemia due to prolonged hypotension after myocardial infarction 10 days before surgery. Note the ulcerated ileum *(left)* and descending colon *(bottom)* superficially resembling Crohn's disease.

enterocolitis by hypertonic formula; colonic necrosis due to the osmotic enema preparation Kayexalate-sorbitol; colitis or ulcers by NSAIDs, sulfasalazine, gold, alpha methyldopa, flucytosine, or methotrexate; and hypotension and ischemia by drugs capable of causing hypotension, vasospasm, or thrombophilia, such as cocaine, amphetamines, catecholamines, ergotamine, methysergide, vasopressin, digitalis, potent diuretics, and estrogens.[98, 119] Bowel wall hematomas may occur after minor trauma or spontaneously in patients taking anticoagulants but are much more frequent in the small bowel than the large.[118] Drugs may cause blood loss. Pseudo-obstruction may be caused by narcotics, anticholinergics, phenothiazines, tricyclic antidepressants, vincristine, and chronic cathartic use.

NSAIDs

Non-steroidal anti-inflammatory drugs (NSAIDs) have been implicated in causing non-specific ulcers of the ileum, ileocecal valve, and ascending colon; mucosal diaphragms; reactivation of quiescent inflammatory bowel disease; hypersensitivity reactions; large numbers of crypt apoptoses; and collagenous or lymphocytic colitis.[100-111] Diclofenac (Volta-

ren), mefenamic acid, and indomethacin are frequent offenders, especially the sustained-release preparations. Patients present with abdominal cramps, diarrhea, or constipation, and laboratory tests reveal iron deficiency anemia and positive fecal occult blood results. Colonic ulcers mainly affect the ascending colon, are located on the crests of mucosal folds, are non-specific histologically, and show submucosal fibrosis with follicular lymphoid aggregates (Fig. 7–9). Colonic diaphragms are stenosing mucosal folds, giving a smooth strictured contour on barium enema.[104] Proctitis with bleeding has been reported with salicylates. Some of the patients had previous ulcerative colitis, but others developed *de novo* proctitis.[100] Proctitis has also been described after suppositories of indomethacin or mefenamic acid. Recurrent inflammatory bowel disease has been described with the use of NSAIDs and confirmed by challenge tests in a small number of cases. The reactivation frequently involved the sigmoid colon.[107]

Bowel Preparation for Endoscopy

Mannitol-induced diarrhea or saline enema produces no change.[112] Fleet's enema and bisacodyl ingestion cause mucosal hyperemia and obliteration of the normal vascular pattern

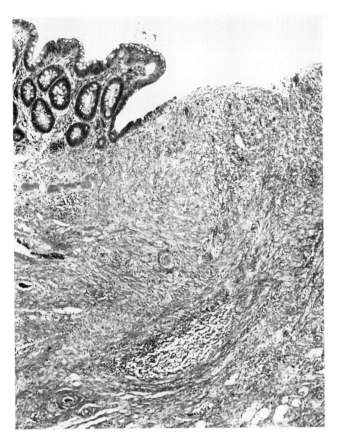

FIGURE 7–9. NSAID ulcer of the ascending colon in a man aged 82 years. Grossly, there were transverse ulcers along the apices of the mucosal folds. The histologic features are non-specific.

on endoscopy and sloughing of the surface epithelium histologically. In addition, bisacodyl caused loss of goblet cell mucus and pallor and homogenization of the epithelial cells on the surface and, to varying depths, within the crypts. The nuclei were pale and lost much of their chromatin. Polymorphonuclear leukocytes were seen in the epithelium and lumina of the crypts in 15% of biopsies.[112] Hypertonic sodium phosphate enemas caused mucin depletion of the glands, increased mucosal fragility, and edema of the lamina propria.[113]

Gold

Eosinophilic infiltration of colonic mucosa has been reported after use of the combination of gold (sodium aurothiomalate) and aspirin for the treatment of seronegative arthritis.[114]

Ampicillin and Penicillins

Transient, acute, right-sided, segmental, hemorrhagic colitis suggestive of ischemia has been associated with penicillins.[115] Pathogenic bacteria were not detected on stool culture. Whether these cases represent true drug-associated disease or coincidental infection or ischemia is unclear. Endoscopic biopsies were not performed. **Antibiotic-related colitis** is a form of infectious colitis due to bacterial overgrowth and altered colonic ecology.

Methyldopa

A handful of cases of transient acute colitis in association with methyldopa treatment have been described.[116] Most presented with bloody diarrhea that remitted on discontinuation of the drug.

Methotrexate

Extensive colonic ulceration and toxic megacolon have been associated with methotrexate therapy, and death has been ascribed to methotrexate colitis.[117] In all of the reported cases, the drug was implicated by temporal association, and other potential contributory factors, particularly hypotension, were not always ruled out. *Oral contraceptives* have been associated with a slight increase in incidence of Crohn's disease as well as with ischemia and ulceration.[119]

5-Fluorouracil

This drug may cause an acute colitis with epithelial necrosis in the acute phase and crypt regenerative features in the healed phase.[120]

Psychotropic Drugs

These have been associated with ischemic-type colitis, and carbamazepine has been linked with eosinophilic colitis.[121]

Pseudomembranous Colitis (PMC)

A pseudomembrane is composed of inflammatory exudate, mucus, and necrotic debris and forms on a mucous membrane in response to epithelial destruction by exotoxins or ischemia. Most cases of PMC follow antibiotic therapy that enhances the proliferation of toxigenic *C. difficile*.[123] Clindamycin, lincomycin, ampicillin, and cephalosporins are strongly associated with PMC development within 4 to 9 days of the onset of antibiotic therapy. Three percent of adults are carriers of *C. difficile,* but not all strains are potentially pathogenic. The patient may either be a preexisting carrier or acquire the organism by ingestion of spores, and nosocomial spread of single strains of *C. difficile* is responsible for most outbreaks.[124] The organism produces two large protein toxins that are responsible for PMC.

PMC presents with watery diarrhea, fever, leukocytosis, and abdominal pain. Occult blood tests are often positive. In severe cases, hypokalemia, hypoalbuminemia, edema, and ascites may develop.[125] Rarely, colonic perforation, toxic megacolon, fulminant colitis without dilatation, and acute reactive arthritis occur.[126, 127] Relapses are common and may be multiple. PMC can be fatal in debilitated patients with preexisting illness,[128] and it may complicate IIBD. Subtotal colectomy and ileostomy may be required for refractory disease, perforation, or toxic megacolon.

Grossly, yellow nodules or plaques of pseudomembrane, from 2 to 20 mm in size, are strewn over the mucosa. The rectum is relatively spared.[128, 129] The mucosa between the pseudomembranes is intact.

Microscopically, PMC displays three lesions of increasing severity.[123] The type 1 lesion consists of ulceration of the surface intercrypt epithelium with a spray of fibrin, mucin, and neutrophils erupting from the erosion (Fig. 7–10). The type 2 lesion is a larger pseudomembrane that covers the mouths of several crypts. The crypts show dilatation and either goblet cell distention or secretory exhaustion. Within the pseudomembrane, neutrophil leukocytes are arrayed in regular files amidst fibrin and mucin. The type 3 lesion consists of pseudomembranes overlying necrotic mucosa with extreme distention of the crypts.[123] The submucosa shows severe edema, fibrin deposition, and capillary thrombi.[128] Candidal overgrowth in the colonic lumen may accompany PMC. Rectosigmoid biopsies are not always diagnostic of PMC, because the distal large bowel is least affected and the mucosa may show only edema, congestion, and neutrophil infiltration similar to any infectious colitis.[129]

DIFFERENTIAL DIAGNOSIS. Conditions that may be confused with plaques of PMC on endoscopy or biopsy include amebiasis, cytomegalovirus infection, chemical colitis caused by endoscope cleaning solution, mucosal prolapse, ulcerated adenoma, acute ischemia, and diversion proctitis. **Mucosal prolapse** exhibits congestion and fibromuscular proliferation in the lamina propria, and the mucosa often has a villiform pattern—features that distinguish it from PMC. The pseudomembranous exudate in amebiasis contains trophozoites, and foci of deep ulceration and necrosis may be present. In **ulcerated adenomas** with surface exudate, the cytologic and architectural dysplasia of the glands allows easy distinction from PMC. **Cytomegalovirus** colitis is occasionally accompanied by surface ulceration covered by a compact fibrinous exudate distinct from the loose mix of mucin, fibrin, and neutrophils in *C. difficile*–related PMC. **Acute ischemia** causes a segmental or diffuse lesion with confluent rather than discrete pseudomembranes. If the underlying mucosa is infarcted, distinction from type 3 lesions of PMC may not be possible. Ischemic mucosa may appear atrophic, and the lamina propria is often hypocellular and collagenous. **Enterohemorrhagic *E. coli* or *Shigella dysenteriae type 1*** may produce pseudomembranes identical to those caused by *C. difficile*.

Granuloma Inguinale

Granuloma inguinale is a venereal disease of the tropics and subtropics caused by *Calymmatobacterium granulomatis*.

It produces anal and genital ulcers, which are typically multiple, painless, red, and elevated. The inguinal nodes are enlarged and tender. Histologically, the ulcers are composed of granulation tissue containing a mixed inflammatory infiltrate of plasma cells, neutrophils, and large, pale histiocytes containing intracellular rod-shaped bacilli (Donovan bodies) that stain positively with silver stains. Antibiotic treatment is curative, but scarring can be extensive.

DIFFERENTIAL DIAGNOSIS. Although this lesion has a distinctive histologic presentation, it is diagnosed and distinguished from **lymphogranuloma venereum** (LGV) by culture of *C. granulomatis*. LGV causes a proctitis, but granuloma inguinale does not.

Rectal Syphilis

Rectal syphilis occurs typically in promiscuous homosexual men as an ulcer or proctitis and may occur concurrently with chancres in the anal canal or at the anal margin. The length of time between infection and presentation may be up to 2 months.[130] Biopsies reveal a heavy infiltrate of plasma cells and lymphocytes, but sometimes there are ill-defined granulomas.[130, 131] Serologic tests may be negative early in the course of the disease.

DIFFERENTIAL DIAGNOSIS. Rectal syphilis can grossly mimic a neoplasm or solitary ulcer syndrome. A case in which rectal biopsy showed confluent nodules of large pleomorphic lymphoid cells in the submucosa mixed with occasional atypical lymphocytes was mistaken for **lymphoma**.[132] The distinction can be made by the absence of clonality on immunostained sections and by identification of treponemes on darkfield examination or on Warthin-Starry stains.

Actinomycosis

Actinomycosis is a chronic suppurative and fibrogenic infection caused by filamentous, gram-positive, anaerobic bacteria, most commonly *Actinomyces israelii*, which is a normal oral and gastrointestinal commensal. ''Sulfur granules'' (colonies of actinomyces) may be seen in pus or colonies may be first observed histologically. On anaerobic culture the

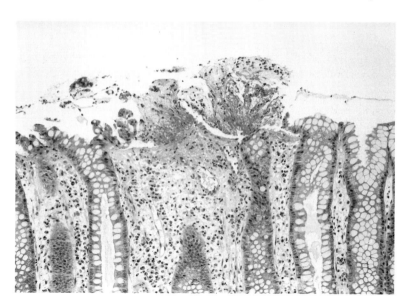

FIGURE 7–10. Pseudomembranous colitis, type 1 lesion. Surface ulceration with spray of exudate and mucosal edema.

colonies have a characteristic radiating filamentous form and are gram-positive but not acid-fast. The infection in the colon often follows surgery (appendectomy) or trauma.[133] Males outnumber females 3 to 1. Intrauterine contraceptive devices predispose to pelvic actinomycosis that can secondarily affect the colon.[134] Diabetes and immunodeficiency also predispose to this infection. Saprophytic colonies may be seen in diverticulitis, in the lumen of the appendix (normal or inflamed), and in suture lines of low rectal anastomoses, but invasive actinomycosis in any of these contexts is rare.[135] Colonic actinomycosis is a great imitator and may present with an abscess, fistula, or tumor-like mass in the retroperitoneum[133, 136] or with non-specific symptoms such as abdominal mass, low-grade fever, malaise, and persisting sinus. When seen as a mass lesion at surgery, it displays a marked fibrotic reaction and contains small pockets of pus with sulfur granules. **Rectal actinomycosis** is rare and is usually seen in the context of anal fistula or stricture,[137–139] but it can occur secondary to ileocecal disease. It can mimic carcinoma.[140] Endoscopic diagnosis of actinomycosis has been made,[141] and biopsies show intact mucosa with submucosal abscess.[139] **Appendiceal actinomycosis** presents as chronic suppurative appendicitis and periappendicitis with fibrosis and sinuses or fistulae to other organs or to the skin. Metastatic abscesses may occur in the liver.

DIFFERENTIAL DIAGNOSIS. Actinomycosis must be considered whenever a visceral mass consists of fibrosis with loculated microabscesses. A thorough examination of the tissue with multiple blocks and levels is indicated because the histologic diagnosis rests on identification of the organisms. *Nocardia* spp. or bacterial colonies may resemble actinomyces. *Nocardia* is acid-fast with the Ziehl-Neelsen method, but *Actinomyces* is not. *Nocardia* can form sulfur granules in the skin but not in the viscera. **Bacterial colonies** are not filamentous, radiating, or gram-positive.[142]

Amebiasis and Ulcerative Postdysenteric Colitis

Infection by *Entamoeba histolytica* may cause acute or chronic colitis or an asymptomatic carrier state. *E. histolytica* infection is relatively common in tropical or subtropical regions but rare in temperate climates, where most new infections are found among foreign travelers, recent immigrants, and homosexual men.[144] Transmission is fecal-oral, but it can also occur through colonic irrigation. The resistant, transmissible form of the organism is a cyst that measures 10 to 20 μm in diameter and contains four nuclei. When released from ingested cysts, trophozoites proliferate by binary fission. Only the trophozoites are seen in tissue; most are 15 to 25 μm in diameter and have a single, round, eccentric nucleus with a single central karyosome.[143] The cytoplasm of the trophozoites contains abundant glycogen. Trophozoites, which contain intracytoplasmic red blood cells, are pathognomonic for *E. histolytica. In vitro* culture of trophozoites is not available in most laboratories, and diagnosis is usually based on stool microscopy. Serologic techniques such as indirect hemagglutination are more specific than stool examination, and less than 1% of the general population of developed countries have antibodies.[144] Twenty-two different isoenzyme patterns (zymodemes) of *E. histolytica* have been distinguished by

electrophoresis, of which 12 zymodemes have never been associated with invasive disease.

Acute Amebic Colitis

Symptoms of acute amebic colitis resemble acute inflammatory bowel disease or dysentery and include diarrhea with blood and mucus, crampy abdominal pain, and tenesmus if there is rectal involvement. There may be tenderness over the cecum or colon and, in the most severe cases, toxic dilatation and fulminant colitis leading to perforation and peritonitis. Massive hemorrhage is rare. Endoscopic features vary: the mucosa may be friable, erythematous, and granular, or there may be small, discrete shallow ulcers or larger, undermined ulcers separated by normal-appearing mucosa. Endoscopic biopsies show a moderate neutrophilic infiltrate, capillary hyperemia, edema of the lamina propria, surface exudate, and hyperplasia of lymphoid follicles. The classic flask-shaped ulcer undermines the muscularis mucosae. In some cases, superficial depression of the mucosal surface with focal erosion of the surface epithelium, mucin depletion, increased numbers of mitotic figures, heavy neutrophilic infiltration, cryptitis, and crypt abscesses can be seen. Invasive lesions display ulcers in which a thin zone of fibrinoid necrosis and an inflammatory exudate separate clusters of amebae from the underlying tissue. Amebae are usually found in the surface exudate or mucus, but they are occasionally found beneath the zone of necrosis within the tissue.[145–149] Plasma cells usually predominate in the inflammatory response in the submucosa; neutrophils may be numerous, but eosinophils are generally rare. The blood vessels show endothelial cell swelling and occasionally thrombosis.

Chronic Amebic Colitis

Chronic amebic colitis is characterized by intermittent diarrhea and abdominal pain with anemia and anorexia. In resected specimens, the cecum is most commonly involved, the ileum rarely. Ulcers may be limited to one region of the colon or spread throughout the colon. They are sharply defined, undermine the adjacent mucosa, and may be associated with a pseudomembranous exudate. Fistulae are a rare complication.[150] Less than 5% of patients develop a localized tumor-like inflammatory mass (pseudotumor) called an ameboma, which leads to obstruction or intussusception. Radiologically and grossly, ameboma resembles carcinoma and may cause an annular constriction. Microscopically, ameboma consists of a florid granulation tissue and fibrotic response with sinuses containing clusters of trophozoites penetrating through it.[151] **Ulcerative postdysenteric colitis** is a persistent chronic diarrhea that follows successful treatment of amebic dysentery. It responds to antibiotics and is therefore probably due to bacterial overgrowth[152] and so may be akin to pouchitis or obstructive colitis. It is associated with colonic strictures due to submucosal scarring after the attack of amebiasis. The strictures are often located at the rectosigmoid junction.[151] Endoscopic and histologic features of chronic colitis with ulceration are reported.[151–153]

DIFFERENTIAL DIAGNOSIS. Amebic colitis can be distinguished from acute infectious colitis, antibiotic-induced colitis, or pseudomembranous colitis by identifying the amebae.

Phlegmonous Colitis

Phlegmonous infection is a rare, potentially lethal, acute, spreading, submucosal bacterial infection caused by streptococci, staphylococci, or gram-negative bacilli.[154, 155] It can affect immunocompetent or immunosuppressed patients. It presents with fever, chills, and neutrophilic leukocytosis. The bowel displays serosal congestion and submucosal edema and hemorrhage. Histologically, the submucosa shows a heavy neutrophilic infiltrate, edema, congestion, hemorrhage, and gram-positive cocci or gram-negative bacilli. Infection by a gas-forming organism is known as emphysematous colitis. Rarely, phlegmonous infection and even death have resulted from excision or banding of hemorrhoids.

DIFFERENTIAL DIAGNOSIS. Like phlegmonous colitis, **acute ischemia** with mucosal infarction may display a heavy neutrophilic infiltrate in the submucosa, but it can be distinguished from phlegmon by the presence of infarct, the absence of bacteria, and the fact that the infiltrate forms a band at the junction of infarcted and viable tissue.

Mesenteric Panniculitis of the Colon

Mesenteric panniculitis is a rare condition that may precede retractile or sclerosing mesenteritis.[156, 157] It usually affects the small bowel mesentery but can sometimes affect the colon, especially the sigmoid. The mean age of patients is 59 years (range, 37–75 years). Male to female ratio is 3:1. Complaints include abdominal pain, diarrhea, abdominal masses, and constipation. Barium enema discloses narrowing and shortening of the bowel, poor distensibility, a ragged or serrated mucosal outline, or, uncommonly, an apple core–like defect. Imaging studies show thickening of the colonic wall with soft-tissue density. At laparotomy, the lesion forms a marked thickening or mass in the mesocolon with a puckered surface and rubbery consistency. Histologic findings include aggregates of lipophages, foreign-body giant cells, lymphocytic infiltration, fibrosis, calcification, and sometimes phlebitis.

Vascular Ectasia

The primary manifestation of vascular ectasia of the colon is angiodysplasia, a telangiectasia of thin-walled capillaries and venules in the mucosa and submucosa that accounts for a large proportion of cases of acute massive colonic bleeding and chronic recurrent bleeding (Fig. 7–11A). Angiodysplasia is associated with von Willebrand's disease, calcific aortic-valve stenosis (15% of cases), cirrhosis, and occlusive vascular disease.[158–161] The mean age at diagnosis is approximately 65 years, but cases have occurred in the young.[162] Two thirds of the lesions are located in the cecum or ascending colon, and one quarter in the left colon, tending to be clustered in specific areas of the bowel.[163] By colonoscopy, they appear as cherry-red congeries of dilated vessels, 5 to 10 mm in diameter. They can be biopsied with impunity and are treated by fulguration.[162, 164, 165] They can sometimes be seen on angiograms,[158, 164] but in resected bowel, the vessels collapse when the specimen is cut open, so gross identification of the lesion becomes impossible by routine methods. Some authors have demonstrated the lesions by making vascular casts with materials such as barium-gelatin. One method that has been used to preserve them in resected specimens has been to fix the specimen by filling the lumen with formalin and then to strip the mucosa and transilluminate it.[166]

DIFFERENTIAL DIAGNOSIS. Telangiectasias are the most common long-term effect of **radiation. Hereditary hemorrhagic telangiectasia** affects younger patients who have a positive family history, recurrent epistaxis, and telangiectasias of the lips and oral mucosa. Histologically, the telangiectasias may have a characteristic sclerotic stromal component,[162] which is not a feature in cases of angiodysplasia. Furthermore, they can involve the muscularis propria and serosa. Sporadic telangiectasias in young patients are very uncommon. **Congestive colopathy** is a newly identified complication of portal hypertension that presents clinically with hematochezia or anemia. Endoscopically, cherry-red spots resembling angiodysplasia[167] or non-specific erythema resembling colitis is seen. Microscopically, there is edema and capillary dilatation.[167, 168] Colorectal varices occur rarely in portal hypertension and may cause massive bleeding. **Hemangiomas** of the colon may be of capillary, cavernous, or mixed types and are usually single, diffusely infiltrative, circumferential lesions that involve a segment of the colon (Fig. 7–11B). Small localized lesions also occur, especially in the **blue rubber bleb-nevus syndrome.**[169] **Congenital arteriovenous malformations** differ from angiodysplasias in having a mixture of thick- and thin-walled abnormal vessels.[170] The mucosal vascular ectasia is the diagnostic component of angiodysplasia; the submucosal venous ectasia is non-specific.[171] Massive colonic bleeding can also arise from **Dieulafoy lesions**—large eroded submucosal arteries.[172] **Fabry's disease** is a rare, sex-linked familial disease of glycosphingolipid metabolism that is caused by a deficiency of lysosomal ceramide trihexosidase. The rectum and small bowel usually reveal characteristic pinpoint angiomas. Chronic intestinal pseudo-obstruction may also occur. Rectal and duodenal biopsies show enlargement and microvesicular vacuolization of ganglion cells of Meissner's plexus, and ultrastructurally, they contain numerous cytoplasmic complex myelin figures or amorphous dense bodies.[173]

Malakoplakia

Malakoplakia is a rare tumor-like disorder in which masses of histiocytes accumulate, accompanied by variable numbers of plasma cells, lymphocytes, and granulocytes. The histiocytes contain Michaelis-Gutmann (MG) bodies, rounded, concentrically laminated, hematoxyphilic intracytoplasmic inclusions, 5 to 8 μm in diameter. The bodies stain positively for phosphorus, calcium, and sometimes iron. The histiocytes also contain PAS-positive granules that correspond ultrastructurally to phagolysosomes, and which include bacilliform organisms in 50% of cases. The basic defect is postulated to be a failure by macrophages to dispose of phagocytosed bacteria or, in cases of extensive disease, a failure of bacterial killing.[174]

The colon is the most common site of malakoplakia outside the urogenital tract and has a bimodal age incidence with one peak in children younger than the age of 13 and a second in middle-aged adults.[174, 175] There is a slight male predominance. Some colonic malakoplakias are incidental foci adjacent to a

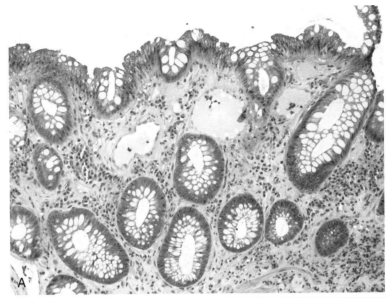

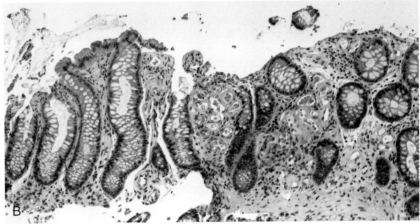

FIGURE 7–11. *A,* Telangiectatic vessels in the colorectal mucosa due to angiodysplasia. Similar appearances can be due to chronic radiation injury or congestive colopathy (as a result of portal hypertension). *B,* Capillary hemangioma of the sigmoid colon (endoscopic biopsy) showing multiple, closely packed capillaries. This was a large angioma and required segmental colectomy.

carcinoma; others are primary and may be associated with immune deficiency or opportunistic infections. Colonic malakoplakia presents with abdominal pain, mass, fever, anemia, diarrhea, or colitis and may simulate Crohn's disease with ulcers and fistulae. Endoscopically, there are ulcerated or umbilicated yellowish mucosal nodules or polyps.[176, 177] Malakoplakia can rarely be an aggressive tumor-like lesion involving several viscera and resulting in fistulae and bowel obstruction, but the bladder is rarely involved concomitantly with large bowel.[178] Intestinal resection sometimes leads to recovery.

DIFFERENTIAL DIAGNOSIS. The main distinction is from nonspecific **xanthogranulomatous** inflammation, **Whipple's disease,** and *Mycobacterium avium–intracellulare* **(MAI)** infection. The histiocytes of xanthogranulomas contain few PAS-positive granules, not the large numbers seen in Whipple's disease. The macrophages of xanthogranulomas never contain MG bodies. The specific bacterium of Whipple's disease, *Tropheryma whippleii,* can now be identified by DNA studies. Ultrastructurally, in untreated Whipple's disease, there are numerous organisms of characteristic morphology in each macrophage. *Mycobacterium avium–intracellulare* (MAI) has been reported once in a case of malakoplakia. Disseminated MAI in AIDS is characterized by large numbers of acid-fast bacilli within the macrophages.

Endometriosis

Endometriosis commonly involves the serosa of the rectosigmoid junction in the pouch of Douglas. Occasionally other parts of the colon are affected. The ectopic endometrium extends into the muscle coat and submucosa, where it may mimic tumor[179, 180] (Fig. 7–12). Symptoms such as altered bowel habit, abdominal pain, and rectal bleeding accompany menstruation. A mass may be palpable on rectal or vaginal examination, and a barium enema may show an obstructing lesion. Endoscopy reveals a nodular mass or stricture. Mucosal ulceration is rare. Cut surface shows marked localized hypertrophy of the muscle coat. Tiny, brown or blood-filled cysts may be visible. Microscopically, the endometriosis may show proliferative, secretory, or inactive appearances. There may be associated endosalpingosis, papillary projections, hobnail cells, hyperplasia, reactive epithelial changes, dysplasia, or neoplasms.

DIFFERENTIAL DIAGNOSIS. Colonic biopsies rarely include endometriosis, but when present, it can be mistaken for **adenocarcinoma**. However, the mucosa overlying endometriosis is usually normal, and the endometrial stroma is quite distinct from the desmoplastic stroma of carcinoma. The cellular dysplasia of adenocarcinoma is not a feature of endometriosis, but endometriotic glands are often hyperchromatic.

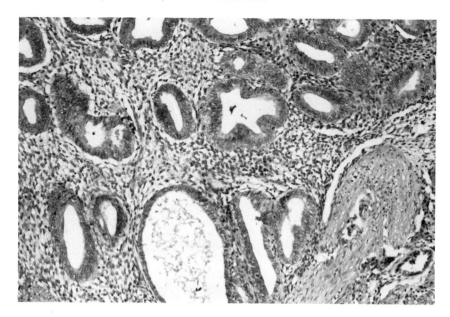

FIGURE 7–12. Endometriosis in a jumbo endoscopic biopsy from the rectosigmoid junction. This must not be mistaken for carcinoma.

Graft-Versus-Host Disease (GVHD)

Acute GVHD is characterized by the triad of dermatitis, diarrhea, and hepatitis. It begins 3 to 4 weeks after bone marrow transplantation in as many as 50% of allograft recipients and uncommonly after solid organ transplantation or blood transfusions.[181–183] The diagnosis of intestinal involvement by GVHD is not usually possible before 20 days post engraftment because the effects of radiation and ablative chemotherapy are morphologically identical to those of GVHD. Watery diarrhea is the main symptom and may be voluminous, but ileus, severe abdominal pain, and signs of peritonitis may also occur. Fecal occult blood tests are usually positive; leukocytes are present in the stool, and protein-losing enteropathy may cause hypoalbuminemia.[181] Intestinal GVHD without skin or liver manifestations is well-recognized but uncommon. Endoscopic findings range from normal through erythema to friability and ulceration.

The earliest lesion is apoptosis of individual crypt cells in the absence of inflammation (Fig. 7–13). Crypt cell loss may lead to flattening of the remaining epithelium, cystic crypt dilatation, regenerative atypia, or loss of entire crypts.[181] Necrotic epithelial cells, which are shed into the lumen, resemble crypt abscesses. Crypt endocrine cells are selectively preserved as small epithelial clusters at the base of the mucosa, detached from the surface epithelium.[184] They are readily identified by their fine eosinophilic granules and can be confirmed by chromogranin immunostaining. Grading of colonic GVHD can be done, as outlined in Table 7–3.

DIFFERENTIAL DIAGNOSIS. The clinical differential diagnosis of diarrhea after bone marrow allograft includes **infectious enterocolitis** and **cecitis due to *Clostridium septicum.*** Apoptotic bodies in the crypt epithelium are the key microscopic finding in GVHD. However, both **CMV infection** and **NSAIDs** also cause crypt cell apoptoses, and, thus, a histologic

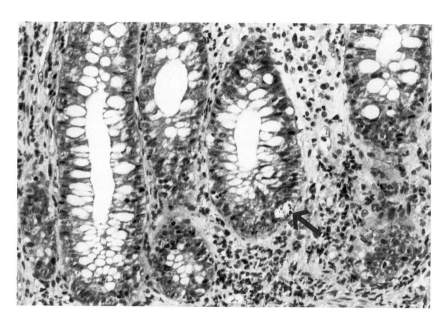

FIGURE 7–13. Colonic biopsy in graft-versus-host disease. Note the apoptoses in crypt epithelium *(arrow).*

Table 7–3. **Grading of Colonic GVHD**

Grade	Histologic Features
1	Individual crypt cell necrosis
2	Crypt abscess, crypt cell flattening, with or without crypt cell degeneration
3	Dropout of one or more whole crypts in a biopsy
4	Total denudation of epithelium

diagnosis of acute GVHD is untenable in the presence of CMV infection.[185]

Mucocele of the Appendix

Mucocele is a sac of mucus that distends the appendix.[186–191] It may be due to obstruction, mucosal hyperplasia, adenoma, or adenocarcinoma. In any mucocele, pools of mucus may dissect into the wall of the appendix, and this finding makes a careful search for carcinoma cells mandatory. When mucoceles rupture, mucus may spread throughout the peritoneal cavity, resulting in a so-called pseudomyxoma peritonei. The mucus elicits a granulation tissue response, causing adhesions. Myxoglobulosis is the formation of small spheres of altered mucus within a mucocele.[192] Rarely, the wall of a mucocele calcifies, the so-called porcelain appendix. Any of the lesions that cause mucocele can be associated with inflammation, torsion, intussusception, or perforation.

DIFFERENTIAL DIAGNOSIS. **Simple mucocele** results from luminal obstruction, rarely exceeds 1 cm in diameter, and is lined by flattened epithelium or granulation tissue. Mucinous adenomas or adenocarcinomas cause larger mucoceles. Mucinous adenomas are usually circumferential villous dysplastic lesions that can have a conventional villous pattern (Fig. 7–14A) or a serrated pattern that is likely the appendiceal equivalent of serrated adenoma of the colon.[190, 191, 193] The distinction between **mucinous adenoma** and **mucinous adenocarcinoma** is based on the presence of invasion and desmoplasia. Extensive sampling is required to exclude focal malignant transformation. Adenomatous epithelium can extend outside the appendix along the track of a ruptured mucocele but can be successfully treated by right hemicolectomy. Simultaneous mucinous neoplasms of the appendix and ovary with pseudomyxoma peritonei are regarded as primary appendiceal tumors.[190] Appendicectomy is the treatment for adenomas that do not involve the resection margin, and right hemicolectomy for adenomas that extend to the margin of resection, ruptured mucoceles, and adenocarcinomas.

Hyperplastic polyp-like change consists of non-dysplastic serrated mucosa with diminished numbers of goblet cells and an expanded proliferative zone that does not extend into the upper third of the crypts (Fig. 7–14B). This change affects the mucosa diffusely and is associated with mild luminal widening but rarely with true mucocele.

Hirschsprung's Disease

Hirschsprung's disease, a congenital absence of parasympathetic ganglion cells from the rectum, affects 1 in 5000 liveborn infants. Males are affected more than females in a ratio of 4:1 in short-segment disease and even more disproportionately in long-segment disease. Ten percent of cases have Down's syndrome. In 90% of patients, the aganglionic segment extends from the anus no farther than the sigmoid colon. This segment fails to relax for the passage of feces and remains spastically contracted. The proximal colon becomes distended, and secondary obstructive enterocolitis or pseudomembranous colitis may ensue. Long-segment Hirschsprung's disease, or total colonic aganglionosis, may give milder symptoms than short-segment disease, and the diagnosis is often delayed.[194] Rarely, the aganglionosis extends into the ileum.

Approximately 7% of the siblings of probands also develop Hirschsprung's disease, indicating an etiologic role for heredity, and mutations of the receptor tyrosine kinase (RET) gene on chromosome 10q11.2 are implicated in familial cases.[195]

The diagnosis is established by demonstrating absence of submucosal ganglion cells on biopsies taken at least 2 cm above the pectinate line. Biopsies should include equal amounts of submucosa and mucosa. Several slides containing ribbons of serial sections stained with H&E should be examined. In affected bowel, ganglion cells are absent from both the submucosal and myenteric nerve plexuses. Increased numbers and size of nerve trunks are consistently present in short-segment disease but are not always seen in total colonic aganglionosis. Hypoganglionosis may occur in the junctional area between the normal bowel and the aganglionic segment. Immunostains for neuron-specific enolase or nitric oxide synthase, which identify ganglion cells, are unnecessary for diagnosis. Acetylcholinesterase histochemistry on frozen sections to display the increased parasympathetic nerve fibers in and around the muscularis mucosae is used routinely in some laboratories.

DIFFERENTIAL DIAGNOSIS. Neonatal constipation and colonic dilatation may be due to **cystic fibrosis** (meconium plug syndrome), **hypothyroidism, intestinal atresia, imperforate anus,** or **small left colon syndrome** (transient functional intestinal obstruction associated with maternal diabetes or use of drugs that inhibit peristalsis). In older children or adults, and rarely in infants, **intestinal pseudo-obstruction** due to visceral myopathy or neuropathy can result in a narrow rectum and dilated colon that mimics Hirschsprung's disease.[197, 198] **Hypoganglionosis** is defined as the presence of only rare ganglion cells, and a full-thickness biopsy is usually necessary to make the diagnosis. **Skip-segment Hirschsprung's disease,** or **zonal aganglionosis,** is a rare variant in which a portion of normal colon is interposed between aganglionic or hypoganglionic segments.[196] **Intestinal neuronal dysplasia** is a rare condition characterized by hyperplasia of the submucosal and myenteric plexuses with giant ganglia, isolated heterotopic ganglion cells in the lamina propria and muscularis mucosae, and increased acetylcholinesterase activity in the parasympathetic fibers of the lamina propria and circular muscle coat.[199–201] It is associated with multiple endocrine neoplasia (MEN) type IIB or neurofibromatosis.[202, 203] MEN IIA and

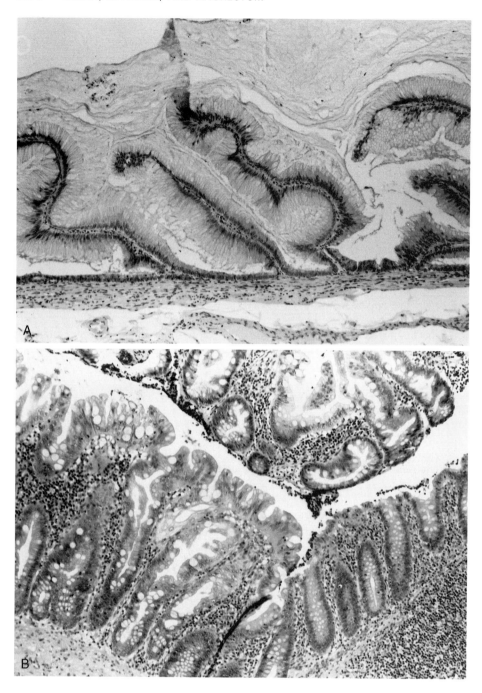

FIGURE 7–14. *A,* Mucinous adenoma of the appendix. *B,* Hyperplastic polyp-like lesion in the appendix.

MEN IIB are caused by different mutations of the receptor tyrosine kinase (RET) gene, the gene that is implicated in Hirschsprung's disease.[195] With time, there may be functional improvement, but not histologic improvement.

Neuronal Hyperplasia of the Anal Canal

Hyperplasia of neuronal and Schwann cells (identified by neuron-specific enolase [NSE] and S-100 stains) is a common observation in hemorrhoidectomy specimens, fibrous polyps, and anal canal resections.[204] The hyperplasia is located beneath squamous epithelium, in the submucosa, and among smooth muscle bundles. The number of ganglion cells is not increased. The etiology is speculative and may be related to scratching or prolapse.

Ehlers-Danlos Syndrome (EDS) and Colon

The most frequent gastrointestinal lesions are inguinal, femoral, and umbilical hernias. Other colorectal complications include spontaneous prolapse of the rectum in childhood, spontaneous perforation, bleeding, and diverticulitis.[205–207] EDS type IV is especially prone to present with rupture of arteries or colonic perforation, and the prognosis is poor because of tissue friability, poor healing, and recurrence.

Elastofibromatous Change of the Rectum

Elastofibromatous change in the submucosa of the rectum can mimic amyloidosis.[208] It consists of sheets of smudgy eosinophilic material in which an occasional fibroblast is embedded. The material may surround small vessels and is negative with Congo red stain, but positive with elastic stains.

POLYPS AND POLYPOSIS SYNDROMES

There are multiple types of colonic polyps and polyposis syndromes, both heritable and acquired. Many of the heritable disorders have overlapping histologic features, and so must be differentiated by their clinical features.

Familial Adenomatous Polyposis

Familial adenomatous polyposis (FAP) is an autosomal dominant condition in which at least 100 adenomas evolve in the large bowel in the early teens and adenocarcinoma supervenes by the fifth decade unless prophylactic colectomy is performed. FAP patients have a germline mutation in the adenomatous polyposis coli (APC) gene, in region 21 of the long arm of chromosome 5 (5q21).[209] More than 126 different APC mutations have been identified. These usually generate stop codons or frameshifts that truncate and inactivate the protein. Attenuated versions of APC with fewer than 100 polyps and delayed disease onset have APC mutations that are clustered at the beginning of the APC gene, and include **hereditary flat adenoma syndrome.**

Gardner's syndrome is familial adenomatous polyposis together with extracolonic manifestations that appear to represent expressions of the APC mutation in multiple tissues.[210]

These include desmoid tumors of the mesentery or abdominal wall, osteomas, dental abnormalities, epidermoid cysts, subcutaneous fibromas, adenomas and carcinomas of the duodenum and periampullary region, fundic polyps of the stomach, and a variety of other tumors. **Turcot's syndrome** is colonic polyposis with malignant tumors of the central nervous system. Although the number of polyps is often less than in FAP,[211] at least some cases do have germline APC mutations.

Flat Adenomas and Flat Adenoma Syndrome

The designation "small flat adenoma" was first used by Muto to describe sessile, nearly flat, adenomas up to 1 cm in diameter.[212] Reportedly, 8.5% of routinely excised adenomas less than 1 cm in diameter are flat.[213] Men are affected more often than women in a ratio of 3.4:1. The average age is about 60 years.[214] On endoscopy, flat adenomas appear reddish and have a central depression when the bowel is well-insufflated. Histologically, all are tubular adenomas, with tubules about twice as long as normal, which tend to spread laterally by proliferating between and on top of normal tubules (Fig. 7–15). Forty-two percent of cases exhibit severe dysplasia (and the majority of these could be designated intramucosal carcinoma at least focally) as compared with 4% in similarly sized pedunculated adenomas.[212, 213] The rate of severe dysplasia increases with the size of the lesion and is significantly higher in women (31.8%) than in men (9.3%).[215] The postulated significance of flat adenomas is that they may be the source of so-called *de novo* adenocarcinomas, which, although discovered while still small, do not display residual adenomatous components. The high rate of severe dysplasia in flat adenomas indicates a higher malignant potential than would be expected from the small size. All severely dysplastic flat adenomas have aneuploid DNA content, and flat adenomas may be precursors of small flat cancers.[216] As isolated lesions, flat adenomas are not a marker for hereditary non-polyposis colonic carcinoma.[217] **Hereditary flat adenoma syndrome** is an attenuated variant of familial adenomatous polyposis in which less than 100 flat adenomas develop and adenocarcinoma evolves at a later age than in conventional FAP.[218]

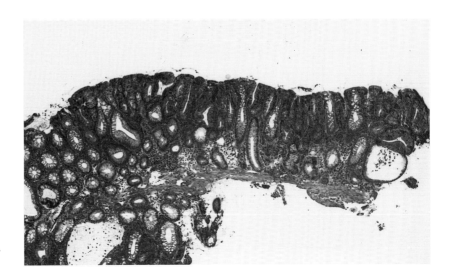

FIGURE 7–15. Flat adenoma showing dysplastic crypts.

Fundic gland polyps of the stomach and small bowel adenomas may be present.

Muir-Torre Syndrome

The Muir-Torre syndrome (MTS) is a rare autosomal dominant condition (only 120 cases had been reported by 1991) characterized by the combination of at least one sebaceous gland tumor and at least one (frequently multiple) visceral neoplasm, of which 50% are colorectal adenocarcinomas.[219] Half of the patients with the syndrome have more than one primary internal malignancy. The sebaceous gland tumor precedes or accompanies the internal malignancy in 63% of cases. The median age for the detection of the internal malignancy is 50 years, a decade earlier than adenocarcinoma of the colon in the general population. Sixty percent of colorectal cancers in this syndrome are at or proximal to the splenic flexure. Colorectal adenomas are found in more than 25% of these patients, being especially prevalent in those with colorectal carcinoma. This syndrome may be a variant of cancer family syndrome (Lynch syndrome).[220]

Peutz-Jeghers Syndrome

Peutz-Jeghers syndrome is characterized by the formation of hamartomatous polyps with a branching skeleton of muscularis mucosae covered by normal mucosa. These polyps are more common in the small bowel than the colon and rarely show focal dysplasia or carcinoma.

Intestinal Ganglioneuromatosis

Intestinal ganglioneuromatosis consists of a diffuse proliferation of nerve fibers and ganglion cells of the enteric nervous system. It may be localized to one part of the gut or generalized (Fig. 7–16). Generalized gastrointestinal ganglioneuromatosis is mainly associated with MEN type IIB. Localized ganglioneuromatosis is sometimes a feature of neurofibromatosis or Cowden's syndrome and has been reported with juvenile polyps and adenocarcinoma of colon also.[202, 221–224] It may affect the mucosa alone, one or both nerve plexuses, or the serosal nerves. Grossly, the bowel may show megacolon, polyps, or tumor-like masses, or it may appear normal. Infants with von Recklinghausen's disease sometimes simulate Hirschsprung's disease. In these infants, the colon may be affected by ganglioneuromatosis with mucosal involvement, which has been designated intestinal neuronal dysplasia.[202] Microscopically, in cases of MEN IIB there is transmural involvement with marked diffuse hypertrophy of the myenteric plexus, lesser prominence of the submucosal plexus, and focal neural proliferation in the mucosa.

Neurofibromatosis

Von Recklinghausen neurofibromatosis type 1 is an autosomal dominant neuroectodermal dysplasia that affects about 1 in 3000 people and men slightly more often than women. The basic defect is in the neurofibrimin gene on chromosome 17. Fifty percent of cases are new mutations. Most patients with gastrointestinal lesions have established cutaneous disease. Ten percent of patients have gastrointestinal lesions, mainly solitary tumors in stomach and small bowel,[225] or microscopic lesions of the nerve plexuses, which induce motility disorders. The tumors may be neurofibromas, leiomyomas, or ganglioneuromas. Gastrointestinal neurofibromas are mainly serosal or submucosal tumors. In most instances they are asymptomatic, but they can be complicated by obstruction, bleeding, intussusception, perforation, or secondary megacolon.[225–229] In children, plexiform neurofibromatosis of the rectosigmoid or ganglioneuromatosis, also called intestinal neuronal dysplasia, can simulate Hirschsprung's disease.[229] The colon shows proliferation of nerve fibers and ganglion cells in the submucosa and mucosa and sometimes also in the myenteric plexus and

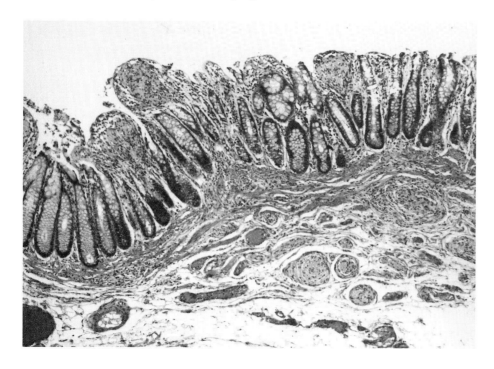

FIGURE 7–16. Ganglioneuromatosis —in this instance an incidental finding adjacent to colonic carcinoma— may be a manifestation of MEN IIB or neurofibromatosis.

serosa. Neurofibromatosis of the colonic mesentery has also been described.[226] Microscopically, neurofibromas are composed of spindle cells, collagen, and mucoid ground substance and display a spectrum of cellularity, from myxoid and paucicellular to highly cellular. The cells have elongated wavy nuclei with pointed ends. The collagen fibers are interspersed between the cells and may be hyalinized. Mast cells, lymphocytes, and rarely xanthoma cells are scattered through the tumor. Some of the cells in neurofibromas are S-100 protein positive, but these tumors are not monoclonal and probably include both Schwann cells and perineurial cells. Malignant transformation is uncommon.[225] Plexiform neurofibromas are similar histologically to those that occur at other sites.

DIFFERENTIAL DIAGNOSIS. Gastrointestinal stromal tumors may arise in von Recklinghausen's disease.[230] They show a fascicular or epithelioid pattern rather than a neurofibromatous one. **Inflammatory fibroid polyps** show an infiltrate of eosinophils and lymphocytes, as well as perivascular onion-skin fibrosis.

Juvenile Polyposis

Juvenile polyposis (JP) is an autosomal dominant disorder, and sporadic new mutations also arise.[231, 232] A practical working definition for the diagnosis of juvenile polyposis proposed by Jass et al. is more than five juvenile polyps of the colorectum, juvenile polyps throughout the gastrointestinal tract, and/or any number of juvenile polyps with a family history of juvenile polyposis.[233] Three forms of the disease are described: (1) a rare sporadic infantile form associated with hemorrhage, intussusception, and death; (2) juvenile polyposis involving only the colon, with onset of symptoms in childhood or early adult life; and (3) generalized juvenile gastrointestinal polyposis involving not only the colon but also the small bowel and stomach, and mainly affecting adults.[234, 235] In this last condition, some of the polyps display focal precancerous dysplasia.[233] These patients are also at increased risk (10%) for colorectal cancer, particularly before the age of 40;[233, 236] they are also at increased risk for stomach cancer.[235] In addition, multiple juvenile polyps have been associated with protein-losing enteropathy. Patients with juvenile polyposis do not have germline APC mutations.

DIFFERENTIAL DIAGNOSIS. Solitary juvenile polyps are pedunculated, smooth-surfaced, rectosigmoid lesions that present with rectal bleeding in children or young adults. They show dilated glands, a wide expanse of lamina propria, surface ulceration, and granulation tissue (Fig. 7–17). When the whole polyp is removed and sectioned, the diagnosis is usually obvious, but individual cases may be difficult to separate from adenoma or inflammatory polyp. **Dysplastic epithelium** does not mature toward the surface and forms sharp junctions with non-dysplastic epithelium. **Inflammatory polyps** have a center of muscularis mucosae and dilated vessels and a covering of nearly normal mucosa with variable inflammation, but no increase of lamina propria volume. Some polyps formerly regarded as solitary juvenile polyps in adults have been distinguished recently as a new entity, **inflammatory myoglandular polyps.** They are characterized by inflammatory granulation tissue, hyperplastic glands with occasional cystic dilatation, and proliferation of smooth muscle in the lamina propria.[237]

The polyps of **Cowden's syndrome** or **Cronkhite-Canada syndrome** may also mimic juvenile polyps.

Cowden's Disease

Cowden's disease is a dominant hereditary syndrome of multiple skin and mucosal hamartomas, which carries a 50% risk of breast cancer in women.[238] This disease presents in the second or third decade with oral mucosal papillomas, multiple facial papular trichilemmomas, and multiple fibroepithelial polyps. The colonic polyps of Cowden's disease resemble hyperplastic polyps endoscopically. Microscopically, they may resemble juvenile polyps, having an excess of lamina propria and normal or elongated crypts, or they may show a core of muscle fibers arising in disorganized muscularis mucosae and a fibrotic lamina propria.

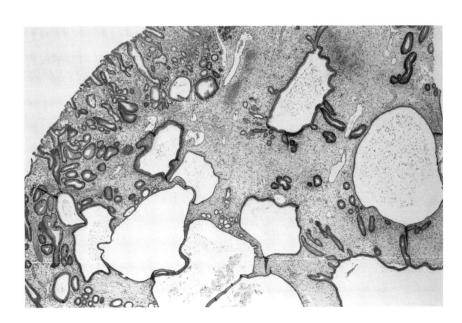

FIGURE 7–17. Juvenile polyp displaying expanded lamina propria, dilated glands, and absence of muscle.

Cronkhite-Canada Polyps

Cronkhite-Canada polyps are a component of this non-familial syndrome of alopecia, onycholysis, skin hyperpigmentation, protein-losing enteropathy, malabsorption, and gastrointestinal polyposis, particularly affecting stomach and colon. The polyps are sessile and have expanded lamina propria and dilated glands; thus, they resemble juvenile polyps except that the latter are pedunculated. They do not have a branching framework of muscularis mucosae as Peutz-Jeghers polyps do, they are not dysplastic, and they occur in older patients between the ages of 34 and 83.[239]

Inflammatory Polyps

There are three main types of inflammatory polyps: granulation tissue polyps, undermined mucosal islands in a sea of ulceration (Fig. 7–18), and mature inflammatory polyps derived from islands after mucosal regeneration.[240] Most cases are manifestations of inflammatory bowel disease, but they may also be caused by severe bacterial colitis, amebic colitis, schistosomiasis, or ischemia. Mature inflammatory polyps can have a variety of gross shapes: threadlike, bulbous, or multi-fingered. Microscopically, they display a non-dysplastic mucosa covering a core of muscularis mucosae with dilated blood vessels. There can be focal crypt occlusion with crypt dilatation or abscess even when the inflammatory bowel disease is quiescent. The epithelial cells may also exhibit hyperplastic/metaplastic change or reparative atypia. True dysplasia is rare in inflammatory polyps; if it occurs, it may be impossible to distinguish from coincidental adenoma. The surrounding flat mucosa must be biopsied for dysplasia. Uncommonly, surface ulceration and excess of lamina propria may make distinction from juvenile polyps difficult, so the clinical history and biopsies of surrounding or adjacent mucosa may be important.

Lymphoid Polyps

Lymphoid polyps may be benign or lymphomatous. The benign form may be a manifestation of immunodeficiency, measure up to 5 mm in diameter, and consist of multiple hyperplastic lymphoid follicles (with germinal centers).[241] Malignant lymphoid polyps are a rare distinctive form of primary gastrointestinal lymphoma and can be much larger than the benign polyps, measuring up to 5 cm in diameter.[242, 243]

Polypoid Prolapsing Mucosal Folds

Polypoid prolapsing mucosal folds (PPMFs) in diverticular disease originate from normal transverse mucosal folds that develop features of mucosal prolapse. Early lesions are brown (hemosiderotic) elevated areas on the mucosal folds. More advanced lesions have full-blown features of mucosal prolapse, including mucosal hyperplasia, muscularization of the lamina propria, surface ulceration, congestion and thrombi in capillaries, crypt hyperplasia, and focal hyperplastic-metaplastic change (Fig. 7–19).[22] These changes appear to result from redundancy of the mucosa, contraction of the muscle coat, and venous congestion. There may be associated non-specific segmental colitis in the diverticular segment.[22]

Inflammatory Myoglandular Polyps

Inflammatory myoglandular polyps, first described in 1992, are idiopathic, solitary, spherical, smooth-surfaced, pedunculated polyps showing surface erosion and redness. The mean age of occurrence is 53 years (range, 15–78 years). Males predominate over females in a ratio of 3 : 1. The most common symptom is bleeding, either occult or overt. The polyps are located in the rectum or sigmoid, descending, or transverse colon. They measure from 0.4 cm to 2.5 cm in diameter. Most are pedunculated; a few sessile. Histologically, they consist of hyperplastic crypts, cystically dilated glands, excess lamina propria, granulation tissue, and proliferation of muscularis mucosae.[237]

DIFFERENTIAL DIAGNOSIS. These polyps lack the tree-like proliferation of the muscularis mucosae that typifies the polyps of the **Peutz-Jeghers syndrome**. In the past, myoglandular polyps were regarded as juvenile polyps, but they differ from juvenile polyps in that they show an abundance of smooth muscle fibers in the cores. Myoglandular polyps differ from **inflammatory cap polyps** in that they are solitary and pedunculated and are rarely covered by a fibrin cap. Myoglandular polyps are also found not only in the rectosigmoid, but in the descending and transverse colon. Mucus, diarrhea, and tenesmus, the most common symptoms of patients with

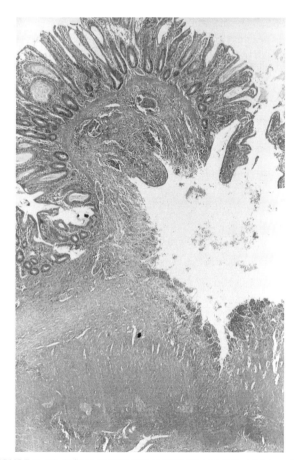

FIGURE 7–18. Inflammatory polyp initially consists of an undermined flap of mucosa.

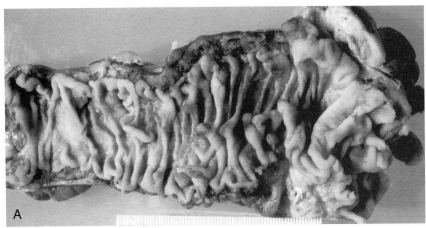

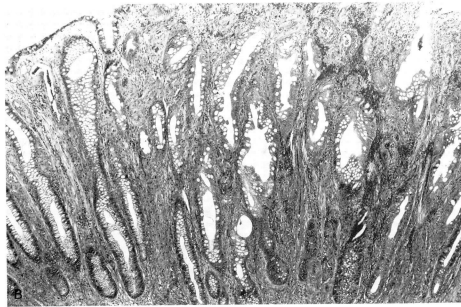

FIGURE 7–19. *A,* Polypoid prolapsing mucosal folds in diverticular disease show congestion or pigmentation. *B,* Histologic changes range from congestion and hemosiderosis to full-blown features of mucosal prolapse (illustrated here), including thickening of mucosa, congestion, muscularization of lamina propria, and serrated change in the crypts.

inflammatory cap polyps, are rare in patients with inflammatory myoglandular polyps.

Polypoid Residual Stalks

Polypoid residual stalks (remnants from previous polypectomy) may alarm the endoscopist but rarely cause histologic difficulty. They are composed of normal mucosa and submucosa, which contains thrombosed or recanalized blood vessels.[244] Rarely, polyps undergo spontaneous autoamputation and bleed profusely. The stalk then may show a small residual focus of adenoma at the ulcerated tip.

Polyps with Atypical Stromal Cells

Polyps with atypical stromal cells occur within granulation tissue or lamina propria in juvenile polyps, adenomas, polypoid prolapsing mucosa in diverticular disease, and the stroma of anal fibroepithelial polyps.[22, 245, 246] The atypical cells may be spindle-shaped, stellate, epithelioid, or rounded, and they often show abundant cytoplasm without mucin or glycogen (Fig. 7–20). The nuclei are vesicular, pleomorphic, and hyper-

chromatic and may have large inclusion-like nucleoli. There are few or no mitotic figures. The cells are usually widely dispersed, although they can be crowded. Immunostains are positive for vimentin, variably positive for smooth muscle actin, and negative for cytokeratin, indicating mesenchymal and possibly myofibroblastic derivation.

DIFFERENTIAL DIAGNOSIS. There is a distinct risk of overdiagnosis of malignancy, especially **sarcoma,** if the atypical cells are crowded. Rarely, the epithelioid variants form round, cohesive clusters resembling acini or vascular structures and can be mistaken for **poorly differentiated carcinoma** or epithelioid variants of **angiosarcoma. CMV** can cause enlarged stromal cells, but the intranuclear inclusions and cytoplasmic granules are distinctive, and if necessary, immunostaining can be performed. Comparable pseudosarcomatous lesions occur in esophageal ulcers, urinary bladder, and vagina.

Hyperplastic Polyps

Hyperplastic polyps (HP) display serrated and hyperplastic crypts with reduced numbers of goblet cells. Oblique sections across the expanded proliferative zone may resemble adenoma and can be misdiagnosed as such when the surface serrated

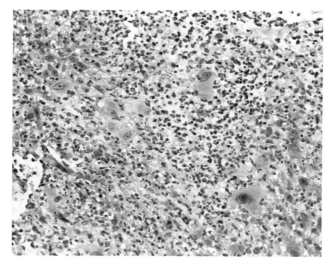

FIGURE 7–20. Bizarre stromal cells in a granulation tissue polyp.

component is not visible. Rarely, in large hyperplastic polyps on the right side of the colon, glands become displaced into the submucosa, mimicking invasion.[247, 248] These polyps occur mainly in women. They can measure up to 2.5 cm in diameter, much larger than the common hyperplastic polyps of the rectum. They tend to surmount the mucosal folds and have a puckered or pitted surface. Histologically, the displaced glands can mimic carcinoma, or can become cystically dilated (localized colitis cystica profunda). Otherwise, in morphology and histochemistry these lesions are identical to other hyperplastic polyps (Fig. 7–21).

Mixed Hyperplastic-Adenomatous Polyps (Serrated Adenomas)

Rarely, features of both adenoma and hyperplastic polyp are present in the same lesion.[193, 249, 250] Adenomas with metaplastic areas, collision or combined tumors in which hyperplastic and adenomatous lesions occur side by side, and serrated adenomas all have been described as mixed hyperplastic-adenomatous polyps. The epithelial cells of the serrated adenoma have eosinophilic cytoplasm, and the mitotic figures extend into the upper zone of the crypts.[193, 250] High-grade dysplasia or intramucosal carcinoma is seen in 10% of mixed polyps,[193] indicating malignant potential (Fig. 7–22).

DIFFERENTIAL DIAGNOSIS. The epithelial cells of serrated adenomas display more nuclear stratification and atypia than **hyperplastic polyps**, and these atypical changes are located near the surface of the polyp. **Goblet cell–rich adenomas** are not serrated and generally contain a much greater number and proportion of goblet cells than do hyperplastic polyps or serrated adenomas.

Mucosal Pseudolipomatosis

Air insufflated at endoscopy can penetrate into the mucosa and produce small clear spaces resembling lipid[251] (Fig. 7–23). Gas cysts may elevate the mucosa in a nodular or polypoid pattern, but in most instances there are no gross lesions.[252] Insufflation pneumatosis is more often seen in inflamed or ulcerated mucosa than in normal mucosa and is often present in lymphoid glandular complexes.

NEOPLASTIC/MALIGNANT LESIONS

Dysplasia in Idiopathic Inflammatory Bowel Disease

Dysplasia is an unequivocally neoplastic condition.[252a–254] The cytologic features include nuclear crowding, stratification, hyperchromatism, pleomorphism, and loss of cytoplasmic differentiation or maturation.[253] In low-grade dysplasia, atypical nuclei remain in the basal portion of epithelial cells, whereas in high-grade dysplasia, the nuclei lose polarity and approach the luminal surface. Architecturally, regular tubules or villi are typical of low-grade dysplasia, whereas more complex structures including glandular budding and back-to-back glands are features of high-grade dysplasia (Fig. 7–24A). Dystrophic goblet cells are seen in either grade of dysplasia. They show reversed polarity with the nucleus on the luminal aspect of the mucin goblet. Variants of dysplasia include those with clear-cell change, serrated change, or large numbers of Paneth, endocrine, or mucinous cells.

Biopsies are classified as "negative for dysplasia," "positive for dysplasia," or "indefinite for dysplasia," the last category divided into "probably negative," "probably positive," and "unknown" categories.[253] The indefinite category includes inflammation, regeneration, hyperplastic-metaplastic change, and metaplasia resembling gastric surface or gallbladder mucosa.

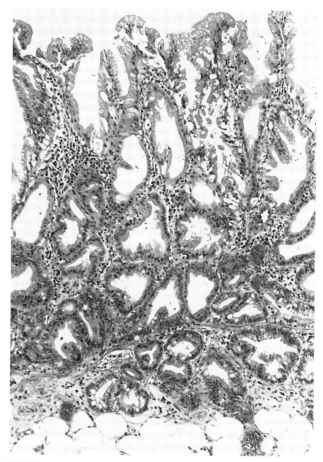

FIGURE 7–21. Hyperplastic polyp with pseudoinvasive displacement of glands below the muscularis mucosae. In poorly oriented biopsies, this can be difficult to distinguish from adenocarcinoma.

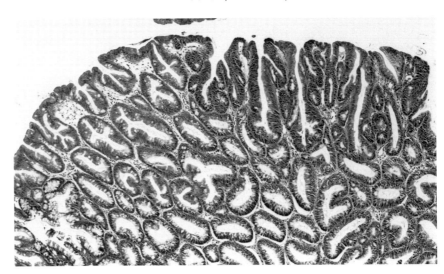

FIGURE 7–22. Serrated adenoma composed of serrated glands with minimal dysplasia *(left)* and with unequivocal dysplasia *(right)*.

Dysplasia is a marker for a high risk of carcinoma, and surveillance colonoscopy is used to try to identify early lesions. If a colectomy specimen is negative for dysplasia after a positive biopsy, the possible explanations include biopsy misinterpretation, sampling error in the resection specimen, or complete removal of the lesion by the biopsy. More often, resection specimens reveal a previously unsuspected infiltrating adenocarcinoma. A minority of these tumors are not associated with dysplasia; this may be due to obliteration of the dysplasia by the carcinoma or development of a *de novo* carcinoma. DNA flow cytometry on colonic biopsy specimens has shown that aneuploidy precedes histologic dysplasia and identifies a subset of patients who are more likely to develop dysplasia and who deserve more intensive colonoscopic surveillance.[255] The dysplasia-carcinoma sequence also occurs in Crohn's disease, but there is little enthusiasm for surveillance colonoscopy in Crohn's disease.

DIFFERENTIAL DIAGNOSIS. Regenerative mucosa poses the greatest diagnostic problem because immature, regenerating epithelial cells can have enlarged, hyperchromatic, crowded nuclei and resemble dysplastic cells. **Inflammation** is associated with rapid epithelial turnover, and a diagnosis of dysplasia is usually not possible when the mucosa is infiltrated by neutrophils. Dysplasia is the defining feature of **adenomas**, but dysplasia differs from adenoma in that it is generally not polypoid but forms an elevated plaque or nodule or no gross lesion. Adenomas can arise in patients with ulcerative colitis, and pedunculated dysplastic lesions are best regarded as adenomas. **Acute radiation damage** is characterized by dilated crypts lined by hyperchromatic cells with pleomorphic hyperchromatic nuclei (Fig. 7–24*B*). The main lesion to distinguish from well-differentiated adenocarcinoma arising in IIBD is **colitis cystica profunda**, non-dysplastic glands displaced into submucosa that show no desmoplastic reaction and do not infiltrate.

Adenoma Containing Invasive Carcinoma (Malignant Polyp)

A malignant polyp is an adenoma that contains a focus of invasive carcinoma. A polypoid carcinoma without residual adenoma can also be regarded as a malignant polyp. A polyp with severe dysplasia/carcinoma *in situ* but without invasion is not classified as malignant. The criteria for invasion are high-grade dysplasia, a desmoplastic response, and penetration through the muscularis mucosae. Most series have included both pedunculated and sessile tumors as malignant polyps, with the sessile group comprised of broad-based or semipedunculated lesions that are also likely to invade the bowel wall directly after invasion of the head of the polyp.[256] A carcinoma arising in a pedunculated adenoma must traverse the stalk before it reaches the plane of the submucosa.

Malignant polyps constitute 2.7% of all adenomas and 5% of all endoscopic polypectomies. Approximately 80% of malignant polyps are removed from the rectosigmoid. More than 90% range from 1 to 3 cm in diameter.[257, 258] The rate of malignancy rises progressively with size.[259] During gross examination of polyps, the stalk, or diathermy burn, should be identified and inked, and the polyp sliced serially and submitted in total to provide optimal histology of the margin of excision. If carcinoma is discovered, step sections are advisable to determine the extent of the tumor.

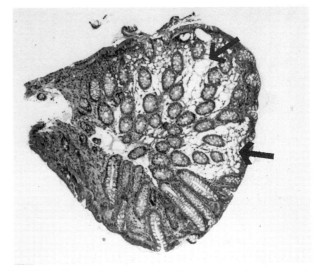

FIGURE 7–23. Pseudolipomatosis. Clear spaces in the mucosa due to permeation of gas insufflated at endoscopy *(arrow)*.

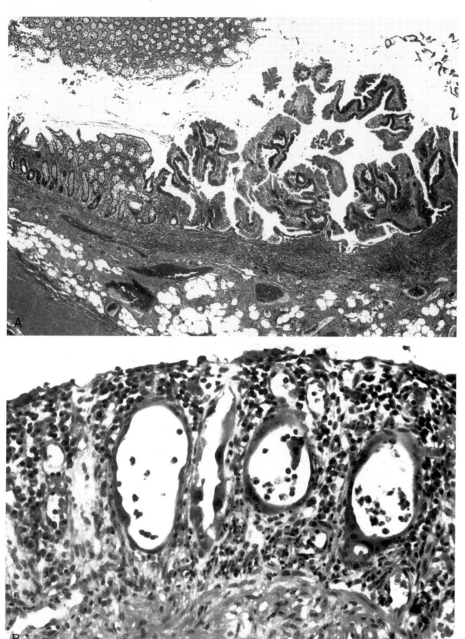

FIGURE 7–24. *A,* Villous dysplasia in chronic ulcerative colitis. *B,* Acute radiation damage mainly affects crypt epithelial cells, which are reduced in numbers, hyperchromatic, and pleomorphic. The crypt lumina are dilated and contain cell debris.

The three adverse prognostic features that warrant segmental colectomy are carcinoma extending to the margin of excision or to cauterized tissue, poorly differentiated carcinoma (grade III),[258] and lymphatic, venous, or microvascular invasion[259, 260] (Fig. 7–25). Comment on these features in your pathology report. Invasion up to or near the cut margin is the most important indication for additional surgery,[256, 257] but the presence of any focus of poorly differentiated carcinoma, regardless of its size or the apparent completeness of excision, is also an indication for surgery.[258] The overall risk of lymph node metastasis is 10% from a sessile malignant polyp[260] and 6% from a pedunculated polyp, but there is virtually no risk of metastasis if the carcinoma is confined to the head, neck, and stalk of the polyp.

DIFFERENTIAL DIAGNOSIS. The principal diagnostic difficulty is in distinguishing carcinoma from **adenomatous glands displaced into the submucosa of the head or stalk** of the polyp (pseudoinvasion).[261, 262] Displaced glands are found in 2% to 10% of pedunculated colorectal adenomas. These glands are usually not severely dysplastic, retain lamina propria, do not show desmoplasia, are associated with hemosiderin deposition, and are generally well circumscribed and non-invasive. Mucin lakes may be present owing to obstruction of glandular drainage. In contrast, carcinomas display invasion, desmoplasia, and severe dysplasia. Desmoplasia is a fibroblastic stromal reaction that is rich in mucosubstances and that replaces the lamina propria. By contrast, lamina propria is a loose connective tissue containing capillaries,

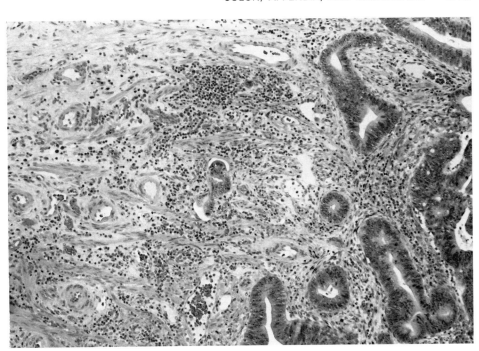

FIGURE 7–25. Microvascular invasion in the stalk of an adenoma, an adverse prognostic feature warranting segmental colectomy.

plasma cells, lymphocytes, and other cells. Glandular displacement into the submucosa is believed to result from torsion. The distinction of splayed fibers of muscularis mucosae from desmoplasia may be difficult. In difficult cases, deeper sections often help.

Mucinous Adenocarcinoma

Mucinous adenocarcinomas are tumors that retain abundant extracellular mucin. The quantity of mucin required to regard the tumor as a mucinous adenocarcinoma has been variously defined as between 50% and 80% by volume. Ten percent to 15% of all colorectal carcinomas are mucinous by this criterion.[263–266] Approximately 30% of colorectal carcinomas contain some mucinous areas.[263] A much greater proportion of mucinous carcinomas than non-mucinous are found in the proximal (right) colon, and more than half of all right-sided carcinomas contain a mucinous component, compared with only a quarter of left-sided tumors.[264, 265, 267] The male:female ratio is approximately equal.[263–265] Several authors report a higher proportion of mucinous tumors in young patients than in older patients,[265] but the converse holds true in Norwegian patients.[263] There is an increased prevalence of mucinous carcinomas in hereditary non-polyposis colonic carcinoma. Many studies that did not apply multivariate analysis concluded that mucinous tumors behave more aggressively and have a poorer prognosis than non-mucinous adenocarcinomas;[264, 265] however, studies that use multivariate analysis do not confirm this and point to two reasons for the perception.[263, 266] First, the signet-ring carcinoma subcategory that is included with mucinous carcinomas has a poorer prognosis; and second, mucinous carcinomas tend to present at a more advanced stage then do non-mucinous carcinomas.[263, 266] Although 15% of non-mucinous carcinomas of the rectum were Dukes stage A, only 3% of mucinous carcinomas were.[266] When site, stage,

and grade of tumor are adjusted for, the presence of a mucinous component does not imply a poorer prognosis unless that predominating component is of signet-ring type.[263]

Mucinous carcinomas arise from adenomas significantly more often than do other types of carcinoma and are associated with polypoid adenomas in other segments of the surgical specimen significantly more often than non-mucinous carcinomas are[266, 268] (Fig. 7–26). Pronounced lymphocytic infiltration is rarely seen in mucinous carcinomas.[266] Mucinous carcinomas possess a diffusely infiltrating invasive margin more often than non-mucinous carcinomas, and mucinous carcinomas feature more perirectal spread.[266] Extramural venous invasion is less frequent in mucinous than in non-mucinous carcinomas.[266]

Signet-Ring Cell Carcinoma

A signet-ring cell carcinoma is a malignant tumor in which more than 50% of the tumor is composed of isolated cells distended with mucus.[269] These tumors are usually regarded as a subtype of mucinous carcinoma. They constitute less than 2% of all colorectal carcinomas.[263, 269] The majority of signet-ring cell carcinomas are located in the right colon, as are other mucinous tumors. There is an increased prevalence of signet-ring cell tumors in hereditary non-polyposis colonic carcinoma.[273] However, the linitis plastica variant is more often located in the left colon or rectum than in the right colon.[263, 270] The male:female ratio is equal. The mean age is 51.8 years (range, 14–79 years), more than a decade younger than with conventional carcinomas. These tumors present at an advanced stage and have a worse prognosis than non-mucinous carcinomas matched for stage.[269] They have a greater propensity for local and peritoneal spread than for distant metastases.[270, 271] Constipation, pain, and rectal bleeding

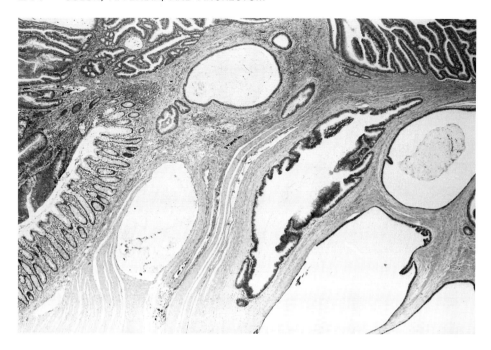

FIGURE 7–26. Mucinous carcinoma invading the muscle coat.

are the main presenting features.[270] About one in five have preexisting ulcerative colitis.

The gross appearance is often that of an exophytic mass with a mucoid cut surface.[269] Tumors composed entirely of signet-ring cells show circumferential thickening and rigidity of the bowel wall with luminal narrowing resembling linitis plastica, and this appearance is more common in the left side of the colon.[269, 270] These tumors may produce an hourglass appearance on barium enema or resemble a stricture of Crohn's disease with nodular, ulcerated, or cobblestoned mucosa. Microscopically, sheets of signet-ring cells or files of cancer cells infiltrate diffusely through all layers of the bowel wall, permeate the muscularis propria in a nondestructive fashion,[270] and elicit a desmoplastic reaction, most prominently in the submucosa and subserosa (Fig. 7–27). These tumors are prone to peritoneal dissemination and can produce Krukenberg-type tumors of the ovaries or obstructive uropathy. Elements of mucinous carcinoma may be admixed.

DIFFERENTIAL DIAGNOSIS. Secondary signet-ring cell carcinoma in the colon is said to be five to ten times more common than the primary type, and the secondaries are derived from the stomach, breast, gallbladder, or prostate, in order of frequency. Secondary signet-ring cell tumors are often associated with diffuse peritoneal spread, multiple lesions, and deposits in the pouch of Douglas, but are occasionally solitary lesions. The intracytoplasmic lumina in lobular carcinoma of the breast show a rim of alcian blue positivity and a central blob of PAS-positive mucin. The gross pattern of linitis plastica can also be caused by diffuse lymphatic permeation by moderately differentiated adenocarcinoma.[270]

Hereditary Non-polyposis Colonic Carcinoma (HNPCC)

The criteria for diagnosing HNPCC are three or more relatives with histologically verified colorectal carcinoma, one of whom is a first degree relative of the other two; colorectal carcinoma involving at least two consecutive generations; and one or more colorectal carcinoma cases diagnosed before age 50.[272] Two forms of HNPCC are known as Lynch syndromes I and II. Lynch syndrome I is characterized by the occurrence of colorectal carcinoma (CRC) at an early age (median, 44 years), a propensity to involve the proximal colon, and an excess of synchronous and metachronous colonic cancers[273] but not an increased incidence of cancers in other organs. Lynch syndrome II features a similar colonic phenotype, but there is a high risk of carcinoma arising in other sites, particularly the endometrium, ovary, kidney and urinary tract, stomach, small bowel, pancreas, biliary tract, or skin. Hematologic malignancies have also been described. The proportion of CRC attributable to HNPCC is variously estimated from 3% to 30% of cases. The genetic defect is a mutation of a mismatch

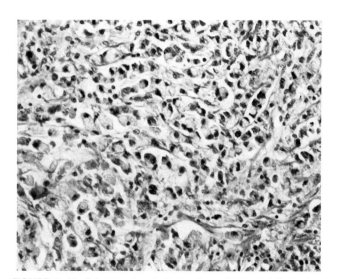

FIGURE 7–27. Primary signet-ring cell carcinoma of the colon. Metastases from stomach and breast must be excluded.

repair gene, one of which is encoded on chromosome 2p16.[274–276] The mutation causes numerous replication errors in short repeated DNA sequences (microsatellites) in the tumors in HNPCC.[274] Identical abnormalities are found in 13% of sporadic cancers. There is a significant correlation between microsatellite instability and tumor location in the proximal colon.

Two thirds of CRCs in HNPCC arise proximal to the splenic flexure. Multiple synchronous carcinomas occur in 7% of patients, and metachronous carcinomas in 8%. There is an increased prevalance of mucinous carcinomas in HNPCC, and a large proportion of mucinous carcinomas occur in particular families, suggesting heterogeneity of colorectal pathology within HNPCC.[273, 277] There is also an increased prevalence of signet-ring cell carcinomas in HNPCC.[273, 277] Approximately 37% of CRC in HNPCC are poorly differentiated when defined as 30% or more of the tumor composed of solid sheets of malignant cells without tubule formation (Fig. 7–28). Most of the poorly differentiated carcinomas are not signet-ring cell carcinomas but are composed of cells with abundant eosinophilic cytoplasm and round, fairly regular nuclei that do not show neuroendocrine differentiation and behave indolently.[273] Despite poor differentiation, survival is good and may by explained by the predominance of diploid tumors and more favorable tumor stage in HNPCC than in control subjects (74% Dukes A versus 45% of control subjects).[273] Adenomas are more prevalant in HNPCC than in the general population and were found in 20% of colons resected for colorectal carcinoma in HNPCC and in 36% of HNPCC patients who were older than 50 years.[278] The adenomas in HNPCC are larger, more often villous, and more often show high-grade dysplasia than in control subjects, suggesting that adenomas are not themselves the result of the HNPCC gene but create the environment in which a mutation in the second mismatch repair allele can occur. The phenotype of multiple replication errors would then be expressed in the adenoma and cause an increased rate of conversion to malignancy.[275, 276]

DIFFERENTIAL DIAGNOSIS. Hereditary flat adenoma syndrome (HFAS), a condition in which colorectal carcinoma develops on a background of flat adenomas concentrated in the proximal colon, is an attenuated variant of familial adenomatous polyposis in which the carcinomas occur later in life than do those arising from usual familial adenomatous polyposis.[212, 279] **Dominantly inherited adenomatous polyps** with colorectal carcinoma is another hereditary form of colonic cancer.[280–282] Patients with **Muir-Torre's syndrome** (sebaceous adenomas or carcinomas of the skin with colorectal carcinoma) may be a subset of Lynch syndrome II.

Melanotic Adenocarcinomas of the Anorectum

Melanotic adenocarcinomas of the anorectum contain melanin and are located at the dentate line, extending beneath the margin of the anal mucosa.[283, 284] In focal areas, the tumor cells phagocytose melanin granules from dendritic melanocytes that are normally resident at the anorectal junction. A nevus, or melanocytic junctional change, is not present. Lymph node metastases do not contain melanin.[284] Ultrastructurally, mucin globules and aggregates of melanosomes in various stages of development are seen in the same cells, and admixed with the epithelial cells are dendritic melanocytes containing individual melanosomes in all stages of development. One case arose in a man who had been treated with arsenicals to the point of toxicity many years earlier.[293]

Adenosquamous Carcinoma

Adenosquamous carcinoma contains malignant glandular and squamous elements intimately admixed with one another, and the term **adenoacanthoma** is used synonymously in the colorectal literature. Many authors exclude tumors within 5 cm of the anal verge, and the main requirement is histologic demonstration of a lack of continuity with squamous or anal transitional mucosa. In reported cases, these tumors are often lumped together with pure squamous carcinomas.[285, 286] They constitute roughly 0.1% of all colonic carcinomas and are distributed evenly around the colon. Men and women are equally affected, and the age range is from 28 to 91 years (mean, 59.5 years). Some cases arise in chronic ulcerative colitis. The 5-year survival is 50% for Dukes B, 33% for Dukes C, and 0% for Dukes D cases. Tumors are usually elevated, annular and ulcerated, and firm and white on cut surface. Histologically, they are mainly high-grade lesions,[285] which show glandular areas with foci of squamous differentiation. Keratinization, intercellular bridges, and positive staining for involucrin are present at least in the best-differentiated areas. Occasional tumors have presented with hypercalcemia and have shown parathormone immunostaining in the squamous elements.[287]

DIFFERENTIAL DIAGNOSIS. Collision tumors composed of adenocarcinoma and squamous carcinomas occurring side by side are not adenosquamous carcinoma. **Small-cell undifferentiated carcinoma** may show foci of squamous differentiation and may arise from adenocarcinoma. These should not be regarded as adenosquamous carcinoma, because squamous foci are a known feature of small-cell carcinomas and the small-cell elements dominate prognostically. **Adenosquamous carcinoma arising in endometriosis,** has been described[288] and must be excluded by careful sampling.

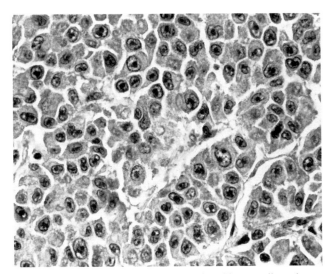

FIGURE 7–28. A form of poorly differentiated large-cell carcinoma in which the cells display abundant cytoplasm and moderate nuclear pleomorphism. This tumor type may occur in HNPCC.

Squamous Cell Carcinomas and Squamous Metaplasia

Pure squamous cell carcinomas of the colon or rectum are rare. Fewer than 40 cases were documented in the English language literature up to 1979.[289] These tumors show squamous cell carcinomatous elements alone, without small-cell undifferentiated or adenocarcinomatous components, and extensive sampling of the tumor to exclude glandular elements is mandatory. The criteria that must be satisfied before a diagnosis of primary squamous carcinoma of the large bowel can be entertained are (1) there must be no evidence of a squamous carcinoma in any other organ that might spread directly into the bowel or provide a source for an intestinal metastasis; (2) the affected bowel should not be involved in any squamous-lined fistula track, a well-recognized site of origin of squamous carcinoma; and (3) when squamous carcinoma occurs in the rectum, tumors arising from the anal squamous epithelium and extending proximally to involve the rectum must be excluded.[289] This can be difficult because the anal squamous epithelium may extend upward into the rectum for a considerable distance. A squamous tumor can only be regarded as arising primarily in the rectum if a lack of continuity between the tumor and the anal epithelium is demonstrated, and such tumors are preferably greater than 5 cm from the pectinate line.[288]

Squamous carcinoma of the colon accounts for approximately 0.1% of all colonic carcinomas and affects two men for every woman. The mean age at diagnosis is 53 years (range, 33–90). Associated conditions include chronic ulcerative colitis, lymphogranuloma venereum, and pelvic irradiation. The tumors are located mainly in the rectosigmoid but have been found throughout the colon in similar distribution to adenocarcinomas. Grossly, the tumors measure from 3 to 8 cm in diameter. They spread to involve the muscular coat and pericolic tissues and metastasize to perirectal or pericolic lymph nodes. Symptoms include rectal bleeding, constipation, and pain. A minority of patients die of their disease.

Most squamous carcinomas of the colon or rectum are thought to arise from adenomas that contain foci of squamous metaplasia (morules). Such foci are found in approximately 0.4% of adenomas[290–292] (Fig. 7–29). Other cases arise from squamous metaplasia of the mucosa or, rarely, from a duplication of the colon.[293] Rectal prolapse, lymphogranuloma venereum, and certain practices may predispose to squamous metaplasia.[291] The cause of squamous metaplasia of the rectum in a psychiatric patient was memorably described by Dukes: "One of the problems of the inmates of institutions is the safe custody of their possessions. During the day they can defend these from covetous neighbours but they have little protection against a thief who steals at night. Faced with these difficulties they have been known to put the rectum to a use not intended by nature and to store their private treasures in its dark recesses each night, bringing them forth again each morning to the light of day. You may have heard the story of the lunatic who was a great admirer of Napoleon and all day carried about a small bust of the emperor which he returned each night to the safety of his back passage."[292]

DIFFERENTIAL DIAGNOSIS. **Adenosquamous carcinomas** must have elements of adenocarcinoma admixed with the squamous. **Small-cell undifferentiated carcinomas** may have small foci of squamous differentiation, but because their prognosis is that of the small-cell elements, they should not be regarded as squamous carcinomas. Squamous carcinomas may arise in **endometriosis,** and this possibility must be excluded by careful gross examination and extensive sampling if the appearances suggest an intramural primary. **Transitional cloacogenic carcinomas** arise from the anorectal junctional region and are more basaloid than squamous.

Basaloid, Transitional, or Cloacogenic Carcinoma

These carcinomas arise at the anorectal margin (transitional zone) and are composed of basaloid cells that form cellular islands with peripheral palisading and central necrosis.[294–296] Focal squamous differentiation with keratin pearl formation is common. A variant with mucin production has been called mucoepidermoid carcinoma, and another variant with regular,

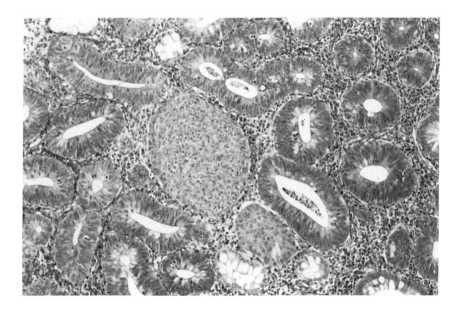

FIGURE 7–29. Squamous morules in an adenoma, the postulated origin of squamous cell carcinomas of colon.

rounded gland-like spaces reminiscent of adenoid cystic carcinoma has been described. Approximately 50% of cases have lymph node metastases at diagnosis. Basaloid carcinoma is histologically distinct from common squamous carcinoma,[294] and it is not associated with human papillomavirus as squamous cell carcinoma is.[297] Basaloid carcinomas have followed radiation for carcinoma of the uterine cervix and occur in homosexual men. Immunostains are positive for cytokeratins, blood group isoantigens, epithelial membrane antigen, and carcinoembryonic antigen but negative for neuron-specific enolase.

DIFFERENTIAL DIAGNOSIS. The main lesions to distinguish from basaloid carcinoma are basal cell carcinoma, small-cell carcinoma, malignant melanoma, and carcinoid tumor. **Basal cell carcinomas** arise from the perianal skin or the skin/anal margin rather than the anorectal margin. They show the typical histologic features of basal cell carcinoma of the skin, with more regular cell shape and size and prominent peripheral palisading.[298] **Small-cell carcinoma** and **anal malignant melanoma** are discussed later. **Carcinoid tumors** may be considered when biopsies of basaloid tumors show cylindromatous or adenoid cystic patterns, but their size and immunostaining usually serve to differentiate the lesions.

Small-Cell Carcinoma

Anaplastic tumors are subdivided into small-cell and non-small-cell carcinomas. The term **small-cell carcinoma** means a tumor resembling small-cell carcinoma of the lung. These tumors may exhibit focal endocrine, squamous, or glandular differentiation, as do their counterparts in the lung, but they are, for the most part, undifferentiated and the small-cell element is the most clinically relevent.[299–304] The term **neuroendocrine carcinoma** is used as a synonym for small-cell undifferentiated carcinoma, but it is also employed in a broader sense to include atypical aggressive endocrine cell neoplasms with intermediate or large cells or carcinoidal architectural features.

Men are affected more often than women. The age range is from 25 to 88 years, but most cases occur between the sixth and eighth decades. Metastases to liver are often present at diagnosis.[299, 303, 305] The clinical course is usually short, with two thirds of patients dead at 5 months.[301, 303] Survival times are now increasing with response to chemotherapy.[301]

Grossly, these carcinomas are usually large, annular, ulcerating masses 4 to 12 cm in diameter, but some are extremely small. Microscopically, they are combined with and appear to arise from an adenoma or adenocarcinomas in 45% of cases,[300, 301, 303, 304] and there is usually a sharp junction between the two components (Fig. 7–30). Architecturally, they are made up of infiltrating cords, clusters, or sheets of cells in a fibrovascular or desmoplastic stroma. The cells are small "oat" cells or intermediate cells that lack distinct cytoplasm and possess dark-staining, fusiform nuclei with dispersed chromatin. Intracytoplasmic mucin is absent. Squamous differentiation is seen focally in 21%, and endocrine differentiation can be identified in most cases if a liberal definition is used (neuron-specific enolase or synaptophysin immunostaining, dense-core granules, or argyrophilia).[301] In some cases there are well-differentiated carcinoid-like areas.[306] Central necrosis may be prominent within sheets of tumor cells.[301, 303, 305] Small rosette-like structures may be present around either an empty space, a vascular lumen, or central fibrillary material.[303, 305] Vascular invasion is often present.[301, 303] Ultrastructurally, there are sparse dense-core granules, desmosomes between a minority of cells, and intracytoplasmic tonofilament bundles and tonofibrils, suggesting squamous differentiation, which may be seen focally. Metastases rarely show squamous or adenocarcinomatous differentiation.[301, 303] Immunostains are positive for EMA, NSE, and neurofilament protein[304] and negative for leukocyte markers.

DIFFERENTIAL DIAGNOSIS. The differential diagnosis includes poorly differentiated adenocarcinoma, lymphoma,

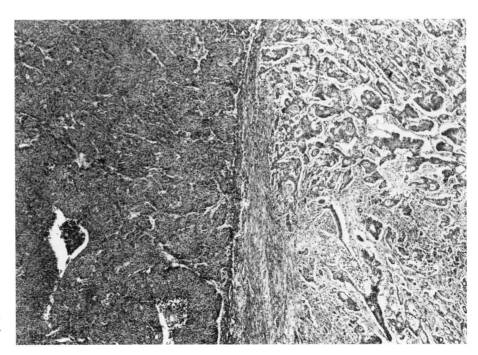

FIGURE 7–30. Small-cell carcinoma *(left)* in association with adenocarcinoma *(right).*

cloacogenic carcinoma, and malignant melanoma. **Adenocarcinomas** form glands and produce mucin, and the cells are large and have abundant cytoplasm. **Lymphomas** do not display rosettes, ribbons, trabeculae, and nests; they show distinct nuclear features depending on type and stain positively for leukocyte common antigen and lymphocyte markers. **Basaloid cloacogenic carcinomas** were discussed previously. **Malignant melanoma** may be an obvious pigmented tumor with epithelioid, spindle cell, and balloon cell areas, or it may be composed of sheets of non-pigmented cells with round nuclei and large, central nucleoli simulating lymphoma or undifferentiated carcinoma (Fig. 7–31). A nested growth pattern is almost always present focally, and junctional change is seen in approximately 75% of cases. Melanoma may contain melanin, reacts positively with S-100 and HMB-45, and is negative for cytokeratin and lymphoma markers.

Undifferentiated Carcinoma

The terms **carcinoma simplex** and **undifferentiated carcinoma** describe an anaplastic carcinoma composed of polygonal or spheroidal cells without any glandular arrangement or mucus secretion.[307, 308] These rare tumors are distinguished by their benign behavior from the notoriously aggressive small-cell carcinomas and constitute approximately 1% of colorectal carcinomas.[308] Many of them contain argyrophilic cells, suggesting that they are large-cell neuroendocrine tumors analogous to those that arise in the lung.[308] Some of these may be cases of HNPCC, because 37% of tumors in HNPCC are reported to contain areas with solid sheets of cells with round, regular nuclei and abundant eosinophilic cytoplasm.[273] Undifferentiated carcinomas show less endocrine and squamous differentiation and fewer liver metastases than small-cell undifferentiated carcinomas.[301]

Grossly, undifferentiated carcinomas range from 2.5 to 10.0 cm in diameter and are crater-like lesions with smooth, ulcerated surfaces that often involve the entire circumference of the bowel and the pericolic tissues.[308] Microscopically, they show a solid pattern of cells with vesicular nuclei, prominent nucleoli, mild pleomorphism, and no abnormal mitoses (see Fig. 7–28). A second cell population with larger nuclei, chromatin clumping, chromatin clearing, and nucleoli is sometimes present. The margins of the tumor are circumscribed with no lymphocytic response.[308] Lymph node metastases are uncommon, and the prognosis is excellent.

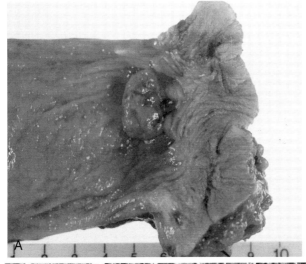

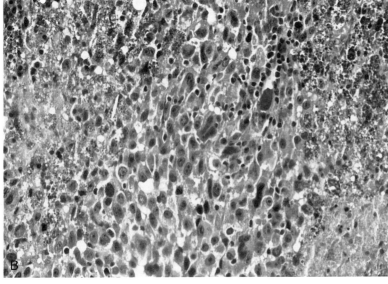

FIGURE 7–31. *A,* Anal malignant melanoma presenting as a sessile polyp 2 cm in diameter. *B,* Anus. An epithelioid and amelanotic variant of malignant melanoma with extensive necrosis.

Rectal and Colonic Carcinoids

Carcinoids are common in the rectum and rare in the colon.[309] Rectal carcinoids are usually discovered incidentally during anorectal examination of asymptomatic patients or for symptoms of unrelated anorectal conditions.[309, 310] They are believed to be derived from extraglandular endocrine cells.[320] Rarely, they are associated with myelofibrosis,[311] ulcerative colitis,[312] or diversion of the fecal stream.[313] Peak incidence is at 40 years of age (range, 20–70).

Grossly, rectal carcinoids appear as firm, pale yellow, polypoid or umbilicated, smooth-surfaced nodules that are covered by mucosa. Approximately 2% of cases are multiple.[314] Two thirds are smaller than 0.4 cm, and the majority are smaller than 2 cm in diameter. Microscopically, carcinoids are located in the lamina propria and submucosa. They are composed of small regular glands and ribbons or sheets of columnar or polygonal cells (Fig. 7–32A). Only a minority resemble classic carcinoids of the appendix or small bowel. About half of all hindgut carcinoids are argyrophilic (Grimelius stain). Three patterns of rectal carcinoid are described: Type 1 is similar to classic midgut carcinoids and is composed of solid nests of tumor cells with some trabecular cords and occasional tubuloacinar differentiation. Type 2 shows a pronounced ribboning pattern, often with an anastomosing configuration and a prominent vascular network. These tumors are non-reactive with silver stains. Type 3 has a mixed pattern with features of type 1 and type 2.[310] Benign carcinoids frequently produce a marked fibroblastic reaction and incorporate smooth muscle (muscularis mucosae) in the stroma of the tumor.[310] Rosettes may be present with small blood vessels occupying their centers. Peripheral nuclear palisading may be prominent. The only consistently reliable criterion of malignancy is invasion of the muscularis propria, but cytologic features of malignancy are usually present: a high mitotic index, pleomorphism, hyperchromatism, and abnormal chromatin patterns.[310] Malignant lesions do not have a type 1 morphology. They are usually larger than 2 cm in diameter.

Rectal carcinoids display positive immunoreactivity for neuron-specific enolase (87%), prostatic acid phosphatase (67%), chromogranin (58%), Leu-7 (53%), serotonin (45%), pancreatic polypeptide (46%), CEA (24%), glucagon (10%), enkephalin (7%), beta-endorphin (3%), gastrin (3%), somatostatin (3%), and ACTH (1%).[315–319]

Tumors reported as carcinoids of the colon (excluding the rectum) constitute a spectrum from small benign lesions to high-grade neuroendocrine carcinomas that are often a component of an adenocarcinoma and that are in fact small-cell carcinomas that have metastasized at the time of diagnosis.[321, 322]

Mixed crypt cell carcinomas (also called goblet cell carcinoids), **composite carcinoid tumors,** and **mucin-secreting carcinoids** are tumors that resemble the goblet cell carcinoids or adenocarcinoids of the appendix. They have a propensity

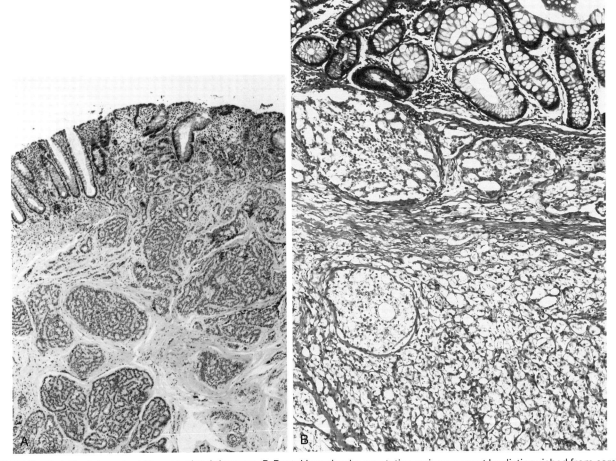

FIGURE 7–32. *A,* Rectal carcinoid tumor, glandular type. *B,* Rectal invasion by prostatic carcinoma must be distinguished from carcinoid.

for deep invasion and transperitoneal spread with a high mortality. The proportion of cells with endocrine differentiation is small, and these tumors are probably better considered carcinomas than carcinoids.[323-326]

DIFFERENTIAL DIAGNOSIS. The term **composite adenocarcinoma-carcinoid tumor** should not be applied to tumors with a small-cell undifferentiated component, because small-cell tumors have a dire prognosis. **Prostatic carcinoma** may directly invade the rectum and infiltrate the mucosa. The prominent nucleoli of prostatic carcinoma and the architectural and cytologic patterns of the tumors usually suffice to distinguish the two lesions (Fig. 7-32B). In cases of difficulty, distinction can be based on immunostains for PSA but not for prostatic acid phosphatase, which rectal carcinoids also contain.

Mucinous (Goblet Cell) Carcinoid of the Appendix and Adenocarcinoma of the Appendix

Mucinous carcinoid, goblet cell carcinoid, adenocarcinoid, crypt cell carcinoma, and **mixed adenocarcinoma-carcinoid tumor** are terms describing distinctive tumors, intermediate between carcinoid and adenocarcinoma, that are more aggressive than conventional carcinoids.[327-334] These tumors resemble carcinoids in their pattern of infiltration of the base of the mucosa, submucosa, and muscle coat, but their histogenesis is controversial. Because they replicate the crypts of the appendix, it is difficult to accept that they arise from laminal or submucosal endocrine cells (subepithelial neurosecretory cells) as conventional carcinoids are postulated to, but equally, they do not show mucosal dysplasia. Grossly, they are ill-defined white tumors and are often found incidental to appendicitis. Microscopically, they are composed of a mixture of goblet or signet-ring cells, endocrine cells, and Paneth cells; they form solid nests, acini, or cords and infiltrate the muscle coat in a carcinoid-like pattern. The endocrine cells are often present only in small numbers and rarely exceed 30% of the total.[329] Tubules or goblet cells may predominate, and the goblet cell type is reputedly more prone to metastasize transperitoneally if it extends to the serosa (Fig. 7-33). The 5-year survival is 80% as compared with almost 100% for conventional carcinoids.[328] The metastasizing tumors are mixed carcinoid-adenocarcinomas that often spread into

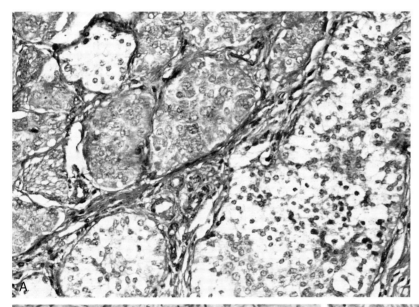

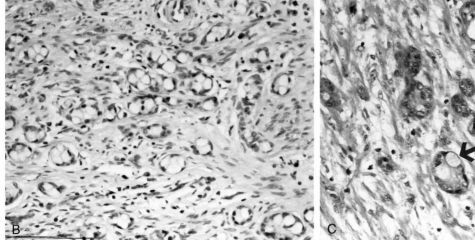

FIGURE 7-33. *A,* Appendix. Classic carcinoid with balloon cells. *B,* Appendix. Goblet cell–rich variant of adenocarcinoid. *C,* Appendix. Adenocarcinoid poor in goblet cells.

cecum or adjacent viscera at the time of diagnosis and have a large carcinomatous pattern (>50%) with areas of mucinous, signet-ring, or single-file pattern, in addition to goblet cell or insular carcinoid.[331] Right hemicolectomy is recommended for tumors that show many mitoses, that reach the peritoneal surface, or that are more than 2 cm in diameter.

Angiosarcoma

Angiosarcomas rarely arise in or involve the colon.[335-339] They present with pain, diarrhea, bleeding, and hematochezia in patients ranging from 34 to 72 years of age. Grossly, they are ill-defined, hemorrhagic, and microcystic or sponge-like and may ulcerate the mucosa. Microscopically, they may be polymorphous or uniform and include anastomosing sinusoids, papillary tufts, giant cells, or plump epithelioid cells. The last may simulate poorly differentiated carcinoma. The prognosis is extremely poor; five of six reported patients were dead at 2 to 23 months, and the sixth was lost to follow-up.[335-339] One case that recovered spontaneously is of questionable authenticity.[336] Immunostaining is positive for Factor VIII–related antigen, *Ulex europeus* lectin, CD-31, and vimentin and negative for cytokeratins, HMB-45, S-100, alpha smooth muscle actin, epithelial membrane antigen (EMA), and leukocyte common antigen (LCA).

DIFFERENTIAL DIAGNOSIS. Epithelioid angiosarcomas can mimic **undifferentiated carcinoma, renal cell carcinoma, melanoma, or epithelioid leiomyosarcoma.** Three cases have been reported of colonic adenocarcinomas with **trophoblastic (choriocarcinoma) differentiation,** and this tumor must be considered in any highly vascular or hemorrhagic epithelioid neoplasm.[340] Choriocarcinoma contains both cytotrophoblast and syncytiotrophoblast and stains positively for cytokeratin and human chorionic gonadotropin (HCG).

Stromal Tumors of the Large Bowel

Stromal tumors, traditionally regarded as smooth muscle tumors, are of uncertain histogenesis and are more common in the rectum than in the colon. Large bowel stromal tumors constituted only 5 of the 100 gastrointestinal cases in the series of Ranchod and Kempson.[341] In the Mayo series of leiomyosarcomas, there were 106 in the small bowel, 26 in the rectum, 15 in the colon, and 2 in the anus.[342] Leiomyomas of the muscularis mucosae are small polypoid submucosal nodules that are invariably benign and are cured by local excision.[343, 344] Deep tumors arising in the muscularis propria are more sinister. A distinction must be drawn between anorectal and colonic tumors. Most **colonic stromal tumors** are malignant, and the microscopic criteria for malignancy are similar to those applied elsewhere in the gut (>5 mitoses/mm², nuclear pleomorphism, high cellularity, invasive borders, confluent necrosis, and size >5 cm). Most are located in the ascending and transverse colon. They are large, round or lobate, and fleshy on cut surface. They tend to metastasize across the peritoneum, and hematogenously to liver, bone, and lungs.[345] Benign stromal tumors are generally firm, whorled tumors, smaller than 5 cm in diameter that show a fascicular pattern of spindle cells, low cellularity, few or no mitoses, and little nuclear pleomorphism. Rarely, multiple leiomyomas (leiomyomatosis) or leiomyosarcomas of the colon and small bowel have been reported.[346, 347] **Anorectal** stromal tumors arise deep in the muscularis propria and are most common within 4 cm of the dentate line. They are usually large symptomatic tumors.[343-345] A distinction between benign and malignant tumors is dubious, and even the low-grade tumors should be considered potentially malignant.[343] Small size is no guarantee of benignity. The cardinal predictor of malignancy is the presence of any mitotic activity, and the other features of malignancy are larger size, nuclear atypia, and zonal necrosis.[344] These tumors have a high rate of local recurrence (60%), but if they are smaller than 2.5 cm in diameter, they can be treated by wide local excision, whereas larger tumors may require abdominoperineal excision.[343, 345] However, there is little evidence that more aggressive treatment prolongs survival.[343] The malignant variants recur locally or with blood-borne metastases.[343-345] Locally recurrent tumors become more cellular, more pleomorphic, and more aggressive with each recurrence. **Anal stromal tumors** are rare and occur predominantly in women.[345, 348]

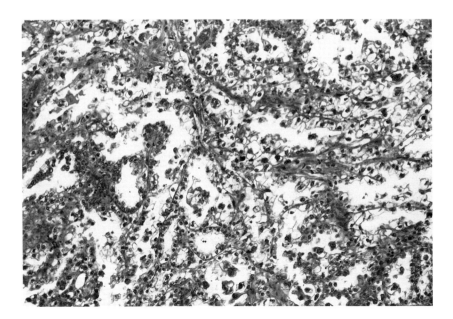

FIGURE 7–34. Clear-cell endometrioid carcinoma arising in endometriosis of the colon.

DIFFERENTIAL DIAGNOSIS. The differential diagnosis includes **neurofibromas** associated with von Recklinghausen disease, **spindle cell carcinomas, spindle cell melanoma, spindle cell (squamous) carcinoma,**[349] **hemangiopericytoma,** other sarcomas, and miscellaneous other lesions. The distinction is made by morphology and immunostaining.

Large Bowel Malignancies Arising from Endometriosis or Endosalpingiosis

A malignancy arising from endometriosis or endosalpingiosis must ideally fulfill three criteria: it must be a tumor that is recognized as being capable of arising from endometriosis or endosalpingiosis; it must grow in continuity with endometriosis or endosalpingiosis; and it must show an *in situ* component in continuity with the endometriosis or endosalpingiosis. If the *in situ* feature is missing, the diagnosis is still valid, but it is presumptive, not proven.

Malignancies rarely arise in endometriosis of the large bowel, but reported examples include **endometrioid carcinoma,**[351, 352] **clear-cell carcinoma**[353] (Fig. 7–34), and **germ cell tumor (with yolk sac, choriocarcinomatous, and teratomatous elements).**[350] Tumors may form large masses on the bowel wall or within the lumen. The full spectrum of malignant neoplasms that are capable of arising in endometriosis also include **sarcoma, mixed mesodermal tumor, squamous cell carcinoma, adenoacanthoma,** and **mucinous cystadenocarcinoma,**[354] but these have not yet been described specifically in colonic endometriosis.

DIFFERENTIAL DIAGNOSIS. Primary colonic carcinomas are morphologically different and arise in the mucosa. The main differential is from **metastatic carcinoma** and depends heavily on the surgical findings. When any unusual colonic malignancy is encountered in a woman, malignancy in endometriosis must be kept in mind, and the tumor should be sampled extensively.

References

1. Day DW, Mandal BK, Morson BC: The rectal biopsy appearance of Salmonella colitis. Histopathology 2:117–131, 1978.
2. Price AB, Jewkes J, Sanderson PJ: Acute diarrhea: Campylobacter colitis and the role of rectal biopsy. J Clin Pathol 32:990–997, 1979.
3. Kumar NB, Nostrant TT, Appelman HD: The histopathologic spectrum of acute self-limited colitis (acute infectious-type colitis). Am J Surg Pathol 6:523–529, 1982.
4. Nostrant TT, Kumar NB, Appelman HD: Histopathology differentiates acute self-limited colitis from ulcerative colitis. Gastroenterology 92:318–328, 1987.
5. Loss RW, Mangla JC, Pereira M: Campylobacter colitis presenting as inflammatory bowel disease with segmental colonic ulcerations. Gastroenterology 79:138–140, 1980.
6. Kelly JK, Pai CH, Jadusingh IH, et al: The histopathology of rectosigmoid biopsies from adults with bloody diarrhea due to verotoxin-producing *Escherichia coli*. Am J Clin Pathol 88:78–82, 1987.
7. El-Meraghi NRH, Mair NS: The histopathology of enteric infection with *Yersinia pseudotuberculosis*. Am J Clin Pathol 71:631–639, 1979.
8. Gleason TH, Patterson SD: The pathology of *Yersinia enterocolitica* enterocolitis. Am J Surg Pathol 6:347–355, 1982.
9. Anand BS, Malhotra V, Bhattacharya SK, et al: Rectal histology in acute bacillary dysentery. Gastroenterology 90:654–660, 1986.
10. Surawicz CM, Belic L: Rectal biopsy helps to distinguish acute self-limited colitis from idiopathic inflammatory bowel disease. Gastroenterology 86:104–113, 1984.
11. Levine JS, Smith PD, Brugge WR: Chronic proctitis in male homosexuals due to lymphogranuloma venereum. Gastroenterology 79:563–565, 1980.
12. Quinn TC, Goodell TC, Mkrtichian E, et al: *Chlamydia trachomatis* proctitis. N Engl J Med 305:195–200, 1981.
13. Hywel-Jones J, Lennard-Jones JE, Morson BC, et al: Numerical taxonomy and discriminant analysis applied to non-specific colitis. Q J Med 42:715–732, 1973.
14. Cooper HS, Raffensperger ED, Jonal L, Fitts WT: Cytomegalovirus inclusions in patients with ulcerative colitis and toxic dilatation requiring colonic resection. Gastroenterology 72:1253–1256, 1977.
15. Surawicz CM, Myerson D: Self-limited cytomegalovirus colitis in immunocompetent individuals. Gastroenterology 94:194–199, 1988.
16. Boulton AJM, Slater DN, Hancock BW: Herpesvirus colitis: A new cause of diarrhea in a patient with Hodgkin's disease. Gut 23:247–249, 1982.
17. Goodell SE, Quinn TC, Mertichian E, et al: Herpes simplex virus proctitis in homosexual men. Clinical, sigmoidoscopic, and histopathological features. N Engl J Med 308:868–871, 1983.
18. Price AB: Overlap in the spectrum of non-specific inflammatory bowel disease—"colitis indeterminate." J Clin Pathol 31:567–577, 1978.
19. Tobi M, Kobrin I, Ariel I: Rectal involvement in sarcoidosis. Dis Colon Rectum 25:491–493, 1982.
20. Pieterse AS, Leong ASY, Rowland R: The mucosal changes and pathogenesis of pneumatosis cystoides intestinalis. Hum Pathol 16:683–688, 1986.
21. Komorowski RA: Histologic spectrum of diversion colitis. Am J Surg Pathol 14:548–554, 1990.
22. Kelly JK: Polypoid prolapsing mucosal folds in diverticular disease. Am J Surg Pathol 15:871–878, 1991.
23. Ament ME, Ochs HD: Gastrointestinal manifestations of granulomatous disease. N Engl J Med 288:382–387, 1973.
24. Roe TF, Coates TD, Thomas DW, et al: Treatment of chronic inflammatory bowel disease in glycogen storage disease Type Ib with colon stimulating factors. N Engl J Med 326:1666–1669, 1992.
25. Vannier JP, Arnaud-Battandier F, Ricour C, et al: Neutropenie primitive et congenitale et maladie de Crohn. A propos de deux observations chez l'enfant. Arch Fr Pediatr 39:367–370, 1982.
26. Abramowsky CR, Sorensen RU: Regional enteritis-like enteropathy in a patient with agammaglobulinemia: Histologic and immunocytologic studies. Hum Pathol 19:483–486, 1988.
27. Depinho RH, Kaplan KL: The Hermansky-Pudlak syndrome: Report of three cases and review of pathophysiology and management considerations. Medicine 64:192–202, 1985.
28. Yang SS, Gibson P, McCaughey RS, et al: Primary Crohn's disease of the appendix. Report of 14 cases and review of the literature. Ann Surg 189:334–339, 1979.
29. Lindhagen T, Ekelund G, Leandoer L, et al: Crohn's disease confined to the appendix. Dis Colon Rectum 25:805–808, 1982.
30. Le Brun HI: Appendicular granuloma. Br J Surg 46:32–40, 1958.
31. Rex JC, Harrison EG, Priestley JT: Appendicitis and ligneous perityphlitis. Arch Surg 82:735–745, 1961.
32. Lee RG: The colitis of Behçet's syndrome. Am J Surg Pathol 10:888–893, 1986.
33. Kasahara Y, Tanaka S, Nishino M, et al: Intestinal involvement in Behçet's disease: Review of 136 surgical cases in the Japanese literature. Dis Colon Rectum 24:103–106, 1981.
34. Thach BT, Cummings NA: Behçet syndrome with "aphthous colitis." Arch Intern Med 136:705–709, 1976.
35. Rams H, Rogers AI, Ghandur-Mnaymneh L: Collagenous colitis. Ann Intern Med 106:108–113, 1987.
36. Sylwestrowicz T, Kelly JK, Hwang WS, Shaffer EA: Collagenous colitis and microscopic colitis: The watery diarrhea-colitis syndrome. Am J Gastroenterol 84:763–768, 1989.
37. Lazenby AJ, Yardley JH, Giardiello FM, Bayless TM: Pitfalls in the diagnosis of collagenous colitis: Experience with 75 cases from a registry of collagenous colitis at the Johns Hopkins Hospital. Hum Pathol 21:905–910, 1990.
38. Lee E, Schiller LR, Vendrell D, et al: Subepithelial collagen table thickness in colon specimens from patients with microscopic colitis and collagenous colitis. Gastroenterology 103:1790–1796, 1992.
39. Gledhill A, Cole FM: Significance of basement membrane thickening in the human colon. Gut 25:1085–1088, 1984.
40. Tanaka M, Mazzoleni G, Riddell RH: Distribution of collagenous colitis: Utility of flexible sigmoidoscopy. Gut 33:65–70, 1992.
41. Lazenby AJ, Yardley JH, Giardiello FM, et al: Lymphocytic ("microscopic") colitis: A comparative histopathologic study with particular reference to collagenous colitis. Hum Pathol 20:18–28, 1988.
42. DuBois RN, Lazenby AJ, Yardley JH, et al: Lymphocytic enterocolitis in patients with "refractory sprue." JAMA 262:935–937, 1989.
43. Breen EG, Coughlan G, Connolly CE, et al: Coeliac proctitis. Scand J Gastroenterol 22:471–477, 1987.
44. Glotzer DJ, Glick ME, Goldman H: Proctitis and colitis following diversion of the fecal stream. Gastroenterology 80:438–441, 1981.
45. Korelitz BI, Cheskin LJ, Sohn N, Sommers SC: Proctitis after fecal diversion in Crohn's disease and its elimination with reanastomosis: Implications for surgical management. Report of four cases. Gastroenterology 87:710–713, 1984.
46. Harig JM, Soergel KH, Komorowski RA, Wood CM: Treatment of diversion colitis with short-chain-fatty acid irrigation. N Engl J Med 320:23–28, 1989.
47. Murray FE, O'Brien MJ, Birkett DH, et al: Diversion colitis. Pathologic findings in a resected sigmoid colon and rectum. Gastroenterology 93:1404–1408, 1987.
48. Yeong ML, Bethwaite PB, Prasad J, Isbister WH: Lymphoid follicular hyperplasia—a distinctive feature of diversion colitis. Histopathology 19:55–61, 1991.
49. Ma CK, Gottlieb C, Haas PA: Diversion colitis: A clinicopathologic study of 21 cases. Hum Pathol 21:429–436, 1990.
50. Warren BF, Shepherd NA, Bartolo DCC, Bradfield JWB: Pathology of the defunctioned rectum in ulcerative colitis. Gut 34:514–516, 1993.

51. Haque S, Eisen RN, West AB: The morphological features of diversion colitis: Studies of a pediatric population with no other disease of the intestinal mucosa. Hum Pathol 24:211–219, 1993.

52. Sladen GE, Filipe MI: Is segmental colitis a complication of diverticular disease? Dis Colon Rectum 27:513–514, 1984.

53. Mathus-Vliegen EMH, Tytgat GNJ: Polyp-simulating mucosal prolapse syndrome in (pre)diverticular disease. Endoscopy 18:84–86, 1986.

54. Peppercorn MA: Drug-responsive chronic segmental colitis associated with diverticula: A clinical syndrome in the elderly. Am J Gastroenterol 87:609–612, 1992.

55. Gore S, Shepherd NA, Wilkinson SP: Endoscopic crescentic fold disease of the sigmoid colon: The clinical and histopathological spectrum of a distinctive endoscopic appearance. Int J Colorectal Dis 7:76–81, 1992.

56. Hughes LE: Post-mortem survey of diverticular disease of the colon. Part I—Diverticulosis and diverticulitis. Gut 10:336–351, 1969.

57. Rodkey GV, Hermann G: Diverticulosis of the right colon. Am J Surg 101:61–65, 1961.

58. Luoma A, Nagy AG: Cecal diverticulitis. Can J Surg 32:283–286, 1989.

59. Salvati E, Hyun BH, Varga CF: Massive hemorrhage from colonic diverticula caused by arterial erosion: A practical theory of its mechanism and causation: Report of two cases. Dis Colon Rectum 10:129–135, 1967.

60. Sugihara K, Muto T, Morioka Y, et al: Diverticular disease of the colon in Japan. A review of 615 cases. Dis Colon Rectum 27:531–537, 1984.

61. Markham NI, Li AK: Diverticulitis of the right colon—experience from Hong Kong. Gut 33:547–549, 1992.

62. Barron ME: Simple non-specific ulcer of the colon. Arch Surg 17:355–407, 1928.

63. Lloyd-Williams K: Acute solitary ulcers and acute diverticulitis of the caecum and ascending colon. Br J Surg 47:351–358, 1960.

64. Himal HS: Benign cecal ulcer. Surg Endosc 3:170–172, 1989.

65. Mahoney TJ, Bubrick MP, Hitchcock CR: Nonspecific ulcers of the colon. Dis Colon Rectum 21:623–626, 1987.

66. Shah NC, Ostrov AH, Cavallero JB, Rogers JB: Benign ulcers of the colon. Gastrointest Endosc 32:102–104, 1986.

67. Grinvalsky HT, Bowerman CI: Stercoraceous ulcers of the colon: Relatively neglected medical and surgical problem. JAMA 171:1941–1946, 1959.

68. Berardi RS, Lee S: Stercoraceous perforation of the colon: Report of a case. Dis Colon Rectum 26:283–286, 1983.

69. Wrenn K: Fecal impaction. N Engl J Med 321:658–662, 1989.

70. Madigan MR, Morson BC: Solitary ulcer of the rectum. Gut 10:871–881, 1969.

71. Rutter KR, Riddell RH: The solitary ulcer syndrome of the rectum. Clin Gastroenterol 4:505–530, 1975.

72. Saul SH, Sollenberger LC: Solitary rectal ulcer syndrome: Its clinical and pathological underdiagnosis. Am J Surg Pathol 9:411–421, 1985.

73. Schweiger M, Alexander-Williams J: Solitary rectal ulcer syndrome: Its association with occult rectal prolapse. Lancet 1:170–171, 1977.

74. du Boulay CE, Fairbrother J, Isaacson PG: Mucosal prolapse syndrome—a unifying concept for solitary ulcer syndrome and related disorders. J Clin Pathol 36:1264–1268, 1983.

75. Womack NR, Williams NS, Holmfield JH, Morrison JF: Ano-rectal function in the solitary rectal ulcer syndrome. Dis Colon Rectum 30:319–323, 1987.

76. Burke AP, Sobin LH: Eroded polypoid hyperplasia of the recto-sigmoid. Am J Gastroenterol 85:975–980, 1990.

77. Lobert PF, Appelman HD: Inflammatory cloacogenic polyp. A unique inflammatory lesion of the anal transitional zone. Am J Surg Pathol 5:761–766, 1981.

78. Saul SH: Inflammatory cloacogenic polyp: Relationship to solitary rectal ulcer syndrome, mucosal prolapse and other bowel diseases. Hum Pathol 18:1120–1125, 1987.

79. Goodall HB, Sinclair ISR: Colitis cystica profunda. J Pathol Bacteriol 73:33–42, 1957.

80. Wayte DM, Helwig EB: Colitis cystica profunda. Am J Clin Pathol 48:159–169, 1967.

81. Magidson JG, Lewin KJ: Diffuse colitis cystica profunda: A case report. Am J Surg Pathol 5:393–399, 1981.

82. Allen DC, Biggert JD: Misplaced epithelium in ulcerative colitis and Crohn's disease of the colon and its relationship to malignant mucosal changes. Histopathology 10:37–52, 1986.

83. Guest CB, Reznick RK: Colitis cystica profunda: Review of the literature. Dis Colon Rectum 32:983–988, 1989.

84. Silver H, Stolar J: Distinguishing features of well differentiated mucinous adenocarcinoma of the rectum and colitis cystica profunda. Am J Clin Pathol 51:493, 1969.

85. Nagasako K, Nakae Y, Kitao Y, Aoki G: Colitis cystica profunda: Report of a case in which differentiation from rectal cancer was difficult. Dis Colon Rectum 20:618–624, 1977.

86. Denton J: Pathology of pellagra. Am J Trop Med 5:173–210, 1925.

87. Whitehead R: The pathology of ischemia of the intestines. Pathol Annu 11:1-52, 1976.

88. Williams LF: Vascular insufficiency of the intestines. Gastroenterology 61:757–777, 1971.

89. Heer FW, Silen W, French SW: Intestinal gangrene without apparent vascular occlusion. Am J Surg 110:231–238, 1965.

90. Boley SJ, Schwartz S, Lash J, Sternhill V: Reversible vascular occlusion of the colon. Surg Gynecol Obstet 116:53–60, 1963.

91. Johnson CC, Baggenstoss AH: Mesenteric vascular occlusion: I: Study of 99 cases of occlusion of veins. Proc Staff Meet Mayo Clin 24:628–636, 1949.

92. Sarage EP, Costa J: Idiopathic enterocolic lymphocytic phlebitis. Am J Surg Pathol 13:303–308, 1989.

93. Romano TJ, Graham SM, Chuong J, et al: Bleeding colonic ulcers secondary to atheromatous microemboli after left heart catheterization. J Clin Gastroenterol 10:693–698, 1988.

94. Gladman DD, Ross T, Richardson B, Kulkarni S: Bowel involvement in systemic lupus erythematosus: Crohn's disease or lupus vasculitis? Arthritis Rheum 28:466–470, 1985.

95. Bienenstock H, Menick R, Rogoff B: Mesenteric arteritis and intestinal infarction in rheumatoid disease. Arch Intern Med 119:359–364, 1967.

96. Kukora JS: Extensive colonic necrosis complicating acute pancreatitis. Surgery 97:290–293, 1985.

97. Duffy TJ: Reversible ischemic colitis in young adults. Br J Surg 68:34–37, 1981.

98. Lillemoe KD, Romolo JL, Hamilton SR, et al: Intestinal necrosis due to sodium polystyrene (Kayexalate) in sorbitol enemas: Clinical and experimental support for the hypothesis. Surgery 101:267–272, 1987.

99. Cappell MS, Simon T: Colonic toxicity of administered medications and chemicals. Am J Gastroenterol 88:1684–1699, 1993.

100. Gibson GR, Whitacre EB, Ricotti CA: Colitis induced by nonsteroidal anti-inflammatory drugs. Report of four cases and review of the literature. Arch Intern Med 152:625–632, 1992.

101. Lee FD: Importance of apoptosis in the histopathology of drug-related lesions of the large intestine. J Clin Pathol 46:118–122, 1993.

102. Lang J, Price AB, Levi AJ, et al: Diaphragm disease: Pathology of disease of the small intestine induced by non-steroidal anti-inflammatory drugs. J Clin Pathol 41:516–526, 1988.

103. Bjarnason I, Price AB, Zanelli G, et al: Clinicopathological features of nonsteroidal antiinflammatory drug-induced small intestinal strictures. Gastroenterology 94:1070–1074, 1988.

104. Halter F, Weber B, Huber T, et al: Diaphragm disease of the ascending colon: Association with diclofenac. J Clin Gastroenterol 16:74–80, 1993.

105. Ravi, S, Keat AC, Keat ECB: Colitis caused by non-steroidal antiinflammatory drugs. Postgrad Med J 62:773–776, 1986.

106. Uribe A, Johanssoon C, Slezak P, et al: Ulcerations of the colon associated with naproxen and acetylsalicylic acid treatment. Gastrointest Endosc 32:242–244, 1986.

107. Rutherford D, Stockdill G, Hamer-Hodges DW, et al: Proctocolitis induced by salicylate. Br Med J 288:794, 1984.

108. Levy N, Gaspar E: Rectal bleeding and indomethacin suppositories. Lancet 1:577, 1975.

109. Giardiello FM, Hansen FC, Lazenby AJ, et al: Collagenous colitis in setting of nonsteroidal antiinflammatory drugs and antibiotics. Dig Dis Sci 35:257–260, 1990.

110. Riddell RH, Tanaka M, Mazzoleni G: Nonsteroidal antiinflammatory drugs as a possible cause of collagenous colitis: A case-control study. Gut 33:683–686, 1992.

111. Bridges AJ, Marshall JB, Diaz-Arias AA: Acute eosinophilic colitis and hypersensitivity reaction associated with naproxen therapy. Am J Med 89:526–527, 1990.

112. Meisel JL, Bergman D, Graney D, et al: Human rectal mucosa: Proctoscopic and morphological changes caused by laxatives. Gastroenterology 72:1274–1279, 1977.

113. Leriche M, Devroede G, Sanchez G, Rossano J: Changes in the rectal mucosa induced by hypertonic enemas. Dis Colon Rectum 21:227–236, 1978.

114. Martin DM, Goldman JA, Gilliam J, Nasrallah SM: Gold-induced eosinophilic enterocolitis: Response to oral cromolyn sodium. Gastroenterology 80:1567–1570, 1981.

115. Sakurai Y, Tsuchiya H, Ikegami F, et al: Acute right-sided hemorrhagic colitis associated with oral administration of ampicillin. Dig Dis Sci 24:910–915, 1979.

116. Graham CF, Gallagher K, Jones JK: Acute colitis with methyldopa. N Engl J Med 304:1044–1045, 1981.

117. Atherton LD, Leib ES, Kaye MD: Toxic megacolon associated with methotrexate therapy. Gastroenterology 86:1583–1588, 1984.

118. Herbert DC: Anticoagulant therapy and the acute abdomen. Br J Surg 55:353–357, 1968.

119. Bernardino ME, Lawson TL: Discrete colonic ulcers associated with oral contraceptives. Dig Dis 21:503–506, 1976.

120. Floch MH, Hellman L: The effects of 5-fluorouracil on rectal mucosa. Gastroenterology 48:430–437, 1965.

121. Larrey D, Lainey E, Blanc P, et al: Acute colitis associated with prolonged administration of neuroleptics. J Clin Gastroenterol 14:64–67, 1992.

122. Beyer KL, Bickel JT, Butt JH: Ischemic colitis associated with dextroamphetamine use. J Clin Gastroenterol 13:198–201, 1991.

123. Price AB, Davies DR: Pseudomembranous colitis. J Clin Pathol 30:1–12, 1977.

124. Johnson S, Clabots CR, Linn FV, et al: Nosocomial *Clostridium difficile* colonisation disease. Lancet 336:97–100, 1990.

125. Rybolt AH, Bennett RG, Laughon BE, et al: Protein-losing enteropathy associated with *Clostridium difficile* infection. Lancet 1:1353–1355, 1989.

126. Snooks SJ, Hughes A, Horsburgh AG: Perforated colon complicating pseudomembranous colitis. Br J Surg 71:291–292, 1984.

127. Templeton JL: Toxic megacolon complicating pseudomembranous colitis. Br J Surg 70:48, 1983.

128. Milligan DW, Kelly JK: Pseudomembranous colitis in a leukemia unit. A report of five fatal cases. J Clin Pathol 32:1237–1243, 1979.

129. Rocca JM, Pieterse AS, Rowland R, et al: Clostridium difficile colitis. Aust N Z J Med 14:606–610, 1984.

130. Bassi O, Cosa G, Colavolpe A, Argentieri R: Primary syphilis of the rectum—endoscopic and clinical features. Report of a case. Dis Colon Rectum 34:1024–1026, 1991.

131. Quinn TC, Lukehart SA, Goodell S, et al: Rectal mass caused by *Treponema pallidum*: Confirmation by immunofluorescent staining. Gastroenterology 82:135–139, 1982.

132. Faris MR, Perry JJ, Westermeier TG, Redmond J: Rectal syphilis mimicking histiocytic lymphoma. Am J Clin Pathol 80:719–721, 1983.

133. Davies M, Keddie NC: Abdominal actinomycosis. Br J Surg 60:18–22, 1973.

134. Asuncion CM, Cinti DM, Hawkins HB: Abdominal manifestations of actinomycosis in IUD users. J Clin Gastroenterol 6:343–348, 1984.

135. Whitaker BL: Actinomycetes in biopsy material obtained from suture line granulomata following resection of the rectum. Br J Surg 51:445–446, 1964.

136. Cowgill R, Quan S: Colonic actinomycosis mimicking carcinoma. Dis Colon Rectum 12:45–46, 1979.

137. Morson BC: Primary actinomycosis of the rectum. Proc R Soc Med 54:723–724, 1961.

138. Ratliff DA, Carr N, Cochrane JPS: Rectal stricture due to actinomycosis. Br J Surg 73:589–590, 1986.

139. Deshmukh N, Heaney SJ: Actinomycosis at multiple colonic sites. Am J Gastroenterol 81:1212–1214, 1986.

140. Mast P, Vereecken L, Van Loon C, Hermans M: Actinomycosis of the ano-rectum: A rare infectious disease mimicking carcinomatosis. Acta Chir Belg 91:150–154, 1991.

141. Piper MH, Schaberg DR, Ross JM, et al: Endoscopic detection and therapy of colonic actinomycosis. Am J Gastroenterol 87:1040–1042, 1992.

142. Robboy SJ, Vickery AL: Tinctorial and morphologic properties distinguishing actinomycosis and nocardiosis. N Engl J Med 282:593–596, 1979.

143. Connor DH, Neafie RC, Meyers WM: Amebiasis. In Binford CH, Connor DH (eds): Pathology of Tropical and Extraordinary Disease. Washington, DC, Armed Forces Institute of Pathology, 1976, pp 308–316.

144. Krogstad DJ: Isoenzyme patterns and pathogenicity in amebic infection. N Engl J Med 315:390–391, 1986.

145. Prathap K, Gilman R: The histopathology of acute intestinal amebiasis. Am J Pathol 60:229–245, 1970.

146. Pittman FE, El-Hashimi WK, Pittman JC: Studies of human amebiasis. Gastroenterology 65:588–603, 1973.

147. Pittman FE, Hennigar GR: Sigmoidoscopic and colonic mucosal biopsy findings in amebic colitis. Arch Pathol 97:155–158, 1974.

148. Kean BH, Gilmore HR, Van Stone WW: Fatal amebiasis: Report of 148 fatal cases. Ann Intern Med 44:831–842, 1956.

149. Brandt H, Tamayo P: Pathology of human amebiasis. Hum Pathol 1:351–385, 1970.

150. Dinner M, Bader E: Internal intestinal fistulae caused by amebiasis. S Afr Med J 35:808–811, 1961.

151. Powell SJ, Wilmot AJ: Ulcerative post-dysenteric colitis. Gut 7:438–443, 1966.

152. Stewart GT: Post-dysenteric colitis. Br Med J 1:405–409, 1950.

153. Fung WP, Monteiro EH, Ang HB, et al: Ulcerative postdysenteric colitis. Am J Gastroenterol 57:341–348, 1972.

154. Rosen Y, Woon OKH: Phlegmonous enterocolitis. Am J Dig Dis 23:248–256, 1978.

155. Blei ED, Abrahams C: Diffuse phlegmonous gastroenterocolitis in a patient with an infected peritoneojugular venous shunt. Gastroenterology 84:636–639, 1983.

156. Adachi Y, Mori M, Enjoji M, et al: Mesenteric panniculitis of the colon. Review of the literature and report of two cases. Dis Colon Rectum 30:962–966, 1987.

157. Kelly JK, Hwang WS: Idiopathic retractile (sclerosing) mesenteritis and its differential diagnosis. Am J Surg Pathol 13:513–521, 1989.

158. Athanasoulis CA, Galdabini JJ, Waltman AC, et al: Angiodysplasia of the colon: A cause of rectal bleeding. Cardiovasc Radiol 1:3–13, 1978.

159. Mitsudo SM, Boley SJ, Brandt LJ, et al: Vascular ectasias of the right colon in the elderly: A distinct pathologic entity. Hum Pathol 10:585–600, 1979.

160. Sebastian-Domingo JJ, Santos-Castro L, Castalomas-Franko D, et al: Angiodysplasia of the colon. Experience in 60 cases. Rev Esp Enferm Dig 72:125–128, 1990.

161. Heer M, Sulser H, Hany A: Angiodysplasia of the colon: An expression of occlusive vascular disease. Hepatogastroenterology 34:127–131, 1987.

162. Santos JCM, Aprili F, Guimaraes AS, Rocha JJR: Angiodysplasia of the colon: Endoscopic diagnosis and treatment. Br J Surg 75:256–258, 1988.

163. Cappell MS: Spatial clustering of simultaneous nonhereditary gastrointestinal angiodysplasia. Dig Dis Sci 37:1072–1077, 1992.

164. Howard OM, Buchannan JD, Hunt RH: Angiodysplasia of the colon. Experience of 26 cases. Lancet 2:16–19, 1982.

165. Stamm B, Heer M, Buhler H, Ammann R: Mucosal biopsy of vascular ectasia (angiodysplasia) of the large bowel detected during routine colonoscopic examination. Histopathology 9:639–646, 1985.

166. Thelmo WL, Vetrano JA, Wibowo A, et al: Angiodysplasia of colon revisited: Pathologic demonstration without the use of intravascular injection technique. Hum Pathol 23:37–40, 1992.

167. Kozarek RA, Botoman VA, Bredfeldt JE, et al: Portal colopathy: Prospective study of colonoscopy in patients with portal hypertension. Gastroenterology 101:1192–1197, 1991.

168. Viggiano TR, Gostout CJ: Portal hypertensive intestinal vasculopathy: A review of the clinical, endoscopic, and histopathologic features. Am J Gastroenterol 87:944–954, 1992.

169. Baker AL, Kahn PC, Binder SC, Patterson JF: Gastrointestinal bleeding due to blue rubber-bleb nevus syndrome. A case diagnosed by angiography. Gastroenterology 61:530–534, 1971.

170. Moore JD, Thompson NW, Appelman HD, et al: Arteriovenous malformations of the gastrointestinal tract. Arch Surg 111:381–389, 1976.

171. Pounder DJ, Roland R, Pieterse AS, et al: Angiodysplasias of the colon. J Clin Pathol 35:824–829, 1982.

172. Barbier P, Luder P, Triller J, et al: Colonic hemorrhage from a solitary minute ulcer. Report of 3 cases. Gastroenterology 88:1065–1068, 1985.

173. O'Brien BD, Shnitka TK, McDougall R, et al: Pathophysiologic and ultrastructural basis for intestinal symptoms in Fabry's disease. Gastroenterology 82:957–962, 1982.

174. McClure J: Malakoplakia. J Pathol 140:275–330, 1983.

175. McClure J: Malakoplakia of the gastrointestinal tract. Postgrad Med J 57:95–103, 1981.

176. Sanusi IS, Tio FO: Gastrointestinal malacoplakia. Report of a case and a review of the literature. Am J Gastroenterol 62:356–366, 1974.

177. Ghosh S, Pattniak S, Jalan R, Maitra TK: Malakoplakia stimulating rectal carcinoma. Am J Gastroenterol 85:910–911, 1990.

178. Lewin KJ, Harell GS, Lee AS, Crowley LG: Malacoplakia. An electron-microscopic study: Demonstration of bacilliform organisms in malacoplakic macrophages. Gastroenterology 66:28–45, 1974.

179. Rowland R, Langman JM: Endometriosis of the large bowel. A report of 11 cases. Pathology 21:259–265, 1989.

180. Forsgren H, Linghagen J, Melander S, Wagermark J: Colorectal endometriosis. Acta Chir Scand 149:431–435, 1983.

181. Sale GE, McDonald GB, Shulman HM, Thomas ED: Gastrointestinal graft-versus-host disease in man: A clinicopathologic study of the rectal biopsy. Am J Surg Pathol 3:291–299, 1979.

182. Roberts JP, Ascher NL, Lake J, et al: Graft versus host disease after liver transplantation in humans: A report of four cases. Hepatology 14:274–281, 1991.

183. Brubaker DB: Transfusion-associated graft-versus-host disease. Hum Pathol 17:1085–1088, 1986.

184. Lanfert IA, Thorpe P, Van Noorden S, et al: Selective sparing of enterochromaffin cells in graft versus host disease affecting the colonic mucosa. Histopathology 9:875–886, 1985.

185. Snover DC: Mucosal damage simulating acute graft versus host reaction in cytomegalovirus colitis. Transplantation 39:669–670, 1985.

186. Higa E, Rosai J, Pizzimbono CA, Wise L: Mucosal hyperplasia, mucinous cystadenoma, and mucinous cystadenocarcinoma of the appendix: A reevaluation of the appendiceal mucocele. Cancer 32:1525–1541, 1973.

187. Qizilbash AH: Hyperplastic polyps of the appendix: Report of 19 cases. Arch Pathol 97:385–388, 1974.

188. Qizilbash AH: Mucoceles of the appendix: Their relationship to hyperplastic polyps, mucinous cystadenomas, and cystadenocarcinomas. Arch Pathol 99:548–555, 1975.

189. Wolff M, Ahmed N: Epithelial neoplasms of the vermiform appendix (exclusive of carcinoid). II: Cystadenomas, papillary adenomas, and adenomatous polyps of the appendix. Cancer 37:2511–2522, 1976.

190. Young RH, Gilks CB, Scully RE: Mucinous tumors of the appendix associated with mucinous tumors of the ovary and pseudomyxoma peritonei. A clinicopathologic analysis of 22 cases supporting an origin in the appendix. Am J Surg Pathol 15:415–429, 1991.

191. Appelman HD: Epithelial neoplasia of the appendix. In Norris HT (ed): Pathology of the Colon, Small Intestine and Anus. New York, Churchill Livingstone, 1983, pp 233–265.

192. Gonzalez JEG, Haan SE, Trujillo YP: Myxoglobulosis of the appendix. Am J Surg Pathol 12:962–968, 1988.

193. Longacre TA, Fenoglio-Preiser CM: Mixed hyperplastic adenomatous polyps/serrated adenomas. A distinct form of colonic neoplasia. Am J Surg Pathol 14:524–537, 1990.

194. Lake BD: Hirschsprung's disease and related disorders. In Whitehead R (ed): Gastrointestinal and Esophageal Pathology. New York, Churchill Livingstone, 1989, pp 257–268.

195. van Heyningen V: One gene—four syndromes. Nature 367:319–320, 1994.

196. Yunis E, Sieber WK, Akers DR: Does zonal aganglionosis really exist? Pediatr Pathol 1:33–49, 1983.

197. Leon SH, Schuffler MD: Visceral myopathy of the colon mimicking Hirschsprung's disease. Diagnosis by deep rectal biopsy. Dig Dis Sci 31:1381–1386, 1986.

198. Kapula L, Haberkorn S, Nixon HH: Chronic adynamic bowel simulating Hirschsprung's disease. J Pediatr Surg 10:885–892, 1975.

199. Meier-Ruge W: Epidemiology of congenital innervation defects of the distal colon. Virchows Archiv A 420:171–177, 1992.

200. Schofield DE, Yunis EJ: Intestinal neuronal dysplasia. J Pediatr Gastroenterol Nutr 12:182–189, 1991.

201. Munakata K, Morita K, Okabe I, Sueoka H: Clinical and histological studies of neuronal intestinal dysplasia. J Pediatr Surg 20:231–235, 1985.

202. Feinstat T, Tesluk H, Schuffler MD, et al: Megacolon and neurofibromatosis: A neuronal intestinal dysplasia. Gastroenterology 86:1573–1579, 1984.

203. Carney JA, Go VLW, Sizemore GW, Hayles AB: Alimentary tract ganglioneuromatosis: A major component of the syndrome of multiple endocrine neoplasia, type 2b. N Engl J Med 295:1287–1291, 1976.

204. Fenger C, Schroder HD: Neuronal hyperplasia in the anal canal. Histopathology 16:481–485, 1990.

205. Sigurdson E, Stern HS, Houpt J, et al: The Ehlers-Danlos syndrome and colonic perforation. Report of a case and physiologic assessment of underlying motility disorder. Dis Colon Rectum 28:962–966, 1985.
206. Sykes EM: Colon perforation in Ehlers-Danlos syndrome. Report of two cases and review of the literature. Am J Surg 147:410–413, 1984.
207. Beighton PH, Murdoch JL, Votteler T: Gastrointestinal complications of the Ehlers-Danlos syndrome. Gut 10:1004–1008, 1969.
208. Goldblum JR, Beales T, Weiss SW: Elastofibromatous change of the rectum. A lesion mimicking amyloidosis. Am J Surg Pathol 16:793–795, 1992.
209. Nishisho I, Nakamura Y, Miyoshi Y, et al: Mutations of chromosome 5-21 genes in FAP and colorectal cancer patients. Science 253:665–669, 1991.
210. Gardner EJ, Richards RC: Multiple cutaneous and subcutaneous lesions occurring simultaneously with hereditary polyposis and osteomatosis. Am J Hum Genet 5:139–147, 1953.
211. Bussey HJR: Extracolonic lesions associated with polyposis coli. Proc R Soc Med 65:294, 1972.
212. Muto T, Kamiya J, Sawada T, et al: Small "flat adenoma" of the large bowel with special reference to its clinicopathologic features. Dis Colon Rectum 28:847–851, 1985.
213. Wolber RA, Owen DA: Flat adenomas of the colon. Hum Pathol 22:70–74, 1991.
214. Adachi M, Muto T, Okinaga K, Morioka Y: Clinicopathologic features of the flat adenoma. Dis Colon Rectum 34:981–986, 1991.
215. Adachi M, Muto T, Morioka Y, et al: Flat adenoma and flat mucosal carcinoma (IIb type)—a new precursor of colorectal carcinoma. Dis Colon Rectum 31:236–243, 1988.
216. Muto T, Masaki T, Suzuki K: DNA ploidy pattern of flat adenomas of the large bowel. Dis Colon Rectum 34:696–698, 1991.
217. Lanspa SJ, Rouse J, Smyrk T, et al: Epidemiologic characteristics of the flat adenoma of Muto. A prospective study. Dis Colon Rectum 35:543–546, 1992.
218. Lynch HT, Smyrk TC, Watson P, et al: Hereditary flat adenoma syndrome: A variant of familial adenomatous polyposis? Dis Colon Rectum 35:411–421, 1992.
219. Cohen PR, Kohn SR, Kurzrock R: Association of sebaceous gland tumors and internal malignancy: The Muir-Torre syndrome. Am J Med 90:606–613, 1991.
220. Lynch HT, Fusaro RM, Roberts L, et al: Muir-Torre syndrome in several members of a family with a variant of the cancer family syndrome. Br J Dermatol 113:295–301, 1985.
221. Snover DC, Weigent CE, Sumner HW: Diffuse mucosal ganglioneuromatosis of the colon associated with adenocarcinoma. Am J Clin Pathol 75:225–229, 1981.
222. Lashner BA, Riddell RH, Winans CS: Ganglioneuromatosis of the colon and extensive glycogenic acanthosis in Cowden's disease. Dig Dis Sci 31:213–216, 1986.
223. d'Amore ESG, Manivel JC, Pettinato G, et al: Intestinal ganglioneuromatosis: Mucosal and transmural types. A clinicopathological and immunohistochemical study of six cases. Hum Pathol 22:276–286, 1991.
224. Donnelly WH, Sieber WK, Yunis EJ: Polypoid ganglioneurofibromatosis of the large bowel. Arch Pathol 87:537–541, 1969.
225. Hochberg FH, Dasilva AB, Galdabini J, Richardson EP: Gastrointestinal involvement in von Recklinghausen's neurofibromatosis. Neurology 24:1144–1151, 1974.
226. Raszkowski HJ, Hufner RF: Neurofibromatosis of the colon: A unique manifestation of von Recklinghausen's disease. Cancer 27:134–142, 1971.
227. Khubchandani IT, Trimpi HD, Sheets JA: von Recklinghausen's disease with involvement of the rectum: Report of a case. Dis Colon Rectum 15:459–460, 1972.
228. Levy D, Khatib R: Intestinal neurofibromatosis with malignant degeneration: Report of a case. Dis Colon Rectum 3:140–144, 1960.
229. Staple TW, McAlister WH, Anderson MS: Plexiform neurofibromatosis of the colon simulating Hirschsprung's disease. Am J Roentgenol Rad Ther Nucl Med 91:840–845, 1964.
230. Schaldenbrand JD, Appelman HT: Solitary solid stromal gastrointestinal tumors in von Recklinghausen's disease with minimal smooth muscle differentiation. Hum Pathol 15:229–232, 1984.
231. Grotsky HW, Rickert RR, Smith WD, Newsome JF: Familial juvenile polyposis coli. A clinical and pathologic study of a large kindred. Gastroenterology 82:494–501, 1982.
232. Veale AMO, McColl I, Bussey HJR, Morson BC: Juvenile polyposis coli. J Med Genet 3:5–16, 1966.
233. Jass JR, Williams CB, Bussey HJR, Morson BC: Juvenile polyposis—a precancerous condition. Histopathology 12:619–630, 1988.
234. Sachatello CR, Hahn IS, Carrington CB: Juvenile gastrointestinal polyposis in a female infant. Report of a case and a review of the literature of a recently recognised syndrome. Surgery 75:107–113, 1974.
235. Sachatello CR, Pickren JW, Grance JT: Generalised juvenile gastrointestinal polyposis. Gastroenterology 58:699–708, 1970.
236. Jarvinen H, Franssila KO: Familial juvenile polyposis coli. Increased risk of colorectal cancer. Gut 25:792–796, 1984.
237. Nakamura S, Kino I, Akaji T: Inflammatory myoglandular polyps of the colon and rectum. A clinicopathological study of 32 pedunculated polyps, distinct from other types of polyps. Am J Surg Pathol 16:772–779, 1992.
238. Starink TM, Van der Veen JP, De Waal LP, et al: The Cowden syndrome: A clinical and genetic study in 21 patients. Clin Genet 29:222–233, 1986.
239. Burke AP, Sobin LH: The pathology of Cronkhite-Canada polyps. Am J Surg Pathol 13:940–945, 1989.
240. Kelly JK: The pathogenesis of inflammatory polyps. Dis Colon Rectum 30:251–254, 1987.
241. Helwig EB, Major JJ: Lymphoid polyps (benign lymphoma) and malignant lymphoma of the rectum and anus. Surg Gynecol Obstet 92:233–243, 1951.
242. O'Briain DS, Kennedy MJ, Daly PA, et al: Multiple lymphomatous polyposis of the gastrointestinal tract. Am J Surg Pathol 13:691–699, 1989.
243. Isaacson PG, Maclennan KA, Subbuswamy SG: Multiple lymphomatous polyposis of the colorectum. Histopathology 8:641–656, 1984.
244. Kelly JK, MacCannell K, Hershfield NB: Residual stalks of pedunculated adenomas—an underrecognized type of colonic polyp. J Clin Gastroenterol 9:227–231, 1987.
245. Berry GJ, Pitts WC, Weiss LM: Pseudomalignant ulcerative change of the gastrointestinal tract. Hum Pathol 22:59–62, 1991.
246. Shekitka KM, Helwig EB: Deceptive bizarre stromal cells in polyps and ulcers of the gastrointestinal tract. Cancer 67:2111–2117, 1991.
247. Sobin LH: Inverted hyperplastic polyps of the colon. Am J Surg Pathol 9:265–272, 1985.
248. Shepherd NA: Inverted hyperplastic polyposis of the colon. J Clin Pathol 46:56–60, 1993.
249. Williams GT, Arthur JF, Bussey HJR, Morson BC: Metaplastic polyps and polyposis of the colorectum. Histopathology 4:155–170, 1980.
250. Gebbers J-O, Laissue JA: Mixed hyperplastic and neoplastic polyp of the colon. An immunohistological study. Virchows Arch [A] 410:189–194, 1986.
251. Snover DC, Sandstad J, Hutton S: Mucosal pseudolipomatosis of the colon. Am J Clin Pathol 84:575–579, 1985.
252. Kozarek RA, Earnest DL, Silverstein ME, Smith RG: Air-pressure induced colon injury during diagnostic colonoscopy. Gastroenterology 78:7–14, 1980.
252a. Morson BC, Pang LSC: Rectal biopsy as an aid to cancer control in ulcerative colitis. Gut 8:423–434, 1967.
253. Riddell RH, Goldman H, Ransohoff DF, et al: Dysplasia in inflammatory bowel disease: Standardized classification with provisional clinical applications. Hum Pathol 14:931–968, 1983.
254. Lennard-Jones JE, Melville DM, Morson BC, et al: Precancer and cancer in extensive ulcerative colitis: Findings among 401 patients over 22 years. Gut 31:800–806, 1990.
255. Rubin CE, Haggitt RG, Burmer GC, et al: DNA aneuploidy in colonic biopsies predicts future development of dysplasia in ulcerative colitis. Gastroenterology 103:1611–1620, 1992.
256. Muto T, Sawada T, Sugihara K: Treatment of carcinoma in adenomas. World J Surg 15:35–40, 1991.
257. Pollard CW, Nivatvongs S, Rojanasakul A, et al: The fate of patients following polypectomy alone for polyps containing invasive carcinoma. Dis Colon Rectum 35:933–937, 1992.
258. Morson BC, Whiteway JE, Jones EA, et al: Histopathology and prognosis of malignant colorectal polyps treated by endoscopic polypectomy. Gut 25:437–444, 1984.
259. Muller S, Chesner IM, Egan MJ, et al: Significance of venous and lymphatic invasion in malignant polyps of the colon and rectum. Gut 30:1385–1391, 1989.
260. Nivatvongs, S, Rohanasakul A, Reiman HM, et al: The risk of lymph node metastasis in colorectal polyps with invasive adenocarcinoma. Dis Colon Rectum 34:323–328, 1991.
261. Muto T, Bussey HJ, Morson BC: Pseudocarcinomatous invasion in adenomatous polyps of the colon and rectum. J Clin Pathol 26:25–31, 1973.
262. Pascal RR, Hertzler G, Hunter S, Goldschmid S: Pseudoinvasion with high-grade dysplasia in a colonic adenoma. Distinction from adenocarcinoma. Am J Surg Pathol 14:694–697, 1990.
263. Halvorsen TB, Seim E: Influence of mucinous components on survival in colorectal adenocarcinomas: A multivariate analysis. J Clin Pathol 41:1068–1072, 1988.
264. Symonds DA, Vickery AL: Mucinous carcinoma of the colon and rectum. Cancer 37:1891–1900, 1976.
265. Umpleby HC, Ranson DL, Williamson RCN: Peculiarities of mucinous colorectal carcinoma. Br J Surg 72:715–718, 1985.
266. Sasaki O, Atkin WS, Jass JR: Mucinous carcinoma of the rectum. Histopathology 11:259–272, 1987.
267. Halvorsen TB: Site distribution of colorectal adenocarcinomas. A retrospective study of 853 tumours. Scand J Gastroenterol 21:973–978, 1986.
268. Sundblad AS, Paz RA: Mucinous carcinoma of the colon and rectum and their relation to polyps. Cancer 50:2504–2509, 1982.
269. Connelly JH, Robey-Cafferty SS, El-Naggar AK, Cleary KR: Exophytic signet-ring cell carcinoma of the colorectum. Arch Pathol Lab Med 115:134–136, 1991.
270. Nakahara H, Ishikawa T, Itabashi M, Hirota T: Diffusely infiltrating primary colorectal carcinoma of linitis plastica and lymphangiosis types. Cancer 69:901–906, 1992.
271. Giacchero A, Aste H, Baracchini P, et al: Primary signet-ring carcinoma of the large bowel. Report of nine cases. Cancer 56:2723–2726, 1985.
272. Vasen HFA, Meklin J-P, Meera-Khan P, Lynch HT: The international collaborative group on hereditary non-polyposis colorectal cancer. Dis Colon Rectum 34:424–425, 1991.
273. Lynch HT, Smyrk TC, Watson P, et al: Genetics, natural history, tumor spectrum, and pathology of hereditary non-polyposis colorectal cancer: An updated review. Gastroenterology 104:1535–1549, 1993.
274. Peltomaki P, Aaltonen LA, Sistonen P, et al: Genetic mapping of a locus predisposing to human colo-rectal cancer. Science 260:810–812, 1993.
275. Fishel R, Lescoe MK, Rao MRS, et al: The human mutator gene homolog MSH2 and its association with hereditary nonpolyposis colon cancer. Cell 75:1027–1038, 1993.

276. Leach FS, Nicolaides NC, Papadopoulos N, et al: Mutations of a mutS homolog in hereditary nonpolyposis colorectal cancer. Cell 75:1215–1225, 1993.
277. Mecklin J-P, Sipponen P, Jarvinen HJ: Histopathology of colo-rectal carcinomas and adenomas in cancer family syndrome. Dis Colon Rectum 29:849–853, 1986.
278. Jass JR, Stewart SM: Evolution of hereditary non-polyposis colorectal cancer. Gut 33:783–786, 1992.
279. Spirio L, Otterud B, Stauffer D, et al: Linkage of a variant or attenuated form of adenomatous polyposis coli to the adenomatous polyposis coli (APC) locus. Am J Hum Genet 51:92–100, 1992.
280. Burt RW, Bishop DT, Cannon LA, et al: Dominant inheritance of adenomatous colonic polyps in colo-rectal cancer. N Engl J Med 312:1540–1544, 1985.
281. Cannon-Albright LA, Skolnik NH, Bishop DT, et al: Common inheritance of colonic adenomatous polyps and associated colo-rectal cancers. N Engl J Med 319:533–537, 1988.
282. Leppert M, Burt R, Hughes JP, et al: Genetic analysis of an inherited predisposition to colon cancer with a variable number of adenomatous polyps. N Engl J Med 322:904–908, 1990.
283. Chumas JC: Melanotic adenocarcinoma of the anorectum. Am J Surg Pathol 5:711–717, 1981.
284. Coma-del-Corral MJ, Perez-Serrano L, Razquin-Lizanaga S: Melanotic adenocarcinoma of the anorectum. J Clin Gastroenterol 12:114–117, 1990.
285. Comer TP, Beahrs OH, Dockerty MB: Primary squamous cell carcinoma and adenoacanthoma of the colon. Cancer 28:1111–1117, 1971.
286. Crissman JD: Adenosquamous and squamous cell carcinoma of the colon. Am J Surg Pathol 2:47–54, 1978.
287. Moll UM, Ilardi CF, Zuna R, Phillips ME: A biologically active parathyroid hormone-like substance secreted by an adenosquamous carcinoma of the transverse colon. Hum Pathol 18:1287–1290, 1987.
288. Grimes DA, Fowler WC: Adenosquamous carcinoma of the cecum arising in endometriosis. Gynaecol Oncol 9:254–255, 1980.
289. Williams GT, Blackshaw AJ, Morson BC: Squamous carcinoma of the colorectum and its genesis. J Pathol 129:139–147, 1979.
290. Lundquist DE, Marcus JN, Thorson AG, Massop D: Primary squamous cell carcinoma of the colon arising in a villous adenoma. Hum Pathol 19:362–364, 1988.
291. Sarlin JG, Mori K: Morules in epithelial tumors of the colon and rectum. Am J Surg Pathol 8:281–285, 1984.
292. Dukes CE: The significance of the unusual in the pathology of intestinal tumours. Ann R Coll Surg 4:90–103, 1949.
293. Hickey WF, Corson JM: Squamous cell carcinoma arising in a duplication of the colon: Case report and literature review of squamous carcinoma of the colon and of malignancy complicating colonic duplication. Cancer 47:602–609, 1981.
294. Grinvalsky HT, Helwig EB: Carcinoma of the anorectal junction. 1: Histological considerations. Cancer 9:480–488, 1956.
295. Pang LSC, Morson BC: Basaloid carcinoma of the anal canal. J Clin Pathol 20:128–135, 1967.
296. Morson BC, Volkstadt H: Mucoepidermoid tumors of the anal canal. J Clin Pathol 16:200–205, 1963.
297. Wolber R, Dupuis B, Thiyagaratnam P, Owen D: Anal cloacogenic and squamous carcinoma. Comparative histologic analysis using in situ hybridization for human papillomavirus DNA. Am J Surg Pathol 14:176–182, 1990.
298. White WB, Schneiderman H, Sayre JT: Basal cell carcinoma of the anus: Clinical and pathological distinction from cloacogenic carcinoma. J Clin Gastroenterol 6:441–446, 1984.
299. Damjanov I, Amenta PS, Bosman FT: Undifferentiated carcinoma of the colon containing exocrine, neuroendocrine and squamous cells. Virchows Arch [A] 301:57–66, 1983.
300. Palvio DHB, Sorensen FB, Klove-Mogensen M: Stem cell carcinoma of the colon and rectum. Dis Colon Rectum 28:440–445, 1985.
301. Burke AB, Shekitka KM, Sobin LH: Small cell carcinomas of the large intestine. Am J Clin Pathol 95:315–321, 1991.
302. Clery AP, Dockerty MC, Waugh JM: Small-cell carcinoma of the colon and rectum: A clinicopathologic study. Arch Surg 83:22–30, 1961.
303. Mills SE, Allen MS, Cohen AR: Small-cell undifferentiated carcinoma of the colon: A clinicopathological study of five cases and their association with colonic adenomas. Am J Surg Pathol 7:643–651, 1983.
304. Wick MR, Weatherby RP, Weiland LH: Small cell neuroendocrine carcinoma of the colon and rectum: Clinical, histologic, and ultrastructural study and immunohistochemical comparison with cloacogenic carcinoma. Hum Pathol 18:9–21, 1987.
305. Gould VE, Chejfec G: Neuroendocrine carcinomas of the colon. Am J Surg Pathol 2:31–38, 1978.
306. Moyana TN, Qizilbash AH, Murphy F: Composite glandular-carcinoid tumors of the colon and rectum. Report of two cases. Am J Surg Pathol 12:607–611, 1988.
307. Dukes CE: The surgical pathology of rectal cancer. J Clin Pathol 2:95–98, 1949.
308. Gibbs NM: Undifferentiated carcinoma of the large intestine. Histopathology 1:77–84, 1977.
309. Jetmore AB, Ray JE, Gathright JB Jr, et al: Rectal carcinoids: The most frequent carcinoid tumor. Dis Colon Rectum 35:717–725, 1992.
310. Burke M, Shepherd N, Mann CV: Carcinoid tumours of the rectum and anus. Br J Surg 74:358–361, 1987.
311. Nelson RL: The association of carcinoid tumors of the rectum with myelofibrosis: Report of two cases. Dis Colon Rectum 24:548–549, 1981.

312. Owen DA, Hwang WS, Thorlakson RH, Walli E: Malignant carcinoid tumor complicating chronic ulcerative colitis. Am J Clin Pathol 76:333–338, 1981.
313. Griffiths AP, Dixon MF: Microcarcinoids and diversion colitis in a colon defunctioned for 18 years. Report of a case. Dis Colon Rectum 35:685–688, 1992.
314. Maruyama M, Fukayama M, Koike M: A case of multiple carcinoid tumors of the rectum with extraglandular endocrine cell proliferation. Cancer 61:131–136, 1988.
315. Federspiel BH, Burke AP, Sobin LH, Shekitka KM: Rectal and colonic carcinoids: A clinicopathologic study of 84 cases. Cancer 65:135–140, 1990.
316. Sobin LH, Hjermstad BM, Sesterhenn IA, Helwig EB: Prostatic acid phosphatase activity in carcinoid tumors. Cancer 58:136-138, 1986.
317. O'Briain DS, Tischler AS, Dayal Y, et al: Rectal carcinoids as tumors of the hindgut endocrine cells: A morphological and immunohistochemical analysis. Am J Surg Pathol 6:131–142, 1982.
318. Alumets J, Falkmer S, Grimelius L, et al: Immunocytochemical demonstration of enkephalin and endorphin in endocrine tumors of the rectum: A survey of 27 colorectal carcinoids. Acta Pathol Microbiol Scand 88(a):103–109, 1980.
319. Fiocca R, Capella C, Buffa R, et al: Glucagon-, glicentin-, and pancreatic polypeptide-like immunoreactivities in rectal carcinoids and related colorectal cells. Am J Pathol 100:81–92, 1980.
320. Stout AP: Carcinoid tumors of the rectum derived from Erspamer's pre-enterochrome cells. Am J Pathol 18:993–1004, 1942.
321. Berardi R: Carcinoid tumors of the colon (exclusive of the rectum): Review of the literature. Dis Colon Rectum 15:383–391, 1972.
322. Ballantyne GH, Saroca PE, Flannery JT, et al: Incidence and mortality of carcinoids of the colon. Data from the Connecticut tumor registry. Cancer 69:2400–2405, 1992.
323. Klappenback RS, Kurman RJ, Sinclair CF, James LP: Composite carcinoma-carcinoid tumors of the gastrointestinal tract: A morphologic, histochemical, and immunocytochemical study. Am J Clin Pathol 84:137–143, 1985.
324. Hernandez FJ, Fernandez BB: Mucus-secreting colonic carcinoid tumors: Light and electron-microscopic study of three cases. Dis Colon Rectum 17:387–396, 1974.
325. Bates HR Jr, Belter LF: Composite carcinoid tumor (argentaffinoma-adenocarcinoma) of the colon: Report of two cases. Dis Colon Rectum 10:467–470, 1967.
326. Watson PH, Alguacil-Garcia A: Mixed crypt cell carcinoma. A clinicopathological study of the so-called "goblet cell carcinoid." Virchows Arch [A] 412:175–182, 1987.
327. Klein HZ: Mucinous carcinoid tumor of the vermiform appendix. Cancer 33:770–777, 1974.
328. Wolff M, Ahmed N: Epithelial neoplasms of vermiform appendix (exclusive of carcinoid). 1: Adenocarcinoma of the appendix. Cancer 37:2493–2510, 1976.
329. Warkel RL, Cooper BH, Helwig EB: Adenocarcinoid, a mucin-producing carcinoid tumor of the appendix. A study of 39 cases. Cancer 42:2781–2793, 1978.
330. Isaacson P: Crypt cell carcinoma of the appendix (so-called adenocarcinoid tumor). Am J Surg Pathol 5:213–224, 1981.
331. Burke AP, Sobin LH, Federspiel BH, et al: Goblet cell carcinoids and related tumors of the vermiform appendix. Am J Clin Pathol 94:27–35, 1990.
332. Edmonds P, Merino MJ, LiVolsi VA, Duray PH: Adenocarcinoid (mucinous carcinoid) of the appendix. Gastroenterology 86:302–309, 1984.
333. Hood IC, Jones AC, Watts JC: Mucinous tumor of the appendix presenting as bilateral ovarian tumors. Arch Pathol Lab Med 110:336–340, 1986.
334. Park K, Blessing K, Kerr K, et al: Goblet cell carcinoid of the appendix. Gut 33:322–324, 1990.
335. Hofman P, Bernard JL, Michiels JF, et al: Primary angiosarcoma of the colon: Anatomo-clinical study of a case. Ann Pathol 11:25–30, 1991.
336. Smith JA, Bhathal PS, Cuthbertson AM: Angiosarcoma of the colon. Report of a case with long-term survival. Dis Colon Rectum 33:330–333, 1990.
337. Taxy JB, Battifora H: Angiosarcoma of the gastrointestinal tract. A report of three cases. Cancer 62:210–216, 1988.
338. Saito R, Bedetti CD, Caines MJ, Kramer K: Malignant epithelioid hemangioendothelioma of the colon. Dis Colon Rectum 30:707–711, 1987.
339. Steiner CA, Palmer LH: Angiosarcoma of the colon. Ann Surg 129:538–542, 1949.
340. Ordonez NG, Luna MA: Choriocarcinoma of the colon. Am J Gastroenterol 79:39–42, 1984.
341. Ranchod M, Kempson RL: Smooth muscle tumors of the gastrointestinal tract and retroperitoneum. Cancer 39:255–262, 1977.
342. Akwari OE, Dozois RR, Weiland LH, Beahrs OH: Leiomyosarcoma of the small and large bowel. Cancer 42:1375–1384, 1978.
343. Walsh TH, Mann CV: Smooth muscle neoplasms of the rectum and anal canal. Br J Surg 71:597–599, 1984.
344. Haque S, Dean PJ: Stromal neoplasms of the rectum and anal canal. Hum Pathol 23:762–767, 1992.
345. Randleman CD, Wolff BG, Dozois RR, et al: Leiomyosarcoma of the rectum and anus. A series of 22 cases. Int J Colorectal Dis 4:91–96, 1989.
346. Vallaeys JH, Cuvelier CA, Bekaert L, Roels H: Combined leiomyomatosis of the small intestine and colon. Arch Pathol Lab Med 116:281–283, 1992.
347. Zornig C, Thoma G, Schroder S: Diffuse leiomyosarcomatosis of the colon. Cancer 65:570–572, 1990.
348. Minsky BD, Cohen AM, Hajdu SI: Conservative management of anal leiomyosarcoma. Cancer 68:1640–1643, 1991.

349. Kalogeropoulos NK, Antonakopoulos GN, Agapitos MB, Papacharalampous NX: Spindle cell carcinoma (pseudosarcoma) of the anus: A light, electron microscopic and immunocytochemical study of a case. Histopathology 9:987–994, 1985.
350. Lankerani MR, Aubrey RW, Reid JD: Endometriosis of the colon with mixed ''germ cell'' tumor. Am J Clin Pathol 78:555–559, 1982.
351. Amano S, Yamada N: Endometrioid carcinoma arising from endometriosis of the sigmoid colon: A case report. Hum Pathol 12:845–848, 1981.
352. Lott JV, Rubin RJ, Salvati EP, et al: Endometrioid carcinoma of the rectum arising in endometriosis: Report of a case. Dis Colon Rectum 21:56–60, 1978.
353. Hitti IF, Glasberg SS, Lubicz S: Clear cell carcinoma arising in extraovarian endometriosis: Report of three cases and review of the literature. Gynecol Oncol 39:314–320, 1990.
354. Heaps JM, Nieberg RK, Beret JS: Malignant neoplasms arising in endometriosis. Obstet Gynecol 75:1023–1027, 1990.

CHAPTER **8**

Diseases of the Pancreas

Carolyn C. Compton, M.D., Ph.D.

LESIONS WITH SIMILAR OR OVERLAPPING HISTOPATHOLOGIC FEATURES

Benign Lesions

Lipomatosis of the Pancreas and Lipomatous Atrophy (Shwachman Syndrome)

Lipomatosis of the pancreas is a misnomer that refers to asymptomatic atrophy of the pancreatic glandular tissue with replacement by fatty infiltration rather than true lipoma formation. It is an entity that is often, but not always, associated with increasing age, obesity, and/or adult onset diabetes mellitus.[1–3] Despite the rather dramatic reduction in pancreatic acinar tissue in pancreatic lipomatosis (Fig. 8–1), pancreatic insufficiency does not usually occur, although cases with steatorrhea have been reported.[4] Perhaps the only important clinical association is the rare occurrence of pancreatic adenocarcinoma within the lesion.[5] Microscopically, the pancreas shows near total atrophy of exocrine tissue and panlobular replacement of acinar cells by fat. Small clusters of acinar cells may remain around ductal structures. The fatty tissue is traversed by thin fibrous septa, and small collections of lymphocytes may appear within the adipose tissue, but there is no real evidence of inflammation and subsequent scarring as the cause of this lesion. Pancreatic islets are typically spared and appear relatively prominent given the paucity of acinar cells. Ductal structures may show widespread mucinous metaplasia but lack cytologic atypia.

Despite the virtually indistinguishable histopathologic appearance of pancreatic lipomatosis and so-called lipomatous atrophy, or Shwachman syndrome, the two entities represent opposite ends of the clinical spectrum. In contrast to lipomatosis, which is an isolated pancreatic lesion, lipomatous atrophy is part of a systemic syndrome with a familial incidence in which the principal manifestations are pancreatic insufficiency, neutropenia, recurrent infections, and a spectrum of skeletal and dermatologic abnormalities.[6] Despite the fact that it is rare, Shwachman syndrome is the second most frequent cause of pancreatic insufficiency in childhood, exceeded in incidence only by cystic fibrosis.[7] Pancreatic insufficiency is the most prominent feature of this syndrome and usually presents as steatorrhea, diarrhea, and failure to thrive in infancy. In molecular studies, a high incidence in chromosome breakage has been found in patients with this

syndrome.[8] As in pancreatic lipomatosis, near total atrophy of the exocrine acinar tissue, sparing of the pancreatic islets, relatively normal appearing ducts, and massive infiltration by fatty tissue are characteristic histopathologic features. The increase in fatty tissue may enormously enlarge the pancreas in both pancreatic lipomatosis and lipomatous atrophy, increasing pancreatic weight severalfold above normal at autopsy.

Non-neoplastic Benign Cystic Lesions

With the exception of pseudocysts, non-neoplastic cystic lesions of the pancreas are rare. These include congenital cysts of various types, retention cysts, and the dyschylic cysts of cystic fibrosis. Unlike mucinous cystic neoplasms (see later discussion), which can occasionally show extensive denudation of their epithelial lining and can be easily mistaken for a pseudocyst, these lesions are almost invariably fully lined by intact epithelium and, though seldom mistaken for pseudocysts, must be distinguished from one another.

CONGENITAL DYSGENETIC CYSTS. These are simple cysts with a fibrous wall lined by monomorphous columnar, cuboidal, or flattened epithelium. They most likely result from focal aberrations in ductal development. Dysgenetic cysts may be solitary or multiple, unilocular or multilocular. They are usually of small diameter and are rarely symptomatic. Stratified squamous epithelium may appear within some cysts, probably as the result of metaplastic change. Occasionally, the cyst wall contains pancreatic acini, islets of Langerhans, and/or intestinal glandular tissue, but usually the fluid content lacks enzymatic activity. The most commonly reported cases of congenital pancreatic cysts have been those seen in association with inherited polycystic disease of kidney, liver, and spleen in pediatric patients.[9] Rarely, large solitary developmental cysts present as abdominal distention in the young child or neonate. However, congenital cysts, unassociated with cysts in any other organ, may be seen in individuals of any age as an incidental finding at autopsy or pancreatic resection.[10, 11]

Occasionally, diagnostic difficulties may arise in differentiating a multilocular dysgenetic cyst in an adult from a cystic neoplasm such as a serous cystadenoma or mucinous cystic neoplasm. Perhaps most helpful in distinguishing between the two is the finding of epithelial tufting. Dysgenetic cysts rarely show papillary tufting of their epithelial lining, whereas papillary tufting is common in cystic neoplasms. Furthermore, dysgenetic cysts rarely show significant mucin production, a feature that, along with epithelial tufting, would strongly sug-

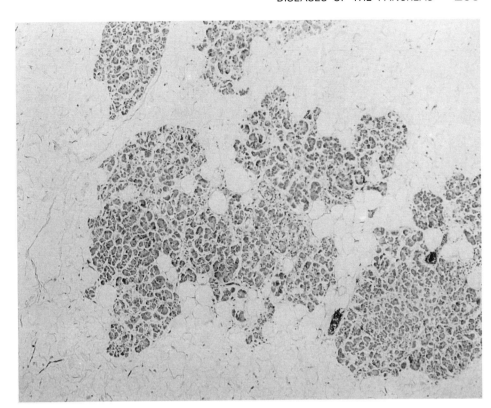

FIGURE 8–1. Pancreatic lipomatosis. The pancreatic parenchyma is markedly atrophic, and remaining acini are surrounded and widely separated by diffuse fatty infiltration of the stroma. (H&E, ×33)

gest a mucinous cystic neoplasm. Definitive differentiation from a serous cystadenoma may be more difficult but is likely to be of little clinical consequence because both would be treated identically and have nearly identical prognoses (the rare exception being serous cystadenoma manifesting aggressive biologic behavior [see later discussion]).

The recently described **multicystic pancreatic hamartoma**[12] may be a multicystic variation of a developmental congenital pancreatic cyst. These lesions contain pancreatic acini within their fibrous walls and are lined by simple ductal-type epithelium. Although fully developed islets of Langerhans apparently are not seen in this entity, endocrine cells are diffusely distributed throughout the exocrine tissue of the wall on immunohistochemical stains. It may be reasonable to classify all congenital cystic lesions that are unassociated with cystic disease in other organs and contain other normal pancreatic elements within their walls as hamartomas instead of "developmental pancreatic cysts."

ENTERIC DUPLICATION CYSTS. Enteric duplication cysts presenting as pancreatic lesions are usually of gastric origin, are lined with gastric- or intestinal-type epithelium, and communicate with their enteric source.[10] Some have ectopic pancreatic tissue within their wall, suggesting development from an enteric diverticulum originating from the pancreatic duct. Patients usually present at an early age with symptoms related to gastric acid secretion or pancreatitis. However, duplication cysts evolving from the caudal foregut (these contain ciliated epithelium) may be asymptomatic. Cyst fluid from these lesions may provide a clue to their diagnosis. Those representing gastric alimentary duplications may be expected to contain acid and enzymes. Those of caudal foregut origin have been shown to contain increased concentrations of carcinoembryonic antigen and to have increased fluid viscosity, overlapping with the biochemical profiles of fluid from mucinous cystic neoplasms. The characteristically well-developed bilayered muscular wall of duplication cysts is a pathognomonic feature that is very helpful in recognizing these lesions. In contrast, their lining epithelium can vary in type and may consist of an admixture of cell types: gastric, serous, mucous, and/or ciliated (foregut) epithelium.[13]

RETENTION CYSTS. These cysts are caused by tumors, stones, or inflammatory strictures that occlude the main duct or one of its tributaries and lead to upstream ductal dilatation and cyst formation. Thus, the proximate cause is usually apparent, either clinically or histopathologically. The cyst itself is usually unilocular, lined by a flattened epithelium, and contains serous pancreatic secretions. When occurring in heterotopic pancreatic tissue within the duodenal submucosa, the cyst may be visualized endoscopically as a polypoid projection into the lumen.

DYSCHYLIC CYSTS OF CYSTIC FIBROSIS. The dyschylic cysts of cystic fibrosis (Fig. 8–2) are always multiple and are seen within a background of marked lobular interstitial fibrosis containing atrophic, ectatic acini.[14] The cystically dilated ducts are filled with retained mucoproteinaceous secretions that form lamellar hyaline plugs within the lumina (see Fig. 8–2). The lobular ductal architecture is maintained so that the anatomic distribution of the affected ducts is usually apparent. The degree of flattening of the ductal epithelium usually depends on the size of the concretions and the degree of ductal dilatation.

INFECTIOUS CYSTS. Infectious cysts such as parasitic pseudocysts caused by *Echinococcus* constitute a rare entity whose diagnosis depends on recognition of its content of parasitic structures.

LYMPHOEPITHELIAL CYSTS. Lymphoepithelial cysts of the pancreas look like cutaneous epidermal inclusion cysts with

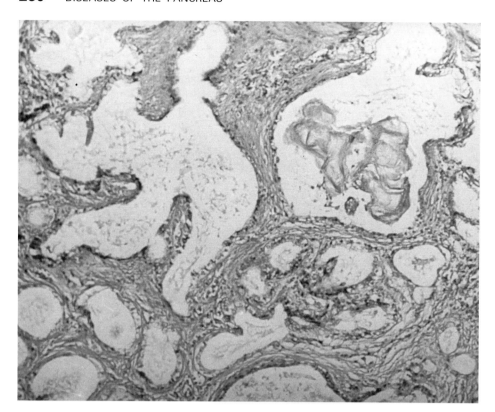

FIGURE 8–2. Cystic fibrosis. Dilated ductal structures in a background of interstitial fibrosis contain inspissated secretions. (H&E, ×33)

lymphocytes in their walls.[15] They are lined by a mature keratinizing squamous epithelium and are filled with keratinaceous debris.[16] In contrast to cystic teratomas (see later discussion), from which it is important to distinguish them, lymphoepithelial cysts contain no epidermal appendageal structures in their walls.[17]

Nesidioblastosis and Adenomatosis

From a histopathologic standpoint, the diagnosis of nesidioblastosis remains ill defined. The major problem surrounding this diagnosis is the broad overlap of normal variation in pancreatic structure with specific changes thought to reflect nesidioblastic endocrine hyperplasia. Several studies of the normal pancreas have shown that features that have been regarded as key diagnostic features of nesidioblastosis,[18, 19] such as ductulo-insular complexes (proliferation of ductules showing buds of epithelium with neuroendocrine differentiation) and scattered insular cells among acini, are found in about 10% of normal pancreases from fetal through adult life.[20, 21] Thus, it is not surprising that the existence of nesidioblastosis as a pathologic entity has been questioned. Various labor-intensive and somewhat complicated histomorphometric techniques have been used to establish reliable criteria for distinguishing this entity from the normal variability of pancreatic endocrine cells. Some investigators have concluded that the nuclear area and DNA content of the pancreatic beta cells in the islets of Langerhans are increased in neonatal hyperinsulinemic hypoglycemia (nesidioblastosis) compared with those of age-matched normal controls. The term **nesidiodysplasia** has been used to describe these enlarged, hyperchromatic neuroendocrine cells both within islets and dispersed throughout the acinar tissue.[22] It has been claimed that the increase in average size and density of islet beta cell nuclei

("macronuclei") constitutes a morphologic criterion for diagnosis of nesidiodysplasia,[23] but this been disputed because macronuclei can be seen in the beta cells of infants of diabetic mothers.

Although the features of nesidioblastosis overlap with those of normal pancreas, the *sine qua non* of this lesion is an increase in the total volume of pancreatic endocrine cells. Thus, it is essential to be able to accurately label all pancreatic endocrine cells within the tissue resected using immunohistochemical labeling for chromogranin, neuron-specific enolase, or synaptophysin and to determine the proportion of beta cells present by immunohistochemical localization of insulin. Immunohistochemistry is also helpful in highlighting the findings regarded as **characteristic of nesidioblastosis, including (1) giant islets of Langerhans (measuring up to 750 μm in diameter, showing a prominent vascular pattern, and containing pleomorphic cells with prominent nucleoli)** (Fig. 8–3); **(2) ductulo-insular lesions (small aggregates of ductular and endocrine elements in which nests of ductal epithelial cells undergoing neuroendocrine differentiation are seen to bud from and to indent proliferating ducts)** (Fig. 8–4); **and (3) diffuse distribution of isolated beta cells among acini and duct epithelium** (Fig. 8–5). These features may be more meaningful in the adult patient than in the young child, because it has been shown that the specific histologic features of nesidioblastosis enumerated here as well as a large endocrine mass in general are also seen in the normal young infant.[20, 24] In any case, it may be helpful to compare immunohistochemically labeled sections of patient specimens with those from normal site-matched control tissues from the head, body, or tail of the pancreas, as appropriate in the specific case. Overall, the diagnosis of nesidioblastosis in neonatal hyperinsulinemic hypoglycemia is best considered a clinicopathologic entity that can seldom, if ever, be made with cer-

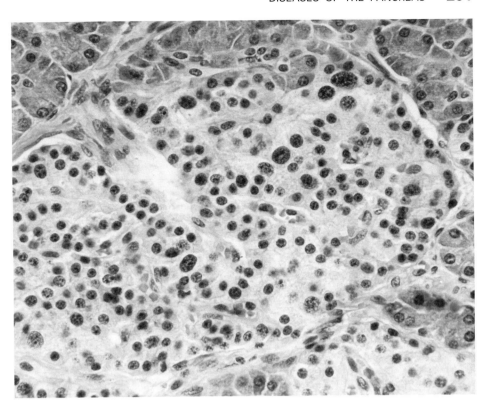

FIGURE 8–3. Nesidioblastosis. The cells within a giant islet of Langerhans show nuclear pleomorphism and nucleolar prominence. (H&E, ×250)

tainty on a tissue basis alone. Yet, despite the lack of a definitive histopathologic counterpart to this physiologic abnormality, reduction of pancreatic endocrine mass by surgical resection remains the treatment of choice,[25] and the pathologist is asked to assess the respective specimen in such cases. **Thus, the findings of lesions in the pancreas consistent with a histopathologic diagnosis of nesidioblastosis plus a positive response to surgical resection remain the most straightforward ways to confirm the diagnosis.** It is well to remember that persistent hypoglycemia in infancy may not be the result of inappropriate insulin secretion at all. Persistent hypoglycemia may occur in infants with a wide variety of

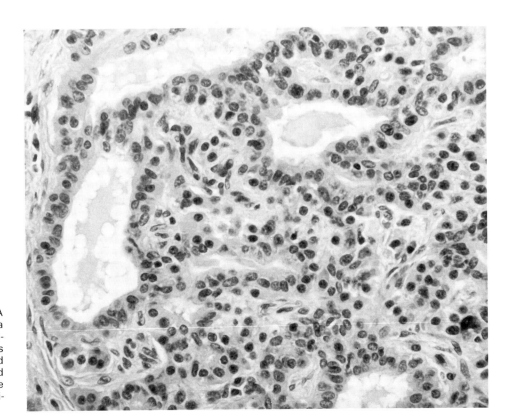

FIGURE 8–4. Nesidioblastosis. A ductulo-insular lesion is seen as a periductal and intraductal proliferation of neuroendocrine cells. Nests of neuroendocrine cells surround and focally indent ducts, and numerous single neuroendocrine cells appear within the ductal epithelium. (H&E, ×250)

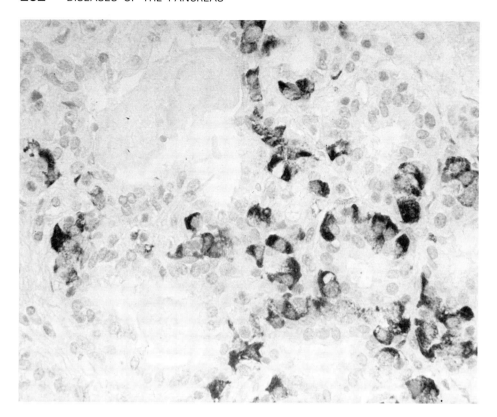

FIGURE 8–5. Nesidioblastosis. An immunohistochemical stain for insulin shows diffuse distribution of beta cells within a ductulo-insular lesion. (H&E, ×250)

disorders, including ketotic hypoglycemia from panhypopituitarism, growth hormone deficiency, Addison's disease, hyperthyroidism, and hepatic enzyme deficiencies (e.g., glycogen storage diseases, disorders of gluconeogenesis).

In summary, the diagnosis of nesidioblastosis on a histopathologic basis alone may not be supportable. The bulk of evidence suggests that this is a hyperfunctioning syndrome that has no definite morphologic counterpart. Further complicating the issue is the fact that the ductulo-insular structures that have been regarded as the hallmark of nesidioblastosis in the past are seen in a variety of other pancreatic disorders, including diabetes mellitus, cystic fibrosis, and chronic pancreatitis.[26, 27] **Proliferation of ductules with periductal neuroendocrine budding is common in adults with intrapancreatic endocrine tumors and in the multiple endocrine neoplasia syndrome type I (MEN I).** It is also important to recognize that the severity of the characteristic features of nesidioblastosis may vary considerably from case to case or from region to region within the same pancreas and that overlap with normal features in any given section may occur. In addition to normal-appearing islets, there is a diffuse intermingling of endocrine cell clusters within the exocrine acini, producing small clusters of endocrine cells at various points throughout the exocrine parenchyma. In contrast, the islets of the normal mature pancreas are largely localized to the center of the pancreatic lobules and show a uniform size range. As discussed previously, large islets and proliferation of single endocrine cells from duct epithelium may be observed in the normal newborn up to 8 months of age. Careful comparisons between age-matched normal and diseased pancreases have revealed no significant differences in the volume density of endocrine tissue in the vast majority of cases. However, a relative decrease of D cells (somatostatin-secreting)[28] or of A cells (glucagon-secreting)[29] has been reported in a small number of individual cases, suggesting that nesidioblastosis may actually be part of a broader syndrome of islet cell dysmaturation.[30]

Given the problems in histologic diagnosis of nesidioblastosis, it is usually comparatively easy to recognize either islet cell adenoma or adenomatosis as a cause of persistent hyperinsulinemic hypoglycemia.[24, 31] The lesion known as **focal or multifocal adenomatosis** is characterized by huge clusters of endocrine cells that surround small ducts. Endocrine cell hypertrophy is often obvious in the lesions of this syndrome, although islets outside of the hyperplastic foci are normal in size, shape, and cell composition in many cases. The findings overlap with diffuse nesidioblastosis in that ductulo-insular complexes are also conspicuous in this disease, and abnormal distribution of endocrine cells in areas remote from the adenomatous foci may also be present. In the infant, focal nesidioblastosis or adenomatosis occurs most commonly in the absence of endocrine abnormalities in other organs. In the adult, however, adenomatosis is seen most commonly in association with MEN I.[32] **The endocrine pancreas is affected in approximately 50% to 85% of patients with MEN I, and the most common pattern of involvement is localized or widespread ductulo-insular lesions, hyperplastic islets, and one or more endocrine tumors that may or may not be seen macroscopically.** The entire pancreas may be studded with microadenomas or show a combination of microadenomatosis with larger discrete, grossly visible pancreatic endocrine tumors. In these patients, it may be difficult to successfully treat the pancreatic disease by any means other than total pancreatectomy. Hyperplasia and/or tumors of the endocrine pancreas may also occur in rare syndromes displaying features of both MEN I and MEN II. Thus, it is important to investigate the adult patient with pancreatic adenomatosis for MEN I (tumors in the adrenal cortex, the pituitary, and the thyroid, and in overlap cases, pheochromocytoma).

True, well-demarcated single pancreatic endocrine tumors in the infant and neonate are relatively rare.[31, 33] Even when found, such proliferations often show a lobulated, irregular structure distinct from the usual smooth-bordered round contour of the pancreatic endocrine tumor in the adult and may represent a variation of focal adenomatosis. In these cases, immunohistochemistry may be helpful in differentiating adenomatosis from true neoplasia, because pancreatic endocrine tumors are most often unihormonal, with multihormonal tumors being less common. Even in multihormonal pancreatic endocrine tumors, however, the spatial distribution and relative proportions of the various hormone-specific cell types within the nodules differ from those of the normal islet. By contrast, in adenomatosis, the distribution and proportions of endocrine cells within the hyperplastic nodules often mimic those of normal islets of Langerhans.[24] This distinction may be important for several reasons. On the one hand, nesidioblastosis and adenomatosis are believed to be benign lesions with no premalignant disposition. Pancreatic endocrine tumors, on the other hand, must always be regarded with suspicion because, with the possible exception of a small number of highly malignant clearly invasive tumors, it is usually impossible to tell whether they are benign or malignant based on histologic criteria alone. The only reliable criteria for malignancy are massive infiltration of adjacent organs and metastasis to regional lymph nodes or the liver.

Tumors with Uncertain Malignant Potential

Serous Cystadenoma

The serous cystadenoma (Fig. 8–6) was long believed to be the only truly benign cystic tumor of the pancreas with no premalignant potential.[34–39] However, in light of reports of the rare occurrence of metastases resulting from these innocuous-looking lesions,[40, 41] it is probably prudent to regard serous cystadenomas as being of uncertain malignant potential. The epithelial cells lining the cystic spaces of these tumors are monotonous in appearance with a flattened to cuboidal shape, glycogen-rich, clear cytoplasm, and small regular nuclei. Pleomorphism and mitotic activity are characteristically lacking. Most commonly these tumors are large in size (mean, 11 cm in greatest dimension), encapsulated, and composed of innumerable tiny cysts that create a sponge-like appearance on cross section. For this reason, they are most commonly known as **microcystic adenomas.** However, this term is somewhat misleading because some tumors may contain large cystic spaces measuring up to 8 cm in diameter that are lined with the same monomorphous glycogen-rich serous cells.[42] Thus, the term serous cystadenoma or **glycogen-rich adenoma,** which refers only to the benign serous epithelial lining and not to the size of the cystic spaces, serves as a more universal moniker for this class of tumors. Although they are almost always completely benign, it is important to keep in mind that in rare cases this lesion has been reported to metastasize to the stomach and liver and to invade the splenic vein, clear-cut evidence of aggressive biologic behavior without evidence of significant cytologic atypicality. In such cases, by defini-

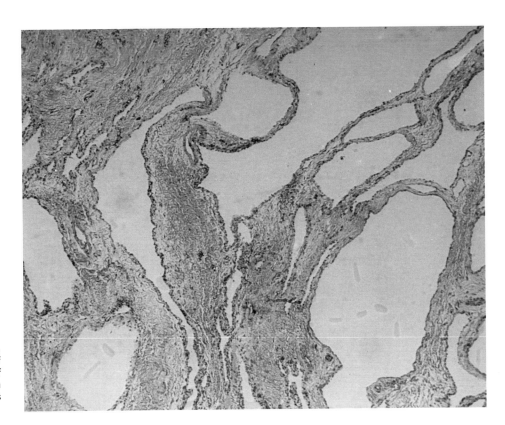

FIGURE 8–6. Serous cystadenoma. The common microcystic variety of serous cystadenoma is made up of multiple small, relative uniform cysts lined by monomorphous cuboidal serous cells. (H&E, ×33)

tion, the entity must be termed a **serous cystadenocarcinoma.**[40]

It is also important to recognize that serous cystadenoma (microcystic adenoma) may coexist with pancreatic ductal adenocarcinoma. By statistical analysis, such coincidence has been estimated to represent more than just a chance association between the two lesions, but it has been thought unlikely that the adenomas were precursors of the carcinomas in such cases.[43] The occasional association with ductal carcinoma and the rare occurrence of aggressive biologic behavior underlie the potential pitfalls in the treatment of serous cystadenomas. The presence of a large benign tumor may overshadow the presence of a coincident adenocarcinoma and lead to undertreatment. Conversely, it may be argued that because postoperative mortality can be significant in the elderly or in other patients who are poor operative risks, serous cystadenomas should be treated conservatively whenever possible. When the tumors occur in the pancreatic body or the tail, they are less likely to cause obstructive problems that require surgical intervention. Because biopsy may be undertaken to identify them,[34] it should be kept in mind that serous cells may be a variable component of mucinous cystic neoplasms, tumors with significantly more malignant potential than serous cystadenomas. Therefore, on finding more than a rare scattered mucin-containing cell in a biopsy specimen of a cystic tumor, the diagnosis of serous cystadenoma cannot be made with confidence.

Two lesions that closely mimic the histologic appearance of microcystic adenomas are the congenital cysts of the von Hippel-Lindau syndrome and lymphangiomas of the pancreas. Recognition of the former is simplified by knowledge of coexistent central nervous system hamartomas that characteristically dominate the clinical presentation. Diagnosis of the latter may depend on immunohistochemical demonstration of the endothelial nature of the lesion with expression of factor VIII or *Ulex europus* antigen. Differentiation from lymphangioma may be especially difficult in the rare case of microcystic adenoma, which manifests glycogen-poor epithelium[44] and is not periodic acid-Schiff (PAS) positive.

Mucinous Cystic Neoplasms

In the past, mucinous cystic neoplasms have been grouped together with serous cystadenomas (microcystic adenomas, glycogen-rich adenomas)[45–50] but have now been recognized to constitute an entity that is histologically, clinically, and prognostically distinct from serous lesions.[10, 47–56] Mucinous cystic neoplasms may be uni- or multilocular and are lined by an admixture of serous and mucin-producing cells in varying proportion. Most commonly, the vast majority of cells show mucin production, either in fine apical vacuoles or, less commonly, within a single large cytoplasmic vacuole that indents the nucleus (goblet-type cells). A wide variation in cell shape may be seen, ranging from flattened or low cuboidal to tall columnar epithelium, and although the cells usually form a simple (single-cell) epithelial layer over the fibrous stroma separating loculi, papillary tufting of epithelium is a variable feature and may be marked in some tumors (Fig. 8–7). Other variable features include the presence of neuroendocrine cells (argentaffin cells) or Paneth's cells within the neoplastic epithelium, a highly cellular so-called ''ovarian'' stroma (predominantly found in female patients), and cellular pleo-

morphism. None of these features as single variables has prognostic significance.

Mucinous cystic neoplasms with severely atypical epithelium but no further evidence of malignancy have been called ''borderline'' lesions (**borderline mucinous cystadenomas**)[56] and are generally regarded as low-grade malignancies. We have found that the feature having the most significant association with aggressive biologic behavior in borderline lesions is the presence of mitotic activity. Such tumors may contain foci of overt carcinoma *in situ* (not uncommonly papillary carcinoma *in situ*) or microinvasive carcinoma when sampled thoroughly. Tumors containing overt evidence of malignancy with cribriform cell growth, extreme pleomorphism, brisk mitotic activity, stromal infiltration, and/or metastasis to peripancreatic lymph nodes may be categorized outright as **mucinous cystadenocarcinomas.** Some cystadenocarcinomas are composed predominantly of overtly malignant epithelium with little evidence of origin from a mucinous cystic neoplasm remaining. Once malignant transformation has taken place, the prognosis for these tumors is guarded but overall appears to be better than that of ductal adenocarcinoma.[53] Unfortunately, however, prospective studies of stage-matched tumors are lacking.

Predicting the behavior of mucinous cystic neoplasms, especially those with atypia, is the major clinical problem associated with these lesions. In a review of our experience with mucinous cystic neoplasms at the Massachusetts General Hospital from 1979 to 1994, we have found that the feature most closely associated with focal malignancy within the neoplasm and/or aggressive biologic behavior with death from disease within the next 7 years is the presence of mitotic activity.[57] Based on this experience, we recommend that the finding of even a single mitotic figure should prompt an aggressive search for focal malignancy within the lesion. We have also found the presence of mitoses to be a reliable indicator of malignancy on intraoperative frozen section. Our more recent studies as well as those of other investigators have shown that analyses of cyst fluids from these tumors may be very helpful in discriminating between benign and malignant lesions.[58–63] Values for CA 125 in cyst fluid are typically high in all malignant cysts (greater than 200 U/ml). In mucinous cystic neoplasms, cyst fluid CA 125 levels are variable but are usually (though not always) less than 200 U/ml. Although other authors have suggested that cyst fluid levels of carcinoembryonic antigen (CEA) are significantly higher in malignant compared with benign tumors,[60, 61] we have found that cyst fluid CEA levels are high (>350 ng/ml) in both benign and malignant mucinous cysts and do not distinguish between the two.[58]

We have also found that cyst fluid levels of CA 15-3 are helpful, but not definitive, in differentiating benign from malignant mucinous cystic tumors.[59] Although concentrations of more than 100 ng/ml (mean, 178 ng/ml; range, 40–392 ng/ml) are typical for cystadenocarcinomas, some overlap exists in the lower concentration ranges with pseudocysts (mean, 15 ng/ml; range, 0–66 ng/ml). Levels of CA 15-3 in benign tumors are consistently less than 35 ng/ml. A more specific marker for discriminating between malignant and non-malignant mucinous cystic neoplasms is CA 72-4 (TAG 72).[62] Levels of this marker are typically markedly elevated in cyst fluid from malignant tumors (>750 U/ml; mean, 10,000 U/ml), whereas levels in fluid from benign

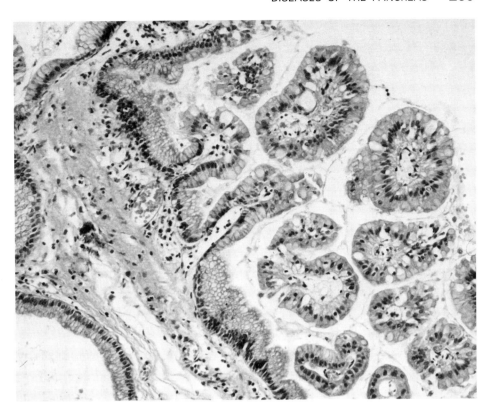

FIGURE 8–7. Mucinous cystic neoplasm. The epithelium is made up of an admixture of nonmucinous and mucin-producing cells, some of which show goblet cell–type differentiation. In some loculi, the epithelial lining is flat (*left*), and in others, papillary projections are prominent (*right*). (H&E, ×100)

tumors are always low (<150 U/ml; mean, 45 U/ml). Unfortunately, a possible pitfall in the use of cyst fluid analysis alone to establish a diagnosis of malignancy or benignity is the innate variability in fluid composition among loculi of a multiloculated tumor.[63] Thus, a combination of cyst fluid analysis and microscopic examination may prove to be the most accurate diagnostic approach to mucinous cystic neoplasms.

Perhaps the most common misdiagnosis associated with mucinous cystic neoplasms is that of **pseudocyst**[64, 65] This is a significant problem for both surgeon and pathologist. From the histopathologic standpoint, the occurrence of extensive epithelial denudation of mucinous cystic neoplasms can closely mimic a pseudocyst. We have experienced a case in which an epithelial lining remnant was discovered in only one of 20 microsopic sections submitted from a single tumor. Misdiagnosis of cystic neoplasms as pseudocysts usually leads to improper surgical treatment, with either consequent recurrence of benign tumor or the more serious consequence of recurrence with malignant transformation. Misdiagnosis occurs both because there are no reliable clinical or radiologic criteria to permit preoperative differentiation of pseudocysts and mucinous cystic neoplasms and because extensive epithelial denudation occurs commonly in mucinous cystic neoplasms and can be a pitfall in pathologic diagnosis either at frozen section or even with ample sampling on permanent section. In this setting, cyst fluid analysis may prove extremely helpful in establishing the identity of the cyst. Cyst fluid amylase and lipase content are generally high in pseudocysts and low in cystic tumors, either benign or malignant.[58] Cyst fluid viscosity is high (greater than serum viscosity) in about 90% of mucinous tumors, but is low (less than serum) in pseudocysts.[58] Epithelial antigen markers such as CEA and CA 125 are low in pseudocysts and are variable to high in mucinous cystic neoplasms. In pseudocysts, CEA values generally do not exceed 25 ng/ml, and CA 125 levels are no greater than 50 U/ml. In contrast, the cyst fluid from mucinous cystic neoplasms, whether benign or malignant, contain more than 300 to 350 ng/ml CEA. Levels of CA 125 in the cyst fluid of mucinous cystic neoplasms may be as low as pseudocyst values, but when greater than 100 U/ml they strongly indicate neoplasia.[58]

Intraductal Papillary and Hyperplastic Lesions of the Pancreas (Including Atypical Papillary Hyperplasia, Papillary Carcinoma, and Mucinous Ductal Ectasia)

Clinicopathologic studies of epithelial proliferative lesions in the pancreatic ductal system have defined a spectrum of lesions of increasing atypicality that are believed to be part of a spectrum of progression to carcinoma *in situ* and, ultimately, invasive carcinoma. The basic histopathologic changes common to all these lesions are epithelial cell enlargement with increased nuclear-to-cytoplasmic ratio, nuclear crowding, nuclear pleomorphism, papillary epithelial tufting, and mucin production. The overlapping nomenclature for these lesions has created confusion in the literature, as to not only their recognition but their clinical importance as well.

Ductal epithelial hyperplasia without cytologic atypia may be found with or without papillary tufting in both normal pancreases and those with obstructive pancreatitis.[66, 67] It is a common lesion characterized cytologically by the presence of tall columnar epithelial cells filled with mucin in their apical region (Fig. 8–8). With papillation formation, delicate infoldings of the duct lamina propria are seen as slender fibrovascular stalks. Typically, nuclei are small, uniform, and

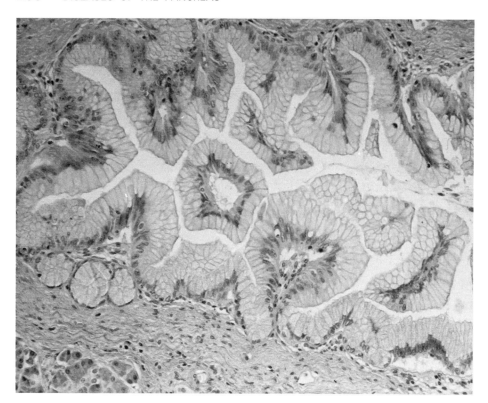

FIGURE 8–8. Typical papillary hyperplasia in chronic pancreatitis. The ductal epithelial cells have undergone mucinous metaplasia and formed papillary infoldings within the ductal lumen. The cells are monomorphic, lacking in atypia or hyperchromasia, and the papillations contain fibrovascular cores. (H&E, ×150)

basally located. It is generally agreed that this change does not signify neoplastic growth.[66] In contrast, intraductal epithelial hyperplasias that show cytologic atypia are found neither in the normal pancreas nor in pancreatitis and are believed to be true precursors of malignancy.[68–71]

Atypical papillary hyperplasias may show varying amounts of mucin production, pleomorphism, and loss of the fibrovascular cores within the epithelial papillations (Fig. 8–9). Discrete, highly arborized, exophytic growths with atypical epithelial cells covering fibrovascular cores are often indistinguishable from adenomas and have been termed papillomas. On biopsy, the distinction between atypical (adenomatous) hyperplasia and a **true adenoma** is moot because they are histopathologically indistinguishable and both are premalignant. If nuclear fragmentation (necrosis), marked pleomorphism, and/or atypical mitotic figures are present, a diagnosis of papillary carcinoma would be warranted. **Papillary adenocarcinoma** diffusely involving a significant proportion of the ductal system has been reported in some cases.[72] Infiltrating carcinoma may also be present in about one third to one half of these cases.[73, 74] Because atypical ductal hyperplasias may be multifocal and are most commonly seen in a background of either non-papillary or papillary hyperplasia without atypia (Fig. 8–10), it is possible that these lesions are part of a pathologic spectrum, i.e., a field effect involving the ductal system regionally or diffusely. Indeed, it is common in cases of atypical hyperplasia to be able to identify cytologic changes ranging from typical hyperplasia to atypical hyperplasia to carcinoma *in situ*.[75, 76]

Clinically, atypical papillary hyperplasia is often highly distinctive because of the extreme dilatation of the involved parts of the ductal system and the copious amounts of mucin produced by the neoplastic cells. Lesions with marked mucin production have been termed **intraductal hypersecreting**

neoplasms of the pancreas. The terms **mucinous ductal ectasia** and **intraductal cystadenoma** have also been coined to reflect the dramatic clinical manifestations of these lesions, which are readily apparent on endoscopic retrograde cholangiopancreatography (ERCP), sonography, and computed tomography (CT) scan.[74, 77–79] Thick tenacious mucus extruding from the patulous orifice of the involved duct or from the papilla of Vater is a typical finding on ERCP. Unlike mucinous cystic neoplasms, mucinous ductal ectasias typically communicate with the main ductal system and can be filled with contrast material by retrograde injection. Because mucinous ductal estasia is more frequent in the head of the pancreas than in the tail, it often presents with symptoms of chronic relapsing pancreatitis. Overall, it appears that atypical epithelial hyperplastic lesions of the pancreatic ducts tend to grow intraluminally for long periods and are either slow to undergo malignant transformation or are slow to invade the duct wall once transformation has occurred. Thus, they have a favorable prognosis.[80, 81] Even with atypia encompassing **carcinoma *in situ***, total pancreatectomy is curative.[74, 79] With the presence of invasive malignancy or lymph node metastases, however, the prognosis is apparently poor, and death from disease within a year of resection in such cases has been reported.[82] Because atypical epithelial hyperplasias may either be multifocal within the ductal system or involve a large segment of the ductal system in a confluent manner, critical evaluation of the ductal tree, especially the ducts at the pancreatic resection margin, is necessary in resection specimens. With the finding of extensive atypicality, carcinoma *in situ*, or even diffuse intraductal papillary adenocarcinoma extending to the margin, resection of the residual pancreatic tissue may be indicated. We have noted that extraductal acellular mucin pools are present in most cases of mucinous ductal estasia and do not necessarily indicate malignancy with invasion. However, in

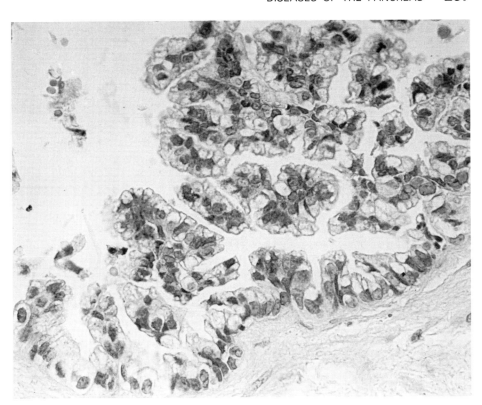

FIGURE 8–9. Atypical papillary hyperplasia. The nuclear-to-cytoplasmic ratio is high, and papillations lack fibrovascular cores. However, nuclear pleomorphism is only mild in degree. (H&E, ×200)

the presence of carcinoma *in situ* within adjacent ducts, atypical cells within the mucin pools and/or microinvasive carcinoma in the stroma should be sought (this may require tissue levels). Cytologically the key to the diagnosis of atypical hyperplastic lesions, whether focal or part of a more diffuse adenomatous dysplasia, is the recognition of the characteristic

cytologic changes (nuclei of varying sizes, hyperchromatism, and pseudostratification). The presence of mitotic figures and/or multinucleation would exceed criteria for adenomatous dysplasia and favor a diagnosis of carcinoma *in situ*. As in adenomas elsewhere in the gastrointestinal tract, complex architecture and epithelial growth associated with its own

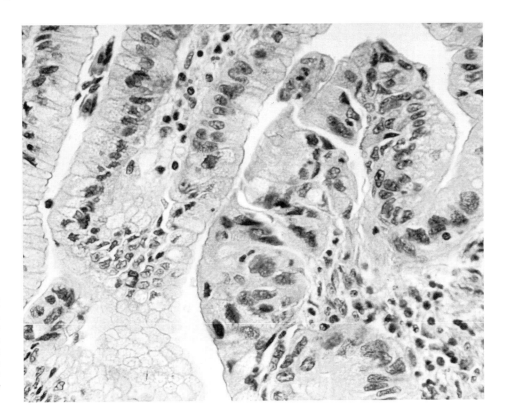

FIGURE 8–10. Concomitant typical and atypical papillary hyperplasia. Adjacent epithelial papillations within the same duct demonstrate a spectrum of cytologic appearances from hyperplasia without atypicality (*far left*), to minimal atypicality (*center*), to severe atypicality (*far right*). (H&E, ×250)

proliferative but benign stroma differentiate a true adenoma from an epithelial hyperplasia in which the ductal epithelial cells use the backbone of the normal ductal structure on which to proliferate.

Solid and Cystic (Papillary Cystic) Tumors

As the name implies, solid and cystic tumors of the pancreas are composed predominantly of cells with a solid growth pattern (Fig. 8–11).[83–95] The papillary or cystic feature by which they can also be recognized is thought to be a secondary phenomenon related to tumor cell degeneration and the formation of cystic spaces filled with myxoid mucopolysaccharide (Fig. 8–12), pseudopapillations of tumor cells grouped around vascular structures, and glandular structures consisting of tumor cells surrounding central collections of myxoid mucopolysaccharide (Fig. 8–13). Because of both their solid growth pattern and their predominant occurrence in pediatric and young adult patients, they may be mistaken for either pancreatic endocrine tumors or pancreatoblastomas. In the adult, acinar cell carcinomas, which may display solid as well as acinar, trabecular, or glandular growth patterns, must be included in a differential diagnosis.

Solid and cystic tumors have been called **infantile-type carcinoma of the pancreas, adenocarcinoma of the pancreas of childhood, papillary epithelial neoplasm, solid and papillary epithelial neoplasm,** and **solid and cystic acinar cell tumor.** They are rare tumors that usually occur in young women (mean age about 25 years) and are typically of large size (mean, 7.5 cm in diameter) when discovered.[88] They are usually well defined, with a capsule of variable thickness that may partially or wholly encompass the tumor, but tumors lacking capsules (so-called infiltrating variety of solid and cystic neoplasm) that invade the pancreatic parenchyma at their periphery have been described.[94] On gross examination, these tumors typically show degenerative changes, including areas of hemorrhage, necrosis, or dystrophic calcification that can sometimes be seen radiologically. They may occur in any region of the pancreas and most frequently present as an otherwise asymptomatic abdominal mass or with vague abdominal pain. This tumor must be suspected in any adolescent girl or young woman with a cystic or partially cystic pancreatic mass, and preoperative or intraoperative diagnosis by fine needle aspiration and cytologic analysis may be helpful.

Cytologically, solid and cystic neoplasms are composed of a monomorphous population of large regular cells with delicately creased or folded nuclei. Some tumor cells contain small hyaline globules that are PAS positive,[84] but there is no evidence of intracellular mucin production, a feature that may help differentiate this tumor from adenocarcinoma. Mitotic activity is rare, and nuclear pleomorphism or atypism is uncommon. Perhaps the most characteristic feature of this lesion and one that can readily help differentiate this tumor from either pancreatic neuroendocrine tumors or acinar cell carcinomas is the formation of pseudopapillary or pseudoglandular formations within a background of solid tumor growth. In solid areas, the tumor is highly vascular, and the regularity of the cells with their centrally placed nuclei and abundant clear to pink cytoplasm may mimic either pancreatic neuroendocrine tumor or acinar cell carcinoma. However, with the stromal myxoid degeneration that is characteristic of this lesion, cystic spaces appear between tumor cells that contain PAS-positive diastase-resistant amorphous material that also stains weakly for alcian blue and mucicarmine. Macrophages and scattered cholesterol granulomas are common in areas of tumor necrosis with hemorrhage. Dystrophic calcifications may be present. Pseudopapillary formations result from viable tumor cells adherent to stromal vessels within a background of necrosis and cystic space formation.

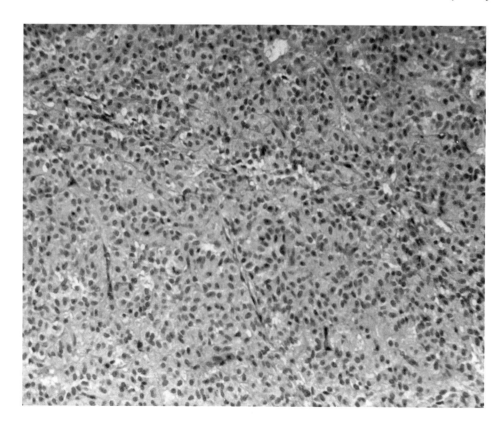

FIGURE 8–11. Solid and cystic tumor. Typically monomorphous tumor cells lacking mitotic activity are seen growing in solid sheets. (H&E, ×100)

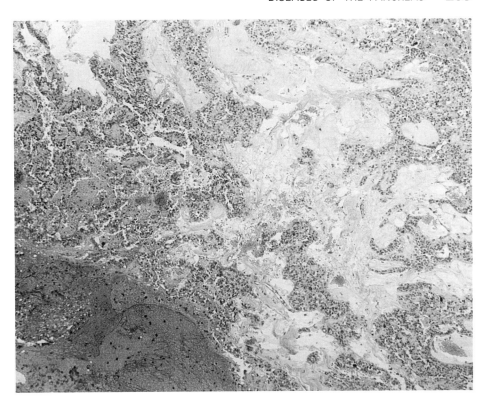

FIGURE 8–12. Solid and cystic tumor. Pseudopapillary projections of viable tumor are seen within cystic spaces filled with myxoid mucopolysaccharide. (H&E, ×33)

It should be pointed out that solid and cystic neoplasms may have a variable immunohistochemical profile suggesting both endocrine and exocrine differentiation within the same tumor. They have been reported to be immunoreactive for alpha-1-antitrypsin, alpha-1-antichymotrypsin, phospholipase A₂, and neuroendocrine markers such as neuron-specific enolase and synaptophysin.[95] Like pancreatic acinar tumors, they

may be positive for amylase[94] but apparently do not make lipase or trypsinogen.[96] In contrast to pancreatic endocrine tumors, solid and cystic neoplasms are usually negative for chromogranin.[95]

Solid and cystic neoplasms are indolent tumors with a good to excellent prognosis and are usually cured by surgical resection. Nevertheless, in a small number of cases, local

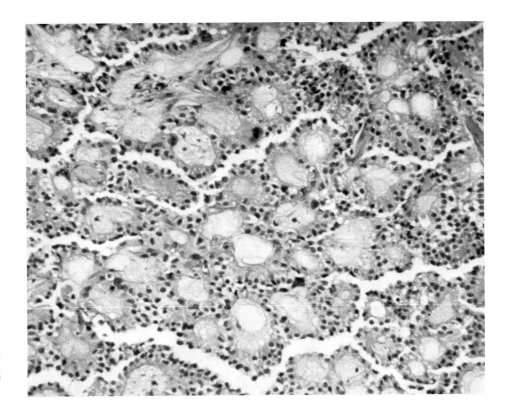

FIGURE 8–13. Solid and cystic tumor. Pseudoglandular structures are formed by accumulations of myxoid mucopolysaccharide around vessels in the centers of tumor papillations. (H&E, ×100)

recurrence or remote metastasis occurs and death from disease ensues.[90] At present, there are no reliable criteria for differentiating benign from malignant solid and cystic tumors. Selective criteria that have been suggested to be indicative of malignant potential include venous invasion, high nuclear grade, necrobiotic nests, and mitotic activity.[97] More recently, nuclear morphometric analyses have suggested that the mean nuclear area and nuclear/non-nuclear ratio of metastasizing papillary cystic tumors are both significantly greater than in nonmetastasizing tumors. However, image analysis has revealed no statistical differences in the nuclear regularity between benign and malignant tumors.[97]

An **oncocytic variant of a solid and cystic tumor has been reported.**[98] Although both the gross and conventional light microscopic appearance of this tumor were consistent with a papillary cystic tumor, densely packed blue granules were found in the cytoplasm of tumor cells stained by phosphotungstic acid–hematoxylin (PTAH) stain, and ultrastructural study revealed the tumor cells to be packed with mitochondria. As the authors discuss, oncocytic change may be seen in other types of pancreatic tumors, including pancreatic endocrine tumors, but tumors composed of greater than 90% oncocytes have been defined as oncocytic carcinomas.[99] Only three cases of **oncocytic carcinoma of the pancreas** have been previously reported, and like papillary cystic tumors, they are large encapsulated tumors composed of uniform cells without evidence of neuroendocrine granule formation[99] or chromogranin immunoreactivity.[100] The reported oncocytic carcinomas of the pancreas further resemble solid and cystic neoplasms in their relatively favorable prognosis as a tumor of low-grade or indefinite malignant potential. Although Lee et al.[98] have suggested that perhaps all oncocytic carcinomas of the pancreas are variants of solid and cystic neoplasms, this remains to be proved. Differences between the two tumors include the occurrence of oncocytic carcinomas exclusively in middle aged to elderly patients (without female predominance) and the lack of immunoreactivity of oncocytic carcinomas for either neuron-specific enolase or alpha-1-antitrypsin so commonly found in solid and cystic tumors. Indeed, in cases in which it has been studied, oncocytic carcinomas have not been shown to react immunohistochemically for any pancreatic endocrine or exocrine cell antigens. Perhaps the most important issue related to oncocytic transformation of solid and cystic neoplasms or even to the diagnosis of oncocytic carcinoma itself is differentiation of both of these tumors from acinar cell carcinoma, which has a poor prognosis in general (see later discussion). In all these tumors, the cells have abundant granular cytoplasm. Thus, in order to make a diagnosis of oncocytic tumor (oncocytic carcinoma or oncocytic variant of solid and cystic tumor), it is important to confirm that the cytoplasmic granules are neither zymogen nor neuroendocrine in type and that they stain positively for PTAH.

Pancreatic Endocrine Tumors (Islet Cell Tumors)

Pancreatic endocrine tumors (PETs) are most often solitary, well-demarcated (often encapsulated) lesions. They may arise in any part of the pancreas and vary in diameter from less than a centimeter to more than 15 cm.[101] Most PETs are secretory and produce hormone-related syndromes that may lead to their clinical recognition before their histopathologic

identification.[102] Both the clinical and histopathologic diagnoses of these tumors are greatly facilitated by immunoreactive assays for their polypeptide product or products.[103–105] A functional classification of PET is usually based on the leading clinical symptom and/or the hormone with the most elevated serum level, and the clinical diagnosis is often known at the time of surgical resection. Arguably, then, the role of the pathologist in identifying and classifying PET is most critical in cases of non-functional, clinically silent tumors.

Histologically, most PETs have a characteristically monomorphic histology with little pleomorphism of cells. Most commonly, they grow in (1) a trabecular, ribbon-like, or gyriform pattern resembling the architecture of the pancreatic islets, (2) a glandular pattern in which the cells arrange themselves in a rosette-like array around blood vessels, (3) small discrete nests (Fig. 8–14), or (4) solid sheets. The growth pattern itself has no prognostic significance and correlates with neither biologic behavior nor hormone output. It is also important to recognize that PETs may show variations in growth pattern that resemble either spindle cell sarcomas or non-endocrine carcinomas. Thus, immunohistochemical staining may be essential not only for identification of their polypeptide tumor product or products but, on a more fundamental level, to definitively identify these tumors as endocrine in type. Non-secretory PETs may only be recognizable by immunostaining for neuroendocrine differentiation antigens such as chromogranin or synaptophysin. Despite its name, neuron-specific enolase (although usually positive in PETs) is the least specific of the markers for neuroendocrine differentiation.

PETs with a predominantly solid growth pattern create the most difficult differential diagnostic problems for the pathologist in that they can be easily confused with other tumors that characteristically show solid growth, including solid and cystic neoplasms, acinar cell carcinomas, oncocytomas, and pancreatoblastomas. From a clinical point of view, this differential diagnosis can usually be narrowed down on the basis of the patient's age and clinical presentation. Acinar cell carcinomas apparently occur exclusively in adults, and pancreatoblastomas occur almost exclusively in children and infants. However, because solid and cystic neoplasms may occur in children as well as adults of any age, distinguishing PETs from these tumors may represent the most common dilemma for pathologists. On frozen section, for example, cell size and shape are usually not helpful in differentiating PETs from solid and cystic neoplasms. Likewise, growth pattern is often unhelpful because both PETs and solid and cystic tumors may show pseudorosette formation or a trabecular, ribbon-like growth. One important distinguishing feature is the presence of mucoid degenerative change; it is characteristic of solid and cystic neoplasms but lacking in PETs. However, this must be distinguished from cystic degeneration occurring as a result of tumor necrosis. Cystification may occur in either PETs or solid and cystic neoplasms and can cause clinical confusion with cystic tumors.[106]

Another feature that, if present, can be helpful in differentiating PETs from other look-alike tumors is the presence of **psammoma bodies** (Fig. 8–15).[107] These have been reported to occur in as many as one third of insulinomas of the pancreas, the most common PET, and are characteristic of duodenal somatostatinomas (those in the periampullary region may arise from pancreatic tissue and be included in the broad category

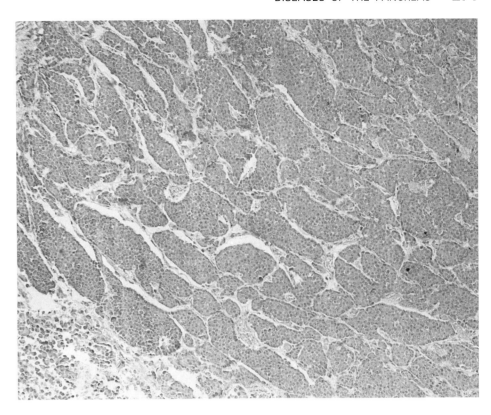

FIGURE 8–14. Pancreatic endocrine tumor. Tumor growth in both discrete nests and trabeculae with sharply defined borders is seen. (H&E, ×33)

of PETs). Although rare in other PETs, psammoma bodies do not occur in other look-alike tumors. Also helpful in the differential diagnosis is the finding of fine hyaline droplets in the cytoplasm of tumor cells, a common feature of solid and cystic neoplasms. Cells with a coarsely granular cyto-

plasm would suggest either acinar cell carcinoma or an oncocytoma rather than a PET or solid and cystic tumor. Accurate diagnosis of PETs is of special importance, not only because their therapy may differ significantly from that of other tumors with which they can be confused but also because their prog-

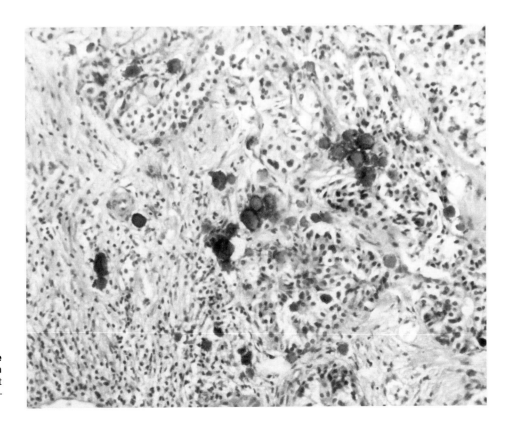

FIGURE 8–15. Pancreatic endocrine tumor. (Insulinoma) Psammoma bodies are scattered throughout tumor nests and stroma of this insulinoma. (H&E, ×100)

nosis may be significantly different. With the exception of pancreatic polypeptide-secreting PET (PP-omas), which are almost always benign, and insulinomas, which are predominately benign, PETs are more likely to behave in a malignant fashion than are solid and cystic neoplasms. Acinar cell carcinomas (see later discussion) are aggressively malignant lesions and do not have benign counterparts like PETs.

The problem of differentiating benign from malignant PETs remains the most problematic aspect of pathologic evaluation of these tumors. **It is generally accepted that there are no reliable histopathologic criteria that allow distinction of benign from malignant PETs.** This includes the presence of mitotic figures, pleomorphism, vascular invasion, and infiltration of peripancreatic structures. Only metastatic disease in local lymph nodes or distant sites confirms a PET as malignant. Although it had been previously reported that human chorionic gonadotrophin (hCG) or its alpha subunit was expressed far more often in malignant than in benign PETs and might serve as a marker for malignancy in functioning PETs,[108] this has not been confirmed as a reliable marker for malignancy.[109] More recently, immunostaining for proliferating cell nuclear antigen (PCNA) has been suggested as a method for predicting aggressive biologic behavior in PETs. A PCNA index of greater than 5% of tumor cells has been reported to correlate with extrapancreatic extension of PETs as well as decreased survival time.[110] Quantification of the number of silver-staining nuclear organizer regions (AgNORs) per tumor cell has also been proposed as a useful predictor of malignancy in PETs. Tumors exhibiting at least 5% of cells with more than six AgNORs per nucleolus were malignant in 96% of cases in one study.[111]

Immunohistochemical staining for neuron-specific enolase does not differentiate PETs from solid and cystic neoplasms because both are typically positive. Immunohistochemical staining for alpha-1-antitrypsin and vimentin may prove more useful, because PETs are typically negative for both of these antigens, whereas solid and cystic neoplasms are usually positive. Alpha-1-antitrypsin, amylase, and lipase are negative in PETs but may be positive in both solid and cystic neoplasms and acinar cell carcinomas. Trypsin may be a more specific marker for acinar cell carcinoma of the pancreas and has been reported in 100% of cases in some studies.[112] Unfortunately, a minor endocrine component recognizable with antibodies against either chromogranin or pancreatic endocrine hormones can be identified in more than one third of acinar cell carcinomas of the pancreas. Furthermore, acinar, solid, trabecular, and glandular patterns of growth can be seen in acinar cell carcinomas, and for this reason, they may closely mimic PETs histologically as well. Because acinar cell carcinoma has also been reported to occur (rarely) in childhood, even the patient's age may not be helpful in distinguishing between acinar cell carcinoma and PET. However, correct diagnosis in such cases is of particular importance because acinar cell carcinomas are uniformly aggressive tumors with half of patients having metastatic disease at presentation and mean survival of all cases being less than 2 years.[112] In contrast, PETs are unpredictable in their biologic behavior and may prove to be either entirely benign or indolent.

In cases of non-secretory PETs, some of which may even lack significant immunostaining for general neuroendocrine differentiation antigens such as chromogranin or synaptophysin, electron microscopy may be needed to confirm the diagno-

sis. By ultrastructural examination, PETs are typically identified by the presence of dense core neurosecretory granules. However, such granules have also been identified in solid and cystic tumors, which may show evidence of neuroendocrine as well as acinar cell differentiation in different foci. The presence of large zymogen granules in tumor cells would eliminate the diagnosis of PET but would not distinguish between solid and cystic tumor and acinar cell carcinoma.

In the context of neuroendocrine tumors and their origin from ductal progenitor cells, it is not surprising that tumors showing a combination of PET-like cells and cells with either ductal[113–116] or acinar cells[117] have been reported. **Carcinomas with cells showing features of both neuroendocrine and glandular differentiation have been called amphicrine carcinomas, mucinous islet cell carcinomas, or mixed ductal-islet tumors.**[116] These tumors are characterized by neurosecretory granule formation as well as gland formation and mucin production by the same tumor cells. Formation of small compact uniform glandular structures without apparent intervening stroma is their most characteristic histopathologic feature. The gland lumina may contain mucinous secretions. The cells are variable in size and typically have scanty cytoplasm. Focal areas of giant cell formation or cribriform growth may be seen, as well as areas of solid growth in which the tumor cells typically show indistinct cell margins and extremely scanty cytoplasm. Areas of tumor necrosis are common, whereas sclerotic stromal responses are usually lacking. Neurosecretory granules can be identified by electron microscopy. Recognition of this tumor type is of great prognostic importance. **Unlike pure PETs, which sometimes behave in a benign fashion, carcinomas with mixed features are apparently always malignant.** In early reports, amphicrine tumors showing both endocrine-type cytologic detail and gland formation within a background of predominantly solid growth (no apparent intervening stroma between glands) were termed **microadenocarcinoma** (solid microglandular carcinoma).[118] It was noted that these tumors were aggressive lesions with a short survival but that they strongly resembled carcinoid tumors histologically.

Perhaps even more rare than amphicrine carcinomas are tumors showing completely separate foci of endocrine and exocrine (ductal) differentiation (Fig. 8–16). Although little is known of the biologic behavior of these lesions, it would appear from our limited experience that their prognosis resembles that of the usual pancreatic ductal carcinoma.

Malignant Epithelial Tumors: Differential Diagnostic Problems

Pancreatoblastoma (Infantile Carcinoma)

Pancreatoblastoma is a rare neoplasm that occurs only in infancy and childhood (age range, 3 weeks to 13 years).[119–123] It is a primitive tumor that may show both epithelial and mesenchymal differentiation. Most pancreatoblastomas are found to arise from the head or body of the pancreas and grossly appear encapsulated. The cut surface of the tumor may show areas of necrosis, hemorrhage, and cystification. Thus, its gross appearance is not distinctive and may resemble that of either a pancreatic endocrine tumor, a solid and cystic neoplasm, or an acinar cell carcinoma, all of which may be

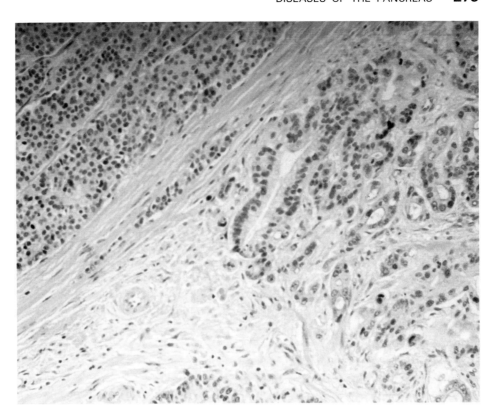

FIGURE 8–16. Combined pancreatic ductal and neuroendocrine carcinoma. This carcinoma shows separate foci of ductal differentiation (*right*) and neuroendocrine differentiation within the same tumor. (H&E, ×100)

included in the differential diagnosis of pancreatoblastoma.[85–123] Histologically, these tumors are comprised of a variable admixture of epithelial and mesenchymal elements (Fig. 8–17). The epithelial cells of pancreatoblastoma are typically polygonal and monomorphic with oval nuclei and occasional nucleoli. They usually show only mild to moderate pleomorphism and may be arranged in an organoid pattern characterized by nests of cells separated by dense fibrous stroma. However, they may manifest one or more additional growth patterns, including formation of solid sheets, acini, or

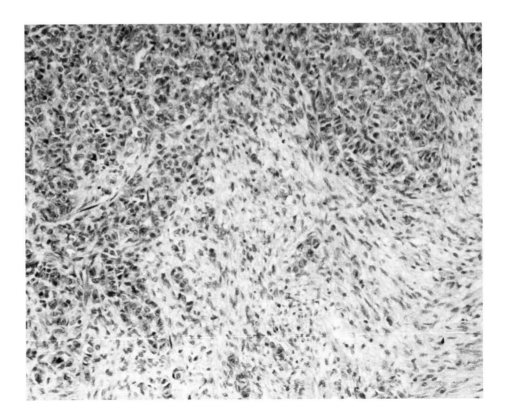

FIGURE 8–17. Pancreatoblastoma. A combination of both epithelial (*top*) and mesenchymal (*bottom*) differentiation is characteristic of pancreatoblastoma. (H&E, ×100)

tubular structures, all of which may resemble PET or acinar cell carcinoma. Mitotic figures are often frequent, a feature that may help distinguish pancreatoblastoma from solid and cystic tumors.[123] The epithelial cells may contain PAS-positive granules in their cytoplasm that resemble those seen in either solid and cystic neoplasms or acinar cell carcinomas. However, a pathognomonic feature that definitively differentiates pancreatoblastoma from any other pancreatic tumor with solid growth is the presence of squamous nests or corpuscles (Fig. 8–18). Mesenchymal differentiation is seen in the form of spindle cell areas with either chondroid or osteoid formation. With the identification of such foci, a diagnosis of pancreatoblastoma can be made more confidently, but teratoma must be excluded (see later discussion). It is important to remember that only the mixed form of pancreatoblastoma contains a mesenchymal component. When present, it is a very helpful diagnostic feature, but it must be distinguished from reactive inflammatory changes that can be seen in this or other tumors. Rare case reports of evolution of pancreatoblastoma with transformation of its histologic features to those of an adult-type well-differentiated adenocarcinoma have been reported.[124] This kind of transformation is well known in neuroblastomas and germ cell tumors and apparently can occur in pancreatoblastoma as well.

The immunohistochemical staining properties of pancreatoblastoma reflect its primitive and pluripotential nature. Positivity for acinar cell products such as lipase, trypsin, chymotrypsin, and alpha-1-antitrypsin may be seen as well as positivity for neuroendocrine markers in some cases.[96, 124, 125] Electron microscopic studies likewise show an admixture of cells with zymogen-like granules and cells with neuroendocrine differentiation (i.e., dense core granules of either glucagon or insulin type). Pancreatoblastomas may also express alpha-fetoprotein, which can be demonstrable by immunohistochemistry.[126, 127] Although expression of alpha-fetoprotein is not unique to pancreatoblastomas, its expression by other pancreatic malignancies such as ductal adenocarcinomas or PETs is rare. However, alpha-fetoprotein expression is not uncommon in acinar cell carcinomas (see later discussion) and may even occur relatively more frequently in these tumors than in pancreatoblastomas.

The prognosis for pancreatoblastoma is difficult to predict. Apparently, pancreatoblastomas are slow to metastasize, and metastatic disease is rarely found at surgical resection despite the typically large size of these tumors at discovery (7–11 cm). Although reported cases are few in number, it appears overall that the prognosis in most patients is poor, but long-term survivors after complete surgical excision have been reported.[123]

Cystic teratomas of the pancreas, although rare, may be included in the differential diagnosis of pancreatoblastoma because both may be cystic, show areas of calcification, and occur in young individuals.[128, 129] Cystic teratomas are composed of tissues derived from any of the three germinal layers and may produce a wide variety of structures with different degrees of differentiation. Whereas solid teratomas are usually undifferentiated and malignant, cystic teratomas are almost always well differentiated and benign. Of the 10 reported cases of this lesion, all patients were younger than 25 years of age, and in four cases, preoperative plain films of the abdomen showed calcification within the cyst wall. Thus, they may be confused radiologically with a pseudocyst, a pancreatoblastoma (calcification of the osteoid within the mesenchymal component), a mucinous cystic neoplasm, or a serous cystadenoma (microcystic adenoma). On preoperative biopsy, cystic teratomas can be easily recognized by their content of hair or sebaceous material and histologic findings of epithelial, mesenchymal, or neural tissues within the cyst

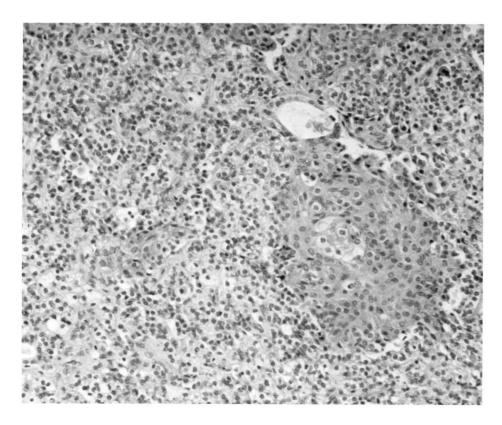

FIGURE 8–18. Pancreatoblastoma. A squamous nest, seen within an epithelial area of a pancreatoblastoma, helps differentiate this tumor from other pancreatic tumors with solid growth patterns. (H&E, ×100)

wall. Mucinous cystic neoplasms or serous cystadenomas, as discussed earlier, would show a pattern of simple ductal epithelium. Pancreatoblastoma would appear as sheets of undifferentiated epithelial cells with a high mitotic rate (see earlier) that may show focal squamous morula formation or be admixed with primitive spindled mesenchymal elements.

Acinar Cell Carcinoma

Acinar cell carcinoma is a rare but distinctive type of pancreatic cancer with a high degree of differentiation (Fig. 8–19) but a characteristically aggressive biologic behavior and poor prognosis (survival is generally less than 1 year). [112, 130–134] Although the majority of affected patients are adults with a mean age of 62 years, acinar cell carcinoma may also occur in children.[112] Because of their predominantly solid growth pattern and uniform cells with abundant cytoplasm, these tumors may resemble pancreatoblastomas, PETs, or solid and cystic neoplasms. Helpful in recognizing acinar cell carcinomas are the aggregation of tumor cells into acinar structures and cords with peripherally oriented nuclei (basal palisading) (Fig. 8–20).[112] However, nuclear palisading can also be seen in PETs. The nuclei of acinar cell carcinomas typically have an open vacuolated appearance with distinct nucleoli, in contrast to the finely stippled nuclei lacking nucleoli characteristic of PETs. Occasionally acinar cell carcinomas show foci of true gland formation with central mucin secretion and thereby resemble ductal adenocarcinoma carcinoma.

A key diagnostic feature in acinar cell carcinoma is the abundant stippled cytoplasm of the cells (see Fig. 8–19), the granules of which are PAS positive and diastase resistant.[112] The size of the granules is uniform and minute, contrasting with the PAS-positive droplets seen in solid and cystic neoplasms and occasionally in pancreatoblastoma. If the tumor

is anaplastic, many of these features may be absent or poorly expressed, and the diagnosis will require immunohistochemical and/or ultrastructural identification of the tumor cells as acinar in differentiation.

Immunohistochemical stains are typically positive for lipase, trypsin, amylase, chymotrypsin, and alpha-1-antitrypsin.[112] In about 20% of cases, elevated serum lipase levels result from tumor secretion, and subcutaneous and marrow fat necrosis, polyarthropathy, and eosinophilia may result.[112] Expression of alpha-fetoprotein may be marked enough to cause increased serum levels.[134, 135] Electron microscopic examination reveals zymogen granules in the cell cytoplasm. It must be kept in mind, however, that acinar differentiation with zymogen granule production may also be seen focally in pancreatoblastomas[119] as well as solid and cystic neoplasms.[95] The acinar cell differentiation in those tumors also results in expression of alpha-1-antitrypsin and alpha-1-chymotrypsin. However, it has been suggested that positive staining for alpha-amylase may help eliminate solid and cystic neoplasm from the differential diagnosis because it is expressed only by acinar cell carcinomas and pancreatoblastomas.[96]

Occasionally, acinar carcinoma may be incorrectly suspected if artifactual eosinophilic granularity of the cytoplasm occurs in either ductal carcinomas or other exocrine or endocrine tumors. Immunohistochemistry often resolves this dilemma. Another diagnostic pitfall is the possible confusion of either pancreatic oncocytomas (see later discussion) or PETs having oncocytic change with acinar cell carcinoma. Electron microscopy reveals the typical mitochondria-packed cytoplasm of oncocytomas, and phosphotungstic acid hematoxylin (PTAH) stains the mitochondria of oncocytes blue. Although immunohistochemical staining reveals the nature of most PETs, it is important to remember that mixed (amphicrine) tumors with a combination of both acinar and endocrine

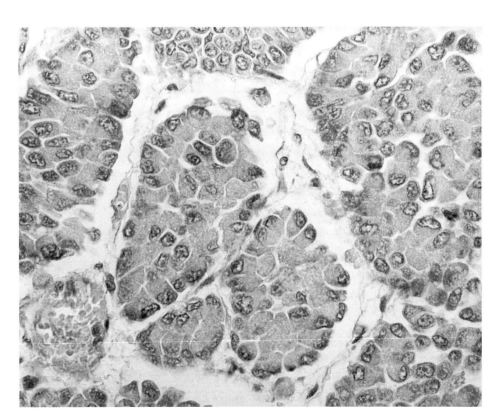

FIGURE 8–19. Acinar cell carcinoma. Tumor cells with eccentric nuclei and abundant amphophilic granular cytoplasm closely resemble normal acinar cells. (H&E, ×250)

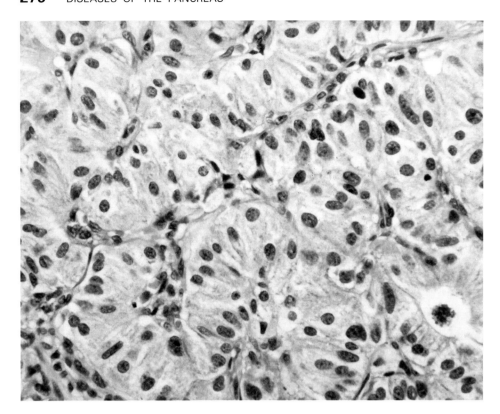

FIGURE 8–20. Acinar cell carcinoma. Growth in trabeculae or nests with peripheral nuclear palisading is typical of acinar cell carcinomas but can also be seen in pancreatic endocrine tumors. (H&E, ×250)

differentiation may be confused with acinar cell carcinomas.[117] Given the common epithelial origin of all ductal, acinar, and endocrine cells of the pancreas, it should not be surprising that tumors with bimodal pathways of differentiation are frequently encountered.

A distinctive subtype of acinar cell carcinoma deserves special mention: **acinar cell cystadenocarcinoma.**[136] This tumor comprises multi-loculated cysts lined by acinar-type cells with abundant eosinophilic granular cytoplasm. Cyst contents are watery and would be likely to contain pancreatic enzymes secreted by the surrounding cells. In the septa between cysts, the cells may form small glands or solid nests that bear a close resemblance to typical acinar cell carcinomas. This tumor is exceedingly rare but appears to have the same aggressive course and poor prognosis of ordinary acinar cell carcinomas. The differential diagnosis of acinar cell cystadenocarcinoma, however, includes other cystic epithelial neoplasms of the pancreas, including serous cystadenoma, mucinous cystic neoplasm, and mucinous cystadenocarcinoma. However, the granularity of the cytoplasm, positivity on PTAH stain, lack of mucin production, presence of zymogen granules on electron microscopy, and immunohistochemical evidence of pancreatic enzyme production should differentiate acinar cell cystadenocarcinoma from all other cystic epithelial neoplasms.

Giant Cell Tumors

Giant cell tumors (also known as **pleomorphic carcinomas, spindle and giant cell carcinomas,** or **sarcomatoid carcinomas**) are rare lesions with a strikingly bizarre histologic appearance.[137–140] The pleomorphic subtype is a highly aggressive tumor that frequently presents with metastatic disease, whereas the osteoclastic subtype has a better progno-

sis.[141–148] Giant cell tumors may occur anywhere in the pancreas and are frequently large (mean of greatest dimension, 11 cm). Their cut surface typically shows multiple areas of hemorrhage and necrosis. Cystification may occur as a secondary phenomenon.

Pleomorphic giant cell tumors are characterized by large, highly pleomorphic tumor cells that may be mononucleated or multinucleated and vary in shape from plump and perfectly round to stellate and spindled.[137–140] Both the multinucleated and mononucleated giant cells within this tumor are clearly malignant with large, bizarre hyperchromatic nuclei. The cytologic appearance of the giant cells in the pleomorphic subtype contrasts with that of the giant cells in the osteoclastic subtype in which the multinucleated giant cells have numerous regular round nuclei with prominent nucleoli and closely resemble osteoclasts.[141–148] The distinction is important because **osteoclastic giant cell tumors** of the pancreas tend to have a better prognosis than pleomorphic giant cell tumors. Otherwise, the two lesions are virtually indistinguishable and are usually regarded as variants of the same tumor. The rare occurrence of mixed tumors containing both pleomorphic and osteoclastic giant cells is supportive evidence of a common origin for both subtypes of giant cell tumor.[148]

Giant cell tumors may show foci of gland formation with mucin production within both the neoplastic glands and some giant cells. The majority of cases of pleomorphic giant cell tumor show perineural invasion, infiltration of lymphatics and veins, and infiltration of arterial walls consistent with aggressive biologic behavior. Survival beyond a few months is unusual. In contrast, osteoclastic-type giant cells are slow to metastasize, and long-term survival has been reported postresection. Osteoclastic giant cell tumors, with their distinctive osteoclast-like giant cells and osteoid formation, are usually easy to recognize and to differentiate from pleomorphic giant cell tumors that lack osteoclastic cells. However, pleomorphic giant cell tumors can be confused histologically with malignant melanoma, rhabdomyosarcoma, choriocarcinoma, sarcomas of connective tissue origin, or even bizarre lymphomas. Thus, immunohistochemical staining may be necessary for definitive identification of these lesions.

Immunohistochemical staining patterns and ultrastructural features in giant cell tumors are erratic and may show evidence of either epithelial[141-143] or mesenchymal[145, 146, 148] differentiation. Staining for low molecular weight keratins and carcinoembryonic antigen has been described in some cases,[143] whereas other reported cases have shown staining for vimentin in the absence of epithelial markers.[144] We have studied a case of mixed giant cell tumor (both osteoclastic and pleomorphic giant cells present) in which no keratin or epithelial membrane antigen expression could be detected immunohistochemically, but stains for alpha-1-antitrypsin, alpha-1-antichymotrypsin, vimentin, neuron-specific enolase, and synaptophysin (focal) all were positive.[148] The reported ultrastructural features of giant cell tumors of the pancreas indicate that this lesion may display either epithelial or mesenchymal differentiation or both in any given case. Thus, it seems reasonable to hypothesize that these tumors may arise from a precursor cell capable of differentiating along divergent lines.

Along with other investigators,[149, 150] we have encountered osteoclastic giant cell tumors arising in association with a mucinous cystic neoplasm, either benign or malignant. At present, the relationship between these two lesions is unclear, but the rare coincidence of these two tumors should be kept in mind when examining fluid aspirates or biopsies from cystic tumors, especially if multinucleate giant cells are observed.

PROBLEMS IN THE DIAGNOSIS OF PANCREATIC DUCTAL CARCINOMA

Frozen Section Diagnosis of Pancreatic Carcinoma

One of the most difficult diagnoses to make by frozen section is that of pancreatic ductal carcinoma,[151-154] and misdiagnoses may occur in as many as 30% of cases.[154] Besides the inevitable artifactual distortion of frozen tissue, several factors complicate the interpretation of pancreatic biopsy. Chronic pancreatitis is almost always present in association with ductal adenocarcinoma, and the fibrosis and glandular distortion of the ductal system in the chronically inflamed pancreas may show marked distortion and association with stromal fibrosis that closely mimic infiltrating carcinoma. Furthermore, mucinous metaplasia and epithelial ductal hyperplasia are common in chronic pancreatitis and may be misinterpreted as neoplastic features. Wedge biopsies may be easier to interpret than needle biopsies because they provide a more adequate panorama of the overall architecture, and it is easier to determine whether ductal structures represent part of the normal duct system. A haphazard proliferation of ducts of different sizes and shapes without lobular orientation (Fig. 8–21) may often be most easily recognized as malignant on low-magnification examination of the section. At higher magnification, haphazard orientation of cells, hyperchromatism, and pleomorphism are helpful in recognizing malig-

nancy, but necrosis within the glands, atypical mitotic figures, perineural infiltration, and vascular invasion remain the most reliable features on which to base a malignant diagnosis. Unfortunately, only vascular invasion is absolutely definitive. Even perineural infiltration may be mimicked by the presence of benign epithelial inclusions in pancreatic nerves[155] or pseudoneoplastic proliferation of endocrine cells in pancreatic fibrosis.[156] **Hyland et al.[151] have suggested three major criteria for diagnosis of pancreatic carcinoma on frozen section based on frequency of occurrence and reproducibility. These include (1) nuclear size variation of 4 : 1 or greater between epithelial cells, (2) incomplete ductal lumina, and (3) disorganized duct distribution. Five minor criteria have also been defined by these authors and include (1) large irregular epithelial nucleoli, (2) necrotic glandular debris, (3) glandular mitosis, (4) glands unaccompanied by connective tissue stroma within smooth muscle bundles, and (5) perineural invasion (Fig. 8–22). In the ampullar region, the presence of atypical glands within fascicles of smooth muscle may be especially helpful in recognizing invasive maligancy.[120]**

Unusual Histologic Types of Ductal Carcinoma

Mucinous Carcinoma (Colloid Carcinoma)

Like mucinous carcinomas occurring elsewhere in the gastrointestinal tract, the uncommon mucinous adenocarcinoma of the pancreas is composed largely of mucinous pools divided by fibrous septa that may or may not contain residual neoplastic cells (Fig. 8–23).[157] When present, the cells are typically found floating within the mucin rather than growing only at the periphery of the mucin lake in contact with the stroma as would be seen in a mucinous cystadenocarcinoma. The cells may vary from polygonal to tall columnar cells filled with apical mucin or forming poorly defined glands. Rarely, fronds of papillary carcinoma are found within the mucin lake. Generally, the tumor may be considered to be moderately differentiated if cords, strands, or clumps of gland-forming epithelium are found within the mucin pools, whereas a predominance of signet ring cells would best be classified as poorly differentiated. The median patient age, distribution of sites of origin, and stage-matched survival resemble those of typical ductal adenocarcinomas. It has been suggested, however, that mucin-producing tumors lacking signet ring cells may have a somewhat better prognosis.

Oncocytic Carcinoma

Oncocytic carcinoma of the pancreas is an ill-defined entity that may represent a group of tumors of varying histogenesis whose common feature is oncocytic change in the majority of the tumor cells.[44, 98-100, 158-162] Both benign[98, 160, 161] and malignant[44, 99, 100, 158, 162] oncocytic tumors have been reported, thus oncocytic change does not correlate directly with biologic behavior. Like oncocytomas elsewhere in the body, those in the pancreas are composed predominantly of cells with abundant mitochondria, giving their cytoplasm a finely granular appearance. Mitotic activity is variable, as is nuclear pleomorphism. In some tumors, ultrastructural evidence of specific

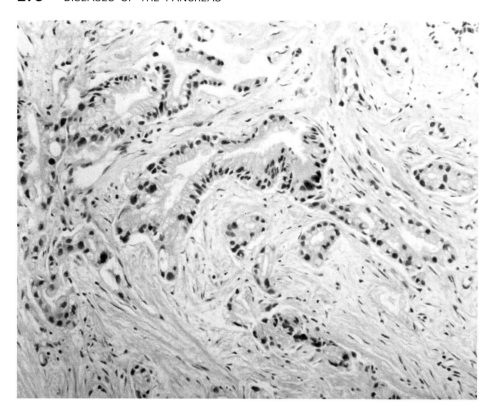

FIGURE 8–21. Pancreatic ductal carcinoma. Proliferation of irregular ductal structures some of which lack lumina or are lined by pleomorphic, hyperchromatic cells and which show no recognizable lobular architecture are characteristic of ductal carcinoma. (H&E, ×100)

differentiation can be found in the form of mucigen, zymogen, or neuroendocrine granules. Some tumors show more than one line of differentiation. Growth patterns in solid sheets arranged around fibrovascular cores, otherwise indistinguishable from solid and cystic neoplasms, have been reported.[44, 98] It has even been suggested that most, if not all, pancreatic oncocytic carcinomas represent variants of solid and cystic neoplasms. However, reports of pancreatic oncocytic carcinomas with growth patterns that include multilocular cysts[44] or completely solid growth with neither cystification

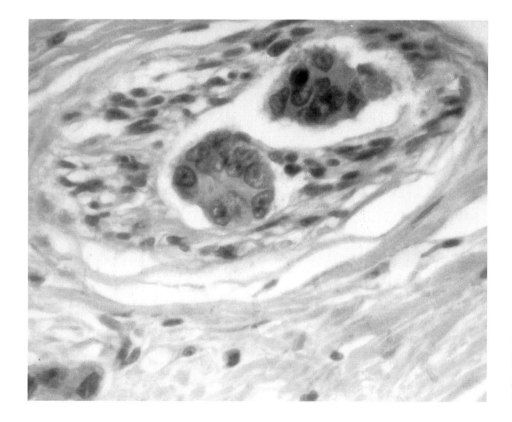

FIGURE 8–22. Pancreatic ductal carcinoma. Perineural infiltration, as shown here, remains one of the most reproducible criteria by which to recognize ductal carcinoma on biopsy. (H&E, ×275)

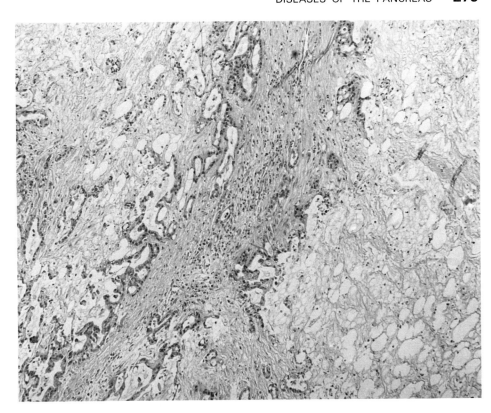

FIGURE 8–23. Mucinous carcinoma of the pancreas. Most of the tumor mass consists of large mucin pools at the periphery of which viable adenocarcinoma cells are seen abutting a fibrous septum. (H&E, ×33)

nor true cyst formation[99] would indicate that resemblance to solid and cystic neoplasms is lacking in many cases. Furthermore, extensive oncocytic change is known to occur in tumors otherwise clearly identifiable both clinically and pathologically as functioning PETs.[158] Thus, it would appear that only those oncocytic tumors of the pancreas with little or no evidence of specific differentiation should be categorized as oncocytic carcinomas. Otherwise, it may have more prognostic value to classify the tumor according to its primary pattern of differentiation (e.g., solid and cystic neoplasm, PET, cystadenocarcinoma) and to subclassify the tumor as an oncocytic variant.

Clear-Cell Carcinoma

This is a very rare variant of pancreatic adenocarcinoma that has been reported both in humans and in experimental animal models of pancreatic cancer. These tumors closely resemble the far more common clear-cell type of renal cell carcinoma or adrenal cortical carcinoma; thus, diagnosis of clear-cell carcinoma of the pancreas requires strict elimination of primary tumors in the kidneys and adrenals. The tumor cells grow in solid sheets through which slender fibrovascular septa run.[163] Fat stains are negative, but stains for mucin may be positive. Because foci of benign clear cells have been identified in the normal human pancreas in histologic studies, this tumor may represent rare differentiation toward that unusual cell type.

Ciliated Cell Carcinoma

Although ciliated cell carcinomas of the pancreas have been described,[164] it is not clear that pancreatic adenocarcinoma

with ciliated cells (even a predominance of ciliated cells) warrants a separate category. Ciliated cells have been identified in the ducts of the normal pancreas, and production of cilia by pancreatic ductal carcinoma cells may represent an uncommon differentiation feature of an otherwise straightforward ductal carcinoma. It should be kept in mind that cancers containing numerous ciliated cells are statistically more likely to represent metastatic lung cancers than primary pancreatic carcinomas.

Oat Cell Carcinoma

Rarely, poorly differentiated small-cell carcinomas of the pancreas histologically and histochemically identical to oat cell carcinoma of the lung may arise in the pancreas.[165–168] They are characterized by a diffuse infiltrative pattern of small cells with hyperchromatic nuclei and a small amount of cytoplasm that is usually Grimelius negative. It is of paramount importance that such tumors be differentiated from malignant lymphomas. This mandates either immunohistochemical and/or electron microscopic analysis.

Large-Cell Undifferentiated Pancreatic Carcinoma

A small group of tumors composed of large anaplastic cells showing no evidence of specific differentiation may occur in the pancreas.[118] These tumors usually show a solid growth pattern with no evidence of gland formation, mucin production, neuroendocrine differentiation, or zymogen granule production. Anaplastic carcinomas can be difficult to distinguish from lymphoma on a morphologic basis alone,[169] and immunohistochemical staining may be needed to differentiate between the two. They are usually aggressive tumors that diffusely infiltrate the pancreas and may be discovered only at autopsy.

Adenosquamous Carcinoma

Adenosquamous carcinoma of the pancreas is an unusual histologic variant of ductal carcinoma[118, 170–173] but has the same clinical presentation and biologic behavior as its typical counterpart. This tumor may show varying proportions of adenocarcinoma and squamous cell carcinoma as well as spindle cell growth with sarcomatoid features. If spindled areas are extensive, documentation of their epithelial nature may be aided by immunohistochemical staining for keratin and other epithelial markers such as epithelial membrane antigen. Very rarely, pure squamous cell carcinomas of the pancreas may occur.

NON-EPITHELIAL TUMORS OF THE PANCREAS

Sarcomas

Primary pancreatic sarcomas are rare.[173] Leiomyosarcoma, fibrosarcoma, rhabdosarcoma, malignant schwannoma, malignant hemangiopericytoma, and malignant fibrous histiocytoma all have been reported to occur in the pancreas. Diagnostic difficulties might arise in differentiating some sarcomas from giant cell tumors, PET with spindle cell growth patterns, adenosquamous (spindle cell) carcinomas, or pancreatoblastomas. Immunohistochemistry and/or electron microscopy may be needed to definitely identify a primary pancreatic sarcoma and to differentiate them from the far more common look-alike epithelial (or pluripotential) pancreatic malignancies.

Lymphoma/Leukemia

Very rarely, the pancreas may be the primary site of a non-Hodgkin's lymphoma, or more commonly, the pancreas may be secondarily involved by a non-Hodgkin's lymphoma, Hodgkin's disease, or leukemia.[173] Reported primary pancreatic lymphomas have included reticulum cell sarcoma (probably corresponding to an immunoblastic sarcoma, B- or T-cell), plasmacytoma, and lymphosarcoma (B-cell lymphoma, small-or large-cleaved follicular center cell). Secondary involvement of the pancreas occurs in about one third of cases of non-Hodgkin's lymphoma. Most commonly, diffuse histiocytic lymphoma and diffuse mixed histiocytic lymphoma are present. Advanced Hodgkin's disease frequently involves the pancreas, as does American Burkitt's lymphoma (pancreas involved in >80% of cases). Rarely, a Burkitt's lymphoma may even present as acute pancreatitis. Any type of acute or chronic leukemia may involve the pancreas, usually as a late occurrence discovered at autopsy.

The major differential diagnostic problem surrounding pancreatic lymphoma or leukemia is the possibility of confusion with a poorly differentiated adenocarcinoma or pleomorphic carcinoma of the small-cell type (oat cell carcinoma) on biopsy. Carcinomas and lymphomas may show similar cytologic features, such as signet-ring cell formation, as well as similar growth patterns including perineural infiltration.

However, leukocytic tumor cells can usually be easily differentiated from epithelial tumor cells by immunohistochemistry. Stains for leukocyte common antigen (CD45) can be performed on paraffin sections, as can stains for epithelial antigens such as keratin, epithelial membrane antigen, and CEA.

Metastatic Disease Involving the Pancreas

Among the most common types of metastatic disease to involve the pancreas are breast, lung, stomach, and colon cancer and malignant melanoma.[173] However, virtually all carcinomas and several types of sarcomas (e.g., osteogenic sarcoma, neuroblastoma, and so on) have been known to metastasize to the pancreas. Strictly speaking, differentiation of metastatic adenocarcinoma from primary pancreatic ductal carcinoma would not necessarily be possible on a histopathologic basis alone unless carcinoma *in situ* in the surrounding pancreatic ducts or differentiation along acinar lines was observed to support a diagnosis of a pancreatic primary.

References

Pancreatic Lipomatosis

1. Kreel L, Sandin B: Changes in pancreatic morphology associated with aging. Gut 14: 962–970, 1973.
2. Bartholomew LG, Baggenstoss AH, Morlock CG, et al: Primary atrophy and lipomatosis of the pancreas. Gastroenterology 36:563–572, 1959.
3. Seifert G, Klöppel G: Diagnostic value of pancreatic biopsy. Pathol Res Pract 164(4):357–384, 1979.
4. Robson HN, Scott GBD: Lipomatous pseudohypertrophy of the pancreas. Gastroenterology 23:74–81, 1953.
5. Salm R: Carcinoma arising in a lipomatous pseudohypertrophic pancreas. BMJ III:293, 1968.

Shwachman Syndrome

6. Goeteyn M, Oranje AP, Vuzevski VD, et al: Ichthyosis, exocrine pancreatic insufficiency, impaired neutrophil chemotaxis, growth retardation, and metaphyseal dysplasia (Shwachman syndrome). Arch Dermatol 127(2):225–230, 1991.
7. Bom EP, van der Sande FM, Tjon RTO, et al: Shwachman syndrome: CT and MR diagnosis. J Comput Assist Tomogr 17(3):474–476, 1993.
8. Tada H, Ri T, Yoshida H, et al: A case report of Shwachman syndrome with increased spontaneous chromosome breakage. Hum Genet 77(3):289–291, 1987.

Non-neoplastic Benign Cystic Lesions

9. Mcgeoch JE, Darmady EM: Polycystic disease of kidney, liver and pancreas: A possible pathogenesis. J Pathol 119(4):221–228, 1976.
10. Howard JM: Cystic neoplasms and true cysts of the pancreas. Surg Clin North Am 69(3):651–665, 1989.
11. Mao C, Greenwood S, Wagner S, et al: Solitary true cyst of the pancreas in an adult. Int J Pancreatol 12(2):181–186, 1992.
12. Flaherty MJ, Benjamin DR: Multicystic pancreatic hamartoma: A distinctive lesion with immunohistochemical and ultrastructural study. Hum Pathol 23(11):1309–1312, 1992.
13. Pins MR, Compton CC, Southern JF, et al: Ciliated enteric duplication cyst presenting as a pancreatic neoplasm: Report of a case with cyst fluid analysis. Clin Chem 38(8):1501–1503, 1992.
14. Oppenheimer EH, Esterly JR: Pathology of cystic fibrosis. Review of the literature and comparison with 146 autopsied cases. Perspect Pediatr Pathol 2:241–278, 1975.
15. Kaiserling E, Seitz KH, Rettenmaier G, et al: Lymphoepithelial cyst of the pancreas. Clinical, morphological, and immunohistochemical findings. Zentralbl Pathol 137(5):431–438, 1991.
16. Cappellari JO: Fine needle aspiration cytology of a pancreatic lymphoepithelial cyst. Diagn Cytopathol 9(1):77–84, 1993.
17. Markovsky V, Russin VL: Fine needle aspiration of dermoid cyst of the pancreas: A case report. Diagn Cytopathol 9(1):66–69, 1993.

Nesidioblastosis and Adenomatosis

18. Heitz PU, Klöppel G, Häcki WH, et al: Nesidioblastosis: The pathological basis of persistent hyperinsulinemic hypoglycemia in infants. Morphological and quantitative analysis of seven cases based on specific immunostaining and electron microscopy. Diabetes 26(7):632–642, 1977.
19. Goossens A, Gepts W, Saudubray J-M, et al: Diffuse and focal nesidioblastosis. A clinicopathological study of 24 patients with persistent neonatal hyperinsulinemic hypoglycemia. Am J Surg Pathol 13(9):766–775, 1989.
20. Witte DP, Greider MH, DeSchryver-Kecskemeti K, et al: The juvenile human endocrine pancreas: Normal vs. idiopathic hyperinsulinemic hypoglycemia. Semin Diagn Pathol 1(1):30–42, 1984.
21. Gould VE, Chejfec G, Shah K, et al: Adult nesidiodysplasia. Semin Diagn Pathol 1(1):43–53, 1984.
22. Ariel I, Kerem E, Schwartz-Arad D, et al: Nesidiodysplasia—a histologic entity? Hum Pathol 19(10):1215–1218, 1988.
23. Gould VE, Memoli VA, Dardi LE, et al: Nesidiodysplasia and nesidioblastosis of infancy. Ultrastructural and immunohistochemical analysis of islet cell alterations with and without associated hyperinsulinaemic hypoglycaemia. Scand J Gastroenterol Suppl 70:129–142, 1981.
24. Jaffe R, Hashida Y, Yunis EJ: Pancreatic pathology in hyperinsulinemic hypoglycemia of infancy. Lab Invest 42(3):356–365, 1980.
25. Schönau E, Deeg KH, Huemmer HP, et al: Pancreatic growth and function following surgical treatment of nesidioblastosis in infancy. Eur J Pediatr 150(8):550–553, 1991.
26. Traverso LW, Bockman DE, Pleis SK, et al: Nesidioblastosis as a mechanism to prevent fibrosis-induced diabetes after pancreatic duct obstruction. Pancreas 8(3):325–329, 1993.
27. Odaira C, Choux R, Payan M-J, et al: Chronic obstructive pancreatitis, nesidioblastosis, and small endocrine pancreatic tumor. Dig Dis Sci 32(7):770–774, 1987.
28. Bishop AE, Polak JM, Chesa PG, et al: Decrease of pancreatic somatostatin in neonatal nesidioblastosis. Diabetes 30(2):122–126, 1981.
29. Barresi G, Inferrera C, deLuca F, et al: Persistent neonatal normoinsulinaemic hypoglycemia. Histopathology 5(1):45–52, 1981.
30. Gabbey KH, Gang DL: Hypoglycemia in a three-month-old girl. N Engl J Med 299:241–248, 1978.
31. Lloyd R, Caceres V, Warner TF, et al: Islet cell adenomatosis. A report of two cases in the literature. Arch Pathol Lab Med 105:198–202, 1981.
32. Vance JE, Stoll RW, Kitabchi AE, et al: Familial nesidioblastosis as the predominant manifestation of multiple endocrine adenomatosis. Am J Med 52(2):211–227, 1972.
33. Fischer GW, Vazquez AM, Buist NR, et al: Neonatal islet cell adenoma: Case report and review of the literature. Pediatrics 53(5):753–756, 1974.

Serous Cystadenoma

34. Compagno J, Oertel JE: Microcystic adenomas of the pancreas (glycogen-rich cystadenomas). A clinicopathologic study of 34 cases. Am J Clin Pathol 69(3):289–298, 1978.
35. Zamora JL, Gunn LC, Manaligod JR: Microcystic adenoma of the pancreas: A newly recognized benign lesion. Curr Surg 41(6):448–452, 1984.
36. Shorten SD, Hart WR, Petras RE: Microcystic adenomas (serous cystadenomas) of pancreas. A clinicopathologic investigation of eight cases with immunohistochemical and ultrastructural studies. Am J Surg Pathol 10(6):365–372, 1986.
37. Torres-Barrera G, Fernández-del Castillo C, Reyes E, et al: Microcystic adenoma of the pancreas. Dig Dis Sci 32(5):454–458, 1987.
38. Itai Y, Ohhashi K, Furui S, et al: Microcystic adenoma of the pancreas: Spectrum of computed tomographic findings. J Comput Assist Tomogr 12(5):797–803, 1988.
39. Alpert LC, Truong LD, Bossart MI, et al: Microcystic adenoma (serous cystadenoma) of the pancreas. A study of 14 cases with immunohistochemical and electron-microscope correlation. Am J Surg Pathol 12(4):251–263, 1988.
40. George DH, Murphy F, Michalski R, et al: Serous cystadenocarcinoma of the pancreas: A new entity? Am J Surg Pathol 13(1):61–66, 1989.
41. Yoshimi N, Sugie S, Tanaka T, et al: A rare case of serous cystadenocarcinoma of the pancreas. Cancer 69(10):2449–2453, 1992.
42. Lewandrowski KB, Warshaw AL, Compton CC: Macrocystic serous cystadenoma of the pancreas: A morphologic variant differing from microcystic adenoma. Hum Pathol 23(8):871–875, 1992.
43. Montag AG, Fossati N, Michelassi F: Pancreatic microcystic adenoma coexistent with pancreatic ductal carcinoma. Am J Surg Pathol 14(4):352–355, 1990.
44. Friedman H: Nonmucinous, glycogen-poor cystadenoma of the pancreas. Arch Pathol Lab Med 114(8):888–891, 1990.

Mucinous Cystic Neoplasms

45. Ayella AS, Howard JM, Grotzinger PJ: Cystadenoma and cystadenocarcinoma of the pancreas. Am J Surg 103:242–246, 1962.
46. Becker WF, Welsh RA, Pratt HS: Cystadenoma and cystadenocarcinoma of the pancreas. Ann Surg 161(6):845–863, 1964.
47. Hodgkinson DJ, ReMine WH, Weiland LH: Pancreatic cystadenoma. A clinicopathologic study of 45 cases. Arch Surg 113(4):512–519, 1978.

48. Friedman AC, Lichtenstein JE, Dachman AH: Cystic neoplasms of the pancreas. Radiological-pathological correlation. Radiology 149(1):45–50, 1983.
49. Hyde GL, Davis JB, McMillin RD, et al: Mucinous cystic neoplasm of the pancreas with latent malignancy. Am Surg 50(4):225–229, 1984.
50. Corbally MT, McAnena OJ, Urmacher C, et al: Pancreatic cystadenoma. A clinicopathologic study. Arch Surg 124(11):1271–1274, 1989.
51. Compagno J, Oertel JE: Mucinous cystic neoplasms of the pancreas with overt and latent malignancy (cystadenocarcinoma and cystadenoma). Am J Clin Pathol 69(6):573–580, 1978.
52. Katoh H, Rossi RL, Braasch JW, et al: Cystadenoma and cystadenocarcinoma of the pancreas. Hepato-gastroenterology 36(6):424–430, 1989.
53. Talamini MA, Pitt HA, Hruban RH, et al: Spectrum of cystic tumors of the pancreas. Am J Surg 163(1):117–124, 1992.
54. Albores-Saavedra J, Angeles-Angeles A, Nadji M, et al: Mucinous cystadenoma of the pancreas. Morphologic and immunocytochemical observations. Am J Surg Pathol 11(1):11–20, 1987.
55. Albores-Saavedra J, Gould EW, Angeles-Angeles A, et al: Cystic tumors of the pancreas. Pathol Ann 25(Pt 2):19–50, 1990.
56. Yamaguchi K, Enjoji M: Cystic neoplasms of the pancreas. Gastroenterology 92(6):1934–1943, 1987.
57. Warshaw AL, Compton CC, Lewandrowski KB, et al: Cystic tumors of the pancreas. New clinical, radiologic, and pathologic observations in 67 patients. Ann Surg 212(4):432–443, 1990.
58. Lewandrowski KB, Southern JF, Pins MR, et al: Cyst fluid analysis in the differential diagnosis of pancreatic cysts. A comparison of pseudocysts, serous cystadenomas, mucinous cystic neoplasms and mucinous cystadenocarcinoma. Ann Surg 217(1):41–47, 1993.
59. Rubin D, Warshaw AL, Southern JF, et al: Cyst fluid CA 15-3 concentration differentiates pancreatic mucinous cystadenocarcinomas from benign pancreatic cysts. Surgery 115(1):52–55, 1994.
60. Yu HC, Shetty J: Mucinous cystic neoplasm of the pancreas with high carcinoembryonic antigen. Arch Pathol Lab Med 109(4):375–377, 1985.
61. Tatsuta M, Iishi H, Ichii M, et al: Values of carcinoembryonic antigen, elastase 1, and carbohydrate antigen determinant in aspirated pancreatic cystic fluid in the diagnosis of cysts of the pancreas. Cancer 57(9):1836–1839, 1986.
62. Alles AJ, Warshaw AL, Southern JF, et al: Cyst fluid CA 72-4 (TAG 72) in the differential diagnosis of pancreatic cysts: A new marker to distinguish malignant from benign pancreatic neoplasms and pseudocysts. Ann Surg 219(2):131–134, 1994.
63. Lewandrowski KB, Warshaw AL, Compton CC, et al: Variability in cyst fluid carcinoembryonic antigen level, fluid viscosity, amylase content, and cytology among multiple loculi of a pancreatic mucinous cystic neoplasm. Am J Clin Pathol 100:425–427, 1994.
64. Sachs JR, Deren JL, Sohn M, et al: Mucinous cystadenoma: Pitfalls of differential diagnosis. Am J Gastroenterol 84(7):811–816, 1989.
65. Warshaw AL, Rutledge PL: Cystic tumors mistaken for pancreatic pseudocysts. Ann Surg 205(4):393–398, 1987.

Intraductal Papillary Lesions

66. Klöppel G, Bommer G, Rückert K, et al: Intraductal proliferation in the pancreas and its relationship to human and experimental carcinogenesis. Virchows Arch [Pathol Anat] 387(2):221–233, 1980.
67. Oertel JE: The pancreas. Nonneoplastic alterations. Am J Surg Pathol 13(Suppl 1):50–65, 1989.
68. Ferrari BT, O'Halloran RL, Longmire WP, et al: Atypical papillary hyperplasia of the pancreatic duct mimicking obstructing pancreatic carcinoma. N Engl J Med 301(10):531–532, 1979.
69. Obara T, Saitoh Y, Maguchi H, et al: Multicentric development of a pancreatic intraductal carcinoma through atypical papillary hyperplasia. Hum Pathol 23(1):82–85, 1992.
70. Kozuka S, Sassa R, Taki T, et al: Relation of pancreatic duct hyperplasia to carcinoma. Cancer 43(4):1418–1428, 1979.
71. Yoshida J, Ozaki H, Yamamoto J, et al: Adenocarcinoma and concomitant intraductal papillary adenoma in the pancreas. Jpn J Clin Oncol 21(6):453–456, 1991.
72. Conley CR, Scheithauer BW, van Heerden JA, et al: Diffuse intraductal papillary adenocarcinoma of the pancreas. Ann Surg 205(3):246–249, 1987.
73. Yamada M, Kozuka S, Yamao K, et al: Mucin-producing tumor of the pancreas. Cancer 68(1):159–168, 1991.
74. Itai Y, Ohhashi K, Nagai H, et al: "Ductectatic" mucinous cystadenoma and cystadenocarcinoma of the pancreas. Radiology 161(3):697–700, 1986.
75. Morohoshi T, Kanda M, Asanuma K, et al: Intraductal papillary neoplasms of the pancreas. A clinicopathologic study of six patients. Cancer 64(6):1329–1335, 1989.
76. Furukawa T, Takahashi T, Kobari M, et al: The mucus-hypersecreting tumor of the pancreas. Development and extension visualized by three-dimensional computerized mapping. Cancer 70(6):1505–1513, 1992.
77. Nickl NJ, Lawson JM, Cotton PB: Mucinous pancreatic tumors: ERCP findings. Gastrointest Endosc 37(2):133–138, 1991.
78. Bastid C, Bernard JP, Sarles H, et al: Mucinous ductal ectasia of the pancreas: A premalignant disease and a cause of obstructive pancreatitis. Pancreas 6(1):15–22, 1991.

79. Rickaert F, Cremer M, Devière J, et al: Intraductal mucin-hypersecreting neoplasms of the pancreas. A clinicopathologic study of eight patients. Gastroenterology 101(2):512–519, 1991.
80. Tian F, Myles J, Howard JM: Mucinous pancreatic ductal ectasia of latent malignancy: An emerging clinicopathologic entity. Surgery 111:109–113, 1992.
81. Kawarada Y, Yano T, Yamamoto T, et al: Intraductal mucin-producing tumors of the pancreas. Am J Gastroenterol 87(5):634–638, 1992.
82. Milchgrub S, Compuzano M, Casillas J, et al: Intraductal carcinoma of the pancreas. Cancer 69(3):651–656, 1992.

Solid and Cystic Tumor

83. Boor P, Swanson M: Papillary-cystic neoplasm of the pancreas. Am J Surg Pathol 3(1):69–75, 1979.
84. Klöppel G, Morohoshi T, John HD, et al: Solid and cystic acinar cell tumor of the pancreas. A tumour in young women with favourable prognosis. Virchows Arch [Pathol Anat] 392:171–183, 1981.
85. Lack EE, Levey R, Cassady JR, et al: Tumors of the exocrine pancreas in children and adolescents. A clinical and pathologic study of eighteen cases. Am J Surg Pathol 7(4):319–327, 1983.
86. Morrison DM, Jewell LD, McCaughey WTE, et al: Papillary cystic tumor of the pancreas. Arch Pathol Lab Med 108(9):723–727, 1984.
87. Matsunou H, Konishi F: Papillary-cystic neoplasm of the pancreas. A clinicopathologic study concerning the tumor aging and malignancy of nine cases. Cancer 65(2):283–291, 1990.
88. Yamaguchi K, Hirakata R, Kitamura K: Papillary cystic neoplasm of the pancreas: Radiological and pathological characteristics in 11 cases. Br J Surg 77(9):1000–1003, 1990.
89. Kamei K, Funabiki T, Ochiai M, et al: Three cases of solid and cystic tumor of the pancreas. Int J Pancreatol 10(3/4):269–278, 1991.
90. Sclafani LM, Reuter VE, Coit DG, et al: The malignant nature of papillary and cystic neoplasm of the pancreas. Cancer 68(1):153–158, 1991.
91. Ueda N, Nagakawa T, Ohta T, et al: Clinicopathological studies on solid and cystic tumors of the pancreas. Gastroenterol Jpn 26(4):497–502, 1991.
92. Pettinato G, Manivel JC, Ravetto C, et al: Papillary cystic tumor of the pancreas. A clinicopathologic study of 20 cases with cytologic, immunohistochemical, ultrastructural and flow cytometric observations, and a review of the literature. Am J Clin Pathol 98(5):478–488, 1992.
93. Nishihara K, Tsunyoshi M: Papillary cystic tumors of the pancreas: An analysis by nuclear morphometry. Virchows Arch A Pathol Anat Histopathol 422(3):211–217, 1993.
94. Matsunou H, Konishi F, Yamamichi N, et al: Solid, infiltrating variety of papillary cystic neoplasm of the pancreas. Cancer 65(12):2747–2757, 1990.
95. Stömmer P, Kraus J, Stolte M, et al: Solid and cystic pancreatic tumors. Clinical, histochemical and electron microscopic features in ten cases. Cancer 67(6):1635–1641, 1991.
96. Morohoshi T, Kanda M, Horie A, et al: Immunocytochemical markers of uncommon pancreatic tumors. Acinar cell carcinoma, pancreatoblastoma, and solid cystic (papillary-cystic) tumor. Cancer 59(4):739–747, 1987.
97. Nishihara K, Nagoshi M, Tsuneyoshi M, et al: Papillary cystic tumors of the pancreas. Assessment of their malignant potential. Cancer 71(1):82–92, 1993.
98. Lee W-Y, Tzeng C-C, Jin Y-T, et al: Papillary cystic tumor of the pancreas: A case indistinguishable from oncocytic carcinoma. Pancreas 8(1):127–132, 1993.
99. Zerbi A, De Nardi P, Braga M, et al: An oncocytic carcinoma of the pancreas with pulmonary and subcutaneous metastases. Pancreas 8(1):116–119, 1993.
100. Huntrakoon M: Oncocytic carcinoma of the pancreas. Cancer 51(2):332–336, 1983.

Pancreatic Endocrine Tumors

101. Larsson L-I: Endocrine pancreatic tumors. Hum Pathol 9(4):401–416, 1978.
102. Friesen SR: Tumors of the endocrine pancreas. N Engl J Med 306(10):580–590, 1982.
103. Hammar S, Sale G: Multiple hormone producing islet cell carcinomas of the pancreas. Hum Pathol 6(3):349–362, 1975.
104. Mukai K, Greider MH, Grotting JC, et al: Retrospective study of 77 pancreatic endocrine tumors using the immunoperoxidase method. Am J Surg Pathol 6:387–399, 1982.
105. Solcia E, Capella C, Buffa R, et al: The contribution of immunohistochemistry to the diagnosis of neuroendocrine tumors. Semin Diagn Pathol 1(4):285–296, 1984.
106. Nojima T, Kojima T, Kato H, et al: Cystic endocrine tumor of the pancreas. Int J Pancreatol 10:65–72, 1991.
107. Greider MH, DeSchryver-Kecskemeti K, Kraus FT: Psammoma bodies in endocrine tumors of the gastroenteropancreatic axis: A rather common occurrence. Semin Diagn Pathol 1:19–29, 1984.
108. Heitz PU, Kasper M, Klöppel G, et al: Glycoprotein-hormone alpha-chain production by pancreatic endocrine tumors: A specific marker for malignancy. Cancer 51:277–282, 1983.
109. Graeme-Cook F, Nardi G, Compton CC: Immunocytochemical staining for human chorionic gonadotrophin subunits does not predict malignancy in insulinomas. Am J Clin Pathol 93(2):273–276, 1990.
110. Pelosi G, Zamboni G, Doglioni C, et al: Immunodetection of proliferating cell nuclear antigen assesses the growth fraction and predicts malignancy in endocrine tumors of the pancreas. Am J Surg Pathol 16(12):1215–1225, 1992.
111. Rüschoff J, Willemer S, Brunzel M, et al: Nucleolar organizer regions and glycoprotein-hormone alpha-chain reaction as markers of malignancy in endocrine tumours of the pancreas. Histopathology 22:51–57, 1993.
112. Klimstra DS, Heffess CS, Oertel JE, et al: Acinar cell carcinoma of the pancreas: A clinicopathologic study of 28 cases. Am J Surg Pathol 16(9):815–837, 1992.
113. Kniffin WD, Spencer SK, Memoli VA, et al: Metastatic islet cell amphicrine carcinoma of the pancreas. Association with an eosinophilic infiltration of the skin. Cancer 62(9):1999–2004, 1988.
114. Ordóñez NG, Balsaver AM, Mackay B: Mucinous islet cell (amphicrine) carcinoma of the pancreas associated with watery diarrhea and hypokalemia syndrome. Hum Pathol 19(12):1458–1461, 1988.
115. Laine VJO, Ekfors TO, Gullichsen R, Nevalainen TJ: Immunohistochemical characterization of an amphicrine mucinous islet-cell carcinoma of the pancreas. APMIS 100(4):335–340, 1992.
116. Permert J, Mogaki M, Andrén-Sandberg A, et al: Pancreatic mixed ductal-islet tumors. Int J Pancreatol 11(1):23–29, 1992.
117. Ulich T, Cheng L, Lewin KJ: Acinar-endocrine cell tumor of the pancreas. Report of a pancreatic tumor containing both zymogen and neuroendocrine granules. Cancer 50(10):2099–2105, 1982.
118. Cubilla AL, Fitzgerald PJ: Morphological patterns of primary nonendocrine human pancreatic carcinoma. Cancer Res 35(8):2234–2248, 1975.

Pancreatoblastoma

119. Ohaki Y, Misugi K, Sasaki Y, et al: Pancreatic carcinoma in childhood. Report of an autopsy case and a review of the literature. Acta Pathol Jpn 35(6):1543–1554, 1985.
120. Lack E: Primary tumors of the exocrine pancreas. Classification, overview, and recent contributions by immunohistochemistry and electron microscopy. Am J Surg Pathol 13(Suppl 1):66–89, 1989.
121. Grosfeld JL, Vane DW, Rescorla FJ, et al: Pancreatic tumors in childhood: Analysis of 13 cases. J Pediatr Surg 25(10):1057–1062, 1990.
122. Jaksic T, Yaman M, Thorner P, et al: A 20-year review of pediatric pancreatic tumors. J Pediatr Surg 27(10):1315–1317, 1992.
123. Horie A, Haratake J, Jimi A, et al: Pancreatoblastoma in Japan, with differential diagnosis from papillary cystic tumor (ductuloacinar adenoma) of the pancreas. Acta Pathol Jpn 37(1):47–63, 1987.
124. Ohaki Y, Misugi K, Fukuda J, et al: Immunohistochemical study of pancreatoblastoma. Acta Pathol Jpn 37(10):1581–1590, 1987.
125. Silverman JF, Holbrook CT, Pories WJ, et al: Fine needle aspiration cytology of pancreatoblastoma with immunocytochemical and ultrastructural studies. Acta Cytol 35(5):632–640, 1990.
126. Isaki M, Suzuki T, Koizumi Y, et al: Alpha-fetoprotein-producing pancreatoblastoma. A case report. Cancer 57(9):1833–1835, 1986.
127. Morohoshi T, Sagawa F, Mitsuya T: Pancreatoblastoma with marked elevation of serum alpha-fetoprotein. An autopsy case report with immunocytochemical study. Virchows Arch A Pathol Anat Histopathol 416(3):265–270, 1990.

Cystic Teratoma

128. Mester M, Trajber HJ, Compton CC, et al: Cystic teratomas of the pancreas. Arch Surg 125(9):1215–1218, 1990.
129. Jacobs JE, Dinsmore BJ: Mature cystic teratoma of the pancreas: Sonographic and CT findings. AJR 160(3):523–524, 1993.

Acinar Cell Carcinoma

130. Webb JN: Acinar cell neoplasms of the exocrine pancreas. J Clin Pathol 30(2):103–112, 1977.
131. Cantrell BB, Cubilla AL, Erlandson RA, et al: Acinar cell cystadenocarcinoma of human pancreas. Cancer 47(2):410–416, 1981.
132. di Sant'Agnese P: Acinar cell carcinoma of the pancreas. Ultrastruct Pathol 15(4–5):573–577, 1991.
133. Hseuh C, Kuo T: Acinar cell carcinoma of the pancreas. Report of two cases with complex histomorphologic features causing diagnostic problems. Int J Pancreatol 12(3):305–313, 1992.
134. Itoh T, Kishi K, Tojo M, et al: Acinar cell carcinoma of the pancreas with elevated serum alpha-fetoprotein levels: A case report and a review of 28 cases reported in Japan. Gastroenterol Jpn 27(6):785–791, 1992.
135. Nojima T, Kojima T, Kato H, et al: Alpha-fetoprotein-producing acinar cell carcinoma of the pancreas. Hum Pathol 23(7):828–830, 1992.
136. Stamm B, Burger H, Hollinger A: Acinar cell cystadenocarcinoma of the pancreas. Cancer 60(10):2542–2547, 1987.

Giant Cell Tumors

137. Alguacil-Garcia A, Weiland LH: The histologic spectrum, prognosis, and histogenesis of the sarcomatoid carcinoma of the pancreas. Cancer 39(3):1181–1189, 1977.

138. Tschang TP, Garza-Garza R, Kissane JM: Pleomorphic carcinoma of the pancreas: An analysis of 15 cases. Cancer 39(5):2114–2126, 1977.
139. Reyes CV, Crain S, Wang T: Pleomorphic giant cell carcinoma of the pancreas: A review of nine cases. J Surg Oncol 15(4):345–348, 1980.
140. Silverman JF, Dabbs DJ, Finley JL, et al: Fine-needle aspiration biopsy of pleomorphic (giant cell) carcinoma of the pancreas. Cytologic, immunocytochemical and ultrastructural findings. Am J Clin Pathol 89(6):714–720, 1988.
141. Rosai J: Carcinoma of pancreas simulating giant cell tumor of bone. Electron microscopic evidence of its acinar origin. Cancer 22(2):333–344, 1968.
142. Jalloh SS: Giant cell tumour (osteoclastoma) of the pancreas—an epithelial tumour probably of acinar origin. J Clin Pathol 36(10):1171–1175, 1983.
143. Berendt RC, Shnitka TK, Wiens E, et al: The osteoclast-type giant cell tumor of pancreas. Arch Pathol Lab Med 111(1):43–48, 1987.
144. Fischer HP, Altmannsberger M, Kracht J: Osteoclast-type giant cell tumor of the pancreas. Virchows Arch A Pathol Anat Histopathol 412(3):247–253, 1988.
145. Suster S, Phillips M, Robinson MJ: Malignant fibrous histiocytoma (giant cell type) of the pancreas. A distinctive variant of osteoclast-type giant cell tumor of the pancreas. Cancer 64(11)2303–2308, 1989.
146. Goldberg RD, Michelassi F, Montag AG: Osteoclast-like giant cell tumor of the pancreas: Immunotypic similarity to giant cell tumor of bone. Hum Pathol 22(6):618–622, 1991.
147. Dworak O, Wittekind C, Koerfgen HP, et al: Osteoclastic giant cell tumor of the pancreas. An immunohistological study and review of the literature. Pathol Res Pract 189(2):228–231, 1993.
148. Lewandrowski KB, Weston L, Dickersin GR, et al: Giant cell tumor of the pancreas of mixed osteoclastic and pleomorphic cell type: Evidence for a histogenetic relationship and mesenchymal derivation. Hum Pathol 21(11):1184–1187, 1990.
149. Posen JA: Giant cell tumor of the pancreas of the osteclastic type associated with a mucous secreting cystadenocarcinoma. Hum Pathol 12(10):944–947, 1981.
150. Mentes A, Yuce G: Osteoclastic giant cell tumor of the pancreas associated with mucinous cystadenoma. Eur J Surg Oncol 19(1):84–86, 1993.

Pancreatic Ductal Carcinoma: Frozen Section Diagnosis

151. Hyland C, Kheir SM, Kashlan MB: Frozen section diagnosis of pancreatic carcinoma. A prospective study of 64 biopsies. Am J Surg Pathol 5(2):179–191, 1981.
152. Lee Y–T: Tissue diagnosis for carcinoma of the pancreas and periampullary structures. Cancer 49(5):1035–1039, 1982.
153. Weiland LH: Frozen section diagnosis in tumors of the pancreas. Semin Diagn Pathol 1(1):54–58, 1984.
154. Campanale RP 2d, Frey CF, Farias LR, et al: Reliability and sensitivity of frozen-section pancreatic biopsy. Arch Surg 120(3):283–288, 1985.
155. Costa J: Benign epithelial inclusions in pancreatic nerves [letter]. Am J Clin Pathol 67(3):306–307, 1977.
156. Bartow SA, Mukai K, Rosai J: Pseudoneoplastic proliferation of endocrine cells in pancreatic fibrosis. Cancer 47(11):2627–2633, 1981.

Mucinous Carcinoma

157. Chen J, Baithum SI: Morphological study of 391 cases of exocrine pancreatic tumours with special reference to the classification of exocrine pancreatic carcinoma. J Pathol 146(1):17–29, 1985.

Oncocytic Carcinoma

158. Radi MJ, Fenoglio-Preiser CM, Chiffelle T: Functioning oncocytic islet-cell carcinoma. Report of a case with electron-microscopic and immunohistochemical confirmation. Am J Surg Pathol 9(7):517–524, 1985.
159. Gotchall J, Traweek ST, Stenzel P: Benign oncocytic tumor of the pancreas in a patient with polyarteritis nodosa. Human Pathol 18(9):967–969, 1987.
160. Bondeson L, Bondeson A–G, Grimelius L, et al: Oncocytic tumor of the pancreas. Report of a case with aspiration cytology. Acta Cytol 34(3):425–428, 1990.
161. Nozawa Y, Abe M, Sakuma H, et al: A case of pancreatic oncocytic tumor. Acta Pathol Jpn 40(5):367–370, 1990.
162. Sadoul J–L, Saint-Paul M-Ch, Hoffman P, et al: Malignant pancreatic oncocytoma. An unusual cause of organic hypoglycemia. J Endocrinol Invest 15(3):211–217, 1992.

Clear-Cell Carcinoma

163. Kanai N, Nagaki S, Tanaka T: Clear cell carcinoma of the pancreas. Acta Pathol Jpn 37(9):1521–1526, 1987.

Ciliated Cell Carcinoma

164. Moriyaga S, Tsumuraya M, Nakajima T, et al: Ciliated-cell adenocarcinoma of the pancreas. Acta Pathol Jpn 36(12):1905–1910, 1986.

Oat Cell Carcinoma

165. Reyes CV, Wang T: Undifferentiated small cell carcinoma of the pancreas: A report of five cases. Cancer 47(10):2500–2502, 1981.
166. Kodama T, Mori W: Morphological behavior of carcinoma of the pancreas. Acta Pathol Jpn 33(3):467–481, 1983.
167. Ibrahim NB, Briggs JC, Corbishley CM: Extrapulmonary oat cell carcinoma. Cancer 54(8):1645–1661, 1984.
168. Motojima K, Furui J, Terada M, et al: Small cell carcinoma of the pancreas and biliary tract. J Surg Oncol 45(3):164–168, 1990.

Large-Cell Undifferentiated Carcinoma

169. Ackerman NB, Aust JC, Bredenberg CE, et al: Problems in differentiating between pancreatic lymphoma and anaplastic carcinoma and their management. Ann Surg 184(6):705–708, 1976.

Adenosquamous Carcinoma

170. Ishikawa O, Matsui Y, Aoki I, et al: Adenosquamous carcinoma of the pancreas: A clinicopathologic study and report of three cases. Cancer 46(5):1192–1196, 1980.
171. Yamaguchi K, Enjoji M: Adenosquamous carcinoma of the pancreas: A clinico-pathologic study. J Surg Oncol 47(2):109–116, 1991.
172. Motojima K, Tomioka T, Kohara N, et al: Immunohistochemical characteristics of adenosquamous carcinoma of the pancreas. J Surg Oncol 49(1):58–62, 1992.

Lymphomas and Metastatic Tumors

173. Cubilla AL, Fitzgerald PJ: Malignant neoplasms. In Hartmann WH, Sobin LH (eds): Tumors of the Exocrine Pancreas. Fascicle 19, Atlas of Tumor Pathology, Second Series. Bethesda, MD, Armed Forces Institute of Pathology, 1984, pp 109–233.

CHAPTER 9

Liver and Gallbladder Pathology

Linda D. Ferrell, M.D.

LIVER

Problems in the Diagnosis of Cirrhosis and Hepatitis

Liver biopsies are not often seen in the surgical pathology laboratories of community hospitals, so the average practicing surgical pathologist may not be familiar with even this organ's most common lesions. Fortunately, the histologic diagnosis of fibrosis, cirrhosis, and hepatitis is usually an easy task, but not always. Many times, the cause of a fibrotic or inflammatory process in the liver can be difficult to recognize because the liver responds to a wide range of injuries in only a limited number of ways. However, certain patterns of injury and other microscopic features, when applied in the appropriate clinical setting, can help differentiate various causes of such processes.

"Hard-to-Diagnose" Cirrhosis

The **first thing to look for when considering a diagnosis of cirrhosis is loss of normal architecture**—that is, loss of normal central-portal relationships. In order to make this observation, the specimen must be large enough to contain several intact portal and central areas. A specimen that is fragmented into small pieces of hepatic parenchyma containing scant connective tissue, no normal portal tracts, and perhaps an irregular pattern of central veins may suggest a cirrhotic process, especially if regenerative cell plates ("twin plates," two cells thick) are present, or if the fragments have rounded edges, suggestive of nodularity. When performing a biopsy on a cirrhotic liver with a cutting core needle, the biopsied tissue may fragment because the cirrhotic nodules are easily extracted from the liver, but the connective tissue component that joins the nodules remains *in situ*. The rounded fragments that are removed can still contain some connective tissue around their edges, which can be visualized more readily on collagen or reticulin stains. The reticulin stain also enhances areas of regeneration by better demonstrating the presence of double cell plates. The atypical enlargement of nuclei with little if any corresponding increase in nucleocytoplasmic ratio, known as **"large-cell change," or "dysplasia,"** is very common in cirrhotic livers, but this cytologic aberration should be used only as an adjunct to the diagnostic clues of regeneration and architectural abnormalities for identifying cirrhosis.

In another rare type of cirrhosis, called **incomplete septal cirrhosis,**[1] extremely thin bands of collagen partially or totally

separate hepatocytic nodules. Some disorganized cell plates or zones resembling foci of nodular regenerative hyperplasia can be seen (see section on this topic later). The main complication of this variant of cirrhosis is portal hypertension; liver function is usually well preserved. Connective tissue is extremely difficult to identify on needle biopsies, and a possible diagnosis of cirrhosis could be missed if areas of regeneration or rounded fragments are not noted by the pathologist.

Wedge biopsies can pose special diagnostic problems because the subcapsular connective tissue can be more prominent (especially on specimens obtained from the sharp anterior border of the liver) and extend into the portal triads within 1 cm of the capsule. In addition, if a fragment or zone of fibrous tissue contains a large artery and large duct, it may represent a normal portal tract rather than scar tissue. Finally, if regeneration without fibrosis is present in a clinical setting of portal hypertension, nodular regenerative hyperplasia might be considered in the differential diagnosis (as discussed later).

For all biopsies though, if the tissue is scant, or if the degree of fibrosis is difficult to determine (i.e., if diffuse disease with portal-portal, central-portal, or central-central bridging fibrosis is not definitively present), a diagnosis of "probable cirrhosis," "suggestive of cirrhosis," "possible cirrhosis," or "cannot exclude cirrhosis" may be made, depending on the degree of suspicion.

Etiologies and Patterns of Injury
Alcoholic Fibrosis and Cirrhosis

When present concurrently, micronodular cirrhosis, Mallory bodies, and fatty change are highly indicative of alcoholic cirrhosis. Fatty change and Mallory bodies, however, can resolve over time (2–4 weeks and 6–12 weeks, respectively), and alcoholic injury can induce a cirrhosis with larger nodules, probably as a result of periodic abstinence from alcohol intake, during which time more regeneration of the hepatocytes can occur. There are other patterns of injury, however, that also suggest an alcoholic cause (Table 9–1). Probably the most reliable of these is perivenular, pericellular fibrosis[2, 3] present as partial or complete obliteration of the central vein (Fig. 9–1). These sclerotic central regions can best be differentiated from portal regions by the absence of arterioles in the central zone. The presence of ductular structures without an arteriole should not be used as a criterion for identifying former portal tracts, because ductular structures can occur outside of the portal zones in cirrhotic livers. Ischemia or other toxic injuries can also cause centrilobular fibrosis, so this finding is not a

Table 9–1. **Features of Alcoholic Cirrhosis**

Often seen in a micronodular pattern
Mallory hyalin, usually in centrilobular location
Fatty change
Centrilobular sclerosis
Pericellular, perivenular fibrosis ("chickenwire" pattern)
Fairly uniform, diffuse process
Paucity of inflammation
Central-central, central-portal bridging prominent

pathognomonic finding; however, when hepatocytes are individually surrounded by collagenous stroma in the centrilobular region, the process is more likely due to alcohol (see Fig. 9–1). This pattern of pericellular fibrosis (or "chickenwire" fibrosis because of its appearance on trichrome or van Gieson stains) can extend throughout the entire lobule. This finding should not be confused with a variant of normal vein structure (Fig. 9–2) consisting of a uniform, dense, thick central vein wall. The centrilobular injury leads to more prominent central zone–central zone and central zone–portal zone bridging than in cirrhosis due to biliary disease and, possibly, chronic hepatitis. Additionally, relatively few inflammatory cells of mononuclear or neutrophilic type are present, unless there is a superimposed viral or alcoholic hepatitis, respectively.

DIFFERENTIAL DIAGNOSIS. It is important to note that conditions other than alcoholism can induce fatty change with fibrosis and mimic alcoholic hepatitis (with Mallory bodies, fat, and neutrophilic infiltrates) or cirrhosis,[4] including obesity, diabetes mellitus, Weber-Christian disease, and drugs such as perhexilene maleate, glucocorticoids, synthetic estrogens, amiodarone,[5] and nifedipine.[6] Some surgical procedures, such as jejunoileal bypass or extensive small bowel resection, may also induce lesions that mimic alcoholic cirrhosis. Such lesions, which can progress to cirrhosis, are categorized as **nonalcoholic steatohepatitis.**[7–9] The swollen hepatocytes in these cases may contain eosinophilic material diagnostic or highly suggestive of Mallory bodies. In this entity, in contrast to alcoholic injury, an inflammatory component of mononuclears (including plasma cells) can be more prominent.[10]

Cardiac Fibrosis (Sclerosis), Ischemia, and Venous Outflow Obstruction

Cardiac disease associated with chronic heart failure or constrictive pericarditis can induce a centrilobular sclerosis similar to that seen with alcoholic injury[11] (Table 9–2); however, with cardiac injury, the sinusoids are often dilated and filled with erythrocytes, which can compress liver cell plates. Hemosiderin- and lipochrome-laden macrophages (resulting from the breakdown of erythrocytes in the sinusoids and hepatocytic necrosis, respectively) and inflammatory cells all can be present. Cholestasis at the edge of the fibrotic zone can also occur. PAS-positive globules, which by light microscopic analysis are morphologically similar to alpha-1-antitrypsin globules, have been reported in ischemic central zones.[12] Cardiac sclerosis (or cirrhosis) rarely involves portal tracts significantly only late in the course. Overall, cardiac sclerosis rarely progresses to a fully developed cirrhosis.

If an **acute ischemic process** has occurred with or without an underlying chronic ischemic process, coagulative hepatocyte necrosis can occur around the central vein. This type of necrosis is not seen with alcohol toxicity.

A distinctive but somewhat uncommon centrilobular lesion associated with ischemic necrosis and congestion consists of loss of hepatocytes within the cell plates and replacement by erythrocytes,[13] the mirror image of that seen in chronic passive congestion, in which the hepatocytes are intact and the sinusoids are congested (Fig. 9–3).

Venous outflow obstruction can also cause an ischemic injury and so must be considered in the differential diagnosis in the appropriate clinical context. A common form of venous outflow obstruction of the liver is the **Budd-Chiari syndrome,** a lesion characterized by occlusion of the large hepatic vein(s) or their entrances into the inferior vena cava. This occlusion is usually caused by a thrombus; thus, it is commonly associated with disorders of blood coagulation as seen in polycythemia vera and myeloproliferative disorders and with oral contraceptive use. Other associated lesions include neoplasia (especially renal carcinoma with invasion of the inferior vena cava) and suppurative infections of the liver

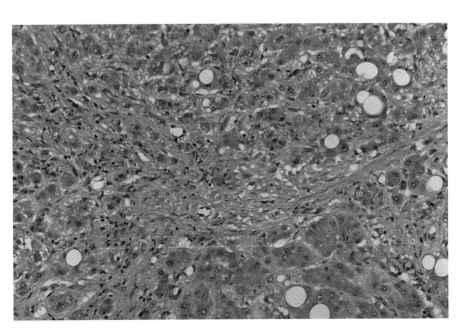

FIGURE 9–1. **Alcoholic cirrhosis** with fat and centrilobular sclerosis. Also note the pericellular fibrosis. (H&E, ×50)

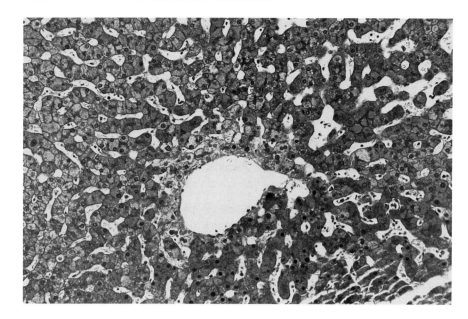

FIGURE 9–2. Normal central vein with thick collagen along wall. (Trichrome stain, ×25)

and/or hepatic veins.[14] Characteristic clinical findings in the Budd-Chiari syndrome include gross ascites as well as abdominal pain, mild jaundice, and/or hepatomegaly. The liver lesions are central and may have an acute or chronic appearance. Acute changes often include severe sinusoidal congestion with necrosis of the centrilobular hepatocytes. In the chronic lesions, fibrosis develops in the centrilobular zone, but periportal regeneration can be prominent, reminiscent of nodular regenerative hyperplasia, causing nodule formation.[14]

Another form of venous outflow obstruction is **veno-occlusive disease (VOD)** secondary to radiation therapy and chemotherapy during bone marrow transplantation. VOD usually develops within 1 to 3 weeks after transplantation, presenting often as hepatomegaly, ascites, and jaundice similar to Budd-Chiari syndrome. During the first few days of therapy, congestion of sinusoids and hemorrhagic necrosis of the central zonal hepatocytes occur.[15] Later, thin strands of loosely aggregated collagen fibers as well as hemosiderin macrophages and fragmented red blood cells can be noted within the central vein. The trichrome stain can help differentiate the dense, somewhat wavy collagen remnants of the original central vein from the newly aggregated, thinner strands of wispy collagen present in early VOD.[15] Over time, these centrilobular collagen deposits become more concentric, resulting in severe congestion. A minimal degree of fibrosis can be found in portal zones as well, and they may show dilated lymphatics and venules.[15]

DIFFERENTIAL DIAGNOSIS. Cardiac fibrosis, ischemia, and VOD can be virtually indistinguishable from one another because the basic pathophysiology of ischemia and central fibrosis are key to all; however, the presence of intravascular occlusive changes with preservation of the original vascular wall is more likely present in VOD and the Budd-Chiari syndrome than in cardiac sclerosis. Correlation of the histologic findings with a history of cardiac disease, bone marrow transplantation with combined therapy, or thrombotic disorders is usually necessary to confirm the diagnosis. As discussed in the previous section, alcohol toxicity is a more common cause of central fibrosis; it usually has a more pericellular pattern of fibrosis and lacks the congestion and the compression of the cell plates that are often seen in vascular outflow lesions.

Chronic Hepatitis and Cirrhosis

The findings pertinent to the diagnosis of cirrhosis due to chronic hepatitis are discussed in detail in the section on Chronic Hepatitis and Tables 9–3, 9–4, and 9–5.

Biliary Tract Disease

Cirrhoses resulting from biliary tract disorders such as primary biliary cirrhosis (PBC), sclerosing cholangitis (primary or secondary), inflammatory changes associated with idiopathic inflammatory bowel disease, and duct obstruction (localized smaller duct versus large duct obstruction) show a spectrum of common histologic findings in their early stages. These changes, together with the clinical and laboratory findings (especially disproportionately elevated levels of alkaline phosphatase), are used to differentiate these lesions from chronic hepatitis (Tables 9–3 and 9–4). Because biliary disease primarily damages the portal tracts, the cirrhosis frequently appears to have a "jigsaw" pattern. That is, the portal-portal bridging fibrosis at low-power light microscopy separates anastomosing bands of hepatocytes. Distinctive, isolated, rounded cirrhotic nodules are not typical, and regeneration with rosette formation or numerous double cell plates is often not prominent. The central veins are either not involved in the fibrotic process or become involved late in the course

Table 9–2. Central Sclerosis

	Cardiac	Alcoholic
Sinusoidal dilatation	Yes	No
Compressed liver plates	Yes	No
Inflammation at edge of lesion	Yes	±
Cholestasis at edge of lesion	++	±
Pigmented macrophages	+++	±
Central necrosis	+++	±
Ballooned hepatocytes	±	+++

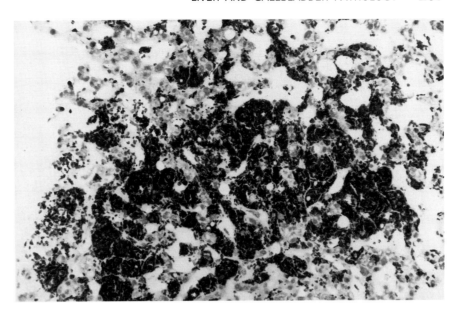

FIGURE 9–3. Cardiac-related ischemia with replacement of hepatocytes by erythrocytes within the confines of the original cell plates. (H&E, ×25)

of the disease, so central-portal relationships are minimally distorted. Chronic cholestatic disorders are also associated with the accumulation of copper in the periportal hepatocytes, which can be visualized with copper stains. The orcein (Fig. 9–4) or Victoria blue stains can also be used effectively. These probably do not stain the copper itself, but rather react with the copper-associated protein; and the staining in each correlates well with quantitative copper measurements in the tissue. Periportal Mallory body formation occurs in chronic, severe, cholestatic disorders and is, perhaps, related to the copper deposition. Bile duct damage of any kind can result in cholangiolar proliferation, portal tract inflammation with neutrophils around the cholangioles, and disruption of the terminal plate by mononuclear inflammatory cells, sometimes referred to as "ductular piecemeal necrosis" (Fig. 9–5).

DIFFERENTIAL DIAGNOSIS. A common difficulty for pathologists lies in distinguishing early biliary disease from mild chronic hepatitis. The inflammation in the periportal zones seen in biliary disease can mimic the disruption of the limiting plate and the piecemeal necrosis of chronic active hepatitis (or chronic hepatitis with mild to moderate inflammatory activity). Ductular piecemeal necrosis usually differs from the piecemeal necrosis of chronic active hepatitis in that while the periportal hepatocytes are surrounded by inflammatory cells, they are usually normal histologically, especially in less cholestatic states, and display no significant swelling, necrosis,

or rosette formation. In addition, the mononuclear cells in ductular piecemeal necrosis do not seem to cuff or encircle the hepatocytes, and the fibrosis does not form thin, holly-leaf like extensions into the nodule as seen in chronic hepatitis.

Other significant problems arise when attempting to differentiate one type of biliary disorder from another. Although many of these disorders have several common features, many other features are unique to the individual lesions and can be used to distinguish one from another. **Sepsis** (so-called cholangitis lenta)[16] produces proliferations of dilated cholangioles containing bile at the periphery of the portal tract in the periportal zone (Fig. 9–6). Features unique to **bile duct obstruction** are bile lakes and infarcts. Bile plugs in canaliculi are a feature of duct obstruction, including large duct obstruction in primary sclerosing cholangitis (PSC), but it is generally not a feature of PBC until late in the course of the disease. Loss of interlobular bile ducts (those located in the small portal tracts adjacent to the arteriole) is a feature of both PBC (Fig. 9–7) and PSC. Increased numbers of mononuclear cells in the sinusoids and spotty hepatocyte necrosis with a hepatitis-like appearance,[17] portal-based, periductal granulomas (see Fig. 9–7), and microgranulomas in the parenchyma are features typical of **PBC** (Table 9–5), especially in the earlier stages. In contrast, **PSC** is usually associated with periductular fibrosis around small and large ducts, with eventual loss of ducts and replacement by a hyalinized scar[18,19] (Fig. 9–8). Thus, a peripheral core biopsy of primary sclerosing cholangitis can show a

Table 9–3. **Biliary Tract Disease (BTD) versus Chronic Active Hepatitis (CAH)**

	BTD	CAH
Disruption of terminal plate ("piecemeal")	++	++
Cholangiolar proliferation	+++	+
Periportal copper deposition	++	−
Periportal hepatocyte rosettes	±	++
Pericellular mononuclear cuffing	±	++
Holly-leaf pattern of fibrosis	±	++
Cholestasis with bile plugs	DO	−
Bile infarcts, bile lakes	LBDO	−

DO, duct obstruction; LBDO, large bile duct obstruction.

Table 9–4. **Primary Biliary Cirrhosis (PBC) versus Chronic Active Hepatitis (CAH)**

	PBC	CAH
Granulomas, portal	++	−
Microgranulomas, parenchymal	++	−
Loss of interlobular ducts	+++	−
Increased sinusoidal mononuclears	+++	±
Lymphoid aggregates	++	+
Plasma cells	++	+
Cholestasis (bile plugs)	rare	rare, periportal
Mallory bodies	rare, periportal	−

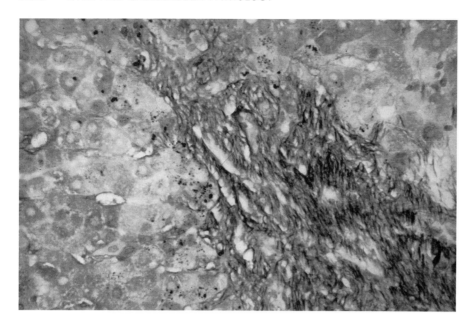

FIGURE 9–4. Primary biliary cirrhosis, orcein stain, showing black granularity of hepatocytes in periportal zone, representing copper-associated protein. (Orcein stain, ×75)

combination of findings, including reduced numbers of ducts, scarring around small ducts, and/or evidence of large bile duct obstruction such as bile lakes or infarcts (when large duct obstruction has occurred), cholestasis, and/or bile ductular proliferation with pericholangitis. In addition, PSC is likely to be a predisposing factor for the development of adenocarcinoma in the liver hilum or upper portion of the extrahepatic ducts,[20] which could also cause findings consistent with large duct obstruction on peripheral core biopsy. The large hilar ducts can also be involved with an active inflammatory process, ulceration, exudation, bile inspissation,[19] and xanthomatous reaction. Laboratory and clinical data can help differentiate PBC from PSC (see Table 9–5).

A newly described entity very similar to PBC is **primary autoimmune cholangitis,** also called autoimmune cholangiopathy.[21–23] This disease may affect women more than men, clinically presents with pruritus, and is associated with other autoimmune manifestations such as arthralgias, sicca syndrome, and Raynaud's phenomenon. However, the antimitochondrial antibody (AMA) is negative and the antinuclear antibody (ANA) is positive, as seen in autoimmune chronic hepatitis. The histopathologic aberrations include ductopenia with bile duct damage similar to that seen in PBC, mild chronic active hepatitis-like portal changes, and bile ductular proliferation.[21, 22] Some descriptions of this entity note the absence of granulomas and the similarities to autoimmune hepatitis,[21, 22] but others note that granulomas may be present and suggest that the entity is more likely a variant of AMA-negative PBC.[23]

Other lesions that can cause obliteration of bile ducts and lead to subsequent cirrhosis include biliary atresia in infants, liver transplant rejection, sarcoidosis, long-standing obstruction or cholangitis, and severe suppurative cholangitis. With **long-standing obstruction or cholangitis,** periductal fibrosis or even the rare disappearance of small ducts can occur, mimicking the small duct lesions of PSC.[19] In **suppurative**

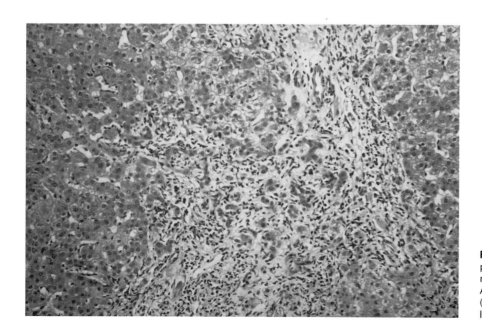

FIGURE 9–5. Primary biliary cirrhosis with prominent portal mononuclear inflammation and disruption of limiting plate. Also note the loss of interlobular bile duct (artery, *upper right*) and prominent ductular proliferation. (H&E, ×25)

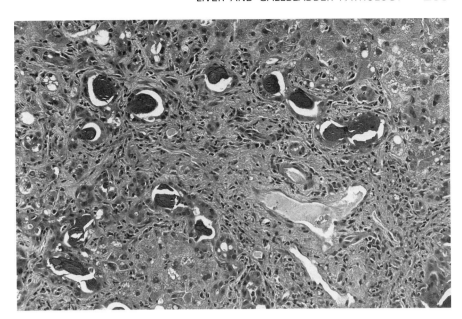

FIGURE 9–6. Sepsis with proliferation and dilation of bile-containing cholangioles in the outer portion of the portal tract. The interlobular duct is not involved. (H&E, ×50)

cholangitis, the larger ducts can be destroyed and replaced by fibrous scars or atretic ducts, again mimicking PSC in late stages. With **sarcoidosis,** the granulomas can coalesce and produce a considerable scar reaction and well-developed reticulin network, suggesting a chronic, organizing process. Nodules of scar can be seen at sites of "healed" granulomas (Fig. 9–9). There is no obvious centering of the granulomas around the ducts, and other types of inflammatory cells are usually few in number. Entities that cause bile duct damage, but which probably do not lead to biliary cirrhosis, include graft-versus-host disease and hepatitis C.

Hepatitis

The diagnosis of hepatitis can be problematic. Because acute hepatitis is not often seen on biopsies, features that can help to differentiate acute from chronic hepatitis are not well known to many pathologists. Most of the biopsies are done to identify chronic hepatitis, and perhaps to grade its level of activity. Thus, the pathologist must be able to differentiate acute from chronic hepatitis, must know when the sample is insufficient or non-diagnostic, and must be able to differentiate hepatitis from other lesions that can mimic it.

Hepatitis can be classified in two main ways: by etiologic agent and by the type of clinical syndrome. Because the morphologic appearances of the various forms of hepatitis are quite similar for many causative agents (Tables 9–6 and 9–7), the pathologist usually needs the clinical history and specific laboratory studies in order to identify a likely cause. Thus, it probably makes more sense for the pathologist to approach the classifications of hepatitis in the setting of clinical syndromes.

Acute Hepatitis

ACUTE VIRAL HEPATITIS. The diagnosis of typical acute viral hepatitis with spotty necrosis is usually a straightforward matter. Such lesions predominantly contain diffuse sinusoidal and portal mononuclear infiltrates (lymphocytes, plasma cells,

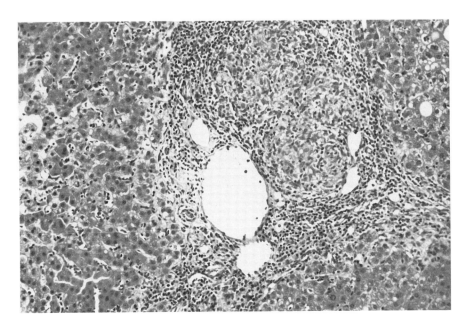

FIGURE 9–7. Primary biliary cirrhosis with portal granuloma and loss of interlobular bile duct. The lymphocytic infiltrate also is present in the sinusoids, mimicking hepatitis. (H&E, ×25)

Table 9–5. **Primary Biliary Cirrhosis (PBC)/ Primary Sclerosing Cholangitis (PSC)**

	PBC	PSC
Similarities		
Disappearing bile ducts		
Chronic inflammatory infiltration		
"Ductular piecemeal"		
Periportal Mallory bodies and copper		
Histology		
Granulomas, bile duct	+++	±
Granulomas, parenchymal	+++	±
Lymphoid aggregates	+++	+
Sinusoidal infiltrate	+++	±
Scarring at bile duct	+	++
Concentric fibrosis	±	++
Portal tracts without ducts	+++	+
Lesions of LBDO	No	Yes
Laboratory/Clinical		
History of UC/Crohn's	−	++
AMA	+++	±
ANA, DSDNA, SMAb	+	±
↑ IgM	+++	−
↑ Alkaline phosphatase	++	++
ERCP findings	+	+++
Long indolent course	+	+++

LBDO, large bile duct obstruction; UC, ulcerative colitis; AMA, antimitochondrial antibody; ANA, antinuclear antibody; DSDNA, double-stranded DNA; SMAb, smooth muscle antibody; ERCP, endoscopic retrograde cholangiopancreatography.

Kupffer cells), swollen hepatocytes, and/or necrotic hepatocytes (also called apoptotic, acidophilic, or Councilman bodies). There can be cholestasis, as evidenced by canalicular bile plugs, but this is not usually prominent except in the acute cholestatic varieties of hepatitis (see later discussion). Generally, low-power light microscopy reveals lobular disarray and increased cellularity. Cell plates and sinusoids may be indistinct in more severe cases as a result of hepatocyte swelling, filling of sinusoids by mononuclear inflammatory cells, and regeneration of hepatocytes. Some piecemeal necrosis as seen in chronic hepatitis may occur. More severe cases can also show prominent hepatocellular necrosis and reticulin condensation around the central vein (zone 3).

RESOLVING HEPATITIS. Although the diagnosis of typical acute hepatitis is relatively straightforward, that of resolving hepatitis can be more problematic. This lesion presents clinically as a late stage of acute hepatitis and so is usually not biopsied. Occasionally, however, a mild hepatitis is noticed on a biopsy from a patient with a subclinical infection of unknown duration; hence, a differential diagnosis consisting of acute, chronic, or resolving hepatitis arises. Also, because the residual histologic effects of a hepatitis seen in resolving stages can occasionally persist for more than 6 months, this lesion can be confused with chronic hepatitis. Thus, clinical follow-up with rebiopsy may be necessary if symptoms persist or the pathologic findings are not clear-cut.

Differential Diagnosis. Prolonged resolving acute hepatitis can be very difficult to distinguish histologically from mild chronic hepatitis. In resolving hepatitis, Kupffer cells with focal microgranulomas (or Kupffer cell nodules) are usually prominent within the sinusoids near central veins but can also be scattered throughout the liver parenchyma. These Kupffer cells may contain iron or lipochrome and are best demonstrated by the PAS digest (PASD) technique. Portal tract inflammation may not be as prominent, and early changes of fibrosis are usually not present as in chronic hepatitis, but both lesions may contain foci of spotty lobular necrosis. Also, residual centrilobular necrosis and inflammation are more prevalent in resolving hepatitis. Cases of severe chronic active hepatitis can have centrilobular necrosis, but these cases are usually not a diagnostic problem because they also display significant portal-based inflammatory changes, piecemeal necrosis, and fibrosis, indicating that the lesion is still quite active and chronic, rather than resolving.

ACUTE CHOLESTATIC HEPATITIS. An unusual form of acute hepatitis is the acute cholestatic variant. This lesion is rarely seen in any of the hepatitides, but when it is, it is usually due to **hepatitis A virus (HAV) or, in endemic areas, hepatitis**

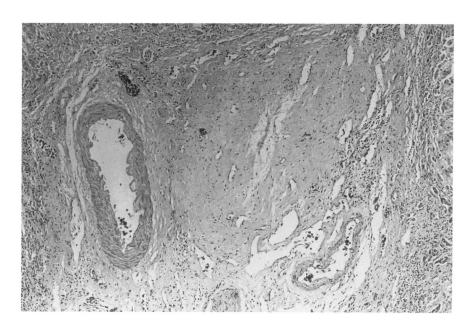

FIGURE 9–8. Primary sclerosing cholangitis with hyaline scar to the right of the large artery at site of previous medium-sized duct. (H&E, ×10)

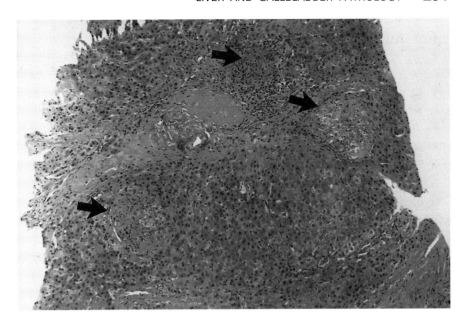

FIGURE 9–9. Sarcoidosis of liver with several epithelioid granulomas *(arrows)* and fibrosis, with focal dense hyaline scar. (H&E, ×25)

E. This pattern of injury mimics obstructive jaundice with bile ductular proliferation, pericholangitis (neutrophils around ducts), and cholestasis. Hepatocyte swelling (ballooning) can be prominent, and "pseudoglands" can form around bile plugs.

Differential Diagnosis. Acute cholestatic hepatitis can be differentiated histologically from obstruction by the presence of necrotic hepatocytes, which are not present in obstruction. The patient's HAV status and results of biliary imaging studies to exclude obstruction would also be important factors to consider in the diagnosis.

ACUTE HEPATITIS WITH SUBMASSIVE OR MASSIVE NECROSIS. Acute hepatitis can present with submassive or massive necrosis in which confluent necrosis extends from portal to portal zone or from portal to central zone (bridging necrosis), usually with an inflammatory reaction similar to typical acute hepatitis (see earlier) when caused by a hepatotropic virus. Submassive cases predominantly involve centrilobular zones (zone 3 of the liver acinus) but can involve the midzonal regions (zone 2 of the liver acinus). The pattern of injury depends on when during the disease course the biopsy is obtained. In early stages, hepatocyte necrosis with replacement by Kupffer cells and fibrin is seen, but the underlying reticulin framework remains intact. Later in the course, regeneration occurs in the zones with preserved hepatocytes (usually the better-oxygenated zone, such as the periportal zone 1 of the liver acinus), leading to the formation of nodules that compress the residual reticular framework; this stage should not be confused with cirrhosis. Trichrome stain reveals the lack of significant, dense collagen deposition, and the reticulin stain demonstrates the collapse of the reticulin framework in these necrotic zones. Subsequently, regeneration may be inhibited, probably as a result of compression of the original residual framework and early scar formation. These later regenerative stages are often called subacute hepatic necrosis, and the regenerative nodules should not be confused with the nodules of long-standing cirrhosis. Obviously, correlation with the time course of the disease can help avoid this error.

Table 9–6. **Hepatotropic Hepatitis Viruses**

Type	Old Name	Clinical Presentation	Specific Histology	Diagnostic Tests
A	Infectious hepatitis agent	AH, ACH, SN, MN, NH, no chronic hepatitis	↑ Plasma cells, ↑ periportal damage, cholestasis±	Anti-HAV IgM or IgG
B	Serum hepatitis agent	AH, SN, MN, NH, chronic hepatitis, cirrhosis, HCC	In chronic hepatitis, ground-glass cells, HBsAg + and HBcAg + on section	HBsAg, HBsAb, HBcAg, HBcAb, PCR
C	Transfusion-associated NANB hepatitis virus	AH, chronic hepatitis, cirrhosis, HCC (?SN,MN,NH)	Fatty change, prominent lymphoid nodules, bile duct inflammatory infiltrate	Anti-HCV IgG, PCR
D	δ agent	AH, SN, MN, chronic hepatitis, cirrhosis	Sometimes microvesicular fat	Anti-δ antigen IgG
E	Enteric NANB hepatitis virus	AH, ACH, others?, no chronic hepatitis	Cholestasis and ↑ PMNs, possible fat	Electron microscopy on tissue

AH, acute hepatitis; ACH, acute cholestatic hepatitis; SN, submassive necrosis; MN, massive necrosis; NH, neonatal hepatitis; HCC, hepatocellular carcinoma; PCR, polymerase chain reaction; NANB, non-A, non-B; PMN, polymorphonuclear neutrophil leukocyte.

Table 9–7. **Non-viral Causes of Hepatitis**

Type	Clinical Presentation	Histology
Drug reaction	Acute or chronic hepatitis	Similar to hepatotropic viruses
Autoimmune	Chronic active hepatitis; can be rapidly progressive	Similar to hepatotropic viruses
Wilson's disease	Acute, including fulminant; chronic active hepatitis	Similar to hepatotropic viruses; copper deposits
Alpha-1-antitrypsin deficiency	Chronic active hepatitis (unusual finding)	Similar to hepatotropic viruses; alpha-1-antitrypsin globules
?Alcoholism	Chronic active hepatitis (may be due to HCV or HBV)	Similar to hepatotropic viruses

Acute hepatitis with massive necrosis usually exhibits extensive involvement, including all zones, with the possible exception of the periportal regions (zone 1). The surviving cells in zone 1 may attempt to proliferate, often in the form of ductules or pseudoglands. The remaining parenchyma is filled with necrotic hepatocytes and/or Kupffer cells, the latter containing lipochrome and cell debris. In early stages, the reticulin framework is intact, but it may partially collapse in later stages if the patient survives long enough. In livers removed at time of transplantation from patients with fulminant hepatic failure, large nodular zones of regeneration can be present, confirming that the extent of necrosis may vary from region to region. Thus, any given liver biopsy sample may not represent the organ's overall functional state and consequently may not be predictive of outcome.[24]

Differential Diagnosis. The major diagnostic problem in differentiating among these hepatitides is in the determination of the etiologic agent, because toxic/drug reactions and viral causes can appear histologically identical. A non-hepatotropic viral infection such as herpes simplex virus (HSV) should be excluded as a possible cause because it would be likely to recur soon after transplantation (see section on Non-hepatotropic Viral Infections).

NEONATAL HEPATITIS. Neonatal hepatitis due to viral agents is a unique form of acute hepatitis. Its morphologic features include cholestasis, giant cell transformation (usually most prominent around the central vein in zone 3), hepatocyte ballooning and necrosis, and sinusoidal and portal-based, predominantly mononuclear, inflammatory infiltrates. Portal fibrosis with some ductular proliferation as well as extramedullary hematopoiesis can also occur. The giant hepatocytes can persist for up to 6 months after the hepatitis has resolved (personal observation). Viral agents associated with neonatal hepatitis include the hepatotropic viruses as well as viruses such as cytomegalovirus (CMV), HSV, varicella, rubella, coxsackievirus, and echovirus. In addition, toxoplasmosis and treponema have also been noted to cause this giant cell hepatitis.

Differential Diagnosis. This lesion can pose diagnostic problems because non-viral causes of giant cell transformation are also commonly seen. The neonatal liver is unique in its capacity to form giant cells in response to any hepatocyte injury. The exact reason for their formation is unknown; perhaps infection or some other injury inhibits cell division. Regardless, giant cells are not specific for infectious causes of liver injury and can be seen frequently in metabolic or cholestatic disorders of the liver, especially in children younger than 1 year. Metabolic disorders associated with

a neonatal hepatitis–like morphology include **alpha-1-antitrypsin (AAT) deficiency,**[25, 26] **fructose intolerance,**[27] and **cortisol deficiency.**[28] The **extrahepatic biliary atresias** can also induce significant proliferations of giant cells as a result of cholestasis; but there should be more portal-based fibrosis, proliferations of bile ductules, and ductular cholestasis without evidence of significant loss of hepatocytes compared with viral hepatitis.

A hepatitis with giant cells has recently been described in association with infection by paramyxovirus;[29] however, giant cell formation is not pathognomonic for paramyxoviral infection.[30] When associated with paramyxovirus, the lesion has been termed ''syncytial giant cell hepatitis'' (or type G hepatitis) and can occur in any age group.[29] The giant cells are usually most prominent in zone 3 of the acinus. Fibrosis and lymphocytic portal inflammation are typical, and some cases show prominent plasma cell infiltrates similar to autoimmune hepatitis. Varying degrees of acinar inflammation, hepatocyte necrosis, rosette formation, and cholestasis can be present.[29]

Chronic Hepatitis

In the past, the term **chronic active hepatitis** (CAH) had been used only for patients who had known liver disease for more than 6 months with the classic histologic findings of portal-based inflammation, fibrosis, disruption of the terminal plate, and piecemeal necrosis. This lesion is now designated as **chronic hepatitis with piecemeal (periportal) necrosis,** with or without fibrosis. The periportal hepatocytic damage in this form of hepatitis probably stimulates regeneration, resulting in periportal hepatocyte rosettes (Fig. 9–10), or clusters of hepatocytes arranged in a circular manner. Ballooned hepatocytes and acidophilic bodies can also be seen in a periportal location. Many times, the mononuclear cells appear to form rings or ''cuffs'' around the swollen hepatocytes. An occasional necrotic hepatocyte (acidophilic body) can often be seen within the lobule. Collagen deposition occurs in the periportal zone, forming septa that extend into the lobule in a holly-leaf pattern (see Table 9–3). Ductular proliferation may be present but is usually not prominent except in the more severe, aggressive lesions. When ductular proliferation is present, neutrophils may be present in the periductal inflammatory infiltrate. The lesions with piecemeal necrosis are thought to more likely progress to cirrhosis, especially if the process shows bridging or confluent necrosis between the central vein and the portal zone.[31–33]

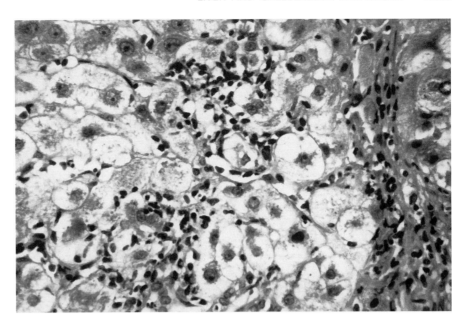

FIGURE 9–10. Chronic active hepatitis with disruption of limiting plate by inflammatory cell infiltrate, swollen hepatocytes, and mononuclear cuffing around hepatocytes. (H&E, ×100)

Chronic persistent hepatitis (CPH) has been used to describe those lesions of chronic hepatitis with no significant periportal necrosis or regeneration but that, nonetheless, had a fairly dense mononuclear portal infiltrate. This lesion is now referred to as **chronic hepatitis without piecemeal necrosis.** Frequently, acidophilic bodies could be seen within the lobule rather than in the periportal zone.

Chronic lobular hepatitis (CLH)[34] was a term infrequently used to describe a form of mild chronic hepatitis that consisted of persistent parenchymal focal hepatocyte necrosis (apoptosis) with mononuclear sinusoidal infiltrates. This lesion is now called **chronic hepatitis without piecemeal necrosis.** CLH mimics mild acute hepatitis in its degree of cell necrosis, but the condition persists longer than 6 months. No bridging necrosis or periportal piecemeal necrosis is present. Because this nomenclature was not readily in use, such lesions had been referred to as CPH with prominent lobular activity.

Another uncommon variant of chronic hepatitis is **chronic septal hepatitis.** Lesions of this type show portal inflammation and fibrous septa but no piecemeal necrosis.[35] Thus, the inflammatory component would suggest CPH, but the fibrosis would suggest a more progressive lesion. This lesion would now be classified as **chronic hepatitis with fibrosis,** and it may represent a stage of CAH in regression, that is quiescent, or that is being treated with immunosuppressive or antiviral therapy. Clinical history and pathologic correlation are important for making this diagnosis.

As noted earlier, the classifications for the two major types of chronic hepatitis, chronic active and chronic persistent hepatitis, as well as the less popular term chronic lobular hepatitis, are now falling into disfavor.[36–38] After the establishment of the old nomenclature,[39, 40] new discoveries were made about the ability of hepatitis B virus (HBV)[41–43] and hepatitis C virus (HCV)[36] to wax and wane in such a manner that an initial diagnosis of CPH might actually develop into end-stage cirrhosis despite a favorable histologic diagnosis. Sampling errors can also contribute to misclassification because foci of necrosis can vary from portal zone to portal zone and any one biopsy may contain more or less necrosis than the remaining

unbiopsied liver tissue. Thus, to base a diagnosis on a single biopsy sample can lead to a misjudgment of the patient's prognosis. Also, the chronic hepatitis of HCV is often very mild. Frequently, even after evaluation of multiple sections, only limited piecemeal necrosis can be seen, so it is very difficult to classify these lesions as either CPH or mild CAH. Yet, with the advent of antiviral therapies for these diseases, more detailed analysis by the pathologist of the severity of the lesions may be needed in order to justify or follow the clinical and histologic response to antiviral therapy. For these reasons, it has been recommended that the CAH/CPH nomenclature be replaced by the more simple terminology of "chronic hepatitis,"[36–38] with the addition of a grading of activity of the hepatitis based on the degree of inflammation, piecemeal or bridging necrosis, and fibrosis[38, 44–46] and including the etiologic agent or cause, if known (Table 9–8). It should be noted that this new scheme includes not only chronic viral and autoimmune hepatitis, but also chronic hepatitis of drug-related or unknown cause, biliary lesions such as PBC, PSC, and autoimmune cholangitis[21] that are similar histologically to chronic hepatitis, Wilson's hepatitis, and alpha-1-antitrypsin deficiency; thus, the term *chronic* is not always applied. In addition, when scoring for portal and lobular inflammatory activity, if the scores are not the same, the more severe score should be used.

DIFFERENTIAL DIAGNOSIS. Unfortunately, the various causes of the chronic hepatitides (see Tables 9–6 and 9–7) can be difficult to distinguish. It is, therefore, very important to correlate clinical information with the pathologic findings. Obviously, the serologic data now available on **HAV, HBV, HCV, and HDV** can be used to identify the viral infections, and autoimmune antibody assays can be used to identify **autoimmune hepatitis** (see later). Other clinical tests can be done to determine the presence of **Wilson's disease or alpha-1-antitrypsin deficiency.** Drug histories should also be investigated to exclude **drugs** as etiologic agents.

Although the histologic patterns of the various chronic hepatitides overlap significantly, some histologic features can help suggest a specific diagnosis. For example, in **hepatitis**

Table 9–8. **Proposal for an Updated Terminology of Chronic Hepatitis**

	Grade of Inflammatory Activity			Stage/Degree of Fibrosis	
Grade	*Portal*	*Lobular*	*Stage*	*Degree of Fibrosis*	
0	None or minimal	None	1	No fibrosis, or confined to enlarged portal tracts	
1	Inflammation	Inflammation without necrosis	2	Periportal fibrosis or portal-portal septa; intact architecture	
2	Mild limiting plate (LP) necrosis	Focal necrosis or acidophilic bodies	3	Septal fibrosis, architectural distortion; no cirrhosis	
3	Moderate LP necrosis	Severe focal necrosis	4	Probable or definite cirrhosis	
4	Severe LP necrosis	Bridging necrosis			

Adapted from Ludwig J: The nomenclature of chronic active hepatitis: An obituary. Gastroenterology 105:274–278, 1993.

A (acute hepatitis), zone 1 (periportal) hepatocytes are more susceptible to injury than those of zone 3, and prominent portal and periportal inflammation with numerous plasma cells can occur.[47, 48] The lack of fibrosis can help differentiate acute hepatitis A from chronic hepatitis with moderate to severe activity.

In **HBV** infections, ground-glass cells containing hepatitis B surface antigen (HBsAg) can be seen on H&E-stained sections, and the presence of HBsAg can be confirmed by positive staining with an immunoperoxidase or orcein stain. HBV can also be identified by immunohistochemical staining for the hepatitis B core antigen (HBcAg) (Fig. 9–11). The staining reaction can vary, depending on sample size and stage of disease. For example, in acute hepatitis, surface antigen staining is usually negative, as the infected cells are effectively cleared from the liver.[49] The positive staining is instead seen in chronic hepatitis, in which the viral proliferation outstrips the immune clearance.[50] Likewise, in late-stage chronic hepatitis or in long-term healthy carriers, HBsAg can be present, but not HBcAg.[49] This is probably because the viral genome is incorporated into nuclear DNA so that HBsAg is coded for, but viral DNA is not. HBcAg is often positive in immuno-compromised patients, and the presence of HBcAg in the cytoplasm of hepatocytes may suggest replication of HBV.[49]

HCV is thought to induce a milder form of disease and to produce more bile duct damage, lymphocyte infiltration of the parenchyma, and reactive changes in the duct epithelium than does HBV (Fig. 9–12). The duct damage is not thought to be severe enough to cause duct loss or cirrhosis. Additionally, lymphocytic aggregates in the portal zones (Fig. 9–13) and fatty change of hepatocytes are more frequent than with HBV.[51–54] At the time of writing of this chapter, immunoperoxidase techniques for staining paraffin-embedded tissues for HCV were not commercially available.

Delta hepatitis can be superimposed on hepatitis B as either acute or chronic clinical exacerbations of disease.[55–57] Submassive or massive hepatic necrosis can occur;[58] thus, delta hepatitis should be suspected in any patient with chronic hepatitis B that suddenly flares up significantly. With HDV, the necro-inflammatory activity of the process is often more pronounced than that seen with HCV or HBV.

Autoimmune forms of hepatitis (AIH) have now been subclassified into three forms characterized by differences in the clinical presentations or the antibodies found.[59, 60] Most

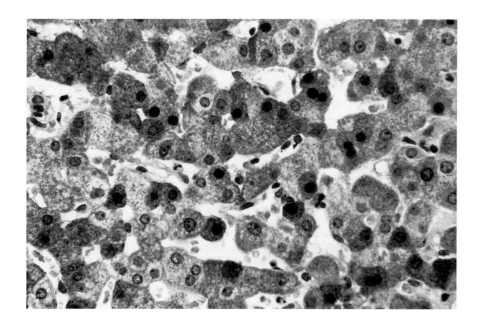

FIGURE 9–11. Hepatitis B core antigen. Immunoperoxidase staining shows nuclear and cytoplasmic positivity (darkly staining cells and nuclei) in a patient with minimal H&E changes of hepatitis. (Immunoperoxidase stain for hepatitis B core antigen, ×83)

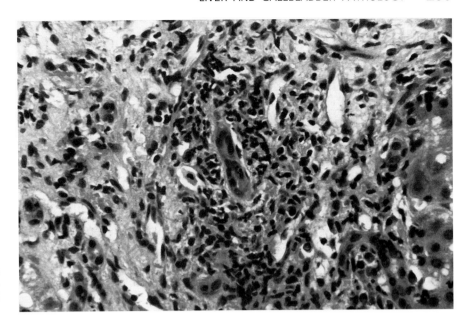

FIGURE 9–12. Chronic active hepatitis C with mononuclear inflammation of inter-lobular bile duct and bile duct epithelial damage. (H&E, ×75)

patients respond favorably to immunosuppressive therapy, with a resultant decrease in the activity of the disease, so the distinction from viral hepatitis or chronic hepatitis due to other causes is important. **Classic type 1 AIH**[59, 60] presents the typical profile of a predominantly female disease occurring primarily from ages 10 to 15 and 45 to 70 years, with positive antinuclear antibody (ANA) titers and some association (approximately 10%) with other autoimmune disorders such as arthralgias and thyroid disease. **Type 2 AIH**[59, 60] seems to present more in children and is frequently associated with other autoimmune disorders (approximately 17%) as well. The anti–liver-kidney microsomal (LKM) antibody is present in these patients, who often present with the clinical picture of acute or fulminant hepatitis. The most recently described variant, **type 3,**[59, 60] also occurs mostly in women, but with later onset. Approximately 25% of these patients have anti-soluble liver antigen (SLA) only. These patients are seronega-

tive for ANA and LKM antibody, but 75% have anti-smooth muscle antibody (SMA) or liver membrane antibody (LMA). In contrast to types 1 and 2, systemic autoimmune manifestations are not typical.

AIH often displays the prominent lymphoid aggregates and duct damage as seen with HCV hepatitis; however, patients with AIH seem to have more diffuse and severe peicemeal necrosis, an increased incidence of bridging and confluent necrosis, and more rapid progression to cirrhosis.[61] In addition, infiltration of mononuclear inflammatory cells tends to be diffuse with AIH and focal with chronic HCV.[61] Plasma cells are usually more prominent in AIH than in HCV.

Other types of chronic hepatitis can have rather characteristic, but not necessarily diagnostic, features. The finding of copper deposits would be necessary to make a diagnosis of **Wilson's disease**; but since these deposits may be focal, a liver core biopsy may not sample them. **Alpha-1-antitrypsin**

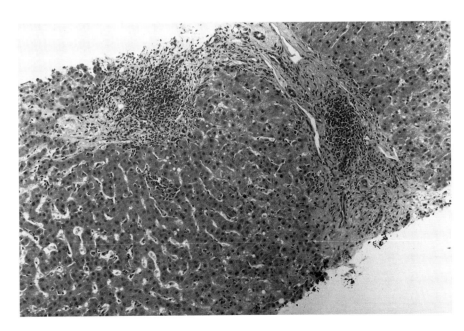

FIGURE 9–13. Chronic active hepatitis C with lymphoid aggregates in portal zones. (H&E, ×33)

(AAT) disease should have eosinophilic globules in periportal zones. PAS digest and AAT immunoperoxidase stains are good for confirming the nature of the globules. Large numbers of AAT globules have also been noted in alcohol-associated disease[62] and with other disorders,[63] so phenotyping is necessary for definitive diagnosis. **Alcohol** may or may not produce a CAH-like picture. Recent studies of alcoholics[64–66] have shown that a large percentage of these patients (possibly 30%) also have HCV antibodies and are positive for HCV by the polymerase chain reaction (PCR). Because typical alcoholic injury involves minimal inflammatory activity, the presence of considerable mononuclear inflammation and the absence of diagnostic evidence of alcohol damage may indicate that a viral infection is the cause of the liver injury.

CAH can also be difficult to distinguish from PBC (see section on Biliary Cirrhosis and Tables 9–3 and 9–4) and resolving acute hepatitis (see section on Acute Hepatitis).

Exacerbations, or sporadic rises in the quantities of liver enzymes, are commonly seen in patients with chronic hepatitis. These exacerbations have been associated with increased hepatocyte necrosis on biopsy, and usually the presence of portal-based fibrosis is the most reliable histologic feature to identify an exacerbation of a chronic disease. The clinical history and/or serum markers may be needed, however, to distinguish this lesion from a *de novo* acute hepatitis. It has been well documented that HBV and HCV can both wax and wane;[41–43, 67] thus, a diagnosis of CPH may not assure the patient of a favorable outcome. Some exacerbations in type B infections can be due to the delta agent (see Table 9–6).[55–58] Other exacerbations of chronic hepatitis could possibly be due to mixed infection of HBV and HCV,[68] or to HAV or CMV superimposed on chronic HBV or HCV.[36, 42] However, more recent studies have also shown that mixed infections of HBV and HCV tend to behave clinically as HBV infection alone.[69, 70]

DIFFERENTIAL DIAGNOSIS OF NON-HEPATOTROPIC VIRAL INFECTIONS. The herpes viruses account for most of the other viral infections of the liver (Table 9–9). **HSV** and **CMV** both can cause acute hepatitis, but, in our experience, HSV is more likely than CMV to cause submassive or massive necrosis. There is usually minimal chronic inflammatory reaction, because these viruses cause a cytopathic form of injury in severe cases. Usually these infections are seen only in immunocompromised patients, neonates, or pregnant women,[71] but they have been rarely seen in immunocompetent patients as well.[72–74] In cases with extensive necrosis, the virus can usually be identified by light microscopy by the presence of inclusion bodies. Definitive confirmation can be made with ultrastructural or immunoperoxidase techniques. The milder forms of hepatitis may or may not have inclusions. CMV is a much more frequent cause of a mild hepatitis, which consists of spotty, focal hepatocyte necrosis. The necrosis can involve multiple hepatocytes at one site, but there is no zonal preference. Kupffer cell hyperplasia and granulomas can be associated with the necrosis. Portal mononuclear infiltrates can also be present.

Epstein-Barr virus (EBV) can cause an infectious mononucleosis syndrome in immunocompetent or immunocompromised hosts (see later). In the liver, these infections can produce a dense, portal, lymphocytic infiltrate, increased numbers of lymphocytes in the sinusoids, and foci of mild hepatocellular necrosis.[75] The lymphocytes can look somewhat atypical, with enlarged nuclei and abundant cytoplasm. Inclusions are not seen, but granulomas can be present.

Liver Dysfunction in the Immunocompromised Patient

In immunocompromised patients, acute and chronic hepatitides can be caused by different agents and have a different histologic presentation than in normal individuals. In profoundly immunocompromised patients, such as those with **human immunodeficiency virus (HIV),** the **hepatotropic viruses** do not appear to cause significant injury. Homosexuals and intravenous drug abusers have increased incidence of **HBV** *and* **HCV** infections, but when HIV is superimposed,

Table 9–9. **Other Viruses Causing Hepatitis**

Type	Clinical Setting	Clinical Presentation	Specific Viral Light Microscopic Findings	Histologic Features
CMV	Infectious mononucleosis; fairly common in IC individuals	Infectious mononucleosis, IC, acute hepatitis	Cytomegaly, nuclear and cytoplasmic inclusions; immunoperoxidase stain	IC—Patchy parenchymal necrosis; ±mononuclear infiltrate of portal tracts; PMN abcesses
HSV	Increased in IC patients, pregnant women	Often acute fulminant liver failure	Intranuclear inclusions, ground-glass nuclei; immunoperoxidase stain	IC—Confluent necrosis
EBV	Infectious mononucleosis, IC host	Infectious mononucleosis	*In situ* hybridization	Minimal single cell necrosis; ↑ sinusoidal mononuclears; portal tract mononuclears; atypical lymphocytes
Adenovirus	Extremely rare	Fulminant liver failure	Intranuclear inclusions, smudge cells; immunoperoxidase stain	Focal or extensive confluent necrosis

CMV, cytomegalovirus; IC, immunocompromised; PMN, polymorphonuclear neutrophil leukocytes; HSV, herpes simplex virus; EBV, Epstein-Barr virus.

no significant hepatitis occurs. Rare exceptions do occur, but these might be due to a cytopathic event in which the virus directly kills the hepatocytes, rather than depending on a host immunologic response to kill the infected liver cell.

Hepatitis B and C can occur in **less-severely compromised individuals,** such as transplant patients or those receiving chemotherapy. HBV is usually a more significant clinical problem in liver transplant patients than is HCV, because nearly all patients who receive a transplant because of chronic hepatitis B develop recurrent infection in the graft.[76] Many of these infections can progress to cirrhosis. Uncommonly, the infection can be rapidly progressive, resembling submassive necrosis.[77] In these more severe cases, cytopathic changes of hepatocyte swelling (ballooning) and necrosis occur associated with a diminished inflammatory response, which suggests a component of direct viral killing. In addition, a fibrosing, cholestatic variant of HBV with large numbers of ground-glass cells, hepatocyte ballooning, and only a mild, mixed inflammatory reaction has been described.[78–80] Recurrent post-transplant HCV is usually manifested as a mild form of chronic hepatitis; however, an aggressive hepatitis that progresses rapidly to cirrhosis can also occur.[81–83] At times, the HCV infection may also present with a component hepatocyte swelling (often centrilobular) or necrosis without significant inflammation,[82] mimicking an ischemic or toxic reaction.

The **non-hepatotropic viruses,** which cause more direct cytopathic damage to hepatocytes, often cause significant problems in immunocompromised patients (see Table 9–9). **CMV** is probably the most common viral infection affecting these patients. It typically causes a mild hepatitis that can progress to fatal systemic infection if not treated early. The CMV infection usually causes spotty necrosis with sinusoidal aggregates of neutrophils (microabscesses)[84, 85] or Kupffer cell hyperplasia. Viral inclusions are frequently seen, not only in association with the neutrophil collections but also as isolated findings in the parenchyma, bile duct, or endothelial cells of the sinusoids.[85] CMV can mimic HBV or HCV when inclusions or microabscesses are absent;[82] however, culture for CMV, immunostaining for HBcAg, or PCR for HCV can help distinguish these lesions histologically. Immunostaining for

CMV can also increase the diagnostic accuracy[85] but for practical purposes is not necessary because anti-CMV therapy is usually begun on immunocompromised patients even if the histologic findings are only suspicious for CMV and no definitive inclusions are immediately identifiable. Furthermore, if the infection responds to ganciclovir treatment, it is most likely CMV; persistence of disease suggests a hepatotropic viral infection. In liver transplant patients, CMV typically occurs earlier, at 3 to 5 weeks post-transplant, whereas HBV and HCV tend to occur usually no sooner than 2 months post-transplant.[78, 82]

EBV can cause infectious mononucleosis[86] as well as a post-transplant lymphoproliferative disorder,[87] which can usually be easily differentiated from mononucleosis syndrome by its more intense lymphoid infiltrate and the presence of atypical lymphocytes invading the lobule and expanding into portal zones. In addition, more prominent confluent necrosis can be seen.[87]

Other opportunistic infections, including a wide variety of fungal, parasitic, and bacterial organisms, can cause liver dysfunction in the immunocompromised host. *Mycobacterium tuberculosis* (Mtb) and *Mycobacterium avium complex* (MAI) infections are now being seen much more frequently in liver, especially in patients with acquired immunodeficiency syndrome (AIDS).[88–91] In AIDS patients (as in non-immunocompromised patients), Mtb in the liver usually presents as isolated, epithelioid, parenchymal granulomas.[92] Caseous necrosis can be present, and only a few organisms can be seen. In contrast, MAI in AIDS patients usually presents in the liver as collections of slighty foamy or striated-appearing histiocytes that are literally stuffed with acid-fast organisms, which are visible on Fite's stain.[88, 90, 91] Isolated Kupffer cells can also harbor the atypical mycobacterium.[88, 90]

Bacillary angiomatosis has been described in the liver.[93] This lesion mimics peliosis hepatis grossly and radiographically. Microscopically, the lesion more closely resembles vascular and edematous granulation tissue than peliosis hepatis, although foci of large dilated, blood-filled spaces are present (Fig. 9–14). The smaller lesions may appear on needle biopsy as loosely aggregated connective tissue containing a few small

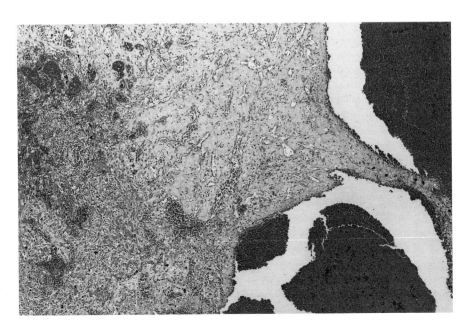

FIGURE 9–14. Bacillary angiomatosis with dilated blood-filled spaces and intervening loose connective tissue. Residual liver cells are in the lower left. (H&E, ×13)

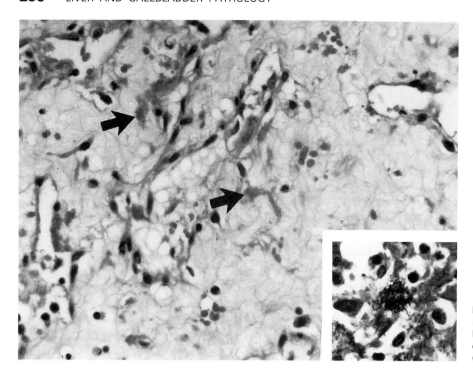

FIGURE 9–15. Bacillary angiomatosis. Loose connective tissue component with blue bodies *(arrows)* consisting of clumps of bacilli on Warthin-Starry stain *(inset).* (H&E, ×100; *inset,* Warthin-Starry, ×132)

capillaries (Fig. 9–15). The typical small blue bodies (which Steiner or Warthin-Starry stains prove to be bacterial rods) should be visible on routine H&E stains (see Fig. 9–15).

Problems in the Diagnosis of Liver Tumors and Tumor-like Lesions

In general, the diagnosis of benign or malignant liver tumors is not a major problem for pathologists, especially when the diagnosis is made on a resection specimen. However, difficulties may arise when the biopsy samples are small, as with core or fine-needle aspiration (FNA) biopsies, or when it is necessary to distinguish between reactive processes and benign or malignant tumors of the same cell type. In these situations, it is important to know the most definitive criteria for making a diagnosis and to understand the pitfalls inherent in core or FNA biopsies so that the most appropriate diagnostic sample can be obtained.

Hepatocellular Tumors

Diagnostic problems usually arise when attempting to differentiate benign proliferative processes from well-differentiated, primary malignant lesions. To do this, it is first necessary to be aware of the usual differential diagnosis for lesions in cirrhotic livers versus non-cirrhotic livers (Table 9–10); thus, reliable information about the background liver is crucial. This information is best obtained by tissue biopsy, as radiographic findings and even a surgeon's impression of the gross appearance of the liver can be in error. Without such definitive information, it may be wise to exercise caution when making a diagnosis.

Hepatocellular Tumors in Cirrhotic Livers

In cirrhotic livers, a mass would most likely represent either a macroregenerative nodule (with or without fatty change)

or a hepatocellular carcinoma (see Table 9–10). Metastatic tumors rarely involve cirrhotic livers.[94] Large nodules with atypical features, such as being a different color from the background cirrhotic nodules (e.g., greener, paler, more yellow), irregular as opposed to uniformly rounded borders, or a tendency to expand or bulge when the initial cut is made through it, should raise suspicions of an early hepatocellular carcinoma (HCC). In addition, any nodule larger than 3 cm most likely represents a true neoplasm; however, a caveat to be aware of is that radiographically or by gross inspection multiple regenerative nodules may appear as a single large mass.

MACROREGENERATIVE NODULES. Macroregenerative nodules (MRN), often referred to as a form of adenomatous hyperplasia,[95–97] measure more than 0.8 cm in diameter and presumably represent regenerative foci of hepatocytes within a cirrhotic liver.[95, 98, 99] On light microscopic examination, MRNs maintain the cell plate architecture and reticulin framework of typical, smaller regenerative nodules, and the hepatocyte morphology is unremarkable (Fig. 9–16). MRNs usually contain portal tracts and central veins, and because they are so

Table 9–10. **Differential Diagnosis for Lesion in Liver, Hepatocellular Type**

With Cirrhosis	Without Cirrhosis
Macroregenerative nodule (MRN)	Adenomatous hyperplasia
Hepatocellular carcinoma (HCC)	Adenoma
	Focal nodular hyperplasia
Dysplasia	Fibrolamellar HCC
	Non-fibrolamellar HCC
Mimics Cirrhosis Clinically	**In Children Without Cirrhosis**
Nodular regenerative hyperplasia	Hepatoblastoma
Partial nodular transformation	Mesenchymal hamartoma

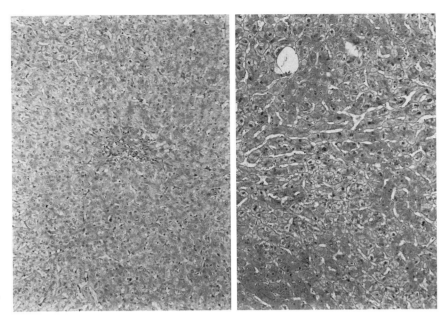

FIGURE 9–16. Macroregenerative nodule with bland cytologic features. H&E on left, reticulin on right, shows intact framework and architecture similar to other cirrhotic nodules. (*left,* H&E, ×25; *right,* Snook's reticulin, ×25)

large, a core biopsy may not reveal the fibrous bands that distinguish them from the rest of the cirrhotic liver; thus, a biopsy sample can resemble normal liver. A reticulin stain, however, may reveal double-layered cell plates and layers of reticulin fibers at the edge of the specimen fragments, both of which are features of cirrhotic nodules. MRNs can also contain increased iron stores,[100] bile, and Mallory bodies,[96, 98] and they may undergo fatty change.[98, 101]

Macroregenerative nodules with borderline or overt malignant changes have been much studied in Japan, where it is felt that the lesions can be preneoplastic or neoplastic,[97] especially when associated with cytologic atypia such as small-cell change (or dysplasia, see later), fat,[102] clear-cell change, or clusters of Mallory hyaline bodies.[96, 103–105] Of these atypical features, small-cell change appears to be a much greater risk factor than large-cell change (dysplasia) for progression to HCC (Table 9–11).[106–108] As the name implies, in small-cell change, the hepatocytes are considerably smaller than normal liver cells and appear as a zone of nuclear crowd-

ing[109] (Fig. 9–17, *right*) or increased nuclear density.[110] The cytoplasm may be more basophilic than in normal hepatocytes, but there is no significant nuclear atypia or enlargement. These smaller cells should be present in clusters rather than as isolated, single cells. Large-cell change (dysplasia),[109, 110] in comparison, consists of scattered foci within a cirrhotic liver of enlarged hepatocytes with large, often irregularly shaped nuclei and nucleoli but with a normal nucleocytoplasmic ratio (Fig. 9–17, *left*). Its preneoplastic nature has never been definitively proven.

BORDERLINE MACROREGENERATIVE NODULES. Borderline macroregenerative nodules,[110] also called atypical adenomatous hyperplasia,[97] type II MRN,[95] atypical macroregenerative nodules,[98] and **dysplastic nodules,** are those macronodules with atypical features not overtly diagnostic of malignancy, but with features of uncertain malignant potential. These nodules may have foci of fat, Mallory bodies, bile, iron, or clear-cell change. There may be foci of small-cell change, which can give an appearance of increased nuclear density in the

Table 9–11. **Diagnostic Features: Macroregenerative Nodules (MRN) versus Well-differentiated, Small Hepatocellular Carcinoma (HCC)**

Morphology	MRN and Borderline Nodule	HCC
Large-cell change	Common	Common
Nuclear density > 2 × normal (small-cell change)	Occasional small foci in borderline lesions	Common, large foci
Cell plates, zone ≥ 3 cells thick (trabecular)	None, rare in borderline lesions, no zones of trabeculae	Common pattern
Decrease or loss of reticulin	Uncommon, focal in borderline lesions	Common, extensive
Fibrous septa separating thick plates	None	Occasional pattern
Irregular, infiltrative edge	Sometimes present in borderline lesions	Occasional
Pseudoglands	Rare in borderline lesions	Occasional
Presence of portal zones	Usually present	None
Increased iron stores	Occasional	Almost always absent
Fatty change	Can be present	Can be present
Bile production	Can be present	Can be present
Mallory hyalin	Can be present	Can be present (clusters)

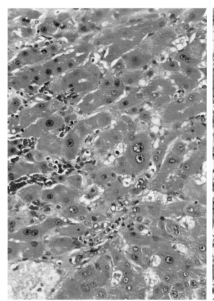 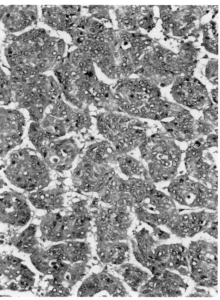

FIGURE 9–17. *Left,* **Large-cell change** in a cirrhotic liver. The larger nuclei are scattered among more normal cells. (H&E, ×50) *Right,* **Small-cell change** in a trabecular hepatocellular carcinoma, showing increased nuclear crowding. (H&E, ×50)

involved zone. In borderline lesions, the nuclear density can focally be up to twice normal without there being a significant concern for HCC.[110] Such nodules can also show more significant focal decreases in the reticulin framework, and liver cell plates may be up to three cells thick, but should not be arranged in uniform groups of trabeculae.[110] The edges of the nodules may protrude irregularly, and isolated gland-like structures (pseudoglands) may be present. Similar borderline foci can also be present in regenerative nodules of less than 0.8 cm diameter.

WELL-DIFFERENTIATED HCC. In well-differentiated HCC (see Table 9–11), cytologic atypia (small- or large-cell change) can be seen, as well as significant architectural abnormalities such as numerous trabeculae at least three cells thick that form zones of irregular cell plates (see Fig. 9–17, *right*).[110] If there are significant degrees of small-cell change present on H&E stain or a greater than two-fold increase in nuclear density, a reticulin stain should be used to examine for abnormal cell plate architecture.[110] Because benign nodules should have a well-developed reticulin framework, the lack of such strongly supports a diagnosis of carcinoma[102, 110] (Fig. 9–18). Angioinvasion may also be diagnostic for HCC, but this may not be evident on small samples or present in small lesions. Additionally, the presence of numerous pseudoglands is another feature usually indicative of carcinoma.[111] However, the most important diagnostic markers of HCC are the architectural features of irregular and thickened cell plates and loss of reticulin.

In some cases of well-differentiated HCC, fibrous septa separating the trabecular cell plates may be present. This has been referred to as the so-called **scirrhous variant of HCC**[102, 110] (Fig. 9–19). These septa stain strongly positive with reticulin, but the cell plates are usually greater than two cells thick as in the more typical trabecular-type lesions without fibrosis.

Differential Diagnosis. Distinguishing cases of well-differentiated HCC from a regenerative nodule can pose diagnostic problems for the pathologist, especially on FNA biopsies. The literature on this subject deals mostly with lesions

of moderate to poor differentiation, which are relatively straightforward.[112, 113] The main problems arise when the pathologist attempts to make the diagnosis on FNA of a well-differentiated hepatocellular lesion without making and examining a cell button preparation, which would allow for architectural evaluation by H&E and reticulin stains. On smears, architectural abnormalities such as abnormally thick trabeculae lined by endothelial cells can be easily disrupted or be difficult to distinguish from regenerative cell plates. Also, it may be impossible to determine whether the hepatocytes sampled represent small-cell change because there may be no normal cells sampled with which to compare them, and furthermore, the smeared cells may be affected by shrinking, drying, or crowding artifacts. Thus, an increased nucleocytoplasmic ratio or increased nuclear density, which usually occurs in HCC, can easily be missed. Large-cell change within a cirrhotic liver can look very similar to a well-differentiated HCC arising in a cirrhotic liver on FNA smears, as both lesions may have only a few atypical cells against a background of more normal-appearing hepatocytes. In addition, if the lesion is small, the surrounding cirrhotic liver is likely to have been sampled, resulting in the presence of ductal epithelium or lipochrome-laden hepatocytes from the adjacent liver appearing on the smear. The presence of bile, fat, or Mallory bodies is not a specific diagnostic criterion, because these can be found in both MRNs and HCCs. Hence, smears alone are often insufficient for rendering a diagnosis, and a cell button should be obtained in order to evaluate architecture. Furthermore, if an FNA sample does not reveal obvious HCC, then a core biopsy would be appropriate in order to further evaluate architecture.

So far, special stains and immunoperoxidase studies have not been much help in differentiating benign hepatocellular proliferations from malignant ones; however, these stains can differentiate HCC from metastatic adenocarcinomas or cholangiocarcinoma. Mucicarminophilic material is present in many adenocarcinomas (including cholangiocarcinomas) and mixed hepatocellular-cholangiocarcinomas. Alphafetoprotein can be focally positive in HCC,[113, 114] but many

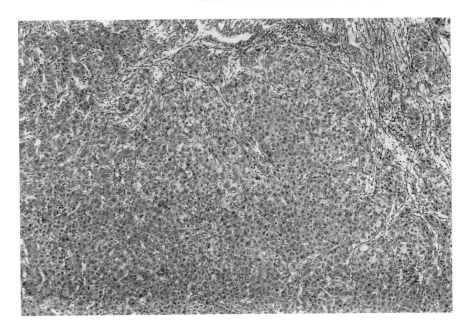

FIGURE 9-18. Hepatocellular carcinoma, reticulin stain, with extensive loss of framework and small-cell change. (Snook's reticulin, ×25)

HCCs will not stain. Keratin stain AE1 (keratin 19) is usually negative in HCC (rare cells may stain)[113, 115] but is positive in adenocarcinoma; CAM 5.2 keratin reacts with most hepatocellular carcinomas[115] and adenocarcinoma. Staining of the bile canaliculi with polyclonal CEA is specific for HCC,[116, 117] whereas cytoplasmic staining with polyclonal CEA and cytoplasmic and membranous monoclonal CEA is typical of adenocarcinomas, but not of HCC.[113, 117] Other markers for adenocarcinoma such as Leu-M1 and B-72.3 are probably not as specific, but tend to be more positive in adenocarcinoma than HCC.[114] Various neuroendocrine stains such as Grimelius[118] and immunoperoxidase stains such as neuron-specific enolase,[118] chromogranin-A,[119] and neurotensin have been reported to be positive in hepatocellular malignancies, including fibrolamellar carcinoma[120] and hepatoblastoma.[119] Thus, a tumor arising in a cirrhotic liver that morphologically appears as a typical HCC but has a positive staining pattern with one of these neuroendocrine markers should likely be viewed as an HCC with neuroendocrine differentiation.

Hepatocellular Tumors in Non-cirrhotic Livers

In a non-cirrhotic liver in an older patient, a tumor mass would more likely be a **metastatic carcinoma** than a primary liver process (Table 9-12) such as **focal nodular hyperplasia, partial nodular transformation, adenoma,** or the **fibrolamellar variant of HCC** (these last two are more commonly seen in young women). **Primary hepatocellular carcinoma of the non-fibrolamellar type** can also occur in the non-cirrhotic liver, although it is much more frequently associated with cirrhosis. Diagnostic possibilities in children include hepatoblastoma versus other rare tumors such as mesenchymal hamartoma if the lesion is hepatocellular in nature.

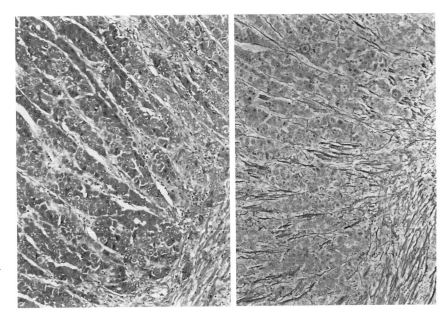

FIGURE 9-19. Hepatocellular carcinoma (HCC). *Left,* HCC with fibrous septa separating thickened trabeculae. (H&E, ×25) *Right,* Reticulin stain shows increased reticulin in the fibrous septa. (Snook's reticulin, ×25)

Table 9–12. **Differential Diagnosis of Hepatocellular Lesions in Non-cirrhotic Livers**

	Focal Nodular Hyperplasia	Adenoma	Nodular Regenerative Hyperplasia	Fibrolamellar HCC
Hepatocellular morphology (large versus small cells)	Normal, no small- or large-cell change	Normal or slightly larger cells, may have fat, glycogen	Normal or slightly compressed, suggesting foci of small-cell change	Larger than normal polygonal shapes, pale bodies, enlarged nuclei, abundant eosinophilic granular cytoplasm
Bile ducts	Present in scar	Not present	Present in portal zones	Not present
Large vessels	Present	Present	Not present	Not typical, variable
Connective tissue	Scar	May be present	Not present	Lamellar fibrosis
Mitoses	None	None	None	Rare
Reticulin stain	Normal pattern sinusoidal staining; may show double cell plates	Normal or slightly decreased sinusoidal staining; may show double cell plates	Normal with regenerative foci (thicker cell plates) compressing single-cell plates	Not used for diagnosis, variable pattern

302

The pathology of metastatic lesions is not considered in this chapter. These lesions, however, account for the majority of all liver tumors, and it is important to obtain a complete patient history that would indicate any previous neoplasms. Metastases should be considered if a tumor shows cytologic features not typical of a primary liver lesion. Immunoperoxidase or other special stains as described earlier should be used, if necessary.

FOCAL NODULAR HYPERPLASIA. Focal nodular hyperplasia (FNH) is thought to be a non-neoplastic tumor that may arise as part of a vascular malformation/hamartoma[121] or hemangioma[122, 123] or as a reaction to a previous localized insult such as ischemia. FNH was originally called focal cirrhosis because of its resemblance to cirrhosis microscopically. It typically contains large bands of fibrous tissue, which may be most prominent in the center of the lesion, the so-called stellate scar, but this gross feature is not always present. Variable numbers of bile ducts or ductules are present in the fibrous tissue. Large, muscular vessels are present in the larger fibrous bands (Fig. 9–20), but no large bile ducts are associated with them, supporting the concept that these vessels are abnormal and the lesion is more likely a hamartomatous one.

Differential Diagnosis. Because FNH may be present as multiple nodules within the same liver, differentiating it from multiple adenomas or metastatic lesions may be difficult by gross examination. A microscopic examination should quickly eliminate metastases from the differential diagnosis, but distinguishing it from adenoma may be difficult on small core biopsies or FNA biopsy. Thus, adequate sampling is the key to identifying the necessary ductular structures in the fibrous stroma present in FNH but not in adenoma.

PARTIAL NODULAR TRANSFORMATION. Partial nodular transformation is a perihilar lesion composed of regenerative hepatocytes without fibrosis. This lesion is likely to be a focal variant of **nodular regenerative hyperplasia,** a diffuse process involving the entire liver, and both can result in portal hypertension. The nodules in both lesions contain regenerating liver cells with thickened cell plates that compress adjacent non-regenerating single cell plates. These regenerative and compressive hepatocytic changes can be observed readily with

the reticulin stain. Portal tracts are present and essentially normal. Nodular regenerative hyperplasia, also known as nodular or micronodular transformation, has been found in association with a variety of disease states, including immune complex diseases,[124–126] lymphoproliferative or myeloproliferative disorders,[124, 125] massive hepatic metastases,[124] immunosuppressive drug therapy,[124, 125] primary biliary cirrhosis,[127] organic cardiac disease,[128] lesions with right-sided cardiac hypertrophy such as pulmonary hypertension,[128, 129] and systemic amyloidosis.[128] The etiology of both lesions is unknown, but a reactive hyperplasia after an ischemic injury or irregular blood flow to the liver has been implicated as a possible factor.

Differential Diagnosis. Clinically and grossly, nodular regenerative hyperplasia is often mistaken for cirrhosis because of clinical evidence of portal hypertension or gross nodularity of the liver. However, liver function tests are usually minimally abnormal, and of course, the biopsy shows no evidence of fibrosis. This lesion can be especially difficult to diagnose on needle biopsy, and only somewhat easier to diagnose on a deep wedge biopsy. A reticulin stain revealing thick regenerating cell plates compressing the intervening ones can at least suggest the diagnosis. One diagnostic problem is to differentiate nodular regenerative hyperplasia from macronodular cirrhosis when the biopsy lacks the characteristic fibrous bands of the latter. Another diagnostic consideration is the macroregenerative nodule, in which normal portal zones are also commonplace. Neither of these lesions, however, would be expected to show the variable pattern of regeneration and compression that nodular regenerative hyperplasia shows.

For partial nodular transformation, the clinical impression is more likely to be that of a tumor within a non-cirrhotic liver, and adequate sampling is again needed to distinguish it from an adenoma or focal nodular hyperplasia. In contrast to partial nodular transformation, adenoma would lack portal zones (see later), and focal nodular hyperplasia would have abnormal portal-like zones with bile duct proliferaton and fibrosis (see earlier).

ADENOMA. An adenoma can appear as a single or as multiple nodules[130] (usually the former). It may or may not be encapsu-

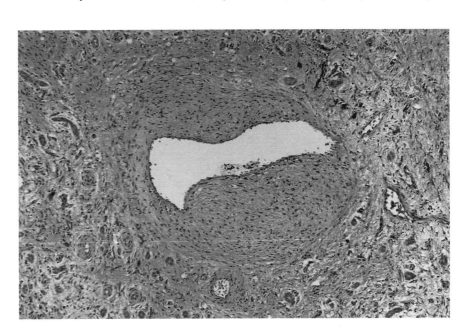

FIGURE 9–20. Focal nodular hyperplasia with scar zone containing bile ductules as well as a large muscular vessel. This vessel is disproportionately large and has an irregular thick wall. There is no corresponding large duct in the zone. (H&E, ×25)

lated and is usually fairly round, with smooth borders. On light microscopy, the cell plates mimic normal liver but can be two to three cells thick. Reticulin formation is present but may be less than that seen in normal (or regenerative) liver. No bile ductules or portal triads are present in the lesion, but central vein-like vessels are present. In addition, large muscular vessels (arteries and/or veins) are typically present. The cytology of the tumor cells is very similar to that of normal liver,[130, 131] although the hepatocytes may be slightly larger than normal. Usually, nuclei are relatively small, round, and uniform and have small nucleoli.[131] Fibrosis,[132] hemorrhage,[130] necrosis,[130, 131] bile production,[133] acinar formation,[133] and fatty change[130, 133, 134] can occur, and glycogen deposits,[132, 133] lipochrome pigment,[133] and Mallory bodies[132, 133] can be present. Mitoses and vascular invasion are not seen.[133] Rarely, a hepatocellular carcinoma has arisen in a lesion that was histologically and clinically an adenoma.[135]

Differential Diagnosis. Adenoma, partial nodular transformation, focal nodular hyperplasia, and even normal liver can be virtually impossible to diagnose on an FNA biopsy sample because their cytologic and architectural features are so similar.[136] A core biopsy is a better method for obtaining a diagnostic sample, but the core must be long enough (1.5–2 cm) to obtain material with distinctive architectural features such as the absence of portal zones in adenoma or a focal cirrhosis-like picture in focal nodular hyperplasia. The presence of abnormally large muscular arteries (or vessels) without a corresponding large duct would be typical of focal nodular hyperplasia or adenoma but not normal liver; however, it may be necessary to do a wedge or excisional open biopsy in order to clearly differentiate the lesions as described earlier. In addition, a well-differentiated HCC must always remain in the differential diagnosis even in a non-cirrhotic liver.

FIBROLAMELLAR VARIANT OF HCC. The fibrolamellar variant of HCC also arises in non-cirrhotic liver but usually occurs in younger individuals than those with cirrhosis and HCC.[137, 138] This tumor, as originally described by Craig et al.,[137] has abundant, dense, fibrous, stromal bands that separate the nests and clusters of tumor cells. The malignant hepatocytes vary in shape, but for the most part, the cells are large and have polygonal, eosinophilic, and granular cytoplasm.

Differential Diagnosis. Because this tumor occurs in non-cirrhotic livers of younger individuals, it must be differentiated from the benign lesions (see earlier) that occur in a similar clinical setting. The cytologic pleomorphism of the lesion is the key to the diagnosis, as normal livers and those with benign hepatocytic tumors lack this feature. The **scirrhous variant of HCC** (see Fig. 9–19) that usually occurs in the cirrhotic liver also contains considerable fibrous tisssue, but it does not have the distinctive lamellar fibrosis and pleomorphic cytologic features seen in the fibrolamellar type. Another fibrosing tumor of the liver, so-called **sclerosing hepatic carcinoma,** associated with hypercalcemia[139] has also been described. This type of carcinoma has extensive fibrosis, can be of hepatocellular or cholangiolar type, and occurs in cirrhotic and non-cirrhotic livers but, again, such a lesion does not have the typical hepatocellular cytologic features of fibrolamellar carcinoma. Thus, because a diagnosis of fibrolamellar HCC implies a favorable prognosis compared with other hepatic carcinomas,[137, 138] adherence to these diagnostic criteria should be applied when making the diagnosis.

Hepatocellular Tumors in Children

In children, the differential diagnosis of hepatocellular tumors is considerably different than it is in adults. Cases of hepatocellular carcinoma are very rare, but when seen, they are usually in the setting of cirrhosis or a metabolic disorder such as tyrosinemia.[140] HCC in children has the same architectural and cytologic features as in adults.

HEPATOBLASTOMA. Hepatoblastoma is the most common hepatocellular tumor of children, usually occurring in children younger than 5 years of age. The most common histologic subtypes are the **epithelial or epithelial-mesenchymal types,**[140–142] followed by the **small-cell undifferentiated (anaplastic) type**[141, 142] and **macrotrabecular type.**[140, 142] The epithelial subtype differentiates into two patterns: the fetal and the embryonal (Fig. 9–21). The fetal differentiation consists of polygonal tumor cells with round, medium-sized nuclei and moderate amounts of eosinophilic cytoplasm. The tumor cells are smaller than normal liver cells and resemble fetal hepatocytes. They are arranged in cords and often contain glycogen or fat appearing as an alternating pink and white cytoplasmic pattern on low-power light microscopy. There is a marked diminution of the reticulin framework in most zones. The embryonal pattern is made up of smaller, darker-staining cells with meager, more basophilic cytoplasm. The cells are often arranged in an acinar or tubular pattern. Some studies indicate a better prognosis for patients with tumors of predominantly fetal differentiation (>75% of the tumor).[143]

The small-cell undifferentiated (anaplastic) type is composed of a fairly uniform population of cells that lack evidence of epithelial or stromal differentiation and could be mistaken for neuroblastoma, lymphoma, or rhabdomyosarcoma. This subtype is also often associated with the fetal epithelial type and, when present, seems to result in a poorer prognosis.[143]

The macrotrabecular type of hepatoblastoma has architectural features similar to those of a trabecular variant of HCC (Fig. 9–22), but the presence of this pattern probably does not worsen the overall prognosis of the tumor. The trabeculae should be at least 10 cells thick and present in a repetitive pattern. Cytologic atypia in this variant may be present, but the cells are usually smaller than normal rather than larger as in many HCCs.[142] According to Haas et al.,[143] this subtype is always associated with the fetal epithelial subtype, so this variant can potentially be distinguished from HCC by thoroughly examining the resected tumor specimen microscopically for the fetal pattern.

Mesenchymal elements, including osteoid, cartilage, and fibrous tissue, can show varying degrees of differentiation. The presence of stromal elements probably does not influence prognosis.[142, 143] Extramedullary hematopoiesis can often be present.

Differential Diagnosis. Diagnostic problems arise when attempting to differentiate the various forms of hepatoblastoma from other tumor types such as hepatic adenoma, hepatocellular carcinoma, embryonal carcinomas, neuroblastoma, lymphoma, or rhabdomyosarcoma on sparse biopsy material. For example, a pure fetal type of differentiation should not be confused with hepatic adenoma, which is extremely rare in children younger than 10 years old. The fetal component of hepatoblastoma should contain smaller than normal liver cells with increased nuclear density (increased nucleocy-

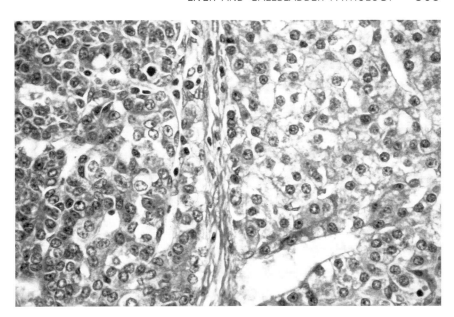

FIGURE 9–21. Hepatoblastoma, embryonal *(left)* and fetal *(right)* zones. The embryonal areas show immature, relatively undeveloped cells, while in the fetal zones, the cells resemble hepatocytes as seen in fetal liver. (H&E, ×83)

toplasmic ratio) and most likely a "light and dark" cytoplasmic change due to the deposition of glycogen and fat as described earlier. The macrotrabecular type of hepatoblastoma usually does not have the variation in cell size or cellular enlargement seen in many HCCs, which only rarely occurs in children with non-cirrhotic livers. But this form of hepatoblastoma could still be impossible to differentiate from HCC by histologic means; thus, further sampling or resection may be necessary. The small-cell variant can be differentiated from lymphoma by leukocyte common antigen and/or B- and T-cell lymphocyte immunohistochemical markers, but differentiation from neuroendocrine tumors is more problematic because hepatoblastomas can demonstrate neuroendocrine differentiation.[119] One might also suspect that focal rhabdomyoblastic differentiation could be present. Again, thorough examination of the biopsy or resection specimen should show other patterns of differentiation in hepatoblastoma.

In hepatoblastoma, as in HCC, alpha-fetoprotein (AFP) levels may be elevated; however, in the former, the patients are usually younger (younger than 2 years of age, compared with older than 5 years of age for HCC), and there is usually no background cirrhosis[142] or underlying metabolic disorder. Alpha-fetoprotein levels may also be elevated in embryonal malignancies such as yolk sac tumor, so this is not specific for HCC or hepatoblastoma. Alpha-fetoprotein levels should not be significantly elevated in benign hepatocellular lesions such as adenoma or focal nodular hyperplasia.

MESENCHYMAL HAMARTOMA. Another rare tumor in children is mesenchymal hamartoma. This benign tumor can be quite large and contains clusters of normal-appearing hepatocytes arranged in cell plates admixed with an abundant myxoid stroma that contains numerous branched bile ducts (Fig. 9–23). Numerous cystic spaces lined by flattened cells are also present, filled with a translucent fluid or gelatinous mate-

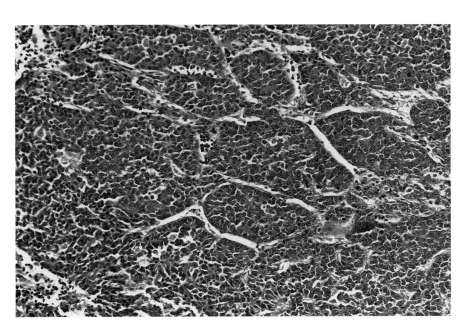

FIGURE 9–22. Hepatoblastoma, macrotrabecular pattern. Large, wide trabeculae with numerous small tumor cells. (H&E, ×50)

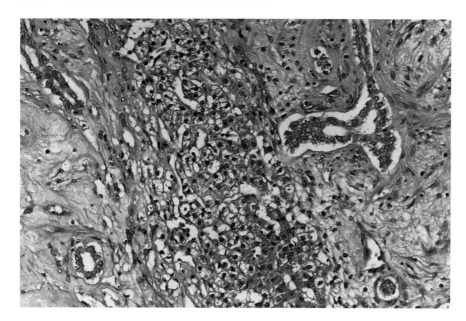

FIGURE 9–23. Mesenchymal hamartoma with ducts embedded in myxoid stroma separating smaller clusters of otherwise normal-appearing liver cells arranged in cell plates. (H&E, ×50)

rial.[140, 144] The stroma often contains smaller lymphatic-like channels.

Differential Diagnosis. When cystic spaces are the most prominent components of the tumor, mesenchymal hamartoma can somewhat mimic polycystic disease of the liver, but the former tumor is a single nodule rather than a multifocal lesion, the stroma (which contains ductules between the cysts) is more prominent and myxoid, and uniform collections of intervening hepatocytes with normal architecture between the cysts can be easily identified. **Infantile hemangioendothelioma** may also contain many ducts separating the vascular slits and stroma throughout the tumor, but this tumor has more prominent vasculature, often with solid areas of endothelial proliferation, than seen with mesenchymal hamartoma.

Differential Diagnosis of Vascular and Mesenchymal Tumors

In the liver, the main problem in diagnosing vascular and stromal tumors is recognizing their mesenchymal natures. This can be especially difficult on small-core or FNA biopsy samples. Even common lesions such as **cavernous hemangiomas,** which pose no diagnostic problem in resected livers, may be unrecognizable on FNA samples because they contain very few cells and yield highly bloody biopsy specimens. Likewise, **Kaposi's sarcoma** (KS) in the liver is usually not a clinical diagnostic problem in a patient with a history of AIDS and KS at other sites, but, again, it can be difficult or impossible to diagnose with FNA. **Hemangioendothelioma** in children, **epithelioid hemangioendothelioma,** and **angiosarcoma** all are uncommon, and a diagnosis of one of these tumors is best made on a biopsy specimen or resected tissue in order to sufficiently examine the cytologic and architectural features.

Vascular Neoplasms

EPITHELIOID HEMANGIOENDOTHELIOMA. Epithelioid hemangioendothelioma is a rare primary vascular tumor with many histologic appearances. The tumor cells can be spindled or dendritic with branching processes, polygonal with epithelioid features, and/or signet ring–like with intracytoplasmic spaces or lumina (Fig. 9–24).[145, 146] The tumor characteristically grows into the venous channels as either solid tufts of epithelial cells or as myxoid/fibrous stroma containing the irregularly shaped cells described previously. The lesion spreads throughout the liver in such an irregular manner that it can spare some zones of residual liver even in the center of the tumor. In addition, the stroma can become densely collagenized over time, and can even calcify and appear radiopaque. Most of the tumor cells (>60%) stain for endothelial markers with immunoperoxidase techniques. This lesion can be multifocal and behaves in a low-grade malignant fashion; overall, it is a much less aggressive tumor than angiosarcoma.

Differential Diagnosis. This is the vascular neoplasm most likely to be misdiagnosed, because its peculiar pattern of spread within the sinusoids, variable cell shape, and the accompanying myxoid/fibrous reaction[145, 146] can mislead the unwary into making a diagnosis of adenocarcinoma, HCC, or even an unusual scar reaction. The polygonal tumor cells can resemble entrapped hepatocytes or duct cells, and the individual vacuolated cells entrapped in the stroma may mimic the signet-ring cells of adenocarcinoma, but mucin stains should be negative. Other immunoperoxidase stains can also easily differentiate the neoplastic processes: many of the polygonal and epithelioid cells should be positive for endothelial markers such as Factor VIII, *Ulex europaeus,* or CD 31 or 34 in epithelioid hemangioendothelioma, whereas AFP, monoclonal CEA, polyclonal CEA, and keratin stains can be used to identify hepatocellular carcinomas or adenocarcinomas.

ANGIOSARCOMA. Angiosarcoma is usually multicentric and also has a variety of histologic appearances. It is similar to epithelioid hemangioendothelioma in that it has a predilection to spread along sinusoids and veins; however, the myxoid/fibrous stroma seen in the latter is either not prominent or absent in angiosarcoma. The tumor cells are usually spindled or polygonal and have a tendency to line the sinusoids adjacent

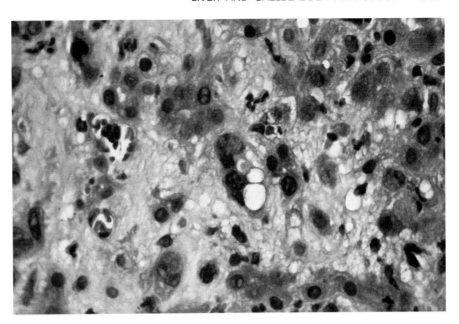

FIGURE 9–24. Epithelioid hemangioendothelioma with typical myxoid stroma, inflammatory cells including neutrophils, and epithelioid cells. The epithelioid tumor cells should not be mistaken for entrapped hepatocytes or bile ductules. The tumor cells can be "vacuolated" as evidence of a capillary luminal space. (H&E, ×100)

to surviving hepatocytes in a scaffold-like pattern, dissecting the cell plates into smaller fragments or expanding the sinusoidal space between cell plates (Fig. 9–25). The tumor cells can also grow in solid sheets and form small and large, irregular vascular spaces or peliotic channels. These larger spaces may contain papillary projections of tumor cells. Extramedullary hematopoiesis is often present. Endothelial markers should show some positivity, but solid, spindled cell areas may be negative. Angiosarcoma has a rapidly progressive course with a much poorer prognosis as compared with epithelioid hemangioendothelioma. Angiosarcoma can occur in children[147] as well as in adults.

Differential Diagnosis. In children, angiosarcoma should be distinguished from **undifferentiated (embryonal) sarcoma,**[148–150] which can contain similar-appearing spindled areas. Embryonal sarcoma, however, more closely resembles malignant fibrous histiocytoma than does angiosarcoma.[149, 150]

Embryonal sarcoma can be distinguished by the presence of large, multinucleated tumor cells and hyaline PAS-digest-positive globules[148] within the cytoplasm of the tumor cells or in the tumor stroma (Fig. 9–26). These globules are negative for alpha-fetoprotein and alpha-1-antitrypsin, and their exact nature is unknown.

Stromal Neoplasms

Primary stromal neoplasms such as lipoma, fibrosarcoma, and malignant fibrous histiocytoma have been described as rare occurrences in the liver. These tumors, when present, are morphologically identical to the soft tissue primaries and do not resemble hepatocellular neoplasms, and so are not discussed further here. However, one lesion that can pose difficult diagnostic problems in the liver is **angiomyolipoma.** This benign lesion typically consists of a triad of well-formed

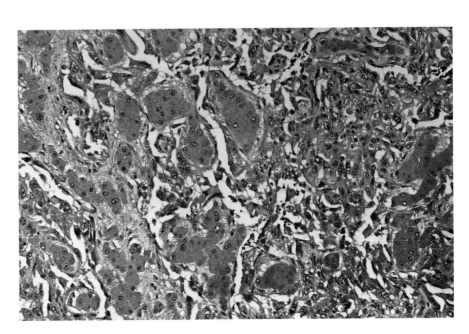

FIGURE 9–25. Angiosarcoma. The infiltrating edge of the tumor shows atypical endothelial cells lining sinusoids and disrupting cell plate architecture. (H&E, ×50)

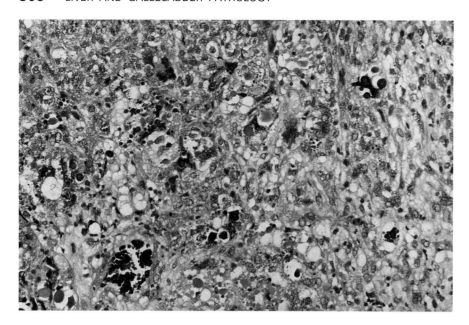

FIGURE 9–26. Embryonal sarcoma. A pleomorphic sarcomatous tumor with large hyaline globules, focal giant cells, and hemorrhagic debris. (H&E, ×50)

vessels, fat, and spindle cells, the last representing the muscle component. Foam cells (histiocytes) and hematopoietic elements can also be present.[151] Mitotic figures are not seen.

DIFFERENTIAL DIAGNOSIS. Unfortunately, angiomyolipomas can often vary from the typical picture. They can demonstrate a very prominent spindle cell or epithelioid type of differentiation, with little or no fat, and lack the prominent vasculature.[151, 152] Trabecular patterns have also been described, which simulate that of HCC,[152] and oncocytic cytoplasmic changes reminiscent of fibrolamellar hepatocellular carcinoma may also be prominent. These lesions can become very large and have significant necrosis. When these atyical patterns are present, immunohistochemical stains may help differentiate these lesions from malignant processes. The characteristic immunohistochemical profile includes positivity for HMB-45[152–154] and smooth muscle actin.[153] Desmin staining is variable,[153–155] and cytokeratin, carcinoembryonic antigen, alpha-fetoprotein, and chromogranin are negative.[154] Factor VIII antigen or other endothelial markers stain only the walls of identifiable vessels within the tumor.[155]

Non-neoplastic Tumor-like Lesions

Two non-neoplastic lesions that can present diagnostic problems are inflammatory pseudotumor[156–158] and focal fatty change.[159–161]

Inflammatory Pseudotumors

Inflammatory pseudotumors are composed of variable amounts of an inflammatory infiltrate composed predominantly of mononuclear cells such as lymphocytes and plasma cells, but eosinophils can also be present and quite prominent. The amount and type of fibrous tissue in the lesion also vary and include a loose, fasciitis-like process, a whorled laminated pattern, and relatively acellular dense sclerosis. This lesion is very uncommon in the liver and can be difficult to biopsy because of its obvious inflammatory and/or fibrous nature; thus, without total excision, it may not be possible to distin-

guish it from a reactive process adjacent to a neoplasm, abscess, or infarct.

Focal Fatty Change

Focal fatty change consists of a focus of liver parenchyma with abundant fat, much more so than the surrounding liver. The diagnostic problem on small samples or FNA biopsy is to determine whether the fat represents the clinical lesion or the surrounding liver; thus, an adequate sampling with the assurance of appropriate needle placement must be done.

GALLBLADDER AND EXTRAHEPATIC BILE DUCTS

Problems in the Diagnosis of Rare Inflammatory and Proliferative Disorders

The gallbladder and extrahepatic bile ducts do not seem to offer as many problems in diagnosis as does the liver, so this discussion focuses only on a few unusual inflammatory and reactive disorders and on variants of adenocarcinoma.

Xanthogranulomatous Cholecystitis

Xanthogranulomatous cholecystitis[162] can form an isolated mass that could be grossly confused with carcinoma. The lesion is composed of foamy macrophages, cholesterol clefts, and a variable number of predominantly chronic inflammatory cells. Michealis-Gutmann bodies have been noted in rare cases, consistent with a diagnosis of malakoplakia.[163]

DIFFERENTIAL DIAGNOSIS. This type of cholecystitis has been seen in association with **adenocarcinoma**,[164, 165] so one must search carefully for atypical epithelial elements in such cases. Keratin stains can help differentiate malignant epithelial components from inflammatory cells. This lesion should also be differentiated from **granular cell tumor** (granular cell myoblastoma),[166] which is a rare lesion that can occur anywhere along the biliary tree. The cells making up the granular cell tumor resemble the foamy macrophages of xanthomatous inflammation. They have small round nuclei and abundant cytoplasm, but cholesterol clefts and chronic inflammatory cells are not present. The tumor cells are often arranged in small clusters separated by collagen bundles and appear to be infiltrative, especially at the tumor margin. The cytoplasm contains PAS-positive diastase-resistant granules, in large part owing to cytoplasmic phagocytic vacuoles or lysosomes,[167] and is S-100 positive.[166]

Other unusual forms of cholecystitis include **eosinophilic,**[168, 169] **CMV, and cryptosporidial cholecystitis.**[170] The etiology of the former is unknown, and the last two have been seen only in AIDS patients, and then only rarely.

Metaplastic and Hyperplastic Mucosal Changes

The gallbladder mucosa can also undergo a variety of **metaplastic and hyperplastic changes associated with cholelithiasis**[171] **or cholecystitis.** The metaplastic changes most commonly seen include antral-type gastric mucosa, intestinal-type mucosa with Paneth cells or goblet cells, and even enterochromaffin cells.[171] These cell types should show no significant cytologic atypia but can cause focal architectural irregularities of the mucosa that should not be confused with carcinoma; however, metaplasia has also been noted in association with adenocarcinoma of the gallbladder (cholangiocarcinoma),[172] suggesting a possible role in the carcinogenesis.

Hyperplastic changes include a variety of morphologies. In one, the so-called **villous**[173] **or papillary**[174] **hyperplasia,** the villi elongate and cytologic smears appear normal or only slightly atypical. This change is usually seen in association with cholesterolosis or chronic cholecystitis. In rare instances, the villi coalesce at various points along their surface, forming enclosed glandular spaces, sometimes called spongiform hyperplasia.[173] The mucosal epithelial elements do not infiltrate into the muscularis. A form of **adenomatous hyperplasia** has been described by Weedon[173] and Christensen and Ishak;[175] however, Weedon describes it as a lesion very similar to gastric antral metaplasia or to adenomyomatosis, whereas Christensen and Ishak compare it with villous or papillary hyperplasia. Thus, to avoid confusion or misunderstanding, it may be best not to use the term.

Adenomyomatosis

Adenomyomatosis is itself another somewhat misunderstood term when applied to the gallbladder. Basically, this lesion is a form of hyperplasia in which Rokitansky-Aschoff sinuses proliferate and ''invade'' the underlying muscularis or beyond.[176, 177] The muscle is often thickened and hyperplastic, and the sinuses can form extramural or intramural glandular cysts. The villi are also often accentuated and thickened. Adenomyoma, usually found in the fundus, can be considered a localized form of this lesion.[176, 177]

DIFFERENTIAL DIAGNOSIS. The pseudo-infiltrating sinuses and glands in adenomyomatosis should not be confused with adenocarcinoma. In the absence of inflammation, the cytology of the glandular cells should be similar to the normal epithelial cells of the gallbladder, and the lesion would thus be similar

to ''cystica profunda'' seen in the small or large intestine. In the setting of cholecystitis, some inflammatory atypia may be present, but the presence of muscle bundles between the glands should help differentiate this lesion from adenocarcinoma, which would more likely elicit a desmoplastic response. In addition, the glands of adenomyomatosis would be uniformly larger and more cystic than in adenocarcinoma, which, although it can have large cystic glands, usually also contains smaller, more angulated glands, often with significant focal cytologic atypia. Adenocarcinomas have been reported to arise in association with adenomyomatosis,[178, 179] but this so rarely occurs that extreme caution must be exercised before making such a diagnosis.

Adenocarcinoma

Making the diagnosis of adenocarcinoma of the biliary tree or gallbladder is usually not a problem on routine sections, but it can pose problems on frozen sections of resected margins, because these tumors are usually well differentiated. It is very important not to confuse glands of the **normal duct and gallbladder wall** with foci of adenocarcinoma. The perimuscular connective tissue of the gallbladder has small, relatively well-circumscribed clusters of glands without significant cytologic atypia arranged in lobules that can be seen microscopically at low magnification.[180] The bile ducts also often have pits that extend into the fibrous wall of the duct, which are usually surrounded by similar ducts.[180] In the presence of inflammation and fibrosis, as seen in chronic cholangitis, these ducts can exhibit cytologic and architectural changes that could be confused with well-differentiated adenocarcinoma; the presence of neural invasion, loss of lobular architecture, formation of back-to-back or cribiform glands (gland within a gland), positive CEA staining, and significant cytologic atypia, including prominent nucleoli, nuclear size variation, and nuclear irregularities, point to a diagnosis of infiltrative adenocarcinoma.[181]

DIFFERENTIAL DIAGNOSIS. The more common variants of adenocarcinoma that arise in the gallbladder include the **intestinal type of adenocarcinoma,** which is morphologically similar to that seen in large intestine,[182] **mucinous adenocarcinoma,**[183] **papillary adenocarcinoma** with or without associated adenoma,[184] and **poorly differentiated adenocarcinoma.**[184] The papillary neoplasms are the most difficult lesions, and most agree that the histologic criteria used to diagnose papillary neoplasms in the colon be used to determine the presence of carcinoma in a papillary neoplasm in the gallbladder. Hence, invasion into the lamina propria or stalk would be representative of invasive carcinoma, and the atypical cytologic or architectural criteria described previously could be used to assist in the diagnosis of invasive or in situ carcinoma.

The **precancerous dysplastic lesions**, or atypical hyperplasias, are not as well defined as invasive adenocarcinoma. Some forms of dysplasia mimic a uniform zone of adenomatous change (as seen in adenoma of the colon) with similar corresponding degrees of atypia, which is graded in the same manner as in colon lesions.[185, 186] This pattern can also be papillary or villous, again mimicking the villous adenoma of the colon; however, it has been our experience that other forms of atypia, which lack the uniformity seen with adenomatous change and have only a few foci of cytologically abnormal cell clusters, can occur. These lesions can show more cellular pleomorphism and cytoplasm and less crowding than those with atypical adenomatous change. The classification of these lesions has not been dealt with consistently. Most agree that an increased nucleocytoplasmic ratio, loss of cell polarity, and hyperchromatism[186–188] would warrant a diagnosis of dysplasia. Atypical mitotic figures and prominent nucleoli[186] can also be present.

The question of when to call a lesion **carcinoma in situ** (CIS) is even less well defined. Many of the lesions described as CIS are reported in association with adenomas, but a few have also been described in the absence of adenoma or invasive carcinoma.[186, 187] Morphologic criteria for the diagnosis include increased nucleocytoplasmic ratio, loss of cell polarity, and hyperchromatism,[186–188] of a more severe degree than would be expected in dysplasia. As in CIS in the colon, a cribriform pattern would be sufficient architectural change for a diagnosis of CIS. Unfortunately, the demarcation of dysplasia versus CIS has not been convincingly established.

References

1. Millward-Sadler GH: Cirrhosis. In MacSween RNM, Anthony PP, Scheuer PJ (eds): Pathology of the Liver. London, Churchill Livingstone, 1987, pp 342–363.
2. Nasrallah S, Nasar V, Galambos J: Importance of terminal hepatic venule thickening. Arch Pathol Lab Med 104:84–86, 1980.
3. Burt A, MacSween RNM: Hepatic vein lesions in alcoholic liver disease: Retrospective biopsy and necropsy study. J Clin Pathol 39:63–67, 1986.
4. Review by an international group: Alcoholic liver disease: Morphological manifestations. Lancet 1:707–711, 1981.
5. Lewis J, Mullick F, Ishak K, et al: Histopathologic analysis of suspected amiodarone hepatotoxicity. Hum Pathol 21:59–67, 1990.
6. Babany G, Uzzan F, Larrey D, et al: Alcoholic-like liver lesions induced by nifedipine. J Hepatol 9:252–255, 1989.
7. Lee R: Nonalcoholic steatohepatitis: A study of 49 patients. Hum Pathol 20:594–598, 1989.
8. Diehl A, Goodman Z, Ishak K: Alcohol-like liver disease in nonalcohol-induced liver injury. Gastroenterology 95:1056–1062, 1988.
9. Wanless I, Lentz J: Fatty liver hepatitis (steatohepatitis) and obesity: An autopsy study with analysis of risk factors. Hepatology 12:1106–1110, 1990.
10. Snover D: The liver in systemic disease. In Snover D: Biopsy Diagnosis of Liver Disease. Baltimore, Williams and Wilkins, 1992, pp 192–194.
11. Arcidi J, Moore G, Hutchins G: Hepatic morphology in cardiac dysfunction: A clinicopathologic study of 1000 subjects at autopsy. Am J Pathol 104:159–166, 1981.
12. Klatt E, Koss M, Young T, et al: Hepatic hyaline globules associated with passive congestion. Arch Pathol Lab Med 112:510–513, 1988.
13. Kanel G, Ucci A, Kaplan M, Wolfe H: A distinctive perivenular hepatic lesion associated with heart failure. Am J Clin Pathol 73:235–239, 1980.
14. Bras G, Brandt K: Vascular disorders. In MacSween RNM, Anthony PP, Scheuer PJ (eds): Pathology of the Liver. London, Churchill Livingstone, 1987, pp 478–502.
15. Shulman H, McDonald G: Liver disease after marrow transplantation. In Sale G, Shulman H (eds): The Pathology of Bone Marrow Transplantation. New York, Masson Publishing, 1984, pp 104–135.
16. Lefkowitch J: Bile ductular cholestasis: An ominous histopathologic sign related to sepsis and cholangitis lenta. Hum Pathol 13:19–24, 1982.
17. Nakanuma Y: Necroinflammatory changes in hepatic lobules in primary biliary cirrhosis with less well-defined cholestatic changes. Hum Pathol 24:378–383, 1993.
18. Harrison R, Hubscher S: The spectrum of bile duct lesions in end-stage primary sclerosing cholangitis. Histopathology 19:321–327, 1991.
19. Ludwig J, MacCarty R, LaRusso N, et al: Intrahepatic cholangiectases and large-duct obliteration in primary sclerosing cholangitis. Hepatology 6:560–568, 1986.
20. Wee A, Ludwig J, Coffey R, et al: Hepatobiliary carcinoma associated with primary sclerosing cholangitis and chronic ulcerative colitis. Hum Pathol 16:719–726, 1985.
21. Taylor S, Dean P, Riely C: Primary autoimmune cholangitis: An alternative to antimitochondrial antibody-negative primary biliary cirrhosis. Am J Surg Pathol 18:91–99, 1994.
22. Ben-Ari Z, Dhillon A, Sherlock S: Autoimmune cholangiopathy: Part of the spectrum of autoimmune chronic active hepatitis. Hepatology 18:10–15, 1993.
23. Goodman Z, McNally P, Davis D, Ishak K: Autoimmune cholangitis—a variant of primary biliary cirrhosis. Hepatology 18:109A, 1993.
24. Ferrell L, Cregan P, Wright T, et al: Predictive value of pretransplant liver biopsy in patients with fulminant/subfulminant hepatitis. Mod Pathol 6:109A, 1993.
25. Hadchouel M, Gautier M: Histopathologic study of the liver in the early cholestatic phase of alpha-1-antitrypsin deficiency. J Pediatr 89:211–215, 1976.
26. Ghishan F, Greene H: Liver disease in children with PiZZ alpha-1-antitrypsin deficiency. Hepatology 8:307–310, 1988.
27. Ishak K, Sharp H: Metabolic errors and liver disease. In MacSween RNM, Anthony PP, Scheuer PJ (eds): Pathology of the Liver. London, Churchill Livingstone, 1987, pp 99–180.
28. Leblanc A, Odievre M, Hadchouel M, et al: Neonatal cholestasis and hypoglycemia: Possible role of cortisol deficiency. J Pediatr 99:577–580, 1981.
29. Phillips M, Blendis L, Poucell S, et al: Syncytial giant cell hepatitis: Sporadic hepatitis with distinctive pathological features, a severe clinical course, and paramyxoviral features. N Engl J Med 324:455–460, 1991.
30. Devaney K, Goodman Z, Ishak K: Postinfantile giant-cell transformation in hepatitis. Hepatology 16:327–333, 1992.
31. Popper H: Changing concepts of the evolution of chronic hepatitis and the role of piecemeal necrosis. Hepatology 3:759–762, 1983.
32. Cooksley W, Bradbear R, Robinson W, et al: The prognosis of chronic active hepatitis without cirrhosis in relation to bridging necrosis. Hepatology 6:345–348, 1986.
33. Chen T, Liaw Y: The prognostic significance of bridging hepatic necrosis in chronic type B hepatitis: A histopathologic study. Liver 8:10–16, 1988.
34. Popper H, Shaffner F: The vocabulary of chronic hepatitis. N Engl J Med 284:1154–1156, 1971.
35. Gerber M, Vernace S: Chronic septal hepatitis. Virchows Arch [A] 363:303–309, 1974.
36. Scheuer PJ: Changing views on chronic hepatitis. Histopathology 10:1–4, 1986.
37. Gerber M: Chronic hepatitis C: The beginning of the end of a time-honored nomenclature? Hepatology 15:733–734, 1992.
38. Ludwig J: The nomenclature of chronic active hepatitis: An obituary. Gastroenterology 105:274–278, 1993.
39. Review by an international group: A classification of chronic hepatitis. Lancet 2:626–628, 1968.
40. Review by an international group: Acute and chronic hepatitis revisited. Lancet 2:914–919, 1977.
41. Davis G, Hoofnagle J, Waggoner J: Spontaneous reactivation of chronic hepatitis B virus infection. Gastroenterology 86:230–235, 1984.
42. Liaw Y, Chen J, Chen T: Acute exacerbation in patients with liver cirrhosis: A clinicopathological study. Liver 10:177–184, 1990.
43. Fattovich G, Brollo L, Alberti A, et al: Spontaneous reactivation of hepatitis B virus infection in patients with chronic type B hepatitis. Liver 10:141–146, 1990.
44. Knodell R, Ishak K, Black W, et al: Formulation and application of a numerical scoring system for assessing histological activity in asymptomatic chronic active hepatitis. Hepatology 1:431–435, 1981.
45. Mattsson L, Weiland O, Glaumann H: Application of a numerical scoring system for assessment of histological outcome in patients with chronic posttransfusion non-A, non-B hepatitis with or without antibodies to hepatitis C. Liver 10:257–263, 1990.
46. Scheuer P: Classification of chronic viral hepatitis: A need for reassessment. J Hepatol 13:372–374, 1991.
47. Teixeira M, Weller I, Murray A, et al: The pathology of hepatitis A in man. Liver 2:52–60, 1982.
48. Kryger P, Christoffersen P: Liver histopathology of the hepatitis A virus infection: A comparison with hepatitis type B and non-A, non-B. J Clin Pathol 36:650–654, 1983.
49. Gerber M, Thung S: The diagnostic value of immunohistochemical demonstration of hepatitis viral antigens in the liver. Hum Pathol 18:771-774, 1987.
50. Ulich T, Anders K, Layfield L, et al: Chronic active hepatitis of hepatitis B and non-A, non-B etiology. Arch Pathol Lab Med 109:403–407, 1985.
51. Lefkowitch J, Apfelbaum T: Non-A, non-B hepatitis: Characterization of liver biopsy pathology. J Clin Gastroenterol 11:225–232, 1989.
52. Scheuer P: Non-A, non-B hepatitis. Virchows Arch [A] 415:301–303, 1989.
53. Scheuer P, Ashrafzadeh P, Sherlock S, et al: The pathology of hepatitis C. Hepatology 15:567–571, 1992.
54. Gerber M, Krawczynski K, Alter M, et al: Histopathology of community acquired chronic hepatitis C. Mod Pathol 5:483–486, 1992.
55. Govindarajan S, DeCock K, Redeker A: Natural course of delta superinfection in chronic hepatitis B virus-infected patients: Histopathologic study with multiple liver biopsies. Hepatology 6:640–644, 1986.
56. Govindarajan S, Valinluck B: Serum hepatitis B virus-DNA in chronic hepatitis B and delta infection. Arch Pathol Lab Med 109:398–399, 1985.
57. Lefkowitch J, Goldstein H, Yatto R, Gerber M: Cytopathic liver injury in acute delta virus hepatitis. Gastroenterology 92:1262–1266, 1987.
58. Govindarajan S, DeCock K, Peters R: Morphologic and immunohistochemical features of fulminant delta hepatitis. Hum Pathol 16:262–267, 1985.
59. Johnson P, McFarlane I, Feddleston A: The natural course and heterogeneity of autoimmune-type chronic active hepatitis. Semin Liver Dis 11:187–196, 1991.
60. Manns M: Cytoplasmic autoantigens in autoimmune hepatitis: Molecular analysis and clinical relevance. Semin Liver Dis 11:205–214, 1991.
61. Bach N, Thung S, Schaffner F: The histological features of chronic hepatitis C and autoimmune chronic hepatitis: A comparative analysis. Hepatology 15:572–577, 1992.
62. Pariente E, Degott C, Martin J, et al: Hepatocytic PAS-positive diastase-resistant inclusions in the absence of alpha-1-antitrypsin deficiency: High prevalence in alcoholic cirrhosis. Am J Clin Pathol 76:299–302, 1981.
63. Ferrell L, Steinkirchner T, Sterneck M, et al: Alpha-1-antitrypsin (AAT) globules in cirrhotic livers. Mod Pathol 6:110A, 1993.

64. Sterneck M, Ferrell L, Wright T, et al: Viral co-factors in patients with alcoholic cirrhosis undergoing liver transplantation. Gastroenterology 100(Suppl):A800, 1991.
65. Takase S, Takada N, Enomoto N, et al: Different types of chronic hepatitis in alcoholic patients: Does chronic hepatitis induced by alcohol exist? Hepatology 13:876–881, 1991.
66. Brillanti S, Masci C, Siringo S, et al: Serological and histological aspects of hepatitis C virus infection in alcoholic patients. J Hepatol 13:347–350, 1991.
67. Berman M, Alter H, Ishak K, et al: The chronic sequelae of non-A, non-B hepatitis. Ann Int Med 91:106, 1979.
68. Papaevangelou G, Tassopoulos N, Roumeliotou-Darayannis A, Richardson C: Etiology of fulminant viral hepatitis in Greece. Hepatology 4:369–372, 1984.
69. Krogsgaard K, Wantzin P, Mathiesen L, Ring-Larsen L: The Copenhagen Hepatitis Acuta Programme. Chronic evolution of acute hepatitis B: The significance of simultaneous infection with hepatitis C and D. Scand J Gastroenterol 26:275–280, 1991.
70. Colombari R, Dhillon A, Piazzola E, et al: Chronic hepatitis in multiple virus infection: Histopathological evaluation. Histopathology 22:319–325, 1993.
71. Jacques S, Qureshi F: Herpes simplex virus hepatitis in pregnancy: A clinicopathologic study of three cases. Hum Pathol 23:183–187, 1992.
72. Miyazaki Y, Akizuki S, Sakaoka H, et al: Disseminated infection of HSV with fulminant hepatitis in a healthy adult: A case report. APMIS 99:1001–1007, 1991.
73. Groza S, Delic D, Zerjav S, et al: Recovery from herpes simplex virus type-1 hepatitis in a female adult. Klin Wochenschr 66:796–798, 1988.
74. McMinn P, Lim I, McKenzie P, et al: Disseminated herpes simplex virus infection in an apparently immunocompetent woman. Med J Aust 151:588–594, 1989.
75. Gowing NFC: Infectious mononucleosis: Histopathologic aspects. Pathol Annu 10:1–20, 1975.
76. Demetris A, Jaffe R, Sheahan D, et al: Recurrent hepatitis B in liver allograft recipients: Differentiation between viral hepatitis B and rejection. Am J Pathol 125:161–172, 1986.
77. Demetris A, Todo S, Van Thiel D, et al: Evolution of hepatitis B virus liver disease after hepatic replacement: Practical and theoretical considerations. Am J Pathol 137:667–676, 1990.
78. Davies S, Portmann B, O'Grady J, et al: Hepatic histological findings after transplantation for chronic hepatitis B virus infection, including a unique pattern of fibrosing cholestatic hepatitis. Hepatology 13:150–157, 1991.
79. Benner K, Lee R, Keeffe E, et al: Fibrosing cytolytic liver failure secondary to recurrent hepatitis B after liver transplantation. Gastroenterology 103:1307–1312, 1992.
80. Harrison R, Davies M, Goldin R, Hubscher S: Recurrent hepatitis B in liver allografts: A distinctive form of rapidly developing cirrhosis. Histopathology 23:21–28, 1993.
81. Wright T, Donegan E, Hsu H, et al: Hepatitis C viral infection in liver transplant recipients: The importance of detection of viral RNA using the polymerase chain reaction. Gastroenterology 103:317–322, 1992.
82. Ferrell L, Wright T, Roberts J, et al: Pathology of hepatitis C viral infection in liver transplant recipients. Hepatology 16:865–876, 1992.
83. Thung S, Shim K, Shieh C, et al: Hepatitis C in liver allografts. Arch Pathol Lab Med 117:145–149, 1993.
84. Snover D, Hutton S, Balfour H, Bloomer J: Cytomegalovirus infection of liver transplant recipients. J Clin Gastroenterol 9:659–665, 1987.
85. Theise N, Conn M, Thung S: Localization of cytomegalovirus antigens in liver allografts over time. Hum Pathol 24:103–108, 1993.
86. Randhawa P, Markin R, Starzl T, Demetris A: Epstein-Barr virus-associated syndromes in immunosuppressed liver transplant recipients: Clinical profile and recognition on routine allograft biopsy. Am J Surg Pathol 14:538–547, 1990.
87. Nalesnik M, Jaffe R, Starzl T, et al: The pathology of post-transplant lymphoproliferative disorders occurring in the setting of cyclosporine A-prednisone immunosuppression. Am J Pathol 133:173–192, 1988.
88. Glasgow B, Anders K, Layfield L, et al: Clinical and pathologic findings of the liver in the acquired immune deficiency syndrome (AIDS). Am J Clin Pathol 83:582–588, 1985.
89. Libovics H, Thung S, Schaffner F, Radensky P: The liver in the acquired immunodeficiency syndrome: A clinical and histologic study. Hepatology 5:293–298, 1985.
90. Gordon S, Reddy R, Gould E, et al: The spectrum of liver disease in the acquired immunodeficiency syndrome. J Hepatol 2:475–484, 1986.
91. Ferrell L: Gastrointestinal pathology of AIDS. Semin Gastroenterol 2:37–48, 1991.
92. Sterneck M, Ferrell L, Ascher N, et al: Mycobacterial infection after liver transplantation: A report of three cases and review of the literature. Clin Transpl 6:55–61, 1992.
93. Perkocha L, Geaghan S, Yen T, et al: Clinical and pathological features of bacillary peliosis hepatis in association with human immunodeficiency virus infection. N Engl J Med 323:1581–1586, 1990.
94. Melato M, Laurino L, Mucli E, et al: Relationship between cirrhosis, liver cancer, and hepatic metastases: An autopsy study. Cancer 64:455–459, 1989.
95. Furuya K, Nakamura M, Yamamoto Y, et al: Macroregenerative nodule of the liver: A clinicopathologic study of 345 autopsy cases of chronic liver disease. Cancer 61:99–105, 1988.
96. Terada T, Hoso M, Nakanuma Y: Mallory body clustering in adenomatous hyperplasia in human cirrhotic livers: Report of four cases. Hum Pathol 20:886–890, 1989.
97. Nakanuma Y, Terada T, Ueda K, et al: Adenomatous hyperplasia of the liver as a precancerous lesion. Liver 13:1–9, 1993.
98. Ferrell L, Wright T, Lake J, et al: Incidence and diagnostic features of macroregenerative nodules vs. small hepatocellular carcinoma in cirrhotic livers. Hepatology 16:1372–1381, 1992.
99. Theise N, Schwartz M, Miller C, Thung S: Macroregenerative nodules and hepatocellular carcinoma in forty-four sequential adult liver explants with cirrhosis. Hepatology 16:949–955, 1992.
100. Terada T, Nakanuma Y: Survey of iron-accumulative macroregenerative nodules in cirrhotic livers. Hepatology 10:851–854, 1989.
101. Terada T, Nakanuma Y, Hoso M, et al: Fatty macroregenerative nodule in nonsteatotic liver cirrhosis: A morphologic study. Virchows Arch [A] 415:131–136, 1989.
102. Nakanuma Y, Ohta G, Sugiura H, et al: Incidental solitary hepatocellular carcinomas smaller than 1 cm in size found at autopsy. Hepatology 6:631–635, 1986.
103. Nakanuma Y, Ohta G: Expression of Mallory bodies in hepatocellular carcinoma in man and its significance. Cancer 57:81–86, 1986.
104. Nakanuma Y, Ohta G: Is Mallory body formation a preneoplastic change? A study of 181 cases of liver bearing hepatocellular carcinoma and 82 cases of cirrhosis. Cancer 55:2400–2404, 1985.
105. Nakanuma Y, Ohta G: Small hepatocellular carcinoma containing many Mallory bodies. Liver 4:128–133, 1984.
106. Kondo F, Wada K, Nagato Y, et al: Biopsy diagnosis of well-differentiated hepatocellular carcinoma based on new morphologic criteria. Hepatology 9:751–755, 1989.
107. Sakamoto M, Hirohashi S, Shimosato Y: Early stages of multistep hepatocarcinogenesis: Adenomatous hyperplasia and early hepatocellular carcinoma. Hum Pathol 22:172–178, 1991.
108. Nagato Y, Kondo F, Kondo Y, et al: Histological and morphometrical indicators for a biopsy diagnosis of well-differentiated hepatocellular carcinoma. Hepatology 14:473–478, 1991.
109. Crawford J: Pathologic assessment of liver cell dysplasia and benign liver tumors: Differentiation from malignant tumors. Semin Diagn Pathol 7:115–128, 1990.
110. Ferrell L, Crawford J, Dhillon A, et al: Proposal for standardized criteria for the diagnosis of benign, borderline, and malignant hepatocellular lesions arising in chronic advanced liver disease. Am J Surg Pathol 17:1113–1123, 1993.
111. Kondo Y, Nakajima T: Pseudoglandular hepatocellular carcinoma: A morphogenetic study. Cancer 60:1032–1037, 1987.
112. Cohen M, Haber M, Holly E, et al: Cytologic criteria to distinguish hepatocellular carcinoma from nonneoplastic liver. Am J Clin Pathol 95:125–130, 1991.
113. Hurlimann J, Gardiol D: Immunohistochemistry in the differential diagnosis of liver carcinomas. Am J Surg Pathol 15:280–288, 1991.
114. Fucich L, Cheles M, Thung S, et al: Primary versus metastatic hepatic carcinoma: An immunohistochemical study of 34 cases. Mod Pathol 6:110A, 1993.
115. Johnson D, Herndier B, Medieros L, et al: The diagnostic utility of the keratin profiles of hepatocellular carcinoma and cholangiocarcinoma. Am J Surg Pathol 12:187–197, 1988.
116. Carrozza M, Calafati S, Edmonds P: Immunocytochemical localization of polyclonal carcinoembryonic antigen in hepatocellular carcinomas. Acta Cytol 35:221–224, 1991.
117. Sebo T, Batts K: Immunohistochemical analysis of carcinoembryonic antigen (CEA) in the differential diagnosis of hepatic neoplasia. Mod Pathol 6:114A, 1993.
118. Wang J, Dhillon A, Sankey E, et al: Neuroendocrine differentiation in primary neoplasms of the liver. J Pathol 163:61–67, 1991.
119. Ruck P, Harms D, Kaiserling E: Neuroendocrine differentiation in hepatoblastoma: An immunohistochemical investigation. Am J Surg Pathol 14:847–855, 1990.
120. Garcia de Davila M, Gonzalez-Crussi F, Mangkornkanok M: Fibrolamellar carcinoma of the liver in a child: Ultrastructural and immunologic aspects. Pediatr Pathol 7:319–331, 1987.
121. Wanless I, Mawdsley C, Adams R: On the pathogenesis of focal nodular hyperplasia of the liver. Hepatology 5:1194–1200, 1985.
122. Ndimbie O, Goodman Z, Chase R, et al: Hemangiomas with localized nodular proliferation of the liver: A suggestion on the pathogenesis of focal nodular hyperplasia. Am J Surg Pathol 14:142–150, 1990.
123. Mathieu D, Zafrani E, Anglade M, Dhumeaux D: Association of focal nodular hyperplasia and hepatic hemangioma. Gastroenterology 97:154–157, 1989.
124. Wanless I: Micronodular transformation (nodular regenerative hyperplasia) of the liver: A report of 64 cases among 2500 autopsies and a new classification of benign hepatocellular nodules. Hepatology 11:787–797, 1990.
125. Stromeyer F, Ishak K: Nodular transformation (nodular regenerative hyperplasia) of the liver: A clinicopathologic study of 30 cases. Hum Pathol 12:660–671, 1981.
126. Nakanuma Y, Ohta G, Sasaki K: Nodular regenerative hyperplasia of the liver associated with polyarteritis nodosa. Arch Pathol Lab Med 108:133–135, 1984.
127. Nakanuma Y, Ohta G: Nodular hyperplasia of the liver in primary biliary cirrhosis of early histological stages. Am J Gastroenterol 82:8–10, 1987.
128. Nakanuma Y: Nodular regenerative hyperplasia of the liver: Retrospective survey in autopsy series. J Clin Gastroenterol 12:460–465, 1990.
129. Yutani C, Imakita M, Ishibash-Ueda H, et al: Nodular regenerative hyperplasia of the liver associated with primary pulmonary hypertension. Hum Pathol 19:726–731, 1988.
130. Kahn H, Manzarbeitia C, Theise N, et al: Danazol-induced hepatocellular adenomas: A case report and review of the literature. Arch Pathol Lab Med 115:1054–1057, 1991.
131. Tao L: Oral contraceptive-associated liver cell adenoma and hepatocellular carcinoma: Cytomorphology and mechanism of malignant transformation. Cancer 68:341–347, 1991.

132. Poe R, Snover D: Adenomas in glycogen storage disease type 1: Two cases with unusual histologic features. Am J Surg Pathol 12:477–483, 1988.

133. Chandra R, Kapur S, Kelleher J, et al: Benign hepatocellular tumors in the young: A clinicopathologic spectrum. Arch Pathol Lab Med 108:168–171, 1984.

134. Heffelfinger S, Irani D, Finegold M: ''Alcoholic hepatitis'' in a hepatic adenoma. Hum Pathol 18:751–754, 1987.

135. Ferrell L: Hepatocellular carcinoma arising in a focus of multilobular adenoma. Am J Surg Pathol 17:525–529, 1993.

136. Tao L, Ho C, McLoughlin M, et al: Cytologic diagnosis of hepatocellular carcinoma by fine-needle aspiration biopsy. Cancer 53:547–552, 1984.

137. Craig J, Peters R, Edmondson H, Omata M: Fibrolamellar carcinoma of the liver: A tumor of adolescents and young adults with distinctive clinico-pathologic features. Cancer 46:372–379, 1980.

138. Berman M, Sheahan D: Fibrolamellar carcinoma of the liver: An immunohisto-chemical study of nineteen cases and a review of the literature. Hum Pathol 19:784–794, 1988.

139. Omata M, Peters R, Tatters D: Sclerosing hepatic carcinoma: Relationship to hypercalcemia. Liver 1:33–49, 1981.

140. Weinberg A, Finegold M: Primary hepatic tumors of childhood. Hum Pathol 14:512–537, 1983.

141. Abenoza P, Manivel C, Wick M, et al: Hepatoblastoma: An immunohistochemical and ultrastructural study. Hum Pathol 18:1025–1035, 1987.

142. Conran R, Hitchcock C, Waclawiw M, et al: Hepatoblastoma: The prognostic significance of histologic type. Pediatr Pathol 12:167–183, 1992.

143. Haas J, Muczynski K, Krailo M, et al: Histopathology and prognosis in childhood hepatoblastoma and hepatocarcinoma. Cancer 64:1082–1095, 1989.

144. Stocker J, Ishak K: Mesenchymal hamartoma of the liver: Report of 30 cases and review of the literature. Pediatr Pathol 1:245–267, 1983.

145. Ishak K, Sesterhenn I, Goodman Z, et al: Epithelioid hemangioendothelioma of the liver: A clinicopathologic and follow-up study of 32 cases. Hum Pathol 15:839–852, 1984.

146. Dean P, Haggitt R, O'Hara C: Malignant epithelioid hemangioendothelioma of the liver in young women: Relationship to oral contraceptive use. Am J Surg Pathol 9:695–704, 1985.

147. Noronha R, Gonzalez-Crussi F: Hepatic angiosarcoma in childhood: A case report and review of the literature. Am J Surg Pathol 8:863–871, 1984.

148. Stocker J, Ishak K: Undifferentiated (embryonal) sarcoma of the liver: Report of 31 cases. Cancer 42:336–348, 1978.

149. Lack E, Schloo B, Azumi N, et al: Undifferentiated (embryonal) sarcoma of the liver: Clinical and pathologic study of 16 cases with emphasis on immunohisto-chemical features. Am J Surg Pathol 15:1–16, 1991.

150. Aoyama C, Hachitanda Y, Sato J, et al: Undifferentiated (embryonal) sarcoma of the liver: A tumor of uncertain histogenesis showing divergent differentiation. Am J Surg Pathol 15:615–624, 1991.

151. Goodman Z, Ishak K: Angiomyolipomas of the liver. Am J Surg Pathol 8:745–750, 1984.

152. Tsui W, Yuen A, Ma K, Tse C: Hepatic angiomyolipomas with a deceptive trabecular pattern and HMB-45 reactivity. Histopathology 21:569–573, 1992.

153. Chan J, Tsang W, Pau M, et al: Lymphangiomyomatosis and angiomyolipoma: Closely related entities characterized by hamartomatous proliferation of HMB-45-positive smooth muscle. Histopathology 22:445–455, 1993.

154. Weeks D, Malott R, Arnesen M, et al: Hepatic angiomyolipoma with striated granules and positivity with melanoma-specific antibody (HMB-45): A report of two cases. Ultrastruct Pathol 15:563–571, 1991.

155. Linton P, Ahn W, Schwartz M, et al: Angiomyolipoma of the liver: Immunohisto-chemical study of a case. Liver 11:158–161, 1991.

156. Chen K: Inflammatory pseudotumor of the liver. Hum Pathol 15:694–696, 1984.

157. Anthony P, Telesinghe P: Inflammatory pseudotumor of the liver. J Clin Pathol 39:761–768, 1986.

158. Shek T, Ng I, Chan K: Inflammatory pseudotumor of the liver: Report of four cases and review of the literature. Am J Surg Pathol 17:231–238, 1993.

159. Kudo M, Ikekubo K, Yamamoto K, et al: Focal fatty infiltration of the liver in acute alcoholic liver injury: Hot spots with radiocolloid SPECT scan. Am J Gastroenterol 84:948–952, 1989.

160. Grove A, Vyberg B, Vyberg M: Focal fatty change of the liver: A review and a case associated with continuous ambulatory peritoneal dialysis. Virchows Arch [A] 419:69–75, 1991.

161. Ishak K: Benign tumors and pseudotumors of the liver. Appl Pathol 6:82–104, 1988.

162. Goodman Z, Ishak K: Xanthogranulomatous cholecystitis. Am J Surg Pathol 5:653–659, 1981.

163. Charpentier P, Prade M, Bognel C, et al: Malacoplakia of the gallbladder. Hum Pathol 14:827–828, 1983.

164. Benbow E: Xanthogranulomatous cholecystitis associated with carcinoma of the gallbladder. Postgrad Med J 65:528–531, 1989.

165. Lopez J, Elizalde J, Calvo M: Xanthogranulomatous cholecystitis associated with gallbladder adenocarcinoma: A clinicopathologic study of 5 cases. Tumori 77:358–360, 1991.

166. Eisen R, Kirby W, O'Quinn J: Granular cell tumor of the biliary tree: A report of two cases and a review of the literature. Am J Surg Pathol 15:460–465, 1991.

167. Lack E, Worsham F, Callihan M, et al: Granular cell tumor: A clinicopathologic study of 110 patients. J Surg Oncol 13:301–316, 1980.

168. Weedon D: Eosinophilic cholecystitis. In Weedon D: Pathology of the Gallbladder. New York, Masson Publishing Company, 1984, pp 121–123.

169. Dabbs D: Eosinophilic and lymphoeosinophilic cholecystitis. Am J Surg Pathol 17:497–501, 1993.

170. Hinnant K, Schwartz A, Rotterdam H, Rudski C: Cytomegaloviral and cryptospori-dial cholecystitis in two patients with AIDS. Am J Surg Pathol 13:57–60, 1989.

171. Albores-Saavedra J, Nadji M, Henson D, et al: Intestinal metaplasia of the gallblad-der: A morphologic and immunocytochemical study. Hum Pathol 17:614–620, 1986.

172. Kijima H, Watanabe H, Iwafuchi M, Ishihara N: Histogenesis of gallbladder carcinoma from investigation of early carcinoma and microcarcinoma. Acta Pathol Jpn 39:235–244, 1989.

173. Weedon D: Mucosal hyperplasias and carcinoma in situ. In Weedon D: Pathology of the Gallbladder. New York, Masson Publishing Company, 1984, pp 212–222.

174. Albores-Saavedra J, Defortuna S, Smothermon W: Primary papillary hyperplasia of the gallbladder and cystic and common bile ducts. Hum Pathol 21:228–231, 1990.

175. Christensen A, Ishak K: Benign tumors and pseudotumors of the gallbladder: Report of 180 cases. Arch Pathol Lab Med 90:423–432, 1970.

176. Weedon D: Adenomyomatosis. In Weedon D: Pathology of the Gallbladder. New York, Masson Publishing Company, 1984, pp 185–194.

177. Ram M, Midha D: Adenomyomatosis of the gallbladder. Surgery 78:224–229, 1975.

178. Katoh T, Nikai T, Hayashi S, Satake T: Noninvasive carcinoma of the gallbladder arising in localized type adenomyomatosis. Am J Gastroenterol 83:670–674, 1988.

179. Aldridge M, Gruffaz F, Castaing D, Bismuth H: Adenomyomatosis of the gallblad-der. A premalignant lesion? Surgery 109:107–110, 1991.

180. Frierson H: The gross anatomy and histology of the gallbladder, extrahepatic bile ducts, Vaterian system and minor papilla. Am J Surg Pathol 13:146–162, 1989.

181. Nakajima T, Kondo Y: Well-differentiated cholangiocarcinoma: Diagnostic sig-nificance of morphologic and immunohistochemical parameters. Am J Surg Pathol 13:569–573, 1989.

182. Albores-Saavedra J, Nadji M, Henson D: Intestinal-type adenocarcinoma of the gallbladder: A clinicopathologic and immunocytochemical study of seven cases. Am J Surg Pathol 10:19–25, 1986.

183. Brandt-Rauf P, Pincus M, Adelson S: Cancer of the gallbladder: A review of forty-three cases. Hum Pathol 13:48–53, 1982.

184. Nakajo S, Yamamoto M, Tahara E: Morphometrical analysis of gallbladder ade-noma and adenocarcinoma with reference to histogenesis and adenoma-carcinoma sequence. Virchows Arch [A] 417:49–56, 1990.

185. Ojeda V, Shilkin K, Walters M: Premalignant epithelial lesions of the gallbladder: A prospective study of 120 cholecystectomy specimens. Pathology 17:451–454, 1985.

186. Albores-Saavedra J, Alcantra-Vazquez A, Cruz-Ortiz H, Herrera-Goepfert R: The precursor lesions of invasive gallbladder carcinoma: Hyperplasia, atypical hyper-plasia and carcinoma. Cancer 45:919–927, 1980.

187. Bivins B, Meeker W, Weiss D, Griffen W: Carcinoma in situ of the gallbladder: A dilemma. South Med J 68:297–300, 1975.

188. Nakajo S, Yamamoto M, Tahara E: Morphometric analysis of gallbladder adeno-carcinoma: Discrimination between carcinoma and dysplasia. Histopathology 416:133–140, 1989.

CHAPTER 10

The Genitourinary Tract

Clara E. Mesonero, M.D., and P. Anthony di Sant'Agnese, M.D.

KIDNEY

Childhood Lesions

Nephroblastomatosis and Nodular Renal Blastema (Nephrogenic Rest) versus Wilms' Tumor

The basic abnormality in **nodular renal blastema (NRB)** and **nephroblastomatosis** consists of abnormal persistence of collections of renal blastemal cells (metanephric tissue) after renal development should be completed.[1, 2] In **NRB** the collections are microscopic (each measuring less than 300 μ in diameter), multiple, and bilateral, and most frequently subcapsular (cortical-perilobular location) (Fig. 10–1). The lesion generally lacks stromal and epithelial differentiation, although small foci of glomerular or tubular differentiation may be encountered.[3] The term **perilobar nephroblastomatosis** (Fig. 10–2) can be applied to a bilateral form of NRB in a more diffuse distribution. The kidneys are enlarged, showing on cut surface subcapsular confluent nodules. Microscopically, it is similar to NRB, and tubular differentiation may be encountered. As in NRB, no mesenchymal component is identified. Nephroblastomatosis can also present as intralobar rests alone or combined with rests in the perilobar location. **Intralobar nephroblastomatosis** can contain fibromyxoid stroma, dilated tubules, dysplastic tubules, and nests of blastemal cells (Figs. 10–3 and 10–4). The stroma can be a predominant tissue that tends to be the rhabdomyomatous type.[4] **Panlobar nephroblastomatosis** is referred to as a widespread failure of nephrogenesis with persistent metanephric tissue diffusely distributed throughout all the kidney, so that the cortex and medulla lack completely matured elements.[2]

NRB presents at birth and in infants younger than 3 months. Nephroblastomatosis can be seen since birth and in children as old as 13 years. These lesions can be seen alone or associated with Wilms' tumor in the same or the opposite kidney. Patients with Wilms' tumors associated with nephroblastomatosis should be followed up carefully after treatment for Wilms' tumor because of a 5% risk of subsequent tumor development in the contralateral kidney. Perilobal nephroblastomatosis has a lower risk (5% probability) for developing a subsequent Wilms' tumor in the contralateral kidney than does intralobar nephroblastomatosis (16% probability).[5] NRB and nephroblastomatosis are considered benign lesions with the potential to develop into malignant lesions. Their malignant counterpart is Wilms' tumor or nephroblastoma.

Wilms' tumor is the most common intra-abdominal malignant tumor in childhood. This tumor presents most commonly in the first 5 years of life, with only 20% to 30% of cases occurring in older children. There is no predilection for either sex. It generally presents as an asymptomatic unilateral mass or with hematuria, fever, and abdominal pain. Bilateral Wilms' tumor has been seen in 2% to 14% of reported cases.[6] It can occur with several dysmorphic syndromes (hemihypertrophy, aniridia, and genitourinary abnormalities). It is the most frequent tumor associated with the Beckwith-Wiedemann syndrome. Some tumors with aniridia show deletion of the p13–14.1 band of the short arm of chromosome 11.[7]

Wilms' tumor usually measures more than 5 cm in diameter at the time of diagnosis and can be larger than 10 cm. Grossly, the affected kidney is enlarged, and on cross section the cut surface shows a pseudoencapsulated, solid, soft to firm, gray to tan lobulated mass. The mass may show areas of hemorrhage, necrosis, or cystic degeneration. Microscopically, there are three components: blastemal, epithelial, and stromal. Heterologous elements consisting of skeletal muscle, smooth muscle, cartilage, bone, and even neuronal tissue may be identified. The components may be proportional in amount (mixed or "classic type") or more frequently one component predominates over the others. In such cases, the tumor might present diagnostic difficulties, some of which are discussed later.

Blastemal Predominant Wilms' Tumor versus Anaplastic Wilms' Tumor, Clear-Cell Sarcoma, and Neuroblastoma

Blastemal cells in Wilms' tumor are small with a high nuclear/cytoplasmic ratio. The nuclei are ovoid and hyperchromatic, and there is very little cytoplasm that may be periodic acid-Schiff (PAS) positive. The cells grow in large sheets, nodules, or anastomosing serpentine bands. Rarely, they can form cords or rosettes (Fig. 10–5). Typically, there is an absence of reticulin fibers surrounding the blastemal cells. In blastemal predominant Wilms' tumor, the blastemal cells show a higher mitotic index than seen in classic Wilms' tumor. The increase in mitotic figures by itself does not qualify the tumor as being of anaplastic type. It is the variant of Wilms' tumor more frequently associated with anaplasia. Focal or diffuse anaplasia in Wilms' tumor indicates a particularly poor prognosis and warrants more aggressive therapy. Three features are required for the histologic diagnosis of **anaplasia:** (1) abnormal multipolar mitotic figures, (2) enlarged nuclei (to three or more times the size of surround-

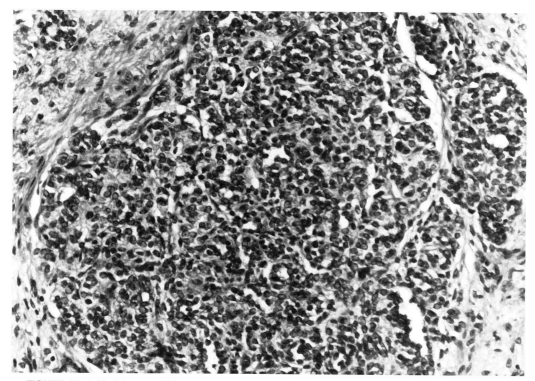

FIGURE 10–1. Nodular renal blastema. Microscopic focus of persistent metanephric tissue. (×660)

ing blastemal cells), and (3) hyperchromasia of the cells.[8] An exception to the prognostic significance of anaplasia is that when it is present in documented stage I Wilms' tumor, it does not appear to alter the prognosis compared with non-anaplastic stage I tumors.[5] ''Anaplasia'' in striated muscle cells does not have the same prognostic significance.

Blastemal predominant Wilms' tumor should be distinguished from **clear-cell sarcoma of kidney (CCSK),** also known as bone-metastasizing renal tumor of childhood.[9–11] Together with the rhabdoid tumor of kidney and anaplastic variant of Wilms' tumor, it is considered as part of the tumors of unfavorable histology included in the National Wilms'

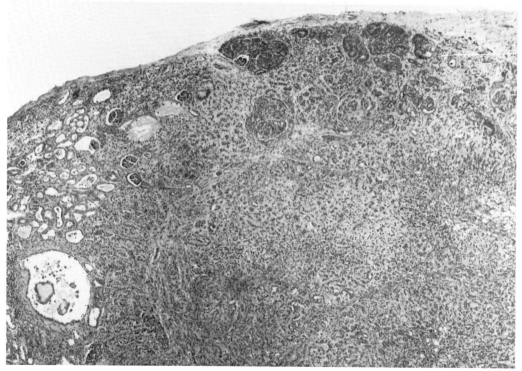

FIGURE 10–2. Perilobar nephroblastomatosis. (×66)

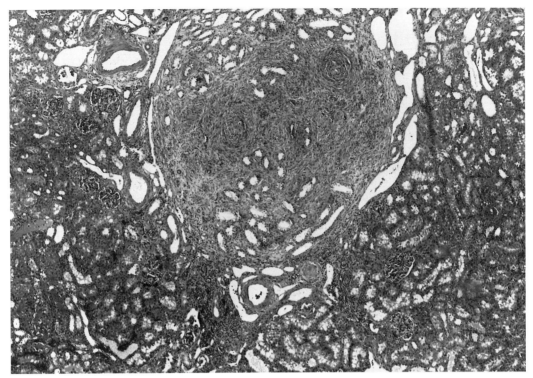

FIGURE 10–3. Intralobar nephroblastomatosis. Note dysplastic tubules and fibrous stroma. (×330)

Tumor Study.[12] CCSK accounts for about 4% of malignant renal tumors in childhood. It presents in children from 1 to 5 years of age, more often in males than in females. This tumor is very aggressive despite its deceptive bland histologic appearance. However, with intense triple-agent chemotherapy treatment, the prognosis has improved significantly as shown in the National Wilms' Tumor Study-3 (NWTS-3).[12] The tumor, as its name indicates, has a predilection for metastasizing to bone. Grossly, CCSK has a bulging cut surface and is sharply demarcated from the adjacent kidney. The cut surface

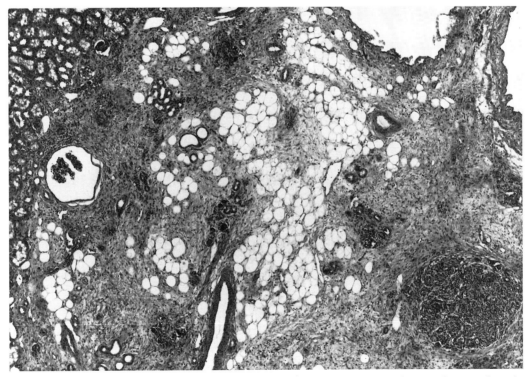

FIGURE 10–4. Intralobar nephroblastomatosis. Note blastemal component in lower right quadrant and mesenchymal components in the center of the figure. (×66)

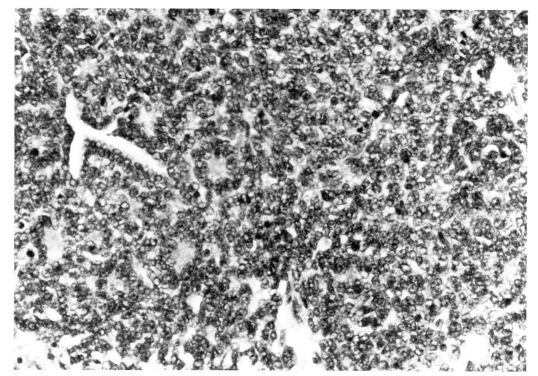

FIGURE 10–5. Blastemal portion of Wilms' tumor forming cords and rosettes simulating neuroblastoma. (×412)

is firm, gray tan, with occasional small isolated cysts. Microscopically, the cells are small and polygonal with an oval "bland" nucleus. The nucleus is classically optically clear (Fig. 10–6). The cells are arranged in cords and columns separated by delicate fibrovascular septa, reminiscent of the "chicken-wire"-like vasculature seen in myxoid liposarco-

mas. The solid pattern and the fact that the tumor tends to infiltrate the adjacent kidney entrapping tubules might cause the observer to confuse it with a blastemal predominant Wilms' tumor. The cytologic features identifying the tubules as non-tumoral but entrapped normal tubules should be helpful in arriving at the correct diagnosis. A reticulin stain may

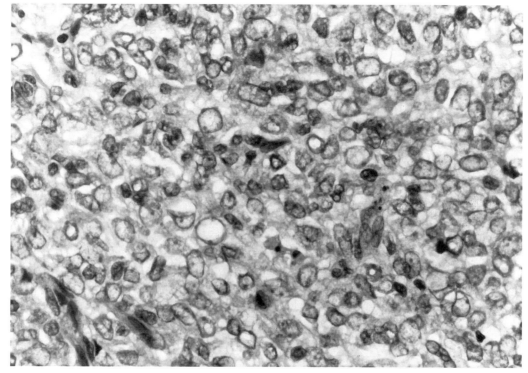

FIGURE 10–6. Clear-cell sarcoma showing "bland" optically clear nuclei. (×990)

also be helpful because there are more reticulin fibers around individual cells in CCSK than in the blastemal portion of a Wilms' tumor.

CCSK can present with a hyalinizing, epithelioid, angiectatic, spindled, cystic, or myxoid pattern. None of these patterns has a particular association with biologic behavior.[13]

CCSK and blastemal predominant Wilms' tumor both can simulate **neuroblastoma,** from which they should be also distinguished. Cells in CCSK can occasionally simulate a neural pattern when there is perivascular palisading of the cells. However, no true tubules are identified in CCSK. Focal positive reaction for cytokeratins and/or a constant positive reaction for vimentin are characteristic for CCSK. Vimentin is negative in neuroblastoma. Sometimes the rosette-like configuration adopted by blastemal cells in a blastemal predominant Wilms' tumor can also suggest the diagnosis of a neuroblastoma (see Fig. 10–5). **Neuroblastomas** arise most commonly in the adrenal medulla, with possible secondary involvement of the kidney. Primary renal neuroblastoma is extremely rare.[14] Adrenal neuroblastomas are usually single and unilateral, although bilateral cases have been reported. Two thirds of the cases present in children younger than the age of 5 and may be seen as early as birth. Grossly, the tumor is very soft owing to hemorrhage and necrosis. It also frequently shows areas of calcification. Microscopically, the tumor is comprised of small round cells with minimal cytoplasm. It grows in nests and sheets. A diagnostic feature is the formation of true rosettes with central areas of neurofibrils. These can be difficult to find or may be absent. Immunohistochemical studies help in the differential diagnosis with the other mimicking lesions. The cells are positive for neuron-specific enolase, PGP 9.5, synaptophysin, and neurofilament protein, among other neural markers. CCSK and the blastemal portion of a Wilms' tumor are negative for these markers.

Stromal Predominant Wilms' Tumors versus Congenital Mesoblastic Nephroma, Malignant Spindle Cell Neoplasm, and Clear-Cell Sarcoma

The stromal component in Wilms' tumor may show different types of differentiation, the most common being the fibrous and myxoid types. When the predominant component is fibrous stroma, the tumor should be distinguished from congenital mesoblastic nephroma (CMN), a malignant spindle cell neoplasm, and a clear-cell sarcoma with spindle cell features.

Congenital mesoblastic nephroma (CMN) constitutes approximately 50% of childhood renal tumor in patients younger than 1 year old. It is typically found in the neonatal period.[15] They can also occur less frequently in older children. CMN presents as a unilateral mass. The mass has the gross appearance of a leiomyoma, but with indistinct borders as a result of infiltration of the adjacent renal tissue by finger-like projections of tumor cells (Fig. 10–7). Microscopically, the tumor cells consist of fibroblasts and myofibroblasts. Foci of cartilage and immature mesenchyme may be identified. Cellularity can vary, but tends to be low or moderate. The cells are plump with generally minimal or no atypia (Fig. 10–8). Cases with increased cellularity, atypia, high mitotic index, and necrosis in children older than 3 months have been called "atypical."[16] These features may have a predictive value for recurrence and metastasis in older patients, but not in infants younger than 3 months. In the neonatal period, these features are seen in 25% to 30% of the cases, with no evidence of association with an aggressive behavior.[5, 17] Of crucial importance for the surgeon is to obtain free surgical margins. Microscopic strands may extend beyond the capsule and into the renal hilum. Incomplete surgical resection is associated

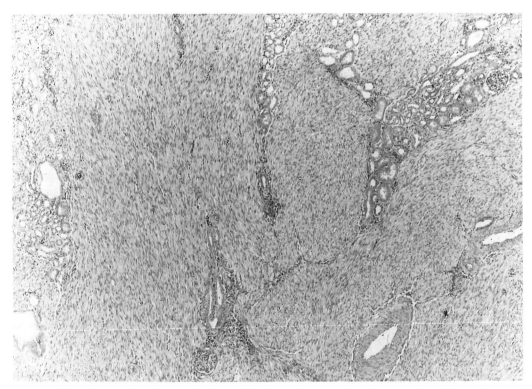

FIGURE 10–7. Advancing border of congenital mesoblastic nephroma entrapping normal renal parenchyma. (×330)

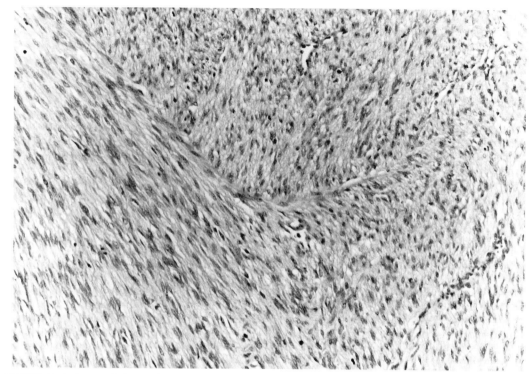

FIGURE 10–8. Congenital mesoblastic nephroma. Note bland cytology and scattered mitotic figures. (×420)

with recurrence of tumor. Rare variants of CMN contain plump clear cells associated with an angiomatous pattern simulating **CCSK** from which it should be distinguished.[18] CMN and stromal predominant Wilms' tumor should be distinguished from malignant spindle cell tumors such as **leiomyosarcoma** and **fibrosarcoma.** The infiltrative margins might suggest malignancy; however, the lack of atypia and generally low mitotic index should favor congenital mesoblastic nephroma. In addition, malignant spindle cell sarcomas such as leiomyosarcomas and fibrosarcomas are extremely rare in young children. Immunohistochemical studies are not very helpful in the differential diagnosis. CMN cells contain vimentin and occasionally desmin. S-100 protein and neuron-specific enolase may also be expressed.[11]

Wilms' Tumor with Predominant Striated Muscle Differentiation versus Rhabdomyosarcoma and Rhabdoid Tumor

Rare cases of Wilms' tumor also known as **rhabdomyomatous nephroblastomas**[19] are composed almost completely by fetal striated muscle (Fig. 10–9), with only small foci of more classic Wilms' tumor. This finding does not indicate a worse prognosis or "sarcomatous" Wilms' tumor. This type of Wilms' tumor tends to affect younger children. There is a male predominance, and 30% are bilateral. Although some authors advocate a better prognosis, cases with aggressive behavior and metastasis have been reported. The tumor has to be differentiated from true rhabdomyosarcoma.[20]

Primary true rhabdomyosarcomas of the kidney are extremely rare. Children's rhabdomyosarcomas of the genitourinary tract are of the embryonal type, often sarcoma botryoides, with the characteristic peripheral cambium layer. It

involves more often other portions of the genitourinary tract other than the kidney.

It is essential to distinguish a Wilms' tumor from a rhabdoid tumor. Wilms' tumor can simulate rhabdoid tumor when presenting with a predominant rhabdomyomatous component, or less commonly when it has a predominance of the blastemal component in which blastemal cells can rarely contain cytoplasmic inclusions.

Rhabdoid tumor is an extremely aggressive neoplasm. It is one of the most malignant tumors of childhood.[21] It presents in young children generally younger than the age of 5 with the mean age of 11 to 13 months. Patients usually die within 1 year of diagnosis, with widespread metastasis. In the National Wilms' Tumor Study-3, the 2-year relapse-free survival and 3-year survival rate of randomized and followed patients with rhabdoid tumor was 19%.[12] Hypercalcemia (due to ectopic parathormone secretion) and a second primary neoplasm of the central nervous system have been associated with this tumor.[22,23] It involves the kidney unilaterally, characteristically the perihilar renal tissue. Most tumors are rounded and poorly demarcated from the adjacent renal tissue. The cut surface is usually gray, with variable foci of hemorrhage and/or necrosis. Microscopically, the tumor is composed of a monotonous population of round to polygonal cells, growing in diffuse sheets, without clearly defined tubule formation. A distribution in nodules or anastomosing bands seen in the blastemal component of Wilms' tumor is not seen in RTK. It has a very infiltrative pattern similar to the pattern seen in CCSK and different from the pushing border of Wilms' tumor. The cells have abundant cytoplasm and a round vesicular nucleus with a prominent large central nucleolus (Fig. 10–10). The latter is not seen in Wilms' tumor or CCSK. Some cells contain hyaline or fibrillary rounded cytoplasmic inclusions. The

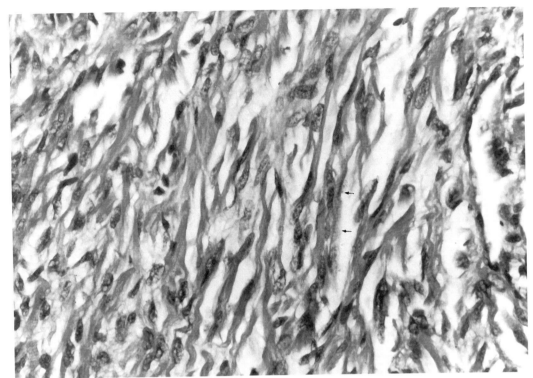

FIGURE 10–9. Fetal striated muscle in rhabdomyomatous Wilms' tumor. Note cytoplasmic striations *(arrows)*. (×990)

cytoplasm tends to be eosinophilic. These cytoplasmic features suggest skeletal muscle differentiation. However, striations are never seen. Immunohistochemical studies show coexpression of vimentin and cytokeratin in some cases, as well as epithelial membrane antigen. It does not show positive reaction for myogenic differentiation.[21] By electron microscopy, the inclusions correspond to whorled arrays of 6- to 9-nm filaments and parallel arrays of 10-nm filaments. Filaments characteristic of striated muscle are not seen by electron microscopy.

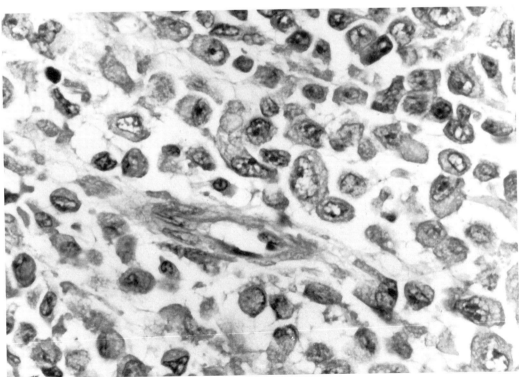

FIGURE 10–10. Rhabdoid tumor of kidney showing cells with abundant cytoplasm and round vesicular nucleus with prominent nucleolus. No cytoplasmic striations are seen. (×990)

Wilms' Tumor with Predominant Heterologous Differentiation (Teratoid Tumor) versus Renal Teratoma

A small subgroup of Wilms' tumors has a predominance of heterologous elements (>50%) which include mature adipose tissue, squamous epithelium, and cartilage. Neural elements have also been described.[24] This type of Wilms' tumor was termed **teratoid Wilms' tumor** by Variend, et al.[25] There are only a few reports of this variant of nephroblastoma. It should be distinguished from true primary renal teratoma of the kidney, which is even more unusual.[13, 26] The lack of attempt of heterotopic organ formation by the heterologous elements, presence of more classic Wilms' triphasic areas, and/or the association with nephroblastomatosis help in the differentiation.

Cystic Wilms' Tumor versus Multilocular Cyst of Kidney (Cystic Nephroma), Cystic Partially Differentiated Nephroblastoma, and Cystic Clear-Cell Sarcoma

Wilms' tumor can frequently show scattered small-to-medium-sized cysts. The cysts do not alter the behavior and clinical outcome of the tumor. These cases should be distinguished from developmental and other neoplastic renal cystic lesions. These include multilocular cyst of kidney (cystic nephroma), cystic partially differentiated nephroblastoma, and cystic clear-cell sarcoma.

Multilocular cyst of kidney[27] is considered by some authors as a developmental anomaly of unknown cause.[28] Other authors support the hypothesis of a differentiated Wilms' tumor and prefer to call the lesion a cystic nephroma.[29] Based on the criteria proposed by Powell et al., the lesion

has to be solitary, unilateral, cystic, and multilocular.[28] The locules do not communicate with one another or with the renal pelvis. They are lined by a simple cuboidal or flattened epithelium. The interlocular septa are devoid of renal parenchyma. The lesion presents generally in children younger than the age of 2. Multilocular cyst of kidney, or cystic nephroma, is a benign lesion that can be treated safely by surgery alone. When the lesion contains microscopically blastemal and other undifferentiated cell types, it is classified as a cystic partially differentiated nephroblastoma (CPDN).[30]

Cystic partially differentiated nephroblastoma (Fig. 10–11) classically shows microscopic islands of blastemal cells beneath the lining epithelium of the locules, islands of blastemal cells in immature mesenchyme, foci of immature skeletal muscle, and immature neoplastic tubules. This lesion has generally a favorable outcome even without adjuvant therapy.

Multilocular cyst (cystic nephroma) and CPDN have similar clinical presentations and gross appearance. If the interlocular septa grossly contain tumor nodules, **cystic clear-cell sarcoma of kidney and Wilms' tumor** should be considered in the differential diagnosis. If the tumor nodules contain blastema, tubules, and mesenchyme, the tumor should be considered a Wilms' tumor (cystic) and treated in accordance with its stage. The distinction with clear-cell sarcoma is also based on cytologic features, previously discussed.

Multicystic Dysplasia versus Multilocular Cyst of Kidney and Infantile Polycystic Disease

Multicystic dysplastic kidney (MDK) is the most common lesion that presents as an abdominal mass in the newborn. It presents sporadically, and the cause is unknown. It is a non-

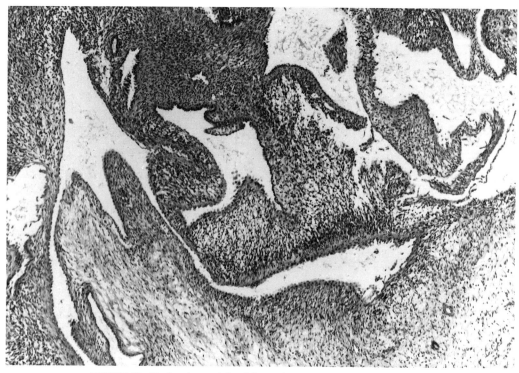

FIGURE 10–11. Cystic partially differentiated nephroblastoma. (×165)

familial maldevelopment of the kidney with no associated cystic lesions of pancreas, liver, or lung.[31] Frequently, it is associated with other lower urinary tract congenital abnormalities such as renal pelvic atresia with involvement of the renal vascular pedicle and ureter. The pathogenesis is unclear. An inhibition of the ampullary inductive activity on the metanephric blastema during renal development appears responsible for the malformation.[32] A suggested mechanism is vascular compromise of the ureter and developing ampullae with subsequent stenosis and urinary tract obstruction that contributes in the development of congenital multicystic dysplastic kidney.[31] It generally presents as a unilateral mass. A few cases are bilateral with total, focal, or segmental involvement. **Unilateral** multicystic dysplastic kidney has to be differentiated from a multilocular cyst (described previously) and chronic pyelonephritis.[33] Most unilateral cases manifest during early childhood, although rare cases might remain undetected and first manifest in adulthood.[34] When **bilateral** with total involvement of the kidneys, the patients die soon after birth as a result of lack of renal function. Bilateral cases need to be distinguished from infantile polycystic kidney.[35] The latter is an inherited form of cystic renal disease that can present with variable severity. The newborn presents also with hepatic abnormalities, such as cysts and bile duct proliferation with portal fibrosis. Accurate diagnosis is crucial for appropriate genetic counseling of the parents and work-up of siblings for possible disease manifestation.

The gross and microscopic appearances of both cystic lesions are quite different. In **MDK,** the affected kidney has totally lost its reniform shape and presents as a multilobulated cystic mass. On cross section, there is no identifiable renal cortex or medulla. A central area of fibrous tissue is identified. This tissue contains microscopically primitive tubules with surrounding concentric fibromuscular tissue (Fig. 10–12) and focal areas of cartilaginous stroma (Fig. 10–13).

In polycystic renal disease, the kidneys are always bilaterally enlarged and retain their reniform shape. On cross section, cortical and medullary areas are usually identified with numerous cysts throughout both areas (Fig. 10–14). The cysts tend to be elongated and radiate toward the pelvic calyx. The intervening renal tissue shows microscopically glomeruli and/or uninvolved collecting tubules.[35] (Fig. 10–15).

Adult Lesions

Renal Cortical Adenoma versus Renal Cell Carcinoma

The differentiation of these two renal cortical tumors is controversial. Renal cortical **adenoma** is a proliferative cortical, generally subcapsular lesion with either tubular or papillary differentiation and no cytologic atypia (Fig. 10–16). It can be found incidentally during work-up of other lesions or at autopsy in as many as 23% of patients. The lesion is generally asymptomatic. Based primarily on Bell's studies,[36] a lesion less than 3 cm in diameter has been arbitrarily called adenoma. Its behavior is usually benign; however, there are rare reports of metastasis from small "adenomas." Bell found that 4.6% of the lesions that metastasized measured less than 3 cm in diameter. Subsequent reports have shown additional small metastasizing lesions that cannot be differentiated on histologic grounds from the non-metastasizing ones.[37] Therefore, they should be considered a neoplasm of low malignant potential or small renal cell carcinoma.[38, 39] With increase in tumor size, there is a higher risk for developing metastasis. We reserve the diagnosis of adenoma for lesions less than 1 cm in size that are subcapsular, with papillary architecture, no clear-cell component, and no cytologic atypia. Both neoplasms, renal cell carcinoma and adenoma, have shown a

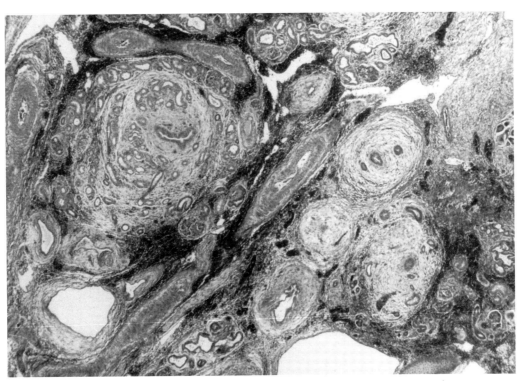

FIGURE 10–12. Renal dysplasia. (×66)

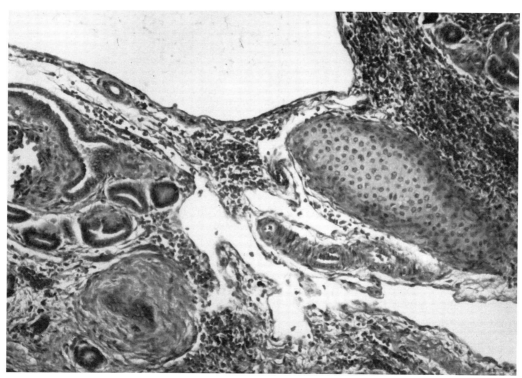

FIGURE 10–13. Renal dysplasia. Note primitive tubules surrounded by concentric fibromuscular layers and focus of cartilage. (×165)

common origin in the tubules of the kidney. With immunohistochemical markers and electron microscopy, features of proximal convoluted tubules are more often found than features of distal tubules.

Renal cell carcinoma (RCC) is the most common primary malignant renal neoplasm in adults (80% to 90%), with rare cases presenting in children and adolescents.[40] The peak incidence occurs in the sixth decade. Males are more commonly affected than females (male:female ratio, 2:1). There is a higher incidence in patients with von Hippel-Lindau syndrome and in patients with long-term dialysis and secondary acquired cystic disease.[41] They are usually solitary masses, but multiple

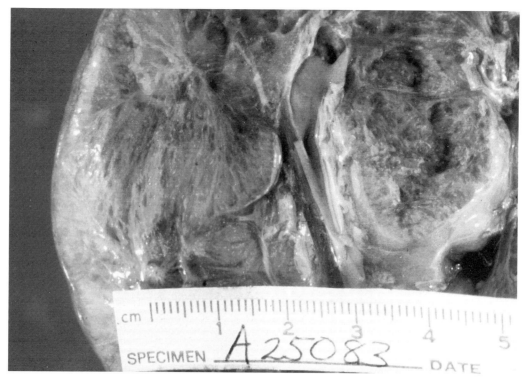

FIGURE 10–14. Cross section of infantile polycystic kidney with elongated cortical and medullary cysts. Note to the left, smooth outer renal contour.

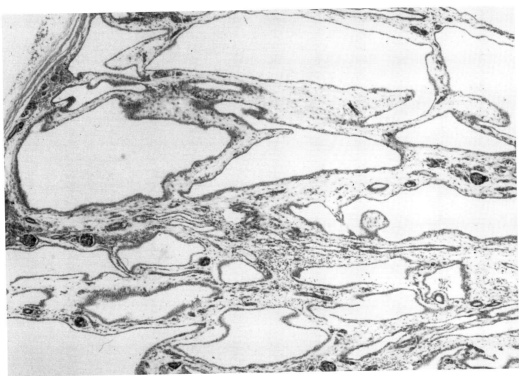

FIGURE 10–15. Infantile polycystic kidney. Elongated cysts with intervening renal tissue. (×66)

or bilateral tumors have been reported, especially in cases with von Hippel-Lindau disease. Rare cases of familiar predisposition with chromosome 3 rearrangement have also been reported.[42] The most frequent presentation of renal cell carcinoma is hematuria. The classic triad of hematuria, flank pain, and flank mass occurs only in few patients and reflects advanced disease. There is, in addition, a series of systemic manifestations that can be associated with the tumor and its metastasis, the most common being anemia, fever, and increased erythrocyte sedimentation rate. In rare occasions,

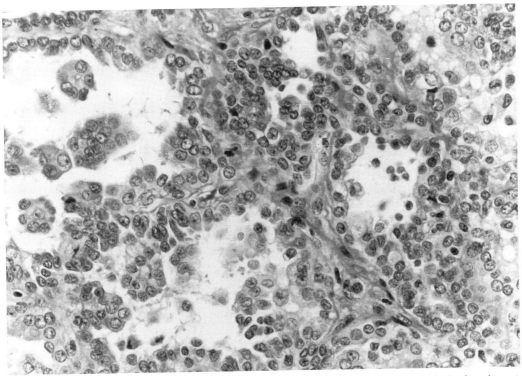

FIGURE 10–16. High power of subcapsular renal adenoma with tubulopapillary architecture. Note lack of nuclear atypia. (×206)

there are findings related to production of substances by the tumor cells (erythropoietin, parathormone-like substance, insulin and so on). In other instances, the first presentation is that of a metastasis from an occult renal cell carcinoma. Grossly, RCC varies generally from 5 to 10 cm in maximum diameter, but they can be smaller or larger. The cut surface is variegated, reflecting necrosis, hemorrhage, lipid content, and variegated histologic patterns. The tumor tends to have a bulging cut surface with "pushing" margins. In the absence of cystic variants or massive necrosis, the tumor tends to have a solid consistency. Microscopically, this tumor can have clear, granular, or spindled cells, with most tumor having a mixture of clear and granular cells with a predominance of one type over the others. Architecturally, the tumor can have an alveolar (nest), solid sheet-like, microcystic, tubular, papillary, or tubulopapillary pattern. A fine vasculature in the solid and alveolar pattern is also very characteristic. (Fig. 10–17). The different histologic and cytologic features do not correlate with prognosis and behavior with the exception of the spindle cell or sarcomatoid renal cell carcinoma (worse prognosis)[43] and the "papillary-cystic variant" (generally better prognosis than non-papillary renal cell carcinoma).[44, 45] However, awareness and recognition of the variegated microscopic appearance are helpful in resolving the diagnostic difficulties that these variants can present. They can masquerade as other entities or tumors from which they should be distinguished. Examples of differential diagnosis are discussed later. In terms of prognosis, the pathologist should be able to assist in assessing tumor stage (evaluating tumor size, renal distortion, capsular invasion, involvement of renal veins and/or vena cava, lymph nodes, and metastasis), tumor grade (nuclear grade), and histologic patterns (sarcomatoid and papillary variants).

Renal Oncocytoma versus Renal Cell Carcinoma with a Predominance of Granular Cells (with Oncocytic Features)

Oncocytoma, as the name implies, is a neoplasm exclusively composed of oncocytes.[46] It was first described in 1976 by Klein and Valensi.[47] Ultrastructurally, their abundant eosinophilic cytoplasm lacks lipid and glycogen and contains numerous mitochondria. Renal cell carcinomas with oncocytic features (granular cell variant) contain an increase in cytoplasmic mitochondria and variable amounts of glycogen and lipid. Many renal oncocytomas were initially classified as renal cell carcinomas. As with renal cell carcinoma, they occur more frequently in males than in females, and their peak incidence overlaps with that of renal cell carcinoma. The majority are asymptomatic and are discovered during the work-up of other abdominal lesions or at autopsy. This tumor tends to be unilateral, although bilateral and multicentric cases have been reported. Symptomatic patients present with pain, hematuria, or flank mass. Its frequency of presentation averages 5% of renal tumors in adulthood. It is known to have characteristic angiographic features that are highly suggestive of oncocytoma. However, renal cell carcinoma cannot be completely ruled out by angiography.[48, 49] Characteristic features include:

1. Uniform blush during nephrogram phase
2. Well-demarcated smooth contours with vessels stretched around the tumor
3. Hypervascularity with lack of pulling of contrast medium
4. "Spoke-wheel" pattern of tumor vascularity
5. Lack of arteriovenous shunting

Renal cell carcinoma, on the contrary, demonstrates neovascularity, tortuous irregular vessels, a diffuse tumor blush, arterio-

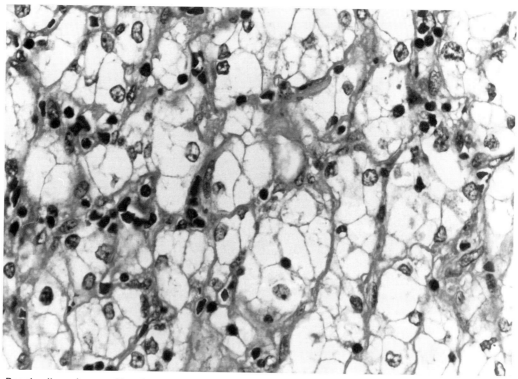

FIGURE 10–17. Renal cell carcinoma. Alveolar pattern with fine intervening vasculature. Note lack of cytoplasmic vacuolation in clear cells. (×825)

venous shunting, pooling of contrast media, and accentuation of capsular vessels.[50] The final differential diagnosis still relies on histopathologic findings. Grossly, oncocytomas average 3 to 7 cm. The typical presentation is that of a well-circumscribed, encapsulated, red-brown tumor on cut surface. A characteristic central fibrous scar is often, but not always, present. Hemorrhage, necrosis, and cystic change are absent or minimal. The tumor lacks gross capsular or renal vein invasion. Microscopically, the tumor is uniformly composed of bright granular eosinophilic cells that lack mitotic activity and nuclear atypia (oncocytoma grade I). The nucleoli are present but not prominent. The cells are arranged in nests, cords, or tubules in a loose edematous stroma (Fig. 10–18). The central scar consists of acellular dense collagen. When the tumor follows the criteria given for a classic oncocytoma with no cytologic atypia, this tumor is considered benign, regardless of size, presence of necrosis, and microscopic vascular or capsular invasion. When there is nuclear atypia, it has been classified as oncocytoma grade II. In a Mayo Clinic study, 14% (4 of 28 patients) of patients with oncocytoma grade II died of metastatic disease.[51] The greater the atypia, the more likelihood of finding clear cells that would classify the tumor as a renal cell carcinoma with oncocytic features. Until more studies are done, it is better to reserve the term *oncocytoma* only for the classic accepted grade I lesion.[52] We prefer to call "oncocytoma grade II" renal cell carcinoma, granular cell variant. Renal cell carcinoma with oncocytic features does not behave differently from more classic renal cell carcinoma with clear cells. It is important to differentiate oncocytomas from renal cell carcinoma because of the different surgical treatment (partial nephrectomy versus radical nephrectomy with possible regional lymph node dissection) and behavior.

Sarcomatoid Renal Cell Carcinoma versus Primary Renal Sarcoma

The term **sarcomatoid renal cell carcinoma** is applied to the renal cell carcinoma with a prominent spindle cell component.[53, 54] Sarcomatoid RCC usually presents in advanced stage, the median survival being 6 months after diagnosis. It generally also contains classic areas of clear and/or granular-type cells. It constitutes approximately 5% of all renal cell carcinomas. The spindle cell component characteristically shows marked nuclear atypia (Fig. 10–19) and can present with several different architectural patterns resembling fibrosarcoma, malignant fibrous histiocytoma, and in rare instances with heterologous differentiation with chondrosarcoma and osteosarcoma differentiation. Careful study of numerous sections are recommended in a "sarcomatous" renal tumor to differentiate a sarcomatoid renal cell carcinoma from renal sarcoma. In sarcomatoid renal cell carcinoma, generally there are areas with more classic epithelial differentiation.

Immunohistochemical studies are not helpful. Sarcomas that have been reported as primary renal tumors in the literature are leiomyosarcomas, liposarcomas, fibrosarcomas, angiosarcomas, malignant fibrous histiocytomas, osteosarcoma, chondrosarcoma, and malignant peripheral nerve sheath tumor. They constitute 4% of adult renal tumors.

Leiomyosarcomas are the most frequent primary renal sarcomas.[55, 56] They arise mainly from the periphery of the kidney, either from the renal capsule or renal pelvic wall. They compress from without and can infiltrate the renal parenchyma with poorly demarcated advancing borders. Grossly and microscopically, they do not differ from leiomyosarcomas at other more common body sites. Vascular invasion is common,

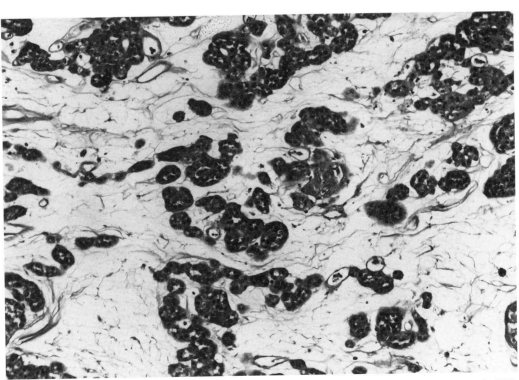

FIGURE 10–18. Oncocytoma. Cells arranged in tubules and nests in a loose edematous stroma. (×165)

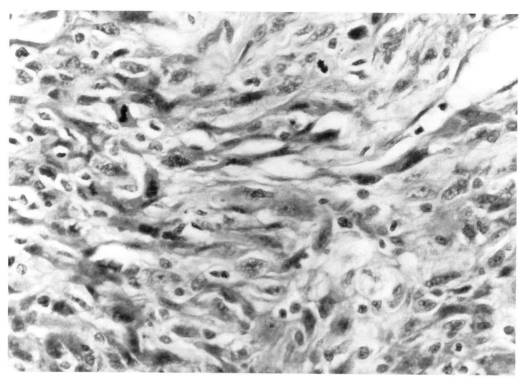

FIGURE 10–19. Sarcomatoid RCC. (×250)

and distant metastases are frequent. The prognosis is very poor. A renal leiomyosarcoma should be differentiated from renal leiomyoma, angiomyolipoma, renal mesoblastic nephroma, and fibrosarcoma.

Cystic Renal Cell Carcinoma versus Other Non-malignant Cystic Renal Lesions

Renal cell carcinoma can have a predominant cystic component (**cystic renal cell carcinoma**) in as many as 15% of cases.[57] In such cases, they can present diagnostic difficulties radiologically and pathologically. It can present as a unilocular cystic mass or as a multiloculated cystic mass. They can be intrinsically loculated or arise in the setting of non-neoplastic cystic renal disease.

When renal cell carcinomas are intrinsically cystic, they can present as a single cyst with central degeneration, necrosis, and recent and old hemorrhage. The remaining mass is formed by a solid tumor. Intrinsically, cystic renal cell carcinoma can also present as a multiloculated mass. In this case, grossly the tumor consists of numerous, non-communicating cysts of variable sizes generally filled with clear fluid or blood. A pseudocapsule separates it from the adjacent uninvolved renal tissue. Microscopically, the cysts are lined by tumor cells that generally are of the clear-cell variant (Fig. 10–20). The stroma in between cysts also contains tumor cells and can be extensively hyalinized with calcifications and even ossification.[58] This tumor should be separated from the generally benign lesion **cystic nephroma** and **cystic partially differentiated nephroblastoma,** which may remain undetected until adulthood. For description, refer to discussion of these entities under ''Childhood Lesions.''

When renal cell carcinoma is associated with a preexisting cystic renal disease such as acquired polycystic kidneys

(patient on chronic hemodialysis)[59] or simple cyst, the most common histologic pattern is that of **tubulopapillary variant.** This tumor variant can be necrotic, accounting for additional cystic degeneration. It has characteristic fibrovascular stalks, which may be distended with foamy lipid-laden macrophages (Fig. 10–21).[60, 61] The papillae are lined by a single layer of cells with variable generally mild cytologic atypia. When arising in the setting of cystic disease, they tend to be well differentiated and associated with a very good prognosis. When RCC tubulopapillary variant presents *de novo* without preexisting cystic disease, it also tends to be well differentiated, even when large masses are encountered. In only rare instances, they have metastasized or have been invasive. In such cases, the cells have shown marked cytologic atypia, and the tumor has been more necrotic.

Collecting Duct Carcinoma (Bellini's Duct Carcinoma) versus Renal Cell Carcinoma

Collecting duct carcinoma (CDC) is a very rare neoplasm that arises from the epithelium of the collecting tubules of the medulla and extends secondarily into the renal cortex. There are only a few cases reported, all of which seem to be associated with aggressive behavior, early metastasis, and poor prognosis.[62] The clinical presentation is similar to that of renal cell carcinoma. However, it presents more frequently at earlier ages than renal cell carcinoma. Histologically, several patterns have been reported, with the papillary and infiltrating tubular patterns (Fig. 10–22) being the most frequently encountered. In those cases, a papillary (tubulopapillary) renal cell carcinoma might be considered in the differential diagnosis. A transitional cell carcinoma component is also frequently seen. The tumor can present in a cystic mass reminiscent also of the relatively common cystic variant of renal cell

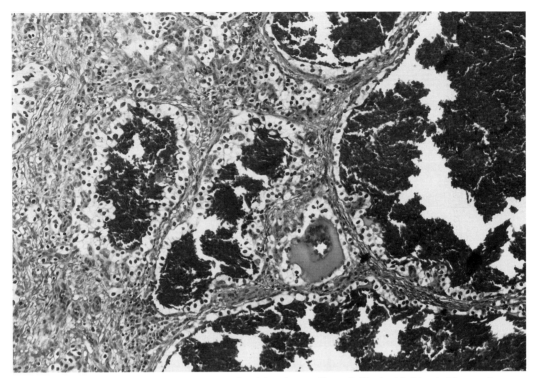

FIGURE 10-20. Cystic renal cell carcinoma. Cystic spaces lined by clear cells and filled with blood. Clear cells are present also in intervening stroma. (×165)

carcinoma. CDC shows characteristically an intense desmoplastic response elicited by the tubular component (Fig. 10–23) which is absent in renal cell carcinoma. Cytologic atypia is most prominent in the tubular component, whereas the papillary areas usually have a less atypical appearance.

Collecting ducts adjacent to the tumor usually show atypical hyperplastic changes in their epithelium (Fig. 10–24). It is important to distinguish CDC from RCC because of the apparently more aggressive behavior of the collecting duct carcinoma compared with the more benign course of renal cell

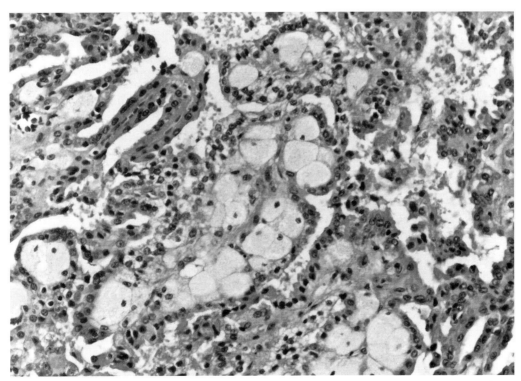

FIGURE 10-21. Tubulopapillary renal cell carcinoma. Note papillary stalks distended by lipid-laden macrophages. (×330)

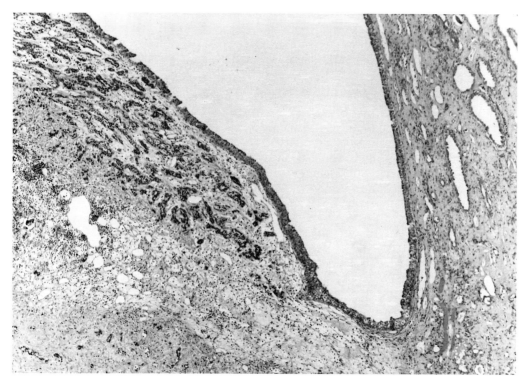

FIGURE 10–22. Infiltrating tubular pattern in collecting duct carcinoma. Note tubules infiltrating through medullary area. (×66)

carcinoma, especially the tubulopapillary variant. Both neoplasms can be distinguished by their different site of origin: collecting tubule/medulla (CDC) versus proximal tubule/cortex (RCC).[63] Immunohistochemical and electron microscopy studies have also supported the origin of this tumor from collecting ducts rather than from proximal tubules. CDC can show positive staining for mucicarmine in tubular areas (Fig. 10–25); by immunohistochemistry, it shows positive staining for epithelial membrane antigen (EMA), high and low molecular weight keratins, vimentin, and peanut lectin.[62, 64] Renal cell

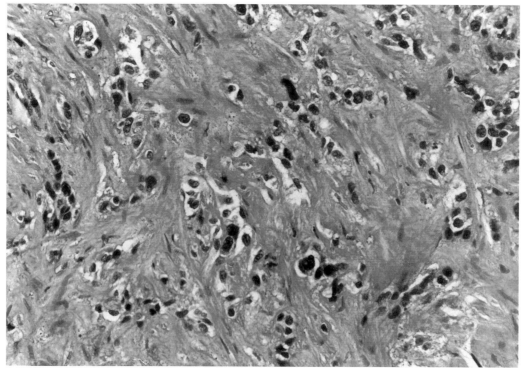

FIGURE 10–23. Desmoplastic stroma elicited by tubular component in collecting duct carcinoma. (×330)

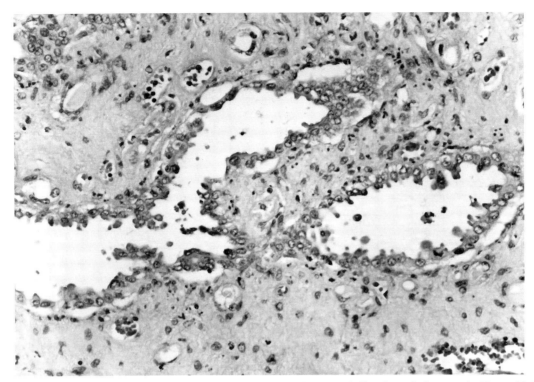

FIGURE 10-24. Atypical hyperplastic epithelium in collecting ducts adjacent to infiltrating tubules seen in Figure 10-22. (×330)

carcinomas stain predominantly for low molecular weight keratin, EMA, and vimentin.[65]

Xanthogranulomatous Nephritis (XGN) versus Renal Cell Carcinoma

XGN is an uncommon, progressive, highly destructive inflammatory process. It occurs more commonly in women (mean age, fifth to sixth decade).[66, 67] The patient presents with a flank mass, possible flank pain, fever, and anemia. It is an inflammatory disorder characterized by numerous foamy histiocytes, which can give the lesion a yellow color. This inflammatory process is frequently associated with culture-positive urinary tract infections (*Escherichia coli, Proteus mirabilis, Aerobacter,* and other gram-negative bacteria). Renal calculi (staghorn type) are encountered in many cases. The process shows grossly a nodular configuration with central areas of necrosis. It can extend into perirenal tissue. These features can mimic renal cell carcinoma of the predominant clear-cell type. The renal pelvis can be largely distorted, simulating also on radiologic grounds a neoplasm. Microscopically, careful sampling shows characteristic features that distinguish this lesion from renal cell carcinoma. The center of the nodule shows necrosis, cholesterol clefts, neutrophils, plasma cells, and scattered histiocytes. This area is surrounded by chronic inflammation and granulation tissue. The outer zone consists mainly of vacuolated lipid-laden histiocytes. Special stains for microorganisms are generally negative. The histiocytes lack cytologic atypia and have fine cytoplasmic vacuolation (Fig. 10–26), which is absent in clear-cell predominant renal cell carcinoma (see Fig. 10–17). The fine vascularity seen in renal cell carcinoma is also absent in XGN.

The importance in making this diagnosis relies in the different clinical significance, behavior, and treatment.

Angiomyolipoma versus Primary Renal Nonepithelial Tumors

Angiomyolipomas are tumors of mixed composition, as the name implies. The tumor consists of prominent thick abnormal vessels admixed with variable amounts of smooth muscle and adipose tissue. This tumor can present associated with the **tuberous sclerosis complex (TSC)**[68] or more frequently in a sporadic manner. When unassociated with TSC, they tend to be single unilateral lesions and occur more frequently in women than in men. It often presents as a flank mass with pain or with massive hemorrhage within the tumor. When associated with TSC, they tend to be smaller, multiple, and more often bilateral. Usually they are discovered at a younger age and as an incidental finding in a patient with neurologic problems related to TSC. As many as 80% of patients with TSC have angiomyolipomas; however, less than 40% of cases with angiomyolipomas have TSC. Angiomyolipomas are generally considered benign tumors, with controversy about the real nature of the lesion (varying from choristoma, hamartoma, to true neoplasm). There are numerous reports of extrarenal angiomyolipomas associated with renal angiomyolipomas.[69, 70] Most authors agree in considering these cases as multicentric tumors rather than as metastatic angiomyolipomas. A single case report by Lowe et al.[71] described sarcomatoid transformation of a preexisting angiomyolipoma. However, to our knowledge, this is the only case of malignant transformation described in the literature. Angiolipomas are generally well-circumscribed lesions. Grossly, depending on the predominant tissue composition,

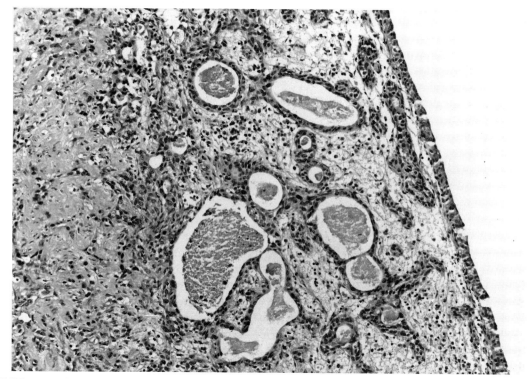

FIGURE 10–25. Collecting duct carcinoma. Note dilated tubules ("glands") filled with mucinous secretions. (×165)

they may be lobulated yellow (adipose tissue) or predominantly tan-gray, firm, and whorled (smooth muscle). There is frequently evidence of recent hemorrhage. Necrosis is seen only in very large tumors. Microscopically, as previously stated, the tumor exhibits prominent thick-walled vessels that are abnormal and resemble those in arteriovenous shunt malformations. Special stains show abnormal internal elastica. The amount of adipose and smooth muscle tissue can vary, and sometimes they predominate, with subsequent pitfalls in the diagnosis of such lesions, causing confusion with **leiomyomas** or **lipomas.** The

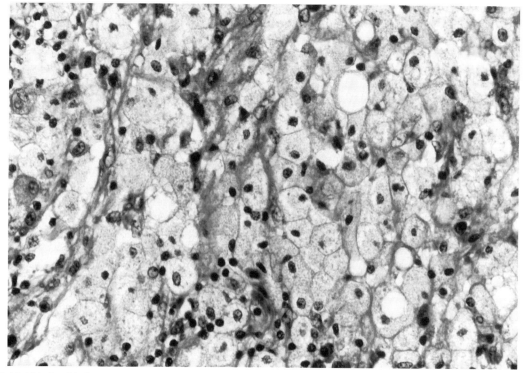

FIGURE 10–26. Lipid-laden histiocytes seen in outer zone of XGN. Note fine cytoplasmic vacuolation and lack of nuclear atypia. (×990)

smooth muscle component in angiomyolipomas seems to blend with the smooth muscle of the vessels, arranging itself around the vessels in a tangential/perpendicular manner. It extends in short bundles into the background admixed with or without adipose tissue (Fig. 10–27). Often the smooth muscle shows pseudosarcomatous features with marked cytologic atypia and occasional mitosis, leading to an additional differential diagnosis of **leiomyosarcoma.** A true sarcoma should show marked atypia and numerous atypical mitoses. The adipose tissue may show fat necrosis, lipophages, and when admixed with a small amount of atypical smooth muscle cells, has also misled occasionally to the diagnosis of **liposarcoma.** Because of the potential pitfalls, thorough sampling of these tumors is recommended.

BLADDER

Papillary Lesions

Transitional Cell Papilloma

Transitional cell papillomas are papillary neoplasms of the bladder lined by histologically and cytologically normal transitional epithelium with seven or less layers of cells. The nuclei show no or only minimal cytologic atypia. Mitotic figures are absent.[72] There are numerous authors who consider papillomas as low-grade papillary carcinomas grade I. This belief is based on reported "papillomas" that later recurred and invaded. The problem is further accentuated because of the use of the term "recurrence."[71] As many as 70% of patients with so-called true papillomas can show "recurrence," and ultimately 7% of the patients can develop invasive carcinoma of the bladder. These lesions occur very frequently in a small area of the bladder dome near the urethral orifices and trigone. This makes it difficult to distinguish among new tumors, incompletely excised tumors, and true recurrences at the site where the original tumor was removed. Two studies[73, 74] have shown that

1. "Recurrences" are in some cases incomplete removal of first tumors, multifocality of the lesion, and new tumors at different sites.
2. Later developed invasive carcinomas were originated from different sites or in a nearby region to the primary so-called papillomas.

The best interpretation of these studies is that, although there is no evidence that true transitional cell papillomas become malignant, they do arise in the urothelial mucosa that is prone to develop other proliferative lesions including invasive papillary transitional cell carcinoma. Careful follow-up of this lesion is recommended. Thirty percent of removed papillomas show no further recurrence or new neoplasms.

Inverted Papilloma

Inverted papilloma can clinically and pathologically be misinterpreted as a papillary transitional cell carcinoma of the superficial invasive and inverted type. They each have similar clinical presentations, with hematuria being the most common sign. They can present in the renal pelvis, ureter, bladder, and urethra, the bladder being the most frequent site of presentation. On cystoscopy, they present as polypoid exophytic masses. However, the inverted papilloma has generally a smoother surface as compared with the more papillary surface of transitional cell carcinoma. Microscopically the inverted papilloma shows an exophytic mass covered by urothelium that shows no atypia and no mitotic figures and frequently retains umbrella cells (Fig. 10–28). From this urothelium, numerous anastomosing cords and nests of cells extend downward into the lamina propria, accounting for a mass that

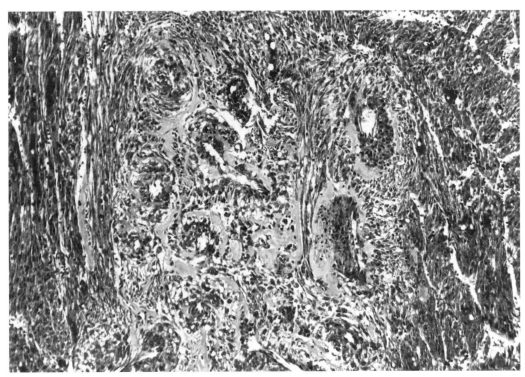

FIGURE 10–27. Angiomyolipoma. Prominent thick abnormal vessels in lower field, surrounded by abnormal smooth muscle cells arranged perpendicularly around vessels. (×330)

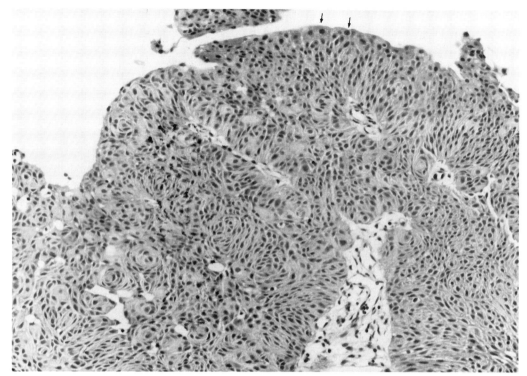

FIGURE 10–28. Inverted papilloma of the urinary bladder. Note "umbrella" cells of the overlying urothelium *(arrows)*. The anastomosing cords show lack of cellular atypia and no mitotic figures. (×250)

projects into the bladder lumen and produces an exophytic polypoid gross appearance. The nests and cords characteristically do not extend into the muscle and remain confined to the lamina propria. The basement membrane of the overlying epithelium is in continuity with the basement membrane surrounding nests and cords in the lamina propria. The nests can show non-keratinizing squamous metaplasia and cystic spaces occasionally filled with mucin (Fig. 10–29). The stroma in between nests and cords tends to be minimal and shows mild or no inflammation. The cells show minimal or no atypia and rare or absent mitotic figures. When mitotic figures are present, they are found adjacent to the basement membrane. Although inverted papillomas in 95% of the cases are benign lesions that do not recur, they are occasionally found in association with true papillary transitional cell carcinoma, and in some instances there have been reports of transitional cell carcinoma arising in inverted papillomas.[72, 75, 76]

Papillary and Polypoid Cystitis

Papillary cystitis and polypoid cystitis are two reactive, non-neoplastic, inflammatory lesions that can simulate low-grade transitional cell carcinoma, grade I.[77] Both inflammatory lesions are closely related and often coexist and can be multiple in the same patient. These lesions frequently occur in patients with a chronic insult such as an indwelling catheter. They regress with the removal of the insulting agent. Microscopically, they both have a papillary configuration without branching of the papillary projections. The lamina propria shows hypervascularity, congestion, and an intense chronic inflammatory infiltrate. Polypoid cystitis has bulbous projections as a result of marked edema in the lamina propria. The overlying epithelium in both lesions shows no hyperplasia

and no anaplasia. Mild reactive atypia may be noted, as well as squamous metaplasia. Umbrella cells are present.

Papillary Transitional Cell Carcinoma (PTCC)

Papillary transitional cell carcinoma usually has an exophytic fine papillary surface. When presenting with inverted features, it can also present with a relatively normal overlying urothelium. However, the endophytic nests tend to have a central fibrovascular core, and there is no basement membrane around the nests or the inverted papillary projections. Atypia and mitoses are present in variable degrees, depending on the grade of the lesion (Fig. 10–30). The stroma shows inflammatory cells, especially with a superficially invasive transitional cell carcinoma. The non-invasive grade I might present diagnostic difficulties with the papillary lesions described earlier.

Papillary transitional cell carcinoma grade I shows hyperplasia of the urothelium and mild cytologic atypia. Umbrella cells may or may not be present. Fine branching of the papillae, a feature not present in benign lesions, is also helpful (Fig. 10–31). The lamina propria has minimal inflammation, edema, and congestion.

Squamous Lesions

Squamous Papillomas and Condyloma Acuminatum

These are two rare squamous lesions that can be occasionally encountered in the bladder, especially in association

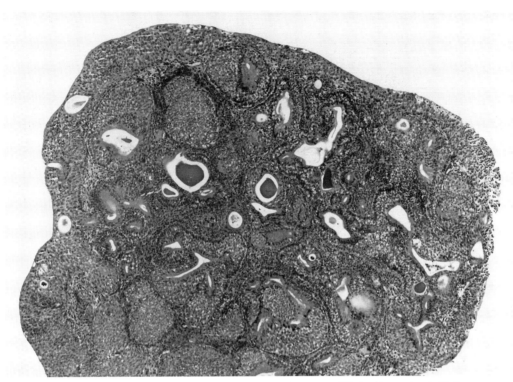

FIGURE 10–29. Inverted papilloma with cystic spaces filled with mucin. (×660)

with viral lesions in the urethra. These lesions have a papillary architecture and are lined by squamous epithelium. They show full maturation of the epithelium, acanthosis, and papillomatosis. Rare dyskeratotic cells can occasionally be identified, as well as mild cytologic atypia and koilo-cytosis in the case of condyloma acuminatum (Fig. 10–32). These lesions should be distinguished from verrucous squamous cell carcinoma, conventional non-verrucous squamous cell carcinoma, and transitional cell carcinoma with squamous differentiation.

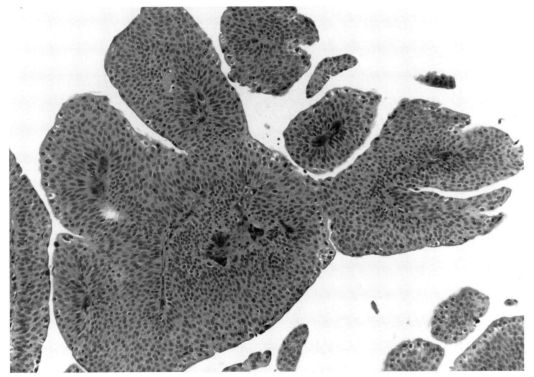

FIGURE 10–30. Papillary transitional cell carcinoma, grade II. There is an increase in urothelial thickness, nuclear overlap, and moderate nuclear atypia. (×660)

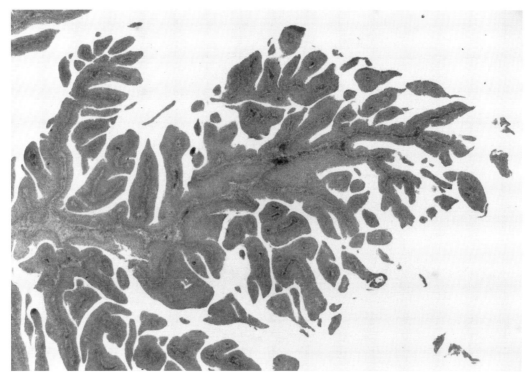

FIGURE 10–31. Low-grade papillary transitional cell carcinoma. Note fine branching of papillae. (×260)

Verrucous Carcinoma (VC)

Verrucous carcinoma of the bladder is extremely rare.[78] In many instances it arises in association with a schistosomal cystitis, as does the more conventional squamous cell carcinoma. It also arises in the absence of schistosomal cystitis, especially in countries outside the Middle East. Grossly, this lesion is warty and exophytic, as the two benign lesions described earlier, but usually considerably larger. However, this invasive neoplasm has a blunt pushing base (Fig. 10–33) compared with the benign non-invasive and non-neoplastic reactive papillary lesions, which show a serrated papillomatous base. Verrucous carcinoma shows marked acanthosis and hyperkeratosis. Characteristically, there is minimal cytologic atypia and rare mitoses can be seen only at the base of the lesion. The underlying stroma may show dense chronic inflammation. To distinguish this lesion from the benign viral squamous papillary lesion or from more aggressive conventional squamous cell carcinoma, it is essential to sample the lesion in its entirety, with full mucosal thickness and assessment of the infiltrating borders. If the latter shows tongue-like and/or finger-like invasive projections of tumor into underlying stroma, the tumor should be classified as a conventional squamous cell carcinoma (Fig. 10–34). Other features that exclude the diagnosis of verrucous carcinoma are marked squamous atypia and mitosis throughout the mucosal thickness. If, during sampling of the tumor, areas of transitional cell carcinoma are encountered, the tumor should be classified as transitional cell carcinoma with squamous differentiation.

Squamous Cell Carcinoma (SCC)

Squamous cell carcinoma constitutes 3% to 12% of bladder carcinomas. These tumors are more frequent in the Middle East, related to the prevalence of schistosomiasis. Otherwise this tumor and transitional cell carcinoma overlap in peak age of presentation, male predominance, and presenting symptoms such as hematuria and dysuria. However, there are distinctive pathologic features.

Grossly, this tumor is highly infiltrative. The surface is more often ulcerated than papillary. Microscopically, most squamous cell carcinomas are moderately differentiated. They usually present at a higher stage than transitional cell carcinoma, often with vascular, lymphatic, and perineural invasion at the time of initial diagnosis.[79]

Transitional Cell Carcinoma (TCC) with Squamous Differentiation

Transitional cell carcinoma shows focal squamous and/or glandular differentiation in 25% of the cases.[80] This finding does not alter the behavior of the tumor. However, when such components are extensive, the lesion should be considered of mixed differentiation. The diagnosis and prognosis are based on the most prevalent histologic component.

Glandular Lesions

Cystitis Cystica and Glandularis versus Adenocarcinoma of the Bladder

Brunn's nests, cystitis cystica, and cystitis glandularis all are considered benign proliferative urothelial lesions. These lesions are all closely related and often coexist in the same specimen. They are best interpreted as a progression in the proliferative changes seen in chronic bladder inflammation. They can occur in the setting of chronic infections and trauma (calculus disease, exotrophic bladder, indwelling catheters, and so on) and in neurogenic bladders. They have been

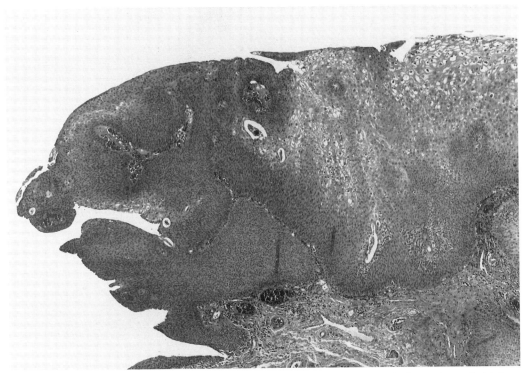

FIGURE 10–32. Condyloma acuminatum of bladder. Papillomatous squamous lesion showing koilocytotic atypia (right upper quadrant). (×66)

described in children and adults, with the incidence increasing with age. They occur more frequently in the area of the trigone. They can be focal or diffuse. The lesions themselves can produce submucosal nodules or even polypoid masses simulating low-grade papillary neoplasms and inverted papillomas.

Inverted papillomas, as previously described, can undergo cystic changes resembling Brunn's nests and cystitis cystica.

In cases of cystitis glandularis, the mucosa shows diffuse involvement by proliferating downgrowth of urothelium that has undergone cystic changes. The cystic spaces are lined by

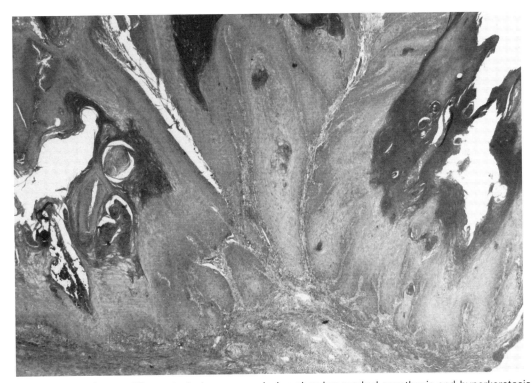

FIGURE 10–33. Verrucous carcinoma. Warty atypical squamous lesion showing marked acanthosis and hyperkeratosis. Compare its blunt pushing base with the finger-like downward projections of a conventional squamous carcinoma as seen in Figure 10–34. (×33)

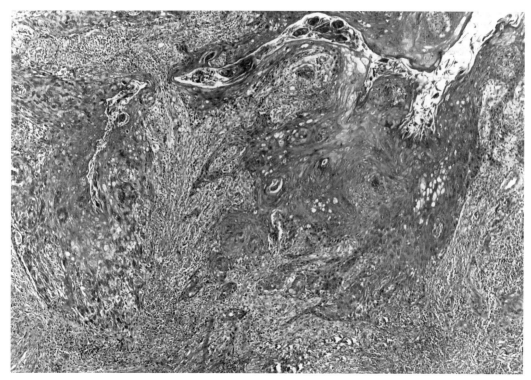

FIGURE 10–34. Infiltrating squamous cell carcinoma of the bladder. (×33)

columnar cells and prominent metaplastic goblet cells (Fig. 10–35). The ''glands'' are often filled with mucin, which can focally extravasate into the surrounding lamina propria and simulate invasive adenocarcinoma.[81, 82] Distinguishing features from adenocarcinoma are those of identifying co-existing Brunn's nests and cystitis cystica, no cytologic atypia, and no invasion of the muscular wall. These lesions remain confined to the lamina propria and do not extend into the muscular wall of the bladder. Reactive atypia may be encountered if there is marked associated chronic inflammation.

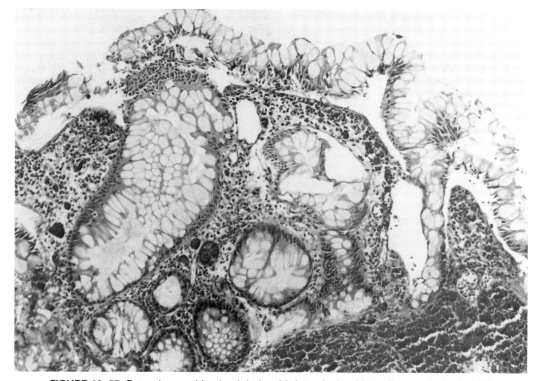

FIGURE 10–35. Extensive cystitis glandularis with intestinal goblet cell metaplasia. (×165)

Nuclei show nucleoli and hyperchromasia. However, the nuclear contours remain smooth.

The frequent association of cystitis glandularis with adenocarcinoma of the bladder (urachal and non-urachal type) has prompted controversy in interpreting the association between these two lesions.[83] Some authors have suggested considering cystitis glandularis as a premalignant lesion.[84-86] Sometimes long-standing cystitis glandularis has shown adenomatous change (Fig. 10–36). However, there is no clear evidence of progressive evolution to carcinoma.[87, 88] What has been accepted is that there is an increase in the risk for developing adenocarcinoma in patients with long-standing cystitis glandularis, more likely owing to a common etiology to the proliferative metaplastic change and the proliferative neoplastic event.[89, 90]

Pure **adenocarcinomas** of the bladder follow in frequency the more common transitional cell carcinoma, squamous cell carcinoma, and poorly differentiated carcinoma. They can be divided into primary vesical, urachal type, and extravesical metastatic to the bladder.[91, 92] They present in a broad range of age, with their peak incidence in the sixth decade. As most of the epithelial neoplasms of the bladder, they are more commonly seen in men, and they present most often in the trigone, anterolateral wall, and dome areas. When arising from the dome or anterosuperior walls, urachal-type adenocarcinoma should be considered. The importance of this distinction lies in the more extensive surgical treatment for urachal adenocarcinoma and the poor prognosis of the urachal carcinoma compared with vesical adenocarcinoma.

Adenocarcinomas can present as localized tumors or less frequently as multiple tumors. In the majority of the cases, the tumor is already invasive at the time of diagnosis. Gross findings include nodular, papillary, or ulcerated lesions.

Microscopically, the tumor may often resemble colonic adenocarcinomas. Other histologic features include papillary, colloid (mucinous), signet-ring cell type (linitis plastica) and clear-cell variants. The signet-ring cell variant (Fig. 10–37) carries the worst prognosis of all.[93] These cases may present diagnostic difficulties because metastatic adenocarcinomas to the bladder are quite common (prostate, colon, breast, ovary, and stomach being the most common primary sites). Immunohistochemical studies have not been very helpful, except for prostate alkaline phosphatase (PAP) or prostate-specific antigen (PSA), which stains metastatic prostatic adenocarcinoma.[87, 92] In a few cases tumor cells have reacted with polyclonal antibodies to PSA, probably owing to cross-reactivity of the antibody with common antigenic sites.

Nephrogenic Adenoma versus Clear-Cell Adenocarcinoma

Nephrogenic adenoma is another less common proliferative lesion encountered in the context of chronic cystitis. It can present at any age but usually presents at a younger age than other benign proliferative lesions and carcinomas.[94, 95] It is more often found in the area of the trigone, although it has also been described at other bladder and extravesical sites of the urinary system. This lesion was termed nephrogenic adenoma, based on the microscopic tubular histology simulating aberrant renal tubules.[96] Other terms applied to this lesion include adenomatoid metaplasia, nephrogenic metaplasia, and hamartoma. Most authors believe that the pathogenesis of this lesion involves metaplasia of the urothelium under the influence of chronic irritation, infection, trauma, or previous surgery. No preneoplastic significance has been attributed to this lesion.

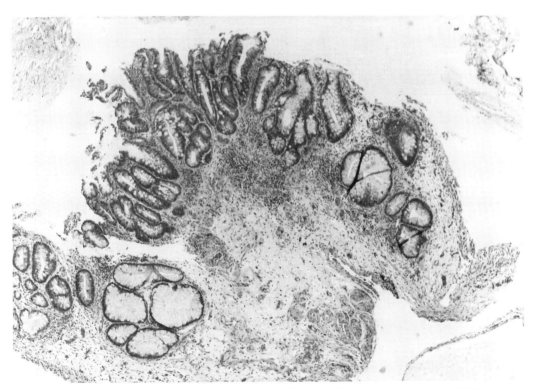

FIGURE 10–36. Extensive cystitis glandularis with focus of adenomatous change. (×66)

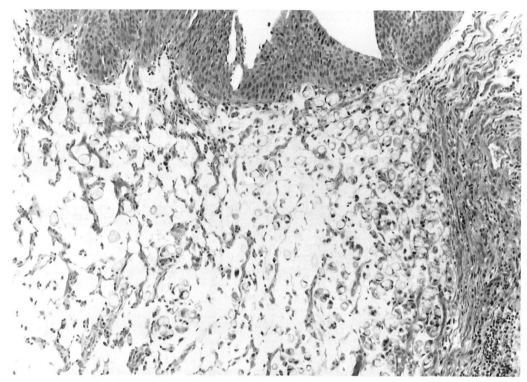

FIGURE 10–37. Primary bladder adenocarcinoma, signet-ring cell type. (×165)

Grossly, it has a polypoid and/or papillary configuration. The lesion can often be superficially ulcerated. Microscopically, the papillary fronds consist of broad inflamed fibrovascular stalks lined by a single layer of cuboidal cells. At the base of the papillary fronds, in the lamina propria and often filling the fronds (Fig. 10–38), there are numerous tubules lined by the same cuboidal cells and limited by a basement membrane. The tubules are often surrounded by inflammatory cells. The tubular lining cells lack significant cytologic atypia and mitoses (Fig. 10–39). This lesion should be differentiated from other benign and low-grade papillary neoplasms and adenocarcinomas. Among the latter, the clear-cell variant merits special discussion.

Clear-cell adenocarcinoma ("mesonephric carcinoma") is a variant of adenocarcinoma frequently encountered in the female genital tract. In the genital tract, it was initially described as of mesonephric origin. However, it has been demonstrated to be derived from mullerian epithelium. In rare instances, it has been described in the urethra and even less commonly in the bladder.[97] Despite the similar histologic features with the genital carcinoma, its cell of origin has yet to be defined at this location. Of interest is its positive staining for PSA and PAP by immunohistochemical studies when arising in the urethra.[98] In the bladder, the immunohistochemical studies for this antigen have been so far negative.[87]

The tumor usually forms a large mass with a nodular, ulcerated surface. Histologically, it is formed by papillary and tubular structures lined by atypical optically clear and "hobnail"-type cells with markedly atypical nuclei protruding into the tubular lumen or from the papillary fronds.

These tumors occur more frequently in women than in men, in contrast to the previously mentioned benign proliferative lesions and carcinomas, which all show a male predominance.

Features that help in the differentiation from nephrogenic adenoma include the larger size (nephrogenic adenoma is usually a small lesion), nuclear and cytologic atypia, and invasive growth pattern. The tumor may, however, have focal areas resembling nephrogenic adenoma. Despite their histologic resemblance, there is no association between nephrogenic adenoma and clear-cell adenocarcinoma.

Endometriosis versus Adenocarcinoma of the Bladder

Endometriosis can present in women at any site of the genitourinary system including the bladder.[99] In rare occasions it has also been described in men treated with estrogen therapy for prostatic adenocarcinoma.[100] Bladder endometriosis may simulate invasive adenocarcinoma when the pathologist lacks clinical history (the patient usually has endometriosis at other more common sites) and the lesion is deep-seeded in the bladder wall with minimal or no apparent stroma or hemosiderin-laden histiocytes (Figs. 10–40 and 10–41). The glands in endometriosis are lined by endometrioid-type cells and rarely by mucin cells with mucinous secretions. Features that help in the differential diagnosis in these cases include (1) lack of nuclear pleomorphism, (2) lack of extravasated mucin, and (3) focality of the lesion. Clinical history and adequate sampling of the tissue are very helpful as well.

Spindle Cell Lesions

Pseudosarcomatous Lesions

There are two benign spindle cell proliferative lesions of the bladder that should be differentiated from malignant spin-

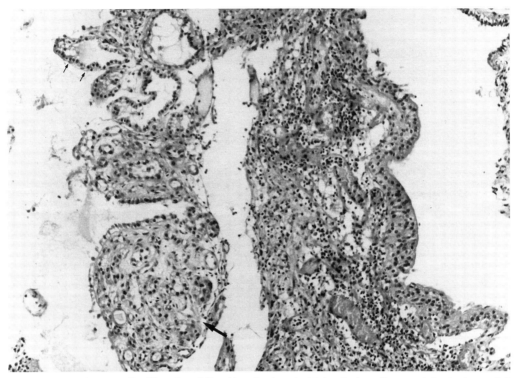

FIGURE 10–38. Nephrogenic adenoma. Papillary frond lined by single cuboidal cells *(small arrows)*. In the lower left quadrant, note closely packed tubules *(large arrow)*. (×165)

dle cell neoplasms. These two lesions (postoperative spindle cell nodule and inflammatory pseudotumor) are histologically very similar, with only slight pathologic differences. The main difference is the different clinical setting in which they present.

Postoperative spindle cell nodule (PSCN), as the name implies, generally develops 3 to 5 months after a surgical intervention on the pelvis. This lesion was first described by Proppe et al. in 1984.[101] It can present at various sites of the lower genitourinary system, with several reports describing

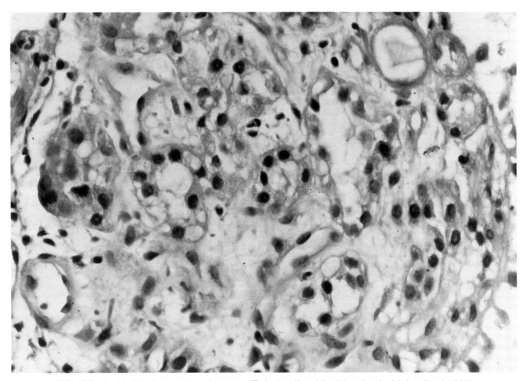

FIGURE 10–39. Nephrogenic adenoma. Tubules lined by bland cuboidal cells. (×660)

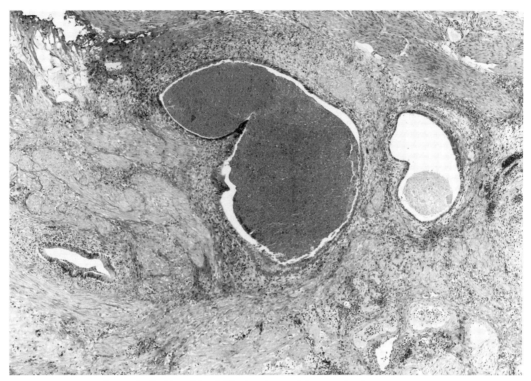

FIGURE 10–40. Bladder endometriosis. Note blood-filled endometrial-type glands and stroma in muscular layer. (×165)

the bladder as one of the sites of development. It can present in both sexes, but it is more commonly seen in the prostate, especially after transurethral prostatic resection. The lesion forms a small mass or nodule that can be superficially ulcerated. Microscopically, there is a proliferation of spindle cells arranged randomly or in poorly defined fascicles (Fig. 10–42). Cellularity can vary from field to field. The cells show a strikingly high number of mitotic figures, ranging from a few to 25 per 10 high-power fields (HPF). However, there are no abnormal mitotic figures, and there is minimal or no nuclear

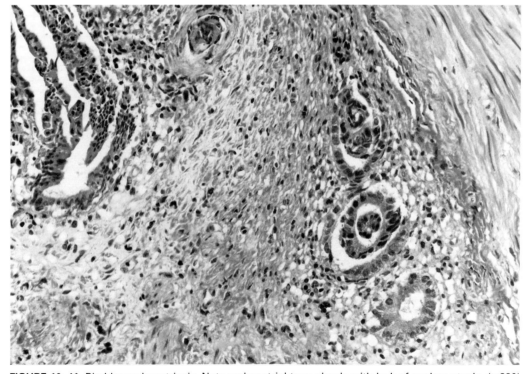

FIGURE 10–41. Bladder endometriosis. Note endometrial type glands with lack of nuclear atypia. (×330)

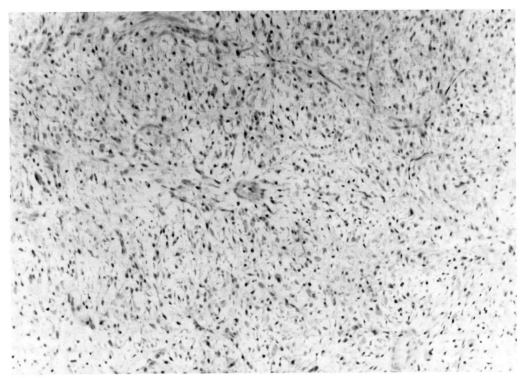

FIGURE 10–42. Postoperative spindle cell nodule. Poorly defined fascicles of spindle cells in an edematous background. Note fine vascularity. (×165)

pleomorphism or hyperchromasia (Fig. 10–43). The background shows prominent thin-walled vessels and variable stromal edema with areas of extravasated red blood cells and interstitial hemorrhage resembling Kaposi's sarcoma. The stroma also contains an acute and chronic inflammatory infiltrate, unrelated to the superficial ulceration. Granulation tissue may or may not be present. The lesion can resemble a leiomyosarcoma, Kaposi's sarcoma, malignant fibrous histiocytoma, or a sarcomatous carcinoma. The clinical history, small size, and benign cytologic features should be helpful in arriving at

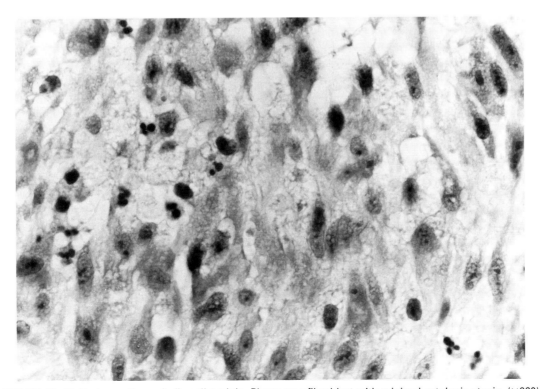

FIGURE 10–43. Postoperative spindle cell nodule. Plump myofibroblast with minimal cytologic atypia. (×660)

the correct diagnosis. Few immunohistochemical studies have been performed with only a small number of cases. PSCN stains positive for vimentin and negative for EMA. Results with desmin and keratin have not been consistent.[102, 103]

The **inflammatory pseudotumor** was first described by Roth.[104] Several reports have followed thereafter. This lesion presents in a broader range of age than PSCN, with an apparent higher incidence in women than in men. Similar lesions have been reported in children.[105] The lesion presents without a known previous history of trauma or surgery to the lower genitourinary area, which makes the differential diagnosis with a sarcoma more difficult. Grossly, the lesions tend to be larger than the PSCN, reaching several centimeters in greatest dimension. The lesion can be a nodular or polypoid mass.[106] Similar to the PSCN, it can be superficially ulcerated. Microscopically, there is a spindle cell proliferation in a loose myxoid and edematous background. These cells are fibroblastic/myofibroblastic with slender elongated eosinophilic or amphophilic cytoplasm. Multinucleated giant cells were reported in one case.[107] The cells show a low mitotic rate ranging from rare to 2 per 10 HPF. The cells can infiltrate superfical smooth muscle cells of the bladder wall. Inflammatory cells are present throughout the lesion. Thin walled vessels are present but not as prominent as in PSCN. This lesion should also be differentiated from leiomyosarcoma (especially the myxoid type)[108, 109] (Figs. 10–44 and 10–45) and the other malignant spindle cell lesions previously mentioned. The lack of nuclear pleomorphism, lack of abnormal mitotic figures, and lack of hyperchromasia should be helpful in making the distinction from malignant neoplasms. Immunohistochemical studies have shown variable results for desmin, muscle-specific actin,

keratin, and vimentin.[110, 111] Ultrastructurally the cells appear to be of a myofibroblastic nature.[106, 110, 111]

Leiomyosarcoma

Leiomyosarcoma is the most frequent bladder sarcoma in adults. However, its occurrence is very rare compared with transitional cell carcinoma. These tumors have been reported over a large age range affecting children and adults (mean age of 49) and in both sexes, with a higher incidence in males.[109, 112] There are reports of leiomyosarcomas of the bladder arising after treatment with cyclophosphamide for Hodgkin's disease.[113, 114] In general, leiomyosarcomas present as solid masses that can superficially ulcerate. In contrast to the previously described benign lesion, the spindle cell proliferation in leiomyosarcoma shows nuclear pleomorphism, abnormal mitotic figures, and often necrosis and hemorrhage. Cellularity tends to be uniform throughout the tumor, and distinct fascicles are present. The background generally lacks inflammatory cells unless associated with ulceration. All tumors have infiltrative margins with invasion of the bladder wall. Benign reactive lesions (PSCN and inflammatory pseudotumor) can occasionally infiltrate, but only superficially.

Sarcomatous Transitional Cell Carcinoma

High-grade transitional cell carcinoma may contain a malignant spindle cell component (**sarcomatous transitional cell carcinoma**).[115] If the component is the predominant one, it might simulate a true sarcoma (Fig. 10–46). A single biopsy may not be sufficient to recognize the epithelial origin of the tumor, and careful sectioning of the tumor or several biopsies

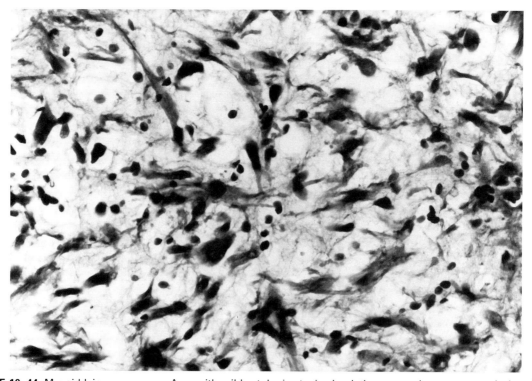

FIGURE 10–44. Myxoid leiomyosarcoma. Area with mild cytologic atypia simulating a pseudosarcomatous lesion. (×495)

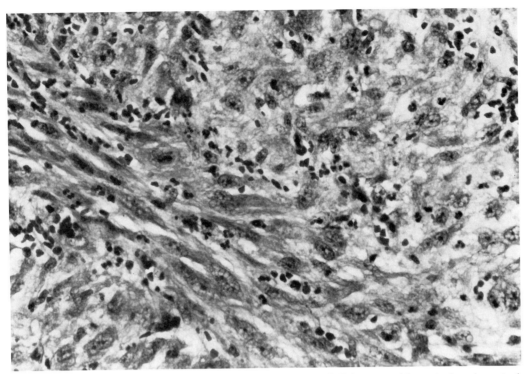

FIGURE 10–45. Myxoid leiomyosarcoma. Same case as in Figure 10–44. Cellular area with marked nuclear atypia. (×330)

may be required to identify an epithelial component (Fig. 10–47).

Immunohistochemical stains assist in the differential diagnosis. The sarcomatous component is positive for keratins and vimentin, whereas the epithelial component is positive for keratin and EMA.[115] If the malignant spindle cell component is only vimentin positive and there is an additional epithelial component, the tumor can be classified as a carcinosarcoma. Sometimes there is evidence of heterologous differentiation (Fig. 10–48).

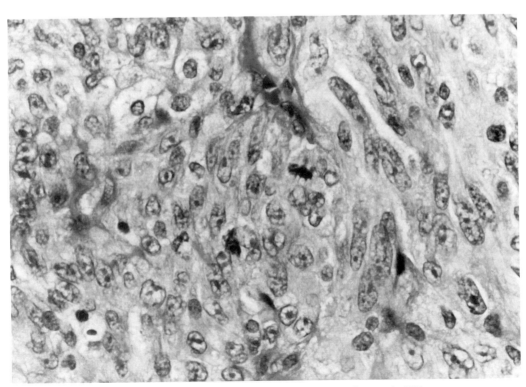

FIGURE 10–46. Sarcomatous transitional cell carcinoma. (×825)

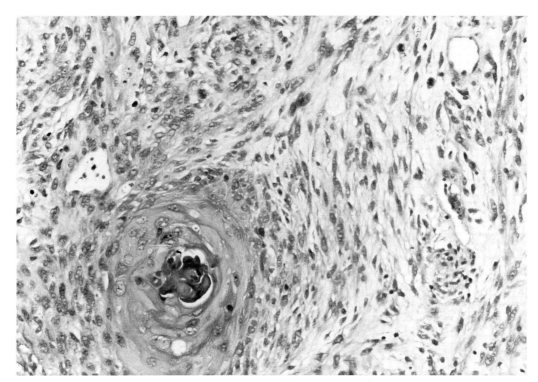

FIGURE 10–47. Sarcomatous carcinoma with squamous differentiation. (×248)

Pseudosarcomatous Stromal Reaction in Urothelial Carcinoma

In rare cases, an invasive urothelial carcinoma is associated with a pseudosarcomatous stromal response. The stromal cells, although atypical with hyperchromatic and pleomorphic nuclei, show no mitotic activity and usually are distributed haphazardly in a loose myxoid stroma,[116] at times resembling a nodular fasciitis-like pattern.[117] The same stromal reaction has been seen in metastatic urothelial carcinoma. These nonmalignant cells are positive for vimentin and negative for keratin.

Intraurothelial Lesions

The bladder urothelium can undergo several non-neoplastic changes that have to be differentiated from carcinoma *in situ* (CIS).

Hyperplasia

Hyperplasia can be defined as flat, thickened urothelium without cytologic atypia.

Atypia (Dysplasia)

There are no strict criteria or grading systems for the urothelial atypias that do not fulfill the criteria for CIS. Mild reactive atypia (due to trauma, infection, non-infectious inflammation, and so forth) cannot be reliably distinguished from mild dysplasia or premalignant change. Atypia that approaches CIS with loss of polarization, hyperchromasia, and nuclear crowding can be more confidently termed dysplasia (Fig. 10–49),

especially when the patient has a history of concurrent CIS or papillary transitional cell carcinoma. When isolated, it is best to classify these lesions as atypical of undetermined significance with a comment stating the degree of atypia. These patients should be closely followed up for possible development of an *in situ* or invasive carcinoma.

Carcinoma In Situ (CIS)

Carcinoma *in situ* was first described by Melicow and Hollowell.[118] This term is applied to flat bladder mucosa replaced (full thickness) by neoplastic cells that have not invaded the basement membrane. The cells show loss of polarity and disorganization, variable high nucleocytoplasmic (N:C) ratio, nuclear irregularities, hyperchromasia, coarse chromatin, and sometimes prominent nucleolus. Mitotic figures are usually present but not necessarily abnormal or numerous.[119]

Treatment-Induced Changes

The bladder urothelium can undergo cytologic changes after radiation or chemotherapy. These changes may mimic carcinoma *in situ*. Clinical history stating previous history of bladder carcinoma and treatment with radiation and/or chemotherapy are essential. Time interval between administration of treatment and biopsy or cytologic examination of urinary specimens are also helpful in the assessment of urothelial atypia. None of the treatment-induced changes are specific for the agent that induces them.

Radiation-induced injury of the bladder can follow radiation to the bladder prior to cystectomy for a bladder neoplasm and radiation to pelvic neoplasms other than bladder (uterine, prostatic, or colonic). Hyperemic changes can be seen within

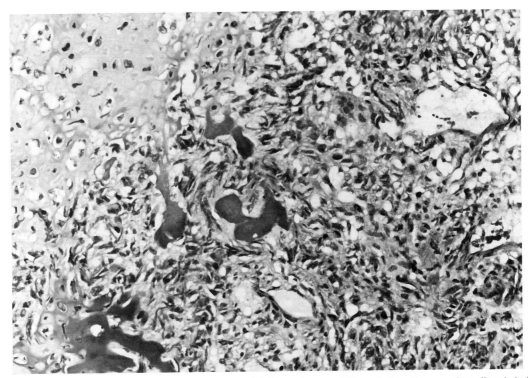

FIGURE 10–48. Sarcomatous carcinoma of bladder with heterologous differentiation (bone and cartilage). (×330)

the first 24 hours; however, pronounced changes follow only several weeks after the radiotherapy has concluded. The changes consist of intense hyperemia, telangiectasia, and edema in the lamina propria with mucosal ulceration.[120] The urothelium can present with marked cytologic atypia. The urothelial cells can become highly pleomorphic, bizarre, and

multinucleated. Features that distinguish these cells from those of CIS include lower N:C ratio, eosinophilic often vacuolated cytoplasm, and degenerated appearance of the nucleus with poorly defined chromatin pattern.[120, 121] With time, chronic changes show stromal edema and fibrosis with markedly atypical myofibroblasts in the lamina propria that should be distin-

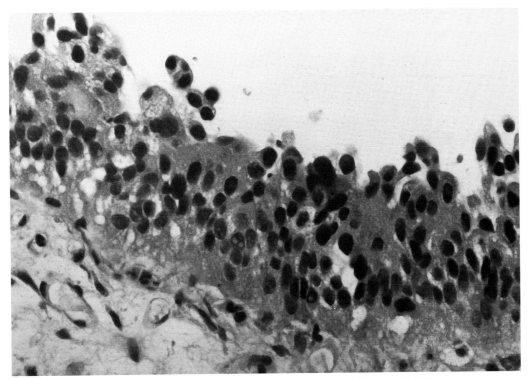

FIGURE 10–49. High-grade dysplasia (moderate) of bladder. (×990)

guished from invasive transitional cell carcinoma.[122] The atypical reactive myofibroblasts can easily be identified as non-epithelial by immunohistochemical studies (cytokeratin negative).

Chemotherapy-induced injury of the bladder follows the systemic or local administration of alkalating agents such as cyclophosphamide, thiotepa, and mitomycin C. These agents can produce cystitis associated with epithelial atypia. In the case of **cyclophosphamide,** the bladder shows marked edema and hemorrhage within the lamina propria. The epithelium can become ulcerated or very thin with atypia. When the epithelium regenerates, there is an intraepithelial increase in mitotic figures and pronounced cytologic atypia.[123] At times when appropriate clinical history is lacking or the patient has concurrent CIS, CIS and cyclophosphamide-induced changes can be very difficult or impossible to distinguish from each other. A helpful feature when present is the lack of a "crisp" nuclear chromatin in cyclophosphamide-treated bladder. Although the cyclophosphamide-induced atypical cells have a high N:C ratio and hyperchromatic nuclei, the latter show a rather pyknotic, glassy, or smudged chromatin pattern. These features are better recognized on urinary cytologic preparations ("Cytoxan cells").[124, 125] The atypia disappears after treatment is discontinued.

In the case of **thiotepa** and **mitomycin C,** which are given for treatment of superficial bladder carcinomas, there is extensive exfoliation and degeneration of the superficial cells.[126] The superficial cells are multinucleated, large, and hyperchromatic. The N:C ratio, however, tends to be smaller than that observed in CIS, and the overall size of the atypical cells is larger than that of malignant cells. The cytoplasm appears often vacuolated.[127, 128] Often both types of atypia can be seen in the same specimen. With time and prolonged therapy, the changes can be accompanied by extensive fibrosis of the bladder.[129]

PROSTATE

Microglandular Lesions

Sclerosing Adenosis versus Microacinar Adenocarcinoma

Sclerosing adenosis (Fig. 10–50) is a relatively recently described entity[130-133] that may be related to atypical adenomatous hyperplasia/adenosis and basal cell hyperplasia. The lesion has some similarities with sclerosing adenosis of the breast. Sclerosing adenosis appears to be associated with benign prostatic hyperplasia and may occur as part or nearly all of a hyperplastic nodule. It is composed of disorganized small glands that are angulated and compressed by a proliferating fibroblastic stroma. The periphery of the lesion is generally circumscribed. Basal myoepithelial cells (not present in the normal prostate) are usually detectable and may be multilayered around glands and cords of epithelial cells. Individual spindled myoepithelial cells may also be seen in the stroma. A thick basement membrane–like material is often seen around groups and even individual epithelial cells. Nuclear atypia including nucleoli may be present but are usually not prominent, and intraluminal mucin may also be occasionally seen. Immunocytochemistry (Fig. 10–51) is helpful in distinguishing this entity from microacinar adenocarcinoma, which it can closely mimic because of its small glands, infiltrating nature, cellular atypia, and mucin production. In sclerosing adenosis, basal myoepithelial cells stain for cytokeratin (EAB

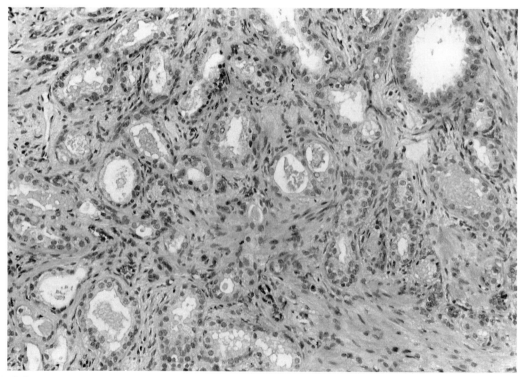

FIGURE 10–50. Sclerosing adenosis of the prostate with variable-sized somewhat angulated glands with an associated spindle cell proliferation. (×165)

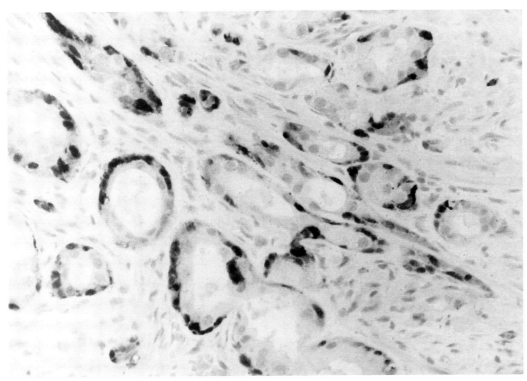

FIGURE 10–51. Sclerosing adenosis of the prostate immunostained for S-100 demonstrating positive staining of myoepithelial cells. (×330)

903) and muscle markers such as muscle-specific actin (HHF 35) as well as more focally with S-100. Neither cytokeratin positive basal cells nor myoepithelial cells are present in prostatic microacinar adenocarcinoma.

Atypical Adenomatous Hyperplasia versus Microacinar Adenocarcinoma

The term **atypical adenomatous hyperplasia** is the most generally accepted term for an entity whose definition is still undergoing refinement and has also been referred to as adenosis, atypical glandular proliferation, atypical hyperplasia small acinar type, and adenomatous pattern of primary atypical hyperplasia[134–137](Fig. 10–52). This microglandular proliferation has been characterized and defined somewhat differently by several different authors, ranging from lesions that many would call well-differentiated microacinar carcinoma to very bland microglandular proliferations without cellular atypia and with the presence of well-defined basal layer. There is probably a continuum from completely benign lesions to well-differentiated microacinar adenocarcinomas that may frequently be seen in the same patient specimen, indicating that separation from cancer may be somewhat arbitrary and intermediate (?evolving) histologic lesions may be seen. These microglandular proliferations often occur in the transition zone, are nodular, are frequently associated with benign prostatic hyperplasia, and are even seen developing within typical nodules of benign prostate hyperplasia (BPH).[138–140] A case could be argued that BPH gives rise to these atypical adenomatous hyperplasias and well-differentiated microacinar carcinomas that are frequently discovered on transurethral resection of the prostate (TURP) specimens (stage A1 and some A2 lesions). Some of these cancers may be biologically less

aggressive (?latent cancers) in contrast to those generally higher grade cancers arising in the periphery of the gland and often associated with high-grade prostatic intraepithelial neoplasia. At the clearly benign end of the spectrum of atypical adenomatous hyperplasia or adenosis are small uniform glands that tend to have some intervening stroma. Only minimal nuclear atypia is seen, and mucin and/or crystalloids are not seen. A distinct basal layer can often be seen but may be focal or discontinuous and is highlighted by cytokeratin EAB 903 immunostaining[141, 142] (Fig. 10–53). At the other end of the spectrum are cases with some of the following features: small back-to-back glands with some nuclear enlargement and nucleoli, intraluminal mucin and/or crystalloids, and a lack of a basal cell layer. If most or all of these features are present, a diagnosis of well-differentiated microacinar carcinoma is warranted. It is easier to distinguish these gradations on transurethral resection of prostate specimens as opposed to needle biopsies. Further studies need to be done to better define atypical adenomatous hyperplasia and its biologic potential.

Prostatic Intraepithelial Neoplasia (PIN)

Precancerous lesions of the prostate (excluding the controversial atypical adenomatous hyperplasia) have been variously termed atypical hyperplasia, duct-acinar dysplasia, intraductal dysplasia, and prostatic intraepithelial neoplasia.[143–148] At a recent consensus conference, the term **prostatic intraepithelial neoplasia** was accepted with a grading system from 1 to 3, which was further subdivided into low grade (PIN 1) and high grade (PIN 2,3).[149] There are a variety of the lines of evidence including histologic, topologic, chronologic, and predictive that indicate that the higher grade peripheral cancers

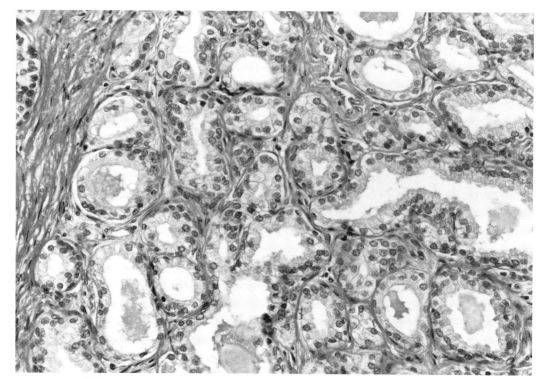

FIGURE 10-52. Focus of atypical adenomatous hyperplasia of the prostate. (×330)

of the prostate develop from a progression of intraepithelial neoplasia.[145, 150] Both prostatic duct/endometrioid carcinoma and tubuloscirrhous carcinoma appear to arise from PIN, whereas well-differentiated transition zone cancers associated with BPH (stage A1 and some A2) may arise from atypical adenomatous hyperplasia (see earlier discussion).

Ductal Hyperplasia versus Low-Grade PIN (PIN 1)

Low-grade PIN (Figs. 10–54 and 10–55) can be distinguished from normal or hyperplastic glands by an increase in the N:C ratio caused mainly by loss of secretory cytoplasm and piling up of epithelial cells to a few layers thick with some intraluminal tufting. Nuclear atypia is generally minimal. The basal cell layer and basal lamina are intact. Generally the easiest way to recognize these areas are relatively low power, where the PIN 1 glands contrast quite clearly with adjacent normal or hyperplastic glands, appearing somewhat more hematoxylinophilic and more "lush." Higher power can confirm the impression.

Low-Grade PIN (PIN 1) versus High-Grade PIN (PIN 2,3) (Fig. 10–56)

PIN 2 is similar to PIN 1, but with more pronounced cellular stratification and tufting, somewhat more nuclear atypia with small nucleoli often noted, and with a higher N:C ratio. PIN 3 should probably be considered synonymous with carcinoma *in situ* and is composed of malignant-appearing cells with prominent nucleoli and a high N:C ratio, marked piling up of cells with loss of polarity, and the formation of papillary and/or cribriform patterns. Basal cells that can be stained with

keratin EAB 903 and basal lamina are usually present, but both may be discontinuous.[141, 151]

PIN 3 (Carcinoma In Situ) versus Invasive Ductal/"Endometrioid"-Type Cancer

The distinction between PIN 3 (carcinoma *in situ*) and invasive cancer of the ductal/"endometrioid" type[152, 153] may be difficult, and frequently both may co-exist. Rather large areas of ductal/"endometrioid" carcinoma may remain within the framework of the co-existing duct system and may in fact represent PIN 3 (carcinoma *in situ*). A clue is that the ductal proliferation follows the contours of the normal duct structures, and the neoplastic units are relatively uniformly separated by stroma.

Cribriform Lesions

There are two benign entities with cribriform features that may be confused with and must be distinguished from cribriform carcinoma *in situ* (PIN 3) and invasive cribriform carcinoma. The first is clear-cell cribriform hyperplasia, and the second is a normal papillary and cribriform morphologic variant seen in the central zone.

Clear-Cell Cribriform Hyperplasia versus Cribriform Carcinoma In Situ (PIN 3)

Clear-cell cribriform hyperplasia[154, 155] (Figs. 10–57 and 10–58) is a variant of benign nodular prostatic hyperplasia with papillary and cribriform glands composed of clear cells without evidence of nuclear atypia, increased N:C ratio, or

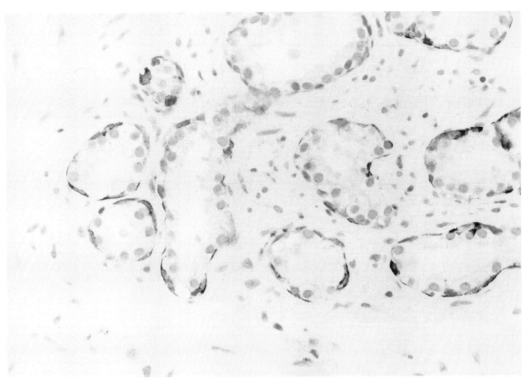

FIGURE 10–53. Atypical adenomatous hyperplasia of the prostate immunostained for keratin EAB 903 demonstrating the presence of the basal cell layer. (×660)

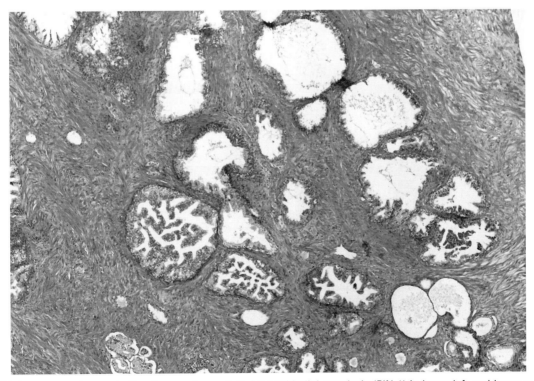

FIGURE 10–54. Low power demonstrating low-grade prostatic intraepithelial neoplasia (PIN 1) in lower left and lower central portion of picture contrasted with normal glands in upper portion of picture. (×66)

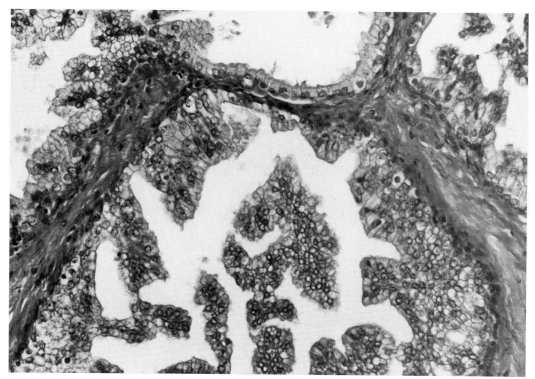

FIGURE 10–55. Low-grade prostatic intraepithelial neoplasia (PIN 1) demonstrating mild enlargement of nuclei with minimal atypia, increased nuclear cytoplasmic ratio of epithelial cells, piling up of cells, and formation of papillary and cribriform structures. (×330)

mitotic figures. A continuous basal layer is present that can be highlighted by cytokeratin EAB 903 staining. In addition to these findings, which help distinguish this entity from carcinoma, clear-cell cribriform hyperplasia occurs in discrete nodular foci with stromal proliferation.

Central Zone Papillary and Cribriform Morphologic Variant versus Cribriform Carcinoma In Situ (PIN 3)

This normal morphologic variant in the central zone of the prostate (Fig. 10–59) is manifested as papillary and cribriform (''Roman Bridge'') foci that may be quite extensive. As with clear-cell cribriform hyperplasia, benign cytologic features and a continuous basal layer can help distinguish this histology from malignant *in situ* and invasive lesions.

Basal Cell Lesions

Basal Cell Adenoma/Hyperplasia versus Adenoid Cystic-like Carcinoma

A variety of neoplastic lesions related to basal cells of the prostate have been described under the following names: basal cell adenoma, basal cell hyperplasia, malignant mixed tumor salivary gland type, adenoid cystic carcinoma, adenoid cystic-like carcinoma, basaloid carcinoma, and adenoid basal cell tumor. Basal cell adenoma and basal cell hyperplasia[156-158] (Fig. 10–60) are synonymous terms for an entirely benign entity that is a variant of benign prostatic hyperplasia and typically occurs as single or multiple nodules with stromal proliferation with nests of basal cells or small glands sur-

rounded by multiple layers of basal cells. The basal cells immunostain for cytokeratin EAB 903 and focally for S-100. The only importance in recognizing this variant of benign prostatic hyperplasia is not to confuse it with adenocarcinoma or with potentially more aggressive basal cell lesions.

The remainder of the terms previously listed describe lesions that are closely related. True classic adenoid cystic carcinomas of the prostate (Fig. 10–61) are very rare. These tumors are generally of uncertain malignant potential.[159-162] Some cases are locally infiltrative, and rare cases with metastases have been described, but generally these lesions have a good prognosis. These tumors may immunostain minimally or not at all for prostatic epithelial proteins (PAP and PSA) and are positive for EAB 903 and S-100.

Neuroendocrine Prostate

Endocrine-paracrine (neuroendocrine, amine precursor uptake and decarboxylation [APUD]) cells are dendritic regulatory cells abundantly present in the normal prostate gland (Fig. 10–62).[163,164] Based on ultrastructural classification of secretory granule morphology, there appear to be a variety of cell types.[165] Chromogranin A, serotonin, calcitonin, somatostatin, and bombesin-like immunoreactivity have been found in these cells.[166-170] Neuroendocrine differentiation in prostatic carcinoma probably reflects, albeit in caricature, the bidirectional differentiation present in the normal prostate gland.

Neuroendocrine Carcinoma versus Non-neuroendocrine Carcinoma

Neuroendocrine differentiation in prostatic carcinoma most frequently occurs as focal neuroendocrine differentiation in

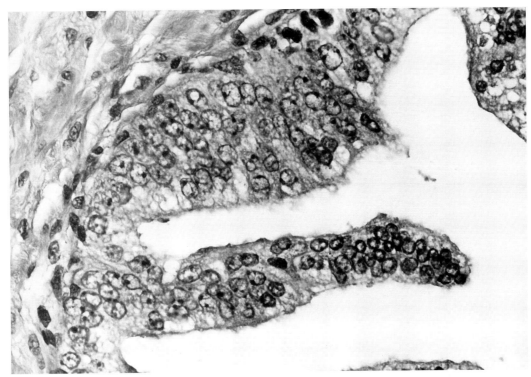

FIGURE 10–56. High-grade prostatic intraepithelial neoplasia (PIN 2,3) with marked enlargement of the nuclei and the presence of nucleoli. (×660)

conventional adenocarcinoma of all grades.[166, 171–174] This phenomenon occurs at least minimally in most, if not nearly all, prostatic adenocarcinomas but is marked in about 10%. With the rare exception of Paneth cell–like metaplasia,[175–177] in which large neurosecretory granules are visible on hematoxylin and eosin (H&E) stain, and the somewhat more frequent phenomenon, in which neoplastic cells appear finely granular and red staining,[178] neuroendocrine differentiation must be assessed by silver stains or immunocytochemistry. Argentaffin and the more sensitive argyrophil stain can be used for these purposes.[178–180] Foci of neuroendocrine differentiation are most frequently stained by chromogranin A, with neuron-specific

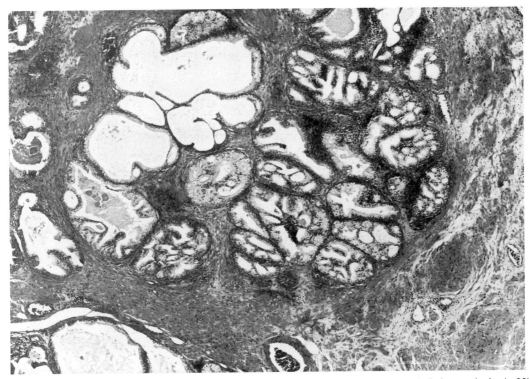

FIGURE 10–57. Clear-cell cribriform hyperplasia in a nodule of benign nodular prostatic hyperplasia. (×66)

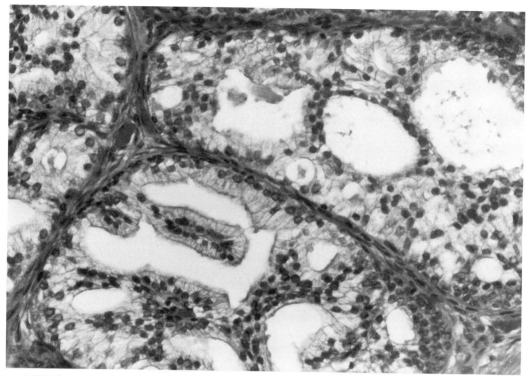

FIGURE 10–58. Higher power of the cribriform clear-cell hyperplasia seen in Figure 10–57. (×330)

enolase and serotonin as additional useful stains.[166, 171, 172, 174] Less frequently immunostaining for a peptide such as calcitonin or bombesin may be seen. Focal neuroendocrine differentiation in prostatic carcinoma appears to influence prognosis, which may be related to, or be in addition to, a tendency toward resis-tance to hormonal manipulation therapy.[166, 171, 181, 182] Recent studies employing chromogranin A and neuron-specific enolase as serum markers have tended to confirm these findings.[183, 184]

Small-cell neuroendocrine carcinoma (Figs. 10–63 to 10–65) is rather rare, with an incidence of 1% to 2% of

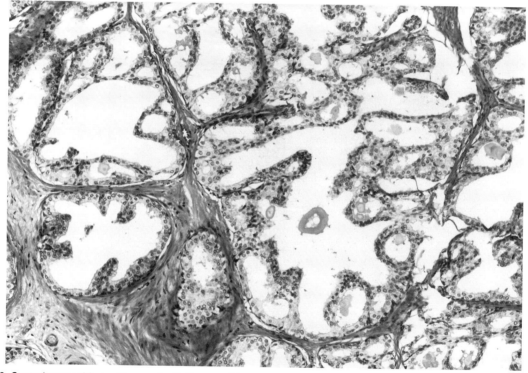

FIGURE 10–59. Central zone with papillary and cribriform architecture, which is a normal variant seen to varying degrees in the central zone of prostates. (×165)

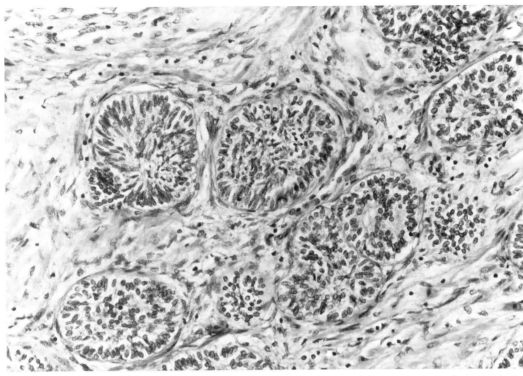

FIGURE 10–60. Basal cell hyperplasia/adenoma arising in association with nodular benign prostatic hyperplasia. (×330)

all prostatic carcinomas. These tumors are aggressive, with the rapid development of widespread metastases and a resistance to hormonal manipulation therapy.[185–187] These tumors frequently produce little, if any, prostatic acid phosphatase and prostatic specific antigen. Histologic criteria are generally the same as for small-cell carcinoma of the lung.

Carcinoid-like tumors (Figs. 10–66 and 10–67) have been described[181, 188–190] but generally do not have the typical appearance of carcinoid tumors elsewhere and tend to be architectur-

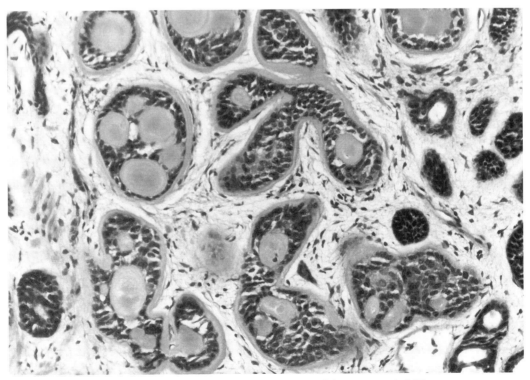

FIGURE 10–61. Adenoid cystic carcinoma of the prostate. (×330)

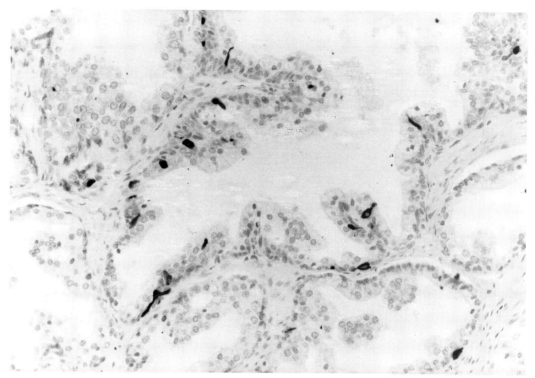

FIGURE 10–62. Focus of prostatic endocrine-paracrine cells immunostained for serotonin. (×330)

ally poorly differentiated adenocarcinomas with rather small uniform nuclei and, at times, rather clear cytoplasm. Marked but focal neuroendocrine differentiation is seen. We classify most of these cases as adenocarcinoma with focal neuroendocrine differentiation.

Paraganglion Cells versus Neuroendocrine Carcinoma

Nests of normal paraganglion cells may be present in close association with nerves in the region of the prostatic capsule

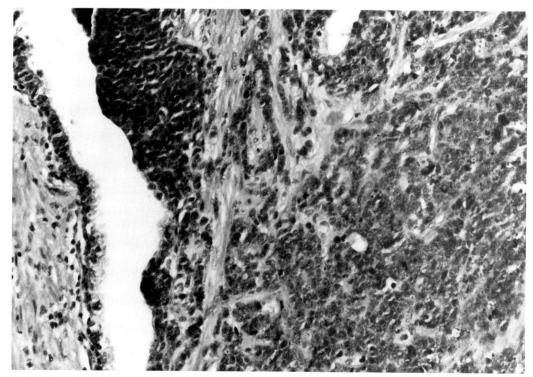

FIGURE 10–63. Small-cell neuroendocrine carcinoma of the prostate that is invasive to the right and has an *in situ* component to the left. (×330)

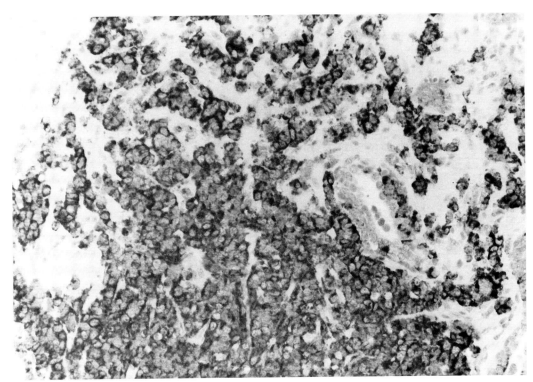

FIGURE 10–64. Same small-cell carcinoma as seen in Figure 10–63 immunostained for chromogranin A. (×330)

and periprostatic tissues (Fig. 10–68). These nests are composed of highly vascularized rather small clear cells that may mimic adenocarcinoma of the prostate.[191] They can generally be distinguished from carcinoma by a morphology that is different from the prostatic carcinoma present in the case, as well as by strong positive immunostaining for synaptophysin and PGP 9.5. Negative immunostaining for serotonin and chromogranin distinguishes paraganglion nest from carcinoma with neuroendocrine differentiation. Neuron-specific enolase (NSE) may be positive in both carcinoma with neuro-

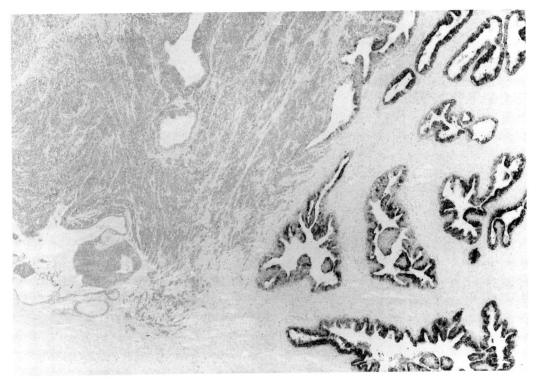

FIGURE 10–65. Same small-cell carcinoma seen in Figures 10–63 and 10–64 immunostained for prostatic specific antigen. Note staining of normal glands to right and negative staining of the small-cell carcinoma. (×66)

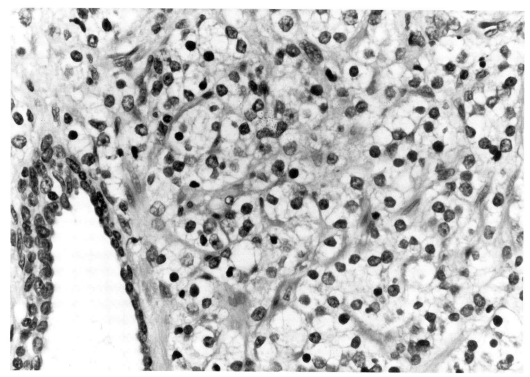

FIGURE 10–66. Carcinoid-like prostatic carcinoma. (×660)

endocrine differentiation and in paraganglion cells. The immunostaining pattern of paraganglion cells also tends to be more diffuse rather than a focal individual cell staining as is usually the case with prostatic carcinoma with neuroendocrine differentiation. The distinction is of considerable importance because lack of recognition of this entity may result in overstaging of the carcinoma. Rarely a true chromaffin paraganglioma or pheochromocytoma may occur in the prostate.[192]

Stromal Neoplasms

Spindle Cell Sarcoma versus Postoperative Spindle Cell Nodule

Sarcomas of the prostate are rare, constituting 0.1% of malignant neoplasms.[193, 194] Rhabdomyosarcomas generally occur in the first decade. The remainder of sarcomas are generally of the spindle cell type and occur in adults and are most frequently leiomyosarcomas[195, 196] and less often malignant fibrous histiocytomas[197, 198] as well as other sarcomas. The diagnostic features are the same as elsewhere, although specific criteria for leiomyosarcoma versus leiomyoma are lacking owing to the small number of cases. It is very important to distinguish spindle cell sarcomas from the entity known as postoperative spindle cell nodule (Fig. 10–69), which can occur in the prostate up to several months or more after surgical instrumentation.[101, 103, 199] The nodules are usually small (at most a few centimeters in size) and composed of cellular non-atypical spindle cells, often with a high mitotic rate. Atypical mitoses are not seen. Areas with hypervascularity, edema, hemorrhage, and inflammation may also be seen. The spindle cells in addition to vimentin may express muscle markers such as muscle-specific tractin (MSA) and desmin.

Postoperative spindle cell nodules may recur but are entirely benign reactive lesions often mistaken for sarcomas.

Mixed Epithelial/Stromal Neoplasms

Fibroadenoma versus Benign Cystosarcoma Phyllodes, Malignant Cystosarcoma Phyllodes, and Carcinosarcoma

Neoplasms closely resembling **fibroadenoma** of the breast have been reported in the prostate and are generally a variant of nodular benign prostatic hyperplasia.[200] Neoplasms that are similar to **cystosarcoma phyllodes** of the breast have been reported in the prostate and are related to nodular benign prostatic hyperplasia. These have also been referred to as phyllodes type of atypical prostatic hyperplasia.[201] These tumors can reach a large size (up to 15 cm) and may occasionally recur but do not metastasize. The stroma may be cellular and atypical, but mitoses are rare. This entity must be distinguished from nodular benign prostatic hyperplasia with bizarre nuclei,[202] which resembles those nuclei seen in symplastic leiomyomas of the uterus. Finally, malignant **cystosarcoma phyllodes** has been reported with pleomorphic stromal cells with numerous mitoses.[203–206] Evolution of malignant cystosarcoma phyllodes from "benign" cystosarcoma has been reported. Another rare entity that can be distinguished from cystosarcoma phyllodes is a giant multilocular prostatic cystadenoma that may or may not be attached to the prostate and is located in the pelvic retroperitoneum.[207] This lesion is composed of rounded cystic spaces lined by prostatic epithelium and a hypocellular fibrous stroma. These lesions are benign but may recur.

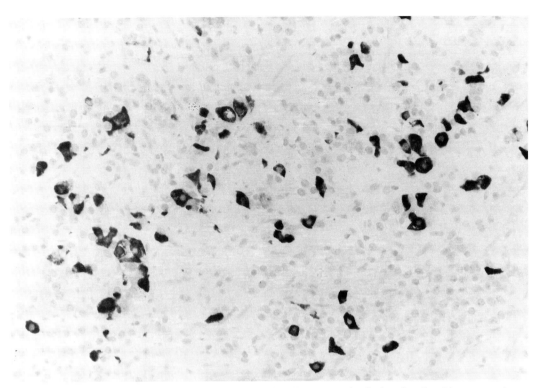

FIGURE 10–67. Same tumor as in Figure 10–66 immunostained for chromogranin A showing focal but extensive neuroendocrine differentiation. (×330)

Carcinosarcomas of the prostate[208–210] are rare mixed epithelial/stromal neoplasms composed of an adenocarcinomatous component that is often poorly differentiated with a sarcomatous stromal component, which may have homologous (i.e., a fibrosarcoma or leiomyosarcoma) or heterologous (with rhabdomyosarcomatous, chondrosarcomatous, osteosarcomatous, and so on) differentiation. The epithelial component is often positive for PSA and PAP by immunocytochemistry. These are rapidly progressive, highly malignant tumors.

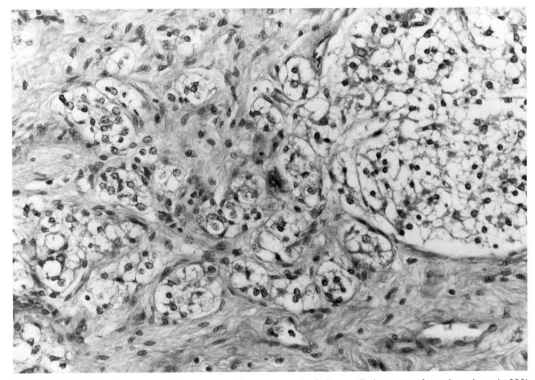

FIGURE 10–68. Small extraprostatic paraganglia composed of clear cells in nests of varying sizes. (×330)

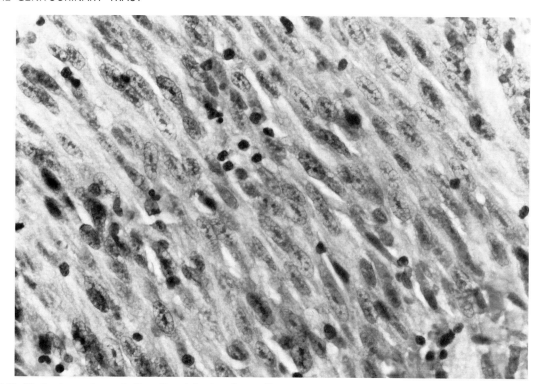

FIGURE 10–69. Postoperative spindle cell nodule showing uniform spindle cells with interspersed inflammatory cells. (×660)

TESTIS

Germ Cell Tumors and Their Differential Diagnosis

Cryptorchid Testis with Sertoli Cell Nodule versus Intratubular Germ Cell Neoplasia

Cryptorchidism is a condition characterized by lack of descent of a testis. It is usually unilateral but can be bilateral. The maldescended testis can be found high in the scrotum, in the inguinal canal, or in the abdomen. The diagnosis can be established clinically by the end of the first year of life. Grossly, in the **postpubertal age,** the testis is smaller than a descended testis. Microscopically, the testis shows a decrease in the diameter of the seminiferous tubules, with increase in the peritubular connective tissue. Sclerosis of the tubules and scarring increase with time in the undescended testis. The tubules show marked decrease or absence of germ cells. The germ cells are less likely to be found in cryptorchid testis from the abdomen than in cryptorchid testis from the inguinal canal or high in the scrotum. The tubules show predominantly Sertoli cells. Occasionally there is Sertoli cell hyperplasia in several tubules, which aggregate and form a nodule—the so-called Sertoli cell nodule or adenoma of Pick, which has no malignant potential[211] (Figs. 10–70 and 10–71). These nodules should not be confused with intraepithelial germ cell neoplasia developing in a cryptorchid testis. The latter does have a malignant potential (discussed later). In the **prepubertal age,** the differences with a testis of a matched age are not as pronounced. There is a mild decrease in the number of germ cells and a decrease in the mean tubular diameter. Thickening and scarring of the tubules are absent. Two percent to

8% of cryptorchid testes have abnormal germ cells within their seminiferous tubules (intratubular germ cell neoplasia).

Intratubular germ cell neoplasia (ITGCN), also known as carcinoma *in situ* of testis, can be seen in patients with cryptorchidism or gonadal dysgenesis and/or associated with invasive germ cell tumors in the ipsilateral or contralateral testis. It is not seen in children with yolk sac tumor or teratoma or in adults with spermatocytic seminoma. More often it is diagnosed in patients undergoing testicular biopsies for work-up or infertility.[212] It is important to recognize this condition because of its potential of developing into an invasive germ cell tumor.[213] Histologically, the abnormal germ cells are distributed through almost all the tubules. These cells may appear adjacent to the tubular basement membrane, leaving Sertoli cells more centrally located, or they may fill the tubules completely (Fig. 10–72). They have abundant clear cytoplasm (PAS positive) and a central large round nucleus with a prominent nucleolus. Mitotic figures may be seen. The chromatin is clumped and coarse. The cells react with placental alkaline phosphatase (PLAP) by immunohistochemistry. This marker is useful for its detection in questionable cases. The cells are usually negative for keratin, alpha-fetoprotein (AFP), and human chorionic gonadotropin (hCG).[214, 215]

"Classic" Seminoma versus Spermatocytic Seminoma

Seminoma is an invasive germ cell tumor seen in young men (mean age, 35) that can be bilateral in 2% of the cases. It is the most frequent germ cell neoplasm arising in cryptorchid testis and the most frequent type of germ cell tumor encountered in bilateral testicular neoplasms. This type of germ cell neoplasm does not develop in infants. It can occur in a pure

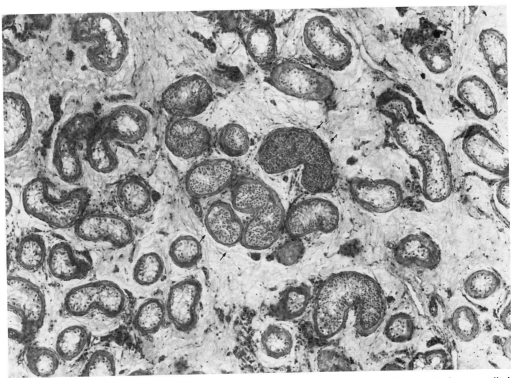

FIGURE 10–70. Cryptorchid testis with Sertoli cell hyperplasia (nodule) in the center *(arrows)*. Note lack of germ cells in tubules. (×99)

form or more frequently associated with other germ cell tumors. In 85% of the cases, the uninvolved tubules show intratubular germ cell neoplasia (Fig. 10–73). Grossly, the tumor forms a well-demarcated, gray-white nodule. It is of variable consistency and can show areas of necrosis when it

reaches large sizes. Histologically, the "classic seminoma" is composed of sheets of large polygonal cells that are compartmentalized by fibrous septa. The septa characteristically show a variable amount of lymphocytic infiltrate in 80% of the cases. The malignant germ cells appear as a monotonous

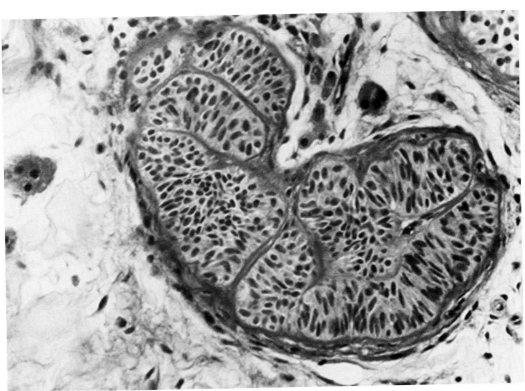

FIGURE 10–71. High power of Sertoli cell hyperplasia seen in Figure 10–70. (×825)

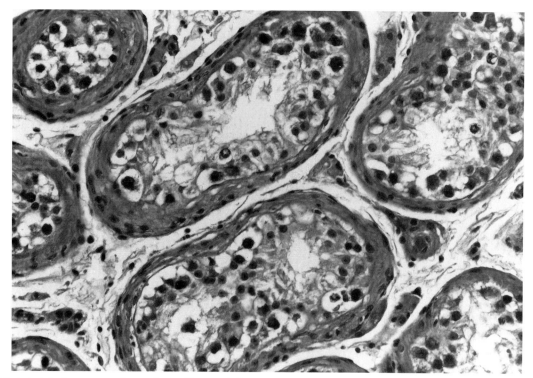

FIGURE 10–72. Intratubular germ cell neoplasia. The seminiferous tubules show atypical enlarged hyperchromatic germ cells with abundant cytoplasm. There is no evidence of spermatogenesis. (×330)

population with abundant pale or clear cytoplasm that is PAS positive as a result of its high cytoplasmic glycogen content. The cell borders are very well demarcated. The nucleus is large, round to polyhedral, and hyperchromatic. It can contain one or two prominent nucleoli (Fig. 10–74). Mitotic activity may be present; however, the "classic seminoma" characteristically has a low number of mitotic figures. Other features that can be seen in this type of seminoma are associated syncytial trophoblastic cells (7% to 35% of cases) and an associated granulomatous inflammation (17% of cases) (Fig.

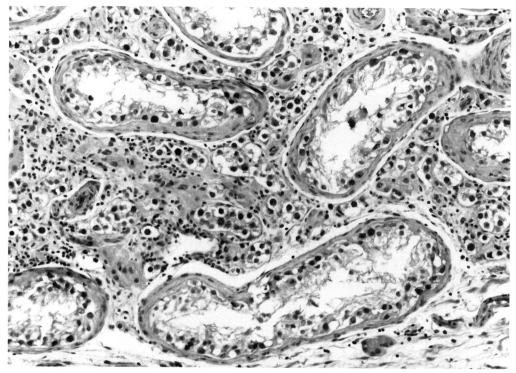

FIGURE 10–73. Intratubular germ cell neoplasia and infiltrating seminoma. (×248)

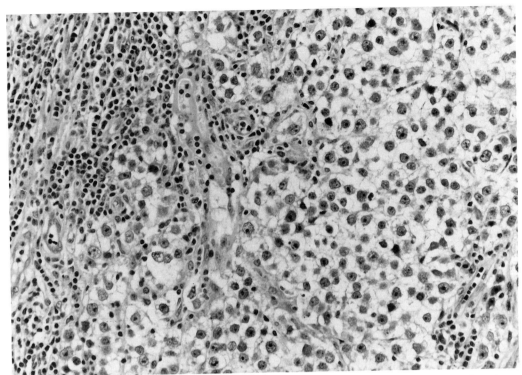

FIGURE 10–74. Seminoma. Monotonous germ cells with abundant well-demarcated clear cytoplasm, round nucleus, and prominent nucleolus. Note lymphocytic infiltrate and delicate fibrous septa that compartmentalize the cells into nests. (×330)

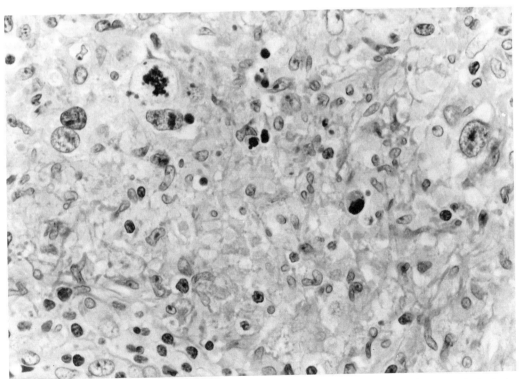

FIGURE 10–75. Granulomatous seminoma. There is an abundance of epithelioid histiocytes and scattered atypical germ cells with abundant clear cytoplasm, nucleus with clumped chromatin, and prominent nucleolus. One abnormal mitotic figure is seen in the upper outer quadrant. (×825)

10–75). Seminoma with its variations in presentation has to be differentiated from the seminoma with choriocarcinoma, granulomatous orchitis, embryonal carcinoma, spermatocytic seminoma, intratesticular lymphomas, plasmacytomas, and poorly differentiated metastatic carcinomas, which can mimic its histologic picture. Their behavior and clinical significance differ considerably.

Spermatocytic seminomas are less frequent germ cell tumors (2% to 3%) that arise at a slightly older age (mean age, 50) and can be more frequently bilateral (10% of cases) as compared with classic seminomas. There are numerous additional features that differentiate this type of seminoma from the classic seminoma. Spermatocytic seminomas characteristically do not arise in undescended or dysplastic testes, but rather in normal testes. They always occur in a pure form, not associated with other germ cell tumors. Rare cases have been reported in association with primary sarcomas of the testis.[216–218] In some cases the patients died from metastatic sarcoma. Spermatocytic seminomas are well circumscribed and demarcated from the adjacent uninvolved testicular parenchyma. The cut surface is pale yellow-gray, with a spongy, edematous, or mucinous appearance. The tumor has edematous areas that can lead to cystic areas or separation of the tumor mass into several tumor nodules. Necrosis and hemorrhage are exceedingly rare. Microscopically, at low power there is lack of compartmentalization. The tumor is composed of a heterogeneous population of cells growing in sheets that can have poorly developed connective tissue septa that lack the lymphocytic infiltrate seen in ''classic seminoma'' (Fig. 10–76). The cellular composition is very characteristic (Fig. 10–77). There are three different cell types based on size, with intermediate cells being the most prevalent type.[219] The other two cell types, smaller and larger in size, respectively,

are present in fewer numbers. The intermediate and large cells have a round nucleus with evenly distributed chromatin and/or a filamentous spireme-like chromatin that is more accentuated in the larger cells. Mitoses are present, but in low numbers. The cytoplasm is scant and eosinophilic. The cell borders are poorly demarcated compared with the well-demarcated ones of classic seminoma. The cytoplasm is characteristically PAS negative. The smaller cells have a hyperchromatic, almost pyknotic nucleus and a very scant cytoplasm. Findings such as lymphocytic and granulomatous inflammation or syncytiotrophoblastic cells are not seen in spermatocytic seminoma. The cells from both types of seminomas, classic and spermatocytic, differ in their immunohistochemical properties. Cells from classic seminomas stain with PLAP and neuron-specific enolase.[214, 220] Staining for keratin and vimentin is occasionally focally positive. Staining for EMA is consistently negative. The spermatocytic seminoma is uniformly negative for vimentin, PLAP, hCG, and AFP.[221] It is important to differentiate both types of seminoma because of their different treatment and prognosis. The spermatocytic seminoma, if not associated with a sarcoma (rare event), is generally cured by orchiectomy. There is only one case report in the literature with metastatic pure spermatocytic seminoma.[222]

Tubular Seminoma versus Sertoli Cell Tumor

A rare and uncommon variant of seminoma is the so-called tubular seminoma. Young et al. in 1989[223] described a case and found three additional descriptions in the literature of invasive seminoma with tubular architecture.[224] In this variant of seminoma, the tumor cells are arranged predominantly in closely packed, solid elongated and branching tubules. These

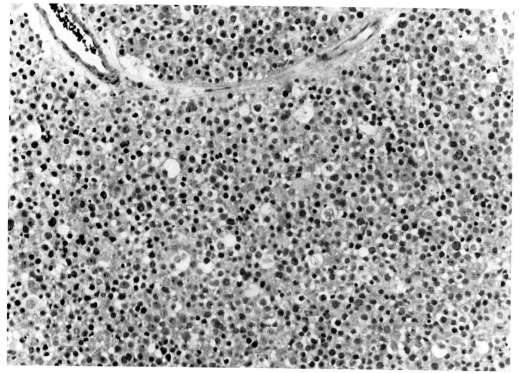

FIGURE 10–76. Spermatocytic seminoma. Heterogeneous population of cells growing in sheets. Note fibrous septum devoid of lymphocytic infiltrate. (×165)

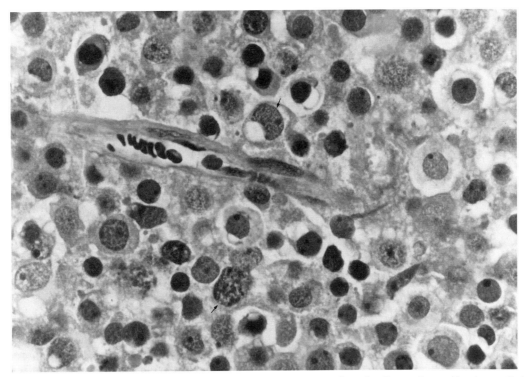

FIGURE 10–77. Spermatocytic seminoma. There are three types of cells based on nuclear size. Note spireme-like chromatin in intermediate and large cells *(arrows)*. Smaller lymphocytic-like cells show hyperchromatic almost pyknotic nuclei. (×825)

tubules are separated by scant acellular fibrous tissue with minimal lymphocytic infiltrate. The tubules are filled with characteristic seminoma cells that are uniformly distributed or arranged in a cribriform pattern. Other features are the finding of occasional balloon cells with large cytoplasmic vacuoles displacing the nucleus, similar to signet-ring cells, and tubules filled with predominantly cytoplasm with nuclei displaced to the periphery of the tubules. These patterns might suggest a Sertoli cell tumor of the lipid rich type. However, the neoplastic tubules in tubular seminoma contain malignant cells with the cytologic features characteristic of seminoma cells. These cells are rich in glycogen and show the same immunohistochemical staining seen in classic seminoma. Sertoli cell tumors are negative for PLAP by immunohistochemistry, and these cells lack cytoplasmic glycogen. Other features that may assist in the diagnosis are the finding of seminiferous tubules with intratubular germ cell neoplasia adjacent to the tubular seminoma, as well as more characteristic foci of infiltrating seminoma in sheets with a more typical compartmentalization arrangement.

Seminoma with Prominent Granulomatous Host Response versus Granulomatous Orchitis

Extensive granulomatous inflammation of the testis can be seen in different clinical settings with different treatment and prognostic implications. A **granulomatous reaction** can be elicited in response to an **infectious agent** (e.g., tuberculosis, syphilis, brucellosis, fungal disease) or in the setting of **sarcoidosis**.[225–227] In the majority of the cases, the testicular involvement is an additional manifestation of disseminated disease. Histologically, the inflammatory granulomatous

response occupies the interstitium and secondarily involves the tubules in advanced disease. The epididymis is also frequently affected. The clinical history, special histochemical stains to visualize organisms, and culture of the affected tissue are helpful in arriving at the correct diagnosis.

Autoimmune or idiopathic orchitis is a granulomatous inflammatory process in which no infectious agent can be demonstrated. There is no evidence of sarcoidosis. It usually presents unilaterally in the fifth to sixth decade. The cause is unknown, although prior trauma and immunologic injury have been proposed as possible mechanisms. Characteristically the granulomatous response starts within the seminiferous tubules, rather than in the interstitium. The interstitium also shows prominent inflammation. Tubular destruction is seen in advanced cases. In the early stages, the inflammatory process is mainly intratubular with destruction of the tubular cellular elements, particularly germ cells. As the disease progresses, the tubules fill with non-caseating granulomas and eventually all merge together, creating a nodular patten.[228, 229]

When encountering a prominent granulomatous process in a testis, it is important to rule out a **seminoma with prominent granulomatous response**[230] (see Fig. 10–75). Careful sampling and examination of the sections will disclose the PAS- and PLAP-positive malignant germ cells.

Seminoma versus Lymphoma

Seminomas can have a variable amount of lymphocytic infiltration, which, if prominent, may occasionally obscure the infiltrating seminoma cells and/or simulate a lymphoma. Testicular lymphomas, primary or as a manifestation of disseminated disease, are generally of the high-grade non-Hodgkin's type. The lymphomatous infiltrate initially fills the interstitium between seminiferous tubules and, with progression, may secondarily surround and invade the tubules. In the case of involvement by leukemia (usually of lymphoblastic type), the cells remain in the interstitium surrounding the seminiferous tubules (Fig. 10–78). Immunohistochemical studies with antibodies directed against PLAP and lymphoid markers for T and B cells and kappa and lambda light chains help in resolving the differential diagnosis. Most of the testicular lymphomas are generally of B-cell phenotype with kappa or lambda light chain restriction. Lymphomas are consistently negative for PLAP. In seminomas, the malignant germ cells are positive for PLAP, and the lymphocytic infiltrate contains a polyclonal mixture of T and B cells with a predominance of B-cell lymphocytes.[231]

Seminoma versus Yolk Sac Tumor

Pure yolk sac tumor of the testis occurs only in children. In adults it is always a component of a mixed germ cell tumor. It is important to distinguish a yolk sac tumor component in an otherwise pure seminoma and in a non-seminomatous germ cell tumor because its presence implicates different treatment and prognosis. Studies looking at long-term disease-free survival and autopsies of patients with metastatic germ cell tumors have shown that yolk sac tumor is less chemosensitive than other germ cell tumors and is responsible for late-development chemoresistant recurrences.[232, 233] Yolk sac tumors can present with numerous histologic patterns, which include the "classic" perivascular pattern with Schiller-Duval bodies (Fig. 10–79), and solid, microcystic, hepatoid, and embryonic-like patterns. Ulbright and Roth[234] described these patterns and immunohistochemical characteristics. The solid pattern of yolk sac tumor can mimic seminoma. These cells can be relatively uniform with well-defined cytoplasmic mem-

branes and arranged in solid sheets. However, fibrous septa with compartmentalization seen in seminoma are not present in yolk sac tumor, and fortunately most of the time, the solid pattern of yolk sac tumor is generally combined with other, easier to identify patterns. Histologic features characteristic of yolk sac tumor that are not present in seminoma or embryonal carcinoma are extracellular basement membrane deposition and hyaline refractile PAS-positive proteinaceous material (Fig. 10–80). Immunohistochemical studies are also helpful. Yolk sac tumors are generally positive for alpha-fetoprotein (AFP) and almost always strongly positive for cytokeratins, whereas seminomas are negative for AFP and negative or only focally or weakly positive for cytokeratins.[234]

Anaplastic Seminoma versus Solid Variant of Embryonal Carcinoma

The term **"anaplastic"** seminoma was proposed in 1968 by Maier et al.[235, 236] In a series of seminomas studied at Walter Reed Hospital in Washington, this variant accounted for 5% of all seminomas and 40% of all seminoma-related deaths. These tumors show marked nuclear atypia, with marked hyperchromasia, nuclear irregularities, two to three nucleoli, and, characteristically, numerous mitotic figures (30/10 HPF). Necrosis is more common than in classic seminoma.[237] At the present time, the significance of these histologic features is unclear. Two groups, Kademian et al. and Bobba et al.[238, 239] also reported the more aggressive behavior of these tumors, with high relapse and death rate. In their studies they also considered the stage-factor of the tumors compared with classic seminomas. Other authors, however, believe that the separation of anaplastic seminoma as a distinct entity is unnecessary. This belief is based on other reports that showed that "anaplastic" seminomas when compared with "classic"

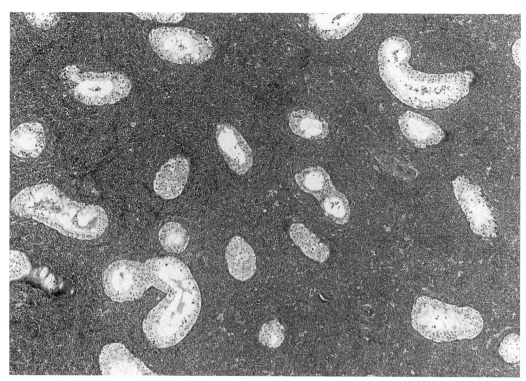

FIGURE 10–78. Acute lymphoblastic leukemia involving the testis. (×66)

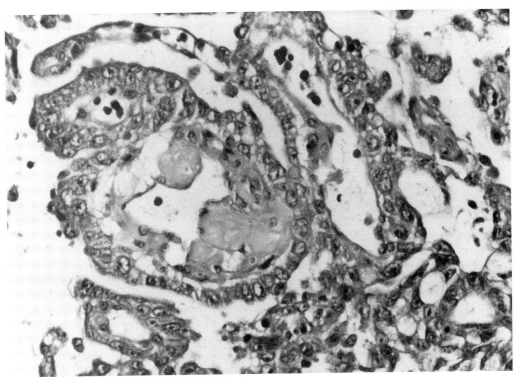

FIGURE 10–79. Yolk sac tumor showing Schiller-Duval bodies. Note extracellular basement membrane–like material. (×99)

seminomas of the same clinical stage showed very similar outcome and prognosis.[240] This type of seminoma is not included in the classification of testicular germ cell tumors (World Health Organization).[241]

It is important to distinguish ''anaplastic'' seminoma from a solid variant of embryonal carcinoma. **Embryonal carci-** **noma** is the second most common germ cell tumor in adults. It is composed of very primitive cells that are frequently arranged in glandular (Fig. 10–81), tubular, papillary, or solid patterns. The most common presentation is that of combined histologic patterns.[237] It usually presents at a somewhat younger age than seminoma. At the time of presentation, many

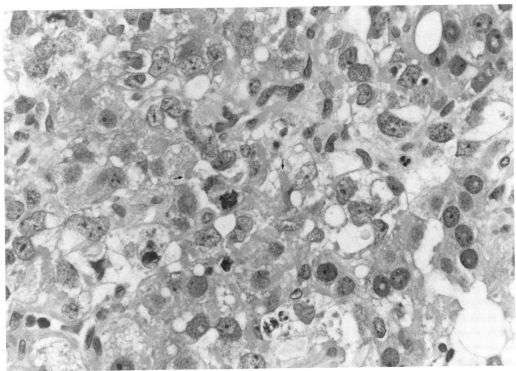

FIGURE 10–80. Yolk sac tumor. Area of solid pattern. Note extracellular and hyaline refractile proteinaceous material *(arrows).* (×660)

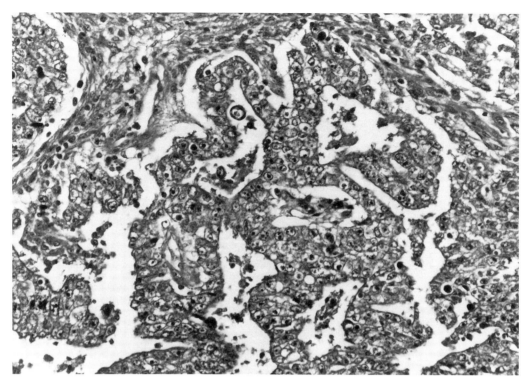

FIGURE 10–81. Embryonal carcinoma arranged in glandular patterns. There is nuclear pleomorphism, some nuclear overlap, and lack of cytoplasmic glycogen (dense cytoplasm). (×330)

of the cases already have metastasized, i.e., they present at a more advanced stage than classic seminoma, similar to "anaplastic" seminoma that also tends to present at a more advanced stage. Grossly, embryonal carcinoma shows characteristically variable hemorrhage and necrosis, which is usually absent in seminoma. The distinction with seminoma is usually easy, based only on the architectural features. However, when the solid pattern predominates, the distinction from seminoma, especially with the anaplastic variant, relies on the lack of cytoplasmic glycogen and strong cytokeratin positivity of the cells by immunohistochemistry in embryonal carcinoma. Both germ cell tumors (seminoma and embryonal carcinoma) react with PLAP.[242, 243]

Germ Cell Tumors with Trophoblastic Cells versus Choriocarcinoma

Seminoma and other germ cell tumors can present with elevated levels of serum beta hCG. Microscopically, many of these tumors show syncytiotrophoblastic giant cells, which can explain the site of production of this hormone.[244] In their absence, immunohistochemical studies often show individual large mononuclear cells with immunoreactivity similar to placental intermediate trophoblastic cells. These cells react with anti-hCG antibodies as well as with cytokeratins, human placental lactogen, and pregnancy-specific beta-1 glycoprotein.[242] Their presence in the absence of cytotrophoblastic cells does not categorize the tumor as having a choriocarcinomatous component and does not alter the course of the disease.[245, 246] For the diagnosis of choriocarcinoma, both syncytial and cytotrophoblastic cells in close association should be present (Fig. 10–82).

Pure choriocarcinoma of the testis is extremely rare.[247] More frequently it occurs associated with other germ cell tumors in the testis or in their metastasis.[237] Grossly pure choriocarcinomas are very hemorrhagic tumors. When associated with other germ cell tumors, these show focal areas of hemorrhage. The prognosis of testicular choriocarcinoma is very poor because of its propensity to metastasize early in the course of the disease.

Sex-Cord Stromal Tumors and Their Differential Diagnosis

Leydig Cell Hyperplasia versus Leydig Cell Nodule and Leydig Cell Neoplasia

Leydig cell hyperplasia is seen in response to hormonal stimulation. It is recognized as a diffuse increase in the number of mature Leydig cells filling the interstitium in between seminiferous tubules (Fig. 10–83). It is often seen in patients with Klinefelter's syndrome or congenital adrenogenital syndrome or with the administration of exogenous hCG. The hyperplasia tends to be bilateral and regresses with cessation of the hormonal stimulation. Occasionally the hyperplastic foci can form multifocal nodules. There is no compression atrophy of the adjacent seminiferous tubules. Leydig cell hyperplasia, diffuse and nodular, has to be differentiated from Leydig cell tumors.

Leydig cell tumor is the most common sex cord stromal tumor in testis.[248] It can present at any age, but more frequently in men older than 40 years old. Children often present with precocious puberty, and adults with gynecomastia. These clinical presentations are related to inappropriate production of

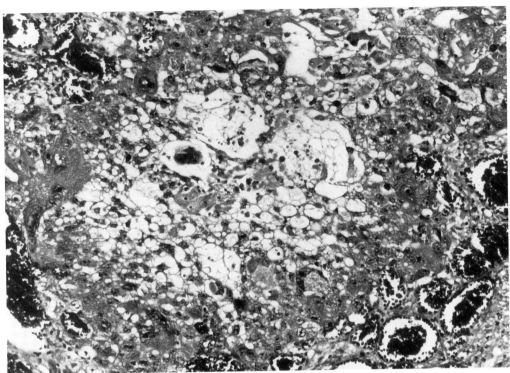

FIGURE 10–82. Focus of choriocarcinoma in a germ cell tumor. Note both components, syncytiotrophoblasts and cytotrophoblasts. (×165)

hormones by the Leydig cells. Hormones that have been reported include testosterone, estradiol, progesterone, corticosterone, and prolactin.[249, 250] Leydig cell tumors can present as testicular masses or with a hormone-related syndrome and no palpable mass that requires studies such as ultrasonography to detect the testicular mass. In children, all Leydig cell tumors are benign, whereas in adults 10% are malignant and metastasize.[251, 252]

Grossly, Leydig cell tumors are well-demarcated yellow to mahogany masses that generally measure 3 to 5 cm in greatest

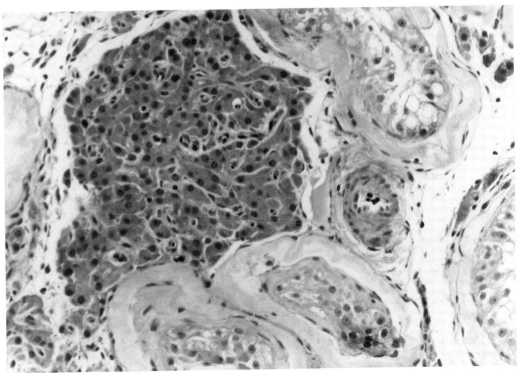

FIGURE 10–83. Leydig cell hyperplasia. Interstitial aggregates of Leydig cells. Note no compression or distortion of adjacent tubules. (×330)

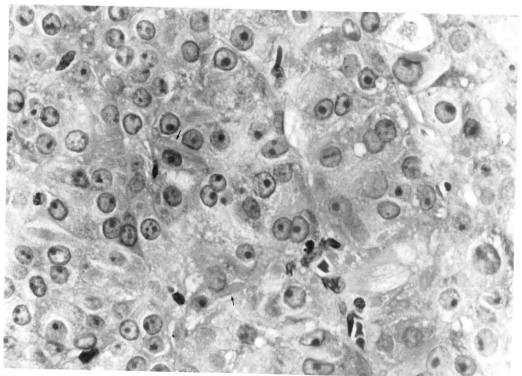

FIGURE 10–84. Leydig cell tumor. Polygonal cells with abundant granular eosinophilic cytoplasm. Note intracytoplasmic Reinke crystals *(arrows)*. Nuclei are round with prominent nucleolus. (×660)

dimension. Small foci of hemorrhage or necrosis can be seen in larger masses. Microscopically, the cells are polygonal with abundant granular, eosinophilic, or clear vacuolated cytoplasm. Frequently there is an admixture of these cells. The cytoplasm often contains lipofuscin, and in 25% to 40% of the tumors Reinke crystals are seen, which are pathognomonic for Leydig cells (Figs. 10–84 and 10–85). Spindle cells and atypical multinucleated large Leydig cells are often scattered through the tumor as well. The presence of atypical large cells by itself is not a reliable feature for malignancy. However,

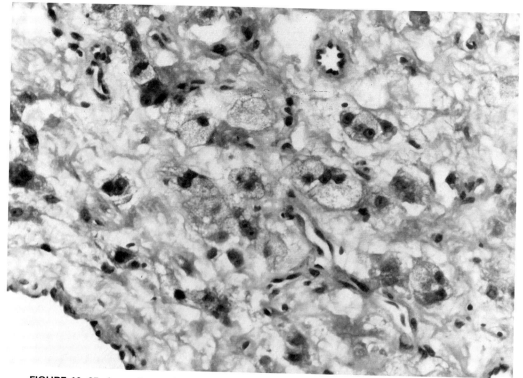

FIGURE 10–85. Area of vacuolated Leydig cells in same tumor shown in Figure 10–84. (×330)

these cells are more often seen in malignant cases. The neoplastic Leydig cells are arranged in sheets, nests, or cords surrounded by fibrous stroma[248] (Fig. 10–86). The tumor, like many endocrine tumors, shows high vascularity of the capillary type.

Aggressive behavior can be suspected when the tumor measures more than 5 cm, has infiltrative margins, extends into adjacent testicular structures, invades vessels, or shows significant mitotic activity and cytologic atypia. However, the only reliable feature for malignancy is distant metastasis. When evaluating the tumor for invasion of adjacent structure, the pathologist should be able to recognize Leydig cells that can normally be found in the spermatic cord and testicular capsule.[237, 253] Leydig cell tumors, unless very poorly differentiated, are hormonally active and can be positive for estrogen and testosterone by immunohistochemistry.[254] They are negative for epithelial markers (EMA and cytokeratin) and positive for vimentin.[255]

Leydig Cell Tumor versus Adrenal Rest

Ectopic adrenal tissue should not be confused with a Leydig cell tumor or Leydig cell nodule. Leydig cell tumors, as previously mentioned, can show clear vacuolated abundant cytoplasm similar to the cells of an adrenal rest. Generally, however, other types of cells are seen in association with eosinophilic and granular cytoplasm in Leydig cell lesions. Adrenal rests are more often seen in children younger than 1 year old than in older children or adults. They can be found anywhere along the tract of gonadal descent to the scrotum, or they may be found within the scrotum but not within the testicular parenchyma. Tumors arising in the substance of the testis should generally be considered of Leydig cell origin. In extratesticular location, helpful differentiating features of the adrenal rests are encapsulation, small size, zonal tissue orientation simulating adrenal cortex, and lack of Reinke crystals.[237]

Benign Sertoli Cell Tumor versus Malignant Sertoli Cell Tumor

Sertoli cell tumors can present at any age, but more often they present in the first decade (30%) and in the 20- to 40-year age range (30%).[256] The patients present with a slow-growing testicular mass and sometimes with gynecomastia. Grossly, small lesions are firm, yellow-tan-gray, and well demarcated. Larger lesions can be cystic. Microscopically, the cells can be highly differentiated with oval vesicular nuclei and small reddish nucleolus (Fig. 10–87) or less differentiated with spindle cell morphology. Architecturally, the cells are arranged in well to poorly defined tubules without lumen and cords surrounded by bands of fibrous tissue serving as basement membrane. Thirty percent of the cases have an admixture of Leydig cells and should be classified as mixed gonadal (Sertoli-Leydig cell) tumors.[257] Sertoli cell tumors are positive for keratin by immunohistochemistry.[255]

Malignant Sertoli cell tumors are rare.[258, 259] They can present at any age, often accompanied by gynecomastia. A diagnosis of malignancy is based on evidence of distant metastasis and invasion of lymphatics and blood vessels and/or adjacent testicular structures. Features that suggest malignancy are increased mitotic activity, marked nuclear atypia, and loss of architectural differentiation.[259]

Malignant Sertoli Cell Tumor versus Large-Cell Calcifying Sertoli Cell Tumor

A variant of Sertoli cell tumor with characteristic clinical and histologic features is the **large-cell calcifying Sertoli cell**

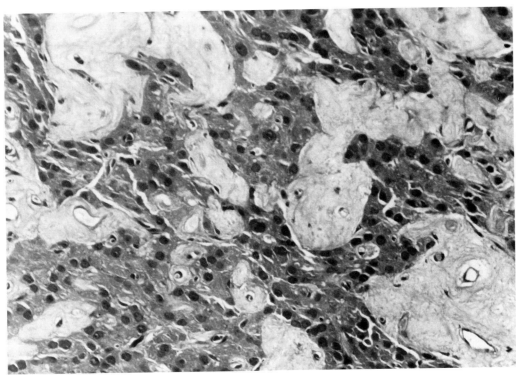

FIGURE 10–86. Leydig cell tumor. Nests and cords of cells surrounded by fibrous stroma. The cells show abundant granular cytoplasm. (×412)

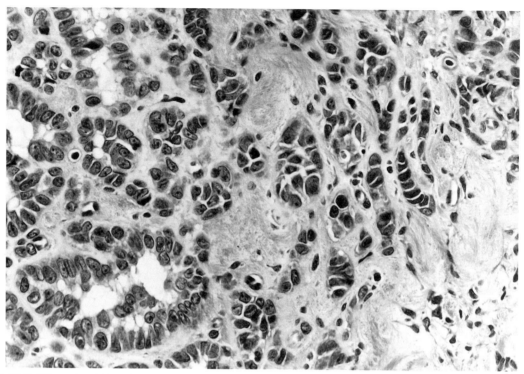

FIGURE 10–87. Well-differentiated Sertoli cell tumor arranged in tubules and cords surrounded by fibrous stroma. The cells show scant cytoplasm and oval nucleus with prominent nucleolus. (×660)

tumor.[260] It usually presents before the age of 20, and it is frequently bilateral and multifocal. Clinically, it has been associated with sexual precocity, gynecomastia, adrenal hyperplasia, cardiac myxoma, and Peutz-Jeghers syndrome.[261]

Microscopically, this tumor is composed of large atypical cells with abundant granular cytoplasm and hyperchromatic nuclei with prominent nucleoli. Multinucleated atypical giant cells are also frequently seen. The cells are arranged in tubules or in interstitial nests. The involved tubules show thickened walls and are separated from other tubules and interstitial nests by fibrous trabeculae or myxoid stroma that can have a lymphocytic infiltrate. Characteristically there are laminated calcified bodies randomly distributed throughout the tumor. Despite the cytologic atypia, these tumors are generally benign. Only one malignant case has been reported.[260] As with other sex cord tumors, invasion of adjacent structures, vasculature, or distant metastasis are required for the diagnosis of malignancy.

PENIS AND SCROTUM

Lesions with Intraepithelial Pagetoid Spread

Extramammary Paget's disease has been described in the penis[262, 263] and inguinal-scrotal area[264, 265] (Fig. 10–88). It has been associated with underlying transitional cell carcinoma of the urethra or bladder[263, 266] and in conjunction with prostatic carcinoma.[267] Jenkins reported a case with adenocarcinoma of the periurethral gland.[262] At times no underlying malignancy is identified. These lesions present in adult men, as do Bowen's disease and superficial spreading melanoma. These three

lesions can show intraepithelial cells in a pagetoid pattern. Usually there are distinctive pathologic features that distinguish these three diseases. Extramammary Paget's disease shows intraepithelial large cells with abundant pale, eosinophilic, basophilic, or vacuolated cytoplasm. The nuclei are large with prominent nucleoli, and scattered mitotic figures are present. No dyskeratotic cells are seen. The cells are seen singly or in nests and generally above the basal cell layer of the epithelium (Figs. 10–88 and 10–89). The surrounding epithelial cells show no atypical features.

In **Bowen's disease,** the cells are distributed singly through the entire epithelial thickness. The cells are often dyskeratotic and show numerous atypical mitoses. The surrounding epithelial cells show atypical features as well (Fig. 10–90).

In **superficial spreading melanoma,** the cells are large with atypical large nuclei, prominent nucleoli, and abundant cytoplasm that may or may not contain melanin. These cells invade the epithelium in nests and singly and are seen predominantly among basal cells above the basement membrane and scattered through the epithelial thickness (Fig. 10–91). The surrounding epithelial cells show no evidence of dyskeratosis or atypical features. Despite the previously described distinguishing features, there are occasions when the distinction between these lesions cannot be made on routine H & E-stained histologic sections. Special stains for mucicarmine and PAS with diastase and immunocytochemistry often resolve the problem. A panel of antibodies to high and low molecular weight cytokeratins, epithelial membrane antigen, carcinoembryonic antigen, S-100 protein, and HMB 45 is recommended. These stains are also helpful for assessment of surgical margins. In Paget's disease, these cells are positive for one or more of the following antibodies: monoclonal low molecular cytokeratins (PKK 1 and 35

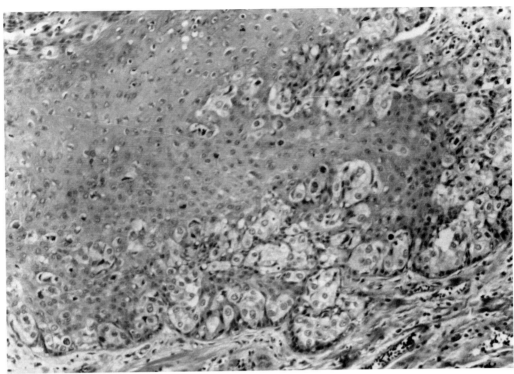

FIGURE 10–88. Scrotum showing extramammary Paget's disease. The neoplastic cells are arranged singly and in nests above the basal cell layer. (×165)

beta H-11), EMA, and CEA. The cytoplasm is often positive for mucicarmine and/or PAS with diastase. The pagetoid cells in Bowen's disease are negative for S-100 protein, HMB 45, CEA, EMA, and low molecular weight cytokeratins (PKK 1 and 35 beta H-11). These cells are positive for high molecular weight cytokeratins (35 beta E 12 and 35 beta 4). The cells are negative for intracytoplasmic mucin. Pagetoid superficial spreading melanoma stains for either S-100 protein or HMB 45, or for both antibodies. Low and high molecular weight cytokeratins are negative.[268–271]

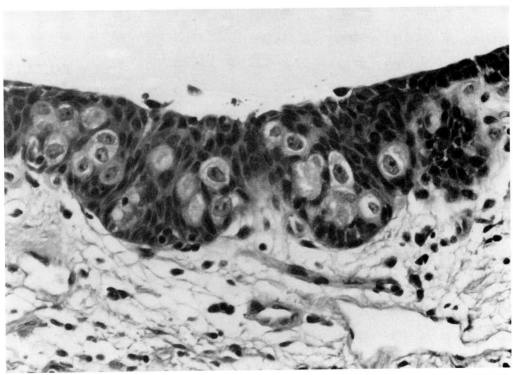

FIGURE 10–89. Prostatic urethra showing metastatic pagetoid spread from bladder transitional cell carcinoma of bladder origin. (×495)

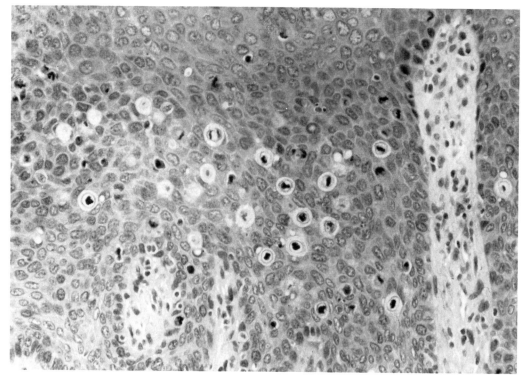

FIGURE 10–90. Penile Bowen's disease. Scattered intraepithelial single pagetoid cells. Note dyskeratotic and atypical surrounding cells. (×330)

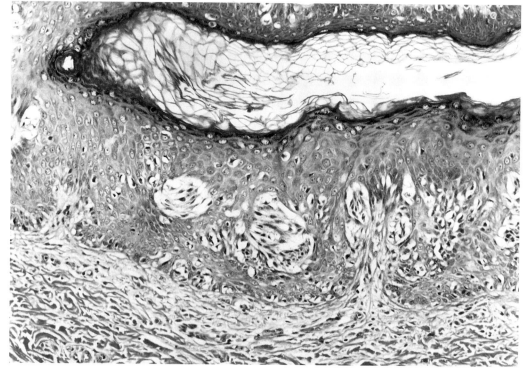

FIGURE 10–91. Superficial spreading melanoma. Pagetoid cells are seen singly and in nests. Note atypical cells among basal cells. (×66)

Squamous Lesions

See description under "Bladder–Squamous Lesions" for verrucous carcinoma and squamous cell carcinoma.

Condyloma

The pathologist is encountering an increasing number of penile biopsies for evaluation of papillomatous and acetowhite flat lesions of partners of women with human papillomavirus (HPV)–associated lesions. Many times we find ourselves as pathologists with lesions inconclusive or only suspicious for human papillomavirus cytopathic effect. Schulz et al.[272] compared the results of histologic examination and nucleic acid hybridization analysis for HPV in 44 patients with acetowhite penile lesions. They found that lesions with minimal nonspecific changes correlate poorly with the presence of HPV nucleic acids and in most cases do not represent disease involving common viral types (types 6, 11, 16, 18, and 51). Hyperkeratosis, parakeratosis, acanthosis, and/or perinuclear halos without cytologic atypia are non-specific findings that should not be called condyloma. The same findings in a papillomatous lesion are insufficient for a definite diagnosis. Strict histologic criteria requiring koilocytotic atypia should be applied when making a positive diagnosis to avoid overtreatment of minor epithelial changes. Immunohistochemical studies and/or nucleic acid hybridization analysis for these non-specific lesions are at this point not recommended for clinical management, because no study has demonstrated that treatment of asymptomatic males and females with positive viral DNA analysis influences the natural course of the disease.[272]

References

1. Bove K, Koffler H, McAdams A: Nodular renal blastema. Definition and possible significance. Cancer 24:323–332, 1969.
2. Hou L, Holman R: Bilateral nephroblastomatosis in a premature infant. Pathol Bacteriol 82(2):249–255, 1961.
3. Hennigar R, Othersen H, Garvin A: Clinicopathologic features of nephroblastomatosis. Urology 32(4):259–270, 1989.
4. Machin G, McCaughey W: A new precursor lesion of Wilms' tumour (nephroblastoma): Intralobular multifocal nephroblastomatosis. Histopathology 8:35–53, 1984.
5. Beckwith J: The John Lattimer Lecture. Wilms' tumor and other renal tumors of childhood: An update. J Urol 136:320–324, 1986.
6. Blute M, Kelalis P, Offord K, et al: Wilms' tumor. Bilateral Wilms' tumor. J Urol 138:968–973, 1987.
7. Koufos A, Hansen M, Lampkin B, et al: Loss of alleles at loci on human chromosome 11 during genesis of Wilms' tumour. Nature 309(10):170–172, 1984.
8. Beckwith J, Palmer N: Histopathology and prognosis of Wilms' tumor. Results from the first national Wilms' Tumor Study. Cancer 41:1937–1948, 1978.
9. Marsden H, Lawler W, Kumar P: Bone metastasizing renal tumor of childhood. Morphological and clinical features, and differences from Wilms' tumor. Cancer 42:1922–1928, 1978.
10. Marsden H, Lawler W: Bone metastasizing renal tumour of childhood. Histopathological and clinical review of 38 cases. Virchows Arch [Pathol Anat] 387:341–351, 1980.
11. Schmidt D, Harms A, Leuschner I: Malignant renal tumors of childhood. Pathol Res Pract 188:1–15, 1992.
12. D'Angio G, Breslow N, Beckwith JB, et al: Treatment of Wilms' tumor. Results of the Third National Wilms' Tumour Study. Cancer 64:349–360, 1989.
13. Beckwith J: Wilms' tumor and other renal tumors of childhood: A selective review from the National Wilms' Tumor Study Pathology Center. Hum Pathol 14:481–492, 1983.
14. Shende A, Wind E, Lanzkowsky P: Intrarenal neuroblastoma mimicking Wilms' tumor. N Y State J Med 79:93, 1979.
15. Boland R, Brough AJ, Izant R: Congenital mesoblastic nephroma of infancy. A report of eight cases and the relationship to Wilms' tumor. Pediatrics 40(2):272–278, 1967.
16. Joshi V, Kasznica J, Walters T: Atypical mesoblastic nephroma. Pathological characterization of a potentially aggressive variant of conventional congenital mesoblastic nephroma. Arch Pathol Lab Med 40:100–106, 1986.
17. Beckwith J, Weeks D: Congenital mesoblastic nephroma. When should we worry? Arch Pathol Lab Med 110:98–99, 1986.
18. Pettinato G, Manivel J, Wick M, Dehner L: Classical and cellular (atypical) congenital mesoblastic nephroma: A clinicopathologic, ultrastructural, immunohistochemical, and flow cytometric study. Hum Pathol 20:682–690, 1989.
19. Wigger H: Fetal rhabdomyomatous nephroblastoma—a variant of Wilms' tumor. Hum Pathol 7(6):613–623, 1976.
20. Mahoney J, Saffos R: Fetal rhabdomyomatous nephroblastoma with a renal pelvic mass simulating sarcoma botryoides. Am J Surg Pathol 5:297–306, 1981.
21. Weeks D, Beckwith J, Mierau G, Luckey D: Rhabdoid tumor of kidney. A report of 111 cases from the National Wilms' Tumor Study Pathology Center. Am J Surg Pathol 13(6):439–458, 1989.
22. Rousseau-Merck M, Nogues C, Nezelof C, et al: Infantile renal tumors associated with hypercalcemia. Characterization of intermediate-filament clusters. Arch Pathol Lab Med 107:311–314, 1983.
23. Howat A, Gonzales M, Waters K, Campbell P: Primitive neuroectodermal tumour of the central nervous system associated with malignant rhabdoid tumour of the kidney: Report of a case. Histopathology 10:643–650 1986.
24. Magee J, Ansari S, McFadden D, Dimmick J: Teratoid Wilms' tumour: A report of two cases. Histopathology 20:427–431 1992.
25. Variend S, Spicer R, Mackinnon A: Teratoid Wilms' tumor. Cancer 53:1936–1942, 1984.
26. Dehner L: Intrarenal teratoma occurring in infancy: Report of a case with discussion of extragonadal germ cell tumors in infancy. J Pediatr Surg 8:369–378, 1973.
27. Castillo O, Boyle E, Kramer S: Multilocular cyst of kidney. A study of 29 patients and review of the literature. Urology 37:156–162, 1991.
28. Powell T, Shackman R, Johnson H: Multilocular cysts of the kidney. Br J Urol 23:142–152, 1951.
29. Bauldauf M, Schulz D: Multilocular cyst of the kidney. Report of three cases with review of the literature. Am J Clin Pathol 65:93–102, 1976.
30. Joshi V, Banerjee A, Yadav K, Pathak I: Cystic partially differentiated nephroblastoma. A clinicopathologic entity in the spectrum of infantile renal neoplasia. Cancer 40:789–795, 1977.
31. DeKlerk D, Marshall F, Jeffs R: Multicystic dysplastic kidney. J Urol 118:306–308, 1977.
32. Bernstein J: The morphogenesis of renal parenchymal maldevelopment (renal dysplasia). Pediatr Clin North Am 18:395–406, 1971.
33. Bernstein J: Developmental abnormalities of the renal parenchyma: Renal hyperplasia and dysplasia. Pathol Annu 3:213–247, 1968.
34. Ambrose S, Gould R, Trulock T, Parrot T: Unilateral multicystic renal disease in adults. J Urol 128:366–369, 1982.
35. Lieberman E, Salinas-Madrigal L, Gwinn J, et al: Infantile polycystic disease of the kidneys and liver: Clinical, pathological and radiological correlations and comparison with congenital hepatic fibrosis. Medicine 50(4):277–318, 1971.
36. Bell E: A classification of renal tumors with observations on the frequency of the various types. J Urol 39:238–243, 1938.
37. Bennington J: Cancer of the Kidney—etiology, epidemiology, and pathology. Cancer 32:1017–1029, 1973.
38. Pfannkuch F, Leistenschneider W, Nagel R: Problems of assessment in the surgery of renal adenomas. J Urol 125:95–98, 1981.
39. Tsukamoto T, Kumamoto Y, Takahashi A, et al: Tumor size of renal cell carcinoma: Its clinical implication. Urol Int 48:378–383, 1992.
40. Lack E, Cassady J, Sallan S: Renal cell carcinoma in childhood and adolescence. A clinical and pathologic study of 17 cases. J Urol 133:822–828, 1985.
41. Hughson M, Hennigar G, McManus F: Atypical cysts, acquired renal cystic disease, and renal cell tumors in end stage dialysis kidneys. Lab Invest 42(4):475–480, 1980.
42. Berger C, Sandberg A, Todd I, et al: Chromosomes in kidney, ureter and bladder cancer. Cancer Genet Cytogenet 13:1–21, 1984.
43. Fuhrman S, Lasky L, Limas C: Prognostic significance of morphologic parameters in renal cell carcinoma. Am J Surg Pathol 6:655–663, 1982.
44. Mydlo J, Bard R: Analysis of papillary renal adenocarcinoma. Urology 30(6):529–534, 1987.
45. Bard R, Lord B, Fromwitz F: Papillary adenocarcinoma of kidney. II. Radiographic and biologic characteristics. Urology 19(1):16–20, 1982.
46. Mei GS, Rendler S, Herskowitz A, Molnar J: Renal oncocytoma. Report of five cases and review of literature. Cancer 45:1010–1018, 1980.
47. Klein M, Valensi Q: Proximal tubular adenomas of the kidney with so-called oncocytic features. Cancer 38:906–914, 1976.
48. Sos T, Gray G, Baltaxe H: The angiographic appearance of benign renal oxyphilic adenoma. Am J Roentgenol 127:717–722, 1976.
49. Ambos M, Bosniak M, Valensi Q, et al: Angiographic patterns in renal oncocytomas. Radiology 129:615–622, 1978.
50. Lang E: Arteriography in the diagnosis and staging of hypernephromas. Cancer 32:1043–1052, 1973.
51. Lieber M, Tomera K, Farrow G: Renal oncocytoma. J Urol 125:481–485, 1981.
52. Delahunt B, Gupta R, Nacey J: Diagnosis of renal oncocytoma. Urology 37:602, 1991.
53. Bertoni F, Ferri C, Benati A, et al: Sarcomatoid carcinoma of the kidney. J Urol 137:25–28, 1987.
54. Ro J, Ayala A, Sella A, et al: Sarcomatoid renal cell carcinoma: Clinicopathologic. A study of 42 cases. Cancer 59: 516–526, 1987.
55. Farrow G, Harrison E, Utz D, ReMine W: Sarcomas and sarcomatoid and mixed malignant tumors of the kidney in adults—Part I. Cancer 22:545–550, 1968.

56. Srinivas V, Sogani P, Hajdu S, Whitmore W: Sarcomas of the kidney. J Urol 132:13–16, 1984.
57. Hartman D, Davis C, Johns T, Goldman S: Cystic renal cell carcinoma. Urology 28:145–153, 1986.
58. Pozo J: Calcified cystic adenocarcinoma of the kidney. J R Soc Med 74:920–921, 1981.
59. Bretan P, Busch M, Hricak H, Williams R: Chronic renal failure: A significant risk factor in the development of acquired renal cysts and renal cell carcinoma. Case reports and review of the literature. Cancer 57:1871–1879, 1986.
60. Fuhrman S, Lasky L, Limas C: Prognostic significance of morphologic parameters in renal cell carcinoma. Am J Surg Pathol 6:655–663, 1982.
61. Mancilla-Jimenez R, Stanley R, Blath R: Papillary renal cell carcinoma. A clinical, radiologic, and pathologic study of 34 cases. Cancer 38:2469–2480, 1976.
62. Kennedy S, Merino M, Linehan W, et al: Collecting duct carcinoma of the kidney. Hum Pathol 21:449–456, 1990.
63. Fleming S, Lewi H: Collecting duct carcinoma of the kidney. Histopathology 10:1131–1141, 1986.
64. Rumpelt H, Storkel S, Moll R, et al: Bellini duct carcinoma: Further evidence for this rare variant of renal cell carcinoma. Histopathology 18:115–122, 1991.
65. Dierick A, Praet M, Roels H, et al: Vimentin expression of renal cell carcinoma in relation to DNA content and histological grading: A combined light microscopic, immunocytochemical and cytophotometrical analysis. Histopathology 18:315–322, 1991.
66. Malek R, Elder J: Xanthogranulomatous pyelonephritis: A critical analysis of 26 cases and of the literature. J Urol 119:589–593, 1978.
67. Parsons M, Harris S: Xanthogranulomatous pyelonephritis: A pathological, clinical and aetiological analysis of 87 cases. Diagn Histophathol 6:203–219, 1983.
68. Bissada N, White H, Sun C, et al: Tuberous sclerosis complex and renal angiomyolipoma. Urology 6:105–113, 1975.
69. Malone M, Johnson P, Jumper B, et al: Renal angiomyolipoma: 6 case reports and literature review. J Urol 135:349–353, 1986.
70. Waisman J: Additional cases of angiomyolipoma with regional lymph node involvement. Hum Pathol 18:206, 1987.
71. Lowe B, Brewer J, Houghton D, Jacobson E: Malignant transformation of angiomyolipoma. J Urol 147:1356–1358, 1992.
72. Eble J, Young R: Benign and low-grade papillary lesions of the urinary bladder: A review of the papilloma-papillary carcinoma controversy, and a report of five typical papillomas. Semin Diagn Pathol 6:351–371, 1989.
73. National Bladder Cancer Collaborative Group A (NBCCGA): Surveillance, initial assessment, and subsequent progress of patients with superficial bladder cancer in a prospective longitudinal study. Cancer Res 37:2907–2910, 1977.
74. Brawn P: The relationship between non-invasive papillary lesions and invasive bladder carcinoma. Cancer 54:620–623, 1984.
75. Mattalaer J, Leonard A, Goddeeris P, et al: Inverted papilloma of bladder: Clinical significance. Urology 32:192–197, 1988.
76. Talbert M, Young R: Carcinomas of the urinary bladder with deceptively benign-appearing foci. A report of three cases. Am J Surg Pathol 13(5):374–381, 1989.
77. Young R: Papillary and polypoid cystitis. A report of eight cases. Am J Surg Pathol 12(7):542–546, 1988.
78. Horner S, Fisher H, Barada J, et al: Verrucous carcinoma of the bladder. J Urol 145:1261–1263, 1991.
79. Faysal M: Squamous cell carcinoma of the bladder. J Urol 126:598–599, 1981.
80. Grace D, Winter C: Mixed differentiation of primary carcinoma of the urinary bladder. Cancer 21:1239–1243, 1968.
81. Emmett J, McDonald J: Proliferation of glands of the urinary bladder simulating malignant neoplasm. J Urol 48:257–265, 1942.
82. Lowry E, Hamm F, Beard D: Extensive glandular proliferation of the urinary bladder resembling malignant neoplasm. J Urol 52:133–138, 1944.
83. Bell T, Wendel R: Cystitis glandularis: Benign or malignant? J Urol 100:462–465, 1968.
84. Shaw J, Gislason J, Imbriglia J: Transition of cystitis glandularis to primary adenocarcinoma of the bladder. J Urol 79:815–822, 1958.
85. Mostofi F: Potentialities of bladder epithelium. J Urol 71:705–720, 1954.
86. Edwards P, Hurm R, Jaeschke W: Conversion of cystitis glandularis to adenocarcinoma. J Urol 108:568–570, 1972.
87. Abenoza P, Manivel C, Fraley E: Primary adenocarcinoma of urinary bladder. Clinicopathologic study of 16 cases. Urology 29:9–14, 1987.
88. Wiener D, Koss L, Sablay B, Freed S: The prevalence and significance of Brunn's nests, cystitis cystica and squamous metaplasia in normal bladders. J Urol 122:317–321, 1979.
89. Heyns S, Dekock M, Kirsten P, Van Velden D: Pelvic lipomatosis associated with cystitis cystica and glandularis and adenocarcinoma of the bladder. J Urol 145:364–366, 1991.
90. Johnston O, Bracken R, Ayala A: Vesical adenocarcinoma occurring in patient with pelvic lipomatosis. Urology 15:280–282, 1980.
91. Burnett A, Epstein J, Marshall F: Adenocarcinoma of urinary bladder: Classification and management. Urology 37(4):315–321, 1991.
92. Grignon D, Ro J, Ayala A, et al: Primary adenocarcinoma of the urinary bladder. A clinicopathologic analysis of 72 cases. Cancer 67:2165–2172, 1991.
93. DeFillipo N, Blute R, Klein L: Signet-ring cell carcinoma of bladder. Evaluation of three cases with review of literature. Urology 29:479–483, 1987.
94. McIntire T, Soloway M, Murphy W: Nephrogenic adenoma. Urology 29:237–241, 1987.
95. Nold S, Terry W, Cerniglia F, et al: Nephrogenic adenoma of the bladder in children. J Urol 142:1545–1547, 1989.
96. Friedman N, Kuhlenbeck H: Adenomatoid tumors of the bladder reproducing renal structures (nephrogenic adenomas). J Urol 64:657–670, 1950.
97. Young R, Scully R: Nephrogenic adenoma. A report of 15 cases, review of the literature, and comparison with clear cell adenocarcinoma of the urinary tract. Am J Surg Pathol 10(4):268–275, 1986.
98. Spencer J, Brodin A, Ignatoff J: Clear cell adenocarcinoma of the urethra: Evidence for origin within paraurethral ducts. J Urol 143:122–125, 1990.
99. Neto W, Lopes R, Cury M, et al: Vesical endometriosis. Urology 24:271–274, 1984.
100. Pinkert T, Catlow C, Straus R: Endometriosis of the urinary bladder in a man with prostatic carcinoma. Cancer 43:1562–1567, 1979.
101. Proppe K, Scully R, Rosai J: Postoperative spindle cell nodules of genitourinary tract resembling sarcomas. A report of eight cases. Am J Surg Pathol 8:101–108, 1984.
102. Vekemans K, Vanneste A, Van Oyen P, et al: Postoperative spindle cell nodule of bladder. Urology 35:342–344, 1990.
103. Wick M, Brown B, Young R, Mills S: Spindle-cell proliferations of the urinary tract. An immunohistochemical study. Am J Surg Pathol 12(5):379–389, 1988.
104. Roth J: Reactive pseudosarcomatous response in urinary bladder. Urology 16:635–637, 1980.
105. Albores-Saavedra J, Manivel C, Essenfeld H, et al: Pseudo Sarcomatous myofibroblastic proliferations in the urinary bladder of children. Cancer 66:1234–1241, 1990.
106. Nochomovitz L, Orenstein J: Inflammatory pseudotumor of the urinary bladder—possible relationship to nodular fasciitis. Two case reports, cytologic observations, and ultrastructural observations. Am J Surg Pathol 9(5):366–373, 1985.
107. Ro J, Ayala A, Ordonez N, et al: Pseudosarcomatous fibromyxoid tumor of the urinary bladder. Am J Clin Pathol 86:583–590, 1986.
108. Young R, Proppe K, Dickerson G, Scully R: Myxoid leiomyosarcoma of the urinary bladder. Arch Pathol Lab Med 111:359–362, 1987.
109. Mills S, Bova S, Wick M, Young R: Leiomyosarcoma of the urinary bladder. A clinicopathologic and immunohistochemical study of 15 cases. Am J Surg Pathol 13(6):480–489, 1989.
110. Coyne J, Wilson G, Sandhu D, Young R: Inflammatory pseudotumour of the urinary bladder. Histopathology 18:261–264, 1991.
111. Hughes D, Biggart J, Hayes D: Pseudosarcomatous lesions of the urinary bladder. Histopathology 18:67–71, 1991.
112. Weitzner S: Leiomyosarcoma of urinary bladder in children. Urology 12(4):450–452, 1978.
113. Thrasher J, Miller G, Wettlaufer J: Bladder leiomyosarcoma following cyclophosphamide therapy for lupus nephritis. J Urol 143:119–121, 1990.
114. Seo I, Clark S, McGovern F, et al: Leiomyosarcoma of the urinary bladder. 13 years after cyclophosphamide therapy for Hodgkin's disease. Cancer 55:1597–1603, 1985.
115. Young R, Wick M, Mills S: Sarcomatoid carcinoma of the urinary bladder. A clinicopathologic analysis of 12 cases and review of the literature. Am J Clin Pathol 90:653–661, 1988.
116. Young R, Wick M: Transitional cell carcinoma of the urinary bladder with pseudosarcomatous stoma. Am J Clin Pathol 90:216–219, 1988.
117. Mahadevia P, Alexander J, Rojas-Corona R, Koss L: Pseudosarcomatous stromal reaction in primary and metastatic urothelial carcinoma. A source of diagnostic difficulty. Am J Surg Pathol 13:783–790, 1989.
118. Melicow M, Hollowell J: Intra-urothelial cancer: Carcinoma in situ, Bowen's disease of the urinary system. Discussion of thirty cases. J Urol 68:763–772, 1952.
119. Melamed V, Voutsa N, Grabstald H: Natural history and clinical behavior of in situ carcinoma of the human urinary bladder. Cancer 17:1533–1545, 1964.
120. Koss L: Tumors of the urinary bladder. In Atlas of Tumor Pathology, Fascicle II, 2nd Series. Washington, DC, Armed Forces Institute of Pathology, 1975, pp 99–102.
121. Fajardo L, Berthrong M: Radiation injury in surgical pathology: Part I. Am J Surg Pathol 2:159–199, 1987.
122. Beyer-Boon M, Voogt H, Schaberg A: The effects of cyclophosphamide treatment on the epithelium and stroma of the urinary bladder. Eur J Cancer 14:1029–1035, 1978.
123. Philips F, Sternberg S, Cronin A, Vidal P: Cyclophosphamide and urinary bladder toxicity. Cancer Res 21:1577–1589, 1961.
124. Koss L: Diagnostic Cytology and its Histopathologic Basis, 3rd ed. Philadelphia, JB Lippincott, 1979, pp 711–817.
125. Forni A, Koss L, Geller W: Cytological study of the effect of cyclophosphamide on the epithelium of the urinary bladder in man. Cancer 17:1348–1355, 1964.
126. Murphy W, Soloway M, Finebaum P: Pathological changes associated with topical chemotherapy for superficial bladder cancer. J Urol 126:461–464, 1981.
127. Murphy W, Soloway M, Crabtree W: The morphologic effects of mitomycin C in mammalian urinary bladder. Cancer 47:2467–2574, 1981.
128. Nieh P, Daly J, Heaney J, et al: The effect of intravesical thio-tepa on normal and tumor urothelium. J Urol 119:59–61, 1978.
129. Wajsman Z, McGill W, Englander L, et al: Severely contracted bladder following intravesical mitomycin C therapy. J Urol 130:340–341, 1983.
130. Jones E, Clement P, Young R: Sclerosing adenosis of the prostate gland. A clinicopathological and immunohistochemical study of 11 cases. Am J Surg Pathol 15(12):1171–1180, 1991.
131. Sakamoto N, Tsuneyoshi M, Enjoji M: Sclerosing adenosis of the prostate. Histopathologic and immunohistochemical analysis. Am J Surg Pathol 15(7):660–667, 1991.

132. Collina G, Botticelli A, Martinelli A, et al: Sclerosing adenosis of the prostate. Report of three cases with electronmicroscopy and immunohistochemical study. Histopathology 20:505–510, 1992.

133. Grignon D, Ro J, Srigley J, et al: Sclerosing adenosis of the prostate gland. A lesion showing myoepithelial differentiation. Am J Surg Pathol 16(4):383–391, 1992.

134. McNeal J: Morphogenesis of prostatic carcinoma. Cancer 18(12):1659–1666, 1965.

135. Kastendiek H. Correlations between atypical primary hyperplasia and carcinoma of the prostate. A histological study of 180 total prostatectomies. Pathol Res Pract 169:366–387, 1980.

136. Brawn P: Adenosis of the prostate: A dysplastic lesion that can be confused with prostate adenocarcinoma. Cancer 49:826–833, 1982.

137. Srigley J: Small-acrinar patterns in the prostate gland with emphasis on atypical adenomatous hyperplasia and small-acinar carcinoma. Semin Diagn Pathol 5(3):254–272, 1988.

138. Greene D, Wheeler T, Egawas, et al: A comparison of the morphological features of cancer arising in the transition zone and in the peripheral zone of the prostate. J Urol 146(4):1069–1076, 1991.

139. Greene D, Wheeler T, Egawa S, et al: Relationship between clinical stage and histological zone of origin in early prostate cancer: Morphometric analysis. Br J Urol 68(5):499–509, 1991.

140. Pagano F, Zattoni F, Vianello F, et al: Is there a relationship between benign prostatic hyperplasia and prostatic cancer? Eur Urol 20 (Suppl 1):31–35, 1991.

141. Hedrick L, Epstein J: Use of keratin 903 as an adjunct in the diagnosis of prostate carcinoma. Am J Surg Pathol 13(5):389–396, 1989.

142. O'Malley F, Grignon D, Shum D: Usefulness of immunoperoxidase staining with high-molecular-weight cytokeratin in the differential diagnosis of small-acinar lesions of the prostate gland. Virchows Arch A Pathol Anat Histopathol 417(3):191–196, 1990.

143. Tannenbaum M: Atypical epithelial hyperplasia or carcinoma of prostate gland. Urol 4(6):758–760, 1974.

144. McNeal J, Bostwick D: Intraductal dysplasia: A premalignant lesion of the prostate. Hum Pathol 17:64–71, 1986.

145. Bostwick D, Brawer M: Prostatic intra-epithelial neoplasia and early invasion in prostate cancer. Cancer 59:788–794, 1987.

146. Kovi J, Mostofi F, Heshmat M, Enterline J: Large acinar atypical hyperplasia and carcinoma of the prostate. Cancer 61:555–561, 1988.

147. McNeal J: Significance of duct-acinar dysplasia in prostatic carcinogenesis. The Prostate 13:91–102, 1988.

148. Brawer M: Prostatic intraepithelial neoplasia: A premalignant lesion. Hum Pathol 23:242–248, 1992.

149. Drago J, Mostofi F, Lee F: Introductory remarks and workshop summary. Urology Supp 34(6):2–3, 1989.

150. Nagle R, Brawer M, Kittelson J, Clark V: Phenotypic relationships of prostatic intraepithelial neoplasia to invasive prostatic carcinoma. Am J Pathol 138:119–128, 1991.

151. Brawer M, Peehl D, Stamey T, Bostwick D: Keratin immunoreactivity in the benign and neoplastic human prostate. Cancer 45:3663–3667, 1985.

152. Dube V, Farrow G, Greene L: Prostatic adenocarcinoma of ductal origin. Cancer 32:402–409, 1973.

153. Christensen W, Steinberg G, Walsh P, Epstein J: Prostatic duct adenocarcinoma. Findings at radical prostatectomy. Cancer 67:2118–2124, 1991.

154. Ayala A, Srigley J, Ro J, et al: Clear cell cribriform hyperplasia of prostate. Report of 10 cases. Am J Surg Pathol 10(10):665–671, 1986.

155. Frauenhoffer E, Ro J, El-Naggar A, et al: Clear cell cribriform hyperplasia of the prostate. Immunohistochemical and DNA flow cytometric study. Am J Clin Pathol 95:446–453, 1991.

156. Dermer G: Basal cell proliferation in benign prostatic hyperplasia. Cancer 41:1857–1862, 1978.

157. Lin J, Cohen E, Villacin A, et al: Basal cell adenoma of prostate. Urology 11(4):409–410, 1978.

158. Cleary K, Choi H, Ayala A: Basal cell hyperplasia of the prostate. Am J Clin Pathol 80:850–854, 1983.

159. Manrique J, Albores-Saavedra J, Orantes A, Brandt H: Malignant mixed tumor of the salivary-gland type, primary in the prostate. Am J Clin Pathol 70:932–937, 1978.

160. Kuhajda F, Mann R: Adenoid cystic carcinoma of the prostate. A case report with immunoperoxidase staining for prostate-specific acid phosphatase and prostate-specific antigen. Am J Clin Pathol 81:257–260, 1984.

161. Young R, Frierson H, Mills S, et al: Adenoid cystic-like tumor of the prostate gland. Am J Clin Pathol 89:49–56, 1988.

162. Denholm S, Webb J, Howard G, Chisholm G: Basaloid carcinoma of the prostate gland: Histogenesis and review of the literature. Histopathology 20:151–155, 1992.

163. di Sant'Agnese P, de Mesy Jensen K: Human prostatic endocrine-paracrine (APUD) cells: Distributional analysis with a comparison of serotonin and neuron-specific enolase immunoreactivity and silver stains. Arch Pathol Lab Med 109:607–612, 1985.

164. Abrahamsson P, Wadstrom L, Alumets J, et al: Peptide-hormone- and serotonin-immunoreactive cells in normal and hyperplastic prostate glands. Pathol Res Pract 181:675–683, 1986.

165. di Sant'Agnese P, de Mesy Jensen K: Endocrine-paracrine cells of the prostate and prostatic urethra: An ultrastructural study. Hum Pathol 15:1034–1041, 1984.

166. Abrahamsson P, Falkmer S, Falt K, Grimelius L: The course of neuroendocrine differentiation in prostatic carcinomas: An immunohistochemical study testing chromogranin A as an "endocrine marker." Pathol Res Pract 185:373–380, 1989.

167. di Sant'Agnese P: Calcitonin-like immunoreactive and bombesin-like immunoreactive endocrine-paracrine cells of the human prostate. Arch Pathol Lab Med 110:412–415, 1986.

168. di Sant'Agnese P, de Mesy Jensen K: Calcitonin, katacalcin and calcitonin gene-related peptide in the human prostate: An immunocytochemical and immunoelectron microscopic study. Arch Pathol Lab Med 113:790–796, 1989.

169. Sunday M, Kaplan L, Motoyama E, et al: Biology of disease: Gastrin-releasing peptide (mammalian bombesin) gene expression in health and disease. Lab Invest 59:5–24, 1988.

170. di Sant'Agnese P, de Mesy Jensen K: Somatostatin and/or somatostatin-like immunoreactive endocrine-paracrine cells in the human prostate gland. Arch Pathol Lab Med 108:693–696, 1984.

171. Abrahamsson P, Wadstrom L, Alumets J, et al: Peptide-hormone and serotonin-immunoreactive tumour cells in carcinoma of the prostate. Pathol Res Pract 182:298–307, 1987.

172. di Sant'Agnese P, de Mesy Jensen K: Neuroendocrine differentiation in prostatic carcinoma. Hum Pathol 18:849–856, 1987.

173. di Sant'Agnese P: Neuroendocrine differentiation and prostatic carcinoma: The concept "comes of age" [editorial]. Arch Pathol Lab Med 112:1097–1099, 1988.

174. di Sant'Agnese P: Neuroendocrine differentiation in prostatic carcinoma. Hum Pathol 23:287–296, 1992.

175. Frydman C, Bleiweiss I, Unger P, et al: Paneth cell-like metaplasia of the prostate gland. Arch Pathol Lab Med 116:274–276, 1992.

176. Weaver M, Abdul-Karim F, Srigley J, et al: Paneth cell-like change of the prostate gland. A histological, immunohistochemical, and electron microscopic study. Am J Surg Pathol 16(1):62–68, 1992.

177. Weaver M, Abdul-Karim F, Srigley J: Paneth cell-like change and small cell carcinoma of the prostate. Two divergent forms of prostatic neuroendocrine differentiation. Am J Surg Pathol 16(10):1013–1016, 1992.

178. Azzopardi J, Evans D: Argentaffin cells in prostatic carcinoma: Differentiation from lipofuscin and melanin in prostatic epithelium. J Pathol 104:247–251, 1971.

179. Kazzaz B: Argentaffin and argyrophil cells in the prostate. J Pathol 112:189–193, 1974.

180. Capella C, Usellini L, Buffa R, et al: The endocrine component of prostatic carcinomas, mixed adenocarcinoma-carcinoid tumors and non-tumor prostate: Histochemical and ultrastructural identification of the endocrine cells. Histopathology 5:175–192, 1981.

181. Dauge M, Delmas V: APUD type endocrine tumor of the prostate: Incidence and prognosis in association with adenocarcinoma. In Murphy GP, Khoury S, Kuss R, et al (eds): Progress in Clinical and Biological Medicine. New York, Alan R. Liss, 1986, pp 529–531.

182. Cohen R, Glezerson G, Haffejee Z, Afrika D: Prostatic carcinoma: Histological and immunohistological factors affecting prognosis. Br J Urol 66:405–410, 1990.

183. Tarle M, Rados N: Investigation on serum neuron-specific enolase in prostate cancer diagnosis and monitoring: Comparative study of a multiple tumor marker assay. Prostate 19:23, 1991.

184. Kadmon D, Thompson T, Lynch G, Scardino P: Elevated plasma chromogranin-A concentrations in prostatic carcinoma. J Urol 146:358–361, 1991.

185. Tetu B, Ro J, Ayala A, et al: Small cell carcinoma of the prostate: Part I. A clinicopathologic study of 20 cases. Cancer 59:1803–1809, 1987.

186. Turbat-Herrera E, Herrera G, Gore I, et al: Neuroendocrine differentiation in prostatic carcinomas: A retrospective autopsy study. Arch Pathol Lab Med 112:1100–1106, 1988.

187. Christopher M, Seftel A, Sorenson K, Resnick M: Small cell carcinoma of the genitourinary tract: An immunohistochemical, electron microscopic, and clinicopathological study. J Urol 146:382–388, 1991.

188. Almagro U, Tieu T, Remeniuk E, et al: Argyrophilic, "carcinoid-like" prostatic carcinoma. Arch Pathol Lab Med 110:916–919, 1986.

189. Fetissof F, Bruandet P, Arbeille B, et al: Calcitonin-secreting carcinomas of the prostate: An immunohistochemical and ultrastructural analysis. Am J Surg Pathol 10:702–710, 1986.

190. Stratton M, Evans D, Lambert I: Prostatic adenocarcinoma evolving into carcinoid: Selective effect of hormonal treatment? J Clin Pathol 39:750–756, 1986.

191. Rode J, Bentley A, Parkinson C: Paraganglial cells of urinary bladder and prostate: Potential diagnostic problem. J Clin Pathol 43(1):13–16, 1990.

192. Dennis P, Lewandowski A, Rohner T, et al: Pheochromocytoma of the prostate: An unusual location. J Urol 141:130–132, 1989.

193. Smith B, Dehner L: Sarcoma of the prostate gland. Am J Clin Pathol 58:43–50, 1972.

194. Tannenbaum M: Sarcomas of the prostate gland. Urology 5(6):810–814, 1975.

195. Witherow R, Molland E, Oliver T, Hind C: Leiomyosarcoma of prostate and superficial soft tissue. Urology 15(5):513–515, 1980.

196. Camuzzi F, Block N, Charyulu K, et al: Leiomyosarcoma of prostate gland. Urology 18(3):295–297, 1981.

197. Bain G, Danyluk J, Shnitka T, et al: Malignant fibrous histiocytoma of prostate gland. Urology 26(1):89–91, 1985.

198. Chin W, Fay R, Ortega P: Malignant fibrous histiocytoma of prostate. Urology 27(4):363–365, 1986.

199. Huang W, Ro J, Grignon D, et al: Postoperative spindle cell nodule of the prostate and bladder. J Urol 143:824–826, 1990.

200. Cox R, Dawson M: A curious prostatic tumor: Probably a true mixed tumor (cystadeno-leiomyofibroma). Br J Urol 32:306–311, 1960.

201. Manivel C, Shenoy V, Wick M, Dehner L: Cystosarcoma phyllodes of the prostate. Arch Pathol Lab Med 110:534–538, 1986.

202. Eble J, Tejada E: Prostatic stromal hyperplasia with bizarre nuclei. Arch Pathol Lab Med 115:87–89, 1991.

203. Gueft B, Walsh M: Malignant prostatic cystosarcoma phyllodes. NY State J Med 75:2226–2228, 1975.

204. McNeal J, Reese, J, Redwine E, et al: Cribriform adenocarcinoma of the prostate. Cancer 58:1714–1719, 1986.

205. Lopez-Beltran A, Gaeta J, Huben R, Croghan G: Malignant phyllodes tumor of prostate. J Urol 35(2):164–167, 1990.

206. Young J, Jensen P, Wiley C: Malignant phyllodes tumor of the prostate. A case report with immunohistochemical and ultrastructural studies. Arch Pathol Lab Med 116:296–299, 1992.

207. Maluf H, King M, DeLuca F, et al: Giant multilocular prostatic cystadenoma: A distinctive lesion of the retroperitoneum in men. A report of two cases. Am J Surg Pathol 15(2):131–135, 1991.

208. Quay A, Proppe K: Carcinosarcoma of the prostate: Case report and review of the literature. J Urol 125:436–438, 1981.

209. Wick M, Young R, Malvesta R, et al: Prostatic carcinosarcomas. Clinical, histologic, and immunohistochemical data on two cases, with a review of the literature. Am J Clin Pathol 92:131–139, 1989.

210. Nazeer T, Barada J, Fisher H, Ross J: Prostatic carcinosarcoma: Case report and review of literature. J Urol 146:1370–1373, 1991.

211. Scully R, Galdabini J, McNeely B: Case records of the Massachusetts General Hospital. N Engl J Med 296:439–444, 1977.

212. Pryor J, Cameron K, Chilton C, et al: Carcinoma in situ in testicular biopsies from men presenting with infertility. Br J Urol 55:780–784, 1983.

213. Skakkebaek N, Berthelsen JG, Müller J: Carcinoma-in-situ of the undescended testis. Urol Clin North Am 9:377–385, 1982.

214. Burke A, Mostofi F: Placental alkaline phosphatase immunohistochemistry of intratubular malignant germ cells and associated testicular germ cell tumors. Hum Pathol 19:663–670, 1988.

215. Reinberg Y, Manivel C, Fraley E: Carcinoma in situ of the testis. J Urol 142:243–247, 1989.

216. True L, Otis C, Delprado W, et al: Spermatocytic seminoma of testis with sarcomatous transformation. A report of fives cases. Am J Surg Pathol 12(2):75–82, 1988.

217. Floyd C, Ayala A, Logothetis C, Silva E: Spermatocytic seminoma with associated sarcoma of the testis. Cancer 1:409–414, 1988.

218. Matoska J, Talerman A: Spermatocytic seminoma associated with rhabdomyosarcoma. Am J Clin Pathol 94:89–95, 1990.

219. Talerman A: Spermatocytic seminoma. Clinicopathological study of 22 cases. Cancer 45:2169–2176, 1980.

220. Kuzmits R, Schernthaner G, Krisch K: Serum neuron-specific enolase. A marker for response to therapy in seminoma. Cancer 60:1017–1021, 1987.

221. Dekker I, Rozeboom T, Delemarre J, et al: Placental-like alkaline phosphatase and DNA flow cytometry in spermatocytic seminoma. Cancer 69:993–996, 1992.

222. Matoska J, Ondrus D, Hornak M: Metastatic spermatocytic seminoma. A case report with light microscopic, ultrastructural, and immunohistochemical findings. Cancer 62:1197–1201, 1988.

223. Young R, Finlayson N, Scully R: Tubular seminoma. Report of a case. Arch Pathol Lab Med 113:414–416, 1989.

224. Collins D, Symington T: Sertoli cell tumor. Br J Urol 36:52–61, 1964.

225. Stein A, Miller D: Tuberculous epididymo-orchitis: A case report. J Urol 129:613, 1983.

226. Emberton H, Ellis B, Duchesne G: Seminoma or sarcoid? Clin Oncol 4:56–57, 1992.

227. Gross A, Heinzer H, Loy V, Dieckman K: Unusual differential diagnosis of testis tumor: Intrascrotal sarcoidosis. J Urol 147:1112–1114, 1992.

228. Fauer R, Goldstein A, Green J, Onofrio R: Clinical aspects of granulomatous orchitis. Urology 12:416–419, 1978.

229. Sporer A, Seebode J: Granulomatous orchitis. Urology 19:319–321, 1982.

230. Nochomovitz L, DeLa Torre F, Rosai J: Pathology of germ cell tumors of the testis. Urol Clin North Am 4:359–378, 1977.

231. Wilkins B, Williamson J, O'Brien C: Morphological and immunohistological study of testicular lymphomas. Histopathology 15:147–156, 1989.

232. Logothetis C, Samuels M, Trindade A, et al: The prognostic significance of endodermal sinus tumor histology among patients treated for stage III nonseminomatous germ cell tumors of the testes. Cancer 53:122–128, 1984.

233. Nseyo U, Englander L, Wajsman Z, et al: Histological patterns of treatment failures in testicular neoplasms. J Urol 133:219–220, 1985.

234. Ulbright T, Roth L: Recent developments in the pathology of germ cell tumors. Semin Diagn Pathol 4:304–319, 1987.

235. Maier J, Sulak M, Mittemeyer B: Seminoma of the testis: Analysis of treatment success and failure. Am J Roentgenol 102(3):596–602, 1968.

236. Maier J, Mittemeyer B, Sulak M: Treatment and prognosis in seminoma of the testis. J Urol 99:72–78, 1968.

237. Mostofi S, Price E Jr: Tumors of the Male Genital System: Atlas of Tumor Pathology, 2nd Series, Fascicle 8. Washington DC, Armed Forces Institute of Pathology, 1973.

238. Kademian M, Bosch A, Caldwell W, Jaeschke W: Anaplastic seminoma. Cancer 40:3082–3086, 1977.

239. Bobba V, Mittal B, Hoover S, Kepka A: Classical and anaplastic seminoma: Difference in survival. Radiology 167:849–852, 1988.

240. Johnson D, Gomez J, Ayala A: Anaplastic seminoma. J Urol 114:80–82, 1975.

241. Mostofi SK: Histological Typing of Testis Tumors. Geneva, World Health Organization, 1976.

242. Manivel J, Niehans G, Wick M, Dehner L: Intermediate trophoblast in germ cell neoplasms. Am J Surg Pathol 11(9):693–701, 1987.

243. Niehans G, Mainvel C, Copland G, et al: Immunohistochemistry of germ cell and trophoblastic neoplasms. Cancer 62:1113–1123, 1988.

244. Kurman R, Scardino P, McIntire R, et al: Cellular localization of alpha-fetoprotein and human chorionic gonadotropin in germ cell tumors of the testis using an indirect immunoperoxidase technique. Cancer 40:2136–2151, 1977.

245. Kuber W, Kratzik C, Schwarz H, et al: Experience with beta-HCG-positive seminoma. Br J Urol 55:555–559, 1983.

246. Javadpour N: Human chorionic gonadotropin in seminoma. J Urol 131:407, 1984.

247. Ramon Y, Cajal S, Pinango L, et al: Metastatic pure choriocarcinoma of the testis in an elderly man. J Urol 137:516–519, 1987.

248. Kim J, Young R, Scully R: Leydig cell tumors of the testis. A clinicopathological analysis of 40 cases and review of the literature. Am J Surg Pathol 9:177–192, 1985.

249. Perez C, Novoa J, Alcaniz J, et al: Leydig cell tumor of the testis with gynaecomastia and elevated oestrogen, progesterone and prolactin levels: Case report. Clin Endocrinol 13:409–412, 1980.

250. Karpf D, Yamashita S, Melmed S, et al: In vitro secretion of deoxycorticosterone by a benign Leydig cell tumor of the testis. J Urol 136:114–116, 1986.

251. Grem J, Robins I, Wilson K, et al: Metastatic Leydig cell tumor of the testis. Report of three cases and review of the literature. Cancer 58:2116–2119, 1986.

252. Kaplan G, Cromie W, Kelalis P, et al: Gonadal stromal tumors: A report of the prepubertal testicular tumor registry. J Urol 136:300–302, 1986.

253. Trainer T: Histology of the normal testis. Am J Surg Pathol 11:797–809, 1987.

254. Kurman R, Andrade D, Goebelsmann U, Taylor C: An immunohistological study of steroid localization in Sertoli-Leydig tumors of the ovary and testis. Cancer 42:1772–1783, 1978.

255. Miettinen M, Wahlstrom T, Virtanen I, et al: Cellular differentiation in ovarian sex-cord-stromal and germ-cell tumors studied with antibodies to intermediate-filament proteins. Am J Surg Pathol 9:640–651, 1985.

256. Gabrilove J, Freiberg E, Leiter E, Nicolis G: Feminizing and non-feminizing Sertoli cell tumors. J Urol 124:757–767, 1980.

257. Perito P, Ciancio G, Civantos F, Politano V: Sertoli-Leydig cell testicular tumor: Case report and review of sex cord/gonadal stromal tumor histogenesis. J Urol 148:883–885, 1992.

258. Talerman A: Malignant Sertoli cell tumor of the testis. Cancer 28:446–455, 1971.

259. Godec C: Malignant Sertoli cell tumor of testicle. Urology 26:185–188, 1985.

260. Proppe K, Scully R: Large-cell calcifying Sertoli cell tumor of the testis. Am J Clin Pathol 74:607–619, 1980.

261. Carney J, Gordon H, Carpenter P, et al: The complex of myxomas, spotty pigmentation, and endocrine overactivity. Medicine 64:270–283, 1985.

262. Jenkins I: Extramammary Paget's disease of the penis. Br J Urol 63:103–104, 1989.

263. Begin L, Deschenes J, Mitmaker B: Pagetoid carcinomatous involvement of the penile urethra in association with high grade transitional cell carcinoma of the urinary bladder. Arch Pathol Lab Med 115:632–635, 1991.

264. Perez M, LaRossa D, Tomaszewski J: Paget's disease primarily involving the scrotum. Cancer 63:970–975, 1989.

265. Hartley E, Nambisan R, Rao U, Karakousis C: Extramammary Paget disease of the inguinoscrotal area. NY State J Med 88:546–548, 1988.

266. Tomaszevski J, Korat O, Livolsi V: Paget's disease of the urethral meatus following transitional cell carcinoma of the bladder. J Urol 135:368–370, 1986.

267. Powell F, Bjornsson J, Doyle J, Cooper A: Genital Paget's disease and urinary tract malignancy. J Am Acad Dermatol 13:84–90, 1985.

268. Ordonez N, Awalt H, Mackay B: Mammary and extramammary Paget's disease. An immunocytochemical and ultrastructural study. Cancer 59:1173–1183, 1987.

269. Shah K, Tabibzadeh S, Gerber M: Immunohistochemical distinction of Paget's disease from Bowen's disease and superficial spreading melanoma with the use of monoclonal cytokeratin antibodies. Am J Clin Pathol 88:689–695, 1987.

270. Reed W, Oppedal B, Larsen T: Immunohistology is valuable in distinguishing between Paget's disease, Bowen's disease and superficial spreading malignant melanoma. Histopathology 16:583–588, 1990.

271. Guarner J, Cohen C, DeRose P: Histogenesis of extramammary and mammary Paget cells. An immunohistochemical study. Am J Dermatopathol 11:313–318, 1989.

272. Schultz R, Miller J, MacDonald G, et al: Clinical and molecular evaluation of acetowhite genital lesions in men. J Urol 143:920–923, 1990.

CHAPTER 11

Adrenal Gland: Tumors and Tumor-Like Lesions

L. Jeffrey Medeiros, M.D., and Lawrence M. Weiss, M.D.

INCIDENTAL ADRENAL CORTICAL NODULES

Cortical nodules without clinical evidence of hyperfunction are commonly detected in the adrenal glands. For example, at autopsy the incidence of cortical nodules in patients without clinical evidence of hyperfunction varies from 1.5% to 37%, dependent on whether the study is retrospective or the nodules are searched for prospectively.[1–3] Some investigators have identified cortical nodules more commonly in patients with systemic hypertension or diabetes mellitus.[2, 4] Dobbie[4] has shown that adrenal capsular blood vessels more often exhibit intimal proliferation and luminal narrowing in patients with cortical nodules. He suggested that local ischemia secondary to vascular disease leads to localized atrophy, followed by regeneration and hyperplasia. However, others[3] have not correlated cortical nodules with hypertension or diabetes mellitus.

With the use of sensitive radiologic imaging studies such as computed tomography, magnetic resonance imaging, and scintigraphy, cortical nodules are being detected more frequently *in vivo*. For example, the incidence of an unsuspected adrenal mass without clinical evidence of hyperfunction is approximately 0.6% to 1.3% in various studies,[5, 6] with a subset of these cases being incidental cortical nodules.

Pathologic Features

Grossly, incidental adrenal cortical nodules are usually defined as smaller than 1 cm. The nodules arise in the cortex but may protrude into the medulla or into the surrounding adipose tissue. These nodules also may be found outside the boundaries of the adrenal gland, either attached to the capsule or free within the adipose tissue.[4, 7] Incidental cortical nodules are often bilateral and may be multiple. Histologically, the nodules are well circumscribed but not encapsulated and are composed of cytologically normal cells of the zona fasciculata.

A subset of incidental adrenal cortical nodules may be pigmented. In an autopsy series of 100 consecutive patients, Robinson et al.[3] identified small pigmented nodules in 37 patients. In this study, the authors considered nodules with any degree of brown or black color visible to the naked eye to be pigmented.[3] Like other cortical nodules, pigmented nodules are small, well-circumscribed but not encapsulated, and corticomedullary.

Histologically, pigmented nodules are composed of zona reticularis cells with abundant lipofuscin. The cells in these nodules are usually cytologically normal; nuclei may contain prominent nucleoli or exhibit mild nuclear atypia.[3]

Differential Diagnosis

INCIDENTAL ADRENAL CORTICAL NODULE VERSUS ADENOMA. Incidental cortical nodules are small, usually defined as less than 1.0 cm, and are found in patients without clinical evidence of hyperfunction.[3, 4, 7] The non-nodular adrenal cortex is normal. By contrast, adrenal cortical adenomas are larger, up to 5 cm in diameter. Adenomas are commonly functional, with suppression of the uninvolved cortex leading to atrophy.

INCIDENTAL ADRENAL CORTICAL NODULE VERSUS NODULAR HYPERPLASIA. In the majority of cases, this distinction is not difficult. Patients with nodular cortical hyperplasia have symptoms of Cushing's syndrome and have multiple, often large, cortical nodules in both adrenal glands.[8, 9] Patients with incidental cortical nodules are without symptoms and usually have a single, relatively small cortical nodule.[4] A problem in differential diagnosis may occur in cases of nodular hyperplasia in which there is one dominant nodule. Again, the nodule in hyperplasia is likely to be larger, and close inspection of the remaining adrenal(s) reveals smaller nodules. Also, the non-nodular cortex is hyperplastic in nodular hyperplasia but normal in patients with an incidental cortical nodule.[4, 10, 11]

ADRENAL CORTICAL ADENOMA

Adrenal cortical adenomas are benign neoplasms of the adrenal cortex. Adults with adenomas may present with symptoms and signs of endocrine dysfunction, usually Cushing's syndrome.[12] Less frequently, adenomas cause primary hyperaldosteronism and, rarely, virilization. Adults with adenomas also may be asymptomatic.

In contrast, almost all children with adenomas present with mixed endocrine syndromes—most often virilization plus Cushing's syndrome.[13] In children, approximately half of all adenomas occur before the age of 3 years, 82% in children younger than 7 years old.[13]

Pathologic Features

Grossly, adenomas are typically solitary, encapsulated and relatively small. Adenomas are rarely larger than 50 g or 5 cm in diameter.[12, 14-16] The size and color of adenomas correlate somewhat with their hormone production. Adenomas found in patients with primary hyperaldosteronism are usually small, often no larger than 2 cm in diameter, and tan or pale yellow.[10] Glucocorticoid-secreting neoplasms are larger, with a bright yellow or orange cut surface secondary to the presence of abundant lipid. Functional adenomas suppress the uninvolved cortex, resulting in atrophy.

Histologically, mineralocorticoid-secreting tumors are composed of cells that may resemble zona glomerulosa cells, but may also resemble cells of the zona fasciculata or cells with hybrid features of both cell types. Cytoplasmic lipid is usually present; glycogen is absent. Nuclear atypia is infrequent, and mitotic figures are rare. Necrosis is usually absent. Mast cells commonly infiltrate these tumors and represent one histologic clue that an adenoma may be secreting mineralocorticoids.[17]

In patients treated with spironolactone, spironolactone bodies may be found in the neoplastic cells (Fig. 11–1) These bodies are eosinophilic globules, 2 to 15 μ, located in the tumor cell cytoplasm.[18, 19] Electron microscopic studies have shown these bodies to be composed of lamellar whorls of membranes thought to be derived from smooth endoplasmic reticulum.[18, 19]

Glucocorticoid-secreting adenomas are composed of lipid-rich cortical cells that usually resemble those of the zona

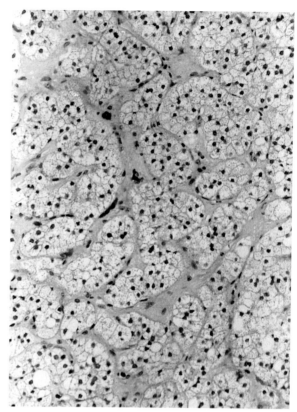

FIGURE 11–2. Adrenal cortical adenoma associated with Cushing's syndrome. A nesting pattern of zona fasciculata–type cells is seen.

fasciculata or zona reticularis, or a mixture of these cell types (Fig. 11–2). Cytoplasmic glycogen is usually absent. Although these tumors may have nuclear atypia (Fig. 11–3), including nucleomegaly and hyperchromasia, mitotic figures are extremely rare or absent.[15, 16] Mast cells are rare in these tumors.[17] Necrosis is usually absent and, if present, only focal. Foci of myelolipomatous change or lymphocytic aggregates may be found. Rarely, a well-developed myelolipoma may coexist within an adenoma.[20]

In some cases, adenomas may contain focal hemorrhage. Extensive hemorrhage is unusual in benign cortical tumors. However, one adrenal adenoma has been reported with extensive hemorrhage, thrombosis, and organization, with some resemblance to a vascular neoplasm.[21]

Black adenomas are cortical adenomas in which the neoplastic cells have abundant cytoplasmic brown pigment.[22] Otherwise, these tumors are similar to typical cortical adenomas both clinically and histologically. Most investigators have concluded that the pigment is most consistent with lipofuscin, although Damron et al.[23] have suggested that it may be neuromelanin. Occasional black adenomas are clinically functional, causing primary hyperaldosteronism or Cushing's syndrome. However, most black adenomas are asymptomatic. Nonfunctional black adenomas may not be true neoplasms, but instead represent extremely large pigmented cortical nodules.[3]

In a recent study, Sasano et al.[24] described three adrenal cortical tumors that they designated as oncocytoma. These neoplasms, all of which followed a benign clinical course, were grossly similar to other adenomas. Histologically, these tumors were composed of lipid-depleted cells with intensely eosinophilic, granular cytoplasm (Fig. 11–4). The tumor cell

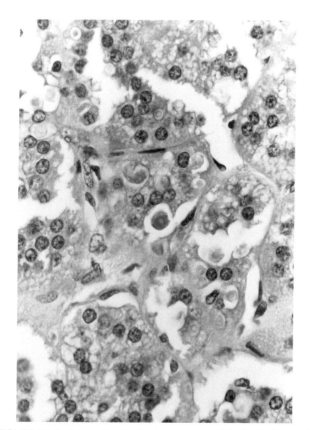

FIGURE 11–1. Adrenal cortical adenoma associated with hyperaldosteronism (Conn's syndrome). Note numerous laminated spironolactone bodies.

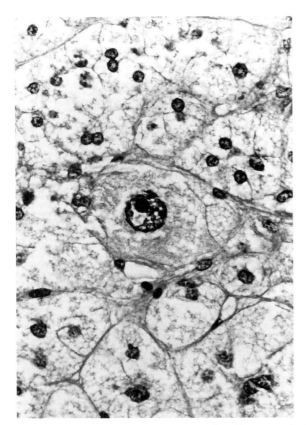

FIGURE 11–3. Adrenal cortical adenoma. Significant cytologic atypia may be seen in otherwise unremarkable tumors.

nuclei were vesicular, some of which were enlarged with prominent nucleoli or hyperchromasia. Mitotic figures were rare or absent. Thus, these tumors resembled oncocytomas as are described at other sites such as the kidney.[25] Immunohisto-chemical studies for steroidogenic enzymes were negative, indicating that the neoplastic cells were non-functional.[24] Electron microscopic analysis of one case revealed abundant mito-chondria as would be expected in oncocytoma.[25]

Immunohistochemical findings in adrenal cortical adeno-mas and adrenal cortical carcinomas are closely related, and are discussed later (see Adrenal Cortical Carcinoma).

Electron microscopic studies of adenomas have revealed findings similar to normal adrenal cortex, although both rough and smooth endoplasmic reticulum and cytoplasmic lipid may be abundant secondary to increased secretory activity.[26] The endoplasmic reticulum may be arranged in parallel arrays, referred to as lamellar or stack-like. Cell junctions, but not desmosomes, are found. Adenoma cells also have distinctive mitochondrial changes that correlate with the secretory activ-ity of the neoplastic cells. In mineralocorticoid-secreting tumors, the mitochondria are relatively small, round or slightly elongated, with sacotubular cristae. By contrast, in glucocorti-coid-secreting tumors, the mitochondria are large, spherical, and contain tubular or vesicular cristae.[27] Some adenomas may have clinical and electron microscopic evidence of both mineralocorticoid and glucocorticoid secretion.[28, 29]

Differential Diagnosis

ADRENAL BLACK ADENOMA VERSUS MALIGNANT MELA-NOMA. Grossly, the dark brown or black color of a cortical

adenoma may raise the possibility of malignant melanoma. Adenomas also may exhibit nuclear atypia, increasing the possibility of confusion. However, black adenomas are gener-ally smaller, lack necrosis and hemorrhage, and do not exhibit the degree of nuclear atypia identified in malignant melanoma. Mitotic figures and atypical mitotic figures, numerous in mela-noma, are absent or very rare in adenoma. Further study of the pigment, either using special stains or electron microscopy, shows that the pigment in the adenoma is lipofuscin, not melanin. Electron microscopy proves the presence of premela-nosomes or melanosomes only in melanoma. Furthermore, although primary malignant melanoma of the adrenal gland has been reported rarely in the literature,[29] in the overwhelm-ing majority of cases malignant melanoma in the adrenal gland is metastatic and the clinical setting of widely disseminated cancer is known.

HEMORRHAGIC ADRENAL ADENOMA WITH ORGANIZATION VERSUS MALIGNANT VASCULAR NEOPLASM. Granger et al.[21] recently described a 20 × 20 × 15 cm cortical adenoma that was composed predominantly of hemorrhage and thrombus with a thin rim of surrounding adenomatous tissue. There was extensive organization with ingrowth of blood vessels into the mass and large areas of fibrin that were surrounded by active, spindle-shaped cells with hyperchromatic nuclei and prominent nucleoli. Mitotic figures were common, up to 5/10 HPF. These histologic findings were reminiscent of a malignant vascular neoplasm. However, the atypical cells were negative for endothelial markers and positive for vimen-tin, and the patient had a benign postoperative course for 16 months.

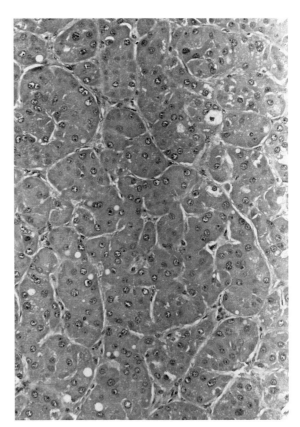

FIGURE 11–4. Adrenal cortical neoplasm with features of oncocy-toma. The cells contain uniform granular, eosinophilic cytoplasm.

ADRENAL CORTICAL CARCINOMA

Adrenal cortical carcinomas are rare; less than 0.05% of all malignant neoplasms arise in the adrenal gland cortex.[30] Similar to adenomas, carcinomas may be the cause of Cushing's syndrome, virilization, or, rarely, hyperaldosteronism.[31] However, unlike adenomas, carcinomas are more often nonfunctional.[32-34]

Adrenal cortical carcinomas in adults are highly malignant neoplasms for which the best current therapy is complete surgical excision. The survival of patients with adrenal cortical carcinoma is poor. The mean or median survival time of patients reported has ranged from 4 to 30 months.[32, 35, 36] These tumors may recur locally or metastasize, most frequently to the liver, regional lymph nodes, lungs, and bones.[32, 37, 38]

Adrenal cortical carcinomas in children are exceptionally rare.[13] The vast majority of childhood carcinomas, unlike those in adults, cause clinical evidence of endocrine hyperactivity; usually mixed virilization and Cushing's syndrome.[13, 34]

Pathologic Features

Grossly, adrenal cortical carcinomas are most often large neoplasms, usually greater than 5 cm and 100 g.[14-16] Very large neoplasms, more than 1000 g are not uncommon.[12, 15, 33] However, small carcinomas do also occur. For example, Gandour and Grizzle[39] reported a 40-g adrenal cortical carcinoma that metastasized.

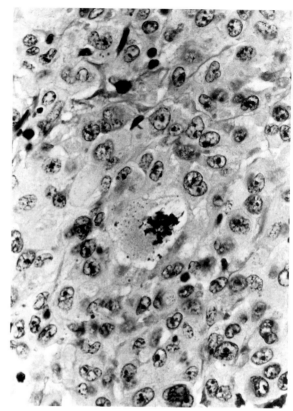

FIGURE 11–6. Adrenal cortical carcinoma. An atypical mitotic figure is seen.

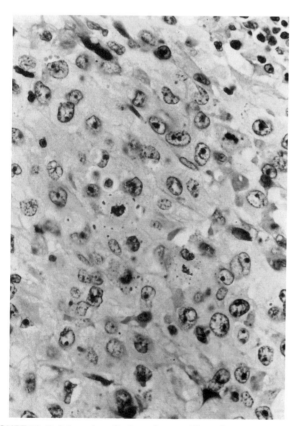

FIGURE 11–5. Adrenal cortical carcinoma. The cells possess highly atypical nuclei and show a high mitotic rate.

Histologically, adrenocortical carcinomas are composed of cells with either eosinophilic or finely reticulated cytoplasm that often exhibit various combinations of the following features: mitotic figures, atypical mitoses, nuclear atypia, capsular or vascular invasion, and necrosis[15, 16, 40, 41] (Figs. 11–5 to 11–9). Rarely, these tumors may be spindled or contain abundant myxoid material[42] (Fig. 11–10). Other pathologic features are discussed in greater detail later, as part of the discussion of the differential diagnosis of adenoma and carcinoma.

Routine histochemical stains are not particularly helpful in the analysis of adrenal cortical carcinoma. The periodic acid-Schiff (PAS) reaction is usually negative, as glycogen is not present. The Grimelius stain does not demonstrate cytoplasmic argyrophilia.[34] Mucin is usually absent, although rare cases have been described with focal cytoplasmic mucin.

Immunohistochemical studies of adrenal cortical neoplasms are more useful. The results of these studies are discussed in two parts: those derived using frozen sections and those obtained using fixed, paraffin-embedded sections.

FROZEN TISSUE. In frozen sections, keratins in low density are commonly detected in adrenal cortical cells and in adrenal cortical neoplasms. The keratins present are those found in relatively simple (non-stratified) epithelia, such as keratins 8 and 18.[43] Furthermore, Gaffey et al.[44] demonstrated keratins in normal adrenal cortex, adenomas, and carcinomas using Western blotting.

Miettinen[43] also has reported that a subset of adrenal cortical carcinomas contains low-density neurofilaments, synaptophysin, and neuron-specific enolase. Chromogranin and three neu-

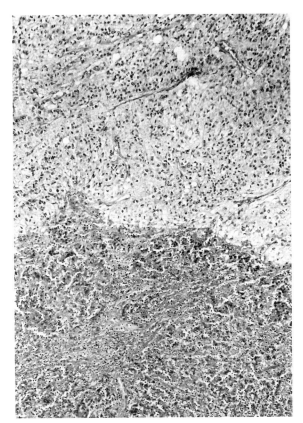

FIGURE 11–7. Adrenal cortical carcinoma. A focus of tumor necrosis is seen at bottom.

and the majority of carcinomas.[49, 51] The c-*myc* protein has been reported to be nuclear in adenomas but nuclear and cytoplasmic in carcinomas.[49]

The monoclonal antibody D11 has been proposed as a marker specific for adrenal cortical cells using fixed, paraffin-embedded sections.[52] Schroder et al.[52, 53] studied 190 neoplasms, including 100 adrenal tumors, and reported nuclear and cytoplasmic staining in normal adrenal cortex, in adenomas secreting either aldosterone or cortisol, and in adrenocortical carcinomas. Normal adrenal medulla and pheochromocytomas were negative. A smaller number of tumors metastatic to the adrenal as well as the majority of primary renal cell and thyroid carcinomas were negative for D11. However, the D11 antibody also reacts with hepatocellular and lung carcinomas.[53]

Electron microscopic examination of adrenal cortical carcinomas, as described previously for adenomas, reveals abundant rough and smooth endoplasmic reticulum that may be present in parallel arrays and numerous mitochondria with unusually shaped cristae (shelf-like, tubular, or tubulovesicular).[26, 54] Intercellular junctions, but not desmosomes, are present. Cytoplasmic lipid is more variable in carcinomas than in adenomas. Lysosomes may be found that may resemble membrane-bound neurosecretory granules.[54] In addition, Miettinen identified true membrane-bound dense core granules in five cases of adrenocortical carcinoma.[43]

Our understanding of the molecular genetic findings in adrenocortical neoplasms is limited. For many years, a genetic component was suspected in the pathogenesis of adrenal cortical tumors. This suspicion was based on the high incidence

ropeptides (calcitonin, gastrin, and somatostatin) were absent.[43]

PARAFFIN-EMBEDDED TISSUE. Most studies using fixed, paraffin-embedded sections have focused on the utility of immunohistochemical results in distinguishing adrenal cortical neoplasms from other morphologically similar tumors.[44–46] Non-neoplastic adrenal cortical cells generally express keratins, whereas carcinomas are negative.[44–46] A subset of adenomas express keratins. The incidence of keratin positivity is greater if either enzyme predigestion is used or monoclonal antibodies reactive with keratins derived from simple epithelium are employed (e.g., CAM 5.2, an antibody that is reactive with keratin 18).[44]

Vimentin expression in benign and malignant adrenal cortical cells appears to have an inverse relationship with keratin expression.[44, 46–49] In non-neoplastic cortex, vimentin is usually not detected. By contrast, a subset of adenomas and the majority of adrenal cortical carcinomas intensely express vimentin.[43, 44, 46–48]

Other antibodies less frequently have been used to study adrenal cortical tumors. Epithelial membrane antigen, carcinoembryonic antigen, alpha-fetoprotein, anti-HMFG-2, and various blood group antigens are generally not expressed by normal or neoplastic adrenal cortical cells.[44, 45] Lectins and beta-2-microglobulin are expressed rarely by adrenal cortical carcinomas.[45, 50] Reports of S-100 staining have been inconsistent: either negative or positive in adrenal cortical tumors.[45, 46] In our experience, S-100 is usually negative in both adenomas and carcinomas. Antibodies specific for epidermal growth factor receptors stain approximately half of adenomas

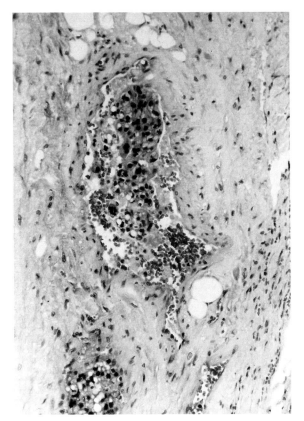

FIGURE 11–8. Adrenal cortical carcinoma. Venous invasion is seen. Note the fibromuscular wall.

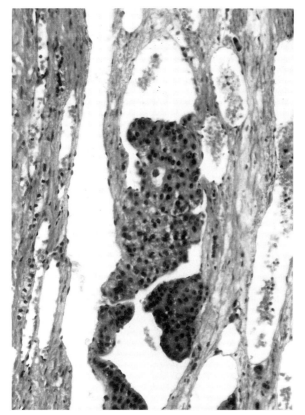

FIGURE 11–9. Adrenal cortical carcinoma. Sinusoidal invasion is seen. The vascular channel lacks a fibromuscular wall.

of adrenocortical neoplasms in the Beckwith-Wiedemann and the Li-Fraumeni (SBLA) syndromes.[55, 56]

More recently, both conventional cytogenetics and Southern blot hybridization techniques have yielded evidence of one or more tumor suppressor genes being involved in the pathogenesis of carcinomas.[57–59] Tumor suppressor genes, inherited in an autosomal recessive fashion, code for proteins that play a role in inhibiting the development of neoplasia.

The inactivation and/or deletion of both alleles of a tumor suppressor gene removes this inhibitory influence, and malignant neoplasms are able to develop. One proposed, but poorly characterized, tumor suppressor gene is located on chromosome 11p15.5. This gene also may be involved in the pathogenesis of other tumors such as Wilms' tumor, hepatoblastoma, and rhabdomyosarcoma.[60] Other tumor suppressor genes also may be involved, located on chromosomes 13q and 17p.[59] In this regard, neoplasia of the adrenal cortex may be a multistep process involving multiple genetic alterations, as has been shown to be the case in other systems such as the pathogenesis of colorectal carcinomas.[61]

Prognostic Indicators of Adrenal Cortical Carcinoma

Certain pathologic features have been shown to have significance in predicting the prognosis of patients with carcinoma. Of these, stage and mitotic rate are most important.

STAGE. A staging system for adrenal cortical carcinoma originally was developed by Macfarlane[62] and has been modified by others.[63, 64] The staging system elaborated by Henley et al.[64] is shown (Table 11–1).

Patients with stage I or II tumors have the best chance of cure with complete surgical excision.[32, 36, 38, 63, 65–67] In fact, in some studies, the stage I or II tumors delineated earlier are grouped together as one stage. As would be expected, patients with distant metastases at the time of diagnosis have the shortest survival time, and resection of the primary tumor has little effect on survival.[64, 65, 68]

MITOTIC ACTIVITY. Although the value of mitotic figures in distinguishing benign from malignant adrenocortical tumors has been stressed by many investigators,[15, 40, 41] few studies have addressed the prognostic significance of the mitotic rate in malignant tumors. In our own study of 42 adrenal cortical carcinomas,[69] we correlated various histologic parameters useful in making the diagnosis of carcinoma with disease-free survival. From this analysis, mitotic rate emerged as a strong predictor of the clinical virulence of adrenal cortical carcino-

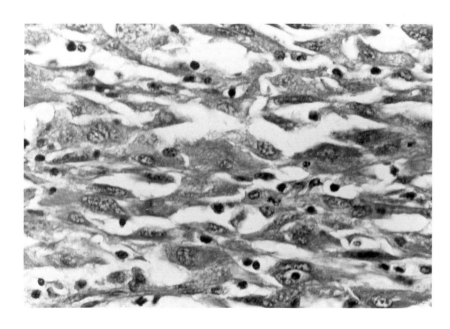

FIGURE 11–10. Adrenal cortical carcinoma. This case shows spindling of the neoplastic cells.

Table 11–1. **Staging System for Adrenal Cortical Carcinoma**

	Staging Criteria
T1	Tumor ≤5 cm, localized
T2	Tumor >5 cm, localized
T3	Tumor any size, locally invading to but not involving adjacent organs
T4	Tumor any size, locally invading into adjacent organs
N0	No positive regional lymph nodes
N1	Positive regional lymph nodes
M0	No distant metastases
M1	Distant metastases

Stage

I	T1 N0 M0
II	T2 N0 M0
III	T1 or T2 N1 M0 or T3 N0 M0
IV	Any T and N with M1, T3 N1, or T4

Table 11–2. **Histopathologic Criteria Proposed by Weiss for Distinguishing Benign from Malignant Adrenocortical Neoplasms***

1. High nuclear grade (criteria of Fuhrman)
2. Mitotic rate greater than 5/50 HPF
3. Atypical mitotic figures
4. Eosinophilic tumor cell cytoplasm (≥75% of tumor cells)
5. Diffuse architecture (≥33% of tumor)
6. Necrosis
7. Venous invasion (smooth muscle in wall)
8. Sinusoidal invasion (no smooth muscle in wall)
9. Capsular invasion

* The presence of three or more criteria highly correlates with subsequent malignant behavior.

mas.[69] Patients with carcinomas with a high mitotic rate had significantly shorter disease-free survival periods than did patients whose carcinomas had a low mitotic rate. In fact, there was a statistically significant negative correlation ($r = -0.666$; $p < .01$) between the number of mitotic figures and disease-free survival. In our study, a critical value of 20 mitoses per 10 HPF divided our 42 cases into two equal groups. Those patients whose tumors had more than 20 mitoses per 10 HPF had a median disease-free survival of 14 months. In contrast, those individuals with carcinomas with 20 or fewer mitoses per 10 HPF had a median disease-free survival of 58 months. Based on these findings, we have suggested that carcinomas may best be divided into two groups, low and high grade, perhaps directing the more toxic medical therapies toward the high-grade group.[69] Van Slooten et al.[41] also have suggested that mitotic rate correlates with the aggressiveness of adrenal cortical carcinoma.

Recently, both the Ki-67 (MIB-1) and proliferating cell nuclear antigen (PC10) antibodies have been used in adrenocortical neoplasms to assess cell proliferation.[49, 70] Both antibodies yielded results that correlated with each other as well as the mitotic rate.[70] Thus, these antibodies appear to be useful in assessing the proliferative rate and prognosis of adrenocortical neoplasms.

Differential Diagnosis

ADRENAL ADENOMA VERSUS CARCINOMA IN ADULTS. The size of an adrenocortical neoplasm is extremely helpful in predicting its subsequent behavior. Large masses are most often malignant, whereas small tumors are usually benign.[15, 40, 41] Nevertheless, the diagnostic value of tumor size can be overemphasized.[14] Only during the past decade have histologic criteria been assessed rigorously in large series of adrenocortical tumors with extensive clinical follow-up and shown to be useful in predicting clinical behavior. Most authors now concur that tumor size, *per se,* should not be used to establish a benign or malignant diagnosis. Very large adrenocortical tumors without metastases[12, 40] and small neoplasms with metastases[15, 36, 37, 39] have been reported. In these instances, application of histopathologic criteria, in contrast with tumor size, more correctly predicted subsequent clinical behavior.

Three separate sets of histologic criteria have been published that reliably distinguish benign from malignant adrenocortical tumors. We focus here primarily on the system proposed previously by Weiss[15] and subsequently modified by us in 1989.[69] Other systems have been proposed by Van Slooten et al.[41] and by Hough et al.[40]

Weiss studied 43 cases of adrenocortical tumors, with a minimum of 5 years clinical follow-up. In this system[15] (Table 11–2), nine histologic findings were found to be associated with adrenal cortical neoplasms that metastasized or recurred locally (i.e., were clinically malignant). In addition, three of these nine histologic findings were found only in malignant tumors: a mitotic rate greater than 5/50 HPF, atypical mitotic figures, and venous invasion.

Using this system, all 24 benign adrenocortical neoplasms studied had two or less of these nine histologic criteria of malignancy. In contrast, 18 of 19 malignant tumors had four or more histologic criteria of malignancy.[15] Subsequently, we slightly modified the system and proposed that the presence of three or more of these histologic findings predicts malignant clinical behavior.[69]

A second system for distinguishing benign from malignant adrenocortical tumors was developed by Van Slooten et al.[41] who analyzed 45 patients with adrenocortical tumors and 10-year clinical follow-up. They proposed a system of seven histologic criteria that are useful for distinguishing benign from malignant neoplasms (Table 11–3).

For an individual neoplasm, the numeric values for each histologic parameter present were combined, yielding a histologic index. In their study, the critical value for the histologic index was 8. Those patients with a histologic index less than

Table 11–3. **System of Van Slooten et al. for Distinguishing Benign from Malignant Adrenocortical Neoplasms***

Histologic Criteria	Numeric Value
1. Extensive regressive changes (necrosis, hemorrhage, fibrosis, calcification)	5.7
2. Loss of normal structure	1.6
3. Nuclear atypia (moderate/marked)	2.1
4. Nuclear hyperchromasia (moderate/marked)	2.6
5. Abnormal nucleoli	4.1
6. Mitotic activity (2/10 HPF)	9.0
7. Vascular or capsular invasion	3.3

* Histologic index >8 correlates with subsequent malignant behavior.

8 more often had smaller neoplasms and remained free of metastases during the 10-year clinical follow-up period. However, using the histologic index did not discriminate completely between the benign and malignant tumors, as demonstrated by the fact that some patients with neoplasms with a high histologic index remained well after surgical extirpation.[41]

Hough et al.[40] have proposed a third system based on their study of 41 patients with adrenocortical tumors who were followed for a minimum of 5 years. They proposed 12 criteria, seven histologic and five non-histologic, that are useful in distinguishing benign from malignant adrenocortical neoplasms[40] (Table 11–4). The numeric values for each criterion were determined using a modification of Bayes' theorem for predicting the likelihood of the presence of metastases in association with each histologic or non-histologic finding. In practice, for an individual case, the numeric indices are combined, yielding two numbers: the histologic index of malignancy and the non-histologic index of malignancy. Regarding the histologic index of malignancy, Hough et al.[40] provided the mean values for the malignant (2.91), indeterminate (1.00), and benign (0.17) tumors in their study. Combining the histologic and non-histologic indices of malignancy provided better separation of benign from malignant adrenocortical tumors than did using either index by itself.

In our experience, all three systems are useful for predicting the subsequent behavior of adrenocortical neoplasms. In fact, as has been discussed by Page et al.,[71] all have excellent predictive value as compared with a malignant diagnosis in other organs (e.g., the breast). Nevertheless, each system has unique aspects, and in some cases, one system may predict a benign or indeterminate clinical course, whereas another system may suggest malignant behavior. In addition, histologic findings common to each system are defined differently or vaguely in these systems, further increasing the chance of disparity among the methods.

Of the three systems described here, we prefer to use the

Weiss system.[15, 69] In large part, our preference is attributed to personal bias. However, we also think that there are objective reasons for favoring this system.

First, the Weiss system is based solely on histologic findings (as is the Van Slooten system). In contrast, the system proposed by Hough et al. is based on clinical and pathologic data. Although we concur with Page et al.[71] that clinical data usually are readily available and are helpful in establishing the diagnosis, in some cases reported in the literature and in our own experience, clinical data were either unavailable or incomplete.

Second, we are not convinced that assigning numeric values to histologic criteria, as is done in the Hough and Van Slooten systems, is more helpful than simply counting the number of histologic findings present, as is done in the Weiss system. Nor do the numeric values make either method easier to use. In the Weiss system, the presence of at least three and usually four or more criteria indicates that the neoplasm is likely to locally recur or metastasize.[69]

Third, the mitotic index may be the single most helpful histologic feature in making the distinction between benign and malignant adrenocortical neoplasms. Accordingly, we prefer the Weiss system[15, 69] because it rigorously assesses the presence and number of mitotic figures. Analogous to the method of mitosis counting used in the evaluation of uterine smooth muscle tumors, in the Weiss system 10 HPF are carefully studied for mitotic figures in each of the five areas that have the highest mitotic rate. In contrast, in the Van Slooten method[41] the mitotic rate is based on 10 HPF, but the total number of fields counted is not specified; and in the approach advocated by Hough et al., 100 HPF are analyzed, but the fields chosen for counting appear to be selected randomly.[40]

Fourth, we suggest that some of the criteria of the Van Slooten system could be subdivided or collated to improve diagnostic accuracy. For example, four histologic findings are combined into one criterion labeled ''regressive changes'': hemorrhage, fibrosis, calcification, and necrosis. Of these four findings, in our experience only extensive tumor necrosis is indicative of malignant behavior; we have commonly observed hemorrhage, fibrosis, and calcification in both benign and malignant tumors. Also, in the Van Slooten system, nuclear atypia, nuclear hyperchromasia, and nucleolar structure are individual criteria that might be incorporated better into one criterion, the equivalent of nuclear grade (Weiss system) or pleomorphism (Hough method).

One potential drawback to the Weiss system may be the application of nuclear grade, which is based on the most high grade areas of the neoplasm. For example, a tumor with a small focus of grade IV nuclear atypia, even if the majority of the tumor is grade I, would be classified as grade IV. Although we have not performed a systematic study, our recent experience has led us to wonder whether nuclear grade as applied by Hough et al.[40] is more predictive. As we understand their system, tumor grade is based on the cytologic features of the majority of the neoplasm and not the worst area.[40] It may be true that a combination of the systems developed by us,[15, 69] Van Slooten et al.,[41] and Hough et al.[40] may be better than only one method. For example, although we use the Weiss system, we still incorporate pertinent clinical data, if available, and gross pathologic findings in reaching our final diagnosis.

Table 11–4. **System of Hough et al. for Distinguishing Benign from Malignant Adrenocortical Neoplasms***

Criteria	Numeric Value
Histologic Criteria	
1. Diffuse growth pattern	0.92
2. Vascular invasion	0.92
3. Tumor cell necrosis	0.69
4. Broad fibrous bands	1.00
5. Capsular invasion	0.37
6. Mitotic index (1/10 HPF)	0.60
7. Pleomorphism (moderate/marked)	0.39
Non-histologic Criteria	
1. Tumor mass ($\geq$100 g)	0.60
2. Urinary 17-ketosteroids (10 mg/g creatinine/24 hours)	0.50
3. Response to ACTH (17-hydroxysteroids increased two times after 50 μg ACTH IV)	0.42
4. Cushing's syndrome with virilism, virilism alone, or no clinical manifestations	0.42
5. Weight loss (10 lb/3 months)	2.00

ACTH, adrenocorticotropic hormone; IV, intravenous.

* In this system both histologic and non-histologic indices are derived. The mean histologic index of malignant tumors was 2.91, indeterminate tumors 1.00, and benign tumors 0.17.

ADRENAL ADENOMA VERSUS CARCINOMA IN CHILDREN. The distinction between adenoma and carcinoma in infants and children is currently more controversial than it is in adults. Cagle et al.[72] studied 23 adrenal cortical neoplasms in children younger than 16 years of age, 17 benign and six malignant. In their study, malignant tumors were "defined clinically as those producing metastases and/or resulting in death from direct effects of the tumor."[72] Using this definition, necrosis, nuclear pleomorphism, mitotic figures, atypical mitotic figures, and either capsular and/or vascular invasion were common in pediatric tumors originally diagnosed as either adenoma or carcinoma but with subsequent benign clinical follow-up. Cagle et al.[72] emphasized the utility of tumor size in predicting subsequent clinical behavior: tumors less than 100 to 150 g rarely metastasize, tumors from 150 to 500 g are indeterminate, and tumors more than 500 g are usually malignant. Furthermore, malignant tumors in childhood more frequently were associated with virilization or feminization than were benign tumors; the latter more often caused Cushing's syndrome.[72]

As is the case in adults, we completely agree that tumor size is very useful in predicting subsequent clinical behavior. However, the approach by Cagle et al.[72] does not address the possibility that a localized adrenal cortical carcinoma may be cured by complete excision. This possibility is certainly the case in other organs, such as the breast and colon, where the predictive value of the diagnosis of carcinoma is approximately 50%.[71] The high frequency of symptoms and physical signs of endocrine hyperfunction in children[13, 72] with adrenocortical neoplasms and the relative ease (as compared with adults) of palpating an abdominal mass in the pediatric population may increase the likelihood that these tumors are detected early, when the tumor is smaller, localized, and more readily completely excised.[73] Furthermore, as has been suggested by others,[74] young children with malignant adrenocortical tumors may have a more benign clinical course than that of adults, as is the case with other tumors (such as malignant lymphomas) that affect both children and adults.

Thus, we believe that tumor size and the same histologic criteria that are used to evaluate adult tumors are the best means of distinguishing adenomas from carcinomas in children. Others also agree with this view.[75, 76] For example, in a study of childhood adrenocortical tumors clustered in Brazil, Bugg et al.[76] also reported that histologic findings were useful in predicting the behavior of adrenal cortical neoplasms in children.

DNA content analysis also has been proposed as an additional means useful for distinguishing benign from malignant adrenal cortical tumors in both adults and children. For example, combining the results of five studies, the majority of adenomas had diploid DNA content, whereas most carcinomas contained aneuploid stem cell lines.[49, 77–80] However, more recent studies have shown that aneuploid DNA content is not uncommon in adenomas; also, a small subset of carcinomas may be diploid.[81, 82] For example, Cibas et al.[81] studied 43 adrenal cortical neoplasms: 30 adenomas and 13 carcinomas. Six of 30 (20%) adenomas had aneuploid DNA content, whereas 4 of 13 (31%) malignant neoplasms had diploid DNA content. With prolonged clinical follow-up (median, 59 months), the patients with aneuploid adenomas had a benign course.[81] Thus, although there is a correlation between aneuploid DNA content and a malignant histologic diagnosis, for an individual case, aneuploid DNA content does not predict the histologic diagnosis or the subsequent clinical behavior of adrenal cortical tumors.

ADRENAL CORTICAL NEOPLASM VERSUS PHEOCHROMOCYTOMA. See later discussion of differential diagnosis of pheochromocytoma.

ADRENAL CORTICAL CARCINOMA VERSUS METASTATIC NEOPLASMS. Malignant neoplasms metastasize frequently to the adrenal glands; the most common tumors are those of breast, lung, and gastrointestinal (GI) tract origin and malignant melanoma.[83] These lesions are usually first documented histologically at autopsy.[83, 84] However, occasionally one (less commonly both) adrenal gland involved by metastatic neoplasm may be initially diagnosed as a surgical specimen.[84] Extensive metastases to the adrenal glands may cause insufficiency.[83]

Histologically, metastatic tumors have features corresponding to their sites of origin. Only rarely do metastatic breast, lung, or GI tract carcinomas or malignant melanomas sufficiently resemble a primary adrenal gland tumor to cause a diagnostic problem. Breast, lung, and GI tract metastases may exhibit evidence of glandular formation. In these tumors, mucin may be present; it is usually absent in adrenal cortical carcinoma.[84] Lung carcinomas also may have evidence of squamous differentiation or, in other instances, be of undifferentiated small-cell type. Acute inflammation is found commonly within metastatic tumors, but is relatively infrequent in adrenal cortical carcinomas. In metastatic melanoma, abundant melanin pigment is usually present.

Immunohistochemical studies demonstrate keratin, epithelial membrane antigen, and HMFG-2 (in breast) in metastatic adenocarcinoma or squamous cell carcinoma, and S-100 protein and/or HMB-45 antigen in metastatic melanoma. Furthermore, metastases to the adrenal glands are usually bilateral,[83] and the clinical setting of widespread cancer is usually known.

Certain neoplasms, although metastatic to the adrenal glands much less often than breast, lung, and GI tract tumors or malignant melanoma, may be much more difficult to distinguish from adrenal cortical carcinoma. Two neoplasms that may closely resemble adrenal cortical carcinoma histologically are renal cell carcinoma and hepatocellular carcinoma. With the relative close proximity of the kidneys, adrenal glands, and liver, the differential diagnosis of a primary large abdominal mass also may include these tumors.

ADRENAL CORTICAL CARCINOMA VERSUS RENAL CELL CARCINOMA. Histologically, renal cell carcinomas of clear-cell type have cells with completely clear or empty cytoplasm, often containing abundant glycogen and a variable amount of lipid. By contrast, the neoplastic cells of adrenal cortical carcinomas of clear-cell type have finely reticulated or "bubbly" cytoplasm, lack glycogen, and usually contain abundant lipid. Thus, the PAS reaction may be very helpful, although a subset of renal cell carcinomas lack glycogen that can be appreciated histologically. Renal cell carcinomas of granular cell type and adrenocortical carcinomas with eosinophilic cytoplasm are even more difficult to distinguish histologically. When present, cytoplasmic hyaline globules favor the diagnosis of adrenal cortical carcinoma. However, cytoplasmic globules rarely have been reported in renal cell carcinoma.[85]

Immunohistochemical studies can be very helpful. Using fixed, paraffin-embedded sections, the vast majority of renal cell carcinomas express keratins, epithelial membrane antigen, and blood group isoantigens,[45, 86] which are usually not found in adrenal cortical carcinomas.[44, 45] Vimentin is expressed commonly by both high-grade renal cell carcinomas and adrenocortical carcinomas.[44, 86]

Although rarely necessary if immunohistochemical studies are used, electron microscopy is also helpful. Glycogen is usually abundant in renal cell carcinoma, lipid is often present but is not abundant, and the mitochondria are relatively normal. Adrenal cortical carcinomas lack glycogen, contain abundant lipid and endoplasmic reticulum, and have distinctive mitochondria with shelf-like or tubulovesicular cristae.[54]

ADRENAL CORTICAL CARCINOMA VERSUS HEPATOCELLULAR CARCINOMA. Histologically, hepatocellular carcinomas typically have abundant eosinophilic cytoplasm, and thus may be difficult to distinguish from adrenal cortical carcinomas with eosinophilic cytoplasm. Hepatocellular carcinomas often contain bile, and canaliculi may be seen; both of these are absent in adrenal cortical carcinoma. Cytoplasmic hyaline globules are commonly present in hepatocellular carcinoma[87] and are of little help in this differential diagnosis.

Immunohistochemical studies using fixed, paraffin-embedded sections are very helpful. Although hepatocellular carcinomas are usually negative for keratins derived from stratified epithelia, they usually express keratins from simple epithelia as detected with the CAM 5.2 antibody.[88] Adrenal cortical carcinomas are usually keratin-negative in fixed sections. Hepatocellular carcinomas also may express a variety of proteins absent in adrenocortical carcinomas. For example, Ganjei et al.[87] studied a large group of hepatocellular carcinomas: 89% expressed an erythropoiesis-associated antigen (ERY-1), 41% alpha-1-antitrypsin, and 17% alpha-fetoprotein. We are not aware of ERY-1 staining in adrenocortical neoplasms. However, both alpha-1-antitrypsin and alpha-fetoprotein are negative in adrenal cortical carcinomas.

ADRENAL PHEOCHROMOCYTOMA

The paraganglion system may be divided into two groups: those arising in the adrenal gland and those arising in extra-adrenal sites. In this discussion, we refer to paragangliomas of the adrenal gland medulla as pheochromocytomas.

Pheochromocytoma is the most common neoplasm of the adrenal gland medulla in adults.[89] Sporadic pheochromocytoma has been referred to as the 10% neoplasm: approximately 10% are malignant, 10% arise outside the confines of the adrenal gland medulla, 10% occur in children (more often bilateral), and 10% are bilateral. In addition, approximately 10% of all pheochromocytomas are familial,[89] and these tumors occur as a component of syndromes such as multiple endocrine neoplasia (MEN) type IIA (medullary carcinoma of thyroid, pheochromocytoma, and parathyroid abnormalities), MEN type IIB (medullary carcinoma of thyroid, pheochromocytoma, marfanoid body appearance, and mucosal neuromas), von Hippel-Lindau syndrome, and neurofibromatosis.[90, 91] In familial syndromes, particularly MEN types IIA and IIB, pheochromocytomas develop in younger patients, are more often bilateral, and commonly arise in the setting of adrenal medullary hyperplasia.[90, 91]

Chromaffin Reaction

The chromaffin reaction is a very helpful method for distinguishing adrenal gland pheochromocytoma from other neoplasms, such as adrenocortical tumors. In the most frequently used chromaffin reaction, fresh tumor tissue is immersed in potassium dichromate, pH 5 to 6. Pheochromocytomas turn dark brown to black; other neoplasms retain their normal color (Fig. 11–11). The histochemical basis for the chromaffin reaction is uncertain. The dark color may be the result of the formation of colored chromium oxides or oxidation products of catecholamines.[90, 92]

In our experience, more than 90% of pheochromocytomas exhibit a positive chromaffin reaction.[98] Because a positive reaction requires a high concentration of catecholamines to be present, the 10% of pheochromocytomas that are negative may be inefficient synthesizers of catecholamines. Although Zenker's fixative contains potassium dichromate, this fixative is suboptimal for the chromaffin reaction, with a much lower rate of positivity.[90, 92] The acetic acid in Zenker's fixative may explain the inefficiency of this fixative for yielding a positive chromaffin reaction.[90]

A variation of the chromaffin reaction is the use of 10% potassium iodate. Fresh pheochromocytoma tissue in this solution results in a brilliant purple or magenta color, the result of an interaction between the solution and norepinephrine.[90]

Pathologic Features

Grossly, pheochromocytomas may be small, weighing only a few grams, or extremely large; we have studied one case that was 3600 g.[92] The neoplasms appear encapsulated, although they are frequently multibosselated, with projections of tumor extending into or through the capsule. The cut surface may be yellow-white, dark red, or red-brown. Hemorrhage, necrosis, and cystic degeneration are frequent and may be extensive.[92, 93] Melicow[93] reported one patient who presented with massive hemoperitoneum secondary to a ruptured pheochromocytoma.

Gross examination of the tumor and attached residual adrenal gland medulla may be helpful in distinguishing sporadic from familial neoplasms. In the former, the pheochromocytoma is usually a single mass and the residual medulla is normal. In familial cases, the neoplasm is often multicentric

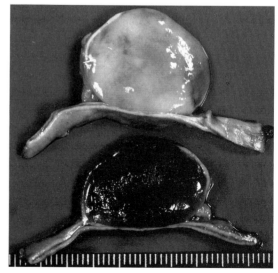

FIGURE 11–11. Pheochromocytoma. A positive chromaffin reaction is seen at bottom.

and the residual medulla may be expanded (hyperplastic), either diffusely or in a nodular pattern.[91, 94]

Histologically, familial and sporadic neoplasms are indistinguishable.[90, 91] Pheochromocytomas may exhibit a variety of histologic patterns. The tumor cells may be arranged in trabecular, diffuse, or alveolar patterns and frequently are arranged in a mixture of these patterns.[92] The German word *zellballen*, meaning balls of cells, has been used to describe the pattern of pheochromocytoma referred to as alveolar in this discussion. Although this pattern is the best-known pattern of growth in pheochromocytoma, various authors disagree regarding its frequency. For example, in some studies the alveolar pattern was observed in virtually all pheochromocytomas, whereas in our own and others' experience, approximately one third to one half of cases exhibit this pattern.[92, 94] Different interpretations of *zellballen* may explain these discrepancies. In this discussion, we regard the pattern to be alveolar when there are groups of tumor cells virtually completely surrounded by fibrovascular septa[92] (Fig. 11–12). When groups of tumor cells are connected in tortuous cords, we consider this to be a trabecular pattern.[92] Using this definition, the alveolar pattern is present more frequently in extraadrenal paragangliomas (such as carotid body tumors) than it is in pheochromocytoma.[92, 94]

In some cases, the neoplasm invades vascular structures or penetrates the tumor capsule. Neither finding correlates with subsequent malignant behavior.[92, 94]

In addition, we have seen cases of pheochromocytoma in which the majority of the neoplasm is located outside the boundaries of the adrenal gland. These tumors possibly represent a paraganglioma of a ganglion located near the adrenal

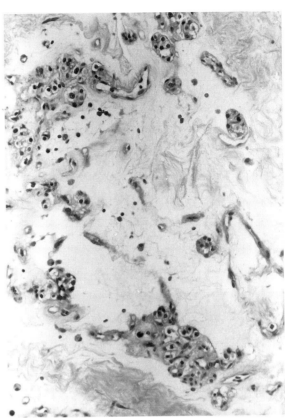

FIGURE 11–13. Pheochromocytoma. Small nests of pheochromocytoma can be seen in a background of an edematous stroma with vascular proliferation.

gland, with secondary invasion of the adrenal gland, rather than truly arising within the adrenal gland medulla.

In neoplasms with marked cystic change, vascular proliferation may be prominent superficially, resembling granulation tissue or a vascular neoplasm[95] (Fig. 11–13).

The neoplastic cells of both benign and malignant tumors have central nuclei, often with prominent nucleoli, and either basophilic or eosinophilic granular cytoplasm (Fig. 11–14). In occasional cases, the neoplastic cells may be oncocytic.[92, 94] Rarely, the neoplastic cells contain abundant cytoplasmic lipid and resemble adrenal cortical cells.[96] In some tumors, a subset of the neoplastic cells may be spindled (Fig. 11–15), although this pattern rarely predominates.[92, 94]

Nucleomegaly and hyperchromasia are the rule, although these findings may be focal. Large tumor cells with nuclear pseudoinclusions are found in approximately one third to one half of cases[90, 92] (Fig. 11–16). These structures represent invagination or protrusion of tumor cell cytoplasm into the nucleus, which in cross section resembles a true nuclear inclusion.[90, 97] Nuclear pseudoinclusions are found in both sporadic and familial tumors, with similar frequency,[92, 94] and their presence is a reflection of the high degree of nuclear irregularity in these tumors.[97] Mitotic figures are infrequent, usually less than 1/10 HPF, in less than half of neoplasms.[92, 94]

Cytoplasmic, eosinophilic hyaline globules also are present in approximately one third to two thirds of pheochromocytomas[90, 92, 94] (Fig. 11–17). The nature of these globules is unknown. They are found in pheochromocytomas as well as in normal adrenal medulla in patients with other diseases and are 2 to 25 μ, acid-fast, PAS-positive, and autofluorescent.[98]

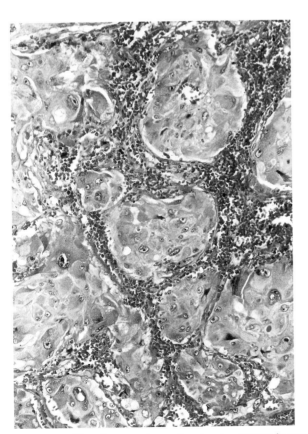

FIGURE 11–12. Pheochromocytoma. An alveolar pattern is seen.

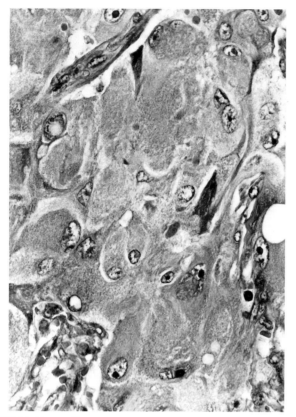

FIGURE 11–14. Pheochromocytoma. The cells have abundant granular cytoplasm.

we systematically analyzed 19 additional pheochromocytomas for amyloid, using Congo red and both polarization and electron microscopy: only two (10.5%) tumors were positive (R. Miranda et al., unpublished observations, 1994).

Formaldehyde-induced fluorescence for catecholamines is a useful technique for detecting catecholamines in pheochromocytoma. Using appropriate conditions, frozen or fixed unstained sections of tumor exposed to formaldehyde vapor emit yellow-green fluorescence through the chemical formation of isoquinolone derivatives.[103]

Immunohistochemical studies using fixed, paraffin-embedded sections have shown that normal medullary and pheochromocytoma cells express abundant chromogranin, neuron-specific enolase,[100, 104] and synaptophysin.[105, 106] Typically, chromogranin is expressed more strongly in normal and hyperplastic medullary cells as compared with pheochromocytomas. It also is common for chromogranin to be expressed by only a subset of the neoplastic medullary cells.[100] Using either frozen or paraffin-embedded sections, pheochromocytomas also commonly express a variety of other peptides, including enkephalins, adrenocorticotropic hormone (ACTH), calcitonin, vasoactive intestinal peptide (VIP), somatostatin, neurotensin, bombesin, pancreatic polypeptide, neurofilaments, substance P, and neuropeptide Y.[106–110] Vasoactive intestinal peptide highlights singly scattered ganglion cells that may be found in a subset (approximately 20%) of pheochromocytomas. Rarely, pheochromocytomas may present with clinical syndromes related to hypersecretion of these products. For example, Berenyi et al.[111] have described a pheochromocytoma that caused Cushing's syndrome secondary

Using electron microscopy, Mendelsohn and Olson[99] described these globules as being composed of neurosecretory granules within a dense, finely granular matrix. Others have observed similar findings but interpreted the globules to be composed of lysosomes, most consistent with end-products of lipid peroxidation.[98]

A second population of cells, representing a small percentage of all cells in the pheochromocytomas, are sustentacular cells. These cells are slender, spindle-shaped, or branching with small hyperchromatic nuclei and dendritic cell processes that are found between and encasing the pheochromocytes. These cells are numerous in hyperplastic adrenal medulla and in pheochromocytomas that arise in patients with the MEN type II syndromes. In contrast, in sporadic pheochromocytomas sustentacular cells are infrequent.[100, 101]

The Grimelius technique is the most valuable routine histochemical stain. Cytoplasmic argyrophilia frequently is identified in pheochromocytomas and is helpful in demonstrating the neuroendocrine nature of the tumor. However, a subset of pheochromocytomas does not exhibit argyrophilia.

Amyloid may be present, and occasionally is abundant, in the fibrovascular stroma and in blood vessel walls of pheochromocytomas. Steinhoff et al.[102] studied 20 pheochromocytomas with Congo red and polarization microscopy and detected amyloid in 14 (70%) cases. Despite these observations, in our own experience amyloid is far less common. In a study of 60 tumors, we observed eosinophilic amyloid-like material in five cases, three of which were positive for Congo red and exhibited apple-green fluorescence.[92] However, we did not routinely stain all cases with Congo red. More recently,

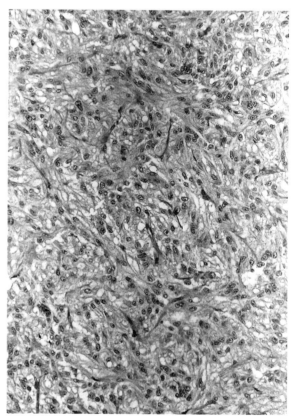

FIGURE 11–15. Pheochromocytoma. Spindling of the tumor cells is seen in this field.

to ACTH secretion. S-100 protein is not expressed by the chromaffin cells of pheochromocytoma. However, the sustentacular cells exhibit both nuclear and cytoplasmic S-100 reactivity.[100-101]

Sporadic and familial pheochromocytomas, both benign and malignant, exhibit a similar immunohistochemical profile. However, anti–S-100 antibodies detect many more sustentacular cells in familial pheochromocytomas as compared with sporadic pheochromocytomas.[100, 101]

Electron microscopic findings in pheochromocytoma include round or oval nuclei with some containing prominent nucleoli, numerous cytoplasmic organelles, and, most importantly, many cytoplasmic membrane-bound, neurosecretory granules.[92, 112] As described in the literature,[92] classic norepinephrine-containing granules contain a central, often eccentric, electron-dense core surrounded by a lucent zone. Epinephrine-containing granules are composed of a much less electron-dense core without a prominent surrounding lucent zone. However, in our experience,[92] the majority of granules in pheochromocytoma cells do not fit these descriptions. For example, less electron-dense cores may be surrounded by a lucent zone, or electron-dense cores may not be surrounded by a lucent zone. These non-classic granules may represent immature granules in various stages of maturation or granules that contain non-catecholamine products.

Brown Fat

Brown fat, in contrast with adult fat, is composed of adipocytes with multilocated or foamy cytoplasm and central nuclei; lipofuscin pigment may be present in the adipocytes.[113]

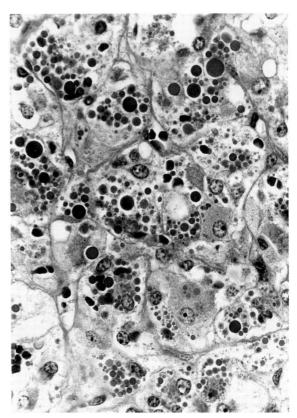

FIGURE 11–17. Pheochromocytoma. Almost all cells show abundant cytoplasmic hyaline globules.

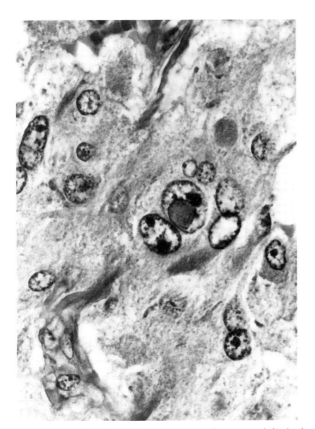

FIGURE 11–16. Pheochromocytoma. A nuclear pseudoinclusion is seen.

Brown fat is present commonly in the periadrenal tissues surrounding pheochromocytoma. This observation led Melicow[114] to suggest that the presence of brown fat may be associated with pheochromocytoma and might be an additional finding helpful in differential diagnosis. However, brown fat also is known to be present surrounding the adrenal glands in patients of all ages at autopsy[113] (Fig. 11–18). Thus, in a previous study, we questioned this association and showed that the prevalence of brown fat surrounding the adrenal glands is not increased in patients with pheochromocytoma as compared with a control population who died without medical illness (medicolegal cases).[113] The possibility that pheochromocytoma might cause hypertrophy of existing brown fat is more difficult to exclude, although we did not find evidence of hypertrophy in our study. Thus, the presence of brown fat is not helpful diagnostically.

Differential Diagnosis

BENIGN VERSUS MALIGNANT ADRENAL PHEOCHROMOCYTOMA. Approximately 5% to 15% of adrenal gland pheochromocytomas are clinically malignant.[92, 94, 115] Distinguishing benign from malignant pheochromocytomas is problematic. Except for the obvious criterion, the presence of distant metastases at sites where chromaffin tissue is not normally found,[93] other criteria for distinguishing benign from malignant pheochromocytomas are either controversial or less well established. For example, we and others consider extensive local invasion evidence of malignancy.[92, 94] Nevertheless, patients

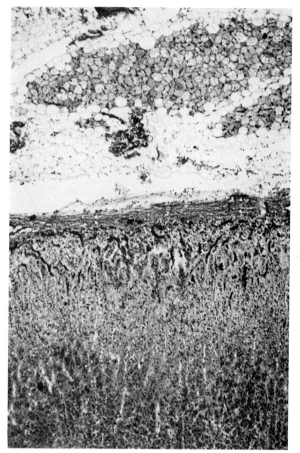

FIGURE 11–18. Normal adrenal gland. Notice brown fat in the periadrenal adipose tissue.

with locally invasive tumors who undergo complete surgical resection may be cured, whereas patients with distant metastases usually have a dismal prognosis.[92] Thus, one could argue that locally invasive tumors, although aggressive, are not truly malignant.

Traditional histologic criteria that are helpful in distinguishing benign from malignant tumors in other organs are not helpful in predicting the clinical behavior of pheochromocytomas.[92, 94] Nucleomegaly, nuclear hyperchromasia, nuclear pseudoinclusions, mitotic figures, and either capsular and/or vascular invasion may occur in both benign and malignant neoplasms.

Some gross and histologic findings have been found to correlate with, although not absolutely predict, subsequent malignant behavior. For example, in a previous study, we suggested that extensive tumor necrosis, large tumor size, and neoplasms composed predominantly of small cells more often were malignant.[92] Prior to our study, others[116, 117] also had reported that necrosis correlated with malignancy. More recently, Linnoila et al.[94, 107] studied a large series of adrenal pheochromocytomas and extra-adrenal paragangliomas. They found that extra-adrenal location, male sex, large tumor size, confluent tumor necrosis, vascular and/or extensive local invasion, and coarse tumor nodularity were present more often in malignant tumors, whereas cytoplasmic hyaline globules and the immunohistochemical demonstration of neuropeptides were commonly absent in malignant pheochromocytomas.[94]

One exceptional aspect of this study is that the authors used logistic regression analysis to analyze the effect of 16 non-histologic and histologic parameters on subsequent clinical behavior. They also proposed a model incorporating four parameters: extra-adrenal location, coarse nodularity of the neoplasm, confluent tumor necrosis, and the absence of cytoplasmic hyaline globules. Using these criteria, the authors could predict the subsequent behavior of 70% of pheochromocytomas and paragangliomas.[94]

Unfortunately, in many studies in the literature, including those by Linnoila et al.,[94] adrenal pheochromocytomas and extra-adrenal paragangliomas (pheochromocytomas) are grouped together for analysis.[94, 107, 115] When analyzing these studies, it is not possible to separate completely adrenal from the extra-adrenal neoplasms. This grouping makes the assumption that the value of these criteria for predicting subsequent behavior is the same, regardless of anatomic site. This assumption may not be correct, as it is known that extra-adrenal paragangliomas have a higher frequency of malignancy.[94]

Immunohistochemical studies also are helpful in distinguishing benign from malignant pheochromocytoma. As compared with benign tumors, malignant pheochromocytomas frequently do not express neuropeptides such as enkephalins or neuropeptide Y, may express chromogranin weakly or have a subset of cells that are completely negative, and typically contain very few S-100–positive sustentacular cells.[100, 101, 110]

DNA content analysis of pheochromocytomas using either flow cytometry or image analysis has yielded contradictory results. In one study, malignant pheochromocytomas, but not benign tumors, were found to commonly contain tetraploid or aneuploid DNA stem cell lines.[126] However, in other studies, aneuploid DNA content has been identified in both benign and malignant pheochromocytomas.[119, 120] Morphometric analysis of pheochromocytomas also has been used to compare benign and malignant tumors. Hoffman et al.[121] have shown that in malignant tumors, the tumor cell nuclei are generally smaller, with a narrow size distribution, as compared with benign tumors, in which the nuclei are generally larger, with a wider distribution of sizes.[121] These results agree with histologic studies that have suggested that tumors composed of small cells are more often malignant.[92]

In summary, currently it is not possible to distinguish malignant from benign pheochromocytomas reliably. However, the following clinical and pathologic findings raise the index of suspicion of malignancy: male sex, large tumor size (gross), coarse nodularity, tumor necrosis, predominantly small tumor cell size, absence of cytoplasmic hyaline globules, and immunohistochemical absence of neuropeptides and/or S-100–positive sustentacular cells.[94, 100, 107] The greater the number of these characteristics in a given tumor, the more likely that the neoplasm will behave in a malignant fashion.

SPORADIC VERSUS FAMILIAL ADRENAL PHEOCHROMOCYTOMA. As is mentioned earlier, this distinction may be made grossly. Sporadic tumors are usually unicentric and are associated with normal residual medullary tissue. Familial neoplasms are usually multicentric and associated with grossly visible hyperplastic residual adrenal medulla.[91] Histologically, with the exception of the presence of hyperplasia in the residual medulla, sporadic and familial neoplasms are indistinguishable in routinely stained sections.[90, 91] Immunohistochemical studies have shown that S-100–positive sustentacular cells are more numerous in familial tumors.[100]

ADRENAL PHEOCHROMOCYTOMA VERSUS MEDULLARY HYPERPLASIA. There is a continuous spectrum between nodular medullary hyperplasia and pheochromocytoma.[122, 123] Carney et al.[122] chose the arbitrary criterion of 1 cm to differentiate nodular medullary hyperplasia ($<$ 1 cm) from pheochromocytoma ($\geq$ 1 cm). This number was chosen because, in most studies of pheochromocytoma published previously, the lower size limit of pheochromocytoma was 1 cm.

ADRENAL PHEOCHROMOCYTOMA VERSUS NEUROBLASTOMA. Both pheochromocytoma and neuroblastoma (including its more mature forms, ganglioneuroblastoma and ganglioneuroma) are derived from neural crest and a common progenitor cell. Thus, it is not surprising that these tumors may occur together as an adrenal compound tumor (described later) and may share histologic and immunohistochemical features. For example, scattered ganglion cells may be found in pheochromocytoma, and, in tissue culture, pheochromocytoma cells may be induced to form cell processes resembling neurites, as do neuroblasts.

Nevertheless, in most cases this distinction is obvious at the histologic level. In neuroblastoma, the neoplastic cells have a high nucleocytoplasmic ratio, with limited evidence of differentiation. Homer Wright rosettes may be found.[124] Otherwise, the neoplastic cells are arranged in sheets. Neurofibrillary stroma is usually present, at least focally, and is often abundant.[124] By contrast, in pheochromocytomas the neoplastic cells have relatively greater cytoplasm and may be arranged in a trabecular or alveolar pattern.[92, 94] Nuclear pseudoinclusions and cytoplasmic hyaline globules are not features of neuroblastoma and are commonly present in pheochromocytomas.[92, 94]

Immunohistochemically, both neuroblastoma and pheochromocytoma cells express abundant neuron-specific enolase and neurofilaments and may be associated with S-100–positive cells. Pheochromocytomas and neuroblastomas with some maturation also may express VIP, particularly in ganglion cells. However, chromogranin is typically weak or absent in neuroblasts and is abundantly expressed in pheochromocytoma cells. Enkephalins also are rare in neuroblastoma but positive in many pheochromocytomas.[108]

ADRENAL PHEOCHROMOCYTOMA VERSUS ADRENAL CORTICAL NEOPLASM. In some circumstances, pheochromocytomas may resemble an adrenal cortical tumor and, not infrequently, adrenal cortical carcinoma. The clinical setting is helpful in this distinction. Pheochromocytomas rarely are associated with Cushing's syndrome and are virtually never associated with excessive sex steroid production, as is common with adrenal cortical tumors. Grossly, the chromaffin reaction is very helpful. More than 90% of pheochromocytomas become dark-brown or black after being immersed in potassium dichromate.[92] Adrenal cortical tumors have a negative reaction.

Histologically, cytoplasmic argyrophilia, when present, occurs in pheochromocytoma but not in adrenal cortical tumors. Although cytoplasmic hyaline globules are more common in pheochromocytoma, these also may be found in adrenal cortical neoplasms. Cytoplasmic lipid favors the diagnosis of an adrenal cortical tumor. However, rare pheochromocytomas have had neoplastic cells with extensive cytoplasmic lipid, perhaps secondary to degeneration.[96]

Formaldehyde-induced fluorescence for catecholamines is very helpful in this distinction. Pheochromocytomas, but not adrenocortical tumors, emit yellow-green fluorescence indicative of catecholamines.

Immunohistochemical studies using fixed paraffin sections also are very useful. As described earlier, pheochromocytomas express synaptophysin, neuron-specific enolase, and chromogranin, as well as numerous other peptides that are not present in adrenal cortical neoplasms. Keratins, absent in pheochromocytomas, may be detected in a subset of adrenal adenomas but usually not in carcinomas using paraffin sections. (Using frozen sections, synaptophysin and keratins have been identified in a large subset of adrenal cortical neoplasms.) The monoclonal antibody D11 may be particularly promising, as it has been reported to stain benign and malignant adrenal gland cortex but not medulla.[52, 53]

Electron microscopy also is helpful. Membrane-bound dense-core granules are characteristic in pheochromocytomas. However, Miettinen[43] has reported membrane-bound granules in a subset of adrenal cortical carcinomas. Abundant endoplasmic reticulum, cytoplasmic lipid, and distinctive mitochondria with shelf-like, tubular, or tubulovesicular cristae are found in adrenal cortical neoplasms.[54]

ADRENAL PHEOCHROMOCYTOMA VERSUS METASTATIC NEOPLASMS. The histologic findings of pheochromocytomas are sufficiently different from most metastatic adenocarcinomas, such as those arising from the lung, breast, and gastrointestinal tract, to allow this distinction. Obvious neoplastic glands are usually found in metastatic tumors and are absent in pheochromocytoma. Nests of cells in pheochromocytoma may undergo central necrosis, forming "pseudoglands" (Fig. 11–19). Pseudoglands, which may be found in a small subset of pheochromocytomas, are histologically distinctive, lack mucin, and usually are not as numerous as are true glands in metastatic adenocarcinoma. Mitotic figures, with atypical forms, are numerous in metastatic carcinomas and infrequent in pheochromocytomas. The nesting of cells surrounded by fibrovascular stroma ("neuroendocrine low-power appearance") also is not a feature of metastatic carcinomas. In the unusual circumstance in which histologic findings may overlap, an adequate clinical history usually precludes the need for other studies. However, if needed, immunohistochemical or electron microscopic studies are very helpful. Poorly differentiated metastatic carcinomas typically express keratin and epithelial membrane antigen and are negative for chromogranin, synaptophysin, or neuron-specific enolase. Neurosecretory granules are not found in most metastatic adenocarcinomas.

Metastatic malignant melanoma to the adrenal gland might also cause confusion with pheochromocytoma. Melanomas often exhibit nucleomegaly with nuclear pseudoinclusions, as are seen frequently in pheochromocytomas. However, abundant melanin pigment, common in melanoma, is rare in pheochromocytoma. Metastatic malignant melanomas also have a high mitotic rate with atypical forms; mitoses are infrequent in pheochromocytomas and usually are not atypical. For cases in which the histologic findings are difficult to interpret, the clinical history and either immunohistochemical or electron microscopic studies are helpful. Malignant melanomas, unlike pheochromocytomas, are S-100– and HMB-45 antigen–positive and lack neurosecretory granules.

The angiomatous pattern that may occur in extensively cystic pheochromocytomas,[95] combined with occasional

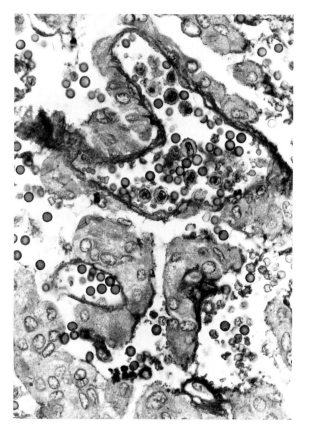

FIGURE 11–19. Pheochromocytoma. "Pseudoglands" are seen, formed by central necrosis and subsequent dropout of the centers of the nests.

mitotic figures in endothelial cells, may lead to confusion with a metastatic (or primary) tumor of vascular origin. However, the angiomatous changes are confined to the boundaries of the pheochromocytoma, and obvious anaplasia is absent.[95]

Neuroendocrine carcinomas metastatic to the adrenal gland medulla may cause a diagnostic dilemma. In the setting of MEN, medullary carcinoma of the thyroid gland (MTC) may metastasize to the adrenal gland. Tumor-to-tumor metastasis, i.e., MTC metastasizing to a pheochromocytoma, also has been reported.[125] Medullary carcinoma of the thyroid is consistently and strongly positive for calcitonin. Pheochromocytomas may express calcitonin, but in less than one third of cases. In this setting, usually the clinical history of MEN is well known, and MTC and pheochromocytoma have sufficiently different histologic features to allow distinction. If there is a history of prior thyroid gland surgery, the findings in the adrenal gland may be compared with a previously excised thyroid neoplasm. If necessary, electron microscopy with the detection of the neurosecretory granules typically seen in pheochromocytoma is very helpful.

COMPOUND NEOPLASMS OF THE ADRENAL GLAND MEDULLA

Tumors of the adrenal gland medulla rarely may be composed of either ganglioneuroma or ganglioneuroblastoma (derived from the sympathetic nervous system) and pheochromocytoma (derived from the chromaffin system). According to Tischler et al.,[126] as of 1987, nine compound tumors of the adrenal medulla had been reported. We are aware of at least nine additional compound adrenal medullary tumors reported subsequently.[94, 127–129] The pheochromocytoma component rarely has been malignant.[130] A subset of patients (approximately 20%) had neurofibromatosis.[126, 128] These tumors also have been associated with cortical neoplasms.[131] Compound tumors of the adrenal medulla may present with symptoms secondary to excessive secretion of either catecholamines or VIP. There is also one case report of a compound adrenal medullary neoplasm composed of pheochromocytoma and malignant nerve sheath tumor.[132]

Although rare, this occurrence of compound tumors in the adrenal gland medulla is not surprising, because both ganglioneuroma and ganglioneuroblastoma as well as pheochromocytoma may be derived from a common precursor cell of neural crest origin. One can hypothesize that neoplastic transformation occurred in this progenitor cell, with bidirectional differentiation.

Pathologic Features

The histologic criteria to diagnose a compound neoplasm of the adrenal gland medulla are a combination of the histologic criteria for pheochromocytoma (described previously) and for either ganglioneuroma or ganglioneuroblastoma (described later). Both components need to be present unequivocally. In 10% to 20% of pheochromocytomas, singly scattered ganglion cells may be identified;[107] their presence alone does not justify the diagnosis of a compound neoplasm.

The immunohistochemical and electron microscopic findings in these tumors are in keeping with the findings of each component. Neuron-specific enolase is strongly expressed in both components of the tumor.[133] Chromogranin and synaptophysin are strongly expressed by the cells of the pheochromocytoma component but are weak or negative in the ganglioneuroma or ganglioneuroblastoma components (weak staining may be seen in the varicosities of nerve cell processes).[126, 128] These results are in agreement with the distribution of neurosecretory granules observed ultrastructurally. S-100 protein is expressed by the sustentacular cells within the pheochromocytoma component and by Schwann and glial cells in the ganglioneuroblastoma or ganglioneuroma components. Vasoactive intestinal peptide is often expressed intensely by ganglion cells.[134] The expression of VIP in pheochromocytomas is variable. In some studies, VIP is weakly expressed or absent in chromaffin cells.[127, 134] However, others have reported VIP to be commonly expressed in approximately 40% of pheochromocytomas.[107]

NEUROBLASTOMA

Neuroblastoma arises from primitive precursor cells of the sympathetic nervous system. Neuroblastoma, ganglioneuroblastoma, and ganglioneuroma represent a continuous spectrum of differentiation, with neuroblastomas representing the undifferentiated and ganglioneuromas representing the differentiated ends of the spectrum.[135–138]

Neuroblastoma is the most common solid tumor of children younger than 1 year of age, and is third only to leukemia/

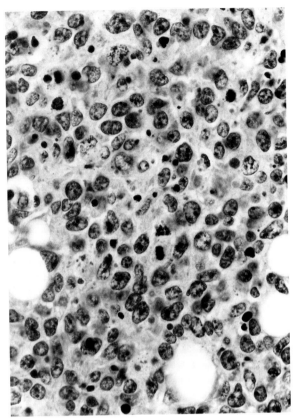

FIGURE 11–20. Undifferentiated neuroblastoma. This retroperitoneal neoplasm shows no differentiating features, and other "small, round, blue cell tumors" must be considered in the differential diagnosis.

lymphoma and central nervous system tumors in children of all ages.[139, 140] More than 50% of cases occur in infants younger than 2 years of age; more than 90% of cases occur in children younger than 10 years old.[140, 141] The adrenal gland is the most common primary site of neuroblastoma in children.

In adults, neuroblastoma is uncommon. In 1986, Allan et al.[142] summarized the clinical and pathologic findings in 34 adult patients with a median age of 34 years. Although the abdomen was a common site of origin (as in children), approximately half of cases arose in the head and neck or thorax. Similarly, Aleshire et al.[143] have shown a high incidence of primary head and neck neuroblastomas in adults. In their study, these tumors were more often low-stage, with a better prognosis than that of neuroblastomas in children.

Pathologic Features

Grossly, neuroblastomas of the adrenal gland may be small or massive. Most tumors are unilateral; rare bilateral cases have been reported.[144] Neuroblastomas are well-circumscribed, but not encapsulated, most easily appreciable in the smaller neoplasms. Their cut surface is lobulated, bulging, and white, gray, or dark red, the last secondary to hemorrhage. Cystic degeneration is common and may be marked.[145] Calcification is frequent and may be palpable.

Histologically, neuroblastomas may exhibit a spectrum of histologic findings. Undifferentiated tumors are composed of

a uniform population of cells with round, hyperchromatic nuclei and speckled nuclear chromatin[124, 135, 136, 138, 143] (Fig. 11–20). Karyorrhexis and mitotic figures, although variable in quantity, are constant.[135, 146] Histologic evidence of neuroblastic differentiation includes increased nuclear size, vesicular nuclei with dispersed chromatin, nucleoli, more visible cell cytoplasm, and tumor cell processes (Fig. 11–21). Neuroblastomas have been subdivided into undifferentiated, poorly differentiated, and differentiated variants, based on the proportion of differentiating neuroblasts (0%, <5%, and >5%, respectively).[136–138] Subtyping should be performed only prior to any therapy (which may induce maturation) and only on adequately sampled specimens (one section for each centimeter of the longest dimension of the resected primary tumor).

Although neuroblasts are usually small cells, a significant proportion of cases may contain larger neuroblasts, either focally or diffusely. Various types of giant cells with single or multiple nuclei, which may exhibit hyperchromasia and pleomorphism, are seen in many cases. Rarely, neuroblastomas may be composed predominantly of these cells.[147] Other rare features of neuroblasts that have been reported include cytoplasmic eosinophilic pseudoinclusions in the nuclei, fusiform to spindle cell change (Fig. 11–22), and focal rhabdoid and pseudorhabdoid change.[138] Abundant black pigment that is histochemically similar to melanin also may be found in neuroblastomas.[137, 148, 149] However, a recent electron microscopic study of one such case did not identify melanosomes. Instead, the pigmented cells contained abundant, variably shaped lysosomes containing electron-dense material more consistent with lipid residues.[149]

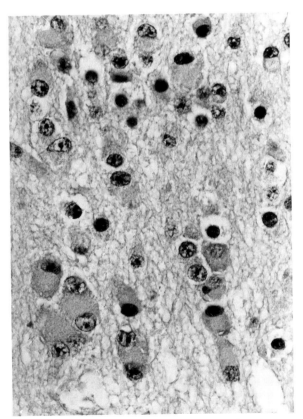

FIGURE 11–21. Differentiating neuroblastoma. Maturing neuroblasts are interspersed among the undifferentiated cells.

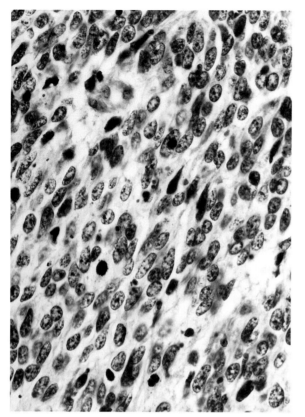

FIGURE 11–22. Neuroblastoma. Spindling of the neoplastic cells was a prominent feature in this case.

Architecturally, most neuroblastomas show a consistent nesting pattern, usually highlighted by the presence of thin fibrovascular septa (Fig. 11–23). Necrosis and calcification are common findings. As maturation occurs, the amount of neuropil increases, manifesting as an increase in intercellular material; the neuropil becomes arranged into parallel arrays, and Homer Wright rosettes are formed[124, 135–139] (Fig. 11–24). In these rosettes, the tumor cell nuclei are organized in a wreath surrounding central neurofibrillary stroma without the formation of a true lumen (see later). Some neuroblastomas may show unusual architectural appearances, including a focal "sclerosing" pattern, a pseudoalveolar pattern, a papillary-like pattern, an angiomatoid pattern, and a starry-sky pattern.[138, 141, 150] Some changes, such as the sclerosing pattern, focal hyalinization of septa, and a focal lymphoplasmacytic infiltration, may be related to regression.[138]

Neuroblastomas contain catecholamines that may be demonstrated by formaldehyde-induced preparations of fine needle aspiration biopsies or in bone marrow aspirate smears when material is limited.

Immunohistochemically, neuroblastomas express a variety of proteins: neuron-specific enolase, protein gene product (PGP) 9.5, neurofilaments, vasoactive intestinal peptide, and microtubule-associated proteins.[146, 152] The presence of S-100 protein–positive spindle cells in the fibrovascular stroma of relatively undifferentiated tumors correlates with greater differentiation.[153]

The electron microscopic findings in neuroblastomas may be very useful in establishing the diagnosis, particularly in undifferentiated neoplasms.[103, 112, 154] The neoplastic cells con-

tain neurosecretory granules, 50 to 200 nm, usually peripherally dispersed in the cell cytoplasm, and form primitive cell processes (neurites). Other less specific features include primitive cell attachments, abundant basal lamina, epithelial-like clusters or molding of tumor cells, well-distributed nuclear chromatin with prominent nucleoli, and occasionally neural tubules or neurofilaments. With increasing maturation, the features associated with mature nerve formation become apparent, such as the Schwann cells and basal lamina.

DNA content analysis has been used to study neuroblastomas.[155, 156] For example, Gansler et al.[156] studied 38 neuroblastomas: 16 of 38 (42%) contained aneuploid stem cell lines. Interestingly, aneuploidy correlated with greater histologic differentiation and lower stage.[156] Thus, aneuploidy in neuroblastomas is a good prognostic sign.[155, 156]

Although a subset of neuroblastomas has been known to be familial,[157, 158] only recently have researchers begun to understand the molecular mechanisms involved in neuroblastoma. For example, classic cytogenetic techniques have shown a high incidence of chromosome 1p deletion in neuroblastoma.[159] Also, the N-*myc* gene, located on chromosome 2p23-24, is commonly amplified in neuroblastoma cell lines and a subset of neuroblastomas.[160, 161] These molecular findings have not been reported in neoplasms that may be histologically confused with neuroblastoma.

Rosettes

Rosettes may be identified in a variety of neoplasms, including tumors of neural (neuroblastoma, medulloblastoma, reti-

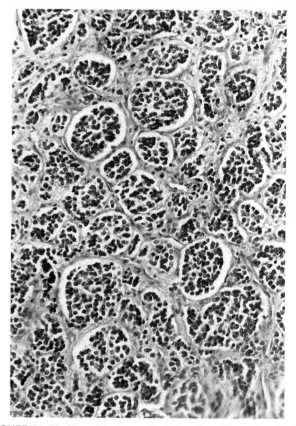

FIGURE 11–23. Neuroblastoma. Packets of undifferentiated cells are seen divided by delicate fibrovascular septa.

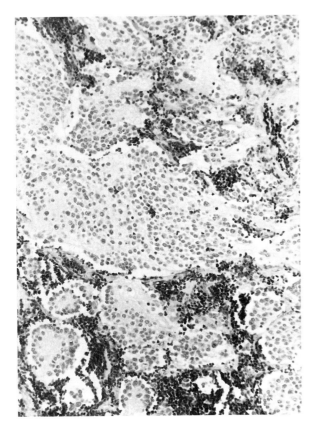

FIGURE 11–24. Neuroblastoma. Abundant neuropil is seen in this tumor. Several Homer Wright rosettes are seen in the lower left corner.

noblastoma, and ependymoma), neuroepithelial (carcinoid, Wilms' tumor), ovarian stromal (granulosa-theca cell tumor), and epithelial (thymoma) origin. Rosettes also are found rarely in malignant lymphomas.[162]

Homer Wright–type rosettes are characteristic of neuroblastoma.[124, 135, 141] In these structures, the neoplastic cells aggregate with the cell nuclei situated peripherally and cell processes and cytoplasm located centrally. In effect, the nuclei encircle the cell cytoplasm and cell processes in wreath-like fashion. A lumen is not present in the center of the rosette. Homer Wright rosettes, which also occur in medulloblastoma, can be distinguished from other types of rosettes, including Flexner-type rosettes and perivascular rosettes (also referred to in the literature as pseudorosettes). Flexner rosettes resemble Homer Wright rosettes except that a lumen is present in the center of the rosette. These rosettes may be found in retinoblastoma and ependymoma, and the epithelial tubules of Wilms' tumor and carcinoid may form structures that may resemble Flexner-type rosettes. In perivascular pseudorosettes, the neoplastic cells aggregate around a blood vessel, with the vessel located centrally. These pseudorosettes are commonly found in thymomas. Rosettes resembling Homer Wright rosettes have been reported in occasional cases of malignant lymphoma.[162] In addition, in poorly fixed malignant lymphomas, the lymphoma cells may appear to aggregate and resemble rosettes.[163]

The primary importance of Homer Wright rosettes is that they are helpful in the differential diagnosis of small round cell tumors. These rosettes do not occur in rhabdomyosarcoma or Ewing's sarcoma, are rare in malignant lymphoma, and are common in neuroblastoma.

Prognostic Indicators in Neuroblastoma

Various clinical, biochemical, histologic, and molecular parameters have been assessed in neuroblastoma. Of these, three parameters are most useful: age, stage, and amplification of the N-*myc* gene. Histologic findings, such as the degree of differentiation and growth rate, are also useful.

AGE. Age independently predicts prognosis in children with neuroblastoma. Approximately 90% of infants younger than 1 year of age have long-term survival.[140, 164] Infants with localized disease need only complete surgical excision. Patients with stage IV disease have been treated with multi-agent chemotherapy. However, the role of therapy in inducing tumor regression in these patients is unclear, because infants exhibit a high rate of spontaneous remission. The mechanism of spontaneous remissions is poorly understood. For infants older than 1 year of age, the possibility of long-term survival is markedly decreased, particularly in those children with high stage disease.[164]

STAGE. Stage also independently predicts survival in children with neuroblastoma. The staging system proposed by Evans et al.[165] as shown in Table 11–5 is the best-known system; no other system has been shown to be more useful. Patients with stage I, II, or IV-S disease have far better survival, often with only surgical excision, than patients with stage III or IV disease. The high rate of long-term survival in infants with stage IV-S disease is remarkable—87% in one series.[166, 167] Young infants (median age, 3 months) present with a stage I or II primary neoplasm, usually involving the adrenal gland, combined with disease present in the liver, bone marrow, or skin. Despite a tumor burden that may be massive, patients often undergo spontaneous remission, and surgical excison alone is adequate; radiation or chemotherapy is often not necessary.[167]

Table 11–5. **Staging System for Neuroblastoma Proposed by Evans et al.**

Stage I	Tumor confined to the organ or structure of origin.
Stage II	Tumors extending in continuity beyond the organ or structure of origin but not crossing the midline. Regional lymph nodes on the homolateral side may be involved.*
Stage III	Tumors extending in continuity beyond the midline. Regional lymph nodes may be involved bilaterally.
Stage IV	Remote disease involving skeleton, organs, soft tissues, or distant lymph node groups, etc.
Stage IV-S	Patients who would otherwise be stage I or II but who have remote disease confined only to one or more of the following sites: liver, skin, or bone marrow (without radiographic evidence of bone metastases on complete skeletal survey).

* For tumors arising in midline structures (e.g., the organ of Zuckerkandl), penetration beyond the capsule and involvement of lymph nodes on the same side are considered stage II. Bilateral extension of any sort is considered stage III.

N-*myc* AMPLIFICATION. The N-*myc* gene is amplified considerably in a subset of neuroblastomas, approximately one third of cases. In cell lines, this gene may be amplified up to 140-fold.[160] N-*myc* gene amplification is highly correlated with advanced stage of disease.[160, 161] Furthermore, within each stage, N-*myc* amplification appears to provide additional prognostic information.[161] For example, Seeger et al.[161] reported that the likelihood of survival at 18 months was 70% for individuals whose tumors did not amplify N-*myc,* 30% for patients with tumors with 3 to 10 copies of the gene, and 5% for children with tumors with more than 10 copies of N-*myc.*

HISTOLOGIC FINDINGS. Shimada et al.[135] have proposed that an index representing both the number of mitotic figures and cells exhibiting karyorrhexis (MKI) is useful in predicting survival. Five thousand cells are observed (the denominator), and the number of mitoses and karyorrhectic cells are tallied (the numerator). Patients with neoplasms that have a low (<100/5000) or intermediate (100–200/5000) MKI have longer survival than patients with tumors that have a high (>200/5000) MKI.[135]

Joshi et al. developed a histologic grading sytem of neuroblastoma based on mitotic rate (≤10/10 HPF) and calcification.[137] Histologic grades 1, 2, and 3 were defined on the basis of the presence of both, any one, or none of these two prognostic features, respectively. Statistically significant differences in survival were observed in the grades after adjusting for age and stage. Joshi et al. have proposed to link age with histologic grade to define two risk groups: a low-risk group, all patients with grade 1 tumors and patients 1 year of age or younger with grade 2 tumors; and a high-risk group, consisting of patients older than 1 year of age with grade 2 tumors and all patients with grade 3 tumors.[137] There is an 84% concordance between these risk groups and the Shimada classification.

In many studies, histologic evidence of differentiation correlates with improved patient survival. Such evidence, as described earlier, includes larger nuclear size, increased cell cytoplasm, mature ganglion cells, and the presence of abundant neurofibrillary stroma with rosette formation.[124, 135–138, 146, 168] However, evidence of differentiation also correlates with age, stage, and histologic grade, as defined previously. Thus, the independent prognostic value of histologic differentiation has been difficult to establish.[137, 146]

Immunohistochemical studies using anti–S-100 have been used as an additional means of demonstrating differentiation, as the number of S-100–positive cells present correlates with differentiation.[146, 153] However, these methods may not have independent prognostic value.[146]

Differential Diagnosis

One of the most difficult problems in surgical pathology is the correct diagnosis of small, round cell tumors, including neuroblastoma.[103]

NEUROBLASTOMA VERSUS RHABDOMYOSARCOMA. Rhabdomyosarcomas, particularly those of alveolar type, histologically may closely resemble neuroblastoma. Often electron microscopy and/or immunohistochemical methods are necessary for correct diagnosis. Using electron microscopy, sarcomere-related structures such as Z, A, H, and M bands may be found. However, in poorly differentiated neoplasms, only 7- to 10-nm cytoplasmic filaments and/or intracytoplasmic phagocytosed collagen fibers may be identified. These structures are not found in neuroblastoma. Unlike neuroblastomas, in rhabdomyosarcomas neurosecretory granules are not identified. Immunohistochemically, muscle-specific proteins such as myoglobin, myosin, muscle-specific actin, and desmin may be detected in rhabdomyosarcoma; neuron-specific enolase is usually absent. Conversely, neuron-specific enolase is usually positive in neuroblastoma[152], and muscle-related proteins are absent.

Formaldehyde-induced fluorescence for catecholamines, present in neuroblastoma, is absent in rhabdomyosarcoma. Cytogenetic studies, if available, are also helpful in distinguishing alveolar rhabdomyosarcoma from neuroblastoma. A chromosomal translocation, t(2;13)(q37;q14), is consistently found in alveolar rhabdomyosarcoma,[169] whereas deletion of the short arm of chromosome 1 (1p) is common in neuroblastoma.[159]

NEUROBLASTOMA VERSUS EWING'S SARCOMA. Neuroblastoma and Ewing's sarcoma histologically may be very similar. Homer Wright rosettes do not occur in Ewing's sarcoma. In the past, the value of the PAS reaction with diastase digestion for glycogen was emphasized. The neoplastic cells of Ewing's sarcoma often contain abundant cytoplasmic glycogen, and many neuroblastomas are negative. However, a subset of Ewing's sarcoma is negative for PAS, and some neuroblastomas may contain cytoplasmic glycogen. Thus, the PAS reaction with diastase digestion provides a clue but is not entirely reliable.[170]

The diagnosis of Ewing's sarcoma can now be established by using immunohistochemical methods and monoclonal antibodies such as HBA71 and 12E7.[171, 172] For example, the HBA71 antibody, which is reactive in formalin-fixed, paraffin-embedded tissues, recognizes the p30/32^{MIC2} cell surface glycoprotein that is present in greater than 90% of cases of Ewing's sarcoma, but is not expressed in neuroblastoma.[171, 173] It should be pointed out that a subset of Ewing's tumor may be positive for neuron-specific enolase, precluding the use of this marker alone for distinguishing neuroblastoma from Ewing's tumor.[152]

If available, cytogenetic studies also are helpful in the distinction between neuroblastoma and Ewing's sarcoma. Deletion of chromosome 1p is common in neuroblastoma, whereas t(11;22)(q24;q12) has been reported in Ewing's sarcoma (and peripheral neuroepithelioma).[159, 174, 175]

NEUROBLASTOMA VERSUS NON-HODGKIN'S LYMPHOMA. Non-Hodgkin's lymphomas, particularly of diffuse type, may histologically resemble neuroblastoma, and rarely rosette-type structures have been reported in lymphomas.[162]

Immunohistochemically, lymphomas are negative for neuron-specific enolase and are positive for lymphoid markers such as CD45 (leukocyte common antigen) and either B-cell or T-cell specific antigens. It should be emphasized that a subset of lymphomas, particularly lymphoblastic lymphomas, express the MIC2 antigen as shown with the 12E7 monoclonal antibody.[172]

Electron microscopy is also useful. Lymphomas do not have neurosecretory granules, external or basal lamina, primitive cell attachments, and clustering or molding of tumor cells.

NEUROBLASTOMA VERSUS WILMS' TUMOR. Neuroblastomas may be confused with Wilms' tumor, particularly in cases of adrenal gland neuroblastoma that secondarily invade the kidney or in rare cases of Wilms' tumor metastatic to the adrenal gland.

Histologically, the majority of Wilms' tumors have three components: undifferentiated blastema, mesenchymal tissue, and epithelial tissue. In tumors with an abundance of undifferentiated blastema, confusion with neuroblastoma is more likely. Epithelial tubules in Wilms' tumor may be confused with the Homer Wright rosettes. Unlike the latter, the tubules of Wilms' tumor may be recognized by their central lumen, a single cell layer of surrounding nuclei, and a distinct basal lamina surrounding the cells.

Immunohistochemical studies are very helpful. The epithelial component of Wilms' tumor reacts with keratin and epithelial membrane antigen, absent in neuroblastoma. If neural elements are present in a Wilms' tumor, these may react with anti–S-100 protein and neuron-specific enolase, as occurs in neuroblastoma. Only neuroblastoma contains catecholamines and neurosecretory granules.

NEUROBLASTOMA VERSUS ADRENAL CORTICAL CARCINOMA. Neuroblastomas, particularly undifferentiated tumors, are unlikely to be confused with adrenal cortical carcinoma. Possibly, a well-differentiated neuroblastoma with abundant neurofibrillary material might be confused with carcinoma. However, in adrenal cortical carcinoma, the neoplastic cells are large with abundant eosinophilic cytoplasm, quite different from neuroblastoma. The clinical presentation of patients with adrenal cortical carcinoma is also very different from neuroblastoma. Most children with adrenocortical carcinoma present with a mixed endocrine syndrome, usually virilization and Cushing's syndrome.

NEUROBLASTOMA VERSUS OTHER MISCELLANEOUS NEOPLASMS. Medulloblastomas closely resemble undifferentiated neuroblastomas. These neoplasms are composed of primitive small cells with hyperchromatic round nuclei. Homer Wright–type rosettes may be found in approximately one third of neoplasms. However, the likelihood of confusing this tumor with adrenal gland neuroblastoma is very low. Medulloblastomas arise in the midline of the cerebellum and uncommonly metastasize outside of the central nervous system. When these neoplasms do exit the central nervous system, they spread to cervical lymph nodes or bones. Spread to the adrenal glands is possible, particularly in patients with a ventriculoperitoneal shunt and extensive tumor spread to the abdominal cavity. However, in this scenario, the clinical setting is known.

Retinoblastomas also may resemble undifferentiated neuroblastoma. However, in this neoplasm the rosettes are different, characterized by a central lumen, and the clinical setting is quite different. Retinoblastomas rarely metastasize to distant sites, usually to bones. We are not aware of any reported case of a retinoblastoma that metastasized to the adrenal glands. The converse, adrenal gland neuroblastoma metastasizing to the retina, is much more likely, but this phenomenon is not the focus of this chapter.

NEUROBLASTOMA VERSUS GANGLIONEUROBLASTOMA. See later discussion in differential diagnosis of ganglioneuroblastoma.

GANGLIONEUROBLASTOMA

Ganglioneuroblastomas are neoplasms that exhibit differentiation intermediate between that of neuroblastoma and gangli-

oneuroma. Shimada et al. use the terminology stroma-rich neuroblastoma to designate these tumors.[135] Most ganglioneuroblastomas occur in young children, most often in the posterior mediastinum or retroperitoneum.[176] These tumors rarely arise in the adrenal gland. The survival of patients with ganglioneuroblastoma is far greater than that of patients with neuroblastoma[135, 137, 177] and is correlated with histologic features (described later).

Pathologic Features

Grossly, ganglioneuroblastomas resemble neuroblastomas, although the areas of maturation tend to be yellow-white and firm.

Histologically, ganglioneuroblastomas are composed of a mixture of immature neuroblasts and maturing elements: ganglion cells, Schwann cells, nerve fibers, and fibrous tissue. These tumors contain pigment, with features of neuromelanin.[178] Ganglioneuroblastomas may be subdivided histologically into three subgroups, designated by Joshi et al.[136] as nodular, intermixed, and borderline. The nodular (also referred to as immature or composite) type of ganglioneuroblastoma is composed of areas of tumor that are completely mature and resemble ganglioneuroma, combined with a single nodule (or a few grossly identifiable nodules) of tumor that resembles neuroblastoma (Fig. 11–25). The boundary between these components is often sharp. Intermixed ganglioneuroblastoma has a few well-defined microscopic neuroblastomatous foci within a neoplasm that otherwise resembles a ganglioneuroma,

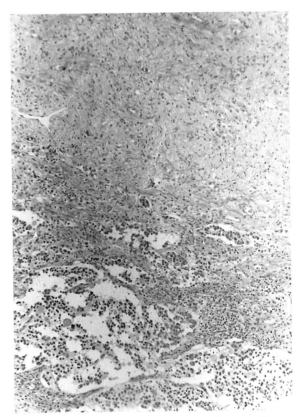

FIGURE 11–25. Ganglioneuroblastoma, nodular type. The upper right shows an area of ganglioneuroma, and a discrete neuroblastomatous nodule is seen in the lower left.

whereas a borderline ganglioneuroblastoma has a few poorly defined neuroblastomatous foci (Fig. 11–26). The intermixed and the nodular subtypes are the most frequent, with the borderline subtype about one half as common as the other two.[136]

Immunohistochemical and electron microscopic findings in ganglioneuroblastomas are similar to neuroblastomas, with greater evidence of differentiation. For example, S-100–positive Schwann cells are more numerous in ganglioneuroblastoma than in neuroblastoma.[153] Vasoactive intestinal peptide is commonly expressed by the ganglion cells. Ultrastructural studies reveal numerous neurosecretory granules, neurotubules, neurons, and Schwann cells.[112]

Prognostic Features

Nodular-type ganglioneuroblastomas may exhibit a malignant behavior and are much more likely to metastasize than intermixed or borderline ganglioneuroblastomas.[136, 177] The latter two variants are best regarded as being of borderline malignancy.[136, 138]

Differential Diagnosis

GANGLIONEUROBLASTOMA VERSUS NEUROBLASTOMA. In
neuroblastoma, neuroblasts and neuropil constitute the predominant or exclusive component of the tumor. The presence of small foci of ganglioneuromatous differentiation does not

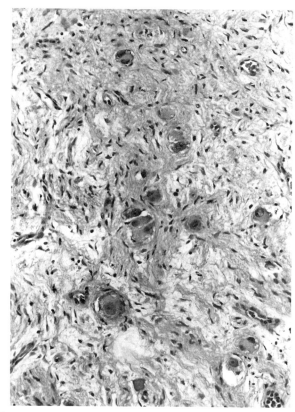

FIGURE 11–27. Ganglioneuroma. The neuronal cells are all mature and completely lacking in atypia. The stroma resembles that of a neurofibroma.

alter the classification. In ganglioneuroblastomas, the ganglioneuromatous component must constitute the majority component. In the adrenal gland, neuroblastomas outnumber ganglioneuroblastomas in a ratio greater than 10:1.

GANGLIONEUROMA

Ganglioneuromas are fully differentiated, benign neoplasms of the sympathetic nervous system. Most of these tumors occur in older adults, usually in the posterior mediastinum or the retroperitoneum. Ganglioneuromas rarely arise in the adrenal gland.

Ganglioneuromas typically are functional, but at the subclinical level. Almost all tumors produce catecholamines, usually precursors such as vanillylmandelic or homovanillic acid.[179] Rarely, ganglioneuromas may be the cause of clinical symptoms owing to hypersecretion. For example, ganglioneuromas may cause hypertension secondary to catecholamines, a diarrheal syndrome secondary to VIP secretion,[180] or virilization secondary to production of sex steroids.[181, 182]

Pathologic Features

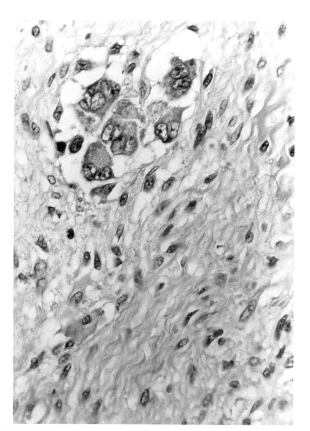

FIGURE 11–26. Ganglioneuroblastoma, borderline type. Most of this tumor consisted of ganglioneuromatous areas, but there were scattered clusters of cytologically atypical neuronal-type cells.

Ganglioneuromas are composed only of mature elements: mature ganglion cells without any atypia, Schwann cells, mature neuritic processes, nerve bundles, and fibrous tissue[135, 182] (Fig. 11–27). Ganglion cells may be numerous and found in clusters. Leydig cells have been identified in a small subset of tumors.[182] There is no evidence of immaturity; in other words, neuroblasts are not identified. The mature neuritic processes are organized into fascicles or bundles, with alignment of Schwann cells along these processes.

Immunohistochemical studies confirm the well-differentiated nature of these neoplasms. Numerous S-100–positive Schwann cells are present. Ganglion cells may express VIP,[180] although only a subset of patients with VIP-positive tumors have a diarrheal syndrome. Ganglion cells may also express testosterone or other sex steroid hormones.[182] Electron microscopic examination of ganglioneuromas demonstrates abundant evidence of maturation and is similar to the findings in normal sympathetic nervous system tissue.[183]

Differential Diagnosis

GANGLIONEUROBLASTOMA VERSUS GANGLIONEUROMA. Although this distinction may be difficult, it is rarely a problem in the adrenal gland, because ganglioneuromas rarely arise at this site.[135] In ganglioneuroma, the neoplasm lacks any neuroblast. The ganglion cells should all be mature and completely lacking in nuclear enlargement, hyperchromatism, or pleomorphism.

GANGLIONEUROBLASTOMA VERSUS NEUROFIBROMA. The presence of ganglion cells distinguishes ganglioneuroblastoma from neurofibroma (Fig. 11–28).

MYELOLIPOMA

Myelolipomas are not truly neoplastic and are composed of mature adipose tissue and a variable mixture of hematopoietic

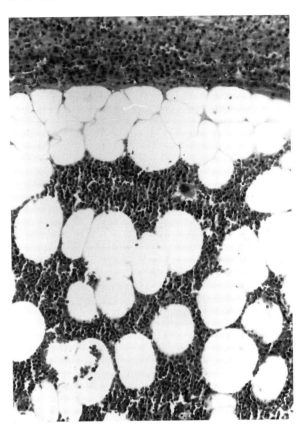

FIGURE 11–29. Adrenal myelolipoma. All three hematopoietic lineages are present and show normal maturation.

elements that may be of myeloid, erythroid, and/or megakaryocytic lineage. Myelolipomas are identified most often in older patients and more commonly occur in nodular adrenal glands.[4, 20] Their pathogenesis is unknown, but may be related to a disturbance of adrenocortical growth, secondary to multiple causes.[20]

The majority of myelolipomas are incidental lesions, usually found at autopsy or by advanced radiologic methods used in the clinical work-up of other diseases. However, occasionally myelolipomas may be of large size and present with abdominal pain.[184] In a previous review of the literature, we found three cases in which an adrenal myelolipoma ruptured, detected clinically as an acute abdomen.[185] Myelolipomas may be found within cortical adenomas and be associated with clinical evidence of hyperfunction.[20] One adrenal gland myelolipoma without cortical adenoma has been reported to be associated with Cushing's syndrome.[186]

Pathologic Features

Myelolipomas are usually small but rarely attain large size. We have seen two cases over 1500 g.[185] The lesions are composed predominantly of adipose tissue and thus are bright yellow and fatty. Red foci mark the areas where hematopoietic elements are abundant. Myeloid, erythroid, and megakaryocytic elements are present in all stages of maturation[185, 186] (Fig. 11–29). Metaplastic bone trabeculae may be present, particularly in large lesions. The lesions are surrounded by a thin rim of histologically unremarkable adrenal cortex.[186, 187]

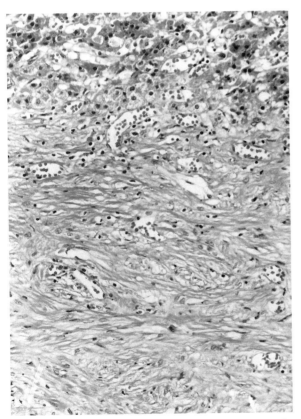

FIGURE 11–28. Adrenal neurofibroma. Note the absence of neurons, differentiating it from ganglioneuroma.

Differential Diagnosis

ADRENAL MYELOLIPOMA VERSUS MYELOLIPOMATOUS FOCI. Small foci of adipocytes associated with lymphocytes and plasma cells, and occasionally with hematopoietic cells of myeloid or erythroid lineage, may be identified in a subset of adrenal glands in normal individuals. Usually, these foci are found in adrenal glands of older patients examined at autopsy. Unlike a true myelolipoma, myelolipomatous foci are microscopic and do not form a mass. Often immature hematopoietic elements are not present or, if present, are not numerous. Metaplastic bone formation is rare. The adrenal glands are not enlarged and are frequently nodular secondary to another cause.[20]

ADRENAL MYELOLIPOMA VERSUS CORTICAL ADENOMA. Histologically, cortical adenomas and myelolipomas are completely different. However, it is not uncommon for an adrenal adenoma to contain a small myelolipoma. These lesions are small but otherwise fulfill all of the histologic criteria of a myelolipoma. Rarely, the adenoma is functional.[20] A myelolipoma also may coexist with an adenoma in the same adrenal gland, but not within the adenoma itself.

In our experience, we have not identified myelolipomatous foci in malignant adrenal cortical carcinomas. Thus, the presence of these foci may have some value in the differential diagnosis of adrenocortical tumors.

ADRENAL MYELOLIPOMA VERSUS LIPOMATOUS NEOPLASMS. Adrenal gland myelolipomas may be confused with other lipomatous neoplasms, either lipomas or well-differentiated liposarcomas arising in the retroperitoneum. Although foci of lymphocytes and plasma cells may be seen in a lipoma or liposarcoma, immature hematopoietic elements of erythroid and myeloid lineage and megakaryocytes are absent. In addition, lipoblasts are present in liposarcoma and absent in myelolipomas.

TUMORS THAT RARELY ARISE IN THE ADRENAL GLAND

Benign

Benign tumors of mesenchymal origin arise rarely in the adrenal gland. Of these, hemangiomas are the most common. According to Vargas in 1980,[188] 12 adrenal gland hemangiomas had been reported, five of which were excised surgically. These lesions may be small or large masses; one reported lesion was 5000 g. The cut surface is red or yellow. Calcification may be grossly apparent and is commonly detected radiologically. Histologically, these tumors are usually cavernous hemangiomas without evidence of cytologic atypia.[188, 189]

Leiomyomas may arise in the adrenal gland, in association with the adrenal vein, and are almost always incidental findings. Most often these tumors are detected at autopsy.

Benign nerve sheath tumors, either schwannoma or neurofibroma, have been described in the adrenal gland, most often in patients with neurofibromatosis[190] (see Fig. 11–28).

Leydig cell adenomas of the adrenal gland have been described.[191] These neoplasms closely resemble cortical adenomas, except that crystalloids of Reinke are found, characteristic of Leydig cell adenomas. However, it may be possible that rare virilizing adrenal cortical adenomas might produce

crystalloids of Reinke. Thus, the relationship of adrenal gland Leydig cell adenomas to cortical adenomas is not clear.

Malignant

Non-Hodgkin's lymphomas and Hodgkin's disease commonly involve the adrenal glands as part of widespread dissemination, detected at autopsy in as many as 20% of patients.[192] Rarely, the destruction of the adrenal glands by lymphoma can cause clinical adrenal insufficiency, which may resolve after chemotherapy.[193] Primary non-Hodgkin's lymphoma of the adrenal glands is extremely rare and is almost always unilateral (Fig. 11–30). In 1990, Choi et al.[194] reported a B-cell diffuse large-cell lymphoma involving the right adrenal gland and summarized the literature. They identified 13 other cases of primary adrenal gland lymphoma—eight bilateral and five unilateral.[194] The histologic subtypes reported were three diffuse mixed small and large cell, six diffuse large cell, one large cell immunoblastic, and four lymphosarcoma, not otherwise specified. Nine cases were analyzed immunophenotypically: seven B-cell and two T-cell.[194] However, in these studies, many cases had relatively short clinical follow-up or less than extensive clinical work-up. In our opinion, in patients presenting with bilateral involvement of the adrenal glands, systemic disease should be suspected and looked for extensively. We are not aware of a well-documented example of Hodgkin's disease arising in the adrenal gland.

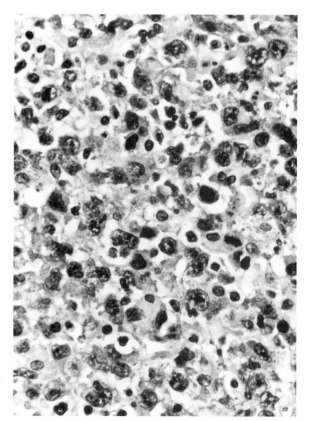

FIGURE 11–30. Malignant lymphoma presenting in the adrenal gland. This anaplastic large-cell lymphoma had a T-cell immunophenotype and also expressed the CD30 antigen.

Primary malignant melanomas of the adrenal gland have been reported.[31, 195] The most important issue in establishing this diagnosis is excluding the possibility of metastasis. Criteria proposed to establish the diagnosis or primary malignant melanoma of the adrenal gland are (1) unilateral adrenal gland involvement; (2) no previous or current pigmented lesions of the skin, mucosa, or retina; (3) melanin in the neoplastic cells; and (4) absence of extra-adrenal site of tumor as determined by autopsy.[195]

Grossly, adrenal gland melanomas may be small or quite large, pigmented, with hemorrhage and necrosis. Histologically, these tumors resemble melanoma at other sites. The prognosis for patients with primary melanoma of the adrenal gland is extremely poor.[31]

Malignant mesenchymal tumors also arise in the adrenal gland. For example, rare examples of angiosarcoma,[196] leiomyosarcoma,[197] and malignant nerve sheath tumor[198] have been described. These tumors are similar to their soft tissue counterparts. Malignant nerve sheath tumors may occur in association with a ganglioneuroma.[198]

Carcinosarcoma of the adrenal gland also has been described. Fischler et al.[199] described a 610-g mass composed of adrenal cortical carcinoma, fibrosarcoma, and rhabdomyosarcoma. An adrenal carcinosarcoma in which the sarcomatous component showed osteosarcomatous and chondroid differentiation has also been reported. In this case, a 79-year-old woman presented with clinical signs of hyperaldosteronism.[200]

Molberg et al.[201] have described a 1048-g neoplasm that arose in the adrenal gland of a 21-month-old child. The tumor was composed of slit-like spaces lined by epithelium, islands of anaplastic epithelial cells, and immature mesenchymal stroma. The authors likened these findings to those of the embryonal adrenal gland cortex. They named this neoplasm adrenocortical blastoma and hypothesized that this neoplasm was the adrenal gland counterpart of Wilms' tumor and hepatoblastoma.

ADRENAL PSEUDOCYSTS

More than 300 cysts and cyst-like lesions of the adrenal gland have been reported in the literature. Others[202] have subdivided these lesions into four general groups: pseudocysts, cystic neoplasms, true cysts, and infectious cysts. Of these, pseudocysts and cystic neoplasms are most common. True cysts of the adrenal gland are exceedingly rare.

Pseudocysts are cyst-like lesions arising within either the adrenal cortex or the medulla that are lined by a fibrous tissue wall devoid of a recognizable layer of lining cells.[202]

Pathologic Features

Grossly, adrenal pseudocysts may be small or extremely large, cyst-like masses containing several liters of brown or bloody fluid. In one study, their median size was reported to be 12 to 13 cm in diameter.[203] Although usually unilateral, approximately 10% of all lesions reported have been bilateral.[203] Pseudocysts often contain abundant necrotic material, hemorrhage, and thrombus. Calcification of the contents and/or the fibrous wall is common. Diffuse calcification of the

wall (so-called eggshell calcification) may be recognized radiologically and is useful diagnostically.[204]

Histologically, pseudocysts are surrounded by a wall composed of well-organized fibrous tissue, without a layer of lining cells (Fig. 11–31).[203, 205] Within the wall, there are often foci of macrophages and blood pigment, either hemosiderin or hematoidin. Elastic tissue and smooth muscle may be found in the wall of some cases, and the latter may be continuous with the adrenal vein muscle.[205] Adrenal cortical cells are commonly entrapped within the wall.[203] Calcification is common, and metaplastic bone formation is not unusual.[205] Surrounding the wall, many sinusoids and small blood vessels may be found. In some cases, analysis of multiple sections suggests that these sinusoids appear to coalesce and form the pseudocyst cavity.[205] An intact lining cell layer is absent. However, in some lesions, small foci of lining cells may be identified that are cuboidal or flattened, without cytologic atypia. The contents of the pseudocyst are composed of a variable mixture of necrotic material, histiocytes laden with lipid and/or either hemosiderin or hematoidin pigment, thrombus, blood-filled spaces, and islands of adrenal cortical cells. Foci of intracystic fat or even myelolipomatous metaplasia also may be present[206] (Fig. 11–32).

Immunohistochemical studies have suggested that many adrenal pseudocysts are of vascular origin.[203, 205, 207] The small foci of residual lining cells in these lesions may express Factor VIII–related antigen, suggestive of blood vessel origin,[205] or may be negative for Factor VIII–related antigen but positive for collagen type IV, suggestive of lymphatic differentia-

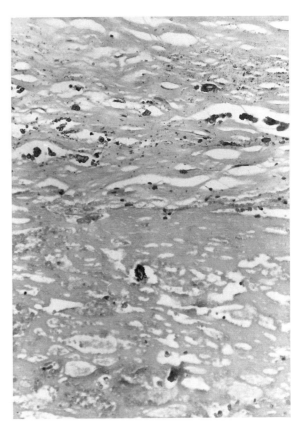

FIGURE 11–31. Adrenal pseudocyst. *Top*, there is a fibrous wall with calcification. *Below*, The cyst contains fibrin, also with calcification.

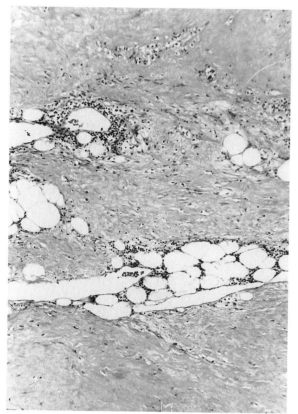

FIGURE 11–32. Adrenal pseudocyst. This pseudocyst shows foci of myelolipomatous transformation. Also note small nests of adrenal cortical cells adjacent to the myelolipomatous foci.

tion.[203] Furthermore, in pseudocysts entirely devoid of any lining cells, the wall of these lesions may stain for laminin or collagen type IV, suggesting derivation from lymphatics.[207] Incze et al.,[208] using electron microscopy, also suggested that these lesions are of lymphatic origin.

In summary, although the origin of adrenal pseudocysts is currently uncertain, at least a subset of these lesions appears to arise from either lymphatic channels or blood vessels (either normal or malformed), with overlapping degenerative changes.

Differential Diagnosis

ADRENAL PSEUDOCYST VERSUS ADRENAL CORTICAL CARCINOMA. It is important not to misdiagnose a pseudocyst as carcinoma. In particular, the presence of abundant necrosis and hemorrhage and the common finding of islands of adrenal cortical cells within the cyst contents have been confused with cortical carcinoma in the past.[203] Although adrenal cortical carcinomas may be cystic, we have not seen a case in which cystic degeneration totally destroyed the neoplastic cortical cells, resulting in a fibrous tissue wall surrounding necrosis. Furthermore, the neoplastic cells demonstrate significant nuclear atypia, mitotic figures, or evidence of invasion.[16] Conversely, the islands of entrapped adrenal cortex present in the fibrous wall and pseudocyst contents do not exhibit significant nuclear atypia or mitotic figures.

ADRENAL PSEUDOCYST VERSUS OTHER CYSTIC ADRENAL TUMORS. Adrenal neoplasms such as adenomas and pheochro-

mocytomas may be cystic, and in some cases the majority of the tumor may be cystic. For example, Melicow[93] described a 32 × 24 cm cystic pheochromocytoma in which only a small area of pheochromocytoma was identified. Nevertheless, extreme examples such as this case are rare, and we have not observed a cystic neoplasm of the adrenal gland in which residual tumor was not easily identifiable. Also, benign adrenal tumors are often clinically functional. Adrenal pseudocysts are almost always clearly non-functional, although rare lesions have been associated with hypertension.[209]

ADRENAL PSEUDOCYST VERSUS METASTATIC CARCINOMA. Carcinomas frequently metastasize to the adrenal glands. Of these, lung, breast, and gastrointestinal tract carcinomas metastasize to the adrenal glands most frequently. Although metastatic lesions may undergo necrosis and cystic formation, the clinical setting is usually well known, and residual metastatic neoplasm is usually readily apparent. However, Gaffey et al.[206] have described one adrenal gland lesion that grossly and histologically resembled a pseudocyst except for the presence of one small focus of anaplastic metastatic carcinoma. Subsequent clinical work-up revealed a primary carcinoma of the breast, histologically similar to the neoplasm in the adrenal gland. The explanation for these findings was unclear. The metastatic tumor and the pseudocyst may have involved the adrenal gland coincidentally. Alternatively, the metastatic neoplasm may have caused the pseudocyst to develop. This case highlights the need for complete sampling of an adrenal cyst-like lesion before concluding that the lesion is a pseudocyst.[206]

Levin et al.[210] also reported an adrenal pseudocyst that was clinically misdiagnosed as metastatic carcinoma. In this case, a 2-month-old child presented with a right chest wall mass destroying the right tenth rib and a 6-cm right upper quadrant mass displacing the kidney inferiorly. Surgical excision revealed a right adrenal gland pseudocyst that dissected superiorly between the chest wall and the pleura to form the right chest wall mass. Although clinically confused with an adrenal tumor with metastasis to the chest wall, the pathologic findings were straightforward.[210]

ADRENAL PSEUDOCYST VERSUS INFECTIOUS CYSTS. A variety of infectious agents may involve and destroy the adrenal gland, with the formation of cavitary lesions in some cases.[211] Radiologically and grossly, these diseases may resemble a pseudocyst. A few of the most common infectious agents include echinococcus, *Mycobacterium tuberculosis,* and fungal infections such as histoplasmosis and blastomycosis.

Histologically, although these lesions are characterized by abundant necrosis and may be surrounded by a fibrous tissue lining wall, the presence of the infectious agent establishes the correct diagnosis. In addition, these lesions most commonly occur in the setting of systemic infection, and, with echinococcus, a travel history or history of exposure to sheep is usually present. Furthermore, these diseases often affect the adrenal glands bilaterally and may cause adrenal insufficiency,[211] a presentation that would be rare for an adrenal gland pseudocyst.

ADRENAL PSEUDOCYST VERSUS NEONATAL MICROCYSTS. In stillborns and young infants, at autopsy small cysts have been commonly identified within the adrenal cortex.[212] These cysts are lined by benign adrenal cortical cells. These lesions are either a normal finding in the development of the adrenal cortex, or more likely, are related to stress. The clinical setting and the histologic features are quite distinct from other cystic lesions of the adrenal gland.

ADRENAL PSEUDOCYST VERSUS OTHER UPPER ABDOMINAL SPACE-OCCUPYING LESIONS. Other lesions that clinically may be confused with adrenal pseudocysts but are pathologically distinct include mesenteric cysts, empyema of the gallbladder, urachal cysts, hepatic hemangiomas, hydronephrosis, multicystic kidneys, and choledochal cysts.[203]

TRUE CYSTS OF THE ADRENAL GLAND

True cysts of the adrenal gland are cystic spaces that are surrounded by a lining layer of cells. In the literature, the term "true" cyst has been used for cysts surrounded by endothelium as well as those surrounded by epithelium or mesothelium. We believe that the former are closely related to pseudocysts (described earlier). Here we discuss true cysts that are not endothelial.

Pathologic Features

True cysts lined by epithelium or mesothelium are rare, small, and usually asymptomatic, and are discovered at the time of autopsy. We have studied one such lesion, a 4.0-cm cyst filled with serous fluid that histologically was shown to be lined by a layer of cytologically bland cuboidal and flattened cells[213] (Fig. 11–33). These cells immunohistochemically were shown to express keratin and to be negative for Factor VIII–related antigen. We concluded that the cyst was most likely lined by cells of mesothelial origin, although true epithelial origin could not be excluded.[213] Rare glandular retention cysts described in the literature may also arise on the basis of mesothelial inclusions.[202]

Differential Diagnosis

TRUE CYST OF ADRENAL GLAND VERSUS ADRENAL PSEUDO-CYST. As described previously, pseudocysts are histologically quite distinct from true cysts. An intact lining layer is not found in pseudocysts, the contents of pseudocysts markedly differ from that of a true cyst, and immunohistochemical studies do not demonstrate keratin-positive lining cells in pseudocysts. Also, pseudocysts are usually larger than true cysts. However, the occurrence of true cysts lined by epithelium/mesothelium raises the possibility that some pseudocysts may also originate from mesothelial inclusions.

TRUE CYST OF ADRENAL GLAND VERSUS CYSTIC ADRENAL NEOPLASMS. In the literature, some investigators have referred to benign adrenal neoplasms with central cystic degeneration as true cysts of the adrenal gland.[214] We do not agree with this designation. Cystic adrenal neoplasms are easily distinguished from true mesothelial cysts in which no evidence of neoplasm is found.

ADENOMATOID TUMOR

Pathologic Features

Two case reports have described adenomatoid tumors involving the adrenal gland.[215, 216] Similar cases were reported previously under the designation of lymphangioma.[217] In both cases, the lesions were small (approximately 3.0 cm and 1.1 cm, respectively) and gray or pale white.

Histologically, these tumors are composed of nests and cords of epithelioid cells with a multicystic component. The lesions diffusely infiltrated the adrenal gland cortex (Fig. 11–34); one lesion was reported to have extended out of the adrenal gland into periadrenal adipose tissue. The borders were not encapsulated.

Electron microscopic examination of one case and immunohistochemical studies in both cases showed evidence supporting mesothelial differentiation. The epithelioid cells had desmosomes and microvilli and expressed keratins.[215]

Differential Diagnosis

ADRENAL ADENOMATOID TUMOR VERSUS ADENOCARCINOMA. The infiltrative borders of an adenomatoid tumor

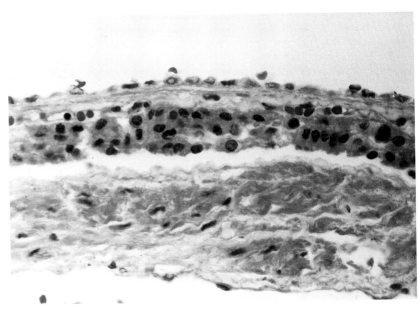

FIGURE 11–33. True cyst of the adrenal. An attenuated lining of epithelial cells is seen at the top overlying a layer of benign adrenal cortical cells.

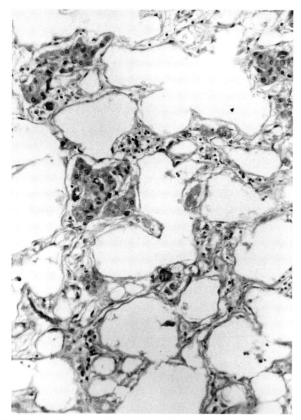

FIGURE 11–34. Adrenal adenomatoid tumor. Dilated spaces are seen between small nests of adrenal cortex. This lesion may be mistaken for a lymphangioma without the appropriate immunohistochemical studies.

should not be misconstrued as evidence of a malignant neoplasm, either primary to the adrenal gland or metastatic. The clinical setting and the small size of these lesions argue against a malignant diagnosis. Furthermore, although the cells are epithelioid, significant cytologic atypia and mitotic figures are absent or very rare in adenomatoid tumors, in contrast with a malignant neoplasm.

ADRENAL ADENOMATOID TUMOR VERSUS TRUE CYST. Unlike adenomatoid tumors, true cysts are much more simple cystic structures, confined to the adrenal gland, and without infiltrative borders. However, because true cysts are also likely to arise from mesothelial inclusions, both true mesothelial cysts and adenomatoid tumors appear to be closely related.

Acknowledgments

The authors thank Roberto N. Miranda, M.D., for his critical review of the manuscript.

References

1. Spain DM, Weinsaft P: Solitary adrenal cortical adenoma in elderly female: Frequency. Arch Pathol Lab Med 78:231–233, 1964.
2. Commons RR, Callaway CP: Adenomas of the adrenal cortex. Arch Intern Med 81:37–41, 1948.
3. Robinson MJ, Pardo V, Rywlin AM: Pigmented nodules (black adenomas) of the adrenal: An autopsy study of incidence, morphology, and function. Hum Pathol 3:317–325, 1972.
4. Dobbie JW: Adrenocortical nodular hyperplasia: The aging adrenal. J Pathol 99:1–18, 1969.
5. Copeland PM: The incidentally discovered adrenal mass. Ann Intern Med 98:940–945, 1983.
6. Prinz RA, Brooks MH, Churchill R, et al: Incidental asymptomatic adrenal masses detected by computed tomographic screening: Is operation required? JAMA 248:701–704, 1982.
7. Boggan JE, Tyrrell JB, Wilson CB: Transsphenoidal microsurgical management of Cushing's disease: Report of 100 cases. J Neurosurg 59:195–200, 1983.
8. Doppman JL, Miller DL, Dwyer AJ, et al: Macronodular adrenocortical hyperplasia in longstanding Cushing's disease. Radiology 166:347–352, 1988.
9. Jessop DS, Cunnah D, Millar JGB, et al: A pheochromocytoma presenting with Cushing's syndrome associated with increased concentrations of circulating corticotropin-releasing factor. J Endocrinol 113:133–138, 1987.
10. Neville AM, Symington T: The pathology of the adrenal gland in Cushing's syndrome. J Pathol Bacteriol 93:19–35, 1967.
11. Cohen RB, Chapman WB, Castleman B: Hyperadrenocorticism (Cushing's disease): A study of surgically resected adrenal glands. Am J Pathol 35:537–561, 1959.
12. Kay S: Hyperplasia and neoplasia of the adrenal gland. Pathol Annu 11:103–137, 1976.
13. Hayles AB, Hahn HB, Sprague RG, et al: Hormone-secreting tumors of the adrenal cortex in children. Pediatrics 37:19–25, 1966.
14. Tang CL, Gray GF: Adrenocortical neoplasms: Prognosis and morphology. Urology 5:691–695, 1975.
15. Weiss LM: Comparative histologic study of 43 metastasizing and nonmetastasizing adrenocortical tumors. Am J Surg Pathol 8:163–169, 1984.
16. Medeiros LJ, Weiss LM: New developments in the pathologic diagnosis of adrenal cortical neoplasms: A review. Am J Clin Pathol 97:73–83, 1992.
17. Aiba M, Iri H, Suzuki H, et al: Numerous mast cells in an 11-deoxycorticosterone-producing adrenocortical tumor: Histologic evaluation of benignancy and comparison with mast cell distribution in adrenal glands and neoplastic counterparts of 67 surgical specimens. Arch Pathol Lab Med 109:357–360, 1985.
18. David DA, Medline NM: Spironolactone (aldactone) bodies: Concentric lamellar formations in the adrenal cortices of patients treated with spironolactone. Am J Clin Pathol 54:22–32, 1970.
19. Shrago SS, Waisman J, Cooper PH: Spironolactone bodies in an adrenal adenoma. Arch Pathol Lab Med 99:416–420, 1975.
20. Vyberg M, Sestoft L: Combined adrenal myelolipoma and adenoma associated with Cushing's syndrome. Am J Clin Pathol 86:541–545, 1986.
21. Granger JK, Houn H-Y, Collins C: Massive hemorrhagic functional adrenal adenoma histologically mimicking angiosarcoma: Report of a case with immunohistochemical study. Am J Surg Pathol 15:699–704, 1991.
22. Macadam RF: Black adenoma of the human adrenal cortex. Cancer 27:116–119, 1971.
23. Damron TA, Schelper RL, Sorensen L: Cytochemical demonstration of neuromelanin in black pigmented adrenal nodules. Am J Clin Pathol 87:334–341, 1987.
24. Sasano H, Suzuki T, Sano T, et al: Adrenocortical oncocytoma: A true nonfunctioning adrenocortical tumor. Am J Surg Pathol 15:949–956, 1991.
25. Medeiros LJ, Gelb AB, Weiss LM: Low grade renal cell carcinoma: A clinicopathologic study of fifty-three cases. Am J Surg Pathol 11:633–642, 1987.
26. Tannenbaum M: Ultrastructural pathology of the adrenal cortex. Pathol Annu 8:109–156, 1973.
27. Osanai T, Konta A, Chui D, et al: Electron microscopic findings in benign deoxycorticosterone and 11-deoxycortisol-producing adrenal tumor. Arch Pathol Lab Med 114:829–831, 1990.
28. Hogan MJ, Schambelan M, Biglieri EG: Concurrent hypercortisolism and hypermineralocorticoidism. Am J Med 62:777–782, 1977.
29. Sasidharan K, Sunderlal Babu A, Pandey AP, et al: Primary melanoma of the adrenal gland: A case report. J Urol 117:663–664, 1977.
30. Third National Cancer Survey: Incidence Data. National Cancer Institute Monograph 41, March 1975 (DHEW publication no. (NIH) 75-787). Bethesda, MD, National Cancer Institute, National Institutes of Health, U.S. Department of Health, Education, and Welfare, Public Health Service, 1975.
31. Alterman SL, Dominguez C, Lopez-Gomez A, et al: Primary adrenocortical carcinoma causing aldosteronism. Cancer 24:602–609, 1969.
32. Didolkar MS, Bescher RA, Elias EG, et al: Natural history of adrenal cortical carcinoma: A clinicopathologic study of 42 patients. Cancer 47:2153–2161, 1981.
33. Heinbecker P, O'Neal LW, Ackerman LV: Functioning and nonfunctioning adrenal cortical tumors. Surg Gynecol Obstet 105:21–33, 1957.
34. Wooten MD, King DK: Adrenal cortical carcinoma. Epidemiology and treatment with mitotane and a review of the literature. Cancer 72:3145–3155, 1993.
35. Greenberg PH, Marks C: Adrenal cortical carcinoma: A presentation of 22 cases and a review of the literature. Am Surg 44:81–85, 1978.
36. Luton J-P, Cerdas S, Billaud L, et al: Clinical features of adrenocortical carcinoma, prognostic factors, and the effect of mitotane therapy. N Engl J Med 322:1195–1201, 1990.
37. Nakano M: Adrenal cortical carcinoma: A clinicopathologic and immunohistochemical study of 91 autopsy cases. Acta Pathol Jpn 38:163–180, 1988.
38. Nader S, Hickey RC, Sellin RV, et al: Adrenal cortical carcinoma: A study of 77 cases. Cancer 52:707–711, 1983.
39. Gandour MJ, Grizzle WE: A small adrenocortical carcinoma with aggressive behavior: An evaluation of criteria for malignancy. Arch Pathol Lab Med 110:1076–1079, 1986.
40. Hough AJ, Hollifield JW, Page DL, et al: Prognostic factors in adrenal cortical tumors: A mathematical analysis of clinical and morphologic data. Am J Clin Pathol 72:390–399, 1979.
41. Van Slooten H, Schaberg A, Smeenk D, et al: Morphologic characteristics of benign and malignant adrenocortical tumors. Cancer 55:766–773, 1985.

42. Tang C-K, Harriman BB, Toker C: Myxoid adrenal cortical carcinoma. Arch Pathol Lab Med 103:635–638, 1979.

43. Miettinen M: Neuroendocrine differentiation in adrenocortical carcinoma: New immunohistochemical findings supported by electron microscopy. Lab Invest 66:169–174, 1992.

44. Gaffey MJ, Traweek ST, Mills SE, et al: Cytokeratin expression in adrenocortical neoplasia: An immunohistochemical and biochemical study with implications for the differential diagnosis of adrenocortical, hepatocellular, and renal cell carcinoma. Hum Pathol 23:144–153, 1992.

45. Wick MR, Cherwitz DL, McGlennen RC, et al: Adrenocortical carcinoma: An immunohistochemical comparison with renal cell carcinoma. Am J Pathol 122:343–352, 1986.

46. Cote RJ, Cordon-Cardo C, Reuter VE, et al: Immunopathology of adrenal and renal cortical tumors: Coordinated change in antigen expression is associated with neoplastic conversion in the adrenal cortex. Am J Pathol 136:1077–1084, 1990.

47. Henzen-Logmans SC, Stel HV, Van Muijen GNP, et al: Expression of intermediate filament proteins in adrenal cortex and related tumors. Histopathology 12:359–372, 1988.

48. Miettinen M, Lehto V-P, Virtanen I: Immunofluorescence microscopic evaluation of the intermediate filament expression of the adrenal cortex and medulla and their tumors. Am J Pathol 118:360–366, 1985.

49. Suzuki T, Sasano H, Nisikawa T, et al: Discerning malignancy in human adrenocortical neoplasms: Utility of DNA flow cytometry and immunohistochemistry. Mod Pathol 5:224–231, 1992.

50. Sasano H, Nose M, Sasano MN: Lectin immunohistochemistry in adrenocortical hyperplasia and neoplasms with emphasis on carcinoma. Arch Pathol Lab Med 113:68–72, 1989.

51. Kamio T, Shigematsu K, Sou H, et al: Immunohistochemical expression of epidermal growth factor receptors in human adrenocortical carcinoma. Hum Pathol 21:277–282, 1990.

52. Schroder S, Niendorf A, Achilles E, et al: Immunocytochemical differential diagnosis of adrenocortical neoplasms using the monoclonal antibody D11. Virchows Archiv A Pathol Anat 417:89–96, 1990.

53. Tartour E, Caillou B, Tenenbaum F, et al: Immunohistochemical study of adrenocortical carcinoma. Predictive value of the D11 monoclonal antibody. Cancer 72:3296–3303, 1993.

54. Silva EG, Mackay B, Samaan NA, Hickey RC: Adrenocortical carcinomas: An ultrastructural study of 22 cases. Ultrastruct Pathol 3:1–7, 1982.

55. Wiedemann HR: Tumors and hemihypertrophy associated with Wiedemann-Beckwith syndrome. Eur J Pediatr 141:129, 1983.

56. Lynch HT, Mulcahy GM, Harris RE, et al: Genetic and pathologic findings in a kindred with hereditary sarcoma, breast cancer, brain tumors, leukemia, lung, laryngeal, and adrenal cortical carcinoma. Cancer 41:2055–2064, 1978.

57. Henry I, Jeanpierre M, Couillin P, et al: Molecular definition of the 11p15.5 region involved in Beckwith-Wiedemann syndrome and probably in predisposition to adrenocortical carcinoma. Hum Genet 81:273–277, 1989.

58. Henry I, Grandjouan S, Couillin P, et al: Tumor-specific loss of 11p15.5 alleles in del11p13 Wilms' tumor and in familial adrenocortical carcinoma. Proc Natl Acad Sci USA 86:3247–3251, 1989.

59. Yano T, Linehan M, Anglard P, et al: Genetic changes in human adrenocortical carcinomas. J Natl Cancer Inst 81:518–523, 1989.

60. Koufos A, Hansen MF, Copeland NG, et al: Loss of heterozygosity in three embryonal tumors suggests a common pathogenetic mechanism. Nature 316:330–334, 1985.

61. Fearon ER, Vogelstein B: A genetic model for colorectal tumorigenesis. Cell 61:759–767, 1990.

62. Macfarlane DA: Cancer of the adrenal cortex: The natural history, prognosis, and treatment in a study of fifty-five cases. Ann R Coll Surg Engl 23:155–186, 1958.

63. Sullivan M, Boileau M, Hodges CV: Adrenal cortical carcinoma. J Urol 120:660–665, 1978.

64. Henley DJ, Van Heerden JA, Grant CS, et al: Adrenal cortical carcinoma—a continuing challenge. Surgery 94:926–931, 1983.

65. Bodie B, Novick AC, Pontes JE, et al: The Cleveland Clinic experience with adrenal cortical carcinoma. J Urol 141:257–260, 1989.

66. Brennan MF: Adrenocortical carcinoma. CA 37:348–365, 1987.

67. Richie JP, Gittes RF: Carcinoma of the adrenal cortex. Cancer 45:1957–1964, 1980.

68. Venkatesh S, Hickey RC, Selin RV, et al: Adrenal cortical carcinoma. Cancer 64:765–769, 1989.

69. Weiss LM, Medeiros LJ, Vickery AL: Pathologic features of prognostic significance in adrenal cortical carcinoma. Am J Surg Pathol 13:202–206, 1989.

70. Goldblum JR, Shannon R, Kaldjian EP, et al: Immunohistochemical assessment of proliferative activity in adrenocortical neoplasms. Mod Pathol 6:663–668, 1993.

71. Page DL, Hough AJ, Gray GF: Diagnosis and prognosis of adrenocortical neoplasms. Arch Pathol Lab Med 110:993–994, 1986.

72. Cagle PT, Hough AJ, Pysher J, et al: Comparison of adrenal cortical tumors in children and adults. Cancer 57:2235–2237, 1986.

73. Medeiros LJ, Weiss LM: Adrenal cortical neoplasms in children. In reply [letter]. Am J Clin Pathol 98:382–383, 1992.

74. Lack EE, Mulvihill JJ, Travis WD, et al: Adrenal cortical neoplasms in the pediatric and adolescent age group: Clinicopathologic study of 30 cases with emphasis on epidemiological and prognostic factors. Pathol Annu 27:1–53, 1992.

75. Humphrey GB, Pysher T, Holcombe J, et al: Overview of the management of adrenocortical carcinoma (ACC). In Humphrey GB, Grindey GB, Dehner LP, et al (eds): Adrenal and Endocrine Tumors in Children. Boston, Martinus Nijhoff Publishing, 1984, pp 349–358.

76. Bugg MF, Ribeiro RC, Roberson PK, et al: Correlation of pathologic features with clinical outcome in pediatric adrenocortical neoplasia: A study of a Brazilian population. Am J Clin Pathol 101:625–629, 1994.

77. Klein FA, Kay S, Ratliff JE, et al: Flow cytometric determinations of ploidy and proliferation patterns of adrenal neoplasms: An adjunct to histologic classification. J Urol 134:862–866, 1985.

78. Bowlby LS, DeBault LE, Abraham SR: Flow cytometric analysis of adrenal cortical tumor DNA: Relationship between cellular DNA and histopathologic classification. Cancer 58:1499–1505, 1986.

79. Taylor SR, Roederer M, Murphy RF: Flow cytometric DNA analysis of adrenocortical tumors in children. Cancer 59:2059–2063, 1987.

80. Camuto P, Schinella R, Gilchrist K, et al: Flow cytometric study of adrenal cortical carcinoma [abstract]. Lab Invest 56:10, 1987.

81. Cibas ES, Medeiros LJ, Weinberg DS, et al: Cellular DNA profiles of benign and malignant adrenocortical tumors. Am J Surg Pathol 14:948–955, 1990.

82. Padberg B-C, Lauritzen I, Achilles E, et al: DNA cytophotometry in adrenocortical tumors: A clinicomorphological study of 66 cases. Virch Arch A Pathol Anat 419:167–170, 1991.

83. Hill GJ, Wheeler HB: Adrenal insufficiency due to metastatic carcinoma of the lung. Cancer 18:1467–1473, 1965.

84. Twomey P, Montgomery C, Clark O: Successful treatment of adrenal metastases from large-cell carcinoma of the lung. JAMA 248:581–583, 1982.

85. Jagirda J, Irie T, French SW, et al: Globular Mallory-like bodies in renal cell carcinoma: Report of a case and review of cytoplasmic eosinophilic globules. Hum Pathol 16:949–952, 1985.

86. Medeiros LJ, Michie SA, Johnson DE, et al: An immunoperoxidase study of renal cell carcinomas: Correlation with nuclear grade, cell type, and pattern. Hum Pathol 19:980–987, 1988.

87. Ganjei P, Nadji M, Albores-Saavedra J, et al: Histologic markers in primary and metastatic tumors of the liver. Cancer 62:1994–1998, 1988.

88. Johnson DE, Herndier BG, Medeiros LJ, et al: The diagnostic utility of the keratin profiles of hepatocellular carcinoma and cholangiocarcinoma. Am J Surg Pathol 12:187–197, 1988.

89. Samaan NA, Hickey RC: Pheochromocytoma. Semin Oncol 14:297–305, 1987.

90. Wilson RA, Ibanez ML: A comparative study of 14 cases of familial and nonfamilial pheochromocytomas. Hum Pathol 9:181–188, 1978.

91. Webb TA, Sheps SG, Carney JA: Differences between sporadic pheochromocytoma and pheochromocytoma in multiple endocrine neoplasia, type 2. Am J Surg Pathol 4:121–126, 1980.

92. Medeiros LJ, Wolf BC, Balogh K, et al: Adrenal pheochromocytoma: A clinicopathologic review of 60 cases. Hum Pathol 16:580–589, 1985.

93. Melicow MM: One hundred cases of pheochromocytoma (107 tumors) at the Columbia-Presbyterian Medical Center, 1926–1976: A clinicopathologic analysis. Cancer 40:1987–2004, 1977.

94. Linnoila RI, Keiser HR, Steinberg SM, et al: Histopathology of benign versus malignant sympathoadrenal paragangliomas: Clinicopathologic study of 120 cases including unusual histologic features. Hum Pathol 21:1168–1180, 1990.

95. Shin W-Y, Groman GS, Berkman JI: Pheochromocytoma with angiomatous features: A case report and ultrastructural study. Cancer 40:275–283, 1977.

96. Ramsay JA, Asa SL, Van Nostrand AWP, et al: Lipid degeneration in pheochromocytomas mimicking adrenal cortical tumors. Am J Surg Pathol 11:480–486, 1987.

97. DeLellis RA, Suchow E, Wolfe JH: Ultrastructure of nuclear ''inclusions'' in pheochromocytoma and paraganglioma. Hum Pathol 11:205–207, 1980.

98. Dekker A, Oehrle JS: Hyaline globules of the adrenal medulla of man. Am J Clin Pathol 91:353–364, 1971.

99. Mendelsohn G, Olson JL: Pheochromocytomas [letter]. Hum Pathol 9:607–608, 1978.

100. Lloyd RV, Blaivas M, Wilson BS: Distribution of chromogranin and S100 protein in normal and abnormal adrenal medullary tissues. Arch Pathol Lab Med 109:633–635, 1985.

101. Unger P, Hoffman K, Pertsemlidis D, et al: S100 protein-positive sustentacular cells in malignant and locally aggressive adrenal pheochromocytomas. Arch Pathol Lab Med 115:484–487, 1991.

102. Steinhoff MM, Wells SA, DeSchryver-Kecskemeti K: Stromal amyloid in pheochromocytomas. Hum Pathol 23:33–36, 1992.

103. Triche TJ, Askin FB: Neuroblastoma and the differential diagnosis of small-, round-, blue-cell tumors. Hum Pathol 14:569–595, 1983.

104. Lloyd RV, Shapiro B, Sisson JC, et al: An immunohistochemical study of pheochromocytomas. Arch Pathol Lab Med 108:541–544, 1984.

105. Gould VE, Wiedenmann B, Lee I, et al: Synaptophysin expression in neuroendocrine neoplasms as determined by immunocytochemistry. Am J Pathol 126:243–257, 1987.

106. Hartmann C-A, Gross U, Stein H: Cushing syndrome-associated pheochromocytoma and adrenal carcinoma: An immunohistological investigation. Pathol Res Pract 188:287–295, 1992.

107. Linnoila RI, Lack EE, Steinberg SM, et al: Decreased expression of neuropeptides in malignant paragangliomas: An immunohistochemical study. Hum Pathol 19:41–50, 1988.

108. DeLellis RA, Tischler AS, Lee AK, et al: Leu-enkephalin-like immunoreactivity in proliferative lesions of the human adrenal medulla and extra-adrenal paraganglia. Am J Surg Pathol 7:29–37, 1983.

109. Trojanowski JQ, Lee VM-Y: Expression of neurofilament antigens by normal and neoplastic human adrenal chromaffin cells. N Engl J Med 313:101–104, 1985.

110. Helman LJ, Cohen PS, Averbuch SD, et al: Neuropeptide Y expression distinguishes malignant from benign pheochromocytoma. J Clin Oncol 7:1720–1725, 1989.
111. Berenyi MR, Singh G, Gloster ES, et al: ACTH-producing pheochromocytoma. Arch Pathol Lab Med 101:31–35, 1977.
112. Misugi K, Misugi N, Newton WA: Fine structural study of neuroblastoma, ganglioneuroblastoma, and pheochromocytoma. Arch Pathol Lab Med 86:160–170, 1968.
113. Medeiros LJ, Katsas GG, Balogh K: Brown fat and adrenal pheochromocytoma: Association or coincidence? Hum Pathol 16:970–972, 1985.
114. Melicow MM: Hibernating fat and pheochromocytoma. Arch Pathol Lab Med 63:367–372, 1957.
115. Scott HW, Halter SA: Oncologic aspects of pheochromocytoma: The importance of follow-up. Surgery 96:1061–1066, 1984.
116. Hosoda S, Suzuki H, Oguri T, et al: Adrenal pheochromocytoma with both benign and malignant components. Acta Pathol Jpn 26:519–531, 1976.
117. King ESJ: Malignant pheochromocytoma of the adrenals. J Pathol Bacteriol 34:447, 1931.
118. Hosaka Y, Rainwater LM, Grant CS, et al: Pheochromocytoma: Nuclear deoxyribonucleic acid patterns studied by flow cytometry. Surgery 10:1003–1009, 1986.
119. Amberson JB, Vaughan ED, Gray GF, et al: Flow cytometric determination of nuclear DNA content in benign adrenal pheochromocytomas. Urology 30:102–104, 1987.
120. Padberg B-C, Garbe E, Achilles E, et al: Adrenomedullary hyperplasia and pheochromocytoma. DNA cytophotometric findings in 47 cases. Virchows Archiv A Pathol Anat 416:443–446, 1989.
121. Hoffman K, Gil J, Barba J, et al: Morphometric analysis of benign and malignant adrenal pheochromocytomas. Arch Pathol Lab Med 117:244–247, 1993.
122. Carney JA, Sizemore GW, Sheps SG: Adrenal medullary disease in multiple endocrine neoplasia, type 2: Pheochromocytoma and its precursors. Am J Clin Pathol 66:279–290, 1976.
123. DeLellis RA, Wolfe JH, Gagel RF, et al: Adrenal medullary hyperplasia: A morphometric analysis in patients with familial medullary carcinoma. Am J Pathol 83:177–196, 1976.
124. Dehner LP: Classic neuroblastoma: Histopathologic grading as a prognostic indicator. The Shimada system and its progenitors. Am J Pediatr Hematol Oncol 10:143–154, 1988.
125. Mendelsohn G, Baylin SB, Eggleston JC: Relationship of metastatic medullary thyroid carcinoma to calcitonin content of pheochromocytomas: An immunohistochemical study. Cancer 45:498–502, 1980.
126. Tischler AS, Dayal Y, Balogh K, et al: The distribution of immunoreactive chromogranins, S-100 protein, and vasoactive intestinal peptide in compound tumors of the adrenal medulla. Hum Pathol 18:909–917, 1987.
127. Schmid KW, Dockhorn-Dworniczak B, Fahrenkamp A, et al: Chromogranin A, secretogranin II and vasoactive intestinal peptide in phaeochromocytomas and ganglioneuromas. Histopathology 22:527–533, 1993.
128. Chetty R, Duhig JD: Bilateral pheochromocytoma-ganglioneuroma of the adrenal in type I neurofibromatosis. Am J Surg Pathol 17:837–841, 1993.
129. Balazs M: Mixed pheochromocytoma and ganglioneuroma of the adrenal medulla: A case report with electron microscopic examination. Hum Pathol 19:1352–1355, 1988.
130. Nakagawara A, Ikeda K, Tsuneyoshi M, et al: Malignant pheochromocytoma with ganglioneuroblastomatous elements in a patient with von Recklinghausen's disease. Cancer 55:2794–2798, 1985.
131. Aiba M, Hirayama A, Fujimoto Y, et al: A compound adrenal medullary tumor (pheochromocytoma and ganglioneuroma) and a cortical adenoma in the ipsilateral adrenal gland: A case report with enzyme histochemical and immunohistochemical studies. Am J Surg Pathol 12:559–566, 1988.
132. Min K-W, Clemens A, Bell J, et al: Malignant peripheral nerve sheath tumor and pheochromocytoma: A composite tumor of the adrenal. Arch Pathol Lab Med 112:266–270, 1988.
133. Tapia FJ, Polak JM, Barbosa AJA, et al: Neuron-specific enolase is produced by neuroendocrine tumours. Lancet 1:808–811, 1981.
134. Kragel PJ, Johnston CA: Pheochromocytoma-ganglioneuroma of the adrenal. Arch Pathol Lab Med 109:470–472, 1985.
135. Shimada H, Chatten J, Newton WA, et al: Histopathologic prognostic factors in neuroblastic tumors: Definition of subtypes of ganglioneuroblastoma and an age-linked classification of neuroblastomas. J Natl Cancer Inst 73:405–416, 1984.
136. Joshi VV, Cantor AB, Altshuler G, et al: Recommendations for modification of terminology of neuroblastic tumors and prognostic significance of Shimada classification. A clinicopathologic study of 213 cases from the Pediatric Oncology Group. Cancer 69:2183–2196, 1992.
137. Joshi VV, Cantor AB, Altshuler G, et al: Age-linked prognostic categorization based on a new histologic grading system of neuroblastomas. A clinicopathologic study of 211 cases from the Pediatric Oncology Group. Cancer 69:2197–2211, 1992.
138. Joshi VV, Silverman JF, Altshuler G, et al: Systematization of primary histopathologic and fine-needle aspiration cytologic features and description of unusual histopathologic features of neuroblastic tumors: A report from the Pediatric Oncology Group. Hum Pathol 24:493–504, 1993.
139. Young JL, Miller RW: Incidence of malignant tumors in U.S. children. J Pediatr 86:254–258, 1975.
140. Rosen EM, Cassady JR, Frantz CN, et al: Neuroblastoma: The Joint Center for Radiation Therapy/Dana-Farber Cancer Institute/Children's Hospital experience. J Clin Oncol 2:719–732, 1984.
141. Kinnier Wilson LM, Draper GJ: Neuroblastoma, its natural history and prognosis: A study of 487 cases. Br Med J 3:301–307, 1974.
142. Allan SG, Cornbleet MA, Carmichael J, et al: Adult neuroblastoma: Report of three cases and review of the literature. Cancer 57:2419–2421, 1986.
143. Aleshire SL, Glick AD, Cruz VE, et al: Neuroblastoma in adults: Pathologic findings and clinical outcome. Arch Pathol Lab Med 109:352–356, 1985.
144. Gonzalez-Crussi F, Hsueh W: Bilateral adrenal ganglioneuroblastoma with neuromelanin: Clinical and pathologic observations. Cancer 61:1159–1166, 1988.
145. Atkinson GO, Zaatari GS, Lorenzo RL, et al: Cystic neuroblastoma in infants: Radiographic and pathologic features. AJR 146:113–117, 1986.
146. Brook FB, Raafat F, Eldeeb BB, et al: Histologic and immunohistochemical investigation of neuroblastomas and correlation with prognosis. Hum Pathol 19:879–888, 1988.
147. Cozzutto C, Carbone A: Pleomorphic (anaplastic) neuroblastoma. Arch Pathol Lab Med 112:621–625, 1988.
148. Mullins JD: A pigmented differentiating neuroblastoma: A light and ultrastructural study. Cancer 45:522–528, 1980.
149. O'Dowd GM, Gaffney EF: Pigmented ganglioneuroblastoma: A tumour cell "storage disease"? Histopathology 22:591–593, 1993.
150. Koppersmith DL, Powers JM, Hennigan GR: Angiomatoid neuroblastoma with cytoplasmic glycogen: A case report with histogenetic considerations. Cancer 45:553–560, 1980.
151. Reynolds CP, Smith RG, Frenkel EP: The diagnostic dilemma of the "small round cell neoplasm." Catecholamine fluorescence and tissue culture morphology as markers for neuroblastoma. Cancer 48:2088–2094, 1981.
152. Tsokos M, Linnoila RI, Chandra RS, et al: Neuron-specific enolase in the diagnosis of neuroblastoma and other small, round-cell tumors in children. Hum Pathol 15:575–584, 1984.
153. Shimada H, Aoyama C, Chiba T, et al: Prognostic subgroups for undifferentiated neuroblastoma: Immunohistochemical study with anti-S100 protein antibody. Hum Pathol 16:471–476, 1985.
154. Taxy JB: Electron microscopy in the differential diagnosis of neuroblastoma. Arch Pathol Lab Med 104:355–360, 1980.
155. Look AT, Hayes FA, Nitschke R, et al: Cellular DNA content as a predictor of response to chemotherapy in infants with unresectable neuroblastoma. N Engl J Med 311:231–235, 1984.
156. Gansler T, Chatten J, Varello M, et al: Flow cytometric DNA analysis of neuroblastoma: Correlation with histology and clinical outcome. Cancer 58:2453–2458, 1986.
157. Kushner BH, Gilbert F, Helson L: Familial neuroblastoma: Case reports, literature review, and etiologic considerations. Cancer 57:1887–1893, 1986.
158. Knudson AG, Meadows AT: Regression of neuroblastoma IV-S: A genetic hypothesis. N Engl J Med 302:1254–1256, 1980.
159. Gilbert F, Feder M, Balaban G, et al: Human neuroblastoma and abnormalities of chromosomes 1 and 17. Cancer Res 44:5444–5449, 1984.
160. Brodeur GM, Seeger RC, Schwab M, et al: Amplification of N-myc in untreated human neuroblastomas correlates with advanced disease stage. Science 224:1121–1124, 1984.
161. Seeger RC, Brodeur GM, Sather H, et al: Association of multiple copies of the N-myc oncogene with rapid progression of neuroblastomas. N Engl J Med 313:1111–1116, 1985.
162. Frizzera G, Gajl-Peczalska K, Sibley RK, et al: Rosette formation in malignant lymphoma. Am J Pathol 119:351–356, 1985.
163. Dorfman RF: Childhood lymphosarcoma in St. Louis, Missouri, clinically and histologically resembling "Burkitt's tumor." Cancer 18:411–417, 1965.
164. Carlsen NLT, Christensen IBJ, Schroeder H, et al: Prognostic factors in neuroblastoma treated in Denmark from 1943 to 1980. Cancer 58:2726–2735, 1986.
165. Evans AE, D'Angio GJ, Randolph J: A proposed staging for children with neuroblastoma: Children's Cancer Study Group A. Cancer 27:374–378, 1971.
166. Evans AE, Chatten J, D'Angio GJ, et al: A review of 17 IV-S neuroblastoma patients at the Children's Hospital of Philadelphia. Cancer 45:833–839, 1980.
167. Evans AE, Baum E, Chard R: Do infants with stage IV-S neuroblastoma need treatment? Arch Dis Child 56:271–274, 1981.
168. Hughes M, Marsden HB, Palmer MK: Histologic patterns of neuroblastoma related to prognosis and clinical staging. Cancer 34:1706–1711, 1974.
169. Wang-Wuu S, Soukup S, Ballard E, et al: Chromosomal analysis of sixteen human rhabdomyosarcomas. Cancer Res 48:983–987, 1988.
170. Triche TJ, Ross WE: Glycogen-containing neuroblastoma with clinical and histopathologic features of Ewing's sarcoma. Cancer 41:1425–1432, 1978.
171. Fellinger EJ, Garin-Chesa P, Glasser DB, et al: Comparison of cell surface antigen HBA71 (p30/32MIC2), neuron-specific enolase, and vimentin in the immunohistochemical analysis of Ewing's sarcoma of bone. Am J Surg Pathol 16:746–755, 1992.
172. Riopel M, Dickman PS, Link MP, et al: MIC2 analysis in pediatric lymphomas and leukemias. Hum Pathol 25:396–399, 1994.
173. Ambros IM, Ambros PF, Strehl S, et al: MIC2 is a specific marker for Ewing's sarcoma and peripheral primitive neuroectodermal tumors. Evidence for a common histogenesis of Ewing's sarcoma and peripheral primitive neuroectodermal tumors from MIC2 expression and specific chromosome aberration. Cancer 67:1886–1893, 1991.
174. Aurias A, Rimbaut C, Buffe D, et al: Chromosomal translocations in Ewing's sarcoma. N Engl J Med 309:496–497, 1983.
175. Whang-Peng J, Triche TJ, Knutsen T, et al: Chromosome translocation in peripheral neuroepithelioma. N Engl J Med 311:584–585, 1984.

176. Adam A, Hochholzer L: Ganglioneuroblastoma of the posterior mediastinum: A clinicopathologic review of 80 cases. Cancer 47:373–381, 1981.

177. Bove KE, McAdams AJ: Composite ganglioneuroblastoma: An assessment of the significance of histological maturation in neuroblastoma diagnosed beyond infancy. Arch Pathol Lab Med 105:325–330, 1985.

178. Hahn JF, Netsky MG, Butler AB, et al: Pigmented ganglioneuroblastoma: Relation of melanin and lipofuscin to schwannomas and other tumors of neural crest origin. J Neuropathol Exp Neurol 35:393–403, 1976.

179. Fernbach DJ, Williams TE, Donaldson MH: Neuroblastoma. In Sutow WW, Vietti TJ, Fernbach DJ (eds.): Clinical Pediatric Oncology, 2nd ed. St. Louis, CV Mosby, 1977, pp 506–537.

180. Hamilton JR, Radde IC, Johnson G: Diarrhea associated with adrenal ganglioneuroma: New findings related to pathogenesis of diarrhea. Am J Med 44:453–463, 1968.

181. Mack E, Sarto GE, Crummy AB, et al: Virilizing adrenal ganglioneuroma. JAMA 239:2273–2274, 1978.

182. Aguirre P, Scully RE: Testosterone-secreting adrenal ganglioneuroma containing Leydig cells. Am J Surg Pathol 7:699–705, 1983.

183. Yokoyama M, Okada K, Tokue A, et al: Ultrastructural and biochemical study of benign ganglioneuroma. Virchows Arch Pathol Anat 361:195–209, 1973.

184. Wilhemus JL, Schrodt R, Alberhasky MT, et al: Giant adrenal myelolipoma: Case report and review of the literature. Arch Pathol Lab Med 105:532–535, 1981.

185. Medeiros LJ, Wolf BC: Traumatic rupture of an adrenal myelolipoma [letter]. Arch Pathol Lab Med 107:500, 1983.

186. Bennett BD, McKenna TJ, Hough AJ, et al: Adrenal myelolipoma associated with Cushing's disease. Am J Clin Pathol 73:443–447, 1980.

187. Plaut A: Myelolipoma in the adrenal cortex. Am J Pathol 34:487–499, 1958.

188. Vargas AD: Adrenal hemangioma. Urology 16:389–390, 1980.

189. Goren E, Bensal D, Reif RM, et al: Cavernous hemangioma of the adrenal gland. J Urol 135:341–342, 1986.

190. Oliver WR, Reddick RL, Gillespie GY, et al: Juxtaadrenal schwannoma: Verification of the diagnosis by immunohistochemical and ultrastructural studies. J Surg Oncol 30:259–268, 1985.

191. Pollock WJ, McConnell CF, Hilton C, et al: Virilizing Leydig cell adenoma of adrenal gland. Am J Surg Pathol 10:816–822, 1986.

192. Rosenberg SA, Diamond HD, Jaslowitz B, et al: Lymphosarcoma: A review of 1269 cases. Medicine 40:31–84, 1961.

193. Carey RW, Harris N, Kliman B: Addison's disease secondary to lymphomatous infiltration of the adrenal glands: Recovery of adrenocortical function after chemotherapy. Cancer 59:1087–1090, 1987.

194. Choi C-HM, Durishin M, Garbadawala ST, et al: Non-Hodgkin's lymphoma of the adrenal gland. Arch Pathol Lab Med 114:883–885, 1990.

195. Carstens PHB, Kuhns JG, Ghazi C: Primary malignant melanoma of the lung and adrenal. Hum Pathol 15:910–914, 1984.

196. Kareti LR, Katlein S, Siew S, et al: Angiosarcoma of the adrenal gland. Arch Pathol Lab Med 112:1163–1165, 1988.

197. Lack EE, Graham CW, Azumi N, et al: Primary leiomyosarcoma of adrenal gland: Case report with immunohistochemical and ultrastructural study. Am J Surg Pathol 15:899–905, 1991.

198. Chandrasoma P, Shibata D, Radin R, et al: Malignant peripheral nerve sheath tumor arising in an adrenal ganglioneuroma in an adult male homosexual. Cancer 57:2022–2025, 1986.

199. Fischler DF, Nunez C, Levin HS, et al: Adrenal carcinosarcoma presenting in a woman with clinical signs of virilization: A case report with immunohistochemical and ultrastructural findings. Am J Surg Pathol 16:626–631, 1992.

200. Barksdale SK, Marincola FM, Jaffe G: Carcinosarcoma of the adrenal cortex presenting with mineralocorticoid excess. Am J Surg Pathol 17:941–945, 1993.

201. Molberg K, Vuitch F, Stewart D, et al: Adrenocortical blastoma. Hum Pathol 23:1187–1190, 1992.

202. Hodges FV, Ellis FR: Cystic lesions of the adrenal glands. Arch Pathol Lab Med 66:53–58, 1958.

203. Gaffey MJ, Mills SE, Fechner RE, et al: Vascular adrenal cysts: A clinicopathologic and immunohistochemical study of endothelial and hemorrhagic (pseudocystic) variants. Am J Surg Pathol 13:740–747, 1989.

204. Costandi YT, Wendel RG, Inaba Y, et al: Calcified adrenal cysts. Urology 5:777–779, 1975.

205. Medeiros LJ, Lewandrowski KB, Vickery AL: Adrenal pseudocyst: A clinical and pathologic study of eight cases. Hum Pathol 20:660–665, 1989.

206. Gaffey MJ, Mills SE, Medeiros LJ, et al: Unusual variants of adrenal pseudocysts with intracystic fat, myelolipomatous metaplasia, and metastatic carcinoma. Am J Clin Pathol 94:706–713, 1990.

207. Groben PA, Roberson JB, Anger SR, et al: Immunohistochemical evidence for the vascular origin of primary adrenal pseudocysts. Arch Pathol Lab Med 110:121–123, 1986.

208. Incze JS, Lui PS, Merriam JC, et al: Morphology and pathogenesis of adrenal cysts. Am J Pathol 95:423–428, 1979.

209. Geelhoed GW, Spiegel CT: "Incidental" adrenal cyst: A correctable lesion possibly associated with hypertension. South Med J 74:626–630, 1981.

210. Levin SE, Collins DL, Kaplan GW, et al: Neonatal adrenal pseudocyst mimicking metastatic disease. Ann Surg 179:186–189, 1974.

211. McMurry JF, Long D, McClure R, et al: Addison's disease with adrenal enlargement on computed tomographic scanning: Report of two cases of tuberculosis and review of the literature. Am J Med 77:365–368, 1984.

212. Rodin AE, Hsu FL, Whorton EB: Microcysts of the permanent adrenal cortex in perinates and infants. Arch Pathol Lab Med 100:499–502, 1976.

213. Medeiros LJ, Weiss LM, Vickery AL: Epithelial-lined (true) cyst of the adrenal gland: A case report. Hum Pathol 20:491–492, 1989.

214. Kearney GP, Mahoney EM, Maher E, et al: Functioning and nonfunctioning cysts of the adrenal cortex and medulla. Am J Surg Pathol 134:363–368, 1977.

215. Travis WT, Lack EE, Azumi N, et al: Adenomatoid tumor of the adrenal gland with ultrastructural and immunohistochemical demonstration of a mesothelial origin. Arch Pathol Lab Med 114:722–724, 1990.

216. Simpson PR: Adenomatoid tumor of the adrenal gland. Arch Pathol Lab Med 114:725–727, 1990.

217. Plaut A: Lymphangioma of the adrenal gland. Cancer 15:1165–1169, 1962.

CHAPTER 12

Diseases of the Ovary and Pelvic Peritoneum

Noel Weidner, M.D., and Ronald L. Goldman, M.D.

The ovary and pelvic peritoneum have been the subject of voluminous literature devoted to their pathology. The morphologic diversity of ovarian and pelvic peritoneal lesions covers a very broad spectrum, and many of the described lesions occurring in these locations are relatively uncommon, especially for those pathologists not practicing at tertiary care medical centers. Thus, many ovarian and pelvic peritoneal lesions could be considered difficult, and we do not wish this chapter to be a summation of all this literature. Nonetheless, we have chosen to discuss some of those lesions that have caused diagnostic problems in our practice.

PRIMARY PERITONEAL PAPILLARY LESIONS

The light microscopic, electron microscopic, and immunohistochemical features of serosal carcinoma and malignant mesothelioma are well described in the medical literature.[1-16] Yet, even experienced diagnostic pathologists occasionally have trouble distinguishing peritoneal mesothelioma from primary peritoneal serosal carcinomas.[16] This can occur not only with the well-differentiated papillary lesions but also with the poorly differentiated examples. Proper diagnosis has considerable prognostic and therapeutic implications to the patient. Thus, it is important to review those light microscopic, electron microscopic, and immunohistochemical features that allow distinction of peritoneal mesothelioma from carcinoma (primary or metastatic).

CLINICOPATHOLOGIC FEATURES. Well-differentiated papillary mesothelioma (WDPM) of the peritoneum is most common in young women in their twenties and thirties,[17] but rare examples may occur in men. Most cases are asymptomatic and discovered incidentally during an operation performed for an unrelated reason. Uncommonly, there is a concomitant history of asbestos exposure, abdominal symptoms, and/or ascites. Clinically, from a few to multiple small nodules, varying from a few millimeters to 2 to 3 cm, cover the pelvic, mesenteric, and/or omental serosal surfaces. Histologically, a well-developed tubulopapillary pattern (Fig. 12–1) is found, sometimes admixed with solid and/or fibrotic areas. Psammoma bodies and surface ovarian involvement may be present. Tumor cells are low cuboidal or flattened and cytologically bland and show few (if any) mitotic figures. The prognosis is extremely good, and, importantly, most fatalities are described in patients who were inappropriately treated with adjuvant therapy. Thus, recognizing this lesion is very important.

Some have reported in North American patients that **diffuse malignant mesothelioma (DMM) of the peritoneum** in women makes up approximately 10% of all malignant mesotheliomas in both sexes and approximately 40% of peritoneal DMMs.[17] Yet, others suggest that when strict criteria are applied, less than 10% of peritoneal mesotheliomas are found in women,[17, 18] often with a history of asbestos exposure and abdominal signs and symptoms. This has been our experience, and we are cautious about making the diagnosis of DMM in a woman. Nonetheless, when it is present, peritoneal surfaces may show multiple nodules, but usually of greater extent than with WDPM and with confluent growth, encasement of organs, and invasion of underlying tissues. Rarely, DMM may cause a single large tumor mass[17] or present as cervical, mediastinal, and/or inguinal lymph nodal metastases.[19] Epithelial, sarcomatoid, biphasic, and poorly differentiated or undifferentiated types occur. Nuclear atypia is greater than that found with WDPM, but low-grade papillary areas may occur (Fig. 12–2) admixed with higher-grade areas (Fig. 12–3), and extensive sectioning may be needed to clearly demonstrate features of malignancy, which are more completely developed in DMM versus WDPM. The prognosis for DMM is generally poor.

Primary **peritoneal serous papillary tumor (PSPT)** presents like a high-stage primary ovarian serous papillary tumor, but the ovaries appear either normal grossly or have only small granules of tumor on their surfaces. Grossly and microscopically they are identical to similar stage and grade ovarian serous tumors, which may extend from borderline (Fig. 12–4) to higher-grade lesions (Fig. 12–5).[20-22] Papillae of serous tumors are lined by columnar to cuboidal cells with varying nuclear atypia and mitotic activity. Often, cellular stratification occurs, and finding detached clusters of similar cells is very helpful in making the diagnosis. Psammoma bodies are frequent, and invasion of underlying viscera may or may not be present. Biscotti and Hart[22] have referred to the borderline serous lesions as **peritoneal serous micropapillomatosis of low malignant potential.** The literature is divided as to whether the prognosis is worse or the same as for patients with ovarian serous cancers with the same degree of differentiation and peritoneal spread.[17]

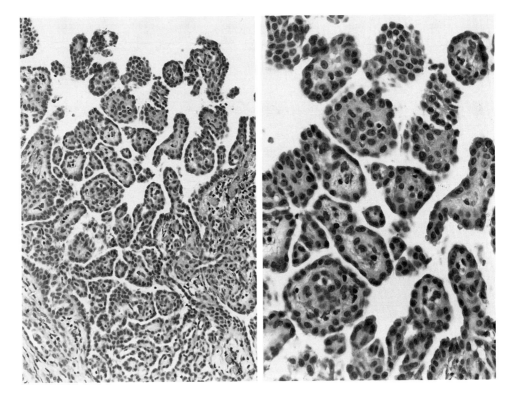

FIGURE 12–1. *Left,* Well-differentiated papillary mesothelioma is shown with a complex branching tubulopapillary pattern. Solid growth areas may also occur. (Hematoxylin and eosin [H&E], original magnification [OM] ×25) *Right,* Papillary tufts are lined by a single layer of cytologically bland low cuboid cells. Very little cytologic atypia is present, and no mitotic figures were present. (H&E, OM ×100)

A variant with close morphologic similarities to borderline SPCP is so-called **serous psammocarcinoma of the ovary and peritoneum,**[17, 23] which is defined as showing invasion of underlying stroma, presence of psammoma bodies in at least 75% of the papillae, no significant solid epithelial component, and only mild to moderate nuclear atypia. Thus far, this lesion has shown a good prognosis. Moreover, peritoneal surfaces may become involved by **ovarian mullerian-type mucinous papillary cystadenomas of borderline malignancy** (Fig. 12–6),[24] and, like **ovarian mixed epithelial papillary cystadenomas of borderline malignancy of mullerian type,**[25] these tumors share more clinicopathologic features with papillary serous borderline tumors than with **intestinal-type mucinous cystadenomas of borderline malignancy**.

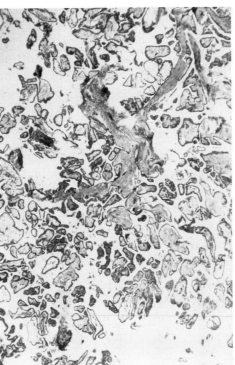
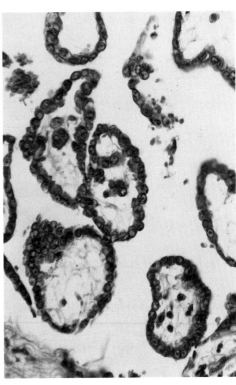

FIGURE 12–2. *Left,* Note exuberant papillary growth of an example of epithelial-type diffuse malignant mesothelioma (DMM). This "well-differentiated" pattern was adjacent to areas with a "higher-grade" invasive glandular growth pattern, which is shown in Figure 12–3, left side. (H&E, OM ×25) *Right,* Note the single row of cuboid mesothelioma cells lining papillae without prominent nuclear crowding. Mesothelial cells are more clearly separated from each other when compared with papillary serous tumors. (H&E, OM ×100)

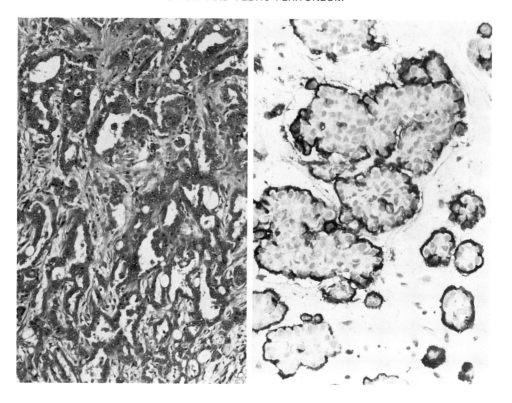

FIGURE 12–3. *Left,* Diffuse malignant mesothelioma is shown forming an invasive glandular pattern. (H&E, OM ×25) *Right,* Clusters of invasive mesothelioma cells are shown stained with human milk-fat globulin-2 (HMFG-2). The clusters show a strong peripheral membranous pattern of immunostaining characteristic of malignant mesothelial cells. Adenocarcinoma cells and benign mesothelial cells may show cytoplasmic granular staining, but the peripheral membranous pattern is unusual. (Diaminobenzidine immunoperoxidase stain [ipox], OM ×100)

Intestinal-type mucinous epithelium contains goblet cells and argentaffin-argyrophilic cells. In the mullerian-type lesions, the mucinous epithelium is of the endocervical type, the peritoneal or omental implants form discrete nodules surrounded by desmoplastic stroma, and the glands are lined by endocervical-like mucinous or indifferent epithelium with focal stratification and tufting. With the mullerian-type lesions, there is no pseudomyxoma peritonei, which is almost always the expression of intestinal-type lesions with peritoneal and/or omental implants.

DIFFERENTIAL DIAGNOSIS. The first consideration in the differential diagnosis of WDPM or PSPT of low malignant potential is exclusion of **mesothelial hyperplasia** and **endosalpingiosis.** Mesothelial hyperplasia is a common reaction

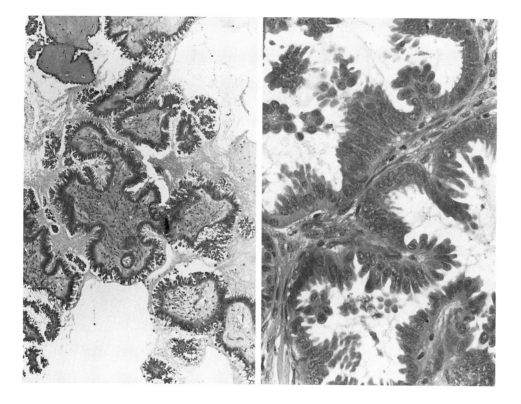

FIGURE 12–4. *Left,* Note papillary growth of a serous borderline papillary tumor of the peritoneum. This pattern also has been referred to as peritoneal serous micropapillomatosis of low malignant potential. (H&E, OM ×25) *Right,* Note the columnar, stratified epithelial cells with cytologic atypia and the detachment of epithelial clusters, which are characteristic of serous papillary tumors. (H&E, OM ×100)

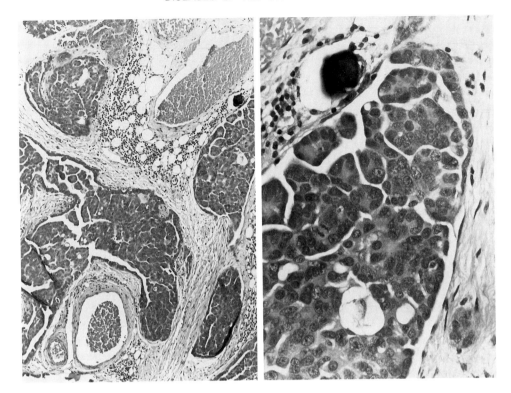

FIGURE 12–5. *Left,* Shown are invasive nests and sheets of well-differentiated, serous papillary carcinoma extending into subperitoneal connective tissues and growing around two medium-sized blood vessels. (H&E, OM ×25) *Right,* Clusters of invasive serous carcinoma cells are shown adjacent to a psammoma body. Note the nuclear crowding and atypia; and, although inconspicuous, a mitotic figure is present. (H&E, OM ×100)

to injury. In mesothelial hyperplasia, nodules are uncommon, atypia is absent or mild, necrosis is most often absent, and macrophages are often admixed. Yet, a diagnostically troublesome **mesothelial hyperplasia may be found in association with ovarian tumors,**[26] wherein the benign mesothelial cells can mimic invasion by forming small nests, cords, and gland-like arrangements of atypical mesothelial cells within cyst walls. Necrosis of these mesothelial cells may occur as well. Overinterpretation of such areas as tumor invasion would lead to improper staging, but awareness of the occasional occurrence of florid mesothelial hyperplasia in patients with ovarian neoplasms should lead to the correct diagnosis. Likewise, **multilocular peritoneal inclusion cysts (benign cystic mesothelioma)** may contain atypical areas of mesothelial

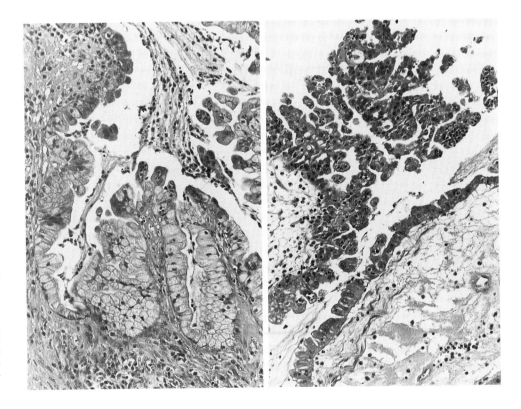

FIGURE 12–6. *Left,* Note the endocervical-like, mucinous epithelium of a mullerian mucinous papillary cystadenoma of borderline malignancy (note inflammatory cell component, which is composed primarily of neutrophils). (H&E, OM ×50) *Right,* Note the complex tufted papillary pattern of the indifferent epithelial component of a mullerian mucinous papillary cystadenoma of borderline malignancy (again note the neutrophilic inflammatory cell component). (H&E, OM ×50)

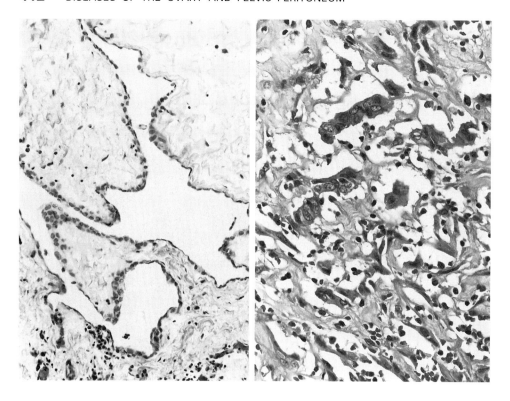

FIGURE 12–7. *Left,* Shown is a multilocular peritoneal inclusion cyst (so-called cystic mesothelioma) composed of locules lined by flat to cuboidal mesothelial cells and separated by collagenous septa containing lymphocytes. (H&E, OM ×10) *Right,* Within the same tumor shown at left, there was an area of mural mesothelial proliferation. Note the inflamed stroma containing pseudoinvasive mesothelial cells arranged in cords, nests, and glands. (H&E, OM ×100)

hyperplasia (Fig. 12–7), which can form tubules, nests, and/or cords simulating adenomatoid tumor, invasive serous carcinoma, or malignant mesothelioma.[27, 28]

Zinsser and Wheeler[29] and Dallenbach-Hellweg[30] have outlined the differential diagnosis of **endosalpingiosis** from malignant cells, such as those from serous tumors (Fig. 12–8). The benign glands of endosalpingiosis are non-infiltrative and lack desmoplastic stromal reaction, although chronic inflam-

mation may be marked. Benign glands have an easily demonstrable basement membrane, papillary features may be seen but are rarely prominent, nuclei are uniform with fine evenly dispersed chromatin and no mitotic figures, cilia are a prominent feature, there is a single well-oriented layer of basal nuclei occurring in columnar and/or cuboidal cells, and there is usually a history of tubal disease or ovarian tumor, but only occasionally associated with malignancy. In contrast,

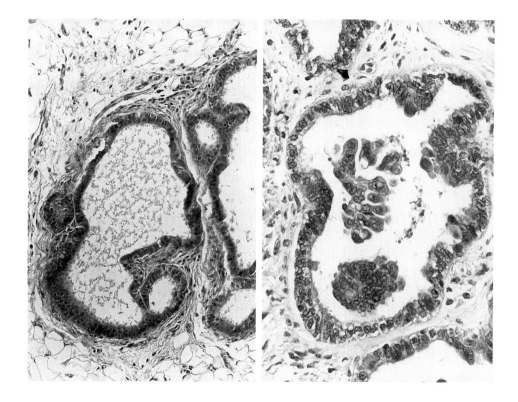

FIGURE 12–8. *Left,* Shown are the benign glands of endosalpingiosis, which are non-infiltrative and lack desmoplastic stromal reaction. Papillary features are not prominent; nuclei are uniform with fine, evenly dispersed chromatin and show no mitotic figures; cilia are present (although difficult to appreciate in this photo). There is a single well-oriented layer of basal nuclei occurring in columnar and/or cuboidal cells, and there is a history of tubal disease in this case. (H&E, OM ×50) *Right,* In contrast, these malignant serous papillary carcinoma glands (low-grade) are surrounded by desmoplastic stroma, papillary features are present with tufting, nuclear atypia is present, cilia are not noted (in this particular case), nuclei are stratified, and there is a history of papillary serous malignancy in the ovary. (H&E, OM ×100)

malignant glands are usually infiltrative with desmoplastic stroma, basal lamina is difficult to demonstrate, papillary features are often prominent (sometimes with detached epithelial clusters, ''tufting''), nuclear atypia and mitotic figures are present, cilia are rare (although cilia are common in serous tumors), nuclei are stratified or piled up, and there is malignancy elsewhere, especially in the ovary. **Endometriosis** is excluded by the absence of surrounding endometrial stroma.

A clear mental picture of the light microscopic features of WDPM and serous carcinoma should lead to a correct diagnosis in most cases. Yet, immunohistochemistry can play a very helpful role in problem cases. Bollinger et al.[8] and Khoury et al.[31] have carefully studied the immunohistochemical features of these two groups of tumors (Table 12–1). Careful selection of a panel of antibodies applied in a good laboratory should lead to the correct diagnosis.

For undifferentiated tumors involving the pleura or peritoneum, the main diagnostic considerations are malignant mesothelioma and poorly differentiated carcinoma (primary or metastatic) (Figs. 12–9 and 12–10). The usual immunohistochemical findings of mesothelioma are strong callus keratin immunoreactivity in a diffuse cytoplasmic distribution and negative staining for carcinoembryonic antigen (CEA) and Leu-M1.[1, 5, 6, 8, 13, 15] Certainly, Leu-M1- and CEA-negative serosal carcinomas occur, but they do not show strong, diffuse cytoplasmic and perinuclear staining with anti-callus keratin. For Leu-M1- and CEA-negative tumors, some authors advocate the use of the additional differentiation markers including immunostaining for B72.3, S-100 protein, placental alkaline phosphatase, CA-125 protein, epithelial membrane antigen, and/or human milk fat globulin-2.[8, 13, 32–34] A peripheral or membranous staining pattern with human milk fat globulin-2 (HMFG-2) or epithelial membrane antigen (EMA) is also

characteristic of mesothelioma. This membranous pattern is reported not to occur in benign, reactive mesothelial cells.[32] Moreover, four separate reports have documented that nuclear immunostaining in formalin-fixed, paraffin-embedded sections for p53 protein is found in malignant (25% to 70% of cases) but not benign reactive mesothelial cells.[35–38] This pattern does not hold up in immunostaining of effusion cytology smears,[39] and remember that p53 protein is also frequently found in metastatic adenocarcinoma cells.[35–39] Also, in our experience, reactive, benign mesothelial cells frequently express desmin immunoreactivity.

Although unusual, non-specific staining for CEA and Leu-M1 antibodies in mesothelioma has been reported in cases with a high content of hyaluronic acid.[11] Furthermore, non-specific CEA immunostaining can occur in areas of tumor necrosis, and non-specific staining of neutrophils and macrophages can occur with polyclonal CEA antibodies owing to the presence of a non-specific cross-reactive antigen (NSCRA). NSCRA reactivity can be eliminated by absorption with human spleen powder or use of a monoclonal antibody to CEA. Yet, monoclonal antibodies can also show peculiar cross-reacting patterns. For example, a monoclonal anti-CEA (Biogenex, San Ramon, CA) was reported to show coarsely granular and/or linear apical staining in 5 (11%) of 45 mesotheliomas,[11] a reactivity not considered related to NSCRA. Significant diffuse or multifocal staining of CEA or Leu-M1 is extremely unusual in mesothelioma, but focal immunostaining can occur for both these antigens in mesothelioma. The cytokeratin reagent AE1/3 tends to be sensitive to low and high molecular weight keratins,[40, 41] and, like mesothelioma, it often strongly stains the cytoplasm of carcinomas in diffuse distribution. In contrast, polyclonal callus keratin reagents tend to react preferentially with higher molecular weight keratins and stain adenocarcinomas weakly and in a peripheral rim pattern (in fact, some adenocarcinomas may be negative for callus keratin).[6] AE1/3 and callus keratin antibodies stain mesothelioma cells strongly, and the diffuse cytoplasmic and/or perinuclear pattern encountered with callus keratin reagents correlates with the diffusely distributed tonofilaments observed by electron microscopy. The finding of one supports the presence of the other. The finding of strong, diffuse, and/or perinuclear staining of tumor cells for callus keratin in suspected mesothelioma has prompted re-examination wherein the characteristic tonofilament pattern was initially missed. Electron microscopic examination of additional blocks leads to discovery of the diffusely distributed cytoplasmic tonofilaments, an experience testifying to the complementary nature of these two techniques.

Unlike mesotheliomas, metastatic carcinomas to serosal surfaces (with the possible exception of metastatic breast or thymic carcinoma) do not show the diffuse and/or perinuclear distribution of tonofilaments[3] (Figs. 12–5 and 12–6). Squamous carcinoma could also show this tonofilament pattern, but squamous carcinomas rarely metastasize to serosal surfaces. The long, thin, and branching microvilli of relatively better differentiated mesotheliomas are often lost in poorly differentiated mesotheliomas.[42–44] However, in these poorly differentiated examples, the diffuse cytoplasmic or perinuclear distribution of tonofilaments often remains a good marker of mesothelial differentiation. Furthermore, not all tumors with long, thin branching microvilli are mesotheliomas; in fact, these features have been described in so-called **''anemone-**

Table 12–1. **Immunohistochemistry of Peritoneal Mesothelioma versus Serous Carcinoma**

Antigen	Mesothelioma (~%)	Serous Carcinoma (~%)
Cytokeratin*	100	100
Leu-M1	10	75
B72.3	0	70
Placental Alkaline Phosphatase	0	65
S-100 Protein	10	85
CA-125	15	90
Carcinoembryonic†	0	15
Human Milk Fat Globulin-2‡	60	90
Epithelial Membrane	80	100
Vimentin	40	30
Amylase	20	35

* Antibodies to high molecular weight keratins (anti-callus keratin) tend to show a strong and diffuse (perinuclear) staining pattern in mesotheliomas, whereas they tend to show weak and peripheral (membrane) staining patterns in carcinomas.

† Antibodies to carcinoembryonic antigen (CEA) should be absorbed with tissue or spleen powder or be monoclonal, because unabsorbed polyclonal antibodies to CEA have non-specific cross-reacting antibody and show reactivity with some mesotheliomas.

‡ The pattern of staining in mesothelioma for antibodies to human milk fat globulin-2 or epithelial membrane antigen (EMA) is a peripheral membranous pattern[32] (see Fig. 12–3, right). This peripheral membranous pattern is not found in carcinoma or benign mesothelial cells, which tend to show a diffuse cytoplasmic and/or granular cytoplasmic pattern. Also, desmin immunoreactivity is frequent in reactive mesothelial cells but less common in malignant mesothelial cells.

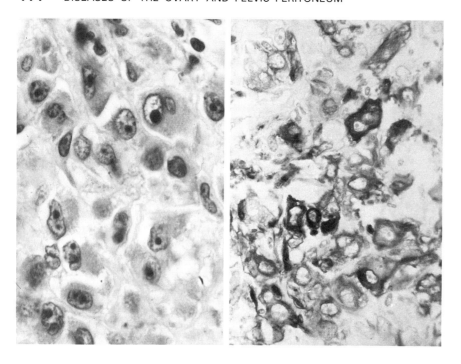

FIGURE 12–9. *Left,* The peritoneal tumor was composed of poorly differentiated, epithelioid cells with eosinophilic cytoplasm and large vesicular nuclei containing prominent nucleoli. (H&E, OM ×100) *Right,* Immunohistochemical staining with polyclonal callus keratin antibody revealed strong, diffuse cytoplasmic or perinuclear staining. (Immunoperoxidase [ipox], OM ×100) (From Weidner N: Malignant mesothelioma of peritoneum. Ultrastruct Pathol 15:515–520, 1991. Reproduced with permission. All rights reserved.)

cell" tumors, which can be either carcinomas or lymphomas.[45–47] It is also worth emphasizing that DMM can occur without a history of asbestos exposure,[48] develop rarely in children as young as 1 year old,[49] undergo osseous and/or cartilaginous differentiation,[50] have a prominent lymphoplasmacytic component causing a striking resemblance to lymphoma,[51] present in a "deciduoid" pattern closely simulating an exuberant, ectopic decidual reaction of pregnancy,[52] be mucin positive,[53] have extensive "small-cell undifferentiated" areas,[54] express desmin ("leiomyoid") and neural marker (neuron-specific enolase [NSE], Leu-7, chromogranin, and S-100 protein) immunoreactivity,[55, 56] and present with a "desmoplastic" pattern.[57, 58] The desmoplastic pattern is apparent when acellular connective tissue dominates (>50% of tumor bulk) and shows anastomosing bands of often hyalinized collagen with a prominent storiform pattern.[57] The differentiation from benign fibrosing peritoneal processes can be very difficult, but **desmoplastic malignant mesothelioma** becomes apparent when there is collagen (infarct-like) necrosis and when hyperchromatic nuclei are present in the proper clinical context.[57] Unfortunately, benign or reactive serosal fibrosing processes, such as pleural plaques and/or scars, contain spindle cells that immunoreact with keratin and epithelial membrand antigen (EMA) antibodies.[58] Given the characteristics of "multipotential subserosal cells," this observation is not surprising.[59] Finally, for the sake of completeness, **des-**

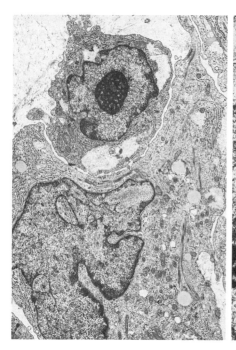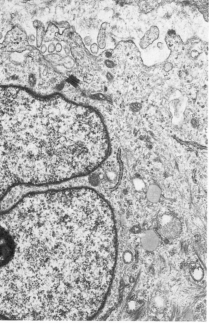

FIGURE 12–10. *Left,* Shown are pleomorphic tumor cells with anaplastic nuclei surrounded by abundant cytoplasm containing glycogen, diffusely distributed cytoplasmic tonofilaments, strands of rough endoplasmic reticulum, mitochondria, and scattered lipid droplets. Note the absence of long, thin, branched microvilli, a common feature of poorly differentiated mesotheliomas. (Lead citrate and uranyl acetate [LCUA], ×2000) *Right,* Shown in greater detail are diffusely distributed, cytoplasmic tonofilaments and a well-developed true desmosome. (LCUA, ×4000) (From Weidner N: Malignant mesothelioma of peritoneum. Ultrastruct Pathol 15:515–520, 1991. Reproduced with permission. All rights reserved.)

moplastic small round-cell tumor of the abdomen or ovary,[60] solitary fibrous tumor of the peritoneum (a lesion in which tumor cells are negative for keratin and EMA),[17] and omental-mesenteric myxoid hamartoma[61] should be considered in the differential diagnosis of this group of lesions. Omental-mesenteric myxoid hamartomas occur in infants and are often overdiagnosed as sarcoma. Of interest, some have suggested that the desmoplastic small round-cell tumor of the abdomen should be considered a form of "mesoblastoma."

UNUSUAL PERITONEAL IMPLANTS, METAPLASIAS, AND LESIONS

There are several distinctly uncommon benign lesions that affect the peritoneum in a multifocal nodular or diffuse manner, imparting a spurious impression of carcinomatosis grossly, and that may cause difficulties in precise histopathologic appraisal.

Gliomatosis Peritonei

This condition, which usually occurs in patients in the first two decades, is characterized by the presence of miliary implants composed of mature glial tissue on the peritoneum or omentum[62-65] (Fig. 12–11). Some authorities believe this results from extrusion of mature glial tissue through spontaneous or surgically induced capsular defects in an ovarian teratoma. The latter is usually of the solid type and may be of any grade; a rare case has been associated with a mature cystic teratoma. There are unusual exceptions to this clinicopathologic picture. Thus, peritoneal gliomatosis has been reported after resection of a congenital gastric teratoma[66] and as a non-neoplastic seeding via a ventriculoperitoneal shunt for infantile hydrocephalus.[67] Of incidental interest, both of those patients were male. Also, gliomatosis peritonei has rarely been reported to occur in association with benign collections of mature glial cells in retroperitoneal lymph nodes,[62, 68] yet there are two cases in which such nodal gliomatosis in the absence of concurrent peritoneal implants was associated with ostensibly unruptured ovarian teratomas,[69, 70] so that putative benign lymphatic spread, rather than direct implantation, may represent an alternative pathogenetic route in some instances.

Grossly, the miliary implants are firm, gray superficial nodules measuring from less than 0.1 cm to 1.5 cm and are generally concentrated on the pelvic peritoneum. In contrast, teratomatous peritoneal metastases are usually few and may be of massive proportions.[63] Microscopically, the nodules are composed exclusively or almost exclusively of mature glial tissue, but in rare instances extensive sampling has also shown mature neurons, foci of keratin debris, mature cartilage and bone, or rare mature epithelial cysts.[63, 71] It is important that thorough sampling be performed in order to exclude the presence of immature neuroepithelial elements, a distinctly ominous prognostic factor if they are present (Fig. 12–11, *right*). Collaterally, when all of the implants are mature, there is, paradoxically, an improved prognosis in those patients with higher-grade teratomas. Alternatively, rare examples of malignant transformation of gliomatosis have appeared, but only one of these stands up to critical scrutiny.[71] Ordinarily, these nodules seem to persist without any clinical symptoms or morphologic changes being detected at second-look operations performed up to 16 years later.[63] Rarely, fibroblastic retrogression ensues.[63]

O'Connor and Norris[71a] analyzed 244 immature ovarian teratomas to evaluate the value of grade in predicting outcome. Grade 1 tumors were defined as having immature neuroepithelium present on any one slide of up to one low-power ($\times 40$) microscopic field. Grade 2 tumors had immature

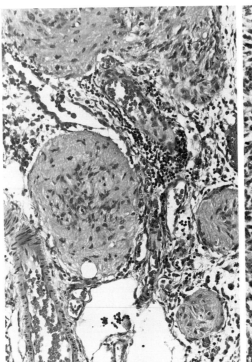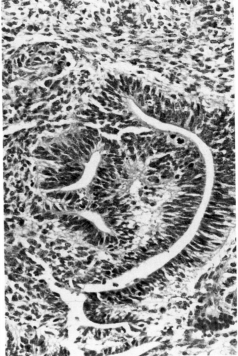

FIGURE 12–11. *Left,* Note multiple nodules of mature glial tissue, which were found over the peritoneal surfaces. (H&E, OM ×50) *Right,* Peritoneal implant is shown composed of immature neurotubular structures (neuroblastoma-like) derived from an immature teratoma of the ovary. (H&E, OM ×50)

neuroepithelium present on any one slide of more than one low-power field but did not exceed three low-power microscopic fields. Grade 3 tumors had immature neuroepithelium present on any one slide exceeding three low-power microscopic fields. Follow-up (mean, 85 months) showed that 18% of patients with high-grade (grades 2 and 3) tumors died of tumor, whereas only 6% of those patients with grade 1 tumors died. Also, this study confirmed that small foci (2 mm or less) of endodermal sinus tumor do not adversely affect the prognosis of immature ovarian teratoma.

Struma Ovarii with Peritoneal Implants

One report describes multiple peritoneal nodules composed of benign thyroid tissue associated with a strumal mass that was unusually situated on the surface of the ovary and that also constituted benign thyroid.[72] Other ovarian teratoid elements were absent, and there was no evidence of tumor involving the cervical thyroid or other regions. The precise nature of the ovarian and peritoneal lesions is unclear, as the authors note. On the basis of topography and lectin histochemistry, they speculated on the possibility that the thyroid tissue may have been the result of mesothelial metaplasia, which seems to be a convenient but implausible concept.

Decidual Metaplasia

Ectopic foci of decidua may occur in the submesothelial stroma of the peritoneum and omentum in pregnancy, and less commonly, within abdominal and pelvic lymph nodes as well.[73] These collections are usually only of microscopic dimension, but may be large and appear as multiple gray to white nodules. They are frequently vascular and hemorrhagic, and they rarely are associated with hemorrhage, sometimes massive and fatal.[74] Especially when associated with similar capsular and intranodal foci,[73, 75] this banal metaplastic phenomenon may simulate metastatic malignancy grossly and microscopically. However, histologically, the decidual cells are usually bland and lack mitotic activity, but focal hemorrhagic necrosis and nuclear atypia, as well as the presence of smooth muscle cells, may occur and complicate the picture. Rarely, some cells may contain cytoplasmic mucinous vacuoles,[76] similar to changes noted in decidual reactions in the endometrium,[77] further simulating malignancy.

Leiomyomatosis Peritonealis Disseminata

This diffuse multifocal process also may simulate malignancy. Like decidual ectopia, it is thought to be a result of metaplasia of submesothelial mesenchyme, in this case into smooth muscle cells.[78] This lesion may also be associated with concurrent leiomyomatous proliferation in regional lymph nodes,[79, 80] simulating metastatic leiomyosarcoma or benign metastasizing leiomyoma. A further similarity is its association with pregnancy or oral contraceptive administration in approximately 70% of cases, although the lesion has occasionally been seen in postmenopausal women. Approximately 40% of the cases have occurred in black women.

Grossly, leiomyomatosis peritonealis disseminata is characterized by a variable number, sometimes very numerous, of firm, solid gray to white peritoneal and omental nodules. Some have measured up to 10 cm, but most are smaller. Microscopically, the nodules are made up of smooth muscle cells having the appearance of a leiomyoma. Fibroblasts and myofibroblasts may be present.[78] In those cases that are associated with pregnancy, plumper deciduoid forms or frank decidual cells may be admixed. Rarely, focal hypercellularity and mitotic activity may be noted.[78] Unique variants have included an epithelioid sex cord–like pattern (analogous to uterine lesions)[81] and vacuolar change that was interpreted as adipocytic differentiation.[82] The natural history is that of partial or complete regression. Finally, rare examples of sarcomatous transformation have been recorded, including one in a male.[83, 84]

Peritoneal Trophoblastic Implants

Persistent trophoblast after salpingostomy for treatment of tubal pregnancy occurs in as many as 7% of cases.[85] Usually, the trophoblast is within the fallopian tube. However, it is important to note that viable implants may ensue on peritoneal and omental surfaces.[85, 86] This complication was reported to follow 1.9% of the cases managed with laparoscopy and 0.6% managed by laparotomy.[85] The implants may cause significant abdominal pain and intra-abdominal hemorrhage. They are usually red, multiple, and average approximately 0.5 cm in diameter. The lesions have been associated with a persistent elevation of beta-human chorionic gonadotropin (β-hCG) level. The appropriate history and histologic features should enable distinction of these implants from metastatic hydatidiform mole and choriocarcinoma.

Miscellaneous Rare Lesions, Implants, and Metaplasias

Peritoneal keratin implants may occur and may be associated with endometrioid adenocarcinoma of the endometrium, ovary, or both, or with squamous cell carcinoma of the cervix.[87] They should be distinguished from viable tumor implants on microscopic examination, because keratin granulomas without viable tumor cells have no prognostic significance. Similar granulomas may also be a result of rupture of an ovarian dermoid cyst.[87] Rare examples of **squamous metaplasia of the peritoneum,**[88] **melanosis peritonei** secondary to spillage of melanin from benign cystic teratomas,[89, 90] and putative primary melanosis peritonei associated with a **melanotic peritoneal cyst**[91] have been recorded. Moreover, the pelvic peritoneum can be the site of almost any of the tumors known to occur in the ovary; indeed, very rarely some can arise from **ectopic ovary.**[92] Usually, they are of the typical ovarian epithelial type, but examples of endometrioid carcinoma, endometrioid stromal sarcoma, mixed mullerian tumors (including adenosarcoma), mucinous tumors, and yolk sac carcinoma occur.[93] Finally, when "stumped" by a difficult lesion, also remember that examples of **fibromatosis, leiomyoma, lipoma, teratoma, adenomatoid tumor, fibrous histiocytoma, neurofibroma, paraganglioma, lymphangioma, hemangioma, hemangiopericytoma, inflammatory pseu-**

dotumor, various sarcomas, cystic mucinous tumors, urogenital mesenteric cysts, and pseudotumors formed from organization of a twisted epiploic fringe (so-called "hard-boiled egg" of the peritoneal cavity) may arise from the peritoneum, omentum, mesentery, and/or retroperitoneum.[93-98]

METASTATIC CARCINOMAS TO THE OVARY

Approximately 5% to 10% of malignant ovarian tumors discovered in surgical specimens are metastatic,[99] and often they mimic primary ovarian tumors clinically, grossly, and/or microscopically. Metastatic tumors to the ovaries can present before, concomitantly, or after the primary has been discovered, but recognition of secondary ovarian malignancy is especially difficult when the ovarian metastasis presents before the primary or when the pathologist does not have complete and/or accurate information. Failure to recognize the metastasis to the ovary can lead to unnecessary radical operation, inappropriate chemotherapy, and/or radiation therapy and delay in identification of the primary tumor.

CLINICOPATHOLOGIC FEATURES. In adults, the more common primary sites of metastatic carcinoma to the ovaries include colon, breast, stomach, uterus, cervix, and appendix. The gallbladder, pancreas, and bladder produce ovarian metastasis less commonly, but the resulting metastases can closely mimic primary ovarian neoplasia. In adults, only rarely do sarcomas metastasize to the ovaries, the most common being endometrial stromal sarcoma or leiomyosarcoma. However, in children (<15 years old) the most common secondary tumors are neuroblastoma, rhabdomyosarcoma, Ewing's sarcoma, malignant rhabdoid tumor of kidney, and carcinoid.[100] Also, melanoma and hematolymphoid malignancies can metastasize to the ovaries and be confused clinically and pathologically with primary tumors.[99]

Some general clinicopathologic features are suggestive of metastatic tumor to the ovaries.[99] First, bilateral ovarian tumors suggest metastatic disease, especially when the tumor histology suggests mucinous, endometrioid, or Sertoli-Leydig cell tumors, because these primary ovarian tumors present with bilateral disease in less than 10% to 15% of cases. However, 25% to 50% of metastatic tumors are unilateral, and primary serous and undifferentiated ovarian carcinomas produce bilateral ovarian disease often enough that bilaterality should not favor metastasis under the latter conditions. Second, ovarian tumor concomitant with similar tumor in the hepatic parenchyma, mesenteric lymph nodes, gastrointestinal tract, pancreas, and/or biliary tract favors metastatic ovarian tumor. Third, the mere presence of concomitant extraovarian tumor, especially when extensive, suggests metastasis to the ovary. Primary, low-grade ovarian mucinous or Sertoli-Leydig cell tumors uncommonly cause peritoneal disease, whereas gastrointestinal tract tumors do so more frequently. Finally, ovarian surface and/or parenchymal multinodular tumor (gross or microscopic), discrete tumor plaques on the ovarian surface, desmoplastic stromal reaction to invasive tumor within or on the surface of the ovary, and/or lymphatic-vascular invasion all suggest metastatic rather than primary ovarian neoplasia. Also, it should be strongly emphasized that extensive cystic change, multiloculation, bland or border-line

cytoarchitectural features, fibromatous stroma, and/or stromal luteinization do not rule out metastatic disease.

DIFFERENTIAL DIAGNOSIS. Certain microscopic findings are associated with certain types of metastatic disease.[99] Metastatic gastrointestinal carcinomas often mimic primary endometrioid and/or less commonly mucinous carcinoma, especially those from the large intestine (Fig. 12–12). On the other hand, some primary mucinous or endometrioid carcinomas of the ovary can closely mimic metastatic gastrointestinal carcinomas (Fig. 12–13). Features suggesting metastasis are a garland and/or cribriform growth pattern, intraluminal "dirty" necrosis, segmental destruction of glands, and absence of squamous metaplasia.[101] These metastatic tumor cells are usually very atypical, show densely eosinophilic cytoplasm, and are poorly differentiated; however, smooth, thin-walled cysts lined by columnar, mucin-producing cells with benign or borderline cytoarchitectural features can be admixed, even when the primary tumors are entirely solid. Please remember that true endometrioid carcinomas can occur concomitantly in the endometrium and ovary. Many of these cases are interpreted as synchronous independent primary tumors,[99] but endometrioid ovarian tumors can be metastatic from the endometrium,[102] and metastasis of ovarian endometrioid carcinoma to the endometrium is rare.[102]

Although most metastases to the ovaries from the large intestine closely resemble the average, moderately differentiated colon carcinoma, some gastrointestinal ovarian metastases closely mimic primary mucinous cystadenocarcinomas or cystic mucinous tumors of borderline malignancy. In these cases, the primary sites might be intestines, appendix, pancreas, biliary tract, and cervix (Fig. 12–14).[99] Metastatic mucinous tumors from the pancreas often show varying degrees of differentiation, containing foci simulating mucinous cystadenoma, mucinous cystic tumor of borderline malignancy, and well-differentiated mucinous cystadenocarcinoma.[103] Clues suggesting metastatic disease include lymphatic-vascular invasion and desmoplastic surface implants, consisting of nodular or plaque-like aggregates of small irregular glands or clusters of carcinoma cells within a prominent fibroblastic stroma.[103] Large, mucinous cystic ovarian tumors covered with mucin, containing mucin extravasated into the ovarian stroma (pseudomyxoma ovarii) (see Fig. 12–14), and abundant intra-abdominal mucin (pseudomyxoma peritonei) are frequently associated with mucinous tumors of the appendix, which are considered the probable primary site of the ovarian tumors.[104] Both the ovarian and appendiceal tumors showed similar features, mucinous cystadenoma and/or cystadenoma of borderline malignancy. When mucinous tumors of the ovary co-exist with mucinous tumors of the cervix, the latter are usually deeply invasive and are of the minimal deviation adenocarcinoma type (so-called adenoma malignum).[105]

Krukenberg tumors are bilateral ovarian tumors characterized by abundant stroma proliferation with admixed, mucin-positive, signet-ring cells (Fig. 12–15). The vast majority are metastatic from the stomach, but other primary sites include breast, large intestine, pancreas, bladder, and gallbladder.[99, 106] Extremely rare, primary Krukenberg tumors have been described, but before this diagnosis is made, a postoperative tumor-free period of at least 10 years and/or a very careful autopsy performed with extensive organ sampling is necessary.[99, 106] The extensive stromal reaction, sometimes with stro-

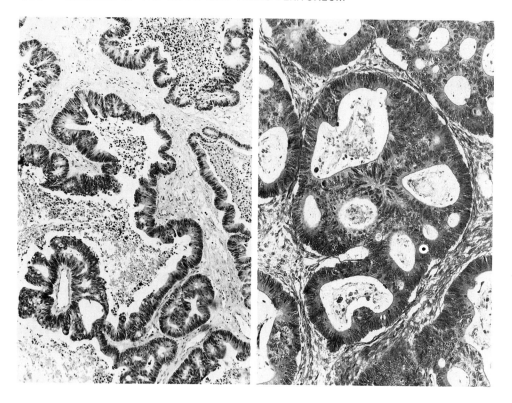

FIGURE 12–12. *Left,* Ovary containing metastatic colon carcinoma. Note the large areas of necrosis with abundant karyorrhectic debris ("dirty" necrosis) outlined by trabeculae of columnar carcinoma cells ("garland" pattern). (H&E, OM ×10) *Right,* Metastatic colonic carcinoma forming cribriform nests and stratified columnar cells reminiscent of patterns often formed in endometrioid adenocarcinoma. The patterns formed by metastatic colonic carcinoma can also mimic primary mucinous ovarian carcinoma. (H&E, OM ×50)

mal luteinization, may mimic ovarian fibroma or fibromathecoma. The signet-ring cells may also simulate primary mucinous carcinoid, which is always unilateral,[107] or Sertoli-Leydig cell tumors with heterologous elements containing mucinous carcinoid.[99] Appendiceal mucinous adenocarcinoid metastatic to the ovaries is almost always bilateral, the appendiceal tumors may be small and inconspicuous, and the ovar-

ian component may show only the mucinous signet-ring cells without the neurosecretory granule-containing carcinoid component.[108] **Sclerosing stromal tumors** (Fig. 12–16),[99] the **signet-ring stromal tumor,**[109] and some **steroid cell tumors** may also contain lipid-laden cells that can mimic signet-ring cells. Tubular Krukenberg tumors show a prominent tubular pattern of metastatic, mucin-producing carcinoma cells, which

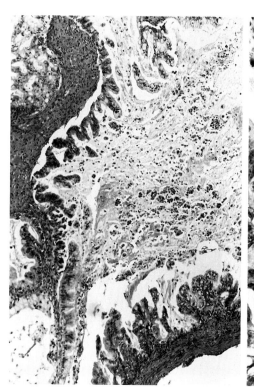
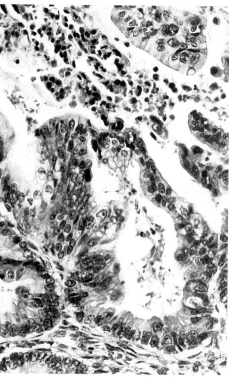

FIGURE 12–13. *Left,* Ovary containing primary mucinous adenocarcinoma. Note the large areas of necrosis with karyorrhectic debris ("dirty" necrosis) outlined by trabeculae of columnar carcinoma cells ("garland" pattern); although in contrast with the case shown in Figure 12–12, a more tufted or papillary pattern is formed. (H&E, OM ×10) *Right,* Shown is primary ovarian mucinous carcinoma forming tufts of stratified columnar, mucin-producing cells, which outline necrotic debris with the "dirty" necrosis pattern. Unfortunately, the distinction between primary mucinous and metastatic adenocarcinoma to the ovary can be difficult in some cases. (H&E, OM ×50)

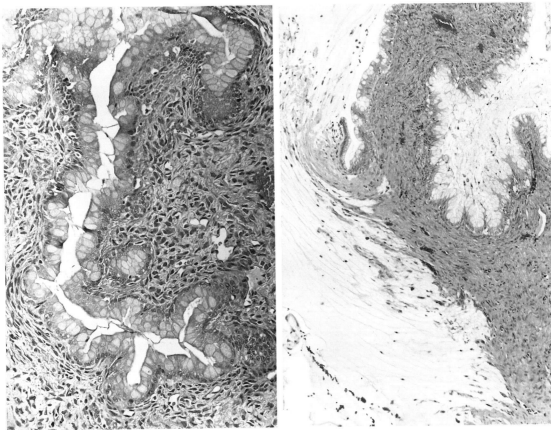

FIGURE 12–14. *Left,* Shown is ovary containing metastatic mucinous cystadenocarcinoma from the appendix. Note the close resemblance to primary low-grade mucinous cystadenocarcinoma of the ovary. (H&E, OM ×40) *Right,* Metastatic mucinous cystadenocarcinoma of the appendix to the ovary showing an area of pseudomyxoma ovarii. (H&E, OM ×10)

mimic Sertoli-Leydig cell tumors, especially when luteinized stromal cells are present.[110] Metastatic clear-cell tumors to the ovary, such as renal carcinoma, are extremely rare but may mimic primary clear-cell carcinoma of the ovary.[99] The highly vascular and organoid or nested pattern of renal cell carcinoma is not a feature of primary clear-cell carcinoma of the ovary. A variety of clear-cell carcinomas from the colon, liver, endometrium, and vagina have been documented to metastasize to the ovaries.[99] Metastatic bladder carcinoma to the ovaries could be confused with proliferating and malignant Brenner tumors, but the presence of benign Brenner tumor makes metastasis unlikely. Before making a diagnosis of primary and pure transitional cell carcinoma of the ovary, a bladder primary should be excluded. Although the pattern of ovarian serous carcinoma is only very rarely produced by metastases from other tumor types, ovarian metastases from serous carcinomas of tubal, peritoneal, or uterine origin should be ruled out. Sometimes determining the site of origin is difficult, and a diagnosis of multiple simultaneous primaries seems most appropriate.

Metastatic carcinoid to the ovaries is frequently bilateral, produces an insular or mucinous adenocarcinoid pattern, often shows a hyalinized hypocellular fibromatous stroma (Fig. 12–17), and may produce a small acinar pattern of growth that can mimic microfollicles of granulosa cell tumors.[99] The abundant fibrous stroma and insular pattern of metastatic carcinoid mimics Brenner tumors, which may also contain argyrophil cells. Breast carcinoma and rarely pancreatic carcino-

mas can also grow in a small acinar pattern. However, breast carcinomas usually produce cords and columns when they spread to the ovaries, especially the lobular variant. Hematolymphoid malignancies may also produce a cords and columns pattern, but usually a diffuse pattern results. Follicle-like spaces and/or a small-cell pattern may be produced by metastatic melanoma, carcinoid, thymic carcinoma, adenoid cystic carcinoma, rhabdomyosarcoma, lymphoma, granulocytic sarcoma, small-cell lung carcinoma, chordoma, and intra-abdominal desmoplastic round cell tumor.[99, 111] The follicle-like space pattern mimics primary small-cell undifferentiated carcinoma and juvenile granulosa cell tumors.

Metastatic tumors showing abundant eosinophilic cytoplasm might include melanoma, breast carcinoma, lung carcinoma, hepatocellular carcinoma, oncocytic carcinoid tumor, adrenocortical carcinoma, malignant rhabdoid tumor, and malignant mesothelioma. Finally, occasional metastatic carcinomas to the ovary (especially breast) may produce a diffuse pattern, and metastatic stromal sarcoma can mimic fibromathecomas as well as adenofibroma when epithelioid (sex-cord stromal) areas of differentiation are present. Metastatic carcinoids and biliary tract carcinomas may also produce an adenofibromatous pattern with innocuous-appearing neoplastic glands, which can simulate primary cystadenofibroma of the ovary.[112]

Finally, as a general point, metastatic tumors can fuse with benign epithelium intrinsic to the organs containing the metastases[113] (Fig. 12–18). Thus, the finding of malignant epithelium

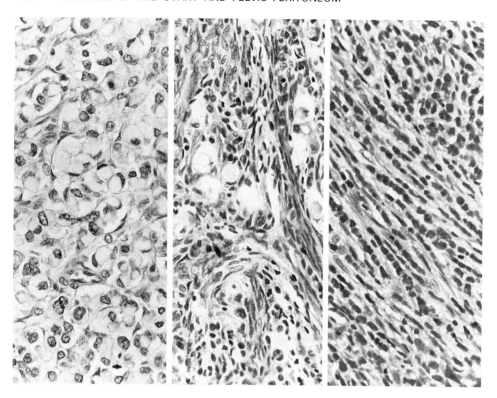

FIGURE 12–15. *Left,* Ovary containing metastatic signet-ring carcinoma of the stomach (Krukenberg tumor). Note numerous signet-ring cells. (H&E, OM ×100) *Middle,* Metastatic signet-ring carcinoma to ovary associated with prominent stromal hyperplasia. Signet-ring cells are inconspicuous and easily missed without careful examination. (H&E, OM ×100) *Right,* Metastatic lobular carcinoma of the breast to ovary. Note single-file infiltrative pattern. (H&E, OM ×100)

in direct continuity with malignant epithelium does not prove origin from that epithelial structure. Some authors have advocated using immunohistochemical panels to distinguish primary ovarian from metastatic carcinomas to the ovary. Fowler et al.[114] report that there was positive immunostaining for **HAM-56 (human alveolar macrophage antigen)** in 85% of ovarian epithelial neoplasms (especially endometrioid, serous, and clear-cell types), whereas only 12% of metastatic gastroin-

testinal cancers were positive for HAM-56 (in the latter, positivity was usually weak). In contrast, **carcinoembryonic antigen (CEA)** was strongly positive in 76% of gastrointestinal cancers and 39% of ovarian cancers; and, of the positive ovarian cancers, the vast majority were mucinous type. All endometrioid carcinomas were negative for CEA. **Cytokeratin 20** has been found to immunostain transitional cell carcinoma of the bladder, gastrointestinal carcinoma, mucinous tumors of the

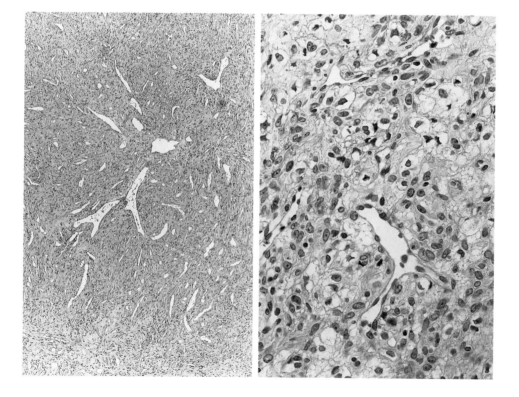

FIGURE 12–16. *Left,* Sclerosing stromal tumor of the ovary showing prominent ectatic vessels in a cellular area. Other areas were more edematous and hypocellular, imparting a pseudolobulated pattern at low-power examination. (H&E, OM ×10) *Right,* The cellular areas were composed of spindle cells admixed with vacuolated cells with shrunken nuclei. The vacuolated cells simulated signet-ring cells, luteinized cells, and/or lipid (steroid-producing) cells. Eighty percent of sclerosing stromal tumors occur in patients younger than 30 years old, a group in whom metastatic carcinoma to the ovary would be uncommon. (H&E, OM ×100)

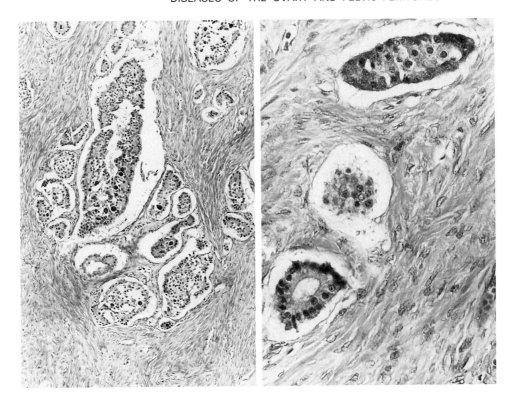

FIGURE 12–17. *Left,* Ovary containing metastatic carcinoid forming an insular pattern with abundant fibrous stroma. Note the prominent clefting artifact from tissue shrinkage during processing. (H&E, OM ×10) *Right,* Metastatic carcinoid forming small nest or tubules of tumor cells. (H&E, OM ×50)

ovary, Merkel cell carcinoma, and pancreaticobiliary carcinoma, whereas other carcinoma types, including those from the breast, lung, and endometrium, are negative.[115]

PRIMARY SARCOMAS OF THE OVARY

In 1987, Shakfeh and Woodruff assiduously reviewed the literature on the subject of primary sarcomas of the ovary, noting 105 previously reported cases and adding 46 pertinent examples from their files.[116] Almost contemporaneously another series was published, but in abstract form,[117] and only a few additional cases have been reported.[118-124] Because primary ovarian sarcoma is usually an unexpected ovarian tumor, it becomes a difficult diagnosis. Awareness of their occasional occurrence in the ovary is the key to proper diagnosis.

CLINICOPATHOLOGIC DIAGNOSIS. Primary ovarian sarcomas are rare, constituting 3% of all ovarian neoplasms.[116] They

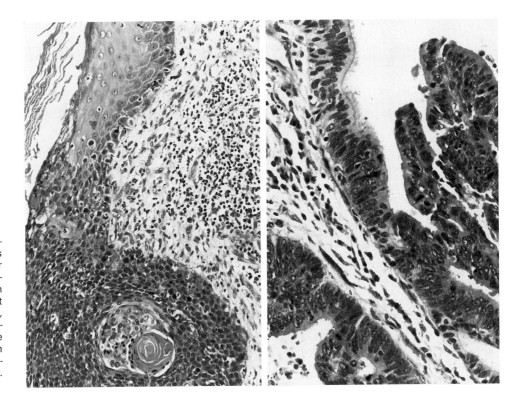

FIGURE 12–18. *Left,* Epidermotrophic metastatic squamous carcinoma is shown in the lower left-hand side of the photograph, growing to fuse with benign squamous epithelium at the upper left-hand side. (H&E, OM ×10) *Right,* Shown is metastatic colonic carcinoma to the lung, which is fusing with benign, ciliated respiratory epithelium (upper left-hand side). (H&E, OM ×50)

usually occur in middle-aged or older women, but they may affect children and adolescents as well.[116, 120] Although such sarcomas could theoretically arise from teratomas and other germinal neoplasms,[125] malignant mixed mullerian tumors, or endometriotic stroma, many ovarian sarcomas are derived from ovarian stromal elements.[122] Importantly, almost all histologic varieties of sarcoma (with their characteristic gross and microscopic features) that have been described in the somatic soft tissues also have been noted in the ovary.[116, 117] Although a detailed itemization and discussion would be otiose, we wish to draw attention to a few tumors that may enter into differential diagnosis.

DIFFERENTIAL DIAGNOSIS. Some ovarian fibromas may be unusually cellular and exhibit some degree of mitotic activity. Prat and Scully[126] compared and contrasted **cellular fibromas and ovarian fibrosarcomas**, and concluded that the former were usually characterized by 1 to 3 mitotic figures per 10 high-power fields (HPF) (average count in 50 HPF), usually behaved in a benign fashion, but rarely recurred locally. On the other hand, the fibrosarcomas contained 4 or more mitoses per 10 HPF and often pursued a frankly malignant course. Similarly, sclerosing stromal tumors of the ovary[127] may contain foci of increased cellularity, with collections of polyhedral and spindle cells with vacuolated or eosinophilic cytoplasm (see Fig. 12–16). However, these lesions usually occur in young women (80% occur in patients younger than 30 years) and microscopically are recognized by pseudolobulation, pronounced diffuse and pericellular sclerosis, prominent vascularity, and only rare mitotic activity. Furthermore, the cells of sclerosing stromal tumor may display positive immunohistochemical reactions for desmin and smooth muscle actin.

As with **myogenic neoplasms of the uterus,** it may be difficult to differentiate benign from malignant smooth muscle tumors of the ovary. Some ovarian ''leiomyomas'' may contain frequent mitoses (6–15 mitotic figures per 10 HPF) but,

if unassociated with nuclear atypism and necrosis, appear to have a good prognosis, analogous to so-called mitotically active leiomyomas of the uterus.[128, 129] Remember, primary ovarian smooth muscle tumors are rare, and most so-called examples are more likely best considered ovarian fibromas.

Endometrioid stromal sarcomas of the ovary often have associated (in ~50% of cases) prior, synchronous, or subsequent endometrioid sarcoma of the uterus. They produce yellow-white, solid and/or cystic, and sometimes necrotic and/or hemorrhagic tumors. They are composed of densely cellular endometrial stroma-like cells (small round or oval cells with scanty cytoplasm) with a variable prominent arteriolar network (spiral arteriole-like), cellular whorling around arterioles, storiform fibromatous patterns, hyaline collagenous bands or plaques, sometimes sex cord–like differentiation, reticulum fibrils around individual cells, extraovarian intravascular growth, and sometimes associated endometriosis (Fig. 12–19).[130] Examples of primary ovarian angiosarcoma (Fig. 12–20),[131] along with other vascular tumors including **capillary and cavernous hemangiomas and epithelioid hemangioendotheliomas (''histiocytoid'' hemangioma),** have been reported.[132] Very rare examples of **ovarian sarcoma resembling telangiectatic osteosarcoma** are now reported,[133] and peculiar cases of **ovarian rhabdomyosarcoma are reported with leukemia-like systemic dissemination[134] and in association with dysgerminoma.**[125] Metastatic sarcomas to the ovary, as discussed elsewhere in this chapter, can almost always be differentiated from primary lesions on clinical grounds, except for endometrial stromal sarcomas.

Also to be considered in the differential diagnosis of primary ovarian sarcoma is **sarcoma-predominant malignant mixed mullerian tumor (carcinosarcoma), metastatic sarcoma to the ovary, heterologous mesenchymal elements occurring in a Sertoli-Leydig cell tumor, sarcomatoid mural nodules occurring in an ovarian epithelial tumor**

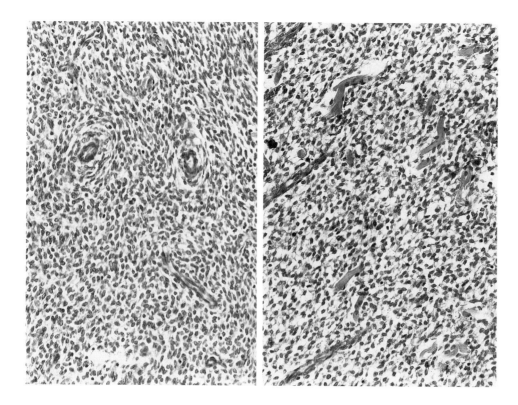

FIGURE 12–19. *Left,* Endometrioid stromal sarcoma of the ovary is shown composed of densely cellular endometrial stroma–like cells (small round or oval cells with scanty cytoplasm) with a variable prominent arteriolar network (spiral arteriole-like) with cellular whorling around arterioles. (H&E, OM ×50) *Right,* Hyaline collagenous bands are shown admixed with the endometrial stroma–like cells. (H&E, OM ×50)

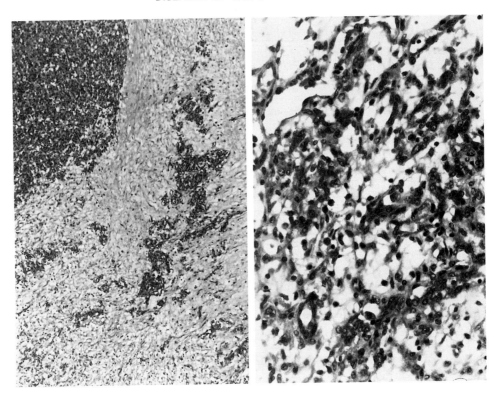

FIGURE 12–20. *Left,* Ovarian stroma is shown containing solid and discontinuous strands of angiosarcoma cells. (H&E, OM ×10) *Right,* Note the anastomosing vascular (capillary-like) channels lined by atypical endothelial cells. (H&E, OM ×100)

(usually mucinous), and **ovarian Wilms' tumor.** Carcinosarcoma is not covered in this chapter, but Sertoli-Leydig cell tumors and metastatic sarcoma to ovary are covered subsequently in this chapter.

In seminal articles,[135–137] the Massachusetts General Hospital group, based on a review of disparate cases from the literature as well as cases from their files, delineated three types of **sarcomatoid mural nodules** that may occur in association with cystic mucinous neoplasms of the ovary. These workers portioned such nodules into an ostensible benign group, sarcoma-like nodules, and two malignant groups, sarcomas and anaplastic carcinomas. The associated mucinous neoplasms, with a rare exception, were all carcinomas or lesions of borderline malignancy. During the succeeding decades, the relevant literature has adhered to this schema; and, whereas there are clinical and prognostic differences between the sarcoma-like nodules on one hand and the malignant varieties on the other, we feel that, especially with the findings of more recent studies that have included immunohistochemical analysis, the anaplastic carcinomas and the sarcomas represent differing expressions of the same neoplastic process. We also suggest that the sarcoma-like nodules may, in fact, also be true neoplasms, albeit with a notably better prognosis.

Grossly, there are no definite distinguishing features among the various subtypes. The cystic component has been unilocular or multilocular, and the cystic lesions have varied from about 5 to 30 cm in greatest diameter. The mural nodules have varied from solitary to multiple and have been of variable size, color, and consistency. Microscopically, the cystic mucinous epithelium, although benign in some areas of some cases, has exhibited the atypia of borderline malignancy and/or features of frank mucinous carcinoma. Although a few of the earlier cases predating the Boston studies included

"mucinous cystadenomas," the extent of sampling appears indefinite, and independent evaluation is difficult. In only two of the more recent cases were mural nodules associated with a mucinous cystadenoma,[135, 138] and only one was stated to have been extensively sampled.[138] It is worthy of note that both of these sarcomatoid lesions were diagnosed as fibrosarcomas, were rapidly aggressive and lethal, and were composed of a dominant monomorphic population, unlike the remainder of the mural nodules to be described. As the authors of both relevant papers note, the histopathologic features were consistent with independent origin of the divergent neoplasms that arose in adjacent areas, and they indicated that this was the most appropriate explanation. Thus, if one excludes these rare examples of monomorphic spindle cell sarcomas, virtually all mural nodules have been associated with borderline or malignant mucinous neoplasms;[139] the case of Bruijn et al.[140] was a non-monomorphic "fibrosarcoma" that did not recur or metastasize.

Mural sarcomatoid areas are characterized by pleomorphic spindle and polyhedral cells, anaplastic mononucleated giant cells, and multinucleated giant cells, the last type varying from pleomorphic to more uniform epulis-like cells. The sarcoma-like nodules were segregated from the others because of their gross and microscopic circumscription and lack of discernible local invasion, including an absence of demonstrable vascular invasion.[136, 137] However, it was noted that these sarcoma-like lesions may be malignant, but that their good prognosis was due to their small size and "encapsulation."[137] The sarcoma-like nodules tended to occur in younger patients than in the other groups, and they were associated with a benign clinical course, contrasting with the unfavorable behavior of the other two groups.

In those nodules that contained anaplastic epithelial elements, the latter were identified by routine microscopy, mucin histochemistry, and, on occasion, supplementary electron microscopy.[141] More recently, sarcomatoid mural nodules have been studied by immunohistochemistry.[142–145] We draw attention to the demonstration of co-expression of epithelial (cytokeratin, EMA) and mesenchymal (vimentin) phenotypes in variable numbers of the sarcomatoid cells because this finding supports the concept that the nodules represent sarcomatoid carcinoma,[146] an entity that many investigators, including ourselves,[148] believe to represent sarcomatous neometaplasia in a carcinoma. The lack of epithelial markers in some examples or the presence of heterologous mesenchymal differentiation[147, 148] certainly does not rule out this pathogenetic route, and sarcomatoid carcinoma fits nicely with a unitarian concept of this subject. We hasten to add that this term should not be confused with ovarian carcinosarcomas of either mixed mesodermal type or of teratoid (biphyletic germinal) derivation. It should be noted that a small number of sarcomatoid lesions have been described in association with ovarian serous tumors.[149] The majority of these cases may represent collision tumors. Yet, a rare case of mural sarcomatoid carcinoma associated with a serous borderline carcinoma has been reported.[139]

There are two well-documented reports of ovarian neoplasms that exhibited the characteristic pattern of **Wilms' tumor.** One example was pure, occurring in a 56-year-old patient who was alive and well 9 years after total abdominal hysterectomy, bilateral salpingo-oophorectomy, and external radiotherapy.[150] The second neoplasm developed in a 20-year-old woman and comprised a dominant component of juvenile granulosa cell tumor with an intralesional nodule of Wilms' tumor. The patient underwent unilateral salpingo-oophorectomy, but details of the follow-up were not supplied.[151] Differentiation of an extrarenal Wilms' tumor from carcinosarcoma is necessary.[150–152] Although both may contain rhabdomyoblasts, additional types of heterologous elements, if present, are much more in favor of carcinosarcoma (malignant mixed mullerian tumor). Characteristically, Wilms' tumors are composed of blastemal cells that are associated with differentiation to typical glomeruloid structures and with a usually bland maturing spindleform stroma, whereas the spindling portions of a carcinosarcoma are frankly sarcomatous, and the differentiating epithelial conformations are of mullerian type.

Finally, in the differential diagnosis of primary ovarian fibrosarcoma and **leiomyosarcoma (including the myxoid variant),**[124] one should consider **ovarian myxoma**[153] and **ovarian fibromatosis,**[154] which may be associated with disseminated intra-abdominal fibromatosis.

METASTATIC SARCOMA AND MELANOMA TO THE OVARY

Sarcomas and melanomas metastatic to the ovary are uncommon and usually present considerable problems in differential diagnosis, particularly if an accurate clinical history has not been provided to the pathologist. Unfortunately, the latter situation is a common and frustrating occurrence. We are constantly reminding clinicians to provide a complete and accurate history, the quality of which often directly increases the quality of the final pathologic diagnoses and comments.

CLINICOPATHOLOGIC FEATURES. The literature contains only sporadic reports of sarcomatous spread to the ovary,[111, 155, 156] often without significant details, except for one study of 21 cases.[157] In that series, 11 tumors were primary in the uterus, and 10 widely divergent histologic types arose from a variety of extragenital sites. The ovarian lesions were generally large, and in 11 instances were discovered at the same time as the primary tumors. But, in seven cases, the ovarian tumor was discovered 7 months to 9 years after diagnosis of the primary neoplasm, and in three cases, the ovarian metastases were discovered 4, 7, and 10 months before detection of the primary. Eleven of the 21 metastatic lesions were bilateral.

DIFFERENTIAL DIAGNOSIS. On microscopic examination, the greatest difficulty was caused by metastatic endometrial stromal sarcomas because of their simulation of various types of ovarian sex cord–stromal tumors, including fibroma, thecoma, and granulosa cell or Sertoli-Leydig cell tumors. Features helpful in distinction from this group include the frequent presence of concurrent extra-ovarian spread, bilaterality, and a characteristic content of small arteries (''spiral'' arteries) exhibited in metastatic stromal sarcoma (see Fig. 12–19). Distinction from primary ovarian stromal sarcoma[130] may be difficult or impossible on purely histologic grounds; yet, the presence of ovarian endometriosis is strongly in favor of primary endometrial stromal sarcoma.

Extragenital metastatic sarcomas to the ovary that pose particularly difficult differential diagnostic problems include epithelioid leiomyosarcoma,[157] as well as the group of ''round cell'' sarcomas comprising rhabdomyosarcoma,[155] Ewing's sarcoma,[157] and desmoplastic peritoneal small-cell tumor with divergent differentiation.[158] Thus, entities to be considered in the differential diagnosis include both primary and metastatic small-cell carcinoma,[99, 155] neuroblastic and primitive neuroectodermal tumors,[159] malignant lymphoreticular neoplasms, and primary ovarian rhabdomyosarcoma,[120] lesions which are discussed elsewhere in this chapter. The clinical history, a variety of features in routinely stained sections, and immunohistochemical and ultrastructural studies may be required to elucidate a particular problem.

The microscopic polymorphism of metastatic malignant melanoma is well known and may cause confusion with a number of primary and metastatic ovarian lesions[99, 160] (Fig. 12–21). Approximately one half of cases of malignant melanoma metastatic to the ovary have a history, sometimes remote, of known malignant melanoma, usually arising from a cutaneous site, and rarely from the choroid. Although the age range of patients has varied from the second to the seventh decades, the majority of examples tend to occur in younger adults. Metastatic lesions are bilateral in approximately 50% of the cases, and some are grossly pigmented, at least to a variable degree, but it is important to note that the majority lack this feature. If pigmented, both endometriosis, particularly that variant with necrotic pseudoxanthomatous nodules, and lipochrome-rich ovarian steroid cell tumor[161] should be given consideration in the differential diagnosis.

Microscopically, the variable features of melanoma raise multiple considerations in differential diagnosis. When dominated by larger eosinophilic cells, metastatic melanoma may be confused with steroid-cell tumor or pregnancy luteoma,[160] hepatoid yolk-sac tumor, hepatoid carcinoma, and metastatic hepatocellular carcinoma,[162] ovarian oncocytoma,[163] and large-cell carcinomas arising from several sites. When follicle-like

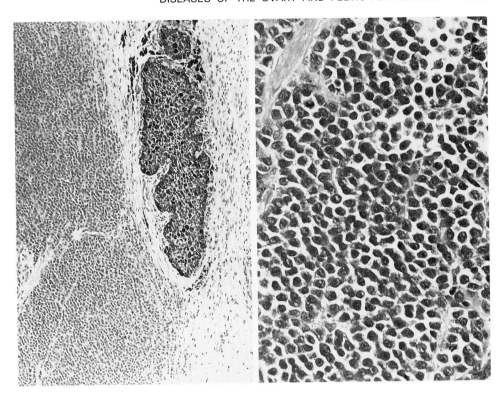

FIGURE 12-21. *Left,* Metastatic melanoma to ovary. Note the black pigment in the melanoma cells and within adjacent melanophages in upper right-hand corner. (H&E, OM ×25) *Right,* Sheets of melanoma cells become apparent at higher magnification. This pattern could mimic a number of poorly differentiated malignant tumors, including lymphoma, carcinoma, and/or sarcoma. (H&E, OM ×100)

spaces are present in metastatic melanoma, confusion with several primary and metastatic tumors may result,[99] particularly juvenile granulosa cell tumors.[160] Pseudonevoid zones in metastatic melanoma may be confused with primary or metastatic insular carcinoid.[99] When the melanoma includes a predominant small-cell population, the differential diagnosis may include primary or metastatic small-cell carcinoma[99, 155, 160] and, less commonly, other types of small cell lesions. When areas of spindling are present,[164] primary or metastatic sarcomas should be included in the differential diagnosis.[111] Differentiation from primary melanomas arising in a cystic teratoma is discussed elsewhere in this chapter. The clinical history and the presence of a unilateral versus a bilateral process are useful initial points of import, as is the microscopic evaluation of nuclear atypia. The presence of cytoplasmic melanin pigment, demonstrated by a Masson-Fontana stain, is very helpful in diagnosing melanoma,[160] but pigment is absent in a significant number of instances. Immunohistochemical staining of melanin using antibodies to S-100 protein and HMB-45, as well as the differential use of alpha-fetoprotein, desmin, cytokeratin, and peptide hormone immunostains, should resolve various diagnostic possibilities. Teratomatous nevi and progonomas and melanosis peritonei are mentioned for the sake of completeness.[160]

HEMATOLYMPHOID LESIONS INVOLVING THE OVARY

Malignant lymphoma with disseminated disease frequently involves the ovaries at the time of autopsy. However, fewer than 1% of patients with malignant lymphoma present with ovarian involvement.[165–171] Collaterally, rare acceptable examples of primary malignant lymphoma of the ovary have

been reported[165, 167, 170, 171] and are supported by clinical follow-up and by documentation of the presence of lymphocytes in normal ovaries.[171] The last two of the foregoing groups of patients are apt to be a source of diagnostic problems.

CLINICOPATHOLOGIC FEATURES. Patients presenting with ovarian lymphoma have ranged widely in age, with a peak incidence in the fourth and fifth decades.[168, 170, 171] Involvement may be unilateral or bilateral with approximately equal frequency. Recent studies suggest that bilateral involvement is a sign of systemic lymphoma.[171] Immunophenotypic analyses have shown that the overwhelming majority of ovarian lymphomas are B-cell neoplasms.[169, 171] With reference to the working formulation, except for **Hodgkin's disease,** which rarely affects the ovary,[170, 171] the lymphomas have been of a variety of types, but the **small non-cleaved lymphomas (Burkitt's or non-Burkitt's types)** have been most common in children and young adults (<20 years), compatible with the concept that this variety of lymphoma preferentially involves the ovaries.[171] Of interest, the non-Burkitt's or undifferentiated type of small non-cleaved lymphoma is called "high-grade B-cell lymphoma, Burkitt-like" in the proposed classification scheme of the International Lymphoma Study Group. This is because they often share morphologic features with large-cell lymphomas, lack c-*myc* rearrangements, but have *bcl*-2 rearrangements, suggesting that these tumors are probably not related to "true" Burkitt's lymphoma.[172] Diffuse large-cell lymphomas are the second most common in the pediatric age group, but they are the most common type in adults. Follicular lymphomas are the second most common type in adults.

DIFFERENTIAL DIAGNOSIS. Microscopically, ovarian lymphomas do not exhibit noticeable cytologic differences in comparison with extraovarian sites. However, in the ovary, the tumor cells not infrequently grow in cords and nests, often with variable degrees of sclerosis.[170, 171] Because of these epithelioid patterns, primary and metastatic undifferentiated carcinoma, primary and metastatic small-cell carcinoma, and metastatic breast carcinoma should be considered in the differential diagnosis.[170] Malignant lymphoma in the ovary may also bear some resemblance to **dysgerminoma** and **granulosa cell tumor.** When considering a diagnosis of ovarian lymphoma, a search for unequivocal glandular differentiation and mucin stains should be performed. Immunohistochemical studies using leukocyte common antigen (CD45) and B- and T-cell associated markers identify the vast majority of lymphomas. Additional differential use of cytokeratins, chromogranin A, and neuron-specific enolase, as well as placental alkaline phosphatase, if dysgerminoma (Fig. 12–22) is suspected, may be needed in selected instances.

Leukemic infiltration of the ovary is also common at autopsy. The only leukemic lesion that may cause a problem in histologic appraisal is **granulocytic sarcoma,**[173, 174] especially when there is no clinical evidence of hematopoietic disease.[175] More commonly, granulocytic sarcoma occurs with known **acute myelogenous leukemia** or **myeloproliferative disease** or as a site of relapse after chemotherapy.[170, 173] It should also be noted that the ovary, as the testis, may also be a site of relapse in **acute lymphoblastic leukemia.**[170] Granulocytic sarcoma, when it affects the ovaries, may be unilateral or bilateral but is rarely green (chloromatous). Granulocytic sarcoma, frequently confused with lymphoma, may contain eosinophilic myelocytes, a helpful differential feature. Stains for chloracetate esterase and/or an immunoperoxidase study for the presence of lysozyme and/or myeloperoxidase are usually diagnostic. **Plasmacytoma** of the ovary is exquisitely rare and may be followed by multiple myeloma.[176] Finally, peculiar cases of lymphoma arising in association with thyroid tissue in mature cystic teratoma[177] or serous carcinoma of low-malignant potential are reported.[178] The report of the thyroid tissue–associated lymphoma suggests that MALT-type lymphomas may arise from the ovary under some circumstances.

SMALL-CELL CARCINOMAS INVOLVING THE OVARY

There are two separate and clinicopathologically distinct varieties of **primary small-cell carcinoma of the ovary, the hypercalcemic type**[179–185] **and the pulmonary type.**[186] These neoplasms must be distinguished from each other, from small-cell carcinomas arising from diverse sites metastatic to the ovary, and from certain other primary and metastatic ovarian neoplasms.

CLINICOPATHOLOGIC FEATURES. The hypercalcemic type was described in the early 1980s.[179] It is usually a highly lethal cancer that affects young women and is associated with hypercalcemia in 62% of cases.[181] Approximately 33% of patients with stage IA disease have long-term survival, whereas nearly all those with more advanced stage disease die from tumor. The age of patients has ranged from 9 to 43, with a mean age of 24.[181, 186] Ninety-nine percent of tumors have been unilateral. The associated hypercalcemia is virtually the sole paraneoplastic syndrome that is associated with this variety of small-cell carcinoma. Although most data suggest this lesion is a form of poorly differentiated carcinoma, the histogenesis of this neoplasm remains unclear.[181, 182] The pathogenesis of the hypercalcemia likely results from secretion of parathyroid hormone–related protein.[181] Essentially no ultrastructural studies of this neoplasm have clearly demonstrated the presence of dense-core granules.[179, 180, 182, 184] Ultrastructural studies show moderate to large amounts of dilated rough endoplasmic reticulum (Fig. 12–23), as well as cell-cell junctions that are sometimes desmosomes.[182] These findings plus

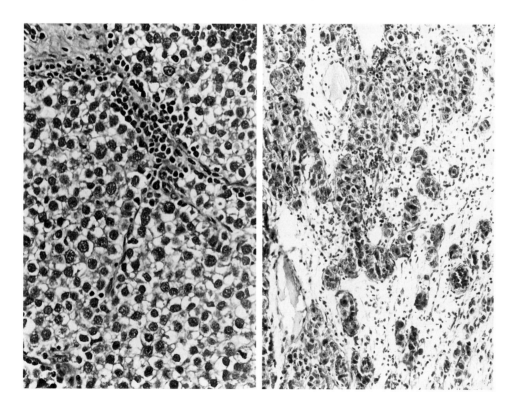

FIGURE 12–22. *Left,* Dysgerminoma is shown with sheets of evenly spaced, vesicular nuclei surrounded by abundant clear cytoplasm. Small lymphocytes and plasma cells are present in a fibrous septa, a feature very helpful in making the diagnosis. (H&E, OM ×50) *Right,* Note this example of dysgerminoma in which the tumor cells form small anastomosing cords of cells mimicking sex cord–stromal tumors, steroid cell tumors, or carcinoma. (H&E, OM ×25)

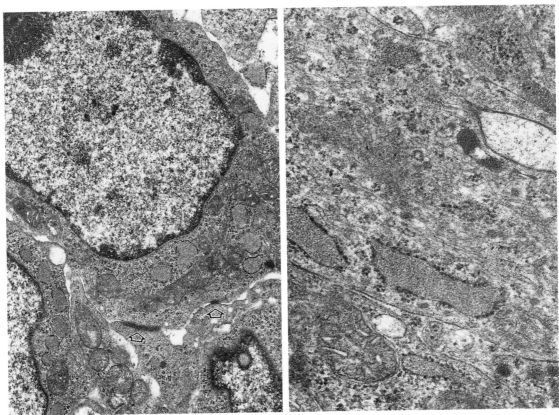

FIGURE 12–23. *Left,* Shown are the ultrastructural features of the tumor cells from a hypercalcemic type of small-cell ovarian carcinoma. Note the dilated rough endoplasmic reticulum and desmosome-like cell-cell junctions *(open arrows).* (LCUA, ×2000) *Right,* Shown in greater detail are the dilated rough endoplasmic reticulum containing protein-like material. Could this be the parathyroid hormone-related protein? (LCUA, ×4000)

the observation that approximately 90% of tumors immunoreact with anti-keratin (most consistently CAM 5.2) favor epithelial differentiation.[181, 182] Nonetheless, other data suggest the possibility of a sex cord–stromal origin,[185] germ cell origin, or neuroendocrine origin.[180–182] Tumor cells also may show immunoreactivity for vimentin (~57%), epithelial membrane antigen (32%), neuron-specific enolase (~58%), chromogranin A (~44%), parathyroid hormone–related protein (~71%), and even parathyroid hormone (~7%).[181] Tumor cells are negative for S-100 protein, B72.3, and desmin.[181]

Alternatively, and more recently delineated,[186] small-cell carcinoma of the ovary of pulmonary type has occurred in women between the ages of 28 and 85. However, most are perimenopausal or postmenopausal, with a mean age of 59. Also, in contrast with the hypercalcemic type, approximately one half of cases are bilateral, and hypercalcemia is absent. Yet, ovarian small-cell carcinomas of the pulmonary type are also highly aggressive, and only 1 of the 11 patients reported by Eichorn et al.[186] was alive and without evidence of disease. The age of affected patients, in addition to some of the findings discerned on histologic examination, strongly suggests that this variety of carcinoma is histogenetically related to and arises on the background of a surface epithelial-stromal tumor, with putative small-cell neoplastic differentiation from neuroendocrine cells contained within such epithelial-stromal neoplasms.

The histologic as well as the immunohistochemical features of both types of small-cell carcinomas may overlap to a certain extent. Both types of neoplasm are composed of small cells with scant cytoplasm. Microscopic features of the hypercalcemic type include diffuse sheets of highly mitotic cells admixed by variable numbers of follicle-like spaces, but the tumor cells can also grow in nests, cords, clusters, or singly. The follicle-like spaces often contain eosinophilic fluid. Glands or cysts lined by mucinous epithelial cells are present in 10% to 15% of cases (Fig. 12–24). Moreover, the hypercalcemic type often contains foci of larger cells with large nuclei, prominent nucleoli, and abundant eosinophilic cytoplasm in as many as 50% of the cases (see Fig. 12–24).[181, 185–187] Although focal in most tumors, these large cells may be moderately abundant in approximately 16% and predominate in approximately 12% of cases.[181, 182] In 1% to 2%, only large cells are present; and in approximately 60%, these cells may contain intracytoplasmic hyaline inclusions, imparting a ''rhabdoid'' appearance. The follicle-like spaces lined by tumor cells are usually present in tumors of the hypercalcemic type, whereas they are rare in the pulmonary type. Appreciation of nuclear details is also of import, as the nuclear chromatin is clumped in the hypercalcemic type and evenly dispersed in the pulmonary type. Nucleoli are single, uniform, and present in most cells of the hypercalcemic type, but they are frequently inconspicuous in the pulmonary type.

Although not exhibiting distinct origin from an epithelial-stromal type of neoplasm, some small-cell carcinomas of pulmonary type have been topographically associated with either endometrioid adenocarcinomas, benign Brenner tumors, or

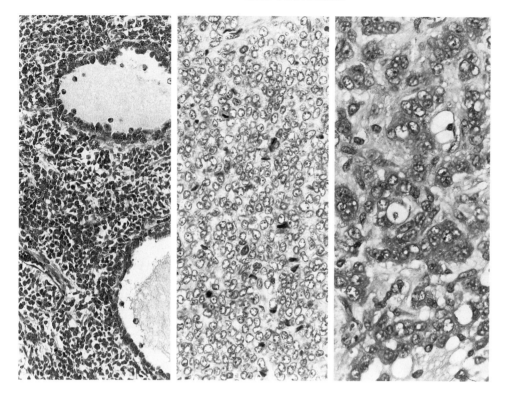

FIGURE 12–24. *Left,* Microscopic features of the hypercalcemic type include diffuse sheets of highly mitotic cells admixed by variable numbers of follicle-like spaces. The follicle-like spaces may appear empty or often contain eosinophilic fluid, as apparent in this case. (H&E, OM ×10) *Middle,* Shown are the nuclear features of the hypercalcemic type of small-cell carcinoma. The nuclear chromatin is clumped, nuclear membranes quite apparent, and nucleoli are single, uniform, and present in most cells. (H&E, OM ×50) *Right,* The hypercalcemic type often contains foci of larger cells with large nuclei, prominent nucleoli, and abundant eosinophilic cytoplasm, as shown here. Although in most cases these large cells are focal, in some they may predominate. (H&E, OM ×50)

mucinous cysts lined by mullerian-type epithelium. Argyrophilic cells are absent in the hypercalcemic type but are sometimes present in the pulmonary type. Both varieties of small-cell carcinoma may be stained for neuron-specific enolase and chromogranin; the positive immunoreactivity in the hypercalcemic type is regarded as a reflection of lack of neuroendocrine specificity.[183, 186] Nevertheless, immunohistochemistry may be helpful, in that vimentin has been demonstrated to be present in approximately one half of the tumors of hypercalcemic type but is absent in pulmonary type carcinomas (Fig. 12–25). Flow cytometry has disclosed that all of the hypercalcemic cases are diploid,[185, 186] whereas five of eight examples of the pulmonary type studied by Eichorn et al. were aneuploid.[186]

DIFFERENTIAL DIAGNOSIS. In terms of additional differential diagnosis, small-cell carcinomas of the lung,[188] lower female genital tract, particularly the cervix,[189] and from elsewhere (gastrointestinal tract, thymus, and skin)[190] may metastasize to the ovary. It is apparent that on a purely histopathologic basis, these metastatic neoplasms cannot be differentiated from primary small-cell carcinoma of the pulmonary type, with the exception of metastatic **Merkel cell carcinomas,** which stain for neurofilament, chromogranin, and cytokeratin 20.[190] Although **metastatic small-cell carcinoma to the ovary** is frequently bilateral, so are primary ovarian small-cell carcinomas of pulmonary type. However, clinical findings are usually sufficient to enable distinction.

A variety of additional primary and metastatic small-cell neoplasms may enter into the differential diagnosis, including **rhabdomyosarcoma, neuroblastoma and primitive neuroectodermal tumors** (Fig. 12–26), **peritoneal (intra-abdominal) small-cell tumor, malignant melanoma, lymphoma-leukemia, and metastatic sarcoma.**[186, 189, 191, 192] When the large-cell population in a hypercalcemic type of primary small-cell carcinoma is preponderant,[185] it may be

difficult or impossible to differentiate such a lesion from the more ordinary undifferentiated large-cell carcinoma of surface mullerian origin.[193]

Given the similar age range of affected patients, it is important to differentiate the hypercalcemic type of small-cell carcinoma from the **granulosa cell tumor** and, in particular, the **juvenile granulosa cell tumor (JGCT)** because of the strikingly different treatment and prognosis between these two lesions. That this is not merely a theoretical exercise in differential diagnosis is illustrated by the fact that several cases of hypercalcemic small-cell carcinoma have been reported in the literature as either benign or malignant granulosa cell tumors.[179] The resemblance between these two disparate neoplasms is furthered at the histologic level by the occasional presence of nuclear atypia and variable, but sometimes high, mitotic activity in JGCT.[194] The JGCT displays follicles that often contain mucicarminophilic material, whereas the follicle-like spaces in the small-cell carcinoma of hypercalcemic type do not contain mucin. The cells of the JGCT have ample eosinophilic cytoplasm and nuclei that are larger than cells of hypercalcemic small-cell carcinoma, which have darker nuclei with scant cytoplasm. However, as previously noted, some of these small-cell carcinomas may harbor a population of larger cells with eosinophilic cytoplasm and thus bear superficial similarity to luteinized granulosa cells. The JGCT contains fibrothecomatous areas, but the small-cell carcinoma does not, and isosexual precocity is usually a feature of JGCT. Immunohistochemically, approximately one third of small-cell hypercalcemic carcinomas express EMA, whereas it is absent in granulosa cell tumors. Conversely, only about one half of the small-cell carcinomas of hypercalcemic type express vimentin, but its presence has been shown in all granulosa cell tumors so studied.[183] Finally, to be considered in the differential diagnosis is **juxtaovarian or ovarian**

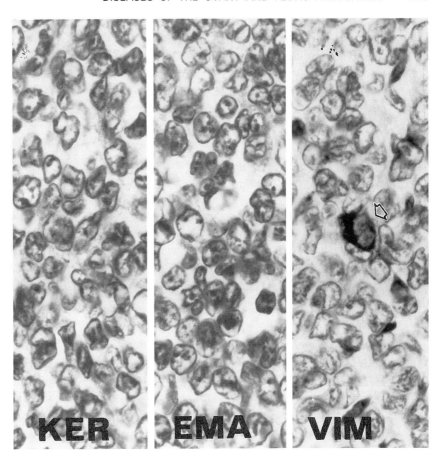

FIGURE 12–25. In this example of small-cell ovarian carcinoma, hypercalcemic type, tumor cells were negative for keratin (KER) (AE1/3) and EMA but positive for vimentin (VIM). (Methanol-fixed tissue, DAB ipox, OM ×25)

tumor of probable wolffian origin, which has been reported to rarely metastasize and cause terminal hypercalcemia.[195] Tumors of this type are discussed in greater detail in the next section.

JUVENILE GRANULOSA CELL TUMORS

Two types of granulosa cell tumors occur in the ovary, the **adult granulosa cell tumor (AGCT) and juvenile granulosa cell tumor (JGCT).** Although both develop over a wide age range, approximately 90% of granulosa cell tumors in prepubertal girls and many of those occurring in women younger than 30 years are of the JGCT type.[194, 196–202] Many JGCTs present as unilateral (stage 1A) adnexal masses associated with features of hyperestrinism, including isosexual pseudoprecocity in girls.[194, 196–202] In fact, more than 80% of the JGCTs in prepubertal girls are associated with isosexual pseudoprecocity. Uncommonly, virilization may also occur. Some are associated with Ollier's disease or Maffucci's syndrome.[196] Rarely, JGCT occurs in the infant testis, often associated with abnormal chromosomes and ambiguous genitalia.[197]

The prognosis for patients with JGCTs is very good, with a recurrence rate of approximately 8% and a mortality rate of approximately 3% for limited-stage tumors.[194, 196–202] Those who die usually do so within 3 years, and stage is the single best predictor of outcome.[194, 196–202] Therapy is usually unilateral salpingo-oophorectomy. Clearly, JGCTs must be distinguished from the more aggressive ovarian tumors with which

they may be confused. This is particularly hazardous because JGCTs may simulate high-grade malignancy (especially germ cell tumors and sometimes small-cell undifferentiated carcinoma) by having hyperchromatic atypical nuclei with numerous mitotic figures.

PATHOLOGIC FEATURES. JGCTs are often large, solid and/or cystic tumors usually measuring in the 10- to 15-cm range, but tumors as large as 32 cm in diameter have been reported. They are usually tan to yellow and may show hemorrhagic or necrotic areas. Microscopically, tumor cells grow in a distinctly nodular and/or diffuse pattern containing irregular follicles, often in the center of the nodules (Fig. 12–27). Call-Exner bodies are not present, and there is often myxoid interstitial material and mucoid fluid within follicles (Fig. 12–28). The myxoid change may be very prominent during pregnancy.[203] In fact, many types of **sex cord–stromal tumors that present during pregnancy** often show atypical microscopic features when compared with their counterparts presenting in the absence of pregnancy. During pregnancy, otherwise specific types of sex cord–stromal tumors display a more disorderly arrangement of their cells, lacking recognizable differentiation in may areas, showing prominent edema, and containing unusually large numbers of lutein or Leydig-like cells. The latter two features seem to be most developed at term. More extensive sampling than usual may be needed to disclose the correct classification.[203]

Classic JGCT cells are poorly differentiated (less mature than in AGCT), epithelioid or spindled, and commonly luteinized, resulting in abundant eosinophilic to pale cytoplasm containing variable intracytoplasmic lipid.[194, 198, 199] Theca cells

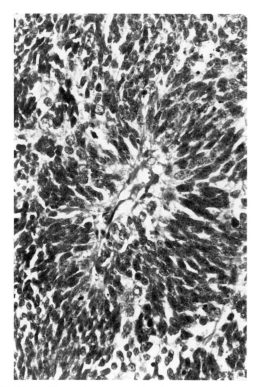

FIGURE 12–26. Shown is an example of monodermal teratoma of the ovary characterized by neuroectodermal differentiation. This example shows ependymoma-like features, but examples occur that resemble medulloblastoma, medulloepithelioma, neuroblastoma, and/or glioblastoma multiforme. Immunostaining for glial fibrillary acidic protein should help in making the correct diagnosis. (H&E, OM ×100)

may be present in varying amounts and also luteinized. Mitotic figures are often numerous and sometimes atypical, and the JGCT cell nuclei are often hyperchromatic (Figs. 12–28 and 12–29). In as many as 15% of cases of JGCT, nuclei are markedly atypical and large (see Fig. 12–29),[195] and flow DNA aneuploidy has been found in approximately 50% of cases.[200] Remember, other sex cord–stromal tumors of the ovary also can display focal areas with bizarre nuclei.[202] JGCT nuclei lack the angular, grooved or folded nuclear membranes found in AGCT.

DIFFERENTIAL DIAGNOSIS. When confronted with a difficult case, extensive sampling of the tumor should reveal areas diagnostic of JGCT. Nonetheless, a number of lesions should be considered in the differential diagnosis of JGCT. **Adult granulosa cell tumors (AGCTs)** may display a variety of morphologic patterns, and familiarity with them should allow separation of AGCTs from JGCTs. The patterns of AGCT include the macrofollicular (Fig. 12–30), microfollicular (Fig. 12–31), diffuse or sarcomatoid (Fig. 12–32), trabecular (Figs. 12–33 and 12–34), insular (see Fig. 12–34), and moiré-silk (watered silk) types (see Fig. 12–33). Sometimes a fibromatous and/or thecomatous stroma is prominent (see Fig. 12–34), rarely tubules with lumina are formed, and "cystic" examples of AGCT develop. Tumor cell nuclei of AGCTs appear "mature," usually show few mitotic figures, contain nuclear grooves, are surrounded by scanty cytoplasm, are haphazardly oriented to one another, and are either somewhat angular, rounded, oval, or slightly spindle-shaped (see Figs. 12–30 to 12–34). As in other sex cord–stromal

tumors, nuclear pleomorphism is lacking, but focally bizarre, degenerative-type nuclei may be found.[201] The latter finding does not predict a poorer prognosis. Biscotti and Hart[199] reported vimentin- and cytokeratin (AE1/3)-positive tumor cells in JGCTs. Moreover, Otis et al.[204] reported characteristic punctate, paranuclear immunoreactivity for cytokeratin antibodies (AE1/3, CAM 5.2, and 35BH11) in AGCTs showing solid, follicular, and/or trabecular patterns, but not in diffuse or sarcomatoid examples. Vimentin was strongly positive, usually in a globoid, paranuclear location, in all patterns of AGCT. Desmin was positive in admixed cortical-type stromal cells; granulosa cells were negative.

Malignant germ cell tumors are common in the same age group as when JGCTs present; and like JGCTs, germ cell tumors can cause isosexual pseudoprecocity or menstrual abnormalities. Perioperative serum human chorionic gonadotropin (hCG) and/or alpha-fetoprotein (AFP) can be very helpful in the distinction of JGCT tumors from a germ cell malignancy, which is usually a **yolk sac tumor (YST).** Dysgerminoma should not be confused with JGCT, unless it is mixed with YST. **Embryonal carcinoma and choriocarcinoma** are very rare in the ovary. **Hyaline bodies,** which are commonly encountered with YST, can be seen in a wide variety of ovarian tumors, including JGCTs, clear-cell carcinomas, serous tumors, mucinous tumors, mixed mullerian (carcinosarcomatous) tumors, Sertoli-Leydig cell tumors, and endometrioid carcinomas.[205] The luteinized cells within JGCT with abundant eosinophilic cytoplasm can simulate **thecomas** and **steroid (lipid) cell tumors,** and focal sclerosis in JGCT tumor can mimic **sclerosing stromal tumor.**

Clear-cell carcinoma sometimes enters the differential diagnosis, but the young ages of the patients and absence of other cytologic features of clear-cell carcinoma make that possibility less likely. More frequently confused with JGCT is the **hypercalcemic type of small-cell carcinoma of the ovary,** especially those examples with well-developed follicles and a "large-cell" component. Frequently, small-cell carcinomas have spread beyond the ovary at presentation, show a "large-cell" component only focally, have "large cells" with a dense sometimes globular cytoplasm, show a more disorderly architecture as compared with JGCT, and have hypercalcemia in approximately 70% of cases. Moreover, undifferentiated carcinomas of other ovarian types are very uncommon in the usual age of presentation of JGCT. Rarely, **metastatic melanoma** to the ovary can very closely mimic JGCT. Prior history of melanoma is crucial in the distinction, but this may not be present. Clues to the diagnosis of melanoma include numerous cytoplasmic intranuclear inclusions, prominent and frequent nucleoli, and melanin pigment. Electron microscopy and immunohistochemistry for expression of S-100 protein and "melanoma-specific" antigen (HMB-45) should clarify the diagnosis in most cases.

Additional lesions that may be confused with JGCTs include **ovarian tumors of probable wolffian origin (OTWO)[206] or female adnexal tumors of probable wolffian origin (FATWO)[207]** (Fig. 12–35). This type of tumor may develop multiple irregular cystic spaces, imparting a follicular or sieve-like appearance, but other areas containing closely packed hollow tubules with compressed lumina by cuboidal or spindled epithelial cells, areas with larger anastomosing tubular glands, and adenomatoid tumor-like areas should disclose the proper diagnosis. Of note, **endometrioid carcinomas (especially of the fallopian tube) may resemble**

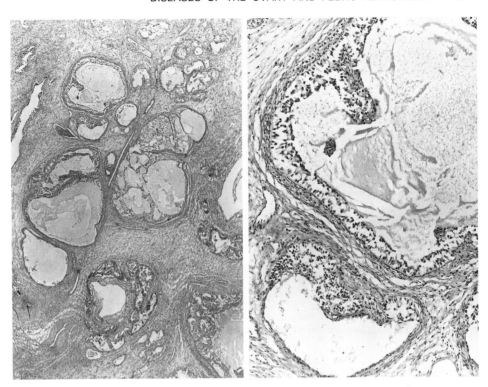

FIGURE 12–27. *Left,* A juvenile granulosa cell tumor (JGCT) is shown with the characteristic nodular or lobulated pattern. (H&E, OM ×5) *Right,* Shown are two nodules separated by fibrous stroma and containing follicles filled with mucin-like extracellular fluid. (H&E, OM ×50)

FATWOs.[208] Finally, peculiar **mixed germ cell–sex cord–stromal tumors of the ovary** occur and cause isosexual precocious puberty,[209] and distinctive ovarian sex cord–stromal tumor has been described as causing the sexual precocity in the **Peutz-Jeghers syndrome.**[210] The clinicopathologic features of these latter two tumors could cause confusion with JGCTs.

SERTOLI-LEYDIG CELL TUMORS

Sertoli-Leydig cell tumors (SLCTs) have been divided into five general categories: **well-differentiated, intermediate-differentiated, poorly differentiated, retiform, and mixed.** Accounting for less than 1% of ovarian tumors, SLCTs can occur in any age group (range, 2 to 75 years), but most occur

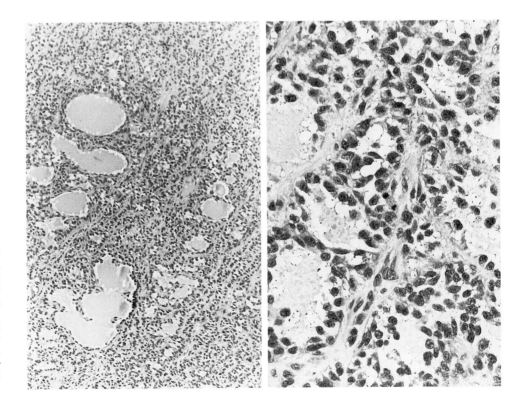

FIGURE 12–28. *Left,* An area of JGCT is shown composed of follicles of varying sizes and shapes separated by cellular areas. (H&E, OM ×10) *Right,* The tumor cells of JGCT contain hyperchromatic nuclei without grooves. Extracellular mucin-like material is focally abundant, imparting a myxoid or edematous appearance. (H&E, OM ×100)

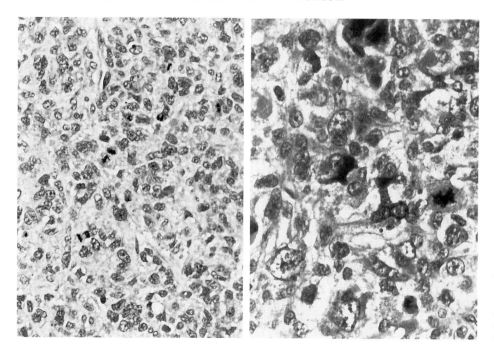

FIGURE 12–29. *Left,* JGCTs may show numerous mitotic figures. In one series, mitotic activity varied from less than 1 to 32 mitotic figures per 10 HPF (mean, 7). (H&E, OM ×50) *Right,* Focally high-grade nuclear atypia with atypical mitotic figures can be found in as many as 15% of cases. (H&E, OM ×100)

in young women at an average age of 25 years.[211–218] Although occasional tumors may produce symptoms of hyperestrinism, approximately 40% of patients with SLCTs present features of excess androgen secretion (amenorrhea, hirsutism, and/or virilization). Approximately 10% to 15% of SLCTs are clinically malignant, almost all have been poorly differentiated, intermediate grade with retiform areas, and/or contained heterologous mesenchymal elements. Classic intermediate-grade SLCTs rarely metastasize. Only 2% of SLCTs are bilateral. Thus, unilateral salpingo-oophorectomy is adequate

treatment for an SLCT in a young woman unless unfavorable prognostic features are present. Unfavorable features include extraovarian spread, poorly differentiated tumor with more than 5 mitotic figures per 10 HPF in stromal cells, heterologous mesenchymal elements, and/or rupture of tumor. Under the latter circumstances and in older women, consideration should be given to total abdominal hysterectomy and bilateral salpingo-oophorectomy. Moreover, chemotherapy should be considered in patients with extraovarian spread and with tumors with heterologous elements.

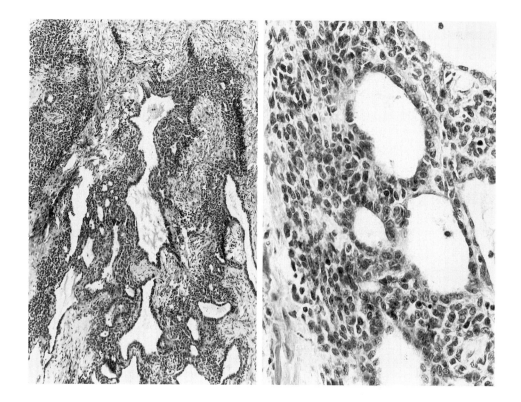

FIGURE 12–30. *Left,* An adult granulosa cell tumor (AGCT) is shown with a macrofollicular pattern. (H&E, OM ×5) *Right,* Shown in greater detail is the macrofollicular pattern of AGCT. (H&E, OM ×50)

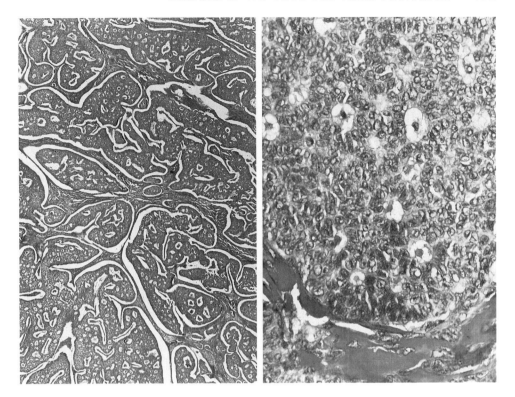

FIGURE 12–31. *Left,* An adult granulosa cell tumor (AGCT) is shown with anastomosing bands and clusters of AGCT cells separated by fibrous stroma forming. (H&E, OM ×5) *Right,* Shown in greater detail are the cells forming the characteristic microfollicular pattern of AGCT. Note the pale monotonous population of grooved nuclei, which are haphazardly oriented one to another. Also, note the microfollicles (Call-Exner bodies), which form tiny cavities containing dense eosinophilic to mucinous or watery material often having a single naked nucleus. (H&E, OM ×100)

The classic examples of well- or intermediate-differentiated SLCTs present only mild diagnostic problems, but the retiform, poorly differentiated, and mixed variants can stump even the very best surgical pathologists. Also, with the exception of the well-differentiated category, all categories of SLCT can be associated with heterologous elements, which can further complicate the diagnosis of SLCT.

PATHOLOGIC FEATURES. SLCTs vary greatly in size, but average approximately 10 cm in diameter. They are lobulated, tan to yellow, solid and/or cystic masses usually covered by a smooth external surface. Cysts are particularly prominent in the retiform variant or in those with heterologous elements. Hemorrhage and necrosis are uncommon, except in the poorly differentiated examples. Well-differentiated SLCTs are com-

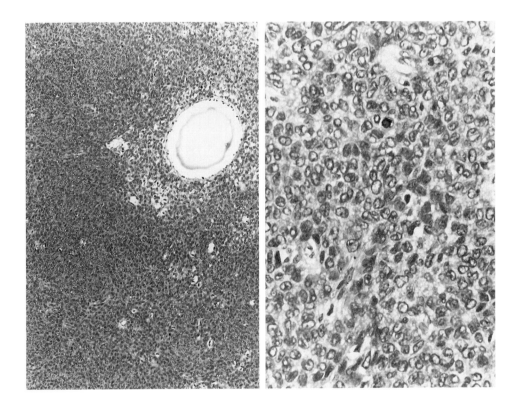

FIGURE 12–32. *Left,* An adult granulosa cell tumor (AGCT) is shown with a diffuse or sarcomatoid pattern. (H&E, OM ×5) *Right,* Shown in greater detail is the diffuse or sarcomatoid pattern of AGCT. Note the pale monotonous population of nuclei, some grooved and many with pale or optically clear nucleoplasm, which are haphazardly oriented one to another. (H&E, OM ×100)

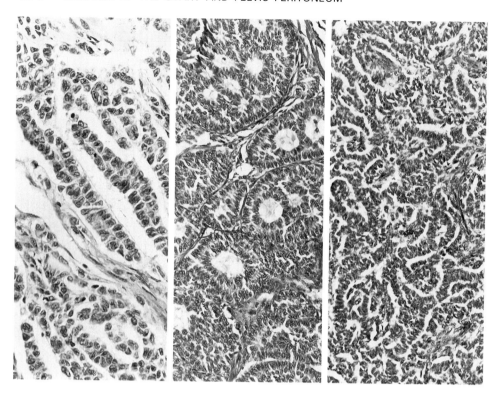

FIGURE 12–33. *Left,* An adult granulosa cell tumor (AGCT) is shown with the characteristic trabecular pattern. (H&E, OM ×100) *Middle,* Shown in greater detail is the microfollicular pattern of AGCT, but developed to such a degree that true glandular or tubular differentiation is simulated. Such a pattern could be confused with endometrioid carcinoma, tubular Krukenberg tumors, Sertoli cell–containing tumors, or sex cord tumors with annular tubules (SCTAT). (H&E, OM ×50) *Right,* Shown in greater detail is the moiré-silk (watered silk) pattern of AGCT. This is a zigzag arrangement of thin winding cords. (H&E, OM ×50)

posed of well-defined tubules (hollow or solid) of Sertoli cells surrounded by stroma containing Leydig cells (Figs. 12–36 and 12–37). The latter only rarely contain Reinke's crystals, but they may become quite lipid-rich and vacuolated. Moreover, the tubules can mimic well-differentiated endometrioid carcinoma glands. Intermediate-grade SLCTs are more lobulated, with densely cellular areas separated by less cellular,

sometimes edematous, connective tissue. The lobules contain nests, clusters, and/or cords of cytoplasm-poor Sertoli cells admixed with nests, clusters, and/or cords of plump eosinophilic Leydig cells. The pattern is distinctive (Fig. 12–38). Variably sized cysts containing eosinophilic material may be present (Fig. 12–39). Remember, SLCTs, granulosa-cell tumors, and thecomas may contain bizarre nuclei, and preg-

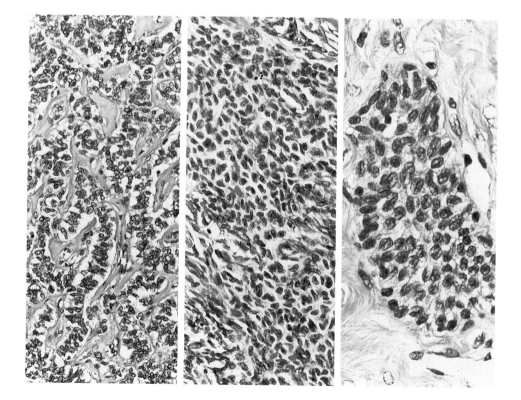

FIGURE 12–34. *Left,* Sometimes in adult granulosa cell tumor (AGCT), fibrosis is more prominent, but a trabecular pattern can still be appreciated. (H&E, OM ×50) *Middle,* In this example of AGCT, the granulosa cells grow in a diffuse or sarcomatoid pattern intimately admixed with a more spindled or thecofibromatous stroma. (H&E, OM ×50) *Right,* Shown is an insular cluster of AGCT cells with the characteristic nuclear features and surrounded by abundant fibrous stroma. (H&E, OM ×100)

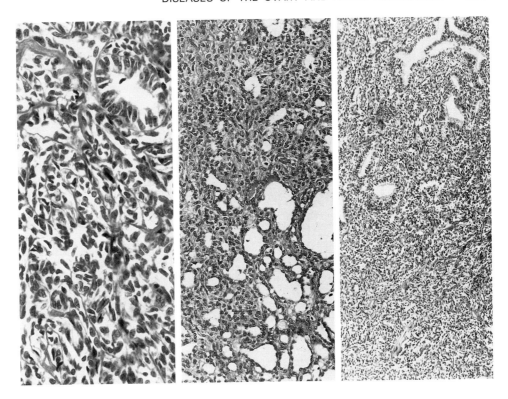

FIGURE 12–35. *Left,* Female adnexal or ovarian tumor of probable wolffian origin (FATWO or OTWO) is shown composed of closely packed tubules; many have compressed lumina lined by columnar, cuboidal, and/or spindled cells. (H&E, OM ×100) *Middle,* Shown is the irregular sieve-like pattern often found in FATWO or OTWO. (H&E, OM ×25) *Right,* In FATWO or OTWO, focally, large tubular glands resembling those of endometrioid carcinoma may be found admixed with the cellular or compact pattern created by areas shown at far left. (H&E, OM ×10)

nant patients may have sex cord–stromal tumors with prominent edema, which can obscure the diagnostic patterns. SLCTs dominated by diffuse growth of atypical, highly mitotic cells suggesting either sarcoma or undifferentiated carcinoma are classified as poorly differentiated, but sex cord–like tubules and/or nests, tubules, and Leydig cells combined with diagnostic patterns of SLCTs are required to establish the diagnosis of poorly differentiated SLCT.

Retiform SLCTs have areas mimicking rete testis (see Fig. 12–39).[213, 216, 218] Retiform SLCTs occur at a younger age (average, 15 years), account for 10% to 15% of SLCTs, are less frequently associated with features of excess androgen production, and may be more aggressive than other SLCTs of the same grade. Retiform patterns show an irregular network of elongated, slit-like tubulocystic structures, which may contain papillae (see Fig. 12–39). The papillae often show

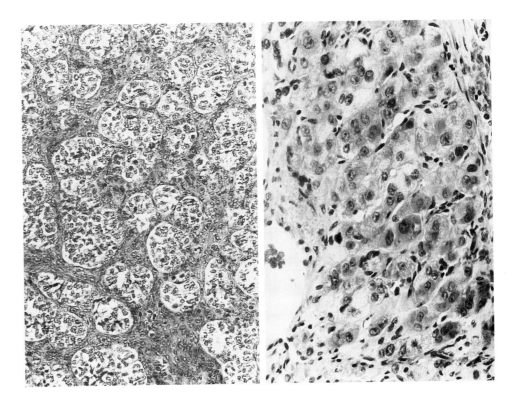

FIGURE 12–36. *Left,* A well-differentiated Sertoli-Leydig cell tumor (SLCT) is shown composed of solid tubules. Leydig cells were found in other fields and are displayed at right. (H&E, OM ×50) *Right,* Leydig cells of SLCT. (H&E, OM ×100)

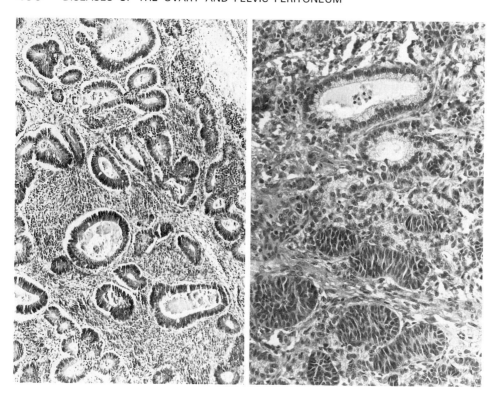

FIGURE 12–37. *Left,* A well-differentiated Sertoli-Leydig cell tumor (SLCT) is shown composed of hollow tubules with interspersed Leydig cells. This pattern could mimic well-differentiated endometrioid tumors. (H&E, OM ×50) *Right,* Tubules of a well-differentiated SLCT are shown with hollow and solid patterns. (H&E, OM ×100)

hyalinized cores. Heterologous elements are found in approximately 20% of SLCTs (Fig. 12–40). The most common heterologous element is gastrointestinal (GI) epithelium (90% of cases), which often contains goblet cells and even neuroendocrine cells. In fact, when the latter are present, small inconspicuous nests of carcinoid may be present. The GI epithelium is benign-appearing in the vast majority of cases, but it may be borderline mucinous tumor, low-grade mucinous carcinoma, or mucinous adenocarcinoid.[212, 217] Less common heterologous elements include cartilage (often fetal-like), skeletal muscle

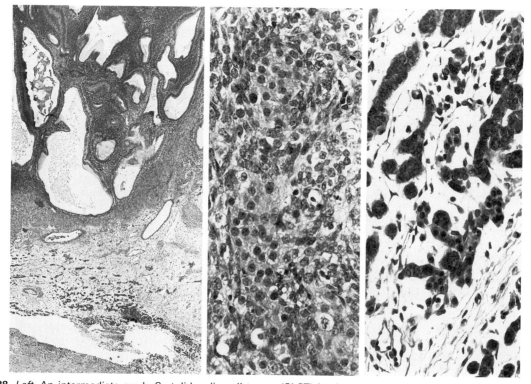

FIGURE 12–38. *Left,* An intermediate-grade Sertoli-Leydig cell tumor (SLCT) is shown with heterologous mucinous elements in the upper portions of the photograph. (H&E, OM ×5) *Middle,* Leydig cells within stroma are shown. (H&E, OM ×100) *Right,* Cords and ribbons of immature Sertoli cells with scanty cytoplasms are shown separated by edematous stroma. These areas frequently contain clusters of Leydig cells, a pattern very helpful in making the diagnosis of intermediate-grade SLCT. (H&E, OM ×100)

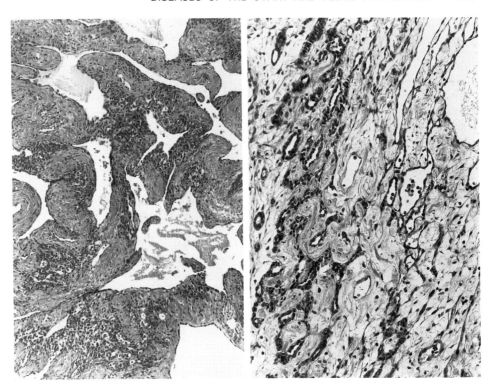

FIGURE 12–39. *Left,* An intermediate-grade Sertoli-Leydig cell tumor (SLCT) is shown composed of multiple cystic spaces. Diagnostic areas were found between the cysts. (H&E, OM ×5) *Right,* SLCT is shown with the retiform pattern. (H&E, OM ×50)

cells (rhabdomyoblast-like or strap cells), hepatocyte-like cells, and neuroectodermal elements. These mesenchymal heterologous elements are usually found in tumors with sarcomatoid (poorly differentiated) background.

DIFFERENTIAL DIAGNOSIS. The differential diagnosis of SLCTs is long and complex,[211–218] but most difficulty occurs with retiform SLCTs, poorly differentiated SLCTs, and SLCTs with heterologous areas. Please remember that,

because SLCTs are almost always unilateral and low-stage, any ovarian tumor that is bilateral and/or high-stage is unlikely to be SLCT. In this situation other diagnostic possibilities must be excluded before a diagnosis of SLCT is made.

Retiform areas can be confused with **papillary serous tumors** (borderline or low-grade) and papillary areas within a **yolk sac tumor (YST).** To complicate matters, some SLCTs have been associated with elevated serum **alpha-fetoprotein**

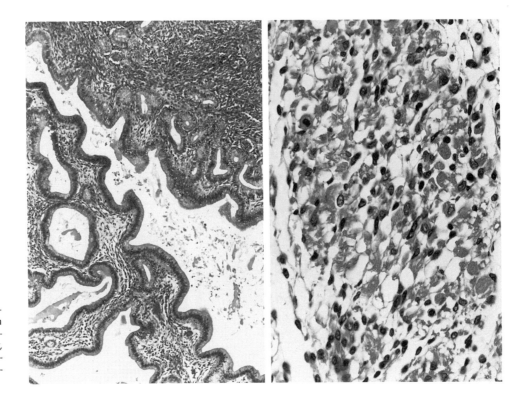

FIGURE 12–40. *Left,* Sertoli-Leydig cell tumor (SLCT) with mucinous heterologous elements. (H&E, OM ×25) *Right,* SLCT with mesenchymal (rhabdomyoblastic) heterologous elements. (H&E, OM ×100)

levels,[219] but this elevation is less than that found with YST. Moreover, serum alpha-fetoprotein has been reported rarely in serous papillary cystadenocarcinoma.[220] The distinction from other ovarian tumors becomes especially problematic when the SLCT is composed almost entirely of the retiform pattern. Extensive tumor sampling and close attention to the tissues between the slit-like, tubulocystic spaces of the retiform areas should reveal areas diagnostic of SLCT. When the heterologous elements dominate and typical SLCT features are minor, diagnostic confusion can occur. Often these tumors are wrongly considered **cystic teratomas,** but squamous epithelium, skin appendages, and respiratory epithelium have not been reported in SLCTs. Also, ovarian neuroectodermal tissues are much rarer in SLCT as compared with teratoma. Pure **cystic mucinous tumors** can be simulated, but extensive tumor sampling to reveal the intercystic SLCT (usually intermediate-grade) yields the proper diagnosis. Extensive mesenchymal heterologous elements can be confused with **primary or secondary ovarian sarcomas or even malignant mixed mullerian tumors (carcinosarcomas),** but these are very rare in young women. Ovarian **endometrioid carcinomas can sometimes show areas closely resembling sex cord–stromal tumors (so-called Sertoli-form endometrioid adenocarcinoma)** (Fig. 12–41) usually of the SLCT type.[221] However, these patients are without symptoms of excess androgen secretion and tend to be older (58 to 86 years) than the average patient with SLCT. Moreover, when enough tumor tissue is examined, areas more characteristic of endometrioid carcinoma are usually found. These areas include large tubular glands of endometrioid carcinoma, foci of squamous differentiation, luminal mucin secretion, and/or an endometrioid adenofibromatous component. **Conditions or lesions associated with luteinized stromal cells** may further complicate the diagnosis in some cases. Other lesions to consider in the differential diagnosis include **metastatic**

adenocarcinoma (tubular Krukenberg variant),[110] **adult granulosa cell tumor (AGCT) with trabecular patterns,**[211] **fibroma with minor sex cord elements,**[211] **sex cord tumors with annular tubules (SCTAT,** a tumor sometimes associated with Peutz-Jeghers syndrome or adenoma malignum of the cervix),[222, 223] **gynandroblastoma** (a tumor composed of substantial amounts of easily recognizable SLCT ["testicular"] and AGCT ["ovarian"] elements),[215] **unclassified sex cord–stromal tumors,**[211, 215] **trabecular carcinoid tumor,**[211, 215] **endometrial stromal sarcoma with ribbons of sex cord–like elements,**[215] **ovarian granulosa cell proliferations of pregnancy,**[224] **gonadoblastoma,**[225] **peculiar mixed germ cell–sex cord–stromal tumors sometimes with heterologous elements (Talerman tumor),**[226] **and the combined germ cell–gonadal stromal–epithelial tumor of the ovary** reported by Tavassoli.[227] Finally, rare examples of Sertoli cell tumors have been described associated with **renin production with hypertension,**[228] and **oxyphilic examples of Sertoli cell ovarian tumors** with abundant eosinophilic cytoplasm are now reported, some in patients with Peutz-Jeghers syndrome.[229] Obviously, the latter considerably expands the differential diagnostic considerations for Sertoli cell tumors, because numerous other ovarian lesions can display large epithelioid cells with abundant eosinophilic cytoplasm. The differential diagnosis of such ovarian lesions is discussed below in heptoid lesions of the ovary.

CLEAR-CELL TUMORS OF THE OVARY

Schiller interpreted a group of ovarian neoplasms, characterized in part by areas of clear cells and papillary structures, as mesonephromas of the ovary.[230, 231] He believed that these tumors represented a neoplastic recapitulation of the embryonic mesonephros and regarded them as of mesonephric deri-

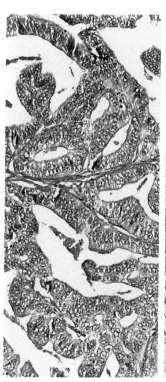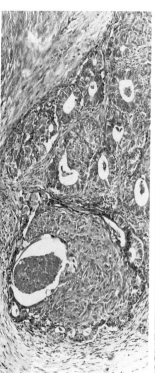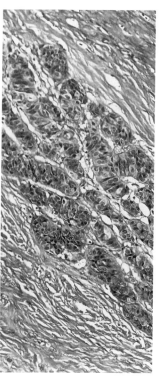

FIGURE 12–41. *Left,* Well-differentiated endometrioid carcinoma with stratified columnar cells is shown. (H&E, OM ×50) *Middle,* Shown are glands with central squamous metaplasia, a finding very helpful in recognizing endometrioid carcinoma. (H&E, OM ×25) *Right,* Shown is an area of Sertoli-form differentiation within the same endometrioid carcinoma displayed in other two parts of the figure. (H&E, OM ×50)

vation. Yet, the term *mesonephroma* was confusing, because Schiller's series was not homogeneous, and Teilum incisively reinterpreted some of these cases as endodermal sinus (yolk sac) tumors.[232, 233] The nature of the remaining examples of ovarian clear-cell carcinoma was the subject of considerable controversy for the next two decades, until Scully and Barlow[234] furnished compelling evidence that they are of surface epithelial origin. This was supported by the frequent association of these neoplasms with ovarian and pelvic endometriosis, an origin in some cases from endometriotic cysts, and the frequent admixture with endometrioid, serous, or mucinous carcinoma.[234-237] It is ironic that the ovarian tumor now interpreted as of likely mesonephric (wolffian) origin does not feature clear cells nor does it usually behave in a malignant fashion.[207] These tumors become diagnostically difficult because they have morphologic features that overlap frequently with other ovarian tumors.

CLINICOPATHOLOGIC FEATURES. Almost all clear-cell tumors of the ovary are malignant. **Clear-cell carcinoma** primarily affects patients in their fifth and sixth decades,[238, 239] and the lesions are bilateral in 10% to 23%[238] of cases. The 5-year survival rate is 35%.[236, 238] Microscopically, clear-cell carcinoma exhibits a number of architectural patterns, including papillary, tubulocystic, diffuse, adenofibromatous, parvilocular, trabecular, and solid, usually with admixtures of these patterns[238, 239] (Fig. 12–42). The papillae often show a dense hyalinized fibrovascular core, a feature of considerable diagnostic utility. The tumor cells are large, with clear, hobnail, cuboidal, flat, signet-ring, and/or oxyphilic (abundant eosinophilic cytoplasm) features, and these types occur in various combinations[235-237, 238, 239] (see Fig. 12–42). Parvilocular areas are characterized by cysts lined by clear or hobnail cells.

Benign and malignant, clear-cell adenofibromas likely represent another form of clear-cell tumor.[240, 241] Benign adenofibromas are rare tumors, constituting less than 1% of all benign ovarian tumors; the incidence of the clear-cell variant of adenofibroma is not "clearly" known, but certainly very rare. In the AFIP series conducted by Kao and Norris, only 3 of 126 cystadenofibromas were reported to be of the clear-cell type.[242] Adenofibromas are less common than cystadenofibromas. Bell and Scully[240, 243] defined as benign those clear-cell adenofibromas with widely spaced simple glands lined by one to two layers of epithelium that showed no significant atypicality. Considered borderline or of low malignant potential are those clear-cell adenofibromatous tumors in which the epithelial cells show cytologic features of low-grade malignancy (grade 1 of 3) according to Bell and Scully[240] or moderate to marked degrees of epithelial atypia according to Roth et al.[241] or Russell[243] but without evidence of stromal invasion (Fig. 12–43). Tumors with stromal invasion are considered malignant. Stromal invasion is defined as the presence of atypical glands, small nests or cords, or single cells extending into fibromatous stroma in a haphazard fashion and causing desmoplasia or myxoid stromal response around the tumor cells. Moreover, because borderline clear-cell tumors often have other areas of overt invasive clear-cell carcinoma, the diagnosis of borderline tumor should not be rendered until the tumor has been extensively sampled. The prognosis of patients with borderline clear-cell tumors has thus far been excellent, even when microinvasion is present.

DIFFERENTIAL DIAGNOSIS. Clear-cell carcinoma involves diverse entities. Clear-cell carcinoma can usually be readily distinguished from **yolk sac tumor** on both clinical and pathologic grounds, but, on occasion, these features may overlap or be less obvious, with a closer resemblance to each other.[244] Clear-cell carcinoma occurs primarily in older women, whereas yolk sac tumor primarily affects patients younger than 30 years of age.[235-237, 239] Solid or tubular areas composed of clear cells may be seen in both types of tumors, but the nuclei of the clear cells in clear-cell carcinoma are more

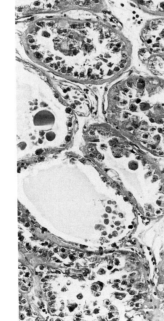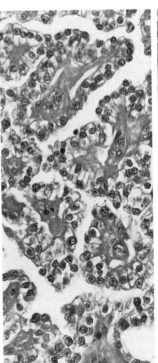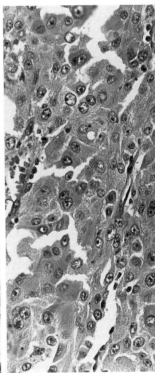

FIGURE 12–42. Left, Clear-cell carcinoma showing the tubulocystic pattern. The spaces are lined by hobnail cells, and hyaline globules are apparent. (H&E, OM ×50) *Middle,* Clear-cell carcinoma showing complex papillae. Note dense (hyalinized) cores. (H&E, OM ×100) *Right,* Oxyphilic cell pattern of clear-cell carcinoma. Note vesicular nuclei and prominent nucleoli. (H&E, OM ×100)

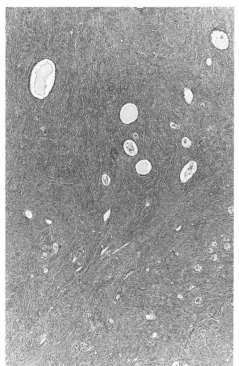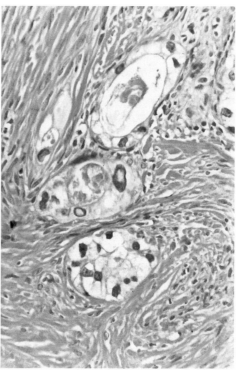

FIGURE 12–43. *Left,* Clear-cell adenofibroma of low malignant potential. Note small cysts and glands within abundant fibromatous stroma. (H&E, OM ×10) *Right,* Higher magnification showing the small glands lined by clear cells with atypical nuclei, features of low malignant potential. (H&E, OM ×100)

regular than the primitive appearance of the nuclei in yolk sac tumor, and the clear-cell foci in yolk sac tumor are usually only a minor component. The papillae in clear-cell carcinoma are multiple, complex, and project into cysts and tubules, and they have dense, hyalinized cores. In contrast, in yolk sac tumors, the papillae (Schiller-Duval bodies), when present, are single and simple, with a central vessel, and extend into a loose reticulated network. The parvilocular zones of clear-cell carcinoma, when present, exhibit only a superficial resemblance to the polyvesicular vitelline areas in yolk sac tumor. PAS-positive, diastase-resistant hyaline globules can be present in both clear-cell carcinoma and yolk sac tumor, as well as many other types of ovarian neoplasms. Also, the presence of **alpha-fetoprotein** in the serum or tumor cells has been demonstrated in many ovarian neoplasms of diverse origin, including clear-cell carcinoma, and alpha-fetoprotein may be absent in some yolk sac tumors.[245] Recent work has shown that approximately 95% of clear-cell carcinomas immunoreact with anti–Leu-M1, whereas approximately 30% of yolk sac tumors immunoreact.[245] In contrast, approximately 86% of yolk sac tumors immunoreact with anti–alpha-fetoprotein, whereas approximatley 18% of clear-cell carcinomas immunoreact. Also, those clear-cell tumors that immunostained only for Leu-M1 all proved to be clear-cell carcinomas, whereas those clear-cell tumors that immunostained only for AFP all proved to be yolk sac tumors.[245] Differentiation of the **oxyphilic variant**[239] **of clear-cell carcinoma** from both **hepatoid yolk sac tumor** and **hepatoid carcinoma of the ovary** is facilitated by the younger age of patients with yolk sac tumor as well as by its more primitive cytologic features and usual association with other typical areas of yolk sac tumor and, conversely in cases of hepatoid carcinoma, by the presence of typical foci of clear-cell carcinoma in the oxyphilic variant.

Both clear-cell carcinoma and yolk sac tumor may be confused with ovarian sex cord–stromal tumors. **Juvenile granu-**

losa cell tumor (JGCT) may contain follicles lined by hobnail cells and resemble the tubulocystic variant of clear-cell carcinoma. Nuclear atypicality and mitotic activity may be seen in JGCT, but the primitive nuclear atypism of yolk sac tumor is absent. **Sertoli-Leydig tumors,**[215] particularly those with a **retiform pattern,**[216] may also resemble clear-cell carcinoma and yolk sac tumor because they may also contain tubules lined by hobnail cells, and the retiform variant may contain papillae with hyalinized centers. Sertoli-Leydig tumors may also be associated with **alpha-fetoprotein** production,[245] although the values are usually not as high as in yolk sac tumor. On the other hand, some examples of yolk sac tumor may display a prominent pattern of rudimentary vacuolated tubules in a mesenchymal[246] stroma that can be extremely difficult to differentiate from poorly differentiated forms[211] of ovarian sex cord–stromal tumors on a purely histopathologic basis.

Clear-cell carcinoma exhibits a strong histopathologic resemblance to **renal cell carcinoma metastatic to the ovary.** This uncommon event may be the initial manifestation of carcinoma of the kidney, compounding diagnostic difficulty. In the small series of Young and Hart,[247] the metastases were composed of a diffuse proliferation of clear cells with a prominent sinusoidal vascular network. Clear-cell carcinoma of the ovary with an exclusive population of clear cells (solid pattern) is uncommon, and the conspicuous vascular pattern is absent in clear-cell carcinoma. In addition, metastatic renal carcinoma lacks hobnail cells and mucin secretion, features that may be present in clear-cell carcinoma. Clear-cell carcinoma of the ovary, particularly when dominated by a solid pattern that is accompanied by necrosis and acute inflammation, may also be confused with **necrotic pseudoxanthomatous nodules of ovarian endometriosis** or with **xanthogranulomatous oophoritis,** analogous to the sometimes perplexing differential diagnosis of xanthogranulomatous pyelonephritis[248] and clear-cell carcinoma of the kidney. Finally, benign and low malignant potential clear-cell adenofibroma also must be distinguished from other benign adenofibromatous tumors, such as **Brenner tumor, mucinous adenofibroma** (Fig. 12–44), **serous adenofibroma** (Fig. 12–45), and **endometrioid adenofibromatous** tumors (Fig. 12–46).[249-252] Remember, all adenofibromatous tumors may be associated with overt invasive carcinoma; thus, these tumors should always be extensively sampled to rule out that possibility.

YOLK SAC TUMOR OF THE OVARY

The **yolk sac tumor (YST)** or **endodermal sinus tumor** is a malignant germ cell tumor differentiating toward extraembryonic endoderm and mesoderm, which recapitulates embryonic development of the yolk sac.[253-259] Most of the characteristic morphologic patterns, including production of **alpha-fetoprotein (AFP),** represent visceral yolk sac differentiation. More than a dozen patterns occur in various combinations within YSTs, and the many different morphologic patterns of YSTs overlap with other primary and secondary ovarian tumors and pose diagnostic problems. Accurate recognition of YST is critical for patient management and prognostication.

CLINICOPATHOLOGIC FEATURES. YSTs of the ovary are somewhat less common than **dysgerminomas** (especially in patients <20 years), occur most commonly in children and adolescents (average age at presentation, 19 years), and are very rare after 40 years. Patients complain of pain, have an unilateral adnexal mass, and show markedly elevated AFP levels. Rarely, patients may present with virilization.[260] YSTs are aggressive tumors, and 30% to 40% of patients present with extraovarian spread. Nonetheless, with modern polyagent chemotherapies at least 80% of stage 1 patients and at least 50% of advance-stage patients achieve long-term survival.[253-259]

YSTs are usually large, with an average diameter of approximately 15 cm. Most are solid and/or mixed cystic, composed of yellow to gray tissue, often show areas of hemorrhage and necrosis, and are usually covered by a smooth glistening capsule. YSTs of the polyvesicular-vitelline variant may show a macroscopic honeycomb appearance. YST cells contain irregular, hyperchromatic nuclei with prominent nucleoli. Tumor cell cytoplasm is moderately abundant and of either clear or granular appearance; glycogen may be present, as well as lipid. Mitotic figures are typically numerous and may be atypical. Intervening stroma often has a primitive, edematous quality.

The various microscopic patterns of YSTs include (1) **endodermal sinus (perivascular, labyrinthine-like, or festoon pattern containing the ''glomeruloid'' or Schiller-Duval bodies)**(Fig. 12–47, left), (2) **microcystic (reticular or honeycomb)**(Fig. 12–47, right), (3) **glandular-alveolar** (Fig. 12–48, left), (4) **myxomatous** (Fig. 12–48, right), (5) **papillary** (Fig. 12–49), (6) **solid** (see Fig. 12–47), (7) **polyvesicular-vitelline** (Fig. 12–50), (8) **hepatoid,** (9) **parietal** (Fig. 12–51), (10) **macrocystic,** (11) **intestinal,** (12) **endometrioid** (Fig. 12–52, left), (13) **clear cell–like** (Fig. 12–52, right), and (13) **sarcomatoid.** In spite of all these complex patterns, almost all YSTs show some areas containing one or more of the following patterns: microcystic, endodermal-sinus, and/or glandular-alveolar, usually with hyaline droplets (see Fig. 12–52). But the less common patterns may cause diagnostic problems. Moreover, a recent study has found that stage I patients with YSTs that show three or four subtype patterns have a better prognosis than those with only one or two subtype patterns.[261] Yet, when all stages were analyzed, FIGO stage, chemotherapeutic regimen, and residual tumor size were most important in predicting outcome.

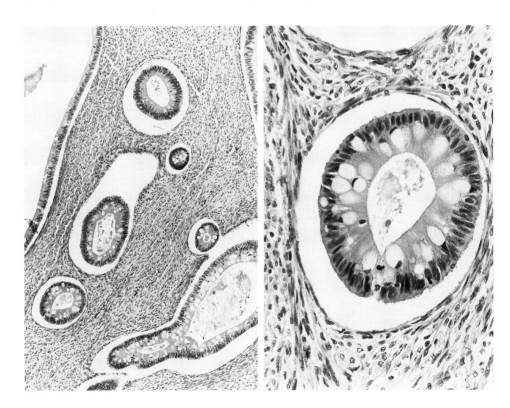

FIGURE 12–44. *Left,* Mucinous adenofibroma. (H&E, OM ×25) *Right,* Mucinous adenofibroma. Note goblet cells. (H&E, OM ×100)

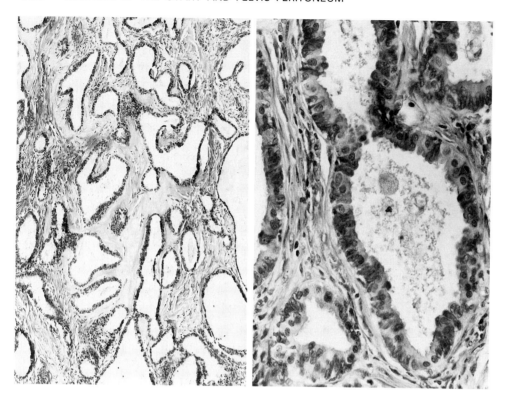

FIGURE 12–45. *Left,* Serous adenofibroma. (H&E, OM ×5) *Right,* Shown are the details of the serous tumor cells. Cilia were easily identified but only faintly visible in this photograph. (H&E, OM ×50)

The parietal pattern is characterized by extracellular basement membrane–like material, analogous to Reichert's membrane of parietal yolk sac origin,[258] and the presence of hepatic and/or enteric differentiation indicates that some YSTs can show embryonal as well as extraembryonal differentiation. This is consistent with the observation that portions of the gastrointestinal tract originate from the yolk sac.[257–259] The

polyvesicular-vitelline (PVV) pattern is composed of small cysts lined by flattened to cuboidal cells separated by spindle cell stroma. These cysts often are eccentrically constricted, simulating the division of the primary yolk sac vesicle in the larger vestigial yolk sac and the smaller precursor of the primitive gut. The hepatoid pattern simulates liver cells and hepatic carcinoma. "Glandular or intestinal" YSTs

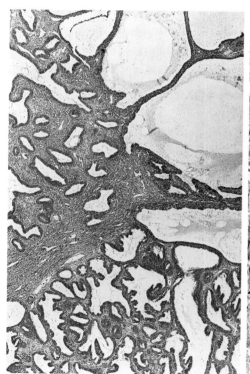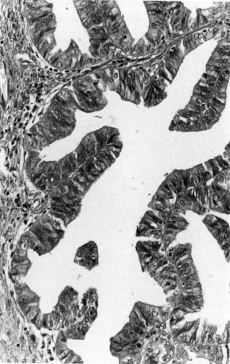

FIGURE 12–46. *Left,* Endometrioid adenofibroma of borderline malignancy of the ovary. Note irregular glandular shapes within fibrous stroma but without evidence of invasion. (H&E, OM ×10) *Right,* The tumor cells of this endometrioid adenofibroma of borderline malignancy show disorganized stratification and low-grade malignant cytologic atypia. (H&E, OM ×100)

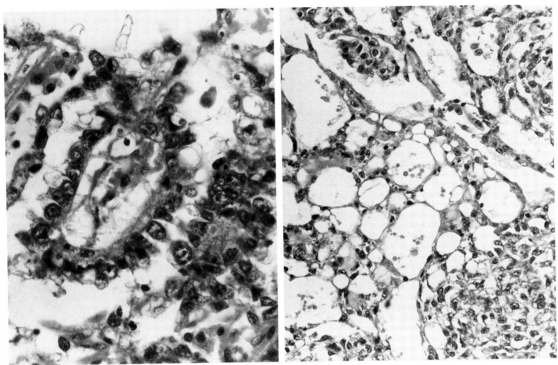

FIGURE 12-47. *Left,* Yolk sac tumor (YST) showing a "glomeruloid" or Schiller-Duval body characteristic of the endodermal sinus pattern (also called perivascular, labyrinthine-like, or festoon pattern). (H&E, OM ×100) *Right,* YST showing the microcystic pattern (also called reticular or honeycomb). Note the solid area at the extreme lower right-hand corner of the photograph. The latter solid pattern can closely mimic dysgerminoma or clear-cell carcinoma. In YST, such areas should be strongly cytokeratin- and alpha-fetoprotein–positive yet negative for epithelial membrane antigen. (H&E, OM ×100)

show intestinal differentiation by electron microscopy;[259] "endometrial-like" YSTs simulate secretory endometrial carcinoma;[262] "parietal" differentiation is characterized by extracellular basement membrane–like material;[246] and the primitive mesenchyme-like components of YSTs may be prominent in some cases, especially after chemotherapy.[263] The last feature may be responsible for some sarcomas arising in the YSTs. Other cellular components occasionally encountered include solid, papillary, myxoid, and/or adenofibromatous areas.[246, 255, 257] Rarely, YST cells may resemble lipoblasts,

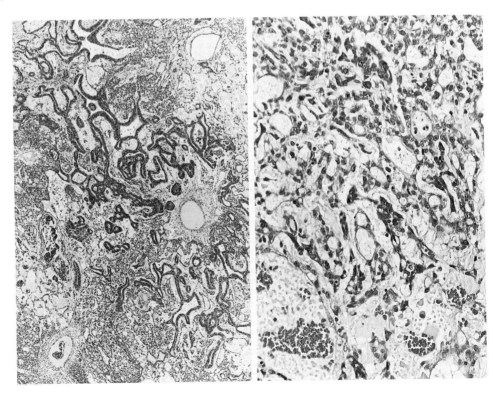

FIGURE 12-48. *Left,* YST showing the glanduloalveolar pattern. (H&E, OM ×10) *Right,* YST showing a reticulated pattern in a myxomatous stroma. (H&E, OM ×50)

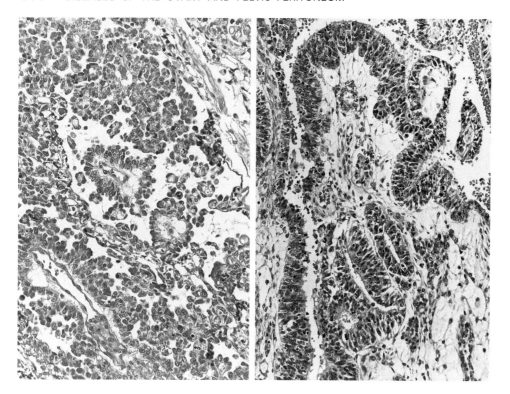

FIGURE 12–49. *Left,* YST showing a papillary pattern as a component of the endodermal sinus pattern. (H&E, OM ×25) *Right,* Embryonal carcinomas may also show papillary areas. Embryonal carcinomas in pure form are very rare in the ovary. Their nuclei are vesicular, overlap in a syncytial pattern within amphophilic cytoplasm, and frequently show marked anisonucleosis, clumped chromatin, and prominent nucleoli. (H&E, OM ×25)

and some YSTs contain mucinous columnar cells, goblet cells, Paneth cells, syncytiotrophoblastic giant cells, luteinized stromal cells, granulomatous inflammation, and/or foci of extramedullary hematopoiesis.[246, 255, 257] Immunohistochemistry shows that the cells of YSTs are positive for AFP, cytokeratin, and placental alkaline phosphatase (PLAP), whereas the hyaline globules are usually negative for AFP.[257, 264] The hyaline globules stain for alpha-1-antitrypsin, but they likely share

features with basement membrane materials by staining in some cases for basement membrane components such as collagen type IV, laminin, and chondroitin sulfate large proteoglycans.[263] Remember, hyaline globules are not specific for YST but may be seen in mixed mullerian tumors, clear-cell carcinomas, serous tumors, mucinous tumors, and rarely endometrioid tumors. The epithelial, glandular, and cystic lining cells of the PVV, hepatoid, and endometrioid patterns are also

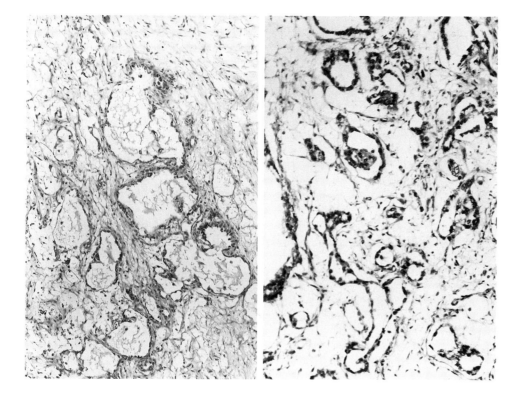

FIGURE 12–50. *Left,* YST showing the polyvesicular-vitellin pattern. Note cytologically bland features and abundant myxomatous stroma. (H&E, OM ×5) *Right,* YST with a microcystic myxomatous area. (H&E, OM ×50)

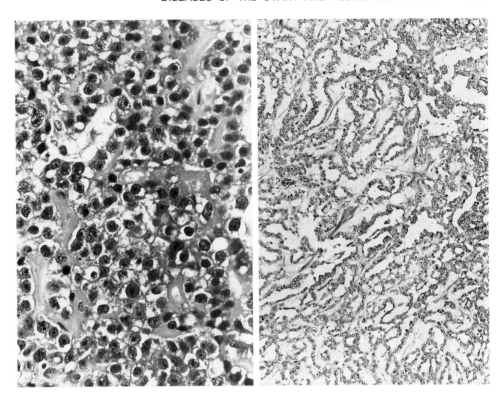

FIGURE 12–51. *Left,* Parietal YST. Note abundant intercellular hyaline basement membrane material. (H&E, OM ×100) *Right,* YST tumor with a predominantly alveolar or labyrinthine-like growth pattern. (H&E, OM ×10)

positive for cytokeratin and alpha-fetoprotein (AFP). The enteric components are usually positive for carcinoembryonic antigen (CEA) and possibly cytokeratin 20.

DIFFERENTIAL DIAGNOSIS. The differential diagnosis of YST includes **juvenile granulosa cell tumor, clear-cell carcinoma** (including the oxyphil variant), **other ovarian carcinomas (especially the endometrioid type), other germ cell** **malignancies (especially embryonal carcinoma), teratoma (especially the immature endodermal type),**[265] **hepatoid carcinoma, steroid (lipid) cell tumors,** and **Sertoli-Leydig cell tumors.** Most of these lesions are discussed in other sections of this chapter. Nonetheless, complete tumor sampling to reveal the entire and "true" characteristics of the tumor, combined with the young patient age, markedly ele-

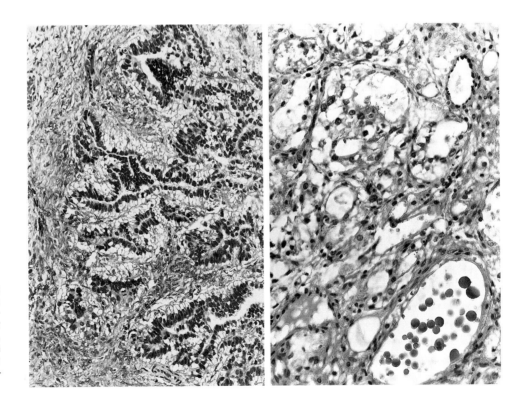

FIGURE 12–52. *Left,* YST showing the endometrioid-like growth pattern. Note the rows of subnuclear vacuoles like early secretory endometrium. (H&E, OM ×50) *Right,* YST with a prominent "clear-cell" pattern with numerous hyaline globules. (H&E, OM ×100)

Table 12–2. **Immunohistochemistry of Germ Cell and Trophoblastic Tumors of the Gonads**

Tumor	Keratin (~%)	EMA (~%)	AFP (~%)	CEA (~%)	PLAP (~%)	A₁-AT (~%)	hCG-β (~%)
Seminoma	10	2	0	0	87	5	5
Embryonal Ca	95	2	33	0	86	11	21
Yolk sac tumor	100	5	74	11	53	42	0
Choriocarcinoma	100	46	0	25	54	33	100

EMA, epithelial membrane antigen; AFP, alpha-fetoprotein; CEA, carcinoembryonic antigen; PLAP, placental alkaline phosphatase; A₁-AT, alpha-1-antitrypsin; β-hCG, beta subunit of human chorionic gonadotropin.

vated serum AFP, primitive appearance of the nuclei lining the glands, immunoreactivity of AFP, and finding of other more characteristic reticular (microcystic), glandular-alveolar, and hyaline globule patterns of YST should lead to the proper diagnosis in the vast majority of cases.

Immunohistochemistry can be useful in sorting out the various types of germ cell malignancies, which may occur in pure or mixed form in the ovary (Table 12–2).[263] Clearly, distinction of dysgerminoma from YST and other higher-grade non-dysgerminomatous tumors of the ovary is very important (Fig. 12–53). From the table, it is apparent that keratin (''cocktail'' of CAM 5.2, MAK-6, +AE1/3) and AFP immunostaining are helpful in distinguishing seminoma or dysgerminoma from other higher-grade, germ cell tumors, although 10% of seminomas or dysgerminomas show less intense foci of diffuse staining for keratin. Also, expression of placental alkaline phosphatase (PLAP) in the absence of epithelial membrane antigen (EMA) immunostaining appears to be a pattern characteristic of germ cell tumors. Primary epithelial malignancies would show concomitant EMA immunoreactivity much more frequently. Neither leukocyte common antigen (CD45) nor S-100 is found in germ cell tumors, an observation that helps rule out lymphoma and melanoma.

Also remember, pure embryonal carcinoma and choriocarcinoma are very rare in the ovary.

A peculiar form of teratoma has been described as **immature endodermal teratoma,** which is closely related to or a variant of YST (Figs. 12–54 and 12–55). These peculiar endodermal teratomas were associated with high serum AFP levels, and epithelia showed exclusively embryologic development of primitive endoderm, ranging from endoderm to tissues similar to esophagus, liver, and intestinal structures.

HEPATOID AND STEROID (LIPID) CELL LESIONS OF THE OVARY

That **hepatoid (hepatic) elements may represent a component of somatic endodermal differentiation in yolk sac carcinomas** was not widely appreciated until the report of Prat et al.,[266] who reported seven cases characterized by masses, nests, and broad bands composed of large epithelial cells with abundant eosinophilic to clear cytoplasm and round central nuclei with prominent single nucleoli, associated with frequent mitotic activity; two cases examined ultrastructurally showed features similar to hepatocellular carcinoma. Numer-

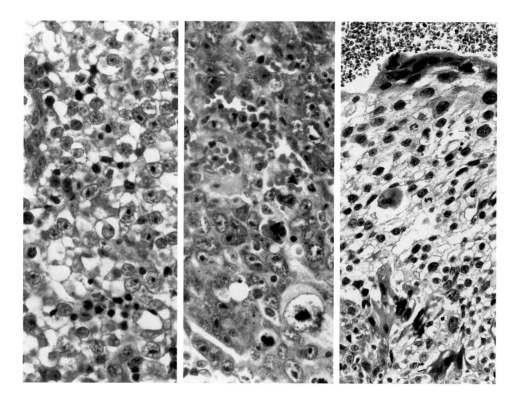

FIGURE 12–53. *Left,* Representative features of dysgerminoma or seminoma. Note evenly spaced vesicular nuclei surrounded by clear cytoplasm. Small lymphocytes are admixed. (H&E, OM ×100) *Middle,* Embryonal carcinoma is shown with nuclei that are vesicular, overlap in a syncytial pattern within amphophilic cytoplasm, and frequently show marked anisonucleosis, clumped chromatin, and prominent nucleoli. (H&E, OM ×100) *Right,* Choriocarcinoma is shown. Note the bilayered arrangement of cytotrophoblasts and syncytiocytotrophoblasts. (H&E, OM ×100)

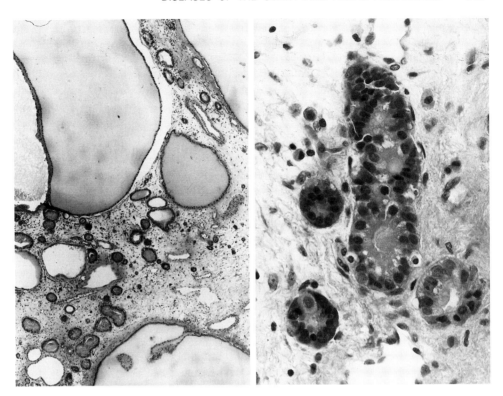

FIGURE 12–54. *Left,* Immature endodermal teratoma is shown with numerous, variably sized microcysts. (H&E, OM ×10) *Right,* Higher magnification showing immature endodermal teratoma with small glands lined by neuroendocrine cells. (H&E, OM ×100)

ous PAS-positive intracytoplasmic and extracellular hyaline bodies of various sizes, a feature of yolk sac carcinoma in general, were also present. The hepatoid pattern was prominent in all instances and was virtually exclusive in four. **Alpha-fetoprotein (AFP)** and alpha-1-antitrypsin (AAT), identified by immunoperoxidase and immunofluorescent techniques, were present in many of the hepatoid cells in four tumors so tested, and albumin was demonstrated in two tumors so tested. The hyaline bodies were essentially devoid of AFP reactivity, but some of the smaller ones contained AAT. Yet, on light microscopic, ultrastructural, and immunohistochemical levels, the **"hepatoid" pattern was that of hepatocellular carcinoma.** Collaterally, the tumors pursued an aggressive course and had a poor prognosis. They occurred in patients with an age range of 7 to 43 years (average, 22). Two patients had gonadal dysgenesis. Subsequently, cases of hepatoid dif-

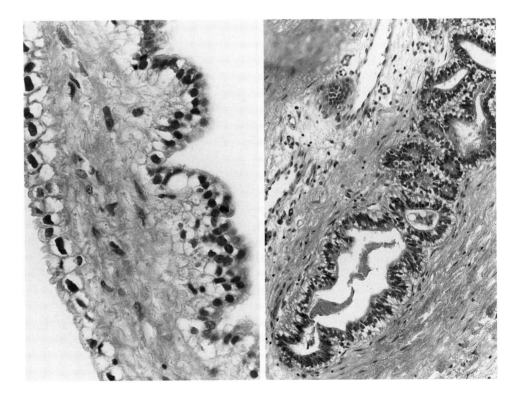

FIGURE 12–55. *Left,* Microcyst of an immature endodermal teratoma is shown lined by indifferent cuboidal cells with subnuclear and apical vacuoles similar to early endodermal derivatives. (H&E, OM ×100) *Right,* Immature endodermal teratoma is shown containing an early intestinal structure. Mitotic figures were apparent within this structure. Immature endodermal teratoma is closely related to YST, and the area shown on the right could be considered a component of YST with endometrioid features. (H&E, OM ×50)

ferentiation exhibiting similar clinical, morphologic, and immunohistochemical features were described in pure ovarian yolk carcinomas or germ cell neoplasms with areas of yolk sac tumor.[267, 268] Approximately 5%[268] to 16%[266] of ovarian neoplasms containing yolk sac areas display hepatoid patterns, although hepatoid differentiation was more frequent in retroperitoneal and sacrococcygeal tumors.[267]

In 1987, Ishikura and Scully described another type of **ovarian carcinoma with hepatoid features.**[269] However, in contrast with hepatoid yolk sac carcinoma, the age of the five affected patients ranged from 42 to 78 years (average, 63), and none had gonadal dysgenesis or associated germ cell components within their tumors. Histologically, the tumor cells of this type also exhibited positive immunohistochemical reactions for AFP and albumin in all cases and for AAT in four of five lesions. These hepatoid neoplasms were similar to the hepatoid foci in yolk sac tumors but displayed a greater degree of cellular pleomorphism. This type of hepatoid carcinoma was felt to be most likely a variant of a common epithelial ovarian carcinoma because they occurred in similar age groups, the abdominal implants that appeared after chemotherapy and radiotherapy in one case had histologic features of a psammomatous serous carcinoma, and two of the tumors stained positively for CA 125, an antigen that is present in a high percentage of cases of serous and endometrioid carcinomas. In addition, **serous carcinomas** may rarely be associated with AFP production.[269] Such carcinomatous hepatocellular metaplasia appears to be analogous to the development of areas of hepatocellular carcinoma in carcinomas of the stomach,[270] duodenum,[271] pancreas,[162, 272] renal pelvis,[273] and lung,[274] none of which have metastasized to the ovary, but the possibility exists that such an extraovarian hepatoid carcinoma might spread to the ovary. Clinical evaluation should usually establish the origin of the tumor in cases of this type.

Hepatocellular carcinoma may rarely metastasize to the ovary. Young et al.[162] reported three pertinent cases, two of which had bilateral ovarian involvement, and the clinicopathologic features either proved or were highly suggestive of metastatic ovarian spread from the liver in all three. However, on a purely histopathologic basis, it is conceivable that metastatic hepatocellular carcinoma would be difficult or impossible to distinguish from primary or metastatic hepatoid carcinoma of the ovary. These varieties of hepatoid carcinomas also involve the differential diagnosis of oxyphil cell tumors involving the ovary in general and, in particular, because of their relative frequency, metastatic malignant melanoma, endometrioid carcinoma of the oxyphilic type,[274a] and the **oxyphilic variant of clear-cell carcinoma of the ovary.**[239] Foci of mature-appearing liver cells have also been described in **ovarian sex cord–stromal tumors,** two **Sertoli-Leydig tumors,**[275, 276] and one **granulosa cell tumor.**[276] These hepatocytic foci might be mistaken for lutein or Leydig cells, but the simulation is superficial. These liver cells are thought to arise by a process of neometaplasia of sex cord mesenchyme.[275, 276]

Also in the differential diagnosis of hepatoid tumors of the ovary are **steroid (lipid) cell tumors of the ovary.** This term is used to describe ovarian tumors composed of large, round, polyhedral, or epithelioid cells that simulate luteinized stromal cells, Leydig cells, or adrenal cortical cells. These frequently highly vascular tumors have cells growing in diffuse sheets and/or cords, columns, or clusters (Fig. 12–56). Although the cells of these tumors may contain fat, approximately 40% do not, and the term "steroid cell" tumor has been proposed to replace "lipid cell" tumor.[277] There are three categories: **stromal luteoma,**[278] **hilus cell tumor,**[279] and **steroid (lipid) cell tumor, not otherwise specified (NOS).**[161] The clinicopathologic features of these lesions are depicted in Table 12–3.

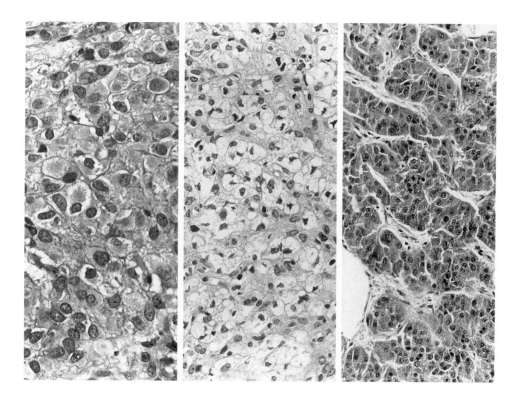

FIGURE 12–56. The many morphologic "faces" of steroid (lipid) cell tumors of the ovary. *Left,* Large polygonal cells with abundant eosinophilic cytoplasm growing in diffuse sheets. Reinke crystals were not present. (H&E, OM ×100) *Middle,* Vacuolated clear cells growing in sheets were shown to contain lipid with fat stains. (H&E, OM ×50) *Right,* Shown are cords of polygonal cells with eosinophilic cytoplasm. (H&E, OM ×50)

Table 12–3. **Clinicopathologic Features of Steroid (Lipid) Cell Tumors of the Ovaries**

Parameter	Stromal Luteoma	Hilus Cell Tumor (Crystal Pos)	Hilus Cell Tumor (Crystal Neg)	Steroid Cell Tumor (NOS)
Age (mean, yr) (range)	58 (28–74)	57 (32–75)	61 (34–82)	43 (2–80)
~% of all cases	20%	11%	9%	60%
Virilization or hirsutism	12%	83%	33%	42%
Estrogenic syndrome	60%	0%	44%	8%
No endocrine syndrome	20%	17%	23%	27%
Cushing's syndrome	0	0	0	6%
Diameter (mean, cm)	1.3	2.4	1.8	8.4
Stromal/nodular hyperthecosis	92%	42%	67%	23%
Endometrial hyperplasia or carcinoma	88%	8%	33%	24%
Incidence of malignancy	0%	0%	0%	20–40%
Important notes	Confined to ovarian stroma by definition; irregular spaces may simulate glands or vessels.	Fibrinoid necrosis in vessel walls in one third; irregular spaces may simulate glands or vessels	Fibrinoid necrosis in vessel walls in one third; irregular spaces may simulate glands or vessels	May cause iso- or heterosexual pseudoprecocity; 20% present with extraovarian spread

Cytoplasm of these tumors varies from eosinophilic to pale to foamy and vacuolated (see Fig. 12–56), and lipochrome pigment may be present. When Reinke crystals are present, the steroid cell tumor can be called a **Leydig cell tumor** (Fig. 12–57). Please note that **stromal or nodular hyperthecosis** (the presence of microscopic or macroscopic luteinized stromal cells in the same or contralateral ovarian stroma) frequently co-exists with steroid (lipid) cell tumors and suggests a stromal origin. Tumors composed of steroid cells arising in a background of spindled cells are closely related sex cord–stromal tumors called **luteinized thecoma** or **stromal Leydig cell tumors** (Fig. 12–58).[280] **Stromal luteomas** are small steroid (lipid) cell tumors (<3.0 cm) that are, by definition,

confined to the ovarian stroma. **Hilus cell tumors** almost always arise in the ovarian hilus from hilar Leydig cells, which can be found in at least 80% of normal ovaries (Fig. 12–59).

Steroid (lipid) cell tumors of NOS type are malignant in 20% to 40%, and 20% present with extraovarian spread. Although usually solid, they may have necrosis, hemorrhage, and show cystic changes. In one series in which there were 2 or more mitotic figures per 10 HPF, 92% of these NOS tumors were malignant; when necrosis was present, 86% were malignant; when larger than 7 cm in diameter, 78% were malignant; when hemorrhage was present, 77% were malignant; and when high-grade nuclear atypia was present, 64%

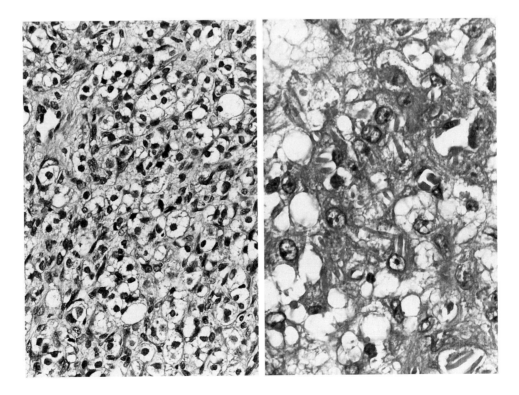

FIGURE 12–57. *Left,* Steroid cell tumor composed of clear cells mimicking renal carcinoma. (H&E, OM ×50) *Right,* Reinke crystals (cigar-shaped) were found in the steroid cell tumor, allowing it to be designated a Leydig cell tumor. (H&E, OM ×100)

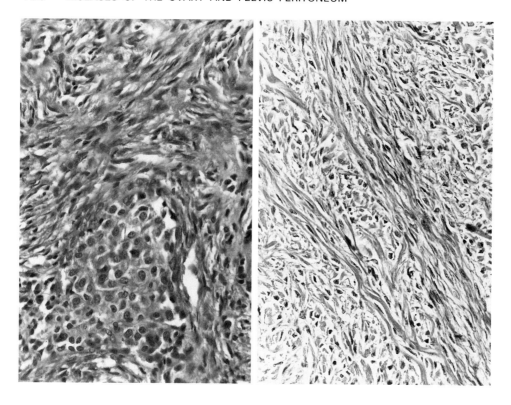

FIGURE 12–58. *Left,* Shown in the bottom half of the photograph is a nest of luteinized cells in a partially luteinized thecoma. (H&E, OM ×100) *Right,* An ovarian fibroma without luteinization is shown for comparison. (H&E, OM ×50)

were malignant.[161] However, cytologically benign tumors may behave in a malignant fashion.

The differential diagnosis of steroid (lipid) cell tumors of the ovary includes extensively **luteinized granulosa-theca cell tumors** (both adult and juvenile types), **lipid-rich Sertoli cell tumors, sclerosing stromal tumor, struma ovarii, strumal carcinoid, primary clear-cell carcinomas (especially the oxyphilic variant), endometrioid carcinomas** with oxyphilic change, hepatoid YSTs, hepatoid carcinoma, and **metastatic carcinomas** from the kidney, adrenal, and liver. **Metastatic melanoma** must also be considered. Moreover, **xanthogranulomatous inflammation** associated with infection or endometriosis (see Fig. 12–59) could be confused with steroid (lipid) cell tumors. Also, remember that extensive stromal luteinization may occur with either metastatic or primary ovarian tumors (Fig. 12–60, left). This

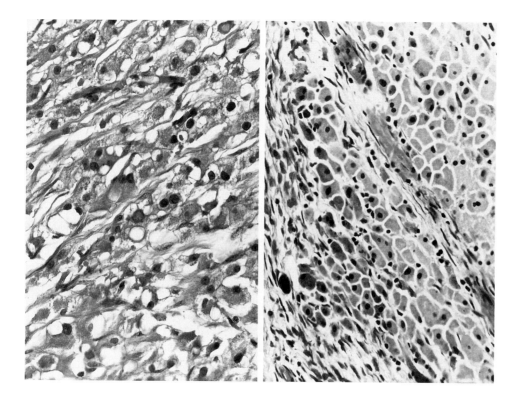

FIGURE 12–59. *Left,* Hilar cells of ovary. (H&E, OM ×100) *Right,* Shown are xanthogranulomatous inflammatory cells associated with endometriosis, but similar inflammatory cells can be found with chronic infection (xanthogranulomatous oophoritis or malakoplakia). These areas could be confused with steroid cell tumors of the ovary. (H&E, OM ×50)

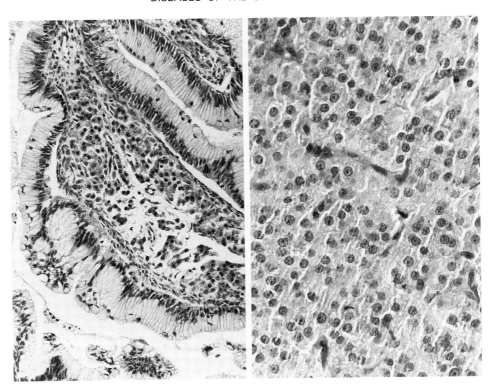

FIGURE 12–60. *Left,* Mucinous ovarian carcinoma is shown with extensive stromal luteinization. The patient also had endometrial hyperplasia. (H&E, OM ×50) *Right,* Shown is a case of pregnancy luteoma. (H&E, OM ×100)

secondary luteinization can be confused with steroid (lipid) cell tumors if the specimen is not adequately sampled. Finally, extensively luteinized tumorous and/or cystic lesions presenting during pregnancy or the puerperium must also be considered. These lesions include **pregnancy luteoma ("nodular theca-lutein hyperplasia of pregnancy")** (Fig. 12–60, right), **hyperreactio luteinalis, intrafollicular granulosa cell proliferations of pregnancy, large solitary luteinized follicle cyst, ectopic decidua,** and **hilus cell hyperplasia.**[281, 282]

STRUMA OVARII AND STRUMAL CARCINOID

It is now generally accepted that the term **struma ovarii** is best reserved for ovarian teratomas in which thyroid tissue is the main component (i.e., constitutes more than 50% of the neoplastic tissue) or those teratomas that demonstrate physiologic activity or pathologic aberration (hyperthyroidism, thyroiditis, adenoma, carcinoma, and so forth).[283–285] The presence of thyroid tissue in a mature cystic teratoma does not, by itself, warrant a diagnosis of struma ovarii, because foci of thyroid tissue may be present in as many as 13% of mature ovarian cystic teratomas.[286] A finding of concomitant thyroid and carcinoid differentiation (often intimately admixed) is referred to as **strumal carcinoid.** These lesions can be confused with a variety of other primary and metastatic ovarian tumors.

CLINICOPATHOLOGIC FEATURES. Struma ovarii is a rare condition. It constitutes approximately 0.3% of ovarian solid tumors and 2.7% of ovarian teratomas.[287] The neoplasm presents in patients ranging from 6 to 74 years of age, with an average age of 42 years. Because this contrasts with the younger average age of presentation of mature cystic teratoma (34 years), it has been speculated that these strumal tumors

are slow-growing, requiring many years of growth before the appearance of symptoms,[285, 288] although rapid growth occurs in some cases.

Most of these tumors are asymptomatic incidental findings discovered during routine pelvic examination or during surgery for some other gynecologic indication.[289] The majority of symptomatic patients have one or more of the following symptoms: abdominal pain, pelvic pressure, backache, urinary retention, constipation, dyspareunia, hematuria, palpable mass, or enlarging abdomen. Thirty-nine percent of women with struma ovarii were reported as presenting with ascites, which can be very marked and associated with hydrothorax in some cases (pseudo-Meigs' syndrome).[285] There are no reports of this neoplasm affecting either menses or fertility.[285] This contrasts with the closely related ovarian strumal carcinoid, in which 8% of the patients in one series exhibited clinical signs of steroid hormone production (endometrial hyperplasia, vaginal bleeding, hirsutism, or virilism).[290]

Of reported cases of struma ovarii, approximately 7% of patients were thought to be clinically hyperthyroid.[291] Unfortunately, some reported patients were seen before the development of precise thyroid function tests; therefore, this reported incidence may be inaccurate. In addition, and as in the case presented, struma ovarii is often not recognized either preoperatively or on gross examination of the operative specimen; and by the time the diagnosis is made, various investigative procedures are no longer possible.[292] These problems are compounded by the observation that patients with struma ovarii may have hyperthyroidism from other causes, including cervical exophthalmic goiter (Graves' disease), cervical adenomatous hyperfunctioning goiter, adenomatous hyperfunctioning tissue in the ovary, or a combination of these conditions.[285] Some patients with struma ovarii (15% to 25%) also have enlargement of the thyroid gland.[285, 293] As might be anticipated, 8% of patients with ovarian strumal carcinoid were reported to have a functioning thyroid component.[8] None of the 50 patients in this latter series of strumal carcinoid had carcinoid syndrome; however, a single patient with strumal carcinoid and carcinoid syndrome has been reported.[294]

The diagnosis of hyperthyroidism secondary to struma ovarii should be considered in any woman with low radioactive iodine uptake over the neck and symptoms of hyperthyroidism. The ovarian lesions are usually palpable, except in the presence of ascites.[285] If the diagnosis is suspected preoperatively, the pelvis can be scanned for radioactive iodine uptake. Both ^{131}I and ^{99m}Tc are reported to be concentrated by struma ovarii.[295] This finding is not specific, because increased ^{131}I uptake in the pelvis has been described in a patient with a hemorrhagic ovarian cyst (pseudostruma ovarii).[296]

Struma ovarii has been reported to be unilateral in approximately 94% of cases.[297] The tumor may be solid or cystic, nodular, hemorrhagic, colloidal or firm. These neoplasms vary greatly in size, ranging from 1.5 to 38 cm in diameter, and may weigh as much as 3400 g. The tumor is usually mahogany- or amber-colored.[297] In approximately 60% of cases, struma ovarii most commonly are combined with components of a mature cystic teratoma.[289] Some have associated mucinous or serous cystadenomas or Brenner tumors. Various authors have estimated that 25% to 50% of struma ovarii are formed solely of thyroid tissue.[284, 298]

Strumal carcinoid and struma ovarii have very similar gross pathologic features, except that strumal carcinoid components tend to be gray, white, or yellow.[290] Strumal carcinoids are usually unilateral, but in 10% of cases, the opposite ovary may contain another type of neoplasm, usually a mature cystic teratoma. This is also occasionally observed in cases of struma ovarii.[283, 290] Struma ovarii is composed of true thyroid tissue and may manifest the entire histologic spectrum of thyroid gland pathology.[297] These features include normal thyroid, toxic and non-toxic nodular goiter, toxic goiter, Hashimoto's struma, non-specific thyroiditis, adenomas, "proliferative changes," oxyphilic change, cystic change, and various carcinomas (Fig. 12–61).[299–301] In most cases, hyperthyroidism from ovarian thyroid tissue appears to be caused by hyperfunctioning adenomatous tissue without the characteristic histologic features.[285]

There is no doubt that malignant change can occur in struma ovarii; however, the true incidence of this event is difficult to estimate, because the criteria used to diagnose malignancy vary among authors.[284] Approximately 45 cases of histologically **malignant struma ovarii** have been reported, and 17 cases (38%) were reported to have metastases.[287, 302] Some authors have estimated that the malignant change in struma ovarii is less than 1%, whereas others have reported it to be as high as 20% to 37%.[283, 285] These markedly different malignancy rates are related to a number of factors. As is characteristic in thyroid lesions of the neck, actual malignancy can be difficult to establish microscopically, especially in follicular neoplasms. Also, the microscopic appearance of metastatic lesions may be that of normal "benign" thyroid (so-called **benign strumosis**).[303] Finally, the prognostic appraisal of "malignant" struma, like that of common thyroid gland carcinomas, is difficult because of long intervals before recurrences and metastases, the known indolent behavior of well-differentiated lesions, inadequate follow-up, and the paucity of cases.[297] Nonetheless, Devaney et al.[299] and Young[300] have recently reviewed the clinical meaning of malignancy and/or atypical findings in struma ovarii. The conclusions reached were that cases of struma ovarii with features that merit a diagnosis of carcinoma in the thyroid gland are rarely clinically malignant, cases of struma ovarii that would be considered benign on histologic grounds in the thyroid gland can rarely be clinically malignant, and spread of struma ovarii may be late and associated with a prolonged clinical course.

A number of carcinoma subtypes have been described as arising in struma ovarii, including **follicular carcinoma** (most common), **papillary carcinoma**, and **anaplastic giant/spin-**

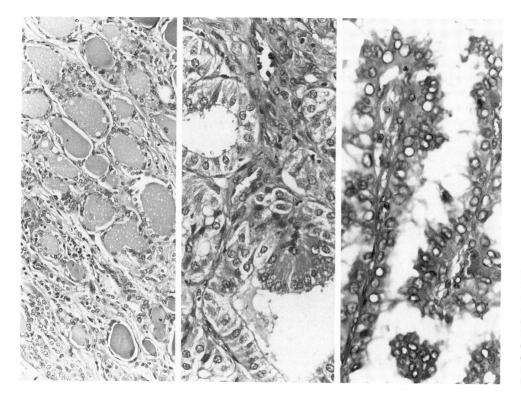

FIGURE 12–61. *Left,* Normal thyroid tissue in a struma ovarii. (H&E, OM ×25) *Middle,* Area of struma ovarii showing oxyphilic change. (H&E, OM ×50) *Right,* Papillary carcinoma with optically clear nuclei and papillary configuration. This thyroid tumor can arise within struma ovarii. (H&E, OM ×100)

dle cell carcinoma.[297] Microscopic diagnosis of the papillary and anaplastic subtypes in most cases should be straightforward; however, follicular tumors should not be diagnosed as malignant unless vascular invasion or metastatic spread is unequivocally present.[283, 304] Assessing capsular invasion in follicular thyroid neoplasms is difficult and very subjective, and therefore it is not a consistently reliable indicator of malignant behavior. This is especially true in struma ovarii because there often is no distinct tumor capsule.[297] Finally, before a diagnosis of primary malignant struma ovarii is made, metastatic carcinoma must be excluded, especially from the thyroid gland.[287]

In **strumal carcinoid,** thyroid follicles co-exist with carcinoid-like cells known to have neurosecretory granules (Fig. 12–62). These latter cells form areas that by light microscopy are identical to trabecular, insular, or mixed trabecular/insular carcinoid tumors found in the gastrointestinal tract.[305] Immunoperoxidase techniques have shown that these cells produce calcitonin or 5-hydroxyindoleacetic acid and are probably of C-cell origin.[287, 294] Some authors have suggested that these lesions may be medullary carcinomas arising in struma ovarii.[305] In the past, strumal carcinoid was included among reported cases of malignant struma ovarii; however, only rare examples have behaved in a malignant fashion.[290, 292] Because of their characteristic carcinoid appearance and indolent behavior, these neoplasms are best considered strumal carcinoid and not medullary carcinoma arising in struma ovarii.

The teratomatous nature of struma ovarii is now generally accepted. The strongest support for this concept stems from the concomitant association with benign mature cystic teratoma. Those struma ovarii that are formed solely of thyroid tissue are thought to be monodermal teratomas or mature cystic teratomas wherein there is a total overgrowth of the thyroid component. It is extremely unlikely that the pure form represents "benign metastases" from the thyroid gland, which

are analogous to the thyroid inclusions sometimes found in cervical lymph nodes.[289]

Some authors regard the intimate admixture of thyroid epithelium and argentaffin cells (with the latter occasionally lining colloid-filled thyroid follicles) in strumal carcinoids as a strong argument against the neuroectodermal origin of argentaffin cells.[292] In one ultrastructural study of two strumal carcinoid neoplasms, neurosecretory granules were found in most, if not all, the follicle lining cells, indicating that the tumor may be a pure carcinoid tumor.[306] Subsequent to the publication of this finding, however, a number of immunohistochemical studies have shown the presence of thyroglobulin and triiodothyronine in the follicles of strumal carcinoid, indicating thyroid differentiation.[284, 298]

The typical benign struma ovarii and strumal carcinoid can be successfully treated with unilateral salpingo-oophorectomy. Although the incidence of bilaterality in struma ovarii is not well established because of the rarity of the disease, it is logical to assume that it may approach the incidence of its more completely studied "cousin," the mature cystic teratoma (13.5%).[288] The incidence of bilaterality in strumal carcinoid has been reported to be 10%.[290] Malignant struma ovarii has been known to metastasize to the contralateral ovary;[287] therefore, contralateral ovarian biopsy should be considered.

Malignant struma ovarii is an indolent tumor in most cases, and the prognosis is good, with 10- to 15-year survivals being common.[283–285, 288, 289, 297] The only apparent exception is the extremely rare struma ovarii with anaplastic giant/spindle cell carcinoma, which has a very poor prognosis.[297] When malignant neoplasms metastasize, they tend to seed the peritoneum and spread within the abdomen to retroperitoneal lymph nodes and the liver. Metastases to bone, brain, lungs, and mediastinum have been described.[287] The treatment of choice for malignant struma ovarii appears to be hysterectomy, bilateral salpingo-oophorectomy, and, on occasion, thyroidec-

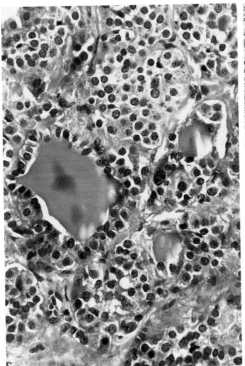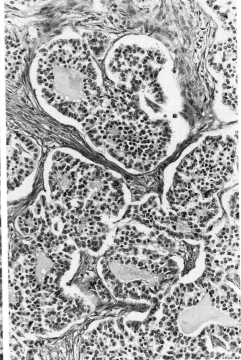

FIGURE 12–62. *Left,* Strumal carcinoma showing carcinoid cells and thyroid follicles. (H&E, OM ×100) *Right,* Shown are nests of strumal carcinoid. (H&E, OM ×25)

tomy. For persistent or metastatic tumor, therapeutic doses of radioactive iodine, preceded by administration of thyroid-stimulating hormone, have been found effective in some cases.[285, 293]

DIFFERENTIAL DIAGNOSIS. In most cases, the diagnosis of struma ovarii should be straightforward. The entity most likely to cause confusion is strumal carcinoid. The diagnosis of strumal carcinoid depends on the findings of thyroid tissue and carcinoid neoplasm, intimately admixed in a portion of the specimen, but occasionally only contiguous.[290] If confusion persists, argentaffin and argyrophil stains should help. As in malignant change in struma ovarii, the carcinoid or thyroid components in strumal carcinoid may be focal, and multiple sections of neoplasm should be examined microscopically. One generous microscopic section for each centimeter of the tumor's diameter seems adequate in most circumstances. Unlike struma ovarii, there appear to be no quantitative or functional requirements for the diagnosis of strumal carcinoid.[290, 292, 298] Strumal carcinoid may be found focally in, or as the predominant component of, a mature cystic teratoma, as one component of another type of neoplasm, or in pure form.[290]

Some strumas are uniformly or predominantly solid and may be misdiagnosed because of the presence of confusing features.[306a] The confusing features include diffuse or pseudo-tubular patterns, a prominent component of oxyphilic or clear cells, a paucity of thyroid follicles, or a combination of these features. When this occurs, differential considerations include **primary ovarian carcinoid** (Fig. 12–63), **clear-cell carcinoma, endometrioid carcinoma, Sertoli-Leydig cell tumor, pregnancy luteoma, metastatic carcinoma or melanoma,** and **granulosa cell tumor.** This group of neoplasms may have areas of colloid-like material in cell-lined spaces.[298] Distinguishing these entities one from another should be easy when sufficient material is available for study; however, dem-onstration of calcium oxalate crystals (relatively specific for thyroid colloid), thyroglobulin, or triiodothyronine by immunoperoxidase techniques is of diagnostic value.[16] Electron microscopy may prove helpful in difficult cases.

BENIGN CYSTIC TERATOMAS WITH MALIGNANT TRANSFORMATION

Benign cystic teratomas are among the most common ovarian tumors encountered in young women. In the vast majority of cases, the gross and microscopic findings are straightforward and offer little diagnostic challenge. Yet, unexpected features can cause diagnostic problems. One of these is malignant change in an otherwise typical benign cystic teratoma.

CLINICOPATHOLOGIC FEATURES. Studies over the last four decades have contributed to clarification of the clinical and pathologic features of this unusual malignant change.[307–311] Malignancy developing in benign cystic teratomas occurs with a frequency of 0.8% to 5% in various series; the most frequently cited figure, however, is approximately 2%. Affected women tend to be older and usually present approximately a decade later than those patients who harbor an uncomplicated lesion, but malignant change has been reported in younger women and in children.

Thus far, all examples have been unilateral, but a banal teratoma is occasionally present in the opposite ovary. Grossly, more than half of the cases show alterations suggesting this complication because of capsular invasion, sometimes associated with infiltration of adjacent structures, or metastases, usually peritoneal. Because of these features, the prognosis is dismal. The most favorable variant is squamous cell carcinoma with an overall survival rate of 77%[312] to 85%[311] in stage I disease, although this figure drops dramatically in stages II to IV. Collaterally, by far the most common malig-

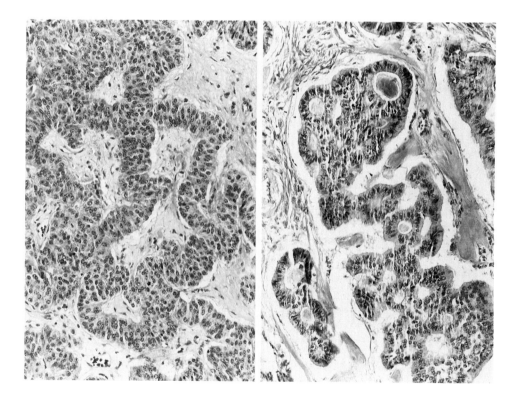

FIGURE 12–63. *Left,* Trabecular pattern of primary ovarian carcinoid tumor. (H&E, OM ×50) *Right,* Primary ovarian carcinoid composed of insular nests. (H&E, OM ×50)

nancy developing in benign cystic teratomas is squamous cell carcinoma, which accounts for approximately 75% of all cases.[311–313] This lesion rarely has been discovered *in situ*[314] but usually is invasive when initially examined. Gross changes suggestive of malignancy include multiple irregular thickenings of the cyst wall, demarcated mural nodules, or an exophytic papillary appearance.[312] Traditionally, malignant transformation has been considered to originate from epidermis at or near the dermoid tubercle. However, 11 of the 28 cases studies by Hirakawa et al.[312] displayed a transition from metaplastic-dysplastic squamous epithelium arising in columnar epithelium, predominantly ciliated (bronchogenic type), but no evidence of direct transition from conventional epidermis to carcinoma was detected in this series. Furthering the resemblance to bronchogenic squamous carcinoma is the presence of hypercalcemia in some cases.[313]

Malignant melanoma has been reported to arise in ovarian cystic teratomas.[319] These secondary neoplasms are usually melanotic but may be devoid of pigment, both grossly and microscopically, after routine and histochemical stains for melanin, their identity being confirmed by immunohistochemical means.[320] Although several types of nevocellular nevi have also been noted in dermoids, junctional activity associated with teratoid melanomas has been demonstrable in only approximately one half of the cases,[319] and it is possible that some melanomas originate from melanocytes that are associated with the neural components of a teratoma. Grossly, this type of malignancy is characterized by one or several pigmented mural nodules. Although local or distant spread has been absent at the time of diagnosis, all patients have died shortly thereafter.[319]

Other malignancies that have been reported to arise in benign cystic teratomas include adenocarcinomas, most of which are poorly differentiated,[307–311] mucinous adenocarcinoma with ''sarcoma-like'' mural nodules,[321] small-cell carcinoma,[322] neuroblastoma,[323] glioblastoma,[324] neuroectodermal tumors,[325] fibrosarcoma,[307, 310] malignant fibrous histiocytoma,[326] leiomyosarcoma,[308] chondrosarcoma,[309] osteogenic sarcoma,[327] and lymphoma.[177] An epithelioid vascular neoplasm of indeterminate malignancy but without overt histologic malignant features has also been reported.[132] Ovarian carcinoid tumors and thyroid carcinoma developing in struma ovarii are discussed elsewhere.

DIFFERENTIAL DIAGNOSIS. Squamous carcinomas of teratomatous origin must be differentiated from other types of primary ovarian squamous cell carcinomas, including endometrioid adenosquamous carcinoma, malignant Brenner tumor, and *de novo* squamous carcinoma (possibly arising from ovarian epidermoid cysts of reputed Walthard rest derivation),[315] and from metastatic squamous cell carcinoma, usually of cervical or vaginal origin.[312] Rarely, extramammary Paget's disease may arise in the teratomatous squamous epithelium,[316, 317] as well as basal cell and sebaceous carcinomas.[311, 318] The differential diagnosis with melanoma developing in teratoma is with metastatic melanoma to the ovary. Bilateral ovarian involvement is strongly in favor of a metastatic process, but unilateral involvement does not exclude a metastasis.[160] Primary (teratomatous) melanomas tend to occur in older patients than those with metastatic melanoma. The history of antecedent removal of a cutaneous lesion, when present, is also helpful. However, in some cases, distinction cannot be made with certainty.[160] For this entire group, finding residual benign cystic teratoma is key to proper diagnosis. Extensive sampling should uncover the teratomatous component to the mass.

BORDERLINE AND MALIGNANT BRENNER TUMOR AND TRANSITIONAL CARCINOMA OF THE OVARY

In 1979, Ober comprehensively reviewed all of the then known aspects of the Brenner tumor[328] and reconfirmed the striking homology of the epithelium of the Brenner tumor and urothelium that had been discerned through histologic studies. Subsequent communications, many of which have used histochemical, immunohistochemical, ultrastructural, and flow cytometric methods, have lent credence to this epithelial propinquity.[329–334] Most investigators strongly favor the concept that Brenner epithelium arises from the pluripotential surface ovarian epithelium through a process of transitional (urothelial) metaplasia. When viewed in this light (and through the microscope), the morphologic spectrum of the Brenner tumor and its variants can be readily appreciated to represent analogues of various transitional cell proliferations of the urinary tract.

CLINICOPATHOLOGIC FEATURES. The spectrum of ''transitional cell'' tumors of the ovary has been amply documented by Roth et al.,[331, 332] who equated the classic Brenner tumor with cell nests of von Brunn. Collaterally, these workers defined the metaplastic variant as one exhibiting mucinous metaplasia of some of the cells in the epithelial nests of a Brenner tumor, thus corresponding to cystitis glandularis, and the proliferating Brenner tumor as a lesion corresponding to papillary non-invasive transitional cell carcinoma, grade 1 or 2 (Fig. 12–64). The Brenner tumor of low malignant potential was deemed to correspond to a papillary non-invasive transitional cell carcinoma, grade 3 (sometimes with foci resembling squamous cell carcinoma *in situ*) that evolved from a proliferating Brenner tumor (Fig. 12–65). The prognosis of all of the foregoing types of Brenner tumor was uniformly excellent. Furthermore, the malignant Brenner tumor was characterized as a neoplasm with a malignant epithelial component, transitional in the better differentiated lesions, but often with an admixture of squamous or undifferentiated carcinoma in poorly differentiated examples, that showed unequivocal stromal invasion and that was associated with a component of benign or proliferating Brenner tumor. Many previous authors had agreed with such a definition of malignant Brenner tumor, requiring the presence of an admixed or adjoining benign Brenner tumor, but others had accepted a less restrictive definition. This divergence was clearly delineated by the clinicopathologic study of Austin and Norris,[335] who drew attention not only to the difference in the histopathologic features of malignant Brenner tumor and transitional cell carcinoma of the ovary but also to their different clinical and prognostic features. Austin and Norris simply stated that transitional cell carcinoma differed from malignant Brenner tumor in its histopathologic appearance only in the absence of an associated benign or proliferating Brenner tumor component. When so defined, malignant Brenner tumors were found to be *less aggressive* than transitional cell carcinoma. Malignant Brenner tumors presented in advanced stage (II–IV) less frequently

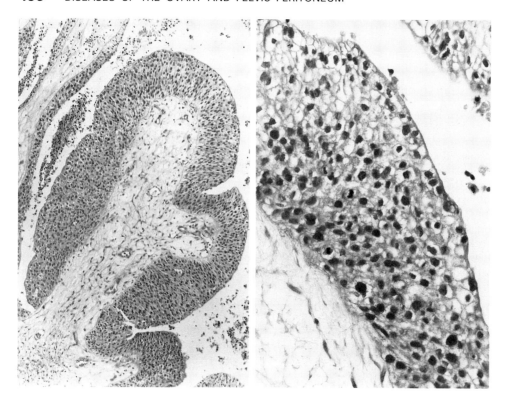

FIGURE 12–64. *Left,* Shown are papillae of a proliferating Brenner tumor. Other areas not shown contained classic Brenner tumor. (H&E, OM ×25) *Right,* Cytologically the lesion showed grade 1 features without invasion of underlying stroma. (H&E, OM ×100)

than transitional cell carcinoma, and a greater percentage of patients with malignant Brenner tumors were tumor-free at last follow-up as compared to those with transitional cell carcinomas, a behavioral difference that persisted when the tumors were compared within the same stage. Histologic grade did not explain the difference because the great majority of tumor type were grade 2 or 3.

Yet, the histologic separation of malignant Brenner tumor from transitional cell carcinoma is not the only distinction of import.[336–338] Several studies indicated that ovarian tumors with a pure or predominant (more than 50%) transitional cell carcinoma component have a better response to chemotherapy and improved patient survival when compared with non-urothelial ovarian carcinomas of the same stage and grade,

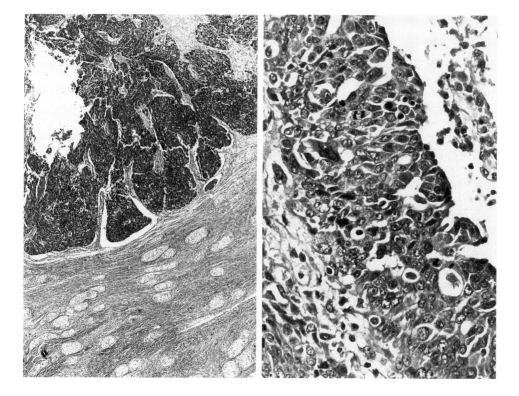

FIGURE 12–65. *Left,* Shown is a Brenner tumor of low malignant potential. Note that there is no stromal invasion and the tumor lies adjacent to classic Brenner tumor. (H&E, OM ×10) *Right,* Note the grade 3 cytologic atypia, yet there was no invasion of underlying stroma. Thus, the diagnosis is low malignant potential Brenner tumor. (H&E, OM ×50)

which had comparable amounts of residual tumor after primary resection and were subjected to similar chemotherapeutic regimens.[336, 337] Such prognostic importance of urothelial differentiation represents a departure from the position that histologic subtype is of little or no significance in malignant epithelial neoplasms of the ovary. In addition, it was shown that patients with transitional cell predominant ovarian carcinoma whose metastases are also composed of predominant transitional cell carcinoma show a distinct 5-year survival advantage over those patients whose metastases are predominantly non-transitional in type.[337]

DIFFERENTIAL DIAGNOSIS. The diagnosis of malignant Brenner tumor as defined by Roth and Czernobilsky[332] and by Austin and Norris[335] is straightforward. The foregoing clinical factors related to transitional cell carcinoma emphasize the importance of its histopathologic recognition. The major difficulty in such appraisal is the problem of "seeing" a urothelial malignancy in an organ outside of the urinary tract, with a resultant tendency to interpret such a neoplasm as an undifferentiated large-cell carcinoma.[336] The presence of undulating papillary folds composed of multilayered epithelium lining cystic spaces in an invasive cystic and solid carcinoma is the most characteristic and helpful feature in the microscopic diagnosis of transitional cell carcinoma of the ovary.[332, 335, 336] The solid areas may be difficult or impossible to distinguish from undifferentiated carcinoma.

The other problem posed by transitional cell carcinoma of an ovary occurs when it is present synchronously or metachronously with a **transitional cell carcinoma of the bladder or ureter,**[339] or, very rarely, the uterine cervix. In such cases it may not be possible to conclusively decide whether the ovarian lesion is primary or metastatic. Fortunately, this clinicopathologic conundrum is represented by only a handful of cases because urothelial tumors are among the neoplasms that spread to the ovary least often[339] and because primary transitional cell carcinoma of the ovary is uncommon. Based on a review of four pertinent cases from the literature and two of their own, Young and Scully[339] considered that features that favored a metastatic nature of the ovarian tumors included deep invasion of the primary (extraovarian) urothelial tumor, metastasis to other sites at the time of ovarian involvement, bilaterality of the ovarian carcinomas, surface implants of the ovarian tumors, and the presence of vascular invasion in either the urothelial or ovarian tumor. Features considered to favor an independent primary transitional cell carcinoma of the ovary were a long interval (3 years or more) between detection of the urothelial and ovarian tumors, absent or only superficial invasion of the urothelial tumor, the presence of only ovarian and urothelial tumors, and absence of extraurinary-tract tumors for 3 years or more after treatment of the ovarian tumor. Nevertheless, these authors noted that after their analysis, some degree of doubt regarding such a differential diagnosis remained in all cases.

GRANULOMATOUS LESIONS OF THE OVARY

Although uncommon, this group includes several entities of import to the surgical pathologist. Those granulomatous lesions that contain considerable numbers of lipid histiocytes must be differentiated from metastatic carcinoma, particularly clear-cell carcinoma, from metastatic melanoma, and from primary ovarian lipid-rich stromal tumors and clear-cell carcinoma. In addition, these "xanthic" variants must be distinguished from other ovarian granulomas.

CLINICOPATHOLOGIC FEATURES AND DIFFERENTIAL DIAGNOSIS. Necrotic pseudoxanthomatous nodules (NPN) of the ovary and peritoneum represent an unusual change in **endometriosis**[340] (see Fig. 12–59, right). Characteristically occurring in older women, NPN cause enlargement of one or both ovaries by cystic nodules of soft yellow to dark tan material. Three of the four cases described by Clement et al.[340] were associated with multiple brown nodules, either attached to the peritoneum of free in the peritoneal cavity. Histologically, all lesional foci were characterized by granulomatous nodules with central spheroidal or stellate necrotic zones composed of eosinophilic and calcific debris and scattered necrotic histiocytes, surrounded by sheets of intact, occasionally palisaded foamy histiocytes. Variable numbers of these last cells contained fine granular pigment that varied from pale yellow to dark brown and that exhibited the staining reactions of lipofuscin (hemofuscin, ceroid). Three of the cases had an associated pseudoxanthomatous salpingitis, and in one, pigmented histiocytes were also present in the omental fat, resulting in a pseudoinfiltrative pattern. Although endometriotic glands and stroma were typically absent in the nodules and their immediate vicinity, in one instance several necrotic nodules lined an endometriotic cyst, and in another, a focus had an appearance transitional between endometriosis and a necrotic nodule.

Differentiation of NPN from metastatic carcinoma, particularly clear-cell carcinomas, and from metastatic melanoma is indicated by the gross and microscopic features. Although metastatic deposits of such tumors may contain necrotic foci, the search for viable malignant tumor cells and the correct identification of the pigment should enable correct differential identification of these various processes. When present in NPN, **pseudoxanthomatous salpingitis,**[341, 342] another manifestation of ovarian endometriotic bleeding,[342] is a helpful ancillary feature. Less likely to be confused with NPN are lipid-rich ovarian stromal lesions and primary clear-cell carcinoma of the ovary. These metastatic and primary lesions are discussed in detail elsewhere.

Rarely, chronic pelvic bacterial infections may be associated with the development of a solid yellow ovarian or tubo-ovarian mass that is dominated histologically by sheets of foamy histiocytes, with lesser numbers of neutrophils, plasma cells, and multinucleated giant cells.[343, 344] This is known as **xanthogranulomatous oophoritis.** Although foci of hemorrhage may occur, pigment deposition is inconspicuous, and necrosis, when present, is punctate, without peripheral histiocytic palisading. This type of oophoritis occurs in younger women and appears morphologically similar to **xanthogranulomatous pyelonephritis.**

Although **malakoplakia** was initially described as a disease of the urinary tract, principally the urinary bladder, almost 100 years ago, and was once thought to be restricted to it, it is now apparent that this peculiar entity, a result of various types of bacterial infection, may occur in a variety of tissues and organs. When it affects the female genital tract, it occurs predominantly in the lower tract (vagina, cervix, and endometrium). Involvement of the ovary is rare and is associated with synchronous lesions in neighboring genital or peritoneal foci.[345–347] The infection is thought to be ascending, but in one instance may have been the result of **diverticulitis.**[347] Ovarian involvement is characterized by a brownish tumor-like mass that may appear infiltrative, and frozen section may suggest lipid cell tumor.[347] Histologically, malakoplakia also contains diffuse collections of histiocytes whose cytoplasm varies from granular and eosinophilic to foamy. However, the pathognomonic feature is the presence of characteristic small, basophilic homogeneous or targetoid mineralized phagolysosomes **(calcospherites),** the **Michaelis-Gutmann bodies,** found within some histiocytes as well as in an extracellular distribution.

Discrete, circumscribed **necrobiotic granulomas, closely resembling rheumatoid granulomas,** but occurring in distinctly unusual sites in the absence of rheumatoid arthritis, were initially described in the urinary bladder, prostate, and cervix.[348] More recently they have been noted in the kidney, and even ''as far'' as the thyroid.[349] Germane to this discussion are identical examples of ovarian granulomas, known as **isolated (palisading) necrobiotic granuloma of the ovary.**[350–352] All instances of extraovarian cases, as well as most of the ovarian cases, have been associated with an antecedent procedure, either diathermy or surgery. However, the two cases of Kernohan et al.[352] as well as one of the four cases of Herbold et al.,[350] the latter slightly unusual histologically, lacked such a history. All patients except those of Kernohan et al.[352] were premenopausal. Isolated palisading granulomas of the ovary, as well as their analogues at other sites, as noted, mimic the structure of rheumatoid granulomas. Obviously, special stains and cultures have revealed no causative organisms. The obvious propinquity of prior surgery and the necrobiotic change is more than fortuitous, in our opinion, and would appear to be the most common pathogenetic mechanism. It is possible that in those instances without such a history, the lesion represents a reaction to unrecognized trauma.

Sarcoid-like granulomas are sometimes encountered in the ovary. Infection always should be ruled out, but **Crohn's disease** may cause ovarian granulomas.[353] They are of the small, non-caseating epithelioid type and are situated within the cortex. One instance of direct suppurative ovarian involvement secondary to a fistulous extension from the bowel, with the formation of a right tubo-ovarian abscess, has been described.[354] The latter type of lesion should be distinguished from left-sided **foreign body granulomatous** ovarian involvement caused by a colo-ovarian fistula secondary to diverticulitis.[355, 356] The cortical epithelioid granulomas of Crohn's disease, which tend to occur in younger women, should be distinguished from the common **superficial cortical granulomas of older women,** thought to be a regression phenomenon of stromal hyperplasia, and which are composed of small, often perivascular collections of lymphocytes, epithelioid-like cells of possible stromal origin, and rare giant cells.[357] The small non-caseating granulomas of true sarcoid may rarely be seen in the ovary[358] and have been associated with known, documented sarcoidosis.

Autoimmune oophoritis is a rare cause of primary ovarian failure[359, 360] and may be associated with other organ-specific autoimmune diseases, particularly **Addison's disease.**[361] In this condition, a pronounced lymphoplasmacytic reaction is present around developing follicles and luteal structures. In some foci, only perifollicular mononuclear cells may be present. In some instances, destruction of the granulosa or thecal

lining ensues, and the central regions of these cellular areas may not be appreciated as follicular or luteal-based. Partial follicular or luteal collapse and resultant stellate configurations, particularly when the cellular infiltrate is predominantly mononuclear, may impart a distinctly granulomatoid picture. The clinical background of ovarian failure in younger women, sometimes associated with other organ-specific deficits, should be appreciated.

Two **infectious granulomatous diseases** merit brief note. Because of its geographic distribution, *Coccidioides* is of potential import in the United States. It may rarely affect the ovary as part of pelvic infection.[362, 363] With the widespread use of the intra-uterine contraceptive device, pelvic infection with **actinomycosis** is not uncommon, and may primarily affect the ovary.[364]

Miscellaneous Pathologic Curiosities

Congenital absence of ovaries[365]
Ectopic ovary (and neoplasms arising therefrom)[92, 366–369]
Ovarian remnant syndrome[370, 371]
Splenic-ovarian fusion[372]
Uterus-like mass[373]
Adipocytic infiltration of the ovary[374]
Ovarian hypoplasia with follicular calcifications[375]
Idiopathic multifocal stromal calcification of the ovary[376]
Yellow ovaries[377]
Arteritis of the female genital tract[378, 379]
Ovarian hemorrhage[380, 381]
Ovarian abscess[382–385]
Abscess (tubo-ovarian, unusual aspects)[386–388]
Cytomegaly in benign ovarian cysts[389]
Foreign body granulomas of the ovaries[390]
Benign cystic teratoma, unusual aspects[391–408]
Unusual mesenchymal neoplasm of the ovary[409–411]

References

1. Suzuki Y: Diagnostic criteria for human diffuse malignant mesothelioma. Acta Pathol Jpn 42:767–786, 1992.
2. Sheibani K, Esteban JM, Bailey A, et al: Immunopathologic and molecular studies as an aid to the diagnosis of malignant mesothelioma. Hum Pathol 23:107–116, 1992.
3. Warhol MJ, Hunter NJ, Corson JM: An ultrastructural comparison of mesotheliomas and adenocarcinomas of the ovary and endometrium. J Gynecol Pathol 1:125–134, 1982.
4. McCaughey WTE, Colby TV, Battifora H, et al: Diagnosis of diffuse malignant mesothelioma: Experience of a US/Canadian mesothelioma panel. Mod Pathol 4:342–353, 1991.
5. Battifora H, Kopinski MI: Distinction of mesothelioma from adenocarcinoma: An immunohistochemical approach. Cancer 55:1679–1685, 1985.
6. Cibas ES, Corson JM, Pinkus GS: The distinction of adenocarcinoma from malignant mesothelioma in cell blocks of effusions. Hum Pathol 18:67–74, 1987.
7. Dardick I, Jabi M, McCaughey WTE, et al: Diffuse epithelial mesothelioma: A review of the ultrastructural spectrum. Ultrastruct Pathol 11:503–533, 1987.
8. Bollinger DJ, Wick MR, Dehner LP, et al: Peritoneal malignant mesothelioma versus serous papillary adenocarcinoma. A histochemical and immunohistochemical comparison. Am J Surg Pathol 13:659–670, 1989.
9. Raju U, Fine G, Greenawald KA, Ohorodnik JM: Primary papillary serous neoplasia of the peritoneum: A clinicopathologic and ultrastructural study of eight cases. Hum Pathol 20:426–436, 1989.
10. Stirling JW, Henderson DW, Spagnolo DV, Whitaker D: Unusual granular reactivity for carcinoembryonic antigen in malignant mesothelioma [correspondence]. Hum Pathol 21:678–679, 1990.
11. Robb JA: Mesothelioma versus adenocarcinoma. False-positive CEA and Leu-M1 staining due to hyaluronic acid [correspondence]. Hum Pathol 20:400, 1989.
12. Daya D, McCaughey WTE: Well-differentiated papillary mesothelioma of the peritoneum. A clinicopathologic study of 22 cases. Cancer 65:292–296, 1990.
13. Wick MR, Mills SE, Swanson PE: Expression of ''myelomonocytic'' antigens in mesotheliomas and adenocarcinomas involving the serosal surfaces. Am J Clin Pathol 94:18–26, 1990.
14. Truong LD, Maccato ML, Awalt H, et al: Serous surface carcinoma of the peritoneum: A clinicopathologic study of 22 cases. Hum Pathol 21:99–110, 1990.

15. Wick MR, Loy T, Mills SE, et al: Malignant epithelioid pleural mesothelioma versus peripheral pulmonary adenocarcinoma: A histochemical, ultrastructural, and immunohistologic study of 103 cases. Hum Pathol 21:759–766, 1990.

16. Fox H: Primary neoplasia of the female peritoneum [invited review]. Histopathology 23:103–110, 1993.

17. Daya D, McCaughey WTE: Pathology of the peritoneum: A review of selected topics. Semin Diagn Pathol 8:277–289, 1991.

18. Kannerstein M, Churg J: Peritoneal mesothelioma. Hum Pathol 8:83–94, 1977.

19. Sussman J, Rosai J: Lymph node metastasis as the initial manifestation of malignant mesothelioma. Report of six cases. Am J Surg Pathol 14:819–828, 1990.

20. Dalrymple JC, Bannatyne P, Russell P, et al: Extra-ovarian peritoneal serous papillary carcinoma. A clinicopathologic study of 31 cases. Cancer 64:110–115, 1989.

21. Bell DA, Scully RE: Serous borderline tumors of the peritoneum. Am J Surg Pathol 14:230–239, 1990.

22. Biscotti CV, Hart WR: Peritoneal serous micropapillomatosis of low malignant potential (serous borderline tumors of the peritoneum). A clinicopathologic study of 17 cases. Am J Surg Pathol 16:467–475, 1992.

23. Gilks CB, Bell DA, Scully RE: Serous psammocarcinoma of the ovary and peritoneum. Int J Gynecol Pathol 9:110–121, 1990.

24. Rutgers JL, Scully RE: Ovarian Mullerian mucinous papillary cystadenomas of borderline malignancy. A clinicopathologic analysis. Cancer 61:3440–348, 1988.

25. Rutgers JL, Scully RE: Ovarian mixed-epithelial papillary cystadenomas of borderline malignancy of Mullerian type. A clinicopathologic analysis. Cancer 61:546–554, 1988.

26. Clement PB, Young RH: Florid mesothelial hyperplasia associated with ovarian tumors: A potential source of error in tumor diagnosis and staging. Int J Gynecol Pathol 12:51–58, 1993.

27. McFadden DE, Clement PB: Peritoneal inclusion cysts with mural mesothelial proliferation. A clinicopathologic study of six cases. Am J Surg Pathol 10:844–854, 1986.

28. Ross MJ, Welch WR, Scully RE: Multilocular peritoneal inclusion cysts (so-called cystic mesotheliomas). Cancer 64:1336–1346, 1989.

29. Zinsser KR, Wheeler JE: Endosalpingiosis in the omentum. A study of autopsy and surgical material. Am J Surg Pathol 6:109–117, 1982.

30. Dallenbach-Hellweg G: Atypical endosalpingiosis: A case report with consideration of the differential diagnosis of glandular subperitoneal inclusions. Pathol Res Pract 182:180–182, 1987.

31. Khoury N, Raju U, Crissman JD, et al: A comparative immunohistochemical study of peritoneal and ovarian serous tumors, and mesotheliomas. Hum Pathol 21:811–819, 1990.

32. Bolen JW, Hammar SP, McNutt MA: Reactive and neoplastic serosal tissue. A light-microscopic, ultrastructural, and immunocytochemical study. Am J Surg Pathol 10:34–47, 1986.

33. Warnock ML, Stoloff A, Thor A: Differentiation of adenocarcinoma of the lung from mesothelioma. Periodic acid-Schiff, monoclonal antibodies B72.3, and leu-M1. Am J Pathol 133:30–38, 1988.

34. Szpak CA, Johnston WW, Roggli V, et al: The diagnostic distinction between malignant mesothelioma of the pleura and adenocarcinoma of the lung as defined by a monoclonal antibody (B72.3). Am J Pathol 122:252–260, 1986.

35. Kafiri G, Thomas DM, Shepherd NA, et al: p53 expression is common in malignant mesothelioma. Histopathology 21:331–334, 1992.

36. Mayall FG, Goddard H, Gibbs AR: p53 immunostaining in the distinction between benign and malignant mesothelial proliferations using formalin-fixed paraffin sections. J Pathol 168:377–381, 1992.

37. Ramel M, Lemmens G, Eerdekens CA, et al: Immunoreactivity for p53 protein in malignant mesothelioma and non-neoplastic mesothelium. J Pathol 168:371–375, 1992.

38. Cagle PT, Brown RW, Lebovitz RM: p53 immunostaining in the differentiation of reactive processes from malignancy in pleural biopsy specimens. Hum Pathol 25:443–448, 1994.

39. Walts AE, Said JW, Shintaku IP, et al: Keratins of different molecular weight in exfoliated mesothelial and adenocarcinoma cells—an aid to cell identification. Am J Clin Pathol 81:442–446, 1984.

40. Weidner N: Malignant mesothelioma of peritoneum. Ultrastruct Pathol 15:515–520, 1991.

41. Otis CN, Carter D, Cole S, Battifora H: Immunohistochemical evaluation of pleural mesothelioma and pulmonary adenocarcinoma. A bi-institutional study of 47 cases. Am J Surg Pathol 11:445–456, 1987.

42. Churg J, Gerber MA: The processing and examination of renal biopsies. Lab Med 10:591–596, 1979.

43. Hammar SP, Bolen JW: Sarcomatoid pleural mesothelioma. Ultrastruct Pathol 9:337–343, 1985.

44. Dardick I, Al-Jabi M, McCaughey WTE, et al: Ultrastructure of poorly differentiated diffuse epithelial mesotheliomas. Ultrastruct Pathol 7:151–160, 1984.

45. Taxy JB, Almanaseer IY: ''Anemone'' cell (villiform) tumors: Electron microscopy and immunohistochemistry of five cases. Ultrastruct Pathol 7:143–150, 1984.

46. Wirt DP, Nagle RB, Gustafson HM, et al: The probable origin of an anemone cell tumor: Metastatic transitional cell carcinoma producing HCG. Ultrastruct Pathol 7:277–288, 1984.

47. Phillips JI, Murray J, Verhaart S: Squamous cell carcinoma with anemone cell features. Ultrastruct Pathol 11:47–52, 1987.

48. Peterson JT, Greenberg SD, Buffler PA: Non-asbestos-related malignant mesothelioma. A review. Cancer 54:951–960, 1984.

49. Fraire AE, Cooper S, Greenberg SD, et al: Mesothelioma of childhood. Cancer 62:838–847, 1988.

50. Yousem SA, Hochholzer L: Malignant mesotheliomas with osseous and cartilaginous differentiation. Arch Pathol Lab Med 111:62–66, 1987.

51. Henderson DW, Attwood HD, Constance TJ, et al: Lympho-histiocytoid mesothelioma: A rare lymphomatoid variant of predominantly sarcomatoid mesothelioma. Ultrastruct Pathol 12:367–384, 1988.

52. Nascimento AG, Keeney GL, Fletcher CDM: Deciduoid peritoneal mesothelioma. An unusual phenotype affecting young females. Am J Surg Pathol 18:439–445, 1994.

53. MacDougall DB, Wang SE, Zidar BL: Mucin-positive epithelial mesothelioma. Arch Pathol Lab Med 116:874–880, 1992.

54. Mayall FG, Gibbs AR: The histology and immunohistochemistry of small cell mesothelioma. Histopathology 20:47–51, 1992.

55. Hurlimann J: Desmin and neural marker expression in mesothelial cells and mesotheliomas. Hum Pathol 25:753–757, 1994.

56. Mayall FG, Goddard H, Gibbs AR: Intermediate filament expression in mesotheliomas: Leiomyoid mesotheliomas are not uncommon. Histopathology 21:453–457, 1992.

57. Wilson GE, Hasteton PS, Chatterjee AK: Desmoplastic malignant mesothelioma: A review of 17 cases. J Clin Pathol 45:295–298, 1992.

58. Epstein JI, Budin RE: Keratin and epithelial membrane antigen immunoreactivity in nonneoplastic fibrous pleural lesions: Implications for the diagnosis of desmoplastic mesothelioma. Hum Pathol 17:514–519, 1986.

59. Bolen JW, Hammar SP, McNutt MA: Serosal tissue: Reactive tissue as a model for understanding mesotheliomas. Ultrastruct Pathol 11:251–262, 1987.

60. Ordonez NG, El-Naggar AK, Ro JY, et al: Intra-abdominal desmoplastic small cell tumor: A light microscopic, immunocytochemical, ultrastructural, and flow cytometric study. Hum Pathol 24:850–865, 1993.

61. Gonzalez-Crussi F, de Mello DE, Sotelo-Avila C: Omental-mesenteric myxoid hamartomas. Infantile lesions simulating malignant tumors. Am J Surg Pathol 7:567–578, 1983.

62. Robboy SJ, Scully RE: Ovarian teratoma with glial implants on the peritoneum: An analysis of 12 cases. Hum Pathol 1:643–653, 1970.

63. Truong LD, Jurco S III, McGavran MH: Gliomatosis peritonei: Report of two cases and review of literature. Am J Surg Pathol 6:443–449, 1982.

64. Nielsen SNJ, Scheithauer BW, Gaffey TA: Gliomatosis peritonei. Cancer 56:2499–2503, 1985.

65. Gratama S, Swaak-Saeys Am, van der Weiden RMF, Chadha S: Low-grade immature teratomas with peritoneal gliomatosis: A case report. Eur J Obstet Gynecol Reprod Biol 39:235–241, 1991.

66. Coulson W: Peritoneal gliomatosis from a gastric teratoma. Am J Clin Pathol 94:87–89, 1990.

67. Lovell MA, Ross GW, Cooper PH: Gliomatosis peritonei associated with a ventriculo-peritoneal shunt. Am J Clin Pathol 91:485–487, 1989.

68. El Shafie M, Furay RW, Chablani LV: Ovarian teratoma with peritoneal and lymph node metastases of mature glial tissue: A benign condition. J Surg Oncol 27:18–22, 1984.

69. Perrone T, Steiner M, Dehner LP: Nodal gliomatosis and alpha-fetoprotein production: Two unusual facets of grade I ovarian teratoma. Arch Pathol Lab Med 110:975–977, 1986.

70. Boehner JF, Gallup DG, Talledo E, et al: Solid ovarian teratoma with neuroglial metastases to periaortic lymph nodes and omentum. South Med J 80:649–652, 1987.

71. Shefren G, Collin J, Soriero O: Gliomatosis peritonei with malignant transformation: A case report and review of the literature. Am J Obstet Gynecol 164:1617–1621, 1991.

71a. O'Connor DM, Norris HJ: The influence of grade on the outcome of stage I ovarian immature (malignant) teratomas and the reproducibility of grading. Int J Gynecol Pathol 13:283–289, 1994.

72. Kragel PJ, Devaney K, Merino MJ: Struma ovarii with peritoneal implants: A case report with lectin histochemistry. Surg Pathol 4:274–280, 1991.

73. Zaytsev P, Taxy JB: Pregnancy-associated ectopic decidua. Am J Surg Pathol 11:526–530, 1987.

74. Richter MA, Choudhry A, Barton JJ, Merrick RE: Bleeding ectopic decidua as a cause of intraabdominal hemorrhage: A case report. J Reprod Med 28:430–432, 1983.

75. Cobb CJ: Ectopic decidua and metastatic squamous carcinoma: Presentation in a single pelvic lymph node. J Surg Oncol 38:126–129, 1988.

76. Clement PB, Young RH, Scully RE: Nontrophoblastic pathology of the female genital tract and peritoneum associated with pregnancy. Semin Diagn Pathol 6:372–406, 1989.

77. Clement PB, Scully RE: Idiopathic postmenopausal decidual reaction of the endometrium: A clinicopathologic analysis of four cases. Int J Gynecol Pathol 7:152–161, 1988.

78. Tavassoli FA, Norris HJ: Peritoneal leiomyomatosis (leiomyomatosis peritonealis disseminata): A clinicopathologic study of 20 cases with ultrastructural observations. Int J Gynecol Pathol 1:59–74, 1982.

79. Hsu YK, Rosenshein NB, Parmley TH, et al: Leiomyomatosis in pelvic lymph nodes. Obstet Gynecol 57(suppl):91–93, 1981.

80. Mazzoleni G, Salerno A, Santini D, et al: Leiomyomatosis in pelvic lymph nodes. Histopathology 21:588–589, 1992.

81. Ma KF, Chow LTC: Sex cord-like pattern leiomyomatosis peritonealis disseminata: A hitherto undescribed feature. Histopathology 21:389–391, 1992.

82. Kitazawa S, Shiraishi N, Maeda S: Leiomyomatosis peritonealis disseminata with adipocytic differentiation. Acta Obstet Gynecol Scand 71:482–484, 1992.

83. Akkersdijk GJM, Flu PK, Giard RWM, et al: Malignant leiomyomatosis peritonealis disseminata. Am J Obstet Gynecol 163:591–593, 1990.

84. Lausen I, Jensen OJ, Andersen E, Lindahl F: Disseminated peritoneal leiomyomatosis with malignant change, in a male. Virchows Archiv A Pathol Anat 417:173–175, 1990.

85. Cartwright PS: Peritoneal trophoblastic implants after surgical management of tubal pregnancy. J Reprod Med 36:523–524, 1991.

86. Beck E, Siebzehnrübl E, Jäger W, et al: Disseminierte intraperitoneale Trophoblast-Aussaat nach laparoskopisch behandelter Extra-uteringraviditä. Geburtshilfe Frauenheilkd 51:939–941, 1991.

87. Kim K-R, Scully RE: Peritoneal keratin granulomas with carcinomas of endometrium and ovary and atypical polypoid adenomyoma of endometrium: A clinicopathologic analysis of 22 cases. Am J Surg Pathol 14:925–932, 1990.

88. Schatz JE, Colgan TJ: Squamous metaplasia of the peritoneum. Arch Pathol Lab Med 115:397–398, 1991.

89. Lee D, Pontifex A: Melanosis peritonei. Am J Obstet Gynecol 122:526–527, 1975.

90. Fukushima M, Sharpe L, Okagaki T: Peritoneal melanosis secondary to a benign dermoid cyst of the ovary: A case report with ultrastructural study. Int J Gynecol Pathol 2:403–409, 1984.

91. Drachenberg CB, Papadimitriou JC: Melanotic peritoneal cyst: Light microscopic and ultrastructural studies. Arch Pathol Lab Med 114:463–466, 1990.

92. Heller DS, Harpaz N, Breakstone B: Neoplasms arising in ectopic ovaries: A case of Brenner tumor in an accessory ovary. Int J Gynecol Pathol 9:185–189, 1990.

93. Thor AD, Young RH, Clement PB: Pathology of the fallopian tube, broad ligament, peritoneum, and pelvic tumors. Hum Pathol 22:856–866, 1991.

94. Gonzalez-Crussi F, Sotelo-Avila C, deMello DE: Primary peritoneal, omental, and mesenteric tumors in childhood. Semin Diagn Pathol 3:122–137, 1986.

95. Young RH, Silva EG, Scully RE: Ovarian and juxtaovarian adenomatoid tumors: A report of six cases. Int J Gynecol Pathol 10:364–371, 1991.

96. Banerjee R, Gough J: Cystic mucinous tumors of the mesentery and retroperitoneum: Report of three cases. Histopathology 12:527–532, 1988.

97. Harpaz N, Gellman E: Urogenital mesenteric cyst with fallopian tube features. Arch Pathol Lab Med 111:78–80, 1987.

98. Vuong PN, Guyot H, Moulin G, et al: Pseudotumoral organization of a twisted epiploic fringe or "hard-boiled egg" in the peritoneal cavity. Arch Pathol Lab Med 114:531–533, 1990.

99. Young RH, Scully RE: Metastatic tumors in the ovary: A problem-oriented approach and review of the recent literature. Semin Diagn Pathol 8:250–276, 1991.

100. Young RH, Kozakevich HPW, Scully RE: Metastatic ovarian tumors in children: A report of 14 cases and review of the literature. Int J Gynecol Pathol 12:8–19, 1993.

101. Lash RH, Hart WR: Intestinal adenocarcinomas metastatic to the ovaries. A clinicopathologic evaluation of 22 cases. Am J Surg Pathol 11:114–121, 1987.

102. Ulbright TM, Roth LM: Metastatic and independent cancers of the endometrium and ovary: A clinicopathologic study of 34 cases. Hum Pathol 16:28–34, 1985.

103. Young RH, Hart WR: Metastases from carcinomas of the pancreas simulating primary mucinous tumors of the ovary. A report of seven cases. Am J Surg Pathol 13:748–756, 1989.

104. Young RH, Gilks CB, Scully RE: Mucinous tumors of the appendix associated with mucinous tumors of the ovary and pseudomyxoma peritonei. A clinicopathologic analysis of 22 cases supporting origin in the appendix. Am J Surg Pathol 15:415–429, 1991.

105. Young RH, Scully RE: Mucinous ovarian tumors associated with mucinous adenocarcinoma of the cervix. A clinicopathologic analysis of 16 cases. Int J Gynecol Pathol 7:99–111, 1988.

106. Holtz F, Hart WR: Krukenberg tumors of the ovary. A clinicopathologic analysis of 27 cases. Cancer 50:2438–2447, 1982.

107. Alenghat E, Okagaki T, Talerman A: Primary mucinous carcinoid tumor of the ovary. Cancer 58:777–783, 1986.

108. Hirschfield LS, Kahn LB, Winkler B, et al: Adenocarcinoid of the appendix presenting as bilateral Krukenberg's tumor of the ovaries. Arch Pathol Lab Med 109:930–933, 1985.

109. Suarez JE, Palacios J, Burgos E, Gamallo C: Signet-ring stromal tumor of the ovary: A histochemical, immunohistochemical, and ultrastructural study. Virchows Archiv A Pathol Anat 422:333–336, 1993.

110. Bullon A, Arseneau J, Prat J, et al: Tubular Krukenberg tumor. A problem in histopathologic diagnosis. Am J Surg Pathol 5:225–232, 1981.

111. Zukerberg L, Young RH: Chordoma metastatic to the ovary. Arch Pathol Lab Med 114:208–210, 1990.

112. Young RH, Scully RE: Ovarian metastases from carcinoma of the gallbladder and extrahepatic bile ducts simulating primary tumors of the ovary. A report of six cases. Int J Gynecol Pathol 9:60–72, 1990.

113. Weidner N, Foucar E: Epidermotropic metastatic squamous cell carcinoma. Report of two cases showing histologic continuity between epidermis and metastasis. Arch Dermatol 121:1041–1043, 1985.

114. Fowler JL, Maygarden SJ, Novotny DB: Human alveolar macrophage-56 and carcinoembryonic antigen monoclonal antibodies in the differential diagnosis between primary ovarian and metastatic gastrointestinal carcinomas. Hum Pathol 25:666–670, 1994.

115. Moll R, Lowe A, Laufer J, Franke WW: Cytokeratin 20 in human carcinomas. A new histodiagnostic marker detected by monoclonal antibodies. Am J Pathol 140:427–447, 1992.

116. Shakfeh SM, Woodruff JD: Primary ovarian sarcomas: Report of 46 cases and review of the literature. Obstet Gynecol Surv 42:331–349, 1987.

117. Prat J, Scully RE: Ovarian sarcomas and related tumors: A clinicopathologic analysis of 98 cases. Lab Invest 54:50A, 1986.

118. Stone GC, Bell DA, Fuller A, et al: Malignant schwannoma of the ovary: Report of a case. Cancer 58:1575–1582, 1986.

119. Anderson B, Turner DA, Benda J: Ovarian sarcoma. Gynecol Oncol 26:183–192, 1987.

120. Chan YF, Leung CS, Ma L: Primary embryonal rhabdomyosarcoma of the ovary in a 4-year-old girl. Histopathology 15:308–311, 1989.

121. Patel T, Ohri SK, Sundaresan M, et al: Metastatic angiosarcoma of the ovary. Eur J Surg Oncol 17:295–299, 1991.

122. Sakata H, Hirahara T, Ryu A, et al: Primary osteosarcoma of the ovary: A case report. Acta Pathol Jpn 41:311–317, 1991.

123. Friedman HD, Mazur MT: Primary ovarian leiomyosarcoma: An immunohistochemical and ultrastructural study. Arch Pathol Lab Med 115:941–945, 1991.

124. Nogales FF, Ayala A, Ruiz-Avila I, Sirvent JJ: Myxoid leiomyosarcoma of the ovary: Analysis of three cases. Hum Pathol 22:1268–1273, 1991.

125. Akhtar M, Bakri Y, Rank F: Dysgerminoma of the ovary with rhabdomyosarcoma: Report of a case. Cancer 64:2309–2312, 1989.

126. Prat J, Scully RE: Cellular fibromas and fibrosarcomas of the ovary: A comparative clinicopathologic analysis of seventeen cases. Cancer 47:2663–2670, 1981.

127. Saitoh A, Tsutsumi Y, Osamura RY, Watanabe K: Sclerosing stromal tumor of the ovary: Immunohistochemical and electron-microscopic demonstration of smooth-muscle differentiation. Arch Pathol Lab Med 113:372–376, 1989.

128. Prayson RA, Hart WR: Primary smooth-muscle tumors of the ovary: A clinicopathologic study of four leiomyomas and two mitotically active leiomyomas. Arch Pathol Lab Med 116:1068–1071, 1992.

129. Prayson RA, Hart WR: Mitotically active leiomyomas of the uterus. Am J Clin Pathol 97:14–20, 1992.

130. Young RH, Prat J, Scully RE: Endometrioid stromal sarcomas of the ovary. A clinicopathologic analysis of 23 cases. Cancer 53:1143–1155, 1984.

131. Ongkasuwan C, Taylor JE, Tang C-K, Prempree T: Angiosarcoma of the uterus and ovary. Cancer 49:1469–1475, 1982.

132. Madison JF, Cooper PH: A histiocytoid (epithelioid) vascular tumor of the ovary: Occurrence within a benign cystic teratoma. Mod Pathol 2:55–58, 1989.

133. Hirakawa T, Tsuneyoshi M, Enjoji M, Shigyo R: Ovarian sarcoma with histologic features of telangiectatic osteosarcoma of the bone. Am J Surg Pathol 12:567–572, 1988.

134. Nunez C, Abboud SL, Lemon NC, Kemp JA: Ovarian rhabdomyosarcoma presenting as leukemia. Cancer 52:297–300, 1983.

135. Prat J, Scully RE: Sarcomas in ovarian mucinous tumors. A report of two cases. Cancer 44:1327–1331, 1979.

136. Prat J, Scully RE: Ovarian mucinous tumors with sarcoma-like mural nodules. A report of seven cases. Cancer 44:1332–1344, 1979.

137. Prat J, Young RH, Scully RE: Ovarian mucinous tumors with foci of anaplastic carcinoma. Cancer 50:300–304, 1982.

138. deNictolis M, diLoreto C, Cinti S, Prat J: Fibrosarcomatous mural nodule in an ovarian mucinous cystadenoma. Report of a case. Surg Pathol 3:309–315, 1990.

139. deRosa G, Donofrio V, deRosa N, et al: Ovarian serous tumor with mural nodules of carcinomatous derivation (sarcomatoid carcinoma): Report of a case. Int J Gynecol Pathol 10:311–318, 1991.

140. Bruijn JA, Smit VT, Que DG, Fleuren GJ: Immunohistology of a sarcomatous mural nodule in an ovarian mucinous cystadenocarcinoma. Int J Gynecol Pathol 6:287–293, 1987.

141. Czernobilsky B, Dgani R, Roth LM: Ovarian mucinous cystadenocarcinoma with mural nodule of carcinomatous derivation: A light and electron microscopic study. Cancer 51:141–148, 1983.

142. Kessler E, Halpern M, Koren R, et al: Sarcoma-like mural nodules with foci of anaplastic carcinoma in ovarian mucinous tumor: Clinical, histological, and immunohistochemical study of a case and review of the literature. Surg Pathol 3:211–219, 1990.

143. Sondergaard G, Kasperson P: Ovarian and extraovarian mucinous tumors with solid mural nodules. Int J Gynecol Pathol 10:145–155, 1991.

144. Matias-Guiu X, Aranda I, Prat J: Immunohistochemical study of sarcoma-like mural nodules in a mucinous cystadenocarcinoma of the ovary. Virchows Archiv A Pathol Anat 419:89–92, 1991.

145. Nichols GE, Mills SE, Ulbright TM, et al: Spindle cell mural nodules in cystic ovarian mucinous tumors: A clinicopathologic and immunohistochemical study of five cases. Am J Surg Pathol 15:1055–1062, 1991.

146. Suurmeijer AJH: Carcinosarcoma-like mural nodule in an ovarian mucinous tumor. Histopathology 18:268–271, 1991.

147. Goldman RL, Weidner N: Pure squamous cell carcinoma of the larynx with cervical nodal metastasis showing rhabdomyosarcomatous differentiation: Clinical, pathologic and immunohistochemical study of a unique example of divergent differentiation. Am J Surg Pathol 17:415–421, 1993.

148. Tsujimura T, Kawano K: Rhabdomyosarcoma coexistent with ovarian mucinous cystadenocarcinoma: A case report. Int J Gynecol Pathol 11:58–62, 1992.

149. Allen C, Stephens M, Williams J: Combined high grade sarcoma and serous ovarian neoplasm. J Clin Pathol 45:263–264, 1992.

150. Sahin A, Benda JA: Primary ovarian Wilms' tumor. Cancer 61:1460–1463, 1988.

151. O'Dowd J, Ismail SM: Juvenile granulosa cell tumour of the ovary containing a nodule of Wilms' tumour. Histopathology 17:468–470, 1990.

152. Casiraghi O, Martinez-Madrigal F, Mostofi FK, et al: Primary prostatic Wilms' tumor. Am J Surg Pathol 15:885–890, 1991.

153. Eichhorn JH, Scully RE: Ovarian myxoma: Clinicopathologic and immunocytologic analysis of five cases and a review of the literature. Int J Gynecol Pathol 10:156–169, 1991.
154. Roche WR, du Boulay CEHD: A case of ovarian fibromatosis with disseminated intra-abdominal fibromatosis. Histopathology 14:101–107, 1989.
155. Young RH, Scully RE: Alveolar rhabdomyosarcoma metastatic to the ovary: A report of two cases and discussion of the differential diagnosis of small cell malignant tumors of the ovary. Cancer 64:899–904, 1989.
156. Swift R, Jalleh R, Patel A, et al: Chondrosarcoma from a rib metastasizing to the ovary. Acta Orthop Scand 62:76, 1991.
157. Young RH, Scully RE: Sarcomas metastatic to the ovary: A report of 21 cases. Int J Gynecol Pathol 9:231–252, 1991.
158. Young RH, Eichhorn JH, Dickersin GR, Scully RE: Ovarian involvement by the intra-abdominal desmoplastic small round cell tumor with divergent differentiation: A report of three cases. Hum Pathol 23:454–464, 1992.
159. Aguirre P, Scully RE: Malignant neuroectodermal tumor of the ovary, a distinctive form of monodermal teratoma: Report of five cases. Am J Surg Pathol 6:283–292, 1982.
160. Young RH, Scully RE: Malignant melanoma metastatic to the ovary: A clinicopathologic analysis of 20 cases. Am J Surg Pathol 15:849–860, 1991.
161. Hayes MC, Scully RE: Ovarian steroid cell tumors (not otherwise specified): A clinicopathological analysis of 63 cases. Am J Surg Pathol 11:835–845, 1987.
162. Young RH, Gersell DJ, Clement PB, Scully RE: Hepatocellular carcinoma metastatic to the ovary: A report of three cases discovered during life with discussion of the differential diagnosis of hepatoid tumors of the ovary. 23:574–580, 1992.
163. Chang A, Harawi SJ: Oncocytes, oncocytosis, and oncocytic tumors. Pathol Annu 27(pt 1):263–304, 1992.
164. Fitzgibbons PL, Martin SE, Simmons TJ: Malignant melanoma metastatic to the ovary. Am J Surg Pathol 11:959–964, 1987.
165. Chorlton I, Norris HJ, King FM: Malignant reticuloendothelial disease involving the ovary as a primary manifestation: A series of 19 lymphomas and 1 granulocytic sarcoma. Cancer 34:397–407, 1974.
166. Rotmensch J, Woodruff JD: Lymphoma of the ovary: A report of 20 new cases and update of previous series. Am J Obstet Gynecol 143:870–875, 1982.
167. Osborne BM, Robboy SJ: Lymphomas or leukemia presenting as ovarian tumors: An analysis of 42 cases. Cancer 52:1933–1943, 1983.
168. Fox H, Langley FA, Goran ADT, et al: Malignant lymphoma presenting as an ovarian tumour: a clinicopathological analysis of 34 cases. Br J Obstet Gynaecol 95:386–390, 1988.
169. Linden MD, Tubbs RR, Fishleder AJ, Hart WR: Immunotypic and genotypic characterization of non-Hodgkin's lymphomas of the ovary. Am J Clin Pathol 89:156–162, 1988.
170. Ferry JA, Young RH: Malignant lymphoma, pseudolymphoma, and hematopoietic disorders of the female genital tract. Pathol Annu 26:227–263, 1991.
171. Monterroso V, Jaffe ES, Merino MJ, Medeiros LJ: Malignant lymphomas involving the ovary: A clinicopathologic analysis of 39 cases. Am J Surg Pathol 17:154–170, 1993.
172. Harris NL, Jaffee ES, Stein H, et al: A revised European-American classification of lymphoid neoplasms: A proposal from the International Lymphoma Study Group. Blood 84:1361–1392, 1994.
173. Yamamoto K, Akiyama H, Maruyama T, et al: Granulocytic sarcoma of the ovary in patients with acute myelogenous leukemia. Am J Hematol 38:223–225, 1991.
174. Magliocco AM, Demetrick DJ, Jones AR, Kossakowska AE: Granulocytic sarcoma of the ovary: An unusual case presentation. Arch Pathol Lab Med 115:830–834, 1991.
175. Pressler H, Horny H-P, Wolf A, Kaiserling E: Isolated granulocytic sarcoma of the ovary: Histologic, electron microscopic, and immunohistochemical findings. Int J Gynecol Pathol 11:68–74, 1992.
176. Cook HT, Boylston AW: Plasmacytoma of the ovary. Gynecol Oncol 29:378–381, 1988.
177. Seifer DB, Weiss LM, Kempson RL: Malignant lymphoma arising within thyroid tissue in a mature cystic teratoma. Cancer 58:2459–2461, 1986.
178. Skodras G, Fields V, Kragel PJ: Ovarian lymphoma and serous carcinoma of low malignant potential arising in the same ovary. A case report with literature review of 14 primary ovarian lymphomas. Arch Pathol Lab Med 118:647–650, 1994.
179. Dickersin GR, Kline IW, Scully RE: Small cell carcinoma of the ovary with hypercalcemia: A report of eleven cases. Cancer 49:188–197, 1982.
180. Ulbright TM, Roth LM, Stehman FB, et al: Poorly differentiated (small cell) carcinoma of the ovary in young women: Evidence supporting a germ cell origin. Hum Pathol 18:175–184, 1987.
181. Young RH, Oliva E, Scully RE: Small cell carcinoma of the ovary, hypercalcemic type. A clinicopathological analysis of 150 cases. Am J Surg Pathol 18:1102–1116, 1994.
182. Dickersin GR, Scully RE: An update on the electron microscopy of small cell carcinoma of the ovary with hypercalcemia. Ultrastruct Pathol 17:411–422, 1993.
183. Aguirre P, Thor AD, Scully RE: Ovarian small cell carcinoma: Histogenetic considerations based on immunohistochemical and other findings. Am J Clin Pathol 92:140–149, 1989.
184. Jensen ML, Rasmussen KL, Jacobsen M: Ovarian small cell carcinoma: A case report with histologic, immunohistochemical and ultrastructural findings. APMIS 23(suppl):126–131, 1991.
185. Eichhorn JH, Bell DA, Young RH, et al: DNA content and proliferative activity in ovarian small cell carcinomas of the hypercalcemic type: Implications for diagnosis, prognosis, and histogenesis. Am J Clin Pathol 98:579–586, 1992.

186. Eichhorn JH, Young RH, Scully RE: Primary ovarian small cell carcinoma of pulmonary type: A clinicopathologic, immunohistologic, and flow cytometric analysis of 11 cases. Am J Surg Pathol 16:926–938, 1992.
187. Young RH: Ovarian tumors other than those of surface epithelial-stromal type. Hum Pathol 22:763–775, 1991.
188. Young RH, Scully RE: Ovarian metastases from cancer of the lung: Problems in interpretation. Gynecol Oncol 21:337–350, 1985.
189. Young RH, Gersell DJ, Roth LM, Scully RE: Ovarian metastases from cervical carcinomas other than pure adenocarcinomas: A report of 12 cases. Cancer 71:407–418, 1993.
190. Eichhorn JH, Young RH, Scully RE: Nonpulmonary small cell carcinomas of extragenital origin metastatic to the ovary. Cancer 71:177–186, 1993.
191. Lack EE, Young RE, Scully RE: Pathology of ovarian neoplasms in childhood and adolescence. Pathol Annu 127(pt 2):281–356, 1992.
192. Young RH, Kozakewich HP, Scully RE: Metastatic ovarian tumors in children: A report of 14 cases and a review of the literature. Int J Gynecol Pathol 12:8–19, 1993.
193. Silva EG, Tornos C, Bailey MA, Morris M: Undifferentiated carcinoma of the ovary. Arch Pathol Lab Med 115:377–381, 1991.
194. Young RH, Dickersin GR, Scully RE: Juvenile granulosa cell tumor of the ovary: A clinicopathological analysis of 125 cases. Am J Surg Pathol 8:575–596, 1984.
195. Abbot RL, Barlogie B, Schmidt WA: Metastasizing malignant juxtaovarian tumor with terminal hypercalcemia: A case report. Cancer 48:860–865, 1981.
196. Tanaka Y, Sasaki Y, Nishihira H, et al: Ovarian juvenile granulosa cell tumor associated with Maffucci's syndrome. Am J Clin Pathol 97:523–527, 1992.
197. Young RH, Lawrence WD, Scully RE: Juvenile granulosa cell tumor—another neoplasm associated with abnormal chromosomes and ambiguous genitalia. A report of three cases. Am J Surg Pathol 9:737–743, 1985.
198. Zaloudek C, Norris HJ: Granulosa tumors of the ovary in children: A clinical and pathologic study of 32 cases. Am J Surg Pathol 6:513–522, 1982.
199. Biscotti CV, Hart WR: Juvenile granulosa cell tumors of the ovary. Arch Pathol Lab Med 113:40–46, 1989.
200. Swanson SA, Norris HJ, Kelsten ML, Wheeler JE: DNA content of juvenile granulosa tumors determined by flow cytometry. Int J Gynecol Pathol 9:101–109, 1990.
201. Young RH, Scully RE: Ovarian sex cord-stromal tumors with bizarre nuclei. A clinicopathologic analysis of seventeen cases. Int J Gynecol Pathol 1:325–335, 1983.
202. Lack EE, Periz-Atayde AR, Murthy ASK, et al: Granulosa theca cell tumors in premenarchal girls. Cancer 48:1846–1854, 1981.
203. Young RH, Dudley AG, Scully RE: Granulosa cell, Sertoli-Leydig cell, and unclassified sex cord-stromal tumors associated with pregnancy: A clinicopathological analysis of thirty-six cases. Gynecol Oncol 18:181–205, 1984.
204. Otis CN, Powell JL, Barbuto D, Carcangiu ML: Intermediate filament proteins in adult granulosa-cell tumors. An immunohistochemical study of 25 cases. Am J Surg Pathol 16:962–968, 1992.
205. Al-Nafussi AI, Hughes DE, Williams ARW: Hyaline globules in ovarian tumours. Histopathology 23:563–566, 1993.
206. Young RH, Scully RE: Ovarian tumors of probable Wolffian origin. A report of 11 cases. Am J Surg Pathol 7:125–135, 1983.
207. Kariminejad MH, Scully RE: Female adnexal tumor of probable Wolffian origin. A distinctive pathologic entity. Cancer 31:671–677, 1973.
208. Daya D, Young RH, Scully RE: Endometrioid carcinoma of the fallopian tube resembling an adnexal tumor of probable Wolffian origin: A report of six cases. Int J Gynecol Pathol 11:122–130, 1992.
209. Lacson AG, Gillis DA, Shawwa A: Malignant mixed germ cell-sex cord-stromal tumors of the ovary associated with isosexual precocious puberty. Cancer 61:2122–2133, 1988.
210. Young RH, Dickersin GR, Scully RE: A distinctive ovarian sex cord-stromal tumor causing sexual precocity n the Peutz-Jeghers syndrome. Am J Surg Pathol 7:233–243, 1983.
211. Zaloudek C, Norris HJ: Sertoli-Leydig tumors of the ovary. A clinicopathologic study of 64 intermediate and poorly differentiated neoplasms. Am J Surg Pathol 8:405–418, 1984.
212. Prat J, Young RH, Scully RE: Ovarian Sertoli-Leydig cell tumors with heterologous elements. II. Cartilage and skeletal muscle: A clinicopathologic analysis of twelve cases. Cancer 50:2465–2475, 1982.
213. Roth LM, Slayton RE, Brady LW, et al: Retiform differentiation in ovarian Sertoli-Leydig cell tumors. A clinicopathologic study of six cases from a gynecologic oncology group study. Cancer 55:1093–1098, 1985.
214. Roth LM, Anderson MC, Govan ADT, et al: Sertoli-Leydig cell tumors: A clinicopathologic study of 34 cases. Cancer 48:187–197, 1981.
215. Young RH, Scully RE: Ovarian Sertoli-Leydig cell tumors. A clinicopathologic analysis of 207 cases. Am J Surg Pathol 9:543–569, 1985.
216. Young RH, Scully RE: Ovarian Sertoli-Leydig cell tumors with a retiform pattern: A problem in histopathologic diagnosis. A report of 25 cases. Am J Surg Pathol 7:755–771, 1983.
217. Young RH, Prat J, Scully RE: Ovarian Sertoli-Leydig cell tumors with heterologous elements. I. Gastrointestinal epithelium and carcinoid: A clinicopathologic analysis of thirty-six cases. Cancer 50:2448–2456, 1982.
218. Talerman A: Ovarian Sertoli-Leydig cell tumor (androblastoma) with retiform pattern. Cancer 60:3056–3064, 1987.
219. Gagnon S, Tetu B, Silva E, McCaughey WTE: Frequency of alpha-fetoprotein production by Sertoli-Leydig cell tumors of the ovary. An immunohistochemical study in eight cases. Mod Pathol 2:63–67, 1989.

220. Higuchi Y, Kouno T, Teshima H, et al: Serous papillary cystadenocarcinoma associated with alpha-fetoprotein production. Arch Pathol Lab Med 108:710–712, 1984.
221. Young RH, Prat J, Scully RE: Ovarian endometrioid carcinomas resembling sex cord-stromal tumors. A clinicopathologic analysis of 13 cases. Am J Surg Pathol 6:513–522, 1982.
222. Hart WR, Kumar N, Crissman JD: Ovarian neoplasms resembling sex-cord tumors with annular tubules. Cancer 45:2352–2363, 1980.
223. Young RH, Welch WR, Dickersin GR, Scully RE: Ovarian sex cord tumor with annular tubules. Cancer 50:1384–1402, 1982.
224. Clement PB, Young RH, Scully RE: Ovarian granulosa cell proliferations of pregnancy: A report of nine cases. Hum Pathol 19:657–662, 1988.
225. Scully RE: Gonadoblastoma. A review of 74 cases. Cancer 25:1340–1356, 1970.
226. Zuntova A, Motlik K, Horejsi J, Eckschlager T: Mixed germ cell-sex cord stromal tumor with heterologous structures. Int J Gynecol Pathol 11:227–233, 1992.
227. Tavassoli FA: A combined germ cell-gonadal stromal-epithelial tumor of the ovary. Am J Surg Pathol 7:73–84, 1983.
228. Korzets A, Nouriel H, Steiner Z, et al: Resistant hypertension associated with a renin-producing ovarian Sertoli-cell tumor. Am J Clin Pathol 85:242–247, 1986.
229. Ferry JA, Young RH, Engel G, Scully RE: Oxyphilic Sertoli-cell tumor of the ovary: A report of three cases, two in patients with the Peutz-Jeghers syndrome. Int J Gynecol Pathol 13:259–266, 1994.
230. Schiller W: Mesonephroma ovarii. Am J Cancer 35:1–21, 1939.
231. Schiller W: Histogenesis of ovarian mesonephroma. Arch Pathol 33:443–451, 1942.
232. Teilum G: Mesonephroma ovarii (Schiller): An extra-embryonic mesoblastoma of germ cell origin in the ovary and testis. Acta Pathol Microbiol Scand 27:249–261, 1950.
233. Teilum G: Classification of endodermal sinus tumour (mesoblastoma vitellinum) and so-called "embryonal carcinoma" of the ovary. Acta Pathol Microbiol Scand 64:407–429, 1965.
234. Scully RE, Barlow JF: "Mesonephroma" of the ovary: Tumor of müllerian nature related to endometrioid carcinoma. Cancer 20:1405–1417, 1967.
235. Kurman RJ, Craig JM: Endometrioid and clear cell carcinoma of the ovary. Cancer 29:1653–1664, 1972.
236. Czernobilsky B, Silverman BB, Enterline HT: Clear cell carcinoma of the ovary: A clinicopathologic analysis of pure and mixed forms and comparison with endometrioid carcinoma. Cancer 25:762–772, 1970.
237. Sherchuk MM, Winkler-Monsanto B, Fenoglio CM, Richart RM: Clear cell carcinoma of the ovary: A clinicopathologic study with review of the literature. Cancer 47:1344–1351, 1981.
238. Montag AG, Jenison EL, Griffiths CT, et al: Ovarian clear cell carcinoma: A clinicopathologic analysis of 44 cases. Int J Gynecol Pathol 8:85–96, 1989.
239. Young RH, Scully RE: Oxyphilic clear cell carcinoma of the ovary: A report of nine cases. Am J Surg Pathol 11:661–667, 1987.
240. Bell DA, Scully RE: Benign and borderline clear-cell adenofibromas of the ovary. Cancer 56:2922–2931, 1985.
241. Roth LM, Langley FA, Fox H, et al: Ovarian clear cell adenofibromatous tumors. Benign, of low-grade malignant potential, and associated with invasive clear cell carcinoma. Cancer 53:1156–1163, 1984.
242. Kao GF, Norris HJ: Unusual cystadenofibromas: Endometrioid, mucinous, and clear cell types. Obstet Gynecol 54:729–736, 1979.
243. Bell DA: Ovarian surface epithelial-stromal tumors. Hum Pathol 22:750–762, 1991.
244. Klemi PJ, Meurman L, Gronroos M, Talerman A: Clear cell (mesonephroid) tumors of the ovary with characteristics resembling endodermal sinus tumor. Int J Gynecol Pathol 1:95–100, 1982.
245. Zirker TA, Silva EG, Morris M, Ordonez N: Immunohistochemical differentiation of clear cell carcinoma of the female genital tract and endodermal sinus tumor with the use of alpha-fetoprotein and Leu-M1. Am J Clin Pathol 91:511–514, 1989.
246. Michael H, Ulbright TM, Brodhecker CA: The pluripotential nature of the mesenchyme-like component of yolk sac tumor. Arch Pathol Lab Med 113:1115–1119, 1989.
247. Young RH, Hart WR: Renal cell carcinoma metastatic to the ovary: A report of three cases emphasizing possible confusion with ovarian clear cell carcinoma. Int J Gynecol Pathol 11:96–104, 1992.
248. Parsons MA, Harris SC, Longstaff AJ, Grainger RG: Xanthogranulomatous pyelonephritis: A pathological, clinical and aetiological analysis of 87 cases. Diagn Histopathol 6:203–219, 1983.
249. Bell DA: Mucinous adenofibroma of the ovary. A report of 10 cases. Am J Surg Pathol 15:27–232, 1991.
250. Bell DA, Scully RE: Atypical and borderline endometrioid adenofibromas of the ovary. A report of 27 cases. Am J Surg Pathol 9:205–214, 1985.
251. Snyder RR, Norris HJ, Tavassoli F: Endometrioid proliferative and low-malignant potential tumors of the ovary. A clinicopathologic study of 46 cases. Am J Surg Pathol 12:661–671, 1988.
252. Roth LM, Czernobilsky B, Langley FA: Ovarian endometrioid adenofibromatous and cystadenofibromatous tumors: Benign, proliferating, and malignant. Cancer 48:1838–1845, 1981.
253. Gershenson DM, Del Junco G, Herson J, Rutledge FN: Endodermal sinus tumor of the ovary: The MD Anderson experience. Obstet Gynecol 61:194–202, 1983.
254. Gonzalez-Crussi F, Roth LM: The human yolk sac and yolk sac carcinoma. Hum Pathol 7:675–691, 1976.

255. Kurman RJ, Norris HJ: Endodermal sinus tumor of the ovary. A clinical and pathologic analysis of 71 cases. Cancer 38:2404–2419, 1976.
256. Takashina T, Kanda Y, Hayakawa O, et al: Yolk sac tumors of the ovary and the human yolk sac. Am J Obstet Gynecol 156:223–229, 1987.
257. Ulbright TM, Roth LM, Brodhecker CA: Yolk sac differentiation in germ-cell tumors. A morphologic study of 50 cases with emphasis on hepatic, enteric, and parietal yolk sac features. Am J Surg Pathol 11:151–164, 1986.
258. Damjanov I, Amenta PS, Zarghami F: Transformation of an AFP-positive yolk sac carcinoma into an AFP-negative neoplasm. Evidence for in vivo cloning of the human parietal yolk sac carcinoma. Cancer 53:1902–1907, 1984.
259. Cohen MB, Mulchahey KM, Molnar JJ: Ovarian endodermal sinus tumor with intestinal differentiation. Cancer 57:1580–1583, 1986.
260. Stewart KR, Casey MJ, Condos B: Endodermal sinus tumor of the ovary with virilization. Light and electron microscopic study. Am J Surg Pathol 5:385–391, 1981.
261. Sasaki H, Furusato M, Teshima S, et al: Prognostic significance of histopathological subtypes in stage 1 pure yolk sac tumor of the ovary. Br J Cancer 69:529–536, 1994.
262. Clement PB, Young RH, Scully RE: Endometrioid-like variant of ovarian yolk sac tumor. A clinicopathologic analysis of eight cases. Am J Surg Pathol 11:767–778, 1987.
263. Nakashima N, Solbue M, Fukata S, et al: Immunohistochemical characterization of extracellular matrix components of yolk sac tumors. Virchows Arch B Cell Pathol 58:309–315, 1990.
264. Niehans GA, Manivel JC, Copland GT, et al: Immunohistochemistry of germ cell and trophoblastic neoplasms. Cancer 62:1113–1123, 1988.
265. Nogales FF, Ruiz Avila I, Concha A, del Moral E: Immature endodermal teratoma of the ovary: Embryologic correlations and immunohistochemistry. Hum Pathol 24:364–370, 1993.
266. Prat J, Bhan AK, Dickersin GR, et al: Hepatoid yolk sac tumor of the ovary (endodermal sinus tumor with hepatoid differentiation): A light microscopic, ultrastructural and immunohistochemical study of seven cases. Cancer 50:2355–2368, 1982.
267. Nakashima N, Fukatsu T, Nagasaka T, et al: The frequency and histology of hepatic tissue in germ cell tumors. Am J Surg Pathol 11:682–692, 1987.
268. Prat J, Matias-Guiu X, Scully RE: Hepatic yolk sac differentiation in an ovarian polyembryoma. Surg Pathol 2:147–150, 1989.
269. Ishikura H, Scully RE: Hepatoid carcinoma of the ovary: A newly described tumor. Cancer 60:2775–2784, 1987.
270. deLorimier A, Park F, Aranha GV, Reyes C: Hepatoid carcinoma of the stomach. Cancer 71:293–296, 1993.
271. Gardiner GW, Lajoie G, Keith R: Hepatoid adenocarcinoma of the papilla of Vater. Histopathology 20:541–544, 1992.
272. Hruban RH, Molina JM, Reddy MN, Boitnott JK: A neoplasm with pancreatic and hepatocellular differentiation presenting with subcutaneous fat necrosis. Am J Clin Pathol 88:639–645, 1987.
273. Ishikura H, Ishiguro T, Enatsu C, et al: Hepatoid adenocarcinoma of the renal pelvis producing alpha-fetoprotein of hepatic type and bile pigment. Cancer 67:3051–3056, 1991.
274. Ishikura H, Kanda M, Ito M, et al: Hepatoid adenocarcinoma: A distinctive histologic subtype of alpha-fetoprotein-producing lung carcinoma. Virchows Arch [A] 417:73–80, 1990.
274a. Pitman MB, Young RH, Clement PB, et al: Endometrioid carcinoma of the ovary and endometrium, oxyphilic cell type: A report of nine cases. Int J Gynecol Pathol 13:290–301, 1994.
275. Young RH, Perez-Atayde AR, Scully RE: Ovarian Sertoli-Leydig cell tumor with retiform and heterologous components: Report of a case with hepatocytic differentiation and elevated serum alpha-fetoprotein. Am J Surg Pathol 8:709–718, 1984.
276. Nogales FF, Concha A, Plata C, Ruiz-Avila I: Granulosa cell tumor of the ovary with diffuse true hepatic differentiation simulating stromal luteinization. Am J Surg Pathol 17:85–90, 1993.
277. Scully RE: Tumors of the ovary and maldeveloped gonads. In Atlas of Tumor Pathology, second series, fascicle 16. Washington, DC, Armed Forces Institute of Pathology, 1979, p 215.
278. Hayes MC, Scully RE: Stromal luteoma of the ovary: A clinicopathologic analysis of 25 cases. Int J Gynecol Pathol 6:313–321, 1987.
279. Paraskevas M, Scully RE: Hilus cell tumor of the ovary: A clinicopathological analysis of 12 Reinke crystal-positive and nine crystal-negative cases. Int J Gynecol Pathol 8:299–310, 1989.
280. Zhang J, Young RH, Arseneau J, Scully RE: Ovarian stromal tumors containing lutein or Leydig cells (luteinized thecomas and stromal Leydig cell tumors): A clinicopathologic analysis of 50 cases. Int J Gynecol Pathol 1:275–285, 1982.
281. Norris HJ, Taylor HB: Nodular theca-lutein hyperplasia of pregnancy (so-called "pregnancy luteoma"). Am J Clin Pathol 47:557–566, 1967.
282. Clement PB: Tumor-like lesions of the ovary associated with pregnancy. Int J Gnecol Pathol 12:108–115, 1993.
283. Woodruff JD, Rauh JT, Markley RI: Ovarian struma. Obstet Gynecol 27:194–201, 1966.
284. Hasleton PS, Kelehan P, Whittaker JS, et al: Benign and malignant struma ovarii. Arch Pathol Lab Med 102:180–184, 1978.
285. Kempers RD, Dockerty MB, Hoffman DL, Bartholomew LG: Struma ovarii—ascitic, hyperthyroid, and asymptomatic syndromes. Ann Intern Med 72:883–893, 1970.

286. Blackwell WJ, Dockerty MB, Mason JC, Mussey RD: Dermatoid cysts of the ovary: Their clinical and pathologic significance. Am J Obstet Gynecol 51:151–172, 1946.
287. Pardo-Mindan FJ, Vazquez JJ: Malignant struma ovarii. Light and electron microscopic study. Cancer 51:337–343, 1983.
288. Beck RP, Latour JPA: Review of 1,019 benign ovarian neoplasms. Obstet Gynecol 16:479–482, 1960.
289. McGoldrick IA: Three rare ovarian tumors: Krukenberg, struma ovarii, and granulosa cell neoplasms. P N G Med J 24:121–126, 1981.
290. Robboy SJ, Scully RE: Strumal carcinoid of the ovary: An analysis of 50 cases of a distinct tumor composed of thyroid tissue and carcinoid. Cancer 46:2019–2034, 1980.
291. Cooper DS, Ridgway EC, Maloof F: Unusual types of hyperthyroidism. Clin Endocrinol Metab 7:199–220, 1978.
292. Scully RE: Ovarian tumors. A review. Am J Pathol 87:686–719, 1977.
293. Adcock LL: Unusual manifestations of benign cystic teratomas. Obstet Gynecol Surv 27:471–474, 1972.
294. Ulbright TM, Roth LM, Ehrlich CE: Ovarian strumal carcinoid. An immunocytochemical and ultrastructural study of two cases. Am J Clin Pathol 77:622–631, 1982.
295. Yeh E, Meade RC, Ruetz PP: Radionuclide study of struma ovarii. J Nucl Med 14:118–121, 1973.
296. Nodine JH, Maldia G: Pseudostruma ovarii. Obstet Gynecol 17:460–463, 1961.
297. Yannopoulis D, Yannopoulis K, Ossowski R: Malignant struma ovarii. In Sommers SC (ed): Pathology Annual. New York, Appleton-Century-Crofts, 1976, pp 403–413.
298. Scully RE: Monodermal and highly specialized teratomas. In Tumors of the Ovary and Maldeveloped Gonads. Washington, DC, Armed Forces Institute of Pathology, 1979, pp 269–285.
299. Devaney K, Snyder R, Norris HJ, Tavassoli FA: Proliferative and histologically malignant struma ovarii: A clinicopathologic study of 54 cases. Int J Gynecol Pathol 12:333–343, 1993.
300. Young RH: New and unusual aspects of ovarian germ cell tumors. Am J Surg Pathol 17:1210–1224, 1993.
301. Szyfelbein WM, Young RH, Scully RE: Cystic struma ovarii: A frequently unrecognized tumor. A report of 20 cases. Am J Surg Pathol 18:785–788, 1994.
302. Scully RE: Case records of the Massachusetts General Hospital case 13-1970. N Engl J Med 282:676–682, 1970.
303. Emge LA: Functional and growth characteristics of struma ovarii. Am J Obstet Gynecol 40:738–739, 1940.
304. Smith FG: Pathology and physiology of struma ovarii. Arch Surg 53:603–626, 1946.
305. Greco MA, LiVolsi VA, Pertschuk LP, Bigelow B: Strumal carcinoid of the ovary. An analysis of its components. Cancer 43:1380–1388, 1979.
306. Ranchod M, Kempson RL, Dorgeloh JR: Strumal carcinoid of the ovary. Cancer 37:1913–1922, 1976.
306a. Szyfelbein WM, Young RH, Scully RE: Struma ovarii simulating ovarian tumors of other types. A report of 30 cases. Am J Surg Pathol 19:21–29, 1995.
307. Peterson, WF: Malignant degeneration of benign cystic teratomas of the ovary: A collective review of the literature. Obstet Gynecol Surv 12:793–830, 1957.
308. Kelly RR, Scully RE: Cancer developing in dermoid cysts of the ovary: A report of 8 cases including a carcinoid and a leiomyosarcoma. Cancer 14:989–1000, 1961.
309. Climie ARW, Heath LP: Malignant degeneration of benign cystic teratomas of the ovary: Review of the literature and report of a chondrosarcoma and carcinoid tumor. Cancer 22:824–832, 1968.
310. Stamp GWH, McConnell EM: Malignancy arising in cystic ovarian teratomas: A report of 24 cases. Br J Obstet Gynaecol 90:671–675, 1983.
311. Chadha S, Schaberg A: Malignant transformation in benign cystic teratomas: Dermoids of the ovary. Eur J Obstet Gynecol Reprod Biol 29:329–338, 1988.
312. Hirakawa T, Tsuneyoshi M, Enjoji M.: Squamous cell carcinoma arising in mature cystic teratoma of the ovary: Clinicopathologic and topographic analysis. Am J Surg Pathol 13:397–405, 1989.
313. Ribeiro G, Hughesdon P, Wiltshaw E: Squamous carcinoma arising in dermoid cyst and associated with hypercalcemia: A clinicopathologic study of six cases. Gynecol Oncol 29:222–230, 1988.
314. Tobon H, Surti U, Naus GJ, et al: Squamous cell carcinoma in situ arising in an ovarian mature cystic teratoma: Report of one case with histopathologic, cytogenetic, and floor cytometric DNA content analysis. Arch Pathol Lab Med 115:172–174, 1991.
315. Chen KTK: Squamous cell carcinoma of the ovary [letter]. Arch Pathol Lab Med 112:114–115, 1988.
316. Randall BJ, Richie C, Hutchison RS: Paget's disease and invasive undifferentiated carcinoma occurring in a mature cystic teratoma of the ovary. Histopathology 18:469–470, 1991.
317. Shimizu S-I, Kobayashi H, Suchi T, et al: Extramammary Paget's disease arising in mature cystic teratoma of the ovary. Am J Surg Pathol 15:1002–1006, 1991.
318. Chumas JC, Scully RE: Sebaceous tumors arising in ovarian dermoid cysts. Int J Gynecol Pathol 10:356–363, 1991.
319. Ueda Y, Kimura A, Kawahara E, et al: Malignant melanoma arising in a dermoid cyst of the ovary. Cancer 67:3141–3145, 1991.
320. Borup K, Rasmussen KL, Schierup L, Moller JC: Amelanotic malignant melanoma arising in an ovarian dermoid cyst. Acta Obstet Gynecol Scand 71:242–244, 1992.
321. Escoffery CT, Kulkarni SK: An unusual malignancy arising in a benign cystic teratoma of the ovary. Aust N`Z J Obstet Gynecol 29:85–87, 1989.

322. Chang DHC, Hsueh S, Soong Y-K: Small cell carcinoma with neurosecretory granules arising in an ovarian dermoid cyst. Gynecol Oncol 46:246–250, 1992.
323. Reid H, van der Walt JD, Fox H: Neuroblastoma arising in a mature cystic teratoma of the ovary. J Clin Pathol 36:68–73, 1983.
324. Shirley RL, Piro AJ, Crocker DW: Malignant neural elements in a benign cystic teratoma: A case report. Obstet Gynecol 37:402–407, 1971.
325. Olah KS, Needham PG, Jones B: Multiple neuroectodermal tumors arising in a mature cystic teratoma of the ovary: Case report. Gynecol Oncol 34:222–225, 1989.
326. Ueda G, Sato Y, Yamasaki M: Malignant fibrous histiocytoma arising in a benign cystic teratoma of the ovary. Gynecol Oncol 5:313–322, 1977.
327. Ngwalle KE, Hirakawa T, Tsuneyoshi M, Enjoji M: Osteosarcoma arising in a benign dermoid cyst of the ovary. Gynecol Oncol 37:143–147, 1990.
328. Ober WB: History of the Brenner tumor of the ovary. Pathol Annu 14:107–124, 1979.
329. Shevchuk MM, Fenoglio CM, Richart RM: Histogenesis of Brenner tumors, I: Histology and ultrastructure. Cancer 46:2607–2616, 1980.
330. Shevchuk MM, Fenoglio CM, Richart RM: Histogenesis of Brenner tumors, II: Histochemistry and CEA. Cancer 46:2617–2622, 1980.
331. Roth LM, Dallenbach-Hellweg G, Czernobilsky B: Ovarian Brenner tumors: I. Metaplastic, proliferating, and of low malignant potential. Cancer 56:582–591, 1985.
332. Roth LM, Czernobilsky B: Ovarian Brenner tumors: II. Malignant. Cancer 56:592–601, 1985.
333. Santini D, Gelli MC, Mazzoleni G, et al: Brenner tumor of the ovary: A correlative histologic, histochemical, immunohistochemical, and ultrastructural investigation. Hum Pathol 20:787–795, 1989.
334. Martin AR, Kotylo PK, Kennedy JC, et al: Flow cytometric DNA analysis of ovarian Brenner tumors and transitional cell carcinomas. Int J Gynecol Pathol 11:188–196, 1992.
335. Austin RM, Norris HJ: Malignant Brenner tumor and transitional cell carcinoma of the ovary: A comparison. Int J Gynecol Pathol 6:29–39, 1987.
336. Robey SS, Silva EG, Gershenson DM, et al: Transitional cell carcinoma in high-grade, high-stage ovarian carcinoma: An indicator of favorable response to chemotherapy. Cancer 63:839–847, 1989.
337. Silva EG, Robey-Cafferty SS, Smith TL, Gershenson DM: Ovarian carcinomas with transitional cell carcinoma pattern. Am J Clin Pathol 93:457–465, 1990.
338. Gersell DJ: Primary ovarian transitional cell carcinoma: Diagnostic and prognostic considerations [editorial]. Am J Clin Pathol 93:586–588, 1990.
339. Young RH, Scully RE: Urothelial and ovarian carcinomas of identical cell types: Problems in interpretation: A report of three cases and review of the literature. Int J Gynecol Pathol 7:197–211, 1988.
340. Clement PB, Young RH, Scully RE: Necrotic pseudoxanthomatous nodules of ovary and peritoneum in endometriosis. Am J Surg Pathol 12:390–397, 1988.
341. Amazon K, Rywlin AM: Ceroid granulomas in a tubo-ovarian cyst. South Med J 73:1067–1069, 1980.
342. Seidman JD, Oberer S, Bitterman P, Aisner S: Pathogenesis of pseudo-xanthomatous salpingiosis. Mod Pathol 6:53–56, 1993.
343. Shalev E, Zuckerman H, Rizescu I: Pelvic inflammatory pseudotumor (xanthogranuloma). Acta Obstet Gynecol Scand 61:285–286, 1982.
344. Pace EH, Voet RL, Melancon JT: Xanthogranulomatous oophoritis: An inflammatory pseudotumor of the ovary. Int J Gynecol Pathol 3:398–402, 1984.
345. Rose G, Morrison EA, Kirkham N, Machling R: Malakoplakia of the pelvic peritoneum in pregnancy. Case report. Br J Obstet Gynaecol 92:170–172, 1985.
346. Chen KTK, Hendricks EJ: Malakoplakia of the female genital tract. Obstet Gynecol 65(suppl):84–87, 1985.
347. Klempner LB, Giglio PG, Niebes A: Malacoplakia of the ovary. Obstet Gynecol 69(pt 2):537–540, 1987.
348. Evans CS, Goldman RL, Klein HZ, Kohout ND: Necrobiotic granulomas of the uterine cervix. A probable post-operative reaction. Am J Surg Pathol 8:841–844, 1984.
349. Manson CM, Cross P, de Sousa B: Post-operative necrotizing granulomas of the thyroid. Histopathology 21:392–393, 1992.
350. Herbold DR, Frable WJ, Kraus FT: Isolated noninfectious granulomas of the ovary. Int J Gynecol Pathol 2:380–391, 1984.
351. Wilson GE, Haboubi NY, McWilliam LJ, Hirsch PJ: Post-operative necrotizing granulomata in the cervix and ovary [letter]. J Clin Pathol 43:1037–1038, 1990.
352. Kernohan NM, Best PV, Jandial V, Kitchener HC: Palisading granuloma of the ovary. Histopathology 19:279–280, 1991.
353. Frost SS, Elstein MP, Latour F, Roth JLA: Crohn's disease of the mouth and ovary. Dig Dis Sci 26:568–571, 1981.
354. Brady K, Yavner DL, Glantz C, Lage JM: Crohn's disease presenting as a tubo-ovarian abscess. A case report. J Reprod Med 33:928–930, 1988.
355. Gilks CB, Clement PB: Colo-ovarian fistula: A report of 2 cases. Obstet Gynecol 69:533–537, 1987.
356. Case Records of the Massachusetts General Hospital: Weekly clinicopathological exercises. Case 13-1988. N Engl J Med 318:835–842, 1988.
357. Janorski NA, Dubrauszky V: Atlas of Gynecologic and Obstetric Diagnostic Histopathology. New York, McGraw-Hill, 1965, pp 308–310.
358. White A, Flaris N, Elmer D, et al: Coexistence of mucinous cystadenoma of the ovary and ovarian sarcoidosis. Am J Obstet Gynecol 162:1284–1285, 1990.
359. Bannatyne P, Russell P, Shearman RP: Autoimmune oophoritis: A clinicopathologic assessment of 12 cases. Int J Gynecol Pathol 9:191–207, 1990.
360. Lonsdale RN, Roberts PF, Trowell JE: Autoimmune oophoritis associated with polycystic ovaries. Histopathology 19:77–81, 1991.

361. Leor J, Levartowsky D, Sharon C: Polyglandular syndrome, Type 2. South Med J 82:374–376, 1989.

362. Parker P, Adcock LL: Pelvic coccidioidomycosis. Obstet Gynecol Surv 36: 225–229, 1981.

363. Bylund DJ, Nanfro JJ, Marsh WL: Coccidioidomycosis of the female genital tract. Arch Pathol Lab Med 110:232–235, 1986.

364. Dawson JML, O'Riordan B, Chopra S: Ovarian actinomycosis presenting as acute peritonitis. Aust N Z J Surg 62:161–163, 1992.

365. Dare FO, Makinde OO, Makinde ON, Odutayo R: Congenital absence of an ovary in a Nigerian woman. Int J Gynecol Obstet 29:377–378, 1989.

366. Lachman MF, Berman MM: The ectopic ovary: A case report and review of the literature. Arch Pathol Lab Med 115:233–235, 1991.

367. Peedicayil A, Sarada V, Jairaj P, Chandi SM: Ectopic ovary in the omentum. Asia Oceania J Obstet Gynaecol 18:7–11, 1992.

368. Barik S, Dhaliwal LK, Gopalan S, Rajwanshi A: Adenocarcinoma of the supernumerary ovary. Int J Gynecol Obstet 34:75–77, 1990.

369. Besser MJ, Posey DM: Cystic teratoma in a supernumerary ovary of the greater omentum: A case report. J Reprod Med 37:189–193, 1992.

370. Price FV, Edwards R, Buchsbaum HJ: Ovarian remnant syndrome: Difficulties in diagnosis and management. Obstet Gynecol Surv 45:151–156, 1990.

371. Brühwiler H, Lüscher KP: Ovarialkarzinom be Ovarian Remnant Syndrome. Geburtshilfe Frauenheilkd 51:70–71, 1991.

372. Meneses MF, Ostrowski ML: Female splenic-gonadal fusion. Hum Pathol 20:486–488, 1989.

373. Rahilly MA, Al-Nafussi A: Uterus-like mass of the ovary associated with endometrioid carcinoma. Histopathology 18:549–551, 1991.

374. Honore LH, O'Hara KE: Subcapsular adipocytic infiltration of the human ovary: A clinicopathologic study of eight cases. Eur J Obstet Gynecol Reprod Biol 10:13–20, 1980.

375. Gloor E, Juillard E, Curchod A, Legeret J-C: Ovarian hypoplasia with follicular calcifications. Am J Clin Pathol 78:857–860, 1982.

376. Clement PB, Cooney TP: Idiopathic multifocal calcification of the ovary stroma. Arch Pathol Lab Med 116:204–205, 1992.

377. Wingfield JG: More yellow ovaries [letter]. JAMA 263:1494, 1990.

378. Womack C: Isolated arteritis of the ovarian hilum [letter]. J Clin Pathol 40:1484–1485, 1987.

379. Lhote F, Mainguene C, Griselle-Wiseler V, et al: Giant cell arteritis of the female genital tract with temporal arteritis. Ann Rheum Dis 51:900–903, 1992.

380. Coulam CB, Field CS, Kempers RD: Spontaneous bilateral ovarian hemorrhages as a cause of premature ovarian failure. Mayo Clin Proc 56:762–764, 1981.

381. Hill JA, Kassam SH: Ovarian hemorrhage in ovulating women receiving anticoagulant therapy: A report of two cases. J Reprod Med 29:205–208, 1984.

382. Evans-Jones JC, French GL: An ovarian cyst infected with Salmonella typhi: Case report. Br J Obstet Gynaecol 90:680–682, 1983.

383. Wetchler SJ, Dunn LJ: Ovarian abscess: Report of a case and a review of the literature. Obstet Gynecol Surv 40:476–485, 1985.

384. Richer E, Vige P: Abces de l'ovaire: A propos de deux observations. J Gynecol Obstet Biol Reprod 20:393–396, 1991.

385. Lipscomb GH, Ling FW, Photopulos GJ: Ovarian abscess arising within an endometrioma. Obstet Gynecol 78(pt 2):951–954, 1991.

386. Ripps B, Muram D, Winer-Muram HT: Large bowel obstruction: An uncommon complication of a tubo-ovarian abscess. J Tenn Med Assoc 85:103–104, 1992.

387. Lipscomb GH, Ling FW: Tubo-ovarian abscess in postmenopausal patients. South Med J 85:696–699, 1992.

388. Hueston WH: A case of tubo-ovarian abscess 6 years after hysterectomy. Kentucky Med Assoc J 90:114–116, 1992.

389. Schuger L, Simon A, Okon E: Cytomegaly in benign ovarian cysts. Arch Pathol Lab Med 110:928–929, 1986.

390. Mostafa SAM, Bargeron CB, Flower RW, et al: Foreign body granulomas in normal ovaries. Obstet Gynecol 66:701–702, 1985.

391. Uzoaru I, Akang EEU, Aghadiuno PU, Nadimpalli VR: Benign cystic ovarian teratomas with prostatic tissue: A report of two cases. Teratology 45:235–239, 1992.

392. McLachlin CM, Srigley JR: Prostatic tissue in mature cystic teratomas of the ovary. Am J Surg Pathol 16:780–784, 1992.

393. Kallenberg GA, Pesce CM, Norman B, et al: Ectopic hyperprolactinemia resulting from an ovarian teratoma. JAMA 263:2472–2474, 1990.

394. Palmer PE, Bogojavlensky S, Bhan AK, Scully RE: Prolactinoma in wall of ovarian dermoid cyst with hyperprolactinemia. Obstet Gynecol 75(pt 2):540–543, 1990.

395. Pruszczynski M, Sporny S, ten Cate LN, Smedts F: Benign cystic ovarian teratoma with lung differentiation. Zentralbl Allg Pathol Anat 134:687–689, 1988.

396. Ulirsch RC, Goldman RL: An unusual teratoma of the ovary: Neurogenic cyst with lactating breast tissue. Obstet Gynecol 60:400–402, 1982.

397. Spaun E, Rix P: Benign cystic monodermal teratoma of neurogenic type. Int J Gynecol Pathol 9:283–290, 1990.

398. McManis JC, Angerine JM: Retinal tissue in benign cystic ovarian teratoma. Am J Clin Pathol 51:508–510, 1969.

399. MacSween RNM: Foetal cerebellar tissue in an ovarian teratoma. J Pathol Bacteriol 96:513–515, 1968.

400. Sahin AA, Ro JY, Chen J, Ayala AG: Spindle cell nodule and peptic ulcer arising in a fully developed gastric wall in a mature cystic teratoma. Arch Pathol Lab Med 114:529–531, 1990.

401. Woodfield B, Katz DA, Cantrell J, Bogard PJ: A benign cystic teratoma with gastrointestinal tract development. Am J Clin Pathol 83:236–238, 1985.

402. Weldon-Linne CM, Rushovich AM: Benign ovarian cystic teratomas with homunculi. Obstet Gynecol 61(suppl):88–94, 1983.

403. Maudsley G, Zakhour HD: Pneumatosis cystoides-like appearances in a mature cystic teratoma of the ovary. Histopathology 14:420–422, 1989.

404. Rubin A: Pneumatosis cystoides-like lesions in ovary [letter]. Histopathology 15:445, 1989.

405. Pantoja E, Noy MA, Axtmayer RW, et al: Ovarian dermoids and their complications: Comprehensive historical review. Obstet Gynecol Surv 30:1–20, 1975.

406. Hardman JM, Schochet SS Jr, Libcke JH, Earle KM: Rosenthal fibers in ovarian teratomas. Arch Pathol 93:448–452, 1972.

407. Yu TJ, Iwasaki I, Teratani T, et al: Primary ovarian pregnancy in a cystic teratoma. Obstet Gynecol 64(suppl):52–54, 1984.

408. Seidman JD, Patterson JA, Bitterman P: Sertoli-Leydig cell tumor associated with a mature cystic teratoma in a single ovary. Mod Pathol 2:687–692, 1989.

409. Pethe VV, Chitale SV, Godbole RN, Bidaye SV: Hemangioma of the ovary: A case report and review of literature. Indian J Pathol Microbiol 4:290–292, 1991.

410. Mira JL: Lipoleiomyoma of the ovary: Report of a case and review of the English literature. Int J Gynecol Pathol 10:198–202, 1991.

411. Hegg CA, Flint A: Neurofibroma of the ovary. Gynecol Oncol 37:437–438, 1990.

CHAPTER 13

Uterus and Fallopian Tubes

John K.C. Chan, M.B.B.S., M.R.C.Path., F.R.C.P.A.,
and William Y.W. Tsang, M.B.B.S., F.R.C.P.A.

This chapter focuses on a number of common and less common problems encountered by the pathologist in assessment of specimens obtained from the uterine corpus and fallopian tubes. The emphasis is on the approach to arriving at a diagnosis; the salient features of the individual entities are summarized in the tables.

DIAGNOSIS OF INTRAUTERINE PREGNANCY IN THE ABSENCE OF CHORIONIC VILLI

Clinical Significance

The pathologist is commonly requested to confirm a diagnosis of intrauterine pregnancy on uterine curetting specimens obtained from women suspected of having abortion. With a positive diagnosis, there is no need to worry about the possibility of ectopic pregnancy should the patient have persistent abdominal pain.

A diagnosis of "products of gestation" is easy to make when chorionic villi or fetal parts are present, or short of that, when isolated syncytiotrophoblastic cells are seen. Otherwise, only the identification of intermediate (placental site) trophoblast is diagnostic of intrauterine pregnancy. Other histologic changes (such as Arias-Stella reaction, ground-glass nuclei in endometrial epithelium mimicking herpes inclusions,[1,2] decidual change, and plump vacuolated endothelium), although they are characteristic and should lead to a search for more conclusive evidence of intrauterine pregnancy, are not pathognomonic, because they can occur in ectopic pregnancy, in hormonal disturbance, and with use of progestogen. Decidual change has even been reported in postmenopausal women as an idiopathic phenomenon.[3]

Recognition of Intermediate Trophoblast

The presence of intermediate trophoblastic cells among decidual cells can be suspected on low-magnification examination, by virtue of the variegated appearance imparted by the large dark nuclei of the former (Fig. 13–1). Intermediate trophoblastic cells are commonly associated with fibrinoid material (Nitabuch fibrin) and prominent ectatic blood vessels. They can be recognized with confidence by their *large nuclei, which typically exhibit multiple deep clefts,* to the extent that they may resemble porcupine quills;[4] this nuclear feature helps distinguish these cells from decidual cells (see Fig. 13–1) (Table 13–1).

A diagnosis of "placental site reaction, indicative of intrauterine pregnancy" is justified on identification of intermediate trophoblast within the decidua. Degenerated decidual cells or endometrial glandular epithelium can occasionally have wrinkled nuclei, but their nuclei are often smaller. In equivocal cases, more tissues, if available, should be embedded for histologic examination. Immunohistochemical staining for cytokeratin is most helpful, by highlighting the isolated trophoblastic cells that are dispersed among the cytokeratin-negative decidual cells.[4–7]

ABNORMAL GLANDULAR ARCHITECTURE IN THE ENDOMETRIUM

Recognition of the Normal Glandular Architecture

Most pathologic conditions of the endometrium, ranging from functional disturbance to malignant neoplasms, are characterized by disturbance of the glandular architecture in one way or another. It is important to be familiar with the morphologic spectrum of the normal endometrium in order to appreciate what constitutes architectural abnormalities.

In the proliferative phase, the glands appear as narrow, loosely coiled tubules with parallel sides (Fig. 13–2A). In the secretory phase, the tubules become dilated and more coiled and therefore appear more crowded and not parallel-sided. In the late secretory and menstrual phases, the glands assume a serrated outline, which can appear stellate in cross sections; intervening stroma can be scanty (Fig. 13–2B). The basalis does not exhibit the cyclic changes that the superficialis does.

Although the single plane of a histologic section almost never includes a gland in its entirety, one can generally trace an imaginary linear course through each individual gland from the surface downward, while making some allowance for the coiling (see Fig. 13–2A). *Failure to trace the linear course or presence of glandular structures not readily explainable by simple coiling suggests presence of architectural disturbance and thus a probable pathologic process* (Figs. 13–3

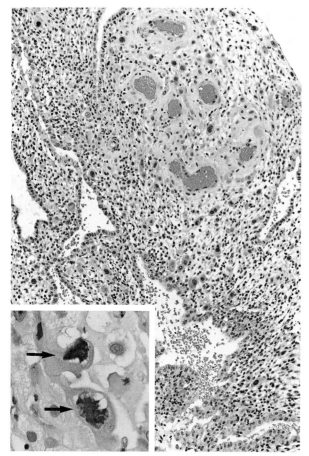

FIGURE 13–1. Placental Site Reaction. The decidua has a variegated appearance owing to the presence of dispersed larger and more darkly stained intermediate trophoblastic cells. *Inset,* The intermediate trophoblastic cells *(arrows)* typically show multiple deep nuclear clefts.

and 13–4). However, the following potential pitfalls have to be kept in mind.

1. Proper assessment should be made only on fragments with satisfactory orientation, that is, with intact surface epithelium. Those pieces without surface epithelium could represent transverse sections of the superficialis (in which the linear arrangement of the glands may not be evident) or could represent the basalis. In the latter, the glands are typically irregular-shaped and weakly proliferative (scanty cytoplasm and few mitoses), and the stroma is often compact, with some thick-walled vessels (Fig. 13–5).

2. Lower segment endometrium may exhibit some irregular-shaped glands; it can be recognized by its stroma, which is more fibrous.

3. Tissue disintegration may bring the glands closer together, giving a false impression of glandular crowding. One should therefore be cautious in assessment of tissue fragments with crumbled stroma.

4. The ''gland-in-gland'' appearance is a common normal phenomenon, probably as a result of telescoping of the gland on itself during curettage.

5. Fragmentation of the stroma by curettage, and particularly by aspiration biopsy, results in pseudocrowding of glands. This phenomenon can be recognized by the empty clefts instead of stroma between the glands and the occurrence of disrupted glands (Fig. 13–6).

Deviations From Normal

Glandular disturbance usually takes one or more of the following forms:

1. Cystic Dilatation—Dilated round glands are not seen in the normal endometrium, but a few small cystic glands are so commonly observed in otherwise normal endometrium of perimenopausal women that they may be viewed as a normal variation. Cysts are commonly seen in senile cystic atrophy, simple hyperplasia, and endometrial polyp (Figs. 13–4, 13–7, and 13–8).

2. Glandular Crowding—Crowding of glands refers to closer apposition of the glands compared with normal (Figs. 13–3, 13–9, and 13–10). It implies an increase in glandular units and is a characteristic feature of endometrial hyperplasia and endometrial carcinoma. The nature of the epithelium should also be taken into consideration: obviously the almost back-to-back arrangement of serrated glands considered normal for late secretory phase endometrium is definitely abnormal if the epithelium is of proliferative type.

3. Abnormal Glandular Shape—Abnormal glandular contour, in excess of that accountable for by simple glandular coiling, is caused by abnormal glandular maturation, abnormal budding, or distortion by an excessive stroma. The extremely narrow atrophic tubular glands widely separated by stroma are characteristic of the effects of oral contraceptives or prolonged progestogen therapy. Abnormal budding, sometimes producing a finger and glove appearance, is commonly observed in endometrial hyperplasia and carcinoma (see Figs. 13–3 and 13–9*B*). Glands with stellate luminal contour but smooth external outline, as characteristic of secretory endometrium and Arias-Stella reaction, should not be mistaken for glandular budding (see Fig. 13–2*B*). Glandular distortion by stroma is common in endometrial polyp (see Fig. 13–8) and mullerian adenofibroma/adenosarcoma; in the latter, the glands often exhibit a phyllodes pattern.

Conditions Associated with Disturbed Glandular Architecture

The diagnosis of the various entities showing abnormal glandular architecture rests on the overall picture and identifi-

Table 13–1. **Comparison Between Intermediate Trophoblast and Decidual Cell**

	Intermediate Trophoblast	**Decidual Cell**
Size	Generally larger	Generally smaller
Nuclei	Mononuclear, sometimes multinucleated. Typically show multiple deep clefts; chromatin often dense, but occasionally vesicular with prominent nucleoli.	Mononuclear. Round to oval nuclei with fine chromatin.
Cytoplasm	Homogeneous eosinophilic cytoplasm without a distinct cell membrane.	Distinct pink-staining cell membrane contrasting with the lightly basophilic cytoplasm.

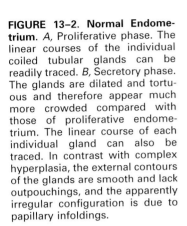
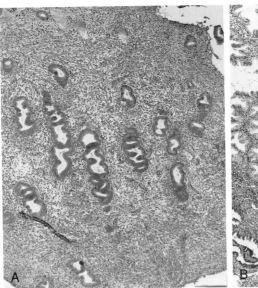
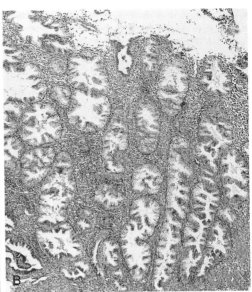

FIGURE 13–2. Normal Endometrium. *A,* Proliferative phase. The linear courses of the individual coiled tubular glands can be readily traced. *B,* Secretory phase. The glands are dilated and tortuous and therefore appear much more crowded compared with those of proliferative endometrium. The linear course of each individual gland can also be traced. In contrast with complex hyperplasia, the external contours of the glands are smooth and lack outpouchings, and the apparently irregular configuration is due to papillary infoldings.

cation of other diagnostic features (Table 13–2). Practically all the listed entities are covered in subsequent sections.

Endometrial polyp is a focal mucosal overgrowth, usually from the basalis, protruding into the uterine cavity.[8, 9] Use of tamoxifen may be associated with an increased risk of developing endometrial polyp;[10–12] these polyps can harbor foci of endometrial hyperplasia or even carcinoma. Polypectomy or hysterectomy is curative for endometrial polyp. However, this benign lesion is associated with a slightly increased risk of developing adenocarcinoma, with a disproportionately high percentage of serous papillary type[13–15] (Fig. 13–11). It is not always easy to recognize endometrial polyp in endometrial curettings, and conversely, the architectural distortion commonly observed in endometrial polyp may lead to an erroneous

diagnosis of endometrial hyperplasia. The following are features essential for a histologic diagnosis of endometrial polyp[8, 9] (see Fig. 13–8):

1. Presence of surface epithelium on at least three sides of the tissue fragment (although this feature is also commonly seen in normal endometrial fragments).
2. Thick-walled vessels.
3. A stroma that is more fibrous than normal.

Almost invariably some glands show abnormal architecture (stellate configuration) or cystic change, but there should not be glandular crowding, which, if present, indicates that there is superimposed endometrial hyperplasia or carcinoma (see Fig. 13–11). The epithelium is usually proliferative or weakly proliferative and often does not show cyclic changes. When-

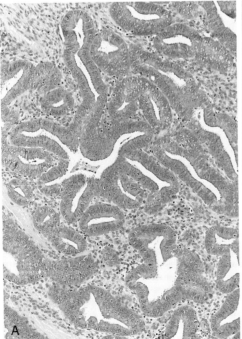
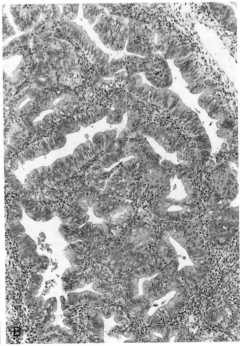

FIGURE 13–3. Abnormal Glandular Architecture. *A,* Complex atypical hyperplasia, with the glands exhibiting marked crowding and complex side-branching, resulting in a pattern that cannot be explained by simple coiling. Cytologic atypia is evident on high magnification (see Fig. 13–20*D*). *B,* Complex hyperplasia. Despite marked glandular crowding, there is still identifiable stroma in between. Some glands form intraluminal papillary infolding without fibrous cores. The epithelium is of proliferative type and lacks atypia.

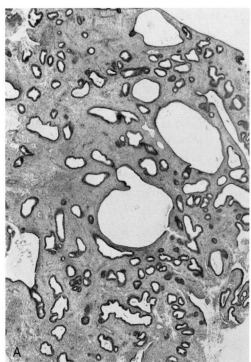

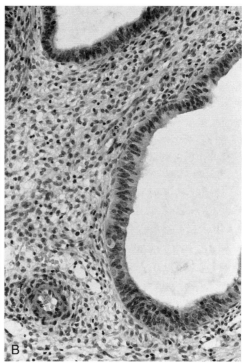

FIGURE 13–4. Simple Hyperplasia. *A,* Abnormally shaped and cystic glands are separated by an appreciable amount of stroma. It is difficult if not impossible to trace the course of the individual glands. *B,* The lining epithelium is of proliferative type.

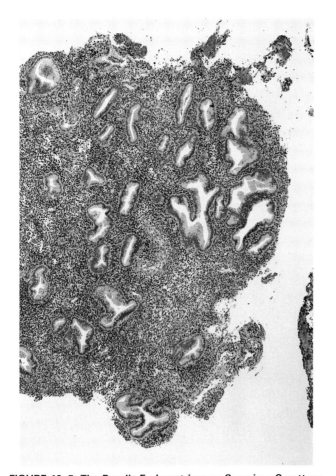

FIGURE 13–5. The Basalis Endometrium as Seen in a Curettage Specimen. It can be recognized by the non-crowded tubular to stellate glands, dense stroma, thick vessels, and frequent absence of surface epithelium.

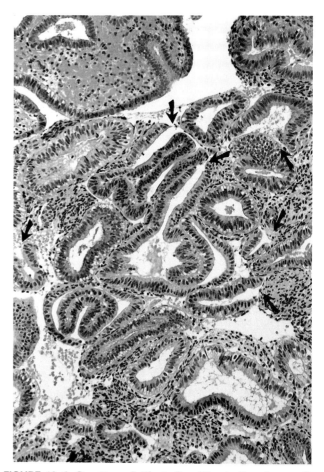

FIGURE 13–6. Curettage Artifacts Resulting in Pseudocrowding of Glands. Note the empty clefts between the glands as well as discontinuities in the glands *(arrows).*

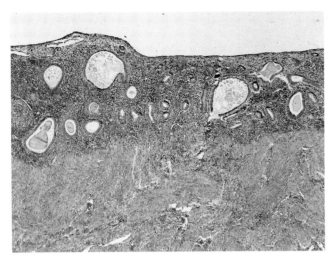

FIGURE 13–7. Senile Cystic Atrophy. Note the thin atrophic endometrium with some cystic glands, which differs from the thickened and voluminous endometrium seen in simple hyperplasia.

ever the stroma shows high cellularity or condensation beneath the epithelium, the possibility of mullerian adenosarcoma must be seriously considered.

BENIGN LESIONS OF THE ENDOMETRIUM POTENTIALLY MISTAKEN FOR ENDOMETRIAL CARCINOMA

A variety of benign lesions may be misinterpreted as endometrial carcinoma:

1. Endometrial metaplasia (Table 13–3)[16–26]
2. Endometrial hyperplasia (Table 13–4)[27–31]
3. Arias-Stella reaction
4. Postcurettage reparative changes
5. Atypical polypoid adenomyoma (Table 13–5)[32–35]
6. Placental site nodule
7. Adenomatoid tumor
8. Radiation changes
9. Adenomyosis with atrophic changes

Problems in Diagnosis

One should be *extremely cautious in rendering a diagnosis of endometrial carcinoma in young patients* (< 40 years), because endometrial carcinomas occur in this age group very infrequently.[33, 36] Therefore, the various mimickers must be seriously considered.

Some benign entities listed previously, such as endometrial hyperplasia, atypical polypoid adenomyoma, adenomatoid tumor, and adenomyosis, show *architectural abnormalities or an infiltrative pattern* that raises a concern for carcinoma. **Adenomatoid tumor** is particularly problematic when it grows predominantly in the form of infiltrative cords and tubular structures (Fig. 13–12). It can be distinguished from endometrial carcinoma by absence of endometrial involvement and lack of cellular atypia. **Adenomyosis,** a diverticular disease of the endometrium with a predilection to involve the uterine fundus, is usually defined by the presence of endometrial islands (glands surrounded by stroma) deeply located in the myometrium, at least one low-power microscopic field (×10 objective) below the endomyometrial junction. In postmenopausal women, the stromal element of the adenomyotic islands may regress, leaving "naked" endometrial glands in the myometrium.[37] These islands can be distinguished from

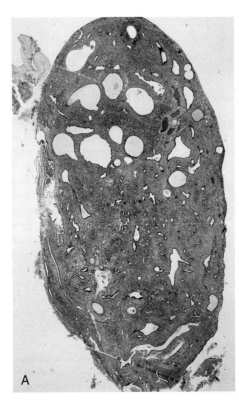

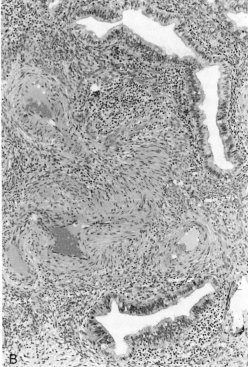

FIGURE 13–8. Endometrial Polyp. *A,* This polypoid fragment is covered by epithelium on all sides. Non-crowded cystic and abnormally shaped glands are evident. *B,* Higher magnification shows a stroma more fibrous than the normal endometrial stroma as well as thick-walled vessels.

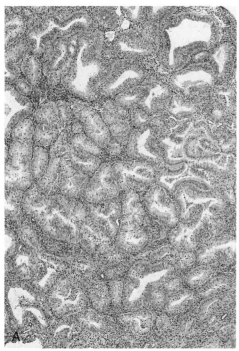
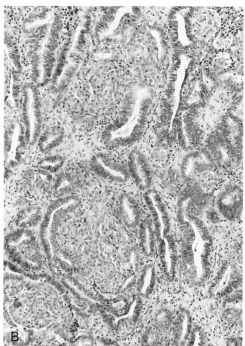

FIGURE 13-9. Complex Atypical Hyperplasia. *A,* There is a striking degree of glandular crowding as well as some degree of glandular complexity. *B,* The glands are markedly crowded and show budding. The pale foci represent squamous (morule) metaplasia, a common occurrence in endometrial hyperplasia. The metaplastic epithelium sometimes appears to bridge adjacent glands.

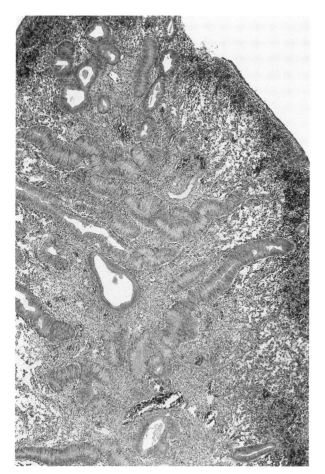

FIGURE 13-10. Simple Atypical Hyperplasia. In this example, although the glands show abnormal architecture with very long narrow tubules assuming a "Sertoliform" appearance, there is only slight crowding and minimal glandular budding. See Figure 13-20*C* for cytologic details.

carcinoma by their atrophic appearance and bland cytology and by the presence of typical adenomyotic foci elsewhere.

Other mimickers of malignancy are characterized by *cellular atypia,* such as atypical hyperplasia, atypical polypoid adenomyoma, Arias-Stella reaction, postcurettage repair, radiation change, and placental site nodule. **Arias-Stella reaction,** an endometrial change occurring in association with pregnancy and trophoblastic disease, can appear alarming owing to glandular crowding, cellular stratification with papillary tuft formation, and nuclear atypia[38,39] (Fig. 13-13). The atypical cells contain enlarged hyperchromatic nuclei that may appear smudgy; occasionally nuclei may even be bizarre. Some cells can assume a hobnail appearance. Features pointing to the benign nature of this lesion are (1) occurrence in reproductive age group, (2) paucity of mitotic figures (although a recent study indicates that mitotic figures, including atypical ones, can sometimes occur),[39a] (3) presence of some normal cells among atypical cells, (4) other histologic evidence of pregnancy, and (5) papillae lacking hyalinized cores. **Postcurettage reparative change,** characterized by scattered cells with enlarged hyperchromatic nuclei and prom-

Table 13-2. **Conditions Associated with Disturbed Glandular Architecture**

Functional disorders and hormonal changes, e.g., abnormal secretory endometrium, oral contraceptive effects
Chronic endometritis
Pregnancy (intrauterine or extrauterine)
Senile cystic atrophy
Endometrial polyp
Polypoid adenomyoma and atypical polypoid adenomyoma
Disordered proliferative endometrium
Endometrial hyperplasia
Endometrial adenocarcinoma
Mixed mullerian tumors (adenofibroma, adenosarcoma, carcinosarcoma)
Metastatic adenocarcinoma

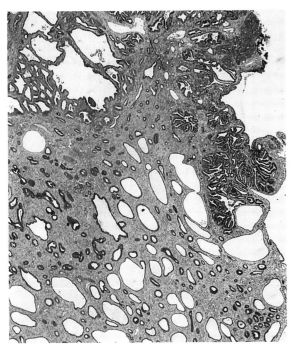

FIGURE 13–11. Endometrial Polyp Complicated by Carcinoma. This polyp shows the typical architectural features of endometrial polyp, but the right upper field shows striking glandular proliferation with areas of invasion, compatible with carcinoma.

inent nucleoli, and occasional hobnail cells, can be recognized by the confinement to the surface epithelium and superficial glands, lack of architectural atypia of the underlying glands, the history of curettage, and lack of evidence of malignancy in the recent curettage.[40] **Radiation** can induce striking cellular atypia in the normal endometrial glands, sometimes accompanied by atypical mitotic figures.[41] Features pointing to the diagnosis are the lack of architectural atypia (the glands often appear widely spaced), random cytologic atypia (normal nuclei interspersed among atypical ones), frequent multinucleated forms, normal nucleocytoplasmic ratio, and the history of radiation (Fig. 13–14).

Atypical polypoid adenomyoma often poses problems in diagnosis because the myoid nature of the mesenchymal cells may not be immediately apparent as a result of the cytoplasm's not being as eosinophilic or abundant as the usual smooth muscle cells (see Table 13–5) (Fig. 13–15). In curettage specimens, this entity can be distinguished from adenocarcinoma showing myometrial invasion by (1) its occurrence in premenopausal age group; (2) cytologic and architectural atypia of only a mild to moderate degree; (3) cellular stroma comprising intersecting fascicles of smooth muscle cells, differing from the more orderly myometrial smooth muscle; and (4) absence of separate fragments of frank carcinoma composed of crowded and coalescent glands. With regard to the last feature, such fragments inevitably are present if the smooth muscle of the problematic lesion truly represents myometrial tissue.

Diagnostic Considerations for Endometrial Epithelial Metaplasia

Endometrial epithelial metaplasia refers to the conversion of the mature specialized cell type to another not normally

present in the endometrium (see Table 13–3). It is a common occurrence, ranging from tiny incidental findings to extensive involvement of the endometrium (Figs. 13–9B and 13–16 to 13–19), and several types of metaplasia commonly co-exist. Endometrial metaplasia *per se* is an innocuous lesion, but it can potentially be mistaken for carcinoma or atypical hyperplasia.[16–23] The key distinguishing features are *lack of cytologic atypia* and paucity of mitotic figures. Because the *various forms of metaplasia occur commonly in endometrial hyperplasia and sometimes in endometrial carcinoma, the most important job is to exclude the presence of these underlying lesions.* Basically, the architecture and cytology of the glandular proliferation should be assessed as if there is no metaplasia (see Figs. 13–9B and 13–17).

Squamous metaplasia must not be mistaken for the squamous component of an endometrioid adenocarcinoma[26] and condyloma acuminatum (a very rare lesion characterized by koilocytosis and papillomatosis).[42, 43] When should one be worried that the squamous proliferation represents a carcinoma? Extensive squamous islands occupying more than half of a low-power field without intervening stroma or presence of significant nuclear atypia should lead to a search for more definite evidence of malignancy.

The problems in assessment of endometrium exhibiting extensive **mucinous metaplasia** are dealt with in a subsequent section (see Fig. 13–19). The possibility of mucinous adenocarcinoma should always be considered whenever the process is extensive.

Papillary syncytial metaplasia may mimic papillary serous carcinoma, but it can be distinguished by its microscopic size, confinement to the surface epithelium and superficial glands, and absence of cellular atypia (see Fig. 13–18).

Problems in Evaluation of Endometrial Hyperplasia and Differential Diagnosis

The classification and terminology of endometrial hyperplasia are fraught with controversies (see Table 13–4).[26, 44–47] The new classification adopted by the World Health Organization is used here.[40, 48, 48a] Use of the term "adenocarcinoma *in situ*" is not advisable.[44] For untreated hyperplasia, more than 50% of the cases will regress, and approximately 20% will persist. Among the various types of hyperplasia, only atypical hyperplasia appears to be a significant precancerous lesion. It should be noted that epithelial metaplasia is commonly superimposed on endometrial hyperplasia.

Simple hyperplasia is usually a generalized process in the endometrium and represents a manifestation of prolonged unopposed estrogen stimulation. Tissues obtained by curettage are typically abundant. Because both the glandular and stromal elements participate in the proliferation, the glands are never very crowded (see Fig. 13–4A). The lining cells are pseudostratified and mitotically active (see Fig. 13–4B). Simple hyperplasia encompasses "cystic glandular hyperplasia" and some cases of mild "adenomatous hyperplasia" by the previous nomenclature (see Fig. 13–10). When features of simple hyperplasia are incompletely developed and areas show a normal proliferative pattern, the term "disordered proliferative endometrium" can be applied; this lesion has no premalignant potential.[46] Senile cystic atrophy may mimic simple

Table 13–3. **Types of Endometrial Metaplasia**[16–26]

Type	Known Etiologic Associations	Salient Histologic Features
Squamous (including morule)	Unopposed estrogen; chronic endometritis; pyometra; foreign body	Squamous metaplasia: replacement of glandular epithelium by stratified squamous epithelium with distinct cell borders and intercellular bridges; keratinization can occur. Rarely, the endometrium is extensively replaced by mature keratinizing squamous epithelium (ichthyosis uteri), a phenomenon mostly secondary to pyometra. Morule metaplasia (immature squamous metaplasia): sheet-like proliferation of bland-looking plump to spindly cells with indistinct cell borders. These cells fill the whole gland or part of the gland; confluence of the adjacent epithelial units and central necrosis can occur.
Mucinous	Usually postmenopausal	Glands lined by columnar cells with abundant cytoplasmic mucin, mimicking endocervical epithelium. Some cases may resemble intestinal epithelium, with interspersed goblet cells.
Papillary syncytial	Regenerative phenomenon, e.g., postcurettage; acute endometrial breakdown and bleeding	Involves only surface epithelium and/or the superficial glands. Cells with eosinophilic cytoplasm and indistinct cell borders form tufts and papillae without stromal support, and occasionally non-papillary sheets. Intraepithelial neutrophils and nuclear debris are common.
Papillary	—	Short papillae with connective tissue cores.
Eosinophilic	—	Glands lined by non-ciliated cells with abundant eosinophilic cytoplasm. Oncocytic variant: the cytoplasm appears granular owing to accumulation of mitochondria.
Ciliated	Unopposed estrogen	The lining cells are ciliated, and cytoplasm is often eosinophilic. Occasionally assuming a cribriform pattern.
Hobnail	Postcurettage regeneration; postabortal	Glands lined by pear-shaped cells with apical nuclei; cytoplasm usually eosinophilic.
Clear-cell	Postabortal	Columnar cells show cytoplasmic clearing.

Table 13–4. **Classification of Endometrial Hyperplasia**[27–29]

Type	Salient Histologic Features	Risk of Subsequent Invasive Carcinoma for "Untreated" Hyperplasia
Simple hyperplasia	Proliferation of both glandular and stromal elements such that the glands are often spaced out. Great variation in glandular size; cysts common. May have areas of mild to moderate glandular crowding but minimal complexity. No cytologic atypia.	1%
Complex hyperplasia	Marked glandular crowding and complexity, but no evidence of stromal invasion. No cytologic atypia.	3%
Atypical hyperplasia (simple or complex)	Defining feature: presence of epithelium with nuclear atypia and loss of polarity. Mild atypia: nuclear enlargement and rounding with fine, dispersed chromatin. Severe atypia: nuclear enlargement, nuclear pleomorphism, prominent nucleoli, irregularly dispersed and clumped chromatin. Architectural features of simple or complex hyperplasia as listed above.	23% (8% for atypical simple hyperplasia; 29% for atypical complex hyperplasia)*

* Some but not all studies have shown that the risk is substantially lower if progestin therapy is given.[28–31]

Table 13–5. **Atypical Polypoid Adenomyoma**[32-35]

Clinical Features

Usually premenopausal (mean, 39 years)
Presentation: abnormal vaginal bleeding
Association: Turner's syndrome on long-term estrogen therapy (uncommon)

Site of Involvement

Usually lower uterine segment, sometimes endocervix or upper uterine corpus

Gross Appearance

Often solitary, <2 cm
Yellow-tan to gray-white polypoid mass with lobulated or bosselated surface
May protrude through cervical os

Salient Histologic Features

Dispersed endometrial glands showing architectural and cytologic atypia (even with formation of cribriform structures); mitotic figures often present.
    Glands may be focally crowded.
Squamous morules often present.
Cellular stroma comprises interlacing bundles of benign-looking and sometimes mildly atypical smooth muscle cells, which can exhibit occasional mitotic
    figures.
In hysterectomy specimens, the interface with the endometrium and myometrium is non-invasive.

Natural History

Hysterectomy is always curative.
For patients treated by endometrial curettage only, follow-up curettage at intervals may reveal no evidence of residual disease, endometrial hyperplasia, or
    persistence of atypical polypoid adenomyoma.
Cautionary note: It is not uncommon to find atypical hyperplasia in the adjacent endometrium; such cases should be managed accordingly.

---

hyperplasia, but can be recognized by the scantiness of tissue and inactive appearance of the epithelium (see Fig. 13–7).

Complex hyperplasia is usually a focal process, and can arise in a background of simple hyperplasia. Because only the epithelial component proliferates, this lesion is characterized by marked glandular crowding, budding, and complexity. The glands show irregular outpouchings not readily explained by simple coiling or sometimes form unusually long narrow tubules (see Figs. 13–3 and 13–9). There may be intraglandular papillary tufting (see Fig. 13–3B). Although crowded, the glands are still separated by at least thin wisps of endometrial stroma (see Figs. 13–3B and 13–9A). Features of stromal invasion should be absent. The lining epithelium is of ordinary proliferative type (see Fig. 13–9B). In curettage specimens,

tissue disintegration or mechanical artifact resulting in deceptive crowding of the glands may mimic complex hyperplasia[49] (see Fig. 13–6). Thus, a diagnosis of endometrial hyperplasia should not be made unless the glands and stroma show intact relationship.[40]

Atypical hyperplasia is usually a focal process. It is characterized by the presence of cytologic atypia in an endometrial proliferation showing architectural features of simple hyperplasia or complex hyperplasia (see Figs. 13–3A, 13–9, and 13–10). There is a significant risk of development of endometrial carcinoma, which is estimated at 23% to 24% according to two studies[28, 46] and a higher rate of 57% according to another study.[50] Distinction from complex hyperplasia can be very difficult for the milder forms of atypical hyperplasia. It

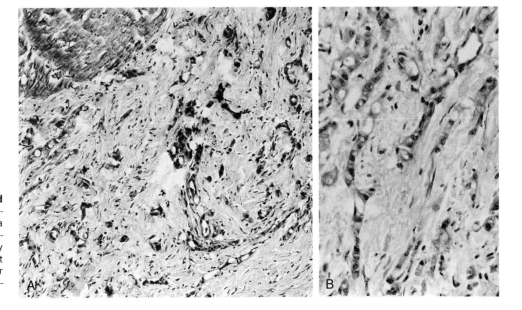

FIGURE 13–12. Adenomatoid Tumor in Uterus. *A,* The occurrence of invasive cords in a fibrous stroma can raise a serious concern for the possibility of carcinoma. *B,* The constituent cells, however, lack nuclear atypia and show frequent vacuolation.

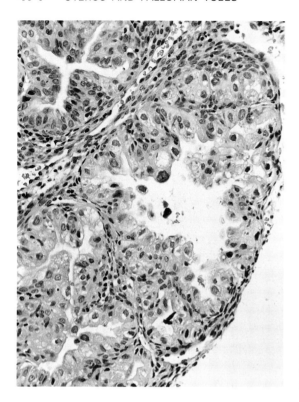

FIGURE 13–13. Arias-Stella Reaction Associated with Intrauterine Pregnancy. Similar to secretory endometrium, the glands show papillary tufts creating a stellate-shaped luminal configuration, but the external contour is smooth. Some cells show nuclear atypia and hyperchromasia, but mitotic figures are not seen.

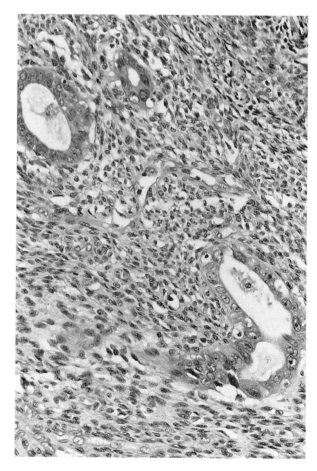

FIGURE 13–14. Endometrium with Radiation Changes. The glands are sparsely distributed and exhibit random cytologic atypia.

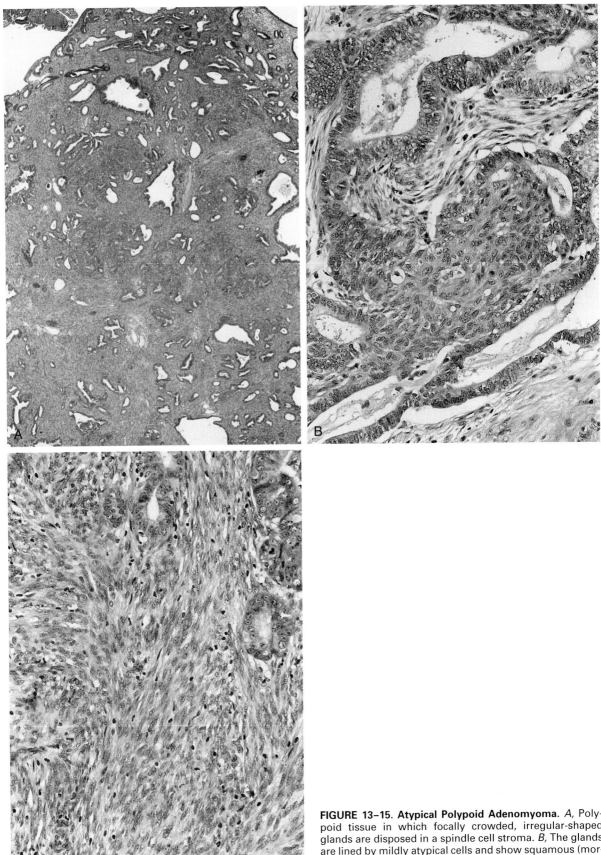

FIGURE 13–15. Atypical Polypoid Adenomyoma. *A,* Polypoid tissue in which focally crowded, irregular-shaped glands are disposed in a spindle cell stroma. *B,* The glands are lined by mildly atypical cells and show squamous (morule) metaplasia. *C,* The glands in this example *(right upper field)* are more atypical. Note the smooth muscle stroma formed by interlacing spindly cells.

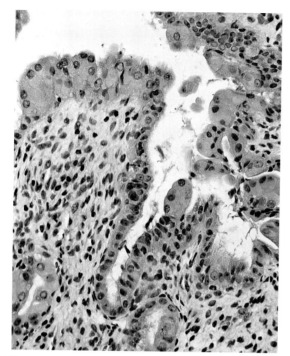

FIGURE 13–16. Eosinophilic Metaplasia. Some epithelial cells are enlarged and contain abundant eosinophilic cytoplasm.

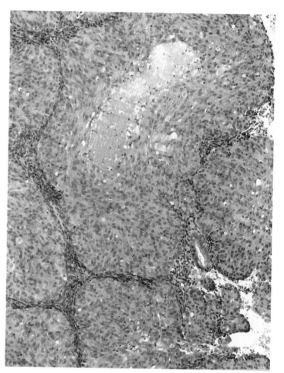

FIGURE 13–17. Complex Hyperplasia with Squamous (Morule) Metaplasia. The individual glands are expanded by bland-looking squamous epithelium. Central necrosis can occur *(upper field).*

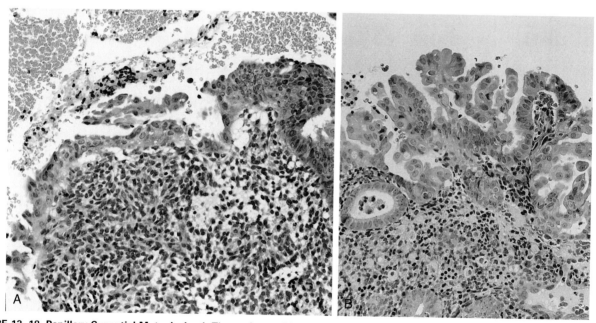

FIGURE 13–18. Papillary Syncytial Metaplasia. *A,* The surface epithelium shows piling up of cells with some papillary tufts. *B,* A more florid example with papillary tuft formation in the surface epithelium. The cells lack nuclear atypia. Foamy cells are seen in the underlying stroma in this case.

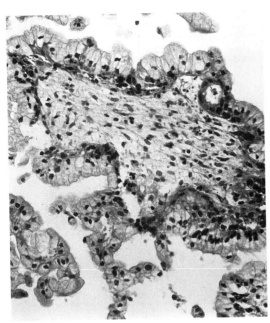

FIGURE 13–19. Mucinous Metaplasia. In this example, papillary processes are formed. The mucinous epithelium shows regular basal nuclei.

is helpful to look for loss of polarity and to compare the cells with those of any residual normal glands. The nuclei often appear rounded and enlarged compared with the oval or elongated nuclei of normal proliferative epithelium (Fig. 13–20). On the other hand, distinction between atypical hyperplasia and well-differentiated adenocarcinoma is even more problematic (see next section). Suffice to say, even if strict criteria are applied, carcinoma is still found in the hysterectomy specimen in a proportion of cases (approximately 18%) performed for a diagnosis of "atypical hyperplasia" made on curettage specimen, although all such carcinomas are well-differentiated and at most superficially invasive.[47, 51–54] Thus, if there is any uncertainty, this should be so stated in the report, such as "consistent with atypical hyperplasia, but the possibility of well-differentiated carcinoma cannot be ruled out." As far as treatment is concerned, hysterectomy is usually performed anyway for postmenopausal women whichever diagnostic label is given—and the diagnosis is certainly clarified in the subsequent hysterectomy specimen. For women in the reproductive age group, the gynecologist has to weigh other factors to decide whether hysterectomy or hormonal therapy with follow-up curettage is more appropriate.

Endometrial Hyperplasia or Well-Differentiated Adenocarcinoma?

Endometrial carcinomas with significant cellular anaplasia or frank invasive features should pose no problems in diagnosis either in a curettage or hysterectomy specimen. It is most difficult to distinguish between complex/atypical hyperplasia and well-differentiated endometrial carcinoma in curettage specimens. The distinction is less critical in a hysterectomy specimen, because in the absence of myometrial invasion, the prognosis of well-differentiated endometrial carcinoma is excellent and hysterectomy is usually curative.

Various authors have proposed different criteria to aid in this distinction.[26, 27, 29, 51, 52] Any of the following features, which reflect the presence of stromal invasion, should point to a *diagnosis of carcinoma.*

1. *Desmoplastic reaction:*[27, 52] The spindly fibroblasts or myofibroblasts in the stroma are readily distinguished from the normal endometrial stroma composed of compact cells with barely visible cytoplasm (Figs. 13–21 and 13–22). The desmoplastic stroma shows some degree of edema and is often sprinkled with inflammatory cells. The fibrous stroma seen in endometrial polyp and lower uterine segment should not be mistaken for desmoplastic stroma; it does not exhibit edema, and the glandular units disposed in it are not crowded.
2. Presence of one or more of the following features in *an extensive fashion,* defined as occupying more than half (2.1 mm) of a low-power field of 4.2 mm diameter.[27, 52]
   a. *Cribriform structures,* with formation of intraglandular bridges devoid of stromal support (Fig. 13–23).
   b. *Papillary pattern,* characterized by multiple branching fibrous processes supporting the epithelium (Fig. 13–24). Intraglandular cellular budding without stromal cores is not counted as papillary pattern.
   c. *Squamous proliferation* in a coalescent pattern.
3. Glands arranged in a *back-to-back pattern* with no stroma in between[47, 48] (Fig. 13–25).

The above-listed criteria help predict those endometrial glandular proliferations that have a significant potential of myometrial invasion as demonstrated in the subsequent hysterectomy specimen.[52, 55] Newer techniques such as morphometry, immunohistochemistry, flow cytometry, and nucleolar organizer region have so far not been shown conclusively to be superior to carefully applied morphologic criteria in making the distinction.[56–63]

These criteria apply only for proliferations that do not exhibit overt malignant features cytologically.[29] If there is frank cytologic anaplasia, a diagnosis of carcinoma can be rendered in the absence of histologic features indicative of stromal invasion.[29, 44]

Subsidiary features suggestive but not diagnostic of endometrial carcinoma are

1. Neutrophils infiltrating the glandular epithelium and lumina[44]
2. Abnormal mitotic figures[44]
3. Foamy stromal cells (although identical cells may also be seen in the normal or hyperplastic endometrium)[47, 48, 64]
4. Focal stromal necrosis (disappearance of stromal cells between the glands and replacement by neutrophils, with or without necrotic cellular debris)[47, 48] (see Fig. 13–22)
5. Stratified epithelium other than squamous/morule change[51]

These features, if present, should lead to more careful search for definite evidence of carcinoma.

PROBLEMS IN ASSESSMENT OF ENDOMETRIAL CARCINOMA

For endometrial carcinoma, the pathologist's role includes not only rendering a correct diagnosis, but also the provision of all information relevant for prognostication and management (Table 13–6).[64a] The presence of adverse prognostic factors

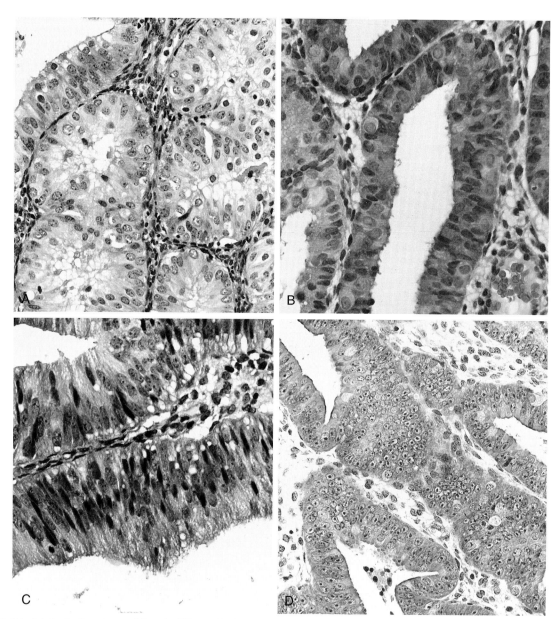

FIGURE 13–20. Cytologic Spectrum of Atypical Hyperplasia. *A,* Mild nuclear enlargement and mild loss of nuclear polarity. *B,* Striking nuclear crowding and loss of polarity. *C,* The cells are unusually elongated with some degree of nuclear hyperchromasia. *D,* Marked nuclear atypia with vesicular chromatin and distinct nucleoli.

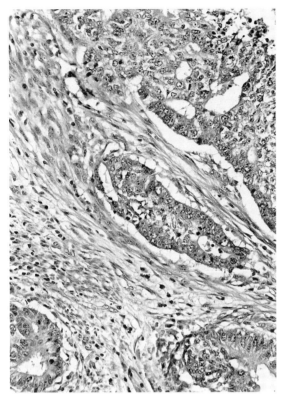

FIGURE 13–21. Endometrioid Adenocarcinoma. The presence of a cellular desmoplastic stroma is an indication of the occurrence of invasion.

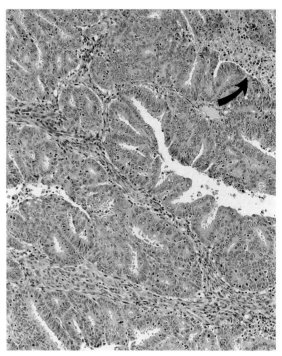

FIGURE 13–22. Endometrioid Adenocarcinoma. The glands are highly complex and crowded and lie in a desmoplastic stroma. The arrow indicates an area of stromal necrosis.

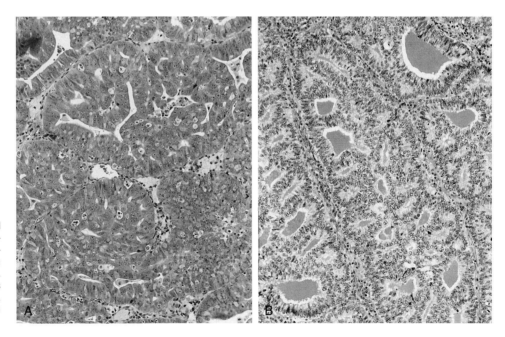

FIGURE 13–23. Endometrioid Adenocarcinoma, in Which Diagnosis of Malignancy is Supported by the Presence of an Extensive Cribriform Pattern. *A,* The cribriform spaces in this case are irregular and slit-like. *B,* In this case, the cribriform spaces are rounded.

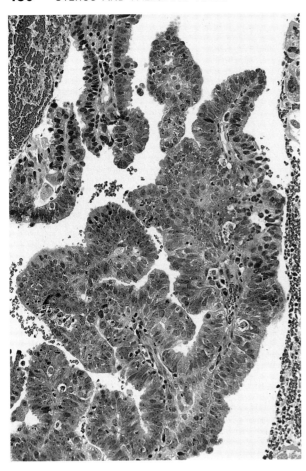

FIGURE 13–24. Papillary (Villoglandular) Variant of Endometrioid Adenocarcinoma. The villous processes are covered by pseudostratified columnar cells. Note the relatively smooth contour of the luminal surface.

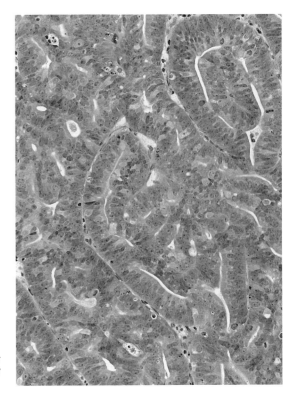

FIGURE 13–25. Endometrioid Adenocarcinoma with a Back-to-Back Glandular Pattern. The glands show extreme complexity and bridging, with no or scarcely any stroma in between.

Table 13–6. **Essential Information to be Included in Pathology Report of Resection Specimen Harboring Endometrial Carcinoma**

1. Diagnosis
2. Histologic subtype
3. Histologic grade
4. Extent of disease
   a. Depth of invasion
   b. Lymphovascular invasion?
   c. Involvement of isthmus/cervix?
   d. Adnexal involvement?
   e. Lymph node status (if relevant)?
   f. Peritoneal washing cytology (if relevant)
5. Status of uninvolved endometrium
6. Other parameters of prognostic importance (if available)
   a. Steroid hormone receptor status
   b. DNA ploidy
   c. Proliferative fraction
   d. Oncogene expression

Synoptic reporting can ensure inclusion of all information.[64a]

in patients with stage I disease may be an indication for adjuvant therapy.

Rendering a Correct Diagnosis of Endometrial Carcinoma

The problems in *distinguishing endometrial carcinoma from various benign lesions* have already been discussed. For any "unusual-looking" carcinoma, the possibility of metastatic carcinoma has also to be considered; the most common primary sites are the breast, colon, and stomach.[65]

It may be difficult to *determine whether the tumor arises from the uterine corpus or endocervix.* Presence of an appreciable amount of intracytoplasmic mucin favors an endocervical primary site, whereas presence of foamy stromal cells favors an endometrial primary site. Particular attention should be paid to the nature of the non-neoplastic glands (endometrial versus endocervical) contiguous to the carcinoma.[40] Although immunohistochemical studies have been considered helpful (such as lower frequency of staining for carcinoembryonic antigen and higher frequency of staining for vimentin in endometrial adenocarcinoma), the significant overlap precludes their practical application in making the distinction. Carefully performed fractional curettage of the endometrial cavity and endocervical canal is most helpful if tumor is detected in only one of these sites.

What is the Histologic Subtype?

There are many subtypes of endometrial carcinoma (Table 13–7), the commonest being endometrioid adenocarcinoma (Tables 13–8 and 13–9)[40, 48, 66–131] (Figs. 13–22 to 13–31). It is most important to recognize **serous papillary adenocarcinoma** because of its aggressive behavior (see Figs. 13–27 and 13–28). A recent study indicates that an endometrial carcinoma with more than 25% component of serous adenocarcinoma behaves as aggressively as pure serous adenocarcinoma;[71] therefore, this component must be reported even if found focally. On the other hand, the non-aggressive **villo-**

glandular variant of endometrioid adenocarcinoma must not be mistaken for serous adenocarcinoma. Features in favor of the former diagnosis are (1) orderly delicate papillae with fibrovascular cores, (2) smooth rather than ragged apical surface, (3) glandular lumina regular and round rather than irregular and slit-like, (4) absence of cellular tufts, (5) pseudostratified columnar cells rather than stratified cuboidal cells, and (6) low nuclear grade (see Fig. 13–24). Admittedly there are instances in which such a distinction can be difficult to make. **Clear-cell carcinoma** shows overlapping histologic features with serous papillary carcinoma, but a distinction is not crucial because both are aggressive tumors of the uterus. Features in favor of the diagnosis of clear-cell carcinoma are (1) papillae with hyalinized cores, (2) tubulocystic pattern, and (3) prominent component of clear cells or hobnail cells[40] (Fig. 13–32).

Among **adenocarcinomas with clear cells,** the possibilities of clear-cell carcinoma (see Fig. 13–32), serous adenocarcinoma, secretory carcinoma, and endometrioid carcinoma with focal clear-cell change have to be considered. It is important not to mistake the last two for the first two, because of differences in prognosis (see Table 13–7). Secretory carcinoma can be distinguished from clear-cell carcinoma and serous adenocarcinoma by (1) the predominant glandular pattern, (2) columnar cells with subnuclear vacuoles, and (3) low nuclear grade[40] (Fig. 13–33). Endometrioid carcinoma with focal clear-cell change can be recognized by the presence of typical endometrioid carcinoma in other areas (see Fig. 13–29).

Mucinous carcinomas of the endometrium are particularly problematic, because they can be difficult to distinguish from endocervical carcinoma and mucinous metaplasia, particularly in curettage specimens. Features favoring a diagnosis of mucinous carcinoma over mucinous metaplasia are (1) epithelial pseudostratification with loss of polarity, (2) areas with nuclear atypia (often subtle), and (3) architectural abnormalities such as glandular crowding, branching, and complex epithelial structures.[90] If uncertain about the nature of a florid mucinous glandular proliferation, particularly in postmenopausal women, hysterectomy is indicated to exclude mucinous

Table 13–7. **Subtypes of Endometrial Carcinoma**

Subtypes with No Proven Prognostic Implication

Endometrioid adenocarcinoma
Variants of endometrioid adenocarcinoma:
   villoglandular
   with squamous differentiation
   with argyrophilic cells
   with ciliated cells (ciliated adenocarcinoma)
   with secretory changes (secretory adenocarcinoma)
Mucinous adenocarcinoma

Subtypes with Worse Prognosis Compared with Endometrioid Adenocarcinoma

Endometrioid carcinoma with trophoblastic differentiation
Endometrioid carcinoma with component of giant cell carcinoma
Serous papillary adenocarcinoma
Clear-cell adenocarcinoma
Pure squamous cell carcinoma
Glassy cell carcinoma
Undifferentiated carcinoma
Small-cell carcinoma

"Mixed" if > 10% of tumor is composed of a second cell type.

(*Text continued on page 488*)

Table 13–8. **Histologic Subtypes of Endometrial Carcinoma**

Histologic Subtype	Frequency and Distinctive Clinical Features	Salient Histologic Features	Prognostic Implications
Endometrioid adenocarcinoma[40, 66, 67]	Commonest (80%). Mean age, 60 years.	Simple, complex, or cribriform glands and occasional papillae, lined by pseudostratified columnar cells with smooth luminal contour. Mucin, if present, is often confined to luminal borders. Focal clear-cell change can occur. Foamy stromal cells common, especially better differentiated tumors.	75% of cases have clinical stage I disease at presentation, and 10% clinical stage II. Crude 5-year survival 70% overall (85% for clinical stage I disease).
Serous papillary adenocarcinoma[68–79]	1.1% to 10%. Older age (mean, 66 years). Less likely to have a history of estrogen use. Some cases arise in endometrial polyp or as late sequela of pelvic radiation.	Broad or narrow complex papillae covered by stratified, tufted epithelium, producing an undulating luminal surface. Irregular slit-like glands also common. Usually high nuclear grade, with macronucleoli and frequent mitoses. May have clear-cell areas. Necrosis and psammoma bodies common. Uninvolved endometrium often atrophic. *Differential diagnosis:* papillary syncytial metaplasia, villoglandular endometrioid carcinoma, clear-cell carcinoma.	Highly aggressive, with a mortality rate of 70%. Often deeply invasive, with lymphovascular permeation. Frequently presenting with high stage disease: 75% show extrauterine spread on pathologic staging. 50% of surgical stage I patients develop recurrence despite use of adjuvant radiotherapy. Presence of myometrial invasion is correlated with a significant risk of recurrence compared with those without, but relapse can develop in the absence of myometrial invasion or for tumors confined to endometrial polyp.
Clear-cell adenocarcinoma[69, 70, 80–87]	1% to 6.6%. Slightly older (mean, 67 years). Clinical and histologic overlap with serous papillary carcinoma.	Tubulocystic, papillary, and/or solid growth; stromal hyalinization. Large polygonal cells with clear glycogen-rich cytoplasm and eccentric nuclei; hobnail cells; attenuated cells; and occasional oxyphilic cells. Nuclei often pleomorphic. Intraluminal mucin and intracytoplasmic mucin common. *Differential diagnosis:* secretory adenocarcinoma, Arias-Stella reaction, serous adenocarcinoma.	Aggressive. One third of cases present with pathologic stage III-IV disease. The reported 5-year survival is 34% to 75%, depending on the proportion of cases with stage I disease.
Mucinous adenocarcinoma[88–92]	1% to 9%. The rare microglandular variant occurs in postmenopausal women who may be taking sex hormones.	Adenocarcinoma with >50% columnar cells rich in cytoplasmic mucin. May show glandular, villoglandular, villous, cribriform, or cystic pattern. Nuclei usually bland-looking; nuclear pseudostratification or atypia is often focal. The microglandular variant is characterized by small glandular spaces and eosinophilic mucinous secretion; neutrophils are found in the lumina and stroma.	Almost all cases have tumor confined to the uterus at presentation. Behavior no different from endometrioid adenocarcinoma.

Table 13–8. **Histologic Subtypes of Endometrial Carcinoma** (*Continued*)

Histologic Subtype	Frequency and Distinctive Clinical Features	Salient Histologic Features	Prognostic Implications
		Differential diagnosis: mucinous metaplasia, endocervical adenocarcinoma, microglandular hyperplasia of cervix.	
Pure squamous cell carcinoma[40, 93–97]	Rare. Some cases associated with cervical stenosis, pyometra, and endometrial squamous metaplasia.	Invasive squamous cell carcinoma in the absence of the following: glandular component, contiguity with cervical squamous epithelium, invasive cervical squamous carcinoma, and connection with *in situ* cervical squamous carcinoma if present. The tumor can be very well differentiated.	Poor prognosis, with 40% of pathologic stage I patients dying of disease within 3 years. Prognosis of the very rare verrucous carcinoma remains to be clarified.[98, 99]
Undifferentiated carcinoma[70, 100]	1.6%. Usually older age (mean, 66 years).	Sheets of large polygonal or spindly cells with pleomorphic nuclei, and no evidence of differentiation. May require immunohistochemistry to confirm its epithelial nature.	Aggressive. Often deeply invasive, with lymphovascular permeation and extrauterine spread. 5-year survival 54% according to one study, and 20% according to another smaller series.
Small-cell carcinoma[100–104a]	Rare. Usually elderly. Tends to spread to lymph nodes and other sites.	Morphologically identical to small-cell carcinoma of other sites; sheets and ribbons of small cells, which often exhibit argyrophilia and ultrastructurally dense-core granules. Sometimes associated with a component of adenocarcinoma, squamous carcinoma, adenosquamous carcinoma, or malignant mixed mullerian tumor. Mimicker: menstrual endometrium with crumbled stroma.	Most cases behave aggressively (median survival, 12 months), although some long-term survivals have also been reported.
Glassy cell carcinoma[105–108]	Rare. No specific clinical features. Variant of adenosquamous carcinoma?	A poorly differentiated neoplasm showing little or no glandular or squamous differentiation. Sheets of polygonal cells with well-defined borders, and granular eosinophilic to amphophilic cytoplasm. Often admixed with abundant inflammatory cells.	Aggressive.

Table 13–9. **Morphologic Variants of Endometrioid Adenocarcinoma of the Uterine Corpus**

Variant	Frequency and Clinical Relevance	Salient Histologic Features
Presence of argyrophilic cells[109–111]	Common finding, especially well-differentiated tumors, but no documented endocrine manifestations.	Variable number of endocrine cells (demonstrated by argyrophilic reaction, immunostaining for chromogranin, or ultrastructural studies) found in otherwise typical endometrioid carcinoma.
Ciliated adenocarcinoma[112, 113]	Rare; more commonly seen in postmenopausal women on estrogen therapy.	Typical endometrioid carcinoma with many ciliated cells. Sometimes growing in sheets punctuated by small lumina, producing a cribriform appearance. Eosinophilic cytoplasm. Low nuclear grade.
Secretory adenocarcinoma[80, 114]	Rare. The secretory change is sometimes attributable to endogenous or exogenous progestogen.	Well-differentiated endometrioid adenocarcinoma with supranuclear and/or subnuclear vacuoles (containing glycogen). Must be distinguished from clear-cell carcinoma.
Villoglandular (papillary) variant*[74, 115, 116]	Rare	A significant component of papillae with delicate fibrovascular cores, but typical endometrioid glands can usually be identified in areas. Must be distinguished from serous adenocarcinoma.
Sex cord–like[117–119]	Very rare	Narrow or solid tubules resembling Sertoli tubules, or cribriform structures resembling Call-Exner bodies.
With squamous differentiation†[48, 120–123]	Common	Endometrioid adenocarcinoma with a squamous component, defined by (1) keratinization, (2) intercellular bridges, or (3) ≥ 3 of the following criteria: sheet-like growth without gland formation or palisading; distinct cell borders; eosinophilic and thick cytoplasm; decreased nuclear-cytoplasmic ratio compared with other foci. The squamous component can assume a spindle cell growth pattern. Traditionally, "adenoacanthoma" refers to adenocarcinomas containing benign-appearing non-invasive squamous elements, and "adenosquamous carcinoma" to those with cytologically malignant, invasive squamous carcinoma. There are, however, cases with intermediate features.
With trophoblastic differentiation‡[124, 125]	Very rare. Often with raised serum human chorionic gonadotropin (hCG) level.	Foci made up of trophoblastic cells (syncytiotrophoblasts), which may assume a choriocarcinomatous pattern.
With giant cell carcinoma‡[126]	Very rare	Foci made up of sheets of large mononuclear or multinucleated epithelial cells with bizarre nuclei. May have a prominent inflammatory infiltrate.

* A recent study suggests that as a group villoglandular endometrioid adenocarcinoma behaves no differently from conventional endometrioid adenocarcinoma, but invasive carcinomas with papillary differentiation in the myometrium are more aggressive than those without.[138a] This finding requires confirmation.

† Although as a group, adenosquamous carcinoma is more aggressive than adenoacanthoma, this is attributable to the higher grade of the tumor (glandular component) in the former.[127–129] The grade of the squamous component generally parallels that of the glandular component. Some studies suggest that low-grade endometrioid adenocarcinoma with squamous differentiation (adenoacanthoma) is associated with a better survival than comparable grade tumor without squamous differentiation.[121, 123, 128–131]

‡ These variants are highly aggressive compared with conventional endometrioid adenocarcinomas of comparable grade.

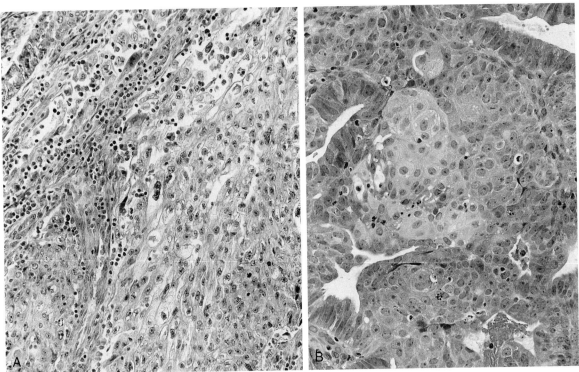

FIGURE 13–26. Endometrioid Adenocarcinoma with Squamous Differentiation. *A,* High-grade (so-called adenosquamous carcinoma). Most of the tumor is formed by polygonal and spindly squamous cells with distinct cell borders and moderate nuclear pleomorphism. The glandular component is evident in the left upper field. *B,* Grade 1 (so-called adenoacanthoma). The squamous component is formed by polygonal cells with bland-looking nuclei.

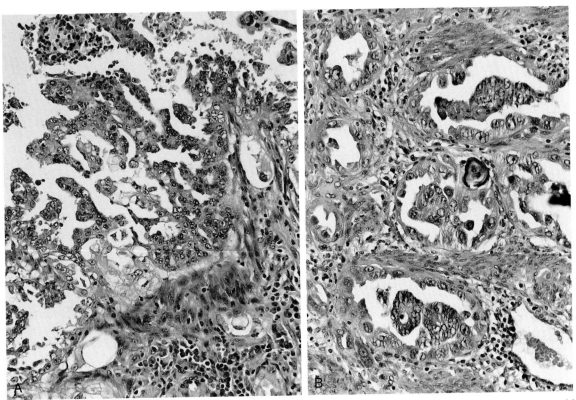

FIGURE 13–27. Serous Papillary Adenocarcinoma. *A,* Papillary tufts are characteristically formed by stratified cells, resulting in an undulating surface. There is significant nuclear pleomorphism. *B,* Papillary tufts are also formed within glands. Note the psammoma body in the central field.

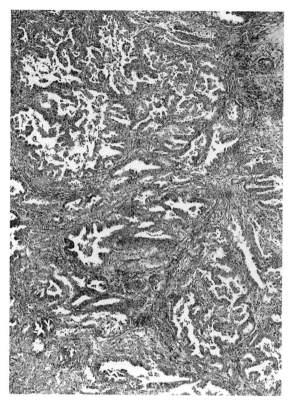

FIGURE 13–28. Serous Papillary Adenocarcinoma. Characteristic growth pattern in the form of irregular complex tubulopapillary glands with narrow cleft-like lumina.

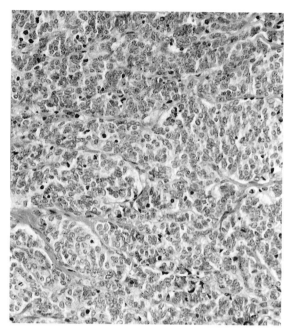

FIGURE 13–30. Small-cell Carcinoma of the Endometrium. The packets of small cells show nuclear molding in areas.

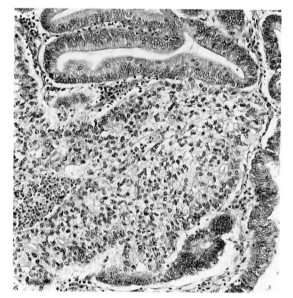

FIGURE 13–29. Endometrioid Adenocarcinoma with Clear-cell Change in the More Solid Foci. Note the characteristic endometrioid appearances of the glandular component.

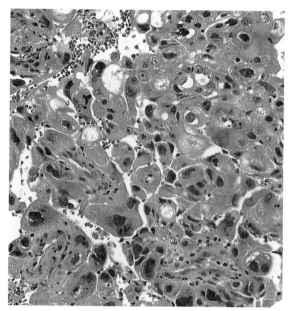

FIGURE 13–31. Giant-cell Carcinoma of the Endometrium. The tumor is composed of very large cells with bizarre nuclei.

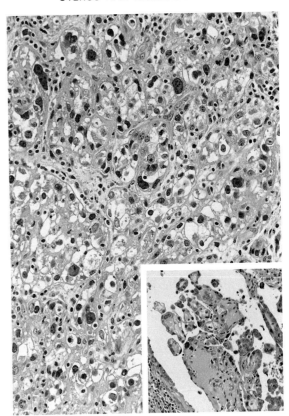

FIGURE 13–32. Clear-cell Carcinoma of the Endometrium. Solid growth comprising polygonal cells with clear cytoplasm. *Inset,* Papillae with hyalinized cores; the cells lining the glands and papillae usually do not have clear cytoplasm.

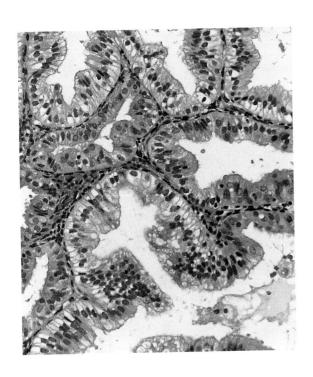

FIGURE 13–33. Endometrioid Adenocarcinoma with Secretory Change (So-called Secretory Carcinoma). Note the subnuclear vacuoles.

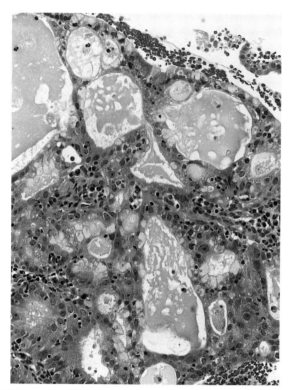

FIGURE 13–34. Mucinous Adenocarcinoma of Endometrium Mimicking Microglandular Hyperplasia. Note the complex small glands with infiltration by neutrophils.

In the previous version (1971) of FIGO grading, in which only architecture is taken into consideration, there is good reproducibility as well as predictability of survival probabilities,[67, 133, 134] with 10-year survival figures for grades 1, 2, and 3 tumors being 78.3%, 61.0%, and 46.2%, respectively.[67] The frequency of lymph node metastasis is also correlated with the histologic grade.[135, 136] In pathologic stage I tumors, grade 3 histology has been shown to be the most accurate predictor of recurrence.[134] The incorporation of the nuclear grade into the revised FIGO grading is based on the demonstration in some studies that the survival is correlated better with the nuclear grade or combined nuclear-architectural grade.[130, 137, 138] Although a large study fails to confirm the value of the new FIGO grading system,[138a] a recent study supports the utility of this system.[138b]

Extent of Disease

Unlike the previously employed clinical staging system, the current recommendation is that the staging should be based on *both surgical and pathologic findings* (Table 13–10). This is a more accurate reflection of the extent of tumor, because more extensive disease is sometimes found on staging of patients with apparently localized (clinical stage I) disease. In reading of reports in the literature, it is most important to ascertain whether the authors are referring to the clinical stage or pathologic stage.

carcinoma. The **microglandular variant** of mucinous carcinoma can be mistaken for microglandular hyperplasia of the cervix, especially in curettage specimens[90] (Fig. 13–34). Its malignant nature is betrayed by the nuclear atypia, which can be subtle and focal.

What is the Histologic Grade?

The revised International Federation of Gynecology and Obstetrics (FIGO) system is predominantly an architectural grading system, but nuclear features are also taken into consideration:[132]

Grade 1—Solid growth ≤5% (see Fig. 13–22)
Grade 2—Solid growth 6% to 50%
Grade 3—Solid growth >50% (Fig. 13–35)

In application of the criteria, a number of rules have to be observed:

1. Areas of morule or squamous differentiation are not counted as solid foci. In such cases, the grading should be performed on the glandular component (see Figs. 13–26*B* and 13–35).

2. Significant nuclear atypia, inappropriate for the architectural grade, raises the grade of a grade 1 or 2 tumor by one (see Fig. 13–21).

3. For serous adenocarcinoma, clear-cell adenocarcinoma, and pure squamous cell carcinoma, nuclear grading should be used instead. Grade 1 tumor shows mild nuclear atypia, even chromatin and inconspicuous nucleoli, whereas grade 3 tumor shows significant nuclear atypia and pleomorphism, with enlarged nucleoli and frequent mitoses.[130]

4. For a mixed carcinoma, a grade should be assigned to each component.

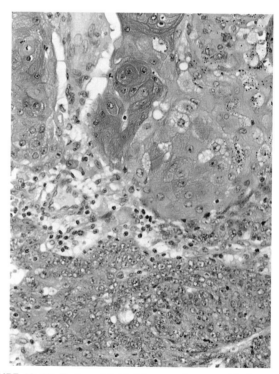

FIGURE 13–35. Endometrioid Adenocarcinoma with Squamous Differentiation, Grade 3. The upper field shows definite squamous differentiation in the form of intercellular bridges and keratohyaline granules; this component should not be counted as "solid growth" for grading purposes. Most of the tumor looks like the lower field, being formed by sheets of tumor cells with scarcely any glandular element. Thus, this tumor qualifies for a grade 3 tumor.

Table 13–10. **FIGO Staging (1988) for Endometrial Carcinoma**

I Tumor confined to uterine corpus
   IA-Tumor limited to endometrium
   IB-Invasion to <1/2 myometrium
   IC-Invasion to >1/2 myometrium

II Presence of cervical involvement
   IIA-Endocervical glandular involvement only
   IIB-Cervical stromal invasion

IIIA Tumor invades serosa and/or adnexa and/or positive peritoneal cytology
IIIB Metastasis to pelvic and/or para-aortic lymph nodes

IVA Tumor invasion of bladder and/or bowel mucosa
IVB Distant metastasis including intra-abdominal and/or inguinal lymph nodes

Depth of Myometrial Invasion

The level of deepest invasion by the endometrial carcinoma has a significant bearing on the prognosis. The mortality rates for intraendometrial carcinoma (stage IA), tumor confined to the inner half of myometrium (stage IB), and tumor with invasion of the outer half of myometrium (stage IC) are 4%, 15%, and 33%, respectively.[137, 138] Some previous studies have categorized tumors as showing invasion of the inner third, middle third, and outer third of the myometrium and have shown similar correlation with mortality.[130] Those with involvement of the serosa are associated with an even worse prognosis.[67, 139] Because deep myometrial invasion is correlated with a higher frequency of vascular invasion and lymph node metastasis,[134–136, 140] some studies have questioned whether the depth of invasion *per se* is an independent prognostic factor.[139, 141]

There may be difficulties in determining the *depth of invasion* if the original endomyometrial junction cannot be properly identified as a result of extensive replacement of the endometrium by tumor or failure to sample the interface with normal tissue (Fig. 13–36). It is helpful to measure the deepest point of invasion from the endomyometrial junction, as well as the *thickness of uninvolved myometrium.* The value of the latter measurement is that tumors reaching to a short distance from the serosa (< 5 mm) are associated with a worse prognosis, irrespective of what proportion of the myometrial wall is involved[142, 143] (Fig. 13–37).

The *invasive fronts* in the myometrium may be pushing or infiltrative (Figs. 13–21 and 13–38). They are accompanied by a desmoplastic reaction (see Fig. 13–21) or no stromal response at all, with the latter causing considerable problems in deciding whether a certain glandular unit is invasive or not (Figs. 13–38 and 13–39).[144] The problem is compounded by the normal irregularity of the endomyometrial junction, which is often accentuated when the endometrium is replaced by tumor. Identification of some residual benign glands and endometrial stroma at the interface between the deep portion of the tumor and the myometrium indicates that there is no myometrial invasion at that focus (Fig. 13–40). If the deep front of the rest of the carcinoma is more or less at this anatomic level, it can be assumed that the carcinoma is confined to the endometrium (see Fig. 13–40A). That is, if there are uncertainties as to whether the tumor has shown superficial myometrial invasion, the tumor can be considered to be intraendometrial, because the prognosis is not different (Figs. 13–36 and 13–41).

Sometimes *carcinoma may extend into islands of adenomyosis* in an *in situ* fashion, which should not be mistaken for myometrial invasion, because the prognosis is identical to intraendometrial carcinoma.[145–147] Features favoring such a process are

1. Smooth-contoured foci without stromal reaction
2. Presence of endometrial stromal cells around the glandular units
3. Presence of benign glands among the neoplastic glands (Fig. 13–42)
4. Presence of typical adenomyosis islands elsewhere

Adenomyotic islands with loss of stroma (usually in postmenopausal women) must not be mistaken for invasive

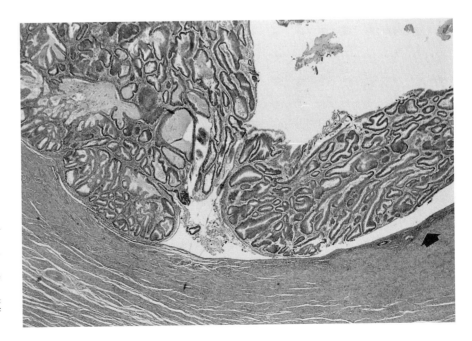

FIGURE 13–36. Endometrial Adenocarcinoma in a Hysterectomy Specimen. The tumor has extensively replaced the endometrium, but it can be recognized as being purely intraendometrial because it does not extend below the level of the residual endometrium *(arrow).* This illustrates the importance of inclusion of the normal endomyometrial junction in histologic sampling for purposes of assessment of depth of invasion.

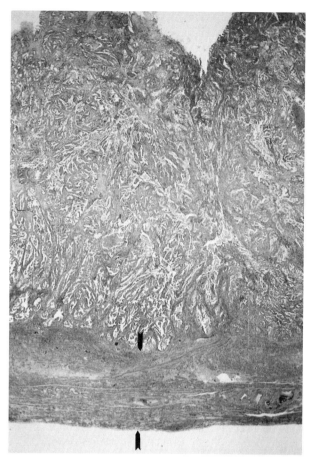

FIGURE 13–37. Endometrial Adenocarcinoma in a Hysterectomy Specimen. This tumor is deeply invasive, with only a thin layer of uninvolved myometrium (indicated between *arrowheads*). The original endomyometrial junction is difficult to discern.

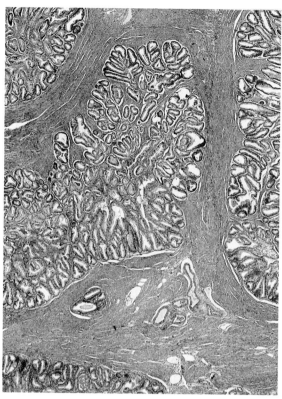

FIGURE 13–38. Endometrial Adenocarcinoma in a Hysterectomy Specimen. In this example, the tumor invades in the form of broad fronts, in the absence of a desmoplastic reaction.

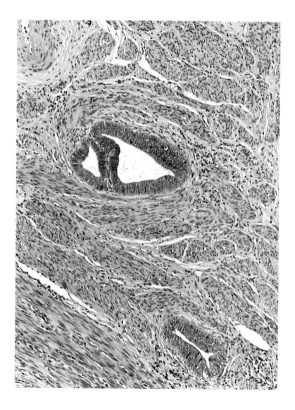

FIGURE 13–39. Endometrial Adenocarcinoma. It invades the myometrium in the form of isolated glands, unaccompanied by a stromal reaction.

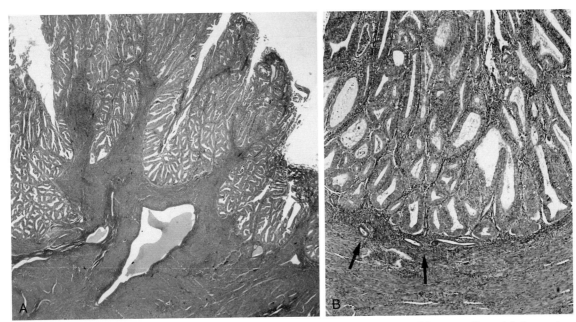

FIGURE 13–40. Endometrial Adenocarcinoma in a Hysterectomy Specimen. *A,* Exaggeration of the normally undulating endomyometrial junction renders it difficult to assess whether superficial myometrial invasion has occurred. *B,* The presence of residual endometrial glands and stroma *(arrows)* at the interface between the tumor and the myometrium indicates that myometrial invasion has not occurred.

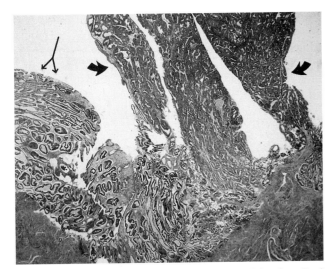

FIGURE 13–41. Endometrial Adenocarcinoma Arising in a Background of Atypical Hyperplasia. The carcinomatous component is on the right and indicated by curved arrows. The background endometrium *(double-head arrow)* shows atypical hyperplasia.

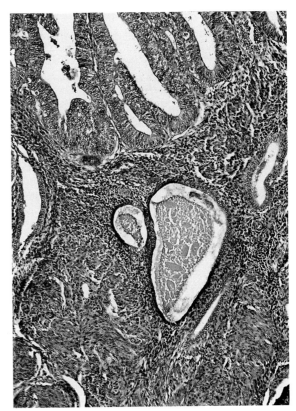

FIGURE 13–42. Endometrial Adenocarcinoma Showing Involvement of an Island of Adenomyosis. This should not be considered myometrial invasion.

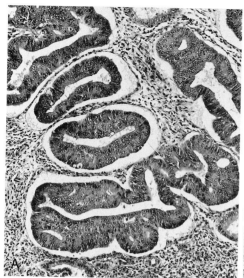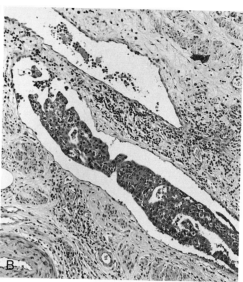

FIGURE 13–43. Endometrial Adenocarcinoma. *A,* Retraction clefts mimicking lymphovascular invasion. *B,* Lymphovascular permeation by serous adenocarcinoma. The space is fully endothelialized. Note also the characteristic lymphoid infiltrate around.

carcinoma within the myometrium; they can be recognized by their atrophic appearance.

Lymphovascular Invasion

Lymphovascular invasion has been shown to be an independent unfavorable prognostic factor.[67, 138, 140, 148–151] This phenomenon is more frequent in high-stage tumor, serous adenocarcinoma, and tumors with adverse prognostic factors. The 5-year survival rates for stage I tumor with and without lymphovascular invasion are 33% to 40% and 94% to 100%, respectively.[138, 149]

It is important not to mistake retraction artifactual spaces around tumor islands as lymphovascular spaces (Fig. 13–43A). To qualify for the latter, there should be a complete endothelial lining around the space; another helpful feature is the frequent presence of a lymphocytic cuff around the involved lymphovascular spaces[140] (Fig. 13–43B). If in doubt, confirmation can be obtained by immunostaining with endothelial markers.[140]

Involvement of the Cervix and Isthmus

The presence of *cervical involvement* worsens the prognosis. The 5-year survival of clinical stage II disease is 52% as compared with 75% for stage I disease.[40] This is at least partly attributable to the associated higher incidence of lymph node involvement (35.5% for clinical stage II versus 10.6% for clinical stage I).[152] Many but not all studies have shown that stage IIB tumor is associated with a much worse prognosis than stage IIA tumor (5-year survival approximately 50% and 80%, respectively).[134, 153–156]

The presence or absence of cervical involvement is best evaluated in hysterectomy specimens. However, endocervical curetting is sometimes performed for preoperative staging purposes. Such specimens cause considerable problems in assessment because of potential artifactual contamination by tumor from the endometrial cavity.[157–160]

Interpretation of endocervical curettings is as follows:

A potential pitfall is mistaking endometrioid metaplasia of endocervical gland for involvement by endometrial carci-

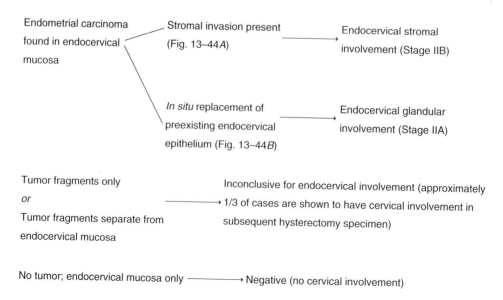

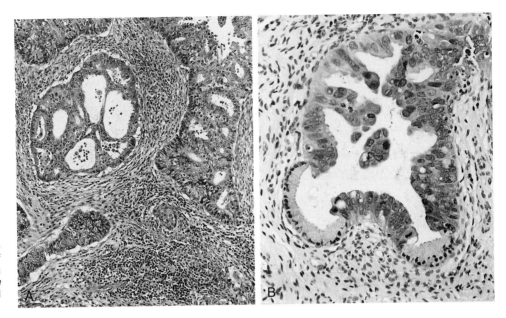

FIGURE 13–44. Endometrial Adenocarcinoma Involving the Cervix. *A,* Invasion of the stroma of the endocervix, associated with desmoplastic reaction. *B, In situ* involvement of an endocervical gland.

noma. The former can be distinguished from the latter by the contour and location conforming to those of normal endocervical glands and the lack of cellular atypia. Similarly, endometriosis of the cervix can be recognized by the presence of endometrial stroma.

A peculiar form of ''cervical implantation metastasis'' has been described by Fanning et al.;[161] the outcome is comparable to that without cervical involvement. It is believed to result from implantation of the endometrial tumor on the denuded endocervix after fractional curettage. The criteria for diagnosis are (1) tumor embedded in the superficial endocervical mucosa and surrounded by granulation tissue and inflammatory cells, (2) tumor in the cervix histologically identical to the uterine corpus tumor, (3) tumor separate from endometrial tumor with no evidence of direct extension, and (4) tumor surrounded by non-neoplastic endocervical glands with no transition between the two.

Because *tumors involving or arising within the lower uterine segment (isthmus)* have prognosis similar to those showing cervical involvement (stage II disease),[135, 162, 163] the isthmic portion of the uterine corpus must be sampled for histologic examination.

Ovarian (Adnexal) Involvement

When there is *simultaneous involvement of the uterine corpus and ovary,* it is difficult to ascertain which is the primary site or whether both are primary tumors. The following chart shows the features that are helpful for distinction of these possibilities.[164–166]

The prognosis of double primary tumors (consistent with two stage I neoplasms) is much better than that of endometrial carcinoma with ovarian metastasis.[164–166] In both situations, atypical hyperplasia is commonly found in the uninvolved endometrium. The possibility of an ovarian primary with uterine metastasis is much less frequent; in such a situation, the ovarian tumor is large, the tumor usually invades the corpus from the serosal side, and there is usually no atypical hyperplasia in the uninvolved endometrium. However, in some cases, a definite conclusion cannot be reached.

Keratin granulomas on the surfaces of the ovary can cause problems in histologic interpretation.[167, 168] Keratin and ghost squamous cells, presumably extruded from the squamous element of endometrial carcinoma through the fallopian tube onto the pelvic serosal surface, are surrounded by histiocytes

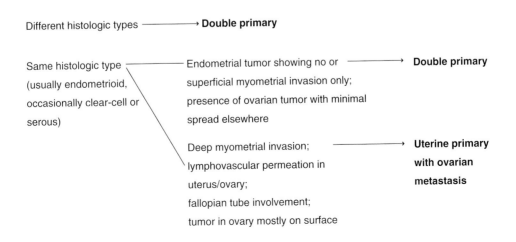

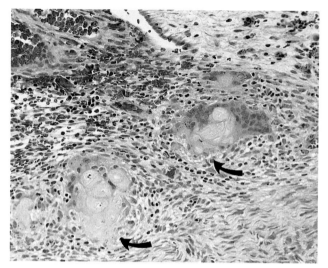

FIGURE 13–45. Keratin Granuloma in Ovary. Ghost squamous cells *(arrows)* are surrounded by histiocytes and multinucleated giant cells.

and foreign body giant cells (Fig. 13–45). The prognosis of cases showing ovarian keratin granulomas is similar to those without ovarian involvement by tumor.[167, 168] Therefore, keratin granuloma should not be considered evidence of ovarian involvement, provided that extensive sampling fails to reveal viable tumor in the ovary. **Endometriosis,** which may exhibit some degree of nuclear atypia, should also not be mistaken for ovarian involvement by tumor. It can be recognized by the associated endometrial-type stroma and frequent presence of siderophages.

Lymph Node Status

Lymph node involvement can occur even in patients with clinical stage I disease (11%).[135] In fact, it has been shown to be one of the most significant adverse prognostic factors.[156] According to one study of clinical stage I endometrial carcinoma, the recurrence rates for tumors with and without lymph node metastases are 47.6% (higher for positive para-aortic than pelvic nodes) and 8.3%, respectively; the 5-year survival rates for these two groups are 54% and 90%, respectively. Therefore, *all* lymph nodes sampled at laparotomy must be examined histologically. Histologic recognition of lymph node metastasis is easy, the only potential mimicker being benign mullerian inclusions (presence of cilia, no cellular atypia, and no desmoplastic reaction).

Peritoneal Washing Cytology

Many[137, 139, 169–171] but not all[172, 173] studies have shown positive findings in peritoneal washings of clinical or pathologic stage I patients to be an independent adverse prognostic factor, with increased risk of tumor recurrence.

Positive results are indicated by the presence of three-dimensional acinar or papillary aggregates with definite nuclear atypia (such as variation in nuclear size and nucleolar prominence). Potential mimickers are reactive mesothelial cells and endosalpingosis/endometriosis.[174] In the former, the cellular sheets are often more monolayered, "windows"

(clefts) are typically found between individual cells, and there is no significant nuclear atypia. In the latter, although cell clusters are formed, the constituent cells have regular nuclei and fine chromatin.

Status of the Adjacent Endometrium

Because presence of endometrial hyperplasia in the adjacent endometrium is a favorable prognostic factor,[175, 176] this feature should be recorded (see Fig. 13–41). In fact, it has been suggested that there are two histogenetically different types of endometrial carcinoma:[177]

1. Estrogen-related (35% of cases): Clinical features of hyperestrinism (such as anovulatory bleeding and infertility); more common in premenopausal women; occurrence of tumor in a background of endometrial hyperplasia; carcinoma often low-grade and only superficially invasive; good prognosis.

2. Non–estrogen-related (65% of cases): No features of hyperestrinism; predominantly in postmenopausal women; uninvolved endometrium atrophic; carcinoma usually high-grade and deeply invasive; poor prognosis.

Other Special Parameters of Prognostic Importance

Hormone Receptor Status

Tumors that are rich in estrogen receptor and/or progesterone receptor have been shown to be associated with a more favorable prognosis.[178–191] Although receptor-rich tumors are usually of endometrioid type, low-grade, low-stage, and not deeply invasive, some studies have shown the hormone receptor status to be an independent prognostic factor.[148, 180, 181, 184, 192] Hormone receptor-negativity may identify subgroups of stage I, grade 1 carcinomas with adverse outcome.[148] The recent availability of reliable monoclonal antibodies reactive in paraffin sections should permit more widespread provision of this parameter to clinicians, who may consider using progestational therapy for adjuvant or treatment purposes.

DNA Ploidy

Most studies have shown aneuploid carcinomas to be more aggressive than diploid ones.[193–201] DNA ploidy has been shown by multivariate analysis in some studies to be one of the best predictors of prognosis.[197–199]

Proliferative Fraction

A high proliferative fraction, as reflected by a high S-phase fraction on flow cytometric analysis, has been shown by some studies to correlate with an unfavorable prognosis.[195, 202]

Oncogene Expression

Some studies have shown *erbB*-2 expression, c-*myc* amplification, K-*ras* mutation, *fms* overexpression, and p53 overexpression/mutation to be associated with a worse prognosis.[203–209]

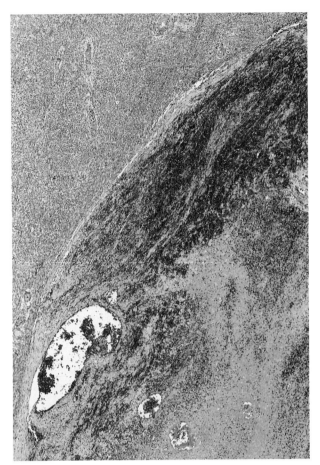

FIGURE 13–46. Apoplectic Leiomyoma. Extensive areas within this benign tumor removed from a pregnant patient show necrosis and hemorrhage.

PURE MESENCHYMAL TUMORS OF THE UTERUS

Diagnostic Clues From Gross Examination

Some mesenchymal tumors of the uterus possess characteristic macroscopic features that permit an almost definitive diagnosis to be made on gross examination alone. Uterine mesenchymal tumors usually arise primarily in the myometrium as mass lesions, but they may also arise primarily in the endometrium, where they often appear polypoid.[210, 211] Circumscribed tumors are usually benign, whereas infiltrative ones are usually malignant, but there can be exceptions.

A circumscribed nodule in the myometrium with or without endometrial involvement may represent a leiomyoma (commonest), endometrial stromal nodule, low-grade endometrial stromal sarcoma, leiomyosarcoma, adenomatoid tumor, or inflammatory pseudotumor.[210, 212–216] The main distinguishing feature is the consistency of the tumor. Leiomyomas are characteristically white, firm, and show a uniform, trabeculated, whorled cut surface, although adenomatoid tumor, inflammatory pseudotumor, and rare leiomyosarcomas may show this appearance. *Any myometrial tumor that deviates from this classic ''fibroid'' appearance warrants thorough sampling to exclude malignancy (at least 1 block per centimeter diameter*

of the tumor). Endometrial stromal tumor and leiomyosarcoma usually show tan, fleshy, bulging cut surfaces with a softer consistency, but some leiomyoma variants (such as cellular and epithelioid types) may have this appearance as well. Although the presence of necrosis and hemorrhage should certainly raise a concern for malignancy, these features can be observed in leiomyomas during pregnancy (red degeneration/ apoplectic leiomyoma)[217] (Fig. 13–46) and associated with hormone usage (oral contraceptives/gonadotropin releasing hormone agonist).[218–220] (Fig. 13–46) Tumors with a gelatinous consistency must be extensively sampled to exclude myxoid leiomyosarcoma (which can appear deceptively circumscribed[221]).

An infiltrative growth in the myometrium is likely to represent a sarcoma, and sometimes adenomatoid tumor, infiltrative leiomyoma, or intravenous leiomyomatosis. The sarcomas are usually fleshy, with or without necrosis and hemorrhage. Low-grade endometrial stromal sarcoma shows serpiginous growth in the periphery, producing the characteristic ''bag of worms'' appearance[210, 211] (Fig. 13–47). In intravenous leiomyomatosis, the myometrial, uterine adnexal, pelvic, or systemic venous channels may be converted into firm, nodular, or cord-like structures by the intravascular extension,[222–225] and the cut surfaces of the involved vessels show occluding plugs of whitish tumor.

Approach to Histologic Growth Patterns

The growth patterns of the uterine mesenchymal tumors are varied, and more than one growth pattern may be observed in a neoplasm (Table 13–11). For pure mesenchymal tumors, the line of differentiation taken up by the tumor cells is of utmost importance in the assessment of their malignant potential, because the *criteria of malignancy differ for smooth muscle and endometrial stromal neoplasms.*[226] Light microscopic examination remains unsurpassed in this aspect, although immunohistochemical and electron microscopic studies may serve as useful adjuncts in selected cases.

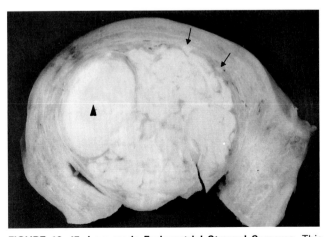

FIGURE 13–47. Low-grade Endometrial Stromal Sarcoma. This tumor is composed of a partly circumscribed oval growth in the myometrium *(arrowhead)* with closely packed serpiginous cords infiltrating the myometrium *(arrows).* Note the lack of the whorled pattern characteristic of leiomyomas.

Table 13–11. **Growth Patterns of Uterine Mesenchymal Tumors**

1. Spindle cell fascicles
2. Endometrial stroma-like
3. Epithelioid cell growth
4. Sex cord–like growth
5. Anaplastic
6. With heterologous elements (fat, cartilage, bone, skeletal muscle)
7. With endometrioid glands/tubules

Spindle cells arranged in sweeping fascicles are most commonly seen in smooth muscle tumors (Fig. 13–48) but may also be seen in some other sarcomas (including sarcomatous component of malignant mixed mullerian tumors and adenosarcomas), inflammatory pseudotumor, and postoperative spindle cell nodule.[227, 228] *Smooth muscle cells* typically possess an appreciable amount of eosinophilic fibrillary cytoplasm (see Fig. 13–48). Their nuclei are cigar-shaped with blunted ends. Sometimes the amount of cytoplasm is scanty and the nuclei appear ''naked'' and closely packed, mimicking endometrial stroma or the postmenopausal myometrium (Fig. 13–49). The myoid nature of such cells can be recognized by the presence of definite cellular fascicles (ovoid or elongated

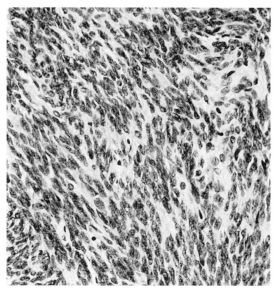

FIGURE 13–49. **Cellular Leiomyoma.** The nuclei of the tumor cells in this growth are closely packed and overlapping, owing to paucity of cytoplasm. Mitotic figures, however, are not found.

nuclei aligned in the same direction), lack of spiral arterioles, and transition with areas showing more typical smooth muscle differentiation. In poorly differentiated leiomyosarcomas in which myoid differentiation is not obvious, electron microscopy may be helpful. Immunohistochemical staining for muscle-specific actin and desmin is usually positive in smooth muscle cells and their neoplasms, but these markers cannot be utilized for distinction from endometrial stromal cells because the latter may show an identical immunophenotype.[229–233] Inflammatory pseudotumor and postoperative spindle cell nodule are predominated by myofibroblasts, the cytoplasm of which is more amphophilic. Squamous (morule) metaplasia may feature spindle cell proliferation, but it can be recognized by its intraglandular location and paucity of reticulin fibers.

Endometrial stromal differentiation is seen in endometrial stromal nodules and low-grade endometrial stromal sarcomas, although occasionally the growth pattern of these tumors may lack even remote resemblance to the normal endometrial stroma, that is, sex cord–like growth. Because the presence of endometrial stromal differentiation in a uterine sarcoma may signify progestogen-responsiveness and therefore influence the choice of treatment, strict morphologic criteria should be applied in its recognition. This requires the presence of two minimum diagnostic features: (*1*) *bland, closely packed stromal cells resembling those of proliferative endometrial stroma, and* (*2*) *regular ramifying spiral arterioles* (Fig. 13–50). The tumor cells usually possess dark-staining nuclei and scanty cytoplasm, although they can appear epithelioid or even foamy. Stromal hyalinization is common (Fig. 13–51A). Hemorrhage, calcification, decidual change, endometrial glands, and heterologous elements can rarely be seen in endometrial stromal tumors.[210, 216, 234–239] Rarely, the stromal cells assume a spindly pattern focally; these spindly cells are short, are often associated with increased collagen, and do not form well-defined intersecting fascicles (Fig. 13–51B). The interspersed spiral arterioles possess small lumina surrounded by pericytes and smooth muscle cells, which are best highlighted

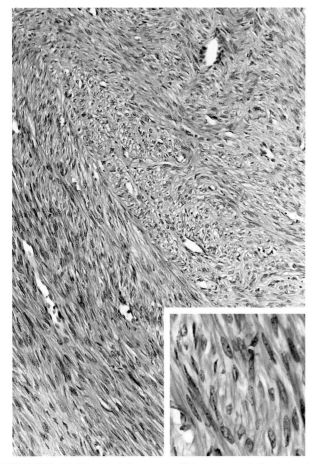

FIGURE 13–48. **Uterine Leiomyoma.** This normocellular tumor is composed of interlacing fascicles of spindle cells with bland elongated nuclei and abundant fibrillary cytoplasm (see *inset*).

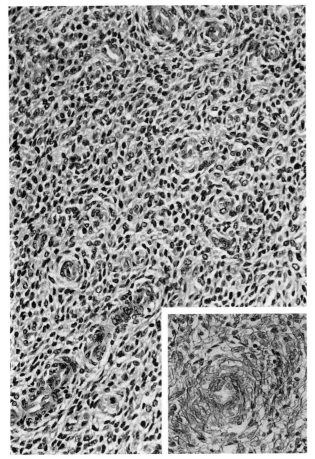

FIGURE 13–50. Low-grade Endometrial Stromal Sarcoma. The bland-looking small ovoid cells together with the spiral arterioles are highly reminiscent of the normal proliferative endometrial stroma. *Inset,* Reticulin fibers surround the pericytes/smooth muscle cells around the arterioles, as well as the individual tumor cells.

by reticulin stain or immunostaining for muscle-specific actin (see Fig. 13–50). They are often surrounded by concentric cuffs of stromal cells. Capillaries, hemangiopericytoma-like staghorn vessels or thick-walled vessels, although often found in typical examples of low-grade endometrial stromal sarcoma, should not be mistaken for the diagnostic arterioles. In fact, most reported examples of uterine ''hemangiopericytoma'' probably represent endometrial stromal sarcoma with prominent pericytomatous vascular channels.[240–242]

Smooth muscle tumors, and occasionally endometrial stromal tumors, may comprise polygonal cells with an appreciable amount of eosinophilic to clear cytoplasm (*epithelioid*) (Fig. 13–52A). The smooth muscle nature of a neoplasm can be recognized by the focal merging of epithelioid cells into typical spindly smooth muscle cells (Fig. 13–52B), and furthermore by immunoreactivity for myoid markers or ultrastructural studies.

Sex cord–like pattern refers to a pattern resembling granulosa cell and Sertoli-Leydig cell tumors[210, 237, 243–245] (Fig. 13–53), with ramifying cords, trabeculae, solid or narrow tubules, and solid nests. The designation ''uterine tumors resembling ovarian sex cord tumors'' has sometimes been applied to these tumors.[245, 246] However, we believe it is more appropriate to classify them as smooth muscle tumor or endometrial stromal nodule/sarcoma with sex cord–like growth if possible (see Fig. 13–53), reserving the term ''uterine tumor resembling ovarian sex cord tumors'' for those tumors lacking specific differentiation on thorough sampling. Although the cells in tumors exhibiting sex cord–like pattern are often epithelioid, this is not always the case (see Fig. 13–53). Thus, ''epithelioid'' feature (a cytologic description) and ''sex–cordlike'' growth (an architectural pattern) are not identical attributes, although they often coexist. Table 13–12 lists the various uterine tumors that may show a sex cord–like growth pattern.

Undifferentiated or anaplastic growth is seen in poorly differentiated leiomyosarcoma, high-grade uterine sarcoma (Fig. 13–54), the sarcomatous component of mixed mullerian

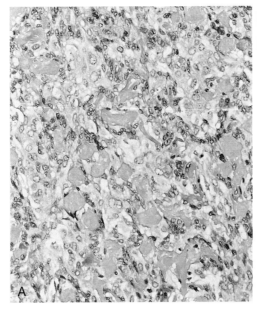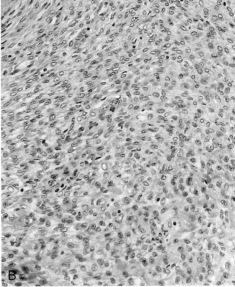

FIGURE 13–51. Low-grade Endometrial Stromal Sarcoma. *A,* Example with prominent hyalinization. *B,* In this example, the cells have slightly more cytoplasm. Focal spindly growth is also evident in the left upper field.

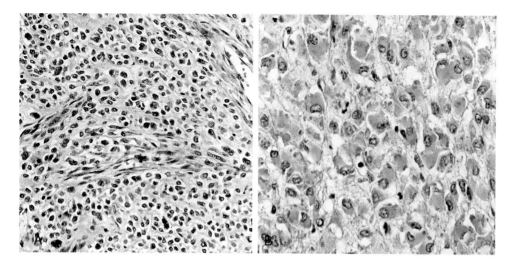

FIGURE 13–52. Epithelioid Leiomyoma (Leiomyoblastoma). *A,* The tumor cells are polygonal and possess abundant eosinophilic cytoplasm. Note absence of mitotic figures. *B,* The polygonal tumor cells blend with spindly cells with typical appearances of smooth muscle. Despite presence of mild nuclear pleomorphism, mitotic figures are not seen. Thus, this case still qualifies for a benign diagnosis.

tumors, and the rare primary sarcomas. The tumor cells are characteristically plump or ovoid and exhibit significant nuclear pleomorphism. In contrast to the sarcomatoid areas of high-grade endometrial carcinoma, these foci are often rich in reticulin fibers.

Heterologous mesenchymal elements can be found in a number of uterine mesenchymal and mixed tumors. Because malignant mixed mullerian tumor is far more common, thorough sampling for epithelial elements should be performed before a diagnosis of primary heterologous sarcoma of the uterus is made.

Rarely, endometrioid glands have been described in otherwise typical endometrial stromal neoplasms[210, 216, 234, 247] (Fig. 13–55). "Leiomyoma with tubules" probably represents a circumscribed adenomatoid tumor associated with a prominent reactive or neoplastic component of smooth muscle,[221, 248] since the tubules have been shown to be mesothelial.

Mitotic Count: Problems and How to Perform the Count

The mitotic count is one of the most important histologic parameters that aids in the distinction between benign and malignant mesenchymal or epithelial-mesenchymal neoplasms of the uterus. This is often expressed as the number of mitotic figures per 10 high-power fields (HPF). Doubts have been raised on the reproducibility and reliability of making mitotic counts, because of the great variabilities of the field size in different microscopes, problems in recognition of mitotic figures versus apoptotic nuclei, and the possible influence of delayed fixation on the mitotic count (with a decrease in the count).[249–257] In future studies, reporting the mitotic count as the number of mitotic figures per unit area (mm²) will perhaps facilitate more proper use of this parameter, because adjustments of the figure can be made according to the microscope used.

While performing mitotic count, it is important to adhere to the guidelines proposed by Kempson and Hendrickson, as follows:[226]

1. Specimens should be promptly and thoroughly fixed.
2. Adequate sampling for tumors other than the typical leiomyoma: at least one block per centimeter of tumor diameter.

3. Histologic sections no thicker than 5 μm.
4. Only convincing mitotic figures (in which at least some chromosome "twigs" are identifiable and in which the cell does not appear to be shrunken) should be counted (see Fig. 13–54). A lighter hematoxylin stain such as periodic acid-Schiff (PAS) preparation may facilitate the distinction from pyknotic nuclei.
5. Use ×40 objective, and ×10 or ×15 eyepiece.
6. Perform counts in areas with highest mitotic activity. Start from a field with a mitotic figure, then move to nine other consecutive fields to give the total count per 10 HPF.
7. Repeat three other sets, and take the highest number.

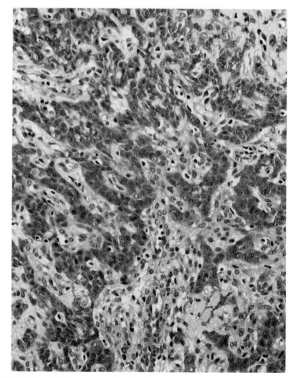

FIGURE 13–53. Low-grade Endometrial Stromal Sarcoma with Sex Cord–Like Growth. Polygonal cells grow in the form of anastomosing cords. Note merging of these larger cells into smaller endometrial-type stromal cells and the rich vasculature.

Table 13–12. **Uterine Tumors with "Sex Cord–Like" Growth**

1. Endometrial stromal nodule/low-grade endometrial stromal sarcoma
2. Smooth muscle tumor
3. Mullerian adenosarcoma
4. Plexiform tumorlet
5. Endometrioid adenocarcinoma with sex cord–like growth

"Uterine tumor resembling ovarian sex cord tumor" is a heterogeneous entity, including low-grade endometrial stromal sarcoma, smooth muscle tumor, and rarely endometrial stromal nodule. It is usually not highly invasive, and the overall prognosis is favorable.

Specific Diagnostic Problems

Criteria of Malignancy for Uterine Smooth Muscle Tumors

Having decided that a mesenchymal tumor shows smooth muscle differentiation, the next job is to determine its likely biologic behavior. Most smooth muscle tumors can be easily assigned to a benign (low cellularity, no atypia, no mitotic figures) or malignant (frankly invasive, significant cellular atypia, high mitotic count) category. However, the behavior of smooth muscle tumors is notoriously difficult to predict from the histologic appearances; some with bizarre cells can behave in a benign fashion, whereas some "bland-looking" tumors can metastasize. The mitotic index remains the most important predictor of outcome, although other histologic parameters should also be taken into consideration. Because the behavior of smooth muscle tumors spans a continuous spectrum, use of two categories (benign versus malignant) to describe them is bound to force tumors with very low risk of malignant behavior into the latter category in order to guarantee a favorable outcome in the former.[226] To partly rectify this situation, the diagnostic label "**smooth muscle tumor of uncertain malignant potential**" (**STUMP**) is applied to those tumors possessing features that have been associated with occasional but far from invariable aggressive behavior.[226] Experience with this group of tumors is limited, but the diagnostic label remains useful in indicating a definite, albeit very low, risk of recurrence and metastasis. Hysterectomy should constitute adequate treatment for such tumors, but if only myomectomy is performed, follow-up without hysterectomy may be justified for those opting to preserve fertility.

Leiomyosarcomas diagnosed on strict morphologic criteria are highly aggressive neoplasms, with survival figures of 15% to 25%.[226, 258–264] They show a high frequency of local recurrence and distant metastasis (especially intra-abdominal and lung). Histologic grading has not been proven useful in segregating groups with less aggressive behavior.

Three levels of stringency of mitotic counts are applied in the assessment of uterine smooth muscle tumors based on a number of architectural and cytologic features (Table 13–13).[226] In the first group, in which the *most lenient criteria* are applied, even tumors showing mitotic count beyond 15/10 HPF are classified as STUMP only. This level of stringency of mitotic count is *applicable only to smooth muscle tumors that show cellularity comparable to or lower than that of the surrounding normal myometrium, with no other*

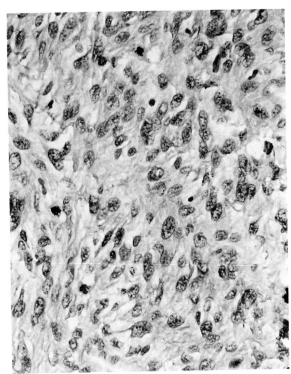

FIGURE 13–54. High-grade Uterine Sarcoma. The plump spindle tumor cells are pleomorphic and mitotically active.

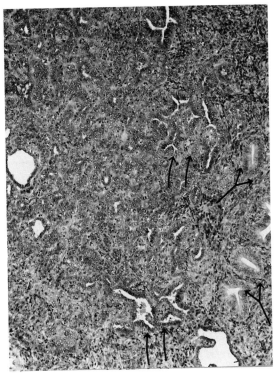

FIGURE 13–55. Low-grade Endometrial Stromal Sarcoma with Sex Cord–Like Growth and Endometrioid Glands. The residual endometrial glands are indicated by double-head arrows; the endometrioid glands, which constitute an integral component of the tumor, are indicated by curved arrows.

Table 13–13. **Assessment of Malignant Potential of the Smooth Muscle Tumors of the Uterine Corpus**

	Mitotic Count/10 HPF				
	0	2	5	10	15
Normocellular, no nuclear atypia	BENIGN				UNCERTAIN MALIGNANT POTENTIAL
Cellular tumor, minimal nuclear atypia *or* invasive margins *or* abnormal mitotic figures	BENIGN		UNCERTAIN MALIGNANT POTENTIAL	LEIOMYOSARCOMA	
Moderate to marked atypia *or* epithelioid morphology *or* intravascular growth *or* coagulative necrosis	BENIGN	UNCERTAIN MALIGNANT POTENTIAL	LEIOMYOSARCOMA		

Beware of myxoid smooth muscle tumors: cases with a low mitotic count should also be regarded as malignant if there is infiltrative growth or vascular invasion.

Modified from Kempson RL, Hendrickson MR: Pure mesenchymal neoplasms of the uterine corpus: Selected problems. Semin Diagn Pathol 5:172–198, 1988.

morphologic predictors of malignant behavior such as cellular atypia or infiltrative growth (Table 13–14)[221, 270–281] (see Fig. 13–48). No tumor in this group possesses a risk of malignant behavior that warrants an unequivocal label of leiomyosarcoma. *Tumors showing mitotic count between 5 and 15/10 HPF are labeled "leiomyomas with increased mitosis" or "**mitotically active leiomyomas**"; besides the mitotic figures, they look otherwise like the usual benign leiomyomas.*[265–269] Such tumors occur almost exclusively in the reproductive years and are associated with pregnancy, progestogen usage, or secretory phase of the menstrual cycle.

In the *intermediate group*, tumors showing mitotic count of 5 to 10/10 HPF are classified as STUMP, and those exceeding and below this range, leiomyosarcomas and leiomyomas, respectively. This level of stringency is *applied to smooth muscle tumors showing cellularity greater than that of the normal myometrium (see Fig. 13–49) and to those showing mild cellular atypia.* Also included in this group are tumors showing *infiltrative growth* and probably those with *abnormal mitotic figures*.

In the third group, in which the *most strict criteria* are applied, tumors showing mitotic count between 2 to 5/10 HPF are classified as STUMP, whereas those beyond this range are leiomyosarcomas. This group *includes tumors with moderate to marked cytologic atypia, epithelioid morphology, and intravascular growth, and also serosal smooth muscle tumors that have detached from the uterus and implanted on omentum, peritoneum, or pelvic wall ("parasitic")*[226, 282] (Figs. 13–52, 13–56, and 13–57). In one study, *coagulative tumor cell necrosis* is found to be the most powerful predictor of poor clinical outcome; thus, smooth muscle tumors showing this feature should also be placed in this group[283, 283a] (see Fig. 13–57A). Coagulative tumor cell necrosis is characterized by *abrupt* transition between necrotic cells and preserved cells. This phenomenon should be distinguished from hyalinizing necrosis, which is not uncommonly seen in benign smooth muscle neoplasms and characterized by a zone of collagen interposed between the dead cells and the preserved cells, reminiscent of organization of an infarct. The novel approach of designating the malignant potential of smooth muscle tumors based predominantly on presence or absence of coagulative necrosis is depicted in Table 13–15.[283a, 283b] **Bizarre leiomyoma** mimics leiomyosarcoma because of presence of highly atypical cells, but can be distinguished from it by the following features: bizarre cells are interspersed among nonatypical cells (whereas leiomyosarcoma usually exhibits generalized cellular atypia), low mitotic count, and lack of coagulative necrosis.

Table 13–14. **Growth Patterns and Cytologic Variants of Uterine Leiomyoma**[*221, 270–281]

1. Cellular†
2. Myxoid†
3. Epithelioid†
   a. With eosinophilic cytoplasm (leiomyoblastoma)
   b. Clear cell
4. With sex cord–like growth pattern
5. Infiltrative†
6. Intravenous†
7. Neurilemoma-like
8. Tubule-containing
9. Lipoleiomyoma
10. With heterologous element (fat, skeletal muscle, cartilage, and bone)
11. Cystic
12. Calcification
13. Apoplectic (cellular, hemorrhagic)
14. With hydropic change
15. Symplastic†
16. Diffuse leiomyomatosis
17. Parasitic leiomyoma

* More than one pattern may coexist in one particular tumor.

† Threshold for diagnosis of leiomyosarcoma has to be lowered for tumors showing such patterns.

Diagnostic Approach to Myxoid Smooth Muscle Tumors

In myxoid smooth muscle neoplasms, a significant proportion of the growth is paucicellular and rich in mucoid matrix (preferably confirmed by histochemical stains to exclude the more commonly seen hydropic degeneration)[212–215, 221, 270,

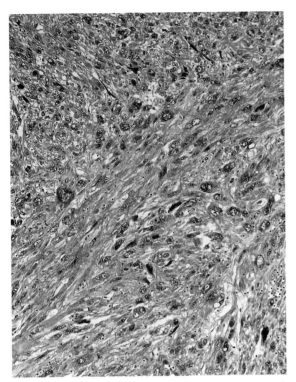

FIGURE 13–56. Bizarre Leiomyoma. The tumor cells possess large, pleomorphic nuclei with coarse chromatin. Many of the nuclei, probably degenerated, appear smudged. Mitotic figures are absent.

[284, 285] (Fig. 13–58). The neoplastic cells often assume a stellate, bipolar, or ''naked'' appearance with scanty cytoplasm, rendering their myoid nature inapparent. It is helpful to search for more cellular areas, where fascicles of spindle cells possessing eosinophilic cytoplasm may be found.[211, 213] Assessment of such areas not only reveals the nature of the growth but also allows proper evaluation of the cytologic features and the mitotic index.

The greatest problem with myxoid smooth muscle tumors is that *malignant behavior can occur in cytologically bland and mitotically inactive (<2/10 HPF) tumors,* although some myxoid leiomyosarcomas may show a high mitotic index similar to their non-myxoid counterparts.[214] The low mitotic count is probably attributable to the low cellularity. However, *all myxoid leiomyosarcomas do exhibit some ''sinister'' histologic features that permit their recognition (such as invasive borders and vascular invasion).* Rarely, myxoid leiomyosarcoma may show significant intravascular growth (Fig. 13–59).

The assessment of myxoid smooth muscle tumors therefore requires thorough sampling of the tumor borders as well as the non-myxoid areas. *A myxoid smooth muscle tumor can be safely labeled benign only if the entire growth is well-circumscribed with no mitotic figures.* The tumor should at least be labeled ''STUMP'' if rare mitotic figures are present, or leiomyosarcoma if it shows invasive borders or contains more than 1 mitosis/10 HPF.

Myxomas identical to those occurring in the somatic tissues have rarely been reported in patients with the syndromal complex of cardiac myxoma, spotty pigmentation, and endocrine hyperactivity (Carney's complex).[286] Uterine myxoma is often

small (< 2 cm), has a uniform appearance, and shows no smooth muscle differentiation.

Approach to Mesenchymal Tumors with Prominent Intravascular Growth

Prominent intravascular growth is most commonly seen in *intravenous leiomyomatosis* (Fig. 13–60), *low-grade endometrial stromal sarcoma* (Fig. 13–61), and very rarely in *mullerian adenofibroma.*[287] Lymphovascular permeation seen in other malignant uterine neoplasms rarely causes diagnostic problems. Non-neoplastic conditions such as adenomyosis and menstrual endometrial tissue can also show intravascular involvement as incidental microscopic findings.[211, 288]

Histologically, uterine tumors with prominent intravascular growth form multiple round, angulated, or serpiginous masses in the myometrium surrounded by narrow clefts that represent the residual vascular lumina (see Fig.13–60A).[289] The tumor masses are usually covered by endothelium, and focal attachment to the vessel wall may be seen. Intravascular growth should be distinguished from artifactual clefts, perinodular hydropic change in leiomyomas[270] (Fig. 13–62), and tumors compressing on the surrounding vessels, by the presence of endothelial lining.

The tumors should be assessed no differently from the non-intravascular neoplasms for the line of differentiation. **Intravenous leiomyomatosis** is characterized by growth of benign-appearing smooth muscle within veins or lymphatics;[222–225, 290–293] it is usually accompanied by myometrial leiomyomas. When the intravascular growth is minor, the term ''leiomyoma with vascular invasion'' is more appropriate.[226, 294] Apart from forming intravascular plaques or polyps, there may also be diffuse smooth muscle proliferation merging with the muscle coat of the involved vessels (see Fig. 13–60A). Hyalinization and hydropic degeneration are common. A characteristic feature is the rich vascularity in the form of thick-walled vessels or dilated cavernous blood spaces, which are particularly prominent in areas with extensive hyalinization (angiomatoid pattern) (see Fig. 13–60A). Many of the morphologic variants observed in uterine leiomyomas can also be seen in intravenous leiomyomatosis (see Table 13– 14).[222, 292, 293] The most stringent criteria of mitotic index must be applied to exclude **leiomyosarcoma with intravascular growth** (see Table 13–13 and Fig. 13–59). Patients with intravenous leiomyomatosis present with symptoms referable to the uterine mass, venous obstruction (e.g., edema), or cardiac extension of the tumor through the pelvic veins and inferior vena cava (e.g., heart failure). Sometimes pulmonary metastasis can develop.[295] The treatment of choice is complete excision of the intra- and extrauterine tumor. Anti-estrogen therapy (oophorectomy or tamoxifen) should be considered for patients with incompletely excised tumors.[223, 224] The prognosis is very favorable.[295] The occasional deaths are usually related to extension of tumor into the heart.

Low-grade endometrial stromal sarcoma is distinguished from intravenous leiomyomatosis by the frequent presence of endometrial involvement, uniform oval tumor cells with scanty cytoplasm arranged in diffuse sheets rather than fascicles, spiral arterioles, and less prominent secondary changes (see Fig. 13–50). In **mullerian adenofibroma with intravascular growth,** the biphasic components are unmistakable. **Adenomyosis** with vascular involvement is often a focal phe-

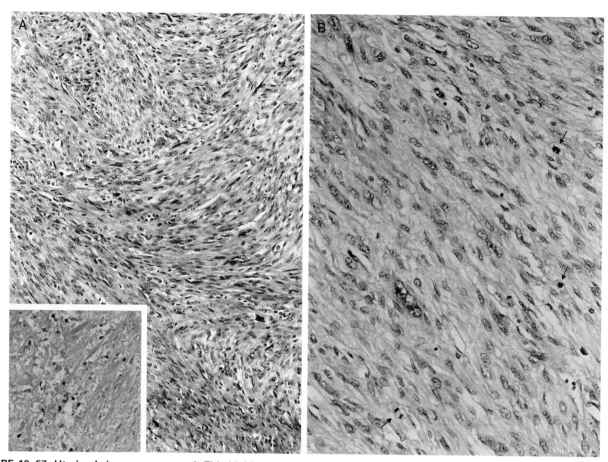

FIGURE 13–57. Uterine Leiomyosarcomas. *A,* This highly cellular tumor is composed of crisscrossing fascicles of spindle cells with pleomorphic, hyperchromatic, and mitotically active nuclei. *Inset,* Coagulative necrosis in foci, characterized by "ghost shadows" of tumor cells. *B,* Bizarre cells and frequent mitotic figures (*arrows*) are found in this growth.

nomenon, and the surrounding myometrium usually shows florid adenomyosis.[211]

Diagnostic Approach to Epithelioid Smooth Muscle Tumors

The designation "epithelioid smooth muscle tumors" should be reserved for growths that are composed predominantly or exclusively of epithelioid cells.[226, 282, 296–301] The tumors are often designated **leiomyoblastoma** when the tumor cells possess abundant eosinophilic cytoplasm[302–304] (see Fig. 13–52), and **clear-cell leiomyoma** when the tumor cells have clear cytoplasm (Fig. 13–63), but the two cell types may co-exist in the same tumor. **Plexiform smooth muscle tumor** is characterized by growth in the form of ramifying cords.[49, 305] The small ones that are often discovered incidentally and located at the endometrial-myometrial junction are often referred to as "plexiform tumorlets" (Fig. 13–64).[301, 306] It should be noted that cases reported in the literature as "plexiform tumors"[221, 298, 307, 308] include both smooth muscle and endometrial stromal tumors with plexiform growth pattern; these tumors show further overlap with uterine tumor resembling ovarian sex cord tumor. Epithelioid smooth muscle neoplasms with bizarre nuclei, intravenous growth, and adipose tissue component have also been described.[276, 292, 309]

For epithelioid smooth muscle tumors, the *most stringent mitotic criteria should be applied* (see Table 13–13).[226, 299, 310] Compared with epithelioid leiomyomas, epithelioid leiomyosarcomas usually show more prominent cytologic atypia, necrosis, and infiltrative borders, but a mitotic count of more than 5/10 HPF may be the only indicator of malignancy in some tumors composed of bland-looking cells. Recently, even this widely adopted approach in diagnosis has been challenged.[311] Based on examination of multiple serial sections of extensively sampled tumor from what would be classified as benign epithelioid leiomyoma on routine sections, the authors identified focal malignant features such as cellular atypia, abnormal mitosis, local infiltration, and vascular invasion in all cases. They therefore proposed viewing *all* epithelioid smooth muscle tumors as low-grade malignancies. However, only three cases were studied, the selection criteria were not known, and the alleged malignancy was not supported by clinical follow-up.

The *differential diagnoses* of epithelioid leiomyosarcoma include poorly differentiated endometrial carcinoma, high-grade uterine sarcoma, malignant mixed mullerian tumor, and placental site trophoblastic tumor (cytokeratin-positive, placental lactogen-positive).[305] Immunostaining for myoid markers and ultrastructural studies are most helpful for confirmation of the smooth muscle nature of the tumor. It

Table 13–15. **Alternative Approach for Evaluation of the Malignant Potential of Uterine Smooth Muscle Tumors**
(Excluding Epithelioid and Myxoid Types)

		Coagulative Tumor Necrosis	
		Absent	**Present**
Diffuse Significant Cellular Atypia	*Absent*	LEIOMYOMA ("Leiomyoma with increased mitoses" if MI ≥ 5)	MI ≥ 10: LEIOMYOSARCOMA MI < 10: SMOOTH MUSCLE TUMOR OF LOW MALIGNANT POTENTIAL (limited experience)
	Present	MI ≥ 10: LEIOMYOSARCOMA MI < 10: ATYPICAL LEIOMYOMA WITH LOW RISK OF RECURRENCE	LEIOMYOSARCOMA

MI, mitotic index (number of mitotic figures per 10 high power fields).
Diffuse significant cellular atypia = Generalized moderate or severe cytologic atypia, which can usually be appreciated on low-magnification examination.
Tumors with focal significant cellular atypia, no coagulative tumor necrosis, and MI <20 are designated "atypical leiomyoma (limited experience)."

should be noted, however, that smooth muscle tumors can also be cytokeratin-positive.[312]

Other Less Common Patterns of Smooth Muscle Tumor Growth

Rarely, smooth muscle tumors may contain *heterologous* elements such as adipose tissue (lipoleiomyoma), skeletal muscle, cartilage, or bone (see Table 13–14). Smooth muscle tumors may harbor abundant *lymphoid cells,* eosinophils, hemopoietic cells, histiocytes, or osteoclast-like giant cells[232, 280, 313–315] (Fig. 13–65). The growth may resemble neurilemoma (Fig. 13–66). Rarely, the tumor cells contain eosinophilic *granular cytoplasm* owing to the accumulation of lyso-somes[316–319] (Fig. 13–67). *Xanthomatous* tumor cells have also been reported in leiomyosarcoma.[232] **Diffuse leiomyomatosis**

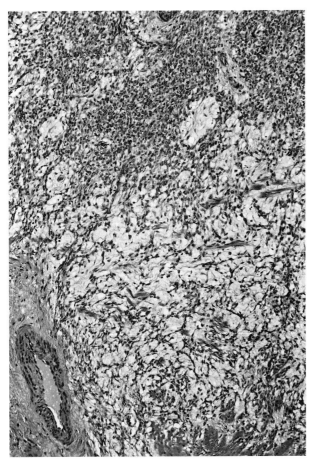

FIGURE 13–58. Myxoid Leiomyosarcoma. In this tumor, myxoid areas merge imperceptibly into cellular areas composed of plump spindly or stellate cells with scanty cytoplasm.

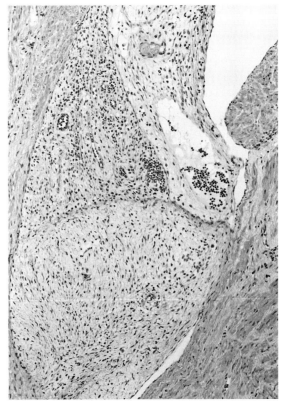

FIGURE 13–59. Intravenous Myxoid Leiomyosarcoma. This innocuous-looking intravascular growth is composed of bland-looking spindle cells in a myxoid background. Mitotic figures, however, are occasionally found, rendering a diagnosis of leiomyosarcoma inevitable.

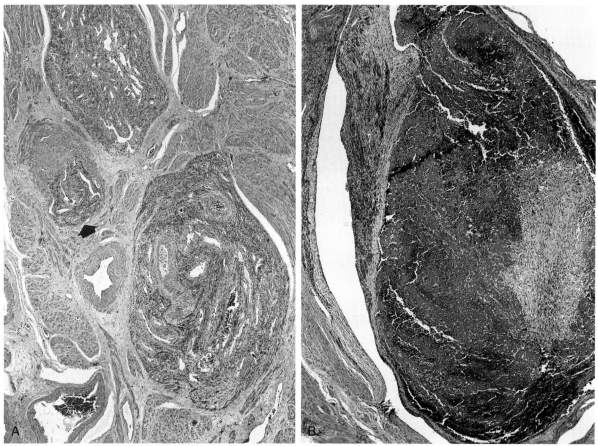

FIGURE 13–60. Intravenous Leiomyomatosis. *A,* The tumor obliterates two vascular spaces, the vascular nature of which is evident only from the residual clefts. A smaller focus of tumor blends with the muscle coat of the involved blood vessel *(arrow).* Note the characteristic rich vascularity of the growth. *B,* A polypoid intravascular growth shows prominent hemorrhage and is associated with thrombus formation.

is a rare condition characterized by numerous leiomyomatous nodules practically replacing the entire myometrium.[320, 321]

Benign metastasizing leiomyoma is defined as the occurrence of benign-looking smooth muscle tumors in lung, lymph node, or rarely other sites, in association with typical uterine leiomyomas, which have often been previously resected.[322–329] This diagnosis can be made only by exclusion, with the uterine tumor thoroughly sampled to rule out leiomyosarcoma, and absence of smooth muscle tumors elsewhere (such as the gastrointestinal tract), which may account for the pulmonary deposits. These "metastatic" nodules show circumscribed growth of bland-looking smooth muscle in fascicles; in the lung, there may be entrapped cleft-like epithelium-lined spaces. Benign metastasizing leiomyoma is often compatible with long-term survival. The proposed pathogeneses include multifocal primary tumor, vascular dislodgement from uterine leiomyoma/intravenous leiomyomatosis, and delayed metastasis from an inadequately sampled low-grade uterine leiomyosarcoma. Benign metastasizing leiomyomas should be distinguished from lymphangiomyomatosis; the latter is characterized by proliferation of morphologically distinctive plump smooth muscle cells with pale ovoid nuclei and abundant pale to clear cytoplasm and by immunoreactivity with HMB-45 in addition to myoid markers.[330]

Diagnostic Approach to Endometrial Stromal Tumors (Including High-grade Uterine Sarcoma)

Low-grade endometrial stromal sarcoma is much more common than **endometrial stromal nodule.** The only distinguishing feature is *lack of invasion in the latter* (Fig. 13–68). Adequate sampling of the tumor-myometrial interface is of utmost importance, which also means that a firm diagnosis can never be made on curettage specimen (Table 13–16). Although endometrial stromal nodules are usually small (a few centimeters), they may measure up to 15 cm.[210, 216, 239] They have pushing, non-invasive borders, but small, 2- to 3-mm, finger-like projections at the edge unaccompanied by inflammatory response are still acceptable. Occasionally, well-formed smooth muscle fascicles can occur within an otherwise typical endometrial stromal nodule, mimicking myometrial invasion by endometrial stromal sarcoma when the specimen is fragmented (such as with curettage).[239] Mitotic index is always low, and all endometrial stromal nodules are cured by complete excision.

Distinction of low-grade endometrial stromal sarcoma from high-grade uterine sarcoma (which lacks definite endometrial stromal differentiation) is most important (Figs. 13–61 and

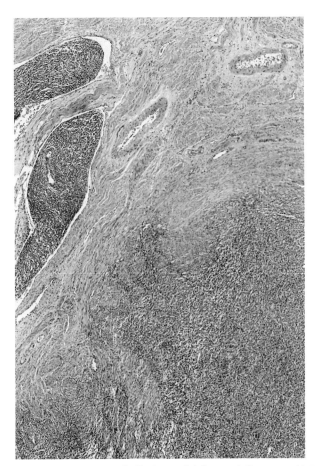

FIGURE 13–61. Low-grade Endometrial Stromal Sarcoma. Note the infiltrative borders and intravascular extension.

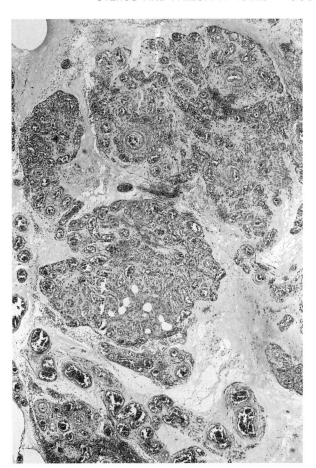

FIGURE 13–62. Leiomyoma with Hydropic Change. Nodules of well-vascularized smooth muscle are separated by edema fluid.

13–69), because the former is indolent and often shows good response to hormonal (progestogen) therapy, whereas the latter is highly aggressive, not responsive to endocrine therapy, and rapidly fatal.[210, 216, 234–237, 245, 331–344] Traditionally, uterine sarcomas other than leiomyosarcomas are designated low-grade endometrial stromal sarcoma and high-grade endometrial stromal sarcoma, using a mitotic index of 10/10 HPF as the dividing line.[210] Evans argues that such a criterion may not be the best predictor to behavior.[334] He further finds *morphologic features far more accurate in predicting the outcome*, in that tumors showing bland cytologic features with interspersed spiral arterioles resembling normal endometrial stroma pursue an indolent and protracted course irrespective of their mitotic count. He proposes reserving the term "endometrial stromal sarcoma" for these neoplasms (see Figs. 13–50 and 13–51). In contrast, tumors showing no morphologic resemblance to normal endometrial stroma are highly aggressive and akin to malignant mixed mullerian tumor and are designated "poorly differentiated endometrial sarcoma." These observations have been supported by subsequent clinical studies[226, 295] as well as flow cytometric studies (morphologic features of endometrial stromal differentiation, but not the mitotic index, predict a low S-phase value and lack of aneuploidy).[345–347] Therefore, invasive tumors showing bland or even mildly atypical cells with the characteristic endometrial stromal cytology should be classified as **low-grade endometrial stromal sarcoma** irrespective of the mitotic count,

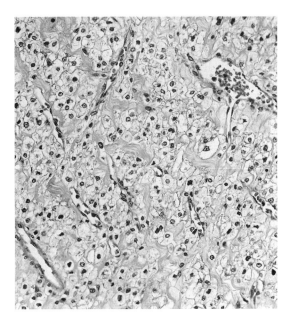

FIGURE 13–63. Clear-cell Epithelioid Leiomyoma. Note the clear cytoplasm of the polygonal cells and absence of mitotic figures.

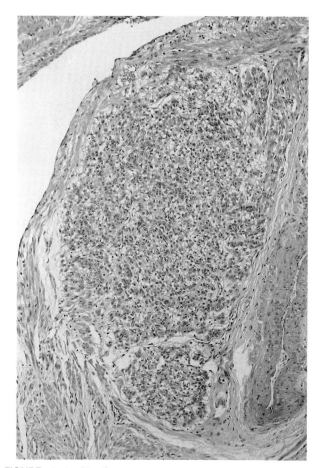

FIGURE 13–64. Plexiform Tumorlet (Leiomyoma) in the Myometrium. This is a small, incidental finding. Note the growth of polygonal cells in cords.

provided that regular spiral arterioles are present. Nevertheless, a high mitotic count of more than 10/10 HPF predicts a more aggressive behavior in patients with high-stage (stage III/IV) disease, but not those with stage I disease.[238] On the other hand, tumors showing marked cellular atypia and lacking the regular vascular pattern are highly malignant, and use of the term **high-grade uterine sarcoma** is justified[48, 226, 334] (Figs. 13–54 and 13–70). What about those tumors with bland cytology resembling normal endometrial stromal cells but lacking the characteristic spiral arterioles? There is little information on this group of neoplasms. One study suggests that these tumors occur in an older age group, have slightly higher frequency of high-stage disease (27%), and are associated with a slightly less favorable prognosis (mean survival 80 months, compared with 97 months for typical low-grade endometrial stromal sarcoma).[238] Until more is known about the behavior of these tumors, it appears appropriate to classify them among the low-grade endometrial stromal sarcomas, with a comment that they lack the typical vasculature. The nomenclature of endometrial stromal tumors and their interconversions are shown in Table 13–17.

Several *differential diagnoses* have to be considered for these endometrial sarcomas besides smooth muscle tumors. Dispersed islands of adenomyosis in the myometrium, when associated with an inconspicuous glandular component (such

as in postmenopausal women), may simulate low-grade endometrial stromal sarcoma but can be recognized by the lack of a definite expansile tumor mass. Lymphoma, leukemia, metastatic lobular carcinoma of the breast, and small-cell carcinoma may also enter into consideration, but these tumors generally show highly permeative growth, more significant cellular atypia, and no ramifying vasculature. Immunohistochemical studies are helpful when there are uncertainties.

Less Common Morphologic Manifestations of Endometrial Stromal Neoplasms

Endometrial stromal neoplasms may show focal foamy change (with accumulation of lipid), decidual change, clear-cell change, rhabdoid appearance, or smooth muscle differentiation.[348, 349] Even focal skeletal muscle differentiation has been reported.[239] There may be focal or extensive sex cord–like growth, also sometimes referred to as "epithelial-like areas" (Figs. 13–53, 13–55, 13–71, and 13–72); foci often demonstrate strong staining for myoid markers and/or cytokeratin and therefore probably represent epithelioid smooth muscle differentiation, with the understanding that myoid cells can express cytokeratin.[210, 230, 237, 243–246, 350–354]

Focally distributed endometrioid glands (which may even exhibit atypia) can sometimes occur in endometrial stromal tumors[247] (see Fig. 13–55). When this phenomenon is extensive, these tumors may be mistaken for endometriosis (so-called aggressive endometriosis) or adenosarcoma. The endometrial glands differ from the sex cord–like areas in that the cells are tall columnar.

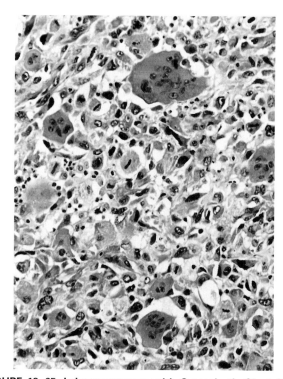

FIGURE 13–65. Leiomyosarcoma with Osteoclastic Giant Cells. The tumor cells have pleomorphic hyperchromatic nuclei and show many mitotic figures. The osteoclastic giant cells have regular nuclei and are reactive in nature.

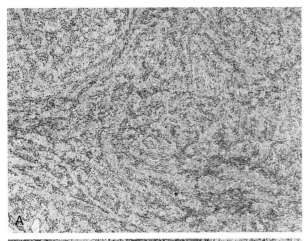

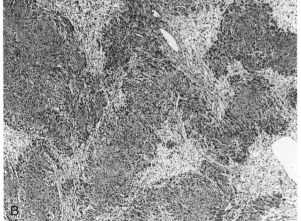

FIGURE 13–66. Neurilemoma-like Leiomyoma. *A,* Nuclear palisading. *B,* Alternating cellularity.

Approach to Uterine Tumors with Mixed Stromal and Smooth Muscle Differentiation

Most mesenchymal tumors of the uterus can be readily classified histologically as smooth muscle or endometrial stromal neoplasms. However, in occasional cases, both endometrial stromal and smooth muscle differentiation co-exist or the line of differentiation is ambiguous. Such tumors are sometimes designated "stromomyoma" or "tumor of mixed endometrial stromal and smooth muscle type."[48, 239, 355, 356] The diagnostic criteria of this mixed category have not been clearly defined, but we believe both components have to be prominent for a case to be so designated. It is well known that endometrial stromal tumors may show small foci of smooth muscle differentiation, and it is pointless to classify these in the mixed category. Nor are immunohistochemical studies helpful in distinction between endometrial stromal and smooth muscle differentiation, because both may show reactivity for muscle-specific actin and desmin, and even occasionally cytokeratin,[229, 230, 232, 233, 312] although there are claims otherwise that endometrial stromal neoplasms are not immunoreactive for myoid markers.[232]

When neoplasms of mixed endometrial stromal and smooth muscle type are well-circumscribed and completely excised,

they would probably have a benign outcome. Problems in treatment arise when the tumor shows infiltrative or intravascular growth. Such a growth pattern, when associated with endometrial stromal differentiation, denotes a malignant, albeit indolent, tumor with possible delayed recurrence and metastasis irrespective of the mitotic index (i.e., low-grade endometrial stromal sarcoma). On the other hand, smooth muscle tumor showing such growth pattern can still be benign (infiltrative leiomyoma or leiomyoma with vascular invasion), of uncertain malignant potential, or malignant, depending on a constellation of features including the mitotic index. Furthermore, adjuvant hormonal therapy is indicated only for endometrial stromal sarcoma but not for leiomyosarcoma. We favor the approach of Kempson and Hendrickson,[226, 238] and consider it safest to regard all infiltrative mesenchymal tumors with definite endometrial stromal differentiation (albeit focal) as low-grade endometrial stromal sarcoma.

MIXED EPITHELIAL-MESENCHYMAL TUMORS OF THE UTERUS

The sometimes confusing nomenclature of uterine tumors with mixed epithelial-mesenchymal elements, along with the pure tumors, is schematically listed in Table 13–18. Table 13–19 attempts to generalize the behavior of these various tumors, which can be broadly grouped into a "low-grade" or a "high-grade" category.[357–370]

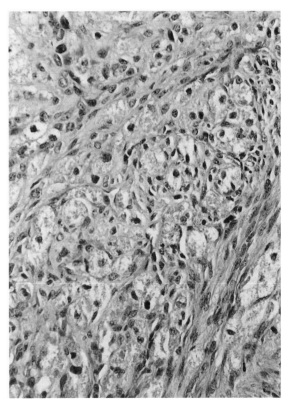

FIGURE 13–67. Granular Cell Leiomyosarcoma. The polygonal tumor cells are rich in cytoplasmic granules. Note merging with spindly cells showing typical smooth muscle features in the right lower field.

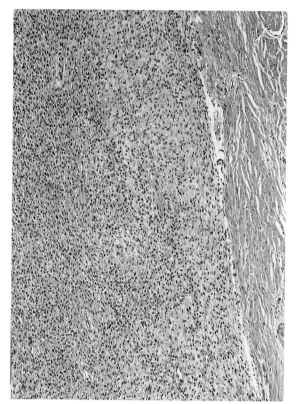

FIGURE 13–68. Endometrial Stromal Nodule. Note the good circumscription of the tumor at the interface with the myometrium *(right)*. Arterioles are evident in the tumor even at this magnification.

Polypoid adenomyoma should pose no problems in diagnosis, and atypical polypoid adenomyoma has been discussed. Although low-grade endometrial stromal sarcoma with sex cord–like growth or endometrioid glandular differentiation and ''uterine tumors resembling ovarian sex-cord tumors'' are often included in the classification of mixed epithelial-mesenchymal tumors,[371, 372] they are not discussed here because the epithelial-like component in such tumors often shows myoid rather than epithelial differentiation.[230, 244]

The mixed tumors are uncommon neoplasms of the uterus. Among them, malignant mixed mullerian tumors (MMMT) vastly outnumber adenofibroma and adenosarcoma,

and carcinofibroma and carcinomesenchymoma are exotic occurrences.[373–375] A diagnosis of carcinofibroma or carcinomesenchymoma should be reserved only for those cases in which the mesenchymal component is convincingly neoplastic.[375]

Diagnostic Approach

Almost all types of mixed tumors of the uterus form polypoid masses in the endometrial cavity.[376, 377] Mullerian adenofibroma and adenosarcoma show solid growth of fleshy tissue with slit-like spaces and cysts representing epithelial clefts. Malignant mixed mullerian tumor is frequently frankly invasive, friable, hemorrhagic, and necrotic; there may be gritty or translucent areas on sectioning as a result of the presence of bone and cartilage, respectively.

Histologic categorization is often straightforward after assessing the epithelial and mesenchymal components (see Table 13–18). The fine points of distinction in the difficult cases are covered in the following sections.

Problems in Diagnosis of Mullerian Adenofibroma and Adenosarcoma

The clinical features of mullerian adenofibroma and adenosarcoma are summarized in Table 13–20.[378–381] These tumors usually arise in the endometrium, although rarely they may involve the cervix or myometrium primarily. Myometrial invasion, usually superficial and in broad fronts, is present in 17% to 50% of adenosarcoma.[370, 382–384] Exceptional examples of adenofibroma showing deep myometrial and vascular invasion have been reported.[287] Myometrial invasion in adenosarcoma is associated with local recurrence after hysterectomy.[383–385] Morphologically, the recurrent tumor may be similar to the original tumor, or may recur as pure sarcoma of a higher grade.[383] Exceptionally, adenosarcoma recurs as heterologous MMMT.[383] **Sarcomatous overgrowth in adenosarcoma** carries a markedly worsened prognosis (mortality 60%, compared with 10% for uncomplicated adenosarcoma)[386] (see Table 13–20), with frequent recurrence and early blood-borne metastasis. It is defined by a significant portion of the tumor (>25%) being composed of pure sarcoma devoid of

Table 13–16. **Diagnostic Criteria of Endometrial Stromal Tumors**

	Criteria for Diagnosis
Endometrial stromal nodule*	Circumscribed. Cells resembling proliferative endometrial stroma, associated with a rich component of arterioles. Mitosis ≤ 10/10 HPF.
Low-grade endometrial stromal sarcoma*	Infiltrative, often with intralymphatic or intravascular growth. Histologically otherwise identical to endometrial stromal nodule. Although mitotic count is often ≤ 10/10 HPF, higher mitotic count is acceptable so long as the characteristic arterioles are present.
High-grade uterine sarcoma	Infiltrative; vascular invasion also common. Moderate to marked cellular atypia; the characteristic arterioles are lacking. Mitosis often > 10/10 HPF.

* May show sex cord–like differentiation.

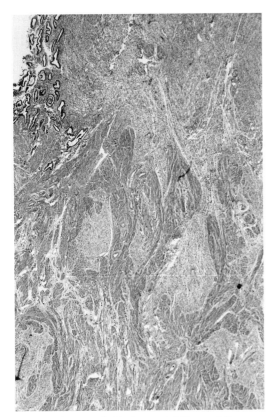

FIGURE 13–69. Low-grade Endometrial Stromal Sarcoma. Note the serpentine growth (pale-staining areas) within the myometrium.

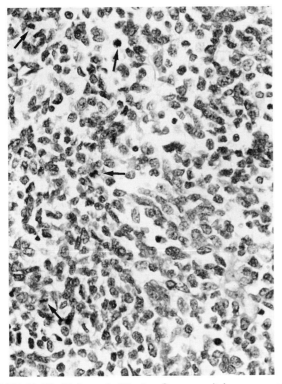

FIGURE 13–70. High-grade Uterine Sarcoma. It is composed of closely packed ovoid cells with pleomorphic hyperchromatic nuclei and scanty cytoplasm. Note the many mitotic figures (*arrows*) and absence of spiral arterioles.

epithelial elements (Fig. 13–73), often associated with increased cytologic atypia and mitotic activity.

Histologically, the benign glandular elements form clefts separating broad fronds of cellular fibrous stromal growth (phyllodes tumor-like), papillary processes, or cysts of variable sizes (Fig. 13–74).[368–371, 387–395] In 10% of adenosarcomas, the glandular elements may form irregular small branching tubules resembling those seen in endometrial hyperplasia (see Fig. 13–74). Although the cuff of hypercellular stroma surrounding the epithelium has been emphasized to be a characteristic feature in adenosarcoma, such phenomenon may not be prominent at all or, conversely, the periglandular zone may appear hypocellular and edematous (Fig. 13–75). Morphologic variations in the epithelial and stromal components in these tumors are listed in Table 13–21[369, 383, 384, 388, 389, 393, 396–402] (Figs. 13–76 to 13–78). The presence of heterologous elements in adenosarcoma probably has no effect on the behavior of the tumor,[383, 384, 393] although some previous studies suggest that it does.[389, 397]

The main diagnostic problem is the *distinction between adenofibroma and adenosarcoma.* The study by Zaloudek and Norris suggested that a mitotic count of 4/10 HPF be the dividing line[385] (see Fig. 13–78). Recent studies, however, have lowered the threshold to 2/10 HPF, because tumors possessing 2 or 3 mitotic figures per 10 HPF have been documented to show extrauterine spread after hysterectomy.[383, 396] It should be noted that adenosarcoma can look deceptively bland, sclerotic, or hypocellular in areas.[383] The difficulty is further compounded by the non-uniformity of the stromal cell distribution; a diagnosis of adenosarcoma should be made instead of adenofibroma even if focal areas reach the threshold mitotic count of 2 or more per 10 HPF. The diagnosis of adenofibroma should be restricted only for thoroughly sampled tumors with mitotic count of less than 2/10 HPF, no significant stromal cell atypia, and no periglandular cellular condensation.[383, 403]

Adenosarcoma can be difficult to *distinguish from benign endometrial polyp* when the latter shows a cellular stroma or bizarre stromal cells.[383, 404] Any uterine polyp showing hypercellular stroma with mitoses, periglandular stromal condensation, or formation of intraglandular stromal papillae with a phyllodes pattern should be diagnosed as adenosarcoma rather than simple polyp.

The *distinction of adenosarcoma from MMMT* is important because of their different prognoses. In MMMT, the epithelial component is often of high cytologic and architectural grade, and squamous differentiation is common; bland-looking glands, if present, are focal. Moreover, the sarcomatous component of MMMT is usually of high grade. Although some adenosarcomas may exhibit architectural and cellular atypia in the glandular component (up to carcinoma *in situ*), such changes are only focal and the rest of the tumor shows benign glands (see Fig. 13–76).

There may be difficulties in distinguishing *low-grade endometrial stromal sarcoma and high-grade uterine sarcoma* from adenosarcoma, because when the former invades the endometrium, intermingling of the tumor with residual glands can give an impression of a mixed mullerian tumor. However, glands are absent in the central portion of the tumor, there is no periglandular condensation of tumor cells, and the tumor is generally more permeative. The last two mentioned features can also help to distinguish low-grade endometrial stromal

Table 13–17. **Classification of Endometrial Stromal Tumors**

Norris and Taylor[210]	Evans[282]	Kempson and Hendrickson[226]	Gynecological Oncology Group[48]
Endometrial stromal nodule	Endometrial stromal nodule	Endometrial stromal nodule	Endometrial stromal nodule
Low-grade ESS (endolymphatic stromal myosis)	ESS	Low-grade ESS	Low-grade ESS
High-grade ESS			High-grade ESS
	Poorly differentiated endometrial sarcoma	High-grade undifferentiated sarcoma	Undifferentiated sarcoma

ESS, endometrial stromal sarcoma.

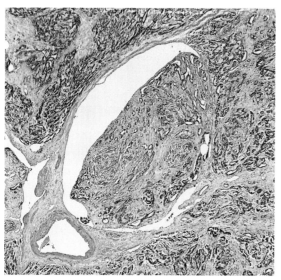

FIGURE 13–71. Low-grade Endometrial Stromal Sarcoma with Sex Cord–Like (Epithelial-like) Growth. This tumor grows in the form of complex anastomosing narrow tubules. Note the intravascular growth.

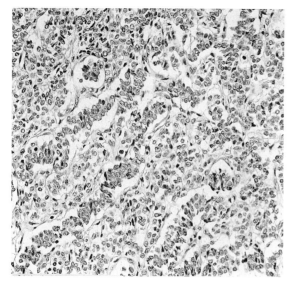

FIGURE 13–72. Low-grade Endometrial Stromal Sarcoma with Sex Cord–Like Growth. The polygonal tumor cells grow in linear cords separated by lighter-staining cells with more cytoplasm, mimicking Sertoli-Leydig cell tumor.

sarcoma with endometrioid glandular differentiation from mullerian adenosarcoma. The distinction is important, because low-grade endometrial stromal sarcoma shows a high risk of recurrence and higher response rate to radiation therapy or progestogen therapy.[238]

Diagnostic Problems of Malignant Mixed Mullerian Tumor

Although the designation "carcinosarcoma" is now recommended by the World Health Organization for this group of

Table 13–18. **Nomenclature of Uterine Corpus Tumors**

Epithelial Element	Mesenchymal Element	Nomenclature of Tumor
Benign	—	(Not applicable)
Malignant	—	Carcinoma
—	Benign	*Homologous:* Endometrial stromal nodule Leiomyoma *Heterologous:* Lipoma, etc.
—	Malignant	*Homologous:* Low-grade endometrial stromal sarcoma High-grade uterine sarcoma Leiomyosarcoma Malignant fibrous histiocytoma *Heterologous:* Liposarcoma, osteosarcoma, etc.
Benign	Benign	Mullerian adenofibroma Adenomyoma
Benign	Malignant	Mullerian adenosarcoma ± sarcomatous overgrowth
Malignant	Benign	Atypical polypoid adenomyoma* Carcinofibroma, carcinomesenchymoma†
Malignant	Malignant	Malignant mixed mullerian tumor Homologous type (carcinosarcoma) Heterologous type (malignant mixed mesodermal tumor)

* The exact category that this entity should fit into is arguable.

† Some cases reported in literature may represent endometrial carcinoma with prominent desmoplastic stroma, or adenofibroma/adenosarcoma with glandular atypia.

Table 13–19. **Grouping of Malignant Mesenchymal and Mixed Tumors of the Uterus by Their Clinical Behavior**

	Low Grade	High Grade
Clinical course	Indolent behavior, compatible with long survival. Tends to show invasion and local recurrence (which may be delayed for many years). Distant metastasis much less common, and often late.	Aggressive; most patients die in 1–2 years. Extensive local infiltration and dissemination in pelvis and peritoneal cavity. Distant metastasis not uncommon.
Entities included	Low-grade endometrial stromal sarcoma Mullerian adenosarcoma	High-grade uterine sarcoma Leiomyosarcoma Mullerian adenosarcoma with sarcomatous overgrowth Malignant mixed mullerian tumor

Table 13–20. **Clinical Features and Diagnostic Criteria of Mixed Mullerian Tumors**

	Clinical Features	Diagnostic Criteria
Mullerian adenofibroma	*Relative frequency:* Adenosarcoma: adenofibroma = 10–20:1. *Age:* Usually postmenopausal, but 1/3 perimenopausal or younger. *Symptoms:* Abdominal pain; vaginal bleeding; may present as recurrent endometrial polyp. Almost always stage I at presentation. *Behavior:* Adenofibroma benign, but some cases may recur.[378, 403] Adenosarcoma indolent; locally recurrent (often delayed) in 25% of cases; hematogenous spread rare (<5%).	1. Glandular component benign; phyllodes pattern common. 2. Stromal component benign, without condensation beneath epithelium. Mitosis < 2/10 HPF.
Mullerian adenosarcoma		1. Glandular component benign or atypical; phyllodes pattern common. 2. Cellular stroma with variable degrees of atypia, often with condensation beneath epithelium. Mitosis ≥ 2/10 HPF. [Some authors recommend also calling tumors with mitotic count <2/10 HPF but showing marked stromal cellularity or atypia ''adenosarcoma'' instead of ''adenofibroma ''].
Mullerian adenosarcoma with sarcomatous overgrowth	Clinical features similar to the above. Aggressive; early postoperative recurrence and early hematogenous spread.	1. As mullerian adenosarcoma. 2. Foci overgrown (>25%) by sarcoma, usually high grade but rarely low grade. Deep myometrial and serosal invasion common.
Adenomyoma	Polypoid lesion of the endometrium, either asymptomatic or presenting with vaginal bleeding.	1. Benign endometrial glands with no architectural complexity or cellular atypia. 2. Stroma composed predominantly or exclusively of benign-looking smooth muscle.
Atypical polypoid adenomyoma	*Age:* Usually premenopausal. *Symptom:* Abnormal vaginal bleeding. *Behavior:* Benign, but may persist after curettage.	1. Complex glands lined by atypical epithelium (even up to carcinoma *in situ*); morule or squamous metaplasia common. 2. Bundles of smooth muscle interdigitating with the glands.
Malignant mixed mullerian tumor (homologous or heterologous)	*Age:* Almost always postmenopausal. *Associations:* May have history of pelvic irradiation; rarely may arise in endometrial polyp.[379–381] *Symptoms:* abdominal pain and vaginal bleeding; 50% have symptoms referable to extrauterine spread. Highly malignant; pelvic tissue and para-aortic lymph node involvement common; hematogenous spread occurs late. 5-year survival, 15% to 40%; median survival, 7 to 22 months. Stage at presentation the most important prognostic factor.	1. Malignant epithelial component, often taking the form of glands or squamous islands. 2. Malignant stromal component. The following elements are considered heterologous: skeletal muscle, fat, cartilage, bone.

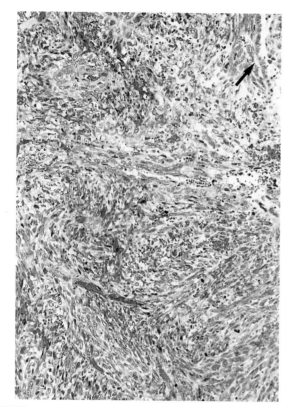

FIGURE 13–73. Mullerian Adenosarcoma with Sarcomatous Overgrowth. The sarcomatous component is formed by highly atypical spindle cells. Residual glandular component is indicated by an arrow.

tumors, we prefer the more popular and succinct designation "malignant mixed mullerian tumor" (MMMT).[48] Furthermore, the term "carcinosarcoma" can cause confusion because it has been used in the older literature only for those tumors with homologous elements;[377] tumors with heterologous elements have often been referred to as "malignant mixed mesodermal tumor."[367, 376, 377, 405–416]

The clinical features of MMMTs are summarized in Table 13–20. As a group, MMMTs after irradiation tend to occur in younger patients at a mean of 11 to 24 years after irradiation, and they are associated with an even worse prognosis.[362, 417, 418] Heterologous elements are also more frequent in postradiation MMMTs. In MMMT, the stage of disease is the most important prognostic factor. Although it has previously been suggested that the presence of heterologous elements in an MMMT signifies a poorer prognosis,[376, 377, 408, 409, 411] recent studies have shown that the difference is unlikely to be significant.[356, 367, 405, 419, 420] Furthermore, the true incidence of heterologous tumor has been underestimated as a result of inadequate sampling.[412]

There is now strong evidence that MMMTs are more related to endometrial carcinoma than sarcoma, although MMMTs have traditionally been grouped with uterine sarcomas—that is, they may be considered metaplastic carcinomas.[367, 419, 421–427] Immunohistochemically, both the epithelial and mesenchymal elements show cytokeratin and vimentin expression,[367, 419, 422] and their immunophenotypic profiles (including p53 protein) in a single tumor are often similar, indicating that they may have derived from the same clone.[419, 427a] Furthermore, the

pattern of spread of MMMTs (pelvic soft tissues, omentum, regional lymph nodes) is similar to that of high-grade endometrial carcinomas rather than endometrial sarcomas (early hematogenous spread). These tumors usually metastasize as pure carcinomas, and it is almost always the carcinomatous component that permeates the lymphovascular spaces in the primary tumor.[419–421] The occurrence of high-grade carcinomatous component, especially with serous and clear-cell subtypes, is associated with a higher frequency of metastasis, whereas no such correlation is found with the sarcomatous component.[367] Thus, the epithelial component within an MMMT dictates the behavior, and therapy regimens developed for endometrial carcinoma may have beneficial effects on patients with MMMT.[421] However, because MMMT is clinically more aggressive than comparable stage high-grade endometrial carcinoma (lower overall survival rate and median survival duration), it should continue to be recognized as a distinct entity.[427b]

Microscopically, the carcinomatous and sarcomatous components of most MMMTs are high-grade, although the epithelial element may appear better differentiated focally (Fig. 13–79). The carcinomatous component is commonly of endometrioid or serous type (see Fig. 13–79), but mucinous, clear-cell, and squamous carcinoma can occur in various combinations.[294] The sarcomatous component is usually an anaplastic nondescript spindle cell growth, or may resemble fibrosarcoma or malignant fibrous histiocytoma (see Fig. 13–79). Heterologous elements can include rhabdomyosarcoma, chondrosarcoma, osteosarcoma, or liposarcoma, in descending order of frequency (Figs. 13–79 and 13–80). Recently, neuroendocrine differentiation has been demonstrated in a significant proportion of MMMTs by immunohistochemical techniques.[419, 428–430]

The diagnosis of MMMT is usually straightforward. **High-grade endometrial adenocarcinoma** may mimic MMMT when there is a significant spindle cell growth associated with squamous differentiation, but these areas usually blend imperceptibly with the carcinomatous element and show sparse reticulin fibers. The demonstration of heterologous element at the light microscopic, immunohistochemical, or ultrastructural level favors a diagnosis of MMMT over high-grade endometrial carcinoma.

When the carcinomatous component in an MMMT is inconspicuous, the tumor overlaps morphologically with **high-grade uterine stromal sarcoma, other sarcomas, and adenosarcoma with sarcomatous overgrowth**[334, 405] (see Fig. 13–73). Thorough sampling is the key to the correct diagnosis. In a uterine curettage that shows a pure sarcomatous growth (with the exception of typical low-grade endometrial stromal sarcoma), MMMT must be excluded. The distinction has a bearing on the choice of treatment, because MMMT is more akin to endometrial carcinoma than sarcoma.

HETEROLOGOUS TISSUE IN THE UTERUS

Entities to be Considered

A variety of conditions can be associated with the presence of heterologous tissue in the uterus, either as the sole lesion

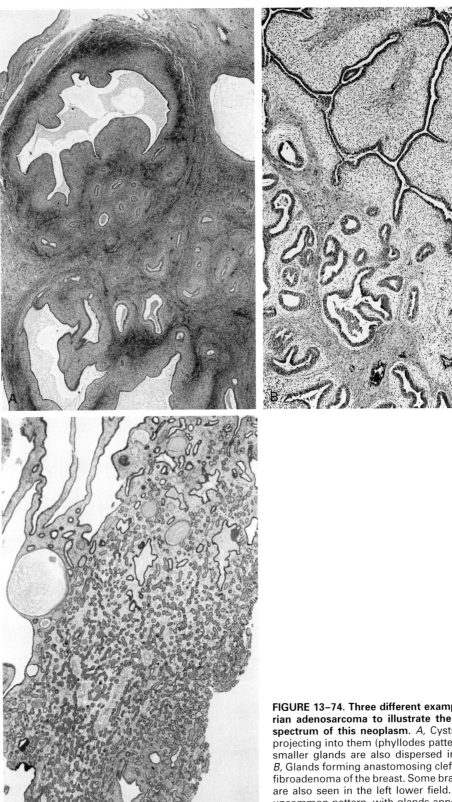

FIGURE 13–74. Three different examples of mullerian adenosarcoma to illustrate the architectural spectrum of this neoplasm. *A,* Cysts with fronds projecting into them (phyllodes pattern). Note that smaller glands are also dispersed in the stroma. *B,* Glands forming anastomosing clefts resembling fibroadenoma of the breast. Some branched glands are also seen in the left lower field. *C,* This is an uncommon pattern, with glands appearing mostly tubular and fairly crowded.

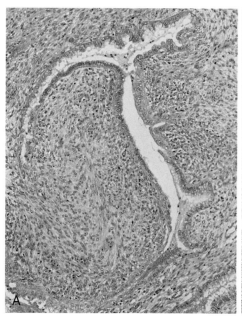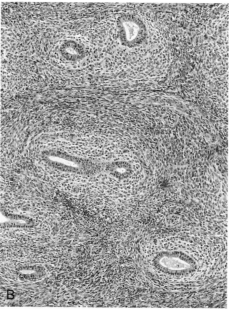

FIGURE 13–75. Mullerian Adenosarcoma. *A,* The stromal component forms fronds projecting into glandular spaces. Note the condensation of the atypical stromal cells immediately beneath the epithelium. *B,* In this example, the cuff of stromal cells around the glands appears hypocellular.

or as a component in a tumor (Table 13–22).[211, 239, 271, 273, 274, 278, 431–451] The commonest situation is the finding of fetal parts in curettage specimens obtained from abortion, but these ''heterologous tissues'' are not embedded within the endometrium or myometrium, and the diagnosis is obvious. Otherwise the commonest cause is mixed mullerian tumor.

Approach to Diagnosis

The heterologous tissue should be assessed as to whether it is mature, immature, or malignant. *Malignant heterologous element* is usually indicative of a diagnosis of mixed mullerian tumor (malignant mixed mullerian tumor or mullerian adenosarcoma), although the rare heterologous sarcomas (chondrosarcoma, osteosarcoma, liposarcoma, rhabdomyosarcoma) are also possibilities (see Figs. 13–79*C* and 13–80). The latter

diagnosis can be rendered with confidence only after extensive sampling to rule out mixed mullerian tumor.

For *mature heterologous tissues,* the possibilities to be entertained are leiomyoma with metaplastic element, stromal metaplasia, fetal part implantation, mature teratoma, and lipoma. Recognition of leiomyomas with metaplastic element, in which fat (lipoleiomyoma), cartilage, bone, or skeletal muscle is present focally or intimately intermingled with the smooth muscle, should be easy because these are well-circumscribed tumors located in the myometrium. The rare lipoma is well-circumscribed and composed entirely of mature adipose cells. Teratoma comprises a multiplicity of mature tissues with an organoid pattern. For the remaining cases, there is no obvious explanation for the occurrence of islands of *heterotopic tissue* (cartilage, bone, skeletal muscle, or glial) in the endometrium or myometrium. Very often they represent incidental findings in curettage or hysterectomy specimens.

Table 13–21. **Morphologic Spectrum of the Epithelial and Stromal Components in Mullerian Adenofibroma and Adenosarcoma**

	Epithelial Element	**Stromal Element**
Adenofibroma	Proliferative endometrial glands (commonest) Secretory glands Mucinous (endocervical type) Serous Metaplastic (non-keratinizing squamous, eosinophilic, papillary, hobnail)	Fibroblastic or endometrial stroma-like (mitotic index < 2/10 HPF) Smooth muscle (rare) Heterologous elements have not been described
Adenosarcoma	Cellular atypia, up to carcinoma *in situ* changes in adenosarcoma Architectural atypia (resembling simple or complex endometrial hyperplasia) in adenosarcoma	Endometrial stromal sarcoma-like (mitotic index ≥ 2/10 HPF) Fibrosarcoma-like Secondary change (hemorrhage, hyalinization, inflammation) Smooth muscle (spindle or epithelioid) Heterologous elements: skeletal muscle (commonest), fat, cartilage Sex cord–like growth Foamy cell Osteoclast-like giant cell (rare) Angiosarcomatous or neuroepithelial-like (rare)

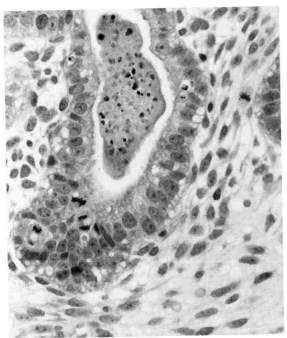

FIGURE 13–76. Mullerian Adenosarcoma with Focal Atypical Change in the Epithelial Element. Mitotic figures are seen both in the glands and the cellular stroma.

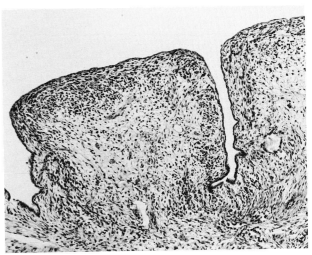

FIGURE 13–77. Mullerian Adenosarcoma with Rhabdomyosarco-matous Component. There is condensation of mesenchymal cells beneath the epithelium of the broad papillary processes, mimicking sarcoma botryoides.

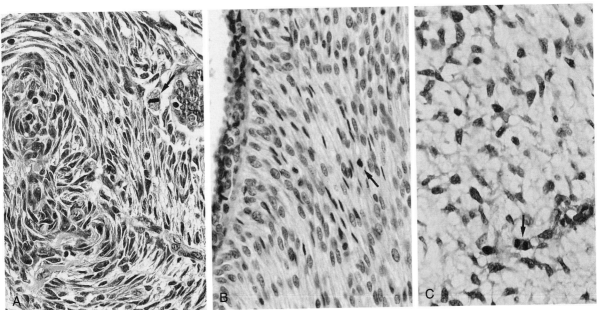

FIGURE 13–78. Mesenchymal Component of Mullerian Adenosarcoma. Mitotic figures are indicated by arrows. *A,* Closely packed spindly cells with mild pleomorphism. *B,* Bland-looking plump spindle cells. Note also the bland-looking epithelium in the left field. *C,* Moderately pleomorphic spindly and stellate cells lying in a myxoid stroma.

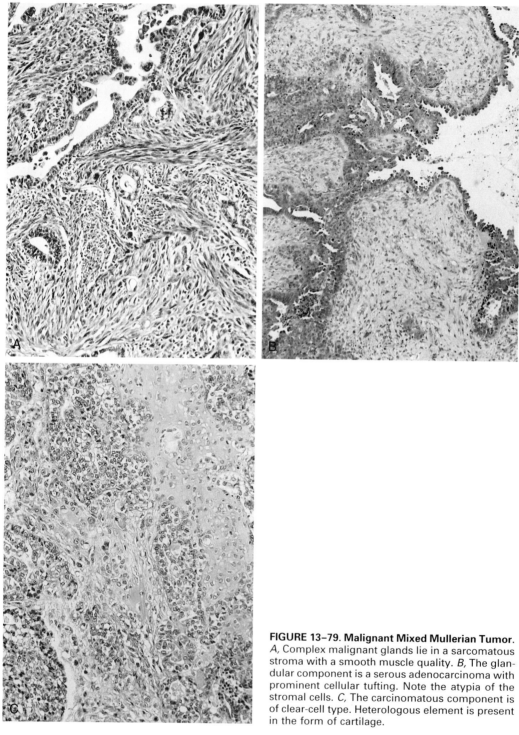

FIGURE 13–79. Malignant Mixed Mullerian Tumor.
A, Complex malignant glands lie in a sarcomatous
stroma with a smooth muscle quality. *B,* The glandular component is a serous adenocarcinoma with
prominent cellular tufting. Note the atypia of the
stromal cells. *C,* The carcinomatous component is
of clear-cell type. Heterologous element is present
in the form of cartilage.

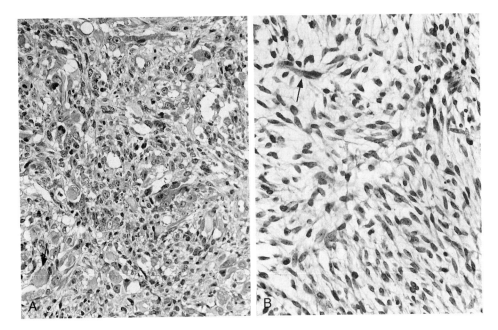

FIGURE 13–80. Malignant Mixed Mullerian Tumor with Heterologous Element. *A,* Larger ovoid cells with eosinophilic cytoplasm and striations *(arrow)* are scattered among pleomorphic stromal cells. *B,* This field appears indistinguishable from embryonal rhabdomyosarcoma. A strap cell is indicated by an arrow.

Their postulated origins include (1) fetal part implantation, as suggested by the frequent history of therapeutic abortion or spontaneous abortion followed by curettage, either recently or in the distant past, and the occasional presence of more than one type of heterotopic tissue; and (2) metaplastic origin,

Table 13–22. **Entities Associated with Presence of Heterologous Tissue**

Cartilage or bone
  Mixed mullerian tumor
  Fetal part implantation/stromal metaplasia[443, 446, 447]
  Leiomyoma with chondroid or osseous metaplasia[221]
  Dystrophic ossification in areas of chronic inflammation[444]
  Teratoma[440, 441]
  Chondrosarcoma, osteosarcoma[434, 435, 438, 439]

Fat*
  Mixed mullerian tumor
  Fetal part implantation/stromal metaplasia[448, 449]
  Lipoleiomyoma and its variant adenomyolipoma[721, 274, 451]
  Omentum included in curettage owing to uterine
    perforation†
  Teratoma
  Lipoma, liposarcoma[273, 437]

Skeletal Muscle
  Mixed mullerian tumor
  Skeletal muscle differentiation in leiomyoma or
    endometrial stromal nodule[239, 450]
  Fetal part implantation/stromal metaplasia
  Rhabdomyosarcoma[431–433, 436]

Glial Tissue
  Fetal part implantation/stromal metaplasia[445, 448]
  Teratoma
  Glioma (invasive tumor with appearances of low-grade fibrillary
    astrocytoma)[442]
  Primitive neuroectodermal tumor

* Foamy stromal cells with finely vacuolated cytoplasm should not be mistaken for fat cells.
† The adipose tissue fragments (omentum) should be separate from the endometrial and/or myometrial tissue.

as suggested by the intimate merging of the heterotopic tissue with the normal stromal or smooth muscle cells in some cases, and the occasional occurrence of such tissue in a very deep location, incompatible with a simple implantation theory. Probably both pathogenetic mechanisms are valid, but it is not possible to tell in an individual case which is the exact cause.

Immature heterologous tissues resemble those derived from the fetus and usually show high cellularity and somewhat small size of the constituent cells but no frank anaplasia. The possibilities of immature teratoma and fetal part implantation have to be considered. The former can be distinguished from the latter by the disorderly disposition of the organoid tissues.

BENIGN LESIONS MIMICKING FALLOPIAN TUBE CARCINOMA

The commonest type of fallopian tube carcinoma is serous adenocarcinoma, which is characterized by papillae and tubules lined by cells showing variable degrees of nuclear pleomorphism; cellular tufting is often prominent. A variety of benign lesions may mimic it by virtue of their unusual growth pattern or artifacts. In **chronic salpingitis,** fusion of mucosal folds results in papillary, complex glandular, and cribriform structures mimicking invasive adenocarcinoma (Fig. 13–81). The problem is further compounded by the occasional occurrence of reactive inflammatory atypia with enlarged vesicular nuclei and extension of the mucosal epithelium into the muscularis. The best clue pointing to the benign nature of the lesion is the presence of cilia, which rarely ever occurs in carcinomas (Fig. 13–82). Furthermore, there is no grossly evident tumor mass, as typical of most fallopian tube carcinomas, and the background is rich in inflammatory cells.

The **metaplastic papillary tumor** is an uncommon, benign, incidental microscopic finding mostly occurring in pregnant or postpartum women; it is controversial whether it is a metaplastic or neoplastic process. It is characterized by segmental

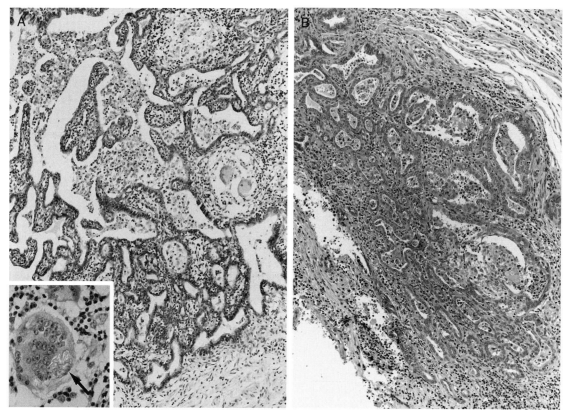

FIGURE 13–81. Chronic Salpingitis. *A,* This example is related to foreign body reaction. See inset for foreign bodies in histiocytes. There is fusion of the mucosal folds, resulting in a complex pattern. *B,* This case is associated with an extremely complex glandular pattern mimicking adenocarcinoma.

replacement of the tubal mucosa by a branching papillary lesion with cellular tufts, reminiscent of borderline tumors of the ovary.[39, 452–455] The pseudostratified epithelial cells are characteristically oncocytic, with or without some interspersed mucin-secreting cells. The nuclei are regular, but mild atypia and prominent nucleoli can be seen in some cells. The benign nature of the lesion is supported by the lack of invasion and mitotic figures. With **cautery artifact,** the epithelial cells appear strikingly elongated, with pseudostratified and streaming nuclei.[456] The artifactual nature is attested to by the lack of chromatin details. **Arias-Stella reaction** involving the fallopian tube can appear worrisome as a result of presence of atypical epithelial cells; its benign nature is supported by the microscopic size and the lack of mitoses.[457] **Epithelial hyperplasia and atypia** can also occur in the absence of inflammation. It is characterized by cellular stratification, mitotic activity, and/or nuclear atypia. Most cases are idiopathic, but some cases are associated with estrogen excess or serous borderline tumor of the ovary.[454, 458–460] There is no current evidence to indicate that these hyperplastic lesions progress to invasive carcinoma. They lack the marked nuclear atypia, brisk mitotic activity, and invasion required for the diagnosis of fallopian tube adenocarcinoma.

The more solid forms of **adenomatoid tumor** can mimic adenocarcinoma by virtue of the lack of circumscription of the tumor and the presence of cords and narrow gland-like structures. However, these lesions are centered on the serosa instead of the mucosa, often show prominent cytoplasmic vacuolation, and do not exhibit nuclear atypia.

Decidual cells occurring in the lamina propria or subserosa of the fallopian tube can be mistaken for primary or metastatic carcinoma because they may exhibit nuclear pleomorphism or even signet-ring forms.[39, 461] The decidual cells typically have distinct pink-staining cell membranes and lack mitotic figures and form only microscopic aggregates.

HISTIOCYTIC INFILTRATE IN THE ENDOMETRIUM OR FALLOPIAN TUBE

Entities to be Considered

The endometrium of fallopian tube can show a prominent infiltrate of histiocytes:

A. *Non-granulomatous*
   Xanthogranulomatous (histiocytic) endometritis/salpingitis
   Pseudoxanthomatous salpingitis/endometritis
   Malakoplakia
   Langerhans' cell histiocytosis (histiocytosis X)
B. *Granulomatous*
   Palisaded granuloma after surgical trauma
   Infective granulomas, e.g., tuberculosis, fungi, actinomycosis, virus
   Foreign body granuloma, e.g., talc, silk suture, Lipiodol (from hysterosalpingography), keratin
   Crohn's disease[462]
   Sarcoidosis[463–465]

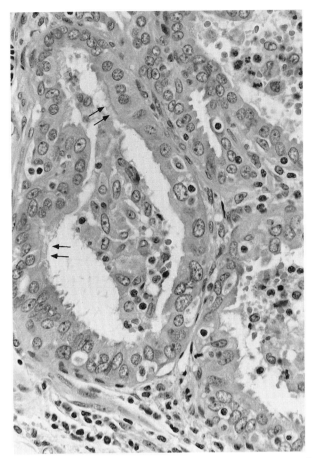

FIGURE 13–82. Chronic Salpingitis (same case as in Fig. 13–81*B*). Some cells exhibit enlarged atypical nuclei. The best clue to the benign nature of the lesion is the presence of cilia *(arrows)* in many epithelial cells.

Approach to Diagnosis

Of prime importance is determining whether the histiocytes form discrete granulomas, because this narrows the differential diagnoses. The appearance of the granuloma further suggests the etiology, although it is always prudent to perform special stains to exclude tuberculosis and fungal infection unless the cause is obvious. It is helpful to examine (including use of polarized light) for foreign bodies that might have been introduced at previous manipulations or for keratin extruded from tumors of the endometrium or ovary (adenocarcinoma with squamous differentiation or atypical polypoid adenomyoma).[466] There are often multinucleated giant cells with haphazardly disposed nuclei in these **foreign body granulomas**[467] (see Fig. 13–81*A*).

Necrobiotic granulomas, characterized by oval, linear, or geographic foci of necrosis surrounded by palisades of histiocytes and fibroblasts, can occur after surgical trauma such as diathermy or biopsy, identical to the palisaded granulomas observed in the prostate after biopsy.[468–470]

Epithelioid granulomas may be observed in tuberculosis, Crohn's disease, sarcoidosis, and rarely in cytomegalovirus infection.[471] In tuberculous infection, the fallopian tube is the preferential site of lodgement in the genital tract, and the uterus is involved through shedding of the organism into the

endometrial cavity. The granulomas in the fallopian tube are often well formed, but those in the endometrium are often poorly formed and associated with variable numbers of neutrophils (Fig. 13–83). The difference is attributable to the cyclical shedding of the endometrium, so that the granulomatous reaction has only a short time to establish itself. The diagnosis of tuberculosis can be confirmed by Ziehl-Neelsen stain and culture.[472] The epithelioid granulomas of sarcoidosis are typically non-necrotizing and, in contrast to tuberculosis, almost always involve the myometrium in addition to the endometrium.[465]

For non-granulomatous histiocytic infiltration of the endometrium or fallopian tube, the diagnosis depends on assessment of the appearance of the histiocytes. Foamy histiocytes predominate in xanthogranulomatous inflammation, although multinucleated giant cells, acute and chronic inflammatory cells, cholesterol crystals, and hemosiderin are often present in variable quantities.[473] **Xanthogranulomatous (histiocytic) endometritis** occurs predominantly in postmenopausal women, often associated with total or partial occlusion of the cervical canal, which probably contributes to the development of hematometra and/or pyometra, with subsequent histiocytic reaction to the breakdown products of the hematoma and pus.[473,474] Some cases have been reported to develop after radiation therapy for endometrial adenocarcinoma, presumably representing an inflammatory reaction to cell injury produced by the radiother-

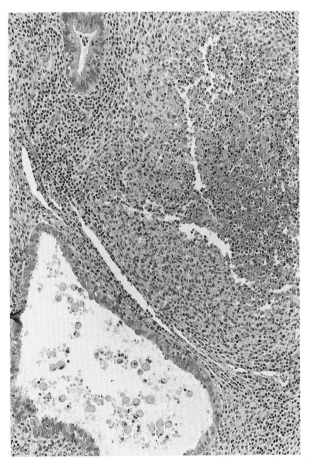

FIGURE 13–83. Tuberculous Endometritis. The granuloma is poorly organized and associated with abundant necrotic material mixed with neutrophils.

apy.[475] On the other hand, **xanthogranulomatous salpingitis** usually occurs in the reproductive age group (Fig. 13–84), and the pathogenetic mechanism is still not known, although some cases may represent foreign body response to oily material (such as lubricants or contrast material).[473]

Pseudoxanthomatous salpingitis is characterized by infiltration of histiocytes with abundant foamy and pigmented cytoplasm. The brown pigment is ceroid. This lesion is associated with pelvic endometriosis or previous pelvic irradiation.[476, 477] Similar histiocytes have also been reported to occur in the endometrium, so-called ''ceroid-containing histiocytic granuloma.''[478]

When histiocytes with eosinophilic granular cytoplasm predominate, **malakoplakia** should be seriously considered; the diagnosis can be confirmed by identification of the diagnostic Michaelis-Gutmann bodies, which are lamellated calcified bodies within the cytoplasm of the histiocytes.[479, 480]

The presence of large numbers of histiocytes with grooved or contorted nuclei, in particular when there are many intermingled eosinophils, points to a diagnosis of **Langerhans cell histiocytosis.** Involvement of the female genital tract by Langerhans cell histiocytosis is rare and occurs mostly in young adults. Either the genital tract is involved alone or the involvement is part of systemic disease.[481]

Exceptionally, **metastatic lobular breast carcinoma** in the uterus may have a histiocyte-like appearance.[484] Its malignant nature can be recognized by the presence of some cells with irregular hyperchromatic nuclei. The diagnosis can be further confirmed by immunostaining for cytokeratin.

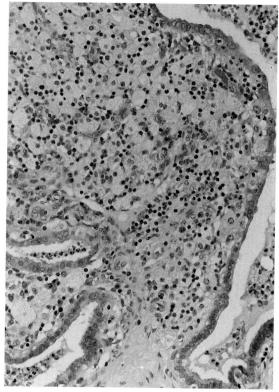

FIGURE 13–84. Xanthogranulomatous Salpingitis. Foamy histiocytes and lymphocytes are increased in the lamina propria.

PROMINENT LYMPHOID INFILTRATE IN THE UTERUS

Entities to be Considered

A variety of conditions can be associated with dense infiltrates of mononuclear lymphoid-looking cells in the uterine corpus (Table 13–23):[485–492]

1. Lymphoma or leukemia[485, 492]
2. Lymphoma-like lesion (reactive lymphoid hyperplasia)
3. Inflammatory pseudotumor
4. Leiomyoma with extensive lymphocytic infiltration mimicking lymphoma

The following entities have to be excluded:

1. Endometrial stromal sarcoma
2. Small-cell carcinoma
3. Primitive neuroectodermal tumor

Approach to Diagnosis

The first step is to ascertain that the infiltrate is indeed hematolymphoid. Hematolymphoid cells rarely show significant nuclear molding as often seen in small-cell carcinoma and primitive neuroectodermal tumor (see Fig. 13–30), usually have distinct cellular outlines, and tend to be diffusely permeative. Furthermore, pseudorosettes, rosettes, and fibrillary matrix as typically seen in primitive neuroectodermal tumor are extremely uncommon in lymphoma.[493] The rich network of arterioles characteristic of endometrial stromal sarcoma is lacking. If in doubt, immunoreactivity for leukocyte common antigen is confirmatory.

If the lymphoid lesion has well-circumscribed borders, the possibilities of leiomyoma with lymphoid infiltrate and inflammatory pseudotumor must be considered instead of malignant lymphoma. Leiomyoma with lymphoid infiltrate can be recognized by identification of a leiomyomatous component in areas and the predominance of non-atypical small lymphocytes. Inflammatory pseudotumor is characterized by spindly cells with features of myofibroblasts mixed with plasma cells and lymphocytes.

Distinction of lymphoma-like lesion from malignant lymphoma can be very difficult, and the presence of many mitotically active large lymphoid cells in the former is particularly worrisome. The former can be distinguished from the latter by the lack of a clinically significant mass lesion, superficial location of the lesion, presence of a heterogeneous cellular infiltrate, and lack of significant atypia in the lymphoid cells (Fig. 13–85).

PROMINENT EOSINOPHILIC INFILTRATE IN THE UTERUS

The endometrium and/or myometrium may be heavily infiltrated by eosinophils in

1. eosinophilic endomyometritis
2. Langerhans cell histiocytosis

Table 13–23. Conditions with a Prominent Lymphoid Infiltrate and Mimickers

Primitive Neuroectodermal Tumor
Very rare.[489–491] Mostly in elderly.
Presentation: Vaginal bleeding.
Outcome: Stage I disease favorable prognosis; stage III/IV disease often proves fatal within 2 years.
Gross: Fleshy polypoid mass in endometrium, often with myometrial invasion.
History: Dense sheets of small primitive, mitotically active cells with scanty cytoplasm. May form pseudorosettes and neuroepithelial tubules.
Probably of mullerian derivation, because some cases are associated with endometrioid adenocarcinoma and endometrial stromal sarcoma.

Leiomyoma with Lymphoid Infiltration
Clinically no different from conventional uterine leiomyoma.[488]
Gross: Typical leiomyoma with whorled appearance; may show softening.
Histology: Moderate to marked infiltrate of lymphocytes in leiomyoma, sometimes obscuring its smooth muscle nature. Occasional large lymphoid cells and plasma cells. Sclerosis common.

Inflammatory Pseudotumor of Uterus
Rare; benign lesion.[487]
Presentation: Lower abdominal pain or incidental finding.
Gross: Well circumscribed mass with a fish-flesh cut surface that may be trabeculated.
Histology: Spindly cells (myofibroblasts or fibroblasts) with fine chromatin and low mitotic count, arranged in interdigitating fascicles. Many plasma cells, some neutrophils, small lymphocytes, and large lymphoid cells. May show areas of hyalinization.

Lymphoma-like Lesion of the Endometrium
Wide age range; benign lesion.[486]
Presentation: Menorrhagia or incidental finding.
Histology: Large activated lymphoid cells in a background of histiocytes, small lymphocytes, plasma cells, and nuclear debris. The large lymphoid cells can form aggregates.

Lymphoma of the Uterus
Rare.[485]
Presentation: Vaginal bleeding.
Gross: Polypoid mass in endometrium.
Histology: Usually high-grade non-Hodgkin's lymphoma.

3. other causes of tissue eosinophilia, e.g., hypereosinophilic syndrome, chronic myeloid leukemia, acute myelomonocytic leukemia with eosinophilia

Eosinophilic endomyometritis is characterized by infiltration of mature eosinophils in the endometrium and/or myometrium, sometimes forming cellular aggregates, and can be accompanied by other inflammatory cells such as small lymphocytes. It apparently does not produce symptoms and is almost always an incidental histologic finding. It can be idiopathic or associated with allergy, but the best known predisposing factor is uterine curettage.[494–496] Such a procedure, performed from less than 1 day to a few weeks before the hysterectomy, is believed to liberate mast cell granules with subsequent recruitment of eosinophils.[494]

Although the histologic changes in hypereosinophilic syndrome are indistinguishable from those of eosinophilic endomyometritis, it can be recognized by the peripheral blood eosinophilia and other systemic manifestations. Similarly, chronic myeloid leukemia can be recognized by the characteristic blood picture and the admixed immature myeloid cells among the cellular infiltrate in the uterus.

MULTICYSTIC LESIONS IN UTERUS OR FALLOPIAN TUBE

Entities to be Considered

When lesions with multicystic pattern are encountered in the uterus or fallopian tube, the following entities may need to be considered (Table 13–24):[497–511]

1. Paratubal cysts
2. Adenomatoid tumor (a benign mesothelial tumor)
3. Multicystic mesothelioma (multilocular peritoneal inclusion cysts)
4. Hemangioma and lymphangioma
5. Cystic Walthard nests
6. Cystic atrophy and cystic glandular hyperplasia (simple hyperplasia) of the endometrium
7. Mullerian adenosarcoma with cystic glands
8. Mature cystic teratoma[510, 511]

Approach to Diagnosis

The last four entities in the list should cause no problems in diagnosis because of the characteristic histopathologic setting and features (see Table 13–24).

Paratubal cysts are common; they are usually solitary but can be multiple. They can be of mullerian (paramesonephric), mesonephric (wolffian), or mesothelial origin. Those of mullerian origin are lined by ciliated epithelium, those of mesonephric origin are lined by cuboidal cells without cilia and

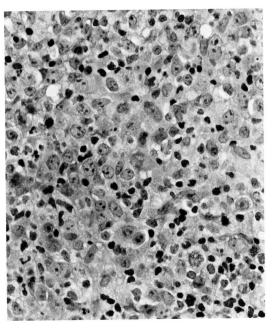

FIGURE 13–85. Lymphoma-like Lesion of the Endometrium. There is a mixture of small lymphocytes, plasma cells, and immunoblasts. The immunoblasts lack atypia such as irregular foldings of the nuclear membrane.

Table 13–24. **Some Entities Characterized by Multicystic Pattern**

Hemangioma and Lymphangioma

Hemangiomas uncommon; lymphangiomas even rarer.[504–506, 508]

Hemangiomas of the uterus are of variable size; they can be subserosal, pedunculated, or intramural.

The proliferated vessels are of capillary or cavernous size and are lined by flat endothelium.

Cystic Walthard Nests

Common incidental findings on the serosal surface of fallopian tube.

They appear as tiny yellow-white nodules, but may form cysts. Always of microscopic size.

The epithelial nests resemble urothelium; the nuclei often exhibit longitudinal grooves. They may form central cystic cavities in which the luminal cells are columnar or mucinous.

Adenomatoid Tumor

Uterine tumors are often small subserosal lesions, but some may be large with a prominent component of cysts.[487–501, 503] Can be circumscribed or ill-defined; cut surfaces have a whorled or trabeculated appearance mimicking leiomyoma.

Fallopian tube tumors are often small lesions causing focal nodular thickening of the wall.[509]

Histologic features: Usually infiltrative, and associated with smooth muscle hyperplasia. Variable proportions of the following elements: (1) polygonal cells with eosinophilic, often vacuolated, cytoplasm and regular nuclei, arranged in solitary units or cords; (2) similar cells forming glandular structures; and (3) cystic spaces lined by attenuated cells. Rarely a papillary pattern is formed. There may be a loose or hyalinized stroma, sometimes with collections with lymphocytes.

Multicystic Mesothelioma (Multilocular Peritoneal Inclusion Cysts)[502, 507]

Usually in reproductive age.

Controversial whether this mesothelial proliferation is reactive or neoplastic.

Presentation: Lower abdominal pain or abdominal mass.

Many patients have history of abdominal operation, pelvic inflammatory disease, or endometriosis.

Approximately 40% develop recurrences, which can be multiple. Rarely lethal.

Gross findings: Multilocular and/or multiple thin-walled cysts loosely attached to or adherent to pelvic peritoneum, including surface of uterus and fallopian tube.

Histology: Variable-sized cysts lined by single layer of flat, cuboidal, or hobnail cells with no atypia. May undergo focal papillary proliferation or squamous metaplasia. The loose fibrovascular septa may be infiltrated by inflammatory cells. Rarely, there is mural mesothelial proliferation of cords and tubules in an inflamed cellular stroma, mimicking carcinoma.

supported by smooth muscle coat, and those of mesothelial origin are lined by flattened cells.

For mass-forming lesions, the possibilities of multicystic mesothelioma, adenomatoid tumor, and lymphangioma have to be considered. The nature of the lining cells, the contents of the cysts, the appearance of the septa, and the other subsidiary features point to the correct diagnosis (Fig. 13–86). In contrast to multicystic mesothelioma, cystic adenomatoid tumor is often centered on the myometrium or fallopian tube wall rather than the serosal surface, exhibits typical features of adenomatoid tumor in some foci (cords and tubules with frequent vacuolated cells), and lacks a prominent inflammatory cell infiltrate (see Fig. 13–86). The possibility of lymphangioma can be virtually excluded if the lining cells show

tufting, budding, and detachment or if basophilic-staining material (acidic mucin) is identified in the lumina (Figs. 13–86 and 13–87). Smooth muscle is often present in the septa and around the cystic spaces in lymphangiomas, but not multicystic mesothelioma. Because adenomatoid tumor is usually infiltrative, smooth muscle of the myometrium or fallopian tube wall is frequently interspersed throughout the lesion (see Fig. 13–86A). In difficult cases, immunohistochemical studies are extremely helpful. The lining cells of multicystic mesothelioma and adenomatoid tumor are cytokeratin-positive, whereas those of lymphangioma are cytokeratin-negative and endothelial marker–positive.

FALLOPIAN TUBE TUMOR WITH A MIXED EPITHELIAL AND SPINDLE CELL PATTERN

Several tumors of the fallopian tube may show a mixture of polygonal epithelial cells and spindly cells, giving an impression of mixed tumor.

1. malignant mixed mullerian tumor, an aggressive tumor with clinical features similar to those of tubal serous carcinoma[512–514]
2. adnexal tumor of probable wolffian origin (Table 13–25)[515–520]
3. endometrioid adenocarcinoma, an uncommon but apparently indolent variant of tubal carcinoma[521]

Malignant mixed mullerian tumor and endometrioid adenocarcinoma grow predominantly intraluminally with or without a polypoid configuration, whereas adnexal wolffian tumor is attached to the serosa of the fallopian tube without mural involvement.

Table 13–25. **Adnexal Tumor of Probable Wolffian Origin**

Age: 18–72 years (mean, 47).

Presentation: Abdominal pain, abdominal swelling, or incidental discovery.

Behavior: Most pursue a benign course, but rare cases show late recurrence after several years and may prove fatal.

Location: Within broad ligament, or attached to broad ligament or fallopian tube by a pedicle.

Gross: Average, 8 cm. Rounded bosselated mass with solid or solid-cystic cut surface. Gray-white, tan, or yellow. Necrosis uncommon.

Histology: Patterns—diffuse, tubular (solid or with small lumina), cystic, or sieve-like. Cuboidal to columnar cells with scanty or occasionally abundant pale cytoplasm. In solid areas, may have a mesenchymal-like spindly appearance; cytoplasmic vacuoles common. Nuclei regular with pale chromatin. Stroma may be hyalinized.

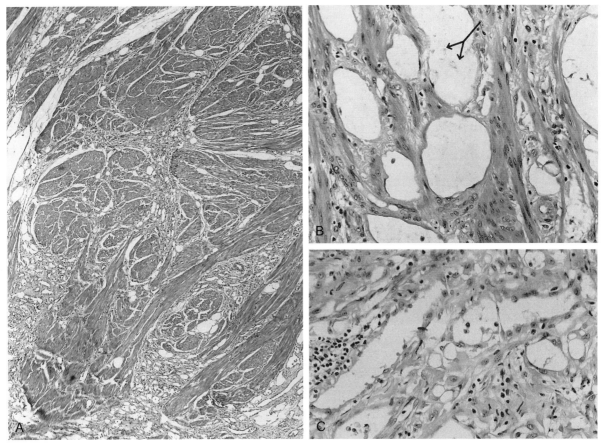

FIGURE 13–86. Adenomatoid Tumor in the Myometrium. *A,* Note the infiltrative growth (mostly in the form of small cysts) among hyperplastic myometrium. *B,* The cysts are lined by attenuated cells. Some contain basophilic material *(double-head arrow)* in the lumen. *C,* The tumor cells form tubules and cords. Cytoplasmic vacuoles are often prominent.

The first tumor shows true mixed epithelial and mesenchymal differentiation, whereas the latter two are pure epithelial neoplasms that exhibit focal pseudomesenchymal growth (with sparse reticulin fibers in contrast to true mesenchymal tissue) (Fig. 13–88). Malignant mixed mullerian tumor usually shows a much greater degree of cellular pleomorphism than the other two tumors, and heterologous elements, if present, provide further support for this diagnosis.

Endometrioid adenocarcinoma can show striking histologic similarity to adnexal wolffian tumor when spindle cells with whorl formation are admixed with microglandular sheets. Features favoring the former diagnosis are (1) predominant intraluminal growth, (2) presence of foci of large tubular glands lined by pseudostratified columnar cells characteristic of endometrioid adenocarcinoma, (3) greater degree of cytologic atypia and mitotic activity, and (4) reticulin fibers surrounding groups of glands instead of single tubules.

UNCOMMON TUMORS AND TUMOR-LIKE LESIONS OF THE UTERUS AND FALLOPIAN TUBE

The following is a list of the very rare tumors and tumor-like lesions that have been reported to occur in the uterus and fallopian tube, but are not covered in the previous sections.

Rare Tumors and Tumor-like Lesions of the Uterine Corpus

- Brenner tumor[522]
- Transitional cell carcinoma[523]
- Paraganglioma (which can be melanotic)[524, 525]
- Pigmented myomatous neurocristoma[526]
- Neurofibroma[232]
- Melanotic schwannoma[232]
- Retinal anlage tumor (pigmented neuroectodermal tumor)[527]
- Yolk sac tumor[527a]
- Wilms' tumor[528]
- Osteoclastic-type giant cell tumor[529, 530]
- Malignant fibrous histiocytoma[531]
- Alveolar soft part sarcoma[532, 533]
- Malignant rhabdoid tumor[534]
- Angiosarcoma[535–538]
- Intravascular lymphomatosis[539]
- Myeloid metaplasia[540]
- Lithiasis[541]

Rare Tumors of the Fallopian Tube

- Serous adenofibroma[542–544]
- Papilloma[545]
- Clear-cell carcinoma[546]
- Adenosquamous carcinoma[547]

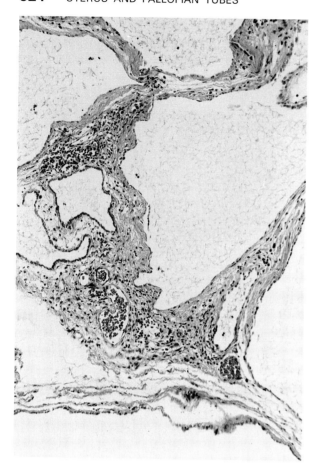

FIGURE 13–87. Cystic Mesothelioma Involving the Serosal Surface of Uterus. The cysts are lined by attenuated cells and separated by delicate fibrous septa often infiltrated by inflammatory cells.

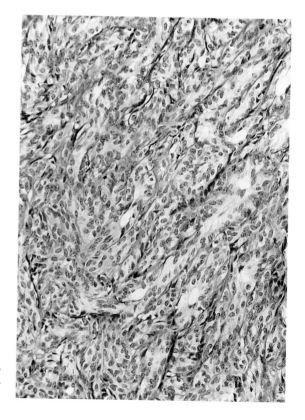

FIGURE 13–88. Adnexal Tumor of Probable Wolffian Origin. Note narrow tubules surrounded by discrete basement membrane and merging into spindly cells in areas.

- Squamous carcinoma[548]
- Transitional cell carcinoma[549, 550]
- Glassy cell carcinoma[551]
- Sex cord tumor with annular tubules[552]
- Leiomyoma[553]
- Neurilemoma[554]
- Lipoma[555]
- Angiomyolipoma[556]
- Ganglioneuroma[557]
- Struma salpingii[558]
- Hydatidiform mole[559]
- Choriocarcinoma[560, 561]

References

1. Yokoyama S, Kashima K, Inoue S, et al: Biotin-containing intranuclear inclusion in endometrial glands during gestation and puerperium. Am J Clin Pathol 99:13–17, 1993.
2. Mazur MT, Hendrickson MR, Kempson RL: Optically clear nuclei: An alteration of endometrial epithelium in the presence of trophoblast. Am J Surg Pathol 7:415–423, 1983.
3. Clement PB, Scully RE: Idiopathic postmenopausal decidual reaction of the endometrium: A clinicopathologic analysis of four cases. Int J Gynecol Pathol 7:152–161, 1988.
4. Wan SK, Lam PWY, Pau MY, Chan JKC: Multiclefted nuclei, a helpful feature for identification of intermediate trophoblastic cells in uterine curetting specimens. Am J Surg Pathol 16:1226–1232, 1992.
5. Daya D, Sabet L: Can one make a diagnosis of intrauterine pregnancy in the absence of chorionic villi? Surg Pathol 3:205–210, 1990.
6. Kurman RJ: The morphology, biology, and pathology of intermediate trophoblast: A look back to the present. Hum Pathol 22:847–855, 1991.
7. Yeh IT, O'Connor DM, Kurman RJ: Intermediate trophoblast: Further immunocytochemical characterization. Mod Pathol 3:282–287, 1990.
8. Schlaen I, Bergeron C, Ferenczy A, et al: Endometrial polyps: A study of 204 cases. Surg Pathol 1:375–382, 1988.
9. Hendrickson MR, Kempson RL: Surgical Pathology of the Uterine Corpus. Major Problems in Pathology, Vol 12. Philadelphia, WB Saunders, 1980.
10. Nuovo MA, Nuovo GJ, McCaffrey RM, et al: Endometrial polyps in postmenopausal patients receiving tamoxifen. Int J Gynecol Pathol 8:125–131, 1989.
11. Corley D, Rowe J, Curtis MT, et al: Postmenopausal bleeding from unusual endometrial polyps in women on chronic tamoxifen therapy. Obstet Gynecol 79:111–116, 1992.
12. De Muylder X, Neven P, De Somer M, et al: Endometrial lesions in patients undergoing tamoxifen therapy. Int J Gynecol Obstet 36:127–130, 1991.
13. Armenia CS: Sequential relationship between endometrial polyp and carcinoma of the endometrium. Obstet Gynecol 30:524–529, 1967.
14. Pettersson B, Adami H, Lindgren A, et al: Endometrial polyps and hyperplasia as risk factors for endometrial carcinoma. Acta Obstet Gynecol Scand 64:653–659, 1985.
15. Silva EG, Jenkins R: Serous carcinoma in endometrial polyps. Mod Pathol 3:120–128, 1990.
16. Gersell DJ: Endometrial papillary syncytial change, another perspective [editorial]. Am J Clin Pathol 99:656–657, 1993.
17. Zaman SS, Mazur MT: Endometrial papillary syncytial change, a nonspecific alteration associated with active breakdown. Am J Clin Pathol 99:741–745, 1993.
18. Hendrickson M, Kempson R: Endometrial epithelial metaplasias: Proliferations frequently misdiagnosed as adenocarcinoma. Report of 89 cases and proposed classification. Am J Surg Pathol 4:525–542, 1980.
19. Lauchlan S: Metaplasias and neoplasias of Mullerian epithelium. Histopathology 8:543–557, 1984.
20. Andersen W, Taylor PJ, Fechner R, et al: Endometrial metaplasia associated with endometrial adenocarcinoma. Am J Obstet Gynecol 157:597–604, 1987.
21. Crum C, Richart R, Fenoglio C: Adenoacanthosis of endometrium: A clinicopathologic study in premenopausal women. Am J Surg Pathol 5:15–20, 1981.
22. Blaustein A: Morular metaplasia misdiagnosed as adenoacanthoma in young women with polycystic ovarian disease. Am J Surg Pathol 6:223–228, 1982.
23. Wells M, Tiltman A: Intestinal metaplasia of the endometrium. Histopathology 15:431–433, 1989.
24. Rorat E, Wallach R: Papillary metaplasia of the endometrium: Clinical and histopathologic considerations. Obstet Gynecol 64:90S–92S, 1984.
25. Bergeron C, Ferenczy A: Oncocytic metaplasia in endometrial hyperplasia and carcinoma [letter]. Int J Gynecol Pathol 7:93–95, 1988.
26. Kraus FT: High-risk and premalignant lesions of the endometrium. Am J Surg Pathol 9(Suppl):31–40, 1985.
27. Norris HJ, Tavassoli FA, Kurman RJ: Endometrial hyperplasia and carcinoma: Diagnostic considerations. Am J Surg Pathol 7:839–847, 1983.
28. Kurman HJ, Kaminski PF, Norris HJ: The behavior of endometrial hyperplasia, a long term study of "untreated" hyperplasia in 170 patients. Cancer 56:403–412, 1985.
29. Kurman RJ, Norris HJ: Endometrium. In Henson DE, Albores-Saavedra J (eds): Pathology of Incipient Neoplasia, 2nd ed. Major Problems in Pathology, Vol 28. Philadelphia, WB Saunders, 1993, pp 268–282.
30. Gal D, Edman CD, Vellios F, et al: Long-term effect of megestrol acetate in the treatment of endometrial hyperplasia. Am J Obstet Gynecol 146:316–320, 1983.
31. Wentz WB: Progestin therapy in endometrial hyperplasia. Gynecol Oncol 2:362–367, 1974.
32. Mazur MT: Atypical polypoid adenomyomas of the endometrium. Am J Surg Pathol 5:473–482, 1981.
33. Young RH, Treger T, Scully RE: Atypical polypoid adenomyoma of the uterus, a report of 27 cases. Am J Clin Pathol 86:139–145, 1986.
34. Clement PB, Young RH: Atypical polypoid adenomyoma of the uterus associated with Turner's syndrome, a report of three cases, including a review of "estrogen-associated" endometrial neoplasms and neoplasms associated with Turner's syndrome. Int J Gynecol Pathol 6:104–113, 1987.
35. Staros EB, Shilkitus WF: Atypical polypoid adenomyoma with carcinomatous transformation: A case report. Surg Pathol 4:157–166, 1991.
36. Lee KR, Scully RE: Complex endometrial hyperplasia and carcinoma in adolescents and young women 15 to 20 years of age: A report of 10 cases. Int Gynecol Pathol 8:201–213, 1989.
37. Clement PB: Tumorlike lesions of the uterine corpus. In Clement PB, Young RH (eds): Tumors and Tumorlike Lesions of the Uterine Corpus and Cervix. Contemporary Issues in Surgical Pathology, Vol 19. New York, Churchill Livingstone, 1993, pp 137–179.
38. Arias-Stella J: Atypical endometrial changes produced by chorionic tissue. Hum Pathol 3:450–453, 1972.
39. Clement PB, Young RH, Scully RE: Non-trophoblastic pathology of the female genital tract and peritoneum associated with pregnancy. Semin Diagn Pathol 6:372–406, 1989.
39a. Arias-Stella J, Arias-Velasquez A, Arias-Stella J: Normal and abnormal mitoses in the atypical endometrial change associated with chorionic tissue effect. Am J Surg Pathol 18:694–701, 1994.
40. Clement PB, Scully RE: Endometrial hyperplasia and carcinoma. In Clement PB, Young RH (eds): Tumors and Tumorlike Lesions of the Uterine Corpus and Cervix. Contemporary Issues in Surgical Pathology, Vol 19. New York, Churchill Livingstone, 1993, pp 181–264.
41. Silverberg SG, DeGiorgi LS: Histopathologic analysis of preoperative radiation therapy in endometrial carcinoma. Am J Obstet Gynecol 119:698–704, 1974.
42. Venkateseshan VS, Woo TH: Diffuse viral papillomatosis (condyloma) of the uterine cavity. Int J Gynecol Pathol 4:370–377, 1985.
43. Roberts PF, Brown JC: Condylomatous atypia of the endometrial cavity, case report. Br J Obstet Gynecol 92:535–538, 1985.
44. Fox H, Buckley CH: The endometrial hyperplasias and their relationship to endometrial neoplasia [invited review]. Histopathology 6:493–510, 1982.
45. Welch WR, Scully RE: Precancerous lesions of the endometrium. Hum Pathol 8:503–512, 1977.
46. Huang SJ, Amparo EG, Fu YS: Endometrial hyperplasia: Histologic classification and behavior. Surg Pathol 1:215–229, 1988.
47. Silverberg SG: Hyperplasia and carcinoma of the endometrium. Semin Diagn Pathol 5:135–153, 1988.
48. Silverberg SG, Kurman RJ: Tumors of the Uterine Corpus and Gestational Trophoblastic Disease. Atlas of Tumor Pathology, 3rd series, Fascicle 3. Washington, DC Armed Forces Institute of Pathology, 1992.
48a. Scully RE, Bonfiglio TA, Kurman RJ, et al: Histological Typing of Femal Genital Tract Tumors. World Health Organization International Histological Classification of Tumours, 2nd ed. Berlin, Springer-Verlag, 1994.
49. Winkler B, Alvarez S, Richart RM, et al: Pitfalls in diagnosis of endometrial neoplasia. Obstet Gynecol 64:185–194, 1984.
50. Sherman AI, Brown S: The precursors of endometrial carcinoma. Am J Obstet Gynecol 135:947–956, 1979.
51. Hendrickson MR, Ross JC, Kempson RL: Toward the development of morphologic criteria for well-differentiated adenocarcinoma of the endometrium. Am J Surg Pathol 7:819–838, 1983.
52. Kurman RH, Norris HJ: Evaluation of criteria for distinguishing atypical endometrial hyperplasia from well differentiated carcinoma. Cancer 49:2547–2559, 1982.
53. Tavassoli F, Kraus FT: Endometrial lesions in uteri resected for atypical endometrial hyperplasia. Am J Clin Pathol 70:770–779, 1978.
54. King A, Seraj IM, Wagner RJ: Stromal invasion in endometrial adenocarcinoma. Am J Obstet Gynecol 149:10–14, 1984.
55. Boronow RC, Morrow CP, Creasman WT, et al: Surgical staging in endometrial cancer: Clinicopathologic findings of a prospective study. Obstet Gynecol 63:825–832, 1984.
56. Tsionou C, Minaretzis D, Papageorgiou I, et al: Expression of carcinoembryonic antigen and ferritin in normal, hyperplastic, and neoplastic epithelium. Gynecol Oncol 41:93–98, 1991.
57. Morse AR, Curran GJ: Distribution of epithelial membrane antigen in normal and abnormal endometrial tissue. Br J Obstet Gynecol 92:1286–1290, 1985.
58. Soderstrom K: Lectin binding into human endometrial hyperplasias and adenocarcinoma. Int J Gynecol Pathol 6:356–365, 1987.
59. Furness PN, Lam EWH: Patterns of basement membrane deposition in benign, premalignant and malignant endometrium. J Clin Pathol 40:1320–1323, 1987.
60. Baak JPA: The use and disuse of morphometry in the diagnosis of endometrial hyperplasia and carcinoma. Pathol Res Pract 179:20–23, 1984.

61. Norris HJ, Becker RL, Mikel UV: A comparative morphometric and cytophotometric study of endometrial hyperplasia, atypical hyperplasia, and endometrial carcinoma. Hum Pathol 20:219–223, 1989.

62. Thornton JG, Quirke P, Wells M: Flow cytometry of normal, hyperplastic, and malignant human endometrium. Am J Obstet Gynecol 161:487–492, 1989.

63. Wilkinson N, Buckley CH, Chawner L, et al: Nucleolar organiser regions in normal, hyperplastic, and neoplastic endometria. Int J Gynecol Pathol 9:55–59, 1990.

64. Dawagne MP, Silverberg SG: Foam cells in endometrial carcinoma. Gynecol Oncol 13:67–75, 1982.

64a. Robboy SJ, Bentley RC, Krigman H, et al: Synoptic reports in gynecologic pathology. Int J Gynecol Pathol 13:161–174, 1994.

65. Clement PB: Miscellaneous primary neoplasms and metastatic neoplasms. In Clement PB, Young RH (eds): Tumors and Tumorlike Lesions of the Uterine Corpus and Cervix. Contemporary Issues in Surgical Pathology, Vol. 19. New York, Churchill Livingstone, 1993, pp 371–418.

66. Kauppila A, Gronroos M, Nieminen U: Clinical outcome in endometrial cancer. Obstet Gynecol 60:473–480, 1982.

67. Abeler VM, Kjorstad KE: Endometrial adenocarcinoma in Norway. Cancer 67:3093–3103, 1991.

68. Silva EG, Jenkins R: Serous carcinoma in endometrial polyps. Mod Pathol 3:120–128, 1990.

69. Lee KR, Belinson JL: Recurrence in noninvasive endometrial carcinoma: Relationship to uterine papillary serous carcinoma. Am J Surg Pathol 15:965–973, 1991.

70. Wilson TO, Podratz KC, Gaffey TA, et al: Evaluation of unfavorable histologic subtypes in endometrial adenocarcinoma. Am J Obstet Gynecol 162:418–426, 1990.

71. Sherman ME, Bitterman P, Rosenshein NB, et al: Uterine serous carcinoma, a morphologically diverse neoplasm with unifying clinicopathologic features. Am J Surg Pathol 16:600–610, 1992.

72. Hendrickson MR, Ross J, Eifel P, et al: Uterine papillary serous carcinoma, a highly malignant form of endometrial adenocarcinoma. Am J Surg Pathol 6:93–108, 1982.

73. Sutton GP, Brill L, Michael H, et al: Malignant papillary lesions of the endometrium. Gynecol Oncol 27:294–304, 1987.

74. Ward BG, Wright RG, Free K: Papillary carcinomas of the endometrium. Gynecol Oncol 39:347–351, 1990.

75. Lauchlan SC: Tubal (serous) carcinoma of the endometrium. Arch Pathol Lab Med 105:615–618, 1981.

76. Jeffrey JF, Krepart GV, Lotocki RJ: Papillary serous adenocarcinoma of the endometrium. Obstet Gynecol 67:670–674, 1986.

77. Abeler VM, Kjorstad KE: Serous papillary carcinoma of the endometrium: A histopathological study of 22 cases. Gynecol Oncol 39:266–271, 1990.

78. Gallion HH, Van Nagell JR Jr, Powell DF, et al: Stage I serous papillary carcinoma of the endometrium. Cancer 63:2224–2228, 1989.

79. Spiegel GW, Cher SS: Endometrial carcinoma in endometrial polyps [abstract]. Mod Pathol 6:78A, 1993.

80. Christopherson WM, Alberhasky RC, Connelly PJ: Carcinoma of the endometrium. I. A clinicopathologic study of clear cell carcinoma and secretory carcinoma. Cancer 49:1511–1523, 1982.

81. Kurman RJ, Scully RE: Clear cell carcinoma of the endometrium, an analysis of 21 cases. Cancer 37:872–882, 1976.

82. Silverberg SG, De Giorgi LS: Clear cell carcinoma of the endometrium. Clinical, pathologic, and ultrastructural findings. Cancer 31:1127–1140, 1973.

83. Eastwood J: Mesonephroid (clear cell) carcinoma of the ovary and endometrium, a comparative prospective clinicopathological study and review of the literature. Cancer 41:1911–1928, 1978.

84. Crum CP, Fechner RE: Clear cell adenocarcinoma of the endometrium, a clinicopathologic study of 11 cases. Am J Diagn Gynecol Obstet 1:261–267, 1979.

85. Abeler VM, Kjorstad KE: Clear cell carcinoma of the endometrium, a histopathological and clinical study of 97 cases. Gynecol Oncol 40:207–217, 1991.

86. Kanbour-Shakir A, Tobon H: Primary clear cell carcinoma of the endometrium: A clinicopathologic study of 20 cases. Int J Gynecol Pathol 10:67–78, 1991.

87. Webb GA, Lagios MD: Clear cell carcinoma of the endometrium. Am J Obstet Gynecol 156:1486–1491, 1987.

88. Tiltman AJ: Mucinous carcinoma of the endometrium. Obstet Gynecol 55:244–247, 1980.

89. Czernobilsky B, Katz Z, Lancet M, et al: Endocervical-type epithelium in endometrial carcinoma, a report of 10 cases with emphasis on histochemical methods for differential diagnosis. Am J Surg Pathol 4:481–489, 1980.

90. Ross JC, Eifel PJ, Cox RS, et al: Primary mucinous adenocarcinoma of the endometrium, a clinicopathologic and histochemical study. Am J Surg Pathol 7:715–729, 1983.

91. Melhem MF, Tobon H: Mucinous adenocarcinoma of the endometrium: A clinicopathological review of 18 cases. Int J Gynecol Pathol 6:347–355, 1987.

92. Young RH, Scully RE: Uterine carcinomas simulating microglandular hyperplasia: A report of six cases. Am J Surg Pathol 16:1092–1097, 1992.

93. Kay S: Squamous cell carcinoma of the endometrium. Am J Clin Pathol 61:264–274, 1974.

94. Jeffers MD, McDonald GSA, McGuinness EP: Primary squamous cell carcinoma of the endometrium. Histopathology 19:177–179, 1991.

95. Abeler V, Kjorstad KE: Endometrial squamous cell carcinoma: A report of three cases and review of the literature. Gynecol Oncol 36:321–326, 1990.

96. Sluijmer AV, Ubachs JMH, Stoot JEGM, et al: Clinical and pathological aspects of benign and malignant squamous epithelium of the corpus uteri: A report of two cases. Eur J Obstet Gynecol Reprod Biol 39:71–75, 1991.

97. Orhon E, Ulgenalp I, Baser I, et al: Primary squamous cell carcinoma of the endometrium. Eur J Cancer 27:946, 1991.

98. Ryder DE: Verrucous carcinoma of the endometrium—a unique neoplasm with a long survival. Obstet Gynecol 59:78S–80S, 1982.

99. Hussain SF: Verrucous carcinoma of the endometrium. APMIS 96:1075–1078, 1988.

100. Abler VM, Kjorstad KE, Nesland JM: Undifferentiated carcinoma of the endometrium, a histopathologic and clinical study of 31 cases. Cancer 68:98–105, 1991.

101. Manivel C, Wick MR, Sibley RK: Neuroendocrine differentiation in Mullerian neoplasms: An immunohistochemical study of a ''pure'' endometrial small cell carcinoma and a mixed Mullerian tumor containing small cell carcinoma. Am J Clin Pathol 86:438–443, 1986.

102. Paz R, Frigerio B, Sundblad A, et al: Small cell (oat cell) carcinoma of the endometrium. Arch Pathol Lab Med 109:270–272, 1985.

103. Huntsman DG, Clement PB, Gilks CB, Scully RE: Small cell carcinoma of the endometrium, a clinicopathological study of 16 cases. Am J Surg Pathol 18:364–375, 1994.

104. Tohya T, Miyaraki K, Katabuchi H, et al: Small cell carcinoma of the endometrium associated with adenosquamous carcinoma, a light and electron microscopic study. Gynecol Oncol 25:363–371, 1986.

104a. van Hoeven KH, Hudock JA, Woodruff JM, Suhrland MJ: Small cell neuroendocrine carcinoma of the endometrium. Int J Gynecol Pathol 14:21–29, 1995.

105. Christopherson WM, Alberhasky RC, Connelly PJ: Glassy cell carcinoma of the endometrium. Hum Pathol 13:418–421, 1982.

106. Arends JW, Willebrand D, DeKoning HJ, et al: Adenocarcinoma of the endometrium with glassy cell features—immunohistochemical observations. Histopathology 8:873–879, 1984.

107. Dawson EC, Belinson JL, Lee K: Glassy cell carcinoma of the endometrium responsive to megestrol acetate. Gynecol Oncol 33:121–124, 1989.

108. Hachisuga T, Sugimori H, Kaku T, et al: Glassy cell carcinoma of the endometrium. Gynecol Oncol 36:134–138, 1990.

109. Bannatyne P, Russell P, Wills EJ: Argyrophilia and endometrial carcinoma. Int J Gynecol Pathol 2:235–254,1983.

110. Inoue M, DeLellis RA, Scully RE: Immunohistochemical demonstration of chromogranin in endometrial carcinomas with argyrophil cells. Hum Pathol 17:841–847, 1986.

111. Inoue M, Ueda G, Yamasaki M, et al: Immunohistochemical demonstration of peptide hormones in endometrial carcinoma. Cancer 54:2127–2131, 1984.

112. Hendrickson MR, Kempson RL: Ciliated carcinoma—a variant of endometrial adenocarcinoma: A report of 10 cases. Int J Gynecol Pathol 2:1–12, 1983.

113. Haibach H, Oxenhandler RW, Luger AM: Ciliated adenocarcinoma of the endometrium. Acta Obstet Gynecol Scand 64:457–462, 1985.

114. Tobon H, Watkins GJ: Secretory adenocarcinoma of the endometrium. Int J Gynecol Pathol 4:328–335, 1985.

115. Chen JL, Trost DC, Wilkinson EJ: Endometrial papillary adenocarcinomas: Two clinicopathologic types. Int J Gynecol Pathol 4:279–288, 1985.

116. O'Hanlan KA, Levine PA, Harbatkin D, et al: Virulence of papillary endometrial carcinoma. Gynecol Oncol 37:112–119, 1990.

117. Fox H, Brander WL: A sertoliform endometrioid adenocarcinoma of the endometrium. Histopathology 13:584–585, 1988.

118. Gernow A, Ahrentsen OD: Adenoid cystic carcinoma of the endometrium. Histopathology 15:197–198, 1990.

119. Chan JKC: Cribriform endometrioid adenocarcinoma, not adenoid cystic carcinoma, of the endometrium [letter]. Histopathology 16:317, 1990.

120. Ng ABP, Reagan JW, Storaasli JP, et al: Mixed adenosquamous carcinoma of the endometrium. Am J Clin Pathol 59:765–781, 1973.

121. Silverberg SG, Bolin MG, DeGiorgi LS: Adenoacanthoma and mixed adenosquamous carcinoma of the endometrium, a clinicopathologic study. Cancer 30:1307–1314, 1972.

122. Haqqani MT, Fox H: Adenosquamous carcinoma of the endometrium. J Clin Pathol 29:959–966, 1976.

123. Alberhansky RC, Connelly PJ, Christopherson WM: Carcinoma of the endometrium. IV. Mixed adenosquamous carcinoma. A clinicopathological study of 68 cases with long-term follow-up. Am J Clin Pathol 77:655–664, 1982.

124. Savage J, Subby W, Okagaki T: Adenocarcinoma of the endometrium with trophoblastic differentiation and metastases as choriocarcinoma: A case report. Gynecol Oncol 26:257–262, 1987.

125. Pesce C, Merino MJ, Chambers JT, et al: Endometrial carcinoma with trophoblastic proliferation, an aggressive form of uterine cancer. Cancer 68:1799–1802, 1991.

126. Jones MA, Young RH, Scully RE: Endometrial adenocarcinoma with a component of giant cell carcinoma. Int J Gynecol Pathol 10:260–270, 1991.

126a. Ambros RA, Ballouk F, Malfetano JH, Ross JP: Significance of papillary (villioglandular) differentiation in endometrial carcinoma of the uterus. Am J Surg Pathol 18:569–575, 1994.

127. Zaino RJ, Kurman RJ: Squamous differentiation in carcinoma of the endometrium: A critical appraisal of adenoacanthoma and adenosquamous carcinoma. Semin Diagn Pathol 5:154–171, 1988.

128. Zaino RJ, Kurman RJ, Herbold D, et al: The significance of squamous differentiation in endometrial carcinoma. Data from a gynaecologic oncology group study. Cancer 68:2293–2302, 1991.

129. Abeler VM, Kjorstad KE: Endometrial adenocarcinoma with squamous cell differentiation. Cancer 69:488–495, 1992.

130. Connelly PJ, Alberhasky RC, Christopherson WM: Carcinoma of the endometrium. III. Analysis of 865 cases of adenocarcinoma and adenoacanthoma. Obstet Gynecol 59:569–575, 1982.

131. Demopoulos RI, Dubin N, Noumoff J, et al: Prognostic significance of squamous differentiation in stage I endometrial adenocarcinoma. Obstet Gynecol 68:245–250, 1986.

132. Shepherd JH: Revised FIGO staging for gynaecological cancer. Br J Obstet Gynaecol 96:889–892, 1989.

133. Sutton GP, Geisler HE, Stehman FB, et al: Features associated with survival and disease-free survival in early endometrial cancer. Am J Obstet Gynecol 160:1385–1393, 1989.

134. Morrow CP, Bundy BN, Kurman RJ, et al: Relationship between surgical-pathological risk factors and outcome in clinical stage I and II carcinoma of the endometrium: A Gynecologic Oncology Group study. Gynecol Oncol 40:55–65, 1991.

135. Creasman WT, Morrow CP, Bundy BN, et al: Surgical pathologic spread patterns of endometrial cancer. A Gynecologic Oncologic Group Study. Cancer 60:2035–2041, 1987.

136. Piver MS, Lele S, Barlow JJ, et al: Paraaortic lymph node evaluation in stage I endometrial carcinoma. Obstet Gynecol 59:97–100, 1982.

137. Hendrickson M, Ross J, Eifel PJ, et al: Adenocarcinoma of the endometrium; Analysis of 256 cases with carcinoma limited to the uterine corpus. Pathology review and analysis of prognostic variables. Gynecol Oncol 13:373–392, 1982.

138. Mittal KR, Schwarz PE, Barwick KW: Architectural (FIGO) grading, nuclear grading and other prognostic indicators in stage I endometrial adenocarcinoma with identification of high-risk and low-risk groups. Cancer 61:538–545, 1988.

138a. Zaino RJ, Silverberg SG, Norris HJ, et al: The prognostic value of nuclear versus architectural grading in endometrial adenocarcinoma: A Gynecologic Oncology Group study. Int J Gynecol Pathol 13:29–36, 1994.

138b. Zaino RJ, Kurman RJ, Diana KL: The utility of the revised FIGO system for the histologic grading of endometrial adenocarcinoma [abstract]. Mod Pathol 7:98A, 1994.

139. Grigsby PW, Perez CA, Kuten A, et al: Clinical Stage I endometrial cancer: Prognostic factors for local control and distant metastasis and implications of the new FIGO surgical staging system. Int J Radiat Oncol Biol Phys 22:905–911, 1992.

140. Ambros RA, Kurman RJ: Combined assessment of vascular and myometrial invasion as a model to predict prognosis in stage I endometrioid adenocarcinoma of the uterine corpus. Cancer 69:1424–1431, 1992.

141. Gal D, Recio F, Zamurovic D: The new International Federation of Gynecology and Obstetrics surgical staging and survival rates in early endometrial carcinoma. Cancer 69:200–202, 1992.

142. Templeton AC: Reporting of myometrial invasion by endometrial cancer. Histopathology 6:733–737, 1982.

143. Lutz MH, Underwood PB, Kreutner A, et al: Endometrial carcinoma: A new method of classification of therapeutic and prognostic significance. Gynecol Oncol 6:83–94, 1978.

144. Mittal KR, Barwick KW: Diffusely infiltrating adenocarcinoma of the endometrium: A subtype with a poor prognosis. Am J Surg Pathol 12:754–759, 1988.

145. Hernandez E, Woodruff JD: Endometrial adenocarcinoma arising in adenomyosis. Am J Obstet Gynecol 138:827–832, 1980.

146. Hall JB, Young RH, Nelson JH: The prognostic significance of adenomyosis in endometrial carcinoma. Gynecol Oncol 17:32–40, 1984.

147. Jacques SM, Lawrence WD: Endometrial adenocarcinoma with variable-level myometrial involvement limited to adenomyosis: A clinicopathologic study of 23 cases. Gynecol Oncol 37:401–407, 1990.

148. Tornos C, Silva EG, El-Naggar A, Burke TW: Aggressive stage I grade I endometrial carcinoma. Cancer 70:790–798, 1992.

149. Gal D, Recio OF, Zamurovic D, et al: Lymphovascular space involvement—a prognostic indicator in endometrial adenocarcinoma. Gynecol Oncol 42:142–145, 1991.

150. Hanson MB, Van Nagell JR Jr, Powell DE, et al: The prognostic significance of lymphovascular space invasion in stage I endometrial cancer. Cancer 55:1753–1757, 1985.

151. Sivridis E, Buckley CH, Fox H: The prognostic significance of lymphatic vascular space invasion in endometrial adenocarcinoma. Br J Obstet Gynaecol 94:991–994, 1987.

152. Morrow CP, DiSaia PJ, Townsend DE: Current management of endometrial carcinoma. Obstet Gynecol 42:399–403, 1973.

153. Bigelow B, Vekshtein V, Demopoulos RI: Endometrial carcinoma, stage II: Route and extent of spread to the cervix. Obstet Gynecol 62:363–366, 1983.

154. Fanning J, Alvarez PM, Tsukada Y, et al: Prognostic significance of the extent of cervical involvement by endometrial carcinoma. Gynecol Oncol 40:46–47, 1991.

155. Reisinger SA, Staros EB, Mohiuddin M: Survival and failure analysis in stage II endometrial cancer using the revised 1988 FIGO staging system. Int J Radiat Oncol Biol Phys 21:1027–1032, 1991.

156. Lurain JR, Rice BL, Rademaker AW, et al: Prognostic factors associated with recurrence in clinical stage I adenocarcinoma of the endometrium. Obstet Gynecol 78:63–69, 1991.

157. Kadar NRD, Kohorn EI, LiVolsi VA, et al: Histologic variants of cervical involvement by endometrial carcinoma. Obstet Gynecol 59:85–93, 1982.

158. Frauenhoffer EE, Zaino R, Wolff TV, et al: Value of endocervical curettage in the staging of endometrial carcinoma. Int J Gynecol Pathol 6:195–202, 1987.

159. Weiner J, Bigelow B, Demopoulos RI, et al: The value of endocervical sampling in the staging of endometrial carcinoma. Diagn Gynecol Obstet 2:265–268, 1989.

160. Caron C, Tetu B, Laberge G, et al: Endocervical involvement by endometrial carcinoma on fractional curettage: A clinicopathologic study of 37 cases. Mod Pathol 4:644–647, 1991.

161. Fanning J, Alvarez PM, Tsukada Y, et al: Cervical implantation metastasis by endometrial adenocarcinoma. Cancer 68:1335–1339, 1991.

162. Tak WK: Carcinoma of the endometrium with cervical involvement (stage II). Cancer 43:2504, 1979.

163. Hachisuga T, Kaku T, Enjoji M: Carcinoma of the lower uterine segment, clinicopathologic analysis of 12 cases. Int J Gynecol Pathol 8:26–35, 1989.

164. Ulbright TM, Roth LM: Metastatic and independent cancers of the endometrium and ovary: A clinicopathologic study of 34 cases. Hum Pathol 16:28–34, 1985.

165. Prat J, Matias-Guiu X, Barreto J: Simultaneous carcinoma involving the endometrium and ovary. A clinicopathologic, immunohistochemical, and DNA flow cytometric study of 18 cases. Cancer 68:2455–2459, 1991.

166. Eifel P, Hendrickson M, Ross J, et al: Simultaneous presentation of carcinoma involving ovary and the uterine corpus. Cancer 50:163–170, 1982.

167. Chen KTK, Kostick ND, Rosai J: Peritoneal foreign body granulomas to keratin in uterine adenoacanthoma. Arch Pathol Lab Med 102:174–177, 1978.

168. Kim K, Scully RE: Peritoneal keratin granulomas with carcinomas of the endometrium and ovary and atypical polypoid adenomyoma of the endometrium. Am J Surg Pathol 14:925–932, 1990.

169. Creasman WT, DiSaia PJ, Blessing J, et al: Prognostic significance of peritoneal cytology in patients with endometrial cancer and preliminary data concerning therapy with intraperitoneal radiopharmaceuticals. Am J Obstet Gynecol 141:921–929, 1981.

170. Harouny VR, Sutton GP, Clark SA, et al: The importance of peritoneal cytology in endometrial carcinoma. Obstet Gynecol 72:394–398, 1988.

171. Turner DA, Gershenson DM, Atkinson N, et al: The prognostic significance of peritoneal cytology for stage I endometrial cancer. Obstet Gynecol 74:775–780, 1989.

172. Yazigi R, Piver MS, Blumenson L: Malignant peritoneal cytology as prognostic indicator in stage I endometrial cancer. Obstet Gynecol 62:359–362, 1983.

173. Hirai Y, Fujimoto I, Yamauchi K, et al: Peritoneal fluid cytology and prognosis in patients with endometrial carcinoma. Obstet Gynecol 73:335–338, 1989.

174. Sidaway MK, Silverberg SG: Endometrial adenocarcinoma, pathologic factors of therapeutic and prognostic significance. Pathol Annu 27:153–185, 1992.

175. Beckner ME, Mori T, Silverberg SG: Endometrial carcinoma: Nontumor factors in prognosis. Int J Gynecol Pathol 4:131–145, 1985.

176. Deligdisch L, Cohen CJ: Histologic correlates and virulence implications of endometrial carcinoma associated with adenomatous hyperplasia. Cancer 56:1452–1455, 1985.

177. Bokhman JV: Two pathogenetic types of endometrial cancer. Gynecol Oncol 15:10–17, 1983.

178. Ehrlich CE, Young PCM, Cleary RE: Cytoplasmic progesterone and estradiol receptors in normal, hyperplastic, and carcinomatous endometria: Therapeutic implications. Am J Obstet Gynecol 141:539–546, 1981.

179. Kauppila A, Kujansuu E, Vihko R: Cytosol estrogen and progestin receptors in endometrial carcinoma of patients treated with surgery, radiotherapy and progestin. Cancer 50:2157–2162, 1982.

180. Martin JD, Hahnel R, McCartney AJ, et al: The effect of estrogen receptor status on survival in patients with endometrial cancer. Am J Obstet Gynecol 147:322–324, 1983.

181. Creasman WT, Soper JT, McCarty KS Jr, et al: Influence of cytoplasmic steroid receptor content on prognosis in early stage endometrial carcinoma. Am J Obstet Gynecol 151:922–932, 1985.

182. Budwit-Novotny DA, McCarty KS, Cox EB, et al: Immunohistochemical analyses of estrogen receptor in endometrial adenocarcinoma using a monoclonal antibody. Cancer Res 46:5419–5425, 1986.

183. Mutch DG, Soper JT, Budwit-Novotny DA, et al: Endometrial adenocarcinoma estrogen receptor content: Association of clinicopathologic features with immunohistochemical analysis compared with standard biochemical methods. Am J Obstet Gynecol 157:924–931, 1987.

184. Chambers JT, MacLusky N, Eisenfield A, et al: Estrogen and progestin receptor levels as prognosticators for survival in endometrial carcinomas. Gynecol Oncol 31:65–77, 1988.

185. Palmer DC, Muir IM, Alexander AI, et al: The prognostic importance of steroid receptors in endometrial carcinoma. Obstet Gynecol 72:388–393, 1988.

186. Brustein S, Fruchter R, Greene GL, et al: Immunocytochemical assay of progesterone receptor in paraffin-embedded specimens of endometrial carcinoma and hyperplasia, a preliminary evaluation. Mod Pathol 2:449–455, 1989.

187. Segreti EM, Novotny DB, Soper JT, et al: Endometrial cancer: Histologic correlates of immunohistochemical localization of progesterone receptor and estrogen receptor. Obstet Gynecol 73:780–785, 1989.

188. Carcangiu ML, Chambers JT, Voynick IM, et al: Immunohistochemical evaluation of estrogen and progesterone receptor content in 183 patients with endometrial carcinoma. Part I: Clinical and histologic correlations. Am J Clin Pathol 94:247–254, 1990.

189. Chambers JT, Carcangiu ML, Voynick IM, et al: Immunohistochemical evaluation of estrogen and progesterone receptor content in 183 patients with endometrial carcinoma. Part II: Correlation between biochemical and immunohistochemical methods and survival. Am J Clin Pathol 94:255–260, 1990.

190. Kleine W, Maier T, Geyer H, et al: Estrogen and progesterone receptors in endometrial cancer and their prognostic relevance. Gynecol Oncol 38:59–65, 1990.

191. Richardson GS, MacLaughlin DT: The staus of receptors in the management of endometrial cancer. Clin Obstet Gynecol 29:628–637, 1986.

192. Ingram SS, Rosenman J, Heath R, et al: The predictive value of progesterone receptor levels in endometrial cancer. Int J Radiat Oncol Biol Phys 17:21–27, 1989.

193. Thornton JG, Quirke P, Wells M: Flow cytometry of normal, hyperplastic, and malignant human endometrium. Am J Obstet Gynecol 161:487–492, 1989.

194. Iversen OE: Flow cytometric deoxyribonucleic acid index: A prognostic factor in endometrial carcinoma. Am J Obstet Gynecol 155:770–776, 1986.

195. Rosenberg P, Wingren S, Simonsen E, et al: Flow cytometric measurements of DNA index and S-phase on paraffin-embedded early stage endometrial cancer, an important prognostic factor. Gynecol Oncol 35:50–54, 1989.

196. Geisinger KR, Kute TE, Marshall RBM, et al: Analysis of the relationship of the ploidy and cell cycle kinetics to differentiation of the female sex steroid hormone receptors in adenocarcinoma of the endometrium. Am J Clin Pathol 85:536–541, 1986.

197. Iversen OE, Utaaker E, Skaarland E: DNA ploidy and steroid receptors as predictors of disease course in patients with endometrial carcinoma. Acta Obstet Gynecol Scand 67:531–537, 1988.

198. Britton LC, Wilson TO, Gaffey TA, et al: Flow cytometric DNA analysis of stage I endometrial carcinoma. Gynecol Oncol 34:317–322, 1989.

199. Britton LC, Wilson TO, Gaffey TA, et al: DNA ploidy in endometrial carcinoma: Major objective prognostic factor. Mayo Clin Proc 65:643–650, 1990.

200. Newbury R, Schuerch C, Goodspeed N, et al: DNA content as a prognostic factor in endometrial carcinoma. Obstet Gynecol 76:251–257, 1990.

201. Symonds DA: Prognostic value of pathologic features and DNA analysis in endometrial carcinoma. Gynecol Oncol 39:272–276, 1990.

202. Konski AA, Myles JL, Sawyer T, et al: Flow cytometric DNA content analysis of paraffin block embedded endometrial carcinomas. Int J Radiat Oncol Biol Phy 21:1033–1039, 1991.

203. Borts MP, Baker VV, Dixon D, et al: Oncogene alterations in endometrial carcinoma. Gynecol Oncol 38:364–366, 1990.

204. Brumm C, Riviere A, Wilckens C, et al: Immunohistochemical investigation and Northern Blot analysis of c-erbB-2 expression in normal, premalignant and malignant tissues of the corpus and cervix uteri. Virchows Arch [Pathol Anat] 417:477–484, 1990.

205. Berchuck A, Rodriguez G, Kinney RB, et al: Overexpression of HER-2/neu in endometrial cancer is associated with advanced stage disease. Am J Obstet Gynecol 164:15–21, 1991.

206. Mizuuchi H, Nasim S, Kudo R, et al: Clinical implications of K-ras mutations in malignant epithelial tumors of the endometrium. Cancer Res 52:2777–2781, 1992.

207. Kacinski BM, Carter D, Mittal K, et al: High level expression of fms proto-oncogene mRNA is observed in clinically aggressive human endometrial adenocarcinomas. Int J Radiat Oncol Biol Phys 15:823–829, 1988.

208. Bur ME, Perlman C, Edelmann L, et al: p53 expression in neoplasms of the uterine corpus. Am J Clin Pathol 98:81–87, 1992.

209. Kohler MF, Berchuck A, Davidoff AM, et al: Overexpression and mutation of p53 in endometrial carcinomas. Cancer Res 52:1622–1627, 1992.

210. Norris HJ, Taylor HB: Mesenchymal tumors of the uterus. I. A clinical and pathologic study of 53 endometrial stromal tumors. Cancer 19:755–766, 1966.

211. Clement PB: Pure mesenchymal tumors. In Clement PB, Young RH (eds): Tumors and Tumor-like Lesions of the Uterine Corpus and Cervix. Contemporary Issues in Surgical Pathology, Vol 19. New York, Churchill Livingstone, 1993, pp 265–328.

212. King ME, Dickersin GR, Scully RE: Myxoid leiomyosarcoma of the uterus. A report of six cases. Am J Surg Pathol 6:589–598, 1982.

213. Chen KTK: Myxoid leiomyosarcoma of the uterus. Int J Gynecol Pathol 3:389–392, 1984.

214. Pounder DJ, Iyer PV: Uterine leiomyosarcoma with myxoid stroma. Arch Pathol Lab Med 109:762–764, 1985.

215. Salm R, Evans DJ: Myxoid leiomyosarcoma. Histopathology 9:159–169, 1985.

216. Tavassoli FA, Norris HJ: Mesenchymal tumours of the uterus. VII. A clinicopathological study of 60 endometrial stromal nodules. Histopathology 5:1–10, 1981.

217. Norris HJ, Hilliard GD, Irey NS: Hemorrhagic cellular leiomyomas ("apoplectic leiomyoma") of the uterus associated with pregnancy and oral contraceptives. Int J Gynecol Pathol 7:212–224, 1988.

218. Fechner RE: Atypical leiomyomas and synthetic progestin therapy. Am J Clin Pathol 49:697–703, 1968.

219. August C, Kepic T, Meier L, Valle J: Histologic findings in uterine leiomyomata of women treated with gonadotropin-releasing hormone agonists [Abstract]. Am J Clin Pathol 97:448, 1992.

220. Colgan TJ, Pendergast S, Leblanc M: The histopathology of uterine leiomyomas following treatment with gonadotropin releasing hormone analogue. Hum Pathol 24:1073–1077, 1993.

221. Mazur MT, Kraus FT: Histogenesis of morphologic variations in tumors of the uterine wall. Am J Surg Pathol 4:59–74, 1980.

222. Clement PB: Intravenous leiomyomatosis. Pathol Annu 23(2):153–183, 1988.

223. Suginami H, Kaura R, Ochi H, Matsuura S: Intravenous leiomyomatosis with cardiac extension: Successful surgical management and histopathologic study. Obstet Gynecol 76:527–529, 1990.

224. Tierney WM, Ehrlich CE, Bailey JC, et al: Intravenous leiomyomatosis of the uterus with extension into the heart. Am J Med 69:471–475, 1980.

225. Rotter AJ, Lundell CJ: MR of intravenous leiomyomatosis of the uterus extending into the inferior vena cava. J Comput Assist Tomogr 15:690–693, 1991.

226. Kempson RL, Hendrickson MR: Pure mesenchymal neoplasms of the uterine corpus: Selected problems. Semin Diagn Pathol 5:172–198, 1988.

227. Gilks CB, Taylor GP, Clement PB: Inflammatory pseudotumor of the uterus. Int J Gynecol Pathol 6:275–286, 1987.

228. Clement PB: Postoperative spindle cell nodule of the endometrium. Arch Pathol Lab Med 112:566–568, 1987.

229. Farhood AI, Abrams J: Immunohistochemistry of endometrial stromal sarcoma. Hum Pathol 22:224–230, 1991.

230. Franquemont DW, Frierson HF, Mills SE: An immunohistochemical study of normal endometrial stroma and endometrial stromal neoplasms. Evidence for smooth muscle differentiation. Am J Surg Pathol 15:861–870, 1991.

231. Azumi H, Ben-Ezra J, Battifora H: Immunophenotypic diagnosis of leiomyosarcomas and rhabdomyosarcomas with monoclonal antibodies to muscle-specific actin and desmin in formalin-fixed tissue. Mod Pathol 1:469–474, 1988.

232. Devaney K, Tavassoli FA: Immunohistochemistry as a diagnostic aid in the interpretation of unusual mesenchymal tumors of the uterus. Mod Pathol 4:225–231, 1991.

233. Binder SW, Nieberg RK, Cheng L, Al Jitawi S: Histologic and immunohistochemical analysis of nine endometrial stromal tumors: An unexpected high frequency of keratin protein positivity. Int J Gynecol Pathol 10:191–197, 1991.

234. Jensen PA, Dockerty MB, Symmonds RE, Wilson RB: Endometrioid sarcoma ("stromal endometriosis"). Report of 15 cases including 5 with metastases. Am J Obstet Gynecol 95:79–94, 1966.

235. Baggish MS, Woodruff JD: Uterine stromatosis. Clinicopathologic features and hormone dependency. Obstet Gynecol 40:487–498, 1972.

236. Hart WR, Yoonessi M: Endometrial stromatosis of the uterus. Obstet Gynecol 49:393–403, 1977.

237. Fekete PS, Vellios F: The clinical and histologic spectrum of endometrial stromal neoplasms: A report of 41 cases. Int J Gynecol Pathol 3:198–212, 1984.

238. Chang KL, Crabtree GS, Lim-Tan SK, et al: Primary uterine endometrial stromal neoplasms. A clinicopathologic study of 117 cases. Am J Surg Pathol 14:415–438, 1990.

239. Lloreta J, Prat J: Endometrial stromal nodule with smooth and skeletal muscle components simulating stromal sarcoma. Int J Gynecol Pathol 11:293–298, 1992.

240. Sooriyaarachchi GS, Ramirez G, Roley EL: Hemangiopericytoma of the uterus: Report of a case with a comprehensive review of the literature. J Surg Oncol 10:399–406, 1978.

241. Buscema J, Klein V, Rotmensch J, et al: Uterine hemangiopericytoma. Obstet Gynecol 69:104–108, 1987.

242. Zaloudek C, Norris HJ: Mesenchymal tumors of the uterus. In Kurman RJ (ed): Blaustein's Pathology of the Female Genital Tract, 3rd ed. New York, Springer-Verlag, 1987, pp 373–408.

243. Yu TJ, Iwasaki I, Teratani T, et al: Circumscribed endometrial stromatosis of the uterus with marked epitheliogenesis. Gynecol Oncol 24:367–372, 1986.

244. Lillemoe TJ, Perrone T, Norris HJ, Dehner LP: Myogenous phenotype of epithelial-like areas in endometrial stromal sarcomas. Arch Pathol Lab Med 115:215–219, 1991.

245. Clement PB, Scully RE: Uterine tumors resembling ovarian sex-cord tumors. Am J Clin Pathol 66:512–525, 1976.

246. Sullinger JC, Scully RE: Uterine tumors resembling ovarian sex-cord tumors: A clinicopathologic study of 92 cases [in preparation].

247. Clement PB, Scully RE: Endometrial stromal sarcomas of the uterus with extensive endometrioid glandular differentiation. A report of three cases that caused problems in differential diagnosis. Int J Gynecol Pathol 11:163–173, 1992.

248. Findley JL, Neill JSA, McCool J, Silverman JF: Uterine leiomyoma with tubules: Light microscopic, immunohistochemical and ultrastructural observations [abstract]. Mod Pathol 6:73A, 1993.

249. Silverberg SG: Reproducibility of the mitosis count in the histologic diagnosis of smooth muscle tumors of the uterus. Hum Pathol 7:451–454, 1976.

250. Scully RE: Mitosis counting. I [editorial]. Hum Pathol 7:481–482, 1976.

251. Kempson RL: Mitosis counting. II [editorial]. Hum Pathol 7:482–483, 1976.

252. Norris HJ: Mitosis counting. III [editorial]. Hum Pathol 7:483–484, 1976.

253. Donhuijsen K: Mitosis counts: Reproducibility of significance in grading malignancy. Hum Pathol 17:1122–1125, 1986.

254. Baak JPA: Mitosis counting in tumors [editorial]. Hum Pathol 21:683–685, 1990.

255. Donhuijsen K, Schmidt U, Hirche H, et al: Changes in mitotic rate and cell cycle fractions caused by delayed fixation. Hum Pathol 21:709–714, 1990.

256. Cross SS, Start RD, Smith JHF: Does delay in fixation affect the number of mitotic figures in processed tissue? J Clin Pathol 43:597–599, 1990.

257. Ellis PSJ, Whitehead R: Mitosis counting—a need for reappraisal. Hum Pathol 12:3–4, 1981.

258. Taylor HB, Norris HJ: Mesenchymal tumors of the uterus. IV. Diagnosis and prognosis of leiomyosarcoma. Arch Pathol Lab Med 82:40–44, 1966.

259. Kempson RL, Bari W: Uterine sarcomas. Classification, diagnosis, and prognosis. Hum Pathol 1:331–349, 1970.

260. Christopherson WM, Williamson EO, Gray LA: Leiomyosarcoma of the uterus. Cancer 29:1512–1517, 1972.

261. Hart WR, Billman JK: A reassessment of uterine neoplasms originally diagnosed as leiomyosarcomas. Cancer 41:1902–1910, 1978.

262. Burns B, Curry RH, Bell MEA: Morphologic features of prognostic significance in uterine smooth muscle tumors: A review of eighty-four cases. Am J Obstet Gynecol 135:109–114, 1979.

263. Barter JF, Smith EB, Szpak CA, et al: Leiomyosarcoma of the uterus: Clinicopathologic study of 21 cases. Gynecol Oncol 21:220–227, 1985.

264. Larson B, Silfversward C, Nilsson B, Pettersson F: Prognostic factors in uterine leiomyosarcoma. A clinical and histopathological study of 143 cases. The Radiumhemmet series 1936–1981. Acta Oncol 29:185–191, 1990.

265. Perrone T, Dehner LP: Prognostically favorable "mitotically active" smooth-muscle tumors of the uterus. A clinicopathologic study of 10 cases. Am J Surg Pathol 12:1–8, 1988.

266. O'Connor DM, Norris HJ: Mitotically active leiomyomas of the uterus. Hum Pathol 21:223–227, 1990.

267. Prayson RA, Hart WR: Mitotically active leiomyomas of the uterus. Am J Clin Pathol 97:14–20, 1992.

268. Tiltman AJ: The effect of progestins on the mitotic activity of uterine fibromyomas. Int J Gynecol Pathol 4:89–96, 1985.

269. Kawaguchi K, Fujii S, Konishi I, et al: Mitotic activity in uterine leiomyomas during the menstrual cycle. Am J Obstet Gynecol 160:637–641, 1989.

270. Clement PB, Young RH, Scully RE: Diffuse, perinodular, and other patterns of hydropic degeneration within and adjacent to uterine leiomyomas: Problems in differential diagnosis. Am J Surg Pathol 16:26–32, 1992.

271. Jacobs DS, Cohen H, Johnson JS: Lipoleiomyomas of the uterus. Am J Clin Pathol 44:45–51, 1965.

272. Willen R, Gad A, Willen H: Lipomatous lesions of the uterus. Virchows Arch [Pathol Anat] 377:351–361, 1978.

273. Pounder DJ: Fatty tumours of the uterus. J Clin Pathol 35:1380–1383, 1982.

274. Sieinski W: Lipomatous neometaplasia of the uterus. Report of 11 cases with discussion of histogenesis and pathogenesis. Int J Gynecol Pathol 8:357–363, 1989.

275. Lin M, Hanai J: Atypical lipoleiomyoma of the uterus. Acta Pathol Jpn 41:164–169, 1991.

276. Brooks JJ, Wells GB, Yeh IT, LiVolsi VA: Bizarre epithelioid lipoleiomyoma of the uterus. Int J Gynecol Pathol 11:144–149, 1992.

277. Novak ER, Woodruff JD: Novak's Gynecologic and Obstetric Pathology with Clinical and Endocrine Relations, 8th ed. Philadelpia, WB Saunders, 1979.

278. Martin-Reay DG, Christ ML, LaPata RE: Uterine leiomyoma with skeletal muscle differentiation. Am J Clin Pathol 96:344–347, 1991.

279. Gisser SD, Young I: Neurilemoma-like uterine myomas: An ultrastructural reaffirmation of their non-Schwannian nature. Am J Obstet Gynecol 129:389–392, 1977.

280. Schmid C, Beham A, Kratochvil P: Haematopoiesis in a degenerating leiomyoma. Arch Gynecol Obstet 248:81–86, 1991.

281. Adany R, Fodor P, Molnar P: Increased density of histiocytes in uterine leiomyomas. Int J Gynecol Pathol 9:137–144, 1990.

282. Evans HL: Smooth muscle neoplasms of the uterus other than ordinary leiomyoma. A study of 46 cases, with emphasis on diagnosis criteria and prognostic factors. Cancer 62:2239–2247, 1988.

283. Bell SW, Kempson RL, Hendrickson MR: Problematic uterine smooth muscle neoplasms. A clinicopathologic study of 212 cases [abstract]. Mod Pathol 6:72A, 1993.

283a. Bell SW, Kempson RL, Hendrickson MR: Problematic uterine smooth muscle neoplasms. A clinicopathologic study of 213 cases. Am J Surg Pathol 18:535–558, 1994.

283b. Tsang WYW, Chan JKC: A novel approach for assessing the malignant potential of uterine smooth muscle tumors. Adv Anat Pathol 1:135–140, 1994.

284. Peacock G, Archer S: Myxoid leiomyosarcoma of the uterus: Case report and review of the literature. Am J Obstet Gynecol 160:1515–1519, 1989.

285. Shroff CP, Deodhar KP, Bhagwat AG: Myxoid leiomyosarcoma of the uterus—a case report with light microscopic and ultrastructural appraisal. Tumori 70:561–566, 1984.

286. Barlow JF, Abu-Gazeleh S, Tam GE, et al: Myxoid tumor of the uterus and right atrial myxomas. South Dakota J Med 36:9–13, 1983.

287. Clement PB, Scully RE: Mullerian adenofibroma of the uterus with invasion of myometrium and pelvic veins. Int J Gynecol Pathol 9:363–371, 1990.

288. Banks ER, Mills SE, Frierson HF: Uterine intravascular menstrual endometrium simulating malignancy. Am J Surg Pathol 15:407–412, 1991.

289. Suzuki M, Aizawa S, Ushigome S: Endometrial stromal sarcoma of low-grade malignancy. Immunohistochemical and three-dimensional reconstruction study with special emphasis on the inadequate terminology of endolymphatic stromal myosis. Acta Pathol Jpn 39:260–265, 1989.

290. Norris HJ, Parmley T: Mesenchymal tumors of the uterus. V. Intravenous leiomyomatosis. A clinical and pathological study of 14 cases. Cancer 36:2164–2178, 1975.

291. Nogales FF, Navarro N, de Victoria JMM, et al: Uterine intravascular leiomyomatosis: An update and report of seven cases. Int J Gynecol Pathol 6:331–339, 1987.

292. Clement PE, Young RH, Scully RE: Intravenous leiomyomatosis of the uterus. A clinicopathological analysis of 16 cases with unusual histologic features. Am J Surg Pathol 12:932–945, 1988.

293. Brescia RJ, Tazelaar HD, Hobbs J, Miller AW: Intravascular lipoleiomyomatosis: A report of two cases. Hum Pathol 20:252–256, 1989.

294. Zaloudek CJ, Norris HJ: Mesenchymal tumors of the uterus. In Fenoglio CM, Wolff M (eds): Progress in Surgical Pathology, Vol III. New York, Masson, 1981, pp 1–35.

295. Mulvany NJ, Slavin JL, Ostor AG, Fortune DW: Intravenous leiomyomatosis of the uterus, a clinicopathologic study of 22 cases. Int J Gynecol Pathol 13:1–9, 1994.

296. Rywlin AM, Recher L, Benson J: Clear cell leiomyoma of the uterus: Report of 2 cases of a previously undescribed entity. Cancer 17:100–104, 1964.

297. Lavin L, Hajdu SI, Foote FW Jr: Gastric and extragastric leiomyoblastomas. Clinicopathologic study of 44 cases. Cancer 29:305–311, 1972.

298. Goodhue WW, Susin M, Kramer EE: Smooth muscle origin of uterine plexiform tumors. Ultrastructural and histochemical evidence. Arch Pathol Lab Med 97:263–268, 1974.

299. Kurman RJ, Norris HJ: Mesenchymal tumors of the uterus. VI. Epithelioid smooth muscle tumors including leiomyoblastoma and clear-cell leiomyoma. A clinical and pathological analysis of 26 cases. Cancer 37:1853–1865, 1976.

300. Chang V, Aikawa M, Druet R: Uterine leiomyoblastoma. Ultrastructural and cytologic studies. Cancer 39:1563–1569, 1977.

301. Kaminski PF, Tavassoli FA: Plexiform tumorlet: A clinical and pathologic study of 15 cases with ultrastructural observations. Int J Gynecol Pathol 3:124–134, 1984.

302. Mazur MT, Priest JE: Clear cell leiomyoma (leiomyoblastoma) of the uterus: Ultrastructural observations. Ultrastruct Pathol 10:249–255, 1986.

303. Hyde KE, Geisinger KR, Marshall RB, Jones TL: The clear-cell variant of uterine epithelioid leiomyoma. An immunohistochemical and ultrastructural study. Arch Pathol Lab Med 113:551–553, 1989.

304. Kurman RJ, Norris HJ: Mesenchymal tumors of the uterus. VI. Epithelioid smooth muscle tumors including leiomyoblastoma and clear-cell leiomyoma. A clinical and pathologic analysis of 26 cases. Cancer 36:1853–1865, 1976.

305. Seidman JD, Yetter RA, Papadimitriou JC: Epithelioid component of uterine leiomyosarcoma simulating metastatic carcinoma. Arch Pathol Lab Med 116:287–290, 1992.

306. Balaton AJ, Vuong PN, Vaury P, Baviera EE: Plexiform tumorlet of the uterus: Immunohistochemical evidence for smooth muscle origin. Histopathology 10:749–754, 1986.

307. Fisher ER, Paulson JD, Gregorio RM: The myofibroblastic nature of the uterine plexiform tumor. Arch Pathol Lab Med 102:477–480, 1978.

308. Nunez-Alonso C, Battifora HA: Plexiform tumors of the uterus: Ultrastructural study. Cancer 44:1707–1714, 1979.

309. Ito H, Sasaki H, Miyagawa K, Tahara E: Bizarre leiomyoblastoma of the cervix uteri. Immunohistochemical and ultrastructural study. Acta Pathol Jpn 36:1737–1745, 1986.

310. Buscema J, Carpenter SE, Rosenshein NB, Woodruff JD: Epithelioid leiomyosarcoma of the uterus. Cancer 57:1192–1196, 1986.

311. Kyriazis AP, Kyriazis AA: Uterine leiomyoblastoma (epithelioid leiomyoma) neoplasm of low-grade malignancy, a histopathologic study. Arch Pathol Lab Med 116:1189–1191, 1992.

312. Miettinen M: Immunoreactivity for cytokeratin and epithelial membrane antigen in leiomyosarcoma. Arch Pathol Lab Med 112:637–640, 1988.

313. Darby AJ, Papadaki L, Beilby JOW: An unusual leiomyosarcoma of the uterus containing osteoclast-like giant cells. Cancer 36:495–504, 1975.

314. Pilon V, Parikh N, Maccera J: Malignant osteoclast-like giant cell tumor associated with a uterine leiomyosarcoma. Gynecol Oncol 23:381–386, 1986.

315. Marshall RJ, Braye SG, Jones DB: Leiomyosarcoma of the uterus with giant cells resembling osteoclasts. Int J Gynecol Pathol 5:260–261, 1986.

316. Suster S, Rosen LB, Sanchez JL: Granular leiomyosarcoma of the skin. Am J Dermatopathol 10:234–236, 1988.

317. Nistal M, Paniagua R, Picazo ML, et al: Granular changes in a vascular leiomyosarcoma. Virchows Arch [Pathol Anat] 386:239–284, 980.

318. LeBoit PE, Barr RJ, Burall S, et al: Primitive polypoid granular cell tumor and other cutaneous granular cell neoplasms of apparent nonneural origin. Am J Surg Pathol 15:48–58, 1991.

319. Sobel HJ, Churg J: Granular cells and granular cell lesions. Arch Pathol 77:132–141, 1964.

320. Clement PB, Young RH: Diffuse leiomyomatosis of the uterus: A report of four cases. Int J Gynecol Pathol 6:322–330, 1987.

321. Lai FM, Wong FWS, Allen PW: Diffuse leiomyomatosis with hemorrhage. Arch Pathol Lab Med 115:834–837, 1991.

322. Boyce CR, Buddhdev HN: Pregnancy complicated by metastasizing leiomyoma of uterus. Obstet Gynecol 42:252–258, 1973.

323. Abell MR, Littler ER: Benign metastasizing uterine leiomyoma with multiple lymph node metastases. Cancer 36:2206–2213, 1975.

324. Horstmann JP, Pietra GG, Harman JA, et al: Spontaneous regression of pulmonary leiomyomas during pregnancy. Cancer 39:314–321, 1977.

325. Tench WD, Dail D, Gmelich JT, Matani N: Benign metastasizing leiomyomas: A review of 21 cases [abstract]. Lab Invest 38:367, 1978.

326. Wolff M, Silva F, Kaye G: Pulmonary metastases (with admixed epithelial elements) from smooth muscle neoplasms. Am J Surg Pathol 3:325–342, 1979.

327. Cramer SF, Meyer JS, Kraner JF, et al: Metastasizing leiomyoma of the uterus. Cancer 45:932–937, 1980.

328. Deppe G, Clachko M, Deligdisch L, Cohen CJ: Uterine fibroleiomyomata with aortic node metastases. Int J Gynaecol Obstet 18:1–3, 1980.

329. Banner AS, Carrington CB, Emory WB, et al: Efficacy of oophorectomy in lymphangioleiomyomatosis and benign metastasizing leiomyoma. N Engl J Med 305:204–209, 1981.

330. Chan JKC, Tsang WYW, Pau MY, et al: Lymphangiomyomatosis and angiomyolipoma: Closely related entities characterized by hamartomatous proliferation of HMB-45-positive smooth muscle. Histopathology 22:445–455, 1993.

331. Yoonessi M, Hart WR: Endometrial stromal sarcomas. Cancer 40:898–906, 1977.

332. Mazur MT, Askin FB: Endolymphatic stromal myosis. Unique presentation and ultrastructural study. Cancer 42:2661–2667, 1978.

333. Smith ML, Faaborg LL, Newland JR: Dedifferentiation of endolymphatic stromal myosis to poorly differentiated uterine stromal sarcoma. Gynecol Oncol 9:108–113, 1980.

334. Evans HL: Endometrial stromal sarcoma and poorly differentiated endometrial sarcoma. Cancer 50:2170–2182, 1982.

335. Paulsen SM, Nielsen VT, Hansen P, Ferenczy A: Endolymphatic stromal myosis with focal tubular-glandular differentiation (biphasic endometrial stromal sarcoma). Ultrastruct Pathol 3:31–42, 1982.

336. Thatcher SS, Woodruff JD: Uterine stromatosis: A report of 33 cases. Obstet Gynecol 59:428–434, 1982.

337. Piver MS, Rutledge FN, Copeland L, et al: Uterine endolymphatic stromal myosis: A collaborative study. Obstet Gynecol 64:173–178, 1984.

338. De Fusco PA, Gaffey TA, Malkasian GD Jr, et al: Endometrial stromal sarcoma: Review of Mayo Clinic experience 1945–1980. Gynecol Oncol 35:8–14, 1989.

339. Dgani R, Shoham Z, Czernobilsky B, et al: Endolymphatic stromal myosis (endometrial low-grade stromal sarcoma) presenting with hematuria: A diagnostic challenge. Gynecol Oncol 35:262–266, 1989.

340. Montag TW, Manart FD: Endolymphatic stromal myosis: Surgical and hormonal therapy for extensive venous recurrence. Gynecol Oncol 33:255–260, 1989.

341. Styron SL, Burke TW, Linville WK: Low grade endometrial stromal sarcoma recurring over three decades. Gynecol Oncol 35:275–278, 1989.

342. Berchuck A, Rubin SC, Hoskins WJ, et al: Treatment of endometrial stromal tumors. Gynecol Oncol 36:60–65, 1990.

343. Larson B, Silfversward C, Nilsson B, Pettersson F: Endometrial stromal sarcoma of the uterus. A clinical and histopathologic study. The Radiumhemmet series 1936–1981. Eur J Obstet Gynecol Reprod Biol 35:239–249, 1990.

344. Mansi JL, Ramachandra S, Wiltshaw E, Fisher C: Endometrial stromal sarcomas. Gynecol Oncol 36:113–118, 1990.

345. August CZ, Bauer KD, Lurain J, Murad T: Neoplasms of endometrial stroma: Histopathologic and flow cytometric analysis with clinical correlation. Hum Pathol 20:232–237, 1989.

346. El-Naggar A, Abdul-Karim FW, Silva EG, et al: Uterine stromal neoplasms: A clinicopathologic and DNA flow cytometric correlation. Hum Pathol 22:897–903, 1991.

347. Hitchock CL, Norris HJ: Flow cytometric analysis of endometrial stromal sarcoma. Am J Clin Pathol 97:267–271, 1992.

248. Lifschitz-Mercer B, Czernobilsky B, Dgani R, et al: Immunocytochemical study of an endometrial diffuse clear cell stromal sarcoma and other endometrial sound sarcomas. Cancer 59:1494–1499, 1987.

349. Fitko R, Brainer J, Schink JC, et al: Endometrial stromal sarcoma with rhabdoid differentiation [letter]. Int J Gynecol Pathol 9:379–382, 1990.

350. Caglar H, Traub B, Jenis EH, et al: Plexiform or sex cord tumors resembling tumors of the uterus. Am J Obstet Gynecol 145:639–640, 1983.

351. Fekete PS, Vellios F, Patterson BD: Uterine tumor resembling an ovarian sex-cord tumor: Report of a case of an endometrial stromal tumor with foam cells and ultrastructural evidence of epithelial differentiation. Int J Gynecol Pathol 4:378–387, 1985.

352. Iwasaki I, Yu TJ, Takahashi A, et al: Uterine tumor resembling ovarian sex-cord tumor with osteoid metaplasia. Acta Pathol Jpn 36:1391–1395, 1986.

353. Kantelip B, Cloup N, Dechelotte P: Uterine tumor resembling ovarian sex-cord tumors: Report of a case with ultrastructural study. Hum Pathol 17:91–94, 1986.

354. Malfetano JH, Hussain M: A uterine tumor that resembled ovarian sex-cord tumors: A low-grade sarcoma. Obstet Gynecol 74:489–491, 1989.

355. Roth LM, Senteny GE: Stromomyoma of the uterus. Ultrastruct Pathol 9:137–143, 1985.

356. Tang CK, Toker C, Anges IG: Stromomyoma of the uterus. Cancer 43:308–316, 1979.

357. Macasaet MA, Waxman M, Fruchter RG, et al: Prognostic factors in malignant mesodermal (mullerian) mixed tumors of the uterus. Gynecol Oncol 20:32–42, 1985.

358. Wheelock JB, Krebs H, Schneider V, et al: Uterine sarcoma: Analysis of prognostic variables in 71 cases. Am J Obstet Gynecol 151:1016–1022, 1985.

359. George M, Pejovic MH, Kramar A, et al: Uterine sarcomas: Prognostic factors and treatment modalities—study in 209 patients. Gynecol Oncol 24:58–67, 1986.

360. Kahanpaa KV, Wahlstrom T, Grohn P, et al: Sarcomas of the uterus: A clinicopathologic study of 119 patients. Obstet Gynecol 67:417–424, 1986.

361. Dinh TV, Slavin RE, Bhagavan BS, et al: Mixed mullerian tumors of the uterus: A clinicopathologic study. Obstet Gynecol 74:388–392, 1989.

362. Gagne H, Tetu B, Blondeau L, et al: Morphologic prognostic factors of malignant mixed mullerian tumor of the uterus: A clinicopathologic study of 58 cases. Mod Pathol 2:433–438, 1989.

363. Gallup DG, Gable DS, Talledo E, Otken LB Jr: A clinical-pathologic study of mixed mullerian tumors of the uterus over a 16-year period—The Medical College of Georgia experience. Am J Obstet Gynecol 161:533–538, 1989.

364. Nielsen SN, Podratz KC, Scheithauer BW, O'Brien PC: Clinicopathologic analysis of uterine malignant mullerian tumors. Gynecol Oncol 34:372–378, 1989.

365. Larson B, Silfversward C, Nilsson B, Pettersson F: Mixed mullerian tumors of the uterus—prognostic factors: A clinical and histopathologic study of 147 cases. Radiother Oncol 17:123–132, 1990.

366. Schweizer W, Demopoulos R, Beller U, Dubin H: Prognostic factors for malignant mixed mullerian tumors of the uterus. Int J Gynecol Pathol 9:129–136, 1990.

367. Silverberg SG, Major FJ, Blessing JA, et al: Carcinosarcoma (malignant mixed mesodermal tumor) of the uterus. A gynecologic oncology group pathologic study of 203 cases. Int J Gynecol Pathol 9:1–19, 1990.

368. Gloor E: Mullerian adenosarcoma of the uterus: Clinicopathologic report of five cases. Am J Surg Pathol 3:203–209, 1979.

369. Fox H, Harilal KR, Youell A: Mullerian adenosarcoma of the uterine body: A report of nine cases. Histopathology 3:167–180, 1979.

370. Ostor AG, Fortune DW: Benign and low grade variants of mixed mullerian tumour of the uterus. Histopathology 4:369–382, 1980.

371. Hilton P: Mullerian adenofibroma. Case report. Br J Obstet Gynecol 91:1261–1265, 1984.

372. Clement PB, Scully RE: Uterine tumors with mixed epithelial and mesenchymal elements. Semin Diagn Pathol 5:199–222, 1988.

373. Thompson M, Husemeyer R: Carcinofibroma—a variant of the mixed mullerian tumor. Br J Obstet Gynaecol 88:1151–1155, 1981.

374. Peters WM, Wells M, Bryce FC: Mullerian clear cell carcinofibroma of the uterine corpus. Histopathology 8:1069–1078, 1984.

375. Chen KTK, Vergon JM: Carcinomesenchymoma of the uterus. Am J Clin Pathol 75:746–748, 1981.

376. Norris HJ, Roth E, Taylor HB: Mesenchymal tumors of the uterus. II. A clinical and pathologic study of 31 mixed mesodermal tumors. Obstet Gynecol 28:57–63, 1966.

377. Norris HJ, Taylor HB: Mesenchymal tumors of the uterus. III. A clinical and pathologic study of 31 carcinosarcomas. Cancer 19:1459–1465, 1966.

378. Seltzer VL, Levine A, Spiegel G, et al: Adenofibroma of the uterus: Multiple recurrences following wide local excision. Gynecol Oncol 37:427–431, 1990.

379. Kahner S, Ferenczy A, Richart RM: Homologous mixed mullerian tumors (carcinosarcoma) confined to endometrial polyps. Am J Obstet Gynecol 121:278–279, 1975.

380. Klomp A, Smith LA, Pounder DJ: Malignant mixed mesodermal tumour of the uterus initially confined to a polyp. Aust N Z J Obstet Gynaecol 22:248–251, 1982.

381. Barwick KW, LiVolsi VA: Heterologous mixed Mullerian tumor confined to an endometrial polyp. Obstet Gynecol 53:512–514, 1979.

382. Oda Y, Nakanishi I, Tateiwa T: Intramural mullerian adenosarcoma of the uterus with adenomyosis. Arch Pathol Lab Med 108:798–801, 1984.

383. Clement PB, Scully RE: Mullerian adenosarcoma of the uterus: A clinicopathological analysis of 100 cases with a review of the literature. Hum Pathol 21:363–381, 1990.

384. Kaku T, Silverberg SG, Major FJ, et al: Adenosarcoma of the uterus: A gynecologic oncology group clinicopathologic study of 31 cases. Int J Gynecol 11:75–88, 1992.

385. Zaloudek CJ, Norris HJ: Adenofibroma and adenosarcoma of the uterus: A clinicopathologic study of 35 cases. Cancer 48:354–366, 1981.

386. Clement PB: Mullerian adenosarcomas of the uterus with sarcomatous overgrowth. A clinicopathological analysis of 10 cases. Am J Surg Pathol 13:28–38, 1989.

387. Abell MR: Papillary adenofibroma of the uterine cervix. Am J Obstet Gynecol 110:990–993, 1971.

388. Vellios F, Ng ABP, Reagan JW: Papillary adenofibroma of the uterus: A benign mesodermal mixed tumor of mullerian origin. Am J Clin Pathol 60:543–551, 1973.

389. Clement PB, Scully RE: Mullerian adenosarcoma of the uterus: A clinicopathologic analysis of ten cases of a distinctive type of mullerian mixed tumor. Cancer 34:1138–1149, 1974.

390. Grimalt M, Arguelles M, Ferenczy A: Papillary cystadenofibroma of endometrium: A histochemical and ultrastructural study. Cancer 36:137–144, 1975.

391. Katzenstein AA, Askin FB, Feldman PS: Mullerian adenosarcoma of the uterus: An ultrastructural study of four cases. Cancer 40:2233–2242, 1977.

392. Baratz M, Gitstein SZ, David MP, et al: Papillary cystadenofibroma of the endometrium. Acta Obstet Gynecol Scand 59:467–470, 1980.

393. Martinelli G, Pileri S, Bazzocchi F, et al: Mullerian adenosarcoma of the uterus: A report of 5 cases. Tumori 66:499–506, 1980.

394. Altaras M, Cohen I, Cordoba M, et al: Papillary adenofibroma of the endometrium: Case report and review of the literature. Gynecol Oncol 19:216–221, 1984.

395. Iwai M, Konishi I, Fujii S, et al: A light and electron microscopic study of mullerian adenofibroma of the uterus. Acta Obstet Gynaecol Jpn 36:44–48, 1984.

396. Czernobilsky B, Hohlweg-Majert P, Dallenbach-Hellweg G: Uterine adenosarcoma: A clinicopathologic study of 11 cases with a reevaluation of histologic criteria. Arch Gynecol 233:281–294, 1983.

397. Hariri J: Mullerian adenosarcoma of the endometrium: Review of the literature and report of two cases. Int J Gynecol Pathol 2:182–191, 1983.

398. Hirschfield L, Kahn LB, Chen S, et al: Mullerian adenosarcoma with ovarian sex cord-like differentiation: A light- and electron-microscopic study. Cancer 57:1197–1200, 1986.

399. Clement PB, Scully RE: Mullerian adenosarcomas of the uterus with sex cord-like elements. A Clinicopathological analysis of eight cases. Am J Clin Pathol 91:664–672, 1989.

400. Lack EE, Bitterman P, Sundeen JT: Mullerian adenosarcoma of the uterus with pure angiosarcoma: Case report. Hum Pathol 22:1289–1291, 1991.

401. Chen KTK: Rhabdomyosarcomatous uterine adenosarcoma. Int J Gynecol Pathol 4:146–152, 1985.

402. Gast MJ, Radkins LV, Jacobs AJ, Gersell D: Mullerian adenosarcoma with heterologous elements: Diagnostic and therapeutic approach. Gynecol Oncol 32:381–384, 1989.

403. Clement PB, Scully RE: Tumors with mixed epithelial and mesenchymal elements. In Clement PB, Young RH (eds): Tumors and Tumor-like lesions of the Uterine Corpus and Cervix. Contemporary Issues in Surgical Pathology, Vol 19. New York, Churchill Livingstone, 1993, pp 329–370.

404. Mills SE, Sugg NK, Mahnesmith RC: Endometrial adenosarcoma with pelvic involvement following uterine perforation. Diagn Gynecol Obstet 3:149–154, 1981.

405. Chuang JT, Van Velden JJ, Graham JB: Carcinosarcoma and mixed mesodermal tumor of the uterine corpus: Review of 49 cases. Obstet Gynecol 35:769–780, 1970.

406. Williamson EO, Christopherson WM: Malignant mixed mullerian tumors of the uterus. Cancer 29:585–592, 1972.

407. Rachmaninoff N, Climie ARW: Mixed mesodermal tumors of the uterus. Cancer 19:1705–1710, 1966.

408. Kempson RL, Bari W: Uterine sarcomas: Classification, diagnosis, and prognosis. Hum Pathol 1:331–349, 1970.

409. Schaepman-van Geuns EJ: Mixed tumors and carcinosarcomas of the uterus evaluated five years after treatment. Cancer 25:72–77, 1970.

410. Mortel R, Koss LG, Lewis JL Jr: Mesodermal mixed tumors of the uterine corpus. Obstet Gynecol 43:238–252, 1974.

411. Barwick KW, LiVolsi VA: Malignant mixed mullerian tumors of the uterus: A clinicopathologic assessment of 34 cases. Am J Surg Pathol 3:125–135, 1979.

412. King ME, Kramer EE: Malignant mullerian mixed tumors of the uterus: A study of 21 cases. Cancer 45:188–190, 1980.

413. Shaw RW, Lynch PF, Wade-Evans T: Mullerian mixed tumour of the uterine corpus: A clinical histopathological review of 28 patients. Br J Obstet Gynaecol 90:562–569, 1983.

414. Lotocki R, Rosenshein NB, Brumbine F, et al: Mixed mullerian tumors of the uterus: Clinical and pathologic correlations. Int J Gynaecol Obstet 20:237–243, 1982.

415. Doss LL, Llorens AS, Henriquez EM: Carcinosarcoma of the uterus: A 40-year experience from the State of Missouri. Gynecol Oncol 18:43–53, 1984.

416. Costa MJ, Khan R, Judd R: Carcinosarcoma (malignant mixed mullerian [mesodermal] tumor) of the uterus and ovary. Correlation of clinical, pathologic, and immunohistochemical features in 29 cases. Arch Pathol Lab Med 115:583–586, 1991.

417. Norris HJ, Taylor MB: Postirradiation sarcomas of the uterus. Obstet Gynecol 26:689–694, 1965.

418. Varela-Duran J, Nochomovitz LE, Prem KA, et al: Postirradiation mixed mullerian tumors of the uterus: A comparative clinicopathologic study. Cancer 45:1625–1631, 1980.

419. George E, Manivel JC, Dehner LP, Wick WR: Malignant mixed mullerian tumors: An immunohistochemical study of 47 cases, with histogenic considerations and clinical correlation. Hum Pathol 22:215–223, 1991.

420. Spanos WJ Jr, Wharton JT, Gomez L, et al: Malignant mixed mullerian tumors of the uterus. Cancer 43:311–316, 1984.

421. Bitterman P, Chun B, Kurman RJ: The significance of epithelial differentiation in mixed mesodermal tumors of the uterus. A clinicopathologic and immunohistochemical study. Am J Surg Pathol 14:317–328, 1990.

422. Meis JM, Lawrence WD: The immunohistochemical profile of malignant mixed mullerian tumor. Overlap with endometrial adenocarcinoma. Am J Clin Pathol 94:1–7, 1990.

423. Ramadan M, Goudie RB: Epithelial antigens in malignant mixed mullerian tumors of endometrium. J Pathol 148:13–18, 1986.

424. Geisinger KR, Dabbs DJ, Marshall RB: Malignant mixed mullerian tumors. An ultrastructural and immunohistochemical analysis with histogenetic considerations. Cancer 59:1781–1790, 1987.

425. Auerbach HE, LiVolsi VA, Merino MJ: Malignant mixed mullerian tumors of the uterus. An immunohistochemical study. Int J Gynecol Pathol 7:123–130, 1988.

426. Chung M, Mukai K, Teshima S, et al: Expression of various antigens by different components of uterine mixed mullerian tumors. Acta Pathol Jpn 38:35–45, 1988.

427. de Brito PA, Silverberg SG, Orenstein JM: Carcinosarcoma (malignant versus Mullerian [mesodermal] tumor) of the female genital tract: Immunohistochemical and ultrastructural analysis of 28 cases. Hum Pathol 24:132–142, 1993.

427a. Mayall F, Rutty K, Campbell F, Goddard H: p53 immunostaining suggests that uterine carcinomas are monoclonal. Histopathology 24:211–214, 1994.

427b. George E, Lillemoe TJ, Twiggs LB, Perrone T: Malignant mixed mullerian tumor versus high-grade endometrial carcinoma and aggressive variants of endometrial carcinoma: A comparative analysis of survival. Int J Gynecol Pathol 14:39–44, 1995.

428. Manivel C, Wick MR, Sibley RK: Neuroendocrine differentiation in mullerian neoplasms. An immunohistochemical study of a ''pure'' endometrial small-cell carcinoma and a mixed mullerian tumor containing small-cell carcinoma. Am J Clin Pathol 86:438–443, 1986.

429. Gersell DJ, Duncan DA, Fulling KH: Malignant mixed mullerian tumor of the uterus with neuroectodermal differentiation. Int J Gynecol Pathol 8:169–178, 1989.

430. Liao SY, Choi BH: Expression of glial fibrillary acidic protein by neoplastic cells of mullerian origin. Virchows Arch [Cell Pathol] 42:185–193, 1986.

431. Siegal GP, Taylor LL, Nelson KG, et al: Characterization of a pure heterologous sarcoma of the uterus: Rhabdomyosarcoma of the corpus. Int J Gynecol Pathol 2:303–315, 1983.

432. Vakiani M, Mawad J, Talerman A: Heterologous sarcomas of the uterus. Int J Gynecol Pathol 1:211–219, 1982.

433. Hart WR, Craig JR: Rhabdomyosarcoma of the uterus. Am J Clin Pathol 70:217–223, 1978.

434. Crum CP, Rogers BH, Anderson W: Osteosarcoma of the uterus: Case report and review of the literature. Gynecol Oncol 9:256–260, 1980.

435. Clement PB: Chondrosarcoma of the uterus: Report of a case and review of the literature. Hum Pathol 9:726–732, 1978.

436. Podczaski E, Sees J, Kaminski P, et al: Rhabdomyosarcoma of the uterus in a postmenopausal patient. Gynecol Oncol 37:439–442, 1990.

437. Bapat K, Brusterin S: Uterine sarcoma with liposarcomatous differentiation: Report of a case and review of the literature. Int J Gynecol Obstet 28:71–75, 1989.

438. Kofinas AD, Suarez J, Calame RJ, et al: Chondrosarcoma of the uterus. Gynecol Oncol 19:231–237, 1984.

439. Piscioli F, Govoni E, Polla E, et al: Primary osteosarcoma of the uterine corpus. Report of a case and critical review of the literature. Int J Gynecol Obstet 23:377–385, 1985.

440. Ansah-Boateng Y, Wells M, Poole DR: Coexistent immature teratoma of the uterus and endometrial adenocarcinoma complicated by gliomatosis peritonei. Gynecol Oncol 21:106–110, 1985.

441. Martin E, Scholes J, Richart RM, et al: Benign cystic teratoma of the uterus. Am J Obstet Gynecol 135:429–431, 1979.

442. Young RH, Kleinman GM, Scully RE: Glioma of the uterus: Report of a case with comments on histogenesis. Am J Surg Pathol 5:695–699, 1981.

443. Roth E, Taylor HB: Heterotopic cartilage in the uterus. Obstet Gynecol 27:838–844, 1966.

444. Waxman M, Moussouris HF: Endometrial ossification following an abortion. Am J Obstet Gynecol 130:587–588, 1978.

445. Zettergren L: Glial tissue in the uterus. Am J Pathol 71:419–426, 1983.

446. Tyagi SP, Saxena K, Rizvi R, et al: Foetal remnants in the uterus and their relation to other uterine heterotopia. Histopathology 3:339–345, 1979.

447. Bhatia NN, Hoshiko MG: Uterine osseous metaplasia. Obstet Gynecol 60:256–259, 1982.

448. Brown LJR, Wells M: Heterotopic adipose and glial tissue in the endometrium with staining for glial fibrillary acidic protein: Case report. Br J Obstet Gynecol 93:637–639, 1986.

449. Nogales FF, Pavcovich M, Medina MT, et al: Fatty change in the endometrium. Histopathology 20:362–363, 1992.

450. Martin-Reay DG, Christ ML, Lapata RE: Uterine leiomyoma with skeletal muscle differentiation: Report of a case. Am J Clin Pathol 96:344–347, 1991.

451. Payne F, Rollason TP, Sivridis E: Adenomyolipoma of the endometrium—a hamartoma? Histopathology 20:357–359, 1992.

452. Bartnik J, Powell S, Moriber-Katz S, et al: Metaplastic papillary tumor of the fallopian tube: Case report, immunohistochemical features, and review of the literature. Arch Pathol Lab Med 113:545–547, 1989.

453. Keeney GL, Thrasher TV: Metaplastic papillary tumor of the fallopian tube: A case report with ultrastructure. Int J Gynecol Pathol 7:86–92, 1988.

454. Thor AD, Young RH, Clement PB: Pathology of the fallopian tube, broad ligament, peritoneum, and pelvic soft tissues. Hum Pathol 22:856–867, 1991.

455. Saffos RO, Rhatigan RM, Scully RE: Metaplastic papillary tumor of the fallopian tube—a distinctive lesion of pregnancy. Am J Clin Pathol 74:232–236, 1980.

456. Cornog JL, Currie JL, Rubin A: Heat artifact simulating adenocarcinoma of the fallopian tube. JAMA 214:1118–1119, 1970.

457. Milchgrub S, Sandstad J: Arias-Stella reaction in the fallopian tube epithelium. Am J Clin Pathol 95:892–894, 1991.

458. Robey SS, Silva EG: Epithelial hyperplasia of the fallopian tube. Its association with serous borderline tumors of the ovary. Int J Gynecol Pathol 8:214–220, 1989.

459. Moore SW, Enterline HT: Significance of proliferative epithelial lesions of the uterine tube. Obstet Gynecol 45:385–390, 1975.

460. Stern J, Buscema J, Parmley T, et al: Atypical epithelial proliferations in the fallopian tube. Am J Obstet Gynecol 140:309–312, 1981.

461. Zaytsev P, Taxy JB: Pregnancy associated ectopic decidua. Am J Surg Pathol 11:526–530, 1987.

462. Brooks JJ, Wheeler JE: Granulomatous salpingitis secondary to Crohn's disease. Obstet Gynecol 49:31S–33S, 1977.

463. Kay S: Sarcoidosis of the fallopian tubes: Report of a case. J Obstet Gynecol Br Emp 63:871–874, 1956.

464. Ho KL: Sarcoidosis of the uterus. Hum Pathol 10:219–222, 1979.

465. DiCarlo FJ, DiCarlo JP, Robboy SJ, et al: Sarcoidosis of the uterus. Arch Pathol Lab Med 113:941–943, 1989.

466. Kim KR, Scully RE: Peritoneal keratin granulomas with carcinomas of endometrium and ovary and atypical polypoid adenomyoma of endometrium, a clinicopathologic analysis of 22 cases. Am J Surg Pathol 14:925–932, 1990.

467. Hofman WI, Shanberge JN, Rubovits WH: Salpingitis due to foreign body reaction to silk sutures following tubal ligation: Report of three cases. Obstet Gynecol 25:112–116, 1965.

468. Roberts JT, Roberts GT, Maudsley RF: Indolent granulomatous necrosis in patients with previous tubal diathermy. Am J Obstet Gynecol 129:112–113, 1977.

469. Evans CS, Klein KZ, Goldman RL, et al: Necrobiotic granulomas of the uterine cervix, a probable postoperative reaction. Am J Surg Pathol 8:841–844, 1984.

470. Mies C, Balogh K, Stadecker M: Palisading prostatic granulomas following surgery. Am J Surg Pathol 8:217–221, 1984.

471. Frank TS, Kimebaugh KS, Wilson MD: Granulomatous endometritis associated with histologically occult cytomegalovirus in a healthy patient. Am J Surg Pathol 16:716–720, 1992.

472. Baziz-Malik G, Maheshwari B, Lal N: Tuberculous endometritis: A clinicopathologic study of 1000 cases. Br J Obstet Gynecol 90:84–86, 1983.

473. Ladefoged C, Lorentzen M: Xanthogranulomatous inflammation of the female genital tract. Histopathology 13:541–551, 1988.

474. Buckley CH, Fox H: Histiocytic endometritis. Histopathology 4:105–110, 1980.

475. Russack V, Lammers R: Xanthogranulomatous endometritis: Report of six cases and a proposed mechanism for development. Arch Pathol Lab Med 114:929–932, 1990.

476. Clement PB, Young RH, Scully RE: Necrotic pseudoxanthomatous nodules of ovary and peritoneum in endometriosis. Am J Surg Pathol 12:390–397, 1988.

477. Herrera GA, Reimann BEF, Greenberg HL, et al: Pigmentosis tube, a new entity: Light and electron microscopic study. Obstet Gynecol 61:80S–83S, 1981.

478. Shintaku M, Sasaki M, Babs Y: Ceroid-containing histiocytic granuloma of the endometrium. Histopathology 18:169–172, 1991.

479. Thomas W, Sadeghich B, Fesco R, et al: Malacoplakia of the endometrium, a probable cause of postmenopausal bleeding. Am J Clin Pathol 79:637–643, 1983.

480. Willen R, Stendahl U, Willen H, et al: Malacoplakia of the cervix and corpus uteri: A light microscopic, electron microscopic and X-ray microprobe analysis of a case. Int J Gynecol Pathol 2:201–208, 1983.

481. Axiotis CA, Merino MJ, Duray PH: Langerhans cell histiocytosis of the female genital tract. Cancer 67:1650–1660, 1991.

481. Lou TY, Teplitz C: Malakoplakia: Pathogenesis and ultrastructural morphogenesis, a problem of altered macrophage (phagolysosomal) response. Hum Pathol 5:191–207, 1974.

482. Damjanov I, Katz SM: Malakoplakia. Pathol Annu 16:103–126, 1981.

484. Allenby PA, Chowdhury LN: Histiocytic appearance of metastatic lobular breast carcinoma. Arch Pathol Lab Med 110:759–760, 1986.

485. Harris NL, Scully RE: Malignant lymphoma and granulocytic sarcoma of the uterus and vagina, a clinicopathologic analysis of 27 cases. Cancer 53:2530–2545, 1984.

486. Young RH, Harris NL, Scully RE: Lymphoma-like lesions of the lower-female genital tract: A report of 16 cases. Int J Gynecol Pathol 4:289–299, 1985.

487. Gilks CB, Taylor GP, Clement PB: Inflammatory pseudotumor of the uterus. Int J Gynecol Pathol 6:275–286, 1987.

488. Ferry JA, Harris NL, Scully RE: Uterine leiomyomas with lymphoid infiltrate simulating lymphoma, a report of seven cases. Int J Gynecol Pathol 8:263–270, 1989.

489. Daya D, Lukka H, Clement PB: Primitive neuroectodermal tumor of the uterus: A report of four cases. Hum Pathol 23:1120–1129, 1992.

490. Molyneux AJ, Deen S, Sundaresan V: Primitive neuroectodermal tumor of the uterus. Histopathology 21:584–585, 1992.

491. Hendrickson MR, Scheithauer BW: Primitive neuroectodermal tumor of the endometrium: Report of two cases, one with electron microscopic observation. Int J Gynecol Pathol 5:249–259, 1986.

492. Kapadia SB, Krause JR, Kanbour AI, et al: Granulocytic sarcoma of the uterus. Cancer 41:687–691, 1978.

493. Tsang WYW, Chan JKC, Tang SK, et al: Large cell lymphoma with fibrillary matrix. Histopathology 20:80–82, 1992.

494. Miko TL, Lampe LG, Thomazy VA, et al: Eosinophilic endomyometritis associated with diagnostic curettage. Int J Gynecol Pathol 7:162–172, 1988.

495. Bjersing L, Borglin NA: Eosinophils in the myometrium of the human uterus. Acta Pathol Microbiol Scand 54:353–357, 1962.

496. Divack DM, Janovski NA: Eosinophilia encountered in female genital tract. Am J Obstet Gynecol 84:761–765, 1962.

497. De Rosa G, Boscaino A, Terracciano LM, et al: Giant adenomatoid tumors of the uterus. Int J Gynecol Pathol 11:156–160, 1992.

498. Marcussen N, Donna A: Adenomatoid tumor of the uterus. Histopathology 13:582–583, 1989.

499. Palacios J, Manrique AS, Villaespesa AR, et al: Cystic adenomatoid tumor of the uterus. Int J Gynecol Pathol 10:296–301, 1991.

500. Quigley JC, Hurt WR: Adenomatoid tumor of the uterus. Am J Clin Pathol 76:627–635, 1981.

501. Bisset DL, Morris JA, Fox H: Giant cystic adenomatoid tumor (mesothelioma) of the uterus. Histopathology 12:555–558, 1987.

502. Weiss SW, Tavassoli FA: Multicystic mesothelioma, an analysis of pathologic findings and biologic behavior in 37 cases. Am J Surg Pathol 12:737–746, 1988.

503. Tiltman AJ: Adenomatoid tumors of the uterus. Histopathology 4:437–443, 1980.

504. Pedowitz P, Felmus LB, Grayzel DM: Vascular tumors of the uterus: Benign vascular tumors. Am J Obstet Gynecol 69:1291–1303, 1955.

505. Sanes S, Warner R: Primary lymphangioma of the fallopian tube. Am J Obstet Gynecol 37:316–321, 1939.

506. Carinelli SG, Cattaneo M, Mussida M: Hemangiomas of the uterus [abstract]. Mod Pathol 6:72A, 1993.

507. Ross MJ, Welch WR, Scully RE: Multilocular peritoneal inclusion cysts (so-called cystic mesotheliomas). Cancer 64:1336–1346, 1989.

508. Joglekar VM: Hemangioma of the fallopian tube. Br J Obstet Gynecol 86:823–825, 1979.

509. Young RH, Clement PB, Scully RE: The fallopian tube and broad ligament. In Sternberg SS (ed): Diagnostic Surgical Pathology. New York, Raven Press, 1989, pp 1735–1751.

510. Mazzarella P, Okagaki T, Richart RM: Teratoma of the uterine tube. A case report and review of the literature. Obstet Gynecol 39:381–388, 1972.

511. Horn T, Jao W, Keh PC: Benign cystic teratoma of the fallopian tube. Arch Pathol Lab Med 107:48, 1983.

512. Manes JL, Taylor HB: Carcinosarcoma and mixed Mullerian tumor of the fallopian tube, report of four cases. Cancer 38:1687–1693, 1976.

513. Hanjani P, Peterson RO, Bonnell SA: Malignant mixed Mullerian tumor of the fallopian tube. Report of a case and review of the literature. Gynecol Oncol 9:381–393, 1980.

514. Buchino JJ, Buchino JJ: Malignant mixed Mullerian tumor of the fallopian tube. Arch Pathol Lab Med 111:386–387, 1987.

515. Kariminejad MH, Scully RE: Female adnexal tumor of probable wolffian origin. Cancer 31:671–677, 1973.

516. Prasad CJ, Ray JA, Kessler S: Female adnexal tumor of Wolffian origin. Arch Pathol Lab Med 116:189–191, 1992.

517. Taxy JB, Battifora H: Female adnexal tumor of probable Wolffian origin: Evidence for a low grade malignancy. Cancer 37:2349–2354, 1976.

518. Sivathondan Y, Salm R, Hughesdon PE, et al: Female adnexal tumor of probable Wolffian origin. J Clin Pathol 32:616–624, 1979.

519. Kao GF, Norris HJ: Juxtaovarian adnexal tumor—a clinical and pathologic study of 19 cases [abstract]. Lab Invest 38:250–251, 1978.

520. Abbott RL, Barlogie B, Schmidt WA: Metastasizing juxtaovarian tumor with terminal hypercalcemia: A case report. Cancer 48:860–865, 1981.

521. Daya D, Young RH, Scully RE: Endometrioid carcinoma of the fallopian tube resembling an adnexal tumor of probably Wolffian origin: A report of six cases. Int J Gynecol Pathol 11:122–130, 1992.

522. Arhelger RB, Bocian JJ: Brenner tumor of the uterus. Cancer 28:1741–1743, 1976.

523. Chen KTK: Extraovarian transitional cell carcinoma of female genital tract [letter]. Am J Clin Pathol 94:670–671, 1990.

524. Young TW, Thrasher TV: Nonchromaffin paraganglioma of the uterus: A case report. Arch Pathol Lab Med 106:608–609, 1982.

525. Tavassoli F: Melanotic paraganglioma of the uterus. Cancer 58:942–948, 1986.

526. Martin PC, Pulitzer DR, Reed RJ: Pigmented myomatous neurocristoma of the uterus. Arch Pathol Lab Med 113:1291–1295, 1989.

527. Schulz DM: A malignant melanotic neoplasm of the uterus, resembling the "retinal anlage" tumor: Report of a case. Arch Pathol 28:524–526, 1957.

527a. Joseph MA, Fellow FG, Hearn JA: Primary endodermal tumor of the endometrium. Cancer 65:297–302, 1990.

528. Bittencourt AL, Britto JF, Fonseca LF: Wilms' tumor of the uterus: The first report of the literature. Cancer 47:2496–2499, 1981.

529. Kawai K, Senba M, Tagawa H, et al: Osteoclast-type giant cell tumor of the endometrium. Zentralb Allg Pathol 135:743–749, 1989.

530. Kindblom L, Seidal T: Malignant giant cell tumor of the uterus. Acta Pathol Microbiol Scand 89:179–184, 1981.

531. Fuji S, Kanzaki H, Konishi I, et al: Malignant fibrous histiocytoma of the uterus. Gynecol Oncol 26:319–320, 1987.

532. Gray GF, Glick AD, Kurtin PJ, et al: Alveolar soft part sarcoma of the uterus. Hum Pathol 17:297–300, 1986.

533. Nolan NPM, Gaffney EF: Alveolar soft part sarcoma of the uterus. Histopathology 16:97–99, 1990.

534. Cho KR, Rosenshein NB, Epstein JI: Malignant rhabdoid tumor of the uterus. Int J Gynecol Pathol 8:381–387, 1989.

535. Ongkasuwan C, Taylor JE, Tang C, et al: Angiosarcoma of the uterus and ovary: Clinicopathologic report. Cancer 49:1469–1475, 1982.

536. Witkin GB, Askin F, Geratz D, et al: Angiosarcoma of the uterus: A light microscopic, immunohistochemical, and ultrastructural study. Int J Gynecol Pathol 6:176–184, 1987.

537. Milne DS, Hinshaw K, Malcolm AJ, et al: Primary angiosarcoma of the uterus: A case report. Histopathology 16:203–205, 1990.

538. Quinonez GE, Paraskevas MP, Diocee MS, et al: Angiosarcoma of the uterus: A case report. Am J Obstet Gynecol 164:90–92, 1991.

539. Davey D, Munn R, Smith LW, et al: Angiotropic lymphoma: Presentation in uterine vessels with cytogenetic studies. Arch Pathol Lab Med 114:879–882, 1990.

540. Ferry JA, Young RH: Malignant lymphoma, pseudolymphoma, and hematopoietic disorders of the female genital tract. Pathol Annu 26(1):227–263, 1991.

541. Alpert LC, Haufrect EJ, Schwartz MR: Uterine lithiasis. Am J Surg Pathol 14:1071–1075, 1990.

542. Silverman AY, Artinian B, Sibin M: Serous cystadenofibroma of the fallopian tube: A case report. Am J Obstet Gynecol 130:593–595, 1978.

543. De La Fuente AA: Benign mixed Mullerian tumor—adenofibroma of the fallopian tube. Histopathology 6:661–666, 1982.

544. Chen KTK: Bilateral papillary adenofibroma of the fallopian tube. Am J Clin Pathol 75:229–231, 1981.

545. Gisser SD: Obstructing fallopian tube papilloma. Int J Gynecol Pathol 5:179–182, 1986.

546. Voet RL, Lifshitz S: Primary clear cell adenocarcinoma of the fallopian tube: Light microscopic and ultrastructural findings. Int J Gynecol Pathol 1:292–298, 1982.

547. Moore DH, Woosley JT, Reddick RL, et al: Adenosquamous carcinoma of the fallopian tube. Am J Obstet Gynecol 157:903–905, 1987.

548. Vega AP, Scharfenberg JC, Schneider GT: Multicentric Mullerian squamous neoplasia. South Med J 78:1360–1363, 1985.

549. Hovadhanakul P, Neurenberger SP, Ritter PJ, et al: Primary transitional cell carcinoma of the fallopian tube with primary carcinoma of the ovary and endometrium. Gynecol Oncol 4:138–143, 1976.

550. Koshiyama M, Konishi I, Yoshida M, et al: Transitional cell carcinoma of the fallopian tube: A light and electron microscopic study. Int J Gynecol Pathol 13:175–180, 1994.

551. Herbold DR, Axelrod JH, Bobowski SJ, et al: Glassy cell carcinoma of the fallopian tube: A case report. Int J Gynecol Pathol 7:384–390, 1988.

552. Griffith LM, Carcangiu ML: Sex cord tumor with annular tubules associated with endometriosis of the fallopian tube. Am J Clin Pathol 96:259–262, 1991.

553. Moore OA, Waxman M, Udoffia C: Leiomyoma of the fallopian tube: A cause of tubal pregnancy. Am J Obstet Gynecol 134:101–102, 1979.

554. Okagaki T, Richart RM: Neurilemoma of the fallopian tube. Am J Obstet Gynecol 106:929, 1970.

555. Dede JA, Janovski NA: Lipoma of the uterine tube: A gynecologic rarity. Obstet Gynecol 22:461–467, 1993.

556. Katz DA, Thom D, Bogard P, et al: Angiomyolipoma of the fallopian tube. Am J Obstet Gynecol 148:341–343, 1984.

557. Weber DL, Fazzini E: Ganglioneuroma of the fallopian tube: A hitherto unreported finding. Acta Neuropathol (Berl) 16:173–175, 1970.

558. Henricksen E: Struma salpingii: Report of a case. Obstet Gynecol 5:833–835, 1955.

559. Westerhout FC Jr: Ruptured tubal hydatidiform mole: Report of a case. Obstet Gynecol 23:138–139, 1964.

560. Ober W, Maier RC: Gestational choriocarcinoma of the fallopian tube. Diagn Gynecol Obstet 3:213–231, 1982.

561. Dekel A, van Iddehinge B, Isaacson C, et al: Primary choriocarcinoma of the fallopian tube. Report of a case with survival and postoperative delivery. Review of the literature. Obstet Gynecol Surv 41:142–148, 1986.

CHAPTER 14

The Vulva, Vagina, and Cervix

Charles Zaloudek, M.D.

VULVA

A variety of inflammatory and hyperplastic conditions occur in the vulva, as do many types of benign and malignant neoplasms. Among the benign tumors or tumor-like conditions the surgical pathologist is most likely to encounter are melanocytic nevi, hidradenoma, and condyloma acuminatum. Fortunately, these rarely pose diagnostic problems. Malignant tumors of the vulva are uncommon, constituting only approximately 1% of all malignant tumors in women. Most of these are typical keratinizing or basaloid squamous cell carcinomas and are readily identified. Unusual variants of squamous cell carcinoma may go unrecognized or cause diagnostic problems, as can Paget's disease, adenocarcinoma, melanoma, and mesenchymal tumors.

Verrucous Carcinoma

Verrucous carcinoma is an extremely well-differentiated variant of squamous cell carcinoma. First described in the upper aerodigestive tract, verrucous carcinoma also arises in the female genital tract.[1] The vulva is the most common primary site, followed by the cervix and, rarely, the vagina.[2]

CLINICOPATHOLOGIC FEATURES. Verrucous carcinoma of the vulva affects a wide age range. The average age at diagnosis is 59 years, but it occurs in women as young as 18.[2] Clinically, patients present with pruritus, pain, or a vulvar lesion. Large ulcerated or infected tumors bleed or produce a discharge. A history of condylomata is obtained from about half the patients.[3] Human papillomavirus (HPV) DNA sequences are present in verrucous carcinoma, suggesting a possible role for HPV infection in the genesis of this type of carcinoma.[4, 5] Verrucous carcinoma is appropriately treated by wide local excision in most instances.[3] Radical vulvectomy is required for adequate excision of some large or central tumors. Clinically suspicious inguinal lymph nodes may be sampled by fine needle aspiration or excised at the time of surgery. The prognosis is related to the stage at diagnosis. The cure rate for all stages, as summarized from the literature, is 64% in women treated by surgery.[2] In the largest reported study, 16% of women with stage I or II verrucous carcinoma of the vulva died of cancer.[3]

The tumors range from small growths that resemble condylomata[2] to large neoplasms more than 10 cm in maximum dimension. Typical examples are exophytic, fungating, or papillomatous tumors that are often described as having a "cauliflower-like" surface.[3] The labia majora are the most frequent primary site, but approximately 25% of verrucous carcinomas are central or extensive. The neoplasm is confined to the vulva (stage I or II) at diagnosis in most patients.[3] Regional lymph nodes are frequently enlarged because of reactive changes, but metastases are virtually never found in them.[2, 3]

Microscopically, verrucous carcinoma has a papillomatous surface with hyperkeratosis and parakeratosis. Perinuclear cytoplasmic clearing, or koilocytosis, is frequently seen in superficial squamous cells. The epithelium is markedly acanthotic, and thick bulbous rete ridges push into the underlying dermis or stroma (Fig. 14–1). The dermal or stromal papillae are thin and inconspicuous. Keratin pearls are occasionally found within verrucous carcinoma, and individual tumor cells have abundant, eosinophilic, keratinized cytoplasm. Cytologic atypia is minimal (Fig. 14–2). Mitotic figures vary in number, but are frequently inconspicuous or absent. When present, they are found in the basal portion of the epithelium. The tumor has a pushing border, and the subjacent connective tissue often contains many chronic inflammatory cells. Features that are not associated with verrucous carcinoma include an infiltrative growth pattern with prongs or finger-like projections of epithelium into the subjacent connective tissue and adjacent foci of high-grade vulvar intraepithelial neoplasia (carcinoma *in situ*).[3] It is difficult to diagnose verrucous carcinoma if the biopsy does not include the full thickness of the tumor, including its interface with the underlying stroma.

DIFFERENTIAL DIAGNOSIS. The differential diagnosis of verrucous carcinoma includes two benign entities, condyloma acuminatum and pseudoepitheliomatous hyperplasia, as well as the well-differentiated keratinizing and condylomatous variants of squamous cell carcinoma.

Condyloma acuminatum is a squamous proliferative lesion caused by infection with the human papillomavirus. Condylomata, typically, are small growths less than 1 cm in diameter, in contrast to verrucous carcinoma, which is a large tumor 2 cm or more in diameter.[3] Multiple condylomata are noted in many patients, whereas verrucous carcinoma forms a solitary tumor. A majority of vulvar condylomata are caused by HPV types 6 and 11.[6] Vulvar condylomata have some features in common with verrucous carcinoma, such as hyperkeratosis, parakeratosis, patchy koilocytosis, slight nuclear atypia, and marked acanthosis. However, they are superficial growths that do not invade the underlying stroma as does verrucous carcinoma (Fig. 14–3).

Pseudoepitheliomatous hyperplasia is a benign, reactive, epithelial proliferation most often found at the edge of an

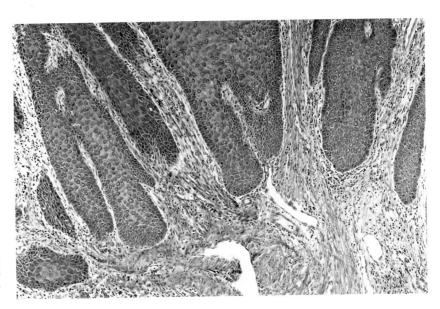

FIGURE 14–1. Verrucous carcinoma of the vulva. Low-power view illustrating bulbous rounded rete ridges pushing into the stroma. (H&E, ×40)

ulcer or in association with a chronic inflammatory process. The superficial epidermis is often edematous and infiltrated by leukocytes. The epidermis is acanthotic, and there is downward extension of irregular nests and tongues of squamous epithelium into the underlying dermis. The hyperplastic epithelium is typically infiltrated by leukocytes, and it lacks the papillomatous surface contour of verrucous carcinoma. Mitotic figures may be numerous, but they are normal. Verrucous carcinoma has a characteristic pattern of invasion into the dermis and does not exhibit the irregular, branching, downward growth seen in pseudoepitheliomatous hyperplasia.

Well-differentiated keratinizing squamous cell carcinoma can have a papillomatous appearance with hyperkeratosis and prominent acanthosis, and it can closely resemble verrucous carcinoma; however, squamous cell carcinoma displays more cytologic atypia than verrucous carcinoma. More mitotic figures are usually present, and some of them may be atypical. The most useful criterion for distinguishing between well-differentiated squamous cell carcinoma and verrucous carcinoma is the presence of irregular, branching, invasive nests of squamous cells surrounded by a desmoplastic and inflamed stroma at the base of the former, which contrasts with the rounded borders of the invasive tumor in verrucous carcinoma.[2]

Condylomatous, or warty, squamous cell carcinoma is a variant of squamous cell carcinoma that bears a gross and microscopic resemblance to condyloma acuminatum.[7, 8] Condylomatous carcinoma differs from verrucous carcinoma in that foci of squamous cell carcinoma alternate with regions reminiscent of condyloma acuminatum. The tumor cells in such areas are koilocytotic, and they have wrinkled, atypical nuclei. Binucleated and multinucleated cells are often present. Irregular nests and prongs of invasive malignant cells are present at the base of the tumor, in contrast to the pattern of pushing invasion by rounded masses of tumor cells seen in verrucous carcinoma.[3, 7, 8]

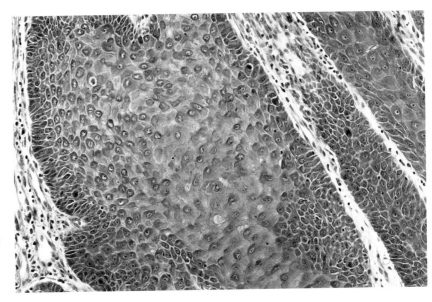

FIGURE 14–2. Verrucous carcinoma of the vulva. There are occasional mitotic figures, but the tumor cells are well differentiated, with abundant keratin production and minimal nuclear atypia and pleomorphism. (H&E, ×200)

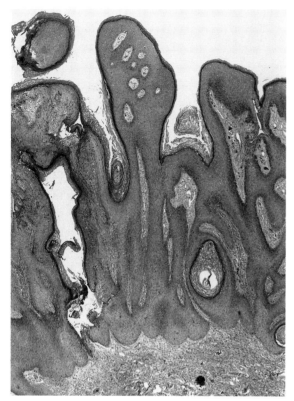

FIGURE 14–3. Condyloma acuminatum of the vulva is papillary and exophytic. In contrast to verrucous carcinoma, it does not grow downward into the underlying dermis. (H&E, ×25)

Paget's Disease

Paget's disease is a type of *in situ* adenocarcinoma. It was originally described in the breast and is most common there. Extramammary Paget's disease occurs at a variety of sites, the vulva being one of the most common. Paget's disease of the vulva differs from mammary Paget's disease in that an underlying carcinoma is not identified in most instances.

CLINICOPATHOLOGIC FEATURES. Paget's disease of the vulva is usually detected after the menopause. The age range is from 40 years to more than 80 years, with an average age at diagnosis of about 65.[9–11] Most patients are white. The most common clinical complaint is pruritus. On physical examination, affected areas are erythematous and eczematous. White areas or ulcers are occasionally present. A mass is present when there is an underlying invasive adenocarcinoma. In most patients, the lesion is unilateral and confined to the labia, but it is not uncommon for Paget's disease to involve both labia, or to extend to the perianal region, the perineum, or the skin of the buttocks, thighs, inguinal area, or mons. The extent of the lesion, as determined by histologic study, is nearly always greater than it appears grossly.[12]

Treatment depends on the extent of the lesion and whether or not there is an underlying adenocarcinoma. Non-invasive Paget's disease is treated by local excision.[9, 13] Local recurrence requiring re-excision is common (approximately 20%), even when the excision margins appear free of Paget's disease by routine histologic study.[9] When concurrent invasive adenocarcinoma and non-invasive Paget's disease are present, the prognosis is unfavorable and treatment is by radical vulvec-

tomy and bilateral inguinal lymphadenectomy.[9, 10, 14] Approximately 30% of women with Paget's disease of the vulva develop carcinoma in other organs.[9, 11]

Paget's disease is composed of tumor cells distributed singly and in variably sized groups in the epidermis. Paget's cells are most numerous in the basal and parabasal zones of the epidermis, but single cells and small groups migrate upward into the superficial epidermis (Fig. 14–4). Paget's cells are large and have vesicular or coarsely granular nuclei and one or more prominent eosinophilic nucleoli. Mitotic figures may be numerous. Tumor cell cytoplasm is abundant and pale and may contain one or more secretory vacuoles. Vulvar Paget's cells are nearly always mucin-positive; only approximately 5% are mucin-negative.[15, 16] Glands are occasionally present within large cell nests along the dermal-epidermal junction. Paget's cells extend downward in the basal zone of the hair follicles, and they are occasionally seen at the periphery of sweat gland ducts, beneath the lining epithelium. Adnexal involvement is typically most prominent just beneath the epidermis. Paget's cells are found within sweat gland acini in as many as 50% of cases.[17] Invasive carcinoma is associated with intra-epithelial Paget's disease in 15% to 30% of patients.[9, 10, 14, 17, 18] Two types of invasive carcinoma are associated with Paget's disease. A minority of cancers are limited to the papillary dermis and are composed of groups of malignant cells similar to those in the overlying epidermis.[11, 18] The infiltrating nests of Paget's cells are surrounded by an inflammatory and fibrous reaction. Most carcinomas associated with Paget's disease are deeply invasive adenocarcinomas. Some exhibit features of apocrine or eccrine differentiation. These are interpreted as invasive Paget's disease by some,[18–20] and as adenocarcinoma of sweat gland origin by others.[17, 21]

Vulvar Paget's disease has a characteristic immunophenotype. Stains for epithelial membrane antigen (EMA), carcinoembryonic antigen (CEA), and B72.3 are generally positive,[16, 22–25] and Paget's cells stain with antibodies to gross cystic disease fluid protein (GCDFP) in a majority of cases.[22, 24–26]

DIFFERENTIAL DIAGNOSIS. The main differential diagnostic considerations are a high-grade vulvar intraepithelial neoplasia (VIN) with pagetoid features and a pagetoid malignant melanoma.

Pagetoid VIN (squamous carcinoma *in situ*, or Bowen's disease), like other forms of VIN, is composed of abnormal squamous cells with enlarged hyperchromatic nuclei and an increased nucleocytoplasmic ratio. The epidermal maturation pattern is disordered, dyskeratotic cells are present, and there are increased numbers of mitotic figures. Scattered dysplastic cells have a pagetoid appearance. These are larger than the cells surrounding them and have abundant pale cytoplasm. The pagetoid cells do not form glands or contain mucin, nor are they found in the stratum corneum. In contrast to Paget's disease, VIN rarely affects adnexal structures. Special stains are helpful in the differential diagnosis. Paget's cells are mucin-positive and are immunoreactive with EMA, CEA, B72.3, and low-molecular-weight cytokeratin. Pagetoid VIN is mucin-negative, does not stain with EMA, CEA, or B72.3, and reacts with antibodies to high-, not low-, molecular-weight cytokeratin. Rarely, VIN and Paget's disease of the vulva are contiguous.[27]

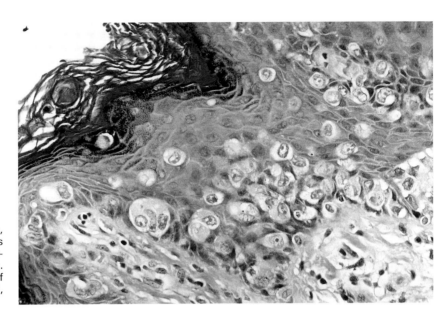

FIGURE 14–4. Paget's disease of the vulva, illustrating the characteristic neoplastic cells with large vesicular nuclei, prominent nucleoli, and abundant amphophilic cytoplasm. Although concentrated in the basal zone of the epidermis, Paget's cells invade upward, reaching the stratum corneum. (H&E, ×200)

Pagetoid melanoma resembles Paget's disease, particularly when no invasive component is present. Melanoma cells are concentrated in nests at the dermal-epidermal junction. Upward migration into the epidermis is common, but the stratum corneum contains few tumor cells. In contrast, a majority of Paget's cells grow singly or in groups in the parabasal zone, with a rim of basal cells separating them from the dermal-epidermal junction. Paget's cells extend throughout the epidermis and are commonly present in the stratum corneum. Melanoma cells have vesicular nuclei and abundant gray cytoplasm that may contain fine or coarse melanin granules. Glands are not present in melanoma. Melanoma cells are negative for mucin, cytokeratin, EMA, CEA, and B72.3. Immunostains for S-100 protein and HMB-45 are positive in melanoma, but negative in Paget's disease.[15, 16, 22, 24, 25, 28]

Melanoma

Melanoma of the vulva is rare; nevertheless, it is the second most common malignant tumor of the vulva after squamous cell carcinoma. Approximately 10% of all vulvar malignancies are melanomas, and 3% to 5% of all melanomas arise in the vulva.[29, 30]

CLINICOPATHOLOGIC FEATURES. Vulvar melanoma can occur at any age, but most are detected in elderly white women.[31, 32] The average age is 60 to 65.[29, 33] The most common presenting complaints are bleeding, pruritus, a vulvar mass, or a change in a preexisting mole.[31, 34] Melanoma is typically centrally located on the mucosal surface of the vulva;[30, 31] a majority involve the clitoris or labia minora. The remainder are lateral lesions that arise in the cutaneous part of the vulva on the labia majora. Most vulvar melanomas measure less than 2 cm in diameter.[31] Although prognosis is related to the depth of invasion (microstage), vulvar melanoma has a poor prognosis because most women have advanced disease at diagnosis.[35–37] The traditional mode of therapy is radical vulvectomy with bilateral inguinal lymph node dissection.[31] There is a recent trend toward more conservative management of women with vulvar melanoma, particularly those with low-risk tumors. Wide local excision is supplanting radical vulvectomy,[32, 36–38] and inguinal lymph node dissection is deferred unless the tumor is deeply invasive or the nodes are clinically positive.[29, 32, 37]

The most common of the three melanoma subtypes is **superficial spreading melanoma.** The light microscopic appearance of this variant includes a prominent junctional component that extends laterally three or more rete ridges beyond the site of dermal invasion (Fig. 14–5). Melanoma cells often invade upward into the epidermis, resulting in a pagetoid appearance. Horizontal growth is absent or limited to less than three rete ridges from the site of vertical growth in **nodular melanoma,** and the invasive component dominates the histologic picture. Nodular melanoma is often ulcerated, and it typically is deeply invasive (level IV or V).[35] Superficial spreading and nodular melanomas are composed of nevoid, epithelioid, or atypical spindle cells with large vesicular nuclei. Nucleoli are often prominent, and intranuclear cytoplasmic inclusions are a characteristic feature (Fig. 14–6). The amount of cytoplasm varies, but it is often moderate to abundant and eosinophilic. Vulvar melanomas may be pigmented or amelanotic. In **acral lentiginous** or **mucous membrane melanoma,** the basal epidermis contains atypical dendritic melanocytes and nests of spindle cells.[30, 31, 38, 39] The invasive component consists of spindle-shaped tumor cells in a desmoplastic stroma. A neurotropic growth pattern is noted in approximately 50% of mucous membrane melanomas.[39] There is usually strong cytoplasmic staining with antibodies to S-100 protein and HMB-45 in superficial spreading and nodular melanomas. Mucous membrane melanoma is generally S-100–positive, but staining with HMB-45 may be weak or negative.

The thickness and microstage of vulvar melanoma should be determined whenever possible. Vulvar melanoma is microstaged like cutaneous melanoma. Some authors use Clark's microstages,[31, 33] but these are difficult to apply in the vulva.[30, 39] Chung et al. proposed an alternative method for microstaging vulvar melanoma in which *in situ* melanoma is level I.[40] A melanoma with 1 mm or less of invasion, measured from the granular layer of the vulvar skin or the outermost

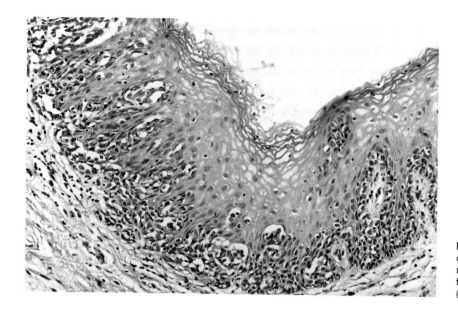

FIGURE 14-5. Superficial spreading melanoma of the vulva, illustrating nests of atypical melanocytes at the dermal-epidermal junction and focal invasion upward into the epidermis. (H&E, ×100)

layer of the vulvar mucosa, is designated as level II. A level III melanoma invades to a depth of 1 to 2 mm, a level IV melanoma invades deeper than 2 mm but does not extend into the subcutaneous fat, and a melanoma that invades the subcutaneous fat is designated as level V. Superficial melanomas are included in most series, but a majority of vulvar melanomas are detected at an advanced stage and are deeply invasive level IV or V tumors more than 3 mm thick.[33]

DIFFERENTIAL DIAGNOSIS. Of prime importance in the diagnosis of melanoma is identification of a junctional *in situ* component adjacent to the invasive melanoma. If the surface is ulcerated or the melanoma is of the nodular type, the *in situ* component may be inconspicuous or absent. Cytoplasmic melanin pigment, intranuclear cytoplasmic inclusions, and a characteristic nevoid or epithelioid cell type are further clues to the diagnosis of melanoma. Immunohistochemical stains are valuable tools in the differential diagnosis of melanoma. The differential diagnosis includes Paget's disease and high-

grade VIN with a pagetoid appearance, as discussed previously, melanosis, spindle cell squamous cell carcinoma, and various types of spindle cell sarcoma.

Melanosis of the vulva is a condition in which there are pigmented patches on the vulva that often clinically mimic melanoma. Microscopic features include hyperpigmentation of the basal layer of the epidermis, a slight increase in the number of single melanocytes in the basal layer, and slight thickening of the papillary dermis with an increase in the number of melanophages.[41] Features of melanoma such as nesting, atypia, mitotic activity, or invasion, are not present.

Spindle cell squamous cell carcinoma is difficult to distinguish from a melanoma with a spindle cell growth pattern, particularly if the surface is ulcerated. Spindle cell squamous cell carcinoma may contain areas of more typical squamous cell carcinoma, or vulvar intraepithelial neoplasia may be present adjacent to the carcinoma, providing a clue to the correct diagnosis. Spindle cell melanoma often contains

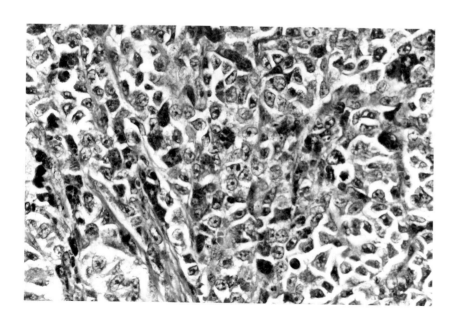

FIGURE 14-6. Melanoma of the vulva. The tumor cells have large vesicular nuclei, prominent nucleoli, and a moderate amount of amphophilic cytoplasm. Some cells contain abundant darkly stained melanin granules in their cytoplasm. (H&E, ×400)

groups of nevoid or epithelioid cells, suggesting the diagnosis. Cytoplasmic melanin pigmentation and intranuclear cytoplasmic inclusions are further evidence in support of a diagnosis of melanoma. Cells of spindle cell squamous cell carcinoma react with cytokeratin and EMA. Melanoma is nonreactive with these antibodies, but reacts with S-100 and/or HMB-45.

A **spindle or epithelioid cell sarcoma** of the vulva can mimic melanoma. Routine light microscopy may provide sufficient information to identify a specific type of sarcoma. Immunohistochemistry may also provide critical evidence for the diagnosis. Leiomyosarcoma is the most common vulvar sarcoma, and the tumor cells react with muscle-specific antibodies. Melanoma and sarcoma both are vimentin-positive. Most sarcomas are S-100–negative, but sarcomas of neural origin and those with chondroid differentiation may be S-100–positive. HMB-45, in contrast, does not react with such sarcomas, but is positive in melanoma.

Aggressive Angiomyxoma

Aggressive angiomyxoma (AAM) is an infiltrative tumor of the pelvic soft tissues.[42] Most develop in young women and are found in the vulva, perineum, vaginal wall, or pelvis. The clinical presentation is with a mass, which may be misinterpreted as a Bartholin's cyst[43] or a hernia.[44, 45] Local recurrence is common, because most examples are inadequately excised, but AAM does not metastasize.[42, 46, 47]

AAM ranges from 3 cm to more than 30 cm in maximum diameter. Most examples appear circumscribed, but AAM extends along tissue planes and may infiltrate adjacent structures, including bone.[46] The consistency varies from soft and fleshy to firm and rubbery. The cut surface is gray or white and is glistening and gelatinous. Microscopically, AAM is composed of small spindle or stellate cells scattered in a myxoid background (Fig. 14–7). The tumor cells have uniform oval nuclei with fine chromatin and inconspicuous nucleoli. The cytoplasm is pale, and the cell borders are ill

defined. No atypical cells are present, and mitotic activity is low. Zones of increased cellularity are present in some neoplasms. The stroma contains numerous blood vessels, including arteries, veins, and dilated small vessels. Immunohistochemical and electron microscopic studies indicate that the spindle cells are fibroblasts or myofibroblasts.[42, 43, 47]

DIFFERENTIAL DIAGNOSIS. The differential diagnosis includes angiomyofibroblastoma and a variety of myxoid soft-tissue tumors.

Angiomyofibroblastoma is a circumscribed tumor composed of spindle and plump stromal cells.[48] The tumor contains numerous thin-walled blood vessels surrounded by zones of hypercellular and edematous hypocellular stroma. The tumor cells exhibit some of the ultrastructural features of myofibroblasts. They are immunoreactive for vimentin and desmin, but not for actin. Based on the limited information available in the literature, angiomyofibroblastoma does not recur after excision. Angiomyofibroblastomas are smaller than AAM, do not infiltrate surrounding tissues, and do not recur after local excision. The stroma is more cellular, and the blood vessels do not have the thick walls that characterize the vessels in AAM. The stroma is edematous, but not myxoid. The immunophenotype is different, as the stromal cells in angiomyofibroblastoma are desmin-positive, whereas reportedly those in AAM are not.

Myxoma is composed of spindle or stellate cells in a myxoid stroma. It is not as cellular as an AAM, and lacks a vascular component. **Myxoid lipoma** has transitional zones between its myxoid and fatty components. A prominent microvascular network and lipoblasts are found in **myxoid liposarcoma,** but not in AAM.[49] **Myxoid neural tumors** generally contain areas that exhibit the typical appearance of a peripheral nerve sheath tumor. They are often associated with nerves, and they are immunoreactive with S-100 protein. The **myxoid variant of malignant fibrous histiocytoma** (MFH) develops in older patients; it contains more abnormal cells than those in AAM, and portions of the tumor exhibit typical features of MFH.

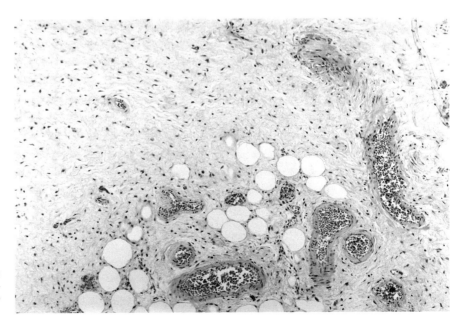

FIGURE 14–7. Aggressive angiomyxoma. Small spindle-shaped or stellate cells grow in a myxoid stroma. Prominent vascularity and infiltration of fat are characteristic findings. (H&E, ×100)

VAGINA

Abnormalities of the vagina that require surgical biopsy are infrequent. A majority of vaginal biopsies are taken to diagnose a squamous intraepithelial lesion (dysplasia or condyloma), or, occasionally, to diagnose cancer. Most malignant tumors of the vagina are secondary and usually represent extensions of cervical or vulvar carcinoma. Bladder, rectal, endometrial, and ovarian carcinoma may also involve the vagina by direct invasion or metastasis. A primary carcinoma of the vagina is almost always squamous cell carcinoma. The conditions that are most likely to cause diagnostic difficulty are diethylstilbestrol (DES)-related abnormalities of the vagina and cervix, such as adenosis and clear-cell carcinoma, and rhabdomyosarcoma of the lower female genital tract.

Adenosis

An abnormality in the formation of the female genital tract, in recent years most often associated with *in utero* exposure to DES, can alter the character of its epithelium, giving rise to foci of glandular epithelium of mullerian type either at the surface or within the superficial stroma in the vagina (adenosis) or on the portio of the cervix (ectropion).[50] Fifty-three percent of the women who participated in a cooperative study of the effect of DES exposure had vaginal epithelial changes on colposcopy or after iodine staining, and 45% of those women had adenosis.[50] Individuals with such abnormalities are at increased risk of developing clear-cell adenocarcinoma of the vagina or cervix.[51]

Adenosis is characterized by the presence of glandular epithelium in the surface mucosa of the vagina, in the superficial stroma, or in both sites.[50, 52, 53] The glandular epithelium is most often composed of tall columnar cells with mucinous cytoplasm, similar to endocervical cells (Fig. 14–8). Endometrial-type and ciliated tubal-type cells are commonly present as well. When similar microscopic findings are noted on the ectocervix, the lesion is called an **ectropion.** Columnar

mucinous epithelium is usually the only type of glandular epithelium found on the portio; tuboendometrial epithelium is seen in only 3% of ectropions.[50]

Adenosis undergoes a process of squamous metaplasia similar to that observed in the transformation zone of the cervix. Early in the metaplastic process, there is an admixture of columnar and squamous metaplastic cells; but later, rare glands or pools of mucin within the metaplastic epithelium are the only evidence of adenosis. Finally, when squamous metaplasia is complete, the epithelium is recognizable as a site of transformed adenosis, because it is composed of immature non-glycogenated metaplastic cells, or because there are pegs of squamous epithelium within the stroma at sites where metaplastic epithelium has replaced adenosis.

DIFFERENTIAL DIAGNOSIS. Adenosis must be differentiated from endometriosis and from mesonephric remnants (discussed in the section on minimal deviation adenocarcinoma of the cervix).

Endometriosis of the vagina may be superficial or it may be located deep in the vaginal wall. It consists of an admixture of endometrial stroma and endometrial glandular epithelium. Fibrosis, inflammation, and macrophages containing hemosiderin pigment frequently surround foci of endometriosis. Adenosis can be differentiated from superficial endometriosis by its lack of a stromal component. Unlike adenosis, endometriosis does not involve the surface epithelium or contain focal or extensive squamous metaplasia.

Clear-Cell Carcinoma of the Vagina and Cervix

Clear-cell carcinoma is an uncommon type of adenocarcinoma of the vagina and cervix. It was reported only rarely prior to 1971,[54] when an association between clear-cell carcinoma and *in utero* exposure to DES was first described.[55] Review of data from several registries of patients with clear-cell carcinoma of the vagina and cervix reveals that 55% to 60% of patients were exposed to DES *in utero* before the

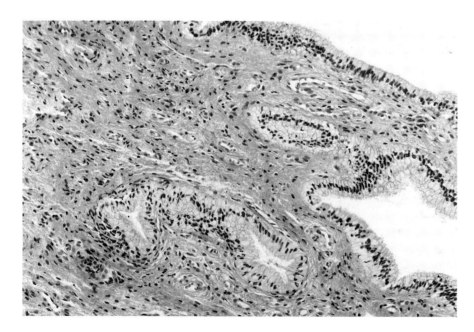

FIGURE 14–8. Adenosis of the vagina. Glands in the vaginal stroma are lined by benign columnar mucinous epithelial cells of endocervical type. (H&E, ×200)

18th week of gestation, and that the mothers of an additional 10% to 12% of patients were treated with another hormone or with an unidentified medication.[56, 57] The peak incidence of DES-associated clear-cell carcinoma was in the mid-1970s, but it will continue to occur until at least the year 2000.[57]

CLINICOPATHOLOGIC FEATURES. Clear-cell carcinoma of the vagina and cervix occurs in patients between 7 and 80 years of age. It is rarely seen in girls younger than 15 years old. There is a plateau of peak incidence in young women 17 to 22 years old, about a quarter of whom have no history of DES exposure.[56–58] The most common clinical presentation is a vaginal discharge or bleeding. Malignant cells are detected in the Pap smear in three quarters of patients.[59] Most vaginal clear-cell carcinomas are localized at diagnosis; 73% are stage I, 21% are stage II, and only 6% are stage III or IV. Among cervical clear-cell carcinomas, 35% are stage I, 29% are stage IIA, 22% are stage IIB, and 14% are stage III.[51] The most common treatment is radical hysterectomy, with partial or total vaginectomy for vaginal neoplasms. The ovaries are conserved in young women with no evidence of metastases. The overall 5-year survival is 78%.[60] Survival in stage I is 87% for women with vaginal neoplasms and 91% for those with cervical neoplasms. The survival for women with stage II vaginal carcinoma is 76%, and that for stage IIA cervical carcinoma is 77%. The overall survival is better than that observed in women with squamous cell carcinoma of the cervix or vagina.

Clear-cell carcinoma varies from a small growth only a few millimeters in diameter to a large tumor mass more than 10 cm in diameter. Most are exophytic polypoid or nodular growths. Microscopically, the tumor cells are cuboidal, columnar, or polygonal, and they have clear or eosinophilic granular cytoplasm. The nuclei are round and bland or large, hyperchromatic, and irregular. The nuclei of some columnar cells bulge into gland lumna (''hobnail cells''). There are three main histologic patterns, which are frequently admixed. The tubulocystic pattern is composed of tubular or cystic glands lined by cuboidal or columnar tumor cells (Fig. 14–9). In the papillary pattern, fibrovascular cores are covered by similar cells. The solid pattern consists of sheets of polygonal clear tumor cells.

The tubulocystic pattern is associated with a more favorable prognosis.[61]

Adenosis is present in more than 95% of DES-exposed patients with clear-cell adenocarcinoma of the vagina.[51] The carcinoma typically arises near the most distal extent of the vaginal epithelial changes.[62] Although mucinous glands are often present, tuboendometrial glands are concentrated in the region around the tumor,[62] and tuboendometrial glands immediately adjacent to the carcinoma may be lined by atypical cells.[63] There is an association between adenosis with tuboendometrial glands and clear-cell carcinoma, but direct transitions between adenosis and clear-cell carcinoma are difficult to demonstrate.[59]

DIFFERENTIAL DIAGNOSIS. The differential diagnosis of clear-cell carcinoma includes hyperplasia and neoplasia of mesonephric remnants (discussed in the section on minimal deviation adenocarcinoma of the cervix), atypical microglandular hyperplasia, yolk sac tumor, and primary and metastatic adenocarcinoma of non–clear-cell type.

Microglandular hyperplasia (MGH) is a common condition that is usually associated with exogenous progesterone administration or pregnancy.[64] It is also occasionally found in women who are exposed only to estrogens or who do not have an altered hormonal milieu. Microglandular hyperplasia is most common in the cervix, but it also develops in the vagina in women with adenosis.[65] Grossly, it may be flat and inconspicuous, or it may form a polyp. Microscopically, microglandular hyperplasia is composed of tightly packed small glands and small cysts lined by low columnar or cuboidal cells (Fig. 14–10). These have round, bland nuclei; mitotic figures are absent or vary rare. Acute inflammatory cells are commonly present in the epithelium, glands, and stroma. The epithelial cells contain intracytoplasmic mucin, and the gland lumen contents are mucinous. The circumscribed nature of the hyperplasia and the absence of significant cytologic atypia and mitotic activity differentiate typical microglandular hyperplasia from adenocarcinoma. Immunohistochemical studies can help distinguish between these lesions, as immunostains for carcinoembryonic antigen (CEA) are negative in MGH but are generally positive in adenocarcinoma.[66] Atypical

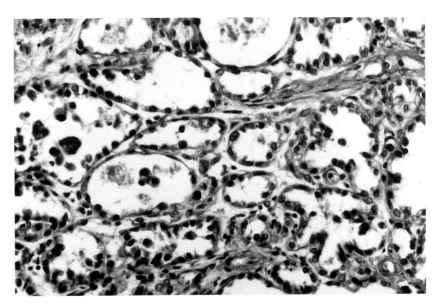

FIGURE 14–9. Clear-cell carcinoma of the vagina, growing in a tubulocystic pattern. The cells have clear cytoplasm and hyperchromatic nuclei, which focally bulge into the lumina. (H&E, ×200)

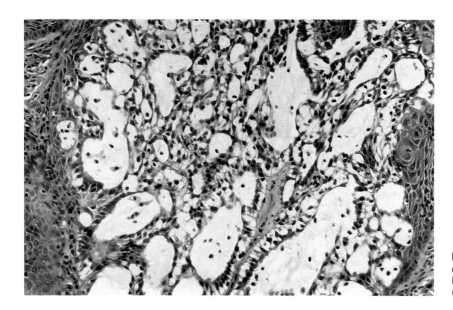

FIGURE 14–10. Microglandular hyperplasia, composed of variably sized small glands lined by cells that contain cytoplasmic mucin. (H&E, ×200)

forms of microglandular hyperplasia that contain areas of solid growth, altered stroma, modest nuclear atypia, or rare mitotic figures may be confused with carcinoma, especially clear-cell carcinoma.[67] The feature that is most helpful in distinguishing atypical MGH from clear-cell carcinoma is the spectrum of changes ranging from atypical foci to typical MGH. In addition, clear-cell carcinoma exhibits greater nuclear atypia and mitotic activity than MGH as well as growth patterns, such as papillae and sheets of cells with abundant clear cytoplasm, that are not seen in atypical MGH.[67]

Yolk sac tumor arises rarely in the vagina or cervix in children younger than 3 years old.[68, 69] Patients present with a bloody vaginal discharge and have a polypoid or sessile tumor that partly or completely fills the vagina. Surgical excision followed by multiagent chemotherapy results in survival of a high percentage of patients.[68, 69] The microscopic features are similar to those of yolk sac tumor of the ovary.[70, 71] The three most common microscopic growth patterns are the reticular pattern, in which a meshwork of microcystic spaces are lined by primitive epithelial cells, the festoon pattern, with trabeculae and glands in a myxoid stroma, and the solid pattern, with solid sheets of primitive epithelial cells. Hyaline eosinophilic bodies are found in a majority of cases, and the tumor cells are immunoreactive with alpha-fetoprotein.[68, 69] Yolk sac tumor enters the differential diagnosis of clear-cell carcinoma, particularly when solid sheets of primitive cells with clear cytoplasm predominate or when the tumor grows in a tubular pattern. The admixture of the typical reticular and festoon patterns and the positive reaction with alpha-fetoprotein serve to differentiate yolk sac tumor from clear-cell carcinoma. The most helpful differential diagnostic feature is the patient's age. Yolk sac tumors of the vagina have not been reported after age 3, and clear cell carcinomas have not been reported before age 6 to 7.

Adenocarcinoma of the vagina of non–clear-cell type may be either primary or metastatic. Adenocarcinoma is reported to constitute 11% to 17% of primary, non–DES-associated vaginal carcinomas, but the histologic appearance of such tumors is poorly documented.[72–74] Only a small number of vaginal adenocarcinomas have been adequately described.

These include an adenocarcinoma *in situ*,[75] a non–clear-cell adenocarcinoma arising in adenosis,[76] an enteric-type adenocarcinoma possibly arising in cloacal remnants,[77] and endometrioid adenocarcinomas arising in vaginal endometriosis.[78] Such tumors are distinctive and are not difficult to differentiate from adenosis or clear-cell carcinoma. The vagina and the ovary are the two most common sites of metastases to the female genital tract.[79] Colorectal carcinoma is the most frequent extragenital tumor, and ovarian and endometrial are the genital tumors most likely to metastasize to the vagina.[79] Adenocarcinoma of the cervix commonly spreads to the vagina as well. The only metastatic adenocarcinoma likely to pose a differential diagnostic problem with clear-cell carcinoma of the vagina is metastatic clear-cell carcinoma of the ovary or endometrium. The histologic features of primary and metastatic clear-cell carcinoma are similar, but knowledge of the clinical history can help differentiate primary from metastatic tumors. Clear-cell carcinoma of the vagina arises in children and young women, whereas clear-cell carcinoma of the ovary or endometrium most often develops in postmenopausal women. In addition, clear-cell carcinoma of the ovary is unlikely to give rise to vaginal metastases in the absence of extensive intraperitoneal tumor spread.

Rhabdomyosarcoma of the Lower Female Genital Tract

Rhabdomyosarcoma is a malignant neoplasm composed of primitive mesenchymal cells that exhibit skeletal muscle differentiation. Approximately 3% of rhabdomyosarcomas arise in the lower female genital tract.[80] The vagina is the most common site, but rhabdomyosarcoma also arises in the uterus and vulva.

CLINICOPATHOLOGIC FEATURES. Rhabdomyosarcoma of the vagina occurs mainly in young children from birth to 4 years old. The average age is slightly younger than 2 years.[80] Patients with uterine (usually cervical) rhabdomyosarcoma are older than those with vaginal neoplasms. In the Intergroup Rhabdomyosarcoma Study (IRS), girls with uterine rhabdomyosarcoma ranged from 4 to 16 years old, with an average age of 13.6 years.[80] Although rhabdomyosarcoma of the cervix is most common in teenagers, it occurs rarely in older women.[81–83] The clinical presentation is with a bloody vaginal discharge, a tumor protruding from the vagina, or because of passage of tumor fragments. Examination reveals a polypoid neoplasm arising from the anterior vagina or cervix. Formerly treated surgically with poor results,[84, 85] rhabdomyosarcoma is now treated by combination therapy, usually including chemotherapy, conservative surgery, and, in some instances, radiation.[80] Contemporary survival rates are higher than 80%.[80–82, 86, 87]

Rhabdomyosarcoma of the vagina and cervix typically grows as one or multiple sessile or pedunculated polypoid masses that project into the vaginal lumen. A minority of cervical rhabdomyosarcomas are endophytic intramural tumors.[88] Microscopically, polypoid vaginal and cervical rhabdomyosarcomas are of the **sarcoma botryoides** subtype, a variant of **embryonal rhabdomyosarcoma** in which the tumor cells grow beneath the mucosal surface of a body cavity or hollow viscus (Fig. 14–11).[89] A hypercellular zone (the "cambium" layer) composed of small spindle-shaped and round cells with fine chromatin, inconspicuous nucleoli, and scanty eosinophilic cytoplasm lies beneath the mucosal surface (Fig. 14–12). The number of mitotic figures is variable. Beneath the hypercellular zone, there is abundant edematous myxoid stroma; the tumor is of low to moderate cellularity, the tumor cells are predominantly spindle-shaped and have eosinophilic cytoplasm, and some of them have cross-striations.[81] Small foci of mature cartilage are occasionally found in sarcoma botryoides of the cervix.[81, 90]

Accurate diagnosis of rhabdomyosarcoma depends on the identification of rhabdomyoblasts. Cells with cross-striations are present in some tumors, but they may be difficult to identify, and most pathologists accept round or polygonal cells with abundant eosinophilic cytoplasm as indicative of rhabdomyoblastic differentiation. Immunohistochemical stains can be of help in making the diagnosis of rhabdomyosarcoma.[91] The most useful antibodies are those against desmin and muscle-specific actin, which stain approximately 80% of

rhabdomyosarcomas.[92] Myoglobin is a highly specific marker, but it stains less than 50% of rhabdomyosarcomas.[92]

DIFFERENTIAL DIAGNOSIS. A variety of small round-cell neoplasms, including lymphoma, neuroblastoma, peripheral neuroectodermal tumor, and Ewing's sarcoma, are generally considered in the differential diagnosis of rhabdomyosarcoma. Fortunately, other small round-cell neoplasms are extremely rare in the lower female genital tract, where the most common diagnostic problems are caused by vaginal polyps and rhabdomyomas.

Fibroepithelial polyps of the lower female genital tract mainly arise in the vulva.[93, 94] Women with polyps may be asymptomatic, or they may have vaginal bleeding or notice a lump or growth.[94–96] The average patient age is 35 to 50 years.[94, 97] Treatment is by simple excision, and recurrences are rare and adequately treated by re-excision.[93] Vulvovaginal polyps are covered by stratified squamous epithelium and have a loose connective tissue core that contains spindle-shaped fibroblastic cells and prominent blood vessels. In some instances, the spindle cells are reactive with vimentin and desmin, which is compatible with myofibroblastic differentiation.[94, 98] Polyps pose a diagnostic problem when their stroma is hypercellular and contains atypical fibroblasts with enlarged, irregular, hyperchromatic nuclei.[93, 96, 97, 99] Mitotic figures are usually absent or rare, but there may be numerous and even atypical mitotic figures in polyps removed from pregnant women.[98, 100, 101] Some polyps contain giant cells with abundant eosinophilic cytoplasm and multiple peripheral nuclei.

The polypoid growth pattern and the presence of spindle cells in an edematous stroma may suggest botryoid rhabdomyosarcoma. Clinical and histologic findings both are important in arriving at the correct diagnosis. Benign vaginal polyps develop almost exclusively in patients older than 5 years and grow slowly. In contrast, rhabdomyosarcoma of the vagina is a rapidly growing tumor that almost always occurs in children younger than 5 years of age. Sarcoma botryoides of the cervix, however, may arise in a teenager or young adult. Microscopic features that distinguish a polyp from a rhabdomyosarcoma are the circumscribed nature of the polyp, the absence of a subsurface hypercellular zone, or cambium layer, the absence

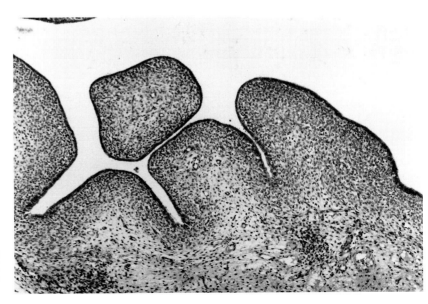

FIGURE 14–11. Rhabdomyosarcoma of the vagina. Note the polypoid surface contour and the hypercellular zone beneath the surface epithelium. (H&E, ×40)

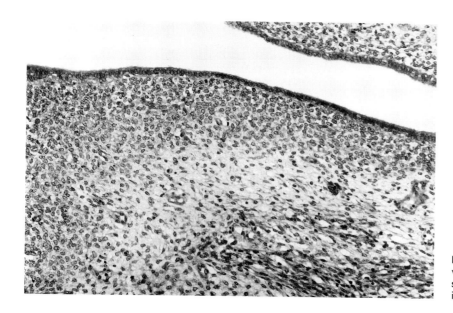

FIGURE 14–12. Rhabdomyosarcoma of the vagina, showing the small round and spindle-shaped tumor cells with scanty cytoplasm and indistinct cell borders. (H&E, ×400)

of tumor cells with cross-striations, the absence of rhabdomyoblasts with prominent eosinophilic cytoplasm, the presence of only a few mitotic figures, and the fibroblastic or myofibroblastic nature of the stromal cells. Desmin- and muscle-specific actin–positive cells are generally prominent in rhabdomyosarcoma but are absent or less conspicuous in a polyp.

Rhabdomyoma is a benign polypoid tumor that arises in the vagina in middle-aged women. There may be no symptoms, or the patient may have abnormal vaginal bleeding or notice a lump. Local excision of the tumor is curative.[99, 102–105]

Rhabdomyoma of the lower female genital tract is a myxoid variant of the fetal type of rhabdomyoma.[106] It is covered by stratified squamous epithelium and is predominantly composed of small, round, oval, or spindle-shaped mesenchymal cells in a loose myxoid stroma (Fig. 14–13).[102, 106, 107] Scattered among the spindle cells are large strap- or racquet-shaped cells with abundant brightly eosinophilic cytoplasm in which there are longitudinal fibrils and, in some cells, cross-

striations. The vesicular nuclei are central or peripheral and have prominent nucleoli. The striated cells are immunoreactive with myoglobin, desmin, and muscle-specific actin. The cytoplasm contains actin and myosin filaments and occasional well-formed sarcomeres with A, I, and Z bands.[103, 107]

The presence of cells with cross-striations in a polypoid tumor of the vagina raises the question of rhabdomyosarcoma. Differential diagnostic features include the older age of patients with rhabdomyoma, the slow growth of the tumor, and, histologically, the absence of a cambium layer, atypical spindle and round tumor cells, and mitotic figures.

CERVIX

Cervical biopsies are the most common female genital tract specimen evaluated in the surgical pathology laboratory. Most are taken during the course of evaluation of an abnormal Pap

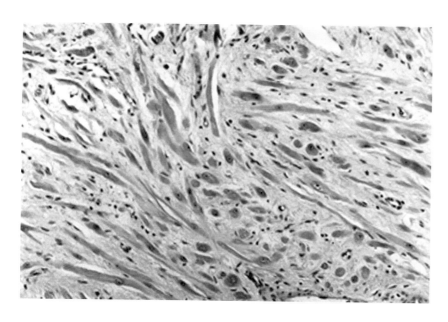

FIGURE 14–13. Rhabdomyoma of the vagina. The tumor is composed of round or strap-shaped cells with abundant eosinophilic cytoplasm. (H&E, ×100)

smear and are colposcopically directed. Other common types of cervical specimens include the endocervical curettage, the loop electrosurgical excision specimen (LEEP), the cone biopsy, and the cervix of the uterus removed by hysterectomy. Pathologists are generally familiar with the morphology of inflammatory changes that occur in the cervix, with dysplasia and condyloma, and with the appearance of typical examples of squamous cell carcinoma and adenocarcinoma. This section concentrates on those variants of squamous cell carcinoma and adenocarcinoma that are likely to cause differential diagnostic problems, either because they are difficult to differentiate from other common conditions or because they are uncommon and pathologists are unfamiliar with them.

Microinvasive Squamous Cell Carcinoma

Microinvasive squamous cell carcinoma, as its name suggests, exhibits minimal stromal invasion. Currently, microinvasion is discovered in fewer than 10% of excisions performed for high-grade squamous intraepithelial lesions (SILs) and in about 15% of hysterectomies performed for stage I cervical cancer.[108, 109] The accurate diagnosis of microinvasive carcinoma often poses a significant problem, with the main difficulty being the overdiagnosis of high-grade SIL with glandular involvement as microinvasive carcinoma. The magnitude of the problem is illustrated by studies in which one third to one half of the potential cases of microinvasive squamous cell carcinoma must be rejected because microinvasion cannot be confirmed on review of the microscopic slides.[110, 111]

The diagnosis of microinvasive carcinoma is also complicated by the fact that a universally accepted definition is yet to be formulated. In the United States, microinvasive carcinoma is variably defined as less than 1 mm of invasion, less than 3 mm of invasion, and less than 5 mm of invasion. Some European authorities measure small carcinomas in three dimensions and define a ''microcarcinoma'' as one with a volume of less than 500 mm³. The International Federation of Gynecology and Obstetrics (FIGO) in 1986 proposed the division of preclinical invasive carcinoma (stage IA) into two categories. A carcinoma with minimal microscopic stromal invasion, less than 1 mm, is designated as stage IA1. A carcinoma with deeper invasion, but where the invasive component is 5 mm or less in depth and 7 mm or less in horizontal spread, is designated as stage IA2.[112] This definition has yet to gain acceptance in the United States, where a definition proposed by the Society of Gynecologic Oncologists (SGO) is widely used. According to the SGO definition, a microinvasive carcinoma is one that invades to a depth of no more than 3 mm and in which capillary–lymphatic space involvement is not identified.

CLINICOPATHOLOGIC FEATURES. Microinvasive carcinoma is, by definition, preclinical. It is asymptomatic, and it is not visible when the cervix is examined with the unaided eye. It is most commonly detected in women 35 to 45 years old, and it is generally found when a woman is evaluated for an abnormal cervical cytology.[113–117] Microinvasive carcinoma has a low risk of pelvic lymph node metastasis, and it seldom recurs or causes the patient's death.[118] The risk of lymph node metastasis or recurrence is less than 1% in patients whose carcinomas invade 3 mm or less and do not involve capillary

lymphatic spaces.[108, 111, 113–115, 117] There is a slightly higher risk of lymph node metastasis (2.6%) and recurrence (4%) in patients with capillary lymphatic space invasion; but when patients are stratified by depth of invasion, there is no significant difference in risk for patients with or without capillary lymphatic space invasion.[113, 117] In one representative series of cervical cancers staged by FIGO criteria, 6 of 309 patients with stage IA1 cancer developed carcinoma *in situ* of the vagina, but none had recurrent invasive carcinoma, and there were no tumor-related deaths. There was recurrence of invasive carcinoma in 5 of 89 (5.6%) stage 1A2 cancers, one patient had dysplasia, and three patients (3%) died of tumor.[119] In a subsequent European series, none of the 232 women with stage IA1 carcinoma died of tumor, and there were only four deaths due to tumor among the 411 women with stage 1A2 carcinoma.[120] The management of microinvasive carcinoma is controversial and ranges from conizatio or simple hysterectomy to radical or modified radical hysterectomy with or without pelvic lymph node dissection. There is general agreement that women whose tumors invade to a depth of less than 3 mm and do not involve capillary lymphatic spaces can be managed by simple hysterectomy or, if conservation of fertility is desired, by conization. In the United States, women whose tumors invade 3 to 5 mm or exhibit capillary-lymphatic space invasion are likely to be treated by radical surgery with pelvic lymph node dissection.[111, 113, 116]

Histologically, microinvasive carcinoma usually arises from epithelium involved by high-grade SIL. Nests of cells with abundant eosinophilic cytoplasm are typically present within the dysplastic epithelium at a site of early stromal invasion. The nuclei of the cells in these nests are larger than those of the surrounding dysplastic cells, and some of the nuclei contain prominent nucleoli. Early invasion is characterized by the presence of irregular tongues of neoplastic cells that break through the basal zone of the epithelium and invade the cervical stroma. In minimal stromal invasion, one or more small, irregular nests of squamous carcinoma cells invade the stroma to a depth of 1 mm or less (Fig. 14–14). Two growth patterns, which are often admixed, are identified in more deeply invasive carcinomas.[118] In the first, multiple discrete tongues of invasive carcinoma extend downward into the stroma. In the second, the carcinoma grows in a confluent pattern as a sheet of malignant cells with an irregular lower margin (Fig. 14–15). Microinvasive carcinoma elicits a stromal reaction in which there is edema, fibroblastic proliferation, and a lymphoplasmacytic cellular infiltrate. The depth of invasion and the lateral extent are best measured with an ocular micrometer. The depth is measured from the basement membrane of the nearest area of uninvolved epithelium to the maximum depth of invasion from the surface epithelium. When invasive carcinoma originates in an endocervical gland, invasion is measured from the basement membrane of the gland to the point of maximum invasion. Other points of possible prognostic significance include the grade of the invasive carcinoma and the presence of capillary-lymphatic space invasion. Tumor cells invade capillary or lymphatic spaces in 10% to 15% of carcinomas that otherwise meet criteria for a diagnosis of microinvasive carcinoma and in as many as 40% of FIGO stage IA2 microcarcinomas (Fig. 14–16).[111, 119] The greater the depth of invasion, the greater the likelihood of vascular invasion.[118, 121] The significance of capillary-lymphatic space invasion is uncertain,[111, 122] although some

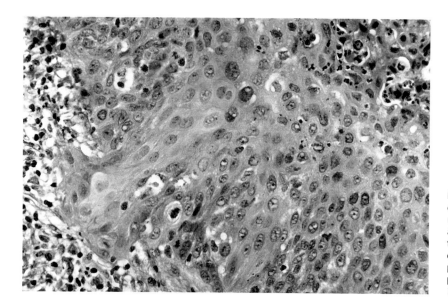

FIGURE 14–14. Microinvasive squamous cell carcinoma of the cervix. A focus of minimal stromal invasion is present *(lower left),* arising from a gland that is replaced by high-grade SIL. Note that the tumor cells at the site of invasion have enlarged nuclei and abundant eosinophilic cytoplasm. The surrounding stroma contains a prominent inflammatory cell infiltrate. (H&E, ×400)

suggest that it signifies an increased risk of metastasis.[109, 117, 120] The presence of capillary-lymphatic space invasion excludes a carcinoma from the microinvasive category as defined by the SGO, but it does not affect the FIGO stage. A diagnosis of microinvasive carcinoma is only appropriate when the entire lesion can be evaluated. Thus, microinvasive carcinoma cannot be diagnosed in a punch biopsy, nor is the diagnosis appropriate when invasive carcinoma or dysplasia extends to the margin of a cone. Further study in such cases may reveal more deeply invasive carcinoma in adjacent tissues.

DIFFERENTIAL DIAGNOSIS. The main differential diagnostic problem is distinguishing microinvasive carcinoma from an unusual pattern of **high-grade SIL (high-grade cervical intraepithelial neoplasia, or CIN III).** This is most difficult when the surface contour is undulating or papillomatous or when high-grade SIL extensively involves the endocervical glands. Tangential sectioning of such areas may suggest stromal invasion and lead to overdiagnosing high-grade SIL as

microinvasive carcinoma. The characteristic cellular changes seen at points of microinvasion, namely abundant eosinophilic cytoplasm, prominent nucleoli, and central necrotic keratinous debris within involved glands, are unlikely to be found in complex or tangentially cut foci of high-grade SIL. Glandular involvement by high-grade SIL has a rounded contour, not the irregular or jagged outline typical of microinvasive carcinoma. Finally, true microinvasion usually incites an inflammatory and fibroblastic stromal response of a type not associated with a purely intraepithelial lesion. Endocervical glands may be found in the stroma at a depth of 5 mm or more from the surface;[123] deep endocervical gland involvement by SIL is not, by itself, an indication of stromal invasion.

Conization, biopsy, and certain obstetric and reconstructive procedures may introduce **nests of benign squamous epithelium** into the cervical stroma. With healing, these nests become completely surrounded by stroma, and may be misinterpreted as foci of microinvasive carcinoma. In contrast to

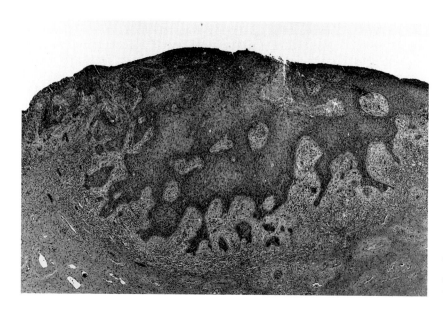

FIGURE 14–15. Microinvasive squamous cell carcinoma of the cervix. Confluent sheets of invasive carcinoma are present centrally, with finger-like prongs extending into the stroma at the periphery. (H&E, ×40)

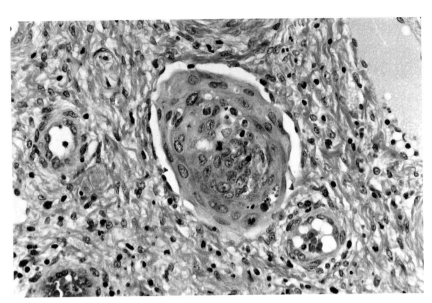

FIGURE 14–16. Capillary-lymphatic space invasion in microinvasive squamous cell carcinoma of the cervix. The tumor lies within a space lined by flattened endothelial cells. (H&E, ×400)

microinvasive carcinoma, misplaced epithelial nests are composed of bland keratinized cells (Fig. 14–17). There is no cytologic atypia, and no desmoplastic stromal response surrounds the nests. Review of the clinical history may be helpful in arriving at the correct diagnosis in such cases.

Squamous Cell Carcinoma with a Sarcoma-like Stroma

Squamous cell carcinomas in this category, which includes spindle cell squamous cell carcinoma, occur within the lower female genital tract in the cervix, vagina, and vulva.[124] Abnormal bleeding is the usual presenting sign. The overall outcome of these tumors in the female genital tract has not as yet been determined, because only a few such cases have been reported.

Grossly, the tumor forms an exophytic mass or polyp. Microscopically, two recognizable elements are present.[124]

Areas of well to moderately differentiated squamous cell carcinoma are often located near the tumor surface. The deeper parts of the tumor are composed of spindled or sarcomatoid cells. The latter cells may be spindle-shaped (Fig. 14–18) or highly pleomorphic with large nuclei, coarse chromatin and one or more prominent nucleoli. They have eosinophilic cytoplasm, which may be fibrillar or foamy. High mitotic activity is noted in sarcoma-like areas. Immunohistochemistry is particularly helpful in the diagnosis of these carcinomas. Not only does it confirm the epithelial nature of the tumor cells, but it highlights inconspicuous foci of well to moderately differentiated squamous carcinoma that are overshadowed by the spindle cell elements. Areas of clear-cut squamous cell carcinoma are strongly immunoreactive for cytokeratin. There is variable immunoreactivity in sarcoma-like or spindle cell areas, but positive cytoplasmic staining is always at least focally present (Fig. 14–19), compatible with the interpretation that these neoplasms are a type of squamous cell carci-

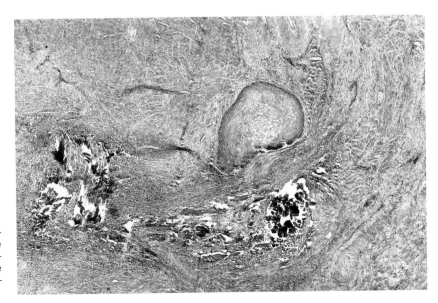

FIGURE 14–17. A nest of benign squamous epithelium in the cervical stroma after a cone biopsy. This should not be confused with invasive squamous cell carcinoma. Note the suture material and inflammation adjacent to the epithelium. (H&E, ×100)

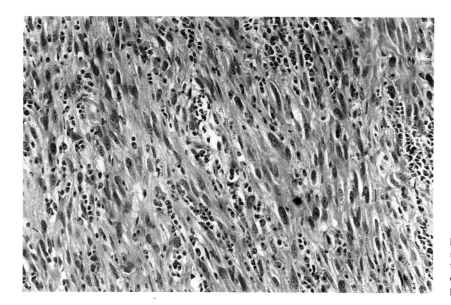

FIGURE 14–18. Spindle cell squamous cell carcinoma. The tumor cells are spindle-shaped with fusiform hyperchromatic nuclei and abundant eosinophilic cytoplasm. Inflammatory cells are present between the tumor cells. (H&E, ×400)

noma. Electron microscopic studies reveal tonofilaments in the cytoplasm of the sarcomatoid cells, which are joined by desmosomes, again supporting the concept that this is a type of spindle cell sarcoma.[124]

DIFFERENTIAL DIAGNOSIS. The differential diagnosis includes malignant melanoma, sarcoma, and carcinosarcoma.

Malignant melanoma poses a diagnostic problem when it grows predominantly in a spindle cell or desmoplastic pattern.[125] Features that are suggestive of melanoma are nests of melanocytes at the epithelial stromal junction above or lateral to an invasive spindle cell tumor, epithelioid or nevoid tumor cells admixed with or adjacent to a spindle cell component, and brown melanin pigment in tumor cell cytoplasm.[126] Immunohistochemical studies are helpful in differentiating melanoma from squamous cell carcinoma with a sarcoma-like stroma. Melanoma gives a positive reaction with S-100 and HMB-45 immunostains.[127] Sarcomatoid squamous cell carcinoma cells give a negative reaction with S-100 and HMB-

45, but they are positive with immunostains for cytokeratin and EMA. Ultrastructural study reveals premelanosomes or melanin granules in melanoma cells, but not in carcinoma cells.

Sarcoma of the cervix is a major consideration in the differential diagnosis of sarcomatoid squamous cell carcinoma. Leiomyosarcoma and endocervical stromal sarcoma pose the greatest diagnostic problems.[128–130] Mesenchymal tumors tend to occur in older women than does squamous cell carcinoma. Microscopically, foci of recognizable squamous cell carcinoma are generally visible in a sarcomatoid carcinoma, usually in the superficial portion of the tumor, but they are absent in a true sarcoma. Immunoreactivity for cytokeratin is present in sarcomatoid squamous cell carcinoma, but sarcoma gives no or only a weak, dot-like reaction. Immunohistochemical reactivity for alpha-smooth muscle actin and muscle-specific actin helps identify a leiomyosarcoma.

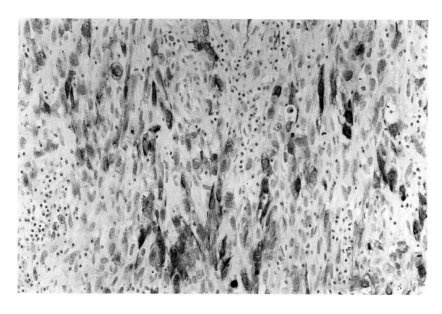

FIGURE 14–19. Spindle cell squamous cell carcinoma. Immunohistochemical stain for cytokeratin, showing strong positive reaction in the cytoplasm of spindle-shaped tumor cells. (Immunostain for cytokeratin, ×400)

Carcinosarcoma may originate in the cervix or, more often, extend from a primary site in the endometrium to the cervix.[131] Carcinosarcoma has malignant epithelial and mesenchymal components.[129, 130, 132] Some, particularly those that arise in the cervix, contain foci of squamous cell carcinoma,[130] either alone or admixed with adenocarcinoma. The tumor is readily identified as a carcinosarcoma when heterologous elements such as cartilage, striated muscle, or bone are present. The distinction from a sarcomatoid squamous cell carcinoma is difficult when the mesenchymal component is a homologous spindle cell sarcoma. The epithelial and mesenchymal components of carcinosarcoma are intimately admixed. A feature that differentiates sarcomatoid squamous cell carcinoma from carcinosarcoma is that in the former the sarcomatoid and differentiated components are often separated, with differentiated carcinoma predominant in the superficial portion of the tumor and spindle cell or sarcoma-like cells most prominent in the deeper parts.[124] Immunohistochemistry is helpful in the differential diagnosis. Strong positive staining of the spindle cell elements with cytokeratin suggests that a tumor is a sarcomatoid squamous cell carcinoma. Immunostains for cytokeratin usually highlight the biphasic nature of carcinosarcoma (Fig. 14–20).

Adenocarcinoma

Adenocarcinoma is a common type of cervical neoplasia, accounting for 10% to 20% of all invasive cervical cancers. The proportion of cervical tumors that are adenocarcinomas is increasing. This is partly due to a decrease in the number of squamous cell cancers as a result of effective cytologic screening and, apparently, an increase in the actual incidence of adenocarcinomas. For the most part, adenocarcinoma poses few diagnostic problems. All of the classic types of mullerian adenocarcinoma (mucinous, endometrioid, serous, and clear-cell) occur in the cervix and are readily recognized. Conditions that are likely to cause differential diagnostic problems include adenocarcinoma *in situ* and glandular dysplasia, which are

being found with increasing frequency in both cytologic and histologic material, and unusual variants of adenocarcinoma.

Adenocarcinoma *In Situ*

Adenocarcinoma *in situ* (ACIS) is a condition in which the endocervical surface and glands are lined by markedly abnormal cells.[133–141] The abnormality is limited to the normal endocervical gland field, and, unlike adenocarcinoma, there is no invasion of the stroma. Lesser degrees of atypia are designated as glandular dysplasia.[142–146]

CLINICOPATHOLOGIC FEATURES. ACIS occurs in young women, with an average patient age of 34 to 37 years.[143, 147–149] It is frequently associated with squamous dysplasia, and many cases are discovered incidentally during the evaluation or treatment of a woman thought to have only CIN. ACIS is undetected prior to conization in as many as 50% of the women who have it.[147] A cone biopsy is required for diagnosis. A large cone biopsy (>25 mm in length) with negative margins is likely to encompass all of the abnormal glandular epithelium. It can be therapeutic as well as diagnostic, particularly in a young woman in whom conservation of fertility is important.[135, 138, 143, 147] Hysterectomy is an alternative definitive treatment in women who have completed childbearing, based on the slight risk of residual ACIS.[147] The percentage of women with residual ACIS in the hysterectomy specimen ranges from 0%[135, 138, 143, 149] to 8%.[147, 148] A significant percentage of women with positive cone margins have residual ACIS,[135, 138, 143, 148] and rare patients have superficially invasive adenocarcinoma.[143] Hysterectomy is the usual treatment in such cases, although repeat conization with negative margins is an alternative when conservation of fertility is a consideration.[147, 148]

Microscopically, glands involved by ACIS are intermixed with normal glands and do not extend deeper into the stroma than the latter. ACIS is found in the transformation zone and in the contiguous endocervical canal. It typically involves the endocervical surface and the underlying glands, although

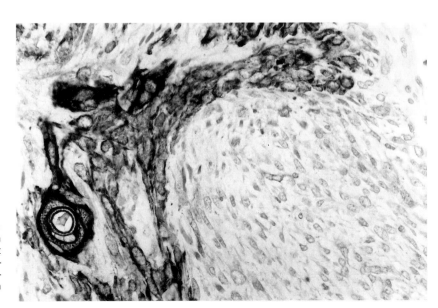

FIGURE 14–20. Carcinosarcoma of cervix. An immunohistochemical stain for cytokeratin shows a strongly reactive epithelial component *(left and upper)*, in this case squamous cell carcinoma, contrasted with a sarcomatous component that does not stain *(right)*. (Immunostain for cytokeratin, ×400)

either site can be involved without the other; ACIS is always present in gland necks.[134] The lining of affected glands may be partly or completely replaced by abnormal columnar cells (Fig. 14–21). These have stratified, enlarged, elongated nuclei and an increased nucleocytoplasmic ratio. The nuclei are hyperchromatic and relatively uniform. Nucleoli are present but not prominent. Epithelial proliferation and stratification may be sufficient to produce intraglandular budding, papillations, or a cribriform appearance. Patterns of differentiation similar to those observed in invasive adenocarcinoma have been described in ACIS. The endocervical type, in which the abnormal cells contain intracytoplasmic mucin demonstrable with the PAS stain, is the most common.[142] The abnormal cells are columnar but do not contain mucin in the endometrioid type of ACIS.[134, 150] Goblet cells with mucin vacuoles characterize the intestinal type of ACIS.[134, 146] Endocrine or Paneth cells are occasionally present. Human papillomavirus DNA, particularly HPV type 18, is frequently present in ACIS.[151–156] There is a concomitant squamous intraepithelial lesion in the cervix in 27% to 90% of cases, and a few patients have microinvasive squamous cell carcinoma.[133, 134, 138, 147, 148]

DIFFERENTIAL DIAGNOSIS. ACIS must be distinguished from glandular dysplasia and benign glandular conditions on one hand, and from invasive adenocarcinoma on the other.

Glandular dysplasia is divided into low and high grades.[142, 144, 146] Criteria for recognizing it and differentiating it from ACIS are evolving and are not yet standardized. Like ACIS, glandular dysplasia is characterized by the presence of atypical columnar cells with enlarged hyperchromatic nuclei. In low-grade dysplasia, the glands are lined by a single layer of cells whose nuclei are slightly enlarged and hyperchromatic. The columnar cell nuclei are larger and more hyperchromatic in high-grade dysplasia, and the nuclei are focally stratified, although not to the degree seen in ACIS. The degree of nuclear atypia is less in high-grade dysplasia than in ACIS, and there are fewer mitotic figures.

Tubal metaplasia is a condition in which normal endocervical glandular epithelium is replaced by tubal type epithelium composed of ciliated, secretory, and intercalated cells (Fig.

14–22).[157–159] Tubal metaplasia is present in a third or more of cervices from women with gynecologic abnormalities.[157] It may suggest ACIS because the metaplastic cells have large nuclei and an increased nucleocytoplasmic ratio. Tubal metaplasia lacks the nuclear hyperchromasia that characterizes ACIS; the nuclei are not stratified, and no mitotic figures are present. Moreover, the three tubal cell types that are present in metaplastic glands, particularly the ciliated cells, are not found in ACIS.

Other benign conditions that must be differentiated from ACIS include **microglandular hyperplasia**,[64] **lower uterine segment type endometrial glands** in the upper endocervix,[150] **endometriosis**, an **Arias-Stella reaction**,[160–162] and **reactive or inflammatory changes** in the endocervical glands.

On the malignant end of the spectrum, the differential diagnosis is with **invasive adenocarcinoma**. Microscopic features indicative of stromal invasion include cytoplasmic eosinophilia of atypical glandular cells with protrusion of buds of epithelial cells into the adjacent stroma, proliferation and budding of small acini, confluent glandular growth, extension of atypical glands deeper into the stroma than surrounding normal glands, formation of complex papillae, and production of inflamed desmoplastic stroma.[163]

Minimal Deviation Adenocarcinoma

Minimal deviation adenocarcinoma (MDAC), also known as ''adenoma malignum,'' is a very well-differentiated form of adenocarcinoma that is difficult to recognize because the malignant glands closely resemble benign endocervical glands.[164–168]

CLINICOPATHOLOGIC FEATURES. Minimal deviation adenocarcinoma occurs over a wide age range, similar to that of typical endocervical adenocarcinoma. The mean age is about 45 years, but a significant number of patients are younger than 40.[166–168] Patients usually present with abnormal bleeding or a vaginal discharge. Malignant or atypical cells are present in the Pap smear in a majority of patients.[165, 168] Treatment is

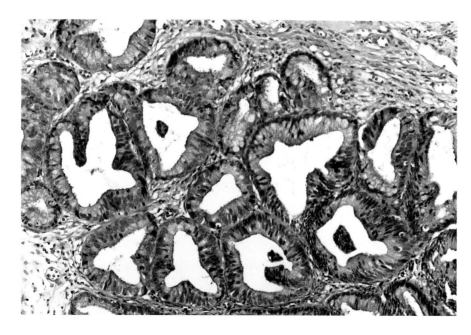

FIGURE 14–21. Adenocarcinoma *in situ* of the cervix. The glands are lined by cells with stratified, hyperchromatic nuclei, and mitotic figures are present. (H&E, ×200)

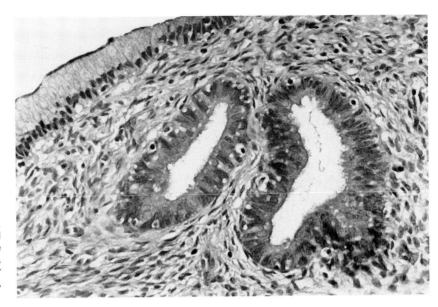

FIGURE 14–22. Tubal metaplasia in the cervix. The metaplastic glands in the stroma are lined by ciliated columnar cells. Their nuclei are larger and their cytoplasm more darkly stained, compared with the normal overlying columnar mucinous endocervical epithelial cells. (H&E, ×400)

with radiotherapy or surgery. Radical hysterectomy with pelvic lymph node dissection is the most appropriate operation, because lymph node metastases are often present.[165, 166] Unfortunately, the diagnosis may not be appreciated until the uterus is removed and examined by the pathologist. Even though MDAC exhibits a well-differentiated growth pattern, a review of the literature revealed that 68% of women with it were dead of tumor or alive with a recurrence at last contact.[166] Despite the overall pessimistic outlook for women with MDAC, several authors have reported favorable survival statistics for women with early-stage tumors.[167, 168] Women with MDAC have two other types of gynecologic tumors more often than expected: mucinous tumors of the ovaries and ovarian sex cord tumors with annular tubules.[166]

The cervix contains an indurated nodular or annular mass. Small, mucus-filled cysts are often noted on cut section. Microscopically, MDAC has a bland appearance. There is an increase in the number of endocervical glands, which vary in size and shape. Many are large and claw-shaped, whereas others have angular projections that extend into the endocervical stroma (Fig. 14–23). There is little atypia, mitotic activity, or nuclear stratification in MDAC, although most tumors contain areas in which these features are present (Fig. 14–24). A key diagnostic feature is the presence of at least an occasional mitotic figure. The stroma ranges from normal to edematous or desmoplastic, and it may contain an inflammatory cell infiltrate. Vascular invasion and perineural growth are helpful diagnostic features, if present. The tumor extends deeply into the endocervical wall, invading beneath the maximum depth of the normal endocervical glands. Immunocytochemical staining for carcinoembryonic antigen is helpful in the diagnosis of MDAC.[166, 169, 170] As is the case in adenocarcinoma of the cervix generally, MDAC is usually immunoreactive for CEA. Staining for CEA is intracytoplasmic, apical, or both. Staining is patchy, and not every gland is positive.[164]

DIFFERENTIAL DIAGNOSIS. The main differential diagnostic problem with MDAC is distinguishing it from benign conditions such as endocervical glandular hyperplasia and deep endocervical glands.

Endocervical glandular hyperplasia is most commonly seen in young women who are pregnant or taking hormones, an atypical setting for MDAC. A type of glandular hyperplasia designated as "diffuse laminar endocervical glandular hyperplasia" may be related to marked chronic cervicitis.[171] Glandular hyperplasias differ grossly from MDAC in that hyperplasia is usually an incidental microscopic finding or, at most, a visible area of cystic change, whereas MDAC forms a visible tumor mass. Microscopically, hyperplasia is limited to the superficial cervical stroma, the glands do not incite a desmoplastic stromal response or infiltrate around nerves or into blood vessels, and the gland cells do not exhibit significant cytologic atypia or mitotic activity. Immunohistochemical stains are helpful in difficult cases, as MDAC is usually CEA-positive, whereas hyperplasias are not.[164, 166, 170]

Deep endocervical glands or nabothian cysts enter the differential diagnosis of MDAC because they are deeper in the endocervical stroma than benign glands are usually seen.[123] These benign glands may extend nearly to the serosa, but they do not have an irregular infiltrative pattern and, unlike MDAC, do not vary markedly in size and shape. Deep benign glands do not incite a desmoplastic stromal response nor do the lining cells exhibit cytologic atypia or mitotic activity.

Cystic endocervical tunnel clusters are circumscribed and superficial.[172] The glands are dilated, filled with mucus, and lined by endocervical cells that show no atypia or mitotic activity.

Mesonephric remnants can be identified in 1% to 22% of cervices, depending on how thoroughly they are searched for.[173] They are located deep within the cervical or vaginal wall and consist of an elongated duct surrounded by small tubules lined by low cuboidal epithelial cells with central round nuclei (Fig. 14–25). The tubular cells do not stain for mucin or with the PAS stain, but their lumina contain dense eosinophilic secretory material that is PAS-positive and diastase-resistant.

Hyperplasia of mesonephric remnants can be difficult to differentiate from MDAC.[174–177] Two patterns of hyperplasia have been described.[174] Lobular hyperplasia is characterized

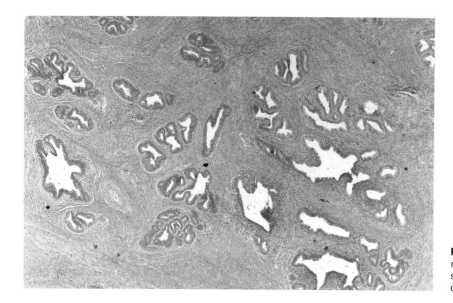

FIGURE 14–23. Minimal deviation adenocarcinoma of the cervix. Low-magnification view showing complex, branching glands deep in the cervical stroma. (H&E, ×25)

by lobules of mesonephric tubules around one or more elongated mesonephric ducts. Hyperplastic mesonephric tubules may be present in the superficial stroma, where they are occasionally admixed with endocervical glands. The other variant, diffuse mesonephric hyperplasia (Fig. 14–26), is rare and can be easily mistaken for adenocarcinoma. It consists of a diffuse proliferation of small mesonephric tubules that may extend to the deep margin of the specimen or even into the vagina or lower uterine segment. Mesonephric ducts are often absent. The hyperplastic tubules do not exhibit the disorderly invasion or back-to-back growth seen in adenocarcinoma, nor is there significant nuclear atypia or mitotic activity.[174, 177]

Mesonephric adenocarcinoma arises within the wall of the cervix or vagina.[174, 176, 178] It is composed of tubules or papillae lined by cuboidal or columnar cells. Areas of solid growth are present in some tumors. Mesonephric adenocarcinoma can be differentiated from hyperplastic mesonephric remnants by its disorderly pattern of infiltration, by back-to-back arrangements of glands, by the presence of nuclear atypia, and by the presence of at least some mitotic figures. Necrosis and a desmoplastic stroma are suggestive of carcinoma.[176] The large, irregular glands that are seen in MDAC are absent in mesonephric carcinoma.

Villoglandular Adenocarcinoma

Villoglandular adenocarcinoma (VGAC) is a form of well-differentiated adenocarcinoma of the cervix in which an exophytic surface papillary component is associated with an underlying *in situ* or invasive glandular component.[179, 180] Villoglandular adenocarcinoma tends to occur in women who are younger than 40 years of age, and it has a favorable prognosis.

CLINICOPATHOLOGIC FEATURES. Villoglandular adenocarcinoma occurs mainly in young women. The average ages in two large series were 33 years and 37 years.[179, 180] Clinically, VGAC often appears papillary or friable. Women with VGAC

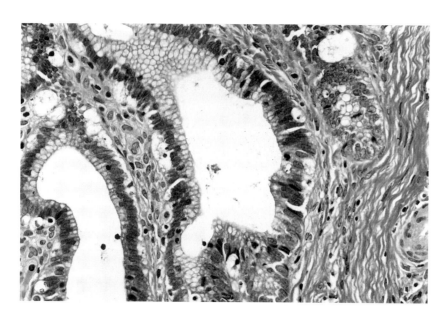

FIGURE 14–24. Minimal deviation adenocarcinoma of the cervix. The glands are lined by cells showing only mild atypia. A rare mitotic figure is present. The stroma *(right)* does not exhibit a desmoplastic change. (H&E, ×400)

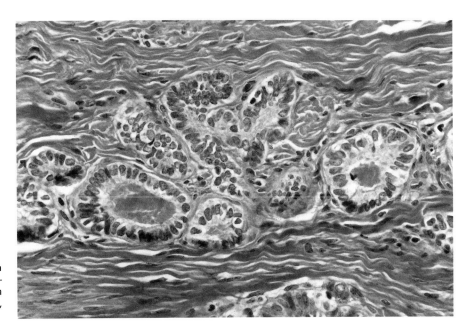

FIGURE 14–25. Mesonephric remnants in the cervix. The tubules are lined by cuboidal cells with bland nuclei. They contain eosinophilic secretory material. (H&E, ×400)

have been treated with a variety of surgical procedures ranging from cone biopsy to radical hysterectomy with pelvic lymph node dissection. Regardless of treatment, all patients studied were alive with no evidence of disease at last contact.[179, 180] Conization can be the definitive treatment in some young women with non-invasive or superficial VGAC when the cone margins are free of tumor.[179, 180]

Villoglandular adenocarcinoma forms a papillary or polypoid mass 0.5 to 3.5 cm in diameter.[179] Microscopically, the superficial portion of the tumor is composed of branching papillae with a fibrovascular core that contains inflammatory cells. The papillae are lined by stratified columnar cells showing mild to moderate nuclear atypia and mitotic activity (Fig. 14–27). Endocervical, endometrioid, and intestinal epithelial differentiation all occur in VGAC.[179] The stroma underlying the papillary component contains *in situ* or, usually, invasive adenocarcinoma. The latter is composed of branching irregular

glands and papillae growing in an abundant fibrous stroma with areas of edema or desmoplasia. Invasion is usually limited to the inner third of the cervix, but occasional examples invade more deeply. Paracervical extension and lymph node metastasis are exceptional.

DIFFERENTIAL DIAGNOSIS. The differential diagnosis of VGAC includes papillary endocervical hyperplasia, mullerian papilloma, papillary adenofibroma, and more aggressive types of adenocarcinoma such as adenocarcinoma with a minor papillary component and papillary serous carcinoma.

In **papillary endocervical hyperplasia,** the villous endocervical architecture is exaggerated as a result of marked chronic inflammation. It differs from VGAC by having a more prominent inflammatory stroma, less prominent papillary growth, and absence of nuclear atypia and mitotic activity.

Mullerian papilloma is a benign papillary process in which fibrovascular stroma is covered by cytologically bland cuboi-

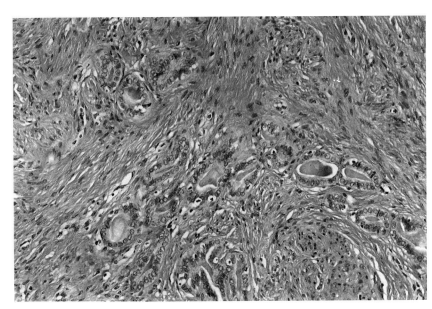

FIGURE 14–26. Hyperplastic mesonephric remnants in the cervix. Note small tubules scattered among the connective tissue bundles. (H&E, ×200)

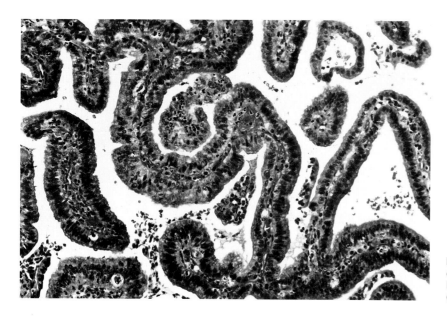

FIGURE 14–27. Villoglandular adenocarcinoma of the cervix. Villous fronds are lined by columnar cells with modest nuclear atypia. (H&E, ×200)

dal epithelium.[181, 182] A major point of distinction from VGAC is that mullerian papilloma occurs in children.

Papillary adenofibroma has a more prominent fibrous stroma than does VGAC, and the epithelial component lacks the atypia, stratification, and mitotic activity seen in VGAC.[183, 184]

Adenocarcinoma may contain foci of superficial papillary growth reminiscent of VGAC. The term *villoglandular adenocarcinoma* is reserved for well to moderately differentiated neoplasms in which a villous pattern predominates in the superficial aspect of the tumor.

Papillary serous carcinoma is uncommon in the cervix.[185, 186] The papillae branch more extensively than do those in VGAC, there is budding of cell groups from the surface, the nuclei are larger and more atypical with prominent nucleoli, mitotic figures are frequent, and psammoma bodies may be present.

Small-Cell Carcinoma

Small-cell carcinoma (SCC) is a neuroendocrine neoplasm morphologically reminiscent of small-cell lung cancer.[187–192] It is biologically aggressive and has an unfavorable prognosis relative to other types of cervical cancer.

CLINICOPATHOLOGIC FEATURES. Small-cell carcinoma constitutes 1% to 2% of all invasive cervical cancers.[193, 194] It occurs in women who are slightly younger (average age, 36–46) than those with typical squamous cell carcinoma or adenocarcinoma.[187, 189, 194] Women with SCC are usually symptomatic, the typical presentation being with vaginal bleeding or discharge. Small-cell carcinoma is rarely diagnosed by cytology.[189] Radical hysterectomy with pelvic lymph node dissection and radiotherapy with or without hysterectomy are the two most common methods of treatment. Small-cell carcinoma is an aggressive neoplasm that is more likely to metasta-

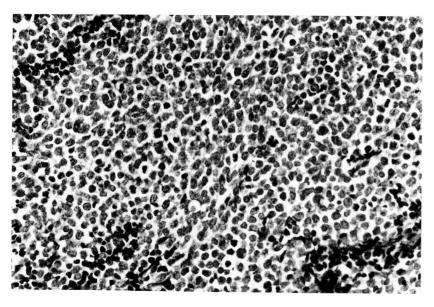

FIGURE 14–28. Small-cell carcinoma of the cervix. There are sheets of uniform small cells with dark nuclei, inconspicuous nucleoli, and poorly defined cell borders. Note the dark smeared nuclear material *(bottom and upper left)*, which is a characteristic finding in small-cell carcinoma. (H&E, ×400)

size to pelvic lymph nodes than other types of cervical carcinoma of comparable stage.[187, 194] The median survival is shorter, and the proportion of women dying of tumor is higher than with other cervical cancers.[189, 191, 193] More than 70% of the patients in several large series died of tumor.[189, 193, 194] Chemotherapy has been added to the treatment regimen in an attempt to improve survival.[195–197]

Small-cell carcinoma does not have a distinctive gross appearance. Microscopically, it is composed of diffusely infiltrating sheets, nests, and cords of small tumor cells with hyperchromatic nuclei and little cytoplasm. The nuclei have uniform finely granular chromatin and inconspicuous nucleoli (Fig. 14–28). Nuclear molding is evident, and there are many mitotic figures. The intermediate cell type of SCC has slightly larger nuclei and coarser nuclear chromatin, and there are nucleoli in some nuclei. Small or large foci of necrosis are common. Vascular invasion is identified in as many as 50% of cases. Minor foci of squamous or glandular differentiation are seen in some tumors. The neuroendocrine nature of SCC was first documented by electron microscopy, which revealed dendritic cell processes and neuroendocrine granules.[188, 189, 194, 198] Some SCCs are argyrophilic,[187, 189, 198, 199] and immunohistochemical staining reveals that most are reactive with one or more neuroendocrine markers.[187, 189, 191, 200, 201] Neuron-specific enolase is typically positive in SCC. Other markers that may be positive include Leu-7, chromogranin, synaptophysin, and various neuropeptides. A majority, but not all, SCCs express cytokeratin and EMA. *In situ* hybridization and polymerase chain reaction studies reveal HPV DNA in SCC.[187, 200, 202] HPV 16 and 18 may be detected, although HPV 18 is the most common.

DIFFERENTIAL DIAGNOSIS. The main differential diagnostic problem is to separate small-cell carcinoma from the small-cell variant of squamous cell carcinoma. Other tumors that need to be distinguished from SCC are the carcinoid tumor and lymphoma.

Squamous cell carcinoma of the small-cell non-keratinizing type must be differentiated from small-cell carcinoma because the latter is more likely to metastasize to pelvic lymph nodes, has a worse prognosis, and requires more aggressive therapy. The distinction can be made by routine light microscopic study in most instances. Small-cell carcinoma infiltrates diffusely or in poorly defined nests, trabeculae, or columns, and it is usually not associated with overlying high-grade SIL. In contrast, small-cell squamous cell carcinoma originates from overlying SIL and invades in cohesive nests of malignant epithelial cells. Squamous cell carcinoma prompts intense inflammatory and desmoplastic host responses, whereas these are usually lacking or minimal around SCC. Finally, nuclear molding is prominent in SCC, but inconspicuous in squamous cell carcinoma. There is some overlap in the immunophenotype of these tumor types. Squamous cell carcinoma is invariably immunoreactive with cytokeratin, but some examples are also reactive with neuroendocrine markers, particularly neuron-specific enolase.[187, 191] A tumor that lacks neuroendocrine markers but is cytokeratin-positive is a squamous cell carcinoma. A tumor that reacts with neuroendocrine markers but is cytokeratin-negative is a SCC.[187] The presence of tonofilaments and desmosomes and the absence of dense core neurosecretory granules, as demonstrated by electron microscopy, indicate that a tumor is a squamous cell carcinoma.

Carcinoid tumors of the cervix are rare neuroendocrine neoplasms that represent the well-differentiated end of the spectrum of neuroendocrine tumors of the cervix.[190, 198, 203] They differ from small-cell carcinoma in that carcinoid cells are larger and have a moderate amount of cytoplasm and vesicular nuclei with coarse, stippled chromatin. Carcinoid tumors grow in sheets, cords, trabeculae, and ribbons. They are less well differentiated than carcinoid tumors of the gastrointestinal tract, and they have an unfavorable prognosis.

Large-cell lymphoma bears some resemblance to SCC, in that the tumor cells are round with a high nucleocytoplasmic ratio and they diffusely infiltrate the cervical stroma.[204] Malignant lymphoid cells do not have the finely granular nuclear chromatin seen in SCC, nuclear molding is absent, and the lymphoma cells may contain prominent nucleoli. The tumor cells are more cohesive in SCC than in lymphoma. Lymphoma is immunoreactive for leukocyte common antigen and other hematopoietic antigens, whereas SCC is not.

References

1. Kraus FT, Perez-Mesa C: Verrucous carcinoma: Clinical and pathologic study of 105 cases involving oral cavity, larynx and genitalia. Cancer 19:26–38, 1966.
2. Crowther ME, Lowe DG, Shepherd JH: Verrucous carcinoma of the female genital tract: A review. Obstet Gynecol Surv 43:263–280, 1988.
3. Japaze H, Dinh TV, Woodruff JD: Verrucous carcinoma of the vulva: Study of 24 cases. Obstet Gynecol 60:462–466, 1982.
4. Rando RF, Sedlacek TV, Hunt J, et al: Verrucous carcinoma of the vulva associated with an unusual type 6 human papillomavirus. Obstet Gynecol 67:70S–75S, 1986.
5. Crowther ME, Shepherd JH, Fisher C: Verrucous carcinoma of the vulva containing human papillomavirus-11. Case report. Br J Obstet Gynaecol 95:414–418, 1988.
6. Crum CP, Nuovo GJ: Genital Papillomaviruses and Related Neoplasms. New York, Raven Press, 1991.
7. Downey GO, Okagaki T, Ostrow RS, et al: Condylomatous carcinoma of the vulva with special reference to human papillomavirus DNA. Obstet Gynecol 72:68–73, 1988.
8. Kurman RJ, Toki T, Schiffman MH: Basaloid and warty carcinomas of the vulva: Distinctive types of squamous cell carcinoma frequently associated with human papillomaviruses. Am J Surg Pathol 17:133–145, 1993.
9. Curtin JP, Rubin SC, Jones WB, et al: Paget's disease of the vulva. Gynecol Oncol 39:374–377, 1990.
10. Taylor PT, Stenwig JT, Klausen H: Paget's disease of the vulva. A report of 18 cases. Gynecol Oncol 3:46–60, 1975.
11. Feuer GA, Shevchuk M, Calango A: Vulvar Paget's disease: The need to exclude an invasive lesion. Gynecol Oncol 38:81–89, 1990.
12. Gunn RA, Gallager HS: Vulvar Paget's disease: A topographic study. Cancer 46:590–594, 1980.
13. Bergen S, Di Saia PJ, Liao SY, et al: Conservative management of extramammary Paget's disease of the vulva. Gynecol Oncol 33:151–156, 1989.
14. Creasman WT, Gallager HS, Rutledge F: Paget's disease of the vulva. Gynecol Oncol 3:133–148, 1975.
15. Glasgow BJ, Wen DR, Al-Jitawi S, et al: Antibody to S-100 protein aids the separation of pagetoid melanoma from mammary and extramammary Paget's disease. J Cutan Pathol 14:223–226, 1987.
16. Helm KF, Goellner JR, Peters MS: Immunohistochemical stains in extramammary Paget's disease. Am J Dermatopathol 14:402–407, 1992.
17. Lee SC, Roth LM, Ehrlich C, et al: Extramammary Paget's disease of the vulva. A clinicopathologic study of 13 cases. Cancer 39:2540–2549, 1977.
18. Jones RE, Austin C, Ackerman AB: Extramammary Paget's disease: A critical reexamination. Am J Dermatopathol 1:101–132, 1979.
19. Hart WR, Millman JB: Progression of intraepithelial Paget's disease of the vulva to invasive carcinoma. Cancer 40:2333–2337, 1977.
20. Parmley TH, Woodruff JD, Julian CG: Invasive vulvar Paget's disease. Obstet Gynecol 46:341–346, 1975.
21. Wick MR, Goellner JR, Wolfe JT 3rd, et al: Vulvar sweat gland carcinomas. Arch Pathol Lab Med 109:43–47, 1985.
22. Olson DJ, Fujimura M, Swanson P, et al: Immunohistochemical features of Paget's disease of the vulva with and without adenocarcinoma. Int J Gynecol Pathol 10:285–295, 1991.
23. Ganjei P, Giraldo KA, Lampe B, et al: Vulvar Paget's disease. Is immunocytochemistry helpful in assessing the surgical margins? J Reprod Med 35:1002–1004, 1990.
24. Ordóñez NG, Awalt H, Mackay B: Mammary and extramammary Paget's disease. An immunocytochemical and ultrastructural study. Cancer 59:1173–1183, 1987.
25. Guarner J, Cohen C, De Rose PB: Histogenesis of extramammary and mammary Paget cells. An immunohistochemical study. Am J Dermatopathol 11:313–318, 1989.

26. Mazoujian G, Pinkus GS, Haagensen DE Jr: Extramammary Paget's disease—evidence for an apocrine origin. An immunoperoxidase study of gross cystic disease fluid protein-15, carcinoembryonic antigen, and keratin proteins. Am J Surg Pathol 8:43–50, 1984.

27. Hawley IC, Husain F, Pryse-Davies J: Extramammary Paget's disease of the vulva with dermal invasion and vulval intra-epithelial neoplasia. Histopathology 18:374–376, 1991.

28. Bacchi CE, Goldfogel GA, Greer BE, et al: Paget's disease and melanoma of the vulva. Use of a panel of monoclonal antibodies to identify cell type and to microscopically define adequacy of surgical margins. Gynecol Oncol 46:216–221, 1992.

29. Tasseron EWK, van der Esch EP, Hart AAM, et al: A clinicopathological study of 30 melanomas of the vulva. Gynecol Oncol 46:170–175, 1992.

30. Johnson TL, Kumar NB, White CD, et al: Prognostic features of vulvar melanoma: A clinicopathologic analysis. Int J Gynecol Pathol 5:110–118, 1986.

31. Podratz KC, Gaffey TA, Symmonds RE, et al: Melanoma of the vulva: An update. Gynecol Oncol 16:153–168, 1983.

32. Trimble EL, Lewis JL Jr, Williams LL, et al: Management of vulvar melanoma. Gynecol Oncol 45:254–258, 1992.

33. Phillips GL, Twiggs LB, Okagaki T: Vulvar melanoma: A microstaging study. Gynecol Oncol 14:80–88, 1982.

34. Jaramillo BA, Ganjei P, Averette HE, et al: Malignant melanoma of the vulva. Obstet Gynecol 66:398–401, 1985.

35. Ronan SG, Eng AM, Briele HA, et al: Malignant melanoma of the female genitalia. J Am Acad Dermatol 22:428–435, 1990.

36. Bradgate MG, Rollason TP, McConkey CC, et al: Malignant melanoma of the vulva: A clinicopathological study of 50 women. Br J Obstet Gynaecol 97:124–133, 1990.

37. Davidson T, Kissin M, Westbury G: Vulvo-vaginal melanoma—should radical surgery be abandoned? Br J Obstet Gynaecol 94:473–476, 1987.

38. Rose PG, Piver MS, Tsukada Y, et al: Conservative therapy for melanoma of the vulva. Am J Obstet Gynecol 159:52–55, 1988.

39. Benda JA, Platz CE, Anderson B: Malignant melanoma of the vulva: A clinical-pathologic review of 16 cases. Int J Gynecol Pathol 5:202–216, 1986.

40. Chung AF, Woodruff JM, Lewis JL Jr: Malignant melanoma of the vulva. A report of 44 cases. Obstet Gynecol 45:638–646, 1975.

41. Sison-Torre EQ, Ackerman AB: Melanosis of the vulva. A clinical simulator of malignant melanoma. Am J Dermatopathol 7 Suppl:51–60 1985.

42. Steeper TA, Rosai J: Aggressive angiomyxoma of the female pelvis and perineum. Report of nine cases of a distinctive type of gynecologic soft-tissue neoplasm. Am J Surg Pathol 7:463–475, 1983.

43. Mandai K, Moriwaki S, Motoi M: Aggressive angiomyxoma of the vulva. Report of a case. Acta Pathol Jpn 40:927–934, 1990.

44. Sutton GP, Rogers RE, Roth LM, et al: Aggressive angiomyxoma first diagnosed as levator hernia. Am J Obstet Gynecol 161:73–75, 1989.

45. Destian S, Ritchie WG: Aggressive angiomyxoma: CT appearance. Am J Gastroenterol 81:711–713, 1986.

46. Smith HO, Worrell RV, Smith AY, et al: Aggressive angiomyxoma of the female pelvis and perineum: Review of the literature. Gynecol Oncol 42:79–85, 1991.

47. Begin LR, Clement PB, Kirk ME, et al: Aggressive angiomyxoma of pelvic soft parts: A clinicopathologic study of nine cases. Hum Pathol 16:621–628, 1985.

48. Fletcher CDM, Tsang WYW, Fisher C, et al: Angiomyofibroblastoma of the vulva: A benign neoplasm distinct from aggressive angiomyxoma. Am J Surg Pathol 16:373–382, 1992.

49. Brooks JJ, Livolsi VA: Liposarcoma presenting on the vulva. Am J Obstet Gynecol 156:73–75, 1987.

50. Robboy SJ, Kaufman RH, Prat J, et al: Pathologic findings in young women enrolled in the National Cooperative Diethylstilbestrol Adenosis (DESAD) Project. Obstet Gynecol 53:309–317, 1979.

51. Herbst AL, Robboy SJ, Scully RE, et al: Clear-cell adenocarcinoma of the vagina and cervix in girls: Analysis of 170 registry cases. Am J Obstet Gynecol 119:713–724, 1974.

52. Hart WR, Townsend DE, Aldrich JO, et al: Histopathologic spectrum of vaginal adenosis and related changes in stilbestrol-exposed females. Cancer 37:763–775, 1976.

53. Antonioli DA, Burke L: Vaginal adenosis: Analysis of 325 biopsy specimens from 100 patients. Am J Clin Pathol 64:625–638, 1975.

54. Herbst AL, Scully RE: Adenocarcinoma of the vagina in adolescence. A report of 7 cases including 6 clear-cell carcinomas (so-called mesonephromas). Cancer 25:745–757, 1970.

55. Herbst AL, Ulfelder H, Poskanzer DC: Adenocarcinoma of the vagina: Association of maternal stilbestrol therapy with tumor appearance in young women. N Engl J Med 284:878–881, 1971.

56. Hanselaar AG, Van Leusen ND, De Wilde PC, et al: Clear cell adenocarcinoma of the vagina and cervix. A report of the Central Netherlands Registry with emphasis on early detection and prognosis. Cancer 67:1971–1978, 1991.

57. Melnick S, Cole P, Anderson D, et al: Rates and risks of diethylstilbestrol-related clear-cell adenocarcinoma of the vagina and cervix: An update. N Engl J Med 316:514–516, 1987.

58. Kaminski PF, Maier RC: Clear cell adenocarcinoma of the cervix unrelated to diethylstilbestrol exposure. Obstet Gynecol 62:720–727, 1983.

59. Robboy SJ, Scully RE, Welch WR, et al: Intrauterine diethylstilbestrol exposure and its consequences. Pathologic characteristics of vaginal adenosis, clear cell adenocarcinoma, and related lesions. Arch Pathol Lab Med 101:1–5, 1977.

60. Herbst AL, Norusis MJ, Rosenow PJ, et al: An analysis of 346 cases of clear cell adenocarcinoma of the vagina and cervix with emphasis on recurrence and survival. Gynecol Oncol 7:111–122, 1979.

61. Herbst AL, Cole P, Norusis MJ, et al: Epidemiologic aspects and factors related to survival in 384 registry cases of clear cell adenocarcinoma of the vagina and cervix. Am J Obstet Gynecol 135:876–886, 1979.

62. Robboy SJ, Welch WR, Young RH, et al: Topographic relation of cervical ectropion and vaginal adenosis to clear cell adenocarcinoma. Obstet Gynecol 60:546–551, 1982.

63. Robboy SJ, Young RH, Welch WW, et al: Atypical vaginal adenosis: Association with clear cell adenocarcinoma in diethylstilbestrol-exposed offspring. Cancer 869:875, 1984.

64. Chumas JC, Nelson B, Mann WJ, et al: Microglandular hyperplasia of the uterine cervix. Obstet Gynecol 66:406–409, 1985.

65. Robboy SJ, Welch WR: Microglandular hyperplasia in vaginal adenosis associated with oral contraceptives and prenatal diethylstilbestrol exposure. Obstet Gynecol 49:430–434, 1977.

66. Speers WC, Picaso LG, Silverberg SG: Immunohistochemical localization of carcinoembryonic antigen in microglandular hyperplasia and adenocarcinoma of the endocervix. Am J Clin Pathol 79:105–107, 1983.

67. Young RH, Scully RE: Atypical forms of microglandular hyperplasia of the cervix simulating carcinoma: A report of five cases and review of the literature. Am J Surg Pathol 13:50–56, 1989.

68. Copeland LJ, Sneige N, Ordóñez NG, et al: Endodermal sinus tumor of the vagina and cervix. Cancer 55:2558–2565, 1985.

69. Young RH, Scully RE: Endodermal sinus tumor of the vagina: A report of nine cases and a review of the literature. Gynecol Oncol 18:380–382, 1984.

70. Kurman RJ, Norris HJ: Endodermal sinus tumor of the ovary. A clinical and pathologic analysis of 71 cases. Cancer 38:2404–2419, 1976.

71. Langley FA, Govan ADT, Anderson MC, et al: Yolk sac and allied tumours of the ovary. Histopathology 5:389–401, 1981.

72. Manetta A, Gutrecht EL, Berman ML, et al: Primary invasive carcinoma of the vagina. Obstet Gynecol 76:639–642, 1990.

73. Eddy GL, Marks RD Jr, Miller MC III, et al: Primary invasive vaginal carcinoma. Am J Obstet Gynecol 165:292–298, 1991.

74. Manetta A, Pinto JL, Larson JE, et al: Primary invasive carcinoma of the vagina. Obstet Gynecol 72:77–81, 1988.

75. Clement PB, Benedet JL: Adenocarcinoma in situ of the vagina: A case report. Cancer 43:2479–2485, 1979.

76. Ray J, Ireland K: Non-clear-cell adenocarcinoma arising in vaginal adenosis. Arch Pathol Lab Med 109:781–783, 1985.

77. Fox H, Wells M, Harris M, et al: Enteric tumors of the lower female genital tract: A report of three cases. Histopathology 12:167–176, 1988.

78. Haskel S, Chen SS, Spiegel G: Vaginal endometrioid adenocarcinoma arising in vaginal endometriosis: A case report and literature review. Gynecol Oncol 34:232–236, 1989.

79. Mazur MT, Hsueh S, Gersell DJ: Metastases to the female genital tract. Analysis of 325 cases. Cancer 53:1978–1984, 1984.

80. Hays DM, Shimada H, Raney RB Jr, et al: Clinical staging and treatment results in rhabdomyosarcoma of the female genital tract among children and adolescents. Cancer 61:1893–1903, 1988.

81. Daya DA, Scully RE: Sarcoma botryoides of the uterine cervix in young women: A clinicopathological study of 13 cases. Gynecol Oncol 29:290–304, 1988.

82. Brand E, Berek JS, Nieberg RK, et al: Rhabdomyosarcoma of the uterine cervix. Sarcoma botryoides. Cancer 60:1552–1560, 1987.

83. Montag TW, d'Ablaing G, Schlaerth JB, et al: Embryonal rhabdomyosarcoma of the uterine corpus and cervix. Gynecol Oncol 25:171–194, 1986.

84. Davos I, Abell MR: Sarcomas of the vagina. Obstet Gynecol 47:342–350, 1976.

85. Hilgers RD: Pelvic exenteration for vaginal embryonal rhabdomyosarcoma. A review. Obstet Gynecol 45:175–180, 1975.

86. Copeland LJ, Gershenson DM, Saul PB, et al: Sarcoma botryoides of the female genital tract. Obstet Gynecol 66:262–266, 1985.

87. Flamant F, Gerbaulet A, Nihoul-Fekete C, et al: Long-term sequelae of conservative treatment by surgery, brachytherapy, and chemotherapy for vulval and vaginal rhabdomyosarcoma in children. J Clin Oncol 8:1847–1853, 1990.

88. Hays DM, Shimada H, Raney RB Jr, et al: Sarcomas of the vagina and uterus: The Intergroup Rhabdomyosarcoma Study. J Pediatr Surg 20:718–724, 1985.

89. Tsokos M, Webber BL, Parham DM, et al: Rhabdomyosarcoma. A new classification scheme related to prognosis. Arch Pathol Lab Med 116:847–855, 1992.

90. Gordon AN, Montag TW: Sarcoma botryoides of the cervix: Excision followed by adjuvant chemotherapy for preservation of reproductive function. Gynecol Oncol 36:119–124, 1990.

91. Parham DM: Immunohistochemistry of childhood sarcomas: Old and new markers. Mod Pathol 6:133–138, 1993.

92. Parham DM, Webber B, Holt H, et al: Immunohistochemical study of childhood rhabdomyosarcomas and related neoplasms. Results of an Intergroup Rhabdomyosarcoma Study project. Cancer 67:3072–3080, 1991.

93. Ostor AG, Fortune DW, Riley CB: Fibroepithelial polyps with atypical stromal cells (pseudosarcoma botryoides) of vulva and vagina: A report of 13 cases. Int J Gynecol Pathol 7:351–360, 1988.

94. Mucitelli DR, Charles EZ, Kraus FT: Vulvovaginal polyps. Histologic appearance, ultrastructure, immunocytochemical characteristics, and clinicopathologic correlations. Int J Gynecol Pathol 9:20–40, 1990.

95. Al-Nafussi AI, Rebello G, Hughes D, et al: Benign vaginal polyp: A histological, histochemical and immunohistochemical study of 20 polyps with comparison to normal vaginal subepithelial layer. Histopathology 20:145–150, 1992.

96. Chirayil SJ, Tobon H: Polyps of the vagina: A clinicopathologic study of 18 cases. Cancer 47:2904–2907, 1981.

97. Norris HJ, Taylor HB: Polyps of the vagina: A benign lesion resembling sarcoma botryoides. Cancer 19:227–232, 1966.

98. Halvorsen TB, Johannesen E: Fibroepithelial polyps of the vagina: Are they old granulation tissue polyps? J Clin Pathol 45:235–240, 1992.

99. Miettinen M, Wahlstrom T, Vesterinen E, et al: Vaginal polyps with pseudosarcomatous features. A clinicopathologic study of seven cases. Cancer 51:1148–1151, 1983.

100. Mitchell M, Talerman A, Sholl JS, et al: Pseudosarcoma botryoides in pregnancy: Report of a case with ultrastructural observations. Obstet Gynecol 70:522–526, 1987.

101. Davies SW, Makanje HH, Woodcock AS: Pseudo-sarcomatous polyps of the vagina in pregnancy. Case report. Br J Obstet Gynaecol 88:566–568, 1981.

102. Gee DC, Finckh ES: Benign vaginal rhabdomyoma. Pathology 9:263–267, 1977.

103. Leone PG, Taylor HB: Ultrastructure of a benign polypoid rhabdomyoma of the vagina. Cancer 31:1414–1417, 1973.

104. Suarez Vilela D, Gimenez Pizarro A, Rio Suarez M: Vaginal rhabdomyoma and adenosis. Histopathology 16:393–394, 1990.

105. Ceremsak RJ: Benign rhabdomyoma of the vagina. Am J Clin Pathol 52:604–606, 1969.

106. Di Sant'Agnese PA, Knowles DM: Extracardiac rhabdomyoma: A clinicopathologic study and review of the literature. Cancer 46:780–789, 1980.

107. Gold JH, Bossen EH: Benign vaginal rhabdomyoma. A light and electron microscopic study. Cancer 37:2283–2294, 1976.

108. Hasumi K, Sakamoto A, Sugano H: Microinvasive carcinoma of the uterine cervix. Cancer 45:928–931, 1980.

109. Sevin B-U, Nadji M, Averette HE, et al: Microinvasive carcinoma of the cervix. Cancer 70:2121–2128, 1992.

110. Sedlis A, Sall S, Tsukada Y, et al: Microinvasive carcinoma of the uterine cervix: A clinical-pathologic study. Am J Obstet Gynecol 133:64–74, 1979.

111. Simon NL, Gore H, Shingleton HM, et al: Study of superficially invasive carcinoma of the cervix. Obstet Gynecol 68:19–24, 1986.

112. FIGO Cancer Committee: Staging announcement. Gynecol Oncol 25:383–385, 1986.

113. Copeland LJ, Silva EG, Gershenson DM, et al: Superficially invasive squamous cell carcinoma of the cervix. Gynecol Oncol 45:307–312, 1992.

114. van Nagell JR Jr, Greenwell N, Powell DE, et al: Microinvasive carcinoma of the cervix. Am J Obstet Gynecol 145:981–991, 1983.

115. Seski JC, Abell MR, Morley GW: Microinvasive squamous carcinoma of the cervix: Definition, histologic analysis, late results of treatment. Obstet Gynecol 50:410–414, 1977.

116. Greer BE, Figge DC, Tamimi HK, et al: Stage IA2 squamous carcinoma of the cervix: Difficult diagnosis and therapeutic dilemma. Am J Obstet Gynecol 162:1406–1411, 1990.

117. Maiman MA, Fruchter RG, DiMaio TM, et al: Superficially invasive squamous cell carcinoma of the cervix. Obstet Gynecol 72:399–403, 1988.

118. Ostor AG: Studies on 200 cases of early squamous cell carcinoma of the cervix. Int J Gynecol Pathol 12:193–207, 1993.

119. Burghardt E, Girardi F, Lahousen M, et al: Microinvasive carcinoma of the uterine cervix (International Federation of Gynecology and Obstetrics Stage IA). Cancer 67:1037–1045, 1991.

120. Kolstad P: Follow-up study of 232 patients with stage Ia1 and 411 patients with stage Ia2 squamous cell carcinoma of the cervix (microinvasive carcinoma). Gynecol Oncol 33:265–272, 1989.

121. Creasman WT, Fetter BF, Clarke-Pearson DL, et al: Management of stage IA carcinoma of the cervix. Am J Obstet Gynecol 153:164–172, 1985.

122. Roche WD, Norris HJ: Microinvasive carcinoma of the cervix. The significance of lymphatic invasion and confluent patterns of stromal growth. Cancer 36:180–186, 1975.

123. Clement PB, Young RH: Deep nabothian cysts of the uterine cervix: A possible source of confusion with minimal-deviation adenocarcinoma (adenoma malignum). Int J Gynecol Pathol 8:340–348, 1989.

124. Steeper TA, Piscioli F, Rosai J: Squamous cell carcinoma with sarcoma-like stroma of the female genital tract. Clinicopathologic study of four cases. Cancer 52:890–898, 1983.

125. Holmquist ND, Torres J: Malignant melanoma of the cervix. Report of a case. Acta Cytol 32:252–256, 1988.

126. Mordel N, Mor-Yosef S, Ben-Baruch N, et al: Malignant melanoma of the uterine cervix: Case report and review of the literature. Gynecol Oncol 32:375–380, 1989.

127. Santoso JT, Kucera PR, Ray J: Primary malignant melanoma of the uterine cervix: Two case reports and a century's review. Obstet Gynecol Surv 45:733–740, 1990.

128. Abdul-Karim FW, Bazi TM, Sorensen K, et al: Sarcoma of the uterine cervix: Clinicopathologic findings in three cases. Gynecol Oncol 26:103–111, 1987.

129. Rotmensch J, Rosenshein NB, Woodruff JD: Cervical sarcoma: A review. Obstet Gynecol Surv 38:456–460, 1983.

130. Abell MR, Ramirez JA: Sarcomas and carcinosarcomas of the uterine cervix. Cancer 31:1176–1192, 1973.

131. Silverberg SG, Major FJ, Blessing JA, et al: Carcinosarcoma (malignant mixed mesodermal tumor) of the uterus. A Gynecologic Oncology Group pathologic study of 203 cases. Int J Gynecol Pathol 9:1–19, 1990.

132. Hall-Craggs M, Toker C, Nedwich A: Carcinosarcoma of the uterine cervix: A light and electron microscopic study. Cancer 48:161–169, 1981.

133. Tobon H, Dave H: Adenocarcinoma in situ of the cervix. Clinicopathologic observations of 11 cases. Int J Gynecol Pathol 7:139–151, 1988.

134. Jaworski RC, Pacey NF, Greenberg ML, Osborn RA: The histologic diagnosis of adenocarcinoma in situ and related lesions of the cervix uteri. Adenocarcinoma in situ. Cancer 61:1171–1181, 1988.

135. Andersen ES, Arffmann E: Adenocarcinoma in situ of the uterine cervix: A clinicopathologic study of 36 cases. Gynecol Oncol 35:1–7, 1989.

136. Quizilbash AH: In situ and microinvasive adenocarcinoma of the uterine cervix: A clinical, cytologic, and histologic study of 14 cases. Am J Clin Pathol 64:155–170, 1975.

137. Gloor E, Ruzicka J: Morphology of adenocarcinoma-in-situ of the uterine cervix: A study of 14 cases. Cancer 49:294–302, 1982.

138. Ostor AG, Pagano R, Davoren RAM, et al: Adenocarcinoma in situ of the cervix. Int J Gynecol Pathol 3:179–190, 1984.

139. Weisbrot IM, Stabinsky C, Davis AM: Adenocarcinoma in situ of the uterine cervix. Cancer 29:1179–1187, 1972.

140. Ayer B, Pacey F, Greenberg M, et al: The cytologic diagnosis of adenocarcinoma in situ of the cervix uteri and related lesions. I. Adenocarcinoma in situ. Acta Cytol 31:397–411, 1987.

141. Betsill WL Jr, Clark AH: Early endocervical glandular neoplasia: I. Histomorphology and cytomorphology. Acta Cytol 30:115–126, 1986.

142. Jaworski RC: Endocervical glandular dysplasia, adenocarcinoma in situ, and early invasive (microinvasive) adenocarcinoma of the uterine cervix. Semin Diagn Pathol 7:190–204, 1990.

143. Cullimore JE, Luesley DM, Rollason TP, et al: A prospective study of conization of the cervix in the management of cervical intraepithelial glandular neoplasia (CIGN)—a preliminary report. Br J Obstet Gynaecol 99:314–318, 1992.

144. Brown LJR, Wells M: Cervical glandular atypia associated with squamous intraepithelial neoplasia: A premalignant lesion? J Clin Pathol 39:22–28, 1986.

145. Luesley DM, Jordan JA, Woodman CBJ, et al: A retrospective review of adenocarcinoma-in-situ and glandular atypia of the uterine cervix. Br J Obstet Gynaecol 94:699–703, 1987.

146. Gloor E, Hurlimann J: Cervical intraepithelial glandular neoplasia (adenocarcinoma in situ and glandular dysplasia). A correlative study of 23 cases with histologic grading, histochemical analysis of mucins, and immunohistochemical determination of the affinity for four lectins. Cancer 58:1272–1280, 1986.

147. Muntz HG, Bell DA, Lage JM, et al: Adenocarcinoma in situ of the uterine cervix. Obstet Gynecol 80:935–939, 1992.

148. Hopkins MP, Roberts JA, Schmidt RW: Cervical adenocarcinoma in situ. Obstet Gynecol 71:842–844, 1988.

149. Bertrand M, Lickrish GM, Colgan TJ: The anatomic distribution of cervical adenocarcinoma in situ: Implications for treatment. Am J Obstet Gynecol 157:21–25, 1987.

150. Noda K, Kimura K, Ikeda M, et al: Studies on the histogenesis of cervical adenocarcinoma. Int J Gynecol Pathol 1:336–346, 1983.

151. Higgins GD, Phillips GE, Smith LA, et al: High prevalence of human papillomavirus transcripts in all grades of cervical intraepithelial glandular neoplasia. Cancer 70:136–146, 1992.

152. Nielsen AL: Human papillomavirus type 16/18 in uterine cervical adenocarcinoma in situ and adenocarcinoma. A study by in situ hybridization with biotinylated DNA probes. Cancer 65:2588–2593, 1990.

153. Farnsworth A, Laverty C, Stoler MH: Human papillomavirus messenger RNA expression in adenocarcinoma in situ of the uterine cervix. Int J Gynecol Pathol 8:321–330, 1989.

154. Tase T, Okagaki T, Clark BA, et al: Human papillomavirus DNA in adenocarcinoma in situ, microinvasive adenocarcinoma of the uterine cervix, and coexisting cervical squamous intraepithelial neoplasia. Int J Gynecol Pathol 8:8–17, 1989.

155. Lee KR, Howard P, Heintz NH, et al: Low prevalence of human papillomavirus types 16 and 18 in cervical adenocarcinoma in situ, invasive adenocarcinoma, and glandular dysplasia by polymerase chain reaction. Mod Pathol 6:433–437, 1993.

156. Leary J, Jaworski R, Houghton R: In-situ hybridization using biotinylated DNA probes to human papillomavirus in adenocarcinoma-in-situ and endocervical glandular dysplasia of the uterine cervix. Pathology 23:85–89, 1991.

157. Jonasson JG, Wang HH, Antonioli DA, et al: Tubal metaplasia of the uterine cervix: A prevalence study in patients with gynecologic pathologic findings. Int J Gynecol Pathol 11:89–95, 1992.

158. Novotny DB, Maygarden SJ, Johnson DE, et al: Tubal metaplasia. A frequent potential pitfall in the cytologic diagnosis of endocervical glandular dysplasia on cervical smears. Acta Cytol 36:1–10, 1992.

159. Suh KS, Silverberg SG: Tubal metaplasia of the uterine cervix. Int J Gynecol Pathol 9:122–128, 1990.

160. Rhatigan RM: Endocervical gland atypia secondary to Arias-Stella change. Arch Pathol Lab Med 116:943–946, 1992.

161. Schneider V: Arias-Stella reaction of the endocervix. Frequency and location. Acta Cytol 25:224–228, 1981.

162. Cove H: The Arias-Stella reaction occurring in the endocervix in pregnancy. Recognition and comparison with adenocarcinoma of the endocervix. Am J Surg Pathol 3:567–568, 1979.

163. Rollason TP, Cullimore J, Bradgate MG: A suggested columnar cell morphological equivalent of squamous carcinoma in situ with early stromal invasion. Int J Gynecol Pathol 8:230–236, 1989.

164. Michael H, Grawe L, Kraus FT: Minimal deviation endocervical adenocarcinoma: Clinical and histologic features, immunohistochemical staining for carcinoembryo-

nic antigen, and differentiation from confusing benign lesions. Int J Gynecol Pathol 3:261–276, 1984.

165. Kaku T, Enjoji M: Extremely well-differentiated adenocarcinoma (''adenoma malignum'') of the cervix. Int J Gynecol Pathol 2:28–41, 1983.

166. Gilks CB, Young RH, Aguirre P, et al: Adenoma malignum (minimal deviation adenocarcinoma) of the uterine cervix: A clinicopathological and immunohistochemical analysis of 26 cases. Am J Surg Pathol 13:717–730, 1989.

167. Kaminski PF, Norris HJ: Minimal deviation adenocarcinoma (adenoma malignum) of the cervix. Int J Gynecol Pathol 2:141–153, 1983.

168. Silverberg SG, Hurt WG: Minimal deviation adenocarcinoma (''adenoma malignum'') of the cervix. Am J Obstet Gynecol 123:971–975, 1975.

169. Rahilly MA, Williams ARW, Al-Nafussi A: Minimal deviation endometrioid adenocarcinoma of cervix: A clinicopathological and immunohistochemical study of two cases. Histopathology 20:351–354, 1992.

170. Steeper TA, Wick MR: Minimal deviation adenocarcinoma of the uterine cervix (''adenoma malignum''). An immunohistochemical comparison with microglandular endocervical hyperplasia and conventional endocervical adenocarcinoma. Cancer 58:1131–1138, 1986.

171. Jones MA, Young RH, Scully RE: Diffuse laminar endocervical glandular hyperplasia: A benign lesion often confused with adenoma malignum (minimal deviation adenocarcinoma). Am J Surg Pathol 15:1123–1129, 1991.

172. Segal GH, Hart WR: Cystic endocervical tunnel clusters. A clinicopathologic study of 29 cases of so-called adenomatous hyperplasia. Am J Surg Pathol 14:895–903, 1990.

173. Friedrich EG Jr, Wilkinson EJ: Vulvar surgery for neurofibromatosis. Obstet Gynecol 65:135–138, 1985.

174. Ferry JA, Scully RE: Mesonephric remnants, hyperplasia, and neoplasia in the uterine cervix: A study of 49 cases. Am J Surg Pathol 14:1100–1111, 1990.

175. Ayroud Y, Gelfand MM, Ferenczy A: Florid mesonephric hyperplasia of the cervix: A report of a case with review of the literature. Int J Gynecol Pathol 4:245–254, 1985.

176. Lang G, Dallenbach-Hellweg G: The histogenetic origin of cervical mesonephric hyperplasia and mesonephric adenocarcinoma of the uterine cervix studied with immunohistochemical methods. Int J Gynecol Pathol 9:145–157, 1990.

177. Jones MA, Andrews J, Tarraza HM: Mesonephric remnant hyperplasia of the cervix: A clinicopathologic analysis of 14 cases. Gynecol Oncol 49:41–47, 1993.

178. Hinchey WW, Silva EG, Guarda LA, et al: Paravaginal wolffian duct (mesonephros) adenocarcinoma: A light and electron microscopic study. Am J Clin Pathol 80:539–544, 1983.

179. Jones MW, Silverberg SG, Kurman RJ: Well-differentiated villoglandular adenocarcinoma of the uterine cervix: A clinicopathological study of 24 cases. Int J Gynecol Pathol 12:1–7, 1993.

180. Young RH, Scully RE: Villoglandular papillary adenocarcinoma of the uterine cervix. A clinicopathologic analysis of 13 cases. Cancer 63:1773–1779, 1989.

181. Selzer I, Nelson HM: Benign papilloma (polypoid tumor) of the cervix uteri in children. Am J Obstet Gynecol 84:165–169, 1962.

182. Janovski NS, Kasdon EJ: Benign mesonephric papillary and polypoid tumors of the cervix in childhood. J Pediatr 63:211–216, 1963.

183. Zaloudek CJ, Norris HJ: Adenofibroma and adenosarcoma of the uterus: A clinicopathologic study of 35 cases. Cancer 48:354–366, 1981.

184. Abell MR: Papillary adenofibroma of the uterine cervix. Am J Obstet Gynecol 110:990–993, 1971.

185. Shintaku M, Ueda H: Serous papillary adenocarcinoma of the uterine cervix. Histopathology 22:506–507, 1993.

186. Gilks CB, Clement PB: Papillary serous adenocarcinoma of the uterine cervix: A report of three cases. Mod Pathol 5:426–431, 1992.

187. Ambros RA, Park JS, Shah KV, et al: Evaluation of histologic, morphometric, and immunohistochemical criteria in the differential diagnosis of small cell carcinomas of the cervix with particular reference to human papillomavirus types 16 and 18. Mod Pathol 4:586–593, 1991.

188. Barrett RJ 2nd, Davos I, Leuchter RS, et al: Neuroendocrine features in poorly differentiated and undifferentiated carcinomas of the cervix. Cancer 60:2325–2330, 1987.

189. Gersell DJ, Mazoujian G, Mutch DG, et al: Small-cell undifferentiated carcinoma of the cervix. A clinicopathologic, ultrastructural, and immunocytochemical study of 15 cases. Am J Surg Pathol 12:684–698, 1988.

190. Ueda G, Yamasaki M: Neuroendocrine carcinoma of the uterus. Curr Top Pathol 85:309–335, 1992.

191. van Nagell JR Jr, Powell DE, Gallion HH, et al: Small cell carcinoma of the uterine cervix. Cancer 62:1586–1593, 1988.

192. Walker AN, Mills SE, Taylor PT: Cervical neuroendocrine carcinoma: A clinical and light microscopic study of 14 cases. Int J Gynecol Pathol 7:64–74, 1988.

193. Miller B, Dockter M, el Torky M, et al: Small cell carcinoma of the cervix: A clinical and flow-cytometric study. Gynecol Oncol 42:27–33, 1991.

194. Sheets EE, Berman ML, Hrountas CK, et al: Surgically treated, early-stage neuroendocrine small-cell cervical carcinoma. Obstet Gynecol 71:10–14, 1988.

195. O'Hanlan KA, Goldberg GL, Jones JG, et al: Adjuvant therapy for neuroendocrine small cell carcinoma of the cervix: Review of the literature. Gynecol Oncol 43:167–172, 1991.

196. Morris M, Gershenson DM, Eifel P, et al: Treatment of small cell carcinoma of the cervix with cisplatin, doxorubicin, and etoposide. Gynecol Oncol 47:62–65, 1992.

197. Tabbara IA, Grosh WA, Andersen WA, et al: Treatment of small-cell carcinoma of the cervix with weekly combination chemotherapy. Eur J Cancer 26:748–749, 1990.

198. Groben P, Reddick R, Askin F: The pathologic spectrum of small cell carcinoma of the cervix. Int J Gynecol Pathol 4:42–57, 1985.

199. Yamasaki M, Tateishi R, Hongo J, et al: Argyrophil small cell carcinomas of the uterine cervix. Int J Gynecol Pathol 3:146–152, 1984.

200. Stoler MH, Mills SE, Gersell DJ, et al: Small-cell neuroendocrine carcinoma of the cervix. A human papillomavirus type 18-associated cancer. Am J Surg Pathol 15:28–32, 1991.

201. Ulich TR, Liao SY, Layfield L, et al: Endocrine and tumor differentiation markers in poorly differentiated small-cell carcinoids of the cervix and vagina. Arch Pathol Lab Med 110:1054–1057, 1986.

202. Wolber RA, Clement PB: In situ DNA hybridization of cervical small cell carcinoma and adenocarcinoma using biotin-labeled human papillomavirus probes. Mod Pathol 4:96–100, 1991.

203. Albores-Saavedra J, Rodriguez-Martinez HA, Larraza-Hernandez O: Carcinoid tumors of the cervix. Pathol Annu 14:273–291, 1979.

204. Harris NL, Scully RE: Malignant lymphoma and granulocytic sarcoma of the uterus and vagina. A clinicopathologic analysis of 27 cases. Cancer 53:2530–2545, 1984.

Placenta and Gestational Trophoblastic Disease

Janice M. Lage, M.D.

LESIONS INVOLVING EARLY PLACENTAL VILLI AND ITS TROPHOBLAST

Hydropic Abortus

Hydropic abortus describes an immature placenta with moderately to markedly swollen villi and attenuated trophoblast.

CLINICOPATHOLOGIC FEATURES. Although this discussion focuses on hydropic abortus, some general comments regarding evaluation of tissues from early pregnancies are appropriate. Early loss of embryonic viability results in spontaneous abortion or clinical signs of missed abortion by the end of the first trimester. Most women with missed abortion present with vaginal bleeding and are diagnosed clinically as "missed abortion," "spontaneous abortion," or "blighted ovum."

Having a single or even a second miscarriage does not affect a couple's reproductive potential. However, couples with frequent pregnancy wastage, i.e., three or more spontaneous abortions, are at increased risk of being carriers of a chromosomal translocation, and fresh villous tissues from a third such pregnancy, whether hydropic or not, should be submitted for cytogenetic analysis.

The pathologist's role in evaluating tissue from a spontaneous abortion is twofold: (1) to confirm intrauterine pregnancy by identifying placental villous tissues (or lacking villous tissue, identification of trophoblast), and (2) in cases of repetitive spontaneous abortion, to submit fresh villous tissues for cytogenetic studies. The entire specimen should be submitted for microscopic examination when the tissue is scant or lacking obvious villi. If no villi or trophoblast is identified on microscopy, the clinician must be notified immediately that an ectopic gestation cannot be excluded.

Grossly, uterine curettings from a spontaneous or hydropic abortus generally contain a small to moderate amount of placental and maternal tissues. Frequently, the entire specimen can be embedded totally in three or four paraffin blocks, and, in many, the entire chorionic vesicle (the villous tissue) fits into one cassette. Rarely, a hydropic abortus has a few very large, grossly visible villi measuring up to 1 cm in diameter. Such villi are more common in chromosomally anomalous conceptions, particularly trisomy 18.[1] By microscopy, the villi of a hydropic abortus are round to oval, resembling slightly deflated balloons, and the overlying trophoblast is markedly attenuated (Figs. 15–1 and 15–2). Fetal blood vessels are inconspicuous, and if present, contain fragmented red blood cells and karyorrhectic debris. Embryonic or fetal tissues are scant, if present at all, and often necrotic. Interestingly, in one study, alcian blue stains at pH 1.2 and 2.5 demonstrated that villous hydrops was due to accumulation of strongly sulfated mucosubstances rather than water.[2] Most hydropic abortuses have diploid DNA content on flow cytometric evaluation, although 10% to 20% may be triploid (Fig. 15–3).

DIFFERENTIAL DIAGNOSIS. The differential diagnosis of hydropic abortus includes partial hydatidiform mole and complete hydatidiform mole (Table 15–1). In partial mole, the villous tissue is abundant and composed of two distinct populations of villi, one small and sclerotic and one large with swollen, scalloped villi containing trophoblastic inclusions and focal trophoblast hyperplasia (Figs. 15–4 to 15–13). In a well-developed complete mole, the markedly enlarged villi exhibit central clear spaces, termed cisterns (Figs. 15–14 and 15–16). Exuberant trophoblast encircles the majority of villi (Figs. 15–14 to 15–17).

The main diagnostic difficulty centers around distinguishing a hydropic abortus from an **early complete mole** (i.e., one of 6–8 weeks' gestational age). Although the villi are enlarged in an early complete mole, they are not cavitated (Figs. 15–18 to 15–20). The striking trophoblastic hyperplasia characteristic of a more mature complete mole is lacking, and in its place is only moderately stratified hyperplastic trophoblast (Figs. 15–18 to 15–21). The increased cytologic atypicality of the **extravillous trophoblast** in an early complete mole is a clue to its diagnosis (Fig. 15–22). In contrast, in a hydropic abortus, the villous trophoblast is thin to inconspicuous and bland cytologically (see Figs. 15–1 and 15–2). Occasionally some villi in a hydropic abortus have central cisterns, and an oblique section of the chorionic vesicle may simulate a cavitated villus with trophoblast hyperplasia. When diagnostic distinction is difficult, it is important to embed the entire specimen to evaluate all of the villi. A key point is this: Always play it safe. If a hydatidiform mole cannot be excluded based on histologic examination of the entire specimen, the pathology report should convey the diagnostic uncertainty so that the clinician may begin hormonal surveillance.

Partial Hydatidiform Mole

A partial hydatidiform mole is a genetically and histologically abnormal placenta containing two populations

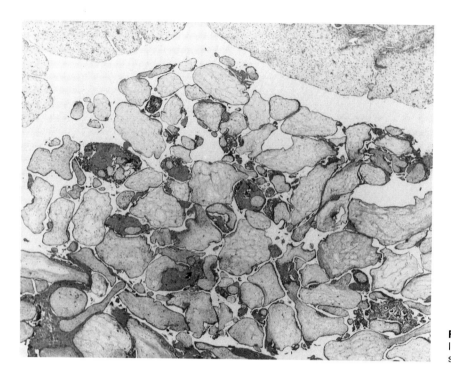

FIGURE 15–1. Hydropic abortus with diffuse villous hydrops resulting in a spectrum of villous sizes.

of villi, some of which have hyperplastic trophoblast. Its genomic DNA is generally **triploid** (69 chromosomes).[3,4]

CLINICOPATHOLOGIC FEATURES. A partial hydatidiform mole results from an abnormal conceptus whose DNA content is one third greater than normal. The extra haploid DNA set is paternally derived, usually a result of dispermy or diplospermy. In 83% to 89% of triploid conceptions, this abnormal DNA content results in a partial hydatidiform mole.[1,5–7] In contrast with complete hydatidiform moles, **fetal tissues** are identified in the vast majority of cases.

A partial hydatidiform mole is one form of gestational trophoblastic disease. The prevalence of partial molar pregnancy is unknown. It occurred at a frequency similar to complete molar pregnancy in one series.[1] The mean age of women with partial mole is near 28 years.[1] Women who have had partial moles have a slight but real risk for persistent gestational trophoblastic disease and, as such, monitoring of serial values of the beta subunit of human chorionic gonadotropin (β-hCG) is warranted.[8] Extremely rare examples of choriocarcinoma after partial hydatidiform mole have been reported.[9]

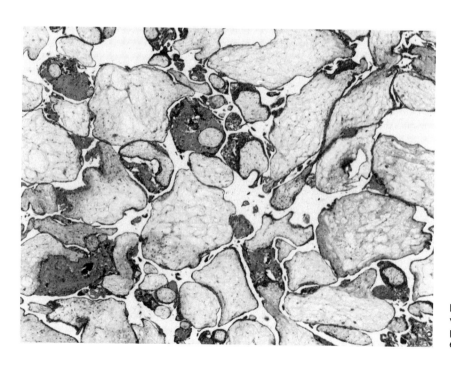

FIGURE 15–2. Hydropic abortus (higher power view of Figure 15–1) showing attenuated trophoblast on villous surfaces, villous stromal expansion, and absence of fetal capillaries.

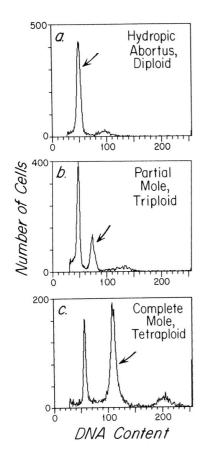

FIGURE 15-3. DNA histogram of (a) diploid hydropic abortus, (b) triploid partial hydatidiform mole, and (c) tetraploid complete hydatidiform mole. Abscissa indicates fluorescence channel number that stoichiometrically corresponds with DNA content. The G0/G1 peak represents non-cycling diploid cells (G0) and cells resulting from recent mitosis now in gap phase (G1). The S peak reflects cells synthesizing DNA for impending mitosis. The G2/M peak represents cells with twice-normal DNA composition (G2) and those undergoing mitosis (M). Note: Arrow indicates diploid G0/G1 peak in a, triploid peak in b, and tetraploid peak in c. (From Lage JM, Popek EJ: The role of DNA flow cytometry in evaluation of partial and complete hydatidiform moles and hydropic abortions. Semin Diagn Pathol 10:267–274, 1993.)

Gross examination of a partial mole reveals abundant villous tissue, noticeably exceeding that expected for the gestational age. Unusually large swollen villi (0.5–1.0 cm in dimension) are admixed with normal-appearing villi.[1] Floating the curetted tissues in saline removes some of the attached blood, making it easier to recognize the dimorphic villous sizes. When villous hydrops is identified macroscopically, consideration should be given to submitting fresh tissue for flow cytometric or cytogenetic analysis, as knowledge of nuclear DNA ploidy may later prove useful in difficult cases.

Microscopically, a partial hydatidiform mole is characterized foremost by **two populations of villi:** one is normal to small and sclerotic; the other, large and hydropic (see Figs. 15–4 to 15–7). Villous cavitation is focal, on average involving between 1% to 15% of the villi. Some examples of partial mole have numerous edematous villi, although cavitated villi may be sparse (see Figs. 15–7 and 15–11). **Trophoblast hyperplasia** involves predominantly the syncytiotrophoblast layer (syncytium) and consists of trophoblastic notches or

finger-like projections (see Figs. 15–6 and 15–9) and/or sheets of syncytiotrophoblast on more than one side of a villus (see Figs. 15–5, 15–7, and 15–10 to 15–13). The trophoblastic hyperplasia involves both small and large villi. The cytotrophoblast generally forms an inconspicuous single layer underneath the syncytium (see Figs. 15–9 to 15–12). The villous outline is scalloped, resulting in villous **stromal trophoblastic inclusions** when sectioned tangentially (see Figs. 15–6 to 15–9). The villous stroma virtually always has blood vessels with viable or degenerating nucleated red blood cells (see Fig. 15–12). Partial moles persisting into the second trimester may have **maze-like[4] villous blood vessels,** constituting a pathognomonic, "one glance" diagnostic feature (see Fig. 15–13). More than 90% of partial moles have fetal/embryonic tissues.

DIFFERENTIAL DIAGNOSIS. The differential diagnosis of partial hydatidiform mole includes hydropic abortus, complete hydatidiform mole, and twin pregnancy with one complete mole and one normal twin. Villi from hydropic abortus exhibit a **spectrum** of villous sizes ranging from small to large (see Figs. 15–1 and 15–2), which contrasts with the dimorphic villous population of partial mole (see Figs. 15–4 to 15–7 and Table 15–1). The trophoblast of a hydropic abortus is attenuated, becoming difficult to recognize, whereas a partial mole has many syncytial knots and definite, though focal, trophoblast hyperplasia (see Figs. 15–7 and 15–9 to 15–13). Villous stromal trophoblastic inclusions are far more frequent in partial mole (see Figs. 15–8 and 15–9) than in complete mole. The complete mole is characterized by very large villi, many to most of which are cavitated and usually, although not always, lack fetal blood vessels (see Figs. 15–14 and 15–16). However, it is the extreme degree of trophoblast hyperplasia, involving cytotrophoblast and syncytiotrophoblast, and intermediately trophoblast with its cytologic atypia that characterize a complete mole (see Figs. 15–16, 15–17, and 15–22).

A **twin pregnancy** with a **normal placenta and a complete mole** may be a diagnostic nightmare (Figs. 15–23 and 15–24). One finds two populations of villi, somewhat similar in sizes to the dimorphic populations in partial mole, but the trophoblast is more exuberant than expected (see Fig. 15–23). This focally marked trophoblast hyperplasia is the clue to diagnosis of complete mole and normal co-twin (see Fig. 15–24). In addition, the extravillous trophoblast (intermediate trophoblast) of the complete hydatidiform mole is composed of markedly enlarged cells with large, hyperchromatic nuclei, far exceeding that of a hydropic abortus or a partial hydatidiform mole (see Fig. 15–22). Absence of a triploid DNA peak on flow cytometric evaluation of fresh or fixed tissues virtually excludes partial mole (see Fig. 15–3).[7] All molar pregnancies, whether partial or complete, need follow-up β-hCG surveillance.

Complete Hydatidiform Mole

A complete hydatidiform mole is a genetically and histologically abnormal placenta characterized by **marked villous swelling and trophoblast hyperplasia.** Its genomic DNA is totally paternally derived.[10]

CLINICOPATHOLOGIC FEATURES. Complete moles result from an abnormal fertilization event in which an "empty

(*Text continued on page 572*)

Table 15–1. **Gross and Microscopic Differences Between Hydropic Abortus, Partial Hydatidiform Mole, and Complete Hydatidiform Mole**

	Hydropic Abortus	**Partial Hydatidiform Mole**	**Complete Hydatidiform Mole**
Amount of Tissue	Scant	Increased for gestational age	Markedly increased
Villous Swelling	Diffuse swelling, involves chorion laeve	Two populations with focal villous swelling	Diffuse swelling
Villous Cavitation	Focal	Focal	Common to extensive
Trophoblast Hyperplasia	None	Focal, involving syncytiotrophoblast	Extensive
Villous Scalloping and Villous Stromal Inclusions	Usually balloon-shaped villi, no scalloping	Focal	Absent
Fetal Tissue	Usually absent, trisomy 18 a notable exception	Usually intact or fragmented fetal parts	Absent
DNA Content	Diploid, often with abnormal karyotype	Triploid, 69,XXX, 69,XXY, rarely 69,XYY	Diploid, paternal 46,XX or 46,XY

From Gompel C, Silverberg SG (eds): Pathology in Gynecology and Obstetrics, 4th ed. Philadelphia, JB Lippincott, 1993.

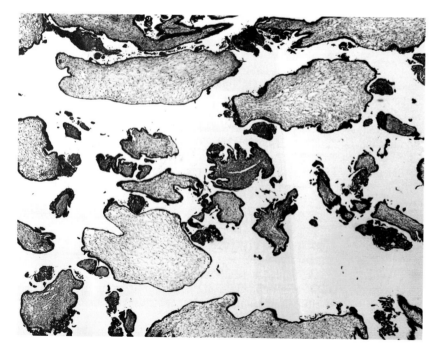

FIGURE 15–4. Partial hydatidiform mole showing two populations of villi; some are large and swollen, and others are small and focally fibrotic. Trophoblast hyperplasia is minimal in this field.

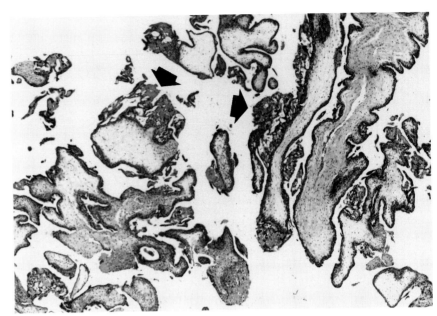

FIGURE 15–5. Partial hydatidiform mole showing enlarged villi with a few smaller villi in background. Trophoblast hyperplasia *(arrowheads)* is more pronounced than in Figure 15–4. Villous stroma is focally clear and loose in some villi and fibrotic in others.

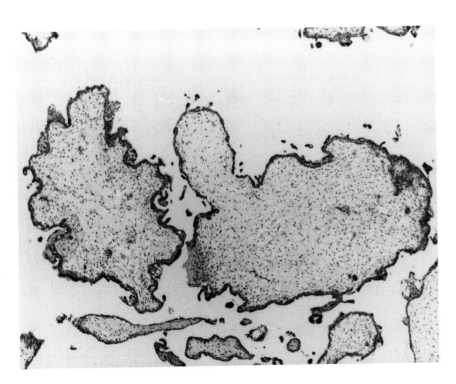

FIGURE 15–6. Partial hydatidiform mole with two enlarged villi and smaller villi in background. Note prominent scalloping of villous outlines and syncytiotrophoblastic knuckles or notches projecting from villous surfaces. Villous stroma is cellular.

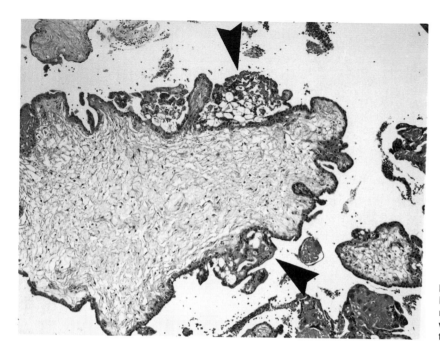

FIGURE 15–7. Partial hydatidiform mole with large, swollen, scalloped villus demonstrating multifocal syncytiotrophoblastic hyperplasia with lacy appearance resulting from vacuolization and scattered trophoblastic notches.

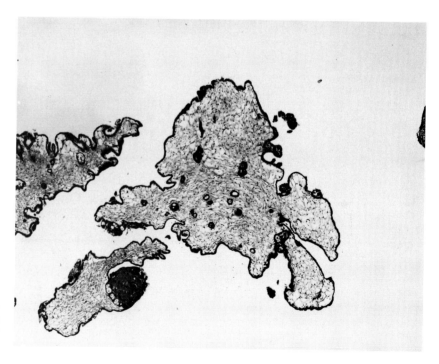

FIGURE 15–8. Partial hydatidiform mole showing a few enlarged villi with scalloped villous outlines resulting in multiple stromal trophoblastic inclusions.

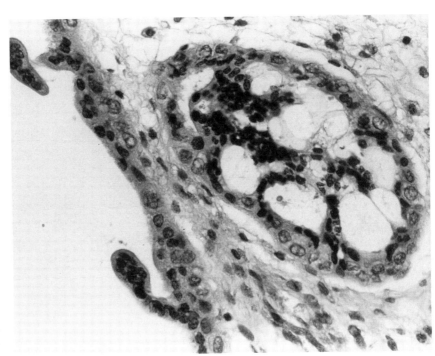

FIGURE 15–9. Partial hydatidiform mole, shown on high-power magnification, illustrating villous stromal trophoblastic inclusion and surface trophoblastic notches.

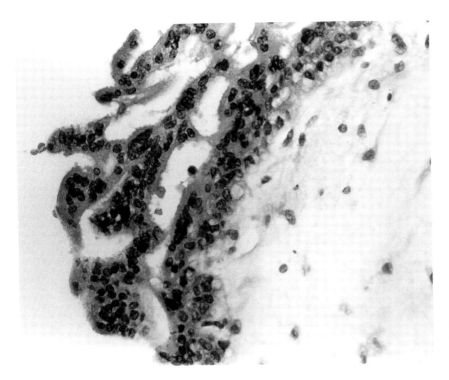

FIGURE 15–10. Partial hydatidiform mole with lacy syncytiotrophoblastic hyperplasia projecting from villous surface. Villous stroma is pale and hypocellular.

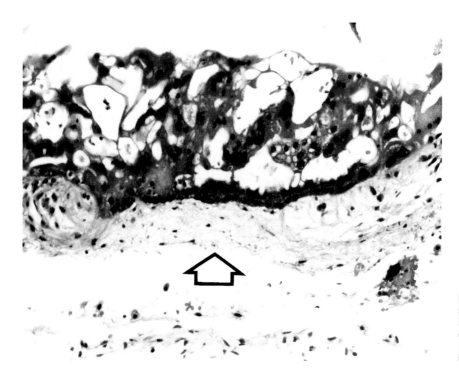

FIGURE 15–11. Partial hydatidiform mole with syncytiotrophoblastic hyperplasia projecting from villous surface. Villous stroma demonstrates early cavitation with a sharp edge *(arrow)* demarcating outline of partially collapsed cistern.

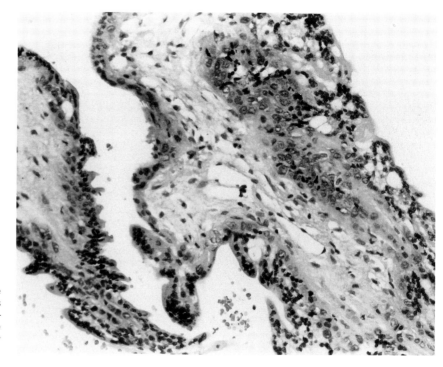

FIGURE 15–12. Partial hydatidiform mole depicting portions of two enlarged villi. Villous trophoblastic hyperplasia involves both syncytiotrophoblast and, to a lesser extent, the cytotrophoblast. Villous stroma contains a few open capillaries.

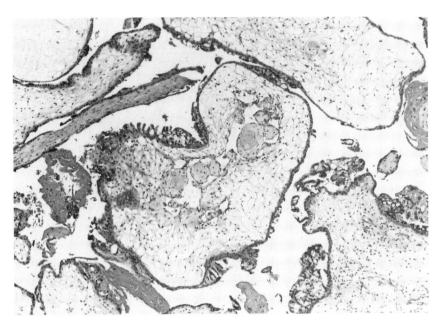

FIGURE 15–13. Partial hydatidiform mole with bizarre villous capillaries characteristic of second trimester partial hydatidiform mole. This unusual capillary architecture of interanastomosing channels with intravascular stromal projections is not seen in normal placentas and suggests partial hydatidiform mole.

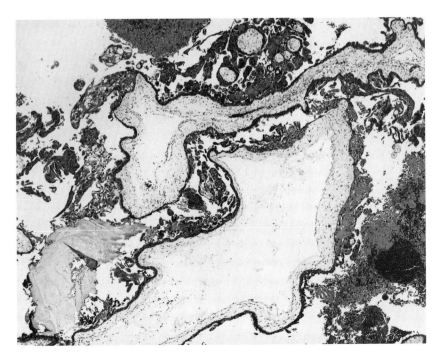

FIGURE 15–14. Complete hydatidiform mole with well-formed cisterns and circumferential trophoblast hyperplasia. A few smaller villi in the background of this mole have hyperplastic trophoblast. (Same magnification as in Figure 15–4.)

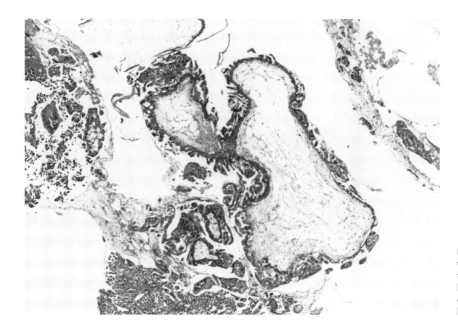

FIGURE 15–15. Complete hydatidiform mole with enlarged villi exhibiting circumferential trophoblast hyperplasia. Stroma of larger villus is loose, but cistern formation has not occurred. Smaller villi in background have hyperplastic trophoblast.

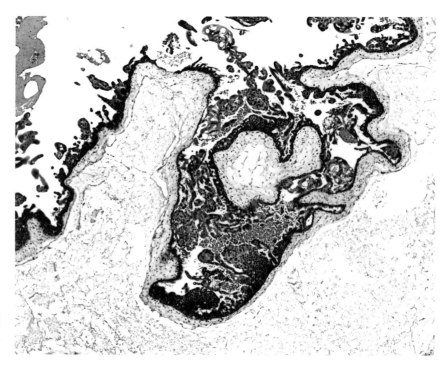

FIGURE 15–16. Complete hydatidiform mole wherein a single villus fills this low-power field. Central cistern contains acellular eosinophilic material.

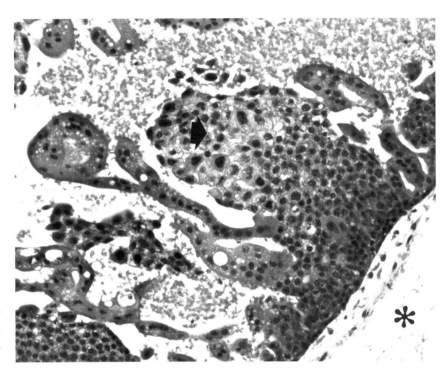

FIGURE 15–17. Complete hydatidiform mole, higher power of trophoblast hyperplasia depicted in Figure 15–16. A portion of the central cistern is just appreciable in the lower right-hand corner (*). The trophoblastic hyperplasia involves both basal cytotrophoblast and the superficial, multinucleated syncytiotrophoblast as well as a nest of larger, hyperchromatic intermediate trophoblast *(arrow)* "maturing" from the underlying cytotrophoblast.

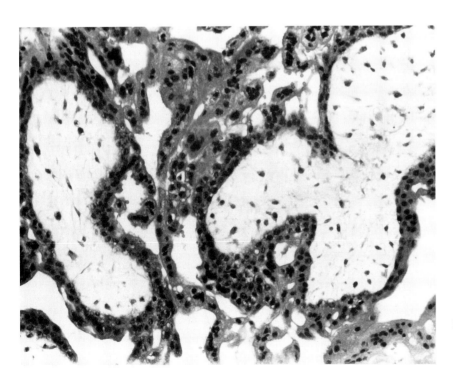

FIGURE 15–18. "Early" complete hydatidiform mole with slightly enlarged villi and focal trophoblastic hyperplasia involving predominantly the syncytiotrophoblast.

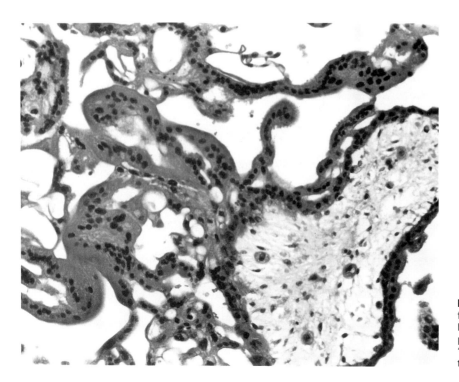

FIGURE 15–19. "Early" complete hydatidiform mole with enlarged villus and focally hyperplastic syncytiotrophoblast. Cytotrophoblast appears more-or-less normal. A few "wandering," slightly vacuolated, trophoblastic cells are present within the villous stroma.

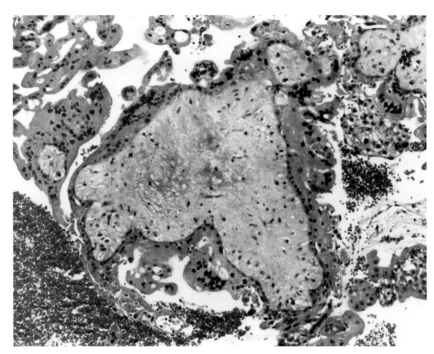

FIGURE 15–20. "Early" complete hydatidiform mole with enlarged, sclerotic villus covered with hyperplastic syncytiotrophoblast.

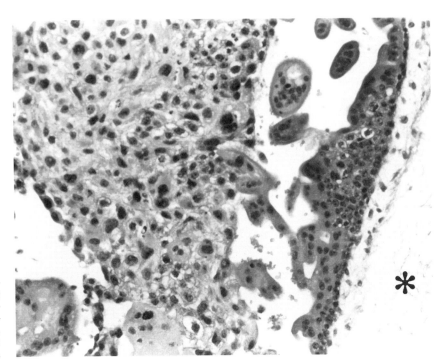

FIGURE 15–21. "Early" complete hydatidiform mole depicting a portion of villus *(right)* with cistern formation (*). The overlying cytotrophoblast and syncytiotrophoblast are moderately hyperplastic, and the intermediate, extravillous trophoblast *(left)* is increased in both quantity and degree of cytologic atypia.

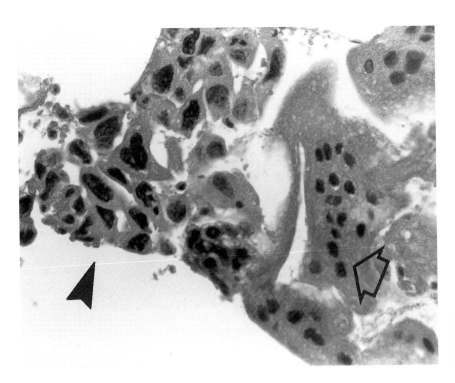

FIGURE 15–22. "Early" complete mole with markedly atypical avillous intermediate trophoblast *(arrowhead)*. Note size of syncytiotrophoblastic nuclei *(open arrow)* for comparison.

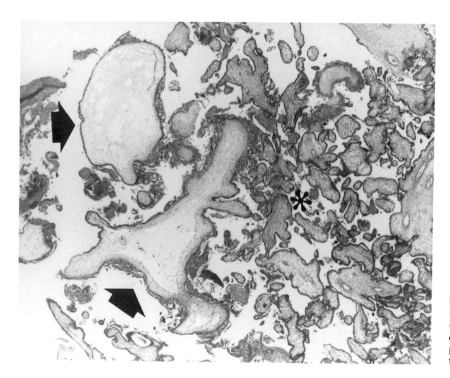

FIGURE 15–23. Twin gestation with complete hydatidiform mole *(arrows)* and normal villi (*). The molar villi are markedly enlarged and cavitated. Thickened, hyperplastic trophoblast proliferates from many areas of the villous surfaces.

ovum'' sans female pronucleus is fertilized by either (1) a haploid spermatozoan, which then duplicates its DNA to diploid content, or (2) two separate spermatozoa fertilizing an ''empty ovum.'' In both, the conceptus forms from paternally derived DNA and lacks all maternal DNA except mitochondrial DNA.[11] It is thought that the paternal DNA allows for placental development, albeit quite abnormal, but is insufficient for embryonic development.[12, 13]

The complete hydatidiform mole constitutes one of the most important forms of gestational trophoblastic disease.

Complete hydatidiform mole occurs in approximately 1 in 4500 deliveries in the United States,[14] 1 in 1300 deliveries in Israel,[15] and in 1 in 95–373 deliveries in Indonesia.[16] The mean age of women with complete mole was 28 years in one series.[1] **Persistent gestational trophoblastic disease** follows 10% to 30% of all complete moles.[1, 17–23] Choriocarcinoma, which previously followed 2% to 5% of complete moles, develops far less commonly today, most likely as a result of advances in assaying β-hCG values and greater efficacy of chemotherapeutic regimens. The risk of a second complete

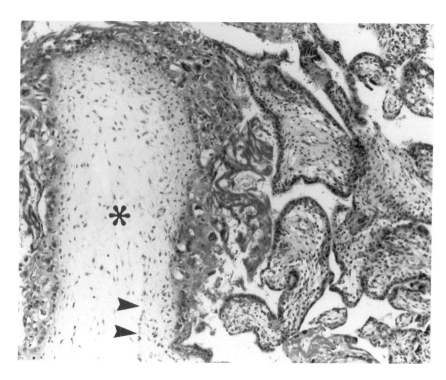

FIGURE 15–24. Higher-power view of Figure 15–23. Molar villus from complete hydatidiform mole (*) illustrating (1) marked disparity of villus size as compared with adjacent normal villi, (2) extreme degree of trophoblastic hyperplasia, and (3) early cistern formation *(arrowheads).*

mole increases significantly in women who have had a previous molar pregnancy. The ultimate reproductive capabilities of women after a single molar pregnancy appear quite good, even when chemotherapy is required to achieve gonadotropin remission.

Because early obstetric ultrasonography is performed frequently, abnormal gestations lacking fetal heart movements are evacuated before clinical signs and symptoms develop. Such uterine curettage specimens necessarily include some complete hydatidiform moles. Although evacuation of an early complete hydatidiform mole at 6 to 9 weeks' gestational age is fortuitous for the patients, interpreting such tissues may be difficult as the diagnostic features are more subtle.

Diagnosis of a fully formed complete hydatidiform mole becomes obvious to all attending the uterine evacuation.[24] The sheer volume alone suggests a molar pregnancy. The villi of a complete mole are grossly visible to the naked eye (Fig. 15–25), measuring approximately 0.75 to 1 cm in greatest dimension.[1] Fetal/embryonic tissues are absent.

Microscopically, a complete hydatidiform mole has markedly enlarged villi with central stromal clearing termed **cavitation** or **cistern formation** (see Figs. 15–14, 15–16, 15–17, and 15–21). A true cistern is sharply demarcated from the surrounding villous stroma. Although extensive cistern formation implies complete mole, **villous trophoblast hyperplasia** must also be present (see Figs. 15–16 and 15–17). This hyperplasia involves both the villous cytotrophoblast and syncytiotrophoblast as well as the extravillous intermediate trophoblast (see Fig. 15–22). The marked stratification of cytotrophoblast (see Fig. 15–17) is distinctly different from the orderly trophoblast proliferations of early villi (Figs. 15–26 and 15–27). The syncytiotrophoblast of complete mole is also stratified, with enlarged, lace-like multinucleated cells forming a loose netting over the villous cytotrophoblast. Apparent trophoblast exfoliation into the intervillous space is both real and artifactual, the latter being derived from tangential sectioning of the villous surfaces. The villous trophoblast may show significant cytologic atypicality characterized by nuclear and cytoplasmic enlargement with nuclear hyperchromasia and increased mitotic activity. Mitotic figures, normal and atypical, are interspersed with occasional bizarre forms. The **implantation site** of a complete mole has prominent intermediate trophoblast with striking nuclear enlargement and hyperchromasia as well as increased amounts of multinucleated syncytiotrophoblast and prominent endovascular trophoblastic proliferation.

Recognition of an "**early**" (young, immature) **complete mole** is far more difficult for both the clinician and the pathologist. In contrast with the fully developed complete mole, there are no obvious clinicopathologic characteristics implying its existence save for the combination of **absence of fetal heart movement** and a **β-hCG value greater than expected for gestational age.**[25] In some instances, one may recognize that the volume of curettings is increased for the gestational age, a subtle and easily overlooked finding. Prospectively, microscopic diagnosis is also difficult. Some of the villi are slightly edematous (see Figs. 15–18 and 15–19) or sclerotic (see Fig. 15–20), and villous cavitation is infrequent (see Fig. 15–21). The trophoblast, although hyperplastic and completely encircling some villi (see Figs. 15–18 to 15–20), does not have the eye-catching exuberance or atypia as in the "fully mature" complete mole. Compared with normal intermediate trophoblast (see Fig. 15–27), the intermediate trophoblast of a complete mole, be it villous or extravillous, displays significant cytologic atypia: the cells are less cohesive and contain abundant eosinophilic cytoplasm and large, hyperchromatic nuclei (see Fig. 15–22). In these situations, it is common for an early complete mole to be misdiagnosed prospectively as hydropic abortus. The correct diagnosis becomes obvious when persistent vaginal bleeding prompts repeat uterine evacuation, at which time fully developed molar villi are found.

DIFFERENTIAL DIAGNOSIS. The differential diagnosis of complete mole chiefly concerns its partner in molar disease, the partial hydatidiform mole (see Table 15–1). The partial mole has two populations of villi, some large and some normal to small (see Figs. 15–4 to 15–7). The trophoblast of partial mole is less exuberant, with syncytiotrophoblast hyperplasia often unaccompanied by cytotrophoblastic hyperplasia (see Figs. 15–7 and 15–9 to 15–12). Stromal trophoblastic inclusions (see Figs. 15–8 and 15–9) and villous blood vessels, both normal (see Fig. 15–12) and ectatic (see Fig. 15–13), may be identified. Cavitated villi (see Fig. 15–11) are uncommon to sparse, with extensive cavitation infrequent. In contrast, the complete mole has many grossly enlarged villi (see Fig. 15–25), which on microscopy have stromal cisterns and significant trophoblastic hyperplasia (see Figs. 15–14 to 15–17).

As the partial mole is almost always triploid,[1, 3, 5–7] flow cytometric analysis of fresh or fixed tissues or cytogenetic analyses can be very helpful (see Fig. 15–3). The majority of complete moles, both "immature" and "mature," are diploid or tetraploid.[1, 7, 17] Additionally, the clinical presentation and β-hCG levels are also different, with partial moles

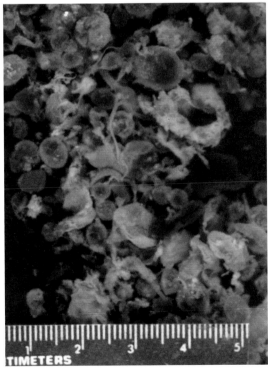

FIGURE 15–25. Complete hydatidiform mole, gross appearance. Molar villi floating in a Petri dish filled with saline. Largest villus is approximately 1.3 cm in diameter. Note that the majority of villi are hydropic. (From Gompel C, Silverberg SG [eds]: Pathology in Gynecology and Obstetrics, 4th ed., Philadelphia, JB Lippincott, 1993.)

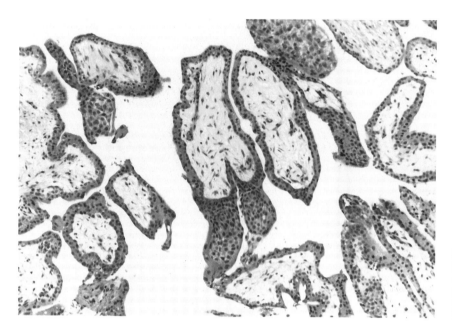

FIGURE 15–26. Normal first trimester villi illustrating organized trophoblastic proliferation of bilaminar cytotrophoblast and syncytiotrophoblast. The base of the central villus has polar trophoblastic proliferation aimed toward the implantation site. (See Fig. 15–27.)

rarely being associated with elevated β-hCG levels above 100,000 mIU/ml or symptoms of excess gonadotropins such as theca lutein cysts, uterine size greater than expected for gestational dates, hyperemesis gravidarum, and thyrotoxicosis. Markedly elevated β-hCG values greater than 100,000 mIU/ml and the previously described clinical signs and symptoms are far more common in complete mole. When a distinction between complete mole and partial mole remains difficult, hormonal surveillance is recommended.

Another occasionally troublesome distinction involves that between the complete mole and a markedly hydropic abortus, particularly when the hydropic abortus has chromo-

somal anomalies such as trisomy 18, and, less commonly, trisomy 13 or 21; 45,XO (Turner's syndrome); or Beckwith-Wiedemann syndrome (Fig. 15–28).[1, 26] The gross and ultrasonographic appearances of these placentas may simulate complete mole because of the extremely large villous sizes, occasionally exceeding 1 to 2 cm in diameter. The presence of fetal tissues or a dysmorphic fetus, however, excludes complete mole. (An exception to this rule are twin gestations in which a normal pregnancy, fetus, and placenta co-exist with a complete hydatidiform mole [Figs. 15–23, 15–24, and 15–29], described previously.) On microscopy, the villi of a hydropic abortus display a spectrum of sizes and its tropho-

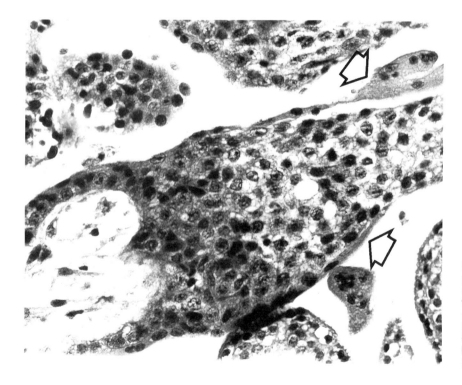

FIGURE 15–27. Higher-power view of normal, proliferating, basally oriented trophoblast. Note the proliferation of cytotrophoblast from the villous tip *(lower left corner)* that merges with intermediate trophoblast. The proliferating mononucleate trophoblast (cytotrophoblast and intermediate trophoblast) is covered by syncytiotrophoblast *(arrows).*

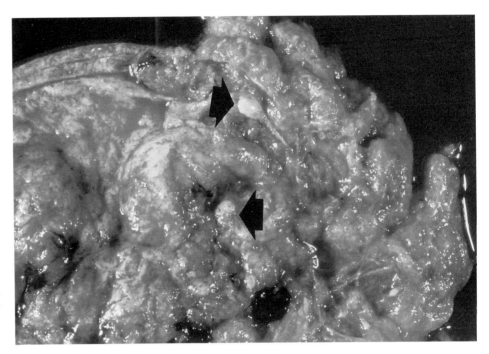

FIGURE 15–28. Beckwith-Wiedemann placenta, maternal surface, depicting scattered hydropic villi *(arrows)*. This gross appearance is indistinguishable from that of a partial hydatidiform mole. (From Lage JM: Placentomegaly with massive hydrops of placental stem villi, diploid DNA content, and fetal omphaloceles: Possible association with Beckwith-Wiedemann syndrome. Hum Pathol 22:591–597, 1991.)

blast is attenuated (see Figs. 15–1 and 5–2). Occasionally, villi with chromosomal anomalies have very bizarre villous vascular proliferations; these may be particularly common in Beckwith-Wiedemann placentas (Fig. 15–30).[26]

Chorangiocarcinoma

Chorangiocarcinoma, a very rare placental villous lesion, forms a **discrete nodule of abnormal villi with stromal vascular proliferation and atypical, hyperplastic villous trophoblast.**

CLINICOPATHOLOGIC FEATURES. Chorangiocarcinoma is a recently described villous lesion of the placenta that seems to be a morphologic hybrid of benign chorangioma and trophoblastic hyperplasia, dysplasia, or neoplasia.[27, 28] It is unclear whether it is a completely benign, premalignant, or intermediate (borderline) malignancy or a frankly malignant lesion. The last possibility seems unlikely, because no instance of metastatic trophoblastic disease has been reported with these

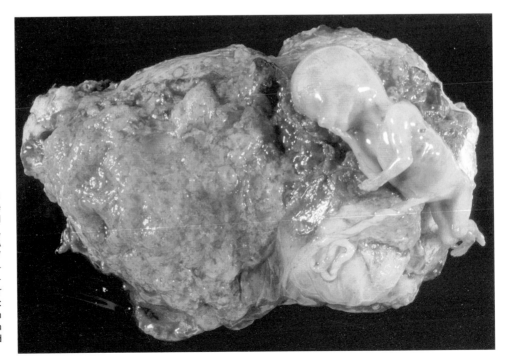

FIGURE 15–29. Twin gestation with complete hydatidiform mole *(left)* and normal twin fetus and placenta *(right)*. (From Lage JM, Mark SD, Roberts DJ, et al: A flow cytometric study of 137 fresh hydropic placentas: Correlation between types of hydatidiform moles and nuclear DNA ploidy. Obstet Gynecol 79: 403–410, 1992. Reprinted with permission from The American College of Obstetricians and Gynecologists.)

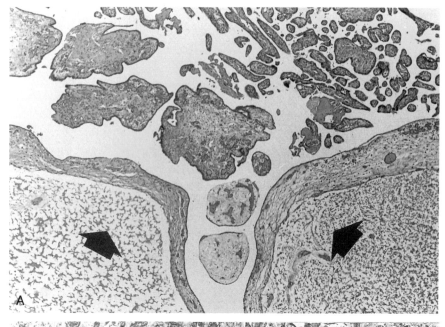

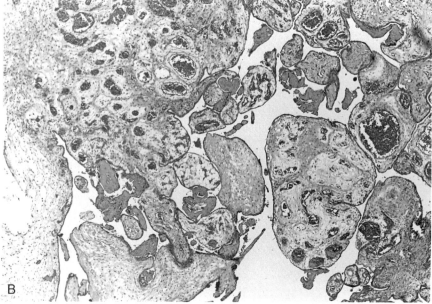

FIGURE 15–30. *A,* Beckwith-Wiedemann placenta. Microscopic appearance of two hydropic, cavitated villi *(arrows)* with intermediate-sized villi in center and small villi *(upper right corner).* The DNA content was diploid. *B,* Beckwith-Wiedemann placenta, illustrating marked vascular proliferation of abnormal villous vessels with cuffing by loose, more myxoid villous stroma. (From Lage JM: Placentomegaly with massive hydrops of placental stem villi, diploid DNA content, and fetal omphaloceles: Possible association with Beckwith-Wiedemann syndrome. Hum Pathol 22:591–597, 1991.)

tumors. A note of caution should be added: Because we know that the biology of other trophoblastic diseases cannot be predicted from histology alone, it may be premature to speculate on the natural history of this lesion given that only a few such cases have been reported.

Grossly, a chorangiocarcinoma forms a **well-circumscribed,** white-tan, villous parenchymal nodule that simulates the gross appearance of a chorangioma embedded in fibrin or an infarct. The two reported cases describe single nodules, although the possibility of multiplicity is not yet excluded. Neither woman developed gestational trophoblastic disease.

Microscopically, both the villous stroma and the villous trophoblast of a chorangiocarcinoma are abnormal (Figs. 15–31 and 15–32). The villi are somewhat enlarged, distended by a proliferation of villous blood vessels simulating chorangiosis or a chorangioma (see Fig. 15–32). The stroma is dense,

similar to that of the equally bizarre ''mesenchymoma'' of placenta. The blood vessels, apart from their number and clustering under the villous surface, appear morphologically normal and are filled with fetal blood. The villous trophoblast is stratified, composed of very large, hyperchromatic mononucleate trophoblast with moderate amounts of violaceous to eosinophilic cytoplasm (see Fig. 15–32). The nuclei are large to enormous, grooved, lobated, and hyperchromatic, with focal chromatin clearing and peripheral condensation leaving a large central eosinophilic nucleolus. In other foci, the trophoblast is bland, simulating the intermediate trophoblast of the chorion. Syncytiotrophoblast, if present, is inconspicuous. Mitoses are common. In the few reported cases, chorangiomas have been single lesions surrounded by infarcted villi. The trophoblast was hCG positive and hPL negative in one case,[27] and, in the other, there was strong staining for keratin, with

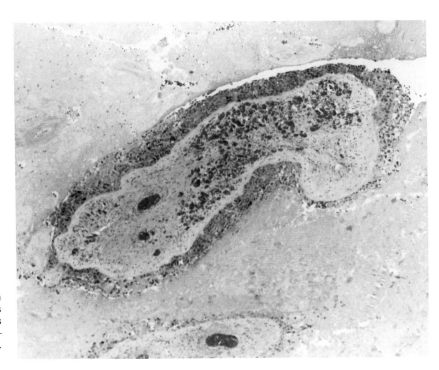

FIGURE 15–31. Chorangiocarcinoma with enlarged villus embedded in fibrin. The villous trophoblast is hyperplastic, and the villous stroma shows an unusual vascular proliferation simulating a chorangioma. (See Fig. 15–32.)

focal hCG and weak to focal human placental lactogen (hPL) staining.[28]

DIFFERENTIAL DIAGNOSIS. Chorangiocarcinoma may be confused with choriocarcinoma developing in a term placenta, a twin gestation with a normal placenta and a complete hydatidiform mole, chorangiosis, and chorangioma. Choriocarcinoma in a term placenta develops from the villous trophoblast of normal-appearing villi[29] (Figs. 15–33 to 15–35). Both cytotrophoblast and syncytiotrophoblast proliferate into the maternal intervillous space, forming large tumor nodules (see Fig. 15–34) that lose their attachment to the underlying villi. The proliferating trophoblast of chorangiocarcinoma is predominantly mononuclear, with moderate cytologic atypia and occasional syncytiotrophoblast. It remains attached to the underlying villi, whose stroma contains proliferating blood vessels simulating a chorangioma. Laboratory studies may be useful because clinically significant choriocarcinomas are always associated with elevated β-hCG values. This finding has not been reported in chorangiocarcinoma.

In a twin gestation with a complete mole and a normal twin, the molar villi are enlarged and cavitated, covered with hyperplastic cytotrophoblast and syncytiotrophoblast (see

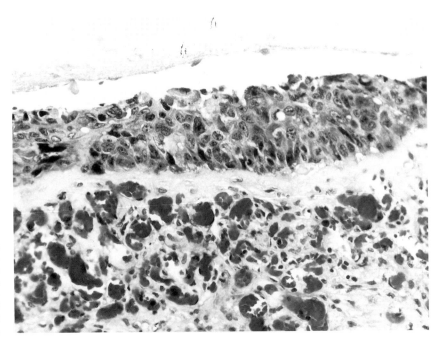

FIGURE 15–32. Higher-power view of villous trophoblast and stroma in a chorangiocarcinoma. The trophoblast is proliferative, being composed of mononucleate trophoblast. A syncytiotrophoblast covering is conspicuously absent. The villous stroma is altered by a proliferation of blood-filled fetal capillaries that are somewhat irregular in size and shape.

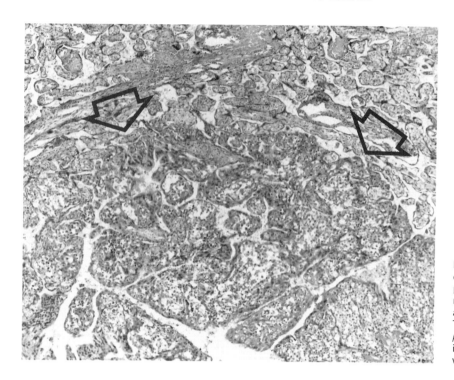

FIGURE 15–33. Choriocarcinoma in a term placenta *(arrows)*. A nest of malignant cytotrophoblast and syncytiotrophoblast displaces normal villi. Larger nodules elsewhere were associated with areas of hemorrhagic necrosis. This woman had a significantly elevated serum β-hCG level and chest metastases when examined post partum. She was successfully treated with chemotherapy.

Figs. 15–23, 15–24, and 15–29). Villous blood vessels are inconspicuous to absent in complete mole. In chorangiosis and chorangioma, villous lesions characterized by increased villous stromal vascularity, the trophoblast covering the villi is normal, composed of only syncytium and minimal cytotrophoblast, and does not show significant atypia, hyperplasia, or mitotic activity (see later discussion).

LESIONS INVOLVING PLACENTAL TROPHOBLAST WITHOUT FORMATION OF VILLI

Placental Site Nodule

A placental site nodule is a **well-circumscribed collection(s) of intermediate trophoblast** remaining *in utero* long after a previous gestation has been expulsed.

CLINICOPATHOLOGIC CORRELATION. A placental site nodule, being of trophoblastic origin, develops in women during their reproductive years.[30–34] The placental site nodule was formerly categorized under the rubric of "subinvolution of the implantation site," a collective term used by obstetricians and pathologists that encompassed all non-malignant uterine pathology relative to retained villous or trophoblastic tissues after parturition. It has been recently revisited, and a subgroup representing a histopathologically distinct category of **non-regressed intermediate trophoblast** has been identified, characterized, and renamed placental site nodule. The mean age of women with placental site nodules was 31.1 years in one large series.[32] Clinically, these patients may be asymptomatic, have abnormal uterine bleeding, infertility, or occasionally an abnormal Papanicolaou (PAP) smear.[32] In some, the antecedent pregnancy occurred quite some time prior to diagnosis, with 2 to 3 years being average, and 8 years, an extreme.[31, 32] Uterine curettage seems effective, with only rare cases persisting after

this treatment. Although initially feared to be a precursor to the deadly placental site trophoblastic tumor, few instances of such progression have been documented, and the relationship between the two entities remains obscure.[33]

As the diagnosis is almost always made on examination of uterine curettings, no characteristic gross appearance is recognized, although, in one series, one fourth of the cases had grossly visible lesions in hysterectomy specimens, the largest measuring 2.9 cm in greatest dimension.[31] Theoretically, placental site nodules could occur at any site of former ectopic implantation—in the fallopian tube, ovary, or elsewhere. The majority of lesions tend to involve non-cycling tissues such as the lower uterine segment or upper endocervical canal. Microscopically, placental site nodules form single to multiple nodules, occurring anywhere in the uterus from the endocervix to fundus (Fig. 15–36). Their most characteristic feature is apparent on low-power scanning: **well-circumscribed,** round or ovoid foci of intermediate trophoblast enmeshed in dense, eosinophilic fibrin (Figs. 15–36 and 15–37). The trophoblast radiates out from a central nidus containing slightly necrotic, eosinophilic debris. Although these nodules displace normal tissues, they do not "invade" surrounding structures. There is minimal to no tissue destruction and scant perinodular chronic inflammation. The intermediate trophoblast composing the nodules has large, polylobated nuclei with nuclear indentations.[35] Mitotic figures are typically absent to sparse. Even after careful searching, one should only rarely encounter mitotic activity as high as 2 mitoses per high-power field (HPF) in an occasional field. There may be a rare atypical mitosis. The overall configuration of a placental site nodule is a virtual mimic of a cell island in the placenta (Fig. 15–38). Immunoperoxidase stains are of help because the intermediate trophoblast is strongly positive for keratin, moderately positive for human placental lactogen (hPL), and weakly or focally positive for hCG. Although rarely found, villi are usually not associated with placental

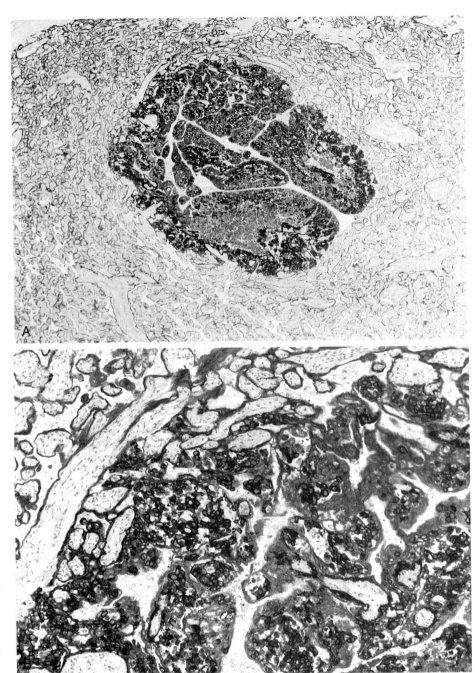

FIGURE 15–34. *A,* Placenta with choriocarcinoma, keratin (AE1/AE3, Boehringer-Mannheim, Indianapolis, IN) immunoperoxidase stain, which highlights the placental nodule of choriocarcinoma. Pale area within tumor is hemorrhagic and necrotic. *B,* Higher-power view of keratin stain showing choriocarcinoma proliferating from the surfaces of normal villi. Some villi even have normal trophoblast on one villous side and choriocarcinoma on the other. (From Lage JM, Roberts DJ: Choriocarcinoma in a term placenta. Pathologic diagnosis of tumor in an asymptomatic patient with metastatic disease. Int J Gynecol Pathol 12:80–85, 1993.)

site nodules.[33] When placental site nodules occur in cycling endometria, the surrounding proliferative or secretory endometrium appears oblivious to their presence. Concomitant gestational endometrium is not a feature of this entity.

DIFFERENTIAL DIAGNOSIS. Placental site nodule is to be distinguished from placental site trophoblastic tumor, choriocarcinoma, invasive squamous cell carcinoma, and normal implantation site. A placental site nodule is a focal lesion, or lesions, **usually superficial** and well-circumscribed, whose orderly columns of intermediate trophoblast radiate from a central core and are enmeshed in fibrin. Placental site trophoblastic tumor is a malignant tumor of intermediate trophoblast that invades the endomyometrium, prompting little tissue reaction or destruction (Fig. 15–39). Differential diagnosis between these two in a hysterectomy specimen offers little

problem. The same is not true in uterine curettings. Uterine curettage of a placental site trophoblastic tumor generally yields a rather generous amount of tumor composed of irregularly shaped cords, small islands, and sheets of bland and monotonous tumor cells (Fig. 15–40), associated with myometrial invasion achieved by splaying apart individual myometrial fibrils. Scattered lymphocytes are admixed with the tumor cells. Necrosis is not too helpful because it tends to be inconspicuous unless the tumor is very large. In contrast, a placental site nodule is formed of a well-circumscribed cluster(s) of intermediate trophoblast radiating out from a paucicellular or hyalinized center (see Fig. 15–37). The trophoblast is confined to the nodule and does not invade surrounding tissues. Mitotic activity and necrosis are minimal. Fibrin (fibrinoid) is a feature of both placental site nodules and

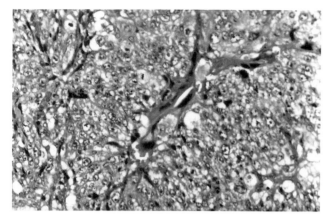

FIGURE 15–35. Choriocarcinoma in a term placenta. Multinucleated syncytiotrophoblast *(center)* lines islands of mononucleate trophoblast.

placental site trophoblastic tumor. Immunoperoxidase stains are of little use, because both are derived from intermediate trophoblast and show similar immunostaining profiles for keratin and hPL. Although scattered hCG immunopositivity is more common in placental site trophoblastic tumors than placental site nodules, this too is non-discriminatory. However, clinical features may be very helpful. Women with placental site trophoblastic tumor usually present with vaginal bleeding

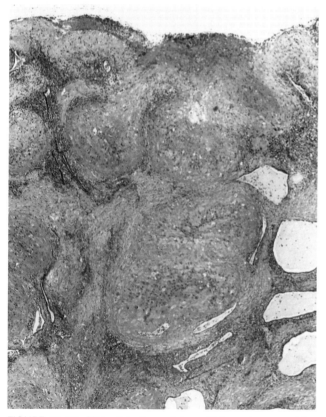

FIGURE 15–36. Placental site nodules within endomyometrium in postpartum uterine curettings. Dilatation and curettage was performed 1 month post partum for persistent vaginal bleeding. Subinvoluted implantation site vessels seen elsewhere may have also contributed to postpartum bleeding.

and an enlarged uterus. Most women with placental site nodules have some menstrual irregularities, but the uterus is not enlarged. Unfortunately, a placental site nodule has been associated with placental site trophoblastic tumor.[33] Because intermediate trophoblastic lesions are uncommon, the pathologist and clinician should discuss the findings, and, if a clear distinction cannot be made, the slides should be submitted for outside consultation.

Choriocarcinoma, a malignant tumor of both syncytiotrophoblast and cytotrophoblast, is a particularly necrotic tumor formed by a proliferation of markedly enlarged, atypical mononuclear trophoblast alternating with foci of recognizable syncytiotrophoblast (Figs. 15–35 and 15–41). Choriocarcinoma extensively invades surrounding normal tissues, and vascular space invasion is an early and constant finding. Because tumor is **incapable of vasculogenesis,** the ensuing **tumor necrosis** is unsurpassed by any other malignancy and becomes the distinguishing feature of choriocarcinoma. Viable tumor is often found only at the "advancing front" of necrotic nodules. Placental site nodules show minimal necrosis and have no syncytiotrophoblast.

Distinguishing a placental site nodule from an invasive, hyalinizing squamous cell carcinoma rests on the nodularity and circumscription of the former and the invasive qualities of the latter. Squamous cell carcinomas demonstrate marked cytologic atypia, invade surrounding normal structures, prompt stromal desmoplasia, and are often associated with overlying squamous carcinoma *in situ* or dysplasia (cervical intraepithelial neoplasia, squamous intraepithelial lesion). Single-cell keratinization or formation of keratin pearls implies a squamous lesion.

Distinguishing a placental site nodule from an implantation site is less difficult. The normal **implantation site,** or one associated with spontaneous abortion, has both stromal trophoblast and intravascular trophoblast. The trophoblast surrounds and invades **large hyalinized vessels.** Most of the trophoblast is intermediate, but some syncytiotrophoblast is present. Fibrin is deposited around the trophoblast in a random, almost haphazard fashion and does not result in the formation of large, eosinophilic nodules as in the placental site nodule. Villous tissue is rarely found with placental site nodules.

Placental Site Trophoblastic Tumor

A placental site trophoblastic tumor is a **malignant tumor of intermediate trophoblast** that **invades myometrium** and is associated with significant maternal morbidity and mortality.[33, 36–40]

CLINICOPATHOLOGIC FEATURES. This rare tumor generally occurs in women in the reproductive age group, although examples in postmenopausal women are described. Most women present with symptoms of **irregular vaginal bleeding,** and on examination the uterus is enlarged. Hysterectomy remains the mainstay of treatment, with adjuvant chemotherapy used for palliation in advanced cases.

Grossly, the tumor may be polypoid, protruding into the endometrium, involve the superficial endomyometrium, or extensively replace the entire uterine corpus. Tumor varies in color and appearance, ranging from small tan-yellow or white nodules to dark-red, bulging tumor masses.

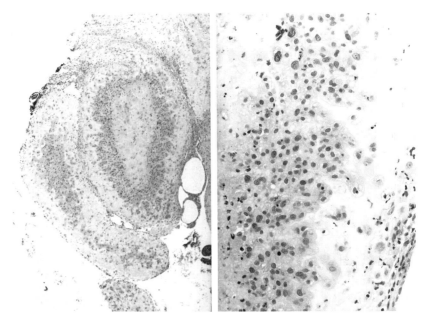

FIGURE 15–37. Placental site nodule. *Left,* Low-power view illustrates two well-circumscribed nodules of mononucleate trophoblast, one of which demonstrates a central fibrin core. *Right,* Higher-power view shows cords of intermediate trophoblast stacked in a somewhat parallel fashion with interspersed fibrin and scattered inflammatory cells. Note benign appearance of trophoblast and lack of mitotic activity.

On microscopy, malignant intermediate trophoblast invades surrounding normal tissues as columns or rows of cells (see Figs. 15–39 and 15–40) **splaying apart myometrial fibrils** without destroying them (Fig. 15–42). The nuclei range from bland and innocuous to enlarged, multilobated, and hyperchromatic. Intranuclear cytoplasmic invaginations are common. The cytoplasm ranges from scant to moderate and is usually clear to amphophilic. Although multinucleated tumor giant cells may be found, only rarely is syncytiotrophoblast present. Mitotic activity is variable, ranging from inconspicuous to moderate. Occasional tumors have large areas of fibrinoid deposition (Fig. 15–43). Some investigators concluded that

numerous mitoses (exceeding 5/10 HPF), extensive necrosis, and strong and diffuse immunostaining for hCG were associated with a poor prognosis.[33, 40] The placental site trophoblastic tumor, being derived from intermediate trophoblast, is **vasculotropic:** The tumor cells appear programmed to transgress the endothelial barrier and somehow remain attached in a parasitic fashion to the endothelium. Neovascularization keeps tumor necrosis at a minimum, although some large tumors have focal necrosis. Recurrences tend to be local, and, in the late stages, tumor grows into contiguous structures and may involve the retroperitoneum and mediastinum. Systemic metastases are generally fatal.[38, 39] Keratin stains are strongly

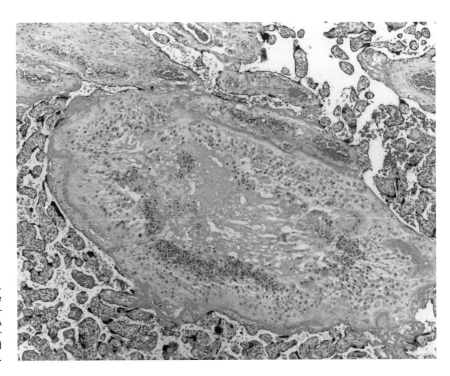

FIGURE 15–38. Cell island of a term placenta. The island is composed of a central loose fibrinoid core, surrounding bland intermediate trophoblast, and outer fibrinoid layer. A few anchoring villi are attached to outer "wall" of this island. Note similarity of cell island to nodules of Figures 15–36 and 15–37.

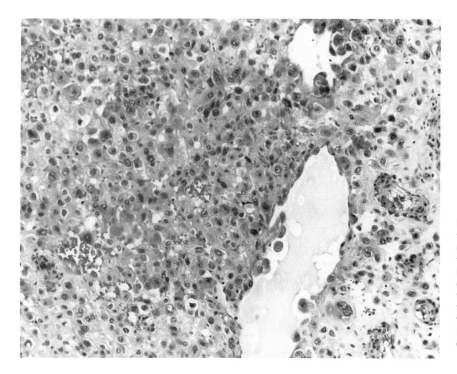

FIGURE 15–39. Placental site trophoblastic tumor, hysterectomy specimen. Tumor is composed of predominantly mononuclear trophoblast, mostly intermediate trophoblast, and possibly some cytotrophoblast with occasional multinucleate cells. No syncytiotrophoblast is present in a placental site trophoblastic tumor. Tumor cells are vasculotropic, attach to the endothelium, and project into the vascular lumina. There is a scattered chronic inflammatory cell infiltrate.

positive; hPL staining is moderate and diffuse, with few hCG-positive cells found. Maternal serum β-hCG levels are only slightly elevated as compared with choriocarcinoma.

DIFFERENTIAL DIAGNOSIS. The differential diagnosis of placental site trophoblastic tumor includes placental site nodule, choriocarcinoma, and, rarely, leiomyosarcoma. Curettings of a placental site nodule show a few to many, eosinophilic, well-circumscribed nodules of intermediate trophoblast enmeshed in fibrin (see Figs. 15–36 and 15–37). These nod-

ules do not invade surrounding structures. That placental site trophoblastic tumor is malignant is undubitable on gross examination of a hysterectomy specimen, but not so in curettings, which may be deceptively bland, composed of sheets and clumps of intermediate trophoblast, some of which is multinucleated, associated with scattered fibrin and lymphocytes. Necrosis tends to be inconspicuous in curettings. No villous tissue is present. Malignancy is recognized by the volume of tumor, lack of circumscription, invasion into sur-

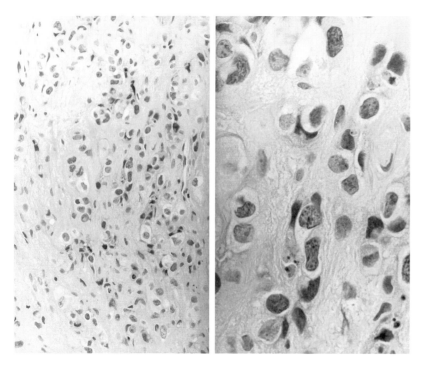

FIGURE 15–40. Placental site trophoblastic tumor, uterine curettings. Tumor is composed of cords of intermediate trophoblast with surrounding fibrin and scattered inflammatory cells. Nuclear detail *(right)* is less than impressive with slight anisocytosis, enlarged nuclei, and inconspicuous to small nucleoli. The fact that this tumor fails to form any rounded structures or nodules, a *sine qua non* for diagnosis of placental site nodule, precludes a benign diagnosis.

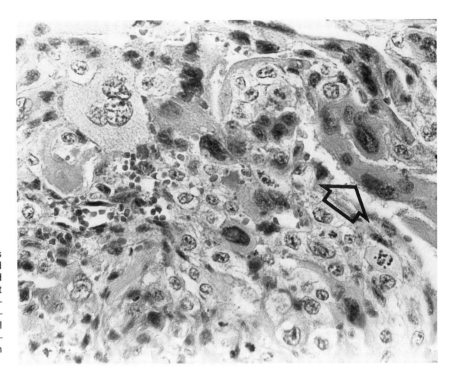

FIGURE 15–41. Choriocarcinoma. Tumor is composed of markedly atypical, gigantic, and bizarre cells that dwarf interspersed red blood cells. Multinucleated syncytiotrophoblast *(arrow)* has striking darkly violaceous cytoplasm, which, although not as easily appreciated in black and white format, is quite helpful in pointing to the correct diagnosis. Spectacular range of cell sizes is not uncommon in gestational choriocarcinoma.

rounding structures, and, in some, increased mitotic activity.

Distinguishing choriocarcinoma from a placental site trophoblastic tumor may be virtually impossible on curettings. Both contain a large proportion of mononuclear trophoblast, much of which is intermediate trophoblast. Choriocarcinoma has admixed syncytiotrophoblast recognized by its multinucleation and violaceous cytoplasm. Choriocarcinoma is far more necrotic and hemorrhagic than placental site trophoblastic tumor. The pattern of uterine wall invasion of these two tumors is different, with placental site trophoblastic tumor invading as single cells, splaying apart myometrial fibrils with little tissue destruction (see Fig. 15–42), and choriocarcinoma replacing and destroying the myometrium. Although placental site trophoblastic tumor may have small necrotic foci, the multifocal widespread necrosis of choriocarcinoma does not occur in placental site trophoblastic tumor. Choriocarcinoma invades vascular spaces but does not cuff around myometrial vessels or attach to endothelium as does placental site trophoblastic tumor. Immunoperoxidase stains may be helpful,

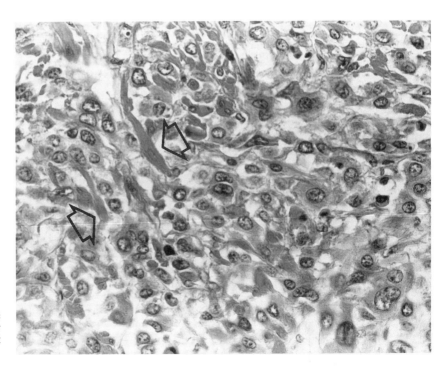

FIGURE 15–42. Placental site trophoblastic tumor. Relatively uniform mononuclear tumor cells infiltrate myometrium, dissecting apart muscle fibrils *(arrows)*. There is no necrosis.

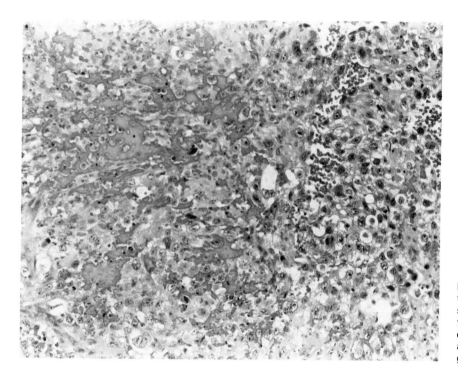

FIGURE 15–43. Placental site trophoblastic tumor. This low-power view of a placental site trophoblastic tumor illustrates abundant fibrin deposition *(left)* and scattered lymphocytic infiltrate. The uniformity of tumor cells and lack of syncytiotrophoblast help distinguish it from choriocarcinoma.

because choriocarcinoma stains strongly for β-hCG and keratin, with some immunostaining for hPL. Likewise, the patient's serum β-hCG level should be quite elevated in choriocarcinoma. A placental site trophoblastic tumor is also keratin-positive, but has more hPL positivity, with only a few rare cells staining for hCG. The patient usually has a low serum β-hCG titer, such as 300 mIU/ml or less. This distinction in practice can be quite difficult, and a clinicopathologic consensus needs to be reached as to the most likely diagnosis, because treatment modalities differ: hysterectomy for placental site trophoblastic tumor and chemotherapy for choriocarcinoma.

Leiomyosarcoma, particularly in its epithelioid form, may mimic the histology of a placental site trophoblastic tumor. It rarely becomes a serious contender, however, because immunoperoxidase stains for smooth muscle markers (such as muscle-specific actin, smooth muscle actin, and desmin) can be used to distinguish myogenous tumors from trophoblast. Trophoblast, be it benign or malignant, is always strongly keratin-positive, and generally far less reactive, if at all, to smooth muscle antibodies.

Gestational Choriocarcinoma

Gestational choriocarcinoma is a malignant tumor of syncytiotrophoblast and cytotrophoblast derived from an initially normal or abnormal conceptus.

CLINICOPATHOLOGIC FEATURES. The incidence of gestational choriocarcinoma varies by geographic location, being highest in women living in Asia. Prevalence rates of 1 in 570 to 1 in 1650 deliveries in Indonesia[16] are much higher than the rate of 1 in 20,000[41] to 1 in 40,000[14] deliveries in the United States. Gestational choriocarcinoma most commonly follows complete hydatidiform mole (as many as 50% of

gestational choriocarcinomas followed complete mole in an older series[42]), although its occurrence subsequent to well-monitored and well-treated complete mole appears to be decreasing.[1,43] As many as one fourth or so follow spontaneous abortion, nearly another one fourth follow normal pregnancy, and a tiny percentage occur after ectopic pregnancies.[42]

Choriocarcinoma usually presents as vaginal bleeding, although a surprising number of other presenting signs and symptoms have been reported. Maternal serum β-hCG level is markedly elevated, and, if the patient is pregnant, its level far exceeds that expected for gestational age. Metastatic lesions are common at time of initial presentation.

Choriocarcinoma after previous molar pregnancy is more chemosensitive than that developing after a previous normal delivery. This may well be a result of the influence of DNA content and parental origin. Choriocarcinoma after normal delivery is usually diploid and heterozygous, having a karyotype quite similar to that of the previous normal gestation,[44–46] whereas that which follows complete mole is completely homozygous and androgenetic (paternal) in origin,[44] just as is the mole, and may be aneuploid.

On gross examination, choriocarcinoma in a uterus forms poorly circumscribed, large dark red to black hemorrhagic nodules that may project into the endometrial cavity or invade deeply into the uterine wall extending through myometrium to the serosa. Multiplicity of nodules and large areas of necrosis are characteristic.

Microscopically, choriocarcinoma is characterized by a proliferation of malignant **mononuclear trophoblast** (usually cytotrophoblast and intermediate trophoblast in various combinations) punctuated by islands of recognizable syncytiotrophoblast (see Figs. 15–35 and 15–41). **Syncytiotrophoblast** has abundant, violaceous to blue cytoplasm, and multiple small and inconspicuous nuclei with occasional eosinophilic nucleoli. Bizarre nuclei within syncytiotrophoblast may be seen. The mononuclear trophoblast is characterized by a moderate amount of pale, clear, or slightly eosinophilic, and slightly granular cytoplasm. Nuclei are large and multilobated, with coarse chromatin and large eosinophilic nucleoli. Choriocarcinoma always leaves its calling card of **widespread hemorrhagic necrosis.** Because the **tumor cannot form blood vessels,** enlarging tumor masses soon become ischemic and necrotic. Viable tumor cells persist at the periphery of large necrotic masses. The early and prominent **vascular invasion** accounts for its proclivity to disseminate systemically. A diagnosis of choriocarcinoma in curettings requires clear-cut endomyometrial and/or vascular space invasion. **Atypical, predominantly mononucleate, trophoblast of a degenerating (previllous) implantation site must be excluded.** Except for tumors arising in ''normal'' placentas, choriocarcinoma is not diagnosed in the presence of villi. Immunoperoxidase stains distinguish choriocarcinoma from other malignant tumors because all trophoblast is strongly keratin-positive; in addition, syncytiotrophoblast is immunopositive for hCG, and intermediate trophoblast is usually reactive for hPL.

DIFFERENTIAL DIAGNOSIS. The differential diagnosis of gestational choriocarcinoma includes placental site trophoblastic tumor (discussed earlier), poorly differentiated carcinoma, leiomyosarcoma, and placental site nodule (discussed elsewhere in this chapter).

A poorly differentiated adenocarcinoma or squamous cell carcinoma sometimes causes diagnostic confusion with trophoblast lesions, particularly when the tumor deeply invades the myometrium and is so poorly differentiated that it lacks gland formation or keratinization. Invasive carcinoma may incite stromal desmoplasia, a feature not observed in trophoblastic tumors. In some instances, examination of multiple sections fortuitously discloses an *in situ* component in the overlying epithelium, clinching the diagnosis. The cervical/uterine carcinomas lack the diagnostic syncytiotrophoblast and extensive tumor necrosis of a choriocarcinoma. Because all these tumors stain for keratin, immunoperoxidase stains for hCG and hPL are often more discriminatory. Thorough evaluation of tumor morphology combined with immunostaining results, patient's serum β-hCG level and previous pregnancy history are usually helpful in formulating a final diagnosis.

Distinguishing a largely mononuclear choriocarcinoma from a leiomyosarcoma, particularly an epithelioid one with copious, dense cytoplasm, may be difficult. Extensive tissue sampling and careful searching for syncytiotrophoblast should be undertaken. The patient's history of recent pregnancy, particularly if molar pregnancy, as well as elevated serum β-hCG level should suggest a trophoblastic tumor. Absent syncytiotrophoblast and the pattern of reactivity to immunoperoxidase stains, including keratin, smooth muscle markers, hCG, and hPL, should be diagnostic (see previous discussion).

The placental site nodule may suggest choriocarcinoma if sampling is limited and the nodule(s) distorted by the curette. In such instances, histology discloses small foci of trophoblast, some of which has mitotic activity, and admixed fibrin. The clinical setting, patient's low or negative β-hCG value, and lack of syncytiotrophoblast and extensive necrosis should point to placental site nodule. Positive serum β-hCG results, presence of syncytiotrophoblast, extensive hemorrhagic

necrosis, and vascular and stromal invasion favor choriocarcinoma.

UNUSUAL INFLAMMATORY AND REACTIVE LESIONS OF THE PLACENTAL VILLI

Chronic Villitis

Chronic villitis is a benign placental villous lesion in which **lymphocytes and mononuclear cells infiltrate villi.**

CLINICOPATHOLOGIC FEATURES. Chronic villitis results from a **chronic fetoplacental infection** or from an **immunologic reaction.**[47-51] Numerous studies suggest that most chronic villitis is immunologic in origin, resulting from inherent abnormalities of normal maternal immune tolerance of the fetoplacental graft. Helper T lymphocytes and activated macrophages that react with monoclonal antibodies to D-related human leukocyte antigen infiltrate the villi.[47] Studies using *in situ* interphase cytogenetics with X and Y chromosome–specific probes suggest that the lymphocytes invading the chronic villi are *maternal* in origin, challenging some of our most basic concepts of maternal-placental interaction.[52]

Chronic villitis involves a small proportion of placentas, with reported incidences of 13.6% and 7.6%.[49] When carefully sought, including examination of as many as 13.4 blocks per case and diagnosis by immunohistochemical means, its incidence is boosted to 76% in normal term placentas.[50] A study from Sweden involving a homogeneous population with good socioeconomic standard found chronic villitis more commonly in placentas of small-for-gestational-age infants (7.5%) as compared with appropriate-for-gestational-age infants (2.8%).[53] Of the known infectious causes, chronic villitis associated with cytomegalovirus (CMV),[54] syphilis,[55, 56] herpes simplex virus (HSV),[57] rubella,[58] and toxoplasmosis[59] is well documented. One study found no association between chronic villitis and hypertension, preeclampsia, smoking, or maternal fever during pregnancy.[53]

Grossly, the **placenta** with chronic villitis is generally **large, pale, and boggy.** It may also be small or have a normal appearance. By microscopy, the involved villi are enlarged, being distended by a stromal infiltrate of **lymphocytes, plasma cells, and mononuclear cells** (Figs. 15–44 to 15–46). As the process progresses, associated findings include villous stromal and trophoblast necrosis, villous scarring with obliteration of fetal vessels, hemosiderin deposition, calcification, and fibrin coating the surface of affected villi (Figs. 15–47 and 15–48).

The first step in the evaluation of chronic villitis is to look for viral inclusions. **Cytomegalovirus** infection (Figs. 15–49 and 15–50) results in focal villous necrosis, lymphoplasmocytic infiltration, and classic **owl-eye inclusions** involving endothelial cells, possibly stromal cells, and/or Hofbauer cells, and, rarely, syncytiotrophoblast.[54] Amnion, amnionic macrophages, and decidual cells may contain viral inclusions.[60] The stromal and/or Hofbauer cells may be enlarged with slightly lobated and cleaved nuclei.[61, 62]

Toxoplasmosis is most easily found in the **placental membranes** and **umbilical cord,** where the encysted organisms, 200 μm in diameter, inhabit macrophages (Fig. 15–51) prior

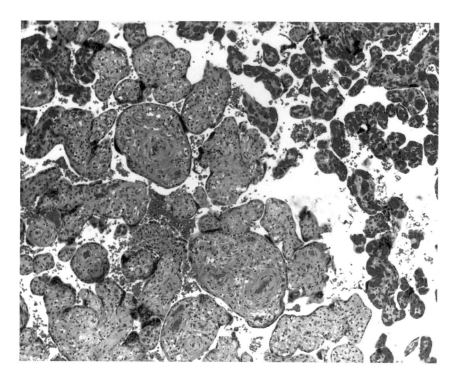

FIGURE 15–44. Chronic villitis is characterized by villous enlargement and hypercellularity. Compare sizes of villi at left and center with the sizes of normal villi in the upper right corner. Villi with chronic villitis are hypercellular, being infiltrated by normal-appearing lymphocytes and macrophages/monocytes. Some villi are fibrotic.

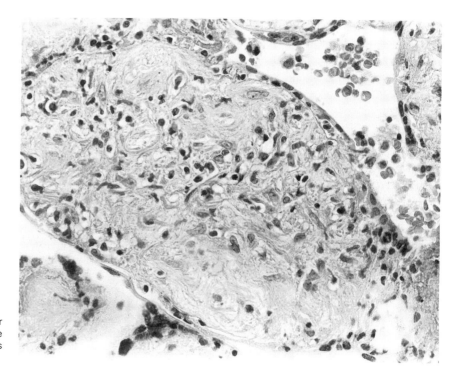

FIGURE 15–45. Chronic villitis, high-power view. Villus is slightly fibrotic, with increase in stromal/mesenchymal cells as well as increase in chronic inflammatory cells.

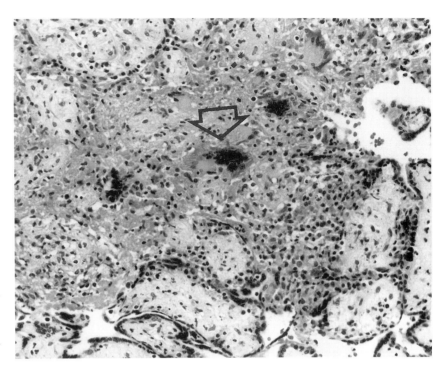

FIGURE 15–46. Chronic villitis. In this instance, the villous architecture is destroyed. The affected villi are fibrotic and agglutinated by intervillous fibrin and a predominantly histiocytic infiltrate that forms multinucleated giant cells *(arrow)*. Villous trophoblast is destroyed. Lymphocytes are also increased. Although these changes may be seen in varicella infection, they are not pathognomonic.

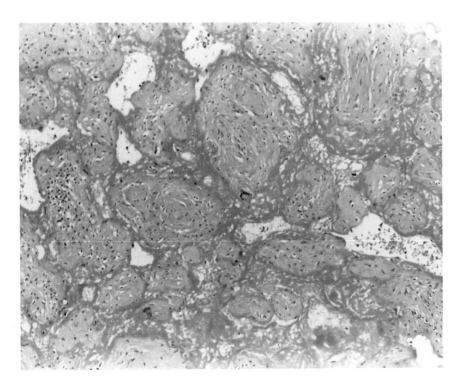

FIGURE 15–47. Chronic villitis, end-stage destruction. Villi are almost completely fibrotic, with residual lymphocytic villous stromal infiltrate appreciated in villi near left side of photograph. The villous trophoblast is destroyed, villous vessels are obliterated, and the intervillous space is filled with fibrin.

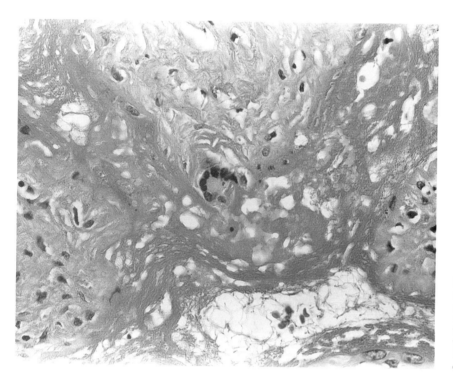

FIGURE 15–48. Chronic villitis, higher-power view of center of Figure 15–47. Villi are coated with dense fibrin. A multinucleated giant cell remains juxtaposed between the fibrin and the villous surface. The villous stroma is fibrotic, with only scattered mononuclear inflammatory cells and villous mesenchymal cells remaining.

to their release as tiny (2–4 μm × 4–8 μm), free organisms. In placentas infected with *Toxoplasma gondii*, the organisms reside freely or within macrophages of the placental membranes, umbilical cord, and amniocytes, where, in most instances, they remain totally unperturbed by any inflamma-

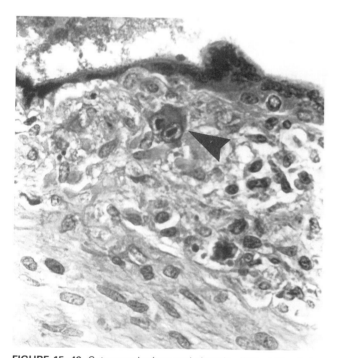

FIGURE 15–49. Cytomegalovirus and chronic villitis. Villus is hypercellular with lymphohistiocytic infiltrate. An infected cell *(center)* displays two nuclei containing large, eosinophilic intranuclear inclusions simulating owl-eye appearance *(arrowhead)* and increased, darkened cytoplasm that contains basophilic cytoplasmic inclusions. There is villous stromal destruction with necrosis.

tory infiltrate.[63] Occasionally, in long-standing lesions, calcification occurs, particularly in the umbilical cord, and is associated with some surrounding chronic inflammation. The placenta tends to be large and pale with a spectrum of villous lesions ranging from slight lymphocytic chronic villitis with minimal fibrosis to a proliferative villitis with prominent lymphocytes, plasma cells, and histiocytes. Villous endarteritis, necrosis, and fibrosis may occur.[59] Villous normoblastemia and erythroblastemia reflect fetal anemia. The decidua has focal chronic deciduitis.

Congenital **syphilitic infections** are characterized by a **large, boggy, pale placenta** and **relative villous immaturity,** with villi being larger and more cellular than expected for gestational age. The chronic villitis of syphilis is lymphoplasmocytic, with **prominent plasma cells** a common hallmark. Early cases tend to have foci of acute villitis as well.[56] But the most striking finding is a **villous endarteritis** with endovascular proliferation resulting in a "buckshot" appearance of the villi, with inflammatory cells radiating outward from the destroyed central vessel and into the surrounding, edematous villous stroma (Figs. 15–52 and 15–53). Villous endovascular proliferation narrows the vessel lumen and impedes blood flow to distal villi. The endothelium and portions of the vessel walls and villous stroma become necrotic. Although villous vasculitis is a striking feature, it is not pathognomonic, because it may be found in other viral infections such as cytomegalovirus and rubella.[64] The **umbilical cord** may be host to a dense, acute or chronic necrotizing perivascular inflammation (funisitis) in which the diagnostic **spirochetes,** highlighted by Warthin-Starry stain, may be identified after diligent searching.[55, 56] In addition, congenital syphilis characteristically causes a **severe fetal anemia,** and the ensuing villous erythroblastemia and normoblastemia may be the first clue to diagnosis of fetal/neonatal congenital syphilis. In a study of histologically confirmed syphilitic placentas by

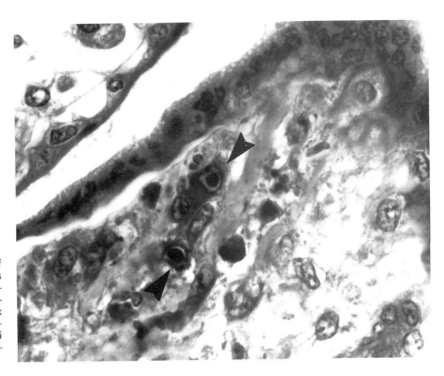

FIGURE 15–50. Cytomegalovirus. Portions of two villi are illustrated. Villous stroma contains cells infected with cytomegalovirus *(arrowheads)* exhibiting large, eosinophilic intranuclear inclusions and abundant dark cytoplasm with basophilic inclusions. Karyorrhectic debris is in background. Elsewhere villi contain plasma cells, and villous stromal calcification is found.

Qureshi et al., the following were characteristic of infected placentas: marked proliferative vascular changes, villous immaturity and hypercellularity, and chronic villitis with or without acute villitis. These investigators did not find chronic chorioamnionitis in any of these specimens.[56]

It is always surprising to me that we have such difficulty identifying **herpes simplex** infection in the placenta. Even in instances of fetal death *in utero* from disseminated herpes infection, the placenta fails to offer any clue as to the existence of congenital herpes infection. Placental herpes simplex infection results from **hematogenous dissemination** or by **ascending infection.** The classic ground-glass inclusions easily identified in other infected sites are rarely found in the placenta. Inclusions in the amnion, chorion, and decidua have been described in H&E-stained material, but infected cells seem to be more easily identified by *in situ* hybridization for HSV-specific DNA than by routine histology.[65-67] Other placental findings in known herpes infections include acute

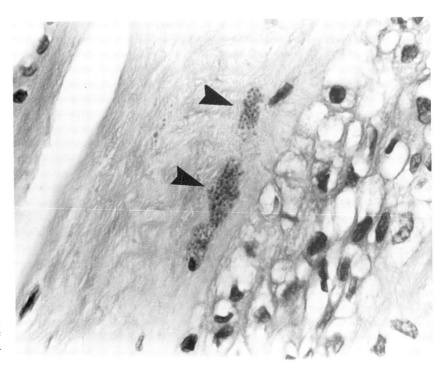

FIGURE 15–51. Toxoplasmosis. Extraplacental membranes (amnion in upper left) containing encysted *Toxoplasma* organisms *(arrowheads).* Note complete absence of associated inflammatory infiltrate. Underlying chorion appears uninvolved.

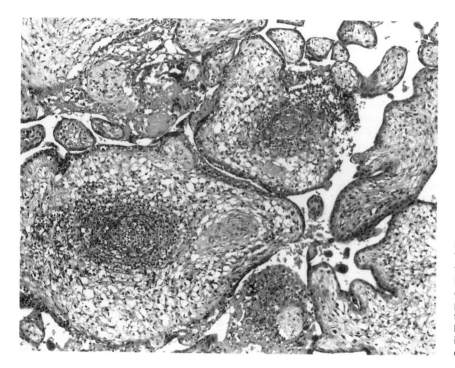

FIGURE 15–52. Congenital syphilis infection. Transverse section of villi exhibits characteristic vasocentric chronic inflammation resulting in buckshot appearance. There is destruction of the endothelium with endovascular and perivascular fibroblastic proliferation and virtual complete obliteration of vessel lumina. Focal subtrophoblastic accumulation of inflammatory cells results in partial avulsion of villous trophoblast *(right of center).*

or subacute chorioamnionitis with amnion necrosis, chronic chorioamnionitis, villous edema, chronic lymphoplasmacytic villitis, villous vasculitis, and villous trophoblast necrosis with surrounding fibrin deposition.[65-68] In a recently reported case, only the maternal-derived cells of the decidua capsularis exhibited immunohistochemical staining with antibodies for herpes simplex virus type 2.[68] Placental villi and trophoblast were negative.

Other more exotic infections such as **coccidioidomycosis, varicella, Epstein-Barr virus,** enteric cytopathogenic human orphan virus 33 (**ECHO 33**) and **ECHO 27,** and *Trypanosoma cruzi* (**Chagas' disease**), among others, have been reported to cause chronic villitis and are well described in textbooks encompassing placental pathology.[64, 69, 70]

DIFFERENTIAL DIAGNOSIS. The differential diagnosis of chronic villitis includes villous abnormalities resulting from fetal artery thrombosis, acute villitis, and secondary villitis due to adjacent infarct. In fetal artery thrombosis, the villi are somewhat enlarged and the villous stroma fibrotic. Lymphocytic infiltrate is minimal and, if prominent, should prompt

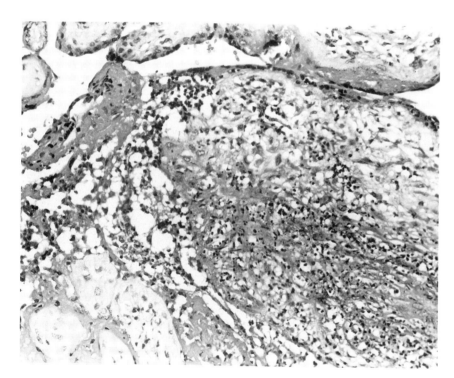

FIGURE 15–53. Congenital syphilis infection, higher-power view. Longitudinal section of villi illustrating the degree of endovascular damage with necrosis of endothelium, obliteration of vessel lumen, and stromal necrosis. Subtrophoblastic inflammatory cells, mostly lymphocytes with some fragmented cells, probably neutrophils, seen at villous surface. Early fibrin deposition. The villi at lower left are fibrotic.

a search for other evidence of chronic villitis. Acute villitis mimics chronic villitis in that inflammatory cells infiltrate villi in both. However, in acute villitis, the inflammatory cells are neutrophils that cap the villous surface and invade the villous stroma from without. In contrast, lymphocytes and mononuclear cells characterize the villous infiltrate in chronic villitis, and the villous surface, though sometimes coated with fibrin, is free of neutrophilic aggregation. The villi surrounding an infarct may also have an inflammatory infiltrate containing a mixture of inflammatory cells with neutrophils usually predominating. In this instance, the villous inflammation results from proximity to an infarct and does not involve villi away from the edge of the infarct.

Acute Villitis

Acute villitis is characterized by a **neutrophilic inflammatory infiltrate involving placental villi.**
CLINICOPATHOLOGIC FEATURES. Most commonly, acute villitis occurs in the setting of **maternal septicemia.** Seeding of either decidua or intervillous space by infectious organisms provides a route for fetal villous infection. Pathogens known to cause acute villitis include *Listeria monocytogenes* and enteric and gram-negative organisms. Cultures of maternal blood or cervix taken antepartum, postpartum placental cultures from the subamnionic tissues in the chorionic plate, or neonatal cultures may yield the infectious agent.

Maternal infection by *L. monocytogenes,* a diphtheroid bacillus, is associated with second trimester spontaneous abortion and may be lethal to newborns.[71-73] The affected fetus often has a pustular skin rash and multiorgan microabscesses, commonly involving adrenals, lung, and liver, as well as acute alveolitis.[72]

Cross-sectioning of the placental parenchyma in acute villitis may expose **macroscopic microabscesses** as well as cloudy, opaque membranes caused by chorioamnionitis. Occasionally the placenta is foul-smelling. Microscopy discloses chorioamnionitis, acute villitis with microabscesses (Fig. 15–54), and occasionally funisitis. The villi display focal subtrophoblastic collections of neutrophils with some admixed fibrin. As these neutrophilic aggregates expand, the trophoblast becomes avulsed, fibrin increases, the intervillous space is obliterated by neutrophils and admixed fibrin, and contiguous villi agglutinate. Adherent maternal neutrophils invade the villous stroma from ''without'' (see Fig. 15–54), and villous destruction ensues. These larger abscesses, generally associated with villous agglutination and necrosis, become macroscopically visible.[74] Villous vascular endarteritis, similar to that of syphilitic infections, develops later, although the vascular infiltrate in listeriosis tends to be purely neutrophilic with less lymphocytes. In **gram-negative infections,** placental villi are also coated with fibrin and neutrophils, producing **microabscesses.** This is accompanied by chorioamnionitis involving the extraplacental fetal membranes, and the chorionic plate and umbilical cord are also inflamed. Gram or Brown-Brenn stains offer clues as to the type of organism(s) involved, with diagnosis confirmed by culture results or serologic tests.
DIFFERENTIAL DIAGNOSIS. Acute villitis is to be distinguished from chronic villitis and villous inflammation at the periphery of an infarct. In chronic villitis, the inflammatory infiltrate is mononuclear, composed of lymphocytes, monocytes, and plasma cells (see Figs. 15–44 to 15–46 and 15–49), whereas in acute villitis, mature maternal neutrophils infiltrate the villous stroma (see Figs. 15–52 to 15–54). Villous inflammation adjacent to a placental infarct is morphologically similar to acute villitis. However, it results from proximity to the infarct and is not found elsewhere in the placenta. True acute villitis is often associated with chorioamnionitis, umbilical vasculitis (funisitis), and sometimes chorionic vasculitis.

Choriangiosis

In 1984, Altshuler defined choriangiosis as a **proliferation of 10 or more fetal blood vessels in 10 villi in 10 fields of non-infarcted and non-ischemic zones in three different areas of the placenta using a ×10 objective.**[75]
CLINICOPATHOLOGIC FEATURES. Choriangiosis consists of a distinct increase in the number of villous blood vessels in a given unit of placenta (Figs. 15–55 and 15–56). Some have challenged this notion by suggesting that choriangiosis represents distention of normal, previously extant, although perhaps collapsed, blood vessels. In one series, choriangiosis was associated with poor perinatal outcome.[75] Altshuler opines that it is ''a manifestation of idiopathic placental malperfusion.''[76] In my experience, true placental choriangiosis (i.e., correctly diagnosed) is extremely uncommon and deserving of further investigation.

This lesion has no grossly recognizable form. Microscopy is required to fulfill the strict criteria defined here (see Figs. 15–55 and 15–56).
DIFFERENTIAL DIAGNOSIS. When these criteria are applied, the differential diagnosis revolves around diffuse choriangiomatosis (diffuse choriangioma) and choriangiocarcinoma. Diffuse choriangiomatosis is rare, being characterized by markedly distended villi containing numerous blood vessels, with or without an increase in the villous mesenchyme (see Fig. 15–31). The vascular proliferation in choriangiomatosis is far greater than in choriangiosis, with some villi in the former containing 30 to 60 blood vessels, whereas the vessel count in the latter just barely meets 10 in some villi, with others having 15 to 20 blood vessels. Choriangiocarcinoma is characterized by villous vascular proliferation (see Figs. 15–31 and 15–32), but, in contrast with choriangiosis, choriangiocarcinoma has trophoblast hyperplasia, which never occurs in choriangiosis (see previous discussion).

Villous Edema

Villous edema describes **increased villous stromal fluid** that forms **multiple, central- and paracentral-cleared spaces** resembling **Swiss cheese.**
CLINICOPATHOLOGIC FEATURES. In 1983, Naeye et al. drew attention to villous edema, which, in their series, correlated with poor neonatal outcome.[77] It is commonly associated with congenital hydrops of various causes, including congenital viral infection, hematologic disorders, and congenital anomalies, particularly those involving thoracic viscera, although, in many instances, the cause remains unknown. Villous edema occurs in preterm placentas affected with **severe necrotizing chorioamnionitis.** In a study of clinically diagnosed chorio-

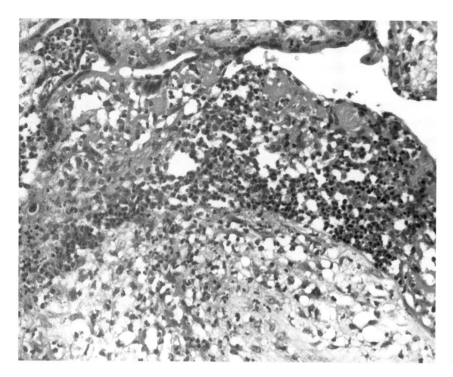

FIGURE 15–54. *Listeria monocytogenes* infection of placenta illustrating acute villitis with villous microabscess. Collections of mature neutrophils and fibrin accumulate between villous trophoblast and the villous stroma. There is early neutrophilic infiltration of villous stroma.

amnionitis, villous edema was present in 62% of placentas and neutrophilic infiltration of the placental plate in 65%.[78] Fox notes that villous edema is difficult to distinguish from villous immaturity and, when found in isolation, discounts its functional significance.[79] Altshuler draws attention to the fact that villous edema in preterm placentas is morphologically different from that observed in term placentas, thus accounting for some of the apparent discrepancies in the reported literature.[76]

A grossly **hydropic placenta** is **heavy for gestational age,** generally **pale, bulky, and thick.** Severely affected placentas may be 5 cm in thickness (chorionic plate to basal plate). Focal villous edema, however, remains a microscopic diagnosis, and unless diffuse, is not recognized on gross examination of the placenta. By microscopy, villous edema produces clear, rounded spaces in the villous stroma, simulating **Swiss cheese** (Figs. 15–57 and 15–58). Some of the "holes" contain macrophages. This sort of Swiss-cheese appearance is most com-

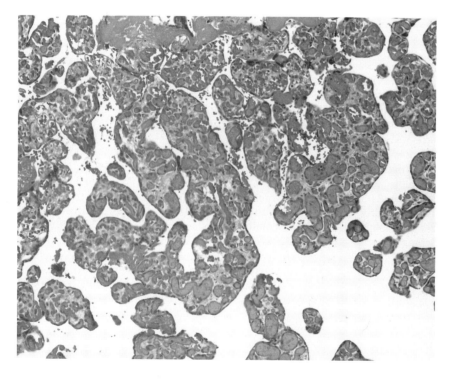

FIGURE 15–55. Chorangiosis. Villi in this field exhibit marked vascular proliferation, with greater than 10 vascular channels in more than 10 villi. Diagnosis requires 10 or more such foci in three different areas of the placenta (see text for formal definition).

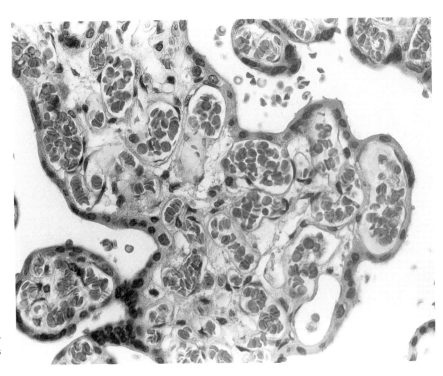

FIGURE 15–56. Chorangiosis, high-power view. This villus is hypervascular and contains more than 10 vascular channels.

monly observed in **preterm villi. Term placentas** exhibit a slightly different form of villous edema in which the edema **"holes" are less rigid** and **more elongate to oblong,** appearing as though the "fluid" has leaked out of whatever space confined it, giving the villous stroma a diffuse "watery" appearance. In some of the edematous villi, the stromal vessels appear collapsed, although larger vessels remain widely patent.

   DIFFERENTIAL DIAGNOSIS. Focal villous edema is to be distinguished from diffuse villous edema and villous immaturity.

The term "villous edema" is often used arbitrarily to connote a *focal* process. As such, it is distinguished from *diffuse* villous edema (hydrops placentalis), in which extensive villous edema (hydrops) involves a large portion of the villi. **Hydrops placentalis** is associated with **placentomegaly** (being heavy for gestational age) (Table 15–2). It is often accompanied by villous normoblastemia and erythroblastemia owing to severe fetal anemia from serious fetal/maternal disorders including hemolytic disease of the newborn such as Rh(D) disease, Kell sensitization, and occasionally ABO incompatibilities. Other

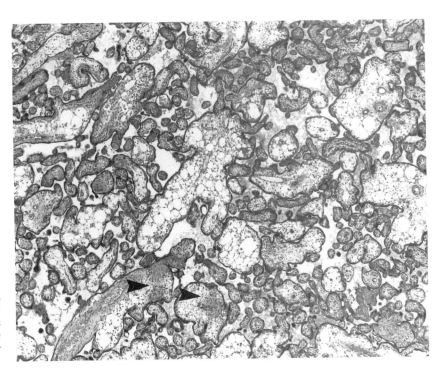

FIGURE 15–57. Villous edema. Immature placenta with marked villous edema associated with cytomegalovirus infection. Focal villous stromal fibrosis and necrosis are due to tissue destruction secondary to active viral replication *(arrows).*

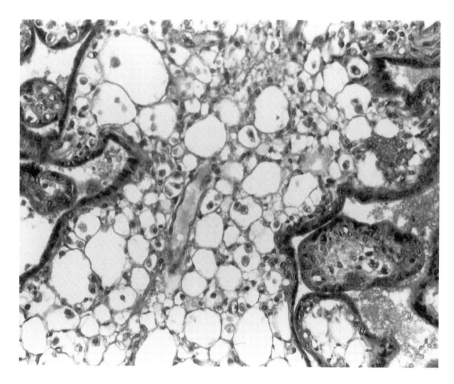

FIGURE 15–58. Villous edema, higher magnification of Fig. 15–57. Villus has open, central vascular channel with innumerable surrounding "Swiss-cheese" holes, many of which contain one or two macrophages.

conditions resulting in diffuse villous edema include alpha-thalassemia, severe fetal-maternal hemorrhage, congenital anomalies including congenital fetal tumors, congenital infections such as parvovirus infection, and congenital nephrotic syndrome (**Finnish nephrosis**). Villous immaturity describes "young," preterm villi that have a loose, pale stroma and numerous Hofbauer cells (macrophages). Although both villous immaturity and villous edema have a clear, loose stroma, the Swiss-cheese appearance characterizing villous edema is not as striking in immature villi.

LESIONS DEFORMING NORMAL PLACENTAL VILLOUS STRUCTURE

Placental Villous Infarct

A placental infarct is an **area of placental tissue that** having lost its maternal perfusion **is dying or dead.**

Table 15–2. **Conditions Associated with Placentomegaly**

Diabetes mellitus, maternal
Blood dyscrasia, fetal-maternal
Neoplasm, fetal or maternal
Storage disorder, fetal
Chronic fetal infection
Fetal macrosomia, including Beckwith-Wiedemann syndrome
Multiple gestations
Anemia, maternal or fetal
Hydrops fetalis, not otherwise specified

Modified from Gompel C, Silverberg SG (eds): Pathology in Gynecology and Obstetrics, 4th ed. Philadelphia, JB Lippincott, 1993.

CLINICOPATHOLOGIC FEATURES. Infarcts are extremely rare in immature placentas. A single infarct in an otherwise normal *term* placenta is common and, by implication, a normal finding.[80] In contrast, **extensive placental infarction** is usually associated with **severe uteroplacental insufficiency** and **poor fetal outcome.** The more extensive the total area infarcted, the greater the perinatal morbidity and mortality. Multiple infarcts reflect serious maternal diseases such as **pre-eclampsia, eclampsia,** and **hypertension.** They are occasionally found in pregnancies complicated by **diabetes mellitus** or **collagen vascular diseases** such as lupus erythematosus. Retroplacental hemorrhage with abruptio is an uncommon but serious condition that may cause extensive placental infarction. As a rule of thumb, placental infarction involving more than 10% of placental villous tissue is considered significant.

Placental infarcts develop when maternal blood flow from the decidual vessels fails to reach the intervillous space. This is usually due to maternal **decidual vasculopathy (acute atherosis,** early atheromatous change), a condition of early atherosis affecting maternal blood vessels of the implantation site and the extraplacental membranes.[81, 82] Decidual vasculopathy is associated with pregnancies complicated by pre-eclampsia,[82] eclampsia, small-for-gestational age infants,[82–85] and hypertension.[86, 87] It is less common in diabetes mellitus[86, 88] and collagen vascular diseases such as lupus erythematosus.[89] **It does not occur in placentas from normal, uncomplicated pregnancies.** Microscopically, decidual vasculopathy has a variety of appearances, all of which are characterized by (1) varying degrees of **luminal and/or concentric fibrin (fibrinoid) deposition** in the vessel walls and (2) infiltration by **macrophages** and **lymphocytes** with occasional plasma cells (Figs. 15–59 to 15–62). Rarely, cholesterol clefts may form (see Fig. 15–62). The similarities of decidual vasculopathy and the vascular changes of allograft transplant rejection suggest a common immunologic etiology.[90]

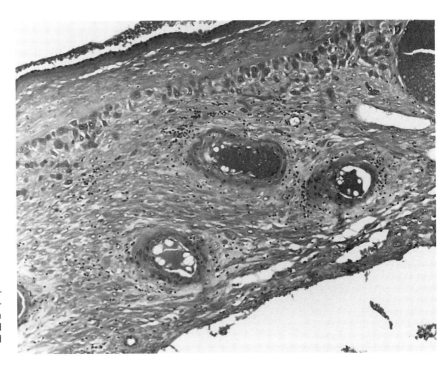

FIGURE 15–59. Decidual vasculopathy. Extraplacental membranes (amnion, *upper left corner*) exhibiting thickened maternal vessels in decidua. Vessel walls have dense fibrinoid deposit and infiltrate of macrophages and lymphocytes.

The gross characteristics of a placental infarct change as it ages. Very fresh infarcts are best identified by palpation rather than by inspection. Recent infarcts are red and well-demarcated from the surrounding parenchyma. As the infarct ages, its color blanches, turning pale to white over time.

On microscopy, the villi of an early infarct crowd together as the maternal intervillous space collapses (Fig. 15–63). Blood from fetal villous vessels may extravasate into the surrounding villous stroma (see Fig. 15–63). Over time, syn-

cytiotrophoblast nuclear and cytoplasmic staining fade, the fetal erythrocytes and vascular endothelium degenerate, and the villous stroma blanches (Fig. 15–64). There may be slight perivillous fibrin deposition. Villi at the edge of the infarct become enshrouded with maternal neutrophils and some fibrinoid. The oldest infarcts are characterized by closely packed "ghost villi" whose outlines alone offer clues as to their original form (Fig. 15–65). For some unknown reason, in infarcts due to abruptio placentae, the dead villi are sur-

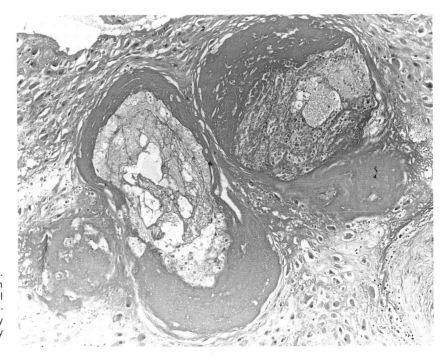

FIGURE 15–60. Decidual vasculopathy. Decidua of extraplacental membranes with markedly enlarged and distended maternal vessels containing concentric fibrinoid deposition in vessel walls. Vessel lumina are virtually obliterated by macrophages and, in one, by partial thrombosis.

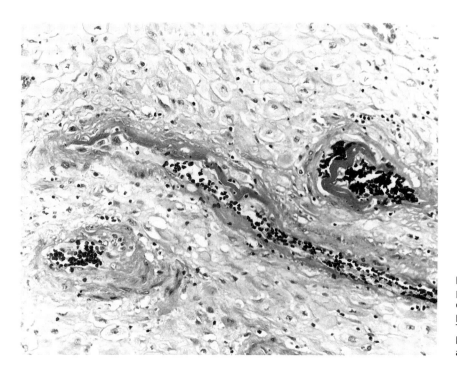

FIGURE 15–61. Decidual vasculopathy. High-power view of extraplacental membranes demonstrating three vessels (central one in profile) affected by decidual vasculopathy. There is fibrin deposition in vessels, which on H&E-stained sections is brightly eosinophilic, and scattered lymphocytes and macrophages.

rounded by wide-open, almost dilated intervillous spaces, in contrast with the collapsed intervillous spaces of infarcts due to decidual vasculopathy.[91]

DIFFERENTIAL DIAGNOSIS. The differential diagnosis of a placental infarct includes intervillous thrombus, fetal artery thrombosis, chorangioma, and metastatic tumor. All of these are somewhat similar, grossly forming a white to cream, slightly firm, wedge-shaped or rounded nodule. An intervillous thrombus is a blood clot or "hemorrhage" that displaces surrounding villi and laminates over time. In a fetal artery thrombosis, the villous stroma is fibrotic, yet the villous syncytiotrophoblast remains viable as maternal perfusion of the intervillous space continues (Fig. 15–66), whereas, even in

a very fresh infarct, loss of maternal blood flow results in pallor to the syncytiotrophoblastic nuclei and its cytoplasm loses its violaceous to amphophilic staining. A chorangioma is a proliferation of fetal blood vessels distending a single villus or nest of villi. When infarcted, a chorangioma loses differential staining, resulting in pallor and faint eosinophilia of all villous components. An infarcted chorangioma is recognized by the outlines of its enlarged villi and numerous empty villous stromal spaces, formerly the capillary lumina. Extramedullary hematopoiesis or erythropoiesis, a common finding in chorangiomas, remains identifiable even in an infarcted chorangioma because the marrow elements retain nuclear staining long after the surrounding cells fade. Hematopoiesis

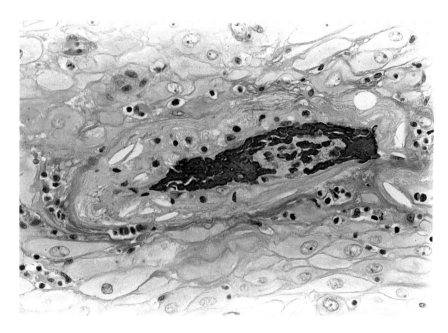

FIGURE 15–62. Decidual vasculopathy. High-power view of decidua from extraplacental membranes exhibiting thickened vessel wall with lymphocytic and macrophage infiltrate and formation of cholesterol clefts.

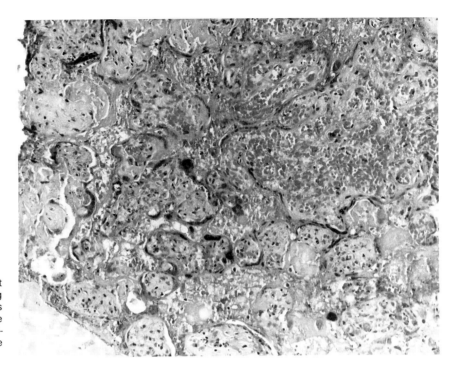

FIGURE 15–63. Fresh (early) placental infarct *(center).* Villi appear crowded together owing to collapse of intervillous space. There is slight pallor to the villous trophoblast. The villous stroma contains extravasated erythrocytes. Villi on the left edge of photograph are sclerotic.

does not occur in an infarct. Metastatic tumors involving the placenta, including adenocarcinoma of the breast, melanoma, and squamous cell carcinoma, are distinguished from an infarct by identification of well-preserved chorionic villi surrounded by viable metastatic tumor filling and distending the intervillous spaces. In an infarct, the pale villi are usually tightly crowded together, obliterating the intervillous space.

Fetal Artery Thrombosis

Cessation of blood flow through a placental fetal artery causes a loss of fetal villous perfusion eventuating in **avascular villi.**

CLINICOPATHOLOGIC FEATURES. **Fetal artery thrombosis** is uncommon in placentas, occurring in 4.5% of carefully examined term placentas.[92] It is probably even less frequently

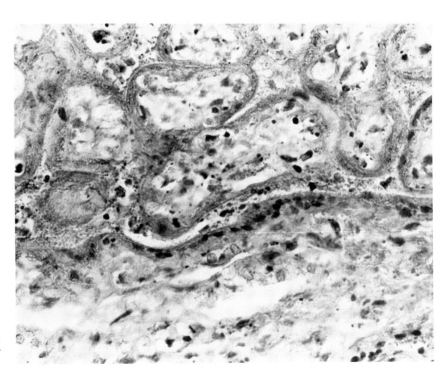

FIGURE 15–64. Fresh (early) placental infarct. Villi are closely approximated and show loss of trophoblastic staining. Villous stroma contains some karyorrhectic debris.

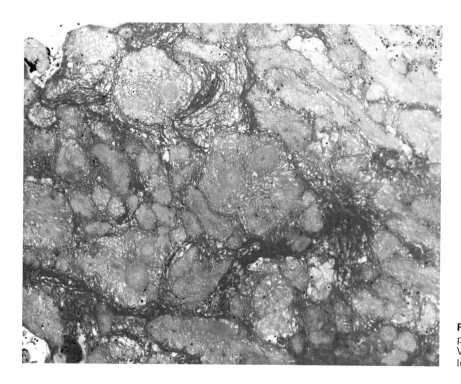

FIGURE 15–65. Older placental infarct. Low-power view of rather large placental infarct. Villi are closely approximated, pale, and acellular. Some are coated with fibrin.

recognized in daily practice. Fetal artery thrombosis is more common in placentas from **diabetic women.**[88, 92] According to Fox, loss of fetal perfusion to a small portion (i.e., <20% to 30%) of villous tissue is generally of no consequence, although extensive involvement results in fetal death *in utero.*[79]

On gross examination, fetal artery thrombosis is a white villous lesion indistinguishable from a placental infarct. It is **triangular in shape,** with its **base facing the basal plate.** On microscopy, the **villi are avascular,** and the villous stroma fibrotic (see Fig. 15–66). The **syncytiotrophoblastic nuclei are well-preserved** as a result of ongoing maternal perfusion of the intervillous space. Often, some of the thrombosed villi are encased in fibrin, and syncytial knots are increased focally.

DIFFERENTIAL DIAGNOSIS. The differential diagnosis of a fetal artery thrombosis is identical to that previously described for a placental infarct.

Fetal Metabolic Storage Diseases Affecting Placental Villi

Fetal metabolic (storage) disorders are **diseases that result in abnormal accumulations of metabolic by-products.** The placental tissues are affected in various ways, depending on the specific disease.

CLINICOPATHOLOGIC CORRELATION. The most common storage disorders affecting the placenta are GM_1 gangliosidosis (type 1),[93] I-cell disease (inclusion cell disease, mucolipidosis type II),[94] mucopolysaccharidosis type IV (Morquio's disease),[95] glycogen storage disease type II,[96] Niemann-Pick disease type A,[97] and sialic acid storage disorder.[98] Accumulation of metabolic by-products eventuates in **cytoplasmic distention** and **vacuolization of affected cells.** The type and extent of placental involvement are determined by the specific

genetic defect. Cytoplasmic alterations are demonstrated in a variety of placental cell types, including syncytiotrophoblast, cytotrophoblast, intermediate trophoblast, amnion, Hofbauer cells, capillary endothelium, and stroma (Figs. 15–67 and 15–68). Enumerating the specific cells involved in each disease is beyond the scope of this chapter. Roberts et al. provide a review of placental findings in storage disorders.[93] A summary of even greater clinical and pathologic detail is furnished by Benirschke and Kaufmann.[69] Readers are referred to these references for assistance in the evaluation of a specific case. Special stains for mucopolysaccharides (periodic acid-Schiff [PAS] with and without diastase, alcian blue at acidic pH levels, and colloidal iron) and lipids (oil red O) may be helpful in demonstrating the abnormal storage product. Clinical, biochemical, and electron microscopic studies are required to confirm the histologic impression of a storage disorder.

DIFFERENTIAL DIAGNOSIS. Abnormal placental cellular morphology consistent with that of a storage disorder must be distinguished from abnormal histomorphology caused by incorrect tissue handling and/or storage conditions, amnionic vacuolization due to fetal gastroschisis or meconium release, and increased Hofbauer cells associated with placental hydrops. Perturbations of normal placental processes, i.e., dropping the placenta in water or soap solutions, and freezing or overheating the tissues, alter cellular appearances and may simulate a storage disorder. Amnionic vacuolization occurs in fetal gastroschisis and meconium release. However, the latter conditions are obvious grossly (gastroschisis) or by associated microscopic findings (pyknosis of amnionic nuclei and pigment-laden macrophages in meconium release). Placental hydrops, also associated with increased number of macrophages, is distinguished from storage disorders by the normalcy of the macrophage cytoplasm, both in quantity and quality, and by its association with other fetoplacental pathology, including villous edema, fetal normoblastemia, chronic

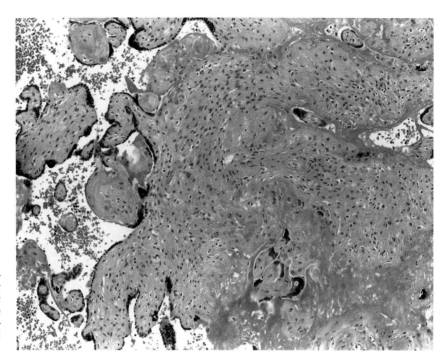

FIGURE 15–66. Fetal artery thrombosis. Occlusion of fetal artery results in fibrotic, avascular villi. Villi right of center are almost completely encased in fibrin, whereas those to the left are fibrotic, with viable surface syncytiotrophoblast and cytotrophoblast due to continued maternal perfusion of the intervillous space.

villitis, fetal anomalies, fetal blood dyscrasias, and chromosomal aberrations.

Placental Thrombus and Hematoma

A **placental thrombus is a blood clot in a placental vascular space.** Thrombi may be subchorionic or intervillous. **Hematomas are hemorrhages developing at marginal, retroplacental, retromembranous, or subamnionic sites.** A marginal or retroplacental hematoma refers to a blood clot at the placental margin in the former or between the (placental) basal plate and the underlying maternal decidua in the latter.

CLINICOPATHOLOGIC FEATURES. Subamnionic hemorrhages develop in the potential space between the amnion and chorion and are visible on inspection of the fetal surface of the placenta. They are of no apparent clinical significance, with the vast majority being caused by umbilical cord traction in an attempt to hasten delivery of the placenta. **Subchorionic thrombus,** called Breus' mole when greater than 1 cm in

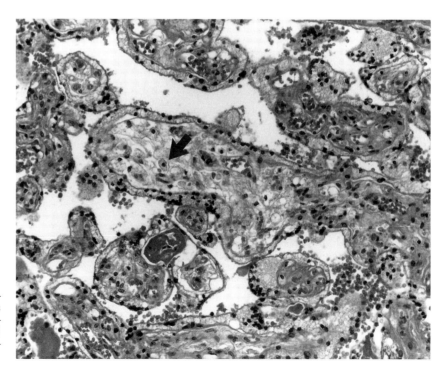

FIGURE 15–67. Placenta with GM$_1$ gangliosidosis (type 1). Term placenta demonstrates enlarged villi with syncytiotrophoblast cytoplasmic distention and vacuolization and increased cytoplasmic vacuolization of stromal Hofbauer cells (macrophages) *(arrow).*

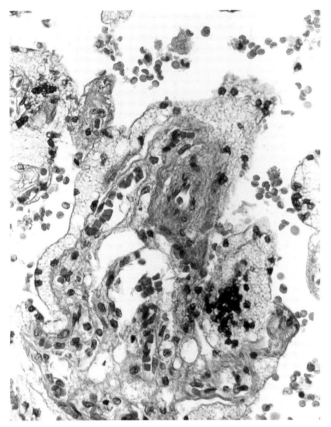

FIGURE 15–68. Placenta with GM₁ gangliosidosis (type 1), higher-power view. Central villous demonstrates marked distention and vacuolization of syncytiotrophoblast cytoplasm. Elsewhere the intermediate trophoblast had vacuolated cytoplasm. In this Bouin's fixed tissue, alcian blue stain at pH 2.5 best highlighted the cytoplasmic accumulation of mucopolysaccharides.

thickness, is thought to be composed of maternal blood.[92, 99, 100] These thrombi involve the space between the overlying chorionic plate and the villous parenchyma proper. When very large, they prolapse with their chorioamnionic covering into the amnionic space. They are visible on antenatal ultrasonographic examination and are associated with spontaneous abortion.

An **intervillous thrombus** is relatively common, occurring in approximately 40% of all placentas,[92] and generally of little clinical significance. As its name implies, it forms in the intervillous space, usually midway between the basal plate and the chorionic plate. Most intervillous thrombi measure 1 to 2 cm in greatest dimension, the larger ones, 3 to 4 cm in greatest dimension (Fig. 15–69). A large intervillous thrombus, or multiple intervillous thrombi may be associated with fetal-maternal transfusion, which, in some instances, causes **fetal anemia**[101] and **maternal sensitization**[102] because some of the blood in the thrombus is of fetal origin. Large intervillous thrombi may obstruct maternal blood flow to the surrounding villi, resulting in villous infarction (Fig. 15–70) and fetal death.

Marginal hematoma occurs at the rim of the placental disk, is crescentic in shape, and may be associated with a placenta previa and antepartum bleeding. It is of little clinical importance unless it enlarges significantly, extends retroplacentally, and causes premature placental separation (abruptio

placentae). **Retroplacental hematomas** are the most dangerous of the placental hematomas and the most likely to be associated with poor fetal outcome. Maternal blood dissecting between the placenta and its attachment to the maternal decidua may cause partial or complete abruptio placentae. Small retroplacental hematomas (i.e., < 2 cm in size) are usually inconsequential. Retroplacental hematomas may remain ''concealed'' until after delivery of the placenta.

Grossly, a fresh thrombus or hematoma is red and gelatinous and may be laminated. With age, the lesion becomes firm and white. By microscopy, non-nucleated red blood cells predominate with scattered admixed white cells (see Figs. 15–69 and 15–70). Fetal nucleated red blood cells can be found on careful screening or by immunostaining for fetal hemoglobin. **Thrombi in the placenta laminate over time but never organize.**

DIFFERENTIAL DIAGNOSIS. Because most pathologists see thrombi and hematomas in many organs, recognition of these lesions in the placenta usually presents little difficulty. Placental thrombi, particularly when old, may pose some diagnostic problems on gross examination because they may simulate an old infarct. Microscopy quickly provides the answer.

Chorangioma

A chorangioma is a proliferation of villous stromal blood vessels that distends a single villus or cluster of villi.

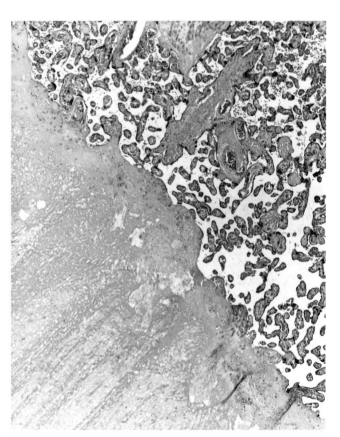

FIGURE 15–69. Intervillous thrombus. Thrombosis in the intervillous space has resulted in a laminated blood clot. Edge of thrombus adjacent to normal villi is composed of fibrin with scattered intermediate trophoblast.

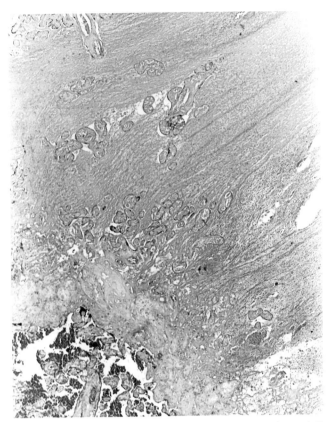

FIGURE 15-70. Intervillous thrombus with entrapped, partially infarcted villi. Laminated thrombus engulfed some villi at its periphery.

CLINICOPATHOLOGIC CORRELATION. A small, solitary chorangioma (chorioangioma, hemangioma) is a common incidental microscopic finding in placentas and is of no clinical significance. Chorangiomas large enough to be recognized on antepartum obstetric sonogram or gross examination are uncommon, but still usually of few sequelae. Although rare, the very **large chorangiomas** (larger than 5 cm) may be associated with both maternal and fetal complications. Maternal complications include **polyhydramnios.**[69] Fetal complications include **cardiomegaly and edema** (probably related to shunting through non–gas-exchanging vessels), **fetal anemia** including microangiopathic hemolytic anemia, and fetal coagulation abnormalities such as **thrombocytopenia** (thought to be related in part to platelet sequestration and destruction within the chorangioma) and disseminated intravascular coagulation. Infarction or destruction of a chorangioma may cause abatement of symptoms.[69] **Chorangiomatosis** describes multiple, diffuse chorangiomas or aberrant villous vascular proliferations (a type of congenital malformation) that involve large portions of the villous system and may affect other fetal organ systems as well.[103]

Most chorangiomas are intraplacental, and the majority are small, usually less than 2 cm in maximum diameter, and tend to be encapsulated and yellow-tan to dark, beefy red. Large lesions may be visible on the fetal surface and attain sizes exceeding 15 cm. Infarction of part or the entire lesion results in a white to tan appearance.

On microscopic examination, a chorangioma contains a stromal component and a vascular component, either of which

may predominate in a particular lesion. Some are virtually a "bag of blood vessels" (Fig. 15–71), whereas a bland stroma containing only scattered fetal blood vessels predominates in others. Larger lesions display a spectrum of histologic patterns ranging from angiomatous to stromal (mesenchymal) forms (Fig. 15–72). A large "feeder" vessel is sometimes identified in a fortuitous section (Fig. 15–73). Large chorangiomas usually have some degree of extramedullary hematopoiesis or erythropoiesis. Although increased mitotic activity may be seen in some chorangiomas, none has resulted in maternal or fetal metastases.

DIFFERENTIAL DIAGNOSIS. The differential diagnosis of chorangioma includes chorangiosis, infarct, chorangiocarcinoma, fetal artery thrombosis, and metastatic tumor. The greatest mimicker of chorangioma is chorangiosis, a diffuse proliferation of fetal blood vessels involving relatively normal appearing villi (see Figs. 15–55 and 15–56) (see previous discussion). In chorangiosis, the villous stroma maintains a relatively normal appearance without increased mesenchyme, and the villi, although slightly enlarged, are not markedly distended as in chorangioma.

An infarct can mimic the gross appearance of some chorangiomas, but on microscopy, the pale, crowded, normal-sized villi of an infarct (see Figs. 15–63 and 15–65) are easily distinguished from the enlarged, hypervascular, and hypercellular villi of a chorangioma. Although a chorangioma may be totally infarcted, outlines of the formerly enlarged villi and some evidence of fetal vascular proliferation remain. Choran-

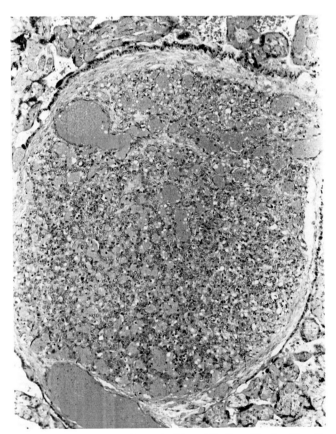

FIGURE 15-71. Chorangioma, incidental finding. Single villus distended by a proliferation of bland fetal capillaries. Surrounding villi are normal.

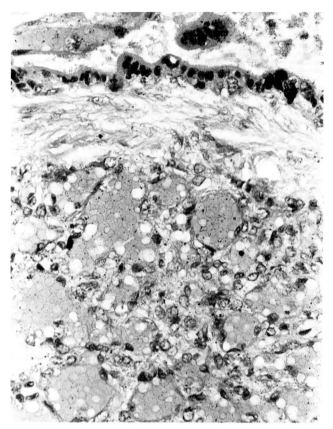

FIGURE 15–72. Chorangioma, higher-power view of Figure 15–71. Note proliferation of villous capillaries and bland overlying cytotrophoblast and syncytiotrophoblast.

giocarcinoma (see Figs. 15–31 and 15–32) is an exceedingly rare lesion characterized by a similar villous vascular proliferation. In contrast with chorangioma, chorangiocarcinoma has marked trophoblastic hyperplasia.[27, 28] A fetal artery thrombosis may also simulate a chorangioma, particularly on gross appearance; but on microscopy, the fetal blood vessels of villi distal to a fetal artery thrombosis are collapsed and difficult to find (see Fig. 15–66), whereas those of a chorangioma are increased. Maternal metastases to placental parenchyma can form grossly nodular lesions. Microscopy, however, demonstrates tumor involving the intervillous spaces. Fetal metastases center around villous blood vessels or perivascular stroma (see later discussion) and are usually revealed only by microscopy.

Septal Cysts

A cyst formed within a placental septum is termed a septal cyst.

CLINICOPATHOLOGIC CORRELATION. The placental villous parenchyma is subdivided by septa that are composed of **fibrin,** trophoblast, predominantly **intermediate trophoblast,** and **decidua from the basal plate.** Anchoring villi are embedded into the sides of the septa. Often the septa contain much fibrinoid material. Occasionally they fill with fluid and/or blood, and the resultant cavitation produces cysts. These cysts may be tiny and recognized microscopically, or large, measuring as much as 5 cm in diameter. Septal cysts may project from the fetal surface into the amnionic cavity or be within the placental parenchyma at any site where the septa lie (Fig. 15–74). They appear to have no clinical significance.

DIFFERENTIAL DIAGNOSIS. Although on gross examination septal cysts may mimic a chorangioma, or, if multiple, a

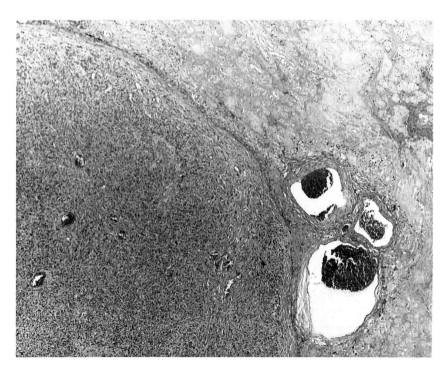

FIGURE 15–73. Chorangioma. Large feeder vessel illustrated at right. Chorangioma *(left)* contains admixed slit-like and well-formed vessels with spindled supporting elements (compare with Fig. 15–72). Surrounding villi are infarcted. Trophoblast of this chorangioma is slightly stratified, but not as hyperplastic, atypical, or mitotically active as in chorangiocarcinoma (see Fig. 15–32).

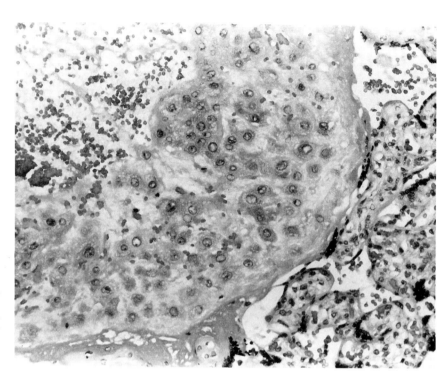

FIGURE 15-74. Septal cyst, intraparenchymal. Septal cyst wall, partially illustrated, is composed of large, mononuclear, intermediate trophoblast, scant decidua, scattered lymphocytes, and fibrin. The center of the cyst *(upper left)* contains fluid and red blood cells. Surrounding villi *(right)* are normal.

partial hydatidiform mole, on microscopy the diagnosis is unequivocal.

LESIONS INVOLVING THE INTERVILLOUS SPACE

Metastatic Tumors of Maternal and Fetal Origin

Placental metastases are malignant tumors from the mother or fetus that secondarily involve the placenta or its adnexa.

CLINICOPATHOLOGIC FEATURES. Maternal malignancies during pregnancy are uncommon, and placental metastases even more infrequent. The literature suggests that **malignant melanoma** is the most common tumor metastasizing to the placenta,[104] but in our hospital practice, **metastatic breast carcinoma** seems more frequent. Metastases from gastrointestinal tumors, squamous cell carcinoma,[105] pulmonary oat cell carcinoma,[106] and adenoid cystic carcinoma of trachea[107] are reported. Although most placental tumors are due to hematogenous metastases, placental involvement via direct extension from a gynecologic malignancy (i.e., from the cervix, endometrium or ovary) can occur. Maternal leukemias/lymphomas tend to involve the decidua and, less frequently, the intervillous space.[108] Because the vast majority of **maternal placental metastases do not invade villi,** fetal metastases develop only rarely.[109] Metastasis of primary fetal malignant tumors to the placenta is very rare. Reported cases include neuroblastoma (generally forming cords of cells in the fetal capillaries)[110] and lymphoma/leukemia, the latter usually associated with trisomy 21. (Choriocarcinoma of the placenta is discussed elsewhere in this chapter.)

Implants of metastatic tumor are infrequently recognized on gross placental examination. Metastatic maternal tumors usually involve the intervillous space, surrounding but rarely invading villi (Figs. 15–75 to 15–77). Vascular ingrowth into these "tumor emboli" is uncommon. Fetal tumors tend to remain intravascularly and only rarely invade the villous stroma. Often, multiple microscopic sections are required in order to identify small micrometastases. Because the treating physician often provides a clinical history of a primary maternal malignancy, elaborate diagnostic studies are seldom required. A careful and thorough evaluation of metastatic foci is indicated, however, if no primary site has been identified.

DIFFERENTIAL DIAGNOSIS. The differential diagnosis of maternal metastases to the intervillous space includes primary placental choriocarcinoma and reactive, hyperplastic intermediate trophoblast.

The most important tumor to exclude is a "primary" choriocarcinoma of the placenta because it is so amenable to treatment when correctly diagnosed and potentially lethal when not (see Figs. 15–33 to 15–35 and 15–41). Choriocarcinoma is a malignant trophoblastic tumor with a biphasic growth pattern. Whereas large foci are hemorrhagic and necrotic, smaller, earlier tumors exhibit only trophoblastic proliferation with minimal necrosis and hemorrhage.[29] A transition from benign, mitotically quiescent trophoblast of normal villi to malignant, proliferating trophoblast with focal necrosis, with or without hemorrhage, should suggest choriocarcinoma. Implants of metastatic breast carcinoma and, to a lesser extent, other metastatic tumors tend to encircle villi without perturbing the normal villous trophoblast. Immunoperoxidase stains including keratin and hCG should offer confirmation. When a definite diagnosis is not possible, the clinician should be notified immediately that the trophoblast is atypical and that the possibility of choriocarcinoma cannot be excluded. Maternal serum β-hCG level should be assayed,

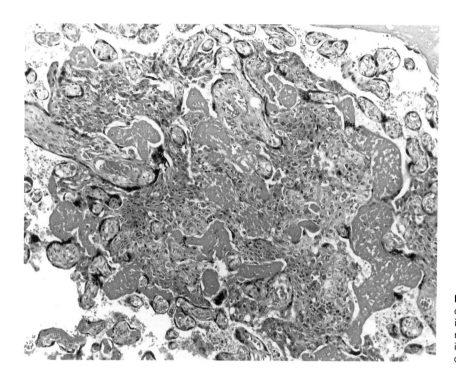

FIGURE 15–75. Placenta with metastatic breast carcinoma. Villi are slightly displaced by an intervillous proliferation of metastatic carcinoma. Tumor surrounds villi but does not invade villous stroma. There is much fibrin deposition in and around the tumor nodule.

and further clinical evaluation is warranted. In metastases from maternal tumors, hCG immunostaining is generally negative and maternal serum β-hCG is low, commensurate with the stage of gestation. Immunoperoxidase studies including HMB-45 antibody and antibodies to S-100 protein and gross cystic disease fluid protein, as well as conventional histochemistry for melanin and mucins, can be applied as appropriate.

Unusually **large nests of intermediate trophoblast** (Fig. 15–78) occasionally simulate maternal metastases, particularly breast carcinoma. Comprised solely of benign intermedi-

ate trophoblast, these lesions lack the biphasic pattern of choriocarcinoma and, in particular, lack syncytiotrophoblast. Necrosis is minimal. Nests of cytologically atypical intermediate trophoblast can be identified in areas of extensive intervillous fibrin deposition. At such sites, the intermediate trophoblast has large, mitotically active nuclei, prominent nucleoli, and cleared chromatin. Intermediate trophoblast is immunopositive for both hPL and keratin; lacks mucin, gland formation, and melanin; and does not stain with antibodies to S-100 protein or with HMB-45. Clinical correlation, particularly absence of known malignancy, is most useful.

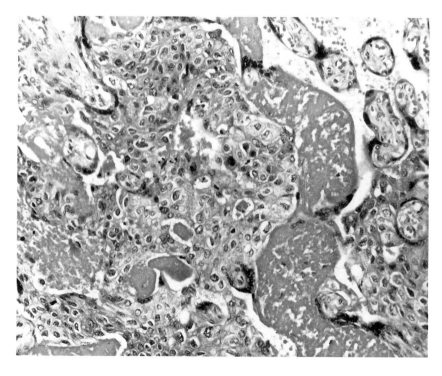

FIGURE 15–76. Placenta with metastatic breast carcinoma. Higher-power view of Figure 15–75. Tumor forms central acini that contain mucin on mucicarmine stain. Immunoperoxidase stains for gross cystic disease fluid protein and keratin are positive. Large cords of intervillous fibrin accompany tumor foci.

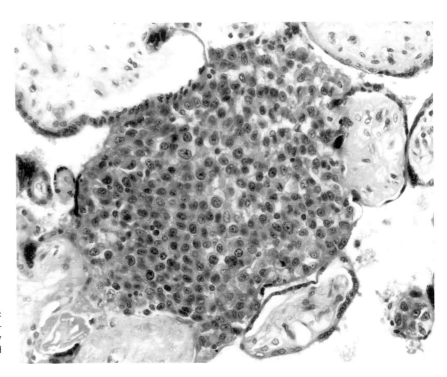

FIGURE 15–77. Placenta with metastatic malignant melanoma. Metastatic tumor nodule in the intervillous space is formed by slightly discohesive cells with large nuclei and finely granular cytoplasm.

The differential diagnosis of fetal metastases to the placenta is simplified by the clinical presentation of the neonate. Usually neuroblastoma is diagnosed clinically before the pathologist reviews slides from the delivered placenta. Occasionally, it is diagnosed at autopsy of a stillborn fetus. The distinction between **congenital leukemias** and **transient myeloproliferative disorder of Down's syndrome infants (myeloid hyperplasia, leukemoid reaction)** is particularly problematic and requires clinical pathologic correlation, including blood cytogenetic studies and evaluation for clonal gene rearrangements.[111, 112]

Acute Intervillositis

Acute intervillositis is characterized by **increased numbers of aggregated neutrophils** in the **maternal intervillous space.** Large collections of maternal neutrophils constitute a **placental abscess.**

CLINICOPATHOLOGIC FEATURES. In most instances, acute intervillositis (microabscess) results from infection by agents such as *Listeria monocytogenes*[72] (see earlier discussion) or other pathogens. Maternal or fetal cultures may demonstrate the infectious agent. Placental infection by *L. monocytogenes*

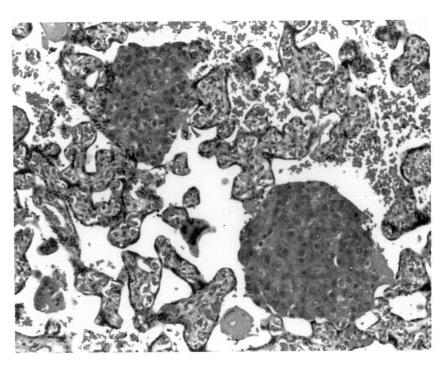

FIGURE 15–78. Nodules of intermediate trophoblast simulating metastatic maternal malignancy. Nodules are composed of mononuclear intermediate trophoblast enmeshed in dense fibrin.

is characterized by collections of subchorionic neutrophils forming abscess pockets associated with acute villitis, villous necrosis, and chorioamnionitis.[72] *Treponema pallidum* (see earlier discussion) results in acute and chronic villitis with acute intervillositis and in focally obliterative villous vasculitis with endovascular and perivascular proliferation.[55, 56] Very rarely, acute intervillositis is found in isolation and suggests **maternal septicemia** with seeding of the intervillous space by a hematogenous pathogen, usually bacterial or spirochetal.

Acute intervillositis is seldom recognized grossly, unless there are microabscesses with associated thrombi, the latter being termed **"septic" intervillous thrombus** (Fig. 15–79). In septic intervillous thrombi, the thrombus is grossly visible, and the neutrophilic aggregates are identified on subsequent microscopy. Microscopically, acute intervillositis is characterized by collections of **maternal neutrophils** within the space between villi (intervillous space) and is most commonly associated with other signs of placental infection, including chorioamnionitis, acute or chronic villitis, and/or funisitis. Occasionally, gram, Dieterle, or Warthin-Starry stains demonstrate pathogens, more commonly in the membranes, cord, or villi as compared with the intervillous space. Interestingly, the bacteria of listeriosis have a predilection for the amnion, though it may be demonstrated elsewhere. Acute intervillositis is rarely encountered in "routine" cases of chorioamnionitis.

DIFFERENTIAL DIAGNOSIS. Acute intervillositis may be confused with chronic intervillositis (see next section). The latter is characterized by a predominance of monocytoid cells, rather than neutrophils, in the intervillous space[47, 50] (see Fig. 15–80).

Chronic Intervillositis

Chronic intervillositis is an uncommon placental finding of a **mononuclear inflammatory infiltrate that fills and distends the maternal intervillous space.**

CLINICOPATHOLOGIC FEATURES. The clinical associations and etiology for chronic intervillositis remain undefined.[47, 50] It has been postulated that chronic intervillositis reflects an immunologic reaction, perhaps pertaining to "placental rejection" or possibly due to an unrecognized infection. Chronic intervillositis may be associated with a form of chronic villitis termed villitis of unknown (or unestablished) origin, a lesion found in 5% to 33.8%[47, 69, 113] of placentas examined and one whose very name confirms our ignorance. When intervillositis is associated with villitis of unknown origin, it tends to correlate with poor reproductive outcome. I have seen examples of isolated chronic intervillositis in otherwise normal pregnancies with normal-appearing liveborn infants. Further investigation of this process is indicated.

A gross appearance of chronic intervillositis is not recognized. Microscopically, the lesion consists of an accumulation of monocytes and histiocytes with scattered lymphocytes and plasma cells that expand the maternal intervillous space (Fig. 15–80). The monocytes are bland and discohesive with kidney bean–shaped nuclei, and the associated histiocytes (macrophages) have round, uniform nuclei.

DIFFERENTIAL DIAGNOSIS. Chronic intervillositis is to be distinguished from acute intervillositis, maternal leukemia, and intervillous metastases. The inflammatory infiltrate of acute intervillositis is neutrophilic, whereas that of chronic intervillositis is mononuclear. Maternal leukemia is virtually never first diagnosed in a placenta because the clinical signs and symptoms of leukemia are recognized before delivery. Putting that aside, absence of peripheral blood abnormalities, the benign cytologic appearance of the histiocytes and lymphocytes, and lack of clonality favor a benign process. When leukemia involves gestational tissues, it often infiltrates the decidua. Maternal placental metastases to the intervillous space from disseminated malignant melanoma or carcinoma were discussed earlier. Briefly, the cytologic atypicality and mitotic activity of metastatic melanoma and the gland forma-

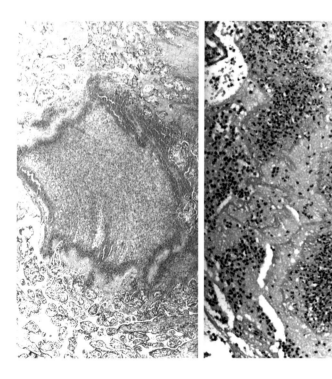

FIGURE 15–79. Acute intervillositis with thrombus formation, so-called septic intervillous thrombus. Low-power view *(left)* illustrates an intervillous thrombus with aggregates of neutrophils collecting in a serpentine fashion at the periphery of the thrombus. Higher-power view *(right)* demonstrates masses of mature neutrophils alternating with layered fibrin.

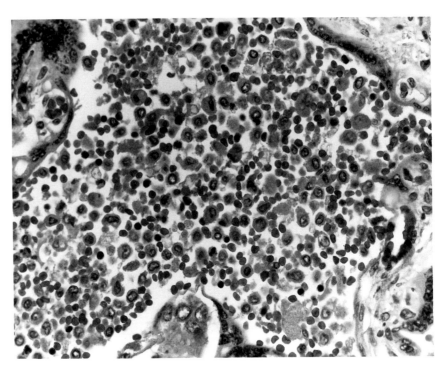

FIGURE 15–80. Chronic intervillositis. Intervillous space is filled with discohesive monocytoid cells, the majority of which are macrophages and lymphocytes, and interspersed red blood cells. The significance of chronic intervillositis remains unclear.

tion and tight cohesion of metastatic carcinoma distinguish metastases from intervillositis.

Fibrin (Fibrinoid) Deposition

Extensive perivillous fibrin accumulation is termed, **"massive intervillous fibrin deposition." Excessive fibrin deposited** in the **basal plate** of the **placenta** is called **"maternal floor infarction."**[114, 115]

CLINICOPATHOLOGIC FEATURES. Acellular fibrin, or fibrinoid (a term preferred by some to describe a "fibrin-like" substance), accumulates in many areas of normal placentas, most commonly around scattered villi and just beneath the chorionic plate. Extensive, dense, concentric perivillous fibrin deposition is pathologic because it sequesters affected villi and deprives them of maternal perfusion. Large basal fibrin accumulations interfere with maternal-placental perfusion. When diffuse and extensive, fibrin deposition leads to fetal growth retardation or fetal death *in utero,* although in some instances, an infant whose placenta was full of fibrin has been delivered healthy. "Maternal floor infarct" is an unfortunate term because the tissue is usually not infarcted, just heavily infiltrated by fibrin. Its etiology is unknown, and it tends to recur in consecutive pregnancies.[114, 115]

Grossly, maternal floor infarction is characterized by a firm placenta with dense, white to yellow, eggshell-like deposits encasing the basal plate. In massive intervillous fibrin deposition, the placenta is quite firm, and on cut section, white serpentine streaks course through the parenchyma.

Microscopically, fibrin (fibrinoid) deposition consists of acellular, amorphous, laminated to stringy eosinophilic material on villous surfaces, around and within villi (Fig. 15–81), under the chorionic plate, and in the basal plate/decidua. In materal floor infarction, accumulation starts in the basal plate (Fig. 15–82) and extends upward into the overlying villous

tissues encasing basal villi, which then become sclerotic. In massive intervillous fibrin deposition, the accumulation is randomly distributed and involves many villous areas.

DIFFERENTIAL DIAGNOSIS. The acellular nature of fibrin (fibrinoid) and its pale pink to light red staining qualities are familiar to most pathologists and are usually not confused with other lesions. Although fibrin may accumulate around villi adjacent to an infarct and simulate excessive intervillous fibrin deposition, villous infarction may occur but is not typical for these lesions; its presence should prompt consideration of other pathologic conditions such as maternal disorders associated with decidual vasculopathy, including preeclampsia, eclampsia, hypertension, diabetes mellitus, and lupus erythematosus. Likewise, although fibrin accumulates around villi with chronic villitis, villous inflammation is usually not featured in massive villous fibrin deposition or maternal floor infarction.

Intervillous Thrombi

See earlier section on Placental Thrombus and Hematoma.

UNUSUAL INFLAMMATORY AND REACTIVE LESIONS OF THE PLACENTAL MEMBRANES

Chronic Chorioamnionitis

Chronic chorioamnionitis is a **chronic inflammatory infiltrate involving placental membranes.**

CLINICOPATHOLOGIC FEATURES. Acute chorioamnionitis, the most frequent placental diagnosis, is characterized by a neutrophilic inflammation of the placental membranes. In

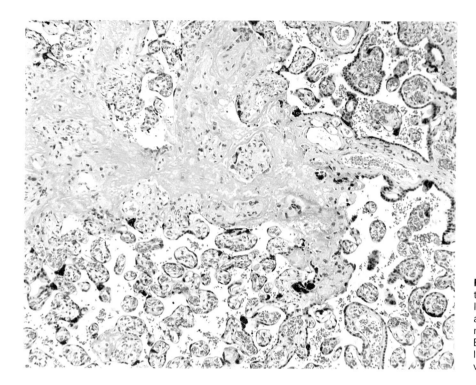

FIGURE 15–81. Intervillous fibrin deposition. Slightly immature placenta with acellular fibrin strands *(center* and *left)* accumulated around villi, precluding maternal perfusion of villous surfaces. Entrapped villi remain viable as fetal villous perfusion continues. Some encased villi become sclerotic and avascular.

chronic chorioamnionitis, lymphocytes and monocytes infiltrate the chorion and amnion. Chronic chorioamnionitis, which has been characterized by Gersell et al,[116] is associated with chronic deciduitis. Although suspected to be of infectious etiology, attempts to identify specific pathogens were unsuccessful in one series.[116]

Unless the inflammatory infiltrate is intense, the gross examination of the placental membranes in chronic chorioamnionitis is unremarkable. Microscopically, a lymphoplasmo-cytic and mononuclear cell infiltrate extends from decidua through chorion and into the amnion (Fig. 15–83). Often, the chronic inflammation is confined to the decidua (chronic deciduitis) and chorion (chronic chorionitis), sparing the amnion. Clearly, further investigation into this area is warranted.

DIFFERENTIAL DIAGNOSIS. Chronic chorioamnionitis is to be distinguished from acute chorioamnionitis. In the latter, the inflammatory infiltrate is acute, whereas in the former, it is chronic.

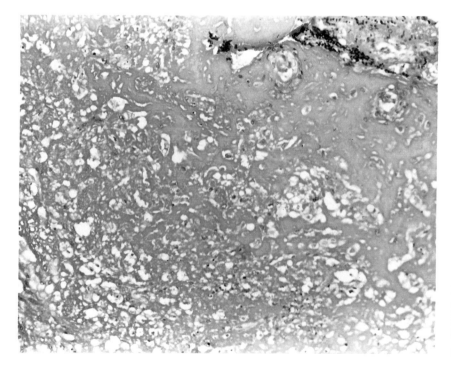

FIGURE 15–82. "Maternal floor infarction," or massive fibrin deposition of maternal floor. Large area of fibrin infiltrates decidua (basal plate) and extends into villous parenchyma. The term "maternal floor infarction" is a misnomer in that no infarct is usually present.

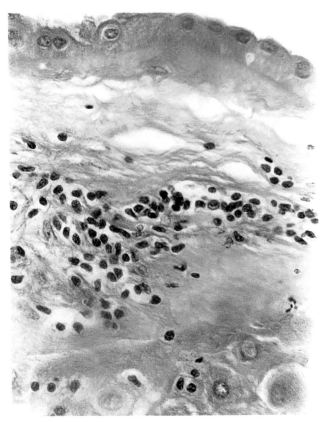

FIGURE 15–83. Chronic chorioamnionitis. Chronic inflammatory cells, predominantly lymphocytes in this case, infiltrate from chorion *(lower right corner)* into subamnionic connective tissues. Chronic deciduitis (not depicted) was also present.

Amnion Nodosum

Amnion nodosum results from **deposition of fetal epithelial cells, hair, and sebaceous material on the amnionic surface.**

CLINICOPATHOLOGIC FEATURES. Amnion nodosum is associated with an extreme degree of **oligohydramnios.** Oligohydramnios is due to prolonged, premature rupture of the membranes with continual loss of amnionic fluid or to a fetal urinary tract anomaly that results in decreased to absent fetal urination. Examples of the latter include bilateral renal agenesis; bilateral cystic/dysplastic kidneys; malformations associated with blockage of the urinary outflow tract at the level of the ureters, bladder, or urethra (i.e., posterior urethral valves); and complex congenital anomalies/tumors that involve large body regions encompassing portions of the genitourinary system (i.e., sirenomelia, fetal tumors). Concomitant **pulmonary hypoplasia** is often responsible for neonatal death in these cases.

Grossly, amnion nodosum consists of nodular deposits of vernix caseosa on the fetal surface of the placenta near the insertion of the umbilical cord. The deposits are numerous, usually more than 100, yellow-white, and elevated, measuring 1 to 5 mm in diameter. They are easily removed by scraping.

Microscopic examination discloses focal erosion or ulceration of the amnion covered by a round to slightly flattened deposit of predominantly acellular eosinophilic debris with admixed fetal squames and hair (Fig. 15–84). Occasionally, amnion grows over the top of the nodule or is preserved at its base.

DIFFERENTIAL DIAGNOSIS. The differential diagnosis of amnion nodosum centers around squamous metaplasia, a benign metaplasia of amnionic epithelium (Figs. 15–85 and 15–86). On gross examination, squamous metaplasia cannot be picked off by gentle rubbing, whereas nodules of amnion nodosum are easily removed. Microscopically, squamous metaplasia is recognized as a transformation of normal columnar amnion into a squamous epithelium with keratohyalin granules and orthokeratosis and parakeratosis (see next section and Fig. 15–86).

Squamous Metaplasia

Squamous metaplasia is a benign transformation of **amnionic epithelium into stratified squamous epithelium** complete with keratohyalin granules.

CLINICOPATHOLOGIC FEATURES. Squamous metaplasia of the amnion appears to be devoid of any relevant clinicopathologic features except that it grossly mimics amnion nodosum.

Grossly, squamous metaplasia consists of innumerable tiny (1 to 2 mm in diameter), elevated, white nodules on the fetal surface of the chorionic plate and umbilical cord. Because they are part of the amnion, they resist removal by gentle scraping.

Microscopically, these lesions are composed of a proliferation of stratified squamous epithelium containing keratohyalin granules and focal orthokeratosis and parakerotosis. The edges of the lesions merge smoothly into surrounding amnion.

DIFFERENTIAL DIAGNOSIS. The differential diagnosis involves amnion nodosum and is discussed in the previous section.

Amnion Vacuolization

Amnion vacuolization represents a very unusual condition of marked vacuolization of the amnionic cytoplasm.

CLINICOPATHOLOGIC FEATURES. Most commonly, amnionic vacuolization is related to **fetal meconium release** and represents a secondary phenomenon. Primary amnion vacuolization is extremely uncommon and is associated with fetal **gastroschisis**[117] or, less often, with fetal omphalocele, although some authors dispute that it occurs in the latter. This controversy probably relates to the difficulty sometimes encountered in distinguishing omphalocele from gastroschisis. Because these congenial abdominal wall defects are recognized by antepartum ultrasonographic examination or immediately at birth, diagnosis of amnionic vacuolization in that setting appears to be of little clinical significance. Isolated amnionic vacuolization has been associated with absence of abdominal wall defects or meconium release, and, apart from indicating extremely rare storage disorders such as mucolipidosis IV[118] and glycogen storage disease type IV (amylopectinase deficiency),[69] its etiology remains unclear.

A gross appearance of vacuolated amnion is not recognized. The lesion is identified microscopically by numerous fine, uniform small to medium-sized clear vacuoles distending the

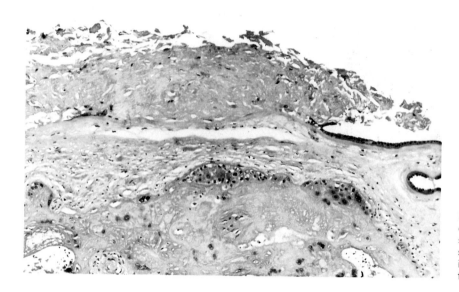

FIGURE 15–84. Amnion nodosum. Section of chorionic plate from fetal surface of placenta showing a large deposit of fetal nucleated squames and acellular debris atop an amnionic ulcer. There is prominent subchorionic fibrin deposition in this example.

amnionic cytoplasm (Fig. 15–87). By electron microscopy, the vacuoles associated with gastroschisis contain lipid.[119]

DIFFERENTIAL DIAGNOSIS. Amnionic vacuolization is a pathologic finding whose etiology relates to anterior abdominal wall defects, meconium release, and congenital metabolic disorders. Most instances of amnion vacuolization identified in routine practice are related to **meconium release.** Amnionic vacuolization from meconium is usually associated with other stigmata reflecting meconium passage, including green to green-brown staining of the fetal surface of the placenta, amnionic columnar metaplasia, ballooning of the amnionic cytoplasm, amnionic nuclear pyknosis, and meconium-laden macrophages in amnion (and/or chorion and decidua). In only

a few congenital metabolic storage disorders, such as mucolipidosis IV[119] and glycogen storage disease type IV (amylopectinase deficiency),[69] is amnion epithelial vacuolization the only placental finding. Benirschke and Kaufmann provide a summary of other placental findings in these extremely rare congenital storage disorders.[69]

Columnar Amnionic Metaplasia

Columnar amnionic metaplasia is an **abnormal state** in which the **cuboidal amnionic epithelium becomes tall and columnar.**

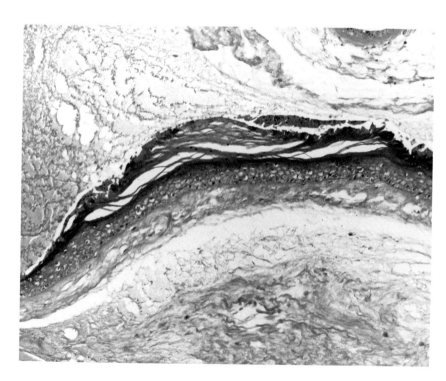

FIGURE 15–85. Squamous metaplasia. Amnionic surface is transformed into metaplastic squamous epithelium with dense orthokeratosis and parakeratosis.

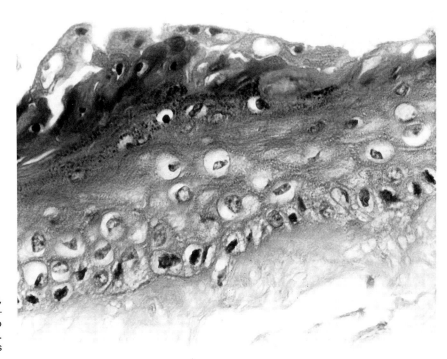

FIGURE 15–86. Squamous metaplasia, higher-power view of Figure 15–85. Transformation of cuboidal amnionic epithelium into squamous epithelium is virtually complete. Dark, slightly coarse, keratohyalin granules present near parakeratotic surface.

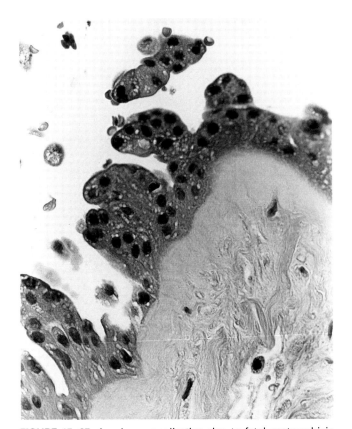

FIGURE 15–87. Amnion vacuolization due to fetal gastroschisis. Amnionic surface epithelium appears stratified, and the cytoplasm contains fine vacuoles. A few macrophages are in the subamnionic connective tissue.

CLINICOPATHOLOGIC FEATURES. Columnar amnionic metaplasia is generally associated with **meconium release.** Less frequently, it results from amnionic irritation from blood products (intra-amnionic or marginal hemorrhages) or may be idiopathic. Meconium is a dark-green to black viscous material within the fetal intestine which, in third-trimester gestations, is not usually passed until after birth. Meconium release before birth is more common in postdate infants[120] and may be associated with fetal distress. In one study, there was no correlation between meconium release and neonatal blood pH values.[121]

Some studies have suggested that inferences pertaining to the timing of meconium release can be drawn from finding macrophages imbued with meconium within the amnion, chorion, and decidua of the extraplacental membranes.[122] These studies were performed *in vitro,* and thus applications to the timing of meconium release *in vivo* remain necessarily speculative.[122]

Grossly, fresh meconium release is associated with green-black staining of the fetal surface of the placenta and the extraplacental membranes. Diluted or metabolized meconium may be green, brown, or light yellow. Apart from its association with meconium staining, columnar amnionic metaplasia is not recognizable grossly.

By microscopy, columnar amnionic metaplasia is characterized by an increase in the height-to-width ratio of amniocytes, ballooning and vacuolization of the cytoplasm, and occasionally by pyknosis and degeneration of amnionic nuclei (Fig. 15–88). (It's as though the amnion were standing up and doing "the wave," like the crowd at a baseball game.) Imbued meconium pigment may be found in the amnion proper and in macrophages of the amnion, chorion, and decidua (Figs. 15–89 and 15–90). There is a marked disparity between the dark-green gross appearance of meconium in the fresh state and its light yellow, finely granular, dusty intracellular appear-

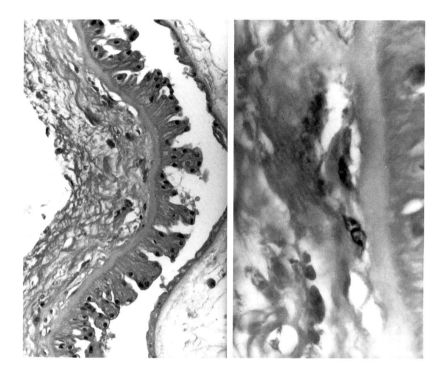

FIGURE 15–88. Columnar amnionic metaplasia, extraplacental membranes. Low-power view *(left)* illustrates tall, columnar amniocytes with slightly vacuolated cytoplasm and subamnionic macrophages imbued with coarsely granular material. Higher-power view *(right)* of macrophages demonstrates imbued dark, coarsely granular material that was positive for iron on Prussian blue stain.

ance in tissue sections (see Fig. 15–90). Its color and texture contrast with the bright yellow clumps of hematoidin and the coarse granularity and dark yellow-brown to brown refractile qualities of hemosiderin (see Fig. 15–88).

DIFFERENTIAL DIAGNOSIS. See discussion of amnion vacuolization.

Amnionic Band Syndrome

Premature rupture of the amnion results in the formation of **bands of amnion and subamnionic connective tissues that entrap, amputate, or otherwise deform developing fetal structures or umbilical cord.**

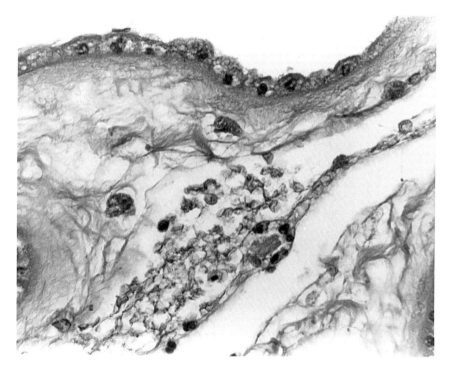

FIGURE 15–89. Amnionic vacuolization due to meconium release. Amniocytes have vacuolated cytoplasm with focally pyknotic nuclei. Underlying macrophages in subamnionic connective tissue contain slightly granular material consistent with meconium.

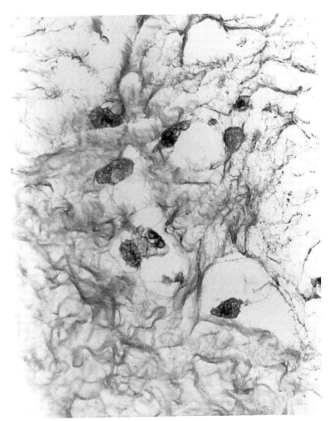

FIGURE 15–90. Meconium in macrophages of amnion. Here meconium appears as tiny, light-yellow to tan, delicate, non-refractile granules within macrophages. Absence of iron staining can be used to confirm this histologic impression if needed.

CLINICOPATHOLOGIC FEATURES. Premature amnion rupture (amnionic band syndrome) destroys the integrity of the amnion, producing strands and cords of amnion and subamnionic connective tissues that float freely within the amnionic cavity. Amnionic bands are more common in previable fetuses, for which the incidence is 1 in 53 as compared with 1 in 2500 to 10,000 live births.[123, 124] Although pregnancy outcome may be normal, in most, the fetus or umbilical cord becomes entwined with one or more of the amnionic bands, resulting in fetal malformations such as encephalocele; large facial clefts; amputation of digits, hands, feet, limbs, head; constriction of umbilical cord; and possibly fetal death.[125] The **sequelae of amnion rupture are related to the timing of the event.** Very early amnion rupture (i.e., first trimester) is more likely to be lethal or cause severe anomalies, including body wall defects, encephaloceles, or facial clefts. Rupture later in gestation may lead to amputation of digits or portions of limbs. Lethal cord constriction may develop at any time. Amnionic bands can be identified antenatally by obstetric ultrasonogram.

The normal amnion is a thin layer of tissue that forms the surfaces of the extraplacental membranes, chorionic plate, and umbilical cord. Avulsion of the amnion from these structures results in roughening of their surface texture and loss of their normal sheen. Irregular strands of subamnionic connective tissues as well as portions of disrupted amnion remain attached to the placenta, particularly at the cord insertion. Amnionic rupture may be focal or diffuse, involving the entire amnionic

sac. Rarely, remnants of an amputated limb or digit are received with the placenta.[126] Even more rarely, both amnion and chorion may rupture, resulting in a gestation that resides "outside" of the amnionic cavity but within the endometrial cavity (extramembranous pregnancy). Constant amnionic fluid loss ensues, because the endometrial cavity is a porous vesicle. Neonatal death is due to pulmonary hypoplasia.

Microscopically, amnionic bands are composed of amnion and paucicellular subamnionic connective tissues (Fig. 15–91). Sections taken at the junction of the amnionic band and the fetal skin in lethal cases of amnionic band syndrome demonstrate amnion in direct continuity with fetal skin (Fig. 15–92).

DIFFERENTIAL DIAGNOSIS. Amnionic band syndrome is to be distinguished from fetal arterial thrombosis and traumatic amnion avulsion. There are very few instances in which *in utero* amputation of fetal parts is not the sequela of amnionic band formation. The most relevant of these is the uncommon **fetal arterial thrombosis syndrome,** in which an occlusive thrombus develops in a main fetal artery. The thrombus completely impedes perfusion, leading to infarction, atrophy, autoamputation, or disappearance of the most distal portion of the affected digit, limb, or portion of intestine. In such cases, placental amnion is intact. Simple traumatic avulsion of the amnion usually occurs during delivery of the placenta and is insufficient for a diagnosis of amnionic band syndrome. The avulsed amnion usually remains attached at the umbilical cord insertion. True amnionic band syndrome exhibits entrapped, amputated, or otherwise deformed fetal parts and amnionic bands.

STRUCTURAL LESIONS OF THE UMBILICAL CORD

Lesions, Remnants, and Tumor-like Conditions of the Umbilical Cord

The most common umbilical cord lesions are **true and false knots, hematomas,** and **cord edema.** Umbilical cord tumors are discussed later. A **true knot** is a complete knot formed by fetal movement through a cord loop. A **false knot** is an aneurysm or vascular dilatation in an umbilical cord vessel. Hematomas of the umbilical cord may be particularly lethal, with 50% mortality reported.[127] Occasionally, marked edema of the cord produces cystic dilatation measuring as large as 15 cm in diameter, which, when transected, oozes clear fluid.

Two remnants of interest are found in term umbilical cords. The first of these is the **omphalomesenteric duct,** originally formed as an outpouching of the primitive yolk sac into the embryonic body stalk (early umbilical cord). As it develops into the secondary yolk sac, it retains its connection to the future embryonic intestinal tract and later serves as a channel for "extracorporeal intraumbilical" rotation of the embryonic intestinal tract. In reviewing sections of a Meckel's diverticulum, we see the morphologic evidence of this early embryonic event.

In the normal umbilical cord, a tiny vestigial remnant of the omphalomesenteric duct is commonly found. The duct itself usually atrophies during the 7th to 16th weeks. The remnant is situated in Wharton's jelly in the periphery of the

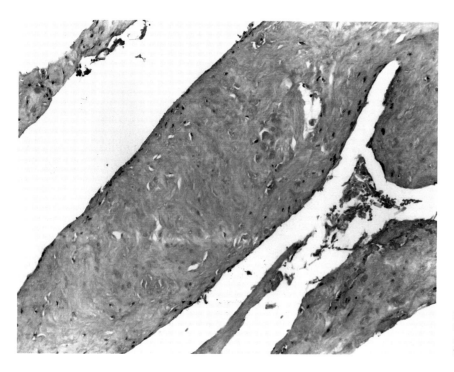

FIGURE 15–91. Amnionic band syndrome. Section of amnionic band revealing amnion and slightly fibrotic subamnionic connective tissue.

cord near the amnionic surface. It is lined by cuboidal to columnar intestinal type epithelium with inconspicuous nuclei and ample clear cytoplasm containing mucin vacuoles. Occasionally remnants of the omphalomesenteric duct house cachets of intestinal-type epithelium, forming miniature gastrointestinal tracts (Fig. 15–93). Rarely gastrointestinal epithelial polyps develop and some prolapse onto the cord surface (Fig. 15–94). Such lesions are extremely rare but interesting to find.

The **allantoic duct** forms as another outpouching of the primitive yolk sac, which eventually connects to the primitive fetal bladder. It is lined by flat to cuboidal transitional-type epithelium with scant clear cytoplasm. The allantoic duct remnant is located between the two umbilical arteries. Rarely, a remnant of the allantoic duct fills with fetal urine, forming a cyst in the cord. "Urination" from a transected cord stump near the fetal abdomen results from continued patency of the allantoic duct to its bladder attachment.

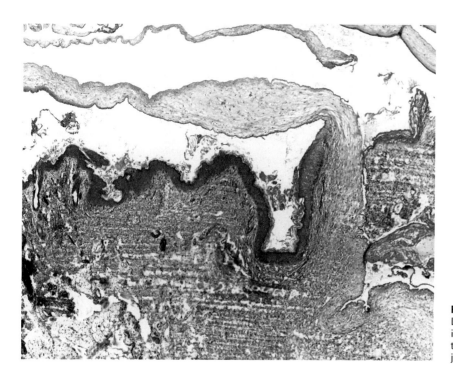

FIGURE 15–92. Amnionic band syndrome. Lethal first-trimester amnion rupture resulted in major facial clefts and encephalocele. Section taken from site where amnionic band joined fetal skin.

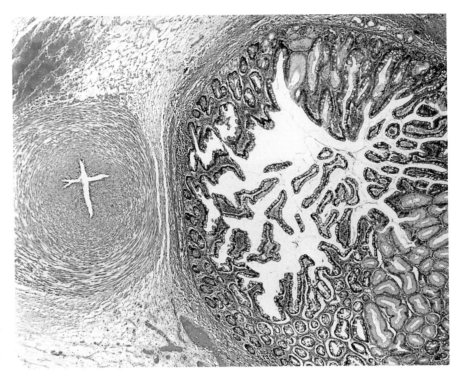

FIGURE 15–93. Umbilical cord with omphalomesenteric duct remnant lined by gastrointestinal-type epithelium. Normal umbilical artery to left. Note preservation of umbilical vitelline vessels in Wharton's jelly at base of intestinal remnant.

Single Umbilical Artery

Presence of only **one umbilical cord artery** is described as single umbilical artery.

CLINICOPATHOLOGIC FEATURES. Because the vast majority of cords contain two fetal arteries, absence of one fetal artery is abnormal. Single umbilical artery occurs in 1% of um-

bilical cords, and its frequency is increased in twins and white infants.[128, 129] It may be identified in an "otherwise" completely normal infant, or be associated with congenital malformations or chromosomal anomalies. Lesions of the genitourinary tract and cardiovascular system tend to associate with single umbilical artery. **Renal anomalies** were found in 19% of the cases with single umbilical artery studied by Leung

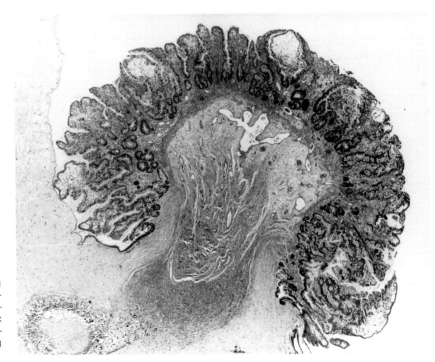

FIGURE 15–94. Umbilical cord with prolapsing intestinal polyp. Lesion developed in omphalomesenteric duct and, upon reaching adequate size, prolapsed out of cord into amnionic cavity. Grossly, it consisted of a 1- to 2-cm lobulated, exophytic, dark red nodule projecting from surface of umbilical cord.

and Robson.[128] Others did not find an association between any specific anomaly and a single umbilical artery.[69] Clearly, further investigation is warranted.

DIFFERENTIAL DIAGNOSIS. Single umbilical artery is generally a straightforward diagnosis. Inaccuracies occur when the umbilical cord is sampled too close to its insertion on the chorionic plate. At that site, the two umbilical arteries fuse, resulting in the appearance of a single umbilical artery. Routine sections of cord should be taken away from the chorionic plate insertion.

Tumors of the Umbilical Cord

Tumors of the umbilical cord are extremely rare, with all reported to date being benign. These include umbilical cord angiomas (hemangiomas), teratomas, hepatic adenomas, and adrenal cortical rests.

Umbilical Cord Angioma

Umbilical cord angiomas are **benign vascular tumors** derived from the umbilical vessels or possibly from angiogenic mesenchyme of the cord.

CLINICOPATHOLOGIC FEATURES. Cord angiomas (hemangiomas, angiomyxomas) are extremely rare tumors. The majority are small and of little clinical significance (Fig. 15–95). Larger lesions obstruct umbilical cord blood flow and may lead to fetal death *in utero*. Umbilical cord angiomas tend to involve the placental end of the cord, and some, particularly the larger ones, evince calcification, bone formation, and myxomatous change[130] (Fig. 15–96). Occasionally, angiomas are associated with an elevated alpha-fetoprotein (AFP) level[131] and, even more rarely, diffuse hemangiomatosis of fetal organs and tissues.

DIFFERENTIAL DIAGNOSIS. The differential diagnosis includes persisting vitelline vessels and umbilical cord hematoma. Persistence of the vitelline vessels may result in a small collection of blood vessels within the cord. True cord angiomas are larger, have a somewhat circumscribed appearance both grossly and microscopically, and contain slightly irregular, ectatic vascular channels. Some angiomas are more diffused and infiltrating. Calcification, bone formation, and myxomatous changes suggest angioma. Umbilical cord hematomas are common and result from traction on the cord at delivery, intrauterine trauma, or rupture of an umbilical venous varicosity. The fresh hemorrhage of a hematoma distends the cord, splays apart normal cells, and lacks the endothelium-lined vascular channels of a true angioma.

Umbilical Cord Teratoma

Umbilical cord teratoma is a **benign tumor** of the cord containing tissue representing **all three germinal layers.**

CLINICOPATHOLOGIC FEATURES. These tumors are extremely uncommon and may occur at any site within the cord as well as between the amnion and chorion of the placental membranes.[132–136] Aberrant migration of germ cells from the yolk sac remains the most plausible explantion for their occurrence in the cord and placental membranes.[134] An alternative hypothesis is that these teratomas represent ''included twins,'' because their dysmorphisms are strikingly similar to those of acardiac ''amorphous'' twins.[135] All cases of placental teratomas have been benign and without malignant sequelae.

DIFFERENTIAL DIAGNOSIS. The differential diagnosis of placental teratoma includes fetus amorphus and benign placental lesions such as hepatic adenoma and adrenal cortical rests. The distinction between an umbilical cord teratoma (mature cystic teratoma, dermoid cyst) and an included twin (fetus amorphus/acardiacus) remains controversial. Some have sug-

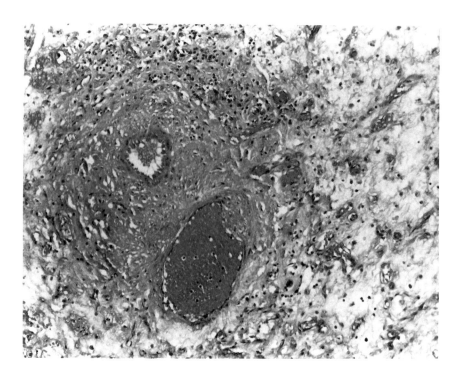

FIGURE 15–95. Umbilical cord hemangioma associated with persistence of vitelline artery and vein. Hemangioma is composed of well-formed vascular channels filled with fetal blood. Stroma contains scattered lymphocytes and macrophages.

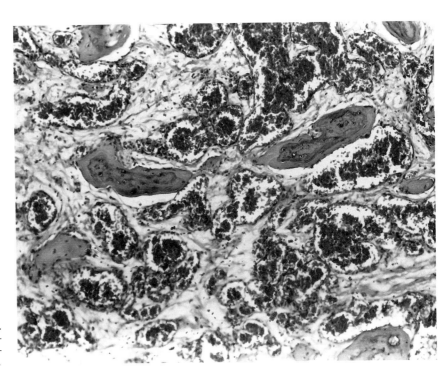

FIGURE 15–96. Umbilical cord angiomyxoma. This benign tumor simulates a cavernous hemangioma with secondary calcification. Surrounding stroma is myxomatous.

gested that the absence of a separate umbilical cord and lack of cranial-caudal organization of fetal tissues distinguish the teratoma from a true included twin.[134, 135] Others believe that a placental teratoma is an included twin, just disorganized. Probably, placental teratoma and fetus acardiacus represent the opposite ends of a continuous spectrum. **Hepatic adenomas** are monodermal, composed solely of benign hepatic parenchyma that usually lacks bile pigments and normally formed bile ducts.[137] **Adrenal cortical rests** are also monodermal and indistinguishable morphologically from those occurring at other sites in the body.[138, 139]

Unusual Inflammatory Processes and Infections Involving Umbilical Cord

In general, inflammation of the umbilical cord, generically termed **funisitis,** first involves the umbilical vein (phlebitis) and then the umbilical arteries (arteritis). As infection continues, fetal neutrophils spread out from the cord vessel walls into Wharton's jelly (perivasculitis). From there they head toward the amnionic surface of the cord. In long-standing inflammation, rings of degenerate inflammatory cells and calcified debris surround the cord vessels, simulating an Ouchterlony immunodiffusion plate (Fig. 15–97). In most instances, umbilical inflammation is associated with chorioamnionitis. Rarely, the pathogen inciting cord inflammation is fungal rather than bacterial and is described in the following section.

Candidal Funisitis

Candidal funisitis denotes inflammation of the umbilical cord due to candidal infection.

CLINICOPATHOLOGIC FEATURES AND DIFFERENTIAL DIAGNOSIS. Candidal infection of the umbilical cord generally involves *Candida albicans,* although infections with *C. parapsilosis* and *C. tropicalis* occur. Signs of fetal/neonatal infection include skin rash, sepsis, pneumonia, and meningitis. Grossly, fungal colonization of the umbilical cord produces tiny, 3- to 4-mm, off-white to creamy yellow nodules just under the amnionic surface. Microscopy discloses neutrophilic inflammation with both hyphal and yeast forms in infections with *C. albicans,* and yeast forms only in *C. parapsilosis* and *C. tropicalis.* The fungi are minimally discernible on routine stains (Fig. 15–98). Both hyphae and yeast forms are enhanced with silver stains or periodic acid-Schiff reaction. Diagnosis of a fetal fungal septicemia requires umbilical cord vascular invasion.[140, 141]

LESIONS RELATED TO TWINNING AND MULTIPLE GESTATION

Determination of Zygosity in Multiple Gestation

Zygosity can be determined from placental examination in monochorionic twin gestations because **monochorionic placentation implies monozygosity.** On the other hand, dichorionic placentation is associated with both monozygous and dizygous twinning.

Monochorionic placentation may be monoamnionic-monochorionic or diamnionic-monochorionic. In the former, there is no dividing septum between the twins, and both share one sac. In the latter, the dividing membrane is composed of two layers of amnion lacking intervening chorion, and each twin resides in its own amnionic sac. Rare instances of separate (bipartite) monochorionic twin placentation[142] remind us that a monochorionic twin placenta may be composed of *two* separate placental disks, just as in bipartite singleton

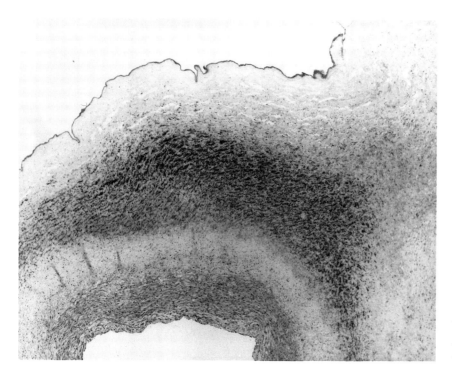

FIGURE 15–97. Umbilical cord depicting portion of umbilical vein partially encircled by a dense band of acute inflammatory cells. There was severe necrotizing chorioamnionitis elsewhere.

placentation (Fig. 15–99). Thus, presence of two placental disks does not always ensure dichorionicity.

Monozygous twins may also have **dichorionic placentas,** i.e., separate or fused placentas in which each twin is encircled in his or her own complete set of amnion and chorion. This results from division of the blastocyst before day 3, and thus each conceptus forms its own amnion and chorion. Whether the placentas remain separate or fuse depends on the proximity of the implantation sites within the uterine cavity. Although

these twins are monozygous, their placentation is indistinguishable from that of dizygous twins. All dizygous twins have dichorionic placentation, either separate or fused.

To determine placentation of twins or multiple births of higher order (triplets, quadruplets, and so on), the only requirements are (1) a carefully drawn diagram and section code indicating where the dividing membranes were sampled, and (2) knowledge that a monochorionic dividing membrane implies monozygosity. In the example shown in Figure

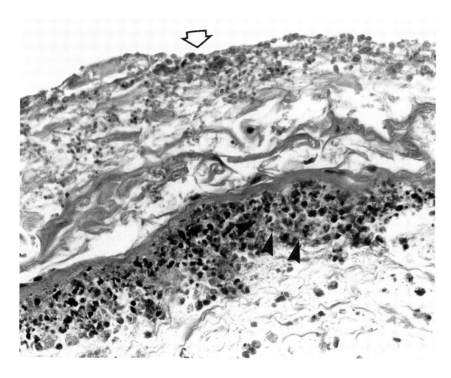

FIGURE 15–98. Candidal funisitis. Umbilical cord coated with hyphal and yeast forms of *Candida albicans (open arrow).* Amnionic surface of cord is disrupted and partially replaced with dense fibrin. Small subamnionic abscesses contain hyphal forms seen here on H&E stain *(closed arrows)* and better demonstrated by silver stain.

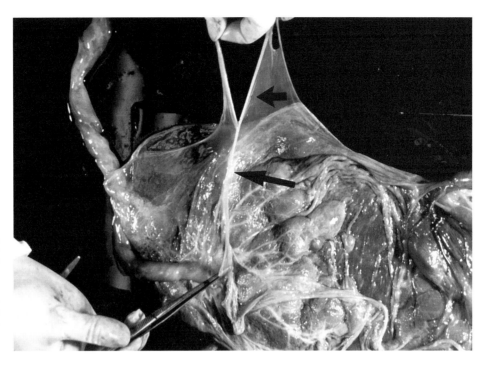

FIGURE 15–99. Separate diamnionic-monochorionic twin placenta (bipartite twin placenta) with two placental disks. Two amnionic sacs are separated by diamnionic dividing membranes *(arrows)*. Majority of second placental disk is out of view. Prosector indicating two layers of diamnionic dividing septum. (From Kim K, Lage JM: Bipartite diamnionic-monochorionic twin placenta with superficial vascular anastomoses. Hum Pathol 22:501–503, 1991.)

15–100, the dividing membranes between all placental disks were diamnionic-dichorionic (Fig. 15–101), thus zygosity could not be determined from placental examination. If any of the twin sets were monochorionic (dividing membranes composed of two layers of amnion only without any intervening chorion) (see Fig. 15–101), then those twins would be monozygous, or identical, to each other.

Twin Transfusion Syndrome

Twin transfusion syndrome results from **passage of blood from one twin to its co-twin via placental vascular anastomoses.**

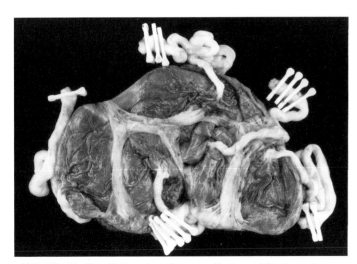

FIGURE 15–100. Quintuplet placenta. Each umbilical cord was sequentially labeled as to birth order. Placenta is penta-amnionic-pentachorionic because all dividing septa are diamnionic-dichorionic.

CLINICOPATHOLOGIC FEATURES. Virtually **all monochorionic placentas have anastomoses that link together the twins' placental circulatory systems.** Such anastomoses generally involve artery-to-artery or vein-to-vein connections with little blood volume exchanged. In the twin (to twin) transfusion syndrome, fetal blood from the donor twin is transfused to the recipient twin via unbalanced placental vascular anastomoses. Such anastomoses are typically vein to artery or artery to vein and usually involve deep villous connections. When the connections are unidirectional, unbalanced shunting (transfusion) of blood ensues. This results in volume overload for the recipient, who develops congestive heart failure, and volume depletion of the donor, who becomes sequentially more and more anemic with each heart beat.[143] At some point, especially if the transfusion begins in the second trimester, one or both twins may succumb, the first often being the recipient twin (Fig. 15–102). The remaining twin may die *in utero* from heart failure or may survive, often severely anemic at birth. Should one twin die *in utero* and the placental vascular anastomoses remain patent, blood flow through the shunts may reverse, resulting in equilibration of blood volumes.[144] Thus, at the time of birth it may be difficult to piece together seemingly contradictory physical and laboratory data.

The twin transfusion syndrome may play a role in the increased rate of cerebral palsy in monochorionic twins.[144] Physical structural defects, such as intestinal atresias, limb defects, or visceral infarcts in monozygous twins are thought to be a result of vascular thromboses[145] somehow related to twin transfusion syndrome. **Twin transfusion syndrome developing in the second trimester is associated with a very high perinatal mortality rate,** approaching 50%. When twin transfusion syndrome develops later in the third trimester, a 5% to 15% mortality rate for both twins is cited.[146, 147]

The twin transfusion syndrome may be diagnosed clinically shortly after delivery: criteria include a 5 g/dl difference in

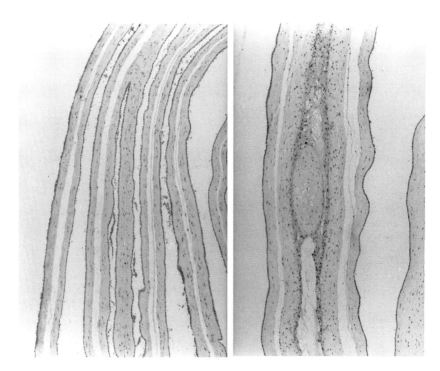

FIGURE 15–101. Composite photograph of dividing membranes in twin placentation. *Left,* Diamnionic dividing membranes imply monochorionic placentation. Note complete absence of chorion and villous tissue. *Right,* Diamnionic-dichorionic dividing membranes imply dichorionic placentation. Residual entrapped villus from chorion laeve noted between the placental membranes. Only in monochorionic placentation is monozygosity ensured.

hemoglobin concentration and 200 g body weight difference. These criteria obviously depend on the age of the fetuses and the duration of the illness. Antepartum obstetric ultrasonographic diagnosis is based on differences in biparietal diameter, associated hydramnios, and other evidence of fetal heart failure such as pleural/pericardial effusions, ascites, and anasarca.

Naeye first called attention to the gross and microscopic features of twin transfusion syndrome in 1965.[143] Grossly, the monochorionic placenta from severe twin transfusion syn-

drome is quite pale and edematous on the **donor's** side and dark, beefy red and somewhat smaller on the **recipient's** side. Although the histologic features may vary depending on degree of transfusion, villi from the donor tend to be large, pale, and edematous, often with "Swiss-cheese" villous stromal edema (Fig. 15–103) and small and inconspicuous vessels.[148] In severely affected fetuses, the villous blood vessels contain foci of intravascular extramedullary erythropoiesis with numerous normoblasts and erythroblasts (Fig. 15–104). The recipient placenta is generally more mature than expected

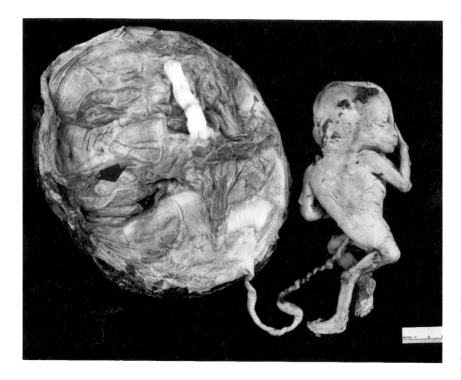

FIGURE 15–102. Twin transfusion syndrome with fetal death *in utero* of one twin, delivered at 27 weeks' gestational age. The macerated twin had no recognizable internal anomalies. Diamnionic dividing septum *(arrow)* was partially removed prior to photography.

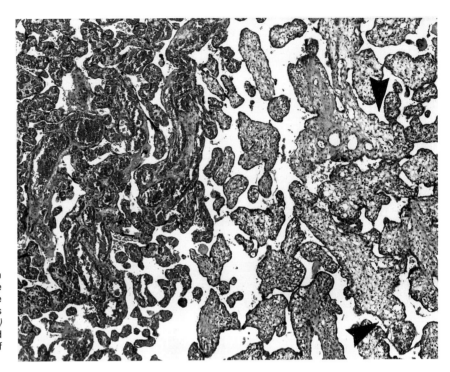

FIGURE 15–103. Twin placentas with twin transfusion syndrome. Junction between the two placental domains is illustrated, with the donor twin *(right)* having large, edematous villi *(arrowheads)* and the recipient twin *(left)* having more mature, small, and congested villi. At birth, one twin had a hematocrit of 24.3%, and the other's was 70.7%.

for gestational age. The villi are normal to small in size with congested blood vessels containing only rare normoblasts, numerous vasculosyncytial membranes with thin trophoblast, and no villous edema.[148]

At autopsy, these neonates have marked visceral size differences, with the recipient's tissues being much larger and darker red than those of the donor, whose organs are smaller and whose tissues, including fetal skin, are pale and lack fat deposits.[143] Signs of congestive heart failure include diffuse hydrops (anasarca), pleural and pericardial effusions, ascites,

visceromegaly for gestational age, in particular, cardiomegaly, and dilated lymphatics in the lungs. Signs of high output cardiac failure and anemia include pallor, small total body and organ weights, absence of effusions, and extreme extramedullary hematopoiesis in all visceral organs.

DIFFERENTIAL DIAGNOSIS. The differential diagnosis revolves around distinguishing twin transfusion syndrome from intrauterine growth retardation of one twin in the setting of a monochorionic twin gestation. Twin transfusion syndrome is suggested by unidirectional or unbalanced placental

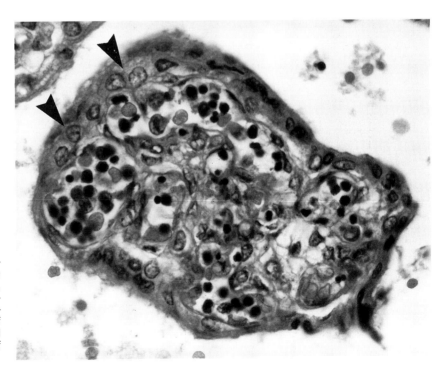

FIGURE 15–104. Villus from donor twin represented in Figure 15–103. Fetal capillaries are site of extensive intravascular erythropoiesis, with erythroblasts and normoblasts predominating. Note overall immaturity of villus characterized by large villous size, persistence of cytotrophoblastic layer *(arrowheads),* and lack of syncytiotrophoblastic giant cells, all of which are abnormal in a term placenta.

vascular anastomoses, villous immaturity, edema and erythroblastemia in the donor twin, and villous hypermaturity and signs of congestive heart failure in the recipient twin. In growth retardation affecting one twin, the uninvolved co-twin is morphologically normal, being of normal weight for gestational age with normal hematologic laboratory values and a normal placenta.

References

1. Lage JM, Mark SD, Roberts DJ, et al: A flow cytometric study of 137 fresh hydropic placentas: Correlation between types of hydatidiform moles and nuclear DNA ploidy. Obstet Gynecol 79:403–410, 1992.
2. Suster S, Robinson MJ: Placental intravillous accumulation of sulfated mucosubstances. A reevaluation of so-called hydropic degeneration of villi. Ann Clin Lab Sci 22:175–183, 1992.
3. Szulman AE, Surti U: The syndromes of hydatidiform mole. I. Cytogenetic and morphologic correlations. Am J Obstet Gynecol 131:665–671, 1978.
4. Szulman AE, Surti U: The syndromes of hydatidiform mole. II. Morphologic evolution of the complete and partial mole. Am J Obstet Gynecol 132:20–27, 1978.
5. Szulman AE, Philippe E, Boue JG, Boue A: Human triploidy: Association with partial hydatidiform moles and nonmolar conceptuses. Hum Pathol 12:1016–1021, 1981.
6. Jacobs PA, Hunt PA, Matsuura JS, et al: Complete and partial hydatidiform mole in Hawaii: Cytogenetics, morphology and epidemiology. Br J Obstet Gynaecol 89:258–266, 1982.
7. Conran RM, Hitchcock CL, Popek EJ, et al: Diagnostic considerations in molar gestations. Hum Pathol 24:41–48, 1993.
8. Rice LW, Berkowitz RS, Lage JM, et al: Persistent gestational trophoblastic tumor after partial hydatidiform mole. Gynecol Oncol 36:358–362, 1990.
9. Gardner HAR, Lage JM: Choriocarcinoma following patial hydatidiform mole: A case report. Hum Pathol 23:468–471, 1992.
10. Kajii T, Ohama K: Androgenetic origin of hydatidiform mole. Nature 268:633–634, 1977.
11. Azuma C, Saji F, Tokugawa Y, et al: Application of gene amplification by polymerase chain reaction to genetic analysis of molar mitochondrial DNA: The detection of anuclear empty ovum as the cause of complete mole. Gynecol Oncol 40:29–33, 1991.
12. Surani MAH, Barton SC, Norris ML: Nuclear transplantation in the mouse: Heritable differences between parental genomes after activation of embryonic genome. Cell 45:127–136, 1986.
13. McGrath J, Solter D: Completion of mouse embryogenesis requires both the maternal and paternal genomes. Cell 37:179–183, 1984.
14. Yen S. MacMahon B: Epidemiologic features of trophoblastic disease. Am J Obstet Gynecol 101:126–132, 1968.
15. Matalon M, Modan B: Epidemiologic aspects of hydatidiform mole in Israel. Am J Obstet Gynecol 112:107–112, 1972.
16. Poen HT, Kjojopranoto M: The possible etiologic factors of hydatidiform mole and choriocarcinoma. Am J Obstet Gynecol 92:510–513, 1965.
17. Lawler SD, Fisher RA, Dent J: A prospective genetic study of complete and partial hydatidiform moles. Am J Obstet Gynecol 164:1270–1277, 1991.
18. Curry SL, Hammond CB, Tyrey L, et al: Hydatidiform mole: Diagnosis, management, and long-term followup of 347 patients. Obstet Gynecol 45:1–8, 1975.
19. Martin DA, Sutton GP, Ulbright TM, et al: DNA content as a prognostic index in gestational trophoblastic neoplasia. Gynecol Oncol 34:383–388, 1989.
20. Lurain JR, Brewer JI, Mazur MT, Torok EE: Natural history of hydatidiform mole after primary evacuation. Am J Obstet Gynecol 145:591–595, 1983.
21. Hatch KD, Shingleton HM, Austin JM Jr, et al: Southern Regional Trophoblastic Disease Center, 1972–1977. South Med J 71:1334–1336, 1978.
22. Morrow CP: Postmolar trophoblastic disease: Diagnosis, management and prognosis. Clin Obstet Gynecol 27:211–220, 1984.
23. Wong LC, Ma HK: The syndrome of partial mole. Arch Gynecol 234:161–166, 1984.
24. Hertig AT: Hydatidiform mole. In Hertig AT: Human Trophoblast. Springfield, IL, CC Thomas, 1968, p 231.
25. Romero R, Horgan D, Kohorn EI, at al: New criteria for the diagnosis of gestational trophoblastic disease. Obstet Gynecol 66:553, 1985.
26. Lage JM: Placentomegaly with massive hydrops of placental stem villi, diploid DNA content, and fetal omphaloceles: Possible association with Beckwith-Wiedemann syndrome. Hum Pathol 22:591–597, 1991.
27. Jauniaux E, Zucker M, Meuris S, et al: Chorangiocarcinoma: An unusual tumour of the placenta. The missing link? Placenta 9:607–613, 1988.
28. Trask C, Lage JM, Roberts DJ: A second case of "chorangiocarcinoma" presenting in a term asymptomatic twin pregnancy. Int J Gynecol Pathol 13:87–91, 1994.
29. Lage JM, Roberts DJ: Choriocarcinoma in a term placenta. Pathologic diagnosis of tumor in an asymptomatic patient with metastatic disease. Int J Obstet Gynecol 12:80–85, 1993.
30. Lee KC, Chan JKC: Placental site nodule. Histopathology 16:193–195, 1990.
31. Young RH, Kurman RJ, Scully RE: Placental site nodules and plaques: A clinico-pathologic analysis of 20 cases. Am J Surg Pathol 14:1001–1009, 1990

32. Huettner PC, Gersell DJ: Placental site nodule: A clinicopathologic study of 38 cases. Int J Gynecol Pathol 13:191–198, 1994.
33. Collins RJ, Ngan HYS, Wong LC: Placental site trophoblastic tumor with features between an exaggerated placental site reaction and a placental site trophoblastic tumor. Int J Gynecol Pathol 9:170–177, 1990.
34. Carinelli SG, Vendola N, Zanotti F, Benzi G: Placental site nodules. A report of 17 cases. Pathol Res Pract 185:30, 1989.
35. Wan SK, Lam PWY, Pau MY, Chan JKC: Multiclefted nuclei: A helpful feature for identification of intermediate trophoblastic cells in uterine curetting specimens. Am J Surg Pathol 16:1226–1232, 1992.
36. Heintz APM, Schaberg A, Engelsman E, van Hall EV: Placental-site trophoblastic tumor: Diagnosis, treatment, and biological behavior. Int J Gynecol Pathol 4:75–82, 1985.
37. Lathrop JC, Lauchlan S, Nayak R, Ambler M: Clinical characteristics of placental site trophoblastic tumor (PSTT). Gynecol Oncol 31:32–42, 1988.
38. Eckstein RP, Russell P, Friedlander ML, et al: Metastasizing placental site trophoblastic tumor: A case study. Hum Pathol 16:632–636, 1985.
39. Finkler NJ, Berkowitz RS, Driscoll SG, et al: Clinical experience with placental site trophoblastic tumor. Int J Gynecol Pathol 9:170–177, 1990.
40. Young RH, Kurman RJ, Scully RE: Proliferations and tumors of intermediate trophoblast of the placental site. Semin Diagn Pathol 5:223–227, 1988.
41. Brinton LA, Bracken MB, Connelly RR: Choriocarcinoma incidence in the United States. Am J Epidemiol 123:1094–1100. 1986.
42. Hertig AT, Mansell H: Tumors of the female sex organs. Part I. Hydatidiform mole and choriocarcinoma. In: Atlas of Tumor Pathology. Sect IX, Fasc 33. Washington, DC, Armed Forces Institute of Pathology.
43. Genest DR, Laborde O, Berkowitz RS, et al: A clinical-pathologic study of 153 cases of complete hydatidiform mole (1980–1990): Histologic grade lacks prognostic significance. Obstet Gynecol 78:402–409, 1991.
44. Fisher RA, Lawler SD, Povey S, Bagshawe KD: Genetically homozygous choriocarcinoma following pregnancy with hydatidiform mole. Br J Cancer 58:788–792, 1988.
45. Chaganti RS, Koduru PR, Chakraborty R, Jones WB: Genetic origin of a trophoblastic choriocarcinoma. Cancer Res 50:6330–6333, 1990.
46. Osada H, Kawata M, Yamada M, et al: Genetic identification of pregnancies responsible for choriocarcinomas after multiple pregnancies by restriction fragment length polymorphism analysis. Am J Obstet Gynecol 165:682–688, 1991.
47. Labarre CA, McIntyre JA, Faulk WP: Immunohistologic evidence that villitides in human normal term placentas is an immunologic lesion. Am J Obstet Gynecol 162:515–522, 1990.
48. Knox WF, Fox H: Villitis of unknown aetiology: Its incidence and significance in placentae from a British population. Placenta 5:395–402, 1984.
49. Russell P: Inflammatory lesions of the human placenta. III. The histopathology of villitis of unknown aetiology. Placenta 1:227–244, 1980.
50. Labarrere CA, Faulk WP, McIntyre JA: Villitis in normal term human placentae: Frequency of the lesion as determined by monoclonal antibody to HLA-DR antigen. J Reprod Immunol 16:127–135, 1989.
51. Mortimer G, MacDonald DJ, Smeeth A: A pilot study of the frequency and significance of placental villitis. Br J Obstet Gynaecol 92:629–633, 1985.
52. Redline RW, Patterson P: Villitis of unknown etiology is associated with major infiltration of fetal tissue by maternal inflammatory cells. Am J Pathol 143:473–479, 1993.
53. Nordenvall M, Sandstedt B: Placental villitis and intrauterine growth retardation in a Swedish population. APMIS 98:19–24, 1990.
54. Muhlemann K, Miller RK, Metlay L, Menegus MA: Cytomegalovirus infection of the human placenta: An immunohistochemical study. Hum Pathol 23:1234–1237, 1992.
55. Jacques SM, Qureshi F: Necrotizing funisitis: A study of 45 cases. Hum Pathol 23:1278–1283, 1992.
56. Qureshi F, Jacques SM, Reyes MP: Placental histopathology in syphilis. Hum Pathol 24:779–784, 1993.
57. Garcia AGP: Maternal herpes-simplex infection causing abortion. Histopathologic study of the placenta. 78:1267–1274, 1970.
58. Driscoll SG: Histopathology of gestational rubella. Am J Dis Child 118:49–53, 1969.
59. Elliott WG: Placental toxoplasmosis: Report of a case. Am J Clin Pathol 53:413–417, 1970.
60. Garcia AGP, Fonseca EF, Marques RL, Lobato YY: Placental morphology in cytomegalovirus infection. Placenta 10:1–18, 1989.
61. Schwartz DA, Khan R, Stoll B: Characterization of the fetal inflammatory response to cytomegalovirus placentitis. Arch Pathol Lab Med 116:21–27, 1992.
62. Blanc WA: Pathology of the placenta, membranes and umbilical cord in bacterial, fungal and viral infections in man. In Naeye RL, Kissane JM (eds): Perinatal Diseases. IAP Monograph Series, No. 22. Baltimore, Williams & Wilkins, 1981, pp 67–132.
63. Werner H, Schmidtke L, Thomascheck G: Toxoplasmose-Infektion und Schwangerschaft: der histologische Nachweis des intrauterinen Infektion-sweges. Klin Wochenschr 41:96–101, 1963.
64. Russell P: Infections of the placental villi (villitis). In Fox H (ed): Haines and Taylor Obstetrical and Gynaecological Pathology, 3rd ed. Vol 2. Edinburgh, Churchill Livingstone, 1987, p 1017.
65. Herzen JL, Benirschke K: Unexpected disseminated herpes simplex infection in a newborn. Obstet Gynecol 50:728–730, 1977.
66. Garcia AGP: Maternal herpes-simplex infection causing abortion. Histopathologic study of the placenta. Hospital 78:1267–1274, 1970.

67. Kaplan C: The placenta and viral infections. Semin Diagn Pathol 10:232–250, 1993.
68. Schwartz DA, Caldwell E: Herpes simplex virus infection of the placenta. The role of molecular pathology in the diagnosis of viral infection of placental-associated tissues. Arch Pathol Lab Med 115:1141–1144, 1991.
69. Benirschke K, Kaufmann P: Pathology of the Human Placenta, 2nd ed. New York, Springer-Verlag, 1990.
70. Lage JM: The placenta. In Gompel C, Silverberg SG (eds): Pathology in Gynecology and Obstetrics, 4th ed. Philadelphia, JB Lippincott, 1993, pp 448–512.
71. Enocksson E, Wretlind B, Sterner G, Anzen B: Listeriosis during pregnancy and in neonates. Scand J Infect Dis Suppl 71:89–94, 1990.
72. Lallemand AV, Gaillard DA, Paradis PH, Chippaux CG: Fetal listeriosis during the second trimester of gestation. Pediatr Pathol 12:665–671, 1992.
73. Khong TY, Frappel JM, Steel HM, et al: Perinatal listeriosis: A report of six cases. Br J Obstet Gynaecol 93:1083–1087, 1986.
74. Gersell DJ: Chronic villitis, chronic chorioamnionitis, and maternal floor infarction. Semin Diagn Pathol 10:251–266, 1993.
75. Altshuler G: Chorangiosis: An important placental sign of neonatal morbidity and mortality. Arch Pathol Lab Med 108:71–74, 1984.
76. Altshuler G: A conceptual approach to placental pathology and pregnancy outcome. Semin Diagn Pathol 10:204–221, 1993.
77. Naeye RL, Maisels J, Lorenz RP, Botti JJ: The clinical significance of placental villous edema. Pediatrics 71:588–594, 1983.
78. Ilagan NB, Elias EG, Liang KC, et al: Perinatal and neonatal significance of bacteria-related placental villous edema. Acta Obstet Gynecol Scand 69:287–290, 1990.
79. Fox H: General pathology of the placenta. In Fox H (ed): Haines and Taylor Obstetrical and Gynaecological Pathology, Vol 2. Edinburgh, Churchill Livingstone, 1987, pp 972–1000.
80. Fox H: The significance of placental infarction in perinatal morbidity and mortality. Biol Neonate 11:87–105, 1967.
81. Robertson WB: Uteroplacental vasculature. J Clin Pathol (Suppl) 10:9–17, 1976.
82. Khong TY, De Wolf F, Robertson WB, Brosens I: Inadequate maternal vascular response to placentation in pregnancies complicated by preeclampsia and small-for-gestational age infants. Br J Obstet Gynaecol 93:1049–1059, 1986.
83. Khong TY: Acute atherosis in pregnancies complicated by hypertension, small-for-gestational age infants, and diabetes mellitus. Arch Pathol Lab Med 115:722–725, 1991.
84. Brosens I, Dixon HG, Robertson WB: Fetal growth retardation and the arteries of the placental bed. Br J Obstet Gynaecol 84:656–663, 1977.
85. Hustin J, Foidart JM, Lambotte R: Maternal vascular lesions in preeclampsia and intrauterine growth retardation: Light microscopy and immunofluorescence. Placenta 4:489–498, 1983.
86. Kitzmiller JL, Watt N, Driscoll SG: Decidual arteriopathy in hypertension and diabetes in pregnancy: Immunofluorescent studies. Am J Obstet Gynecol 141:773–779, 1981.
87. Brosens I: A study of the spiral arteries of the decidua basalis in normotensive and hypertensive pregnancies. J Obstet Gynaecol Br Comm 71:222–230, 1964.
88. Driscoll SG: The pathology of pregnancy complicated by diabetes mellitus. Med Clin North Am 49:1053–1067, 1965.
89. Abramowsky CR, Vegas ME, Swinehart IG, Gyves MT: Decidual vasculopathy of the placenta in lupus erythematosus. N Engl J Med 303:668–672, 1980.
90. Labarre CA: Acute atherosis. A histopathological hallmark of immune aggression. Placenta 9:95–108, 1988.
91. Blanc WA: Circulatory lesions of the human placenta in abruptio. Verh Dtsch Ges Pathol 60:386–392, 1976.
92. Fox H: Pathology of the Placenta. Major problems in pathology series, Vol 7. Philadelphia, WB Saunders, 1978.
93. Roberts DR, Ampola MG, Lage JM: Diagnosis of unsuspected fetal metabolic storage disease by routine placental examination. Pediatr Pathol 11:647–656, 1991.
94. Powel HC, Benirschke K, Favara BE, Pflueger OH: Foamy changes of placental cells in fetal storage disorders. Virchows Arch [A] 369:191–196, 1976.
95. Applegarth DA, Toone JR, Wilson RD, et al: Morquio disease presenting as hydrops fetalis and enzyme analysis of chorionic villus tissue in a subsequent pregnancy. Pediatr Pathol 7:593–599, 1987.
96. Bendon RW, Hug G: Morphologic characteristics of the placenta in glycogen storage disease type II (alpha-1, 4-glucosidase deficiency). Am J Obstet Gynecol 152:1021–1026, 1985.
97. Schoenfeld A, Abramovici A, Klibanski C, Ovadia J: Placental ultrasonographic biochemical and histochemical studies in human fetuses affected with Niemann-Pick disease type A. Placenta 6:33–43, 1985.
98. Jauniaux E, Vamos E, Libert J, et al: Placental electron microscopy and histochemistry in a case of sialic acid storage disorder. Placenta 8:433–442, 1987.
99. Benirschke K, Driscoll SG: The Pathology of the Human Placenta. New York, Springer-Verlag, 1967.
100. Shanklin DR, Scott JS: Massive subchorial thrombo-haematoma. (Breus' mole). Br J Obstet Gynaecol 82:476–487, 1975.
101. Kaplan C, Blanc WA, Elias J: Identification of erythrocytes in intervillous thrombi: A study using immunoperoxidase identification of hemoglobins. Hum Pathol 13:554–557, 1982.
102. Batcup G, Tovey LAD, Longster G: Fetomaternal blood group incompatibility studies in placental intervillous thrombosis. Placenta 4:449–454, 1983.
103. Caldwell C, Purohit DM, Levkoff AH, et al: Chorangiosis of the placenta with persistent transitional circulation. Am J Obstet Gynecol 127:435–436, 1977.
104. Potter JF, Schoeneman M: Metastasis of maternal cancer to the placenta and fetus. Cancer 25:380–388, 1970.
105. Orr JW, Grizzle WE, Huddleston JF: Squamous cell carcinoma metastatic to placenta and ovary. Obstet Gynecol 59:81S–83S, 1982.
106. Delerive C, Locquet F, Mallart A, et al: Placental metastasis from maternal bronchial oat cell carcinoma. Arch Pathol Lab Med 113:556–558, 1989.
107. Schmitt FC, Zelandi FC, Bacchi MM, et al: Adenoid cystic carcinoma of trachea metastatic to the placenta. Hum Pathol 20:193–195, 1989.
108. Tsujimura T, Matsumoto K, Aozasa K: Placental involvement by maternal non-Hodgkin's lymphoma. Arch Pathol Lab Med 117:325–327, 1993.
109. Heite HJ, Kaden G: Matastasierung bosartiger Tumoren, insbesondere des malignen Melanomas, in Plazenta und Kind. Munchen Med Wochenschr 114:1909–1913, 1972.
110. Strauss L, Driscoll SG: Congenital neuroblastoma involving the placenta. Reports of two cases. Pediatrics 34:23–31, 1964.
111. Hayashi Y, Eguchi M, Sugita K, et al: Cytogenetic findings and clinical features in acute leukemia and transient myeloproliferative disorder in Down's syndrome. Blood 72:15–23, 1988.
112. Foucar K, Friedman K, Llewellyn A, et al: Prenatal diagnosis of transient myeloproliferative disorder via percutaneous umbilical blood sampling. Report of two cases in fetuses affected by Down's syndrome. Am J Clin Pathol 97:584–590, 1992.
113. Altshuler G: Placental infection and inflammation. In Perrin EVDK (ed): Pathology of the Placenta. New York, Churchill Livingstone, 1984, pp 141–163.
114. Katz VI, Bowes WA, Sierkh AE: Maternal floor infarction of the placenta associated with elevated second trimester serum alpha-fetoprotein. Am J Perinatol 4:225–228, 1987.
115. Nickell RE: Maternal floor infarction: An unusual cause of intrauterine growth retardation. Am J Dis Child 142:1270–1271, 1988.
116. Gersell DJ, Phillips NJ, Beckerman K: Chronic chorioamnionitis: A clinicopathologic study of 17 cases. Int J Gynecol Pathol 10:217–229, 1991.
117. Ariel IB, Landing BH: A possible distinctive vacuolar change of the amniotic epithelium associated with gastroschisis. Pediatr Pathol 2:283–289, 1985.
118. Kohn G, Livni N, Ornoy A, et al: Prenatal diagnosis of mucolipidosis IV by electron microscopy. J Pediatr 90:62–66, 1977.
119. Grafe MJ, Benirschke K: Ultrastructural study of the amniotic epithelium in a case of gastroschisis. Pediatr Pathol 10:95–101, 1990.
120. Usher RH, Boyd ME, McLean FH, Krames MS: Assessment of fetal risk in postdate pregnancies. Am J Obstet Gynecol 158:259–264, 1988.
121. Rogers BB, Widness JA, Coustan DR, Singer DB: Fetal acidosis and placental pathology [abstract]. Mod Pathol 3(1):498, 1990.
122. Miller PW, Coen RW, Benirschke K: Dating the time interval from meconium passage to birth. Obstet Gynecol 66:459–462, 1985.
123. Kalousek D: Amniotic band syndrome in previable fetuses. Pediatr Pathol 7:488, 1987.
124. Kalousek DK, Bamforth S: Amnion rupture sequence in previable fetuses. Am J Med Genet 31:63–73, 1988.
125. Seidman JD, Abbondanzo SL, Watkin WG, et al: Amniotic band syndrome: Report of two cases and review of the literature. Arch Pathol Lab Med 113:891–897, 1989.
126. Lage JM, vanMarter LJ, Bieber FR: Questionable role of amniocentesis in the formation of amniotic bands. J Reprod Med 33:71–73, 1988.
127. Ruvinski Ed, Wiley TL, Morrison JC, Blake PG: In utero diagnosis of umbilical cord hematoma by ultrasonography. Am J Obstet Gynecol 140:833–834, 1981.
128. Leung AKC, Robson WLM: Single umbilical artery: A report of 159 cases. Am J Dis Child 143:108–111, 1989.
129. Byrne J, Blanc WA: Malformations and chromosomal anomalies in spontaneously aborted fetuses with single umbilical artery. Am J Obstet Gynecol 151:340–342, 1985.
130. Yavner DL, Redline RW: Angiomyxoma of the umbilical cord with massive cystic degeneration of Wharton's jelly. Arch Pathol Lab Med 113:935–937, 1989.
131. Resta RG, Luthy DA, Mahony BS: Umbilical cord hemangioma associated with extremely high alpha-fetoprotein levels. Obstet Gynecol 72:488–491, 1988.
132. Nickell KA, Stocker JT: Placental teratoma: A case report. Pediatr Pathol 7:645–650, 1987.
133. Unger JL: Placental teratoma. Am J Clin Pathol 92:371–373, 1989.
134. Fox H, Butler-Manual R: A teratoma of the placenta. J Pathol Bacteriol 88:137–140, 1964.
135. Stephens TD, Spall R, Urfer AG, Martin R: Fetus amorphus or placental teratoma. Teratology 40:1–10, 1989.
136. Svanholm H, Thordsen C: Placental teratoma. Acta Obstet Gynecol Scand 66:179–180, 1987.
137. Chen KT, Ma CK, Kassel SH: Hepatocellular adenoma of the placenta. Am J Surg Pathol 10:436–440, 1986.
138. Cox JN, Chavrier F: Heterotopic adrenocortical tissue within a placenta. Placenta 1:131–133, 1980.
139. Labarrere CA, Caccamo D, Telenta M, et al: A nodule of adrenocortical tissue within a human placenta: Light microscopic and immunocytochemical findings. Placenta 5:139–144, 1984.
140. Bittencourt AL, dos Santos WLC, de Oliveira CH: Placental and fetal candidiasis: Presentation of a case of an abortus. Mycopathologia 87:181–187, 1984.
141. Schwartz DA, Reef S: Candida albicans placentitis and funisitis: Early diagnosis of congenital candidemia by histopathologic examination of umbilical cord vessels. Pediatr Infect Dis J 9:661–665, 1990.
142. Kim K, Lage JM: Bipartite diamnionic monochorionic twin placenta with superficial vascular anastomoses. Hum Pathol 22:501–503, 1991.

143. Naeye RL: Organ abnormalities in human parabiotic syndrome. Am J Pathol 46:829–842, 1965.

144. Benirschke K: Intrauterine death of a twin: Mechanisms, implication for surviving twin, and placental pathology. Semin Diagn Pathol 10:222–231, 1993.

145. Hoyne HE, Higginbottom MC, Jones KL: Vascular etiology of disruptive structural defects in monozygous twins. Pediatrics 67:288–291, 1981.

146. Robertson EG, Neer KJ: Placental injection studies in twin gestation. Am J Obstet Gynecol 147:170–174, 1983.

147. Rausen AR, Seki M, Strauss L: Twin transfusion syndrome. J Pediatr 66:613–628, 1965.

148. Sala MA, Matheus M: Placental characteristics in twin transfusion syndrome. Arch Gynecol Obstet 246:51–56, 1989.

CHAPTER 16

Breast Diseases

Noel Weidner, M.D.

It has been estimated that approximately one in nine women (living to age 85 years) in the United States will develop breast cancer at some time in their lives; hence, the interpretation of breast biopsies has become a large and important component of the surgical pathologist's practice. This high incidence, increased public awareness of breast disease, greater use of screening mammography to detect early carcinomas, development of multiple therapeutic options (which is often determined by tumor pathology), and a harsh medicolegal climate have placed great pressure on surgical pathologists to make accurate diagnoses of breast lesions. The focus of this chapter is to define the clinicopathologic features of breast lesions that may present diagnostic problems to the general surgical pathologist.

The chapter is divided into four categories: (1) common lesions that mimic other benign or malignant neoplasms; (2) uncommon presentations of common lesions, (3) uncommon lesions worth knowing about, but not otherwise covered, and (4) miscellaneous pathologic curiosities.

COMMON LESIONS THAT MIMIC OTHER BENIGN OR MALIGNANT NEOPLASMS

Several typical breast lesions have morphologic features in common with others. This can create confusion and diagnostic uncertainty; hence, these lesions should be clearly distinguished. The first step in the proper interpretation of a breast biopsy is to distinguish benign from malignant lesions. Usually, this is not a problem; however, diagnostic difficulties develop because some benign lesions clearly share features with malignant tumors.

Benign Breast Lesions

Sclerosing Adenosis

Sclerosing adenosis has a broad spectrum of presentations that can mimic carcinoma both clinically and pathologically. Sclerosing adenosis usually cannot be specifically detected on clinical examination except as a component of a breast mass caused by lesions of fibrocystic change (or disease). Yet, when these lesions present as localized masses large enough to mimic carcinoma, they have been referred to as **adenosis tumors.**[1] Sclerosing adenosis can also involve fibroadenoma.[2]

It is important to recognize sclerosing adenosis; not just to distinguish it from malignant breast disease, but also, as Jensen et al.[3] have shown, because well-developed examples of sclerosing adenosis are associated with a 1.7-fold increased risk for the development of invasive breast cancer. These authors include sclerosing adenosis in the group of histopathologically defined lesions termed **proliferative breast disease (or changes) without atypia,** which implies a relative invasive cancer risk of 1.5 to 2.0.[3]

Although most examples of sclerosing adenosis are easily diagnosed, this lesion is misinterpreted as invasive carcinoma more than any other benign breast lesion.[3, 4] This diagnostic pitfall is amplified when sclerosing adenosis is involved by apocrine metaplasia, presents in a more dispersed (less lobulocentric) form, demonstrates perineural or vessel involvement, and contains foci of lobular or ductal carcinoma *in situ.*

CLINICOPATHOLOGIC FEATURES. Sclerosing adenosis occurs most commonly in the child-bearing and perimenopausal years,[1–4] with most patients presenting in the fourth and fifth decades (only rarely in second or eighth decades). Although it is firm, sclerosing adenosis (even the aggregate or tumoral form) does not have the gritty, hard, or scirrhous texture of invasive carcinoma. When presenting as a mass, sclerosing adenosis usually is multinodular and gray-white to tan-brown. Adenosis tumors are reported to average 2 to 3 cm in diameter, but lesions 6 to 7 cm in diameter have been reported.

Sclerosing adenosis is composed of a cellular proliferation of both duct luminal cells that form acini and spindled myoepithelial cells that impart a sclerotic quality. A very important diagnostic feature is that sclerosing adenosis grows within and expands lobules (often in multiple adjacent foci to form an aggregate), while maintaining the circumscribed, lobulocentric pattern of benign breast lobules (Fig. 16–1). This lobulocentric growth has a whorled and pseudoinvasive quality. Peripheral acini of the lobulocentric aggregates tend to be patent or ectatic; intraluminal calcifications are frequently present. The lobulocentric qualities of sclerosing adenosis are best appreciated at lower magnification. In fact, the cytoarchitectural features of sclerosing adenosis can be especially misleading at higher magnification and can suggest invasive carcinoma; hence, care not to overdiagnose sclerosing adenosis is indicated, especially on frozen sections.

DIFFERENTIAL DIAGNOSIS. Sometimes, however, this lobulocentric pattern can be distorted or dispersed by an admixture of fibrofatty breast tissue that causes the duct luminal and myoepithelial cells to form a pattern mimicking invasive carci-

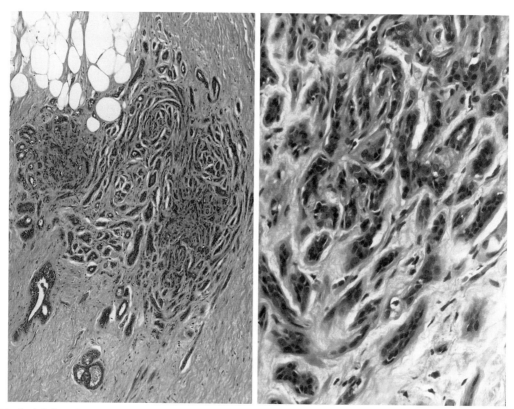

FIGURE 16-1. Typical Sclerosing Adenosis. *Left,* Shown is the whirled, lobulocentric pattern of sclerosing adenosis with relatively circumscribed borders. (H&E) *Right,* Sclerotic, pseudoinvasive pattern of sclerosing adenosis becomes apparent at higher magnification. (H&E)

oma (Fig. 16–2), especially **tubular carcinoma or lobular carcinoma;** however, careful observation at low magnification reveals the general lobulocentric pattern, and, in contrast with invasive carcinoma, there are few mitotic figures, no necrosis, and no desmoplastic stromal reaction. Like invasive carcinoma, **sclerosing adenosis may show perineural "invasion" and involve vessel walls.**[5]

Occasionally foci of sclerosing adenosis can merge with areas consistent with **microglandular adenosis,** a related lesion that shows a more haphazard proliferation of benign glands.[6] Both sclerosing and microglandular adenosis maintain basal lamina around glands; a feature that can be highlighted by immunohistochemical stains for type IV collagen or laminin.[7] Moreover, in sclerosing adenosis, duct luminal cells are surrounded by myoepithelial cells, which bind with antibodies to S-100 protein, high-molecular-weight keratin, and actin.[7] Whether or not the presence of myoepithelial cells is characteristic of microglandular adenosis remains controversial.[7]

One of the most treacherous diagnostic pitfalls for overdiagnosing malignancy is a finding of **apocrine metaplasia within sclerosing adenosis.**[8] The apocrine metaplasia often contains **cytologic atypia** that can be confused with infiltrating carcinoma (Fig. 16–3). The significance of this atypia, which can also occur in cystic examples of apocrine metaplasia (Fig. 16–4, left), remains undetermined.[9] Yet, Page and Anderson[9] appear to regard such lesions as benign, and the report by Carter and Rosen[8] supports this position, because carcinoma did not develop in the 47 women in their series. Apocrine metaplasia can also rarely occur as well-circumscribed adeno-

matous lesions,[10, 11] sometimes with mitotic activity and mild atypia (personal observation).

Nonetheless, sclerosing adenosis with apocrine change should be examined very carefully, because the findings of frequent mitotic figures (especially atypical ones), irregular nuclear membranes, hyperchromatic nuclei, coarse chromatin pattern, multiple nucleoli, and/or necrosis suggest carcinoma, which may be *in situ* within sclerosing adenosis.[12] Also, **apocrine carcinomas** are rarely seen (Fig. 16–4, right), including one reported case in which a breast biopsy 10 months earlier from the same site showed florid apocrine metaplasia intermingled with atypical apocrine cells.[13] Thus, apocrine carcinoma must be included in the differential diagnosis when sclerosing adenosis contains foci of atypical apocrine change.[14, 15] However, difficult or borderline apocrine *in situ* lesions occur, and recently O'Malley et al.[16] have proposed criteria to define apocrine lesions on the borderline between those definitely benign and those indisputably malignant. The clinical utility of their criteria needs to be tested by long-term follow-up studies. Moreover, separating benign atypia from fully malignant atypia in the setting of all types of *in situ* breast lesions can be difficult. Rosai[17] illustrated this problem with borderline epithelial lesions. In a study of 17 cases with atypia, Rosai and a panel of five experts in breast pathology rendered diagnoses that ranged from benign hyperplasia (without atypia) to carcinoma *in situ* in 33% of the cases.

When **sclerosing adenosis is involved by carcinoma *in situ*** (most commonly, lobular carcinoma *in situ* [LCIS], but may be duct carcinoma *in situ* [DCIS]), the pattern mimics

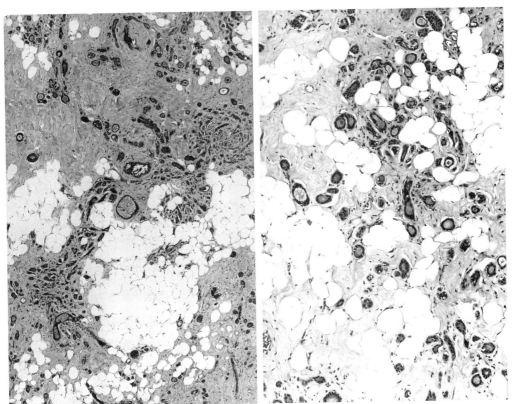

FIGURE 16–2. Sclerosing Adenosis Distorted by Fibrofatty Tissue. *Left,* Shown is sclerosing adenosis with the lobulocentric pattern distorted and dispersed by admixed fibrofatty breast tissues. (H&E) *Right,* Acinar structures of sclerosing adenosis are separated by fibrofatty tissue—a pattern that mimics tubular carcinoma. (H&E)

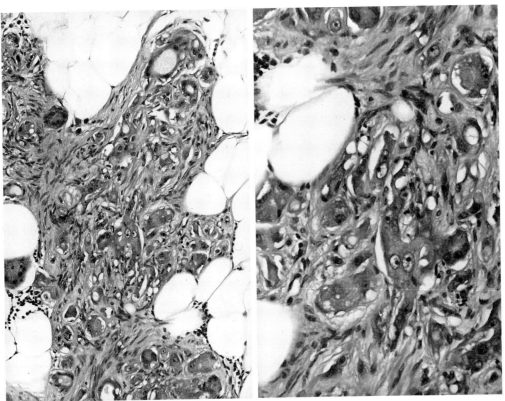

FIGURE 16–3. Sclerosing Adenosis Showing Apocrine Metaplasia. *Left,* The lobulocentric pattern of sclerosing adenosis is apparent. (H&E) *Right,* Atypical apocrine metaplasia is apparent within the sclerosing adenosis because individual cells have large vesicular nuclei, prominent nucleoli, and abundant granular cytoplasm—a treacherous cytoarchitectural pattern that mimics invasive carcinoma. (H&E)

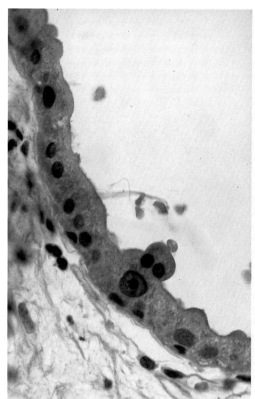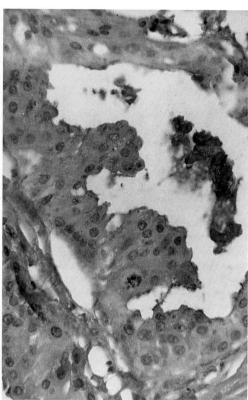

FIGURE 16–4. Apocrine Metaplasia with Benign and Malignant Atypia. *Left,* Cystic apocrine metaplasia showing focal cytologic atypia. (H&E) *Right,* Apocrine carcinoma showing an atypical mitotic figure, nuclear stratification, and necrotic calcified debris within the lumen. (H&E)

invasive carcinoma.[18] Foci of carcinoma *in situ* (CIS) within sclerosing adenosis without invasion can be recognized when the CIS is accompanied by the maintenance of the lobulocentric pattern characteristic of sclerosing adenosis; the presence of peripherally dilated, centrally attenuated ducts; the absence of fat invasion; and the preservation of the myoepithelial layers (Fig. 16–5). Eusebi et al.[19] recommended using anti-actin and periodic acid-Schiff (PAS) stains to demonstrate the intact myoepithelial cells and basal lamina to assist in distinguishing CIS within sclerosing adenosis from invasive carcinoma. Also, immunostains for high molecular weight keratins are useful in highlighting an intact myoepithelial layer.

Microglandular Adenosis

Microglandular adenosis is a proliferation of small, uniform glands that grow in a haphazard fashion in the breast parenchyma[6, 20–23] (Fig. 16–6). Although currently considered benign in most instances, some investigators believe that microglandular adenosis may be a precancerous lesion.[6, 23] This lesion has features of both benign sclerosing adenosis and invasive **well-differentiated (tubular) carcinoma,** with which it might be confused[6, 20–23] (Figs. 16–7 to 16–9). In one series of 11 patients with microglandular adenosis, two patients were inappropriately treated with mastectomy.[22] Typical microglandular adenosis is treatable with excision biopsy, because no metastasis of microglandular adenosis has yet been documented.[22] However, atypical examples of microglandular

adenosis have been described, and rarely invasive carcinoma can evolve in association with microglandular adenosis.[6, 23]

CLINICOPATHOLOGIC FEATURES. In two series,[6, 22] ages of patients have ranged from 28 to 82 years (most patients are in the sixth decade).[6, 22] Patients usually present with a breast mass that has existed for several weeks to years before biopsy. Mammogram findings are non-specific and are often interpreted as abnormal or suspicious. There may or may not be a family history of breast carcinoma.[6, 22]

Microglandular adenosis resembles normal breast or an ill-defined, indurated area of gray-white, fibrofatty breast (essentially identical to that of fibrocystic changes, not otherwise specified). Most lesions are 3 to 4 cm in diameter, but can range from an incidental microscopic focus to 20-cm lesions.[6, 20–23]

Microscopically, microglandular adenosis is characterized by a haphazard proliferation of fairly uniform, small, round glands in either fibrous connective tissue or fat (see Fig. 16–6). The growth pattern is distinctly not lobulocentric and without an intervening spindle cell component, as observed with sclerosing adenosis. The glands are lined by a single layer of monotonous, cuboidal cells with clear (vacuolated) to eosinophilic cytoplasm. Nuclei are bland, and nucleoli are small and indistinct; mitotic figures are uncommon. Gland lumina often contain deeply eosinophilic (colloid-like) secretions. Like tubular carcinoma, a basement membrane around the glands is not easily recognizable by light microscopy. Apical "snouts," like those frequently seen in tubular carcinoma, are not present.

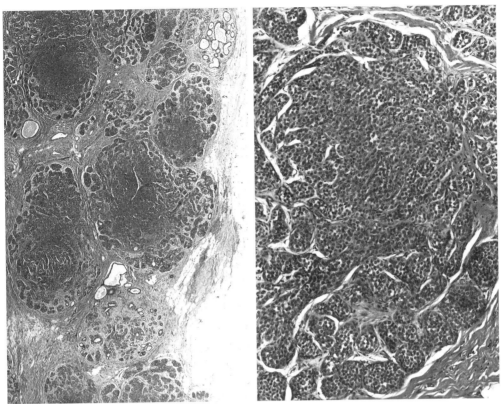

FIGURE 16–5. Sclerosing Adenosis Containing Lobular Carcinoma *In Situ*. *Left,* Note the maintenance of the lobulocentric pattern of each lobular unit of sclerosing adenosis, in spite of the fact that benign epithelial cells have been replaced by LCIS cells. (H&E) *Right,* Cells characteristic of LCIS fill the distorted glands of sclerosing adenosis—a pattern that mimics invasive carcinoma, especially the alveolar variant of invasive lobular carcinoma. (H&E)

With electron microscopy, glands of microglandular adenosis are usually lined by a single layer of luminal epithelial cells that are surrounded by a multilayered basement membrane, although some authors report that the myoepithelial layer is poorly formed.[22] Nonetheless, the ultrastructural demonstration of basement membrane around glands in microglandular adenosis, but not in tubular carcinoma, can be helpful in differentiating these two lesions in difficult cases.[24] More recently, Diaz et al.[7] reported that myoepithelial cells were a consistent finding in microglandular adenosis. They found a rim of myoepithelial cells around the ducts of microglandular adenosis, which was best demonstrated with anti-actin (monoclonal "muscle-specific" actin, HHF-35). Also, these authors were able to consistently demonstrate type IV collagen immunostaining (monoclonal CIV22) around the glands of microglandular adenosis but not tubular carcinoma.

DIFFERENTIAL DIAGNOSIS. Microglandular adenosis can mimic invasive **well-differentiated (tubular) carcinoma,** an invasive carcinoma that should be excised with clear margins combined with axillary node dissection[20, 25–29] when clinically indicated (see Figs. 16–7 to 16–9). The following features are most helpful in distinguishing microglandular adenosis from tubular carcinoma: (1) the distribution of glands in microglandular adenosis at low magnification appears random rather than stellate (as in tubular carcinoma); (2) the glands in microglandular adenosis appear uniform and round rather than having angular protrusions, which seem to dissect desmoplastic stroma; (3) the epithelium in microglandular adenosis is flatter and without apocrine snouts; and (4) cribriform,

micropapillary, or "clinging" intraductal carcinoma frequently accompanies tubular carcinoma but not microglandular adenosis (see Figs. 16–8 and 16–9).[20, 25–29] Indeed, when the cribriform growth pattern makes up the majority of the infiltrating component (tubular component less than 50%), the neoplasm is called **invasive cribriform carcinoma,** which has a better prognosis than infiltrating duct carcinoma, not otherwise specified,[30, 31] and a prognosis like that of tubular carcinoma (see Fig. 16–8). Also, microglandular adenosis needs to be differentiated from **invasive lobular carcinoma, tubulolobular variant.**[32] This should not be difficult, because the invasive components of the latter neoplasm form not only small tubules but also cords of cells more characteristic of invasive lobular carcinoma.

James et al.[23] reported on 14 patients with microglandular adenosis who also developed peculiar, yet "distinctive," invasive carcinomas in association with the adenosis (23% of cases in the authors' files). These carcinomas were associated not only with typical microglandular adenosis but also with a form of **atypical microglandular adenosis** that suggested transitions from microglandular adenosis to invasive carcinoma.[23] Atypical microglandular adenosis is a more pleomorphic form of microglandular adenosis that is characterized by its more complex architecture, formation of trabecular bridges in glandular lumina, cellular expansion and crowding of these lumina, and the presence of vesicular nuclei. Although more clinical follow-up is necessary to characterize these distinctive invasive carcinomas, some patients had a favorable outcome in spite of the fact that each carcinoma had a high-grade

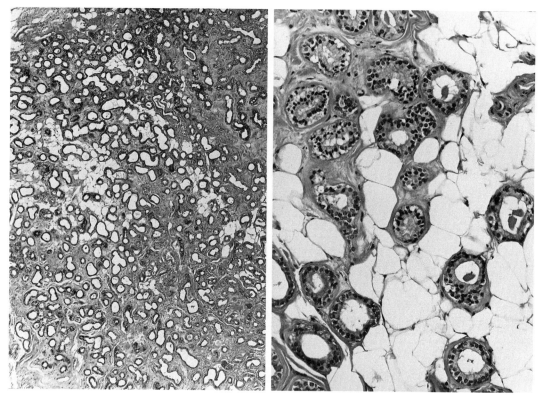

FIGURE 16–6. Microglandular Adenosis. *Left,* Microglandular adenosis shows a dispersed, pseudoinvasive pattern of small round glands permeating through both fat and fibrous tissues. (H&E) *Right,* Note round glands lined by what appears to be a single layer of luminal epithelial cells. Lumina contain colloid-like secretion products. (H&E) (From Weidner N: Benign breast lesions that mimic malignant tumors: Analysis of five distinct lesions. Semin Diagn Pathol 7:90–101, 1990.)

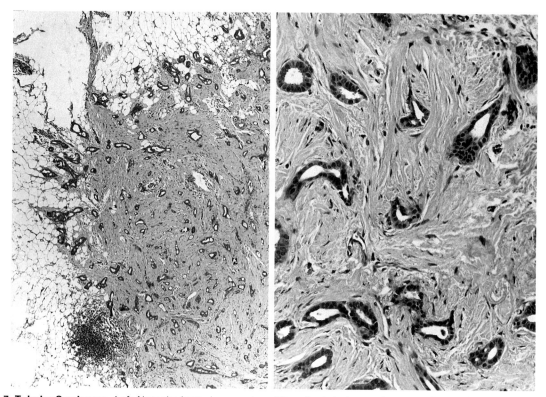

FIGURE 16–7. Tubular Carcinoma. *Left,* Note the irregular margins of invasive tubular carcinoma and central desmoplastic stroma. (H&E) *Right,* Tubular carcinoma glands show irregular, sharply angulated contours, and they are surrounded by desmoplastic stroma. (H&E) (From Weidner N: Benign breast lesions that mimic malignant tumors: Analysis of five distinct lesions. Semin Diagn Pathol 7:90–101, 1990.)

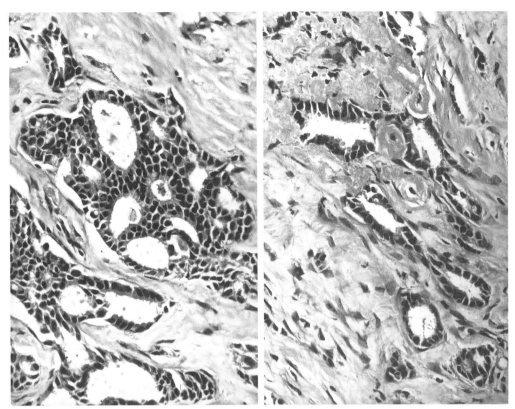

FIGURE 16–8. Cribriform Carcinoma. *Left,* More than 50% of the tumor shows invasive cribriform islands; thus, this carcinoma qualifies as invasive cribriform carcinoma. (H&E) *Right,* Other areas of the same tumor show features of invasive tubular carcinoma. (H&E)

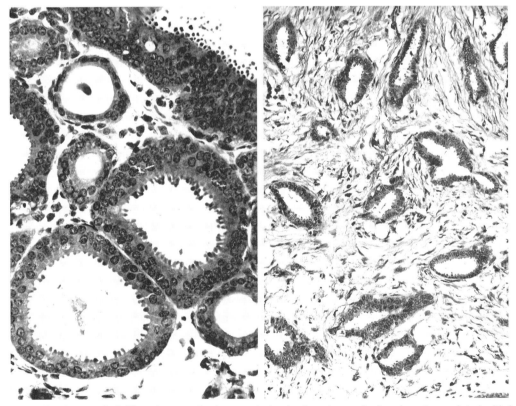

FIGURE 16–9. Tubular Carcinoma. *Left,* Note the peculiar low-grade *in situ* ''carcinoma,'' often found associated with invasive tubular carcinoma. (H&E) *Right,* Tubular carcinoma is admixed with the low-grade *in situ* areas shown at left. (H&E) (From Weidner N: Malignant breast lesions that may mimic benign tumors. Semin Diagn Pathol 12:2–13, 1995.)

component. Atypical microglandular adenosis should be widely excised and followed as a form of atypical hyperplasia.

Because the glandular lumina of microglandular adenosis contain eosinophilic secretions, microglandular adenosis can be mistaken for **secretory carcinoma** of the breast[33–35] (Fig. 16–10). Although initially described in young patients and called juvenile carcinoma, secretory carcinoma has not only been found in children younger than 10 years of age but also in adults as old as 73 years.[33, 34] In a review, Rosen and Cranor[35] found that 37% of patients were younger than 20 years old, 31% were in their twenties, and the remainder were over 30. Although secretory carcinomas have been reported to be more aggressive in adults, Rosen and Cranor[35] failed to find any clinicopathologic difference with age, except for a greater delay in diagnosis in younger patients. Secretory carcinomas are usually well circumscribed, white or brown, and measure from 0.6 to 12 cm. The tumor is characterized by large amounts of extra- and intracellular secretions, which are strongly PAS and mucicarmine positive, and by granular, clear, signet-ring, and/or vacuolated cytoplasm, sometimes with an apocrine appearance. Yet, secretory carcinomas are negative for gross cystic disease fluid protein-15 [GCDFP-15], an apocrine marker.[35, 36] Histologic patterns include varying proportions of secretory microacini, solid areas, and foci of cystic papillary formations. Fibrous stroma may be focally prominent (especially centrally) and contain irregular tubules or ducts, simulating microglandular adenosis or tubular carcinoma.[37, 38] Nuclei are monotonous and cytologically bland; mitotic figures are uncommon; and DCIS may be present in adjacent breast.

Sclerosing Papillary Proliferations

Fibrocystic changes containing florid intraductal hyperplasia may undergo sclerosis, distortion, and entrapment of distorted ducts. This benign lesion has been variously referred to as **sclerosing papillary proliferation,**[39] scleroelastotic lesion simulating malignancy,[40] non-encapsulated sclerosing lesion,[41] indurative mastopathy,[42] complex sclerosing lesion,[43] invasive epitheliosis,[44] and **radial scar**.[45, 46] They are common lesions that can be mistaken for invasive carcinoma, not only by mammogram but also by gross appearance and light microscopy. Indeed, Fenoglio and Lattes[39] stated in their classic report that "unfortunately, radical or modified mastectomies are still occasionally performed because a distorted sclerosed benign papillary proliferation was misinterpreted as a carcinoma, especially on frozen section."

CLINICOPATHOLOGIC FEATURES. In one series of 32 patients with sclerosing papillary proliferation,[45] patients' ages at diagnosis ranged from 30 to 57 years (mean, 43 years). After being observed from 15 to 24.5 years (mean, 19.5 years), only 1 of the 32 patients developed breast carcinoma, a rate comparable to a control population. Furthermore, a subsequent autopsy study failed to show a higher malignant potential for sclerosing papillary proliferations (other than that expected in patients having fibrocystic changes). These investigators suggested that only those sclerosing papillary proliferations containing high-risk epithelial changes such as atypical hyperplasia and carcinoma *in situ* are associated with increased risk of subsequent breast cancer development.[46] Eighty-eight percent of patients with sclerosing papillary proliferations also have fibrocystic changes and/or duct ectasia; in only 9% did

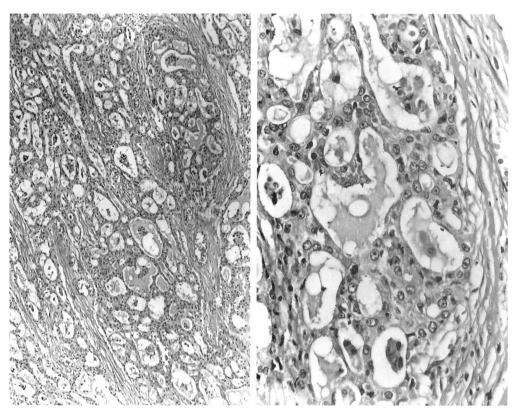

FIGURE 16–10. Secretory Carcinoma. *Left,* Note the fibrous stroma admixed with invasive cribriform nests. (H&E) *Right,* Luminal secretions are prominent, and nuclei are monotonous and cytologically bland; mitotic figures are uncommon. (H&E)

sclerosing papillary proliferation occur as a single lesion without fibrocystic changes.[45] Multicentricity of sclerosing papillary proliferations has been noted in 44% of cases.[45] On mammogram, these lesions can have an irregular stellate appearance; and by gross examination, the lesions are gray-white to yellow, stellate firm densities sometimes with spiculated margins, features easily confused with scirrhous carcinoma.

Sclerosing papillary proliferations display a central, relatively hypocellular core composed of dense hyalinized connective tissue, rich in elastic fibers (Fig. 16–11). The connective tissue fibers seem to radiate toward the periphery, where fibrocystic changes are arranged circumferentially and characterized by varying combinations of duct hyperplasia, cyst formation, sclerosing adenosis, and apocrine metaplasia. The central scleroelastotic core may contain small epithelial nests and glands, which appear distorted and entrapped within the connective tissue, resulting in a pattern simulating invasive carcinoma (**"pseudoinvasion"**).

DIFFERENTIAL DIAGNOSIS. Sclerosing papillary proliferations are most frequently confused with invasive, **well-differentiated (tubular) carcinomas** (see Figs. 16–7 to 16–9). Invasive tubular carcinomas can,[20] but usually do not, display the zonal character of sclerosing papillary proliferation (central hypocellular core surrounded by proliferative fibrocystic changes in a radial fashion). In addition, the **pseudoinvasive glands of sclerosing papillary proliferations** may display a double row of cells (myoepithelial cell layer adjacent to luminal epithelial cells) encased in a hyalinized, elastic tissue–rich stroma. Glands of invasive tubular carcinoma are composed of a single row of atypical cells encircled by relatively loose, desmoplastic stroma. Furthermore, the pseudoinvasion of sclerosing papillary proliferations is limited to the immediate periductal zone; involvement of the interlobular fat would suggest a true carcinoma. Both microglandular adenosis and sclerosing adenosis can involve fat.[1, 2, 4, 39–46] Finally, sclerosing papillary proliferations (like other forms of fibrocystic changes) can occur concomitantly with atypical hyperplasia, carcinoma *in situ,* and invasive carcinoma. A recent study has reported that atypical hyperplasia and/or carcinoma are very uncommonly associated with sclerosing papillary lesions in women younger than 40 years old and when the lesions are less than 6 cm in size.[47] Usual histologic criteria for atypia and carcinoma should be applied in making the latter diagnoses.

Finally, **duct adenoma of the breast** is a benign lesion that should be considered in the differential diagnosis of sclerosing papillary lesions[48, 49] (Fig. 16–12). Lammie and Millis[49] concluded that ductal adenomas evolved by sclerosis of benign intraductal papillary lesions, although sclerosing adenosis and duct ectasia showed similarities. Azzopardi[47] noted similarities between papilloma and salivary-type adenoma. Duct adenomas are adenomatous nodules occurring in small to medium-sized ducts surrounded by densely fibrous walls. These lesions have a circumscribed, variably lobated outline, often with a central scar. Fibrous distortion leads to pseudoinvasion of central or adjacent tissues (Fig. 16–13). Worrisome atypia can also occur, especially when apocrine metaplasia is present.

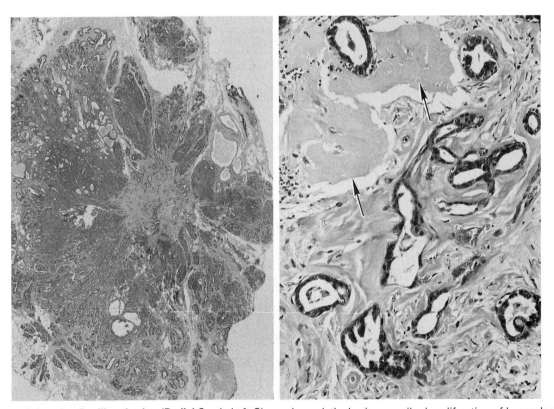

FIGURE 16–11. Sclerosing Papillary Lesion (Radial Scar). *Left,* Shown is a relatively circumscribed proliferation of hyperplastic lobules and ducts with a central, hypocellular scar (also known as radial scar or complex sclerosing lesion). (H&E) *Right,* The central scar shows distorted glands with predominantly rounded contours and admixed granular elastic tissue *(arrows)*—a pattern that mimics invasive carcinoma. (H&E) (From Weidner N: Benign breast lesions that mimic malignant tumors: Analysis of five distinct lesions. Semin Diagn Pathol 7:90–101, 1990.)

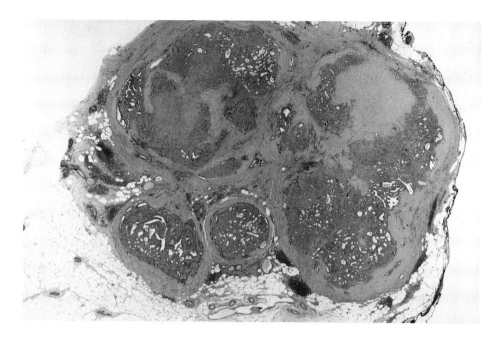

FIGURE 16–12. Duct Adenoma. Shown are the well-circumscribed, fibrotic margins of so-called duct adenoma. These lesions also often appear lobular and may have adjacent intraductal papilloma and/or ductal hyperplasia. (H&E) (From Weidner N: Benign breast lesions that mimic malignant tumors: Analysis of five distinct lesions. Semin Diagn Pathol 7:90–101, 1990.)

But the well-circumscribed outline and the biphasic epithelial-myoepithelial differentiation are reliable criteria for recognizing this lesion as benign.[47, 49]

Intraductal Papilloma

Intraductal papillomas are benign fibroepithelial lesions. Most occur in large ducts where they are usually *single,* but they also arise in peripheral smaller ducts where they are *multiple* in about 10% of cases.[50-53] In two large series, approximately 10% of the benign papillomas had been misdiagnosed as malignant, sometimes resulting in inappropriate radical surgery.[50, 51]

CLINICOPATHOLOGIC FEATURES. In the report of Kraus and Neubecker,[51] patients with benign papilloma ranged from 16 to 71 years (average, 39 years). In contrast, patients with papillary carcinoma tended to be slightly older, with ages at diagnosis ranging from 29 to 78 years (average, 50 years).

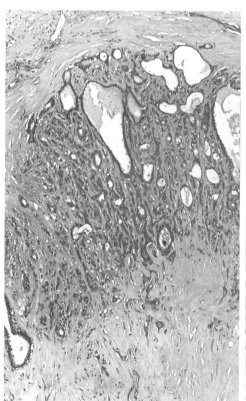

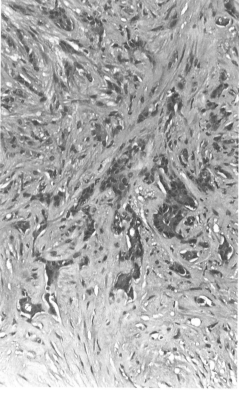

FIGURE 16–13. Duct Adenoma. *Left,* Note the sclerosing adenosis-like and/or radial scar–like qualities of duct adenoma. (H&E) *Right,* The central scarred regions show considerable distortion of glands and myoepithelial cells, imparting a pseudo-invasive pattern. In problematic cases, actin or high-molecular-weight keratin (E903) immunostain is helpful in highlighting the associated benign myoepithelial component. (H&E) (From Weidner N: Benign breast lesions that mimic malignant tumors: Analysis of five distinct lesions. Semin Diagn Pathol 7:90–101, 1990.)

Benign papillomas, like papillary carcinomas, present as masses, often near the nipple, and are sometimes associated with a bloody discharge from the nipple.

These lesions are soft, friable tumors, usually found within dilated cysts (ectatic ducts). The cysts contain fluid, which may be bloody or yellow-brown. Focal necrosis can occur. In one series, they measured from 0.5 to 8.0 cm (mean, 2.3 cm).[51] Grossly, papillary carcinomas can appear similar to intraductal papillomas.[51, 54]

Microscopically, intraductal papillomas show a prominent arborescent, fibrovascular core lined by a double layer of epithelial cells, which is at least focally present in all papillomas (Figs. 16–14 and 16–15). Typically, the core has a prominent collagenous and/or spindled myoepithelial component. The lining epithelial cells have normochromatic nuclei and may have areas of apocrine metaplasia and/or typical duct hyperplasia. Adjacent ducts often have these same features, as well as areas of sclerosing adenosis.

Solitary subareolar papillomas uncommonly display adjacent duct hyperplasia, atypical duct hyperplasia, and/or carcinoma *in situ*;[52, 53] whereas, papillomas that are peripheral and multifocal are frequently associated with duct hyperplasia, sometimes atypical and/or carcinomatous (see Fig. 16–14, left).[52, 53] In fact, some investigators feel strongly that peripheral duct papillomas are highly susceptible to cancerous change.[52–56] In a detailed three-dimensional reconstruction study of intraductal papillomas, Ohuchi et al.[53] "accidentally" discovered that 6 of 16 patients (37%) with peripheral duct papillomas had carcinomas in "close anatomic continuity" to the benign papillomas, whereas none of the 9 patients with

central duct papillomas had cancers. Thus, these observations suggest that multiple peripheral duct papillomas may be a form of "benign" breast disease deserving of complete, yet conservative, local excision, especially when palpable and/or cytoarchitectural atypia is present. Indeed, Haagensen[54] advised that "when local excision of the lesion is carried out, the surgeon must take great care to try to remove all of the grossly evident disease."

Standard histologic criteria for atypia and/or malignancy should be used in evaluating areas of duct hyperplasia that occur in conjunction with intraductal papilloma. Finally, it is important to add that in and around the bases of papillomas there may be considerable fibrosis and epithelial entrapment, resulting in a **pseudoinvasive pattern** (see Fig. 16–14, right). When the glands in these pseudoinvasive areas have a double cell layer cytologically identical to those found in the papilloma, their benign nature is secure. Overdiagnosing the pseudoinvasive areas as invasive carcinoma (especially on frozen sections) must be avoided. But, please remember that true **invasive papillary carcinoma**[57] and **invasive micropapillary carcinoma**[58] occur in the breast and should not be underdiagnosed as benign. If there is any doubt, defer the final diagnosis until permanent sections are available, when special studies can be performed and/or consultation can be obtained from a trusted colleague or an expert in breast pathology.

DIFFERENTIAL DIAGNOSIS. Papillary carcinoma of the breast can closely mimic intraductal papilloma clinically and macroscopically.[51, 59–61] The distinction, therefore, depends on careful light microscopic examination. Although variable, the arborescent fronds of papillary carcinoma are usually com-

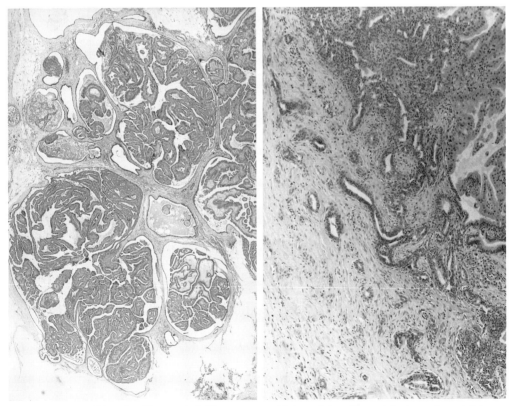

FIGURE 16–14. Multiple Peripheral Duct Papillomas. *Left,* Shown are multiple peripheral breast ducts, each containing a small intraductal papilloma. (H&E) *Right,* At the edge of one of the intraductal papillomas is fibrous tissue containing entrapped distorted glands—a pattern that can be mistaken for invasive carcinoma, especially at frozen section examination. (H&E)

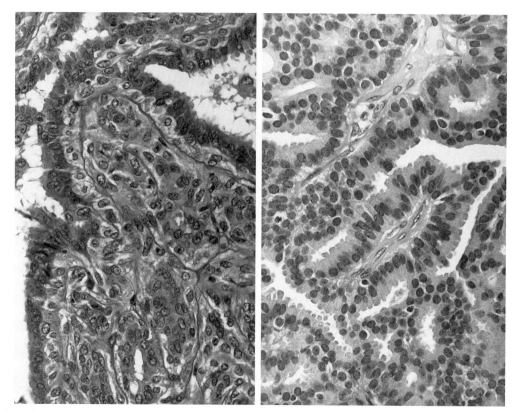

FIGURE 16–15. Intraductal Papilloma Compared with Papillary Carcinoma. *Left,* Benign intraductal papilloma showing two cell layers—columnar duct luminal cells and underlying myoepithelial cells with clear cytoplasm. (H&E) *Right,* Non-invasive papillary carcinoma showing single layer of stratified, columnar epithelial cells covering a fibrovascular core—a pattern similar to adenomatous polyps of the colon. (H&E)

posed of a more delicate fibrovascular core; indeed, the fibrous component may be inconspicuous. The lining epithelial cells are of a single type, showing high nucleocytoplasmic ratios, increased mitotic activity, and uniform, hyperchromatic nuclei (Figs. 16–15, right, and 16–16). Furthermore, the tumor cells may show stratification and resemble the adenomatous epithelium of a tubular adenoma of the gastrointestinal tract. Apocrine metaplasia and sclerosing adenosis are usually absent, and when solid areas of epithelial proliferation are present in adjacent ducts, they often show features of duct carcinoma *in situ* rather than typical duct hyperplasia, which is associated with intraductal papilloma. Obviously, the presence of invasive duct carcinoma makes benign intraductal papilloma less likely.

Although these criteria may seem straightforward, controversial and/or borderline cases do arise. In some cases, the double cell layer may be inconspicuous. To delineate the double cell layer, Papotti et al.[60] proposed using immunohistochemical staining with carcinoembryonic antigen (CEA) and actin. Benign papillomas have a basal layer of actin-rich myoepithelial cells; the cytoplasm of the luminal epithelial cells are CEA-negative. Papillary carcinomas lack the myoepithelial layer, except in areas where multiple papillomas are present and there is often invasion. CEA was detected in 85% of the papillary carcinomas in Papotti et al.'s study. Two of their cases of ''suspected'' carcinoma lacked myoepithelial cells and were interpreted as carcinomas. In another immunohistochemical study of papillomas and papillary carcinomas, Raju et al.[61] found that antibodies to muscle actin (HHF-35) were

reliable markers for myoepithelial cells (better than an antibody to high molecular weight keratin [34BE12] and antiserum to S-100 protein). Furthermore, they found that the presence of a few myoepithelial cells alone did not exclude a malignant diagnosis in the less characteristic papillary lesions such as micropapillary duct carcinoma *in situ* and peripheral papillomas with cancerization. Clearly, experience is always very helpful, and good judgment must be applied in difficult cases.

Pseudoangiomatous Hyperplasia of Mammary Stroma

Pseudoangiomatous hyperplasia of mammary stroma (PHMS) is a benign proliferation of keloid-like fibrosis within which are slit-like pseudovascular spaces. Its main importance is its similarity to low-grade angiosarcoma.[62, 63] Indeed, a diagnosis of angiosarcoma was seriously considered in three of the initial nine cases reported by Vuitch et al.,[62] and a fourth patient had bilateral subcutaneous mastectomies when the PHMS was initially diagnosed as an ''atypical vasoformative process.'' Ibrahim et al.[63] subsequently reported an additional case of PHMS that was overdiagnosed as low-grade angiosarcoma, resulting in inappropriate mastectomy. These workers also analyzed 200 consecutive breast specimens and found foci of PHMS in 23% of them. They concluded that PHMS is a common histologic finding in breast biopsy specimens, and that PHMS represents a clinicopathologic spectrum that ranges from focal, insignificant microscopic changes to cases

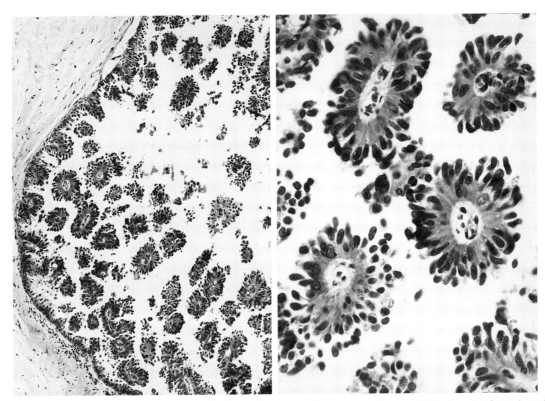

FIGURE 16–16. Non-invasive Papillary Carcinoma. *Left,* Shown is an ectatic duct containing multiple fronds of non-invasive papillary carcinoma. (H&E) *Right,* The delicate papillae of papillary carcinoma contain delicate fibrovascular cores. Tumor cells are pseudostratified, show hyperchromatic nuclei, have increased nucleocytoplasmic ratios, and have no myoepithelial layer. (H&E) (*Left,* from Weidner N: Benign breast lesions that mimic malignant tumors: Analysis of five distinct lesions. Semin Diagn Pathol 7:90–101, 1990. *Right,* from Weidner N: Malignant breast lesions that may mimic benign tumors. Semin Diagn Pathol 12:2–13, 1995.)

in which it produces a distinct breast mass. The importance of distinguishing PHMS from angiosarcoma may have become even greater as there are now reports of the development of secondary angiosarcoma after tylectomy and postoperative radiation therapy and after segmental mastectomy complicated by lymphedema.[64, 65]

CLINICOPATHOLOGIC FEATURES. PHMS usually presents as a painless, well-circumscribed mass; however, rarely, a patient may present with a diffusely enlarged breast and *peau d'orange* changes in the overlying skin, thus mimicking inflammatory breast carcinoma.[62, 63] Thus far, patients having clinically significant disease have been premenopausal; however, focal PHMS changes occur commonly and involve a wide age group (range, 17 to 76 years; mean, 40; 2.5% of patients are older than 50).[63] The overwhelming majority have occurred in women, but Seidman et al.[66] reported a rapidly growing case in axillary gynecomastia in an immunosuppressed man.

Clinically significant PHMS appears as an edematous fibroadenoma, i.e., gray-white, rubbery, and, if fibrocystic changes are present, cystic. In contrast with angiosarcoma, they are not hemorrhagic, necrotic, or ill-defined.[67] Microscopically, clinically significant PHMS is dominated by abundant interlobular stroma characterized by keloid-like fibrosis containing irregular, interconnected spaces resembling capillaries (Fig. 16–17, left). The slit-like spaces are empty and appear to be lined by endothelial-like spindle cells (Fig. 16–17, right), which have been shown to be fibroblasts by ultrastructural and immunocytochemical studies. These fibroblasts may show

mild cytologic atypia, but there are no mitotic figures or "tufting" as noted in angiosarcomas.[67, 68] The lobular architecture is generally maintained within the pseudoangiomatous stroma. The lobules are clearly separated by increased interlobular stroma, and there may be fewer, mildly ectatic ducts. The slit-like spaces in the interlobular stroma may merge with identical spaces of the intralobular stroma.

As an incidental finding in routine breast specimens, PHMS appears much less alarming. Usually, it occurs in areas of stromal fibrosis, often immediately surrounding breast lobules in a concentric fashion. Otherwise, incidental PHMS is histologically identical to PHMS that forms a detectable mass. PHMS changes can occur in association with fibrocystic changes, in fibroadenomas, in gynecomastia, in normal breast, and in **sclerosing lobular hyperplasia**.[63]

DIFFERENTIAL DIAGNOSIS. Mammary angiosarcoma is characterized by open anastomosing vascular channels that infiltrate all components of breast tissue[67, 68] (Fig. 16–18, left). Invasive angiosarcoma does not "respect" normal anatomic boundaries, and when it invades lobules, it produces vascular channels within the intralobular stroma, resulting in separation and atrophy of the terminal duct lobular units. Tufted papillary structures form and are capped by atypical endothelial cells that have enlarged, hyperchromatic nuclei (Fig. 16–18, right). Malignant endothelial cells can be flat, inconspicuous, and negative for Factor VIII–related antigen and *Ulex europaeus*-1 lectin. This pattern can be found in at least some areas in all angiosarcomas. Distinction of low-grade angiosarcomas from PHMS might be difficult in individual cases; however, the

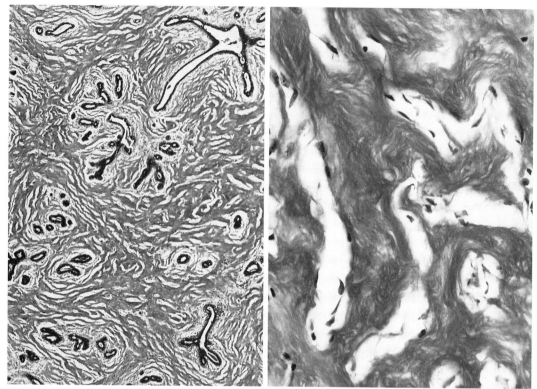

FIGURE 16–17. Pseudoangiomatous Hyperplasia of Mammary Stroma (PHMS). *Left,* Multiple slit-like spaces of PHMS course through the keloid-like fibrotic breast stroma. The pseudovascular spaces involve intralobular as well as interlobular stroma. (H&E) *Right,* These spaces are lined by spindled cells resembling endothelial cells (actually fibroblasts). (H&E) (From Weidner N: Benign breast lesions that mimic malignant tumors: Analysis of five distinct lesions. Semin Diagn Pathol 7:90–101, 1990.)

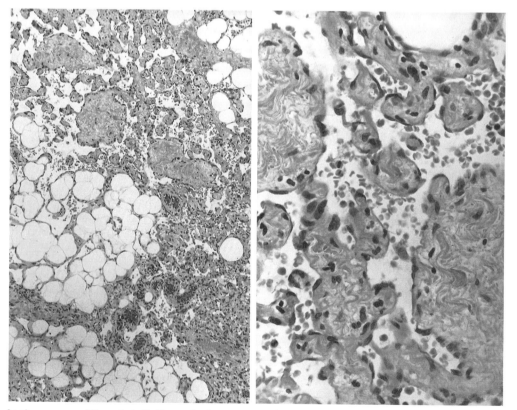

FIGURE 16–18. Angiosarcoma of Breast. *Left,* Shown is the anastomosing network of invasive vessels of angiosarcoma; they dissect through the breast without regard to anatomic structures. (H&E) *Right,* Multiple tufts of fibrous tissue are lined by hyperchromatic, atypical endothelial cells. (H&E)

capillary-like spaces of PHMS are slit-like rather than open, do not cause acinar atrophy, and while involving inter- and intralobular stroma, do not involve fat. Certainly, if the lesion in question shows necrosis, hemorrhage, solid spindle cell areas, and papillary endothelial growth, the diagnosis of angiosarcoma becomes secure.

Diffuse cystic angiomatosis of the breast,[69] **perilobular hemangiomas, venous hemangioma,** and other benign hemangiomas also need to be distinguished from PHMS and angiosarcoma. Rosen et al.[70-74] have described the spectrum of vascular lesions encountered in breast tissues, even some **benign hemangiomas with atypical histologic features**.[70] Careful consideration of the typical features of PHMS and angiosarcoma should lead to the correct diagnosis.

Mammary hamartoma should also be considered in the differential diagnosis of PHMS.[75-78] Mammary hamartomas are well-circumscribed masses presenting as fibroadenoma-like lesions that contain various combinations of fat and fibrous tissue within which are ducts and lobules in an architecturally distorted distribution (Fig. 16–19, left). Smooth muscle differentiation may be present focally, and 25 of 35 breast hamartomas (71%) described by Fisher et al.[75] contained significant amounts of PHMS. Terms such as **adenolipoma** and **fibroadenolipoma** have also been applied to these breast lesions.[75-78] Although benign and of minimal clinical consequence, breast hamartomas continue to cause diagnostic problems. **Tubular adenomas** also present as fibroadenoma-like masses, share features with this group of lesions, and should be considered in the differential diagnosis[2, 75-78] (Fig. 16–19, right).

Collagenous Spherulosis

Collagenous spherulosis is a recently described benign breast lesion composed of a proliferation of duct luminal cells and myoepithelial cells, which make abundant basement membrane material.[79, 80] The fact that collagenous spherulosis can be overdiagnosed as a malignant neoplasm was demonstrated by Clement et al.[79] who reported that one of their initial 15 cases of collagenous spherulosis had been inappropriately called adenoid cystic carcinoma, and three others, intraductal signet-ring carcinoma.

CLINICOPATHOLOGIC FEATURES. Typically, to date, patients with collagenous spherulosis are women from 39 to 55 years of age (mean, 41 years) who have had a breast biopsy or simple mastectomy because of the presence of a palpable mass, abnormal mammogram, or both. Collagenous spherulosis is an incidental microscopic finding, which can be unifocal or multifocal. The lesions occur in duct lumina and consist of intraductal hyperplastic cells containing focal aggregates of well-circumscribed, acellular spherules ranging in size from 20 to 100 μm (Fig. 16–20). At low power, collagenous spherulosis resembles a form of cribriform intraductal carcinoma. The spherules are usually discrete but can coalesce and can range from a few to up to 50 within any given focus. The spherules stain pink-red and appear fibrillar with hematoxylin and eosin (H&E) (see Fig. 16–20, right); many have a pale center and more darkly staining periphery. The fibrillar components are arranged in a concentric laminated pattern, radiate in a star-shaped configuration, or both. Outlining the spherules in

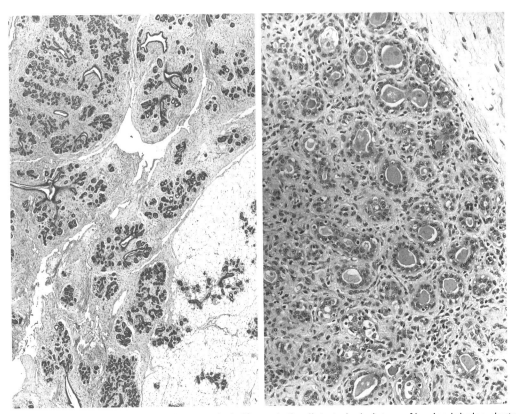

FIGURE 16–19. Breast Hamartoma and Tubular Adenoma. *Left,* Shown is the distorted admixture of benign lobules, ducts, and fibrofatty tissue characteristic of breast hamartoma, a lesion that presents in the breast as a fibroadenoma-like mass and that may contain considerable stroma showing PHMS. (H&E) *Right,* Shown is the well-circumscribed margin of a tubular adenoma, a lesion with features that overlap with adenomyoepithelioma. (H&E)

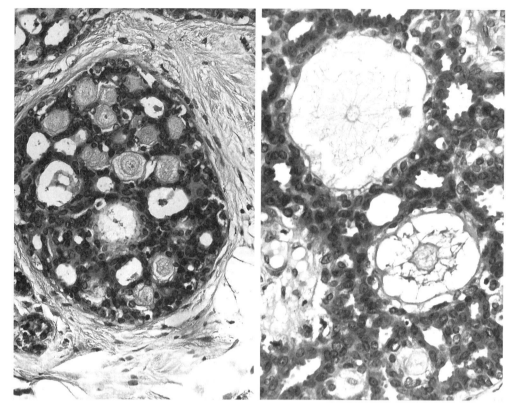

FIGURE 16–20. Collagenous Spherulosis. *Left,* Shown is a duct containing collagenous spherulosis; note the cribriform-like pattern mimicking DCIS. (H&E) *Right,* Within each cribriform-like space is a variably hyalinized spherule surrounded by hyperplastic duct epithelial cells; note the fibrillary and/or targetoid quality of the spherules, which are composed of basal lamina–like material. (H&E)

all cases seen are cells (actually myoepithelial cells) that appear to be stretched or flattened around them in some areas. Epithelial cells identical to those found in typical duct hyperplasia can also be seen.[80] Adjacent breast tissue frequently contains fibrocystic changes with duct hyperplasia, sclerosing adenosis, and/or intraductal papilloma.

DIFFERENTIAL DIAGNOSIS. The differential diagnosis for collagenous spherulosis includes **adenoid cystic carcinoma** and **intraductal signet-ring carcinoma.**[81, 82] Adenoid cystic carcinoma of the breast closely resembles adenoid cystic carcinoma of salivary gland origin;[81] however, in breast it is an extremely rare tumor accounting for approximately 1 in 1000 breast carcinomas. Typically, in adenoid cystic carcinoma, the stroma is infiltrated by cell clusters containing features of smaller epithelium-lined spaces and larger myoepithelium-lined cystic spaces (Fig. 16–21). The tumor cells do not form apical snouts, but have low-grade nuclei, and often form delicate arches. Adenoid cystic carcinoma must have intercellular cystic spaces lined by basement membrane material and biphasic cellularity with myoepithelial cells intermixed with duct luminal epithelial cells.

Intraductal signet-ring carcinoma is a rare lesion composed of large, malignant cells that are vacuolated.[82] The vacuoles are PAS-positive (as are the spherules of collagenous spherulosis), but in contrast with collagenous spherulosis, they are negative with collagen stains. A clear understanding of collagenous spherulosis makes it possible to distinguish it from intraductal signet-ring carcinoma.

Malignant Breast Lesions

Invasive Lobular Carcinoma

Infiltrating lobular carcinoma, **classic type,** is a well-recognized invasive breast lesion[83–96] (Fig. 16–22); but other forms of this,[32, 83–96] including **pleomorphic** (Fig. 16–23), **solid, alveolar, mixed, apocrine, signet-ring, histiocytoid, and tubulolobular variants,** are less well recognized. Some studies have focused on the clinicopathologic significance of these infiltrating lobular carcinoma variants, indicating that solid, alveolar, mixed, and signet-ring forms have a worse prognosis than classic infiltrating lobular carcinoma.[85–94] Fisher et al.[32] reported that the short-term treatment failure rates in patients with tubulolobular invasive carcinoma were intermediate between those of tubular carcinoma and infiltrating lobular carcinoma, suggesting that the tubulolobular variant of infiltrating lobular carcinoma had a better overall prognosis than some others (Fig. 16–24). Too few cases of the histiocytoid (Fig. 16–25) and/or apocrine variants of infiltrating lobular carcinoma have been reported to make firm conclusions regarding their behavior relative to other variants of infiltrating lobular carcinoma.[90, 91] Admittedly, one study suggests that the apocrine variant may be an aggressive variant of breast cancer.[95]

Page et al.[94] have emphasized a **pleomorphic variant** of infiltrating lobular carcinoma that has the infiltrating pattern of classic infiltrating lobular carcinoma, but in which the nuclei are more pleomorphic and there is a tendency for the

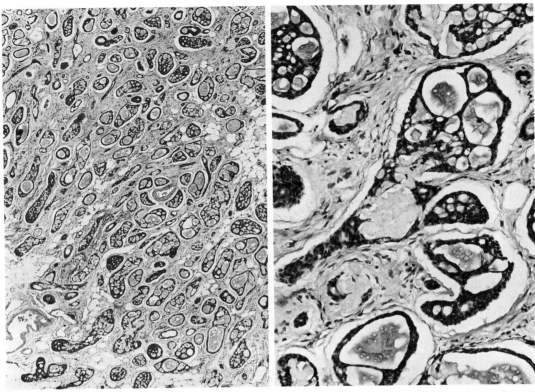

FIGURE 16–21. Adenoid Cystic Carcinoma of the Breast. *Left,* Shown are the invasive cribriform islands of adenoid cystic carcinoma. (H&E) *Right,* The invasive nests or islands are of variable size, shape, and contour, and they show cribriform spaces of "microcysts" filled with mucin. The islands are variably surrounded by hyaline basal lamina–like material and/or desmoplastic stroma. (H&E) (From Weidner N: Benign breast lesions that mimic malignant tumors: Analysis of five distinct lesions. Semin Diagn Pathol 7:90–101, 1990.)

tumor cells to aggregate. Dixon et al.[85-87] included the pleomorphic infiltrating lobular carcinomas in their **mixed category,** which also included infiltrating lobular carcinomas showing various combinations of classic, solid, and/or alveolar patterns. Also, DiCostanzo et al.[88] studied the mixed variant of infiltrating lobular carcinoma, but their study included only cases of infiltrating lobular carcinoma with classic cytologic features (small and uniform cells), thus excluding breast carcinomas with pleomorphic nuclei.

Eusebi et al.[95] presented a series of 10 patients with apocrine-type, pleomorphic infiltrating lobular carcinoma, of which six died of disease within 42 months of diagnosis. Three other patients developed recurrence or distant metastases within a short period of time. In contrast, only 2 of 22 control patients with classic infiltrating lobular carcinoma died of disease after 48 months of follow-up. The authors concluded that pleomorphic infiltrating lobular carcinoma was a very aggressive variant of infiltrating lobular carcinoma. All their cases of pleomorphic infiltrating lobular carcinoma showed the linear, single-file, and targetoid invasive pattern of classic infiltrating lobular carcinoma, but the cytologic features were considered pleomorphic to a degree that contrasted with classic infiltrating lobular carcinoma and highlighted the difficulty of distinguishing pleomorphic infiltrating lobular carcinoma from infiltrating duct carcinoma. Furthermore, their 10 cases often showed eosinophilic, slightly granular, and/or foamy cytoplasm, and all showed immunoreactivity with gross cystic disease fluid protein-15 (GCDFP-15), a known apocrine marker.[96] In this series, 22 classic infiltrating lobular carcinomas failed to react with GCDFP-15.

Weidner and Semple[97] showed that pleomorphic infiltrating lobular carcinoma had a significantly shorter relapse-free survival than classic infiltrating lobular carcinoma ($p \leq .05$, when followed for at least 30 months). Node-negative patients with pleomorphic infiltrating lobular carcinoma were four times more likely to experience recurrence than node-negative patients with classic infiltrating lobular carcinoma. Also, those with positive nodes and pleomorphic histology were 30 times more likely to experience recurrence. Although there appeared to be a trend toward decreased overall survival for those patients with pleomorphic infiltrating lobular carcinoma when compared with those with classic infiltrating lobular carcinoma, this difference did not achieve statistical significance.

CLINICOPATHOLOGIC FEATURES. The gross presentation of infiltrating lobular carcinoma can be most deceptive when it fails to form a discrete mass. In these cases, infiltrating lobular carcinoma can have a doughy consistency by palpation and closely mimic benign breast disease. This gross presentation, plus the often bland cytologic features of classic infiltrating lobular carcinoma, makes the frozen-section diagnosis of infiltrating lobular carcinoma very treacherous and the evaluation of resection margins with frozen section difficult.

The classic pattern of infiltrating lobular carcinoma is characterized by diffusely and/or multifocal infiltrating tumor cells that are small, round, and regular (see Fig. 16–22). They form single files between collagen bundles, which sometimes encircle ducts in a targetoid or onion-skin fashion. Occasional

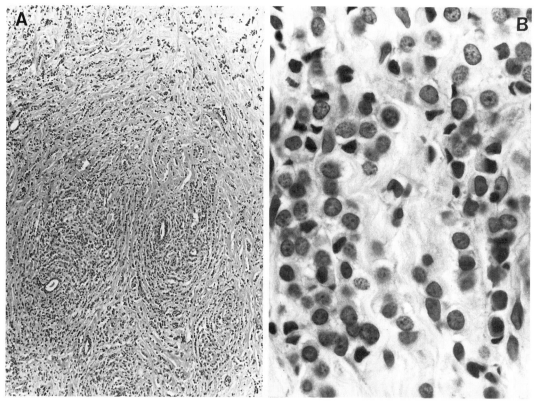

FIGURE 16–22. Infiltrating Lobular Carcinoma, Classic Variant. *Left,* Shown is the characteristic infiltrative pattern of lobular carcinoma produced by invasion of tumor cells in single file and periductal, targetoid, or onion-skin fashion. (H&E) *Right,* Typical infiltrating lobular carcinoma is composed of uniform, small cells with bland nuclei (nuclear grade 1 or type A–like cells) and small amounts of cytoplasm. (H&E)

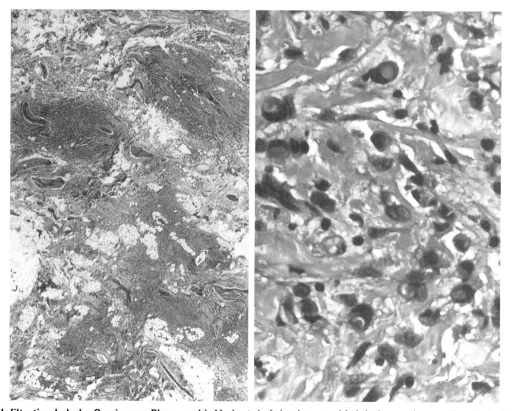

FIGURE 16–23. Infiltrating Lobular Carcinoma, Pleomorphic Variant. *Left,* In pleomorphic lobular carcinoma, the single file and targetoid invasive patterns are well maintained and best appreciated at low magnification. (H&E) *Right,* In contrast with classic lobular carcinoma, the nuclei of pleomorphic lobular carcinoma show greater nuclear irregularities and variation in size (nuclear grade 2 to 3 or type B–like cells). Also, cytoplasm is usually more abundant. This particular case also shows signet ring change. (H&E)

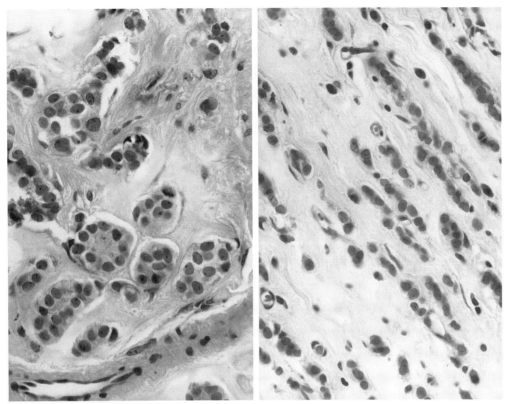

FIGURE 16–24. Invasive Lobular Carcinoma, Tubulolobular Variant. *Left,* Small tubules of invasive carcinoma with cytologic features of classic lobular carcinoma. (H&E) *Right,* Classic invasive lobular carcinoma showing invasive, single-file pattern with grade 1 nuclear features. This pattern was admixed with the invasive tubular pattern shown on the left. (H&E)

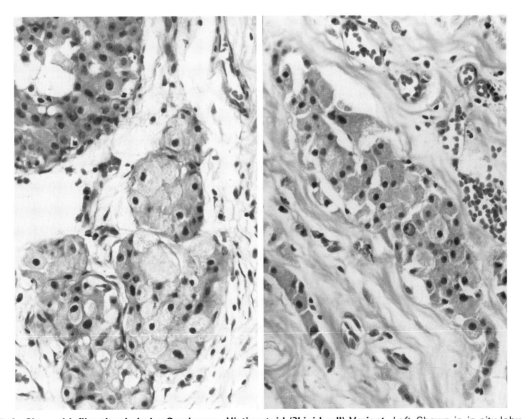

FIGURE 16–25. *In Situ* **and Infiltrating Lobular Carcinoma, Histiocytoid (?Lipid-cell) Variant.** *Left,* Shown is *in situ* lobular carcinoma with abundant foamy to finely granular cytoplasm, characteristic of the histiocytoid (?also lipid-cell) variant. (H&E) *Right,* Area containing invasive histiocytoid (?also lipid-cell) variant of lobular carcinoma. This pattern can be underdiagnosed as benign foamy histiocytes. (H&E)

cases form foci of small tubules, referred to as the tubulolobular variant of infiltrating lobular carcinoma (see Fig. 16–24).

Pleomorphic infiltrating lobular carcinoma shows the infiltrating pattern of classic infiltrating lobular carcinoma (best appreciated at low magnification) (see Fig. 16–23, left); however, the nuclei are more pleomorphic than in classic infiltrating lobular carcinoma, and they display varying degrees of contour irregularity, more prominent nucleoli, greater hyperchromaticity, increased chromatin clumping, increased mitotic activity, and/or greater nuclear size (see Fig. 16–23, right). The degree of nuclear atypia can approach that found in infiltrating duct carcinomas; but the invasive pattern characteristic of the classic lobular variant is always well maintained. Signet ring cytology can be found in both the classic and pleomorphic variants.

To be considered pleomorphic infiltrating lobular carcinoma, pleomorphic nuclei must be present in at least half the tumor cells composing the lesion. Also, if portions of the tumor (more than one low-magnification field, ×40) show alveolar (small, rounded, invasive cell clusters or islands composed of at least 20 tumor cells) and/or solid (cell-to-cell sheets of invasive tumor) areas of invasion, the tumor should not be considered invasive pleomorphic lobular carcinoma, but rather alveolar or solid variants, respectively.

DIFFERENTIAL DIAGNOSIS. The diagnosis of the classic form of infiltrating lobular carcinoma is seldom difficult, and experienced diagnostic pathologists concur in the vast majority of cases. Yet, some invasive breast carcinomas show features of both infiltrating lobular carcinoma and **infiltrating duct carcinoma,** and those invasive tumors maintaining the invasive pattern of infiltrating lobular carcinoma yet having nuclear features approaching that of duct carcinoma represent the pleomorphic variant of lobular carcinoma. Infiltrating duct carcinomas have a more solidly cohesive invasive pattern, without the diffuse, single-file, multifocal, and periductal targetoid pattern of infiltrating lobular carcinoma. Occasional cases of infiltrating lobular carcinoma contain considerable foamy, **histiocytoid, and/or "lipid-rich" cytoplasm** (see Fig. 16–25). The malignant cells resemble foamy histiocytes, a cell-type they can be distinguished from by positive cytokeratin immunostaining, concomitant lobular carcinoma *in situ,* and/or positive mucicarmine staining.

Lobular Carcinoma In Situ

Lobular carcinoma *in situ* (LCIS) is usually an incidental finding in biopsies taken for other reasons, usually for fibrocystic changes.[83, 98–105] Although most common in pre- and perimenopausal women, LCIS can occur in postmenopausal women. LCIS is a multicentric, bilateral lesion that has a well-established association with the subsequent development of invasive carcinoma,[98–100, 104] and both breasts are at risk. (In a review article, Elston and Ellis[99] reported a 10- to 11-fold increased risk for the subsequent development of invasive breast carcinoma, with a 25% absolute risk in 10 years. But it is very important to add that absolute risk is highly dependent on patient age at initial diagnosis, because the incidence of invasive breast carcinoma varies considerably with age.[100])

The distinction of LCIS from **atypical lobular hyperplasia (ALH)** is quantitative, because individual cells of both lesions are essentially identical.[102, 104] Indeed, LCIS and ALH have been collectively referred to as **lobular neoplasia**.[102, 104] ALH

has a reported four- to five-fold increased risk for the subsequent development of invasive breast carcinoma, with a 10% absolute risk in 10 years.[98–104] ALH with duct involvement has a seven-fold increased risk, and ALH and a positive family history of breast carcinoma in a first-degree relative increase the risk eight- to 11-fold.[98–100, 104]

CLINICOPATHOLOGIC FEATURES. LCIS has no distinctive gross appearance, nor does it have a specific microcalcification pattern. Indeed, when calcospherites are present, they are usually in adjacent benign structures or apparently "overrun" by ingrowth of LCIS cells.[101] Classic LCIS is characterized by a group of acini and/or ductules filled by a monotonous (often discohesive) population of small cells with regular nuclei, evenly dispersed chromatin, and inconspicuous nucleoli (Fig. 16–26). The cytoplasm is scant and finely granular to clear; mitotic figures are rare.

As Page et al.[102] state, "consistency in diagnosis of LCIS is fostered by requiring that each of the following criteria be fulfilled: (1) the characteristic and uniform cells must comprise the entire population of cells in a lobular unit, (2) there must be filling of all the acini (no interspersed, intercellular lumina), and (3) there must be expansion and/or distortion of at least one-half the acini in the lobular unit. . . . Lesser degrees of involvement are diagnosed as ALH, a diagnosis carrying a lesser risk of subsequent carcinoma"[102] (Fig. 16–27). Extension of the cells characteristic of ALH/LCIS (lobular neoplasia) into segmental ducts does not allow the diagnosis of LCIS, unless the stated criteria are met in at least one lobular unit (Fig. 16–28).[102] Yet, ALH with duct involvement should initiate a careful search for LCIS by ordering level sections, submitting additional tissue, and/or slide re-examination.

DIFFERENTIAL DIAGNOSIS. Variant patterns of LCIS occur that can be mistaken for ductal carcinoma *in situ* (DCIS). In the most common variant pattern, the entire population of LCIS cells are not **small and uniform (type A cells)** but, rather, admixed with tumor cells with more abundant cytoplasm and **larger, more pleomorphic nuclei sometimes containing nucleoli (type B cells)**[98] (Fig. 16–29). The large-cell variant can develop apocrine differentiation[90] (Fig. 16–30) or sometimes form signet-ring cells of varying sizes[94, 95] (Fig. 16–31). In these instances, DCIS enters the differential diagnosis. Also, the diagnostic problem is complicated by well-documented examples of DCIS plus LCIS occurring within the same biopsy (Fig. 16–32) and even the same duct[103] (Fig. 16–33). Moreover, occasional microacini may form in ducts involved by cells with all the cytologic features of classic LCIS (Fig. 16–34). Indeed, Page et al.[104] presented a photograph they designated as depicting the "gold standard" LCIS (their Figure 2), which contained some of these tiny microacini. Also, Fechner describes both cribriform and papillary patterns of duct extension of LCIS.[105] It is difficult for this author to accept that a few tiny microacini in an otherwise solid area of LCIS totally alters the biologic characteristics of the lesion to render it DCIS.

Nonetheless, for examples of CIS that share features of ductal and lobular types, a diagnosis of DCIS should be favored to encourage adequate local excision of the lesion. Mention should also be made of the concomitant LCIS patterns to emphasize the possible greater risk of bilateral breast carcinoma. This encourages adequate follow-up studies of the contralateral breast. That **intermediate forms of CIS** exist is

(*Text continued on page 649*)

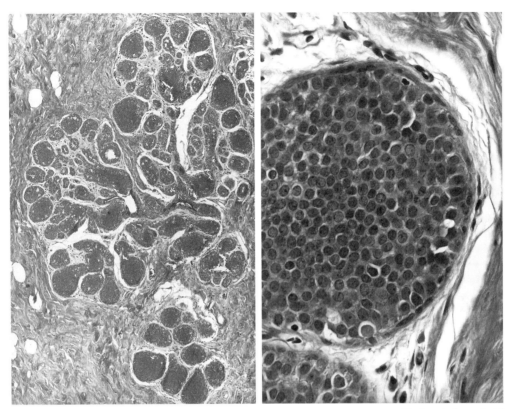

FIGURE 16–26. Lobular Carcinoma *In Situ,* Classic Variant. *Left,* All the acini of this lobule are filled and distended by uniform small (type A) cells characteristic of lobular neoplasia. (H&E) *Right,* Note that this acinus is filled and distended by a uniform population of small cells with grade 1 or small (type A) nuclear features and scant cytoplasm. (H&E)

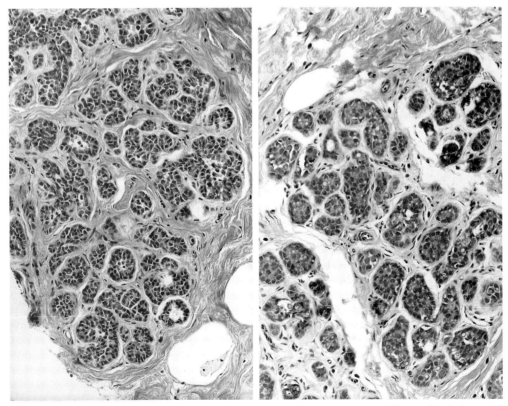

FIGURE 16–27. Atypical Lobular Hyperplasia. *Left,* When fewer than half of the acini of a lobule are filled, distended, or distorted by cells characteristic of lobular neoplasia (most often shown by the presence of residual lumina), then a diagnosis of atypical lobular hyperplasia (ALH) is made. (H&E) *Right,* Another example of atypical lobular hyperplasia. Criteria for LCIS are not met. (H&E)

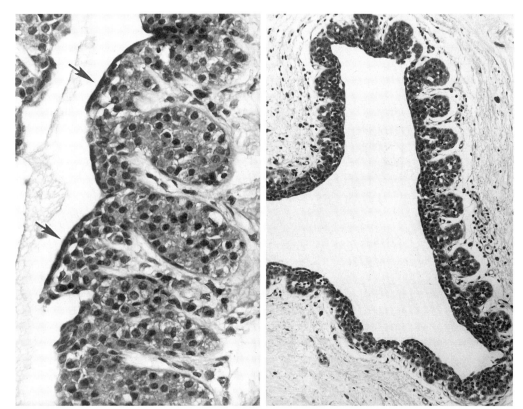

FIGURE 16–28. Duct Extension of Cells Characteristic of Lobular Neoplasia (ALH or LCIS cells). *Left,* Note the proliferation of cells characteristic of lobular neoplasia along the duct lumen, undermining residual duct luminal epithelial cells *(arrows).* (H&E) *Right,* The lobular neoplasia cells produce a cauliflower-like pattern of outpouchings. (H&E)

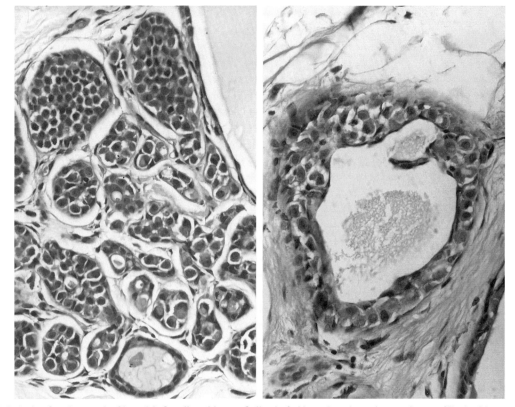

FIGURE 16–29. Lobular Carcinoma *In Situ* with Small and Large Cells. *Left,* Note that the acinar units are filled with small (type A) cells at the top of the field, whereas acinar units toward the bottom are filled with larger (type B) cells. (H&E) *Right,* Segmental duct shows pagetoid spread of LCIS cells (larger variant) undermining a narrow rim of residual duct epithelium. (H&E)

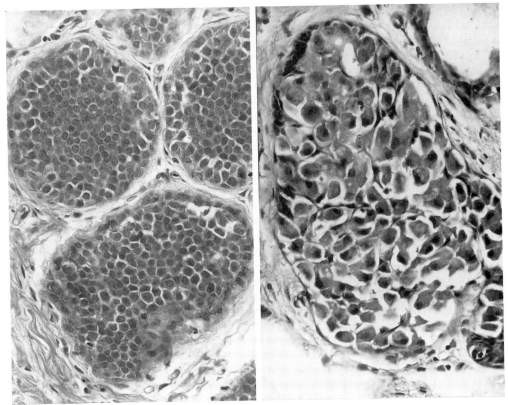

FIGURE 16–30. Classic LCIS Compared with LCIS, Apocrine Variant. *Left,* Classic LCIS. (H&E) *Right,* Note abundant finely granular cytoplasm of LCIS, apocrine variant. (H&E)

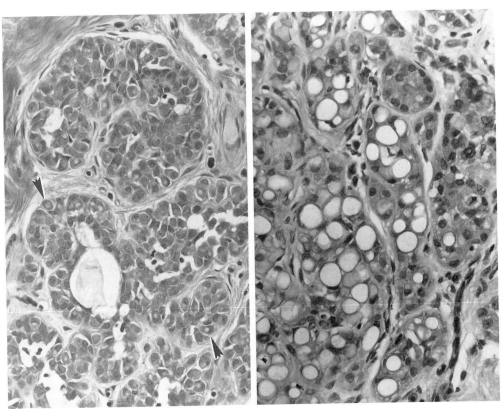

FIGURE 16–31. LCIS with Signet-Ring Features. *Left,* Lobular neoplasia cells showing small cytoplasmic vacuoles of early signet-ring change. (H&E) *Right,* Well-developed signet-ring change is noted in this example of LCIS. (H&E)

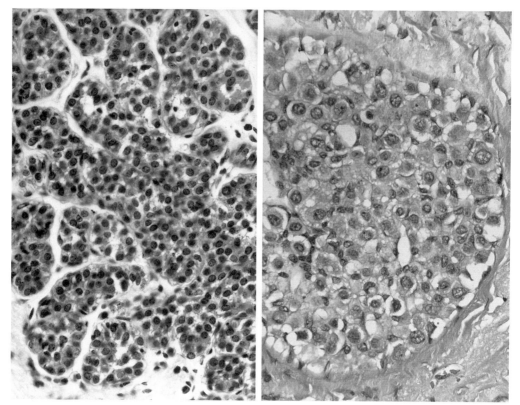

FIGURE 16–32. LCIS and DCIS in Adjacent Areas. *Left,* Classic LCIS in lobules. (H&E) *Right,* Solid DCIS was present within a few millimeters of the LCIS shown at left. (H&E)

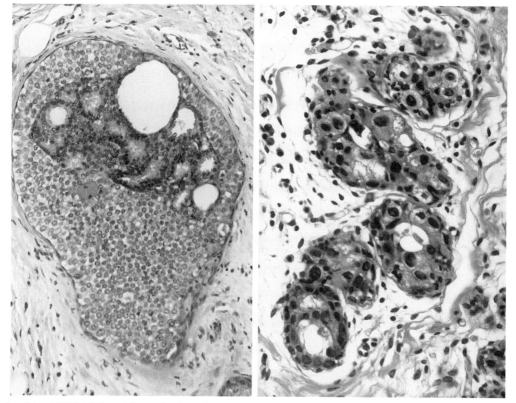

FIGURE 16–33. Combined DCIS-LCIS and Cancerization of Lobules by DCIS. *Left,* Shown is a duct containing low-grade DCIS surrounded by LCIS. Within a few millimeters of this duct there were ducts containing well-developed DCIS and lobules showing classic LCIS. (H&E) *Right,* Shown is a lobule containing DCIS (i.e., cancerization). Note larger cell size, greater nuclear irregularity, and lumen formation by tumor cells. (H&E)

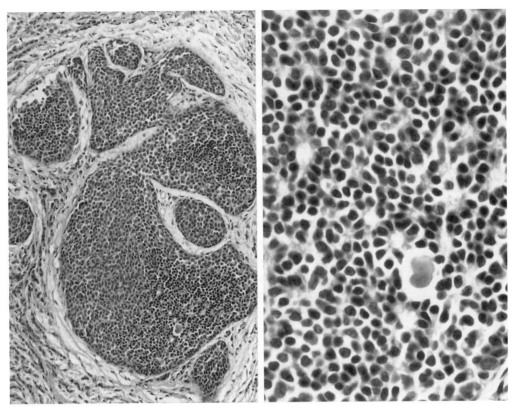

FIGURE 16–34. LCIS Containing Tiny Microacinar Structures. *Left,* Shown is an invasive breast carcinoma with features characteristic of infiltrating lobular carcinoma. Also present were areas of carcinoma *in situ* with cytologic features of classic LCIS; yet, small microacinar structures were present. (H&E) *Right,* Shown are the microacinar structures within a duct containing otherwise classic LCIS. (H&E)

no surprise, especially if Wellings and Jensen are correct that the terminal duct lobular unit complex (lobule) is the site of origin of not only LCIS but also the bulk of DCIS.[106] Of importance in this regard, Ottesen et al.[107] have shown that examples of LCIS composed of larger (type B) cells (i.e., cells with features overlapping with DCIS), and/or when 10 or more lobules are involved by LCIS, there is a significantly greater likelihood of recurrence. Also these recurrences were ipsilateral rather than contralateral.

Cancerization of lobules by duct carcinoma may have features that overlap with the large-cell, apocrine-type, and/or pleomorphic variants of LCIS (see Fig. 16–33, right). Admittedly, it would be very difficult to distinguish cancerization of lobules by DCIS from these variants of LCIS, especially if there were no ''classic'' areas of LCIS present in the biopsy specimen. Furthermore, how could one rule out the concomitant presence of LCIS and DCIS? Cancerization of lobules by high-grade DCIS is usually quite easy to recognize, because the lesion contains large pleomorphic cells, areas of necrosis, and mitotic figures; lumina are also often present (see Fig. 16–33, right). Yet, distinguishing LCIS from cancerization of lobules by a low-grade, non-comedo, or small-cell DCIS could be problematic. Such distinctions are not easy, likely arbitrary, and of uncertain clinicopathologic significance, because the two disease processes may be more alike than different. When in doubt, it is best to favor low-grade DCIS and mention the LCIS patterns, so as to optimize both surgery and patient follow-up.

Benign lesions that may be confused with LCIS (especially the signet-ring form) are **lactational changes** (Fig. 16–35,

left) and so-called **clear-cell metaplasia** of lobules (Fig. 16–35, right). Clear-cell metaplasia can also be confused with clear-cell variants of duct carcinoma.[108] The cause of focal lactational changes and clear-cell metaplasia remains unclear, but the cytologic features are benign and once understood should not cause diagnostic confusion.[108]

When considering the diagnosis of recurrent *in situ* breast carcinoma in patients with prior radiation therapy, **radiation-induced atypia** should be considered.[109] The most characteristic radiation effects produce atypical epithelial cells in the lobules associated with lobular sclerosis and atrophy (Fig. 16–36). Epithelial atypia in larger ducts, stromal changes, and vascular changes are less frequent but are always accompanied by prominent lobular changes. Mitotic figures in radiation-induced atypia are rare to absent. A final area of potential confusion is overdiagnosing **reactive foamy histiocytes** when present either adjacent to areas of duct ectasia (Fig. 16–37, left) or when insinuating themselves between epithelial cells (Fig. 16–37, right). These patterns mimic infiltrating histiocytoid and/or lipid-cell carcinoma or pagetoid spread of lobular neoplasia into segmental ducts.

Low-Grade (Non-Comedo/Small-Cell) Duct Carcinoma In Situ

Duct carcinoma *in situ* (DCIS) is a non-invasive breast lesion that affects ectatic segmental ducts. It is composed of intermediate to large cells (at least relative to that of LCIS), and forms comedo, solid, cribriform, and/or papillary patterns.[102] In contrast with LCIS, DCIS tends to be unilateral

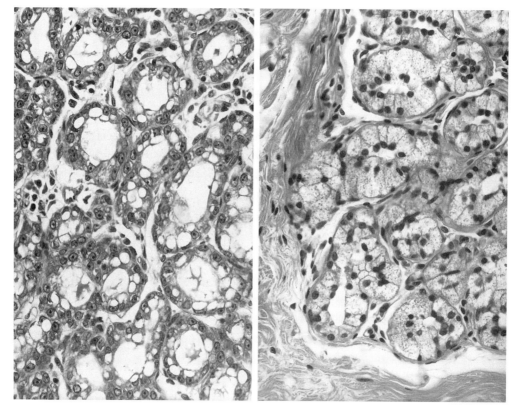

FIGURE 16–35. Lactational Change and Clear-cell Metaplasia. *Left,* Shown is lactational change present in a lactating adenoma. The cells have vacuolated cytoplasm and vesicular nuclei with prominent nucleoli. The latter features can be mistaken for carcinoma, especially at frozen section examination. (H&E) *Right,* A lobule is shown containing clear-cell metaplasia; a pattern that mimics histiocytoid or lipid-rich carcinoma. (H&E)

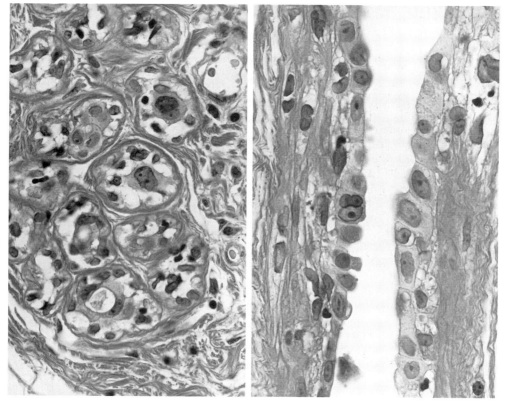

FIGURE 16–36. Breast with Radiation Atypia. *Left,* Breast after radiation showing sclerotic, atrophic lobules containing atypical epithelial cells. (H&E) *Right,* Same breast as shown at left, but also demonstrating atypical cells in segmental duct. (H&E)

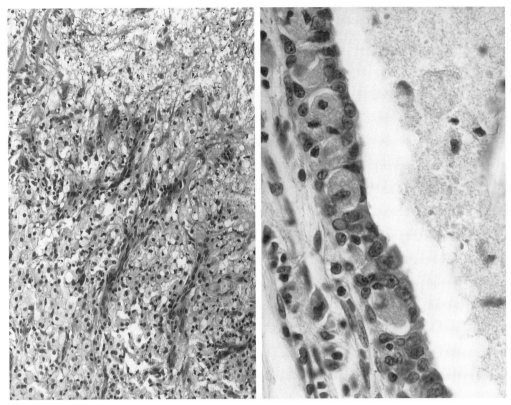

FIGURE 16–37. Foamy Histiocytes in Breast. *Left,* Shown is a breast infarct surrounded by abundant foamy histiocytes—a pattern that can mimic invasive histiocytoid or lipid-rich carcinoma. (H&E) *Right,* Duct luminal cells are shown containing intraepithelial foamy histiocytes—a pattern that may be confused with pagetoid spread of carcinoma. (H&E)

and regional and, thus, amenable to regional surgical therapies.[102, 110] Mammographic screening programs and heightened awareness of the importance of breast self-examination have increased the incidence of CIS relative to invasive carcinoma. Thus, the proper diagnosis of all forms of CIS has assumed greater importance for surgical pathologists.

Low-grade, small-cell, or non-comedo forms of DCIS have a well-documented association with increased risk for the subsequent development of invasive breast cancer, which is usually ipsilateral in the region of the biopsied DCIS.[110] This risk is 10- to 11-fold above that in the general population, with an absolute risk of approximately 25% in 10 years.[99, 100] (Please remember that this absolute risk is dependent on the patient's age at diagnosis.) The **high-grade, large-cell, or comedo forms of DCIS** are composed of large pleomorphic cells, often with abundant cytoplasm and numerous mitotic figures. Marked central necrosis is characteristic, and when all features are present, the diagnosis is fairly easy. Often, a periductal stromal reaction occurs that is associated with contour irregularities and discontinuities of the basal lamina. These latter features often complicate the interpretation of so-called microinvasion (Fig. 16–38), a diagnostic problem amplified by the occasional finding of metastases to regional lymph nodes without apparent invasion.[111-113] Low axillary lymph node dissections may be justified for high-grade, comedo forms of DCIS, especially those that are "extensive" or large (i.e., greater than 2.5 cm in diameter), show areas suspicious for microinvasion, and/or have marked periductal, myxoid, or desmoplastic stromal reaction (features often asso-

ciated with a palpable mass). This ensures proper staging and therapy.

High-grade or large-cell, comedo DCIS is generally considered a more aggressive lesion than the localized, small-cell or low-grade examples of DCIS studied by Page et al.[110] Unfortunately, there are fewer definitive follow-up data for high-grade DCIS, because the vast majority have been treated with extensive surgery. Nonetheless, Lewis and Geschickter[114] followed a few cases diagnosed as "comedo carcinoma." Most were palpable and showed no or inconspicuous invasion of fat or fibrous tissue, and six of eight (75%) women developed subsequent carcinoma within 4 years. **Intermediate grades of DCIS** have also been described,[111-113] and, until additional information is obtained for therapeutic decision-making, they are best considered equivalent to the high-grade, comedo forms of DCIS and treated accordingly, especially when "extensive" within the breast. I have encountered cases of intermediate-grade DCIS that have followed an aggressive course much like that of high-grade DCIS. Furthermore, some investigators have suggested that necrosis in the absence of pure classic comedo cytology is a marker for increased local recurrence equivalent to pure types of comedo DCIS[115] and that micropapillary DCIS is significantly more likely than other patterns to involve multiple quadrants of breast, irrespective of nuclear grade or necrosis.[116]

CLINICOPATHOLOGIC FEATURES. Like LCIS, low-grade DCIS does not usually present as a palpable mass. It is usually picked up incidentally by mammogram in an area containing fibrocystic changes or abnormal calcifications. The calcifica-

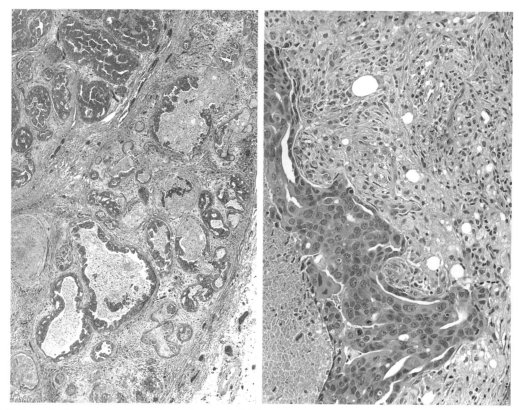

FIGURE 16–38. High-grade, Large-cell, or Comedo Carcinoma. *Left,* Shown is comedo carcinoma (mostly *in situ*) with marked desmoplastic stromal reaction around the ducts—a pattern often associated with a palpable breast mass. (H&E) *Right,* High magnification shows irregular contours to the ducts occupied by comedo carcinoma, suggesting early microinvasion. This pattern is more frequently associated with nodal metastases. (H&E)

tions associated with low-grade DCIS are usually laminated and psammoma-like or rarely amorphous, which are finely granular on X-ray examination. Low-grade DCIS tends to be more localized than the high-grade comedo type of DCIS. The calcifications associated with high-grade DCIS are usually amorphous, occurring within comedo necrotic debris, which present as a linear branching and/or coarse-granular pattern.

By the criteria of Page et al.,[117, 118] making the diagnosis of DCIS requires that at least two duct spaces (both surrounded by basement membrane) be filled entirely (without doubt) with a round or cuboidal proliferation of ductal cells, which are usually evenly spaced with distinct cell borders (Fig. 16–39). Nuclei are round or oval and monotonous throughout the involved duct. Also, it is helpful, but not necessary, that the nuclei are hyperchromatic. The pattern could be solid, cribriform, and/or papillary. In the cribriform pattern, the glandular spaces or lumina are usually round, regular, and smooth and appear as if they were "punched out with a cookie-cutter." Malignant micropapillae have a narrow base, and cellular "bridges" extending across the duct space lack attenuation and form so-called Roman arches[120] (Fig. 16–40). Overall, the patterns produced in low-grade (non-comedo) DCIS have a "rigid" and/or geometric configuration. No swirls or streaming are present like those found in the usual form of duct hyperplasia. Necrosis can be present, but it is spotty, variable, and not as abundant as that found in high-grade, comedo or intermediate-grade forms of DCIS. Azzopardi presents similar morphologic criteria for the diagnosis of low-grade, non-comedo DCIS.[120]

Observations of Bartkova et al.[121] and Lilleng et al.[122] show that low-grade (small-cell) DCIS stains with neuron-specific enolase but not with c-*erb*B2 oncoprotein, whereas high-grade (large-cell) comedo-type DCIS stains with c-*erb*B2 oncoprotein but not with neuron-specific enolase. These markers may prove helpful in determining prognosis and choosing appropriate therapy. Also, the incidence of Ki-67 protein and p53 protein immunostaining increases with increasing histologic grade in DCIS cells.

DIFFERENTIAL DIAGNOSIS. The low-grade, non-comedo forms of DCIS are sometimes difficult to diagnose, especially when attempting to distinguish them from so-called **atypical duct hyperplasia (ADH)**.[110, 111] Rosai[17] demonstrated the difficulty in reproducing these distinctions among experts in breast pathology, and Rosen has stressed that "atypical" proliferative breast disease remains an unresolved diagnostic dilemma.[119] Yet, Page's approach to this difficult diagnostic area appears useful and reasonably applicable.[117, 118] Also, Page has supplemented his diagnostic criteria for the morphologic spectrum from benign proliferative disease without atypia, to proliferative disease with atypia, to low-grade DCIS with extensive follow-up data to define their relative meanings.[110, 117, 118]

Page has histologically defined ADH as having some, but not all, of the features of DCIS as outlined in the prior section. This definition of ADH may seem vague and incomplete, but given the broad spectrum of morphologic presentations of usual duct hyperplasia, ADH, and DCIS, I believe this definition remains practical and useful.[110, 117, 118]

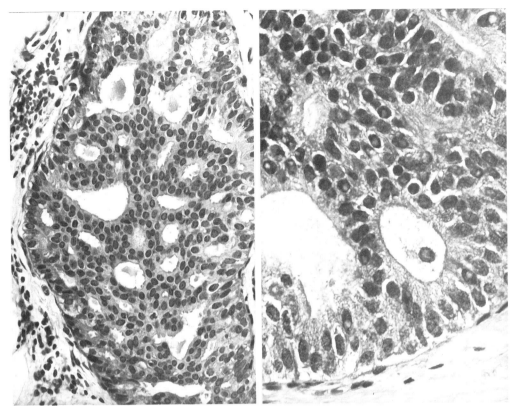

FIGURE 16–39. Low-grade (Small-cell or Non-comedo) DCIS. *Left,* Low-grade DCIS showing a cribriform growth pattern composed entirely of evenly distributed, small, uniform cells with hyperchromatic nuclei. The gland lumina are round, imparting a "punched out with a cookie-cutter" appearance. (H&E) *Right,* High magnification of the cribriform pattern shown at left. Note the radial (right angle) orientation of the columnar cells around the gland lumina, a feature highly suggestive of DCIS. (H&E) (From Weidner N: Malignant breast lesions that may mimic benign tumors. Semin Diagn Pathol 12:2–13, 1995.)

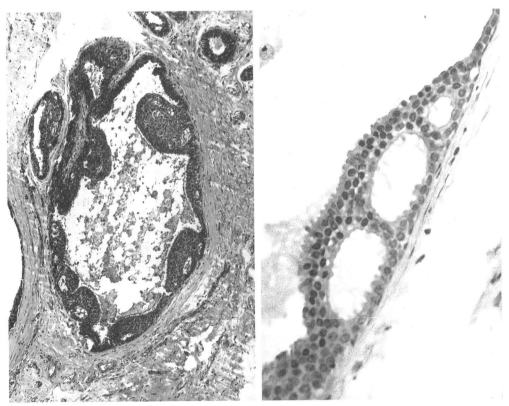

FIGURE 16–40. Low-grade DCIS with "Clinging" or Micropapillary Pattern. *Left,* Shown is a duct lined by a monomorphous population of small cells forming small projections. (H&E) *Right,* High magnification shows the small, round cells of micropapillary or clinging carcinoma forming a structure sometimes referred to as a "Roman" arch. (H&E) (From Weidner N: Malignant breast lesions that may mimic benign tumors. Semin Diagn Pathol 12:2–13, 1995.)

To understand ADH, it is important to understand the criteria for the diagnosis of **benign duct hyperplasia without atypia.**[117, 118] Florid examples of usual duct hyperplasia, no matter how florid, do not qualify as ADH[117, 118] (Figs. 16–41 and 16–42). Many of these florid examples of duct hyperplasia show no features of DCIS and should be diagnosed as **proliferative fibrocystic changes (or disease) without atypia.** In usual duct hyperplasia, nuclei are mostly oval and ''swirled,'' appear to overlap (cell boundaries are indistinct, imparting a syncytial appearance to the cellular proliferation), run parallel, and have evenly distributed chromatin. Yet, florid duct hyperplasia without atypia can show a few cells with cell membranes, occasional nucleoli, and normal mitotic figures. Gland spaces are formed that are ragged, irregular, variably sized and shaped, often slit-like, and often arranged in a ring-like manner at the periphery (see Fig. 16–42, left). This pattern is called ''fenestrated,'' rather than cribriform as found in DCIS.[120] Necrosis and/or atypical mitotic figures in florid hyperplasia are extraordinary; finding either should prompt a vigorous search for DCIS.

This author does not make a diagnosis of ADH unless a diagnosis of low-grade DCIS is being seriously considered and yet the lesion does not qualify for a diagnosis of DCIS because of a lack of uniform and characteristic features throughout the duct space (Figs. 16–43 and 16–44). Page and Rogers[118] reported that ADH exhibits partial involvement of the basement membrane–bound space by a cell population of the type defined for DCIS, non-comedo type. Usually, the second (non-atypical) cell population consists of columnar, polarized cells of the type usually seen in the ductal luminal positions immediately above the basement membrane (see Fig. 16–43, left). The bothersome cell population in ADH usually, but not always, has hyperchromatin nuclei, and they need to constitute an entire bar crossing a space or at least a cell population of six or seven cells across. This avoids calling usual duct hyperplasia without atypia ADH. Also, when in doubt between ADH and DCIS, it is usually best to favor the more benign designation; but only after a vigorous search (i.e., level sections, submitting more tissue, etc.) has failed to reveal areas clearly diagnostic of DCIS.

Moreover, ADH is almost always a very small lesion, measuring less than 3 mm.[118] Indeed, Page et al.[110, 117, 118] have imposed a quantitative criterion for the diagnosis of this low-grade, non-comedo DCIS (there must be at least two duct spaces completely involved by DCIS before that diagnosis can be made). Thus, low-grade DCIS in only one duct space is considered ADH. Likewise, Tavassoli and Norris[123] impose a quantitative criterion for the diagnosis of low-grade, non-comedo DCIS. They state: ''A proliferation may have both the cytologic and architectural features of one of the non-necrotic forms of intraductal carcinoma and the changes may involve two or more ducts or ductules; however, if the

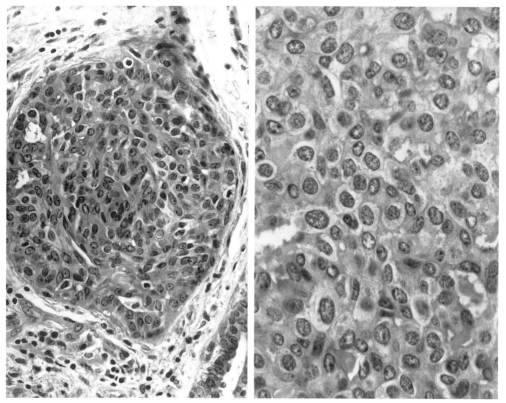

FIGURE 16–41. Florid Duct Hyperplasia Without Atypia. *Left,* Shown is a duct with florid duct hyperplasia without atypia. The duct space is filled by cells with round or oval nuclei that swirl, ''run'' side-by-side or parallel to one another, and overlap or touch with adjacent nuclei. Cell margins are usually inconspicuous, imparting a syncytial appearance to the proliferation. (H&E) *Right,* Although cell margins are usually unclear, occasional cells of duct hyperplasia without atypia may show cell membranes. Nuclear chromatin is fine and fairly regular; nucleoli may be present, as are occasional mitotic figures, but they should not be atypical. Necrosis is very rare. Indeed, finding necrosis should prompt a vigorous search for DCIS. (H&E) (*Left,* from Weidner N: Benign breast lesions that mimic malignant tumors: Analysis of five distinct lesions. Semin Diagn Pathol 7:90–101, 1990. *Right,* from Weidner N: Malignant breast lesions that may mimic benign tumors. Semin Diagn Pathol 12:2–13, 1995.)

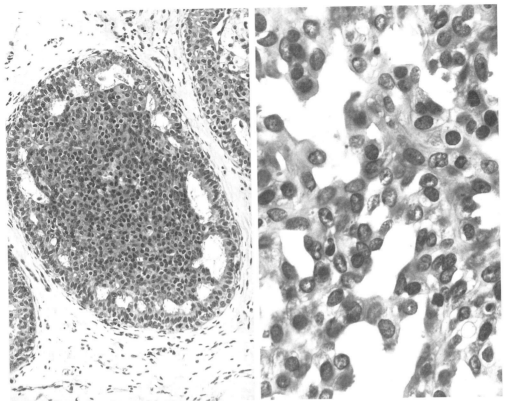

FIGURE 16–42. Florid Duct Hyperplasia Without Atypia. *Left,* Spaces are ragged, slit-like, irregular, vary in size, and orient to the periphery in a ring-like pattern—a pattern referred to as fenestrated rather than as cribriform. (H&E) *Right,* Higher magnification shows the syncytial pattern of growth with irregular or ragged gland lumina, the pattern associated with hyperplasia without atypia. (H&E) (From Weidner N: Malignant breast lesions that may mimic benign tumors. Semin Diagn Pathol 12:2–13, 1995.)

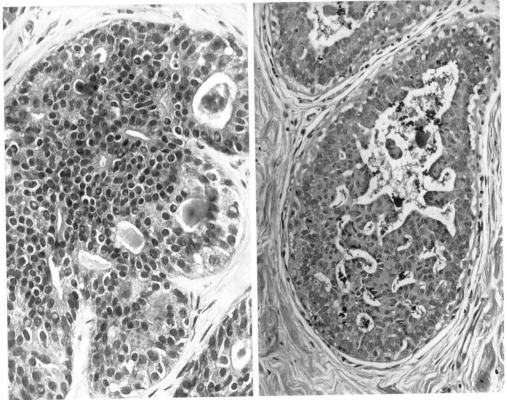

FIGURE 16–43. Atypical Duct Hyperplasia. *Left,* Shown is duct hyperplasia with some but not all the features of DCIS. Note the central uniform round cell proliferation typical of low-grade DCIS; yet, at the periphery a columnar proliferation of duct luminal cells remains, suggesting that the duct space has not been entirely replaced by malignant cells. Thus, this proliferation has some but not all the features of DCIS (H&E). *Right,* Atypical duct hyperplasia is shown with a peculiar slit-like glandular pattern with features of both the fenestrated and cribriform patterns. This was the only duct space in this biopsy occupied by these cells forming this pattern. (H&E) (*Left,* from Weidner N: Malignant breast lesions that may mimic benign tumors. Semin Diagn Pathol 12:2–13, 1995. *Right,* from Weidner N: Benign breast lesions that mimic malignant tumors: Analysis of five distinct lesions. Semin Diagn Pathol 7:90–101, 1990.)

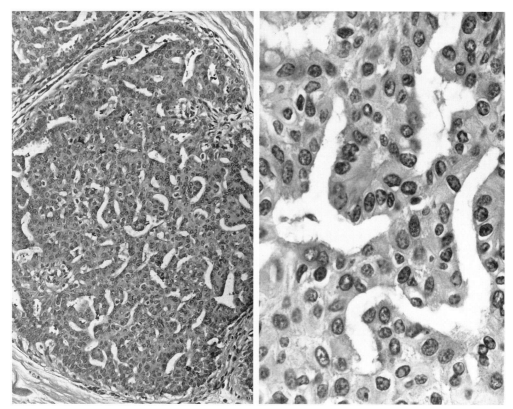

FIGURE 16–44. Atypical Duct Hyperplasia. *Left,* Atypical duct hyperplasia is shown with a semi-rigid-appearing, slit-like, glandular pattern formed by a relatively uniform population of cells. (H&E) *Right,* Irregular gland pattern is shown at higher magnification. Lining cells are variably hyperchromatic and show a tendency to orient at right angles to the lumen. Yet, in aggregate, the cytomorphologic features fall short of DCIS, and a confident diagnosis of DCIS cannot be made. (H&E) (*Left,* from Weidner N: Benign breast lesions that mimic malignant tumors: Analysis of five distinct lesions. Semin Diagn Pathol 7:90–101, 1990. *Right,* from Weidner N: Malignant breast lesions that may mimic benign tumors. Semin Diagn Pathol 12:2–13, 1995.)

involved ducts/ductules measure less than 2 mm in aggregate diameter, the lesion is regarded as atypical intraductal hyperplasia (the involved ducts/ductules may be present in one slide or multiple slides).'' Certainly, this is a controversial diagnostic approach, because a cancer cell should be able to exist as a single cell or as a few adjacent cells.

According to the follow-up data from both studies using both criteria, ADH has a prognosis somewhere between duct hyperplasia without atypia and low-grade, non-comedo DCIS. Women with duct hyperplasia without atypia are twice as likely to develop invasive carcinoma, whereas women with ADH are four to five times as likely or have a 10% absolute risk in 10 years.[98–100] Adding a family history of breast carcinoma in a first-degree relative doubles the risk for ADH patients to eight- to 10-fold.[98–100] These findings are also consistent with the observation that a small DCIS has a better prognosis than a large, extensive DCIS.[111–113] Although it may be unpleasant for some cytomorphologists to impose quantitative criteria on the qualitative recognition of carcinoma cells, current data suggest that these criteria are practical for patient management purposes.

Other lesions should be considered in the differential diagnosis of low-grade DCIS. These are **mucocele-like tumor of the breast** (Fig. 16–45), **cystic hypersecretory hyperplasia, cystic hypersecretory duct carcinoma** (Fig. 16–46), **gynecomastoid hyperplasia** (a mimicker of low-grade micropapillary duct carcinoma)(Fig. 16–47), and **duct extension of LCIS forming a solid pattern** (Fig. 16–48).[124–128]

Rosen initially described mucocele-like tumor of the breast as a benign condition characterized by extravasated mucin in the mammary stroma (a constant feature) accompanied by multiple cysts filled with mucin and lined by flat or cuboidal columnar epithelium devoid of significant papillary or other proliferative features.[124] Subsequently, it was shown that the typical mucinous cysts were lined with hyperplastic ducts and could contain foci of low-grade papillary carcinoma (see Fig. 16–45).[126–128] Mucocele-like tumors appear to represent a morphologic continuum from benign lesions to carcinoma *in situ* with abundant mucous production to invasive mucinous or colloid carcinoma.[129, 130] These lesions must be carefully and completely examined and the patients followed up because they may already have or develop low-grade papillary and mucinous carcinomas.[126–130] True connective-tissue myxomas can arise in the breast,[131] and these myxomas are distinct from mucocele-like tumors.

Mucocele-like tumor of the breast and examples of atypical duct hyperplasia (especially papillary examples) need to be distinguished from cystic hypersecretory hyperplasia and carcinoma. Cystic hypersecretory hyperplasia and carcinoma are characterized by ectatic ducts filled with eosinophilic, colloid-like secretion (see Fig. 16–46). The colloid-like secretion does not extravasate into adjacent stroma.[125] The cysts of hypersecretory carcinoma are lined by highly atypical malignant cells that form micropapillary projections (see Fig. 16–46), whereas hypersecretory hyperplastic cysts are lined by cytologically benign cells. Furthermore, benign duct cells

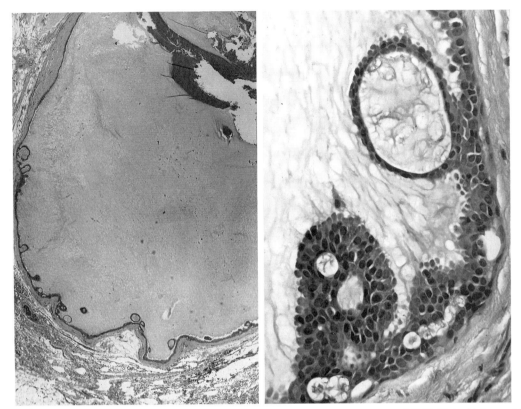

FIGURE 16–45. Mucocele-like Tumor of the Breast. *Left,* Large cyst is shown filled with mucus. (H&E) *Right,* Lining epithelial cells are composed of small uniform cells forming micropapillae similar to micropapillary or clinging carcinoma *in situ.* The findings are consistent with atypical duct hyperplasia/borderline low-grade or clinging carcinoma *in situ.* (H&E) (From Weidner N: Malignant breast lesions that may mimic benign tumors. Semin Diagn Pathol 12:2–13, 1995.)

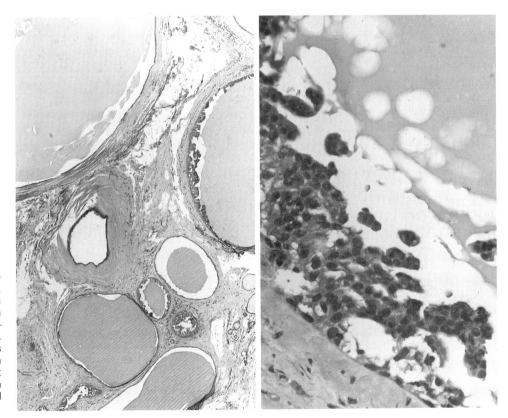

FIGURE 16–46. Cystic Hypersecretory Carcinoma of the Breast. *Left,* Shown are multiple cysts filled with colloid-like secretion characteristic of cystic hypersecretory carcinoma. (H&E) *Right,* Micropapillary carcinoma lines the cystic spaces. (H&E) (From Weidner N: Malignant breast lesions that may mimic benign tumors. Semin Diagn Pathol 12:2–13, 1995.)

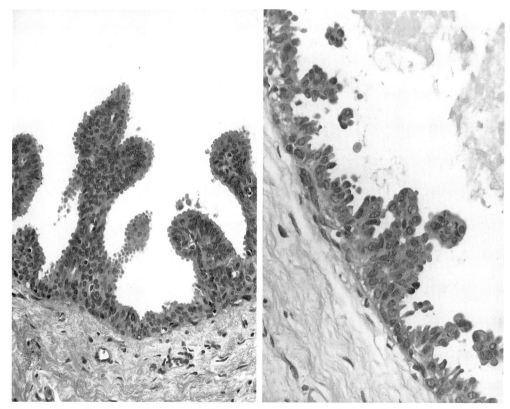

FIGURE 16–47. Micropapillary Carcinoma Compared with Gynecomastoid Hyperplasia. *Left,* Shown are the delicate projections of micropapillary carcinoma. Note the small uniform cell population with hyperchromatic nuclei. (H&E) *Right,* Gynecomastoid hyperplasia is characterized by delicate, yet irregular, projections of duct luminal cells. Note that the cytologic features and syncytial growth pattern are like those of duct hyperplasia without atypia. (H&E) (From Weidner N: Malignant breast lesions that may mimic benign tumors. Semin Diagn Pathol 12:2–13, 1995.)

occasionally form tapered micropapillary structures suggesting low-grade, micropapillary DCIS (see Fig. 16–47). This pattern is common in gynecomastia but may occur in females, hence it is called gynecomastoid hyperplasia.

Finally, this author has observed classic examples of LCIS associated with extensive duct extension by cytologically identical cells, which form solid masses sometimes with central cystic degeneration and calcification (see Fig. 16–48). The pattern mimicked a solid variant of a low-grade, small-cell DCIS or peculiar variant of comedo carcinoma. If doubt remains as to the proper diagnosis, both DCIS and LCIS should be diagnosed to optimize therapy.

UNCOMMON PRESENTATIONS IN THE BREAST OF COMMON LESIONS

Benign Lesions

Granular Cell Tumor

Granular cell tumor is an uncommon tumor that may occur at almost any site in the body, but it is most common in the oral cavity, where (as in other sites) it induces pseudoepitheliomatous hyperplasia (PEH) in the overlying squamous mucosa. Although not a problem in the breast, the secondary PEH can be overdiagnosed as invasive squamous carcinoma. Nevertheless, in the breast, granular cell tumor mimics scirrhous carci-

noma not only clinically but also in its firm, gritty, irregular gross features and by infiltrating collagen with poorly defined margins.[132, 133]

CLINICOPATHOLOGIC FEATURES. Granular cell tumors of the breast usually present in women in their thirties, more commonly in African-Americans. These tumors are gray-white, gritty, firm (secondary to productive fibrosis), and 1 to 3 cm in size, and are composed of polygonal to spindled cells with round nuclei (inconspicuous nucleoli and rare mitoses) and abundant cytoplasm (Fig. 16–49). The cytoplasm contains numerous, variably sized granules that stain brightly with periodic-acid Schiff (PAS) and show S-100 protein immunoreactivity. The S-100 immunoreactivity and ultrastructural features are most consistent with neural differentiation, but a myogenous origin is favored in some cases. Recently, granular cell tumors have been reported to react with CD68 (Kp-1 monoclonal), a presumed histiocyte marker but also apparently a non-specific lysosome marker.[134] In fact, in addition to myelomonocytic cells of hematologic origin, Kp-1 has also been observed to react with hepatocytes, glomeruli, renal tubules, mast cells, malignant melanoma cells, and angiomatoid malignant fibrous histiocytoma (MFH).[134] This author has found Kp-1 to react with renal cell carcinoma and occasional breast carcinomas as well. Clearly, caution is indicated when using this reagent as a "specific" marker for macrophages. Almost always, benign granular cell tumors are cured by local excision. Recurrences are unlikely; yet, very rarely, granular cell tumors metastasize and are therefore considered malig-

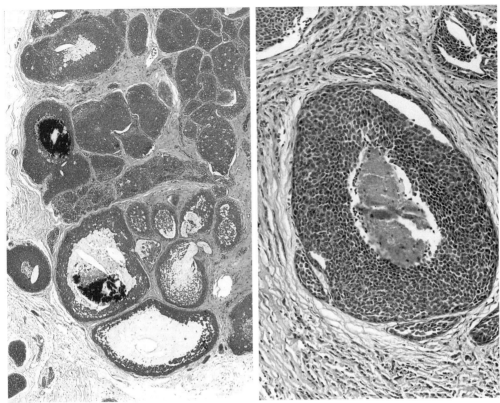

FIGURE 16–48. Carcinoma *In Situ* with Features of Both LCIS and DCIS. *Left,* Ducts and lobules are filled with small cells showing features consistent with lobular neoplasia; yet, large ducts show central cystic degeneration with calcium deposition. (H&E) *Right,* Higher magnification of the lesion at left shows a large duct with central necrosis, mimicking comedo carcinoma. Classification of this case is problematic, but is best considered a variant of CIS showing features of both LCIS and DCIS. This should ensure that the patient is managed properly. (H&E)

nant. Malignant examples usually show greater nuclear atypia and increased mitotic activity.[132, 133]

DIFFERENTIAL DIAGNOSIS. In addition to **scirrhous carcinoma**, the differential diagnosis of granular cell tumors includes **fat necrosis, duct ectasia, and sclerosing adenosis.**[132, 133] The presence in the cytoplasm of a heterogeneous population of variably sized, PAS- and S-100–positive lysosomal granules should make the diagnosis apparent. Invasive lipid cell or **histiocytoid breast carcinoma** could be underdiagnosed as granular cell tumor, but PAS or cytokeratin immunostains should prevent this. **Malignant granular cell tumors** tend to be larger than average (>9 cm) and show rapid growth, extensive local invasion, variable cell size and shape, hyperchromatic plump nuclei, mitotic activity, and disordered cell arrangement.[132, 133]

Salivary and Sweat Gland–like Tumors

Although many varieties of cutaneous adnexal tumors can arise in the skin and subcutis overlying the breast, two lesions deserve special mention because of their propensity for occurring within the breast. These are the **infiltrating syringomatous adenoma of the nipple**[135–137] and **mixed salivary-type (pleomorphic) adenoma** of the breast.[138–141] Given the common embryologic origin of the sweat, salivary, and mammary glands, finding similar tumors in these sites is not surprising.

Infiltrating syringomatous adenoma is closely related to tumors described in other locations, such as **microcystic**

adnexal carcinoma, sclerosing sweat duct (syringomatous) carcinoma, and syringomatous tumor of minor salivary gland.[135–137] Although locally recurrent in 50% of cases, infiltrating syringomatous adenoma should be recognized as a "benign" yet locally aggressive tumor. When infiltrating syringomatous adenoma occurs outside the nipple and within the breast parenchyma, it has been described as **low-grade adenosquamous carcinoma.**[142]

Pleomorphic adenoma of the breast occurs rarely, but it closely resembles its counterparts in salivary glands and skin, where it is also known as chondroid syringoma. Other authors consider pleomorphic adenomas of breast to be variants of intraductal papilloma with myxomatous osteocartilaginous stromal metaplasia.[143] Recognition of pleomorphic adenoma in breast is important, because it can be overdiagnosed as malignant and result in inappropriate surgery. Indeed, Chen[140] reported two new cases and reviewed 24 previously reported ones. He found that inappropriate mastectomy was performed in 42% of cases of pleomorphic adenoma of the breast. Appropriate therapy is local excision with a rim of uninvolved breast. Pleomorphic adenomas of breast show little tendency to recur and even lesser tendency to metastasize.

CLINICOPATHOLOGIC FEATURES. Infiltrating syringomatous adenoma presents as a firm mass in the nipple or subareolar region (1–3 cm diameter). The patient population covers a wide age group, from 11 to 76 years (mean, approximately 40 years). This neoplasm is composed of small ducts two cell layers thick, solid epithelial strands, and small keratin cysts

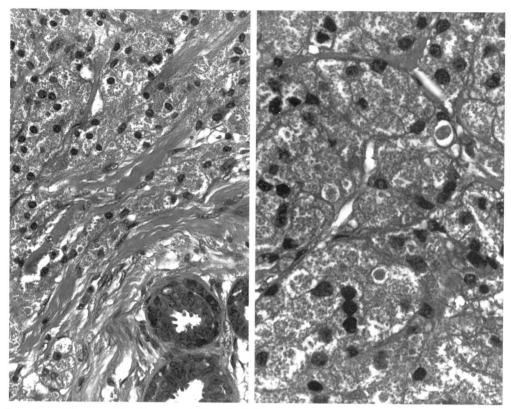

FIGURE 16–49. Granular-cell Tumor of the Breast. *Left,* Note the infiltrate of cells between collagen bundles. The cells show abundant granular cytoplasm and bland uniform nuclei. (H&E) *Right,* Higher magnification shows the variably sized granules characteristic of granular cell tumor. (H&E)

that extend into smooth muscle, dermis, perineural spaces, and underlying breast parenchyma (Fig. 16–50). Local excision with clear margins is the preferred curative therapy, although recurrences have occurred in as many as 50% of cases. The term *infiltrating syringomatous adenoma* is preferred over carcinoma, to avoid excessive surgery and patient anxiety. Yet, adequate treatment may require nipple resection.[135–137]

The clinicopathologic features of pleomorphic adenomas of the breast have been reviewed by Ballance et al.[144] Patients developing pleomorphic adenomas of breast have ranged from 19 to 78 years, with most tumors ranging from 0.8 to 4.5 cm (mean, 2 cm). Yet, one pleomorphic adenoma that was present for 30 years grew to 17 cm. Although pleomorphic adenomas can occur anywhere within the breast, they have a predilection to develop near the areola. Most are well-circumscribed, but can show multifocal growth or satellite lesions. Histologically, pleomorphic adenomas are composed of two cell types: duct epithelial cells and myoepithelial cells. The epithelial cells produce hyperplastic nests with focal duct differentiation (squamous metaplasia can also occur) that merges and display varying degrees of osteocartilaginous metaplasia (Fig. 16–51). Cytologic atypia, mitotic activity, and invasive growth pattern are minimal. Surrounding breast tissue can appear relatively normal or show features of proliferative fibrocystic change, including intraductal papillomas, or of non-continuous invasive carcinoma. The histologic and immunohistochemical features suggest that pleomorphic adenomas arise from a single cell type capable of divergent differentiation;[141] that is, cytokeratin, vimentin, glial fibrillary acidic

protein, muscle-specific actin, S-100 protein, epithelial membrane antigen, and gross cystic disease fluid protein-15 expression all are variably conserved within the bimorphic population of cells found in pleomorphic adenomas.[141]

DIFFERENTIAL DIAGNOSIS. Infiltrating syringomatous adenoma needs to be separated from **tubular carcinoma, florid papillomatosis of nipple ducts,** and **nipple adenoma.**[135–137, 145] Tubular carcinoma has already been discussed. Nipple duct adenoma or florid duct papillomatosis[145] is a circumscribed complex proliferation of ducts of varying sizes with occasional squamous and apocrine metaplasia and keratin cysts. In contrast with infiltrating syringomatous adenoma, nipple duct adenoma often ulcerates the skin and is better circumscribed than infiltrating syringomatous adenoma. It displays a papillomatous pattern that is associated with lactiferous ducts and is closely linked to proliferative fibrocystic changes and intracystic papilloma of the breast. Nipple duct adenoma does not invade perineural or smooth muscles. Rosen and Caicco have described three distinct patterns: (1) sclerosing papillomatosis, (2) papillomatosis, and (3) adenosis.[145]

Pleomorphic adenoma of breast may be overdiagnosed as **metaplastic breast carcinoma.** Most metaplastic breast carcinomas, however, are high-grade malignancies with invasive margins, marked cytologic atypia, increased mitotic activity, regional necrosis, and an associated ductal carcinoma (*in situ* and/or invasive). Other pleomorphic adenomas of breast have been mistaken for **adenoid cystic carcinoma, malignant phyllodes tumor, or primary breast sarcoma.**[141] Overdiagnosis of pleomorphic adenomas based on recognition of suspicious clinical findings, a malignant frozen section appearance,

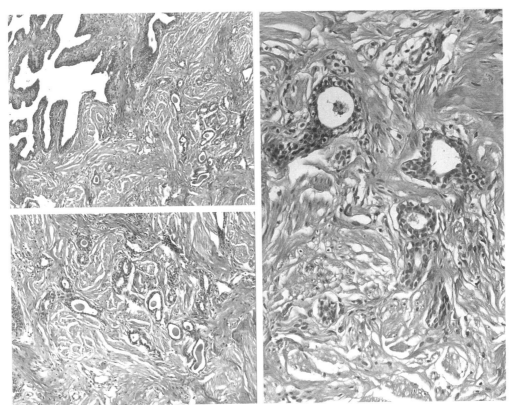

FIGURE 16–50. Infiltrating Syringomatous Adenoma of Nipple. *Upper left,* Adjacent to a large lactiferous duct are multiple small glands. (H&E) *Lower left and right,* At higher magnification, the glands are extending through periductal collagen and form small syringoma-like glands. Closer to the epidermis these glands formed small keratin cysts. (H&E)

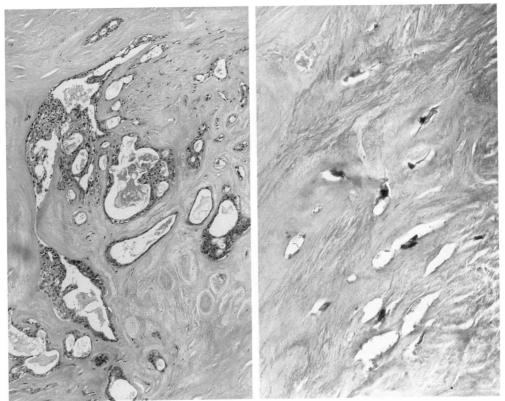

FIGURE 16–51. Pleomorphic Adenoma of Breast. *Left,* Shown are the irregular glands of a pleomorphic adenoma set within a chondroid matrix. (H&E) *Right,* Chondrocyte-like cells are within lacunae of the chondroid matrix characteristic of pleomorphic adenoma. (H&E)

or overinterpretation of fine-needle aspiration (FNA) biopsy as cystosarcoma phyllodes has resulted in unnecessary mastectomies. Recognition of the characteristic invasive patterns and significant cytologic atypia, when present, should lead to the proper diagnosis of these malignancies.

Adenomyoepithelioma has been considered in the differential diagnosis, but this distinction seems arbitrary, because pleomorphic adenomas of breast, including those arising in skin or salivary gland, can be conceptualized as ''adenomyoepitheliomas with osteocartilaginous metaplasia.'' Obviously, this distinction is not quite as critical as the distinction of pleomorphic adenoma from the malignant tumors mentioned previously. **Clear-cell hidradenoma and eccrine spiradenoma-like tumors,** both known to occur rarely in the breast, should be considered in the differential diagnosis of pleomorphic adenoma.[146, 147]

Malignant Lesions

Metastatic Tumors

Primary breast carcinoma currently ranks as the leading cause of death for malignant diseases in women. In contrast, **metastasis to the breast** as part of a disseminated cancer is rarely seen, except at autopsy. Nonetheless, a metastasis to the breast can be the first sign of a clinically occult tumor, and its proper diagnosis will lead to a search for the primary tumor and the avoidance of unnecessary breast surgery.

CLINICOPATHOLOGIC FEATURES. Besides **hematolymphoid malignancies,** and excluding a **metastasis from contralateral breast carcinoma,** most series show that **metastatic melanoma and lung carcinoma** account for most cases (greater than 50%) of metastatic disease in the breast.[148] Ovarian, gastric, renal, and pancreatic carcinomas constitute most of the remaining tumor types. In men, prostate carcinoma has a predilection for metastasizing to the breast.[149] Diffuse-type (signet-ring cell) **gastric carcinoma can spread to the breast and mimic invasive lobular carcinoma;**[148] likewise, **invasive lobular carcinoma can spread to the stomach and produce linitis plastica.**[150] Obviously, the distinction would be very difficult, but immunostaining with GCDFP-15 can help because, like S-100, GCDFP-15 is positive in approximately 60% of breast carcinomas. (GCDFP-15 and S-100 are also positive in salivary and sweat gland carcinomas, and the melanoma marker HMB-45 has now been reported to be immunoreactive with breast carcinomas.[151]) Worth noting is that occult **breast carcinoma can be diffusely metastatic to the spleen and present as ''idiopathic thrombocytopenic purpura,''**[152] and that extramammary carcinoid can initially present as a breast mass, simulating primary breast carcinoma with neuroendocrine differentiation.[153]

DIFFERENTIAL DIAGNOSIS. The absence of an *in situ* component in the breast should always raise the possibility of a metastatic tumor, but the presence of an *in situ* component does not always indicate a breast primary. **Ovarian carcinomas metastatic to the breast can simulate DCIS by growing within the ducts and lobules and producing microcalcifications mimicking primary carcinoma on mammogram.**[154, 155] Obtaining a complete clinical history and judicious application of immunohistochemistry should aid in the proper identification of metastasis to the breast, thus avoiding unnecessary surgery.

UNCOMMON LESIONS WORTH KNOWING ABOUT, BUT NOT COVERED ELSEWHERE

Benign Lesions

Zuska's Disease (Squamous Metaplasia of Lactiferous Ducts)

Although initially described by Zuska et al.[156] in 1951, the association of squamous metaplasia of the lactiferous ducts (SMOLD) and recurrent subareolar abscess remains underrecognized. Proper diagnosis of **SMOLD** abscess or **SMOLDering disease of the breast** is important, because simple incision and drainage is inadequate therapy and is often followed by recurrence.[157] Cure requires excision of all the diseased duct(s) and abscess cavity *in toto.*[158] Although clearly capable of causing considerable anxiety, Zuska's disease is not known to predispose to malignant transformation.

CLINICOPATHOLOGIC FEATURES. Patients with squamous metaplasia of the lactiferous ducts often present with the clinical triad of recurrent subareolar abscess, intermittent periareolar discharge, and (possibly) nipple inversion.[159] Additional findings may be lactiferous duct fistulae, and the discharge can often have a malodorous, pasty quality. Patients are usually of child-bearing age, and symptoms may develop with pregnancy and lactation. SMOLD abscesses are bilateral in about one third of patients.

Although the cause of SMOLDering disease is unclear, apparently squamous metaplasia of one or more ducts leads to keratinous desquamation (Fig. 16–52, left) and plugging by the epithelial debris. Resulting inflammation and infection eventually lead to epithelial denudation, extension of inflammatory debris into surrounding soft tissues, chronic-active abscess formation, and spontaneous drainage along the areolar border and fistula formation. The disease is cured by complete excision of the entire length of the diseased (metaplastic) ducts. Definitive surgery may consist of excision of the fistula and associated ducts, excision of the terminal portions of all ducts, or excision of the nipple/areolar complex if necessary. The last is almost always curative.

DIFFERENTIAL DIAGNOSIS. Carcinoma is rarely seen in periareolar abscesses and should be regarded as coincidental when found.[160] Yet, **cutaneous squamous carcinoma** should be ruled out, and the very rare primary squamous carcinomas of the breast can appear deceptively ''benign.''[161] As in lung and prostate, **squamous metaplasia of breast** can also occur after infarction, especially when it occurs with intraductal papilloma.[162]

It is worth noting that **''tumors'' resembling syringocystadenoma papilliferum** arise from the major lactiferous ducts.[163] In these lesions, dilated ducts contain papillary processes and keratinizing squamous epithelial lining (Fig. 16–52, right). Like SMOLD abscesses, the ducts contain keratin, squamous debris, and inflammatory cells. The papillary processes are lined by two cell layers (outer cuboidal row and inner columnar row) and partly by squamous epithelium. Plasma cells are numerous in the stalks of the papillary processes; and, like SMOLDering breast disease, a fibrinopurulent exudate may be present in response to keratin debris released from ruptured ducts. Whether syringocystadenoma papilliferum–like lesions have a similar natural history to

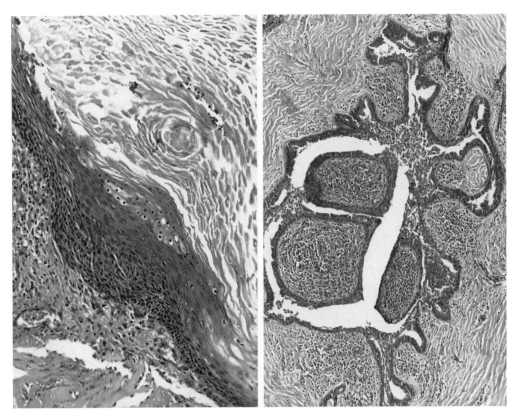

FIGURE 16–52. SMOLDering Breast Disease and Syringocystadenoma Papilliferum-like Lesion of the Breast. *Left,* In SMOLDering (Zuska's) breast disease, large lactiferous ducts are lined by squamous epithelium. Keratinous debris fills the lumina, causing obstruction, suppuration, and eventually fistula formation. (H&E) *Right,* Syringocystadenoma papilliferum-like tumor of the nipple. Note the broad papillae lined by two cell layers and containing numerous plasma cells. (H&E)

SMOLDering breast disease remains unclear; clinical experience with the syringocystadenoma papilliferum–like lesions is limited.

Granulomatous Lobular Mastitis

Granulomatous lobular mastitis causes a breast mass in women of child-bearing age that mimics carcinoma; it is characterized by multiple, chronic-active, necrotizing, granulomatous abscesses centered on the segmental ducts and attached lobules yielding a lobulocentric disease pattern. There is a strong tendency for persistence or recurrence in more than half of the cases, and the cause remains unknown (obstruction and/or hypersensitivity reaction have been suggested).[164] Awareness of this condition is important, because surgical therapy is suboptimal for recurrent disease, which requires antibiotics and even corticosteroids before resolution occurs. In fact, resolution may require several years of therapy.

CLINICOPATHOLOGIC FEATURES. Women with granulomatous lobular mastitis are usually parous (often within 5 years of pregnancy) or receiving oral contraceptive therapy.[165–167] It presents as a mass lesion, and the inflammatory changes are characterized by destructive, necrotizing, granulomatous inflammation involving numerous polymorphonuclear leukocytes, multinucleated giant cells, and focal lipogranuloma-like changes (Fig. 16–53). Lobulocentric abscesses develop in adjacent segmental ducts and terminal duct lobular units, with relative sparing of interlobular stroma.

DIFFERENTIAL DIAGNOSIS. Granulomatous lobular mastitis is distinct from variants of **duct ectasia or periductal masti-** **tis,** which involve dilated large ducts rather than lobules. Yet, **infection** must always be considered with necrotizing granulomatous disease. Indeed, **histoplasmosis** has recently been shown to cause a granulomatous lobular mastitis–like pattern of inflammation.[168] **Mycobacterial, fungal, parasitic, and cat-scratch disease** should also be considered and ruled out with appropriate stains.[168]

Sarcoidosis can involve the breast, but does not contain the necrosis and polymorphous inflammatory infiltrate of granulomatous lobular mastitis.[169, 170] A peculiar lesion called **granulomatous angiopanniculitis** of the breast has been described.[171] This lesion contains multiple, non-necrotic, non-caseous granulomas with a giant-cell component and lymphocytic angiitis, which predominantly involves the subcutis, but can extend into the breast tissue without affecting lobules or ducts.[171] This pattern is quite distinct from granulomatous lobular mastitis. Finally, **giant-cell arteritis, localized polyarteritis noda,** and **Wegener's granulomatosis** can involve the breast, causing a large-vessel necrotizing arteritis or a necrotizing granulomatous angiitis with necrosis.[172–174] Vasculitis is not a usual component of granulomatous lobular mastitis.

Sclerosing Lymphocytic Lobulitis

Sclerosing lymphocytic lobulitis (Fig. 16–54) of breast is an inflammatory breast lesion thought to be of autoimmune origin, much like Sjogren's syndrome, Hashimoto's thyroiditis, and pancreatic insulinitis.[175] A very similar, if not identical, lesion was initially reported by Soler and Khardori[176] as fibrous

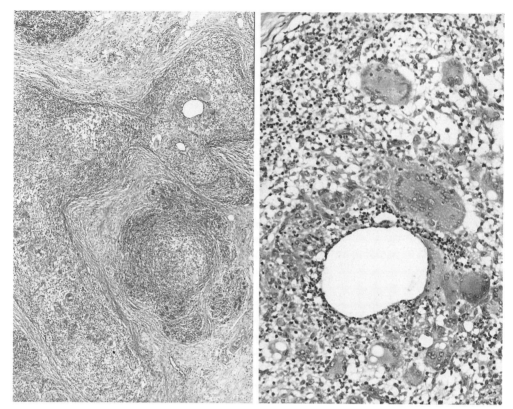

FIGURE 16–53. Granulomatous Lobular Mastitis. *Left,* In granulomatous lobular mastitis the necrotizing inflammation follows the lobules and subsegmental ducts. (H&E) *Right,* Within the lobules there is necrosis, lipid vacuole formation, suppuration, and granulomatous inflammation, often with multinucleated giant cells. Stains for infectious organisms are negative. (H&E)

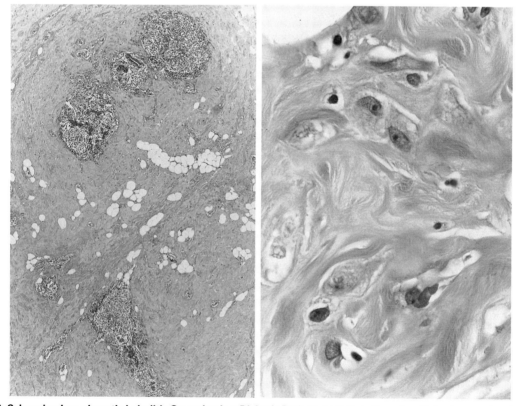

FIGURE 16–54. Sclerosing Lymphocytic Lobulitis Occurring in a Diabetic Patient. *Left,* Note the sclerotic background and atropic lobules closely surrounded by small lymphocytes. (H&E) *Right,* Epithelioid stromal cells are apparent, which could be mistaken for infiltrating carcinoma cells. (H&E)

disease of the breast. Subsequent reports emphasized the **association of sclerosing lymphocytic lobulitis with diabetes**;[177–179] but Schwartz and Strauchen[180] and Lammie et al.[175] reported very similar pathologic features in non-diabetic patients, often with other evidence, however, of autoimmune disease (Hashimoto's thyroiditis or circulating autoantibodies).

CLINICOPATHOLOGIC FEATURES. Diabetic patients with sclerosing lymphocytic lobulitis have early-onset, long-standing, insulin-dependent diabetes, which developed premenopausally. Their breasts contain hard, painless, irregularly contorted, moveable masses, which are often bilateral but may be solitary. Mammography reveals dense tissue suggestive of malignancy. FNA biopsy of these hard masses yields insufficient material for diagnosis in approximately 50% of cases. Histologically, the masses show lymphocytic lobulitis (mature lymphocytes and plasma cells surrounding acini and invading across basement membranes) (see Fig. 16–54), lymphocytic vasculitis (mature lymphocytes surrounding a small venule), and dense keloid-like fibrosis, which, in 75% of cases, contains peculiar epithelioid cells embedded in the dense fibrous tissue[179] (see Fig. 16–54). According to Tomaszewski et al.,[179] the lobulitis and vasculitis can be found in non-diabetic patients, but the epithelioid fibroblasts appear to be unique to the diabetic condition. Lammie et al.[175] believe that the lobular lesions progress through stages, starting with initial dense inflammation, followed by increasing lobular sclerosis and acinar atrophy as the inflammation resolves. At first, an occasional neutrophil and/or multinucleated giant cell may be present.

Immunologic studies of sclerosing lymphocytic lobulitis show a predominance of B lymphocytes in the vast majority of cases, and expression of HLA-DR antigen in involved lobular epithelium. These immunologic features are very much like those found in benign lymphoepithelial lesions of salivary gland and in Hashimoto's thyroiditis. Five of seven patients studied by Lammie et al.[175] had the HLA-DR 3, 4, or 5 phenotype, which is associated with a higher incidence of autoimmune disease (type 1 diabetes and Hashimoto's thyroiditis).

DIFFERENTIAL DIAGNOSIS. Schwartz and Strauchen[180] speculated about a possible association of sclerosing lymphocytic lobulitis with an increased incidence of **lymphoma** development, much like that observed with Sjogren's syndrome and Hashimoto's thyroiditis. The resulting lymphomas are thought to be related to **mucosa-associated lymphoid tissue (MALT)**. However, with insufficient follow-up, these authors were unable to reach a conclusion. Aozasa et al.,[181] Lamovec and Jancar,[182] Hugh et al.,[183] and Mattia et al.[184] all concluded that primary breast lymphomas may show features characteristic of MALT lymphomas (i.e., presence of lymphoepithelial lesions [Fig. 16–55], tendency to remain localized or recur at other MALT sites, low-grade cytology, and indolent behavior) arising from other organs, such as the stomach, salivary glands, and thyroid. Moreover, Aozasa et al.[181] found enough histologic and immunologic evidence to suggest that most mammary lymphomas are B-cell tumors and are associated with co-existing or antecedent lymphocytic mastopathy. In fact, histologic evidence of lymphocytic mastopathy in mammary tissue apart from lymphomas could be evaluated in 11 of 19 patients, and evidence of lymphocytic mastopathy was confirmed in 10 of the 11 patients (>90%). The so-called

lymphoepithelial lesion, a characteristic finding for MALT lymphomas, was observed in 42% of their breast lymphomas. Other observers have not been able to document MALT features in breast lymphoma.[185, 186]

When primary breast lymphomas develop, they are most commonly of the diffuse, large-cell type with B-cell differentiation,[187] but virtually any of the morphologic types defined by the ''working formulation'' can occur. This author has observed a diffuse small cleaved cell lymphoma of the breast that presented with numerous spindle forms and sclerosis, which closely mimicked a **primary sarcoma** (Fig. 16–56). The diffuse small cleaved cell variety is the second most frequent lymphoma type reported in the breast. Also, lymphomas can infiltrate in a single-file pattern like **infiltrating lobular carcinoma** (see Fig. 16–55, right), and the lymphoepithelial lesion–like spread can mimic **pagetoid spread of a breast carcinoma** (see Fig. 16–55, left). Breast lymphomas can mimic **solid variants of infiltrating lobular carcinoma,** and likewise **metastatic lobular carcinoma in lymph nodes can simulate primary lymphoma.**

A variety of **pseudolymphomas (lymphoid hyperplasias)** of the breast have been reported, but they may actually represent either florid cases of sclerosing lymphocytic lobulitis or undetected examples of early, low-grade, B-cell MALT lymphomas.[184, 188, 189] Indeed, Lin et al.[189] concluded their report of five pseudolymphomas of the breast by stating that ''the microscopic picture of pseudolymphoma of the breast greatly resembles that seen in the salivary gland in Sjogren's syndrome.'' Yet, none of the patients actually had Sjogren's syndrome.

Because sclerosing lymphocytic mastitis ''ends'' with lobular atrophy and sclerosis, so-called **megalomastia** should be considered in the differential diagnosis.[190] Megalomastia is a rare entity characterized by enlargement of one or both breasts. Most cases occur in children, and there is often a family history of the disease. The main histologic features are isolated, small, atrophic lobules embedded in abundant, hypocellular collagenous stroma. Some of these fibrotic breasts may show so-called juvenile units, which are composed of branching ducts without lobules surrounded by a rim of myxomatous, alcian blue–positive stroma. Juvenile units resemble mammary tissue during early breast development.

Sometimes the epithelioid stromal cells in sclerosing lymphocytic lobulitis can be so prominent and abundant that the possibility of an infiltrating carcinoma or granular cell tumor can be seriously considered.[191] Ashton et al.[191] reported that the stromal cells have features of myofibroblasts, reacting with anti-actin. These cells were negative for antibodies to keratin (AE1/3), S-100, desmin, Mac 287, Factor XIIIa, CD20 (L26), and CD45RO (UCHL-1); but they reacted with anti-CD68 (Kp-1), suggesting some lysosome formation. Using these immunostains is important because **lymphoepithelioma-like carcinoma of the breast** occurs occasionally, wherein the lymphoid infiltrate could simulate lymphocytic lobulitis and obscure the underlying carcinoma.[192]

Adenomyoepithelioma

Myoepithelial cells are contractile cells located between the luminal epithelial cells and the basal lamina of glandular tissues derived from ectoderm (eccrine, apocrine, lacrimal, Bartholin, salivary, and mammary glands).[193, 194] Myoepithelial

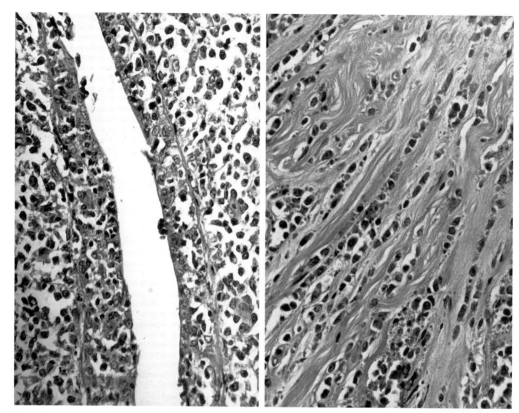

FIGURE 16–55. Lymphoma of the Breast. *Left,* Lymphoma cells are shown infiltrating ductal epithelium, features consistent with a lymphoepithelial lesion (LEL) noted to occur in lymphomas arising in association of mucosa-associated lymphoid tissue (so-called MALT lymphomas). (H&E) *Right,* Breast lymphoma can also infiltrate collagen in a single-file fashion like infiltrating lobular carcinoma. (H&E)

cells are intermediate in differentiation between epithelial cells and smooth muscle cells. They have desmosomes, tonofilaments, and basal lamina and show cytokeratin immunoreactivity (epithelial features), while simultaneously forming microfilaments, fusiform densities, and numerous subplasmalemmal pinocytotic vesicles. They are also immunoreactive to actin and vimentin (smooth muscle features).[195–201] In addition, myoepithelial cells are immunoreactive to S-100 protein and neuron-specific enolase.[202, 203]

Cells with myoepithelial differentiation are known to be components of both benign and malignant tumors of sweat, salivary, and mammary gland origin.[194–218] In these tumors, **myoepithelial cells can demonstrate squamous, chondromyxoid, plasmacytoid, clear-cell, and myoid spindle cell differentiation.**[194–218] For identification purposes, some authors insist that neoplastic myoepithelial cells have all the ultrastructural features of non-neoplastic myoepithelial cells,[199–201] but others require less strict criteria.[195–198, 202–205] Like the latter group, this author accepts that neoplastic myoepithelial cells can lose a few of their non-neoplastic characteristics and still be considered to show myoepithelial cell differentiation. Cameron et al.[194] proposed that pure myoepithelial cell tumors be called myoepitheliomas and that those also containing glandular elements be called **adenomyoepitheliomas.**

CLINICOPATHOLOGIC FEATURES. Adenomyoepitheliomas of the breast have been well documented in the English-language literature;[206–218] other authors refer to anecdotal cases.[193] Furthermore, some of these tumors are described as either myoepithelioma or leiomyosarcoma.[194, 219] Zarbo and Oberman[206]

described a cellular adenomyoepithelioma of breast that was well-circumscribed and bicellular, with cytologic features suggestive of low-grade cancer. In addition, Cameron et al.[194] reported a malignant adenomyoepithelioma composed of glands and myoid spindle tumor cells (''leiomyosarcoma'') that invaded fat and skeletal muscle. Kiaer et al.[207] observed a low-grade malignant adenomyoepithelioma arising (over a time span of 18 years) from a benign proliferation breast gland, which they termed adenomyoepithelial adenosis. Likewise, Eusebi et al.[208] reported two cases of low-grade malignant adenomyoepitheliomas that were identical to that described by Kiaer. These lesions had cytologic evidence of low-grade malignancy with nuclear atypia, high mitotic activity, and progression from an adenosis-like picture to a solid, cellular, and sheet-like growth pattern. However, they neither recurred nor metastasized, and the authors admitted that further studies were needed to clarify their biologic behavior and the unique type of adenosis associated with them. Rosen[213] described 18 cases and emphasized that, in most, myoepithelial cells were polygonal and had clear cytoplasm. Myoid, spindle cell differentiation was rarely prominent but was present focally in most cases. In addition, Rosen believed his cases to be benign breast tumors, which could be treated adequately with complete local excision. Furthermore, Jabi et al.[214] (one case) and Young and Clement[215] (three cases) reported four additional adenomyoepitheliomas of breast. Both groups emphasized that the myoepitheliomatous component was composed of polygonal clear cells. Jabi et al.[214] categorized their lesion as benign, whereas Young and Clement stated that limited experience precluded definitive conclusions regarding biologic behavior.

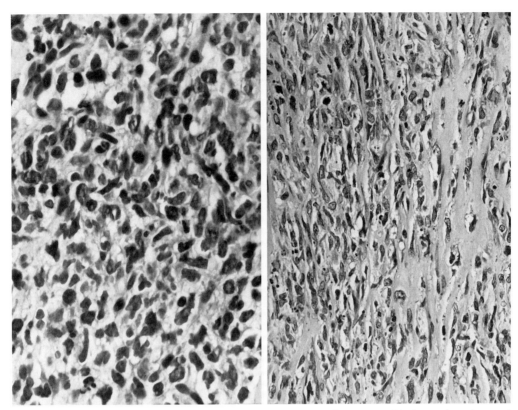

FIGURE 16–56. **Small Cleaved-Cell Lymphoma Mimicking Stromal Sarcoma.** *Left,* In areas this breast lymphoma showed cytologic features entirely consistent with small cleaved-cell lymphoma. (H&E) *Right,* In most areas the same breast lymphoma as shown on the left formed spindled cells with sclerosis mimicking stromal sarcoma. Indeed, this case was initially considered a "stromal sarcoma of the breast." (H&E)

Indeed, one of the cases of Young and Clement[215] recurred three times, and they recommended wide local resection as initial treatment for adenomyoepithelioma of breast. Weidner and Levine[217] reported on two cases of spindle cell adenomyoepitheliomas that followed a benign course. These spindle cell tumors were well-circumscribed and showed no necrosis, cytologic atypia, or mitotic activity, which suggests a benign rather than malignant course. There was no associated adenosis, although areas of proliferative fibrocystic change were adjacent to foci of intraductal carcinoma in case 2. Although these findings may appear unique, Toth[209] described a very similar case. Even though he called his case a myoepithelioma, his histologic description and figures showed a biphasic tumor composed of both glandular elements and surrounding bundles of myoid spindled tumor cells. He also did not observe features suggesting malignant behavior. Tavassoli's[216] study of 27 adenomyoepitheliomas confirmed that these tumors were composed of two populations of cells: tubular cells and spindled or epithelioid myoepithelial cells with clear, pink, and/or amphophilic cytoplasm. Only 2 of the 27 cases recurred, and none metastasized; however, 9 of the 27 patients had mastectomy, eight with excision of axillary nodes, because of an overdiagnosis of carcinoma.

Thus, the bulk of the English-language literature indicates that adenomyoepitheliomas present as breast masses (average, 2–3 cm) in the same age range as patients with breast carcinoma. They are firm to rubbery and can mimic carcinoma grossly. They have a biphasic cytoarchitecture composed of tubular structures lined by duct luminal epithelial cells sur-

rounded by myoepithelial cells that have spindle cell and/or polygonal cell shapes (the latter often with clear cytoplasm) (Fig. 16–57). The myoepithelial cells may predominate, necrosis may be present, and mitotic activity can be brisk, measuring up to 10 mitotic figures per 10 high-power fields (HPF). The vast majority have been benign, but local recurrences can occur; however, Loose et al.'s[218] report of six cases included two malignant examples, one of which metastasized to the lung and brain following multiple local recurrences and caused death. Both malignant examples had high mitotic rates (11–14 per 10 HPF) and cytologically malignant cells. The metastasizing example showed the biphasic features of typical adenomyoepithelioma; the other showed spindle cell morphology in the malignant "sarcomatous" component.

DIFFERENTIAL DIAGNOSIS. It is important to note that **sclerosing adenosis** contains myoid spindled cells admixed with tubuloglandular elements and is, therefore, a form of adenomyoepitheliomatosis. Indeed, the myoid spindled cells of sclerosing adenosis react with S-100 protein, consistent with their myoepithelial nature.[219] Furthermore, McDivitt et al.[220] described and illustrated rare examples of sclerosing adenosis in which the myoid spindled cells multiplied, producing substantial fascicles. In these more exaggerated cases, the authors suggested that Hamperl's term, "myoepithelial tumor," is more appropriate. Indeed, some of the spindle cell adenomyoepithelial tumors reported could be thought of as peculiar and rare variants of sclerosing adenosis; but because they are morphologically distinct from typical sclerosing adenosis, they deserve separate designation as a form of benign adenomyoepithelioma[217] (Fig. 16–58).

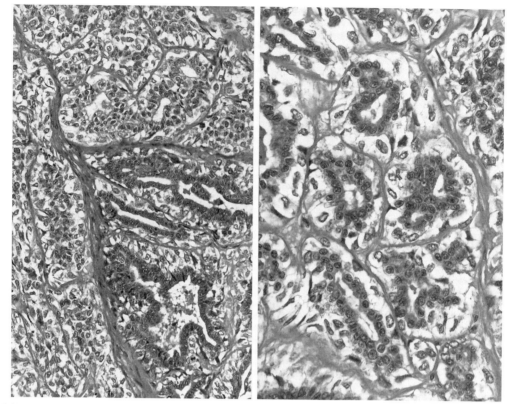

FIGURE 16–57. Adenomyoepithelioma, Clear-Cell Variant. *Left,* Biphasic adenomyoepithelioma is shown composed of clear myoepithelial cells surrounding duct luminal cells forming glands. (H&E) *Right,* Higher magnification shows greater detail of the glands lined by duct luminal epithelial cells surrounded by clear myoepithelial cells. (H&E)

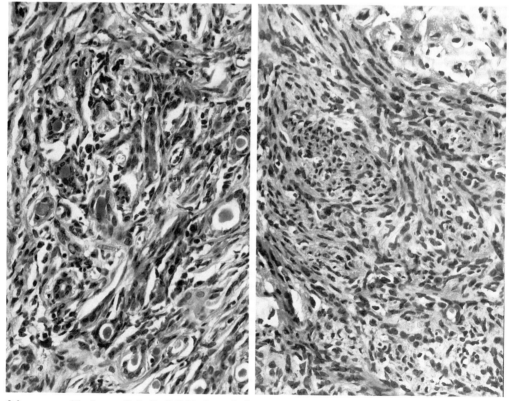

FIGURE 16–58. Adenomyoepithelioma, Spindle-Cell Variant. *Left,* Admixed glands surrounded by spindled myoepithelial cells are apparent. (H&E) *Right,* Other areas were composed almost exclusively of spindled myoepithelial cells. (H&E)

Myofibroblastoma of breast, a tumor showing myofibroblastic differentiation without epithelial features, simulates spindle cell adenomyoepithelioma and other spindle tumors of the breast (Fig. 16–59).[221] Myofibroblastomas have a predilection for occurring in men, but in either sex they are benign tumors.

Diaz et al.[7] maintain that **microglandular adenosis** is actually a biphasic lesion (epithelial and myoepithelial cells) and therefore a type of predominantly tubular or glandular adenomyoepithelial adenomatosis, like that reported by Kiaer et al.[207] Yet, the myoepithelial component is more readily apparent by light microscopy in adenomyoepitheliomas than it is in microglandular adenosis. Lesions with features intermediate between microglandular adenosis and adenomyoepithelioma exist and likely have been variably categorized as one or the other, based on the views of the reporting authors. Also, **cellular angiolipoma** of the breast could simulate the spindle cell variant of adenomyoepithelioma or myofibroblastoma.[222]

Because of the marked differences in tumor aggressiveness and therapy, typical adenomyoepithelioma should be clearly distinguished from the **spindle cell variant of metaplastic breast carcinoma.** Yet, examples of "**malignant myoepithelioma**" or "**myoepithelial carcinoma**" or "**adenomyoepithelioma with undifferentiated carcinoma**" are scattered throughout the literature.[211, 212, 216, 218, 223] Histologic,

ultrastructural, and immunohistochemical features of some malignant adenomyoepitheliomas overlap greatly with those reported for the spindle cell variant of metaplastic breast carcinoma. As is shown in the subsequent discussion of spindle cell breast carcinoma, both lesions show myoepithelial differentiation, and their distinction may have more academic than practical value. Finally, a **peculiar DCIS variant** has been described that is characterized by the intraductal growth of carcinoma cells having clear-cell and spindle cell myoepithelial differentiation.[224]

Malignant Lesions

Phyllodes Tumors

Phyllodes tumors (cystosarcoma phyllodes) are rare breast neoplasms (0.3% of all tumors) that constitute as much as 2.5% of all fibroadenomatous breast lesions.[225] Phyllodes tumors are composed of mixed epithelial and stromal elements, which makes it difficult to clearly distinguish them from typical fibroadenoma at one end of the spectrum and from soft-tissue sarcomas at the other. Furthermore, the spectrum of morphologic features found within the phyllodes tumors is difficult to correlate with clinical behavior. Yet, some generalizations can be made that are useful in managing patients afflicted with these diseases.

CLINICOPATHOLOGIC FEATURES. Phyllodes tumors of the breast present as circumscribed, slow-growing masses ranging widely from 1 to 30 cm or more. Reported average sizes vary from 4 to 8 cm, with malignant forms being larger.[226] In one series, patient ages ranged from 9 to 88 years (mean of 44 years, with 80% between 31 and 60).[225] Like fibroadenoma, phyllodes tumors occur very rarely in men.[227, 228]

Macroscopically, phyllodes tumors are more or less circumscribed and are composed of connective tissue and ductal epithelium, as are fibroadenomas; however, in the former, the connective tissue shows greater cellularity (Fig. 16–60). They are fleshy tumors with spaces filled with leaf-like (phyllodes) projections leaving residual cleft-like spaces. The connective tissue component can contain foci of myxoid, adipose, osseous, chondroid, and even rhabdomyomatous cells.[229, 230] Often the increased cellularity is noted immediately adjacent to the cleft-like spaces lined by epithelium, but this area of stromal condensation may be somewhat separated from the epithelium by a "Grenz" zone (see Fig. 16–60).[231]

Although predicting biologic behavior by histologic criteria is difficult with phyllodes tumors, the World Health Organization (WHO) considers it useful to separate cases into three categories (benign, borderline, and malignant) based on the extent of mitotic figures, infiltrative margins, cellular atypia, and cellularity. Local recurrences are much more frequent than distant metastases. In a review of 187 cases, Grimes[226] reported an overall local recurrence rate of 28%, which was independent of the degree of malignancy (benign 27%, borderline 32%, malignant 26%). No morphologic features predicted recurrence. In this series, distant metastases occurred in 8 of 100 cases with follow-up (two borderline and six malignant). Stromal overgrowth, mitotic rate greater than 15 per 50 HPF, and cytologically atypical cells characterized seven of the eight metastasizing tumors (Fig. 16–61). The high local recurrence rate of phyllodes tumors suggests multifocal growth as

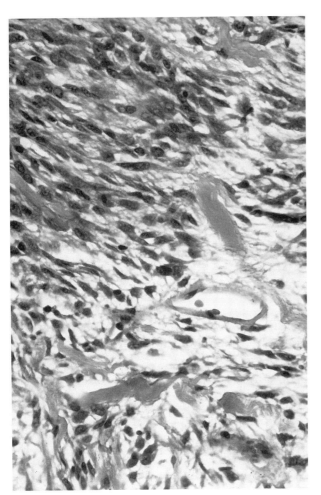

FIGURE 16–59. Myofibroblastoma. Spindled myofibroblasts are shown admixed with thick collagen bands. (H&E)

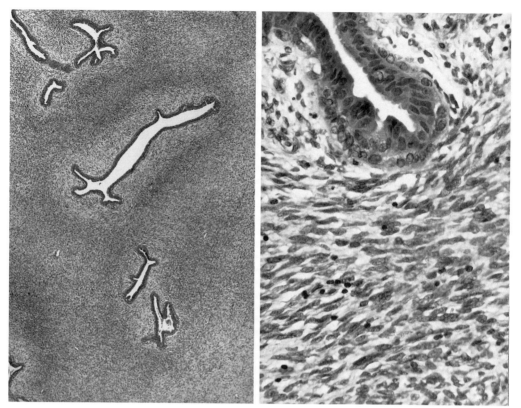

FIGURE 16–60. Phyllodes Tumor, Low-grade Variant. *Left,* Ducts are shown surrounded by densely cellular stroma. Note the "Grenz" zone around the ducts—a pattern sometimes noted in phyllodes tumors. (H&E) *Right,* Higher magnification of the cellular stroma. Mitotic figures are apparent. (H&E)

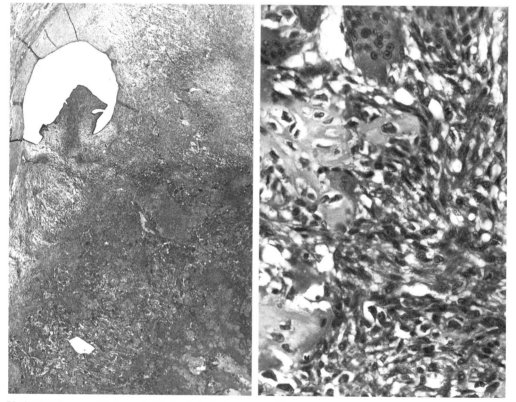

FIGURE 16–61. Phyllodes Tumor, High-grade Variant. *Left,* Large cyst-like space is shown in the upper left containing a protruding tongue ("leaf") of epithelium-lined stroma. Note the stromal overgrowth filling the middle and lower right portions of the illustration. (H&E) *Right,* Highly cellular stroma is shown composed of atypical, hyperchromatic cells forming osteoid and containing osteoclast-like giant cells. (H&E)

reported by Salm.[232] Similar, multifocal fibroadenomas can occur in women and men; and, when florid, they are referred to as **fibroadenomatoid hyperplasia.**[233]

In a review of 26 cases, Ward and Evans[231] studied a number of clinicopathologic features (tumor size, stromal overgrowth, tumor necrosis, mitotic rate, stromal cellularity, nuclear size, nuclear pleomorphism, specialized stroma, and initial therapy) and correlated their ability to predict local recurrence, uncontrolled local recurrence, and distant metastases. Seven of the 26 tumors caused death (five from metastases and two from extensive local recurrence), and six of the seven had stromal overgrowth (defined as mesenchymal proliferation with complete absence of a ductal epithelial element in an area greater than one low-power [×40] field, excluding occasional broad stromal portions of epithelium-lined papillary structures that could, by carefully selecting a given field, fulfill this criterion). With the exception of tumor necrosis (not infarct), which appeared dependent on stromal overgrowth, all the other studied factors were not significantly related to clinical behavior. Likewise, Hart et al.[234] stress the importance of stromal overgrowth in predicting metastasis. Some tumors may have to be extensively sampled to find the focal area of stromal overgrowth.[231]

While acknowledging that there were no consistently reliable morphologic landmarks for predicting outcome, Azzopardi[235] stated that features favoring benign behavior include (1) pushing or well-demarcated tumor border at the microscopic level, (2) even distribution of epithelial tissues within the tumor, (3) fewer than 3/10 HPF, and (4) bland cytologic features with low cellularity. In contrast, features favoring malignant behavior include (1) infiltrating tumor margin, (2) connective-tissue growth outstripping epithelium-lined structures, (3) more than 3/10 HPF, and (4) pronounced cellular atypia with high cellularity.

It is important to add that, when phyllodes tumors occur in women younger than 20 years of age, they are almost always benign, despite clinical and histologic features of malignancy.[236, 237] Flow ploidy or S-phase fraction determinations do not appear to reliably predict behavior.[238]

Proper initial therapy (wide local excision) is helpful in controlling local recurrence but appears irrelevant in preventing distant metastases.[226] Simple mastectomy should be reserved for very large tumors that, for all practical purposes, preclude breast conservation and for cases with multiple recurrences, because some recurrent tumors may progress to higher grade tumors or cause death by invasion of the chest wall. Axillary metastases are very rare.

DIFFERENTIAL DIAGNOSIS. Distinguishing **cellular fibroadenoma** from benign phyllodes tumor may be more of an academic exercise than a practical one, because both are easily managed by conservative local therapy, even with recurrence.[239, 240] Yet, borderline and malignant phyllodes tumors can develop uncontrolled local recurrence and/or distant metastases and should be distinguished from cellular fibroadenoma. Careful application of the criteria outlined earlier should avoid a misdiagnosis. Worth noting is that, like mammary stroma,[241] **fibroadenomas may contain multinucleated stromal giant cells,** which can be mistaken for malignant cells[242] (Fig. 16–62). Also, some fibroadenomas have been mistaken for phyllodes tumors because they show prominent

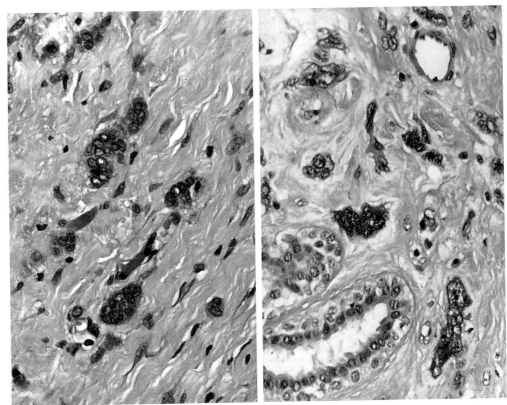

FIGURE 16–62. Atypical Benign Mammary Stromal Cells. *Left,* Multinucleated and/or hyperlobated stromal giant cells are noted in mammary stroma. No mitotic figures are present. (H&E) *Right,* Similar atypical stromal giant cells can occur in the stroma of fibroadenomas. (H&E)

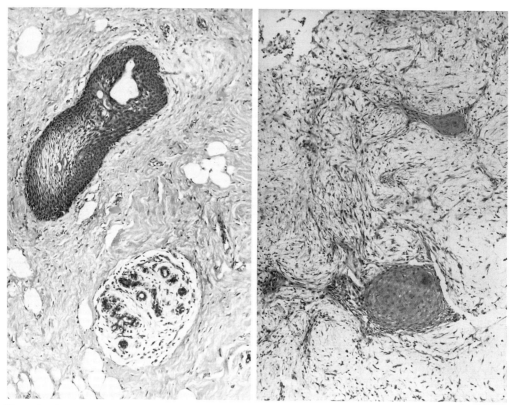

FIGURE 16–63. Metaplastic Breast Carcinoma, Spindle Cell Variant. *Left,* Large duct is shown containing bland-appearing squamous metaplasia. (H&E, original magnification OM ×10) *Right,* In other areas of the same tumor shown at left, cytologically bland spindle cells appear to peel off into a loose myxoid stroma. (H&E)

smooth muscle differentiation,[243] fatty tissue metaplasia,[244] and/or *carcinomatous transformation.*[245] Hiraoka et al.[246] have described a phyllodes tumor of the breast containing the intracytoplasmic inclusion bodies identical with infantile digital fibromatosis.

While extensive tumor sampling may be necessary to reveal stromal overgrowth in a phyllodes tumor, extensive sampling may also be necessary to find the epithelial component amid that stromal overgrowth. Although most recurrent phyllodes tumors have both epithelial and stromal elements, some may recur entirely as stromal sarcomas. Nonetheless, so-called **stromal sarcoma** of the breast should be differentiated from malignant phyllodes tumor. Indeed, the term "stromal sarcoma" of the breast ought to be discarded, and primary sarcomas designated by their pattern of differentiation (**fibrosarcoma, malignant fibrous histiocytoma, osteosarcoma, liposarcoma,** and so on). Jones et al.[247] have reviewed 32 cases of fibrosarcoma and/or malignant fibrous histiocytoma of the breast. They were able to separate them into low- and high-grade tumors. Whereas none of the low-grade tumors metastasized, 25% of the high-grade tumors spread to distant sites (a rate higher than for malignant phyllodes tumors). Also, breast sarcomas with giant cells and osteoid (osteogenic sarcoma) are reported to cause death in most patients with these high-grade sarcomas.[248]

Metaplastic breast carcinomas usually have a component of invasive carcinoma and/or *in situ* carcinoma. Remember, at least focal cytokeratin immunoreactivity can be found in some soft-tissue sarcomas;[249] diffuse and strong immunostaining in a spindle cell lesion suggests true epithelial differentiation.

Spindle Cell Carcinoma of the Breast

Metaplastic breast carcinomas can display squamous, spindle cell, and/or heterologous mesenchymal growth patterns. Although some authors have separated these tumors into a variety of categories,[250–256] others have found little reason to make these distinctions, but rather refer to all mixed carcinomas of the breast as **metaplastic carcinomas,** regardless of whether the metaplastic element is epithelial or mesenchymal.[257, 258] Indeed, Oberman states "the lack of correlation of the microscopic pattern of these neoplasms with prognosis, as well as the presence of apparent overlapping microscopic findings, supports the concept that they are variants of a single entity."[257]

Most of these metaplastic carcinomas are clearly high-grade tumors and easily recognizable as malignant; however, some varieties of so-called **spindle cell carcinoma** of the breast can appear deceptively benign.[251, 255] These tumors are often misdiagnosed as fibrosarcoma, low-grade sarcoma, nodular fasciitis, fibromatosis, granulation-tissue reaction, or squamous metaplasia. Yet, spindle cell carcinomas appear to have the same aggressive biologic behavior as infiltrating duct carcinomas. This discussion focuses on the morphologically **bland variants of spindle cell (metaplastic) breast carcinoma.**[251, 255]

CLINICOPATHOLOGIC FEATURES. Spindle cell carcinoma of the breast presents in the same manner and age group as

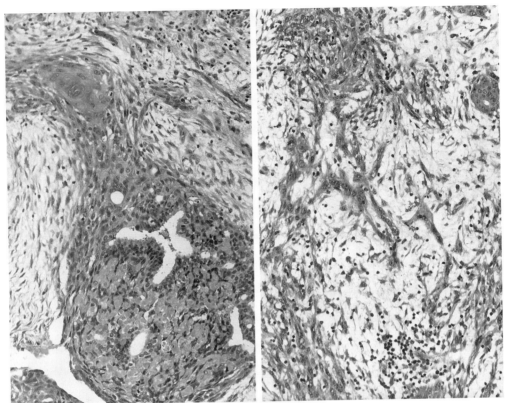

FIGURE 16–64. Metaplastic Breast Carcinoma, Spindle Cell Variant. *Left,* This residual duct within spindle cell breast carcinoma is surrounded by a proliferation of myoepithelial-like cells forming admixed basal lamina material. Note how the island merges with an area showing squamous metaplasia. (H&E) *Right,* Aggregates of spindle stromal cells are shown forming capillary-like structures within a loose myxoid stroma (so-called angioid areas). (H&E)

the common varieties of infiltrating breast carcinoma. Their special qualities lie in their histologic appearance. Spindle cell carcinomas of the breast are composed of sheets of bland spindle cells, variably sized nests of squamous cells (Figs. 16–63 and 16–64), and cysts lined by squamous carcinoma, which may appear deceptively benign. Foci of spindle cells can resemble well-differentiated fibrosarcoma, low-grade malignant fibrous histiocytoma, nodular fasciitis, fibromatosis, and/or granulation tissue. The last pattern is produced by a tracery of numerous branching filaments of spindled carcinoma cells that resemble capillaries of granulation tissue (angioid areas) (see Fig. 16–64, right). These structures can be seen branching off of the squamous epithelial islands. Sometimes the tumor cells form a ring-like or cuff-like proliferation around residual ducts (see Fig. 16–64, left), representing myoepithelial differentiation, a common finding in this variant evident on ultrastructural and immunohistochemical preparations. Minor areas of osteocartilaginous differentiation and/or osteoclast-like giant cells may be present.[251]

In fact, the various patterns of differentiation found in metaplastic breast carcinomas could be explained as a tendency of some breast carcinomas to develop myoepithelial differentiation rather than the more common ductal or lobular epithelial-cell differentiation. Thus, metaplastic breast carcinomas could be conceptualized as carcinomas showing varying amounts of adenomyoepithelial differentiation. It has long been known that myoepithelial cells in the salivary glands differentiate toward spindle cell, squamoid, and osteocartilaginous types.

Indeed, Erlandson and Rosen[199] have already described one case of spindle cell carcinoma of the breast as **infiltrating myoepithelioma.** Also, a case of spindle cell carcinoma of the breast has been described in association with myoepithelial hyperplasia.[259] Moreover, Reddick et al.[260] and Raju[261] have presented histologic, ultrastructural, and immunohistochemical evidence that squamous metaplasia of the breast is derived from myoepithelial cells.

The cumulative 5-year survival rate for spindle cell carcinoma of the breast has been reported at 64%, which is a better survival rate than is usually reported for cytologically high-grade metaplastic breast carcinomas.[251] Although large tumors are more likely to recur, other histologic features such as grade, cellularity, mitotic activity, differentiation of the carcinoma, presence of squamous epithelium, or degree of inflammation do not correlate with outcome.[251]

DIFFERENTIAL DIAGNOSIS. Clearly, the main differential diagnostic pitfall is underdiagnosing spindle cell carcinoma as **fibromatosis, nodular fasciitis, reactive granulation tissue, spindle cell adenomyoepithelioma, low-grade phyllodes tumor, or benign squamous metaplasia.** The best defense against making this mistake is having a high index of suspicion for spindle cell carcinoma and a keen awareness of its histopathologic presentation. Immunohistochemical staining should be very helpful, because the spindle cells are frequently positive for cytokeratin.[251] Electron microscopy shows the myoepithelial features as well.[255] Fibromatosis of the breast resembles fibromatosis occurring elsewhere; fasciitis rarely occurs in the breast parenchyma; and the **angioid areas of**

spindle cell carcinoma should be positive for cytokeratin and negative for Factor VIII–related antigen.

Spindle cell carcinoma can be mistaken for other lesions of the breast that contain squamous components. These include a small number of **infiltrating ductal or medullary carcinomas with focal squamous differentiation** (<5% of such cases), **high-grade metaplastic breast carcinomas with marked mesenchymal differentiation and focal squamous differentiation, pure squamous carcinomas of ductal origin but which lack spindle cell metaplasia, acantholytic variant of squamous carcinoma,**[262, 263] and **mucoepidermoid carcinoma** (both low- and high-grade types).[263–265] Some breast carcinomas with squamous and myoepithelial differentiation can also have **foci of sebaceous differentiation** (Fig. 16–65).[266]

Not all squamous lesions in the breast are malignant, as shown by reports of **post-traumatic lobular squamous metaplasia,**[267] **mixed squamous-mucous cysts,**[268] **squamous metaplasia in gynecomastia,**[269] **infarction with squamous metaplasia of intraductal papilloma,**[162] and **squamous metaplasia in phyllodes tumors and fibroadenomas.**[270]

Extensive sampling of a suspected lesion should lead to discovery of the associated squamous components and/or duct carcinoma (either invasive or *in situ*). The lack of an associated epithelial component in a sarcomatous breast tumor makes it more likely that the neoplasm is a pure sarcoma.[271] Yet, a finding of axillary node metastases composed of malignant cells that stain strongly and diffusely with reliable antikeratin antibodies and/or have ultrastructural features of myoepithelial differentiation should allow the diagnosis of spindle cell "metaplastic" carcinoma. However, metaplastic breast carcinomas may not metastasize as frequently to axillary lymph nodes as other breast carcinomas of similar poorly differentiated nature.[272] In the absence of these features, the diagnosis becomes primary breast sarcoma, which usually but not always has features of fibrosarcoma and/or malignant fibrous histiocytoma. Also, primary breast **leiomyosarcomas, osteosarcomas, and chondrosarcomas** have been reported.[273–275] Christensen et al.[276] reported that metaplastic carcinomas display intense fibronectin immunoreactivity between tumor cells, whereas primary breast sarcomas and stroma of phyllodes tumors stain weakly, especially when compared with surrounding stroma (in this series, unfixed frozen tissues were necessary for fibronectin staining). The importance of the distinction of metaplastic breast carcinoma from its mimickers, using immunohistochemical stains, has been stressed by Christensen et al.,[272] especially for proper prognostication and postoperative therapy.

MISCELLANEOUS PATHOLOGIC CURIOSITIES

A variety of miscellaneous pathologic curiosities have been reported to occur in the breast. Although some obscure lesions are likely missing, the following list is presented for complete-

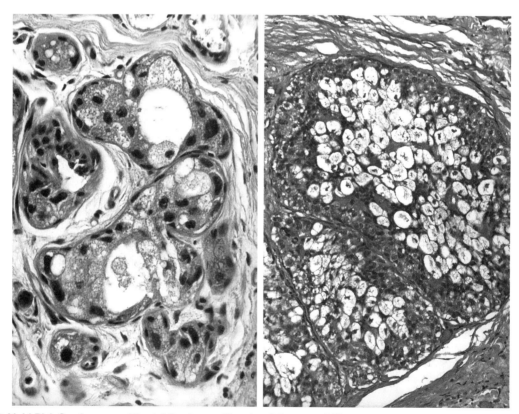

FIGURE 16–65. Lipid-Rich Carcinoma and Ductal Carcinoma Showing Sebaceous Differentiation. *Left,* Carcinoma cells are shown within acini and have abundant foamy cytoplasm, which was lipid-rich as shown by oil red O–positive staining. (H&E) *Right,* Duct carcinoma is shown with focal sebaceous differentiation. (H&E)

ness. Besides, there is always the chance that the general surgical pathologist will encounter an example of one of these unusual lesions.

Benign Lesions

Mondor's disease (thrombophlebitis) and breast cancer[277]
Gynecomastia with lobules and acini[278]
Epidermal cysts of the breast[279]
Breast nodule caused by *Dirofilaria tenuis*[280]
Dirofilaria repens causing breast mass[281]
Chondrolipoma (choristoma) of the breast[282]
Neurilemoma of the breast[283]
Fibrocystic disease in the male breast[284]
Amyloid tumor of the breast[285]
Plasmacytoma of the breast[286]
Inflammatory pseudotumor (plasma cell granuloma) of the breast[287]
Myospherulosis of the breast[288]
Hemangiopericytoma of breast[289]
Papilloma of male breast after phenothiazine therapy[290]
Cholesterol granulomas mimicking breast carcinoma[291]
Signet-ring cell, sinus histiocytosis mimicking metastatic adenocarcinoma in axillary lymph nodes[292]
Nevus cell aggregates in axillary lymph nodes[293]
Myeloid metaplasia presenting as a breast mass[294]
Muscular pseudotumor of the breast after doxorubicin and radiation therapy[295]
Cystic hygroma of breast[296]
Benign epithelial inclusions in axillary lymph nodes[297]
Synovial metaplasia in periprosthetic breast capsule[298]
Calcium oxalate associated with benign breast tissue[299]

Malignant Lesions

Lipid cell carcinoma and variants in breast (see Fig. 16–65, left)[300]
Breast carcinoma with sebaceous differentiation (see Fig. 16–65, right)[301]
Small-cell carcinoma of the breast[302]
Invasive carcinoma with granulomatous reaction[303, 304]
Neural invasion in intraductal carcinoma of breast[305]
Carcinoma with ''choriocarcinomatous'' features[306]
Leiomyosarcoma of breast[307]
Glycogen-rich, clear-cell carcinoma of breast[308]
Oncocytic carcinoma of breast[309]
Skin angiosarcoma aftter radiation for breast carcinoma[310]
Intramyofiber metastasis from breast carcinoma[311]
Unusual giant cell tumor of male breast with myoepithelial and myofibroblastic differentiation[312]
Mammary carcinoma with osteoclast-like giant cells[313, 314]
Neuroendocrine differentiation in breast carcinoma[315]
Lack of diagnostic consistency for medullary carcinoma[316]
Anaplastic variant of Paget's disease[317]

References

1. Nielsen BB: Adenosis tumour of the breast—a clinicopathological investigation of 27 cases. Histopathology 11:1259–1275, 1987.
2. Azzopardi JG: Fibroadenoma. In Azzopardi JG (ed): Problems in Breast Pathology. Philadelphia, WB Saunders, 1979, pp 39–56.
3. Jensen RA, Page DL, Dupont WD, Rogers LW: Invasive breast cancer risk in women with sclerosing adenosis. Cancer 64:1977–1983, 1989.
4. Urban JA, Adair FE: Sclerosing adenosis. Cancer 2:625–634, 1949.
5. Eusebi V, Azzopardi JG: Breast disease. J Pathol 118:9–16, 1976.
6. Rosen PP: Microglandular adenosis: A benign lesion simulating invasive mammary carcinoma. Am J Surg Pathol 7:137–144, 1983.
7. Diaz NM, McDivitt RW, Wick MR: Microglandular adenosis of the breast. Arch Pathol Lab Med 115:578–582, 1991.
8. Carter DJ, Rosen PP: Atypical apocrine metaplasia in sclerosing lesions of the breast: A study of 51 patients. Mod Pathol 4:1–5, 1991.
9. Page DL, Anderson TJ: Adenosis. In Page DL, Anderson TJ (eds): Diagnostic Histopathology of the Breast. Edinburgh, Churchill Livingstone, 1987, pp 51–61.
10. Tesluk H, Amott T, Goodnight JE: Apocrine adenoma of the breast. Arch Pathol Lab Med 110:351–352, 1986.
11. De Potter CR, Cuvelier CA, Roels HJ: Apocrine adenoma presenting as gynaecomastia in a 14-year-old boy. Histopathology 13:697–699, 1988.
12. Oberman HA, Markey BA: Noninvasive carcinoma of the breast presenting in adenosis. Mod Pathol 4:31–35, 1991.
13. Yates AJ, Ahmed AA: Apocrine carcinoma and apocrine metaplasia. Histopathology 14:228–231, 1988.
14. Abati AD, Kimmel M, Rosen PP: Apocrine mammary carcinoma. Clinicopathologic study of 72 cases. Am J Clin Pathol 94:371–377, 1990.
15. Eusebi V, Millis RR, Grazia M, et al: Apocrine carcinoma of the breast. A morphologic and immunocytochemical study. Am J Pathol 123:532–541, 1986.
16. O'Malley FP, Page DL, Nelson EH, Dupont WD: Ductal carcinoma in situ of the breast with apocrine cytology. Definition of a borderline category. Hum Pathol 25:164–168, 1994.
17. Rosai J: Borderline epithelial lesions of the breast. Am J Surg Pathol 15:209–221, 1991.
18. Fechner RE: Lobular carcinoma in situ in sclerosing adenosis. A potential source of confusion with invasive carcinoma. Am J Surg Pathol 5:233–239, 1981.
19. Eusebi V, Collina G, Bussolati G: Carcinoma in situ in sclerosing adenosis of the breast: An immunocytochemical study. Semin Diagn Pathol 6:146–152, 1989.
20. Weidner N: Benign breast lesions that mimic malignant tumors: Analysis of five distinct types. Semin Diagn Pathol 7:90–101, 1990.
21. Rosen PP: Microglandular adenosis. A benign lesion simulating invasive mammary carcinoma. Am J Surg Pathol 7:137–144, 1983.
22. Tavassoli FA, Norris HJ: Microglandular adenosis of the breast. Am J Surg Pathol 7:731–737, 1983.
23. James BA, Cranor ML, Rosen PP: Carcinoma of the breast arising in microglandular adenosis. Am J Clin Pathol 100:507–513, 1993.
24. Nesland JM, Holm R, Lunde S, et al: Diagnostic problems in breast pathology: The benefit of ultrastructural and immunocytochemical analysis. Ultrastruct Pathol 11:293–311, 1987.
25. Taylor HB, Norris HJ: Well-differentiated carcinoma of the breast. Cancer 25:687–692, 1970.
26. Cooper HS, Patchefsky AS, Krall RA: Tubular carcinoma of the breast. Cancer 42:2334–2342, 1978.
27. Oberman HA, Fidler WJ: Tubular carcinoma of the breast. Am J Surg Pathol 3:387–395, 1979.
28. Deos PH, Norris HJ: Well-differentiated (tubular) carcinoma of the breast. Am J Clin Pathol 78:1–7, 1982.
29. Parl FF, Richardson LD: The histologic and biologic spectrum of tubular carcinoma of the breast. Hum Pathol 14:694–698, 1983.
30. Page DL, Dixon JM, Anderson TJ: Invasive cribriform carcinoma of the breast. Histopathology 7:525–536, 1983.
31. Venable JG, Schwartz AM, Silverberg SG: Infiltrating cribriform carcinoma of the breast: A distinctive clinicopathologic entity. Hum Pathol 21:333–338, 1990.
32. Fisher ER, Gregorio RM, Redmond C, et al: Tubulo-lobular invasive breast cancer: A variant of lobular invasive cancer. Hum Pathol 8:679–683, 1977.
33. McDivitt RW, Stewart FW: Breast carcinoma in children. JAMA 195:388–390, 1966.
34. Krauz T, Jenkins D, Grontoft O, et al: Secretory carcinoma of the breast in adults: Emphasis on late recurrence and metastasis. Histopathology 14:25–36, 1989.
35. Rosen PP, Cranor ML: Secretory carcinoma of the breast. Arch Pathol Lab Med 115:141–144, 1991.
36. Tavassoli FA, Norris HJ: Secretory carcinoma of the breast. Cancer 45:2404–2413, 1980.
37. Oberman HA: Secretory carcinoma of the breast in adults. Am J Surg Pathol 4:465–470, 1980.
38. Akhtar M, Robinson C, Ashraf M, Godwin JT: Secretory carcinoma of the breast in adults. Cancer 51:2245–2254, 1983.
39. Fenoglio C, Lattes R: Sclerosing papillary proliferations in the female breast. A benign lesion often mistaken for carcinoma. Cancer 33:691–700, 1974.
40. Eusebi V, Grassigli A, Grosso F: Lesioni focali scleroelastotiche mammarie simulanti il carcinoma infiltrante. Pathologica 68:507–518, 1976.
41. Fisher ER, Palekar AS, Kotwal N, et al: A nonencapsulated sclerosing lesion of the breast. Am J Clin Pathol 71:240–246, 1979.
42. Rickert RR, Kalisher L, Hutter RVP: Indurative mastopathy: A benign sclerosing lesion of breast with elastosis which may simulate carcinoma. Cancer 47:561–571, 1981.
43. Page DL, Anderson TJ: Radial scars and complex sclerosing lesions. In Page DL, Anderson TJ (eds): Diagnostic Histopathology of the Breast. Edinburgh, Churchill Livingstone, 1987, pp 89–103.
44. Azzopardi JG: Over diagnosis of malignancy. In Azzopardi JG (ed): Problems in Breast Pathology. Philadelphia, WB Saunders, 1979, pp 167–191.
45. Andersen JA, Gram JB: Radial scar in the female breast. A long term follow up study of 32 cases. Cancer 53:2557–2560, 1984.
46. Nielsen M, Christensen L, Andersen J: Radial scars in women with breast cancer. Cancer 59:1019–1025, 1987.
47. Azzopardi JG: Ductal adenoma of the breast: A lesion which can mimic carcinoma. J Pathol 144:15–23, 1984.

48. Sloane JP, Mayers MM: Carcinoma and atypical hyperplasia in radial scars and complex sclerosing lesions: Importance of lesion size and patient age. Histopathology 23:225–231, 1993.

49. Lammie GA, Millis RR: Ductal adenoma of the breast—a review of fifteen cases. Hum Pathol 20:903–908, 1989.

50. Haagensen CD, Stout AP, Phillips JS: The papillary neoplasms of the breast. I. Benign intraductal papilloma. Ann Surg 133:18–36, 1951.

51. Kraus FT, Neubecker RD: The differential diagnosis of papillary tumors of the breast. Cancer 15:444–455, 1962.

52. Murad TM, Contesso G, Mouriesse H: Papillary tumors of the large lactiferous ducts. Cancer 48:122–133, 1981.

53. Ohuchi N, Rikiya A, Kasai M: Possible cancerous change of intraductal papillomas of the breast. A 3-D reconstruction study of 25 cases. Cancer 54:605–611, 1984.

54. Haagensen CD: Solitary intraductal papilloma; and Multiple intraductal papilloma. In Haagensen CD: Diseases of the Breast, 3rd ed. Philadelphia, WB Saunders, 1986, pp 136–175 and 176–191.

55. Haagensen CD, Bodian C, Haagensen DE Jr: Breast Carcinoma: Risk and Detection. Philadelphia, WB Saunders, 1981.

56. Carter D: Intraductal papillary tumors of the breast. A study of 78 cases. Cancer 39:1689–1692, 1977.

57. Fischer ER, Palekar AS, Redmond C, et al: Pathologic findings from the National Surgical Adjuvant Breast Project (Protocol No. 4): VI. Invasive papillary cancer. Am J Clin Pathol 73:313–321, 1980.

58. Siriaunkgul S, Tavassoli FA: Invasive micropapillary carcinoma of the breast. Mod Pathol 6:660–662, 1993.

59. Carter D, Orr SL, Merino J: Intracystic papillary carcinoma of the breast. Cancer 52:14–19, 1983.

60. Papotti M, Eusebi V, Gugliotta P, Bussolati G: Immunohistochemical analysis of benign and malignant papillary lesions of the breast. Am J Surg Pathol 7:451–461, 1983.

61. Raju RB, Lee MW, Zarbo RJ, et al: Papillary neoplasia of the breast: Immunohistochemically defined myoepithelial cells in the diagnosis of benign and malignant papillary breast neoplasms. Mod Pathol 2:569–576, 1989.

62. Vuitch MF, Rosen PP, Erlandson RA: Pseudoangiomatous hyperplasia of mammary stroma. Hum Pathol 17:185–191, 1986.

63. Ibrahim RE, Sciotto CG, Weidner N: Pseudoangiomatous hyperplasia of mammary stroma. Some observations regarding its clinicopathologic spectrum. Cancer 63:1154–1160, 1989.

64. Edeiken S, Russo DP, Knecht J, et al: Angiosarcoma after tylectomy and radiation therapy for carcinoma of the breast. Cancer 70:644–647, 1992.

65. Benda JA, Al-Jurf AS, Benson AB: Angiosarcoma of the breast following segmental mastectomy complicated lymphedema. Am J Clin Pathol 87:651–655, 1987.

66. Seidman JD, Borkowski A, Aisner SC, Sun CCJ: Rapid growth of psuedoangiomatous hyperplasia of mammary stroma in axillary gynecomastia in an immunosuppressed patient. Arch Pathol Lab Med 117:736–738, 1993.

67. Donnell RM, Rosen PP, Lieberman PH, et al: Angiosarcoma and other vascular tumors of the breast. Pathologic analysis as a guide to prognosis. Am J Surg Pathol 5:629–642, 1981.

68. Merino MJ, Carter D, Berman M: Angiosarcoma of the breast. Am J Surg Pathol 7:53–60, 1983.

69. Morrow M, Berger D, Thelmo W: Diffuse cystic angiomatosis of the breast. Cancer 62:2392–2396, 1988.

70. Hoda SA, Cranor ML, Rosen PP: Hemangiomas of the breast with atypical histological features. Further analysis of histological subtypes confirming their benign behavior. Am J Surg Pathol 16:553–560, 1992.

71. Jozefczyk MA, Rosen PP: Vascular tumors of the breast. II. Perilobular hemangiomas and hemangiomas. Am J Surg Pathol 9:491–503, 1985.

72. Rosen PP: Vascular tumors of the breast. III. Angiomatosis. Am J Surg Pathol 9:652–658, 1985.

73. Rosen PP, Jozefczyk M, Boram L: Vascular tumors of the breast. IV. The venous hemangioma. Am J Surg Pathol 9:659–665, 1985.

74. Rosen PP: Vascular tumors of the breast. V. Nonparenchymal hemangiomas of mammary subcutaneous tissues. Am J Surg Pathol 9:723–729, 1985.

75. Fisher CJ, Hanby AM, Robinson L, Millis RR: Mammary hamartoma—a review of 35 cases. Histopathology 20:99–106, 1992.

76. Oberman HA: Hamartomas and hamartoma variants of the breast. Semin Diagn Pathol 6:135–145, 1989.

77. Arrigoni MC, Dockerty MB, Judd ES: The identification and treatment of mammary hamartoma. Surg Gynecol Obstet 133:577–582, 1971.

78. Daroca PJ, Reed RJ, Love GL, Kraus SD: Myoid hamartomas of the breast. Hum Pathol 16:212–219, 1985.

79. Clement PB, Young RH, Azzopardi JG: Collagenous spherulosis of the breast. Am J Surg Pathol 11:411–417, 1987.

80. Grignon DJ, Mackay BN, Ordonez NG, et al: Collagenous spherulosis of the breast. Immunohistochemical and ultrastructural studies. Am J Clin Pathol 91:386–392, 1989.

81. Ro JY, Silva EG, Gallager HS: Adenoid cystic carcinoma of the breast. Hum Pathol 18:1276–1281, 1987.

82. Fisher ER, Brown R: Intraductal signet ring carcinoma: A hitherto undescribed form of intraductal carcinoma of the breast. Cancer 55:2533–2537, 1985.

83. Wheeler JE, Enterline HT: Lobular carcinoma of the breast in situ and infiltrating. Pathol Annu 2:161–188, 1976.

84. Martinez V, Azzopardi JG: Invasive lobular carcinoma of the breast: Incidence and variants. Histopathology 3:467–488, 1979.

85. Dixon JM, Anderson TJ, Page DL, et al: Infiltrating lobular carcinoma of the breast. Histopathology 6:149–161, 1982.

86. Dixon JM, Anderson TJ, Page DL, et al: Infiltrating lobular carcinoma of the breast: An evaluation of the incidence and consequences of bilateral disease. Br J Surg 70:513–516, 1983.

87. Dixon JM, Page DL, Anderson TJ, et al: Long-term survivors after breast cancer. Br J Surg 72:445–448, 1985.

88. DiCostanzo D, Rosen PP, Gareen I, et al: Prognosis in infiltrating lobular carcinoma. An analysis of "classical" and variant tumors. Am J Surg Pathol 14:12–23, 1990.

89. Shousha S, Backhous CM, Alaghband-Zadeh J, Burn I: Alveolar variant of invasive lobular carcinoma of the breast. A tumor rich in estrogen receptors. Am J Clin Pathol 85:1–5, 1986.

90. Eusebi V, Betts C, Haagensen DE, et al: Apocrine differentiation in lobular carcinoma of the breast. A morphologic, immunologic, and ultrastructural study. Hum Pathol 15:134–140, 1984.

91. Walford N, Velden JT: Histiocytoid breast carcinoma: An apocrine variant of lobular carcinoma. Histopathology 14:515–522, 1989.

92. Marino MJ, Livolsi VA: Signet-ring carcinoma of the female breast: A clinicopathologic analysis of 24 cases. Cancer 48:1830–1837, 1981.

93. Frost AR, Terahata S, Tien Yeh I, et al: The significance of signet ring cells in infiltrating lobular carcinoma of the breast. Arch Pathol Lab Med 119:64–68, 1995.

94. Page DL, Anderson TJ, Sakamoto G: Infiltrating lobular carcinoma. In Page DL, Anderson TJ (eds): Diagnostic Histopathology of the Breast. New York, Churchill Livingstone, 1987, pp 219–226.

95. Eusebi V, Magalhaes F, Azzopardi JG: Pleomorphic lobular carcinoma of the breast: An aggressive tumor showing apocrine differentiation. Hum Pathol 23:655–662, 1992.

96. Mazoujian G, Pinkus GS, Davis S, Haagensen DE: Immunohistochemistry of a gross cystic disease fluid protein (GCDFP-15) of the breast. A marker of apocrine epithelium and breast carcinomas with apocrine features. Am J Pathol 110:105–112, 1983.

97. Weidner N, Semple JP: Pleomorphic variant of invasive lobular carcinoma of the breast. Hum Pathol 23:1167–1171, 1992.

98. Rosen PP, Lieberman PH, Braun DW, et al: Lobular carcinoma in situ of the breast. Detailed analysis of 99 patients with average follow-up of 24 years. Am J Surg Pathol 2:225–251, 1978.

99. Elston CW, Ellis IO: Pathology and breast screening. Histopathology 16:109–118, 1990.

100. Dupont WD, Page DL: Relative risk of breast cancer varies with time since diagnosis of atypical hyperplasia. Hum Pathol 20:723–725, 1989.

101. Sonnenfeld MR, Frenna TH, Weidner N, Meyer JE: Lobular carcinoma in situ detected in needle directed breast biopsies: Radiology-pathology correlation. Radiology 181:363–367, 1991.

102. Page DL, Anderson TJ, Rogers LW: Carcinoma in situ (CIS). In Page DL, Anderson TJ (eds): Diagnostic Histopathology of the Breast. New York, Churchill Livingstone, 1987, pp 157–192.

103. Rosen PP: Coexistent lobular carcinoma in situ and intraductal carcinoma in a single lobular-duct unit. Am J Surg Pathol 4:241–246, 1980.

104. Page DL, Kidd TE, DuPont WD, et al: Lobular neoplasia of the breast: Higher risk for subsequent invasive cancer predicted by more extensive disease. Hum Pathol 22:1232–1239, 1991.

105. Fechner RE: Epithelial alterations in extralobular ducts of breast with lobular carcinoma. Arch Pathol Lab Med 93:164–171, 1972.

106. Wellings SR, Jensen HM: On the origin and progression of ductal carcinoma in the human breast. J Natl Cancer Inst 50:1111–1118, 1973.

107. Ottesen GL, Graversen HP, Blichert-Toft M, et al., and Danish Breast Cancer Cooperative group: Lobular carcinoma in situ of the female breast. Short term results of a prospective national study. Am J Surg Pathol 17:14–21, 1993.

108. Tavassoli FA, Yeh IT: Lactational and clear cell changes of the breast in nonlactating, nonpregnant women. Am J Clin Pathol 87:23–29, 1987.

109. Schnitt SJ, Connolly JL, Harris JR, Cohen RB: Radiation-induced changes in the breast. Hum Pathol 15:545–550, 1984.

110. Page DL, Dupont WD, Rogers LW: Intraductal carcinoma of the breast. Follow-up after biopsy only. Cancer 49:751–758, 1982.

111. Lagios MD, Westdahl PR, Margolin Fr, Rose MR: Duct carcinoma in situ. Relationship of extent of noninvasive disease to the frequency of occult invasion, multicentricity, lymph node metastases, and short-term treatment failures. Cancer 50:1309–1314, 1982.

112. Lagios MD, Westdahl PR, Margolin FR, Rose MR: Mammographically detected duct carcinoma in situ. Frequency of local recurrence following tylectomy and prognostic effect of nuclear grade on local recurrence. Cancer 63:618–624, 1989.

113. Holland R, Peterse JL, Mills RR, et al: Ductal carcinoma in situ: A proposal for a new classification. Semin Diag Pathol 11:167–180, 1994.

114. Lewis D, Geschickter CF: Comedo carcinomas of the breast. Arch Surg 36:225–244, 1938.

115. Poller DN, Silverstein MJ, Galea M, et al: Ductal carcinoma in situ of the breast: A proposal for a new simplified histological classification association between cellular proliferation and c-erbB-2 protein expression. Mod Pathol 7:257–262, 1994.

116. Bellamy COC, McDonald C, Salter DM, et al: Noninvasive ductal carcinoma of the breast: The relevance of histologic categorization. Hum Pathol 24:16–23, 1993.

117. Page DL, Dupont WD, Rogers LW, Rados MS: Atypical hyperplastic lesions of the female breast. A long term follow-up study. Cancer 55:2698–2708, 1985.
118. Page DL, Rogers LW: Combined histologic and cytologic criteria for the diagnosis of mammary atypical ductal hyperplasia. Hum Pathol 23:1095–1097, 1992.
119. Rosen PP: Proliferative breast ''disease.'' An unresolved diagnostic dilemma. Cancer 71:3798–3807, 1993.
120. Azzopardi JG: Epitheliosis and in situ carcinoma; and Under diagnosis of malignancy. In Azzopardi JG (ed): Problems in Breast Pathology. Philadelphia, WB Saunders, 1979, pp 113–149 and 192–239.
121. Bartkova J, Barnes DM, Millis RR, Gullick WJ: Immunohistochemical demonstration of c-erbB2 protein in mammary ductal carcinoma in situ. Hum Pathol 21:1164–1167, 1990.
122. Lilleng R, Hagmar BM, Nesland JM: C-erbB-2 protein and neuroendocrine expression in intraductal carcinomas of the breast. Mod Pathol 5:41–47, 1992.
123. Tavassoli FA, Norris HJ: A comparison of the results of long-term follow-up for atypical intraductal hyperplasia and intraductal hyperplasia of the breast. Cancer 65:518–529, 1990.
124. Rosen PP: Mucocele-like tumors of the breast. Am J Surg Pathol 10:464–469, 1986.
125. Guerry P, Erlandson RA, Rosen PP: Cystic hypersecretory hyperplasia and cystic hypersecretory duct carcinoma of the breast: Pathology, therapy, and follow-up of 39 patients. Cancer 61:1611–1620, 1988.
126. Ro JY, Sneige N, Sahin AS, et al: Mucocelelike tumor of the breast associated with atypical ductal hyperplasia or mucinous carcinoma. Arch Pathol Lab Med 115:137–140, 1991.
127. Fisher CJ, Millis RR: A mucocele-like tumor of the breast associated with both atypical ductal hyperplasia and mucoid carcinoma. Histopathology 21:69–71, 1992.
128. Komaki K, Sakamoto G, Sugano H, et al: The morphologic feature of mucus leakage appearing in low papillary carcinoma of the breast. Hum Pathol 22:231–236, 1991.
129. Weaver MG, Abdul-Karim FW, Al-Kaisi: Mucinous lesions of the breast: A pathological continuum. Pathol Res Pract 189:873–876, 1993.
130. Fischer ER, Palekar AS, Stoner F, Costantino J: Mucocele lesions and mucinous carcinoma of the breast. Int J Surg Pathol 1:213–220, 1994.
131. Arihiro K, Inai K, Kurihara K, et al: Myxoma of the breast: Report of a case with unique histological and immunohistochemical appearances. Acta Pathol Jpn 43:340–346, 1993.
132. DeMay RM, Kay S: Granular cell tumor of the breast. Pathol Annu 19:121–148, 1984.
133. Damiani S, Koerner FC, Dickersin GR, et al: Granular cell tumor of the breast. Virchows Arch A Pathol Anat Histopathol 420:219–226, 1992.
134. Tsang WYW, Chan JKC: Kp1(CD68) staining of granular cell neoplasms: Is Kp1 a marker for lysosomes rather than the histiocytic lineage? Histopathology 21:84–86, 1992.
135. Jones MW, Norris HJ, Snyder RC: Infiltrating syringomatous adenoma of the nipple. A clinical and pathologic study of 11 cases. Am J Surg Pathol 13:197–201, 1989.
136. Ward BE, Cooper PH, Subramony C: Syringomatous tumor of the nipple. Am J Clin Pathol 92:692–696, 1989.
137. Rosen PP: Syringomatous adenoma of the nipple. Am J Surg Pathol 7:739–745, 1983.
138. McClure J, Smith PS, Jamieson GG: Mixed salivary type adenoma of the human female breast. Arch Pathol Lab Med 106:615–619, 1982.
139. Moran CA, Suster S, Carter D: Benign mixed tumors (pleomorphic adenomas) of the breast. Am J Surg Pathol 14:913–921, 1990.
140. Chen KTK: Pleomorphic adenoma of the breast. Am J Clin Pathol 93:792–794, 1990.
141. Diaz NM, McDivitt RW, Wick MR: Pleomorphic adenoma of the breast: A clinicopathologic and immunohistochemical study of 10 cases. Hum Pathol 22:1206–1214, 1991.
142. Van Hoeven KH, Drudis T, Cranor ML, et al: Low-grade adenosquamous carcinoma of the breast. A clinicopathologic study of 32 cases with ultrastructural analysis. Am J Surg Pathol 17:248–258, 1993.
143. Smith BH, Taylor HB: The occurrence of bone and cartilage in mammary tumors. Am J Clin Pathol 51:610–618, 1969.
144. Ballance WA, Ro JY, El-Naggar AK, et al: Pleomorphic adenoma (benign mixed tumor) of the breast. Am J Clin Pathol 93:795–801, 1990.
145. Rosen PP, Caicco JA: Florid papillomatosis of the nipple. Am J Surg Pathol 10:87–101, 1986.
146. Finck FM, Schwinn CP, Keasbey LE: Clear cell hidradenoma of the breast. Cancer 22:125–135, 1968.
147. Hertel BF, Zaloudek C, Kempson RL: Breast adenomas. Cancer 37:2891–2905, 1976.
148. Di Bonito L, Giarelli L, Falconieri G, Viehl P: Metastatic tumors to the female breast. An autopsy study of 12 cases. Pathol Res Pract 187:432–435, 1991.
149. Green LK, Klima M: The use of immunohistochemistry in metastatic prostate adenocarcinoma to the breast. Hum Pathol 22:242–246, 1991.
150. Cormier WJ, Gaffey TA, Welch JM, et al: Linitis plastica caused by metastatic lobular carcinoma of the breast. Mayo Clin Proc 55:747–753, 1980.
151. Bonetti F, Colombari R, Manfrin E, et al: Breast carcinoma with positive results for melanoma marker (HMB-45). HMB-45 immunoreactivity in normal and neoplastic breast. Am J Clin Pathol 92:491–495, 1989.
152. Cummings OW, Mazur MT: Breast carcinoma diffusely metastatic to the spleen. A report of two cases presenting as idiopathic thrombocytopenic purpura. Am J Clin Pathol 97:484–489, 1992.
153. Warner TFCS, Seo IS: Bronchial carcinoid appearing as a breast mass. Arch Pathol Lab Med 104:531–534, 1980.
154. Di Bonito L, Royen PM, Ziter FMH: Ovarian carcinoma metastatic to the breast. Br J Radiol 47:356–357, 1974.
155. Frauenhoffer EE, Ro JY, Silva EG, El-Naggar A: Well-differentiated serous ovarian carcinoma presenting as a breast mass: A case report and flow cytometric DNA study. Int J Gynecol Pathol 10:79–87, 1991.
156. Zuska JJ, Crile G, Ayres W: Fistulas of lactiferous ducts. Am J Surg 81:312–317, 1951.
157. Crile G, Chatty EM: Squamous metaplasia of lactiferous ducts. Arch Surg 102:533–534, 1971.
158. Habif DV, Perzin KH, Lipton R, Lattes R: Subareolar abscess associated with squamous metaplasia of lactiferous ducts. Am J Surg 119:523–526, 1970.
159. Powell BC, Maull KI, Sachatello CR: Recurrent subareolar abscess of the breast and squamous metaplasia of the lactiferous ducts: A clinical syndrome. South Med J 70:935–937, 1977.
160. Watt-Boolsen S, Rasmussen NR, Blichert-Toft M: Primary periareolar abscess in the nonlactating breast: Risk of recurrence. Am J Surg 153:571–573, 1987.
161. Eggers JW, McChesney T: Squamous cell carcinoma of the breast: A clinicopathologic analysis of eight cases and review of the literature. Hum Pathol 15:526–531, 1984.
162. Flint A, Oberman HA: Infarction and squamous metaplasia of intraductal papilloma: A benign breast lesion that may simulate carcinoma. Hum Pathol 15:764–767, 1984.
163. Subramony C: Bilateral breast tumors resembling syringocystadenoma papilliferum. Am J Clin Pathol 87:656–659, 1987.
164. Murthy MSN: Granulomatous mastitis and lipogranuloma of the breast. Am J Clin Pathol 60:432–433, 1973.
165. Kessler E, Wollach Y: Granulomatous mastitis. A lesion clinically simulating carcinoma. Am J Clin Pathol 58:642–646, 1972.
166. Going JJ, Anderson TJ, Wilkinson S, Chetty U: Granulomatous lobular mastitis. J Clin Pathol 40:535–540, 1987.
167. Brown KL, Tang PH: Postlactational tumoral granulomatous mastitis: A localized immune phenomenon. Am J Surg 138:326–329, 1979.
168. Osborne BM: Granulomatous mastitis caused by histoplasma and mimicking inflammatory breast carcinoma. Hum Pathol 20:47–52, 1989.
169. Banik S, Bishop PW, Ormerod LP, O'Brien TEB: Sarcoidosis of the breast. J Clin Pathol 39:446–448, 1986.
170. Gansler TS, Wheeler JE: Mammary sarcoidosis. Two cases and literature review. Arch Pathol Lab Med 108:673–675, 1984.
171. Wargotz ES, Lefkowitz M: Granulomatous angiopanniculitis of the breast. Hum Pathol 20:1084–1088, 1989.
172. Clement PB, Senges H, How AR: Giant cell arteritis of the breast: Case report and literature review. Hum Pathol 18:1186–1190, 1987.
173. Pambakian H, Tighe JR: Breast involvement in Wegener's granulomatosis. J Clin Pathol 24:343–349, 1971.
174. Ng WF, Chow LTC, Lam PWY: Localized polyarteritus nodosa of the breast: Report of two cases and a review of the literature. Histopathology 23:535–539, 1993.
175. Lammie GA, Bobrow LG, Staunton MDM, et al: Sclerosing lymphocytic lobulitis of the breast—evidence for an autoimmune pathogenesis. Histopathology 19:13–20, 1991.
176. Soler NG, Khardori R: Fibrous disease of the breast, thyroiditis and cheiroarthropathy in type 1 diabetes mellitus. Lancet i:193–194, 1984.
177. Bryd BF, Harmann WH, Graham LS, Hogle HH: Mastopathy in insulin-dependent diabetics. Ann Surg 205:529–532, 1987.
178. Logan WW, Hoffmann NY: Diabetic fibrous breast disease. Radiology 172:667–670, 1989.
179. Tomaszewski JE, Brooks JS, Hicks D, Livolsi VA: Diabetic mastopathy: A distinctive clinicopathologic entity. Hum Pathol 23:780–786, 1992.
180. Schwartz IS, Strauchen JA: Lymphocytic mastopathy. An autoimmune disease of the breast? Am J Clin Pathol 93:725–730, 1990.
181. Aozasa K, Ohsawa M, Saeki K, et al: Malignant lymphoma of the breast. Immunologic type and association with lymphocytic mastopathy. Am J Clin Pathol 97:699–704, 1992.
182. Lamovec J, Jancar J: Primary malignant lymphoma of the breast. Lymphoma of the mucosa-associated lymphoid tissue. Cancer 60:3033–3041, 1987.
183. Hugh JC, Jackson FI, Hanson J, Poppema S: Primary breast lymphoma. An immunohistologic study of 20 new cases. Cancer 66:2602–2611, 1990.
184. Mattia AR, Ferry JA, Harris NL: Breast lymphoma: A B-cell spectrum including the low grade B-cell lymphoma of mucosa associated with lymphoid tissue. Am J Surg Pathol 17:574–587, 1993.
185. Bobrow LG, Richards MA, Happerfield LC, et al: Breast lymphomas: A clinicopathologic review. Hum Pathol 24:274–278, 1993.
186. Arber DA, Simpson JF, Weiss LM, Rappaport H: Non-Hodgkin's lymphoma involving the breast. Am J Surg Pathol 18:288–295, 1994.
187. Brustein S, Filippa DA, Kimmel M, et al: Malignant lymphoma of the breast. A study of 53 cases. Ann Surg 205:144–150, 1972.
188. Fisher ER, Palekar AS, Paulson JD, Golinger R: Pseudolymphoma of breast. Cancer 44:258–263, 1979.
189. Lin JJ, Farha GJ, Taylor RJ: Pseudolymphoma of the breast. I. In a study of 8,654 consecutive tylectomies and mastectomies. Cancer 45:973–978, 1980.

190. Anastassiades OT, Choreftaki T, Ioannovich J, et al: Megalomastia: Histological, histochemical and immunohistochemical study. Virchows Arch A [Pathol Anat Histopathol] 420:337–344, 1992.

191. Ashton MA, Lefkowitz M, Tavassoli FA: Epithelioid stromal cells in lymphocytic mastitis: A source of confusion with invasive carcinoma. Mod Pathol 7:49–54, 1994.

192. Kumar S, Kumar C: Lymphoepithelioma-like carcinoma of the breast. Mod Pathol 7:129–131, 1994.

193. Hamperl H: The myothelia (myoepithelial cells). Normal state; regressive changes; hyperplasia; tumors. Curr Top Pathol 53:161–220, 1970.

194. Cameron HM, Hamperl H, Warambo W: Leiomyosarcoma of the breast originating from myothelium (myoepithelium). J Pathol 114:89–96, 1974.

195. Dardick I, Van Nostrand AWP, Jeans MTD, et al: Pleomorphic adenoma, II: Ultrastructural organization of ''stromal'' regions. Hum Pathol 14:798–809, 1983.

196. Dardick I: A role for electron microscopy in salivary gland neoplasms. Ultrastruct Pathol 9:151–161, 1985.

197. Dardick I, Van Nostrand AWP: Myoepithelial cells in salivary gland tumors: Revisited. Head Neck Surg 7:395–408, 1985.

198. Lam RM: An electron microscopic histochemical study of the histogenesis of major salivary gland pleomorphic adenoma. Ultrastruct Pathol 8:207–223, 1985.

199. Erlandson RA, Rosen PP: Infiltrating myoepithelioma of the breast. Am J Surg Pathol 6:785–793, 1982.

200. Erlandson RA, Cardon-Cardo C, Higgins PJ: Histogenesis of benign pleomorphic (mixed tumor) of the major salivary glands: An ultrastructural and immunohistochemical study. Am J Surg Pathol 8:803–820, 1984.

201. Chaudry AP, Satchidanand S, Peer R, Cutler LS: Myoepithelial cell adenoma of the parotid gland: A light and ultrastructural study. Cancer 49:288–293, 1982.

202. Rode L, Nesland JM, Johannssen JV: A spindle cell breast lesion in a 54-year-old woman. Ultrastruct Pathol 10:421–425, 1986.

203. Kahn HJ, Baumal R, Marks A, et al: Myoepithelial cells in salivary gland tumors. Arch Pathol Lab Med 109:190–195, 1985.

204. Kahn LB, Schoub L: Myoepithelioma of the palate: Histochemical and ultrastructural observation. Arch Pathol 95:209–212, 1973.

205. Sciubba JJ, Brannon RB: Myoepithelioma of salivary glands: Report of 23 cases. Cancer 49:562–572, 1982.

206. Zarbo RJ, Oberman HA: Cellular adenomyoepithelioma of the breast. Am J Surg Pathol 7:863–870, 1983.

207. Kiaer H, Nielsen B, Paulsen S, et al: Adenomyoepithelial adenosis and low-grade malignant adenomyoepithelioma of the breast. Virchows Arch [A] 405:55–67, 1984.

208. Eusebi V, Casadei GP, Bussolati G, Azzopardi JG: Adenomyoepithelioma of the breast with a distinctive type of apocrine adenosis. Histopathology 11:305–315, 1987.

209. Toth J: Benign human mammary myoepithelioma. Virchows Arch [Pathol Anat] 374:263–269, 1977.

210. Dardick I: Malignant myoepithelioma of parotid salivary gland. Ultrastruct Pathol 9:163–168, 1985.

211. Schurch W, Potvin C, Seemayer TA: Malignant myoepithelioma (myoepithelial carcinoma) of the breast: An ultrastructural and immunocytochemical study. Ultrastruct Pathol 8:1–11, 1985.

212. Thorner PS, Kahn HJ, Baumal R, et al: Malignant myoepithelioma of the breast: An immunohistochemical study by light and electron microscopy. Cancer 57:745–750, 1986.

213. Rosen PP: Adenomyoepithelioma of the breast. Hum Pathol 18:1232–1237, 1987.

214. Jabi M, Dardick I, Cardigos N: Adenomyoepithelioma of the breast. Arch Pathol Lab Med 112:73–76, 1988.

215. Young RH, Clement PB: Adenomyoepithelioma of the breast: A report of three cases and review of the literature. Am J Clin Pathol 89:308–314, 1988.

216. Tavassoli FA: Myoepithelial lesions of the breast. Myoepitheliosis, adenomyoepithelioma, and myoepithelial carcinoma. Am J Surg Pathol 15:554–568, 1991.

217. Weidner N, Levine JD: Spindle-cell adenomyoepithelioma of the breast. A microscopic, ultrastructural, and immunocytochemical study. Cancer 62:1561–1567, 1988.

218. Loose JH, Patchefsky AS, Hollander IJ, et al: Adenomyoepithelioma of the breast. A spectrum of biological behavior. Am J Surg Pathol 16:868–876, 1992.

219. Egan MJ, Newman J, Crocker J, Collard M: Immunohistochemical localization of S-100 protein in benign and malignant conditions of the breast. Arch Pathol Lab Med 111:28–31, 1987.

220. McDivitt RW, Stewart FW, Berg JW: Tumors of the breast. In Atlas of Tumor Pathology, 2nd Series, Fascicle 2. Washington, DC, Armed Forces Institute of Pathology, 1968.

221. Wargotz ES, Weiss SW, Norris HJ: Myofibroblastoma of the breast. Sixteen cases of a distinctive benign mesenchymal tumor. Am J Surg Pathol 11:493–502, 1987.

222. Yu GH, Fishman SJ, Brooks JSJ: Cellular angiolipoma of the breast. Mod Pathol 6:497–499, 1993.

223. Michal M, Baumruk L, Burger J, Manhalova M: Adenomyoepithelioma of the breast with undifferentiated carcinoma component. Histopathology 24:274–276, 1994.

224. Tamai M: Intraductal growth of malignant mammary myoepithelioma. Am J Surg Pathol 16:1116–1125, 1992.

225. Salvadori B, Cusumano F, Del Bo R, et al: Surgical treatment of phyllodes tumors of the breast. Cancer 63:2532–2536, 1989.

226. Grimes MM: Cystosarcoma phyllodes of the breast: Histologic features, flow cytometric analysis, and clinical correlations. Mod Pathol 5:232–239, 1992.

227. Hilton DA, Jameson JS, Furness PN: A cellular fibroadenoma resembling a benign phyllodes tumour in a young male with gynaecomastia. Histopathology 18:476–477, 1991.

228. Ansah-Boateng Y, Tavassli FA: Fibroadenoma and cystosarcoma phyllodes of the male breast. Mod Pathol 5:114–116, 1992.

229. The World Health Organization: The World Health Organization histological typing of breast tumors—second edition. Am J Clin Pathol 78:806–816, 1982.

230. Barnes L, Pietruszka M: Rhabdomyosarcoma arising within a cystosarcoma phyllodes. Case report and review of the literature. Am J Surg Pathol 423–429, 1978.

231. Ward RM, Evans HL: Cystosarcoma phyllodes. A clinicopathologic study of 26 cases. Cancer 58:2282–2289, 1986.

232. Salm R: Multifocal histogenesis of a cystosarcoma phyllodes. J Clin Pathol 31:897–903, 1978.

233. Nielsen BB: Fibroadenomatoid hyperplasia of the male breast. Am J Surg Pathol 14:774–777, 1990.

234. Hart WR, Bauer RC, Oberman HA: Cystosarcoma phyllodes. A clinicopathologic study of twenty-six hypercellular periductal stromal tumors of the breast. Am J Clin Pathol 70:211–216, 1978.

235. Azzopardi JG: The differentiation of benign from malignant cystosarcoma. In Azzopardi JG (ed): Problems in Breast Pathology. Philadelphia, WB Saunders, 1979, pp 355–357.

236. Nambiar R, Kutty MK: Giant fibroadenoma (cystosarcoma phyllodes) in adolescent females—a clinicopathologic study. Br J Surg 61:113–117, 1974.

237. Andersson A, Berghahl L: Cystosarcoma phyllodes in young women. Arch Surg 113:742–744, 1978.

238. Keelan PA, Myers JL, Wold LE, et al: Phyllodes tumor: Clinicopathologic review of 60 patients and flow cytometric analysis in 30 patients. Hum Pathol 23:1048–1054, 1992.

239. Fekete P, Petrek J, Majmudar B, et al: Fibroadenomas with stromal cellularity. A clinicopathologic study of 21 patients. Arch Pathol Lab Med 111:427–432, 1987.

240. Pike AM, Oberman HA: Juvenile (cellular) adenofibromas. Am J Surg Pathol 9:730–736, 1985.

241. Rosen PP: Multinucleated mammary stromal giant cells. A benign lesion that simulates invasive carcinoma. Cancer 44:1305–1308, 1979.

242. Berean K, Tron VA, Churg A, Clement PB: Mammary fibroadenoma with multinucleated stromal giant cells. Am J Surg Pathol 10:823–827, 1986.

243. Goodman Z, Taxy JB: Fibroadenomas of the breast with prominent smooth muscle. Am J Surg Pathol 5:99–101, 1981.

244. Oberman HA, Nosanchuk JS, Finger JE: Periductal stromal tumors of breast with adipose metaplasia. Arch Surg 98:384–387, 1969.

245. Diaz NM, Palmer JO, McDivitt RW: Carcinoma arising within fibroadenomas of the breast. A clinicopathologic study of 105 patients. Am J Clin Pathol 95:614–622, 1991.

246. Hiraoka H, Mukai M, Hosoda Y, Hata J: Phyllodes tumor of the breast containing intracytoplasmic inclusion bodies identical with infantile digital fibromatosis. Am J Surg Pathol 18:506–511, 1994.

247. Jones MW, Norris HJ, Wargotz ES, Weiss SW: Fibrosarcoma-malignant fibrous histiocytoma of the breast. A clinicopathologic study of 32 cases. Am J Surg Pathol 16:667–674, 1992.

248. Mufarrij AA, Feiner HD: Breast sarcoma with giant cells and osteoid. A case report and review of the literature. Am J Surg Pathol 11:225–230, 1987.

249. Mentzel T, Kosmehl H, Katenkamp D: Metastasizing phyllodes tumour with malignant fibrous histiocytoma-like areas. Histopathology 19:557–560, 1991.

250. Wargotz ES, Norris HJ: Metaplastic carcinomas of the breast. I. Matrix producing carcinoma. Hum Pathol 20:628–635, 1989.

251. Wargotz ES, Norris HJ: Metaplastic carcinomas of the breast. II. Spindle cell carcinoma. Hum Pathol 20:732–740, 1989.

252. Wargotz ES, Norris HJ: Metaplastic carcinomas of the breast. III. Carcinosarcoma. Cancer 64:1490–1499, 1989.

253. Wargotz ES, Norris HJ: Metaplastic carcinomas of the breast. IV. Squamous cell carcinoma of duct origin. Cancer 65:272–276, 1990.

254. Wargotz ES, Norris HJ: Metaplastic carcinomas of the breast. V. Metaplastic carcinoma with osteoclastic giant cells. Hum Pathol 21:1142–1150, 1990.

255. Gersell DJ, Katzenstein ALA: Spindle cell carcinoma of the breast. A clinicopathologic and ultrastructural study. Hum Pathol 12:550–560, 1981.

256. Foschini MP, Dina RE, Eusebi V: Sarcomatoid neoplasms of the breast: Proposed definitions for biphasic and monophasic sarcomatoid mammary carcinomas. Semin Diagn Pathol 10:128–136, 1993.

257. Oberman HA: Metaplastic carcinoma of the breast. A clinicopathologic study of 29 patients. Am J Surg Pathol 11:918–929, 1987.

258. Pitts WC, Rojas VA, Gaffey MJ, et al: Carcinomas with metaplasia and sarcomas of the breast. Am J Clin Pathol 95:623–632, 1991.

259. Raju GC, Wee A: Spindle cell carcinoma of the breast. Histopathology 16:497–499, 1990.

260. Reddick RL, Jennette JC, Askin FB: Squamous metaplasia of the breast. An ultrastructural and immunologic evaluation. Am J Clin Pathol 84:530–533, 1985.

261. Raju GC: The histological and immunohistochemical evidence of squamous metaplasia from the myoepithelial cells in the breast. Histopathology 16:272–275, 1990.

262. Eusebi V, Lamovec J, Cattani MG, et al: Acantholytic variant of squamous-cell carcinoma of the breast. Am J Surg Pathol 10:855–861, 1986.

263. Bauer TW, Rostock RA, Eggleston JC, Baral E: Spindle cell carcinoma of the breast: Four cases and review of the literature. Hum Pathol 15:147–152, 1984.

264. Fisher ER, Palekar AS, Gregoria RM, Paulson JD: Mucoepidermoid and squamous

cell carcinomas of breast with reference to squamous metaplasia and giant cell tumors. Am J Surg Pathol 7:15–17, 1983.

265. Toikkanen S: Primary squamous cell carcinoma of the breast. Cancer 48:1629–1632, 1981.

266. Prescott RJ, Eyden BP, Reeve NL: Sebaceous differentiation in a breast carcinoma with ductal, myoepithelial, and squamous elements. Histopathology 21:181–184, 1992.

267. Hurt MA, Diaz-Arias AA, Rosenholtz MJ, et al: Posttraumatic lobular squamous metaplasia of breast. An unusual pseudosarcomatous metaplasia resembling squamous (necrotizing) sialometaplasia of the salivary gland. Mod Pathol 1:385–390, 1988.

268. Shousha S: An unusual cyst (of the breast). Histopathology 14:423–425, 1989.

269. Gottfried MR: Extensive squamous metaplasia in gynecomastia. Arch Pathol Lab Med 110:971–973, 1986.

270. Azzopardi JG: Fibroadenoma; and Cystosarcoma phyllodes. In Azzopardi JG (ed): Problems in Breast Pathology. Philadelphia, WB Saunders, 1979, pp 40 and 354.

271. Kaufman MW, Marti JR, Gallager HS, Hoehn JL: Carcinoma of the breast with pseudosarcomatous metaplasia. Cancer 53:1908–1917, 1984.

272. Christensen L, Schiodt T, Blichert-Toft M: Sarcomatoid tumours of the breast in Denmark from 1977 to 1987. A clinicopathological and immunohistochemical study of 100 cases. Eur J Cancer 29A:1824–1831, 1993.

273. Chen KTK, Kuo TT, Hoffmann KD: Leiomyosarcoma of the breast. Cancer 47:1883–1886, 1981.

274. Going JJ, Lumsden AB, Anderson TJ: A classical osteogenic sarcoma of the breast: Histology, immunohistochemistry and ultrastructure. Histopathology 10:631–641, 1986.

275. Beltaos E, Banerjee TK: Chondrosarcoma of the breast. Report of two cases. Am J Clin Pathol 71:345–349, 1979.

276. Christensen L, Nielsen M, Holund B, Clemmensen I: Differentiation between metaplastic carcinomas and sarcomas of the human female breast by fibronectin. Virchows Arch [A] 407:465–476, 1985.

277. Catania S, Zurrida S, Veronesi P, et al: Mondor's disease and breast cancer. Cancer 69:2267–2270, 1992.

278. Haibach H, Rosenholtz MJ: Prepubertal gynecomastia with lobules and acini: A case report and review of the literature. Am J Clin Pathol 80:252–255, 1983.

279. Kowand LM, Verhulst LA, Copeland CM, Bose B: Epidermoid cyst of the breast. Can Med Assoc J 131:217–219, 1984.

280. Gutierrez Y, Paul GM: Breast nodule produced by *Dirofilaria tenuis*. Am J Surg Pathol 8:463–465, 1984.

281. MacDougall LT, Magoon CC, Fritsche TR: *Dirofilaria repens* manifesting as a breast nodule. Am J Clin Pathol 97:625–630, 1992.

282. Marsh WL, Lucas JG, Olsen J: Chondrolipoma of the breast. Arch Pathol Lab Med 113:369–371, 1989.

283. van der Walt JD, Reid HA, Shaw JHF: Neurilemoma appearing as a lump in the breast. Arch Pathol Lab Med 106:539–540, 1982.

284. Banik S, Hale R: Fibrocystic disease in the male breast. Histopathology 11:214–216, 1987.

285. Silverman JF, Dabbs DJ, Norris HT, et al: Localized primary (AL) amyloid tumor of the breast. Am J Surg Pathol 10:539–545, 1986.

286. Marino MJ: Plasmacytoma of the breast. Arch Pathol Lab Med 108:676–678, 1984.

287. Pettinato G, Manivel JC, Insabato L, et al: Plasma cell granuloma (inflammatory pseudotumor) of the breast. Am J Clin Pathol 90:627–632, 1988.

288. Ferrell LD: Myospherulosis of the breast. Diagnosis by fine needle aspiration. Acta Cytol 28:726–728, 1984.

289. Arias-Stella J, Rosen PP: Hemangiopericytoma of the breast. Mod Pathol 1:98–103, 1988.

290. Sara AS, Gottfried MR: Benign papilloma of the male breast following chronic phenothiazine therapy. Am J Clin Pathol 87:649–650, 1987.

291. Wilhelmus JL, Schrodt GR, Mahaffey LM: Cholesterol granulomas of the breast. A lesion which clinically mimics carcinoma. Am J Clin Pathol 77:592–597, 1982.

292. Gould E, Perez J, Albores-Saavedra J, Legaspi A: Signet ring cell sinus histiocytosis. A previously unrecognized histologic condition mimicking metastatic adenocarcinoma in lymph nodes. Am J Clin Pathol 92:509–512, 1989.

293. Erlandson RA, Rosen PP: Electron microscopy of a nevus cell aggregate associated with an axillary lymph node. Cancer 49:269–272, 1982.

294. Brooks JJ, Krugman DT, Damjanov I: Myeloid metaplasia presenting as a breast mass. Am J Surg Pathol 4:281–285, 1980.

295. Wergowski G, Chang JC, Marger D: Muscular pseudotumor of the breast following doxorubicin and radiation therapy for oat cell carcinoma of the lung. Cancer 50:2275–2278, 1982.

296. Sieber PR, Sharkey FE: Cystic hygroma of the breast. Arch Pathol Lab Med 110:353, 1986.

297. Holdworth PJ, Hopkinson JM, Leveson SH: Benign axillary epithelial lymph node inclusions—a histologic pitfall. Histopathology 13:226–228, 1988.

298. Raso DS, Crymes LW, Metcalf JS: Histological assessment of fifty breast capsules from smooth and textured augmentation and reconstruction mammaplasty prostheses with emphasis on the role of synovial metaplasia. Mod Pathol 7:310–316, 1994.

299. Winston JS, Yeh IT, Evers K, Friedman AK: Calcium oxalate is associated with benign breast tissue: Can we avoid biopsy? Am J Clin Pathol 100:488–492, 1993.

300. van Bogaert LJ, Maldague P: Histologic variants of lipid-secreting carcinoma of the breast. Virchows Arch A [Pathol Anat] 375:345–353, 1977.

301. Tavassoli FA, Norris HJ: Mammary adenoid cystic carcinoma with sebaceous differentiation. A morphologic study of the cell types. Arch Pathol Lab Med 110:1045–1053, 1986.

302. Wade PM, Mills SE, Read M, et al: Small cell neuroendocrine (oat cell) carcinoma of the breast. Cancer 52:121–125, 1983.

303. Oberman HA: Invasive carcinoma of the breast with granulomatous response. Am J Clin Pathol 88:718–721, 1987.

304. Coyne J, Haboubi NY: Micro-invasive breast carcinoma with granulomatous stromal response. Histopathology 20:184–185, 1992.

305. Tsang WYW, Chan JKC: Neural invasion in intraductal carcinoma of the breast. Hum Pathol 23:202–204, 1992.

306. Saigo PE, Rosen PP: Mammary carcinoma with ''choriocarcinomatous'' features. Am J Surg Pathol 5:773–778, 1981.

307. Arista-Nasr J, Gonzalez-Gomez I, Angeles-Angeles A, et al: Primary recurrent leiomyosarcoma of the breast. Am J Clin Pathol 92:500–505, 1989.

308. Toikkanen S, Joensuu H: Glycogen-rich clear-cell carcinoma of the breast. Hum Pathol 22:81–83, 1991.

309. Costa MJ, Silverberg SG: Oncocytic carcinoma of the male breast. Arch Pathol Lab Med 113:1396–1399, 1989.

310. Moskaluk CA, Merino MJ, Danforth DN, Medeiros LJ: Low-grade angiosarcoma of the skin of the breast: A complication of lumpectomy and radiation therapy for breast carcinoma. Hum Pathol 23:710–714, 1992.

311. Lasser A, Zacks SI: Intraskeletal myofiber metastasis of breast carcinoma. Hum Pathol 13:1045–1046, 1982.

312. Lucas JG, Sharma HM, O'Toole RV: Unusual giant cell tumor arising in a male breast. Hum Pathol 12:840–844, 1981.

313. Agnantis NT, Rosen PP: Mammary carcinoma with osteoclast-like giant cells. Am J Clin Pathol 72:383–389, 1979.

314. Holland R, van Haelst UJGM: Mammary carcinoma with osteoclast-like giant cells. Cancer 53:1963–1973, 1984.

315. Scopsi L, Andreola S, Pilotti S, et al: Argyrophilia and granin (chromogranin/secretogranin) expression in female breast carcinomas: Their relationship to survival and other disease parameters. Am J Surg Pathol 16:561–576, 1992.

316. Rigaud C, Theobald S, Noel P, et al: Medullary carcinoma of the breast: A multicenter study of its diagnostic consistency. Arch Pathol Lab Med 117:1005–1008, 1993.

317. Rayne SC, Santa Cruz DJ: Anaplastic Paget's disease. Am J Surg Pathol 16:1085–1091, 1992.

Diagnostic Challenges in Soft Tissue Pathology: A Clinicopathologic Review of Selected Lesions

Michael Kyriakos, M.D., Cheryl M. Coffin, M.D., and Paul E. Swanson, M.D.

Despite cries of despair from the innocent, here defined as most general diagnostic pathologists, the field of soft tissue pathology continues to expand, if not logarithmically, at least arithmetically, with the publication of newly described tumors or tumor-like lesions. With the exception of hematopathology, in no other field of pathology have the "splitters" more decisively won the battle of tumor classification than in soft tissue pathology. The surgical pathologist is now faced with the burden of being knowledgeable about more than 100 diagnostic soft tissue entities. The histopathologic criteria that define this apparently ever-expanding nosology place diagnostic demands on experienced and novice pathologists alike that are compounded by the rarity of most of these entities, be they old or newly described. Indeed, even pathologists at tertiary care or referral institutions may encounter some of these lesions only once or twice during the course of a career. Unfortunately, the lack of experience that most surgical pathologists have with these lesions frequently leads to misdiagnoses; specific diagnostic designations are often erroneous, and, on a more fundamental plane, even the determination that a given case is malignant or benign all too often proves to be inaccurate.

With the development of immunohistochemical techniques that were applicable to routinely processed tissues, diagnostic surgical pathology entered the "Brown Age," an epochal transformation that was expected to herald the illumination of human neoplasia by imposing an objective biochemical structure on the art of histopathologic diagnosis. Indeed, the pace of development of immunohistochemical markers easily outstripped the number of newly described soft tissue tumors. Seemingly, every week brought forth the description of new antibodies, each touted as "highly specific and highly sensitive," capable of distinguishing sarcomas from carcinomas, melanomas, and lymphomas and able to discern patterns of differentiation in mesenchymal neoplasms. In some instances, these claims proved to be accurate, but all too often further studies would indicate that not only was the new antibody not very sensitive but not very specific either. Indeed, as experience with these sophisticated diagnostic tools accumu-

lated, it became obvious that not only did many soft tissue tumors share overlapping immunophenotypes but some expressed immunohistochemical profiles that were discordant to native, non-neoplastic mesenchymal elements, thus requiring the use of a panel of different antibodies to various mesenchymal and non-mesenchymal determinants in order to arrive at an accurate histologic diagnosis.

In the face of persistent limitations in the immunohistochemical analysis of some soft tissue tumors, electron microscopy, which had become relegated to a more or less secondary rank in the diagnostic armamentarium, has once again assumed importance in helping to distinguish among those soft tissue lesions that share similar light microscopic and immunohistochemical features. Hence, when faced with a diagnostically difficult soft tissue tumor, the surgical pathologist must often resort to immunohistochemical, electron microscopic, and, in some cases, even cytogenetic studies, in order to reach a correct diagnosis.

Despite this somewhat pessimistic introduction to the subject at hand, all is not gloom and doom for the surgical pathologist. Fortunately, the vast majority of the major soft tissue tumors are fairly easily diagnosed by the examination of conventional hematoxylin and eosin sections. Well-differentiated liposarcoma with its component of lipoblasts, embryonal rhabdomyosarcoma with cross-striated acidophilic rhabdomyoblasts, and classic biphasic synovial sarcoma all are tumors that do not require either immunohistochemical or electron microscopic studies for their accurate diagnosis, and they are not reviewed in this chapter. We have chosen to concentrate on a highly select group of soft tissue lesions that either have only relatively recently been described or have, in our experience, proved to be diagnostic problems. Our choice of entities is based solely on personal preference, and others would no doubt choose different lesions. This chapter is not an encyclopedic survey of all difficult soft tissue tumors, or even of those we chose to discuss. No attempt was made to include every publication extant on every lesion described; however, an extensive review of the English-language medical literature was undertaken so as to ensure a comprehensive evaluation of each lesion in terms of its clinical parameters; light microscopic, immunohistochemical, and electron microscopic features; and clinical course. Rather than include only those immunohistochemical results that typify each of these lesions, we also mention the uncommon and unexpected results that may create confusion in what would otherwise be a straightforward interpretation of the lesion in question. We hope by providing these data, together with a discussion of pertinent differential diagnostic considerations involved in each lesion, that they may, despite their rarity, be confidently analyzed and diagnosed by pathologists with no special interest in soft tissue pathology.

MALIGNANT PERIPHERAL NEUROECTODERMAL TUMOR

A discourse on malignant peripheral neuroectodermal tumor (MPNET) of the soft tissues from the viewpoint of a diagnostic surgical pathologist is analogous to the task of dividing a silk scarf floating in air by the stroke of a sword— although it can no doubt be done, it is a frustrating experience. Part of this frustration is engendered by the fact that, based on the literature, one feels that the subject matter has been appropriated by those principally concerned with the cytogenetics, molecular biology, and biochemistry of this relatively rare neoplasm. Although such studies are of considerable importance for the understanding of fundamental issues in tumor cell biology, they are for the most part beyond the pale of the surgical pathologist trying to arrive at a histologic diagnosis and who would consider himself or herself fortunate to have access to immunohistochemical or electron microscopic facilities let alone tissue culture, cytogenetic, and molecular biology laboratories.

The frustration is further enhanced by the fact that the concept of a primitive neuroectodermal tumor is still an evolving one; indeed, the precise criteria for its diagnosis are still unsettled.

The story of MPNET as a diagnostic entity apparently begins with the 1918 report by Stout, who described a small-cell tumor, with rosette formation, that arose in the ulnar nerve of a 42-year-old man.[1] Stout later classified this lesion as a ''malignant neuro-ectodermal tumor of the peripheral nerve,'' and to which Penfield, in consultation, applied the name ''neuroepithelioma,''[2] a term subsequently adopted by Stout and Murray for these tumors.[3] Although a report of a tumor of the sciatic nerve had been published by Garrè[4] in 1892, and accepted by Stout[2] as a ''malignant neuro-ectodermal tumor,'' this lesion is, by its description and illustrated drawings, consistent with a glandular schwannoma.[5] Isolated case reports of peripheral nerve tumors histologically similar to that described by Stout subsequently appeared; however, similar tumors were also reported that arose in the soft tissues without any apparent connection with a nerve. Over the ensuing years, a host of terms have been used to designate these neural or soft tissue tumors, most being modifications of those put forth by Stout and Penfield. These include neuroepithelioma,[3, 6–8] malignant neuroepithelioma (peripheral neuroblastoma),[9] peripheral neuroepithelioma,[10–19] neuroectodermal tumor,[20–23] peripheral neuroectodermal tumor,[24] primitive neuroectodermal tumor,[25–33] malignant neuroectodermal tumor,[34] peripheral primitive neuroectodermal tumor (peripheral neuroepitheli-

oma),[15] peripheral neuroectodermal sarcoma (peripheral neuroepithelioma),[35] peripheral primitive neuroectodermal tumor,[36–38] and malignant peripheral neuroectodermal tumor.[39–42]

Some small-cell tumors such as the paravertebral tumors described by Tefft et al.,[43] the thoracopulmonary tumors described by Askin et al.,[44] the extraskeletal form of Ewing's sarcoma described by Angervall and Enzinger,[45] and skeletal Ewing's sarcoma[21–23, 40, 46–48] have been reevaluated using light microscopy, immunohistochemistry, and electron microscopy. The results of these studies have shown that many of these tumors now fall either entirely, or in part, within the concept of MPNET because of features indicative of neural differentiation as manifested by the light microscopic presence of rosettes, ganglion cells, or cells with Schwann cell–like features in these various tumors, their immunohistochemical reactivity for neural markers, and/or an electron microscopic cellular morphology consistent with neural differentiation.[8, 14, 31, 47, 49–60] Thus, the demographics, histomorphologic patterns, and prognostic implications of these small-cell tumors have become muddled when the older literature is used as a guide for diagnosis and prognosis. A summary of the historical development of MPNET as a diagnostic entity, and its relationship with Ewing's sarcoma, has been provided by Dehner.[27]

Some semblance of rationality was brought to the concept of MPNET in a proposed classification of primitive neuroectodermal tumors by Dehner,[37] who broadly divided them into (1) central: those arising in the brain or spinal cord; (2) germ cell–derived: those arising in the gonads or in teratomas; and (3) peripheral: those arising in all other locations, mainly the peripheral soft tissues or bone. Although objections were immediately raised over the classification of the central lesions,[61] few have been raised against the peripheral scheme. Within the category of peripheral neuroectodermal tumors, Dehner included classic neuroblastoma, peripheral malignant primitive neuroepithelial tumor, peripheral neuroepithelioma (neuroblastoma), malignant small-cell tumor of thoracopulmonary origin (Askin's tumor), extrathoracopulmonary neuroepithelioma, pigmented neuroectodermal tumor (melanotic progonoma, retinal anlage tumor), ectomesenchymoma, and intraosseous neuroectodermal tumor. Tentatively included as a possible member of this group was Ewing's sarcoma.[37]

In this section, we use the term *malignant peripheral neuroectodermal tumor* in a more restricted sense as the *diagnostic* term for those tumors, exclusive of neuroblastoma, that arise in the soft tissues or peripheral nerves and whose cells have the general features of those found in the so-called malignant, small, round, blue-cell tumors,[62] but which have by light microscopy, immunohistochemistry, or electron microscopy, evidence of neural differentiation. For the purposes of this section, we combine all the entities listed in Dehner's classification[37] as peripheral malignant primitive neuroepithelial tumor, peripheral neuroepithelioma (neuroblastoma), and extrathoracopulmonary neuroepithelioma under the diagnostic term ''MPNET.'' Those primitive neuroectodermal tumors arising in the thoracopulmonary area, as well as those in the bone, are not separately categorized, as they differ from other malignant peripheral neuroectodermal tumors only by location. We do not include within the category of MPNET those tumors whose only evidence of neural differentiation is the immunohistochemical presence of the enzyme neuron-specific enolase (NSE). In our view, the proven non-specificity of this marker[63-65] precludes its use as the sole evidence of neural differentiation (see later discussion).

Although MPNET has been reported in newborns[25, 26, 42] and in patients as old as 81 years,[29] the tumor mainly affects children and young adults. Among those reports we reviewed, there were 189 patients with individual age data.* The average age was 14.8 years (median, 14.0 years); 92% were younger than age 30 years, with 78% younger than age 20 years. Children younger than 5 years of age were not common, accounting for only 14% (26/189) of cases. Among 325 patients for whom gender information was provided, male and females were approximately equally affected, with 167 males (51.4%) and 158 females (48.6%).†

Clinically, MPNET usually manifests itself as a mass that is frequently painful.‡ Because of its occasional origin from a major nerve trunk, secondary neurologic signs or symptoms, including extremity weakness, paresthesias, and loss of motor function, may be present.[1, 3, 6, 10] Patients with chest wall tumors may have pleural effusions with associated dyspnea and fever.[8, 41, 44, 67] MPNET usually develops and grows rapidly, with a relatively short interval from clinical onset to diagnosis. Excluding newborns, the duration of these clinical manifestations before diagnosis ranged from several days[9, 44, 72] to 1.5 years,[9] with the average duration in 32 patients in which this information was individually reported§ being 3.8 months (median, 1.0 month).

In contrast with classic **neuroblastoma,** a tumor with which MPNET may be confused histologically and which characteristically has elevated serum or urinary levels of catecholamines, MPNET is seldom associated with such elevations;[10, 18, 19, 21, 28, 39, 41, 44] most of the patients studied for these biochemical markers had normal levels.‖ However, the true prevalence of elevated levels of these substances in MPNET is difficult to assess because some authors specifically excluded from their series of peripheral neuroectodermal tumors any case in which they were elevated.[29, 38, 41, 42]

Exclusive of those of skeletal origin, MPNET has a wide anatomic distribution, but with a predilection for the trunk, especially the paraspinal and chest wall regions. Among 347 cases with specific site data,¶ the trunk/chest wall was involved in 161 cases (46%), with the chest wall accounting for 42% (146/347) of all cases; the paraspinal area was involved in 35 cases (10%). The extremities accounted for 21% (71 cases), the abdomen/pelvis for 17% (58 cases), and the head and neck region for only 6% (22 cases). Rare examples of MPNET are reported in the ovary and testis.[34, 38] Despite its historical initial description as a tumor originating within major peripheral nerves, such an origin was noted in only 24 of the cases (7%). However, at least some of the large thoracopulmonary tumors may have arisen from intercostal nerves, the origin being obscured by the bulk of the tumor. At times, especially

in these chest wall tumors, the underlying ribs may be either eroded or invaded by the tumor such that an arbitrary choice must be made as to whether it arose within the soft tissue or the bone.[9, 44, 52, 66]

Despite the short clinical duration of disease prior to diagnosis, primitive neuroectodermal tumors tend to be large, with a range in the literature of from 1 to 2 cm[52] to 40 cm.[25] Of 50 cases with size data,* the average maximum size was 8.7 cm (median, 8.5 cm); 82% were equal to or greater than 5.0 cm, with 40% equal to or larger than 10.0 cm.

MPNET is usually deeply situated within the soft tissue or skeletal muscle, although occasional examples occur in the subcutaneous tissue.[9] The tumors are multinodular or lobulated masses that usually appear well circumscribed,[9, 25, 26, 28, 44, 72] but some appear infiltrative.[9, 25] On section, they are soft to fleshy, with a cut surface that varies from gray-white to yellow or reddish-tan; foci of necrosis and hemorrhage are frequently present.† When originating within a large nerve, the tumor causes its fusiform expansion.

As mentioned, MPNET histologically[9, 10, 12, 25, 29, 35, 41, 71] falls within the category of neoplasms generally referred to as round, blue cell tumors.[62] The morphologic pattern of MPNET is characterized by small (10–14 nm), round to oval, or somewhat elongated cells (Fig. 17–1). These may vary in size and shape, with some tumors composed of cells half again as large as those in the classic ''small'' size variety.[28, 31, 74] Nuclei are round or somewhat elongated, may have infoldings, and appear dense with coarse or clumped chromatin that may be either uniformly distributed or concentrated at the periphery of the nucleus with central clearing.[9, 25, 41] Nucleoli are usually either small or absent.[8-10, 35, 41, 69, 71] The cytoplasm is scanty, pale, or finely granular with ill-defined borders.[8-10, 41] The cells are closely packed and may be divided into nests, lobules, cords, or diffuse sheets by fibrovascular septa.‡ Depending on the degree of differentiation, MPNET in its most ''primitive'' form may completely, or in part, mimic **Ewing's sarcoma** by light microscopy.§ Here the nuclei are round and uniform, with an evenly dispersed powdery chromatin, with either absent or small and inconspicuous nucleoli. The pattern of principal and dark cells, found in classic skeletal Ewing's sarcoma, may also be present (Fig. 17–2). The diagnosis of these Ewing's-like tumors as primitive neuroectodermal tumors rests on the demonstration of neural differentiation by immunohistochemistry or electron microscopy. Some of the so-called **large-cell or atypical Ewing's sarcomas,** which are composed of large cells that display coarse nuclear chromatin and possess a central prominent nucleolus, are probably examples of MPNET.[28, 31, 33, 74, 76, 77]

In those MPNETs with a greater degree of neural differentiation, a diagnostic feature is the presence of rosettes (Fig. 17–3). These most frequently take the form of so-called **''pseudorosettes,''** i.e., **Homer Wright rosettes,**‖ in which a circular array of tumor cells has centrally distributed, interdigitating, fibrillary cytoplasmic projections (Fig. 17–4). So-called true rosettes (**Flexner-Wintersteiner** type), in which the cytoplasmic projections are arranged about a central lumen

* References 1, 3, 6, 8–10, 14, 17–19, 24, 26, 28, 30, 35, 38, 41, 43, 44, 52, 66–72.

† References 1, 3, 6, 8–10, 12, 14, 18, 19, 24–26, 28–30, 33, 35, 38, 39, 41, 43, 44, 52, 67, 69–72.

‡ References 9, 14, 17, 19, 24, 26, 30, 43, 44, 52, 66, 67, 70–72.

§ References 1, 3, 6, 8, 41, 43, 44, 55, 66, 67, 72, 73.

‖ References 6, 9, 14, 17, 25, 26, 35, 39, 52, 59, 67, 72.

¶ References 1, 3, 6, 8–10, 12, 14, 17–19, 24–26, 28–30, 33, 35, 38, 39, 41, 43, 44, 52, 66, 68–73.

* References 3, 6, 9, 10, 17, 18, 26, 28, 30, 35, 43, 44, 70, 72.

† References 8–10, 25, 26, 28, 35, 44, 70, 72.

‡ References 8, 9, 26, 29, 35, 41, 44, 66, 69.

§ References 12, 29, 31, 42, 46, 48, 54, 69, 75.

‖ References 9, 10, 12, 26, 35, 42, 59, 66, 69, 70, 74.

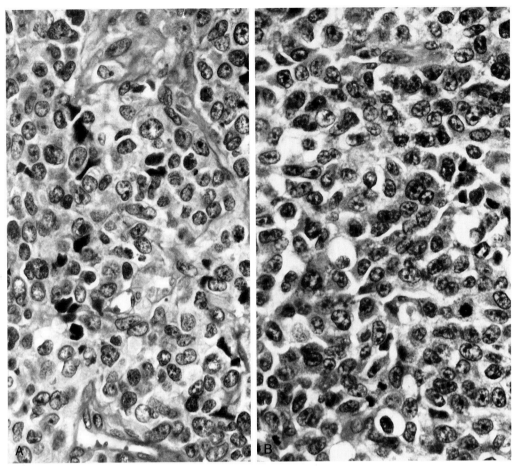

FIGURE 17–1. Views of malignant peripheral neuroectodermal tumor (MPNET) show "small" cells with oval to round, vesicular nuclei. Some variation in cell size is present, and some nuclei have notches or infoldings. The cytoplasm is scant and ill-defined.

(Fig. 17–5), are less commonly found.[9, 12, 69] However, some authors describe as **"pseudorosettes"** structures in which the tumor cells are less conspicuously arranged and the cytoplasmic projections are less clearly seen (Fig. 17–6) than in definitive Homer Wright rosettes.[35] Such structures are also referred to as **"abortive"** rosettes,[56, 57] a designation that at least has the advantage of not being confused with "pseudorosette," used by many as a synonym for a Homer Wright rosette but by others for only rosette-like structures.[47, 54] In our view, the presence of "abortive" rosettes alone is insuffi-

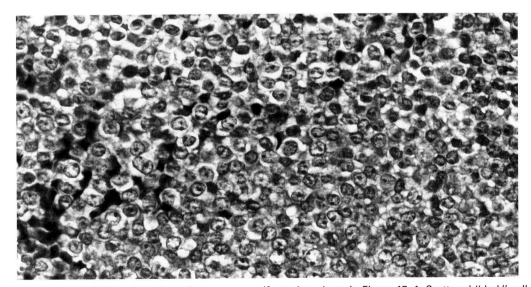

FIGURE 17–2. Example of MPNET in which the cells are more uniform than those in Figure 17–1. Scattered "dark" cells are present. The pattern is similar to that of Ewing's sarcoma.

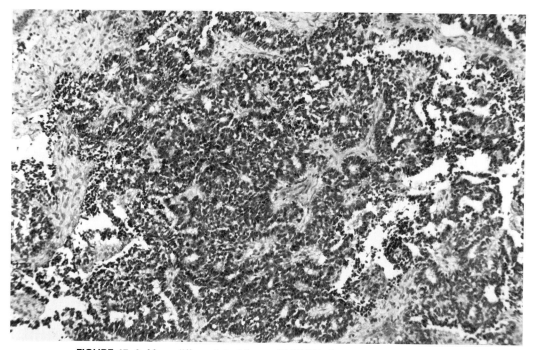

FIGURE 17–3. More differentiated form of MPNET shows numerous rosettes.

cient to designate a tumor as showing neural differentiation. However, the finding of these rosette-like structures should prompt a careful search for the presence of more definitive rosettes. Neural differentiation in MPNET may also be manifested by the presence of small ganglion cells or Schwann-like spindle cell areas.[10, 28, 31, 69, 74] Examples of MPNET are described in which epithelial-like structures mimicking the neural tube are found and to which the name peripheral medulloepithelioma has been applied.[72]

Mitotic figures are usually moderate or numerous in number[6, 8, 26, 35, 41] in MPNET, as are focal areas of necrosis that may contain dystrophic calcification.[8, 9, 25] The tumors are well vascularized and tumor cells may be arranged about these blood vessels creating **"perivascular rosettes."**[9, 10, 12] Stains for cytoplasmic glycogen were positive in more than 50% (89/171) of the cases in our review.* The absence of glycogen was one of the defining criteria for the diagnosis of the so-called **"Askin"** tumor of the chest wall, but subsequent

---

* References 8, 9, 12, 17, 24, 28, 31, 35, 41, 43, 52, 55, 59, 66, 67, 71, 73.

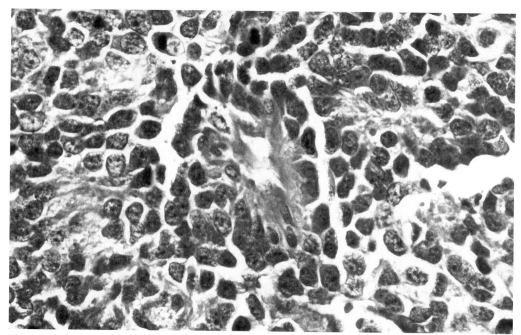

FIGURE 17–4. Higher magnification shows a Homer Wright rosette. Cytoplasmic extensions radiate from the cells toward the center of the aggregate.

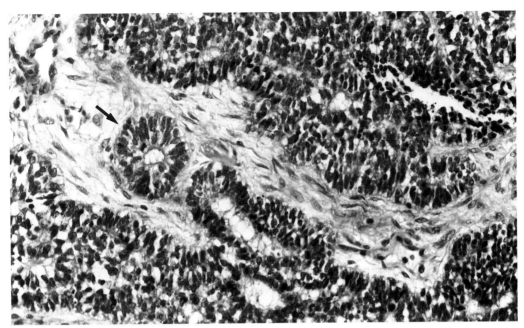

FIGURE 17–5. MPNET with small dark cells and rosettes. A Flexner-Wintersteiner rosette is shown *(arrow)* where the cytoplasmic cell projections converge about a well-defined central lumen.

studies established the presence of glycogen within these tumors as well.[24, 52, 66]

Despite the relative rarity of MPNET, there is an abundant literature on its electron microscopic features, with more than 100 cases so examined.* As one might expect in dealing with a tumor that has a variable range of differentiation by light microscopy, there are some differences in the reported results, but the majority of studies have yielded a fairly consistent pattern of fine structural features for this lesion. The tumor cells vary from round to ovoid, with nuclei that are similarly shaped but frequently irregular or indented, with a peripheral rim of clumped or coarse chromatin. Cytoplasmic organelles tend to be abundant, with numerous ribosomes, polyribosomes, mitochondria, profiles of rough endoplasmic reticulum, and a prominent Golgi zone. Glycogen is usually present and may be abundant. Microfilaments and intermediate filaments, the latter frequently perinuclear, may be found. In the majority of cases, dense-core neurosecretory-type granules are present that may appear atypical or pleomorphic; microtubules are variably present. A distinctive feature of the tumor cells is their broad or narrow cytoplasmic processes that interdigitate with each other and with those from adjacent cells. These projections may contain neurosecretory granules, microtubules, and intermediate filaments. Most studies of MPNET either fail to mention the presence of a basal lamina or specifically indicate its absence,[8, 18, 30, 73, 78] with only a few studies indicating its presence.[12, 28, 35, 69, 71] The latter studies are not reflective of our own experience. Cell junctions of variable type are usually present, from primitive forms to zonula adherens type,† to desmosome or desmosome-like.[26, 35, 38, 41, 66]

A relatively large number of MPNETs have been the object of immunohistochemical studies,* most of which have involved the investigation of neural and mesenchymal markers. The most frequently studied of these markers is neuron-specific enolase (NSE). Although this enzyme was initially thought to be a specific neural marker subsequent immunohistochemical studies indicated that a wide variety of nonneural lesions may stain for this enzyme.[63–65] Despite this nonspecificity, NSE is almost invariably reported in the analysis of MPNET. Indeed, a positive result for NSE has been used by some as part of the criteria for inclusion of a tumor within the category of MPNET.[11, 25, 39, 52, 69, 84] In our review, 272 tumors were studied for NSE reactivity, 239 of which (88%) were positive.† Reactivity for vimentin‡ was found in 76% of cases (107/140); neuron surface antigen[31, 33, 59] in 62% (18/29); synaptophysin[12, 28, 30, 35, 38, 66, 67] in 46% (34/74); neurofilament protein§ in 41% (59/144); Leu-7 antigen‖ in 40% (54/135); S-100 protein¶ in 36% (64/177); and chromogranin[12, 35, 38, 66, 67] in 22% (17/77). Beta-2-microglobulin, the invariant chain associated with HLA (human leukocyte antigen) class I antigens, was found in 74% (63/85) of the tumors.[12, 16, 30, 35, 38] Similarly, reactivity with the anti–B lymphocyte marker MB2 typifies most examples of MPNET, with positive results found in 12 of 15 cases (80%)—six of these were ''Askin'' tumors, all of which were positive.[84, 85] Results for other antigens in MPNET have been less commonly positive and at times have yielded seemingly disparate results. Stains for glial fi-

---

* References 8, 10, 12, 14, 17, 18, 24, 26, 28, 30, 35, 38, 41, 44, 52, 66, 67, 69, 71–73, 78, 79.
† References 10, 17, 18, 24, 28, 30, 44, 52, 71, 73, 78, 79.

* References 8, 9, 12, 16, 17, 24, 28–31, 35, 36, 38, 39, 41, 52, 55, 59, 66, 67, 69, 71, 73, 74, 79–84.
† References 8, 12, 17, 24, 28, 30, 31, 33, 35, 38, 39, 41, 52, 55, 59, 63, 66, 67, 69, 71, 73, 83, 84.
‡ References 12, 17, 28, 30, 31, 35, 41, 66, 67, 73, 83, 84.
§ References 12, 28, 30, 31, 33, 35, 41, 59, 66, 83, 84.
‖ References 12, 35, 38, 40, 66, 67, 69, 79, 83.
¶ References 12, 17, 24, 28, 30, 31, 33, 35, 41, 55, 59, 63, 66, 67, 73, 83, 84.

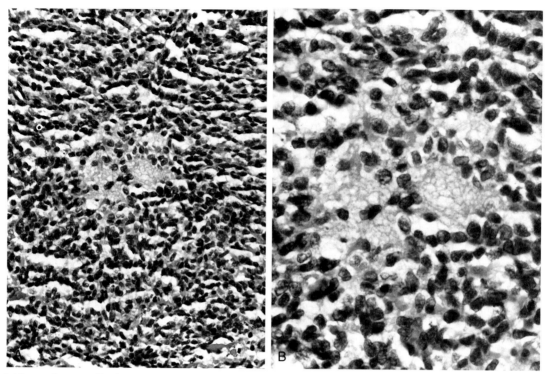

FIGURE 17–6. Views of rosette-like focus in a small-cell tumor that lacks the structured appearance of either a Homer Wright or Flexner-Wintersteiner rosette. Such rosette-like structures are termed "abortive," and although not diagnostic of neural differentiation, their presence should prompt a careful search for definitive rosettes.

brillary acidic protein[17, 35, 41, 66, 83] were positive in 7% of cases (4/56), cytokeratin[12, 17, 30, 31, 38, 66, 73, 83] in 8% (9/119), epithelial membrane antigen[17, 28, 30, 38, 73] in 4% (1/25), and desmin[12, 17, 30, 38, 73, 84] in 3% (2/63). The implications of these latter staining patterns, in light of the polyphenotypic nature of some small, round cell tumors, including desmoplastic small round cell tumor, is unclear. Stains for leukocyte common antigen (CD45) were negative in nine cases,[17, 55, 84] and for myoglobin five cases.[55]

The newly introduced antibody HBA-71, raised against Ewing's sarcoma cell lines and recognizing the pseudoautosomal gene product p30/32 MIC2,[36, 80, 81, 86] has proved to be a sensitive marker for MPNET. Positive results were obtained in 93% (91/98) of primary soft tissue and osseous malignant neuroectodermal tumors.[16, 31, 36, 86] However, this reactivity is not specific for MPNET, being found in a like percentage of Ewing's sarcomas.[36, 80, 86] Like beta-2-microglobulin and MB2,[16, 84, 85] HBA-71 is absent in neuroblastoma, providing a reliable immunohistochemical means of separating this tumor from MPNET. Reactivity is also lacking in most, but not all cases of **rhabdomyosarcoma,** and only occasional examples of non-Hodgkin's lymphomas, including **lymphoblastic lymphoma,** are reactive.[36, 80, 81, 87]

The differential histologic diagnosis of MPNET includes those tumors generally described as small, blue, round cell tumors, including neuroblastoma, embryonal rhabdomyosarcoma, malignant lymphoma, and extraskeletal Ewing's sarcoma. Patients with **neuroblastoma** are usually very young, with most cases occurring within the first 2 years of life.[88–91] Anatomically, neuroblastoma occurs in regions with sympathetic neural tissue, the majority arising in the adrenal gland, retroperitoneum, and mediastinum.[57, 89, 92–94] In contrast,

patients with MPNET tend to be older than those with neuroblastoma, and the tumor has a wider anatomic distribution.[57] However, there is enough overlap in terms of patient age and tumor location so that these parameters are not diagnostically useful in separating these tumors. In classic neuroblastoma, more than 90% of patients have elevated serum or urinary levels of catecholamines or their precursors or metabolites.[62, 94] However, because some primitive forms of neuroblastoma may not be secretory,[62] and some examples of MPNET have had serum or urinary elevations of these biochemical products, their presence or absence alone is not sufficient to distinguish these tumors. They may also be indistinguishable by light and electron microscopy, the differential problem being especially acute between MPNET and the more poorly differentiated neuroblastomas.[12–14, 62, 95] Both neuroblastoma and MPNET are immunohistochemically reactive for a variety of neural markers, including NSE;[49, 59, 95–97] however, as noted previously, neuroblastoma is negative for HBA-71, beta-2-microglobulin, and MB2, three markers frequently detected in MPNET.* Other ancillary methods have been used to distinguish these two tumors. MPNET shares with Ewing's sarcoma the chromosomal translocation (11;22) (q24;q12). This translocation is absent in neuroblastoma which has its own genetic abnormality, a deletion in chromosome 1.[32] Proto-oncogene differences also exist, with MPNET showing amplification of the proto-oncogene c-*myc* and no amplification of N-*myc,* whereas neuroblastoma may show amplification of N-*myc* and no amplification of c-*myc.*[7, 32, 54, 98] Neural transmitters found in neuroblastoma are adrenergic and cholinergic versus the purely cholinergic nature of those in MPNET.[57, 99]

---

* References 11, 12, 16, 35, 36, 57, 80, 81, 84–86.

Malignant **non-Hodgkin's lymphoma** is always a diagnostic consideration when evaluating a small, blue cell tumor, despite its rarity as a primary tumor in the soft tissue.[100, 101] Lymphoblastic and non-cleaved small-cell lymphoma may be cytologically confused with MPNET. The presence of rosettes would generally eliminate lymphoma as a possible diagnosis, but in their absence, electron microscopy may be diagnostically helpful because lymphomas lack the cytoplasmic filaments, neurosecretory granules, cell attachments, and, in the majority of cases, the glycogen found in the cells of MPNET.[14] Immunohistochemically, MPNET lacks leukocyte common antigen (CD45), which is consistently found in almost all lymphomas; and lymphomas, with the rare exception of some non-Hodgkin's lymphomas, as alluded to earlier, lack positivity for HBA-71.

Primitive forms of **rhabdomyosarcoma** lacking acidophilic rhabdomyoblasts or cells with cross-striations may be difficult or impossible to distinguish from MPNET by light microscopy alone.[9, 42, 62, 78, 95, 102] This difficulty is compounded by the reports of positive results for NSE,[14, 27, 64, 95–97, 103] Leu-7 antigen,[27, 79] and HBA-71[27, 36, 80] in some examples of rhabdomyosarcoma. However, with rare exceptions, MPNET lacks reactivity for desmin or muscle-specific actin, markers found in most rhabdomyosarcomas.[95, 103, 104] By electron microscopy, MPNET lacks thick and thin myofilaments, z-band structures, or ribosome-myosin complexes, features characteristic of skeletal muscle differentiation.[55, 62, 78, 102]

True extraskeletal or skeletal **Ewing's sarcoma** may also be impossible to distinguish from MPNET at the light microscopic level.* Clinically, these tumors have overlapping age characteristics and site locations, both have the genetic (11;22)(q24;q12) translocation,[8, 19, 32, 67, 106, 107] and both stain with the HBA-71 antibody.[31, 36, 80, 86] We restrict the diagnosis of Ewing's sarcoma to those tumors that are composed of a homogeneous population of small cells that have regular, round to oval nuclei with a fine, diffuse chromatin pattern, inconspicuous or absent nucleoli, scant cytoplasm, and ill-defined cytoplasmic borders (Fig. 17–7). In contrast, the cells of MPNET usually have more irregular-appearing nuclei, with indentations or infoldings, and may appear more pleomorphic with a coarse and clumped chromatin pattern. Some examples of MPNET show areas with larger nuclei having prominent nucleoli as found in what has been termed ''atypical'' or ''large-cell'' Ewing's sarcoma (Fig. 17–8).[76, 77, 108] We exclude tumors with definitive rosettes, be they Homer Wright or Flexner-Wintersteiner type, from the category of Ewing's sarcoma, and, in terms of this differential diagnosis, their presence would suggest either MPNET or neuroblastoma. As mentioned previously, examples of MPNET occur whose light microscopic cytologic features are indistinguishable from classic Ewing's sarcoma, as defined earlier, but in which electron microscopic or immunohistochemical studies show the neural nature of the tumor. Interestingly, a monoclonal mouse antibody, 5C11, directed against a cell surface antigen in Ewing's sarcoma, was reported to be reactive in 15 of 16 cases of Ewing's sarcoma, and absent in neuroblastoma, rhabdomyosarcoma, and in three cases of MPNET.[82] Whether this antibody will prove specific enough to separate Ewing's sarcoma from MPNET awaits the analysis of more cases.

By electron microscopy, the cells of **extraskeletal Ewing's sarcoma** are similar to their osseous counterparts.[57, 102, 108–113] The cells appear primitive, having few organelles and usually an abundant amount of glycogen, frequently in pools. Unlike the cells of MPNET, those of Ewing's sarcoma lack a basal lamina, microtubules, intermediate filaments, neurosecretory granules, and cytoplasmic projections. For purposes of classification, Ewing's sarcoma also should not demonstrate neural or myogenic markers. In essence, we view Ewing's sarcoma, in both its osseous and extraosseous forms, as a totally primitive or undifferentiated tumor.[114] Although some authors believe Ewing's sarcoma to be an undifferentiated or immature form of MPNET, we believe such terminology to be inappropriate.[22, 59, 115, 116] An undifferentiated neoplasm cannot be assigned to any specific tumor category or lineage, and such usage is no more accurate than would be a diagnosis of undifferentiated adenocarcinoma. By our strict definition, those cases of supposed skeletal and soft tissue Ewing's sarcomas that have been reported with rosettes are more properly diagnosed as MPNETs.[9, 14, 45, 47, 49–51, 56, 57] In sum, the diagnosis of MPNET must depend, at least in some cases, not only on light microscopy but electron microscopic and immunohistochemical evaluation as well.

Although the light microscopic presence of definitive rosettes or the electron microscopic presence of neural differentiation would be, in the proper clinical context, sufficient for a diagnosis of MPNET, the immunohistochemical criteria for the diagnosis are not as firmly established. As suggested earlier, we agree that in cases in which electron microscopic analysis is not available, the immunohistochemical diagnosis of MPNET cannot rely exclusively on reactivity for NSE.[42] Instead, in a lesion having immunohistochemical characteristics that strongly suggest the possibility of MPNET (such as one with positivity for vimentin and HBA-71, as well as for beta-2-microglobulin or MB2), the reactivity for any two neural markers such as Leu-7 antigen, neurofilament protein, chromogranin, S-100 protein, or neuron-surface antigen would, in the appropriate clinical and histologic context, serve as the minimal criteria for the immunophenotypic diagnosis of MPNET. We would further propose that because of its specificity, and relative sensitivity for neuroendocrine or neuroectodermal differentiation, the presence of synaptophysin reactivity alone would, in the same context, be sufficient evidence for a diagnosis of MPNET. Because of its non-specificity, an unresolved question is whether reactivity for NSE should be acceptable as one of the pieces of evidence for neural differentiation. At this time, we are inclined to dismiss NSE as a useful marker in the differential diagnosis of MPNET and to employ other markers in the manner outlined previously.

MPNET is an aggressive tumor with a poor prognosis.* In several of the larger series, mortality has ranged from 60% to approximately 85%.[9, 12, 29, 35, 42, 44, 66, 69] Among 134 patients in our review with individual survival data,† 82 (61.2%) died of tumor, 16 (11.9%) were alive with recurrent or persistent tumor, and 36 (26.9%) were alive and well following therapy. However, among the last group only 13 patients (36%) had

---

* References 29, 31, 39, 42, 45, 48, 54, 69, 105.

---

* References 9, 12, 27, 29, 35, 39, 40, 42, 44, 47, 69, 74, 105.

† References 6, 8–10, 17–19, 24, 26, 28, 30, 31, 35, 38, 41, 43, 44, 52, 55, 66, 67, 70–74.

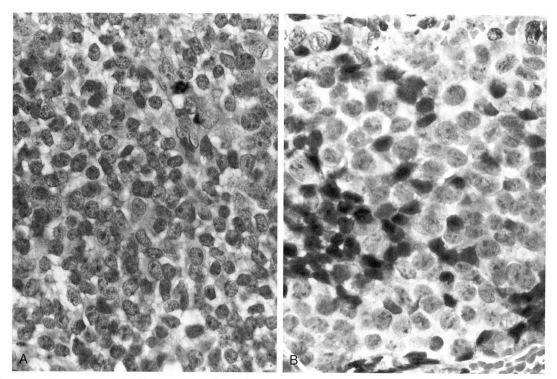

FIGURE 17–7. Ewing's sarcoma. *A,* Uniform tumor cell nuclei, some with small nucleoli, are shown. *B,* The dusty, uniform chromatin pattern and ill-defined cytoplasmic boundaries of Ewing's tumor cells as well as the presence of "dark" cells are shown. Although the uniformity of the nuclei is in contrast to the more irregular nuclei of MPNET, some cases with these features have proved to be examples of MPNET by immunohistochemical or electron microscopic studies.

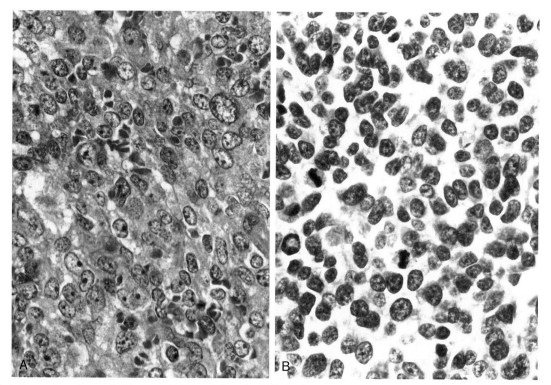

FIGURE 17–8. Examples of so-called large-cell *(A)* and "atypical" Ewing's sarcoma *(B).* The cells in *A* are larger, with more atypical nuclei and more cytoplasm than in the cells of classic Ewing's sarcoma. The cells in *B,* although of similar size to Ewing's tumor cells, have more variation in nuclear size and shape and a denser chromatin pattern. These cytologic features should suggest MPNET as a possible diagnosis rather than Ewing's sarcoma.

survived for 5 or more years. The interval from diagnosis until death ranged from 1 to 71 months, with an average of 18 months (median, 14 months). It has recently been reported that forms of MPNET composed of larger cells than found in ''conventional'' small-cell MPNET have an even poorer prognosis.[31, 33] Although there are some contrary opinions,[15, 56, 57, 117] the survival in MPNET appears to be worse than for Ewing's sarcoma, both osseous and extraskeletal, and hence it is more than just an intellectual exercise at the present time to distinguish between these two tumors.[22, 23, 29, 42, 83, 105]

DESMOPLASTIC SMALL-CELL TUMOR

Desmoplastic small-cell tumor (DSCT),[118, 119] a newcomer to the class of small, round, blue cell tumors, is characterized by an almost specific location in the soft tissues of the abdomen and pelvis and a divergent immunohistochemical profile. Despite its short descriptive history, DSCT has had almost as many terms applied to it as there are reports about it, including desmoplastic small-cell tumor with divergent differentiation,[118] malignant small-cell epithelial tumor of the peritoneum,[119] intra-abdominal desmoplastic small-cell tumor with divergent differentiation,[120–122] intra-abdominal neuroectodermal tumor,[123] desmoplastic primitive neuroectodermal tumor,[124] desmoplastic small-cell tumor of the peritoneum,[125, 126] and intra-abdominal desmoplastic small round-cell tumor.[127–130]

Among 61 patients in our review,[119–125, 127–135] ages ranged from 9 months[124] to 38 years,[128] with a mean of 20.6 years (median, 21 years); 21 patients (46%) were younger than age 20 years, with eight (13%) younger than 10 years of age. Male patients were involved in 47 (77%) of the cases.

Virtually all DSCTs occur intra-abdominally, where they involve the peritoneal surface, omentum, mesentery, or retroperitoneum, with a predilection for the pelvic soft tissues. Examples are reported involving the paratesticular area or the tunica vaginalis,[132, 134] the ovaries,[135] and the cerebellum.[124]

Although examples of DSCT as small as 1.0 cm are reported,[120] most are discovered as large, bulky masses, some as large as 40 cm.[128] The tumor may occur in the form of multiple nodules distributed throughout the abdomen, as a single mass occupying the entire abdominal cavity, or as a single large dominant mass with numerous smaller peritoneal nodules. The masses, which may be multinodular or multilobulated, have smooth or bosselated contours and a gray-white cut surface that may be myxoid with areas of hemorrhage and necrosis.

Histologically,[118–125, 127, 128, 130–133, 135] DSCT is characterized by the presence of a well-vascularized, desmoplastic stroma, which occasionally may be myxoid or loose in character, in which are sharply delimited nests, strands, clusters, or sheets of small, compact, uniform epithelial-like cells (Figs. 17–9 and 17–10).[120, 121, 128] The cells have uniform, oval to round nuclei, with a fine, hyperchromatic chromatin pattern; nucleoli are small or inconspicuous (Fig. 17–9). The cytoplasm is usually scant and ill-defined, but in some cases cells are present with a more abundant cytoplasm that contains a dense eosinophilic inclusion that imparts to them the appearance of rhabdoid cells.[118, 128, 131, 132] In some cases, the cells form tubular or gland-like structures, some containing mucinous material,[119–123, 133, 135] or they elongate to form spindle cells

arranged in streams or whorls.[119, 121, 132] A variable amount of cytoplasmic glycogen may be present but is not abundant. Rosette-like structures, some of Homer Wright type, are described,[122, 123, 131, 132] as are foci having carcinoid or transitional cell carcinoma-like features.[132] Mitotic activity in DSCT is usually frequent. Cytogenetic studies of a single example of DSCT demonstrated a reciprocal 11;22 translocation similar to that in Ewing's sarcoma and malignant peripheral neuroectodermal tumor but involving a different breakpoint on chromosome 22.[129]

Thirty-nine cases of DSCT in our survey were studied electron microscopically, with somewhat variable results.[119–123, 125, 127–132, 135] Most cases showed primitive small cells with round or irregular nuclei, numerous free ribosomes, prominent Golgi, smooth and rough endoplasmic reticulum, and cytoplasmic glycogen. Many cells contained cytoplasmic intermediate filaments that were often aggregated in a paranuclear location.[119, 121, 122, 128, 131, 132, 135] A basal lamina was found in some studies[125, 128, 129, 131, 132, 135] but not in others.[120–122, 127] Cell attachments varied from poorly developed, scanty, simple intercellular junctions to desmosome-like junctions. Cytoplasmic dense-core granules were only rarely found;[122, 123, 128, 131, 135] microvillous-like plasma membrane projections were reported in some cases[120, 132] but not in others.[122, 128] Cytoplasmic processes with microtubules have been described.[122, 131, 132, 135] Groups of cells may be found with intracellular lumina that are rimmed by microvillous projections.[119, 123, 132] The cells of the desmoplastic stroma have features of myofibroblasts.[121, 122]

Immunohistochemically, DSCT has a diverse phenotype, with the co-expression of cytokeratin, vimentin, and desmin being a characteristic feature.[119–132, 134, 135] Tumor cells were immunoreactive for cytokeratin in 96% (51/53), and for vimentin in 88% (35/40) of cases.[119–123, 125–132, 134, 135] Epithelial membrane antigen[119, 121–123, 126–128, 130–132, 135] was present in 97% (34/35), and desmin[119–123, 125–128, 130–132, 134, 135] in 92% (48/52), the latter reactivity being paranuclear and dot-like. Muscle-specific actin[119, 126–132, 134, 135] was found in only 1 of 29 cases (3%), smooth muscle actin[121, 131, 132, 135] in 2 of 13 (15%), whereas myoglobin was not detected in 6 cases.[119, 121, 131, 133] Results for neural and neuroendocrine markers have varied: S-100 protein[119–123, 127, 128, 130–132, 135] was found in 15% (5/33) of cases, Leu-7[120, 125, 132, 135] in 75% (12/16), neuron-specific enolase[120–123, 125–132, 134, 135] in 67% (26/39), synaptophysin[119–121, 123, 125, 128, 131, 132, 135] in 22% (5/23), and chromogranin[119–121, 125, 127–132, 135] in 11% (4/37). Negative results were reported for neurofilament protein[119, 121–123, 125, 127–132, 134, 135] in 27 cases, leukocyte common antigen[127–131] in 12 cases, placental alkaline phosphatase[130, 132] in 9 cases, HMB-45 antigen[130, 132] in 13 cases, carcinoembryonic antigen[119, 125, 130, 131, 134, 135] in 10 cases, and HBA-71[122] in 5 cases. Stains for Leu-M1[130, 132, 134, 135] were positive in 9 of 13 cases (69%); alpha-1-antitrypsin[130, 131] was found in two of the cases studied, and only 1 of 25 cases was reactive for glial fibrillary acidic protein,[121, 123–125, 128, 132, 135] the lone positive tumor originating in the cerebellum.[124]

The differential light microscopic diagnosis of DSCT includes a variety of small, blue cell tumors, including embryonal rhabdomyosarcoma, malignant lymphoma, malignant peripheral neuroectodermal tumor, extrarenal malignant rhabdoid tumor, extraskeletal Ewing's sarcoma, neuroendocrine tumor, malignant small-cell mesothelioma, and metastatic small-cell carcinoma.[118, 120, 121, 125, 128]

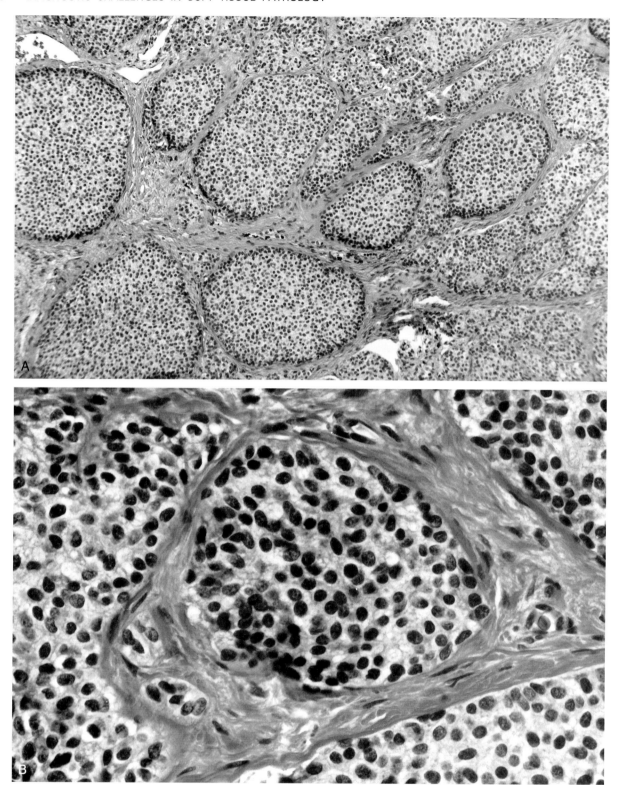

FIGURE 17–9. *A,* Low-power view of desmoplastic small-cell tumor (DSCT) shows variably sized cellular nodules within a dense fibrotic stroma. *B,* Higher-magnification view of nodules shows cells with oval to round uniform nuclei, with ill-defined cytoplasmic borders.

Embryonal rhabdomyosarcoma (ERMS) may be a differential diagnostic problem, not only because of its small blue cell content, but also because its occasional paratesticular location overlaps the anatomic distribution of DSCT. However, in contrast to DSCT, the microscopic pattern of ERMS is not that of large separated nests of tumor cells, but one that has a more diffuse proliferation of cells that are more frequently spindle-shaped than those of DSCT. Although "rhabdoid" cells may occur in DSCT, the eosinophilic rhabdomyoblasts and cross-striated cells of rhabdomyosarcoma

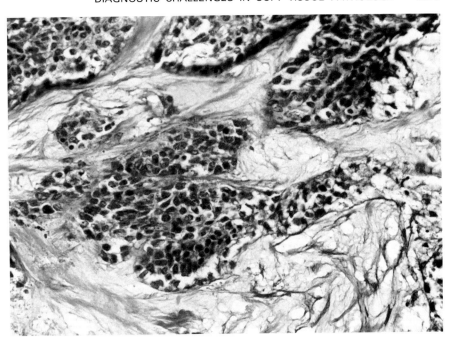

FIGURE 17-10. View of another example of DSCT in which the stroma has a loose myxoid character.

are absent in DSCT. Some rhabdomyosarcomas reportedly contain cytokeratin-positive cells, which may lead to some confusion with DSCT; however, they lack the epithelial membrane antigen reactivity of DSCT and have a considerably higher incidence of positivity for muscle-specific actin. Finally, and most important in this differential diagnosis, the electron microscopic features of skeletal muscle differentiation in rhabdomyosarcoma are absent in the cells of DSCT.

Malignant lymphoma lacks the nesting quality and the pronounced desmoplastic stroma of DSCT and in almost all cases contains leukocyte common antigen (CD45), which is uniformly absent in the cells of DSCT. Lymphoma also lacks the co-expression of desmin and epithelial markers as present in DSCT, as well as the intermediate filaments, neurosecretory granules, and glycogen content of DSCT.

The cells of **extraskeletal Ewing's sarcoma** usually contain more glycogen than those of DSCT, and they lack desmin or epithelial membrane antigen reactivity. In addition, the cells of Ewing's sarcoma are positive for HBA-71, which, to date, has not been found in DSCT.[136] By electron microscopy, Ewing's sarcoma cells lack the aggregates of intermediate filaments, lumina formation, and organelle content as found in DSCT.

Malignant peripheral neuroectodermal tumor (MPNET) may affect the same patient age group as does DSCT and also occurs in intra-abdominal and pelvic locations. Morphologically, MPNET has cells whose features, by light and electron microscopy, overlap those of DSCT. However, in its more differentiated form, the cells of MPNET commonly form rosettes, a pattern that is infrequently found in DSCT, and the desmoplastic stroma of the latter tumor is not present in MPNET. In contrast with DSCT, the cells of MPNET generally lack co-expression of cytokeratin, epithelial membrane antigen, and desmin and are reactive for HBA-71.

Because of the occurrence of rhabdoid cells in some examples of DSCT, **extrarenal malignant rhabdoid tumor** (ERMRT) may be a diagnostic consideration. Although there is some overlap in the ages of the patients affected by these two tumors,

ERMRT usually affects younger patients. However, despite some shared electron microscopic features and a similar immunohistochemical profile, with reactivity for epithelial and mesenchymal markers including cytokeratin, epithelial membrane antigen, vimentin, and desmin, their overall light microscopic patterns differ. The cells of ERMRT have a greater amount of cytoplasm, more vesicular nuclei, and more prominent nucleoli than the cells of DSCT, and are in monomorphic sheet-like arrangements without the characteristic nesting quality found in DSCT. The rhabdoid-like cells in DSCT constitute a minority of the total cells, whereas in ERMRT they usually occur in abundance. However, the illustrations of some cases reported as DSCT certainly strongly resemble those of ERMRT.[131] Of importance in the histologic separation of these two tumors is that the pronounced desmoplastic stroma of DSCT is absent in ERMRT.

By light microscopy, carcinoma metastatic to the abdomen, especially **small-cell carcinoma,** may be difficult to distinguish from DSCT. Clinical information is essential in clarifying this differential diagnosis by indicating the presence of a known primary tumor.[120] Metastatic small-cell carcinoma to the abdomen in a young person is rare, especially in the absence of a known primary tumor. Although the cells of metastatic small-cell carcinoma may have an associated fibrous stroma and contain cytokeratin and epithelial membrane antigen, they lack desmin reactivity. Electron microscopy may not be helpful, because the cells of DSCT have some epithelial features.[132]

Mesothelioma is only rarely found in the age group most frequently affected by DSCT, being predominantly a tumor of older adults.[136, 137] The small-cell variety of mesothelioma also occurs most commonly in the pleura, in contrast with the intra-abdominal location of DSCT. Histologically, **small-cell mesothelioma** lacks the nesting quality of DSCT; furthermore, when sufficient sections are taken, areas of conventional mesothelioma are usually found.[138] Immunohistochemically, the cells of small-cell mesothelioma share with DSCT cytokeratin, Leu-7, and neuron-specific enolase reactivity, but they are negative for desmin. The desmoplastic form of mesothelioma has very dense bundles of hyalinized collagen, which may show bland necrosis, unlike the looser, myxoid stroma of DSCT. Cellular sarcomatoid foci, present in the majority of these mesotheliomas, lack the island-like pattern of DSCT.[139] Electron microscopy may serve to separate mesothelioma from DSCT, with the former showing the characteristic long, slender surface microvilli of mesothelial cells. However, poorly differentiated mesotheliomas may lack microvilli, and microvilli have been noted in some cases of DSCT, although this is uncommon.

Abdominal **neuroendocrine tumors** usually arise in the gastrointestinal tract, but may also develop in extra-intestinal sites. They lack the desmoplastic stroma of DSCT, and by electron microscopy more frequently have neurosecretory granules than do the cells of DSCT. In addition, neuroendocrine tumor cells are more consistently positive for neural markers, such as chromogranin, synaptophysin, and neurofilament protein, than are the cells of DSCT. Like most non-myogenic neoplasms in the differential diagnosis, neuroendocrine tumors also lack desmin reactivity.

Although the precise histogenesis of DSCT remains in question,[128, 132] its clinical aggressiveness does not. Of 55 patients with clinical follow-up information, 37 (67%) died of tumor, 14 were alive with persistent or metastatic tumor (26%), and only 4 (7%) were alive and well. However, the patient with the longest survival had been followed up for only 4 years.[119-125, 127-132, 134, 135] In the two largest series of cases of DSCT, the interval from diagnosis until death ranged from 6 months to 4.5 years, with a mean of 1.7 years (median, 1.25 years) in one,[128] and from 8 to 50 months (mean, 25 months; median, 25.5 months) in the other,[132] despite intense chemotherapy.

EXTRARENAL MALIGNANT RHABDOID TUMOR

In 1978, Beckwith and Palmer[140] described a renal tumor of infants and young children that was characterized by cells with eccentric nuclei, an abundant eosinophilic cytoplasm, and, in some, a large, hyaline-type perinuclear cytoplasmic inclusion. These cells, which resembled rhabdomyoblasts, caused the tumor to be considered as a rhabdomyosarcomatoid variant of Wilms' tumor. Subsequently, however, this tumor type was reclassified as distinct from both Wilms' tumor and rhabdomyosarcoma, and the appellation malignant rhabdoid tumor (MRT) was given to it.[141, 142] The cells with the large hyaline inclusions have since been referred to as "rhabdoid cells." Reports of extrarenal malignant rhabdoid tumor (ERMRT) originating in the soft tissues and visceral organs soon appeared in such an abundance that the lesion was in danger of becoming the malignant fibrous histiocytoma of the 1980s, with "rhabdoid" tumors being found almost everywhere.[143-162] However, a brake to the rapid rise in its diagnostic popularity occurred when Tsuneyoshi et al. showed that a variety of conventional malignant soft tissue tumors, including such tumors as epithelioid sarcoma, synovial sarcoma, extraskeletal myxoid chondrosarcoma, and malignant mesothelioma, could contain "rhabdoid" cells cytologically similar to those in MRT,[163] thus leading to confusion with MRT.

Compounding the problem of what actually constitutes an ERMRT[164] is the immunohistochemical diversity of these lesions, whose cells co-express epithelial and mesenchymal markers. Some authors have questioned whether these extrarenal rhabdoid tumors are true counterparts of the renal tumors, or whether they represent a variety of phenotypically similar lesions with a different histogenesis.[165] The data presented in this section are based on those cases in the medical literature described as ERMRT, with the caveat that some may actually represent other sarcomas in which there was such an abundance of rhabdoid cells that the correct diagnosis was obscured.

In common with its renal counterpart, ERMRT primarily affects young children, although the age range of patients is broader and the average age older than for patients with renal MRT. Among 111 cases of renal MRT, almost all patients were younger than 2 years of age (mean, 16.8 months; median, 11.0 months); only three patients were older than age 5 years, and the oldest age was 8.8 years.[166] However, among 76 patients with ERMRT in our review with individual age information,[143, 144, 146-162, 168, 169, 171, 172] the mean age at diagnosis was 11.3 years (median, 7.3 years), with a range from newborns[152, 159] to 75 years.[172] Approximately 60% of the patients were younger than age 10 years, with 32% younger than 1 year of age. However, in contrast with patients with renal MRT, approximately 13% of the patients with ERMRT were older than age 30 years. As with renal MRT,[166] male patients with ERMRT were slightly more common than females, accounting for 53% of the cases. A familial occurrence of ERMRT, involving two sisters, has been reported.[155] Unlike renal MRT, in which there is a significant incidence of associated primary brain tumors,[159, 166, 173, 174] this has only rarely been reported in patients with ERMRT.[157]

ERMRT has a diverse anatomic distribution, with no single site overwhelmingly dominant. The trunk, including the chest wall and paraspinal areas, accounted for 29% of the 76 cases reviewed, the extremities for 28% (upper 8%; lower 20%), the head and neck region and the intra-abdominal soft tissues for 11% each, and parenchymal organs for 22%, the last category including the brain,[146, 152, 153, 159, 175] liver,[156, 159] prostate,[149, 168] thymus,[168, 169] heart,[158] uterus,[172] and bladder.[142]

ERMRT may arise in the skin, subcutaneous tissue, or deep soft tissues. It is soft, fleshy, and unencapsulated with infiltrating margins and has a cut surface that is gray to yellow-white and frequently has foci of necrosis and hemorrhage.[148, 154, 159, 162, 168] ERMRT tends to be large, most being more than 5 cm in maximum dimensions, with a range of 1.3 cm to 18 cm.[168] In our review, specific size data were given in 17 cases;* the mean maximum dimension was 7.6 cm (median, 6.0 cm).

The basic histologic and cytologic pattern of ERMRT[150, 152, 157, 159, 162, 167-169] is quite similar to its renal counterpart.[140, 141] Although a recent report documented a wide morphologic spectrum in renal MRT,[166] with as many as nine different histologic patterns described, such diversity has so far not been encountered in the extrarenal tumors. ERMRT is typically composed of loosely cohesive round to polygonal

---

* References 143,150, 152, 154, 158, 159, 161, 162, 169, 170.

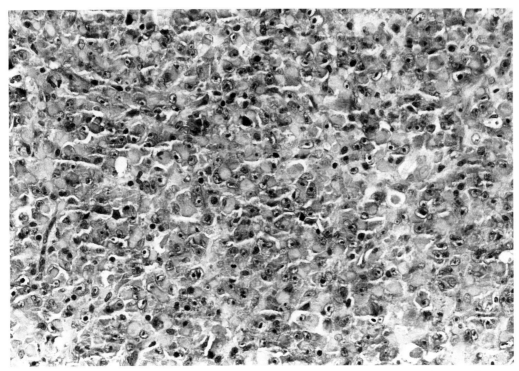

FIGURE 17–11. Sheets of loosely cohesive, round to polygonal epithelioid-type cells characterize the growth pattern of malignant rhabdoid tumor (MRT).

cells, with distinct cell borders, that are most commonly arranged in diffuse sheets (Fig. 17–11). The tumor cells usually have an abundant eosinophilic cytoplasm with central to eccentric vesicular nuclei. Although the nuclei lack significant pleomorphism, the nuclear membranes are often quite prominent owing to marginated condensed heterochromatin, and characteristically contain a prominent central eosinophilic or basophilic nucleolus (Fig. 17–12). A variable number of cells contain a large intracytoplasmic, spherical or round, paranuclear hyaline mass that may have a "glassy" appearance (Fig. 17–12). The number of these "rhabdoid" cells varies from case to case, being abundant in some, whereas in others they may be so infrequent as to require an extensive search to find. The inclusions may be so large as to occupy most or all of the cytoplasm, compressing and eccentrically displacing the nucleus. The inclusions are usually periodic acid-Schiff (PAS)–positive and diastase-resistant,* although some are PAS-negative.[150, 153, 156, 160, 169] Masson trichrome stains may highlight the inclusions, staining them a variety of colors from light green to orange-red or blue.[143, 148, 150, 162, 172] Cross-striations are not found in the cells of MRT.

A fibrovascular stroma may divide the tumor into small nests or clusters.[159, 162] The cells may also occur in pseudoalveolar or trabecular patterns[157, 162, 168] and, in some cases, may be spindle-shaped and arranged in short bundles.[144, 146, 162] In occasional cases of ERMRT, the abundant eosinophilic cytoplasm may be lacking, the cells having only a small amount of eosinophilic or amphophilic cytoplasm (Fig. 17–13), the

appearance of the tumor mimicking a small, round blue cell tumor.[150, 151, 153, 157, 168] Mitoses are variable in number from case to case, but tend to be frequent.

The light microscopic diagnosis of ERMRT should not depend solely on the presence of rhabdoid cells. The overall histologic pattern of a monomorphic sheet-like proliferation of cells with vesicular nuclei, dense marginated nuclear borders, and prominent nucleoli is an equally important diagnostic feature. However, supportive electron microscopic and immunohistochemical information is required to rule out other tumors that may contain rhabdoid cells. Clinical information is important in distinguishing ERMRT from other potentially confusing tumors.

Despite its relatively recent description, the electron microscopic features of ERMRT have been fairly extensively described and are similar to those of renal MRT. In our review, there were 35 cases of soft tissue MRT,* 10 non-renal visceral cases,† and 28 renal examples that had been studied by this modality.[142, 152, 157, 166, 174–177] Electron microscopically, the cells of ERMRT feature the presence of cytoplasmic whorled or stacked arrays of closely packed intermediate filaments that are frequently paranuclear and curve about the nucleus, although in some cells they are more haphazardly arranged in the cytoplasm. These filaments account for the hyaline masses noted by light microscopy. Lipid droplets and cell organelles may be found entrapped within the filament bundles. Sheaves of cytoplasmic tonofilaments may also be present.[160, 162] Although a basal lamina has been reported by some

* References 143, 146, 147, 149, 152, 154–156, 159–162.

* References 148, 150–152, 154, 155, 159–162, 168, 171.
† References 146, 147, 149, 152, 153, 156, 158, 167.

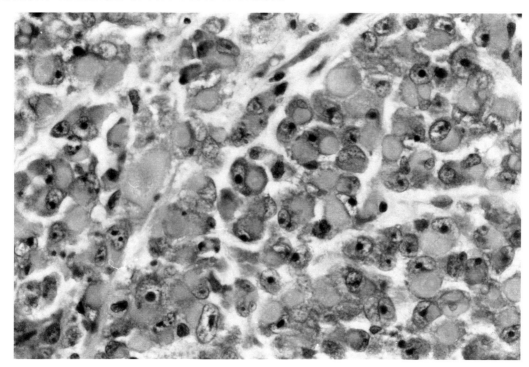

FIGURE 17–12. Cells of MRT have eccentric vesicular nuclei with prominent nucleoli. The cytoplasm is dense and in some cells contains a distinct round, paranuclear hyaline mass.

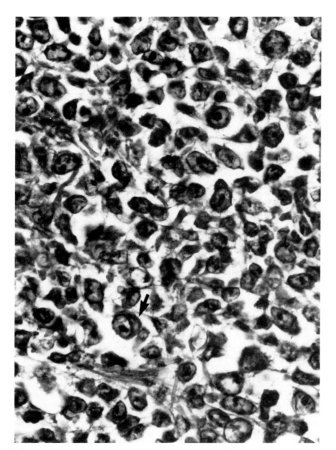

FIGURE 17–13. Example of MRT composed of cells that lack overt intracytoplasmic hyaline inclusions and resemble the cells of other "small, round, blue cell" tumors. A few cells have prominent nucleoli and a small cytoplasmic inclusion *(arrow)*.

workers,[160] in most studies it was absent.[148, 151, 152, 159, 168, 171] Microvilli may be found on the cell surfaces. Significantly, no thick or thin filaments or other morphologic evidence of skeletal muscle differentiation is present.

Immunohistochemically, rhabdoid tumors are characterized by the co-expression of mesenchymal and epithelial markers.* Among the cases of ERMRT, vimentin reactivity† was present in 96% (27/28), cytokeratin‡ in 79% (38/48), and epithelial membrane antigen[149, 156, 157, 160–162, 171, 172, 181] in 78% (36/46). The reactivity for vimentin and cytokeratin often accentuates the perinuclear hyaline masses, a pattern that confirms the electron microscopic character of these cells. The cells also express, to a greater or lesser degree, a wide variety of immunohistochemical markers. Neuron-specific enolase[143, 157, 167, 172, 181] was present in 46% (15/33), alpha-1-antitrypsin[143, 156, 162, 181] in 29% (8/28), desmin[157, 160–162, 167, 171, 172, 181] in 23% (10/43), and myoglobin[143, 149, 157, 160–162, 167, 181] in 10% (4/40); 2 of 34 cases were positive for neurofilament protein,[157, 162, 167, 172, 181] two of eight for alpha-1-antichymotrypsin,[162, 171] two of four for carcinoembryonic antigen,[149, 171] 1 of 23 for glial fibrillary acidic protein;[167, 181] and S-100 protein[143, 157, 161, 162, 167, 171, 172, 181] was found in 3 of 42 cases. Notably, muscle-specific actin was detected in only 1 of 20 cases in one study.[181] These immunohistochemical results roughly parallel those found in renal MRT.[157, 160, 166, 176–180]

Some of these diverse immunohistochemical results may in part be artifactual and reflect entrapment of immunoreagents within the tightly packed cytoplasmic intermediate filaments, or reflect cross-reactivity between different intermediate fil-

---

* References 143, 148, 149, 156, 157, 160–162, 166–168, 171, 172, 176–180.
† References 143, 148, 149, 156, 157, 160–162, 167, 171, 172.
‡ References 143, 148, 149, 156, 157, 160–162, 167, 171, 172, 181.

aments. However, the diffuse cytoplasmic pattern of reactivity for both epithelial and mesenchymal determinants argues for true phenotypic complexity in these lesions. Perhaps the immunophenotype of ERMRT reflects a "final common pathway" of differentiation for a high-grade neoplasm that was orginally mesenchymal or epithelial in nature.

The differential light microscopic diagnosis of ERMRT is, in many cases, a process of exclusion because of the long list of epithelial and mesenchymal tumors whose cells may, at least in part, have "rhabdoid" features.[150, 157, 165] These include epithelioid sarcoma,[163] rhabdomyosarcoma,[181] synovial sarcoma,[163, 182] extraskeletal myxoid chondrosarcoma,[163] malignant melanoma,[183] malignant mesothelioma, salivary gland plasmacytoid myoepithelioma, anaplastic thyroid carcinoma, basal cell carcinoma, hepatocarcinoma, adenocarcinoma of the lung, epidermoid carcinoma, and neuroendocrine carcinoma.[150] Small blue cell tumors, including extraskeletal Ewing's sarcoma, neuroblastoma, malignant lymphoma, and malignant peripheral neuroectodermal tumor, also enter the differential diagnosis when the cells of ERMRT have minimal cytoplasm and rhabdoid cells are scarce. Such a diversity of neoplasms has, in the minds of some, further brought into question the concept of ERMRT as a distinct entity.[164, 165, 168] However, in many of the aforementioned tumors, rhabdoid cells are only focally or rarely present, and most of these tumors are easily separated from ERMRT based on clinical information and their anatomic location. Of course, the finding of specific diagnostic areas by light microscopy or evaluation of the lesion with adjunctive techniques helps minimize confusion with ERMRT.

Among the more difficult of tumors to distinguish from ERMRT is **epithelioid sarcoma**.[150, 164, 168, 170, 171] These two tumors share an overlapping immunohistochemical and electron microscopic profile as well as cytologic features that may be indistinguishable, with rhabdoid cells found in both. However, epithelioid sarcoma occurs in young to middle-aged adults, an older patient population than that usually affected by ERMRT. Furthermore, epithelioid sarcoma occurs predominantly in the dermis and subcutaneous tissue of the distal extremities, most frequently the hand, wrist, or forearm, and histologically consists of multiple nodules of epithelioid cells, often with central necrosis, separated by collagenous bands, creating a pseudogranulomatous pattern. In contrast, ERMRT has a more diverse anatomic distribution, with the upper extremity involved in only 8% of cases, and histologically it has a diffuse growth pattern, without nodularity, and the number of rhabdoid cells is greater than their occasional occurrence in epithelioid sarcoma. Clinically, epithelioid sarcoma also differs from ERMRT, being characterized by a protracted course dominated by multiple local recurrences, in contrast with the usually rapidly aggressive and lethal outcome of ERMRT.

Because of the presence of eosinophilic cells that may superficially resemble rhabdomyoblasts, and the occurrence of smaller tumor cells mimicking a small blue cell tumor, the diagnosis of **rhabdomyosarcoma** (RMS) may be a diagnostic consideration. A differentiating embryonal rhabdomyosarcoma may contain cells, with hyaline inclusions, that are cytologically identical to rhabdoid cells.[181] ERMRT lacks the basic spindle-cell pattern of RMS; the nuclei of RMS cells are coarser and more irregular and pleomorphic than the vesicular bland nuclei of ERMRT; the prominent nucleoli found in

ERMRT are absent in RMS; and cells with cross-striations do not occur in ERMRT. The cells of ERMRT may, like rhabdomyosarcoma, be desmin- and myoglobin-positive, whereas some cases of rhabdomyosarcoma are reported to show cytokeratin positivity;[184, 185] however, unlike RMS, the cells of ERMRT are virtually never positive for muscle-specific actin. Most important in the differential diagnosis between these two tumors is the lack of skeletal muscle differentiation in ERMRT by electron microscopy.

Another soft tissue tumor whose cells co-express cytokeratin and vimentin and in which rhabdoid cells may occasionally be seen is **synovial sarcoma**.[163, 182] This differential, however, should not present a major problem because the classic biphasic pattern of spindle cells and epithelioid foci in synovial sarcoma is not present in ERMRT, and the spindle-cell component of monophasic synovial sarcoma is far more abundant than the spindle-cell areas found in ERMRT. Only occasional rhabdoid cells are present in synovial sarcoma, and it lacks the prominent nucleoli of ERMRT.

Finally, the recently described **intra-abdominal desmoplastic small-cell tumor** may resemble ERMRT because of its immunohistochemical co-expression of cytokeratin, vimentin, and desmin. The potential confusion is heightened by the tendency for the intermediate cytoplasmic filaments in desmoplastic round cell tumor to aggregate in a perinuclear location as they do in ERMRT. However, the intra-abdominal location of desmoplastic small-cell tumor, the nesting quality of its tumor cells, and its prominent desmoplastic stroma serve to distinguish it from ERMRT.

Malignant rhabdoid tumor of the kidney is a highly aggressive and lethal lesion. Approximately one quarter of patients have metastases at the time of diagnosis, and approximately 80% die of tumor.[166] Similarly, ERMRT also pursues a highly aggressive course with frequent metastases and death. Of 58 patients in our review with non-visceral soft tissue tumors and follow-up information, 43 (74%) died of tumor, one was alive with tumor (1.7%), and 14 (24%) were alive and well. However, only three of the surviving patients had been followed up for 5 or more years, with most of the others having relatively short follow-up intervals, indicating that the ultimate fatality rate will equal or exceed that of renal MRT.*

EPITHELIOID SARCOMA

Although first described in 1961 by Lakowski in the Polish medical literature[186] under the designation "aponeurotic sarcoma," epithelioid sarcoma (ES) was given its current designation and brought to widespread recognition as a distinct entity by Enzinger in 1970.[187]

Epithelioid sarcoma is mainly a disease of young adult life. In our survey of 180 patients for whom individual age data were given,[186, 188–233] the average age was 31.9 years (median, 29 years), with a range from 43 months[229] to 90 years.[233] Among 421 patients for whom either individual ages or age groups[233] were reported, approximately 60% were between 20 and 49 years of age; the tumor was uncommon in those younger than age 10 years (4%) and in those older than age

---

* References 143, 150, 152, 154, 155, 157, 159–162, 168–171.

50 years (12%). Sixty-four percent of the 485 patients in our review with gender information were male.

Clinically, ES is characterized by the development of single or multiple soft tissue nodular masses that slowly enlarge.[186, 187, 220, 224, 230, 233] These masses are painful in 25% to 65% of the patients.[186, 187, 233, 234] Although symptoms may be present for as short as 1 week prior to diagnosis,[233] most patients have their lesions for several years before seeking medical attention.[186, 194, 203, 207, 212, 223, 226, 233] In 95 patients for whom symptoms were specified,* their average prediagnosis duration was 3.2 years (median, 2.0 years); almost 20% of the patients had symptoms or lesions for 5 or more years, some for as long as 28 years.[224]

ES primarily affects the extremities. Among the 450 cases with specific site data,† 91% were extremity based, with 65% in the upper and 26% in the lower extremity. ES tends to involve the distal extremities, principally the extensor and volar aspects of the hands,[186, 187, 233] fingers, and feet; the hand, fingers, and wrist accounted for 42%, and the foot, toes, and ankle for 8% of the total cases. The trunk, including the penis[197, 206, 217] and vulva,[200, 202, 214, 222, 233] was the site of origin in 6%, and the head and neck region in only 2% of the cases.

ES may be either superficial or deeply situated.[187, 191, 224, 226, 233, 234] The superficial tumors are located in the subcutaneous tissue or dermis and tend to eventually ulcerate the overlying skin.[187, 191, 203, 207, 226, 229, 233, 234] The deeper tumors are attached to tendons or fascia, as well as to nerve and vascular sheaths.[186, 187, 224, 233, 234] ES occurs as a solitary, hard mass or as multiple separate nodules that may eventually coalesce. Among 80 tumors for which dimensions were given,‡ the sizes ranged from 0.5 cm[217, 225] to 22.0 cm,[237] with an average of 3.8 cm (median, 3.0 cm); approximately 75% were smaller than 5.0 cm.

Histologically, ES has a variety of patterns.§ In its classic form, nodules are present that have irregular undulating borders and contain large, round, polygonal cells that have a relatively abundant and densely eosinophilic cytoplasm that imparts to them an "epithelioid" appearance (Fig. 17–14). The cells are either loosely separated from each other by an intervening dense, hyalinized collagenous stroma, or in small nests or loosely aggregated large clusters. Nuclei tend to be vesicular, and although prominent nucleoli may be found in some cells, most nucleoli are small and inconspicuous (see Fig. 17–14). In general, the nuclei appear bland; significant nuclear or cytologic atypia is absent in ES.[203, 236] Because of their size, shape, and deeply eosinophilic cytoplasm, some tumor cells may resemble acidophilic rhabdomyoblasts (Fig. 17–15); however, cross-striations are absent.[186, 194, 233] ES may have cells with clear cytoplasmic vacuoles creating signet-ring cells (Fig. 17–16) that resemble lipoblasts, mesenchymal cells with primitive vasoformative lumina, or cells of a mucinous adenocarcinoma.[215, 233] The tumor cells may also contain perinuclear, glassy, cytoplasmic condensations or inclusions

creating rhabdoid-like cells (see Fig. 17–15) similar to those of malignant rhabdoid tumor.[194, 234, 240]

Fusiform-shaped tumor cells are a potentially confusing finding in ES, and such cells are found admixed with the epithelioid cells.[186, 191, 212, 224, 229, 233] These fusiform cells tend not to have the same amount of cytoplasm as the round or polygonal cells and may be arranged in bundles or fascicles yielding a fibrosarcomatous appearance (Fig. 17–17). One can appreciate gradual transitions between these spindle cells and the epithelioid cells; however, the sharp biphasic demarcation of spindle-shaped tumor cells from epithelial-like cells as noted in synovial sarcoma is not a feature of ES.[187, 203, 207, 233] Although most epithelioid sarcomas have the round or polygonal epithelioid cells as their major component, examples exist in which the spindle cells predominate.[196, 212, 223, 224]

An important diagnostic feature of ES is the variable presence of central necrosis within the tumor nodules (Fig. 17–18A). Although these necrotic foci may contain residual "ghost" tumor cells, in most cases one sees only necrotic collagen with viable-appearing tumor cells only at the periphery of the nodule (Fig. 17–18B). Small nodules with necrotic foci may coalesce to form large, necrotic, serpiginous areas that are sharply demarcated from the surrounding normal soft tissue. Because of the central necrosis and the abundant eosinophilic cytoplasm of the tumor cells, such foci may superficially resemble a necrobiotic granulomatous process in which the tumor cells of ES are misconstrued as epithelioid histiocytes.[186, 187, 191, 203, 233, 238] However, this highly distinctive necrobiotic granuloma-like appearance may not always be present, with the tumor cells arranged instead in a sheet-like fashion without necrosis.[233]

Epithelioid sarcoma is an infiltrative tumor with a marked propensity to grow along tendons and vascular and nerve sheaths; here the tumor cells may assume a cord-like or indian-file pattern.[186, 187, 194, 220, 234, 241] Binucleate and multinucleated tumor cells may occur within the tumor,[186, 208, 224, 229, 233] and calcification or bone formation is found in as many as 30% of cases.[194, 233] As mentioned, the more superficially located tumors frequently ulcerate the overlying skin.[186, 187, 191, 226, 227]

The dense desmoplastic stromal collagen of ES may, because of the effects of fixation, shrink and split apart, forming slit-like spaces that appear lined by the tumor cells (Fig. 17–19). These spaces resemble vascular channels and impart to the tumor an angiomatous appearance.[194, 199, 203, 226, 236] Similar shrinkage artifacts may cause central spaces to form within the small tumor nests, creating a gland-like pattern reminiscent of adenocarcinoma.[226]

Mitotic activity in ES is variable from tumor to tumor, with some having abundant activity; however, in most cases it is infrequent.* Despite the presence of signet-ring type cells or pseudoglandular areas, mucin stains are negative in ES;[215, 233] however, PAS stains for cellular glycogen may be positive.[187, 198, 223, 233]

A fibroma-like variant of ES has been described that contains fibrohistiocytic/dermatofibroma-like cutaneous nodules. These are predominantly spindle cell lesions with storiform or desmoid-like regions without necrobiotic-type areas; how-

---

* References 186, 189, 191, 194, 198, 203, 207–213, 217, 220, 223–226, 230.

† References 186, 188–191, 193–195, 197–204, 206–230, 232, 233, 236–238.

‡ References 186, 189, 194, 198, 199, 210, 212–215, 217, 218, 220, 222, 224, 225, 230, 232, 237, 239.

§ References 186, 187, 194, 203, 212, 215, 224, 226, 230, 233, 236.

---

* References 187, 188, 190, 197, 203, 207, 212, 219, 223, 229, 232, 234, 236.

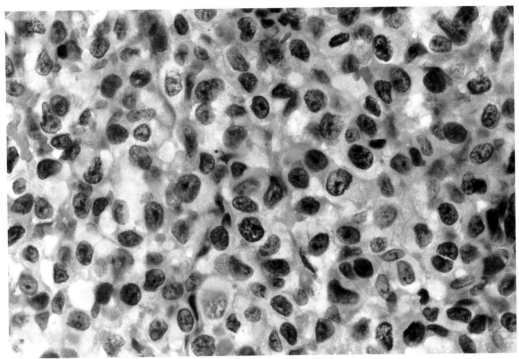

FIGURE 17–14. Epithelioid sarcoma (ES) composed of polygonal and round cells with abundant cytoplasm, some of which have small nucleoli. Significant pleomorphism is absent.

ever, plumper cells with eosinophilic cytoplasm as well as "rhabdoid" cells are also found. This variant of ES apparently has a predilection to also involve bones even at its initial presentation.[216]

Numerous electron microscopic studies of ES are reported,* most of which consist of single cases; the largest series contains 11 cases.[212] Common to most of the 68 cases in our review so studied were round, oval, or polygonal cells, as well as spindle forms, with transitions between them. Nuclei are characteristically irregular in outline with indentations and cytoplasmic invaginations. Nucleoli vary from small to large and prominent. The cytoplasm contains an array of organelles, usually including numerous mitochondria; an abundant and occasionally dilated rough endoplasmic reticulum; free ribosomes and polyribosomes; occasional pinocytotic vesicles; a well-developed Golgi zone; and scattered lipid droplets. The cell membrane is ruffled with either short, blunt filopodia or elongated microvilli, both of which may interdigitate with similar processes from adjacent cells. A distinct and important diagnostic feature is the presence of large aggregates of tightly compacted cytoplasmic intermediate filaments arranged in a whorled or concentric array about the nucleus or in bundles that run parallel to the cell membrane. Dense bodies, similar to those that interrupt microfilament arrays in myofibroblasts and smooth muscle cells, are at times present along these filaments.[189, 196, 197, 210, 223] Tonofilament-like structures are described in occasional cases.[197, 223] Glycogen is either absent, or present in small amounts.[189, 198, 215, 221, 242] The number and extent of the organelles may lead to the appearance of two populations of cells, described as dark and light (clear), with

the latter differing from the former by having fewer organelles and intermediate filaments.[186, 190, 221, 239] With some exceptions,[189, 193, 197, 223, 242, 244] most studies show an absence of a basement membrane or basal lamina. Cell attachments are described as primitive or poorly formed without true desmosomes,* but desmosome or desmosome-like junctions have been reported in some cases.† Gland-like or pseudoglandular spaces lined by microvilli or filopodia are described,‡ but not mentioned in most studies. Because of this spectrum of fine structural features, no concensus exists as to the nature of the tumor cells in ES, with claims made that they are fibrocytic,[198] histiocytic,[187, 220, 245] fibrohistiocytic,[186] myofibroblastic,[189, 196, 197] synovial,[187, 190, 193, 210, 239] or myoepithelial-like.[223]

Epithelioid sarcoma has been extensively studied immunohistochemically.§ With the exception of a report describing three examples of ES that were vimentin-negative,[188] this intermediate filament protein was present in all the remaining 82 cases in our review. The tumor cells of ES express epithelial markers mainly in the large epithelioid cells and, to a lesser extent, in the spindle cells. A variety of markers have been employed in the analysis of these cells. Cytokeratin positivity was present in 86% (146/170) of cases;‖ epithelial membrane antigen in 83% (53/64);[188, 194, 197, 207, 223, 229, 236, 238] human milk fat globulin proteins I and II in 57% (4/7) and 92% (12/13), respectively;[223, 229] tissue polypeptide antigen[194] in 100% (8/8); and carcinoembryonic antigen[194, 196, 207, 212, 233, 236] in

---

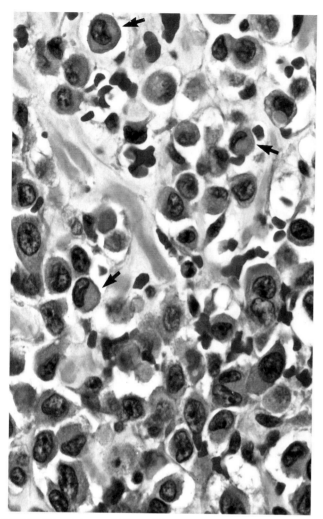

FIGURE 17–15. Area within an ES composed of loosely cohesive tumor cells whose cytoplasm appears denser than that of the cells in Figure 17–14. Such cells may resemble acidophilic rhabdomyoblasts or rhabdoid cells *(arrows).*

29% (18/62). The cells of ES show a diverse immunophenotype in their reactions to a variety of other antibodies: S-100 protein* was found in 11% of cases (8/70), neurofilament protein[201, 243] in 50% (5/10), neuron-specific enolase[201, 229, 243] in 88% (14/16), desmin[188, 196, 207, 229, 236, 243] in 19% (8/43), actin[223, 236] in 52% (11/21), alpha-1-antitrypsin[218, 229, 233, 236] in 36% (17/47), alpha-1-antichymotrypsin[218, 229, 233, 236] in 46% (18/39), *Ulex europaeus* I lectin[236, 248] in 75% (12/16), and CD34 antigen[188, 244] in 58% (11/19). The last, a marker for human hematopoietic progenitor cells, has also been found in a variety of vascular neoplasms.[244] Stains for Factor VIII–related antigen in 36 cases,[188, 233, 236, 248] CD31 antigen in five cases,[247] leukocyte common antigen in 25 cases,[236, 238] and melanoma-associated antigen (HMB-45) in 4 cases[188, 201] were negative. The positive reactions to diverse markers in ES may reflect the same situation that occurs in malignant rhabdoid tumor, in which the variety of positive immunohistochemical results has been attributed by some authors to the density of the intermediate filaments in these tumors, with the possible trapping of the immunoreagents within them, leading to arti-

factual false-positive results. We have doubts about the validity of this explanation.

The clinical course of ES is marked by recurrence rates after local resections of between 65% and 85%, with many of the recurrences characterized by the development of skin ulcers with draining sinus tracts.[220, 224, 226, 229, 233] These high recurrence rates are explained by the marked tendency of ES to microscopically spread along fascial planes, tendon sheaths, and blood vessels such that it is more widespread than can be grossly appreciated at the time of operation. Metastatic disease usually develops only after repeated local recurrences, and occurs in from 40% to 45% of patients.[186, 187, 220, 233] Five-year survival rates are between 60% and 70%,[224, 233, 234] however, ES may have a protracted course, with some patients developing delayed recurrences or metastases 15 to 20 years after therapy.[186, 227, 233, 234]

The histologic description of ES as originally provided by Enzinger[187] has not been signficiantly improved upon, and, based on it, the diagnosis of ES would appear to be straightforward. However, subsequent to the introduction of ES as a diagnostic entity, a variety of other soft tissue sarcomas were described that may, in whole or in part, contain ''epithelioid'' tumor cells similar to those in ES. Furthermore, a variety of both epithelial and mesenchymal lesions exist whose immunohistochemical phenotypes are similar to ES, and a number of mesenchymal soft tissue lesions contain abundant intermediate filaments by electron microscopy such that the cytologic, electron microscopic, and immunohistochemical characteristics of ES are not diagnostically specific. A diagnosis of epithelioid sarcoma must depend on clinical information in combination with morphologic and immunohistochemical evaluation.[212]

Because of its relatively indolent and protracted clinical course, ulcerative skin nodules associated with draining sinus tracts, and a histologic pattern that may suggest a granulomatous reaction with necrobiosis, ES may be confused with an inflammatory process such as **granuloma annulare, necrobiosis lipoidica,** or **rheumatoid disease.** As mentioned, the epithelioid histiocytes present in these necrobiotic lesions may be confused with the epithelioid cells of ES. However, the necrotic nodules with remnant ghost tumor cells seen in ES are distinct from the areas of purely necrotic collagen that occur in these inflammatory conditions. Immunohistochemical studies may be helpful in this differential diagnosis. The cells of ES are positive for epithelial markers such as cytokeratin and epithelial membrane antigen and negative for leukocyte common antigen, whereas the cells in necrobiotic granulomas are negative for epithelial markers and positive for leukocyte common antigen.[238]

Similarly, the clinical presentation of superficially located epithelioid sarcomas may raise the question of **epidermoid carcinoma, cutaneous adnexal carcinoma,** or **malignant melanoma.**[186, 187, 191, 226, 227] Epidermoid and adnexal carcinomas and ES may have tonofilament structures by electron microscopy, although these appear to be the exception in ES; all these tumors are positive for epithelial markers, and some epidermoid carcinomas may co-express vimentin. However, non-keratinizing epidermoid carcinoma is more pleomorphic than ES and tends to be more mitotically active. The absence of hyperplasia or cytologic atypia in the epidermis adjacent to the ulcerating lesion of ES contrasts significantly with their presence in ulcerative epidermoid carcinoma.

* References 188, 196, 197, 201, 212, 223, 229, 233, 236.

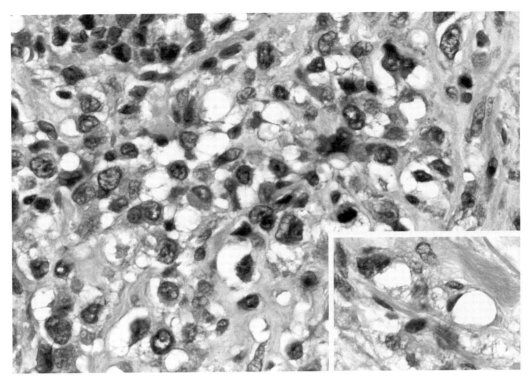

FIGURE 17–16. Chondroid-like region within an ES where the tumor cells have vacuolated cytoplasm and resemble lipoblasts or cells with primitive vasoformative lumina. *Inset* shows tumor cells with signet-ring configuration.

The nodular pattern of malignant melanoma, as well as the presence in melanoma of cells that appear epithelioid, may suggest the possibility of an amelanotic melanoma rather than ES. However, junctional activity, a nesting pattern, and significant cytologic atypia are features of malignant melanoma and not of ES. In addition, stains for S-100 protein are more strongly and frequently positive in melanoma than they are in ES, and melanoma-associated antigen (HMB-45) is absent in ES. Although melanomas are almost always cytokeratin-negative, reactivity for cytokeratin in some recurrent and metastatic melanomas is reported,[249] and thus may complicate the differential diagnosis between ES and melanoma. However,

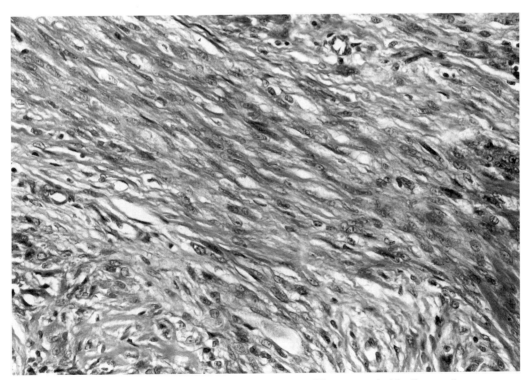

FIGURE 17–17. Fibrosarcomatous area within an ES composed of fusiform cells.

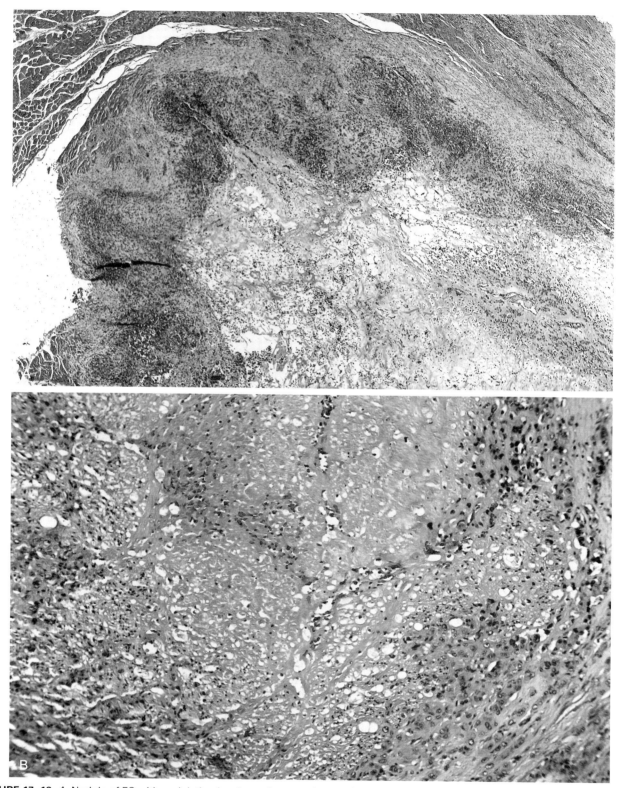

FIGURE 17–18. *A,* Nodule of ES with undulating border and a central area of necrosis. *B,* Central necrotic area contains "ghost" tumor cells. Viable-appearing epithelioid cells are present at the periphery of the necrotic area.

by electron microscopy, melanomas contain premelanosomes and lack the abundant intermediate filament content of ES.

Metastatic poorly differentiated carcinoma may be difficult to distinguish from ES because some carcinomas co-express epithelial and mesenchymal markers.[188, 197, 207, 212, 235] Mucin is absent in ES, but may be present in poorly differentiated carcinoma and thus be helpful in distinguishing between these two diagnostic possibilities. As with epidermoid carcinoma and malignant melanoma, the cells of most metastatic carcinomas are more atypical than those of ES, and the abundant

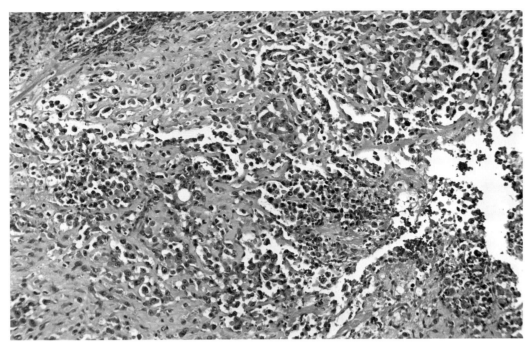

FIGURE 17–19. Artifactual splitting of the dense stroma in ES creates slit-like spaces that resemble vascular channels.

cytoplasmic intermediate filament content in the cells of ES is not usually present in carcinomas. Antibody to CD34 antigen has been advocated as a possible immunohistochemical aid in this diagnostic problem.[188, 244] Approximately one half of all epithelioid sarcomas are positive for CD34 antigen, whereas this antigen is only rarely found in epithelial tumors. These data appear to confirm the suggestion that conjoint reactivity for vimentin, cytokeratin, and CD34 is sufficient for the diagnosis of ES.[188] Perhaps as important as any of the above considerations in aiding the pathologist faced with this diagnostic differential is the clinical history of a previous or existing carcinoma in the patient. To date, we have not detected CD34 in 18 examples of primary cutaneous adnexal carcinomas.

Synovial sarcoma shows the same immunophenotype as ES, with the co-expression of cytokeratin and vimentin, and they may have overlapping electron microscopic features, including the presence of intercellular spaces surrounded by microvilli or filopodia, and cell junctions. Epithelioid-type cells and spindle cells are present in classic synovial sarcoma, as they are in ES; however, in synovial sarcoma these components are more sharply delineated from each other, creating the well-defined biphasic pattern of classic synovial sarcoma, versus their gradual transition in ES. However, the distinction between monophasic synovial sarcoma and spindle cell–dominant ES may be especially difficult without consideration of clinical or electron microscopic evidence. Synovial sarcoma is uncommonly a superficial tumor, being located adjacent to large joints, does not ulcerate the overlying skin, and by electron microscopy does not usually have the abundant intermediate filament content of ES. The cells of synovial sarcoma have a basal lamina, which is absent in most cases of ES.

Because of the presence of pseudovascular slit-like spaces in some cases of ES, as well as cells with cytoplasmic vacuoles that suggest vasoformative foci, **epithelioid angiosarcoma** may be a diagnostic consideration. Epithelioid angiosarcoma lacks the pattern of nodular masses with central necrosis, growing instead in a sheet-like configuration; however, the latter pattern may also exist in some examples of ES. Epithelioid angiosarcomas occur in older patients more often than does ES, with most patients being older than 60 years of age, an age group uncommonly involved by ES. Some epithelioid angiosarcomas are reportedly cytokeratin-positive, but doubts have been expressed about the validity of these results. Both epithelioid angiosarcoma and ES are positive for the vascular markers CD34 antigen and *Ulex europaeus* I lectin, but neither Factor VIII–related antigen nor CD31 are present in ES. By electron microscopy, Weibel-Palade bodies may occur in epithelioid angiosarcoma but are absent in ES.

The presence of vacuolated cells in ES may raise the diagnostic possibility of **epithelioid hemangioendothelioma** (EHE).[248] Unlike epithelioid sarcoma, EHE is angiocentric, being frequently positioned about large veins, has a myxochondroid stroma in contrast with the dense desmoplastic stroma of ES, and has cells that are less densely eosinophilic than those of ES; its vasoformative vacuoles may contain red blood cells, which are never present in the vacuoles found in ES. Although reactivity for *Ulex europaeus* I lectin occurs in both of these tumors, EHE lacks the epithelial membrane antigen reactivity of ES and is positive for Factor VIII–related antigen and CD31, in contrast with their absence in ES.

Because of its extremity location, close association with tendons, and its epithelioid cells, **clear-cell sarcoma** (CCS) is also included in the differential diagnosis with ES. Both ES and CCS affect the same general age group of patients; however, CCS is usually located in the distal extremity about the foot and ankle in contrast with the predominant upper extremity location of ES with its involvement of the hands and fingers. CCS does not involve the skin and has a nesting quality that is absent in ES; its cells have prominent nucleoli and a clear or granular rather than a densely eosinophilic cytoplasm. Multinucleated cells may occur in both tumors, but are more common in CCS. Stains for melanin are frequently positive in CCS but negative in ES. Electron microscopically, premelanosomes are found in CCS and not in ES, whereas CCS lacks the intermediate filament content of ES. Immunohistochemically, the cells of CCS lack epithelial markers and are frequently reactive for S-100 protein and for melanoma-associated antigen (HMB-45), the latter absent in ES.

Although **aponeurotic fibroma** (AF) usually occurs in younger patients than does ES, with approximately one half of the patients younger than 10 years of age, older patients with AF are reported. The slow clinical development of AF, its propensity to occur in the hands or wrist, its infiltrative character and close association with tendons and aponeuroses, and its focal calcification all are features shared with ES, as is its tendency for recurrence following local excision. However, AF is a fibroblastic lesion that has chondroid-like areas and a characteristic flowing pattern of its component fibroblasts, and it lacks epithelioid cells, zones of necrotic collagen, and epithelial markers.

The tumor that causes the most difficulty in the differential diagnosis of ES is **extrarenal malignant rhabdoid tumor** (ERMRT).[207, 222, 243, 250, 251] Both tumors contain "rhabdoid" cells, although they are less frequent in ES than in ERMRT, and both exhibit a diverse immunophenotype with conjoint expression of mesenchymal and epithelial markers. They also share overlapping fine structural features with abundant cytoplasmic intermediate filaments. Clinical parameters help distinguish these entities. ERMRT occurs mainly in children younger than 10 years of age, an uncommon age for the occurrence of ES, and ERMRT is more anatomically diverse than ES, occurring less often in the extremities than does ES. Histologically, ERMRT lacks the central necrosis and nodularity of ES, growing instead in broad sheets. The clinical course of these two tumors is also distinctly different—ERMRT is a rapidly growing, aggressive and lethal tumor, in contrast with the usually long-term indolent course of ES characterized by recurrences and metastases that may take several years to develop.

EPITHELIOID ANGIOSARCOMA

Conventional angiosarcoma most commonly occurs as a cutaneous tumor in the head and neck region of elderly patients. The epithelioid variant of angiosarcoma (EA) is also predominantly a tumor of older adults; however, it is more uncommon than its conventional counterpart. The largest single reported series in the English-language medical literature contains only eight patients.[252]

In our review of 27 cases of EA,[252–259] the average patient age was 61 years (median, 62 years), with a range of 32[252] to 86 years;[259] approximately 80% were older than age 50 years, and men constituted almost three quarters of the patients. In contrast with conventional angiosarcoma, EA has a more widespread anatomic distribution, with cases not only in the skin and soft tissue[252, 253, 255, 257–260] but in such diverse sites as the adrenal, thyroid, bone, pharynx, prostate, and seminal vesicles.[254, 256, 259] Soft tissue EA is a deeply seated tumor most frequently located in the extremities.[252, 253, 260] Among 18 skin

and soft tissue tumors,[252, 253, 255, 257–260] only five arose in the head and neck region.[255, 257–259]

Grossly, EA has varied from 4 cm[254] to 15 cm[252] in maximum size and appears as a poorly defined, hemorrhagic, spongy mass with areas of necrosis.[252, 254, 256] Microscopically,[252–254, 256–258, 260] EA may have a variety of patterns, including areas of conventional angiosarcoma with intercommunicating vascular channels (Fig. 17–20) lined by atypical endothelial cells,[252, 254, 256–258, 260–262] but, most commonly, it is composed of a sheet-like proliferation of large epithelioid cells that have an abundant eosinophilic cytoplasm (Figs. 17–21 and 17–22). The nuclei are large, frequently vesicular, and characteristically contain a basophilic or amphophilic, round to oval, central nucleolus.[252, 254, 256, 258, 262] Overall, the cells have a monotonous uniform appearance, and, in general, they lack significant pleomorphism,[252] although some cases of EA have cells with prominent nuclear pleomorphism.[253] Foci may be present in which the cells are spindle-shaped rather than epithelioid.[257, 260] Mitotic activity is frequent (see Fig. 17–21), with abnormal forms easily found.[252, 254, 256, 260] A diagnostic feature of EA is the presence of vasoformative areas where the cells have cytoplasmic vacuoles (Fig. 17–23) that fuse to form channels, some of which contain whole or fragmented red blood cells.[252, 254, 256–258, 260, 262] Such vasoformative regions may be infrequent and require a prolonged search to find. Rectulin stains are helpful by outlining uncanalized vascular channels within the solid compact zones of the tumor.[252]

Electron microscopic studies of 11 cases of EA[252, 254, 255, 257, 258, 260] showed tumor cells with external lamina, desmosome-like junctions, prominent nucleoli, pinocytotic vesicles, and prominent aggregates of intermediate filaments.[252, 254, 258, 260] The cells may be arranged about small lumina. Weibel-Palade bodies, a morphologic marker of endothelial cell differentiation, have been found in some cases of EA and not in others.[255, 257] Distinctive and peculiar organelles were found in one case of EA. These so-called vesicular rosettes consist of round, moderately dense masses, 300 to 600 nm in diameter, bordered by smaller (50 nm) round bodies or vesicles, associated with cisternae of rough endoplasmic reticulum.[255]

Immunohistochemical studies of EA[252, 254–260] have yielded somewhat controversial results, especially as they pertain to cytokeratin reactivity. Vimentin was found in all nine cases of EA tested for this intermediate filament protein.[254, 256, 257, 260] Several authors report cytokeratin reactivity in all examples of EA.[252, 254, 260, 262] Given the epithelioid appearance of the cells by light microscopy, such a result might lead to a diagnosis of carcinoma. However, other workers have not confirmed cytokeratin positivity in these tumors.[256, 257, 259, 263] It has been suggested that the positive results might be spurious, brought about by the use of inappropriately concentrated cytokeratin antibodies.[259, 263, 264] Factor VIII–related antigen, a highly specific marker for endothelial differentiation, was found in 24 of 26 (92%) epithelioid angiosarcomas.[252, 254–260] This degree of staining with Factor VIII–related antigen is apparently peculiar to the epithelioid variant of angiosarcoma,[252] as other angiosarcomas are notorious for their lack of reactivity for this marker, being absent in as many as 75% of cases.[265, 266] CD31, a platelet cell adhesion molecule (PCAM) present in hematopoietic and endothelial cells, has been a specific and sensitive marker for vascular lesions.[265] It was detected in all of the seven epithelioid angiosarcomas

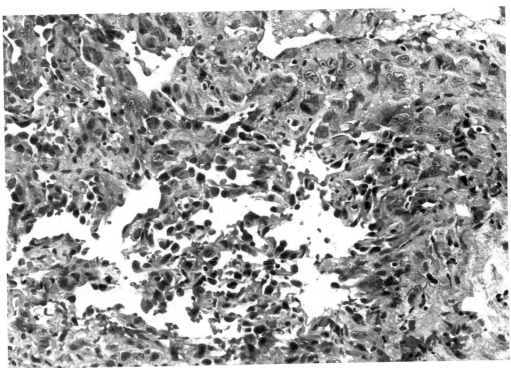

FIGURE 17–20. Epithelioid angiosarcoma (EA) with area of intercommunicating vascular spaces lined by small tumor cells. Larger epithelioid-type tumor cells are shown in the upper right of the field.

tested.[255, 265] Antibodies to CD34, a transmembrane glycoprotein present in endothelial cells, were reactive in 12 of 15 cases (80%) of EA;[252, 259] however, CD34 is not specific for endothelial neoplasms, as it has been found in several other tumors, including other sarcomas that contain epithelioid

cells.[266, 267] The lectin *Ulex europaeus* I is a sensitive marker of endothelial differentiation and was detected in 23 of 25 cases (92%) of EA.[252, 254–257, 259, 260] Like CD34, however, *Ulex europaeus* is not specific, being present in carcinomas and some non-vascular sarcomas, including those that contain epi-

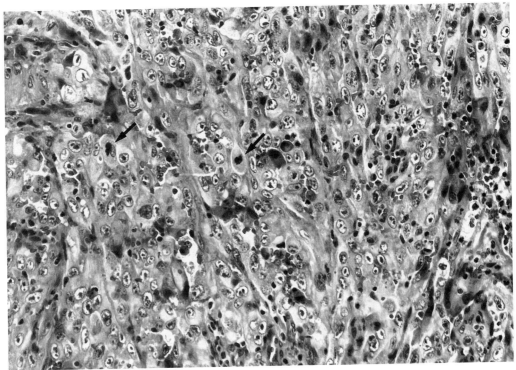

FIGURE 17–21. More typical growth pattern of soft tissue EA consists of tumor cells arranged in broad sheets without evident vascular channels. Mitotic figures are easily found *(arrows)*.

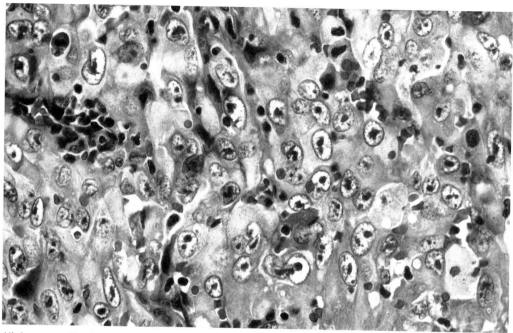

FIGURE 17–22. Higher magnification shows tumor cells with an abundant cytoplasm and ill-defined cell borders. Nuclei are vesicular and contain large, prominent, irregular nucleoli.

thelioid cells.[266, 268] B72.3, a putative marker of epithelial neoplasms, was found in five of seven (71%) epithelioid angiosarcomas and not in other vascular neoplasms or epithelioid-type soft tissue sarcomas.[259] Epithelial membrane antigen was found in only one of nine primary cases of EA[252, 260] and in a single metastasis.[252] A single case of EA was reportedly positive for S-100 protein.[255]

The histologic differential diagnosis of EA includes **metastatic carcinoma, metastatic malignant melanoma,** and other sarcomas that contain epithelioid cells. Some carcinomas, especially those arising in the breast, thyroid, or skin, may have a pseudoangiomatoid appearance, with interconnecting vascular channels and even cells with cytoplasmic vacuoles.[264, 269, 270] Compounding the diagnostic problem is that some of these tumors may immunohistochemically overlap EA,[264, 269, 271] demonstrating cytokeratin, vimentin, CD31, CD34, *Ulex europaeus* I lectin, or Factor VIII–related antigen reactivity. Electron microscopy is an important diagnostic adjunct in separating such carcinomas from EA, with the former showing true desmosomes and tonofilaments, features not present in EA.[269]

The separation of EA from other sarcomas that contain epithelioid cells depends on the lack of vasoformative areas in the latter tumors and the immunohistochemical absence of endothelial cell marker reactivity or Weibel-Palade bodies by electron microscopy. The use of antibody to CD31 antigen may be especially useful in this regard, as it appears, to date, to be a specific marker for vascular differentiation and hence capable of separating EA from these other sarcomas.

Although **malignant melanoma** may assume a variety of morphologic patterns, some of which simulate a vascular neoplasm,[264, 272] it can be distinguished from EA by its nesting pattern, melanin content, reactivity for S-100 protein and HMB-45 antigen, absence of endothelial markers, lack of vasoformative areas, and the electron microscopic presence of premelanosomes.

Another entity that must be distinguished from EA is **epithelioid hemangioendothelioma** (EHE). Unlike EHE, which frequently arises or is centered around large veins, EA is not angiocentric and has a more diffuse cellular proliferation. Intracytoplasmic vacuole formation is more common in EHE, whereas large vascular channels are more common in EA. Cytologically, the tumor cells of EA are larger than those in EHE and have more prominent nucleoli.[252] The antibody B73.2 apparently does not react with the cells of EHE as it does with those of EA,[259] and may be useful in this differential diagnosis when only small biopsy tissue is available for diagnosis.

Analysis of the clinical outcome in EA is hampered by the few cases so far reported. Among 14 patients with follow-up data,[252–254, 256–258] including those with visceral or cutaneous primaries, 11 developed metastatic disease at some time during their course, some even presenting with pulmonary or bone metastases.[252, 256, 257] Six patients died of tumor, three were alive with tumor, and five were alive and well, only one for longer than 5 years.

EPITHELIOID HEMANGIOENDOTHELIOMA

In 1979, Rosai et al.[273] introduced the concept of the existence of vascular lesions whose component blood vessels are lined not by flat, spindle-shaped endothelial cells, but by large, round, oval or cuboidal cells that bulge into the vessel lumina. These lining cells have an abundant eosinophilic cytoplasm and nuclei that have irregular outlines, often with deep indentations, folds, or grooves. These same cells may also occur in the stroma outside of recognizable vessels, either individually or aggregated in small nests. Here, their cytoplasm frequently contains vacuoles that coalesce to form lumina containing red blood cells. These vascular lesions frequently

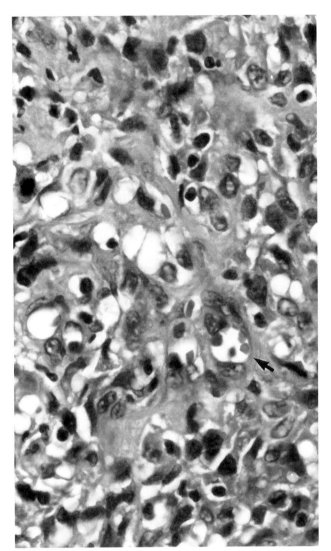

FIGURE 17–23. View of EA in which the cells show primitive vasoformative vacuoles, some of which contain red blood cells *(arrow).*

contain an associated inflammatory infiltrate composed of lymphocytes, plasma cells, neutrophils, and, most prominently, eosinophils.

Cutaneous lesions with these characteristics had been previously reported under a variety of designations, the most frequent being **angiolymphoid hyperplasia with eosinophilia** (AHE). This lesion most commonly occurs in adult women as a dermal or subcutaneous nodule in the head and neck region, especially about the ear, and although it is usually solitary, multiple nodules may occur.[274–277] The large eosinophilic cells of AHE had been shown by electron microscopy to have many of the features of endothelial cells; however, histochemically, they lacked the alkaline phosphatase of normal endothelial cells, but instead contained high levels of respiratory and hydrolytic enzymes as in histiocytes.[273, 278] Based on these latter findings, as well as their cytology and vasoformative features, Rosai et al.[273] concluded that these large eosinophilic cells were a peculiar form of endothelial cell having histiocyte-like properties. They appended the name ''histiocytoid'' to these cells, and to the lesion containing them the name ''histiocytoid hemangioma.'' **Histiocytoid**

hemangioma (HH) was an indolent lesion, although cases exhibiting locally aggressive behavior and local recurrence following operative removal did occur.

Within this seminal report, the authors made the case that some low-grade skeletal angiosarcomas, which had, paradoxically for a malignant vascular tumor, an indolent behavior and an excellent long-term prognosis, were actually examples of histiocytoid hemangioma. They also separated AHE (histiocytoid hemangioma) from **Kimura's disease,** a cutaneous lesion that occurs mainly in young Asian men and which had been erroneously equated with AHE.[273]

The cases of HH described by Rosai et al. occurred in the skin, soft tissue, and bone, but the authors indicated that they had seen similar cases in the spleen, oral cavity, external auditory canal, mediastinum, penis, and aorta.[273] Subsequent to this report, the appellation ''histiocytoid'' for the cells described by Rosai et al. was abandoned by some authors [279] in favor of the term ''epithelioid,'' with the use of the diagnostic term **''epithelioid hemangioma.''**

In 1982, Weiss and Enzinger[280] expanded the concept of vascular tumors containing epithelioid endothelial cells by their description of a distinctive vasoformative soft tissue tumor that was clinically a more aggressive lesion than epithelioid hemangioma and which they designated as epithelioid hemangioendothelioma (EHE). They pointed out that at least some of the cases originally reported by Rosai et al., as well as lesions of the lung previously designated as **intravascular bronchioloalveolar tumor** (IVBAT), and some hepatic tumors diagnosed as sclerosing cholangiosarcomas were examples of EHE. Cases of EHE were subsequently reported in the bone,[281, 282] brain, lymph nodes, and breast.[279] Although the basic morphologic features of EHE are similar in all these locations, here we confine our discussion to those within the soft tissue.

Among the 53 patients with soft tissue EHE in our review,[280, 283–289] ages ranged from 4[284] to 78[286] years; approximately 77% were older than age 30 years.[280, 283–289] The mean age among 21 patients with individual age data was 41.9 years (median, 40 years). The tumor is uncommon in children or adolescents, who accounted for less than 10% of cases. Male patients were involved in 56% of the cases.

Clinically, EHE usually manifests as a single, painful or tender mass[280, 283, 284, 288, 289] that is present for only a few weeks or as long as 4 to 5 years before diagnosis.[280, 283, 284, 286, 288, 289] Patients may have only non-specific pain[287] or symptoms of edema or thrombophlebitis.[280]

Among 50 cases with specific site location,[280, 283–289] the extremities were involved in 24 (48%), with the lower extremity in 15 (30%) and the upper extremity in 9 cases (18%). The head and neck region was involved in 15 cases (30%), the trunk in six (12%), the penis in three (6%), and the mediastinum in two (4%). EHE may be located in the subcutaneous tissue or deep within skeletal muscle; approximately one half are intimately associated with a large blood vessel, most commonly a vein.[279, 280, 285, 288] Here, the tumor either surrounds the vessel or arises within it, extending outward from the lumen toward the adventitial soft tissue, thereby causing an overall fusiform expansion of the vessel.[280] On section, these vessel-associated tumors are reddish-white and may grossly resemble an organizing thrombus; those cases of EHE unassociated with a visible blood vessel have a gray-white solid surface without evidence of hemorrhage.[279, 280, 283] Most examples of

EHE are less than 2.0 cm in maximum dimension,[280, 283, 286, 288, 289] although some as large as 5.5 cm are reported.[285]

Histologically,[280, 283, 286, 288–290] EHE is composed of large, round, polygonal to slightly elongated fusiform cells having a relatively abundant eosinophilic cytoplasm (Figs. 17–24 and 17–25). The cells are frequently arranged in strands, cords, or small nests and are characteristically embedded in a basophilic hyaline to myxoid stroma (see Fig. 17–25A) that may resemble chondroid tissue (Fig. 17–26); its staining reactions are consistent with a sulfated acid mucopolysaccharide content. Cell nuclei are round, oval, and regular, but may show folds or grooves, and contain one or two small nucleoli. When associated with a vessel, the tumor fills the lumen and exhibits a centrifugal growth pattern in which it destroys the muscle and elastic fibers of the wall and extends into the adjacent soft tissue.[279, 180]

Actual blood vessel formation by the epithelioid cells is uncommon in EHE and difficult to discern; reticulin stains may be necessary to outline nests of cells that may show small central lumina. Most commonly, however, the lesion exhibits primitive vasoformation characterized, at the cellular level, by the presence of cytoplasmic vacuoles (see Fig. 17–26) that may become so large as to eccentrically bulge and distort the cell, creating a blister-like effect.[279, 280, 284] Although these vacuolated cells may resemble the signet-ring cells of an adenocarcinoma (see Fig. 17–26), the vacuoles do not contain mucin, but may contain red blood cells. The cells lack glycogen by PAS stains; mitotic figures are usually few in number or totally absent. A lymphocytic or lymphoplasmacytic inflammatory component may be found at the periphery of the lesion, but this is not prominent. Examples of EHE are reported in which numerous osteoclast-type giant cells are found.[285, 288]

In approximately one quarter of cases, EHE has cells that are spindle-shaped, more frequent mitoses, and areas of necrosis.[279] Such cases are associated with a more aggressive clinical behavior, including metastases, and have been designated as "malignant" EHE.[279, 280] However, rare examples of EHE without these features have also behaved aggressively, with metastases, such that there is no histologic means for predicting the course of these more conventional-appearing tumors.[279]

Among nine cases of soft tissue EHE in our review that were studied electron microscopically,[280, 283, 285–287, 289] the tumor cells had many of the features of normal endothelial cells, possessing basal lamina, numerous pinocytotic vesicles, junctional cell attachments (some desmosome-like), small amounts of rough endoplasmic reticulum, and mitochondria. In addition, cytoplasmic vacuoles, at times containing flocculent amorphous material and surrounded by microvilli, were found. Weibel-Palade bodies, characteristic of endothelial cells, were variably present and not found in every case. The feature that distinguishes normal endothelial cells from those of EHE is the presence of abundant cytoplasmic intermediate filaments in the latter, which imparts to the cell its "epithelioid" quality when viewed by light microscopy.[279]

Immunohistochemical studies on EHE of the soft tissue[280, 283–289, 291–293] show reactivity in the tumor cells for a variety of endothelial cell markers: Factor VIII–related antigen[280, 283–289, 291–293] was present in 34 of 42 cases (81%); all 17 of the cases stained with *Ulex europaeus* I lectin[283, 286, 288, 291, 292] were positive, as were 13 cases stained for CD34 antigen.[291, 293] In our experience with three cases of EHE, CD31 was also a sensitive marker, being present in all. Cytokeratin was not detected in any of the 11 soft tissue examples of EHE in our review.[279, 285, 288, 292] However, two studies have reported reactivity for cytokeratin in EHE of bone.[294, 295] In one of

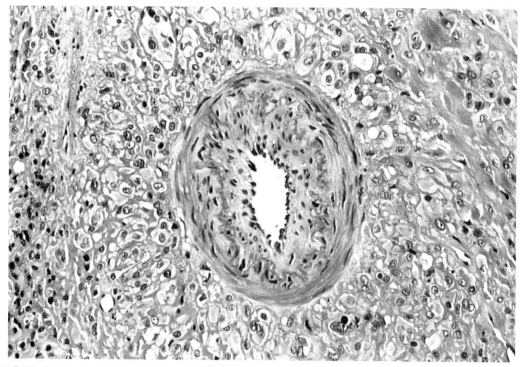

FIGURE 17–24. Epithelioid hemangioendothelioma (EHE) in which a medium-sized artery is surrounded by a proliferation of large polygonal cells.

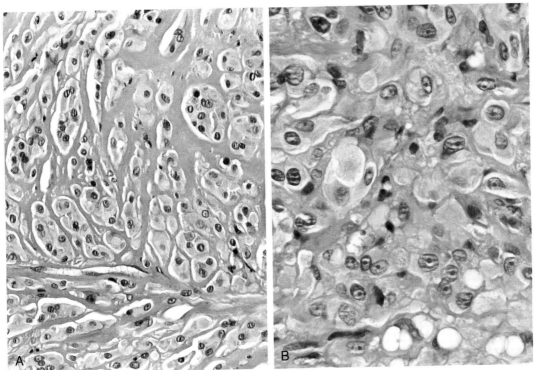

FIGURE 17–25. *A,* Cells of EHE arranged in small nests and individually within a dense hyalinized stroma. *B,* The cells of EHE are polygonal to round with an abundant cytoplasm that imparts to them an epithelioid appearance. Nuclei contain small nucleoli. Cells in the lower right of the field show cytoplasmic vacuolization.

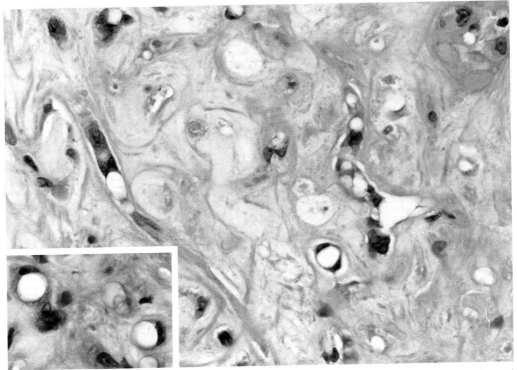

FIGURE 17–26. Chondroid-like matrix of EHE in which are dispersed tumor cells that contain primitive vasoformative cytoplasmic vacuoles. *Inset* shows blister-like cytoplasmic vacuolization that creates a signet-ring appearance.

these,[294] frozen sections yielded positive results for cytokeratin in a single case; another case of osseous EHE, for which only paraffin sections were available, was non-reactive for cytokeratin. In the second study, paraffin sections from four cases of osseous EHE were used, and all four were positive for cytokeratin.[295] The antibody concentrations used in this latter study were not stated; in the former study, two of the three antibodies employed were relatively highly concentrated. As mentioned in the discussion of epithelioid angiosarcoma, positive cytokeratin immunostaining may in some instances be due to the use of highly concentrated antibodies and may not reflect the true presence of cytokeratin. Alternatively, if these results are valid, there may be some inherent differences between EHE that originates in bone and those that arise in the soft tissue.

B72.3 antibody, an epithelial marker that is reactive in some epithelioid angiosarcomas, was not reactive in nine cases of EHE.[292] Studies for vimentin were done in only two cases, both of which were positive;[286, 289] a single case studied for S-100 protein was negative.[288]

Most patients with EHE of the soft tissue have a benign course after excision of the tumor;[279, 280, 283, 286, 288] however, local recurrences develop in 10% to 15% of cases,[279, 280, 286] and in one series metastatic disease occurred in 31% of the patients.[279] Although many of these metastatic lesions involved only regional lymph nodes,[279, 284] some patients developed systemic metastases[279, 280, 283, 289] and died of their tumor.[279, 280] Some of these metastatic tumors assumed the histologic features of epithelioid angiosarcoma.[280]

Because of its fairly distinctive morphology, the differential histologic diagnosis of EHE is limited. The presence of signet-ring type epithelioid cells may raise the possibility of **metastatic carcinoma.** However, the lack of significant cell atypia and mitotic activity in EHE, the lack of epithelial mucin, and the presence of endothelial specific markers, such as Factor VIII–related antigen and CD31, make the distinction between EHE and carcinoma fairly straightforward in most cases.

The basophilic myxoid and chondroid-like stroma of EHE, with its content of sulfated acid mucopolysaccharide, and the dispersed pattern of the tumor cells may suggest a diagnosis of **extraskeletal myxoid chondrosarcoma** (EMCS). Grossly, myxoid chondrosarcoma is multilobular and not angiocentric and characteristically is gelatinous or myxoid, in contrast with the solitary, firm, gray-white to hemorrhagic appearance of EHE. In common with the cells of EHE, those of EMCS are frequently vacuolated, have an eosinophilic cytoplasm, and may even appear epithelioid. However, the cells of EMCS contain glycogen versus its absence in those of EHE. In contrast to EHE, the cells of EMCS are reactive for S-100 protein but not for Factor VIII–related antigen. By electron microscopy, the cells of EMCS show dilated rough endoplasmic reticulin, at times with microtubules, irregular cytoplasmic processes, lipid droplets, and long spacing collagen, all of which are absent in the cells of EHE: Weibel-Palade bodies are also not present in EMCS.

The epithelioid character of the cells of EHE with their cytoplasmic vasoformative vacuoles that contain red blood cells may suggest the possibility of an **epithelioid angiosarcoma** (EA). Indeed, as noted earlier, some examples of "malignant" EHE have had metastases with the morphology of EA, and both tumors share common immunohistochemical and electron microscopic features. However, unlike EHE, epi-

thelioid angiosarcoma is not angiocentric and usually grows as a solid sheet of cells that have large prominent nucleoli versus the small nucleoli in the cells of EHE; epithelioid angiosarcoma also lacks the chondroid-like stroma of EHE. Although primitive cytoplasmic vasoformative features are found in both of these tumors, this is far more frequent in EHE. Epithelioid angiosarcoma may contain areas of conventional angiosarcoma with well-formed intercommunicating vascular channels lined by atypical endothelial cells, a feature never found in EHE. Reactivity with the antibody B72.3 has been found in some epithelioid angiosarcomas but not in EHE,[292] and thus may prove a useful adjunct in this differential diagnosis.

The cytoplasmic vacuolization with signet-ring features and the epithelioid character of the cells of EHE may suggest the possibility of a **chordoma.** However, the presence of physaliferous cells, mucin, glycogen, S-100 protein, cytokeratin, and epithelial membrane antigen in chordoma cells should enable one to easily distinguish between these two lesions.

Epithelioid sarcoma has similar epithelioid-type tumor cells as does EHE. However, the nodular pattern of epithelioid sarcoma with central collagen necrosis is not found in EHE. Although the cells of both tumors have numerous intermediate filaments, the cells of epithelioid sarcoma usually lack a basal lamina, have distinct irregular ruffled cytoplasmic borders and, in most cases, only primitive to poorly formed cell attachments. Immunohistochemically, both tumors may stain with *Ulex europaeus* I lectin, but the cells of epithelioid sarcoma are cytokeratin- and epithelial membrane–positive, markers that are absent in EHE.

In any discussion of the histologic distinction between **histiocytoid hemangioma (epithelioid hemangioma)** and EHE, one is confronted by the existing controversy over the correct terminology for these lesions. Rosai et al. claim that the lesion described as EHE is but one form of histiocytoid hemangioma, the only difference being the name.[296, 297] Weiss and Enzinger take an opposite view and point out that a variety of different entities may contain histiocytoid endothelial cells, including granulation tissue, pyogenic granuloma, organizing thrombi, and angiosarcomas, and believe that the term "histiocytoid hemangioma" should not be used as an all-encompassing diagnostic term.[298] They view "histiocytoid hemangioma" more as a unifying concept or umbrella phrase, rather than as a strict diagnostic term, under which EHE is but one of several distinct entities. Cooper[290] has addressed the issue of the specificity of HH as a diagnostic entity and its distinction from EHE. He observed that EHE and HH share overlapping morphologic features, the only distinct exception being that the myxochondroid stroma of EHE is absent in the cutaneous or soft tissue lesion described as angiolymphoid hyperplasia with eosinophilia, i.e., the histiocytoid hemangioma of Rosai and the epithelioid hemangioma of Weiss and Enzinger. A study by Fetsch and Weiss[299] makes a strong argument for the reactive nature of epithelioid hemangioma, resulting from some vascular injury, in contrast with the neoplastic character of EHE. In line with their general view of EHE as separate from epithelioid (histiocytoid) hemangioma, the authors outlined the diagnostic features they believe separate these two lesions.

In diagnostic terms, the lesion of soft tissue described under the rubric of EHE has a less definitive vascular pattern than occurs in HH (epithelioid hemangioma), in which well-formed

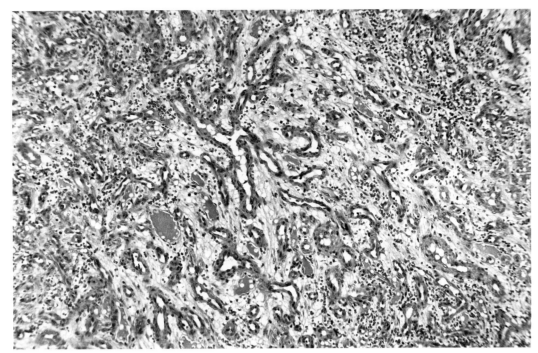

FIGURE 17–27. Histiocytoid (epithelioid) hemangioma shows an abundant proliferation of blood vessels, which contrasts with their rarity in EHE.

vascular channels are present, versus the infrequent formation of distinct vascular channels in EHE, where individual cell vasoformation is more common (Figs. 17–27 to 17–29). EHE contains a lesser degree of inflammation, including significantly fewer eosinophils, tends to occur less often in the head and neck region, and is more angiocentric than HH. The small cords and strands of cells without extensive vascular channel formation in EHE are not found in HH, and the cytoplasmic

lumina are more distinct in EHE than they are in HH. Finally, the myxoid hyaline stroma in which the cells of EHE are embedded is not found in HH.

Whatever one's view of this semantic controversy, it is important to recognize that there does exist a vascular tumor of the soft tissue, composed of epithelioid vasoformative cells within a hyaline chondroid-type stroma, that has the potential for aggressive clinical behavior. The choice of whether to call this histiocytoid hemangioma,[273] histiocytoid hemangioendothelioma,[296] or epithelioid hemangioendothelioma[280] we leave to the reader.

MALIGNANT EPITHELIOID SCHWANNOMA

Malignant epithelioid schwannoma (MES) is a rare tumor, even among soft tissue sarcomas, with fewer than 75 cases reported in the English-language medical literature.[300–311] Only two series of MES exist,[304, 305] which contain only 26 and 14 patients, respectively, with the remainder of the literature consisting of individual case reports. Malignant epithelioid schwannomas are claimed to represent from 5% to 27% of all malignant peripheral nerve sheath tumors, with the lower figure perhaps closer to the true incidence.[302, 304] One reason for the scarcity of reports on this tumor may be that the criteria for its diagnosis are not well established.[302, 304] The strongest evidence for the nerve sheath nature of these tumors is their direct association with a major nerve; however, in one series this was noted in only approximately 60% of cases.[304] In the absence of such evidence, one must use ancillary information such as the presence of von Recklinghausen's disease or the prior removal of a benign peripheral nerve sheath tumor at the site of the tumor. Electron microscopic and immunohisto-

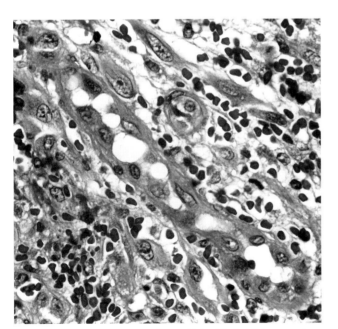

FIGURE 17–28. Vessels in histiocytoid (epithelioid) hemangioma contain lining cells with an abundant vacuolated cytoplasm that bulges into the lumina. The cytoplasmic vacuoles coalesce to create a vascular lumen.

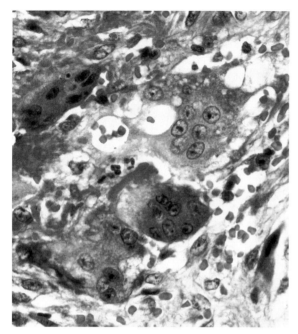

FIGURE 17–29. Multinucleated stromal giant cells, a common finding in histiocytoid hemangioma, show vacuolated cytoplasm. These vacuoles fuse to form lumina that contain red blood cells as present in one of the giant cells.

chemical studies are frequently required to support an interpretation of nerve sheath differentiation.

MES affects patients over a broad age range. Among 51 patients in our review with individual age data,[300–309, 311] ages ranged from 6 to 81 years,[304] with a mean of 38.6 years (median, 34 years); only six (12%) were younger than age 20 years. Male patients accounted for 55% of the cases.

The clinical symptoms induced by MES are variable;[300–309, 311] most patients complain of a mass, which may or may not be painful or tender. At times the mass is associated with neurologic symptoms such as paresthesia or muscle dysfunction;[302–306] in some, neurologic symptoms or pain without a clinically defined mass is the presenting complaint.[305, 306] The duration of symptoms in 22 patients in our survey ranged from 2 weeks[306] to 20 years,[311] with an average of 3.2 years (median, 12 months); four patients had symptoms for longer than 5 years, and in nine the duration was less than 1 year.

The anatomic distribution of MES is diverse. Among 52 tumors in 51 patients, the upper and lower extremities, and the major nerves in these areas, accounted for 83% of the cases, with the thigh, arm, and forearm the most common sites. Other sites included the cheek,[308] mandibular region,[301] chest wall,[304, 305, 307] abdominal wall,[305] and retroperitoneum.[309] Although most malignant epithelioid schwannomas involve the deep soft tissues, they also occur as cutaneous lesions.[304, 308] Thirty-two tumors (62%) were associated with a major or minor nerve trunk, with the sciatic nerve the most commonly involved, but nerves from superficial cutaneous to the brachial plexus have been affected. Some malignant epithelioid schwannomas have arisen within a neurofibroma or neurilemoma.[304, 305, 307, 311]

Macroscopically, MES varies greatly in size. Among 47 cases with size information,[301–308, 311] tumors ranged from 0.9 cm[304, 308] to 20 cm,[307] with an average of 5.6 cm (median, 7.0 cm); 20 (43%) were larger than 5.0 cm, and nine (19%)

were equal to or larger than 10 cm. The superficial tumors tend to be smaller, but even here tumors as large as 14 cm are reported.[304] MES is usually firm, with a white to gray-white surface that may show yellow to tan-brown areas of necrosis and hemorrhage and cystic foci.

Histologically,[300–307, 309–311] MES most frequently occurs as multiple, variably sized nodules that at times are set apart by bands of fibrous tissue. The nodules contain large, round to polygonal cells with an abundant eosinophilic to amphophilic cytoplasm (Fig. 17–30). Nuclei are large, tend to be vesicular, and characteristically have a prominent eosinophilic or basophilic central nucleolus. The cells are arranged either in compact masses or, more frequently, in rows, cords, strands, or small tight clusters within a myxoid stroma that stains with alcian blue, the reactivity being abolished by pretreatment with hyaluronidase. Necrosis and hemorrhage are frequently present, and mitotic activity varies from abundant to minimal. Intracytoplasmic fat droplets may be present, giving some cells a signet-ring appearance;[304] rare examples containing clear and rhabdoid-like cells are reported.[304] The overall general appearance of the tumor cells in MES has led several authors to describe them as "melanoma-like" (Fig. 17–31); however, melanin pigment is absent.[301, 303, 304, 306, 310] Glycogen, demonstrated by PAS stains, may be present.[303–305, 307] MES occurs in either pure form or mixed (Fig. 17–32) with the spindle cells of conventional malignant peripheral nerve sheath tumor.[300, 305] In these latter cases, one finds transitions between the spindle and the epithelioid tumor cells, with the spindle cell nuclei cytologically similar to those of the epithelioid cells.[301, 305, 308, 311]

In contrast with deep-seated malignant epithelioid schwannomas, those that arise in the dermis or subcutaneous tissue usually lack multinodularity and grow as a single mass circumscribed by the capsule of either a preexisting nerve or a benign nerve sheath tumor. Although the cells are more tightly packed in these superficial tumors, with more cell-to-cell molding, they are cytologically similar to their more deeply situated counterparts.[304]

How one classifies malignant nerve sheath tumors that have a mixture of spindle and epithelioid components is not clearly defined in the literature, with some authors stating only that a "significant" number of epithelioid cells be present in order for a tumor to qualify as an MES.[302] A reasonable course, until enough cases are accumulated to determine whether the amount of epithelioid component is prognostically important, might be to require that at least half of the tumor be composed of epithelioid cells in order to designate it as an epithelioid schwannoma.

Although some differences exist among the descriptions of the 23 cases of MES in our review that were studied by electron microscopy,[300, 302–305, 308, 309, 311] most cases contain cells that show the presence of a continuous or discontinuous basal lamina, cytoplasmic projections or processes, fat droplets, intermediate filaments, primitive junctional complexes, and, in some cases, extracellular long spacing collagen. Significantly, premelanosomes are not present.

In only a few cases of MES have immunohistochemical studies been reported.[301–305, 307, 308, 311] In the two large series of MES, reactivity for S-100 protein varied from 50%[305] to 80%[304] of the cases; among 46 cases in our review, 34 (74%) were positive for this antigen.[301–305, 307, 308, 311] Reactivity for neuron-specific enolase was found in 44% (14/32),[303–305] and Leu-7

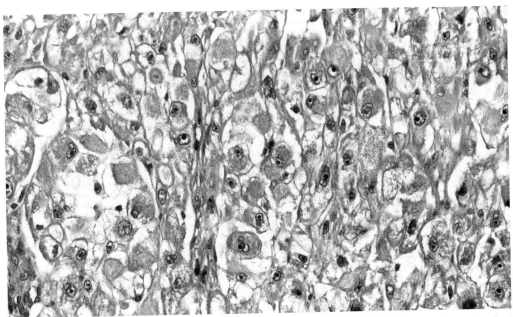

FIGURE 17–30. View of malignant epithelioid schwannoma (MES) shows loosely cohesive large cells with an abundant cytoplasm and irregular nuclei with prominent nucleoli.

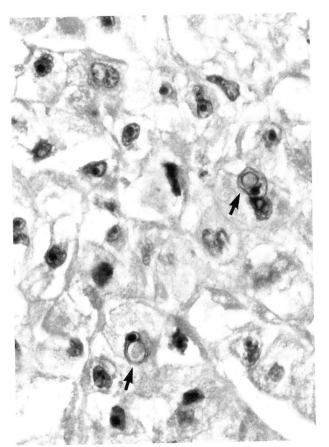

FIGURE 17–31. Melanoma-like appearance of cells of MES because some contain intranuclear cytoplasmic inclusions *(arrows)*.

was absent in the single case studied for this marker.[303] However, in our experience with MES, focal or heterogeneous reactivity for Leu-7 antigen was found in a minority of cases. Stains were negative for HMB-45 antigen in 15 cases,[304] and for cytokeratin in 18 cases,[302, 304, 307] whereas reactivity for vimentin was found in the three cases studied.[303, 307, 308] Type IV collagen was found in 17 (80%) and laminin in 12 (60%) of 20 cases.[304] Most examples of MES stained for type IV collagen show well-defined linear staining around cells and cell clusters, a feature that mirrors the electron microscopic presence of a basal lamina.

Unlike conventional malignant peripheral nerve sheath tumor, only rarely has MES been associated with von Recklinghausen's disease,[305, 307] such that the absence of the latter condition does not help in the differential diagnosis of MES. When located within a nerve or in association with a peripheral nerve sheath tumor, the histologic diagnosis of MES is greatly simplified. However, because a fair number of cases of MES occur in the absence of this association, other tumor types enter into the differential diagnosis, including **malignant melanoma, metastatic carcinoma, malignant sweat gland carcinoma,** and **myxoid chondrosarcoma.**

Desmoplastic or neurotropic malignant melanoma may be exceedingly difficult to distinguish from MES because it may lack melanin pigment and have epithelioid-like cells that contain S-100 protein. Furthermore, desmoplastic melanoma may assume a nerve-sheath appearance and may, unlike typical epithelioid variants of melanoma, acquire a collagen type IV reactive basal lamina. Typically, a scar-like fibrotic background is present in desmoplastic malignant melanoma in contrast with the myxoid stroma of MES. The cells of conventional malignant melanoma not only express S-100 protein but also HMB-45 antigen, which is absent in MES. By electron microscopy, premelanosomes are present in malignant melanoma but not in MES. However, metastatic malignant melanoma may lose evidence of its melanocytic differentiation, and the differential diagnosis with MES then depends on

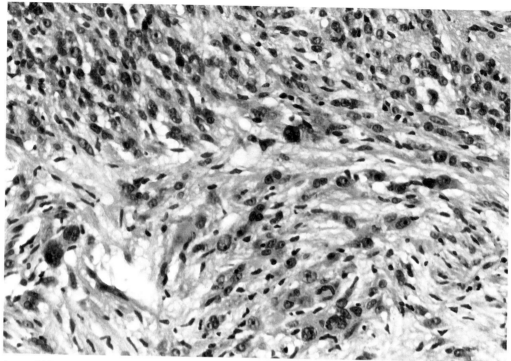

FIGURE 17–32. Area within a conventional malignant peripheral nerve sheath tumor with scattered epithelioid cells shown in the lower portion of the field.

accurate clinical information concerning the presence of a prior melanoma.[304]

Most **metastatic carcinoma** cells are positive for cytokeratin and, with the exception of breast and salivary gland carcinomas, are usually negative for S-100 protein, a phenotypic pattern the reverse of what is expected in MES. The lack of electron microscopic features of epithelial differentiation in MES also argues against a diagnosis of metastatic carcinoma. Although the cells of primary **sweat gland carcinoma** may contain S-100 protein, they are, unlike MES, also cytokeratin positive. Mucin stains may be helpful in the differential diagnosis, being positive in some metastatic carcinomas but negative in MES.

Because of its nodular array, the occasional orientation of the tumor cells in cords or strands, and its myxoid stroma, MES may be confused with **myxoid chondrosarcoma.** However, the cells of myxoid chondrosarcoma are rarely epithelioid and lack the abundant cytoplasm and prominent nucleoli of those in MES. In contrast with MES, the myxoid stroma of myxoid chondrosarcoma contains chondroitin sulfate and not hyaluronic acid as its major component. Although the cells of myxoid chondrosarcoma are S-100 protein–positive, their dilated rough endoplasmic reticulum, dense nuclear lamina, and aggregates of microtubules in association with the rough endoplasmic reticulum are features not found in MES.

MES is an aggressive neoplasm. Among 46 patients with follow-up data,[300, 301, 303–309, 311] 22 (48%) had either died of tumor (16 cases), usually with pulmonary metastases, or were alive with metastatic disease (six cases). Of the remaining 24 patients, all were alive and well, with the exception of a single patient who had died of other causes 18 years after tumor excision. Although 10 of the 23 patients had survived for 5 or more years, nine others had been followed up for only 1

year. Some authors have indicated that superficial MES has a better prognosis than those within the deep soft tissues. However, because the majority of those patients with superficial tumors had been followed up for only 1 year, and deaths from metastatic MES have occurred after 5 years,[305, 306] this conclusion may be premature.

CLEAR-CELL SARCOMA

Despite efforts to rename it **malignant melanoma of soft parts,**[312–315] for some, "clear-cell sarcoma" remains the most commonly used appellation for the unique tumor first described by Enzinger in 1965.[316] Clear-cell sarcoma (CCS) manifests itself as a mass or swelling that is painful or tender in from one third to one half of patients.[313, 315–318] The duration of symptoms until diagnosis is highly variable, with intervals as short as 1 week[313] to as long as 30 years.[319] In our review of 207 patients in whom clinical duration was specified,[312, 314, 315, 317–331] 23% had manifestations of their tumor for 5 or more years, whereas in an approximately equal percentage the duration was 1 year or less; the average interval in two large series of CCS varied from 20 months[318] to 3.5 years.[316]

The largest single series of cases of CCS, reported from the Armed Forces Institute of Pathology (AFIP), consisted of 141 patients whose ages ranged from 7 to 83 years, with a mean of 32 years (median, 27 years).[313] Among 154 additional patients in the literature for whom individual age data were supplied,[312, 314–316, 318–323, 325–341] the average age was 34.1 years (median, 28.5 years), with a range from 9[315] to 82[319] years. Combining these data, approximately 70% of patients with CCS are between 10 and 39 years of age, with one half younger than age 30 years. The tumor is uncommon in those younger than age 10 years, with only four such patients[313, 315, 317] among the total 295 cases (1.4%) in our review. Female patients accounted for 54% of 271 patients with gender information.[312, 314, 315, 318–341]

CCS is overwhelmingly an extremity based tumor. Among 292 cases,[312–315, 317–339, 341] the extremities were involved in 275 (94%), with the lower extremity accounting for 72% of the total cases. The tumor has a predilection for the foot and ankle, a region that alone accounted for 40% (116/292) of all cases. Other common sites included the knee region (15%), the thigh (10%), and the hands and fingers (9%). The trunk and the head and neck region are uncommon locations for CCS, accounting for only 4% and 1.4% of the cases, respectively; exceptional examples of CCS are reported in the penis[330] and in bone.[331]

Within the extremities, CCS is deeply situated and, characteristically, tends to involve tendons, aponeuroses, and the fascia. Although it may extend to the subcutaneous tissue or lower dermis, it does not involve the superficial skin.[313, 316, 317, 329] Grossly, CCS appears as a nodular or lobulated mass that may appear infiltrative or well-circumscribed.[313, 316, 317, 325] Its cut surface is gray-white but may exhibit tan to black areas.[313, 314, 316, 321, 322, 329, 341] Although clear-cell sarcomas as large as 15 cm are reported,[313] most are less than 5.0 cm. Among 131 examples of CCS with tumor dimensions, the mean maximum size was 4.4 cm (median, 4.0 cm); approximately two thirds were less than 5.0 cm, 40% between 2.0 and 3.9 cm in maximum dimension.*

In its usual form, the histologic appearance of CCS is fairly distinctive. A homogeneous proliferation of fusiform to polygonal epithelioid-like cells are arranged in clusters, nests, or short fascicles set off by delicate fibrous septa (Figs. 17–33 and 17–34), the latter well illustrated by reticulin stains.[313, 316–318, 322, 325, 329] These septa are frequently in continuity with denser and broader collagenous bundles in continuity with adjacent tendons, aponeuroses, or fascial elements.[313, 316, 318] The tumor cells generally have a pale to clear cytoplasm with indistinct cell borders; however, belying its name, the cells of some clear-cell sarcomas may have a granular eosinophilic cytoplasm (see Figs. 17–33 to 17–35) that does not appear ''clear.''[316] Nuclei are round to oval and, characteristically, have a large, usually single, prominent basophilic or eosinophilic nucleolus (Fig. 17–35).[313, 316–318, 325] Significant cellular or nuclear pleomorphism is lacking in most examples of CCS;[313, 315, 316, 318, 325, 331] however, in some reports cell pleomorphism was found in as many as one third of cases,[315, 318, 331] most notably in recurrences or metastases where it may be of such a degree that the tumor is no longer recognizable as a CCS.[313, 316, 325, 337] Less often, the cells of CCS may assume spindle shapes[318, 319, 325, 337, 341] and be arranged in large fascicles creating a fibrosarcomatous appearance (Fig. 17–36). However, careful search of the sections usually discloses the more classic areas. CCS tends to grow along nerves and tendon sheaths in a cord-like fashion, with the cells residing within a desmoplastic stroma.[313, 316, 317, 325] A common histologic feature is the presence of multinucleated giant cells, of the Touton or osteoclast type (Fig. 17–37), that occur in one half to two thirds of cases.[313, 316–319, 322, 325, 334, 340] Mitotic activity

is variable. Most examples of CCS have only a scarce number of mitotic figures; however, in some, mitoses may be numerous.[313, 315–318, 325, 331, 334]

The clear tumor cell cytoplasm is due to the presence of abundant glycogen, demonstrable by PAS stains, in virtually all examples of CCS.[312, 313, 319, 325, 334] Both melanin and hemosiderin pigment may also be found on routine hematoxylin and eosin sections.* Special stains for melanin, such as the Fontana-Masson or the more sensitive Warthin-Starry, are positive in the majority of cases of CCS. In 158 cases in which melanin stains were done,† 89 (56%) were positive; however, in the large series from the AFIP in which the Warthin-Starry stain was used, approximately 75% of the cases were positive.[313]

In our review, 35 cases of CCS were studied by electron microscopy, and, with minor differences, the results have been fairly consistent.‡ The tumor cells contain smooth or irregularly shaped convoluted nuclei and, most characteristically, a large prominent nucleolus. The cytoplasm is rich in organelles, with numerous, sometimes dilated mitochondria; prominent Golgi zones; and a granular endoplasmic reticulum. Free ribosomes and polyribosomes are frequently present, as is cytoplasmic glycogen in particulate or aggregate form. An important diagnostic feature is the presence of premelanosomes or melanosomes; however, their number is variable, and, as in malignant melanoma, an extensive search may be required for their discovery. Whorled cytoplasmic microfilaments and intermediate filaments are reported in a few cases.[320, 325, 341] The cell membrane may exhibit irregular cytoplasmic processes that interdigitate with those from neighboring cells. An external basal lamina is present, and although there are no true desmosomes, there may be primitive or intermediate type cell junctions.

Immunohistochemical studies of CCS§ showed the absence of cytokeratin[318, 331, 334, 338, 340] and epithelial membrane antigen[331, 334] in 35 and 11 cases, respectively, whereas vimentin[318, 331, 334] was detected in 83% (29/35). Stains for S-100 protein‖ were positive in 77% (65/84), and reactivity for HMB-45 antigen[318, 331, 334, 338] was found in a similar percentage of cases (27/35). Neuron-specific enolase[331, 338] was present in 71% (5/17), and Leu-7[331, 334, 338] in 42% (5/12), whereas synaptophysin[331, 338] was found in only one of seven cases (14%). Stains for muscle-specific actin[331] in six cases, and for desmin[331, 338] in seven cases, were negative.

Despite the characteristic light microscopic appearance of CCS, a number of other diagnostic entities enter into the differential diagnosis because of the epithelioid appearance of the tumor cells, the occasional spindle cell patterns, and the presence of melanin or premelanosomes by electron microscopy.

The occurrence of spindle cell areas in CCS may raise the question of **synovial sarcoma.** This should pose no diagnostic problem if the tumor in question shows the classic biphasic

---

* References 312, 314–316, 318–325, 329–333, 336, 338, 340, 341.

* References 313, 314, 316–319, 321, 322, 324, 328, 333, 334.
† References 312–314, 319–322, 324, 325, 327, 328, 330, 333–337, 340, 341.
‡ References 312, 314, 319–322, 324, 325, 327, 329, 330, 333–336, 339–341.
§ References 312–314, 316, 318–322, 324, 325, 327, 328, 330, 331, 333–338, 340, 341.
‖ References 312, 313, 318, 320, 325, 327, 330, 331, 334, 338, 340.

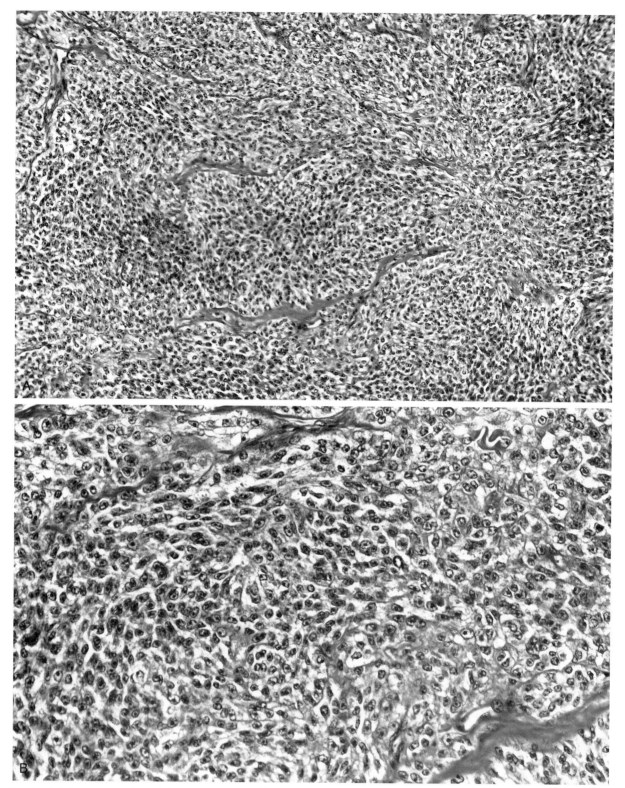

FIGURE 17–33. *A,* Low-power view of clear-cell sarcoma (CCS) shows tumor cells traversed by thin fibrous septa. *B,* Higher magnification of tumor cells shows uniform nuclei with prominent nucleoli. The cytoplasm varies from pale to granular.

pattern of synovial sarcoma. However, when the epithelial component of a synovial sarcoma is scarce or absent, its histologic distinction from CCS may be problematic. However, the large amount of glycogen in CCS contrasts with its absence in synovial sarcoma. Similarly, the presence of epithelial markers and the absence of S-100 protein and HMB-

45 antigen in synovial sarcoma serve to distinguish it from CCS. In addition, the electron microscopic features of CCS, with its large prominent nucleoli and premelanosomes, are absent in synovial sarcoma.

In the same vein, there should be no significant diagnostic difficulty in distinguishing **epithelioid sarcoma** from CCS.

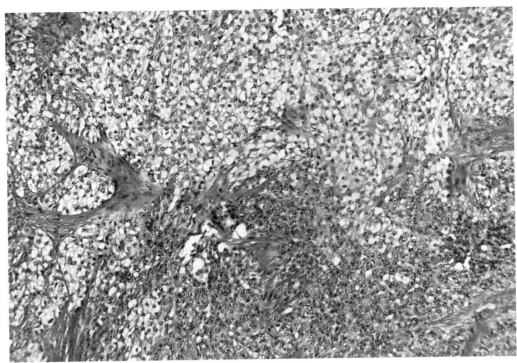

FIGURE 17–34. Clear-cell sarcoma with juxtaposition of cells having clear cytoplasm and those with a dark and granular cytoplasm.

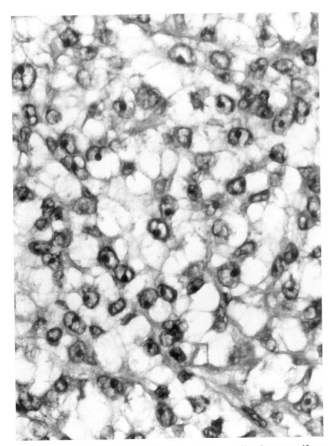

FIGURE 17–35. Higher magnification of clear cells shows uniform oval nuclei with prominent nucleoli.

Epithelioid sarcoma is predominantly an upper extremity tumor that is superficially located and frequently extends into the skin with ulceration. In contrast, CCS is a deeply situated, lower extremity tumor that does not involve the superficial skin. The cells of epithelioid sarcoma have a more eosinophilic cytoplasm than those of CCS and tend to be arranged in nodular aggregates about a central collagenous stroma that shows central necrosis. The cells of epithelioid sarcoma are positive for cytokeratin and epithelial membrane antigen, and although some are reported to be S-100 protein–positive, the cells lack reactivity for HMB-45 antigen. Electron microscopically, the abundant perinuclear whorled arrays of cytoplasmic intermediate filaments in epithelioid sarcoma are absent in CCS, and epithelioid sarcoma lacks premelanosomes.

Epithelioid leiomyosarcoma contains round epithelioid-type cells that have a clear cytoplasm. However, the lack of large prominent nucleoli in epithelioid leiomyosarcoma, the presence of muscle-specific actin and desmin, the absence of S-100 protein and HMB-45 antigen, and the variable presence of electron microscopic features of smooth muscle differentiation reliably distinguish it from CCS.

Metastatic **clear-cell carcinoma** may also be a diagnostic consideration, but the lack of epithelial markers in CCS, or clinical evidence of a known primary carcinoma, helps eliminate this diagnostic alternative.

The presence of osteoclast-type giant cells, hemosiderin pigment, and the intimate relationship to tendons may, rarely, cause confusion between CCS and **giant cell tumor of tendon sheath.** However, the latter lesion is more nodular, lacks a nesting pattern, may have a dense fibrous stroma that harbors foamy histiocytes, and does not display immunohistochemical or electron microscopic evidence of melanocytic differentiation.

Because of its nesting quality, **alveolar soft part sarcoma** may be a histologic consideration. As in CCS, the cells of

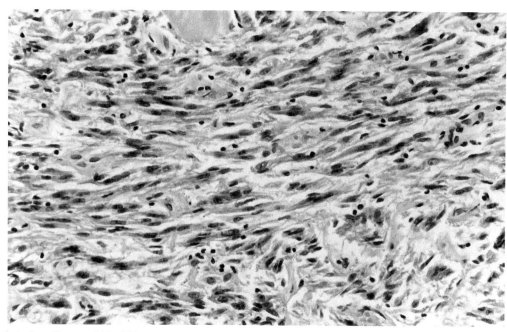

FIGURE 17–36. Spindle cell area within CCS. This pattern may cause diagnostic confusion, especially in small biopsy tissue, as the cells give no clue as to the correct diagnosis.

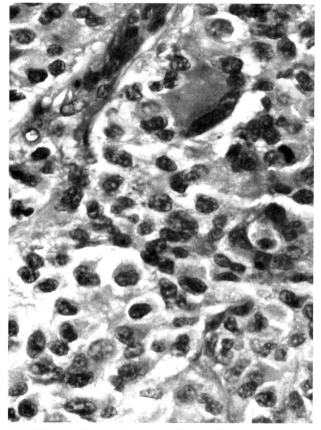

FIGURE 17–37. Clear cell sarcoma with multinucleated giant cell.

alveolar soft part sarcoma are set off in an organoid pattern by fine fibrous septa. However, the eosinophilic cytoplasm of the cells in alveolar soft part sarcoma is denser and more granular than that of CCS. Unlike the cells of CCS, those of alveolar soft part sarcoma contain cytoplasmic PAS-positive, diastase-resistant crystalline material, and the cell nests have an intimate relationship to blood vessels, a feature absent in CCS. Immunohistochemically, alveolar soft part sarcoma lacks S-100 protein and may contain muscle markers such as muscle-specific actin, desmin, and MyoD1. By electron microscopy, the cells of alveolar soft part sarcoma contain diagnostic cytoplasmic rhomboid crystalloids that are not found in CCS.

Malignant epithelioid schwannoma may contain epithelioid polygonal cells with prominent nucleoli. However, these cells reside in a myxoid stroma that is absent in CCS, and despite being positive for S-100 protein, the cells of malignant epithelioid schwannoma lack HMB-45 antigen, and premelanosomes by electron microscopy.

The tumor that is most difficult to distinguish from CCS is **malignant melanoma.** Both CCS and melanoma have a nesting quality and contain S-100 protein, HMB-45 antigen, melanin, and premelanosomes. However, the cells of malignant melanoma are usually more pleomorphic and anaplastic, have a denser eosinophilic cytoplasm, and are more mitotically active than those of CCS. The prolonged clinical course of CCS patients (see later) also argues against a diagnosis of metastatic melanoma. Malignant melanoma is typically more superficially located and only rarely contains osteoclast-like or Touton giant cells. The lack of involvement of the overlying skin argues against a primary diagnosis of malignant melanoma, although in metastatic sites melanoma often is devoid of an epidermal component. There are some who believe that CCS is in actuality the soft tissue counterpart of cutaneous or visceral malignant melanoma,[313–315, 319, 333, 340] a view reflected in the appellation ''malignant melanoma of soft parts.''[312, 313, 315, 326, 333] This subtle semantic argument, however, is of little consequence. The most important point is to establish that one is dealing with a primary sarcoma and not an example of metastatic melanoma. For this determination, accurate and complete clinical information is of critical importance.

CCS is a highly malignant tumor that, however, may have a long clinical course prior to the development of local or systemic recurrences or death. In some of the larger series of CCS, the mortality rate has been 44%,[313] 53%,[325] 54%,[318] 59%,[315] and 62%.[319] Among 256 patients with follow-up data,[312–315, 318–329, 331–338, 340, 341] 127 died of tumor (49.6%), 43 were alive with tumor (16.8%), and 86 were alive and well (33.6%). Local recurrences after excision are frequent and may be multiple;[313, 319] however, the time to first recurrence may take several years.[315, 318, 333, 338] In some patients intervals as long as 17 or 18 years have been reported.[313, 317, 337] Similarly, metastases, most commonly to lymph nodes or lung, may be delayed for many years;[318, 325] metastatic disease has developed in some patients 30 years after therapy.[313, 316] Thus, 5-year survival rates underestimate the ultimate poor prognosis of CCS.[318]

SPINDLE CELL HEMANGIOENDOTHELIOMA

Spindle cell hemangioendothelioma (SCH) was first described by Weiss and Enzinger in 1986 as a distinctive low-grade angiosarcoma with histologic characteristics that combine the features of cavernous hemangioma and Kaposi's sarcoma.[342] SCH is uncommon, with fewer than 75 cases reported in the English-language medical literature.[342–350] Clinically, SCH develops as a painless nodule in the superficial soft tissue or dermis,[342, 344, 345, 348, 349] although the deep soft tissue and muscle may also be the site of origin.[342, 344] SCH is notable for its slow evolution; some patients have a history of having their lesions for 25 to 30 years, during which time multiple lesions may develop.[342, 344–350] Among 61 patients in our review for whom the number of lesions was documented, 32 (53%) had multiple lesions at the time of presentation. Some patients with SCH have had other associated conditions including Maffucci's syndrome, congenital lymphedema, and Klippel-Trenaunay syndrome.[342, 345, 347, 349]

SCH affects patients of any age from newborns[345, 349] to those in the eighth decade of life,[344] but it predominantly occurs in young adults. Among 43 patients, for whom individual age data were reported,[343–350] the average age at diagnosis was 31 years (median, 29 years); 56% were younger than age 30 years. However, some of these adult patients had developed their lesions in infancy or early childhood, which emphasizes the slow development of this tumor. SCH has an approximately equal sex distribution, with 36 male and 35 female patients in our review.[342–350]

SCH has a diverse anatomic distribution. Including patients with multiple lesions, there were 83 tumors with specific site information in our review.[342–350] The extremities were involved in 81%, with the upper extremity in 32 and the lower in 35 cases. The hands and feet accounted for approximately 60% of all the cases. Other sites included the vulva,[347, 349] penis,[349]

trunk and chest wall,[342, 344, 345, 349] and bone.[347] The head and neck region was only rarely involved.[349] Grossly, SCH appears as a well-demarcated, reddish-purple, hemorrhagic nodule. Most are small,[342, 344, 345, 348, 350] less than 2.0 cm in maximum size, although some as large as 11.0 cm are reported.[345]

Histologically,[344–351] SCH is characterized by a biphasic pattern of large, thin-walled cavernous-type blood vessels, which frequently contain organized thrombi or phleboliths, between which are solid cellular Kaposi sarcoma–like areas (Figs. 17–38 and 17–39A). These cellular areas contain spindle-shaped cells whose nuclei are round or elongated without atypia or pleomorphism (Figs. 17–39B and 17–40). The spindle cells form a network of slit-like vascular spaces, among which extravasated red blood cells are frequently present. (see Fig. 17–40), or short interlacing fascicles without vascular spaces. Some of the slit-like spaces are lined by plump, epithelioid (histiocytoid) cells with a pale eosinophilic cytoplasm and oval to round nuclei;[342, 344–347, 349] similar epithelioid cells are found within the cellular areas either singly or in small clusters. The epithelioid cells frequently contain either multiple or single cytoplasmic vacuoles, the latter producing signet-ring cells with compressed nuclei.[342, 344, 345, 347, 349] Such cells are similar to the vacuolated vasoformative epithelioid cells of **epithelioid hemangioendothelioma (histiocytoid hemangioma)**. Occasional cases of SCH appear to arise in the wall or lumen of a large blood vessel.[343, 349] Here, the tumor may have a papillary character with projecting fronds covered by endothelial cells, creating a pattern similar to that seen in **intravascular papillary endothelial hyperplasia of Masson.**[346] Smooth muscle cells are found in SCH distributed either at the periphery of the large cavernous vessels or haphazardly as fascicles within the cellular zones of the tumor.[345] Large, malformed, thick and thin-walled blood vessels, resembling arteriovenous malformations, may occur at the margins of the tumor nodules.[343, 345] The occurrence of such vascular areas has led to speculation that SCH represents a reactive process rather than a true neoplasm.[343, 345] Mitotic activity in SCH is rare to absent.[342, 344, 347–350]

The electron microscopic features of SCH have been described in six cases.[342, 344–346, 349] The cells lining the thin-walled vessels have the features of endothelial cells, including the presence of Weibel-Palade bodies, but, unlike normal endothelial cells, they may contain abundant cytoplasmic intermediate filaments. The epithelioid cells show abundant aggregates of intermediate cytoplasmic filaments, pinocytotic vesicles, subplasmalemmal dense bodies, and interdigitating junctional complexes or desmosome-like junctions. The spindle cells between the vessels have features of macrophages, pericytes, fibroblasts, or smooth muscle cells. Some of these cells also have Weibel-Palade bodies, as well as abundant intermediate filaments and pinocytotic vesicles.

Immunohistochemically,[343–350] the endothelial cells of the large cavernous spaces are reactive for vimentin, Factor VIII–related antigen, and *Ulex europaeus* I lectin. The spindle cell elements, although also reactive for vimentin, are not stained with the latter endothelial markers,[342, 344, 345, 347, 348, 350] but were reactive for smooth muscle actin, muscle-specific actin, and desmin in four of seven cases.[344] The epithelioid cells have been less well characterized in these lesions. In five cases they were positive for Factor VIII–related antigen, for *Ulex europaeus* I lectin in four of the cases, and for vimentin in all five; all were negative for cytokeratin, muscle-

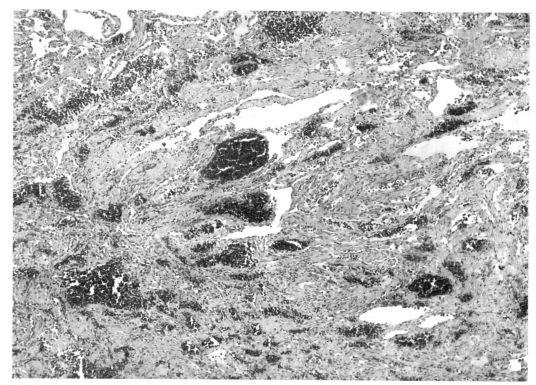

FIGURE 17–38. Spindle cell hemangioendothelioma (SCH) shows large cavernous blood vessels between which is a proliferation of spindle cells.

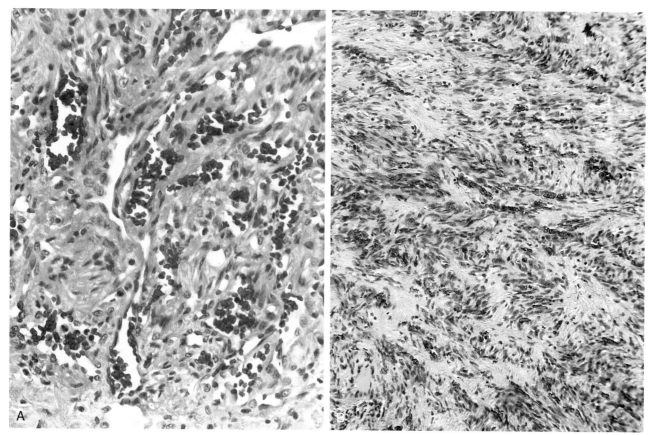

FIGURE 17–39. *A,* Thin-walled engorged capillaries traverse a spindle cell stroma. *B,* Spindle cell area in SCH in which there are slit-like compressed capillaries.

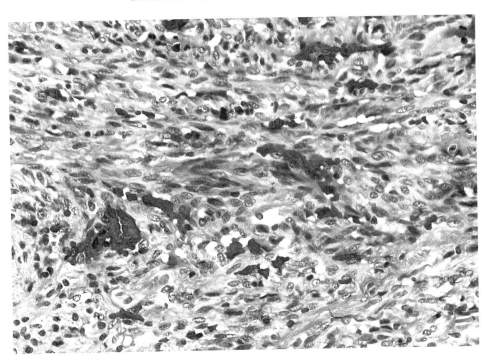

FIGURE 17–40. Higher magnification of SCH with Kaposi-like spindle cell area and extravasated red blood cells. The spindle cells lack the atypia of those in Kaposi's sarcoma.

specific and smooth muscle actin, desmin, and epithelial membrane antigen.[344]

The lesion that most resembles SCH histologically is **Kaposi's sarcoma.** Both lesions may be multifocal and affect the distal extremities, and both contain spindle cells forming slit-like spaces with extravasated red blood cells. However, with the exception of its occurrence in AIDS patients, Kaposi's sarcoma usually affects much older individuals than does SCH. The cells of Kaposi's sarcoma are cytologically more atypical than those of SCH, and the cavernous blood spaces with thrombi found in SCH are lacking in Kaposi's sarcoma, as are the epithelioid endothelial and stromal cells with their cytoplasmic vacuolization. The hyaline globules of Kaposi's sarcoma are not found in SCH.[344, 347, 349]

Because of the occasional location of SCH in a large blood vessel, **Masson's intravascular papillary endothelial hyperplasia** may be a diagnostic consideration. However, the multifocality of SCH and histiocytoid endothelial cells are lacking in intravascular papillary endothelial hyperplasia.

Epithelioid hemangioendothelioma shares with SCH the presence of histiocytoid (epithelioid) endothelial cells with prominent cytoplasmic vacuolization and intracellular lumen formation. However, epithelioid hemangioendothelioma is more frequently angiocentric than is SCH, has a chondroid-like stroma that is absent in SCH, and does not have spindle cell areas with slit-like vascular spaces or cavernous blood vessels. That these two entities share a close relationship is emphasized by the occurrence in some SCH patients of separate lesions of epithelioid hemangioendothelioma.[342, 345, 350]

Although initially introduced as an example of a low-grade angiosarcoma,[342] subsequent studies have shown that SCH is an indolent lesion characterized by either the development of local recurrences after excision or the onset of new lesions unrelated to the site of the original mass over the course of many years.[342, 343, 345, 349] The absence of deaths directly attributable to SCH lends some credence to those who believe that SCH is a peculiar non-neoplastic reactive vascular lesion.[343–346] Conventional angiosarcoma has developed in some patients with SCH.[342, 345]

ANGIOMATOID MALIGNANT FIBROUS HISTIOCYTOMA

Since its original description in 1979 by Enzinger,[352] approximately 150 cases of angiomatoid malignant fibrous histiocytoma (AMFH) have been reported in the English-language medical literature.[353–361] Although initially believed to be a variant of malignant fibrous histiocytoma (MFH), subsequent authors have considered AMFH to be vascular,[356, 360] histiocytic,[359, 361] fibrohistiocytic,[358] myogenic, or myofibroblastic,[354, 362] or a pleuripotential lesion able to differentiate into a variety of mesenchymal tissues.[357] Notwithstanding these divergent views, it is generally agreed that AMFH does not fit the usual mold of MFH in terms of its age incidence, location, microscopic pattern, or relatively indolent clinical behavior.

AMFH has occurred in newborns[358] and in patients 70 years of age,[353] but predominantly affects children and adolescents. In our review of 33 cases in which individual patient ages are reported,[354–358, 360, 361] approximately 80% were younger than 20 years of age, with 36% younger than age 10 years; the mean age was 14.2 years (median, 11.0 years). Female patients accounted for 53% of 141 patients in whom gender was stated.[352, 353, 355–357, 360, 361]

Clinically, AMFH is a slowly growing tumor[352, 353] that is associated with constitutional signs or symptoms in from 14% to 25% of patients, the most common being anemia, often of severe degree; others include weight loss, fever, night sweats, and an increased serum gamma globulin level.[352–354, 357, 358]

AMFH most commonly occurs in the subcutaneous tissue, but may extend to involve the underlying muscle or the lower dermis.[352–354] Among 140 patients in whom the site of the tumor was stated,[352–358, 360, 361] the upper extremity was involved in 43%, the lower extremity in 28%, the trunk in 24%, and the head and neck region in 6% of cases. Grossly, AMFH appears well-circumscribed or sharply delimited[352, 353, 361] and has varied in size from 0.7 cm[352] to 12 cm.[353, 358] In 26 cases with specific size information,[355, 356, 358, 360, 361] the mean maximum dimension was 3.7 cm (median, 3.0 cm). On section, the cut surface is tan to brown and either contains cystic spaces, which are filled with fresh or clotted blood, or has solid hemorrhagic foci.[352, 353, 355, 358, 360, 361]

Histologically,[352–354, 356–358, 360, 361] AMFH consists of a nodular mass delimited by dense, often hyalinized, fibrocollagenous tissue (Fig. 17–41). The nodule contains whorls or fascicles of spindle cells that have elongated, bland vesicular nuclei and pale eosinophilic cytoplasm (Fig. 17–42). In some cases, scattered cells may have pleomorphic nuclei.[352, 353, 356] Characteristically, cystic spaces are present that contain fresh or clotted blood (Fig. 17–43). These spaces, which are more prominent centrally, lack an endothelial lining and are surrounded by plump, histiocyte-like cells that have a pale eosinophilic cytoplasm (Fig. 17–44). Another histologic feature of AMFH is the presence of peripheral aggregates of lymphoplasmacytic cells (Figs. 17–42B and 17–45). These aggregates may have germinal centers such that at low-power examination it may appear that the mass represents a lymph node with metastatic tumor.[352, 356, 358, 360] However, these lymphoplasmacytic aggregates lack the peripheral sinuses of lymph nodes. Similar aggregates of lymphocytes and plasma cells may extend into the tumor, dividing the spindle and histiocyte-like areas into lobules. Small capillaries may permeate the spindle cell areas, and large ectatic blood spaces lined by endothelial cells may be an integral part of the tumor. Associated with this extensive vascularity is the presence, in the majority of cases, of diffuse and abundant extracellular and intracellular hemosiderin deposits and stromal hemorrhages.[352, 356–358, 361] Multinucleated giant cells and foam cells may be present.[352, 354, 356–358] Despite an overall general fibrohistiocytic appearance, storiform foci are rarely found in AMFH.[352, 357, 358]

In some examples of AMFH, the hemorrhagic cystic spaces either are lacking or constitute only a minor aspect of the lesion.[353] In such cases, the tumor is composed almost entirely of sheets of spindle and histiocyte-like cells (see Fig. 17–45). Myxoid foci may occur in which the tumor cells are irregularly dispersed. In general, mitotic activity in AMFH is minimal, although exceptions exist in which there is brisk activity.[352–354, 357, 361] Despite its usual well-circumscribed borders, some examples of AMFH have irregular infiltrating margins and extend from the subcutaneous tissue into the underlying skeletal muscle or the lower dermis.[352–354]

Only a few examples of AMFH have been studied by electron microscopy,[356–358, 360, 361, 363] the results of which have yielded disparate views as to the nature of the constituent tumor cells. Such fine structural features as basal lamina, desmosomes, bundles of intermediate filaments, pinocytotic vesicles, lipid droplets, lysosomes, well-developed rough endoplasmic reticulum, complex cytoplasmic projections, myofilaments, Z-lines, and Weibel-Palade bodies all have been described in one case or another, leading to opinions, based on these findings, that the tumor is endothelial, myogenic, histiocytic, fibroblastic, or myofibroblastic in nature.

Immunohistochemical studies[354, 356, 358, 359, 361] have only partly clarified this situation. To date, the endothelial cell markers Factor VIII–related antigen and *Ulex europaeus* I lectin have been uniformly negative in 23[354, 356, 358, 359, 361] and 10 cases,[358, 359] respectively, making a vascular derivation of this

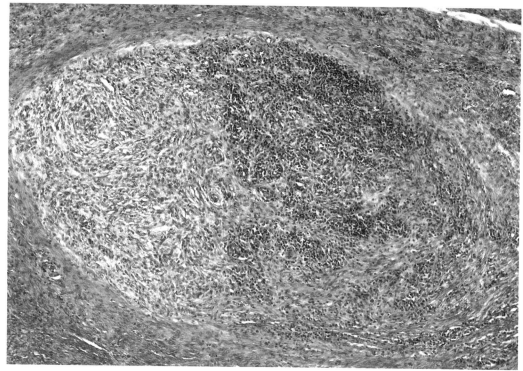

FIGURE 17–41. Nodular lesion of angiomatoid malignant fibrous histiocytoma (AMFH) is surrounded by fibrocollagenous tissue. One half of the nodule is composed of chronic inflammatory cells.

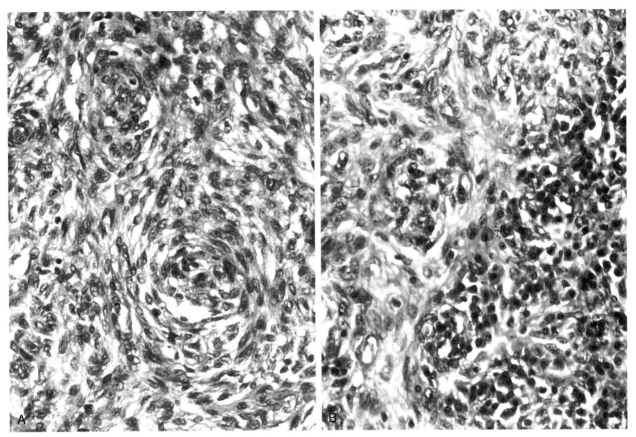

FIGURE 17–42. *A,* Focus within AMFH where uniform spindle cells are arranged in a swirling pattern. *B,* Juxtaposition of plasma cells and lymphocytes to the spindle cells.

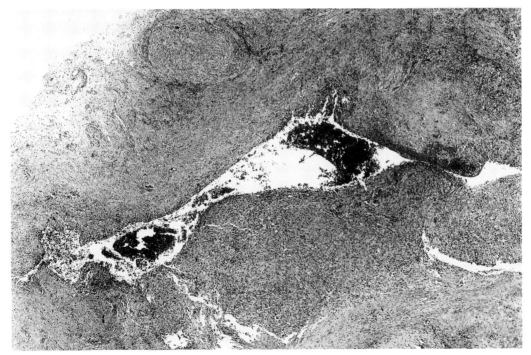

FIGURE 17–43. Large, ectatic blood-filled cystic space in AMFH.

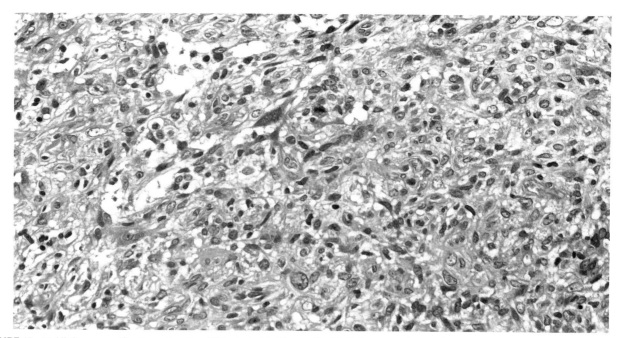

FIGURE 17–44. Higher magnification of cyst wall illustrated in Figure 17–43. Cells are oval, round, and spindle-shaped with pale, granular cytoplasm. Some have large and mildly atypical nuclei. Overall appearance of the cells creates a "fibrohistiocytic" aura.

tumor unlikely. Negative results have also been obtained for cytokeratin[354, 358, 359] and epithelial membrane antigen.[358] Vimentin was found in all cases,[354, 358] as well as alpha-1-antichymotrypsin[358, 361] and alpha-1-antitrypsin, although the latter was reported to be only focally present.[358] Stains for CD68 antigen, a putative macrophage marker, using KP antibody,[359, 362] were positive in 23 of 33 cases (70%), but stains for muramidase were negative in six cases.[359] Another putative histiocytic marker, MAC387, was absent in all 25 cases studied;[354, 359] smooth muscle actin was not found in four cases,[354] but muscle-specific actin[354, 358] was present in 11 of 15 (73%) and desmin[354, 358, 359, 362] in 10 of 24 cases (42%). The

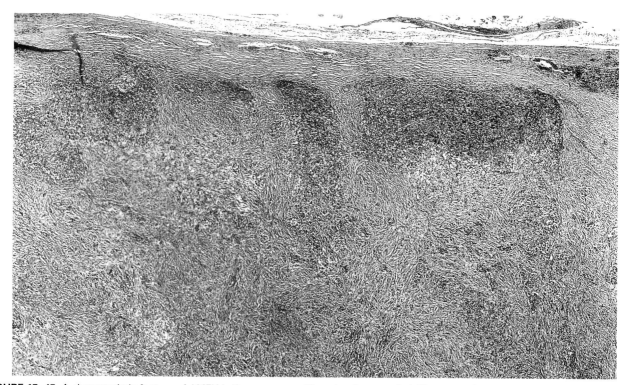

FIGURE 17–45. A characteristic feature of AMFH is the presence of lymphoplasmacytic infiltrates at the periphery of the tumor nodules as illustrated. At low-power magnification, there is a superficial resemblance to a lymph node, but a peripheral sinus is absent.

results of these immunohistochemical studies have led some to propose that AMFH, rather than being a fibrohistiocytic lesion, is a myogenous or myofibroblastic lesion,[354, 362] with the suggestion that the tumor be renamed "**angiomatoid myosarcoma.**"[354] Others take a more neutral stance, suggesting a mesenchymal derivation or differentiation but unable to support either a histiocytic or myogenic differentiation based on the currently available evidence.[353]

Several diagnostic entities enter the light microscopic differential diagnosis of AMFH, including **Kaposi's sarcoma, cutaneous aneurysmal fibrous histiocytoma, sclerosing hemangioma,** and **angiosarcoma.** Kaposi's sarcoma occurs in older patients than does AMFH and, unlike AMFH, is primarily a dermal tumor that has spindle cells, with hyaline cytoplasmic globules, among which are slit-like vascular spaces. Kaposi's sarcoma lacks the nodularity, lymphoplasmacytic aggregates, and the reactivity for histiocytic or smooth muscle markers of AMFH.

Aneurysmal fibrous histiocytoma is a dermal lesion that occurs in older patients than does AMFH. Although its ectatic pseudovascular spaces, abundant hemosiderin deposition, and chronic inflammatory cells are features shared with AMFH, aneurysmal fibrous histiocytoma characteristically has storiform spindle cell areas, which are only rarely present in AMFH, and foci of classic dermatofibroma.

Primary vascular lesions such as **angioma** or **angiosarcoma** are unlikely to be confused with AMFH in view of their usual immunohistochemical reactivity with various endothelial cell markers. However, poorly differentiated angiosarcomas may yield negative results with stains for Factor VIII–related antigen or with *Ulex europaeus* I lectin. In contrast to AMFH, angiosarcoma affects a significantly older population, is more ill defined grossly, microscopically contains intercommunicating vascular channels, has more cellular pleomorphism, and lacks lymphoplasmacytic aggregates.

The clinical course of AMFH is usually indolent, although local recurrences develop in from 12% to 25% of cases. Most such recurrences have been attributed to inadequate local excision.[353, 354, 357, 358] AMFH is considerably less aggressive than conventional MFH, with the majority of patients alive and well after only local excision.[353–355, 357, 358, 360, 361] However, many of the individual reports and small series include patients with short follow-up intervals. Among 94 patients with extended follow-up from the Armed Forces Institute of Pathology (AFIP),[353] only one patient died of disease, although five developed local lymph node metastases, a phenomenon also noted in other studies.[354, 357, 358] Based on the occurrence of lymph node metastases, and three patient deaths due to tumor,[353, 354, 358] at least one of whom had distant metastases,[353] AMFH is considered to be a low-grade aggressive neoplasm. In light of the debate over its histogenesis, and its relatively indolent behavior, the ultimate classification of AMFH as a variant of MFH remains controversial.

PLEXIFORM FIBROHISTIOCYTIC TUMOR

Plexiform fibrohistiocytic tumor (PFHT) was first described in 1988 by Enzinger and Zhang[364] in a series of 65 patients from the AFIP. The rarity of the lesion can be appreciated by the fact that these cases were selected from material received in consultation over a 20-year period. A smaller series of 14 patients was subsequently reported from England by Hollowood et al.[365]

Although patients with PFHT as old as 71 years of age are reported,[364] the tumor is predominantly one of children and young adults. Among the 79 patients in the two series mentioned here, 86% were younger than 30 years of age, with 41% younger than age 10 years. In the AFIP series, 71% of the patients were female,[364] whereas in the series by Hollowood et al., there were an equal number of male and female patients.[365]

PFHT predominantly occurs in the extremities, with a predilection for the upper extremity, which was involved in 64% of the total cases, the lower extremity accounting for 15% of the cases. The head and neck region and the trunk were each involved in approximately 10% of cases. The shoulder, forearm, and hands are the most frequently involved areas. PFHT arises most often in the lower dermis or superficial subcutaneous tissue, with occasional examples extending into the underlying skeletal muscle. The tumor is poorly demarcated and has ranged from 0.3 to 6.0 cm in maximum size, with the majority smaller than 3.0 cm.[364, 365]

The histologic pattern of PFHT varies somewhat from case to case, depending on the presence or absence of its fibrohistiocytic and fibroblastic elements.[364, 365] Under low-power magnification, one usually sees a combination of multiple nodular aggregates of cells interspersed between fascicles or trabeculae of fibroblastic spindle cells (Figs. 17–46 and 17–47). The nodular aggregates have a variable cellular composition. Most frequently they contain epithelioid histiocytic-type cells that have round to oval nuclei and a pale eosinophilic cytoplasm (Figs. 17–48 and 17–49). Interspersed among these histiocytic-type cells are a variable number of multinucleated osteoclast-type giant cells that have basophilic cytoplasm. Transition forms exist between the giant cells and the histiocytic-type cells. Also within the nodules are spindle cells that are similar to those within the adjacent trabeculae; in occasional nodules the spindle cells may constitute the majority of the cells (Fig. 17–50).

The spindled areas contain cells that have vesicular fusiform nuclei and eosinophilic cytoplasm and reside within a collagenized stroma. Some trabeculae are broad, resembling foci of fibromatosis (Fig. 17–51), and they ramify within and entrap intervening normal soft tissue, creating a plexiform pattern. A storiform spindle cell pattern, as found in many fibrohistiocytic tumors, is absent in PFHT.

Microhemorrhages, frequently associated with abundant deposits of hemosiderin pigment, are also commonly present within the nodular aggregates. Some of the fascicles and nodules may be densely hyalinized (Fig. 17–52). Mitotic activity is rare, but occasional cases have a high mitotic rate.[364] Cellular pleomorphism or anaplasia is absent.

Although the majority of cases of PFHT contain fibrohistiocytic aggregates, either alone or in combination with the fibroblastic fascicles, some cases lack them, being instead composed almost exclusively of the plexiform fibroblastic fascicles.

Electron microscopy of seven cases of PFHT has shown primitive mesenchymal cells, fibroblasts, and myofibroblasts, with occasional cells containing cytoplasmic focal densities or dense bodies.[364, 365] Some cells are described with prominent cell processes, thus resembling Schwann cells, but they lacked a well-formed basal lamina.[365]

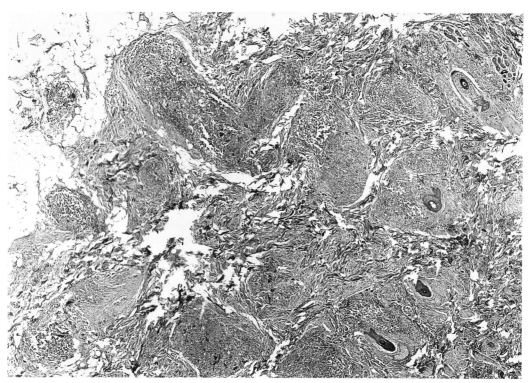

FIGURE 17–46. Low-power view of plexiform fibrohistiocytic tumor (PFHT) shows scattered nodules within the dermis and superficial subcutaneous tissue.

In immunohistochemical studies, Hollowood et al. found smooth muscle actin in the spindle cells of the fibroblastic trabeculae in 10 of 14 cases, as well as in some of the epithelioid and spindle cells within the nodular aggregates.[365] The multinucleated giant cells were positive for CD68 antigen in eight of nine cases, as were occasional spindle cells within the aggregates, but this antigen was absent in the spindle cells within the fibroblastic trabeculae. Our own experience with three cases corroborates these findings. Alpha-1-antitrypsin and alpha-1-antichymotrypsin were found in 3 of 16 (19%) and 4 of 17 (24%) cases, respectively; stains for S-100 protein, desmin, cytokeratin, Factor VIII–related antigen, leukocyte common antigen (CD45), Leu-M1 (CD15), and HLA-DR have been negative.

The differential histologic diagnosis of PFHT includes fibrous hamartoma of infancy, plexiform neurofibroma, fibromatosis, giant cell tumor of tendon sheath, dermatofibroma, and malignant fibrous histiocytoma.

Fibrous hamartoma of infancy affects a similar age group as PFHT and has plexiform fascicles of fibroblasts involving the dermis and subcutaneous tissue. However, it lacks multinodular aggregates and contains distinctive loosely textured, pale-staining foci of immature-appearing stellate to spindle cells that are intimately associated with more mature spindle cell trabeculae.

Unlike PFHT, **plexiform neurofibroma** shows electron microscopic evidence of nerve sheath differentiation and is commonly positive for S-100 protein and Leu-7 antigen (CD57). Selected examples of plexiform neurofibroma are also reactive for glial fibrillary acidic protein (GFAP), a feature that appears to be unique to peripheral nerve sheath tumors among dermal-based neoplasms and also serves to distinguish it from PFHT. Neither fibrous hamartoma nor plexiform neurofibroma contains osteoclast-type giant cells or histiocytic-type cells.

Although the fibroblastic fascicles of PFHT may cytologically resemble areas of **fibromatosis,** the latter is a more deeply situated lesion involving skeletal muscle and is not a dermal lesion. Fibromatosis also lacks a plexiform pattern, giant cells, or micronodular aggregates of histiocytic-type cells. **Giant cell tumor of tendon sheath** may be a diagnostic consideration because, like PFHT, it occurs in the region of the hand and has osteoclast-type giant cells and histiocyte-like cells. However, giant cell tumor of tendon sheath occurs in older patients, is a solid lesion composed of nodules without a plexiform pattern, and may contain pleomorphic cells with atypical nuclear features that are distinct from the bland nuclei found in PFHT.

Although it contains multinucleated giant cells, **dermatofibroma** is a dermal rather than a subcutaneous lesion and has a storiform pattern that is frequently associated with foamy histiocytes, both elements of which are absent in PFHT, and dermatofibroma lacks the multinodular pattern of PFHT.

Conventional malignant fibrous histiocytoma is easily distinguished from PFHT not only by the much older population of patients in which it occurs but by its deeper location in the soft tissues and its vascularity, mitotic activity, cellular pleomorphism, and anaplasia.

Plexiform fibrohistiocytic tumor may be locally aggressive, with local recurrence rates after excision of approximately 40%.[364, 365] Two of the patients reported by Enzinger and Zhang[364] developed local lymph node metastases; however, to date, no deaths due to PFHT have occurred. The exact classification of this lesion as fibrohistiocytic,[364] myofi-

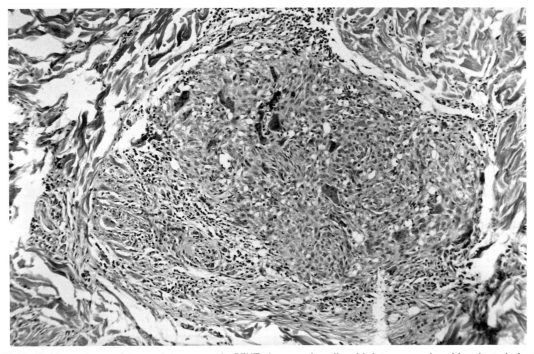

FIGURE 17–47. View of one of the nodular arrays in PFHT shows pale cells with interspersed multinucleated giant cells.

broblastic,[365] or of some other cell type is still unclear and awaits analysis of additional cases.

GIANT CELL FIBROBLASTOMA

Giant cell fibroblastoma (GCF) is an unusual and uncommon soft tissue lesion that was first described in the early 1980s.[366–368] Fewer than 60 cases exist in the English-language

medical literature;[366, 369–381] the largest single series consists of 28 patients from the AFIP.[381]

GCF is a slowly growing, usually painless, lesion located predominantly in the subcutaneous tissue, although it may extend to involve the dermis or superficial skeletal muscle.[369, 371, 372, 374–377, 381, 382] In our review of 56 patients,[366, 368–380] the age at diagnosis ranged from 4 months[381] to 64 years[375] (mean, 9.3 years; median, 3.1 years); 57% were younger than age 5 years. However, GCF can be present for several years before

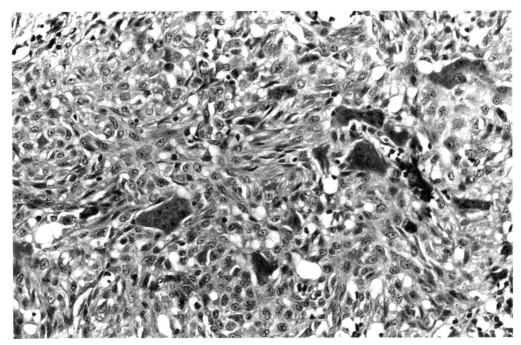

FIGURE 17–48. The nodules of PFHT are usually composed of bland-appearing, round to fusiform (fibrohistiocytic) cells admixed with osteoclast-type giant cells, as shown.

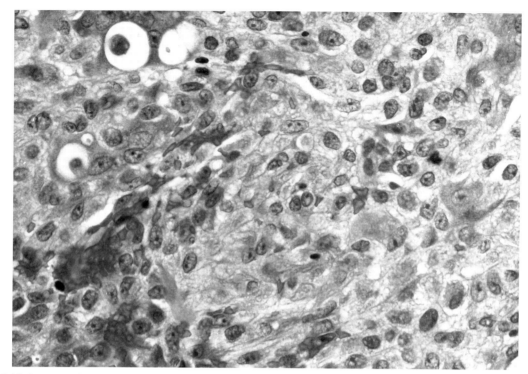

FIGURE 17–49. Higher magnification of one of the nodules in PFHT shows cells that appear histiocytic, with an abundant pale cytoplasm and bland-appearing nuclei.

diagnosis. The age at first manifestation ranged from birth to 64 years,[375, 381] with almost 75% of patients younger than age 10 years and approximately 65% younger than age 5 years. Only a few patients with GCF have been older than age 20 years.[371, 373, 375, 381] Male patients accounted for approximately 70% of cases.

GCF has a wide anatomic distribution: the trunk was involved in 30 cases (54%), the extremities in 21 (38%), with 18 of these in the lower extremity, and the head and neck area in 5 cases (9%). The most frequently involved sites were the chest wall, thigh, inguinal region, axilla, and back. Among the 40 cases with size data,[366, 369, 371, 372, 374, 376–378, 380, 381] GCF ranged

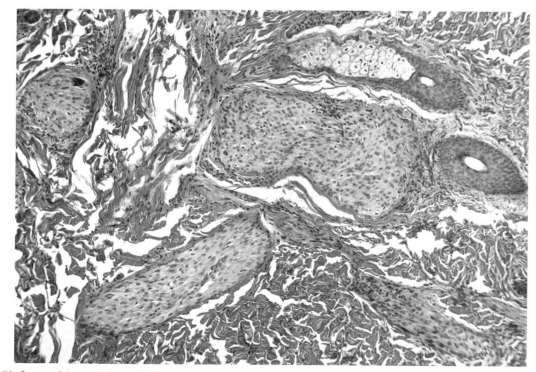

FIGURE 17–50. Some of the nodules in PFHT lack a giant cell component and are composed of only fusiform cells, as illustrated here.

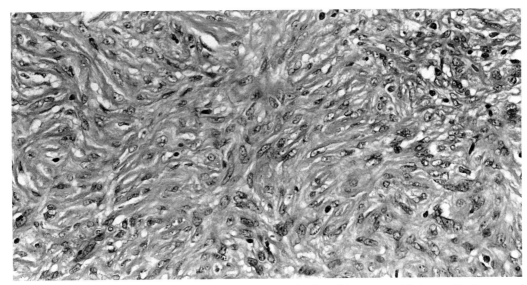

FIGURE 17–51. Fibromatosis-like area in PFHT. Such foci may be found interspersed between the tumor nodules.

from 0.8 to 8.0 cm in maximum dimension,[381] with a mean of 3.6 cm (median, 3.6 cm); 75% were smaller than 5.0 cm.

Grossly, GCF is an unencapsulated, firm mass that has infiltrative borders and a gray-white to gray-tan gelatinous or mucoid surface.[366, 369, 374, 375, 377, 380, 381]

Histologically,[366, 369, 371, 372, 374–377, 379–381] GCF is characterized by collagenous areas in which stellate to spindle-shaped fibroblasts are either arranged in broad or loose fascicles or haphazardly arrayed (Fig. 17–53); at times they form a storiform pattern.[368, 376, 377, 381] The diagnostic histologic feature of GCF is the combined presence of hyperchromatic, multinucleated giant cells that have a peripheral wreath-like arrangement of their nuclei, thus resembling Touton giant cells or floret cells, arranged in a fibrous or myxoid stroma (Figs. 17–54 and 17–55), and "angiectoid" or pseudovascular spaces.[366, 372, 374, 375, 381] These spaces (Figs. 17–56 and 17–57), which are lined by either the stromal giant cells or pleomorphic spindle cells and not by endothelial cells, may contain either red blood cells (see Fig. 17–57) or gray-blue acellular granular material that is rich in hyaluronic acid. The spaces appear to arise in areas where the myxoid stroma condenses and then splits to form pseudovascular areas. Also present within the stroma are spindle cells that have wavy, hyperchromatic, irregular nuclei and slender cytoplasmic extensions. The myxoid stroma gives a positive staining reaction for hyaluronic acid. Mitotic activity in GCF is minimal, and necrosis is absent.

Based on 14 cases studied by electron microscopy,[366, 372, 374, 377–381] the basic tumor cell is a spindle-shaped fibroblast with a well-developed rough endoplasmic reticulum. Some cells have prominent long, intertwining cytoplasmic processes. Their nuclei, which vary from one to several per cell, have a characteristic septate or convoluted cerebriform appearance. Basement membranes, cell junctions, dense bodies, and Weibel-Palade bodies are absent.

Immunohistochemical studies were done on 28 of the cases of GCF in our review,[366, 371, 372, 374–377, 379, 380, 383] with only vimentin being consistently found in the 15 cases studied.[372, 375–377, 379, 380] Negative results were reported for Factor VIII–related antigen,[366, 371, 372, 374–377, 379, 380] *Ulex europaeus* I lectin,[366, 372, 375–377] S-100 protein,[371, 375–377, 379, 380] desmin,[375, 376, 379, 380] myoglobin,[375,

376, 379] neurofilament protein,[375] lysozyme,[372, 379] and epithelial membrane antigen.[376, 379] Four of 12 cases had cells that were reactive for alpha-1-antichymotrypsin,[371, 375–377, 379, 380] one of five for alpha-1-antitrypsin,[372, 377, 379] and four of six for muscle-specific actin.[372, 376, 377, 379] In these last studies, the actin staining was reportedly only weakly or mildly positive. However, three additional cases of GCF are described in which the tumor cells were positive for muscle actin; in one of these cases more than 50% of the cells were reactive, whereas in the other two cases only a few of the stromal cells were reactive.[383]

Because of its hyperchromatic giant cells and myxoid stroma, GCF may be confused with a sarcoma, especially **myxoid malignant fibrous histiocytoma** (MHF) and **myxoid liposarcoma.**[381] However, GCF lacks the cellular pleomorphism, mitotic activity, and plexiform capillary network of myxoid MFH and occurs in younger patients than does myxoid MFH, which predominantly involves patients in the sixth to seventh decades of life. Unlike GCF, myxoid liposarcoma is seldom found in children younger than 10 years of age and virtually never originates as a subcutaneous lesion. GCF lacks the lipoblasts, mucinous pools, and capillary network of myxoid liposarcoma, and myxoid liposarcoma lacks wreath-like giant cells.

A variety of benign conditions are included in the differential light microscopic diagnosis of GCF, including subcutaneous pleomorphic lipoma, pleomorphic fibroma, atypical pseudosarcomatous dermatofibroma, and rudimentary meningocele. Subcutaneous **pleomorphic lipoma** occurs in patients older than 40 years of age, is predominantly located in the neck or upper shoulder region and, unlike the infiltrative pattern of GCF, is well-circumscribed. Although it contains floret-type giant cells and myxoid areas, pleomorphic lipoma lacks the pseudovascular spaces of GCF and contains lipoblasts.

Pleomorphic fibroma of the skin contains atypical pleomorphic stromal cells whose electron microscopic features are similar to those of GCF.[384, 385] However, unlike GCF, pleomorphic fibroma is a polypoid or dome-shaped dermal lesion that histologically lacks pseudovascular spaces.

The cutaneous tumor designated as **pseudosarcomatous dermatofibroma, atypical cutaneous fibrous histiocytoma,** or **dermatofibroma with monster cells** contains atypical stro-

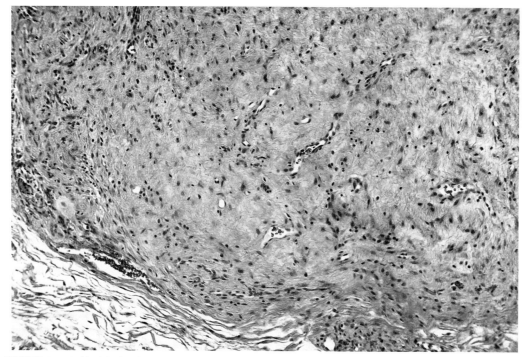

FIGURE 17–52. Nodule in PFHT that is densely hyalinized, resembling a collagenized area of fibromatosis.

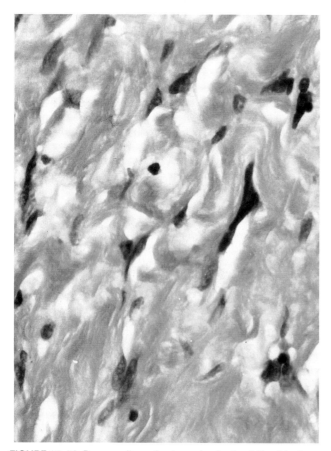

FIGURE 17–53. Dense collagenized area in giant cell fibroblastoma (GCF) shows hyperchromatic spindle to stellate fibroblasts.

mal cells mixed with giant cells. However, this is a dermal lesion that occurs most frequently on the trunk and limbs of middle-aged women and invariably contains areas of conventional dermatofibroma.[386–389]

Finally, **rudimentary meningocele** or **meningothelial hamartoma** may contain pseudovascular spaces as in GCF.[383] This lesion is located almost exclusively in the scalp, a rare location for GCF, and histologically contains a mixture of fibrous, adipose, and vascular elements. Unlike GCF, the cells of rudimentary meningocele contain epithelial membrane antigen and have electron microscopic features of meningothelial cells.[383]

Occasional cases of **dermatofibrosarcoma protuberans** (DFSP) are reported to contain foci of GCF,[381, 386, 390] although in what percentage of cases this occurred is not specified. Nevertheless, these foci, combined with the facts that rare cases of GCF have recurred locally as DFSP,[369, 370] that a case of DFSP has recurred as a GCF,[373] and that storiform areas are found in GCF, have led some to the hypothesis that GCF represents a juvenile form of DFSP.[368, 381] However, other workers did not find any GCF-like areas in a study of 131 examples of DFSP, other than the focal occurrence of multinucleated giant cells, similar to those in GCF, in 6 of 24 cases studied in detail.[391] There are also major clinical and histologic differences between these two entities. DFSP only rarely occurs in patients younger than 10 years of age; it is dermally based, in contrast with the predominant subcutaneous location of GCF; it lacks the pleomorphic cells and angiectoid spaces of GCF; and only rarely does it contain giant cells. Although uncommon, metastases have occurred in DFSP that, to date, have not developed in patients with GCF.

Although the lack of metastases supports the benign nature of GCF, the lesion has a high local recurrence rate after excision. Among 38 patients in our review with follow-up

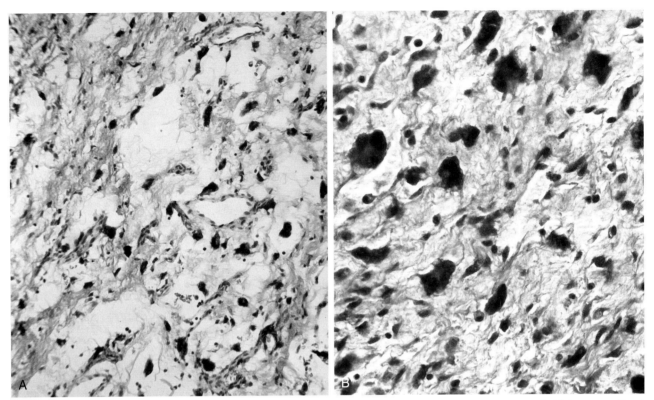

FIGURE 17–54. *A,* Myxoid area in GCF in which reside numerous hyperchromatic multinucleated giant cells. *B,* Higher magnification shows a loose stroma with multinucleated giant cells. Between the giant cells the stroma contains small spindle cells.

data,[366, 369–372, 374–378, 380, 381] 17 (45%) developed a local recurrence, six of whom developed a second recurrence, with some of the recurrences developing as long as 5 years after excision.[366, 372]

POSTOPERATIVE SPINDLE CELL NODULE

First described in 1984 by Proppe et al.,[392] postoperative spindle cell nodule (PSCN) is unique not only for its temporal association with previous operative procedures but also for a histologic appearance that may be mistaken for sarcoma.

PSCN is relatively rare, with only a few cases so far reported.[392–397] It occurs mainly in the genitourinary tract, with the bladder,[392, 394, 397] prostate,[394, 395] prostatic urethra,[392, 394] and the vagina[392] the principal sites of involvement; isolated cases are reported in the endocervix[396] and the endometrium.[395] Similar lesions have also occurred in the larynx and gingiva.[392]

PSCN has developed after transurethral resections, either for benign or malignant prostatic disease or for bladder carcinoma, and after vaginal hysterectomy, episiotomy procedures, and endometrial curettage.[392–397] PSCN is notable for its rapid onset, developing within 2[396] to 12 weeks[392] (mean, 6 weeks; median, 5 weeks) of these operative procedures.[392–394, 396] Although some patients present because of recurrent symptoms for which the original operative procedure was done, for the most part PSCN is incidentally detected at follow-up examinations or in tissue subsequently removed for other reasons. The ages of the 19 patients in our review[392–397] ranged from 29 to 79 years[392] (mean, 57 years; median, 60 years), with all but two older than age 40 years. Males accounted for 13 of the 19 patients (68%).

Macroscopically, PSCN is usually only a few millimeters in size, although occasionally it has been as large as 4.0 cm.[392] Histologically,[392–394, 396, 398] PSCN is characterized by interlacing fascicles of plump to tapering spindle cells (Fig. 17–58) that have a moderate to abundant amount of eosinophilic to amphophilic cytoplasm. Nuclei are fusiform and appear bland without significant atypia; nucleoli may be present but are not prominent (Fig. 17–59). Mitotic activity varies from cases with few[396] to those with numerous mitotic figures;[392–394, 398] however, abnormal mitoses are not present. Interspersed among the spindle cells is a delicate, plexiform capillary network. The stroma may have prominent edematous zones in which are scattered acute and chronic inflammatory cells (see Fig. 17–58). PCSN is infiltrative, and within the bladder and prostate it may destroy the smooth muscle[392] and frequently ulcerate the overlying mucosa.[392, 395, 397]

The significance of immunohistochemical studies of PSCN is restricted by the small number of cases so far analyzed.[394, 395, 397] Wick et al., in a study of two cases, demonstrated reactivity in the spindle cells for cytokeratin, vimentin, desmin, and muscle-specific actin, whereas epithelial membrane antigen and S-100 protein were not detected.[397] Huang et al.,[394] in a study of three patients, found focal vimentin positivity in the spindle cells of all the cases, with two also demonstrating reactivity for desmin; however, cytokeratin was not found in the single case that they studied for this protein. Hughes et al.[395] found vimentin and cytokeratin reactivity in the spindle cells of one case, without reactivity for desmin.

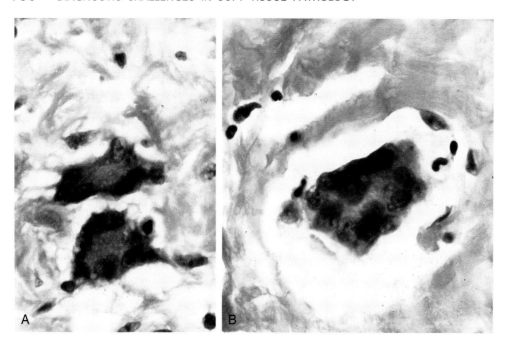

FIGURE 17–55. Views of the multinucleated giant cells found in GCF. The peripheral orientation of their nuclei creates a floret-like appearance.

In a lone case of PSCN examined by electron microscopy, the cells appeared fibroblastic without pinocytotic vesicles, microfilaments, dense bodies, or basal lamina.[392]

The occurrence in PSCN of fascicles of plump spindle cells associated with abundant mitotic activity and infiltrating margins may suggest a diagnosis of sarcoma, but the bland cytologic appearance of the spindle cell nuclei, the lack of atypical mitotic figures, and the associated inflammatory component are features that argue against such a diagnosis. However, **leiomyosarcoma** of the bladder, especially the myxoid variant that is characterized by a prominent edematous myxoid stroma that contains spindle cells, may be impossible to distinguish from PSCN when one has access to only small biopsy specimens. Because some leiomyosarcomas are reported to be reactive for cytokeratin and, like PSCN, are also positive for desmin and muscle-specific actin, immunohistochemical studies are not useful in distinguishing between these two entities. Electron microscopy may be helpful if clear-cut features of smooth muscle differentiation are found.

Sarcomatoid carcinoma must also be considered in the differential histologic diagnosis of PSCN, especially in light of the above-mentioned data that some cells in PSCN may

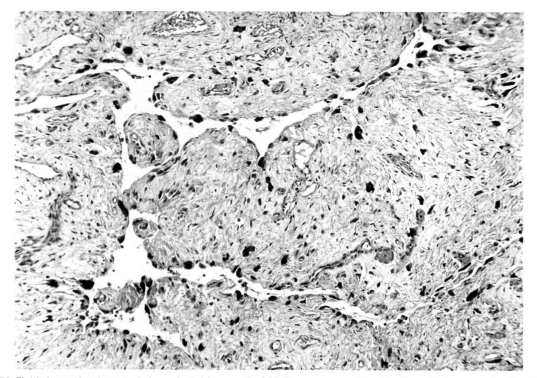

FIGURE 17–56. Field shows the characteristic angiectoid spaces in GCF. The spaces are lined by the spindle stromal cells and multinucleated giant cells.

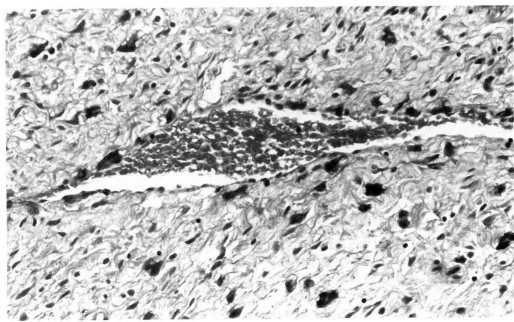

FIGURE 17–57. Illustrated is an angiectoid (pseudovascular) space filled with red blood cells. The space is lined by spindle stromal cells and giant cells and not by endothelial cells.

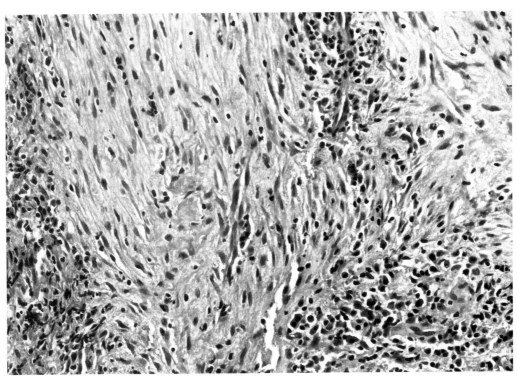

FIGURE 17–58. Postoperative spindle cell nodule of bladder. Fusiform cells are present within a stroma that contains scattered chronic inflammatory cells.

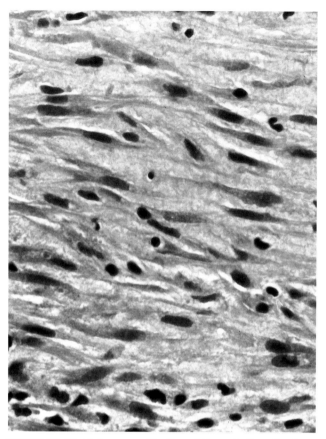

FIGURE 17–59. Higher magnification of the spindle cells shows hyperchromatic nuclei but a lack of significant atypia.

be cytokeratin-positive. However, the lack of epithelial membrane antigen positivity in PSCN, a marker consistently present in cases of sarcomatoid carcinoma,[397] and the lack of muscle-specific actin and desmin in the latter, help distinguish these two tumors. Electron microscopy may be diagnostic by showing features of epithelial differentiation in sarcomatoid carcinoma.

Despite its sarcomatoid appearance, the most useful criterion for establishing a diagnosis of PSCN is the clinical information of a relatively recent operative procedure in the involved area.

Although occasional local recurrences are reported after excision,[392] to date no patient with a diagnosis of PSCN has died as a result of the lesion, despite operative procedures that would be less than adequate if the lesions were sarcomatous,[392, 394, 395, 397] thus supporting the view that PSCN is a reactive rather than a neoplastic condition.

INFLAMMATORY PSEUDOSARCOMA OF THE GENITOURINARY TRACT

Inflammatory pseudosarcoma (IPS) of the genitourinary tract is an uncommon, benign fibroblastic/myofibroblastic lesion first described by Roth in 1980.[399] The lesion is closely related to, if not identical with, postoperative spindle cell nodule,[392] differing from the latter mainly by its lack of a temporal association with a previous operative procedure. As with other relatively recently described soft tissue tumors, the

number of names applied to IPS closely rivals the actual number of reports describing it. These appellations include pseudosarcomatous fibromyxoid tumor,[400, 401] atypical fibromyxoid tumor,[402, 403] reactive pseudosarcomatous response,[399] inflammatory pseudotumor,[404–407] pseudosarcoma,[395, 408] pseudosarcomatous myofibroblastic proliferation,[409, 410] inflammatory myofibroblastic pseudotumor,[407] atypical myofibroblastic tumor,[411] myofibroblastoma,[412] inflammatory pseudosarcoma,[413] myofibroblastic pseudotumor,[414] and sclerosing inflammatory pseudotumor.[415] We have no overriding preference for any of these terms and have arbitrarily chosen to use "inflammatory pseudosarcoma" as the designation for this lesion.

Patients with IPS of the genitourinary tract seek medical attention for a variety of reasons. Among 50 patients in our review with clinical data,[395, 399–402, 404–416] gross or microscopic hematuria, either alone or in combination with urinary frequency, dysuria, or nocturia, was the initial presenting feature in 60%. Other urinary tract symptoms or signs, including urinary retention, urethral irritation, and urinary tract infections, were present in approximately 25% of patients; the remaining patients included those with painless spermatic cord masses[412] or testicular swelling[414] or those in whom the lesion was found during the clinical work-up for an unrelated problem or incidentally discovered within hernia repair tissue.[402, 410]

IPS occurs in patients over a broad age range from children to elderly adults. Among 53 patients with individual age data in our survey,[395, 399–402, 404–407, 409–416] ages ranged from 4 months[414] to 76 years,[410] with an average of 32.3 years (median, 32 years). More than one half of the patients (55%) were between 20 and 59 years of age; one third were younger than age 20 years. Female patients accounted for 56% of the cases.

The bladder is the most frequent site of IPS, accounting for 76% (40/53) of the cases. Other sites included the tunica albuginea of the testis,[412] the epididymis,[414] prostate,[401, 408] urethra,[408] and spermatic cord.[410] Grossly, IPS is a firm, rubbery, pink-tan to gray-white nodular mass with a cut surface that is frequently mucoid and slimy.[395, 405–410] The bladder lesions are frequently exophytic and polypoid, although others are intramural and not only infiltrate the bladder wall but may extend into the perivesical soft tissue.[404, 406, 407, 409, 411, 413] In 33 cases in which specific tumor size was given, IPS ranged from 0.9 cm[408] to 8.0 cm,[413] with a mean of 3.4 cm (median, 3.0 cm); however, between 25% and 30% were equal to or larger than 5.0 cm.[399–401, 404, 406–416]

Microscopically,[395, 398–402, 404–416] IPS features large, elongated spindle or bipolar cells scattered within an abundant myxoid stroma. The cells have an eosinophilic cytoplasm with long, tapering cytoplasmic processes and large, oval to spindle-shaped nuclei that vary from vesicular to moderately hyperchromatic; a single prominent nucleolus may be present (Figs. 17–60 and 17–61). The cells tend to be haphazardly arranged within the stroma, but may be grouped within small fascicles (see Fig. 17–61A). At times, somewhat larger, polygonal and strap-like cells are present that have a dense eosinophilic cytoplasm and resemble rhabdomyoblasts, but without cross-striations.[395, 400, 402, 407] Polygonal cells with an amphophilic cytoplasm, some having a ganglion cell–like appearance, are also found.[395, 407, 409–411] Significant nuclear atypia and pleomorphism are not usual in IPS, although cells with larger and more atypical nuclei (see Fig. 17–61B) may occasionally be

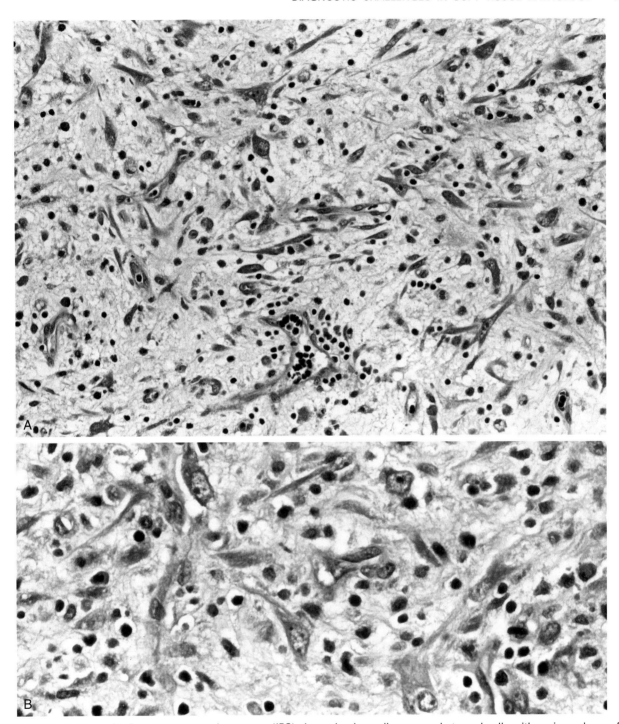

FIGURE 17–60. *A,* View of inflammatory pseudosarcoma (IPS) shows haphazardly arranged stromal cells with various shapes from spindle forms to those that are stellate and ganglion-like. The stroma is loose and myxomatous and well vascularized. Scattered chronic inflammatory cells are present. *B,* Higher magnification shows the stromal cells with vesicular mildly atypical nuclei and small nucleoli.

seen.[400, 401, 408, 414] The mitotic rate varies considerably from case to case, with some having few if any mitotic figures,[399, 401, 402, 407, 408, 410–415] whereas in others numerous mitoses are present;[400, 409, 414, 416] abnormal mitotic figures are notable by their absence.

The myxoid stroma is well vascularized with numerous capillaries and small blood vessels, many with slit-like lumina. Extravasated red blood cells are commonly present. The myxoid stroma stains positively with alcian blue, the stain being abolished by pretreatment with hyaluronidase.

A characteristic histologic feature of IPS is the diffuse presence of inflammatory cells consisting usually of lymphocytes, plasma cells, and mast cells (see Figs. 17–60 and 17–61*B*). However, in some cases, especially those in the bladder, the lesion ulcerates the overlying mucosa, and acute inflammatory cells then become mixed with the chronic inflammatory component.[395, 399, 400, 407, 409] The cells of IPS may insinuate themselves between the smooth muscle of the bladder wall (Fig. 17–62) without appearing to destroy the muscle;[395, 399, 400, 402, 404, 411, 416] as mentioned, the process may extend through the wall into the soft tissue and involve adjacent organs.[400, 409, 413, 416]

Electron microscopic evaluation was done in 22 cases of IPS in our review.* The spindle cells of IPS had features of fibroblasts/myofibroblasts, with bipolar cytoplasmic extensions; numerous cytoplasmic organelles, including an abundant and frequently dilated rough endoplasmic reticulum; a prominent Golgi zone; pinocytotic vesicles; myofilaments with dense bodies; and an external basal lamina.

Immunohistochemical studies† show that in almost all cases the cells of IPS contain vimentin, which was found in 94% (31/33) of cases.[395, 400–402, 406, 408–410, 412, 415] Muscle-specific actin[406, 409, 412] was present in 86% (18/21), and smooth muscle actin [401, 406, 410, 412, 414, 415] in 53% (10/19). Reactivity for desmin‡ was found in only 5 of 37 cases (14%), and then only focally in a few cells.[406, 409, 412] Similar results were reported for cytokeratin,§ for which 5 of 38 cases (13%) yielded positive results,[406, 409, 412] although here too some of the staining was present in only a few cells. Focal epithelial membrane antigen[402, 406, 409, 410] was found in only 2 of 20 (10%) cases.[406] Stains for S-100 protein[401, 402, 406, 408–410, 412, 414, 415] and myoglobin[400–402, 406, 408, 409] were negative in 29 and 22 cases, respectively; reactivity for CD68 antigen, using KP-1 antibody, was absent in 10 cases,[406] and carcinoembryonic antigen was lacking in 11 cases.[406, 412]

The overall light microscopic pattern of IPS suggests reactive-type granulation tissue with an inflammatory background in which the cells lack significant cytologic atypia. However, because of the site involved, the gross appearance, and the myxoid component, a number of other benign and malignant entities enter the differential diagnosis, including myxoid leiomyosarcoma, rhabdomyosarcoma, postoperative spindle cell nodule, aggressive angiomyxoma, inflammatory fibrosarcoma, sarcomatoid carcinoma, and nodular fasciitis.

Both IPS and **myxoid leiomyosarcoma** (MLMS) have in common the presence of bland spindle cells within a myxoid stroma, a mitotic rate that may be low, and spindle cells that may be focally aggregated into fascicles. However, IPS is more cellular than MLMS, and its cells are more haphazardly arranged, in contrast with the more diffuse and uniform distribution of the cells in MLMS. IPS lacks the pools of mucin found in MLMS, and its stroma is more vascular than that of MLMS. Significantly, the prominent inflammatory component of IPS is absent in MLMS. Conventional leiomyosarcomas may contain focal myxoid areas and thus be confused with IPS; however, their cells are more atypical than those of IPS, and they may have abnormal mitotic figures, which are lacking in IPS, as well as areas of necrosis and tissue destruction, in contrast with the infiltrating but non-destructive pattern of IPS. Immunohistochemical studies cannot solve this differential diagnostic problem because muscle markers are present in all three of these entities. Electron microscopy may be of some value if the lesion in question shows clear-cut smooth muscle differentiation. However, when only small biopsy tissue is available, it may be impossible to distinguish between IPS and leiomyosarcoma by light microscopy. Indeed, in some cases, only the examination of resection material will enable the pathologist to arrive at an accurate diagnosis.[404] Unfortunately, this has led to some patients undergoing radical operative procedures, based on a biopsy diagnosis of sarcoma,[395, 403, 409, 413, 415] before the true nature of the lesion was discovered.

Because of the polypoid configuration of many bladder inflammatory pseudosarcomas and the presence of a myxoid stroma and spindle cells, **rhabdomyosarcoma,** in particular **botryoid embryonal rhabdomyosarcoma** (ERMS), is a diagnostic consideration, especially in young patients. However, IPS lacks the cambium layer of botryoid rhabdomyosarcoma, and the cells of the latter are more round or oval than spindle-shaped and demonstrate nuclear irregularity and atypism. Non-botryoid ERMS does contain spindle-shaped tumor cells, as well as densely acidophilic cells of various shapes, including strap-like cells that show cross-striations. Although, as mentioned, such rhabdomyoblastic-like cells are also occasionally found in IPS, cross-striations are absent and immunohistochemical stains for myoglobin are negative. Although the cells of IPS and ERMS may both contain muscle-specific actin and desmin, the latter is relatively infrequent in IPS, and when present, it is found only focally, in contrast with its usually strong and diffuse presence in almost all cases of rhabdomyosarcoma. Electron microscopy may be of help in distinguishing between IPS and ERMS if features of skeletal muscle differentiation can be found.

Sarcomatoid (spindle cell) carcinoma of the urinary tract may contain spindle cells haphazardly arranged in a myxoid stroma and, because of mucosal ulceration, be associated with an inflammatory component. However, sarcomatoid carcinomas tend to be cytologically high-grade tumors with significant cellular atypia and abnormal mitotic activity. Although not always found, the presence of a carcinoma *in situ* mucosal component, or even a focus of obvious invasive carcinoma, easily settles the diagnostic issue between IPS and sarcomatoid carcinoma. Immunohistochemically, the cells of both IPS and sarcomatoid carcinoma express vimentin, and although infrequent, the reported presence of cytokeratin and epithelial membrane antigen in the cells of at least some cases of IPS may lead to a misdiagnosis of sarcomatoid carcinoma. However, the finding of smooth muscle actin or muscle-specific actin in the tumor cells eliminates spindle cell carcinoma from consideration. Electron microscopic evidence of fibroblastic/myofibroblastic differentiation in IPS is also in contrast with the epithelial differentiation expected in sarcomatoid carcinoma.

By light microscopy, **aggressive angiomyxoma** (AA) of the pelvis and perineum shares with IPS the presence of an abundant myxoid stroma. In general, the cellularity of IPS is greater than that found in AA, and IPS tends to be more mitotically active than is AA. The cells of AA are small, monotonous, and spindle to stellate shaped; they are more uniformly distributed within the stroma, in contrast with the more haphazard arrangement of the cells in IPS. Although both of these entities have a prominent vascular component, AA possesses, in addition to thin-walled ectatic capillaries, regions that contain small thick-walled blood vessels that are not found in IPS; AA also lacks the prominent inflammatory component of IPS. Electron microscopic and immunohistochemical studies cannot reliably distinguish between these entities, because the cells of both share electron microscopic features of myofibroblastic or fibroblastic differentiation, and

---

* References 395, 399–401, 404, 406, 407, 409, 411, 412, 415.

† References 395, 400–402, 404, 406–410, 412, 414, 415.

‡ References 395, 400–402, 404, 406, 408–410, 412, 414.

§ References 395, 400–402, 404, 406–410, 412, 414, 415.

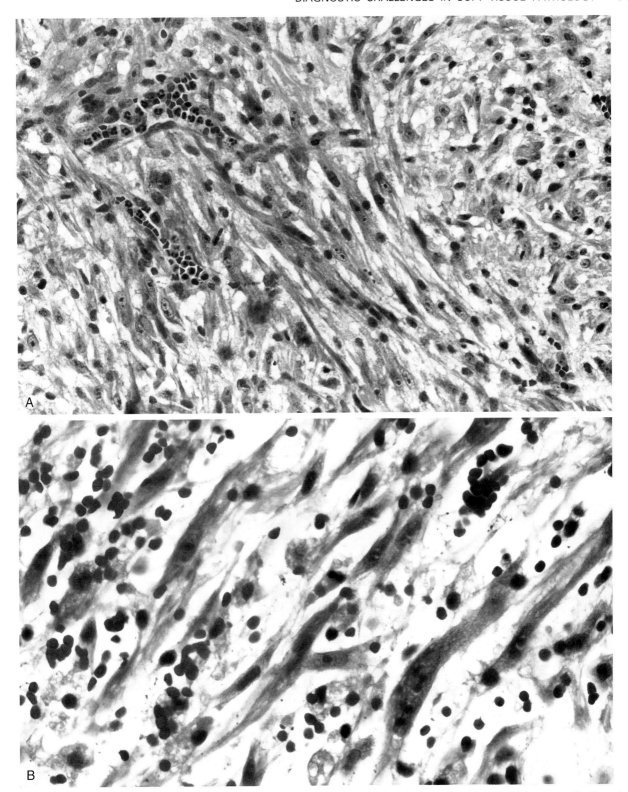

FIGURE 17–61. *A,* The stromal spindle cells of IPS may be found, as illustrated here, in loose fascicles. *B,* Higher magnification shows stromal cells, with long tapering cytoplasm, separated by a myxoid stroma. Nuclei are somewhat atypical, with hyperchromasia and variable size; some contain prominent nucleoli. Inflammatory cells are admixed throughout the field.

immunohistochemically their cells contain vimentin, actin, and even desmin.

Postoperative spindle cell nodule (PSCN) differs significantly from IPS only in its clinical association with a recent operative procedure. In general, PSCN is histologically a more compact lesion than is IPS, with its component spindle cells arranged in interlacing fascicles. Both lesions share prominent vascular and inflammatory components, and both may infiltrate smooth muscle. The myxoid stroma of IPS is, in general, more abundant than in PSCN. The few immunohistochemical

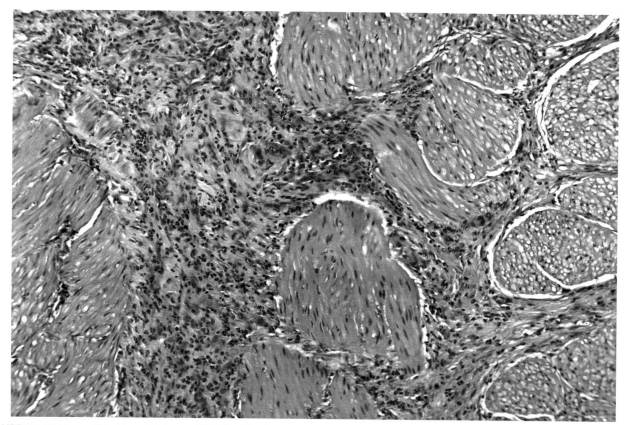

FIGURE 17–62. View of bladder wall shows IPS infiltrating between the smooth muscle bundles of the wall without evidence of necrosis.

studies of PSCN show an overlap in results with those of IPS. In agreement with others,[395, 406, 407, 409] we feel that PSCN and IPS represent a spectrum of response to an inciting event that just happens to be an identifiable one in PSCN, and that no significant differences exist between these two lesions once it is recognized that both are fibroblastic/myofibroblastic reactive responses. Indeed, similar statements may also be made for **nodular fasciitis,** which histologically shows the same major histologic features as does IPS;[417–420] and although occasional subtle features have been used to separate nodular fasciitis from IPS,[409] we see no clear histologic distinction between them. Whether one wishes to designate the genitourinary lesions as visceral forms of nodular fasciitis or as IPS is to us a matter of personal preference,[400, 407, 410, 416, 421] as long as one recognizes their benign reactive character.

The recently described entity **inflammatory fibrosarcoma** (IFS) of the mesentery and retroperitoneum closely resembles IPS histologically because of its spindle and inflammatory cell components.[422] IFS tends to occur in younger patients than does IPS, i.e., mean patient age of 15.0 years in IFS versus 32 years in IPS, although the latter also occurs in young patients. In contrast with IPS, patients with IFS not infrequently have associated systemic symptoms, including anemia, fever, and weight loss, and may also have increased erythrocyte sedimentation rates and increased serum immunoglobulin levels. Grossly, although there is some overlap in size, IFS tends to be larger than IPS, with 90% of the tumors larger than 5.0 cm. Although most examples of IFS are multiple, hard or rubbery masses, a few are soft and slimy, as is IPS. Histologically, the cells of IFS reside in a myxoid stroma

in which chronic inflammatory cells, mainly plasma cells, are present. The predominant tumor cells are spindle shaped; these are arrayed in sweeping fascicles and whorled formations, unlike the haphazard arrangement of the spindle cells in IPS. Nuclei are large, vesicular, and irregular, with large inclusion-type nucleoli. In addition, IFS contains round histiocytoid-like cells that have prominent inclusion-type nucleoli and a foamy to granular cytoplasm such that some have a ganglion cell-like appearance. Most important in this differential diagnosis is that the cells of IFS are irregular and pleomorphic in contrast with the bland cells of IPS. As with IPS, the cells of IFS have electron microscopic features of myofibroblasts/fibroblasts. Immunohistochemically, 90% of the cases of IFS are positive for smooth muscle actin, 83% for muscle-specific actin and vimentin, and 77% of the cases have shown cytokeratin reactivity, a percentage far greater than that found in IPS. The major histologic distinction between IFS and IPS, however, is the nuclear and cytologic atypia of the cells of IFS and their more frequent association within compact fascicles.

Many of the reported patients with IPS have been followed up for relatively short times. Among 46 patients with follow-up information, only 13 (28%) had been followed up for 3 or more years, and only 7 (15%) for more then 5 years. However, despite its "pseudosarcomatous" light microscopic picture, the benign nature of IPS is supported by the fact that although some patients have developed local recurrences after less than radical procedures, such as transurethral resections,[410, 413] no patient has died or developed metastases attributable to IPS.[395, 400–402, 404–416, 423] In contrast, IFS has shown locally aggressive behavior with invasion of the gastrointestinal tract and visceral organs, and approximately one third of those with IFS developed local recurrences. Metastases to the lung or brain developed in several patients with IFS, with death due to tumor in five patients (18%).

EXTRASKELETAL MYXOID CHONDROSARCOMA

Relative to its frequency in bone, chondrosarcoma is an uncommon soft tissue tumor, and, unlike its hyaline osseous counterpart, the soft tissue variant tends to be myxoid in type. Despite its relative rarity, extraskeletal myxoid chondrosarcoma (EMCS) is well-represented in the literature.[424–452]

EMCS is predominantly a tumor of adult life. In our review of 114 patients with individual age data,* the mean age was 49.1 years (median, 50.5 years), with a range from 1[435] to 92 years.[427] Approximately 70% of the patients were 40 years of age or older; only 5% were younger than 20 years. Among 115 patients for whom gender information was reported, males accounted for approximately 60% of the cases.†

Clinically, EMCS develops as a slowly growing, painful or painless mass‡ that may be present for many years before the patient seeks medical attention. In 58 patients in whom the preoperative duration of symptoms was given,§ the average was 14.6 months (median, 6 months), with a range of from 6 days[427] to 10 years;[449] one third had symptoms for 1 year or longer, with 20% for 2 or more years.

EMCS is a tumor that overwhelmingly occurs in the extremities. Among the 114 cases, the extremities were involved in 86%, with the lower extremity involved in 74% and the upper in 12% of cases; the thigh was the single most common site, accounting for almost one third of the cases. The trunk, including the chest wall, was involved in 8%, whereas the head and neck region was an uncommon location, accounting for 4% of cases. EMCS has occurred in the abdomen,[442] retroperitoneum,[427, 433] and thyroid.[448]

Grossly, EMCS is deeply situated within or between skeletal muscle groups, and appears as a fairly well circumscribed, soft, lobular or multinodular tumor with a characteristically gelatinous or mucoid gray-white surface. Hemorrhage, as well as cystic areas of degeneration, is frequently present.[426, 429, 439, 444, 445, 449, 456] In 60 cases in which specific dimensions were given‖ the tumors ranged from 1[449] to 26 cm,[427] with a mean of 8.5 cm (median, 7.0 cm); approximately one third were larger than 10 cm.

Histologically, EMCS is characterized by multiple lobules that contain an abundant myxoid stroma (Figs. 17–63 to 17–66), in which reside polygonal, spindle-shaped or stellate tumor cells that have round to oval, usually bland nuclei and a scant to moderate amount of deeply eosinophilic cytoplasm[427, 429, 444, 451, 456] The cytoplasm is frequently vacuolated, creating either signet-ring cells or, in those with multiple

vacuoles, a bubbly appearance similar to physaliferous cells (Fig. 17–67) of **chordoma**.[429, 437, 441, 449] Within the center of the nodules, the cells are diffuse and loosely arranged (see Fig. 17–64), with some forming small clusters and nests, whereas toward the periphery (see Fig. 17–63), the cells assume a radial pattern of columns, cords, and strands.[427, 429, 451, 456] Occasional cases of EMCS contain more cellular zones, which may constitute the majority of the lesion, with a corresponding decrease in the amount of myxoid stroma.[427, 429] Some examples of EMCS contain tumor cells that are larger than usual, with a more abundant cytoplasm (see Fig. 17–67), giving them an epithelioid appearance.[429, 441, 442, 449] Such cells may contain round, dense, cytoplasmic inclusions similar to those present in the cells of **malignant rhabdoid tumor.** Chondroid-like islands may occur in EMCS and, in rare instances, mature cartilage as well.[427, 431, 449] Cellular pleomorphism is not a feature of EMCS,[431] and although hemorrhage may be frequent, necrosis is only rarely present.[429, 444] Mitotic activity is uncommon in the classic form of EMCS[429, 431, 444, 449, 456] but may be quite numerous in the more cellular variant.[427, 429]

The cells of EMCS are positive for glycogen,[429, 431, 441, 445, 456] and the myxoid stroma is strongly reactive with alcian blue, colloidal iron, and mucicarmine stains. The effect of prior treatment with hyaluronidase on these stromal stains has yielded conflicting results, with some tumors showing either a total elimination or a decrease in the intensity of the stain, thus indicating the presence of a large component of hyaluronic acid.[431, 445, 449] However, in other cases the stromal staining was reportedly hyaluronidase-resistant.[429, 435, 436, 442, 456] The resistant cases demonstrate a critical electrolyte concentration for stain extinction of 0.65 to 1.0 M $MgCl_2$, indicating the presence of chondroitin or keratan sulfate, an indication of cartilaginous differentiation.[431, 438]

Only a few cases of EMCS have been analyzed immunohistochemically.[430, 431, 433, 435, 436, 447, 452] All examples studied for S-100 protein (17 cases) were positive,[431, 433, 435, 436, 447, 452] as were four cases analyzed for vimentin;[436, 452] four of six cases stained for Leu-7 antigen.[435, 436, 452] Stains for cytokeratin and epithelial membrane antigen were negative in six cases,[435, 436, 452] as were five cases studied for carcinoembryonic antigen.[435, 452]

In the 30 cases of EMCS in our review studied by electron microscopy,* the tumor cells showed evidence of cartilaginous differentiation. The most prominent feature was the presence of a well-formed, dilated, rough endoplasmic reticulum with a dense granular matrix. The cells contained glycogen, a well-developed Golgi apparatus, pinocytotic vesicles, lipid droplets, aggregates of microfilaments, and a scalloped irregular cytoplasmic border with long and short cytoplasmic processes. A focal basal lamina and desmosome-like junctions were also present. In approximately one third of cases, parallel microtubules within the cisternae of the rough endoplasmic reticulum were found, a feature rarely found in tumors other than myxoid chondrosarcomas.[427, 428, 436, 447, 452] The extracellular matrix may show long spacing collagen and deposits of flocculogranular material.

Cytogenetic studies of EMCS showed a reciprocal translocation involving chromosomes 9 and 22 in one case[450] and between chromosomes 2 and 13 in another case.[453]

---

* References 424, 426–429, 431, 433, 435–438, 441, 442, 444–455.

† References 424, 426–429, 431, 433, 435–438, 441, 442, 444–452, 454, 455.

‡ References 424, 428, 429, 435–438, 441, 443, 445, 454.

§ References 424, 427–429, 433, 436–438, 442, 443, 445, 447, 449, 451, 454.

‖ References 424, 427–429, 435–437, 444–446, 448, 449, 451, 453, 454.

---

* References 427–429, 435–438, 442, 443, 445, 447–449, 451, 452, 457.

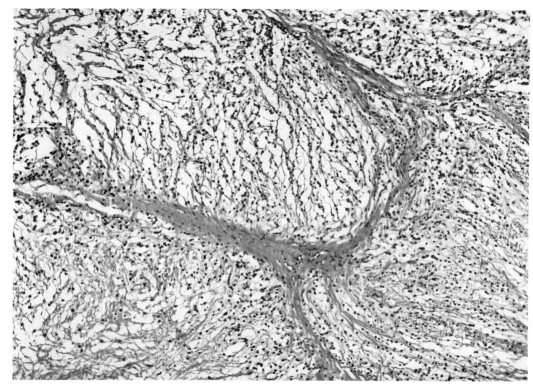

FIGURE 17–63. Low-power view of extraskeletal myxoid chondrosarcoma (EMCS) shows several myxoid lobules separated by thin fibrous septa. One can appreciate the radial arrangement of the cells, in cords or chains, in some of the lobules.

In the light microscopic differential diagnosis, **chordoma** is the tumor whose features most closely resemble those of EMCS. Indeed, because of this apparent morphologic similarity, some myxoid soft tissue tumors were designated as **"chordoid" sarcomas** before it became clear that they were actually examples of EMCS and unrelated to chordoma.[427, 441–443, 451, 452] Both EMCS and chordoma have an alcian blue–positive stroma and contain eosinophilic cells, arranged in cords, strands, or nests, which have cytoplasmic vacuolization and form physaliferous cells. However, chordoma differs from EMCS in its electron microscopic morphology, which shows more extensive cytoplasmic vacuolization, juxtaposition of granular endoplasmic reticulum and mitochondria, the absence of microtubular-rough endoplasmic reticulum complexes, or a basal lamina. Although chordoma cells contain S-100 protein, they are positive for cytokeratin and epithelial membrane antigen, both of which are absent in the cells of EMCS.

Chondroid syringoma of the skin may be histologically indistinguishable from EMCS. However, this adnexal tumor is superficially located within the dermis or subcutaneous tissue in contrast with the deep-seated location of EMCS and is frequently found in the head and neck region, an uncommon location for EMCS. Microscopically, chondroid syringoma has tubular, acinar, or duct-like structures that are lacking in EMCS; however, these may not be present in those chondroid syringomas arising in the extremities. Although the cells of chondroid syringoma are positive for S-100 protein, they also contain cytokeratin. Finally, the electron microscopic morphology of chondroid syringoma differs from that of EMCS in showing epithelial and myoepithelial features.[428, 438]

Myxoid malignant fibrous histiocytoma may enter the differential diagnosis of EMCS because of its abundant myxoid stroma. Microscopically, myxoid malignant fibrous histiocytoma is far more pleomorphic than EMCS, it lacks a radial arrangement of its cells, and, in contrast with EMCS, its cells lack glycogen. Furthermore, the stroma of myxoid malignant fibrous histiocytoma contains hyaluronic acid and lacks the chondroitin or keratan sulfate of EMCS.

Myxoid liposarcoma shares with EMCS vacuolated cells that are S-100 protein–positive, but, unlike those of EMCS, they contain relatively little glycogen. Myxoid liposarcoma has a characteristic plexiform capillary pattern that is absent in EMCS, and its stroma lacks chondroitin or keratan sulfate. Dilated rough endoplasmic reticulum and microtubular rough endoplasmic reticulum aggregates, as present in EMCS, are not found in the cells of liposarcoma.

Although **nerve sheath tumors** may have myxoid areas that contain chondroitin sulfate and have S-100 protein– and Leu-7–positive cells, they typically lack the cytoplasmic glycogen of EMCS.[431, 440] Furthermore, their cells show electron microscopic features of Schwann cells, perineurial cells, or fibroblasts, which is unlike the electron microscopic findings in EMCS.

Soft tissue chondroma consists of lobules of hyaline-type cartilage usually lacking the myxomatous features of EMCS.[458] However, some soft tissue chondromas may appear less mature and contain myxoid areas with eosinophilic chondroblasts that may be arranged in rows or cords such that the distinction from EMCS may be difficult. However, the cells of soft tissue chondroma tend to be larger than those of EMCS, have a more abundant cytoplasm, and are less likely to show

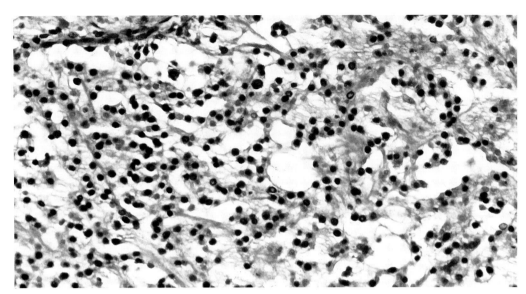

FIGURE 17–64. Higher magnification of the center of one of the lobules of EMCS shows cells, with small, round, uniform nuclei and a scant amount of cytoplasm, uniformly dispersed within the myxoid stroma.

row or cord-like configurations. Myxoid chondrosarcomas are also larger and more deeply located tumors than chondromas, which are typically found in the soft tissues of the hands and feet closely apposed to the bones.

In any case of possible soft tissue EMCS, a primary tumor originating in the adjacent bone must be ruled out by roentgen-

ographic studies, despite the fact that osseous chondrosarcomas are uncommonly of myxoid type.

It was thought that EMCS was a less aggressive tumor than conventional skeletal chondrosarcoma,[445] but a study of 10 patients, with long-term follow-up, indicated its highly aggressive nature.[444] In this series, lung metastases developed in nine

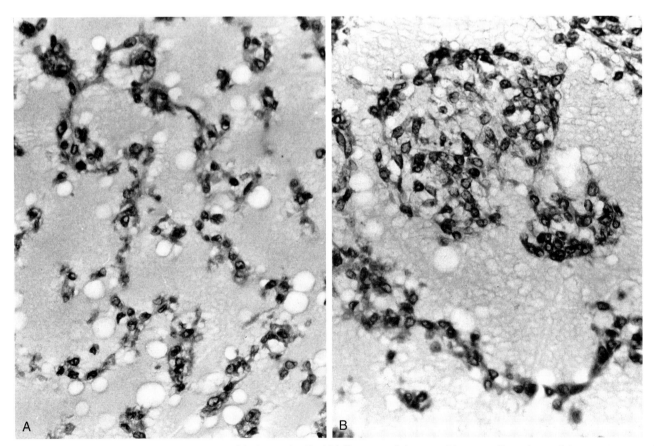

FIGURE 17–65. *A,* View of another lobule in EMCS shows the "bubbly" nature of the myxoid stroma. Here the nuclei are not as round or as dense as those in Figure 17–64; the cells appear to link to form meandering strings. *B,* Higher magnification shows the bland appearance of the nuclei and their loose aggregation.

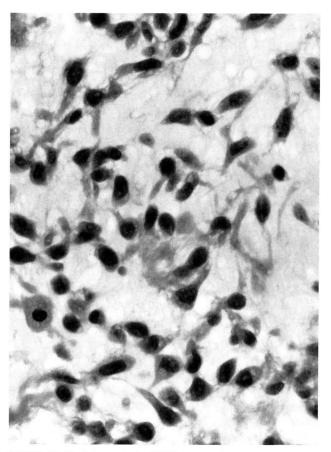

FIGURE 17–66. Other cells in EMCS have stellate to short spindle configurations with interconnecting cytoplasmic extensions.

patients; seven died, and the remaining three were alive with tumor. In our survey of 84 other patients with follow-up data,* 51% either had died of tumor (39%) or were alive with persistent tumor (12%). Of the patients alive without tumor, many had been followed up for relatively short periods. In light of the fact that metastases have developed in some patients more than 10 years after resection,[444, 447, 451] and that patients with metastases may live for many years without symptoms,[429, 444, 451] it is important that patients with EMCS be followed up indefinitely for the possibility of late-developing recurrences. Although some studies indicate that the cellular variety of EMCS has a poorer prognosis than the more myxoid type,[427, 429] others have not found any prognostic difference between them.[444]

MYXOID DERMATOFIBROSARCOMA PROTUBERANS

In 1983, Frierson and Cooper described two adult patients, one man and one woman, with a primary form of dermatofibrosarcoma protuberans (DFSP) that was predominantly myxoid.[459] These cutaneous tumors were located in the suprapubic area in one patient, and in the other on the dorsum of the foot. In contrast with conventional dermatofibrosarcoma, in

which spindle tumor cells are tightly compacted and arranged in a classic storiform pattern (Fig. 17–68), these tumors were characterized by sparsely cellular nodules composed of haphazardly arranged stellate and spindle cells with elongated, bland-appearing nuclei (Fig. 17–69). Cytoplasmic processes extended from the cells to intermix with delicate collagen fibers present within a myxoid, basophilic stroma (see Fig. 17–69). Blood vessels, including venules, capillaries, and arterioles, were scattered throughout the lesions, and subcutaneous fat and skin adnexa were entrapped within them. Mitotic figures were uncommon. At the periphery of the nodules the tumor cells had a more orderly and parallel arrangement, and at the interface with the subcutaneous fat there were tentacular extensions of tumor into the fat (Fig. 17–70). The classic cartwheel or storiform pattern of conventional DFSP was not present within the myxoid zones; however, on careful search of other nodules, or the examination of additional tissue, such conventional foci were discovered and served as an important clue to the diagnosis of DFSP. The myxoid stroma was stained by alcian blue and colloidal iron, the reactivity being abolished by pretreatment with hyaluronidase.

Myxoid foci similar to those in primary myxoid DFSP may be found as a minor component in otherwise conventional dermatofibrosarcomas. Such foci are most commonly found in recurrences or in the rare metastases of conventional dermatofibrosarcomas.[459–466]

Immunohistochemical studies have not been reported in cases of pure myxoid DFSP. However, in conventional DFSP the results of such studies have varied, with some

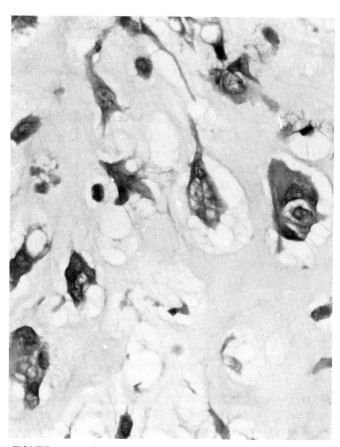

FIGURE 17–67. Occasional foci occur in EMCS where, as shown here, the cells assume an epithelioid appearance and have a vacuolated cytoplasm such that they simulate physaliferous cells.

* References 424, 426, 427, 429, 431, 433, 435, 436, 441, 442, 444, 446, 447, 449, 451, 452, 455.

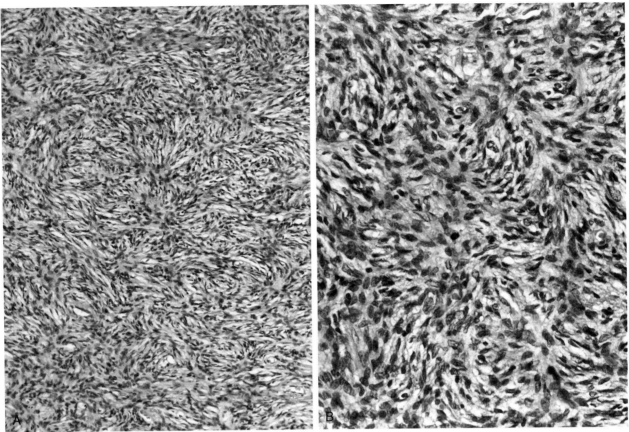

FIGURE 17–68. Low-power *(A)* and high-power *(B)* views of conventional dermatofibrosarcoma show highly cellular foci consisting of tightly compacted spindle cells arranged in a mat-like or storiform pattern.

reports of occasional cell reactivity for the proteolytic enzymes alpha-1-antitrypsin, alpha-1-antichymotrypsin, and lysozyme,[467–469] whereas in others there was an absence of these markers.[462, 470] Similar disparate results have been obtained for muscle-specific actin.[468, 470, 471] However, epithelial determinants, including epithelial membrane antigen and cytokeratin,[470, 472] are absent, as are S-100 protein, desmin, and CD68 antigen.[462, 470, 471] In most studies, stains for Factor XIIIa have been negative,[473, 473a] but others report reactivity in some cases of DFSP.[473b] One report indicates reactivity in DFSP for the human progenitor cell antigen CD34,[473] a pattern of reactivity that is not shared by other "fibrohistiocytic" lesions of the skin and is thought to be definitive for the diagnosis of DFSP. However, a recent report casts doubt on the diagnostic usefulness of CD34 for the diagnosis.[473c]

Electron microscopic analysis has not been done on cases of myxoid DFSP, but conventional DFSP contains fibroblastic spindle cells that have a well-developed rough endoplasmic reticulum, a prominent Golgi apparatus, pinocytotic vesicles, numerous mitochondria, and long cytoplasmic processes. The nuclei are indented and lobulated with a characteristic cerebriform appearance. In some studies, interrupted basal lamina–like material and primitive intercellular junctions are found.[474–479] Based on these electron microscopic studies, there is a general consensus that the cells of DFSP are fibroblastic in nature,[474, 476, 479] and, in some cases, may simulate perineurial cells;[474, 475, 477] however, some authors maintain that the cells have Schwann cell,[475] fibrohistiocytic, or histiocytic features.[464, 469, 473, 478, 479]

The diagnosis of myxoid DFSP is not difficult when one is able to find foci having the characteristic cellular storiform pattern of classic DFSP. In the absence of such areas, particularly in small biopsy specimens, other myxoid lesions, including myxoid neurofibroma, myxoid malignant fibrous histiocytoma, myxoid liposarcoma, nerve sheath myxoma, nodular fasciitis, and myxoid malignant melanoma, may be diagnostic considerations.

Neurofibroma contains spindle cells within a myxoid background, but also has short, thick strands of collagen fibers dispersed throughout it, which are absent in myxoid DFSP. S-100 protein is present in most neurofibromas, in contrast with its absence in DFSP, and muscle-specific actin, as sometimes found in DFSP, is lacking in the cells of neurofibroma. Electron microscopy may not be useful in separating DFSP from neurofibroma, because the cells of the latter may have many features of perineurial cells, such as long cytoplasmic processes, incomplete basal lamina and pinocytotic vesicles, as sometimes found in cells of DFSP.[480] However, the finding of axons in association with the tumor cells favors a diagnosis of neurofibroma, as axons are not present in DFSP.

Myxoid malignant fibrous histiocytoma (MFH) may, like myxoid DFSP, be a superficial tumor involving the subcutaneous tissue and dermis. However, the marked cellular pleomorphism, abundant and frequently abnormal mitotic figures, and the plexiform capillary network of myxoid MFH easily distinguish it from myxoid DFSP.

Myxoid liposarcoma contains stellate or bipolar cells embedded within an abundant myxoid stroma, but rarely

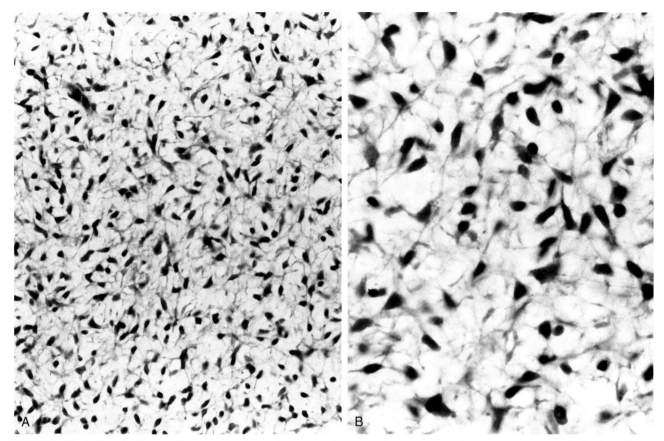

FIGURE 17–69. *A,* Myxoid dermatofibrosarcoma shows loose myxoid stroma in which are well-separated, but evenly distributed, small cells. *B,* Higher magnification shows hyperchromatic cells with stellate to spindle shapes. Cytoplasmic extensions from the cells interconnect to form a loose meshwork. (Prepared from case material provided by Dr. Philip H. Cooper, Department of Pathology, University of Virginia.)

occurs as a superficial tumor. The presence of a plexiform-capillary network, defined pools of mucin, lipoblasts, and immunohistochemical reactivity for S-100 protein serve to distinguish myxoid liposarcoma from myxoid DFSP.

Nerve sheath myxoma is a dermal lesion in which stellate and spindle cells are embedded in a myxoid stroma. However, unlike DFSP, nerve sheath myxoma has distinct lobulation and contains epithelioid-like and multinucleated-type giant cells, and its stroma contains chondroitin sulfate. **Nodular fasciitis** may have extensive myxoid areas, but the characteristic pattern of spindle cells arranged in curving or S-shaped configurations, the presence of brisk mitotic activity, and microcystic areas with extravasated red blood cells help distinguish it from myxoid DFSP.

A primary cutaneous form of **amelanotic malignant melanoma** has been described that is characterized by a predominantly myxoid stroma containing spindle and stellate cells.[481, 482] In contrast with myxoid DFSP, this lesion contains pleomorphic cells and typically has an intraepidermal component. Further, its cells are reactive for S-100 protein and HMB-45 antigen, and melanosomes can be identified by electron microscopy.

Follow-up information on the two patients described by Frierson and Cooper[459] indicated that both developed local recurrences at 26 months and 8.5 years, respectively, after the initial excision of their lesions. After re-excision of the recurrences, the patients were alive and well at 18 and 20 months, respectively. In one of the patients, the recurrent lesion contained areas of conventional DFSP. It is not known whether this rare myxoid variant of DFSP behaves clinically any differently from conventional DFSP, for which recurrence rates have ranged from approximately 10% to 50%,[462, 465, 466] with metastases in from 2% to 6% of cases.[460, 465]

NERVE SHEATH MYXOMA

Nerve sheath myxoma (NSM) is an uncommon benign neoplasm first described by Harkin and Reed in 1969.[483] Despite its relative rarity, this tumor has enjoyed a rich nomenclature with a multiplicity of appellations given it, including pacinian neurofibroma,[484] bizarre cutaneous neurofibroma,[485] neurothekeoma,[486–490] dermal nerve sheath myxoma,[491, 492] myxomatous perineuroma,[493] plexiform myxoma,[494] cutaneous lobular neuromyxoma,[495] perineurial myxoma,[496] cellular neurothekeoma,[497–500] and, most commonly, nerve sheath myxoma.[483, 493, 501–505]

Clinically, NSM is notable for its slow evolution. Although one half of the 30 patients in our review for whom the clinical duration of disease was stated had their lesions for 1 year or less,* and some for less than a month,[504] many patients had

---

* References 484–486, 488, 490–493, 495, 497–499, 501, 504–511.

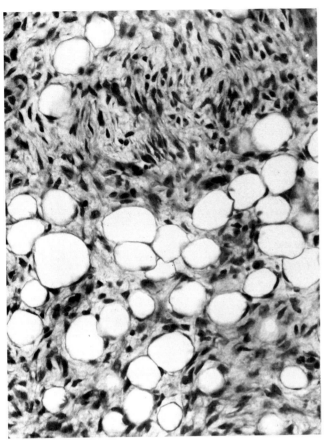

FIGURE 17–70. Deep portion of myxoid dermatofibrosarcoma shows entrapment of subcutaneous fat by tumor cells that are more compact and in an infiltrating pattern similar to that which occurs in conventional dermatofibrosarcoma. (Prepared from case material provided by Dr. Philip H. Cooper, Department of Pathology, University of Virginia.)

their lesion for long periods, some for over 50 years.* With few exceptions, NSM develops as an asymptomatic mass that occasionally becomes painful. Female patients accounted for approximately 70% of the 195 patients in our review.

Among 65 patients with NSM for whom individual age data were given,† the mean age was 30 years (median, 29 years), with a range of 3[514] to 84[491] years. Two thirds of 112 patients were between 10 and 39 years of age; NSM is uncommon in children younger than age 10 years, this age group accounting for only 11% of cases, or in patients older than age 60 years, who accounted for 4% of the cases. The so-called cellular variant of NSM tends to occur more commonly in younger patients than the more conventional myxomatous variety. The mean age of 23 patients with the cellular variant[497–500, 506] was 24.2 years (median, 20 years; range, 8–65 years), whereas in 43 patients with conventional NSM, the mean age was 33.3 years (median, 30 years; range, 10–84 years).

NSM most commonly arises in upper body sites. Among 188 cases with specific site data,‡ the head and neck region

was involved in 36% of the cases, with a predilection for the face and jaw, including the buccal mucosa, lips, tongue, nose, and retromolar region.[488, 492, 500, 504, 508–511] The upper extremities were involved in 37% of cases, with the shoulder and arm the most commonly affected areas; the lower extremities were the site of tumor in only 9% of cases, and the trunk was involved in 18%. NSM tends to be small, the average maximum size in the 40 cases in our review with tumor dimensions was 1.6 cm (median, 1.3 cm), with a range of 0.3[504] to 6.0 cm;[505] 90% were less than 3.0 cm.*

As mentioned, two forms of NSM are histologically described, a conventional myxomatous form and a cellular variant, with the former the more common. Conventional NSM† is predominantly a dermal lesion that is typically separated from the epidermis by normal tissue; it may also extend into the subcutis. The characteristic feature of conventional NSM is its nodularity, a feature that is created by thin collagen septa that divide the tumor into variably sized lobules or nests (Fig. 17–71). The perimeter of the tumor may be surrounded by coarsely condensed dermal collagen.[510, 514] The individual lobules are composed of loosely and haphazardly arranged stellate, spindle, round, and bipolar cells that reside within a myxoid stroma (Fig. 17–72). Tumor cell nuclei are small, round or irregularly shaped, and may be vacuolated; hyperchromasia and moderate nuclear pleomorphism may be prominent.[486, 487, 491, 492, 494, 495, 507] The cytoplasm is acidophilic and may also be vacuolated. Fine wispy projections extend from the cells and intermingle (Fig. 17–73), creating a meshwork pattern of fibers.[484, 491, 510] Frequently, the cells are arrayed in a whorled pattern superficially resembling pacinian corpuscles.[484, 494] Multinucleated cells, many of the osteoclast-type, are found scattered within the lobules,‡ as are mast cells, which may be numerous.[486, 492, 504, 510, 511] Larger cells are sometimes present that have an abundant pale to dense eosinophilic cytoplasm and round to oval nuclei, giving them an epithelioid or histiocytic appearance.[484, 485, 490, 495, 510, 513] Mitotic activity may be frequent, but abnormal mitotic figures are absent.[487, 492, 504, 513] Examples of conventional NSM occur that contain more cellular zones where the myxoid stroma is sharply reduced in quantity.[484–486, 492, 495, 504, 513, 514] Although the myxoid stroma of NSM has been found to contain hyaluronic acid, most cases show staining reactions consistent with the presence of chondroitin sulfate.[485–487, 491, 492, 507] In the normal tissue adjacent to the tumor, small dermal nerves may be found that show a myxomatous stromal change with plump atypical cells.[483, 487, 492]

The cellular form of NSM has been described only since 1986.[497–500, 506, 514] In contrast with the circumscription and lobularity of conventional NSM and its loosely dispersed cells, cellular NSM is an ill-defined and non-lobulated tumor whose cells insinuate and dissect through the dermal collagen (Figs. 17–74 and 17–75). This cellular variant is composed of fascicles or nests of plump spindle-shaped to epithelioid cells that may be found in linear arrays or, less commonly, concentrically arranged. The cells have a relatively abundant pale to densely eosinophilic cytoplasm and vesicular oval to round

* References 484, 485, 490–493, 495, 498, 499, 501, 508.
† References 485, 486, 488, 491, 492, 494, 495, 497–501, 505, 507–512, 514.
‡ References 484–488, 490–495, 497–501, 504–511, 513, 514.

* References 484–486, 488, 490, 491, 493, 494, 497, 499, 501, 504–510.
† References 484, 485, 487, 490–492, 494, 495, 504, 506, 507, 510, 513, 514.
‡ References 485, 491, 492, 494, 504, 506, 510, 511, 513, 514.

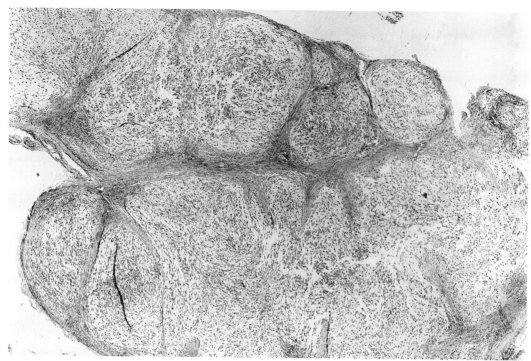

FIGURE 17–71. Low-power view of conventional nerve sheath myxoma (NSM) shows lobular pattern created by collagenous septa.

nuclei. Nuclear pleomorphism and hyperchromasia are common, as is the presence of multinucleated giant cells (Fig. 17–76). Significantly, the myxoid stroma of conventional NSM is absent or minimally present in the cellular variant. Similar hypercellular areas may also be focally found in conventional NSM, but here they constitute only a minor aspect of the tumor in contrast with their diffuse presence in the cellular variant.

Fifteen cases of conventional NSM in our review were examined electron microscopically, with variable results.* Spindle cells are present that have long, interdigitating cell processes and a basal lamina[486, 487, 490, 491, 507, 510, 511] that in some cases has been discontinous[493, 501, 504] and in others duplicated;[491, 510] however, in other studies, a basal lamina was not found.[488, 505] Pinocytotic vesicles, abundant microfilaments, variable amounts of rough endoplasmic reticulum, and myelinoid figures[486–488] are also found; desmosome-like or tight junctions were found in some cases[488, 491, 493, 504] but not in others.[490, 505] Based on these electron microscopic results, there exists no consensus as to the nature of the tumor cells, with opinions divided between considerations that they represent Schwann cells,[486, 487, 490, 507] perineurial cells,[491, 493, 504] or fibroblasts; a combination of all three cell types has also been found.[505, 510] Only one example of cellular NSM has been examined by electron microscopy.[506] The component cells of this lesion were oval to elongated with short filopodia and small junctions at sites of cell contact. The cells lacked a basal lamina, had only rare pinocytotic vesicles and microfilaments, and had an abundant dilated rough endoplasmic reticulum. No dense bodies or other evidence of smooth muscle differentiation was present. Cells with fibroblastic features were found throughout the lesion.

Immunohistochemical studies of conventional NSM* have yielded positive results for S-100 protein[488, 490, 492, 501, 504, 505, 511–515] in 24 of 28 cases (86%). Only 1 of 11 cases studied for Leu-7 antigen was positive;[490, 505, 506, 514] seven cases were nonreactive for neuron-specific enolase,[486, 488, 514] whereas one was positive.[511] Neurofilament protein was absent in four cases from three separate studies;[490, 505, 511] but in a single series of 34 cases, it was found in 40% of the cases, although the number of examined cases was not stated. In this same study, myelin basic protein was found in 70% of the cases examined for this antigen, but again the number of these cases was not given.[489]

In contrast with conventional NSM, none of 32 cases of cellular NSM studied for S-100 protein were positive.[497–500, 506, 514] Reactivity for neuron-specific enolase was present in 12 of 16 cases (75%), although the reaction was only weakly positive in the majority of the cases;[498, 499, 514] stains for Leu-7 in 12 cases[506, 514] and neurofilament protein in three cases[500] were negative. In one study, three of nine cases were positive for smooth muscle actin, and intense staining was also found in all nine for NK1/C3, a putative melanoma-specific marker.[498] However, the significance of the latter results is in question because of the relatively low specificity of this antibody. In this same study, six of the cases examined for HMB-45 antigen were negative. An additional study of cellular NSM showed reactivity for smooth muscle actin in two of four cases, and negative results for HMB-45 antigen.[514] To date, neither the conventional nor the cellular forms of NSM have

* References 486–488, 490, 491, 493, 501, 504, 505, 507, 510, 511.

* References 486, 488–490, 492, 501, 504–506, 511, 513–514.

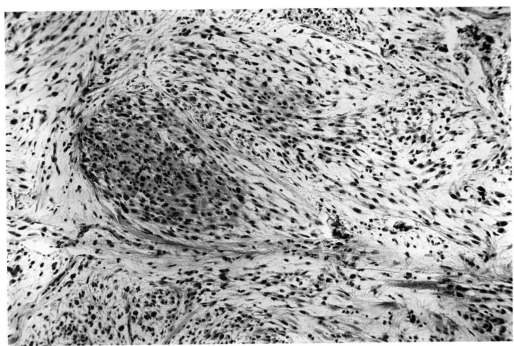

FIGURE 17–72. Central portion of one of the lobules of NSM shows a myxoid stroma in which spindle and stellate cells are dispersed. A more compact cellular focus *(left of center)* is present where the cells have a more abundant cytoplasm.

yielded positive results for epithelial membrane antigen in 61 cases studied,[489, 490, 497–499, 501, 506, 514, 515] or for desmin in 12 cases.[490, 497, 498]

The electron microscopic and immunohistochemical studies have not helped pinpoint the exact histogenesis of NSM. Based on some electron microscopic features and the S-100 protein reactivity of its cells, the consensus view is that con-

ventional NSM appears to exhibit nerve sheath differentiation. As noted earlier, the tumor cells of conventional NSM lack reactivity for epithelial membrane antigen (EMA), normally present in perineurial cells.[502, 515–518] However, EMA-reactive perineurial elements are present that outline the tumor nodules and lobules in some cases,[514] suggesting that, like other benign nerve sheath neoplasms, these lesions arise within peripheral

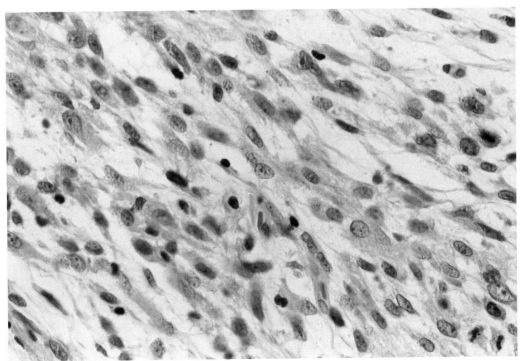

FIGURE 17–73. Cells of conventional NSM are elongated with cytoplasmic extensions that interdigitate. Nuclei vary somewhat in size and shape, but significant pleomorphism is absent.

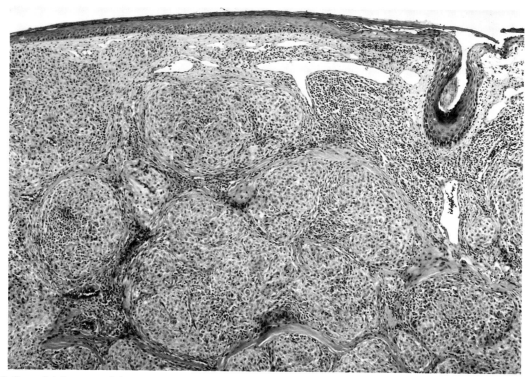

FIGURE 17–74. Superficial aspect of the cellular variant of NSM shows a flattened epidermis with ectasia of dermal lymphatics and a chronic inflammatory infiltrate. The tumor is transected by collagenous septa creating small nests. (Prepared from case material provided by Dr. Zsolt B. Argenyi, Department of Pathology, University of Iowa.)

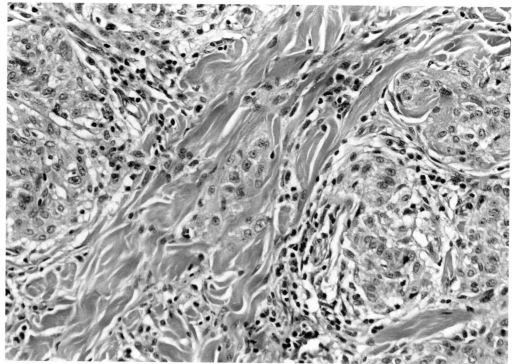

FIGURE 17–75. Small islands of epithelioid-type cells infiltrate the thickened dermal collagen in cellular NSM. (Prepared from case material provided by Dr. Zsolt B. Argenyi, Department of Pathology, University of Iowa.)

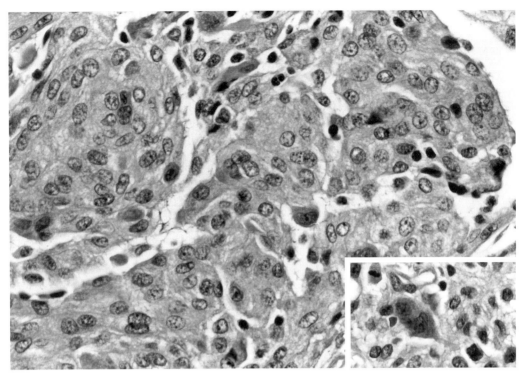

FIGURE 17–76. Cells of cellular NSM have an epithelioid/histiocytic appearance. In this example, no cellular pleomorphism was present. *Inset* shows a multinucleated giant cell. (Prepared from case material provided by Dr. Zsolt B. Argenyi, Department of Pathology, University of Iowa.)

nerves. The presence of myxomatous change and atypical cells within dermal nerves adjacent to some examples of NSM[483, 487, 492] adds support to this view. It has been suggested that the cellular variant of NSM may represent an epithelioid variant of a pilar leiomyoma,[498] although to date the one electron microscopic study of this variant did not show smooth muscle differentiation,[506] and the number of cases immunohistochemically demonstrating smooth muscle actin have been few.[498] Based on their light microscopic and immunohistochemical differences, the question exists as to whether or not the myxoid and cellular lesions are truly different variants of the same tumor or two different entitities.[514]

The differential diagnosis of NSM includes a variety of neural, melanocytic, and fibrohistiocytic lesions. Among the neural lesions, conventional **neurofibroma** and its myxoid variant[487, 503, 504] are diagnostic considerations because they share with NSM a myxoid stroma that contains sulfated acid mucopolysaccharides, S-100 protein–positive cells, and some electron microscopic evidence of Schwann cell differentiation. However, the cells of neurofibroma are not arranged in lobules or nests, epithelioid and osteoclast-type giant cells are not present in neurofibroma, and the wavy bands of collagen and the neurites of neurofibroma are absent in NSM. The cellular variant of NSM is also considerably more cellular than the usual conventional neurofibroma.

The cellular form of NSM may be mimicked by a variety of melanocytic lesions, including **malignant melanoma,** Spitz nevus, spindle cell nevus, and plexiform spindle cell nevus.[512] However, cellular NSM lacks certain important features of melanoma, including junctional activity, marked cellular atypia, premelanosomes or melanin pigment, expression of S-100 protein or HMB-45 antigen, and melanocytic features by electron microscopy.

Because of the histiocytic appearance of the tumor cells in NSM and the presence of multinucleated giant cells, dermatofibroma and myxoid malignant fibrous histiocytoma are possible but unlikely diagnostic possibilities. **Dermatofibroma** has a storiform pattern and foamy histiocytes, lacks a myxoid stroma, and is not lobulated. Although **myxoid malignant fibrous histiocytoma** may be superficially located in the subcutaneous tissue and invade the dermis, its vascularity, pleomorphism, anaplasia, and lack of lobulation easily distinguish it from NSM.

Another diagnostic consideration is **solitary circumscribed neuroma** of the skin (**palisaded encapsulated neuroma**).[519–521] Like NSM, this is an intradermal lesion with a propensity for the face. It is well-circumscribed and composed of fascicles of bland spindle cells. However, unlike NSM, it contains axons by neurofilament staining and lacks the lobulation and myxoid stroma of conventional NSM and the infiltrative character of cellular NSM.

Because the cells of some examples of NSM show electron microscopic features consistent with perineurial cells, **perineuroma** becomes a diagnostic consideration.[515, 522] Perineuroma arises in the subcutaneous or deep soft tissues of the extremities and trunk of middle-aged patients who, like those with NSM, are predominantly women. Although perineuroma has a myxoid stroma and is composed of spindle cells, their nuclei are bland, without the mild to moderate pleomorphism or atypia of the cells of NSM. In addition, and in contrast with NSM, the cells of perineuroma are S-100 protein–negative and typically strongly reactive for epithelial membrane antigen.

The pacinian-like whorled pattern of cells found in NSM also raises the diagnostic possibility of **digital pacinian neuroma.**[523] Digital pacinian neuroma is a rare lesion that occurs in the digits of middle-aged adults. Unlike NSM, it is painful and is composed of abnormal aggregates of mature-appearing pacinian corpuscles and small nerves, unlike the pseudopacinian pattern focally created by the whorled arrangement of cells in NSM. Pacinian neuroma also lacks the epithelioid and giant cells of NSM.

The clinical course of both conventional and cellular NSM has been benign, with all patients alive and well after local resection.* Although a few patients have had local recurrences, these appear to be the result of inadequate initial excision.[487, 495, 496, 504, 506]

AGGRESSIVE ANGIOMYXOMA

Originally described by Steeper and Rosai in 1983 as a soft tissue neoplasm involving the pelvis and perineum of young women,[524] aggressive angiomyxoma (AAM) has subsequently also been reported in men.[525, 526] To date, fewer than 50 cases of AAM have been reported in the English-language medical literature.[524, 525, 527–532]

Most patients with AAM are young adults in the third and fourth decades of life. In our review of 33 patients with individual age data,[524–530, 532–534] the mean age was 36.5 years (median, 36 years), with a range from 18[525] to 70 years;[526] 82% were between 20 and 49 years of age. A similar percentage of the patients were women.

In both men and women, AAM appears to be restricted to pelvic and perineal locations. In women, the vulva and vagina are common sites, as are the pelvic soft tissues. In the few cases of AAM reported in men, the lesion involved the spermatic cord, groin, scrotum, pelvis, and perianal and perineal regions.[525, 526] Aggressive angiomyxomas tend to be large, ranging in size from 3 to 60 cm.[524] Among 27 tumors with individual dimensions,[524–527, 530, 532–534] the mean size was 12.5 cm (median, 10 cm). Grossly, AAM appears circumscribed but is an infiltrating tumor that is firm and fleshy, with a glistening gelatinous cut surface.[524–526, 530, 532–534]

Histologically,[524–526, 528, 530, 533] AAM has irregular margins and infiltrates into fat and skeletal muscle. It is characterized by a monotonous population of small round, spindle, or stellate mesenchymal cells (Figs. 17–77 to 17–79), from which bipolar cytoplasmic extensions traverse a loose myxoid and fibrillar alcian blue–positive stroma (see Fig. 17–79). For the most part, the cells are scarce and widely separated within the stroma; however, focal areas of increased cellularity may be found, especially in recurrent tumors. Nuclei are small and bland with small inconspicuous nucleoli (see Fig. 17–79A); mitotic figures are rare or absent.

A distinctive histologic feature of AAM is its vascularity. Non-arborizing, thin-walled, ectatic capillaries or, more commonly, small thick-walled vessels are dispersed throughout the tumor (see Figs. 17–77 and 17–78). The latter feature is due either to thick smooth muscle in the walls of the vessels or to their investiture by a periadventitial condensation of eosinophilic fibrillar material (see Fig. 17–78B). Stromal mast cells and extravasated red blood cells are frequently found.[524–526, 528, 530, 533, 534]

Only a few examples of AAM have been studied by electron microscopy.[524, 525, 530, 532] The spindle- and stellate-shaped tumor cells show delicate and irregular cytoplasmic processes; a prominent rough endoplasmic reticulum, which may show cisternal dilatation; plasmalemmal pinocytotic vesicles; moderate numbers of mitochondria; and well-developed Golgi zones. Thin actin filaments, at times with focal condensations, are present, as well as intermediate cytoplasmic filaments; some cells have a basal lamina.[525] Based on the electron microscopic features, some have concluded that the cells show myofibroblastic differentiation,[524] whereas others support fibroblastic differentiation.[525]

Immunohistochemical studies of AAM are equally scarce.[525, 526, 530–532] The tumor cells showed universal positivity for vimentin in 16 cases;[526, 530–532] actin reactivity[525, 530–532] was found in 15 of 17 cases (88%). A study of four cases also showed focal positivity for muscle-specific actin.[526] Desmin positivity is less consistently reported; in a study of ten cases, desmin was found in all cases,[531] whereas in other studies, totalling six cases, reactivity for desmin was absent.[526, 531, 532] Studies for S-100 protein,[525, 526, 531, 532] cytokeratin,[525, 532] epithelial membrane antigen,[531] Factor VIII–related antigen,[525, 526, 531, 532] alpha-1-antichymotrypsin and alpha-1-antitrypsin,[531] and *Ulex europaeus* I lectin[524] have been negative.

In the differential histologic diagnosis of AAM, the soft tissue tumor that most closely resembles it is conventional **myxoma.** However, myxoma most commonly is an intramuscular lesion of the extremities and is uncommon in the pelvis. The most important feature that serves to separate these two lesions is the absence of conspicuous stromal blood vessels in myxoma in contrast with their abundance in AAM.

Because of its myxoid stroma and infiltrative character, AAM may be confused with a variety of myxoid sarcomas. **Myxoid liposarcoma** contains an abundant, hyaluronic acid–rich stroma and a prominent vascular network. However, the vessels in myxoid liposarcoma are thin-walled capillaries arranged in a plexiform pattern, unlike the non-arborizing and thick-walled vessels of AAM. In contrast with AAM, myxoid liposarcoma tends to occur in older patients, is uncommon in the pelvis, contains lipoblasts, and is reactive for S-100 protein, which is absent in AAM; smooth muscle markers are absent in liposarcoma.

Myxoid malignant fibrous histiocytoma, like liposarcoma a tumor primarily of older adults, also contains a prominent vascular component; however, it is of the plexiform capillary type. The cell pleomorphism, anaplasia, and the high mitotic rate of myxoid malignant fibrous histiocytoma is in sharp contrast with the bland cells and low mitotic activity of AAM.

Myxoid leiomyosarcoma occurs in the pelvic soft tissues and may be confused with AAM; however, its cells are larger and more atypical than those of AAM. Immunohistochemical stains may be unrewarding in separating these two tumors, because AAM may contain cells reactive for smooth muscle actin or desmin. However, electron microscopy may be of considerable aid in this differential, because the cells of myxoid leiomyosarcoma typically show smooth muscle features rather than the fibroblastic or myofibroblastic character of the cells of AAM.

Because of its myxoid stroma, **botryoid rhabdomyosarcoma** might be a diagnostic consideration. However, botryoid rhabdomyosarcoma occurs in young children and adolescents in contrast with the adult population of those with AAM. The small, irregular character of the tumor cells of rhabdomyosarcoma, the occurrence of rhabdomyoblasts, and the characteris-

---

* References 485, 487, 488, 490, 492, 495, 498–500, 504, 508, 510.

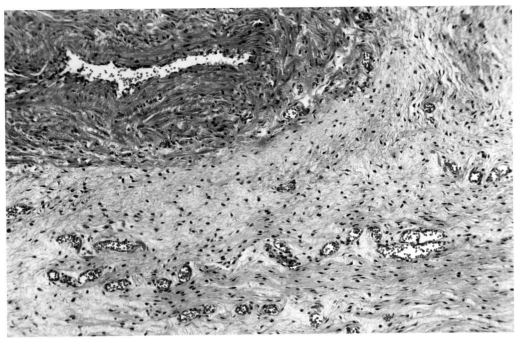

FIGURE 17-77. View of aggressive angiomyxoma (AAM) shows large thick-walled blood vessel within a loose-appearing stroma in which small capillary vessels are dispersed.

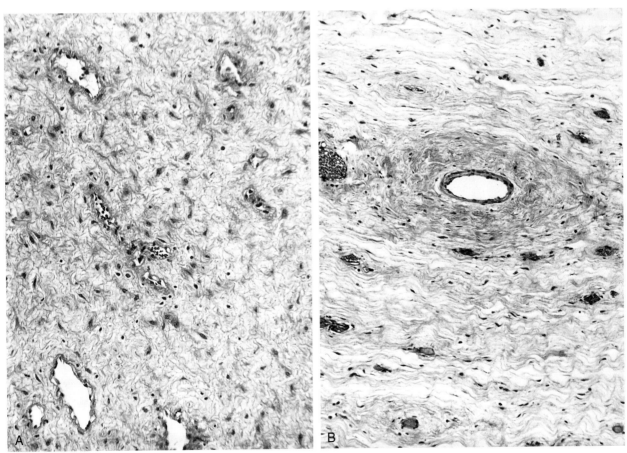

FIGURE 17-78. *A,* Throughout the stroma of AAM are thin-walled vessels. *B,* Similar vessels are also present in which there is a condensation of the surrounding stroma forming a cuff about the vessel.

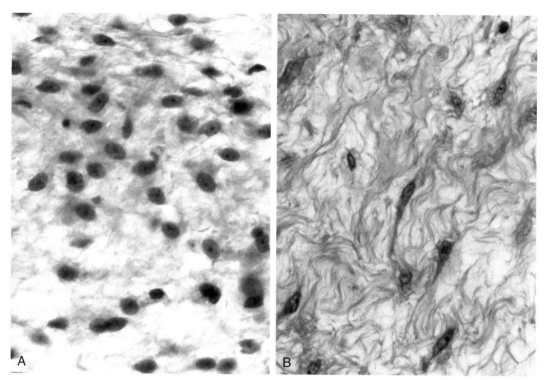

FIGURE 17–79. *A,* Stromal cells in AAM may be round, oval, stellate, or spindle-shaped. Nuclei are bland, some with small nucleoli. *B,* Connecting bipolar cytoplasmic extensions from the spindle cells are illustrated.

tic cambium layer of botryoid rhabdomyosarcoma should reliably separate rhabdomyosarcoma from AAM. However, when dealing with diminutive biopsy specimens in which all of these diagnostic features may not be present, electron microscopic examination may be helpful by demonstrating evidence of skeletal muscle differentiation.

Because of its loose collagenous myxoid stroma, **myxoid neurofibroma** may simulate AAM. However, in contrast with AAM, myxoid neurofibroma lacks prominent vascularity, and its cells are frequently positive for S-100 protein and other neural markers. Electron microscopy also demonstrates the nerve sheath nature of neurofibroma.

AAM should not be equated with **superficial angiomyxoma.**[535] The latter is a subcutaneous lesion, usually of small size, that is most commonly located in the trunk or lower extremities. Histologically, superficial angiomyxoma shows a multinodular proliferation of spindle cells and small to medium-sized thin-walled blood vessels. The nodules may also harbor epithelial elements in the form of epithelial-lined cysts or epithelial strands. Despite their similar names, AAM and superficial angiomyxoma are distinct and separate entities.

A lesion histologically closely related to AAM was described by Fletcher et al.[536] under the rubric of **angiomyxofibroblastoma** (AMF). Of the 11 patients reported, 10 were women, all of whom had vulvar lesions; the single male patient had a scrotal tumor. Patients ranged in age from 25 to 54 years (mean, 36.3 years). In contrast with the diffuse proliferation of the cells in AAM, AMF displays alternating hypo- and hypercellular areas. The cells, which vary from spindle to oval or round, either aggregate about blood vessels or form compact masses where the cells may have a plasmacytoid hyaline appearance similar to the cells of some salivary gland myoepitheliomas. In the hypocellular areas, the cells are dis-

persed in an edematous matrix that contains thin and thick strands of collagen. Unlike the stroma of AAM, that of AMF is not stained by alcian blue. Blood vessels are distributed throughout AMF, but, in contrast with those in AAM, they are thin-walled. AMF is well circumscribed, tends to be superficially located, and, unlike AAM, is not infiltrative. Electron microscopy of three cases of AMF showed a well-developed endoplasmic reticulum and Golgi apparatus, a discontinuous basal lamina, abundant cytoplasmic intermediate filaments, and frequent pinocytotic vesicles. No microfilaments or plasmalemmal plaques were found. The tumor cells were positive for vimentin and desmin in all cases, but negative for muscle-specific actin, smooth muscle actin, S-100 protein, cytokeratin, and myoglobin. The authors distinguished AMF and AAM on both morphologic and clinical grounds, AMF being a superficial, non-infiltrating tumor that was adequately treated by simple excision. The authors also separated AMF from AAM on the basis of the desmin positivity of AMF. However, as already noted, desmin positivity has been reported in some cases of AAM, so that this immunohistochemical distinction may not be valid.

AAM is a locally aggressive tumor that is prone to local recurrence, sometimes of massive degree, after excision.[524, 525, 528, 529] Among 30 patients for whom there was follow-up data,[524–530, 532–534] 15 (50%) had local recurrences, some multiple. To date, with limited follow-up intervals, no deaths or metastases from AAM have been reported.

MYXOID LEIOMYOSARCOMA

The myxoid variant of leiomyosarcoma is an extremely rare neoplasm with only a few cases in the English-language medical literature;[537-542] the largest series contains only 13 patients.[541] Although this tumor occurs mainly in the pelvic region, with the uterus[538] and bladder[539, 542] the most common sites, it has also been reported in the vagina, vulva, prostate, stomach, retroperitoneum, esophagus, parotid, and maxillary antrum,[541] as well as the paravaginal[537] and retrovesicle soft tissues.[540]

Myxoid leiomyosarcoma (MLMS) most commonly affects adults. In our review of 28 patients,[537-542] ages ranged from 16[542] to 88 years,[541] with a mean of 55 years (median, 58.5 years); slightly more than 80% of patients were older than age 40 years. Women are more commonly affected than men in a ratio of 2.5 to 1.

Grossly, MLMS varies greatly in size, from 1.5[542] to 16 cm,[541] but most are large; among the 19 cases with tumor dimensions in our review,[537-542] the mean size was 7.5 cm (median, 8.0 cm). MLMS appears well-circumscribed or even encapsulated and has a soft, jelly-like consistency with a characteristically mucoid cut surface.

As the macroscopic appearance suggests, the histologic pattern of MLMS is marked by the presence of an abundant myxoid stroma (Figs. 17–80 and 17–81). However, because conventional smooth muscle tumors may also contain focal myxoid areas, the amount of such stroma that must be present in order to classify a tumor as "myxoid" has not been established. Mills et al.,[539] in a study involving bladder leiomyosarcomas, required that at least 75% of the tumor be myxoid before designating it as an MLMS. In our view, an MLMS

should obviously have a predominant myxoid component, and we would suggest that, as required for the diagnosis of myxoid malignant fibrous histiocytoma, 50% or more of the lesion be myxoid in order for it to qualify as an MLMS.

With routine hematoxylin and eosin sections, the stroma has an eosinophilic or basophilic hue[538, 542] and contains areas that appear "bubbly" because of vacuoles within it.[541] Pools of mucinous material, similar to those found in myxoid liposarcoma, may be focally present, with their walls formed by compact stromal tumor cells.[538, 541] Periodic acid-Shiff and mucicarmine stains of the myxoid stroma are either weakly positive or negative;[538, 540, 542] alcian blue and colloidal iron stains are positive and not abolished by pretreatment with hyaluronidase.[538, 540, 542]

Haphazardly distributed, and widely dispersed within this stroma, are spindle, round, or polygonal tumor cells (see Figs. 17–80 and 17–81), although most tend to be spindle-shaped and have an eosinophilic and at times fibrillar cytoplasm.[537-542] Nuclei are oval to elongated, at times cigar-shaped, with some containing small nucleoli.[538, 541, 542] Paranuclear vacuoles, as found in conventional leiomyosarcoma, may be present.[541] As a rule, significant nuclear atypia or pleomophism is not a feature of MLMS, the nuclei being pale and bland in appearance (see Fig. 17–80B); however, some cases of MLMS are reported that focally contain pleomorphic cells.[538, 539, 541] Even in relatively pure myxoid leiomyosarcomas, areas are present where the spindle cells either form thin intersecting fascicles (Figs. 17–81 and 17–82), or are aggregated around small,

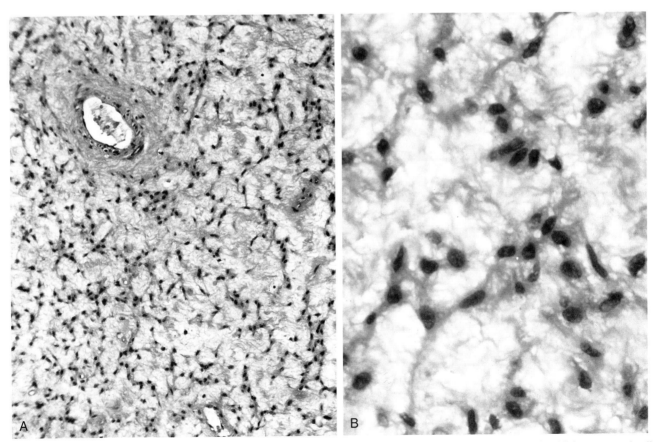

FIGURE 17–80. *A,* Low-power view of myxoid leiomyosarcoma (MLMS) shows a myxomatous stroma in which widely separated cells are dispersed. Blood vessels are present. The pattern is similar to that seen in aggressive angiomyxoma. *B,* Higher magnification shows fibrillar myxoid stroma, and the bland nature of the component stellate to short spindle cells.

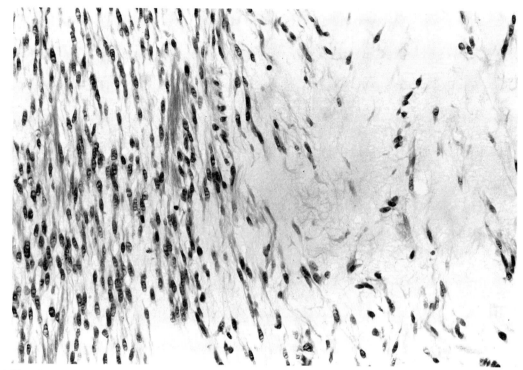

FIGURE 17–81. Myxoid zone to the right of the field is juxtaposed to loose fascicular arrangement of spindle cells with elongated nuclei in MLMS.

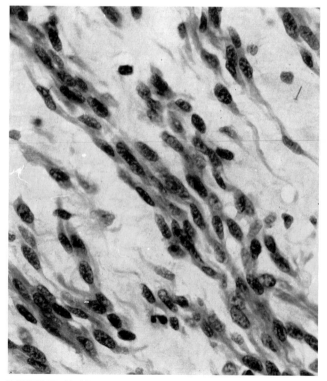

FIGURE 17–82. Higher magnification of the spindle cells in Figure 17–81 shows nuclei that are oval to spindle-shaped, with most having rounded ends and a lack of nuclear atypia.

thin-walled blood vessels that are distributed throughout the tumor.[538–542] Although this vascular component is not prominent, extravasated red blood cells are commonly present within the stroma. Mast cells are also common and may be numerous.[539] Necrosis is not a feature of MLMS. In those myxoid leiomyosarcomas that are not totally myxoid, areas of conventional leiomyosarcoma are found.[540] Despite the usual well-delimited gross appearance of MLMS, the tumor is microscopically infiltrative and may invade blood vessels.[538, 539, 541, 542]

Unlike conventional leiomyosarcomas, in which high mitotic counts are the rule, the mitotic activity in MLMS varies considerably from case to case, with most having either none or only 1 to 2 mitoses/10 HPF,[538, 540, 542] although cases with from 10 to more than 20 mitoses/10 HPF are reported.[539, 541] However, the apparent low mitotic activity of MLMS may be spurious and caused by the wide dispersal of the individual tumor cells within the myxoid stroma, which leads to artificially low values when the counts are based on evaluation of a specific number of individual fields.[539, 541]

Only a few cases of MLMS have been subjected to immunohistochemical analysis. Mills et al. studied four cases, all of which were positive for vimentin and muscle-specific actin and, in three, for desmin.[539] In our own experience, smooth muscle actins are also present. All four tumors in Mills' series were negative for cytokeratin, epithelial membrane antigen, and S-100 protein.

Similarly, only a few examples of MLMS have been examined electron microscopically.[537, 538, 540, 542] In these cases, the cells contained features characteristically found in smooth muscle cells, including a basal lamina, abundant cytoplasmic microfilaments containing dense bodies, intercellular junctions, and plasmalemmal pinocytotic vesicles. However, in one reported case, the cells lacked a basal lamina and pinocytotic vesicles were few in number.[542]

The histologic differential diagnosis of MLMS includes any myxoid soft tissue tumor containing spindle or stellate cells. **Myxoid liposarcoma** can usually be easily distinguished from MLMS by its plexiform capillary vascular pattern, lipoblasts, reactivity for S-100 protein, and the absence of immunohistochemical or electron microscopic features of smooth muscle differentiation. **Myxoid malignant fibrous histiocytoma** is more vascular than MLMS, contains significant cellular anaplasia and pleomorphism, and has a greater degree of mitotic activity. Neither myxoid liposarcoma nor myxoid malignant fibrous histiocytoma are tumors that commonly occur in the pelvic soft tissues, bladder, or uterus, all common sites for MLMS.

The diagnosis of MLMS is particularly difficult when it occurs in the bladder, especially when one is dealing with small biopsy specimens. The most problematic differential diagnostic considerations in this site are **postoperative spindle cell nodule** (PSCN) and its closely related counterpart, **inflammatory pseudosarcoma** (IPS).

Both PSCN and MLMS are infiltrative lesions that may destroy normal tissue. PSCN contains acute and chronic inflammatory cells, but if MLMS ulcerates an overlying mucosa, it may also contain inflammatory cells. Although PSCN contains fascicles of plump to tapering spindle cells within an edematous stroma, it usually lacks the abundant myxoid stroma that is characteristic of MLMS; it has more abundant mitotic activity than does MLMS and a delicate plexiform capillary network that is absent in MLMS. Occasional cases of PSCN have had cells immunoreactive for cytokeratin as well as for muscle-specific actin and desmin. However, because conventional leiomyosarcomas of the bladder may also occasionally contain cytokeratin-positive cells, the use of such a result for the separation of PSCN from MLMS must be regarded as tentative until more myxoid leiomyosarcomas are studied by immunohistochemistry. Electron microscopic analysis may be of diagnostic value in confirming a diagnosis of MLMS if smooth muscle differentiation is present. However, it must be admitted that when only small biopsy specimens are available, the distinction between PSCN and MLMS may be impossible. Of critical importance in solving this problem is the clinical information of a recent operative procedure in the region under question, thus indicating the likelihood of the diagnosis of PSCN.

Inflammatory pseudosarcoma (IPS) is composed of spindle cells within an abundant myxoid stroma and, like MLMS, is infiltrative. However, IPS is more cellular than MLMS, having nodular fasciitis-like foci; the cells of IPS also tend to be more haphazardly arranged than those in MLMS, where the cells are more diffuse and uniformly distributed. IPS lacks the myxomatous pools of MLMS, is more vascular than MLMS, and characteristically has a prominent inflammatory component that is usually lacking in MLMS. Because smooth muscle markers are found in both IPS and MLMS, immunohistochemical studies are of no value in distinguishing between these two lesions. Electron microscopy may be helpful for this distinction if fibroblastic or myofibroblastic cells are found, as in IPS, or if smooth muscle cells are found, as in MLMS. However, as with PSCN, the examination of small biopsy specimens may not allow the pathologist to clearly

distinguish between these two entities, and specimens from larger resections may be needed.

Despite the absence of significant mitotic activity, necrosis, and cellular pleomorphism in most myxoid leiomyosarcomas, several of these deceptively bland-appearing tumors have behaved aggressively, with high local recurrence rates and metastases.[537–539, 541] However, the true biologic behavior of these tumors and how they compare with conventional leiomyosarcoma is unclear owing to the few long-term follow-up studies of patients with MLMS. Of equal importance to the diagnosis of these myxoid lesions as being smooth muscle in nature is the criteria for establishing them as malignant, because leiomyomas may also contain myxoid regions. Such criteria have yet to be defined, but the large size of most myxoid leiomyosarcomas and their microscopically infiltrative margins correlate with their aggressive behavior.[539, 541, 542]

OSSIFYING FIBROMYXOID TUMOR

Ossifying fibromyxoid tumor (OFMT) is a recently described entity for which relatively scant information is available in the literature, with fewer than 100 cases reported.[543–548] The largest, as well as the original, series describing this entity consists of 59 cases from the AFIP.[545]

Although some patients have symptoms or signs of a mass for less than a year before seeking medical attention, OFMT is usually characterized by slow growth, with some patients having had the lesion for 20 to 40 years.[543, 545, 549] The tumor primarily affects adults older than the age of 40 years. In the series from the AFIP,[545] the mean age was 47 years (median, 50 years), with a range of 14 to 79 years. Among the 20 additional patients in our review,[543, 544, 546–548] the mean age was 53.7 years (median, 46 years), with only five younger than age 40 years. The oldest reported patient was 86 years of age.[546] Males accounted for 63% of the 79 patients in our review.[543–548]

OFMT has a propensity to involve the upper and lower extremities, which were involved in two thirds of the cases. The head and neck region and the trunk each accounted for 17% of cases. The shoulder, upper arm, buttock, thigh, and chest wall were the most common sites of involvement, as were the hands and feet, which accounted for 14% of the cases. The tumor has occurred in the scalp, cheek, neck, lip, and abdomen.[547] Occasional patients have had more than one site involved.[548]

Although the deep subcutaneous tissue is most commonly involved by OFMT, it not infrequently extends to involve the deep dermis, fascia, or tendons, as well as skeletal muscle, with some apparently originating within the muscle.[543, 545–548]

Macroscopically, OFMT is a well-circumscribed and pseudoencapsulated tumor that has varied from 1.5 to 17 cm in maximum dimension.[543, 545, 547] It is usually firm or hard and may have a calcified or ossified shell.[545–548] The cut surface shows a multinodular or lobulated pattern of gray-white stroma that contains mucoid or gelatinous foci. Focal hemorrhage and cystic change are occasionally present.

Microscopically (Figs. 17–83 to 17–86), OFMT is composed of uniform, oval to round or stellate cells that reside in a mucoid, fibromyxoid, or fibrous stroma (see Figs. 17–85 and 17–86). The cells usually have an eosinophilic cytoplasm,

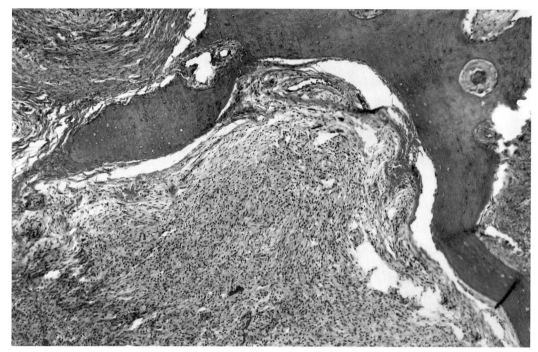

FIGURE 17–83. Low-power view of ossifying fibromyxoid tumor (OFMT) shows peripheral rim of mature lamellar bone encasing a moderately cellular tumor nodule.

indistinct cell borders, and bland-appearing, pale, oval to round vesicular nuclei containing small nucleoli (see Fig. 17–85). The cells are frequently arranged in small lobules set off by thick collagenous septa (see Fig. 17–84). Within the lobules, the cells either are diffusely distributed or are arranged in linear or cord-like arrays (see Fig. 17–85).[545-548] In some areas the cells assume spindle shapes or have clear-cell features (Figs. 17–86 and 17–87) produced by the presence of intracytoplasmic vacuoles.[545-547] Some cases of OFMT are described that contain more compact cellular areas where the cells have distinct cell borders and are arranged in a pavement-type pattern creating a "glomoid" appearance, as well as in fascicular zones composed of elongated cells.[547] Mitotic activity in OFMT is infrequent.[544-548]

A distinctive histologic feature of OFMT is the presence of a thick collagenous capsule that in approximately 80% to 90% of cases contains well-formed trabecular bone (see Fig. 17–83). This bone usually forms an incomplete ring about the tumor and may extend centrally into it along the fibrous septa that arise from the capsule and penetrate into the tumor.[543-548] This ossification may be evident on clinical roentgenograms.[543, 545, 548] The capsular aspect of the tumor may contain well-formed nodules outlined by dense collagenous tissue or have irregular aggregates of tumor cells in a plexiform array. OFMT is richly vascular, with many of the blood vessels having hyalinized walls.[544-548] The myxoid stroma stains with alcian blue, colloidal iron, and mucicarmine stains, the positivity being abolished by pretreatment with hyaluronidase.[545, 547, 548] However, sulfated glycosaminoglycans have also been found in some cases.[545] Significantly, PAS stains for glycogen are negative in the tumor cells.[545-548]

Electron microscopic examination of 18 cases of OFMT in our survey yielded variable results.[544-548] The cells have irregular borders with elongated cell processes.[544-548] A partial or discontinuous basal lamina, reduplicated in some instances, was found in some examples.[544-547] In one series, scarce and small mitochondria, numerous microfilaments, and a few pro-

files of endoplasmic reticulum were found, whereas microtubules, pinocytotic vesicles, desmosomes, and intercellular junctions were absent.[545] However, other workers have described numerous profiles of rough endoplasmic reticulum, occasional pinocytotic vesicles, moderate numbers of mitochondria, prominent arrays of intermediate filaments, and primitive cell junctions, but no microfilaments.[544, 546, 548] Extracellular collagen is generally present, but long-spaced collagen fibrils (Luse bodies) are not encountered.[544, 548] Aggregates of microtubules in association with the rough endoplasmic reticulum were not found.[545]

Only a few cases of OFMT have been studied immunohistochemically.[544-548] The tumor cells are vimentin positive[544, 546-548] and, in about 80% of cases (50/64), reactive for S-100 protein.[544-548] Cytokeratin[544-547] was reported in only 2 of 21 cases (10%), and stains for epithelial membrane antigen,[544, 546, 547] HMB-45 antigen,[544, 546] muscle-specific actin,[544, 546, 547] Factor VIII–related antigen,[547, 548] neurofilament protein,[544] alpha-1-antitrypsin,[548] alpha-1-antichymotrypsin,[548] and CD34 antigen[547] were negative. Glial fibrillary acidic protein[544-547] was found in 3 of 13 cases (23%), Leu-7 in 4 of 8,[544, 546, 547] desmin in 8 of 16,[544, 546-548] smooth muscle actin in 4 of 8 cases,[547] and neuron-specific enolase in the one case examined for this protein.[544] Type IV collagen was found in two of three cases studied, with the positive stain located along the membrane of the tumor cells.[547]

Because of its lobular pattern, myxoid stroma, linear and cord-like arrangement of cells, and S-100 positivity, OFMT may be confused with **myxoid chondrosarcoma.** However, the presence of a basal lamina about the cells of OFMT is not usually found in chondroid cells, and the absence of aggregates of microtubules in association with the rough endoplasmic reticulum in OFMT, as present in myxoid chondrosarcoma, argues against such a diagnosis. However, basal lamina has been found in some cases of myxoid chondrosarcoma, and microtubular aggregates within the rough endoplasmic

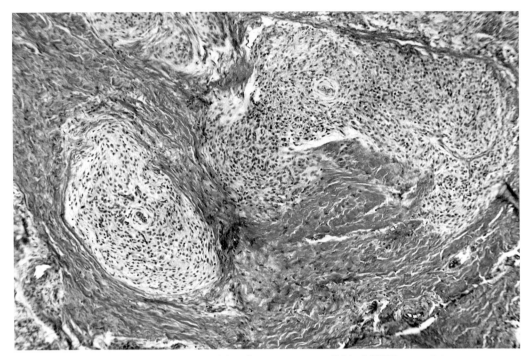

FIGURE 17–84. Peripheral thick collagenous septa divide OFMT into nodules.

reticulum are not always found in myxoid chondrosarcomas. Of more importance to the differential diagnosis is the presence of trabecular bone in OFMT, a feature virtually never found in myxoid chondrosarcoma. In addition, the absence of cellular glycogen in OFMT, a cardinal feature of cartilaginous cells, is strong evidence against a diagnosis of myxoid chondrosarcoma.

Chondroid syringoma, which may have a myxoid stroma, a linear or cord-like arrangement of cells, and, rarely, bone formation, is ruled out as a diagnostic possibility because of its cytokeratin positivity and epithelial or myoepithelial differentiation by electron microscopy.

The clear cytoplasm of some cells in OFMT, combined with the S-100 protein positivity, may raise the possibility of clear-cell sarcoma. However, unlike clear-cell sarcoma, OFMT lacks reactivity for HMB-45 antigen and does not have prominent nucleoli, multinucleated giant cells, or premelanosomes by electron microscopy; bone formation is also not a feature of clear-cell sarcoma.

The possibility that OFMT is a nerve sheath or related tumor is raised by the presence of S-100 protein, Leu-7, and glial fibrillary acid protein in some cases. Indeed, the lobular pattern of OFMT is evocative of a **nerve sheath myxoma.** Although it has a myxoid lobular pattern, nerve sheath myx-

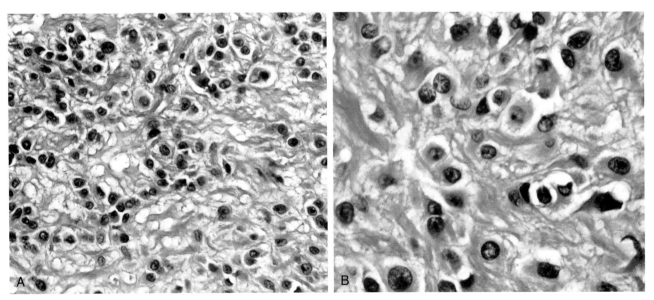

FIGURE 17–85. *A,* Area from OFMT shows round tumor cells dispersed in a fibrous stroma. The cells either are arranged individually or appear loosely attached to form rows or cords. *B,* Higher magnification shows the dense fibrous stroma with dispersed cells having round to oval nuclei, some with small nucleoli; cytoplasmic borders appear to fade into the fibrous stroma.

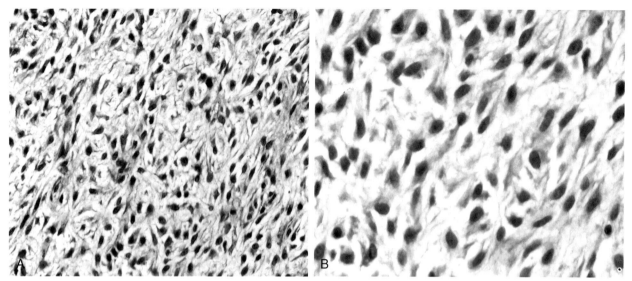

FIGURE 17–86. *A,* View of another example of OFMT shows spindle- to stellate-shaped tumor cells that are diffusely and uniformly distributed within a myxoid stroma. *B,* Higher magnification shows hyperchromatic stellate- to spindle-shaped cells with cytoplasmic projections. Nuclear pleomorphism is absent.

oma lacks ossification, and the electron microscopy of OFMT is not strictly typical of Schwann cell differentiation, which usually shows a continuous basal lamina, mesaxon inclusions, absence of pinocytotic vesicles, and cell processes with microtubules and microfilaments. The lack of epithelial membrane

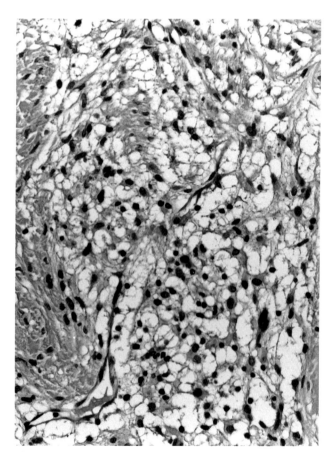

FIGURE 17–87. Area within OFMT in which the cells have clear-cell features produced by extensive cytoplasmic vacuolization.

antigen in OFMT, a marker for perineurial cells, also argues against its being a primary perineurial cell tumor.

Because of the glomoid appearance in some examples of OFMT, **glomus tumor** has been considered a diagnostic possibility, but the clinical absence of the typical pain pattern of a glomus tumor, the deep location of OFMT and its lobulation, and its S-100 protein content are sufficient evidence to distinguish OFMT from this diagnostic alternative.

The exact nosologic classification of OFMT is still unclear and awaits the reporting of further cases. The biologic significance of this lesion is similarly unclear. Of 41 patients in the AFIP series with follow-up information, 27% developed a local recurrence, some with multiple recurrences, with malignant transformation or metastases in two patients.[545] In 14 other patients in our review with follow-up data, locally aggressive behavior that resulted in death occurred in one patient,[548] whereas the remaining patients were without metastases or local recurrence.[543, 546, 547] To date, one would advocate wide local excision for this potentially aggressive tumor of undetermined histogenesis or differentiation.

References

Malignant Peripheral Neuroectodermal Tumor

1. Stout AP: A tumor of the ulnar nerve. Proc NY Pathol Soc 18:2–12, 1918.
2. Stout AP: The malignant tumors of the peripheral nerves. Am J Cancer 25:1–36, 1935.
3. Stout AP, Murray MR: Neuroepithelioma of the radial nerve with a study of its behaviour in vitro. Rev Can Biol 1:651–659, 1942.
4. Garrè C: Ueber sekundar maligne neurome. Beitr Z Klin Chir 9:465–495, 1892.
5. Woodruff JM: Peripheral nerve tumors showing glandular differentiation (glandular schwannomas). Cancer 37:2399–2413, 1976.
6. Harper PG, Pringle J, Souhami RL: Neuroepithelioma—a rare malignant peripheral nerve tumor of primitive origin: Report of two cases and a review of the literature. Cancer 48:2282–2287, 1981.
7. McKeon C, Thiele CJ, Ross RA, et al: Indistinguishable patterns of protooncogene expression in two distinct but closely related tumors: Ewing's sarcoma and neuroepithelioma. Cancer Res 48:4307–4311, 1988.
8. Seemayer TA, Vekemans M, de Chadarévian J-P: Histological and cytogenetic findings in a malignant tumor of the chest wall and lung (Askin tumor). Virchows Arch (A) 408:289–296, 1985.

9. Hashimoto H, Enjoji M, Nakajima T, et al: Malignant neuroepithelioma (peripheral neuroblastoma). A clinicopathologic study of 15 cases. Am J Surg Pathol 7:309–318, 1983.

10. Bolen JW, Thorning D: Peripheral neuroepithelioma: A light and electron microscopic study. Cancer 46:2456–2462, 1980.

11. Cavazzana AO, Ninfo V, Montesco M, et al: Peripheral neuroepithelioma: Morphologic and immunologic criteria for diagnosis. Mod Pathol 1:17A, 1988.

12. Cavazzana AO, Ninfo V, Roberts J, Triche TJ: Peripheral neuroepithelioma: A light microscopic, immunocytochemical, and ultrastructural study. Mod Pathol 5:71–78, 1992.

13. Cavazzana AO, Santopietro R, Sforza V, et al: Morphometry and the differential diagnosis between peripheral neuroepithelioma and neuroblastoma. Mod Pathol 4:615–620, 1991.

14. Mierau GW: Extraskeletal Ewing's sarcoma (peripheral neuroepithelioma). Ultrastruct Pathol 9:91–98, 1985.

15. Miser JS, Kinsella TJ, Triche TJ, et al: Treatment of peripheral neuroepithelioma in children and young adults. J Clin Oncol 5:1752–1758, 1987.

16. Pappo AS, Douglass EC, Meyer WH, et al: Use of HBA 71 and anti-β^2-microglobulin to distinguish peripheral neuroepithelioma from neuroblastoma. Hum Pathol 24:880–885, 1993.

17. Shinoda M, Tsutsumi Y, Hata J, Yokoyama S: Peripheral neuroepithelioma in childhood. Immunohistochemical demonstration of epithelial differentiation. Arch Pathol Lab Med 112:1155–1158, 1988.

18. Voss BL, Pysher TJ, Humphrey GB: Peripheral neuroepithelioma in childhood. Cancer 54:3059–3064, 1984.

19. Whang-Peng J, Triche TJ, Knutsen T, et al: Chromosome translocation in peripheral neuroepithelioma. N Engl J Med 311:584–585, 1984.

20. Isayama T, Iwasaki H, Kikuchi M, et al: Neuroectodermal tumor of bone. Evidence for neural differentiation in a cultured cell line. Cancer 65:1771–1781, 1990.

21. Jaffe R, Santamaria M, Yunis EJ, et al: The neuroectodermal tumor of bone. Am J Surg Pathol 8:885–898, 1984.

22. Rousselin B, Vanel D, Terrier-Lacombe MJ, et al: Clinical and radiologic analysis of 13 cases of primary neuroectodermal tumors of bone. Skeletal Radiol 18:115–120, 1989.

23. Tsuneyoshi M, Yokoyama R, Hashimoto H, Enjoji M: Comparative study of neuroectodermal tumor and Ewing's sarcoma of the bone. Histopathologic, immunohistochemical and ultrastructural features. Acta Pathol Jpn 39:573–581, 1989.

24. Gonzalez-Crussi F, Wolfson SL, Misugi K, Nakajima T: Peripheral neuroectodermal tumors of the chest wall in childhood. Cancer 54:2519–2527, 1984.

25. Coffin CM, Dehner LP: Peripheral neurogenic tumors of the soft tissues in children and adolescents: A clinicopathologic study of 139 cases. Pediatr Pathol 9:387–407, 1989.

26. Das L, Chang C-H, Cushing B, Jewell P: Congenital primitive neuroectodermal tumor (neuroepithelioma) of the chest wall. Med Pediatr Oncol 10:349–358, 1982.

27. Dehner LP: Primitive neuroectodermal tumor and Ewing's sarcoma. Am J Surg Pathol 17:1–13, 1993.

28. Hasegawa T, Hirose T, Kudo E, et al: Atypical primitive neuroectodermal tumors. Comparative light and electron microscopic and immunohistochemical studies on peripheral neuroepitheliomas and Ewing's sarcomas. Acta Pathol Jpn 41:444–454, 1991.

29. Kushner BH, Hajdu SI, Gulati SC, et al: Extracranial primitive neuroectodermal tumors. The Memorial Sloan-Kettering Cancer Center experience. Cancer 67:1825–1829, 1991.

30. Parham DM, Dias P, Kelly DR, et al: Desmin positivity in primitive neuroectodermal tumors of childhood. Am J Surg Pathol 16:483–492, 1992.

31. Shishikura A, Ushigome S, Shimoda T: Primitive neuroectodermal tumors of bone and soft tissue: Histological subclassification and clinicopathologic correlations. Acta Pathol Jpn 43:176–186, 1993.

32. Stephenson CF, Bridge JA, Sandberg AA: Cytogenetic and pathologic aspects of Ewing's sarcoma and neuroectodermal tumors. Hum Pathol 23:1270–1277, 1992.

33. Ushigome S, Shimoda T, Nikaido T, et al: Primitive neuroectodermal tumors of bone and soft tissue with reference to histologic differentiation in primary or metastatic foci. Acta Pathol Jpn 42:483–493, 1992.

34. Aguirre P, Scully RE: Malignant neuroectodermal tumor of the ovary, a distinctive form of monodermal teratoma. Am J Surg Pathol 6:283–292, 1982.

35. Llombart-Bosch A, Terrier-Lacombe MJ, Peydro-Olaya A, Contesso G: Peripheral neuroectodermal sarcoma of soft tissue (peripheral neuroepithelioma): A pathologic study of ten cases with differential diagnosis regarding other small, round-cell sarcomas. Hum Pathol 20:273–280, 1989.

36. Ambros IM, Ambros PF, Strehl S, et al: MIC2 is a specific marker for Ewing's sarcoma and peripheral primitive neuroectodermal tumors. Evidence for a common histogenesis of Ewing's sarcoma and peripheral primitive neuroectodermal tumors from MIC2 expression and specific chromosome aberration. Cancer 67:1886–1893, 1991.

37. Dehner LP: Peripheral and central primitive neuroectodermal tumors. A nosologic concept seeking a consensus. Arch Pathol Lab Med 110:997–1005, 1986.

38. Swanson PE, Jaszcz W, Nakhleh RE, et al: Peripheral primitive neuroectodermal tumors. A flow cytometric analysis with immunohistochemical and ultrastructural observations. Arch Pathol Lab Med 116:1202–1208, 1992.

39. Jürgens H, Bier V, Harms D, et al: Malignant peripheral neuroectodermal tumors. A retrospective analysis of 42 patients. Cancer 61:349–357, 1988.

40. Llombart-Bosch A, Lacombe MJ, Peydro-Olaya M, et al: Malignant peripheral neuroectodermal tumours of bone other than Askin's neoplasm: Characterization of 14 new cases with immunohistochemistry and electron microscopy. Virchows Arch (A) 412:421–430, 1988.

41. Schmidt D, Harms D, Burdach S: Malignant peripheral neuroectodermal tumours of childhood and adolescence. Virchows Arch (A) 406:351–365, 1985.

42. Schmidt D, Herrmann C, Jürgens H, Harms D: Malignant peripheral neuroectodermal tumor and its necessary distinction from Ewing's sarcoma. A report from the Kiel Pediatric Tumor Registry. Cancer 68:2251–2259, 1991.

43. Tefft M, Vawter GF, Mitus A: Paravertebral "round cell" tumors in children. Radiology 92:1501–1509, 1969.

44. Askin FB, Rosai J, Sibley RK, et al: Malignant small cell tumor of the thoracopulmonary region in childhood. A distinctive clinicopathologic entity of uncertain histogenesis. Cancer 43:2438–2451, 1979.

45. Angervall L, Enzinger FM: Extraskeletal neoplasm resembling Ewing's sarcoma. Cancer 36:240–251, 1975.

46. Kawaguchi K, Koike M: Neuron-specific enolase and Leu-7 immunoreactive small round-cell neoplasm. The relationship to Ewing's sarcoma in bone and soft tissue. Am J Clin Pathol 86:79–83, 1986.

47. Llombart-Bosch A, Lacombe MJ, Contesso G, Peydro-Olaya A: Small round blue cell sarcoma of bone mimicking atypical Ewing's sarcoma with neuroectodermal features. An analysis of five cases with immunohistochemical and electron microscopic support. Cancer 60:1570–1582, 1987.

48. Schmidt D, Mackay B, Ayala AG: Ewing's sarcoma with neuroblastoma-like features. Ultrastruct Pathol 3:143–151, 1982.

49. Carter RL, Al-Sams SZ, Corbett RP, Clinton S: A comparative study of immunohistochemical staining for neuron-specific enolase, protein gene product 9.5 and S-100 protein in neuroblastoma, Ewing's sarcoma and other round cell tumours in children. Histopathology 16:461–467, 1990.

50. Dierick AM, Roels H, Langlois M: The immunophenotype of Ewing's sarcoma. An immunohistochemical analysis. Pathol Res Pract 189:26–32, 1993.

51. Kissane JM, Askin FB, Foulkes M, et al: Ewing's sarcoma of bone: Clinicopathologic aspects of 303 cases from the Intergroup Ewing's Sarcoma Study. Hum Pathol 14:773–779, 1983.

52. Linnoila RI, Tsokos M, Triche TJ, et al: Evidence for neural origin and PAS-positive variants of the malignant small cell tumor of thoracopulmonary region ("Askin tumor"). Am J Surg Pathol 10:124–133, 1986.

53. Lizard-Nacol S, Lizard G, Justrabo E, Turc-Carel C: Immunologic characterization of Ewing's sarcoma using mesenchymal and neural markers. Am J Pathol 135:847–855, 1989.

54. Llombart-Bosch A, Carda C, Peydro-Olaya A, et al: Soft tissue Ewing's sarcoma. Characterization in established cultures and xenografts with evidence of a neuroectodermic phenotype. Cancer 66:2589–2601, 1990.

55. Mierau GW, Berry PJ, Orsini EN: Small round cell neoplasms: Can electron microscopy and immunohistochemical studies accurately classify them? Ultrastruct Pathol 9:99–111, 1985.

56. Pinto A, Grant LH, Hayes FA, et al: Immunohistochemical expression in neuron-specific enolase and Leu 7 in Ewing's sarcoma of bone. Cancer 64:1266–1273, 1989.

57. Shimada H, Newton WA Jr, Soule EH, et al: Pathologic features of extraosseous Ewing's sarcoma: A report from the Intergroup Rhabdomyosarcoma Study. Hum Pathol 19:442–453, 1988.

58. Stuart-Harris R, Wills EJ, Philips J, et al: Extraskeletal Ewing's sarcoma.: A clinical, morphological and ultrastructural analysis of five cases with a review of the literature. Eur J Cancer Clin Oncol 22:393–400, 1986.

59. Ushigome S, Shimoda T, Takaki K, et al: Immunocytochemical and ultrastructural studies on the histogenesis of Ewing's sarcoma and putatively related tumors. Cancer 64:52–62, 1989.

60. Yunis EJ: Ewing's sarcoma and related small round cell neoplasms in children. Am J Surg Pathol 10(Suppl 1):54–62, 1986.

61. Rubinstein LJ: "Primitive neuroectodermal tumors." Arch Pathol Lab Med 111:310–311, 1987.

62. Triche TJ, Askin FB: Neuroblastoma and the differential diagnosis of small-, round-, blue-cell tumors. Hum Pathol 14:569–595, 1983.

63. Haimoto H, Takahashi Y, Koshikawa T, et al: Immunohistochemical localization of γ-enolase in normal human tissues other than nervous and neuroendocrine tissues. Lab Invest 52:257–263, 1985.

64. Leader M, Collins M, Patel J, Henry K: Antineuron specific enolase staining reactions in sarcomas and carcinomas: Its lack of neuroendocrine specificity. J Clin Pathol 39:1186–1192, 1986.

65. Vinores SA, Bonnin JM, Rubinstein LJ, Marangos PJ: Immunohistochemical demonstration of neuron-specific enolase in neoplasms of the CNS and other tissues. Arch Pathol Lab Med 108:536–540, 1984.

66. Contesso G, Llombart-Bosch A, Terrier P, et al: Does malignant small round cell tumor of the thoracopulmonary region (Askin tumor) constitute a clinicopathologic entity? An analysis of 30 cases with immunohistochemical and electron-microscopic support treated at the Institute Gustave Roussy. Cancer 69:1012–1020, 1992.

67. Füzesi L, Heller R, Schreiber H, Mertens R: Cytogenetics of Askin's tumour. Case report and review of the literature. Pathol Res Pract 189:235–241, 1993.

68. Lagerkvist B, Ivemark B, Sylvén B: Malignant neuroepithelioma in childhood. A report of three cases. Acta Chir Scand 135:641–645, 1969.

69. Marina NM, Etcubanas E, Parham DM, et al: Peripheral primitive neuroectodermal tumor (peripheral neuroepithelioma) in children. A review of the St. Jude experience and controversies in diagnosis and management. Cancer 64:1952–1960, 1989.

70. Nesbitt KA, Vidone RA: Primitive neuroectodermal tumor (neuroblastoma) arising in sciatic nerve of a child. Cancer 37:1562–1570, 1976.

71. Nesland JM, Sobrinho-Simões MA, Holm R, Johannessen JV: Primitive neuroectodermal tumor (peripheral neuroblastoma). Ultrastruct Pathol 9:59–64, 1985.

72. Seemayer TA, Thelmo WL, Bolande RP, Wiglesworth FW: Peripheral neuroectodermal tumors. Perspect Pediatr Pathol 2:151–172, 1975.

73. Fujii Y, Hongo T, Nakagawa Y, et al: Cell culture of small round cell tumor originating in the thoracopulmonary region. Evidence for derivation from a primitive pluripotent cell. Cancer 64:43–51, 1989.

74. Ushigome S, Shimoda T, Nikaido T, Takasaki S: Histopathologic diagnostic and histogenetic problems in malignant soft tissue tumors. Reassessment of malignant fibrous histiocytoma, epithelioid sarcoma, malignant rhabdoid tumor, and neuroectodermal tumor. Acta Pathol Jpn 42:691–706, 1992.

75. Kudo M: Neuroectodermal differentiation in "extraskeletal Ewing's sarcoma." Acta Pathol Jpn 39:795–802, 1989.

76. Llombart-Bosch A, Peydro-Olaya A: Scanning and transmission electron microscopy of Ewing's sarcoma of bone (typical and atypical variants). An analysis of nine cases. Virchows Arch (A) 398:329–346, 1983.

77. Nascimento AG, Unni KK, Pritchard DJ, et al: A clinicopathologic study of 20 cases of large-cell (atypical) Ewing's sarcoma of bone. Am J Surg Pathol 4:29–36, 1980.

78. Erlandson RA: The ultrastructural distinction between rhabdomyosarcoma and other undifferentiated "sarcomas." Ultrastruct Pathol 11:83–101, 1987.

79. Michels S, Swanson PE, Robb JA, Wick MR: Leu-7 in small cell neoplasms. An immunohistochemical study with ultrastructural correlations. Cancer 60:2958–2964, 1987.

80. Fellinger EJ, Garin-Chesa P, Triche TJ, et al: Immunohistochemical analysis of Ewing's sarcoma cell surface antigen p30/32MIC2. Am J Pathol 139:317–325, 1991.

81. Hamilton G, Fellinger EJ, Schratter I, Fritsch A: Characterization of a human endocrine tissue and tumor-associated Ewing's sarcoma antigen. Cancer Res 48:6127–6131, 1988.

82. Hara S, Ishii E, Tanaka S, et al: A monoclonal antibody specifically reactive with Ewing's sarcoma. Br J Cancer 60:875–879, 1989.

83. Harms D, Schmidt D: Critical commentary to "Cytogenetics of Askin's tumour." Pathol Res Pract 189:242–244, 1993.

84. Kahn HJ, Thorner PS: Monoclonal antibody MB2: A potential marker for Ewing's sarcoma and primitive neuroectodermal tumor. Pediatr Pathol 9:153–162, 1989.

85. Swanson PE, Dehner LP, Wick MR: Small round cell tumors in children: A lectin histochemical and immunohistochemical analysis of 30 cases. Surg Pathol 5:5–16, 1993.

86. Fellinger EJ, Garin-Chesa P, Glasser DB, et al: Comparison of cell surface antigen HBA71 (p30/32MIC2), neuron-specific enolase, and vimentin in the immunohistochemical analysis of Ewing's sarcoma of bone. Am J Surg Pathol 16:746–755, 1992.

87. Riopel MA, Dickman PS, Link M, Perlman EJ: MIC2 analysis in pediatric lymphomas. Mod Pathol 6:128A, 1993.

88. Dehner LP: Pediatric Surgical Pathology, 2nd ed. Baltimore, Williams & Wilkins, 1987, pp 562–574.

89. deLorimier AA, Bragg KU, Linden G: Neuroblastoma in childhood. Am J Dis Child 118:441–450, 1969.

90. Enzinger FM, Weiss SW: Soft Tissue Tumors, 2nd ed. St. Louis, CV Mosby, 1988, pp 816–828.

91. Thomas PRM, Lee JY, Fineberg BB, et al: An analysis of neuroblastoma at a single institution. Cancer 53:2079–2082, 1984.

92. Dehner LP: Whence the primitive neuroectodermal tumor? Arch Pathol Lab Med 114:16–17, 1990.

93. Kaye JA, Warhol MJ, Kretschmar C, et al: Neuroblastoma in adults. Three case reports and a review of the literature. Cancer 58:1149–1157, 1986.

94. Romansky SG, Crocker DW: Neuroblastoma. Prog Surg Pathol 5:67–93, 1983.

95. Leong AS-Y, Kan AE, Milios J: Small round cell tumors in childhood: Immunohistochemical studies in rhabdomyosarcoma, neuroblastoma, Ewing's sarcoma, and lymphoblastic lymphoma. Surg Pathol 2:5–17, 1989.

96. Osborn M, Dirk T, Käser H, et al: Immunohistochemical localization of neurofilaments and neuron-specific enolase in 29 cases of neuroblastoma. Am J Pathol 122:433–442, 1986.

97. Tsokos M, Linnoila RI, Chandra RS, Triche TJ: Neuron-specific enolase in the diagnosis of neuroblastoma and other small, round-cell tumors in children. Hum Pathol 15:575–584, 1984.

98. Thiele CJ, McKeon C, Triche TJ, et al: Differential protooncogene expression characterizes histopathologically indistinguishable tumors of the peripheral nervous system. J Clin Invest 80:804–811, 1987.

99. Triche TJ: Neuroblastoma and other childhood neural tumors: A review. Pediatr Pathol 10:175–193, 1990.

100. Lanham GR, Weiss SW, Enzinger FM: Malignant lymphoma. A study of 75 cases presenting in soft tissue. Am J Surg Pathol 13:1–10, 1989.

101. Travis WD, Banks PM, Reiman HM: Primary extranodal soft tissue lymphoma of the extremities. Am J Surg Pathol 11:359–366, 1987.

102. Dickman PS, Triche TJ: Extraosseous Ewing's sarcoma versus primitive rhabdomyosarcoma: Diagnostic criteria and clinical correlation. Hum Pathol 17:881–893, 1986.

103. Parham DM, Webber B, Holt H, et al: Immunohistochemical study of childhood rhabdomyosarcomas and related neoplasms. Results of an Intergroup Rhabdomyosarcoma Study project. Cancer 67:3072–3080, 1991.

104. Miettinen M, Rapola J: Immunohistochemical spectrum of rhabdomyosarcoma and rhabdomyosarcoma-like tumors. Expression of cytokeratin and the 68-kD neurofilament protein. Am J Surg Pathol 13:120–132, 1989.

105. Hartman KR, Triche TJ, Kinsella TJ, Miser JS: Prognostic value of histopathology in Ewing's sarcoma. Long-term follow-up of distal extremity primary tumors. Cancer 67:163–171, 1991.

106. Gorman PA, Malone M, Pritchard J, Sheer D: Cytogenetic analysis of primitive neuroectodermal tumors. Absence of the t(11;22) in two of three cases and a review of the literature. Cancer Genet Cytogenet 51:13–22, 1991.

107. Turc-Carel C, Aurias A, Mugneret F, et al: Chromosomes in Ewing's sarcoma. I. An evaluation of 85 cases and remarkable consistency of t(11;22) (q24;q12). Cancer Genet Cytogenet 32:229–238, 1988.

108. Llombart-Bosch A, Blache R, Peydro-Olaya A: Ultrastructural study of 28 cases of Ewing's sarcoma: Typical and atypical forms. Cancer 41:1362–1373, 1978.

109. Gillespie JJ, Roth LM, Wills ER, et al: Extraskeletal Ewing's sarcoma. Histologic and ultrastructural observations in three cases. Am J Surg Pathol 3:99–108, 1979.

110. Hashimoto H, Tsuneyoshi M, Daimaru Y, Enjoji M: Extraskeletal Ewing's sarcoma. A clinicopathologic and electron microscopic analysis of 8 cases. Acta Pathol Jpn 35:1087–1098, 1985.

111. Mahoney JP, Alexander RW: Ewing's sarcoma. A light- and electron-microscopic study of 21 cases. Am J Surg Pathol 2:283–298, 1978, 1978.

112. Navas-Palacios, JJ, Aparicio-Duque R, Valdés MD: On the histogenesis of Ewing's sarcoma. An ultrastructural, immunohistochemical, and cytochemical study. Cancer 53:1882–1901, 1984.

113. Považil C, Matějovský Z: Ultrastructure of Ewing's tumour. Virchows Arch A Pathol Anat Histol 374:303–316, 1977.

114. Moll R, Lee I, Gould VE, et al: Immunocytochemical analysis of Ewing's tumors. Patterns of expression of intermediate filaments and desmosomal proteins indicate cell type heterogeneity and pluripotential differentiation. Am J Pathol 127:288–304, 1987.

115. Cavazzana AO, Magnani JL, Ross RA, et al: Ewing's sarcoma is an undifferentiated neuroectodermal tumor. Prog Clin Biol Res 271:487–498, 1988.

116. Cavazzana AO, Miser JS, Jefferson J, Triche TJ: Experimental evidence for a neural origin of Ewing's sarcoma of bone. Am J Pathol 127:507–518, 1987.

117. Ladanyi M, Heinemann FS, Huvos AG, et al: Neural differentiation in small round cell tumors of bone and soft tissue with the translocation t(11;22) (q24;q12): An immunohistochemical study of 11 cases. Hum Pathol 21:1245–1251, 1990.

Desmoplastic Small-cell Tumor

118. Gerald WL, Rosai J: Case 2. Desmoplastic small cell tumor with divergent differentiation. Pediatr Pathol 9:177–183, 1989.

119. Ordóñez NG, Zirkin R, Bloom RE: Malignant small-cell epithelial tumor of the peritoneum coexpressing mesenchymal-type intermediate filaments. Am J Surg Pathol 13:413–421, 1989.

120. Gonzalez-Crussi F, Crawford SE, Sun C-CJ: Intraabdominal desmoplastic small-cell tumors with divergent differentiation. Observations on three cases of childhood. Am J Surg Pathol 14:633–642, 1990.

121. Nikolaou I, Barbatis C, Laopodis V, et al: Intra-abdominal desmoplastic small-cell tumours with divergent differentiation. Report of two cases and review of the literature. Pathol Res Pract 188:981–988, 1992.

122. Norton J, Monaghan P, Carter RL: Intra-abdominal desmoplastic small cell tumour with divergent differentiation. Histopathology 19:560–562, 1991.

123. Variend S, Gerrard M, Norris PD, Goepel JR: Intra-abdominal neuroectodermal tumour of childhood with divergent differentiation. Histopathology 18:45–51, 1991.

124. Yachnis AT, Rorke LB, Biegel JA, et al: Desmoplastic primitive neuroectodermal tumor with divergent differentiation. Broadening the spectrum of desmoplastic infantile neuroepithelial tumors. Am J Surg Pathol 16:998–1006, 1992.

125. Layfield LJ, Lenarsky C: Desmoplastic small cell tumors of the peritoneum coexpressing mesenchymal and epithelial markers. Am J Clin Pathol 96:536–543, 1991.

126. Schröder S, Padberg B-C: Desmoplastic small-cell tumor of the peritoneum with divergent differentiation: Immunocytochemical and biochemical findings. Am J Clin Pathol 99:353–355, 1993.

127. Cheung NYA, Khoo US, Chan KW: Intra-abdominal desmoplastic small round-cell tumour. Histopathology 20:531–534, 1992.

128. Gerald WL, Miller HK, Battifora H, et al: Intra-abdominal desmoplastic small round-cell tumor. Report of 19 cases of a distinctive type of high-grade polyphenotypic malignancy affecting young individuals. Am J Surg Pathol 15:499–513, 1991.

129. Sawyer JR, Tryka AF, Lewis JM: A novel reciprocal chromosome translocation t(11;22) (p13;q12) in an intraabdominal desmoplastic small round-cell tumor. Am J Surg Pathol 16:411–416, 1992.

130. Setrakian S, Gupta PK, Heald J, Brooks JJ: Intraabdominal desmoplastic small round cell tumor. Report of a case diagnosed by fine needle aspiration cytology. Acta Cytol 36:373–376, 1992.

131. Asano T, Fukuda Y, Fukunaga Y, et al: Case report. Intra-abdominal desmoplastic small cell tumor in an adolescent suggesting a neurogenic origin. Acta Pathol Jpn 43:275–282, 1993.

132. Ordóñez NG, El-Naggar AK, Ro JY, et al: Intra-abdominal desmoplastic small cell tumor: A light microscopic, immunocytochemical, ultrastructural, and flow cytometric study. Hum Pathol 24:850–865, 1993.

133. Outwater E, Schiebler ML, Brooks JJ: Intraabdominal desmoplastic small cell tumor: CT and MR findings. J Comput Assist Tomogr 16:429–432, 1992.

134. Prat J, Matias-Guiu X, Algaba F: Desmoplastic small round-cell tumor. Am J Surg Pathol 16:306–308, 1992.

135. Young RH, Eichhorn JH, Dickersin GR, Scully RE: Ovarian involvement by the intra-abdominal desmoplastic small round cell tumor with divergent differentiation: A report of three cases. Hum Pathol 23:454–464, 1992.
136. Fraire AE, Cooper S, Greenberg SD, et al: Mesothelioma of childhood. Cancer 62:838–847, 1988.
137. Coffin CM, Dehner LP: Mesothelial and related neoplasms in children and adolescents: A clinicopathologic and immunohistochemical analysis of eight cases. Pediatr Pathol 12:333–347, 1992.
138. Mayall FG, Gibbs AR: The histology and immunohistochemistry of small cell mesothelioma. Histopathology 20:47–51, 1992.
139. Wilson GE, Hasleton PS, Chatterjee AK: Desmoplastic malignant mesothelioma: A review of 17 cases. J Clin Pathol 45:295–298, 1992.

Extrarenal Malignant Rhabdoid Tumor

140. Beckwith JB, Palmer NF: Histopathology and prognosis of Wilms' tumor. Results from the First National Wilms' Tumor Study. Cancer 41:1937–1948, 1978.
141. Beckwith JB: Wilms' tumor and other renal tumors of childhood: A selective review from the National Wilms' Tumor Study Pathology Center. Hum Pathol 14:481–492, 1983.
142. Haas JE, Palmer NF, Weinberg AG, Beckwith JB: Ultrastructure of malignant rhabdoid tumor of the kidney. A distinctive renal tumor of children. Hum Pathol 12:646–657, 1981.
143. Balaton AJ, Vaury P: Paravertebral malignant rhabdoid tumor in an adult. A case report with immunocytochemical study. Pathol Res Pract 182:713–716, 1987.
144. Batsakis JG, Manning JT: Malignant rhabdoid tumor. Ann Otol Rhinol Laryngol 97:690–691, 1988.
145. Biegel JA, Rorke LB, Emanuel BS: Monosomy 22 in rhabdoid or atypical teratoid tumors of the brain. N Engl J Med 321:906, 1989.
146. Biggs PJ, Garen PD, Powers JM, Garvin AJ: Malignant rhabdoid tumor of the central nervous system. Hum Pathol 18:332–337, 1987.
147. Carter RL, McCarthy KP, Al-Sam SZ, et al: Malignant rhabdoid tumour of the bladder with immunohistochemical and ultrastructural evidence suggesting histiocytic origin. Histopathology 14:179–190, 1989.
148. Dervan PA, Cahalane SF, Kneafsey P, et al: Malignant rhabdoid tumour of soft tissue. An ultrastructural and immunohistological study of a pelvic tumour. Histopathology 11:183–190, 1987.
149. Ekfors TO, Aho HJ, Kekomaki M: Malignant rhabdoid tumor of the prostatic region. Immunohistological and ultrastructural evidence for epithelial origin. Virchows Arch (A) 406:381–388, 1985.
150. Frierson HF, Jr, Mills SE, Innes DJ Jr: Malignant rhabdoid tumor of the pelvis. Cancer 55:1963–1967, 1985.
151. Gaffney EF, Breatnach F: Diverse immunoreactivity and metachronous ultrastructural variability in fatal primitive childhood tumor with rhabdoid features. Arch Pathol Lab Med 113:1322, 1989.
152. Gonzalez-Crussi F, Goldschmidt RA, Hsueh W, Trujillo YP: Infantile sarcoma with intracytoplasmic filamentous inclusions. Distinctive tumor of possible histiocytic origin. Cancer 49:2365–2375, 1982.
153. Jakate SM, Marsden HB, Ingram L: Primary rhabdoid tumour of the brain. Virchows Arch (A) 412:393–397, 1988.
154. Kent AL, Mahoney DH Jr, Gresik MV, et al: Malignant rhabdoid tumor of the extremity. Cancer 60:1056–1059, 1987.
155. Lynch HT, Shurin SB, Dahms BB, et al: Paravertebral malignant rhabdoid tumor in infancy. In vitro studies of a familial tumor. Cancer 52:290–296, 1983.
156. Parham DM, Peiper SC, Robicheaux G, et al: Malignant rhabdoid tumor of the liver. Evidence for epithelial differentiation. Arch Pathol Lab Med 112:61–64, 1988.
157. Schmidt D, Leuschner I, Harms D, et al: Malignant rhabdoid tumor. A morphological and flow cytometric study. Pathol Res Pract 184:202–210, 1989.
158. Small EJ, Gordon GJ, Dahms BB: Malignant rhabdoid tumor of the heart in an infant. Cancer 55:2850–2853, 1985.
159. Sotelo-Avila C, Gonzalez-Crussi F, deMello D, et al: Renal and extrarenal rhabdoid tumors in children: A clinicopathologic study of 14 patients. Semin Diagn Pathol 3:151–163, 1986.
160. Tsokos M, Kouraklis G, Chandra RS, et al: Malignant rhabdoid tumor of the kidney and soft tissues. Evidence for a diverse morphological and immunocytochemical phenotype. Arch Pathol Lab Med 113:115–120, 1989.
161. Tsujimura T, Wada A, Kawano K, et al: A case of malignant rhabdoid tumor arising from soft parts in the prepubic region. Acta Pathol Jpn 39:677–682, 1989.
162. Tsuneyoshi M, Daimaru Y, Hashimoto H, Enjoji M: Malignant soft tissue neoplasms with the histologic features of renal rhabdoid tumors: An ultrastructural and immunohistochemical study. Hum Pathol 16:1235–1242, 1985.
163. Tsuneyoshi M, Daimaru Y, Hashimoto H, Enjoji M: The existence of rhabdoid cells in specified soft tissue sarcomas. Histopathological, ultrastructural and immunohistochemical evidence. Virchows Arch (A) 411:509–514, 1987.
164. Chase DR: Rhabdoid versus epithelioid sarcoma. Am J Surg Pathol 14:792–794, 1990.
165. Weeks DA, Beckwith JB, Mierau GW: Rhabdoid tumor. An entity or a phenotype? Arch Pathol Lab Med 113:113–114, 1989.
166. Weeks DA, Beckwith JB, Mierau GW, Luckey DW: Rhaboid tumor of kidney. A report of 111 cases from the National Wilms' Tumor Study Pathology Center. Am J Surg Pathol 13:439–458, 1989.
167. Cossu A, Massarelli G, Manetto V, et al: Rhabdoid tumours of the central nervous system. Report of three cases with immunocytochemical and ultrastructural findings. Virchows Arch (A) 422:81–85, 1993.
168. Kodet R, Newton WA Jr, Sachs N, et al: Rhabdoid tumors of soft tissue: A clinicopathologic study of 26 cases enrolled on the Intergroup Rhabdomyosarcoma Study. Hum Pathol 22:647–684, 1991.
169. Lemos LB, Hamoudi AB: Malignant thymic tumor in an infant (malignant histiocytoma). Arch Pathol Lab Med 102:84–89, 1978.
170. Molenaar WM, DeJong B, Dam-Meiring A, et al: Epithelioid sarcoma or malignant rhabdoid tumor of soft tissue? Epithelioid immunophenotype and rhabdoid karyotype. Hum Pathol 20:347–351, 1989.
171. Perrone T, Swanson PE, Twiggs L, et al: Malignant rhabdoid tumor of the vulva: Is distinction from epithelioid sarcoma possible? A pathologic and immunohistochemical study. Am J Surg Pathol 13:848–858, 1989.
172. Ushigome S, Shimoda T, Nikaido T, Takasaki S: Histopathologic diagnostic and histogenetic problems in malignant soft tissue tumors. Reassessment of malignant fibrous histiocytoma, epithelioid sarcoma, malignant rhabdoid tumor, and neuroectodermal tumor. Acta Pathol Jpn 42:691–706, 1992.
173. Bonnin JM, Rubinstein LJ, Palmer NF, Beckwith JB: The association of embryonal tumors originating in the kidney and in the brain. A report of seven cases. Cancer 54:2137–2146, 1984.
174. Howat AJ, Gonzales MF, Waters KD, Campbell PE: Primitive neuroectodermal tumour of the central nervous system associated with malignant rhabdoid tumour of the kidney: Report of a case. Histopathology 10:643–650, 1986.
175. Wakely PE Jr, Giacomantonio M: Fine needle aspiration cytology of metastatic malignant rhabdoid tumor. Acta Cytol 30:533–537, 1986.
176. Mierau GW, Weeks DA, Beckwith JB: Anaplastic Wilms' tumor and other clinically aggressive childhood renal neoplasms: Ultrastructural and immunocytochemical features. Ultrastruct Pathol 13:225–248, 1989.
177. Seo IS, Min KW, Brodhecker C, Mirkin LD: Malignant renal rhabdoid tumour. Immunohistochemical and ultrastructural studies. Histopathology 13:657–666, 1988.
178. Fischer H-P, Thomsen H, Altmannsberger M, Bertram U: Malignant rhabdoid tumour of the kidney expressing neurofilament proteins. Immunohistochemical findings and histogenetic aspects. Pathol Res Pract 184:541–547, 1989.
179. Rutledge J, Beckwith JB, Benjamin D, Haas JE: Absence of immunoperoxidase staining for myoglobin in the malignant rhabdoid tumor of the kidney. Pediatr Pathol 1:93–98, 1983.
180. Vogel AM, Gown AM, Caughlan J, et al: Rhabdoid tumors of the kidney contain mesenchymal specific and epithelial specific intermediate filament proteins. Lab Invest 50:232–238, 1984.
181. Kodet R, Newton WA Jr, Hamoudi AB, Asmar L: Rhabdomyosarcomas with intermediate-filament inclusions and features of rhabdoid tumors. Light microscopic and immunohistochemical study. Am J Surg Pathol 15:257–267, 1991.
182. Oda Y, Hashimoto H, Tsuneyoshi M, Takeshita S: Survival in synovial sarcoma. A multivariate study of prognostic factors with special emphasis on the comparison between early death and long-term survival. Am J Surg Pathol 17:35–44, 1993.
183. Bittesini L, Dei Tos AP, Fletcher CDM: Metastatic malignant melanoma showing a rhabdoid phenotype: Further evidence of a non-specific histologic pattern. Histopathology 20:167–170, 1992.
184. Coindre J-M, De Mascarel A, Trojani M, et al: Immunohistochemical study of rhabdomyosarcoma. Unexpected staining with S100 protein and cytokeratin. J Pathol 155:127–132, 1988.
185. Miettinen M, Rapola J: Immunohistochemical spectrum of rhabdomyosarcoma and rhabdomyosarcoma-like tumors. Expression of cytokeratin and the 68-kD neurofilament protein. Am J Surg Pathol 13:120–132, 1989.

Epithelioid Sarcoma

186. Dabska M, Koszarowski T: Clinical and pathologic study of aponeurotic (epithelioid) sarcoma. Pathol Annu 17(Pt 1):129–153, 1982.
187. Enzinger FM: Epithelioid sarcoma. A sarcoma simulating a granuloma or a carcinoma. Cancer 26:1029–1041, 1970.
188. Arber DA, Kandalaft PL, Mehta P, Battifora H: Vimentin-negative epithelioid sarcoma. The value of an immunohistochemical panel that includes CD34. Am J Surg Pathol 17:302–307, 1993.
189. Blewitt RW, Aparicio SGR, Bird CC: Epithelioid sarcoma: A tumour of myofibroblasts. Histopathology 7:573–584, 1983.
190. Bloustein PA, Silverberg SG, Waddell WR: Epithelioid sarcoma. Case report with ultrastructural review, histogenetic discussion, and chemotherapeutic data. Cancer 38:2390–2400, 1976.
191. Bryan RS, Soule EH, Dobyns JH, et al: Primary epithelioid sarcoma of the hand and forearm. A review of thirteen cases. J Bone Joint Surg (Am) 56:458–465, 1974.
192. Chase DR, Enzinger FM, Weiss SW, Langloss JM: Letter to the editor. Coexpression of keratin and vimentin in epithelioid sarcoma. Am J Surg Pathol 9:462–463, 1985.
193. Cooney TP, Hwang WS, Robertson DI, Hoogstraten J: Monophasic synovial sarcoma, epithelioid sarcoma and chordoid sarcoma: Ultrastructural evidence for a common histogenesis, despite light microscopic diversity. Histopathology 6:163–190, 1982.
194. Daimaru Y, Hashimoto H, Tsuneyoshi M, Enjoji M: Epithelial profile of epithelioid sarcoma. An immunohistochemical analysis of eight cases. Cancer 59:134–141, 1987.

195. DeLuca FN, Neviaser RJ: Epithelioid sarcoma involving bone. Clin Orthop 107:168–170, 1975.

196. Eyden BP, Harris M, Banerjee SS, McClure J: The ultrastructure of epithelioid sarcoma. J Submicrosc Cytol Pathol 21:281–293, 1989.

197. Fisher C: Epithelioid sarcoma: The spectrum of ultrastructural differentiation in seven immunohistochemically defined cases. Hum Pathol 19:265–275, 1988.

198. Fisher ER, Horvat B: The fibrocytic derivation of the so-called epithelioid sarcoma. Cancer 30:1074–1081, 1972.

199. Frable WJ, Kay S, Lawrence W, Schatzki PF: Epithelioid sarcoma. An electron microscopic study. Arch Pathol 95:8–12, 1973.

200. Gallup DG, Abell MR, Morley GW: Epithelioid sarcoma of the vulva. Obstet Gynecol 48(Suppl):14S–17S, 1976.

201. Gerharz CD, Moll R, Meister P, et al: Cytoskeletal heterogeneity of an epithelioid sarcoma with expression of vimentin, cytokeratins, and neurofilaments. Am J Surg Pathol 14:274–283, 1990.

202. Hall DJ, Grimes MM, Goplerud DR: Epithelioid sarcoma of the vulva. Gynecol Oncol 9:237–246, 1980.

203. Heenan PJ, Quirk CJ, Papadimitriou JM: Epithelioid sarcoma. A diagnostic problem. Am J Dermatopathol 8:95–104, 1986.

204. Heppenstall RB, Yvars MF, Chung SMK: Epithelioid sarcoma. Two case reports. J Bone Joint Surg (Am) 54:802–806, 1972.

205. Hoopes JE, Graham WP III, Shack RB: Epithelioid sarcoma of the upper extremity. Plast Reconstr Surg 75:810–813, 1985.

206. Iossifides I, Ayala AG, Johnson DE: Epithelioid sarcoma of penis. Urology 14:190–191, 1979.

207. Ishida T, Oka T, Matsushita H, Machinami R: Epithelioid sarcoma: An electron-microscopic, immunohistochemical and DNA flow cytometric analysis. Virchows Arch (A) 421:401–408, 1992.

208. Linell F, Myhre-Jensen O, Östberg G, Carstam N: Epithelioid sarcoma. Review and report of two cases. Acta Pathol Microbiol Scand (A) Suppl 236:21–26, 1973.

209. Lo H-H, Kalisher L, Faix JD: Epithelioid sarcoma: Radiologic and pathologic manifestations. AJR 128:1017–1020, 1977.

210. Machinami R, Kikuchi F, Matsushita H: Epithelioid sarcoma. Enzyme histochemical and ultrastructural study. Virchows Arch (A) 397:109–120, 1982.

211. Mackay B, Rashid RK, Evans HL: Epithelioid sarcoma. Ultrastruct Pathol 5:329–333, 1983.

212. Meis JM, Mackay B, Ordóñez NG: Epithelioid sarcoma: An immunohistochemical and ultrastructural study. Surg Pathol 1:13–31, 1988.

213. Miettinen M, Lehto V-P, Vartio T, Virtanen I: Epithelioid sarcoma. Ultrastructural and immunohistologic features suggesting a synovial origin. Arch Pathol Lab Med 106:620–623, 1982.

214. Miettinen M, Virtanen I, Damjanov I: Coexpression of keratin and vimentin in epithelioid sarcoma. Am J Surg Pathol 9:460–462, 1985.

215. Mills SE, Fechner RE, Bruns DE, et al: Intermediate filaments in eosinophilic cells of epithelioid sarcoma. A light-microscopic, ultrastructural, and electrophoretic study. Am J Surg Pathol 5:195–202, 1981.

216. Mirra JM, Kessler S, Bhuta S, Eckardt J: The fibroma-like variant of epithelioid sarcoma. A fibrohistiocytic/myoid lesion often confused with benign and malignant spindle cell tumors. Cancer 69:1382–1395, 1992.

217. Moore SW, Wheeler JE, Hefter LG: Epithelioid sarcoma masquerading as Peyronie's disease. Cancer 35:1706–1710, 1975.

218. Mukai M, Torikata C, Iri H, et al: Cellular differentiation of epithelioid sarcoma. An electron-microscopic, enzyme-histochemical, and immunohistochemical study. Am J Pathol 119:44–56, 1985.

219. Nelson FR, Crawford BE: Epithelioid sarcoma. A case report. J Bone Joint Surg (Am) 54:798–801, 1972.

220. Padilla RS, Flynn K, Headington JT: Epithelioid sarcoma. Enzymatic histochemical and electron microscopic evidence of histiocytic differentiation. Arch Dermatol 121:389–393, 1985.

221. Patchefsky AS, Soriano R, Kostianovsky M: Epithelioid sarcoma. Ultrastructural similarity to nodular synovitis. Cancer 39:143–152, 1977.

222. Perrone T, Swanson PE, Twiggs L, et al: Malignant rhabdoid tumor of the vulva: Is distinction from epithelioid sarcoma possible? A pathologic and immunohistochemical study. Am J Surg Pathol 13:848–858, 1989.

223. Persson S, Kindblom L-G, Angervall L: Epithelioid sarcoma. An electron-microscopic and immunohistochemical study. Appl Pathol 6:1–16, 1988.

224. Prat J, Woodruff JM, Marcove RC: Epithelioid sarcoma. An analysis of 22 cases indicating the prognostic significance of vascular invasion and regional lymph node metastasis. Cancer 41:1472–1487, 1978.

225. Ratnam AV, Naik KG: Epithelioid sarcoma—a case report. Br J Dermatol 99:451–453, 1978.

226. Santiago H, Feinerman LK, Lattes R: Epithelioid sarcoma. A clinical and pathologic study of nine cases. Hum Pathol 3:133–147, 1972.

227. Saxe N, Botha JBC: Epithelioid sarcoma. A distinctive clinical presentation. Arch Dermatol 113:1106–1108, 1977.

228. Schiffman R: Epithelioid sarcoma and synovial sarcoma in the same knee. Cancer 45:158–166, 1980.

229. Schmidt D, Harms D: Epithelioid sarcoma in children and adolescents. An immunohistochemical study. Virchows Arch (A) 410:423–431, 1987.

230. Seemayer TA, Dionne PG, Tabah EJ: Epithelioid sarcoma. Can J Surg 17:37–42, 1974.

231. Soule EH, Enriquez P: Atypical fibrous histiocytoma, malignant fibrous histiocytoma, malignant histiocytoma, and epithelioid sarcoma. A comparative study of 65 tumors. Cancer 30:128–143, 1972.

232. Sugarbaker PH, Auda S, Webber BL, et al: Early distant metastases from epithelioid sarcoma of the hand. Cancer 48:852–855, 1981.

233. Chase DR, Enzinger FM: Epithelioid sarcoma. Diagnosis, prognostic indicators and treatment. Am J Surg Pathol 9:241–263, 1985.

234. Bos GD, Pritchard DJ, Reiman HM, et al: Epithelioid sarcoma. An analysis of fifty-one cases. J Bone Joint Surg (Am) 70:862–870, 1988.

235. Kudo E, Hirose T, Fujii Y, et al: Undifferentiated carcinoma of the vulva mimicking epithelioid sarcoma. Am J Surg Pathol 15:990–1001, 1991.

236. Manivel JC, Wick MR, Dehner LP, Sibley RK: Epithelioid sarcoma. An immunohistochemical study. Am J Clin Pathol 87:319–326, 1987.

237. Shimm DS, Suit HD: Radiation therapy of epithelioid sarcoma. Cancer 52:1022–1025, 1983.

238. Wick MR, Manivel JC: Epithelioid sarcoma and isolated necrobiotic granuloma: A comparative immunocytochemical study. J Cutan Pathol 13:253–260, 1986.

239. Gabbiani G, Fu Y-S, Kaye GI, et al: Epithelioid sarcoma. A light and electron microscopic study suggesting a synovial origin. Cancer 30:486–499, 1972.

240. Tsuneyoshi M, Daimaru Y, Hashimoto H, Enjoji M: The existence of rhabdoid cells in specified soft tissue sarcomas. Histopathological, ultrastructural and immunohistochemical evidence. Virchows Arch (A) 411:509–514, 1987.

241. Fletcher CDM, McKee PH: Sarcomas—a clinicopathological guide with particular reference to cutaneous manifestation. I. Dermatofibrosarcoma protuberans, malignant fibrous histiocytoma and the epithelioid sarcoma of Enzinger. Clin Exp Dermatol 9:451–465, 1984.

242. Lombardi L, Rilke F: Ultrastructural similarities and differences of synovial sarcoma, epithelioid sarcoma, and clear cell sarcoma of the tendons and aponeuroses. Ultrastruct Pathol 6:209–219, 1984.

243. Ushigome S, Shimoda T, Nikaido T, Takasaki S: Histopathologic diagnostic and histogenetic problems in malignant soft tissue tumors. Reassessment of malignant fibrous histiocytoma, epithelioid sarcoma, malignant rhabdoid tumor, and neuroectodermal tumor. Acta Pathol Jpn 42:691–706, 1992.

244. Traweek ST, Kandalaft PL, Mehta P, Battifora H: The human hematopoietic progenitor cell antigen (CD34) in vascular neoplasia. Am J Clin Pathol 96:25–31, 1991.

245. Pisa R, Novelli P, Bonetti F: Epithelioid sarcoma: A tumour of myofibroblasts, or not? Histopathology 8:353–355, 1984.

246. Chase DR, Enzinger FM, Weiss SW, Langloss JM: Keratin in epithelioid sarcoma. An immunohistochemical study. Am J Surg Pathol 8:435–441, 1984.

247. De Young BR, Wick MR, Fitzgibbon JF, et al: CD31. An immunospecific marker for endothelial differentiation in human neoplasms. Appl Immunohistochem 1:97–100, 1993.

248. Wick MR, Manivel JC: Epithelioid sarcoma and epithelioid hemangioendothelioma: An immunocytochemical and lectin-histochemical comparison. Virchows Arch (A) 410:309–316, 1987.

249. Zarbo RJ, Gown AM, Nagle RB, et al: Anomalous cytokeratin expression in malignant melanoma: One- and two-dimensional western blot analysis and immunohistochemical survey of 100 melanomas. Mod Pathol 3:494–501, 1990.

250. Chase DR: Rhabdoid versus epithelioid sarcoma. Am J Surg Pathol 14:792, 1990.

251. Molenaar WM, DeJong B, Dam-Meiring A, et al: Epithelioid sarcoma or malignant rhabdoid tumor of soft tissue? Epithelioid immunophenotype and rhabdoid karyotype. Hum Pathol 20:347–351, 1989.

Epithelioid Angiosarcoma

252. Fletcher CDM, Beham A, Bekir S, et al: Epithelioid angiosarcoma of deep soft tissue: A distinctive tumor readily mistaken for an epithelial neoplasm. Am J Surg Pathol 15:915–924, 1991.

253. Byers RJ, McMahon RFT, Freemont AJ, et al: Epithelioid angiosarcoma arising in an arteriovenous fistula. Histopathology 21:87–89, 1992.

254. Eusebi V, Carcangiu ML, Dina R, Rosai J: Keratin-positive epithelioid angiosarcoma of thyroid. A report of four cases. Am J Surg Pathol 14:737–747, 1990.

255. Eyden B, Prescott R, Curry A, Haboubi N: Unusual organelles in an epithelioid angiosarcoma. Ultrastruct Pathol 17:153–159, 1993.

256. Livaditou A, Alexiou G, Floros D, et al: Epithelioid angiosarcoma of the adrenal gland associated with chronic arsenical intoxication? Pathol Res Pract 187:284–289, 1991.

257. Marrogi AJ, Hunt SJ, Santa Cruz DJ: Cutaneous epithelioid angiosarcoma. Am J Dermatopathol 12:350–356, 1990.

258. Perez-Atayde AR, Achenbach H, Lack EE: High-grade epithelioid angiosarcoma of the scalp. An immunohistochemical and ultrastructural study. Am J Dermatopathol 8:411–418, 1986.

259. Sirgi KE, Wick MR, Swanson PE: B72.3 and CD34 immunoreactivity in malignant epithelioid soft tissue tumors. Adjuncts in the recognition of endothelial neoplasms. Am J Surg Pathol 17:179–185, 1993.

260. Gray MH, Rosenberg AE, Dickersin GR, Bhan AK: Cytokeratin expression in epithelioid vascular neoplasms. Hum Pathol 21:212–217, 1990.

261. Maddox JC, Evans HL: Angiosarcoma of skin and soft tissue: A study of forty-four cases. Cancer 48:1907–1921, 1981.

262. Tsang WYW, Chan JKC, Fletcher CDM: Recently characterized vascular tumours of skin and soft tissues. Histopathology 19:489–501, 1991.

263. Swanson PE: Heffalumps, jagulars, and cheshire cats. A commentary on cytokeratins and soft tissue sarcomas. Am J Clin Pathol 95(Suppl 1):S2–S7, 1991.

264. Nappi O, Wick MR, Pettinato G, et al: Pseudovascular adenoid squamous cell carcinoma of the skin. A neoplasm that may be mistaken for angiosarcoma. Am J Surg Pathol 16:429–438, 1992.

265. DeYoung BR, Wick MR, Fitzgibbon JF, et al: CD31. An immunospecific marker for endothelial differentiation in human neoplasms. Appl Immunohistochem 1:97–100, 1993.
266. Leader M, Collins M, Patel J, Henry K: Staining for factor VIII related antigen and Ulex europaeus agglutinin I (UEA-I) in 230 tumours. An assessment of their specificity for angiosarcoma and Kaposi's sarcoma. Histopathology 10:1153–1162, 1986.
267. Traweek ST, Kandalaft PL, Mehta P, Battifora H: The human hematopoietic progenitor cell antigen (CD34) in vascular neoplasia. Am J Clin Pathol 96:25–31, 1991.
268. Ramani P, Bradley NJ, Fletcher CDM: QBEND/10, a new monoclonal antibody to endothelium: Assessment of its diagnostic utility in paraffin sections. Histopathology 17:237–242, 1990.
269. Banerjee SS, Eyden BP, Wells S, et al: Pseudoangiosarcomatous carcinoma: A clinicopathological study of seven cases. Histopathology 21:13–23, 1992.
270. Cox NH, Long ED: Pseudoangiosarcomatous squamous cell carcinoma of skin. Histopathology 22:295–296, 1993.
271. Mills SE, Gaffey MJ, Watts JC, et al: Angiomatoid carcinoma and ''angiosarcoma'' of thyroid gland. A spectrum of endothelial differentiation? Mod Pathol 6:40A, 1993.
272. Nakhleh RE, Wick MR, Rocamora A, et al: Morphologic diversity in malignant melanomas. Am J Clin Pathol 93:731–740, 1990.

Epithelioid Hemangioendothelioma

273. Rosai J, Gold J, Landy R: The histiocytoid hemangiomas. A unifying concept embracing several previously described entities of skin, soft tissue, large vessels, bone, and heart. Hum Pathol 10:707–730, 1979.
274. Castro C, Winkelmann RK: Angiolymphoid hyperplasia with eosinophilia in the skin. Cancer 34:1696–1705, 1974.
275. Olsen TG, Helwig EB: Angiolymphoid hyperplasia with eosinophilia. A clinicopathologic study of 116 patients. J Am Acad Dermatol 12:781–796, 1985.
276. Wells GC, Whimster IW: Subcutaneous angiolymphoid hyperplasia with eosinophilia. Br J Dermatol 81:1–15, 1969.
277. Wilson Jones E, Marks R: Papular angioplasia; vascular papules of the face and scalp simulating malignant tumors. Arch Dermatol 102:422–427, 1970.
278. Eady RAJ, Wilson Jones E: Pseudo-pyogenic granuloma: Enzyme histochemical and ultrastructural study. Hum Pathol 8:653–668, 1977.
279. Weiss SW, Ishak KG, Dail DH, et al: Epithelioid hemangioendothelioma and related lesions. Semin Diagn Pathol 3:259–287, 1986.
280. Weiss SW, Enzinger FM: Epithelioid hemangioendothelioma. A vascular tumor often mistaken for a carcinoma. Cancer 50:970–981, 1982.
281. Mirra JM, Kameda N: Myxoid angioblastomatosis of bones. A case report of a rare, multifocal entity with light, ultramicroscopic, and immunopathologic correlation. Am J Surg Pathol 9:450–458, 1985.
282. Tsuneyoshi M, Dorfman HD, Bauer TW: Epithelioid hemangioendothelioma of bone. A clinicopathologic, ultrastructural, and immunohistochemical study. Am J Surg Pathol 10:754–764, 1986.
283. Arnold G, Klein PJ, Fischer R: Epithelioid hemangioendothelioma. Report of a case with immuno-lectinhistochemical and ultrastructural demonstration of its vascular nature. Virchows Arch (A) 408:435–443, 1986.
284. Ellis GL, Kratochvil FJ: Epithelioid hemangioendothelioma of the head and neck: A clinicopathologic report of twelve cases. Oral Surg Oral Med Oral Pathol 61:61–68, 1986.
285. Lamovec J, Sobel HJ, Zidar A, Jerman J: Epithelioid hemangioendothelioma of the anterior mediastinum with osteoclast-like giant cells. Am J Clin Pathol 93:813–817, 1990.
286. Meister P, Hoede N, Rumpelt H-J: Epithelioid hemangioendothelioma of the scalp. A case report with immunohistochemical and ultrastructural study. Pathol Res Pract 180:220–226, 1985.
287. Verbeken E, Beyls J, Moerman P, et al: Lung metastasis of malignant epithelioid hemangioendothelioma mimicking a primary intravascular bronchioalveolar tumor. A histologic, ultrastructural, and immunohistochemical study. Cancer 55:1741–1746, 1985.
288. Williams SB, Butler BC, Gilkey FW, et al: Epithelioid hemangioendothelioma with osteoclastlike giant cells. Arch Pathol Lab Med 117:315–318, 1993.
289. Zagzag D, Yang G, Seidman J, Lusskin R: Malignant epithelioid hemangioendothelioma arising in an intramuscular lipoma. Cancer 71:764–768, 1993.
290. Cooper PH: Is histiocytoid hemangioma a specific pathologic entity? Am J Surg Pathol 12:815–817, 1988.
291. Ramani P, Bradley NJ, Fletcher CDM: QBEND/10, a new monoclonal antibody to endothelium: Assessment of its diagnostic utility in paraffin sections. Histopathology 17:237–242, 1990.
292. Sirgi KE, Wick MR, Swanson PE: B72.3 and CD34 immunoreactivity in malignant epithelioid soft tissue tumors. Adjuncts in the recognition of endothelial neoplasms. Am J Surg Pathol 17:179–185, 1993.
293. Traweek ST, Kandalaft PL, Mehta P, Battifora H: The human hematopoietic progenitor cell antigen (CD34) in vascular neoplasia. Am J Clin Pathol 96:25–31, 1991.
294. Gray MH, Rosenberg AE, Dickersin GR, Bhan AK: Cytokeratin expression in epithelioid vascular neoplasms. Hum Pathol 21:212–217, 1990.
295. van Haelst UJGM, Pruszczynski M, Cate LN, Mravunac M: Ultrastructural and immunohistochemical study of epithelioid hemangioendothelioma of bone: Coex-

pression of epithelial and endothelial markers. Ultrastruct Pathol 14:141–149, 1990.
296. Rosai J: Angiolymphoid hyperplasia with eosinophilia of the skin. Its nosological position in the spectrum of histiocytoid hemangioma. Am J Dermatopathol 4:175–184, 1982.
297. Rosai J, Gold J, Landy R: Letter to the editor. Vascular disorder. Am J Surg Pathol 11:651–652, 1987.
298. Weiss SW, Enzinger FM: Letter to the editor. Am J Surg Pathol 11:654, 1987.
299. Fetsch JF, Weiss SW: Observations concerning the pathogenesis of epithelioid hemangioma (angiolymphoid hyperplasia). Mod Pathol 4:449–455, 1991.

Malignant Epithelioid Schwannoma

300. Alvira MM, Mandybur TI, Menefee MG: Light microscopic and ultrastructural observations of a metastasizing malignant epithelioid schwannoma. Cancer 38:1977–1982, 1976.
301. Chu T-A, Shmookler BM: Malignant epithelioid schwannoma: A light microscopic and immunohistochemical study. J Surg Oncol 39:68–72, 1988.
302. DiCarlo EF, Woodruff JM, Bansal M, Erlandson RA: The purely epithelioid malignant peripheral nerve sheath tumor. Am J Surg Pathol 10:478–490, 1986.
303. Honma K, Watanabe H, Ohnishi Y, et al: Epithelioid malignant schwannoma. A case report. Acta Pathol Jpn 39:195–202, 1989.
304. Laskin WB, Weiss SW, Bratthauer GL: Epithelioid variant of malignant peripheral nerve sheath tumor (malignant epithelioid schwannoma). Am J Surg Pathol 15:1136–1145, 1991.
305. Lodding P, Kindblom L-G, Angervall L: Epithelioid malignant schwannoma. A study of 14 cases. Virchows Arch (A) 409:433–451, 1986.
306. McCormack LJ, Hazard JB, Dickson JA: Malignant epithelioid neurilemoma (schwannoma). Cancer 7:725–728, 1954.
307. Molenaar WM, Ladde BE, Koops HS, Dam-Meiring A: Two epithelioid malignant schwannomas in a patient with neurofibromatosis. Cytology, histology and DNA-flow-cytometry. Pathol Res Pract 184:529–534, 1989.
308. Morgan KG, Gray C: Malignant epithelioid schwannoma of superficial soft tissue? A case report with immunohistology and electron microscopy. Histopathology 9:765–775, 1985.
309. Taxy JB, Battifora H: Epithelioid schwannoma: Diagnosis by electron microscopy. Ultrastruct Pathol 2:19–24, 1981.
310. Tsuneyoshi M, Enjoji M: Primary malignant peripheral nerve tumors (malignant schwannomas). A clinicopathologic and electron microscopic study. Acta Pathol Jpn 29:363–375, 1979.
311. Yousem SA, Colby TV, Urich H: Malignant epithelioid schwannoma arising in a benign schwannoma. A case report. Cancer 55:2799–2803, 1985.

Clear-cell Sarcoma

312. Benson JD, Kraemer BB, Mackay B: Malignant melanoma of soft parts: An ultrastructural study of four cases. Ultrastruct Pathol 8:57–70, 1985.
313. Chung EB, Enzinger FM: Malignant melanoma of soft parts. A reassessment of clear cell sarcoma. Am J Surg Pathol 7:405–413, 1983.
314. Raynor AC, Vargas-Cortes F, Alexander RW, Bingham HG: Clear-cell sarcoma with melanin pigment: A possible soft-tissue variant of malignant melanoma. J Bone Joint Surg (Am) 61:276–280, 1979.
315. Sara AS, Evans HL, Benjamin RS: Malignant melanoma of soft parts (clear cell sarcoma). A study of 17 cases, with emphasis on prognostic factors. Cancer 65:367–374, 1990.
316. Enzinger FM: Clear-cell sarcoma of tendons and aponeuroses. An analysis of 21 cases. Cancer 18:1163–1174, 1965.
317. Eckardt JJ, Pritchard DJ, Soule EH: Clear cell sarcoma. A clinicopathologic study of 27 cases. Cancer 52:1482–1488, 1983.
318. Lucas DR, Nascimento AG, Sim FH: Clear cell sarcoma of soft tissues. Mayo Clinic experience with 35 cases. Am J Surg Pathol 16:1197–1204, 1992.
319. Tsuneyoshi M, Enjoji M, Kubo T: Clear cell sarcoma of tendons and aponeuroses. A comparative study of 13 cases with a provisional subgrouping into the melanotic and synovial types. Cancer 42:243–252, 1978.
320. Azumi N, Turner RR: Clear cell sarcoma of tendons and aponeuroses: Electron microscopic findings suggesting Schwann cell differentiation. Hum Pathol 14:1084–1089, 1983.
321. Bearman RM, Noe J, Kempson RL: Clear cell sarcoma with melanin pigment. Cancer 36:977–984, 1975.
322. Boudreaux D, Waisman J: Clear cell sarcoma with melanogenesis. Cancer 41:1387–1394, 1978.
323. Epstein AL, Martin AO, Kempson R: Use of a newly established human cell line (SU-CCS-1) to demonstrate the relationship of clear cell sarcoma to malignant melanoma. Cancer Res 44:1265–1274, 1984.
324. Hoffman GJ, Carter D: Clear cell sarcoma of tendons and aponeuroses with melanin. Arch Pathol 95:22–25, 1973.
325. Kindblom L-G, Lodding P, Angervall L: Clear-cell sarcoma of tendons and aponeuroses. An immunohistochemical and electron microscopic analysis indicating neural crest origin. Virchows Arch (A) 401:109–128, 1983.
326. Morishita S, Onomura T, Yamamoto S, Nakashima Y: Clear cell sarcoma of tendons and aponeuroses (malignant melanoma of soft parts) with unusual roentgenologic findings. Case report. Clin Orthop 216:276–279, 1987.

327. Ohno T, Park P, Utsunomiya Y, et al: Ultrastructural study of a clear cell sarcoma suggesting Schwannian differentiation. Ultastruct Pathol 10:39–48, 1986.
328. Pavlidis NA, Fisher C, Wiltshaw E: Clear-cell sarcoma of tendons and aponeuroses: A clinicopathologic study. Presentation of six additional cases with review of the literature. Cancer 54:1412–1417, 1984.
329. Sartoris DJ, Haghighi P, Resnick D: Case report 423: Clear-cell sarcoma plantar aspect of right foot. Skeletal Radiol 16:325–332, 1987.
330. Saw D, Tse CH, Chan J, et al: Clear cell sarcoma of the penis. Hum Pathol 17:423–425, 1986.
331. Swanson PE, Wick MR: Clear cell sarcoma. An immunohistochemical analysis of six cases and comparison with other epithelioid neoplasms of soft tissue. Arch Pathol Lab Med 113:55–60, 1989.
332. Dutra FR: Clear-cell sarcoma of tendons and aponeuroses. Three additional cases. Cancer 25:942–946, 1970.
333. Ekfors TO, Rantakokko V: Clear-cell sarcoma of tendons and aponeuroses: Malignant melanoma of soft tissues? Report of four cases. Pathol Res Pract 165:422–428, 1979.
334. Hasegawa T, Hirose T, Kudo E, Hizawa K: Clear cell sarcoma. An immunohistochemical and ultrastructural study. Acta Pathol Jpn 39:321–327, 1989.
335. Huntrakoon M: Premelanosomes in clear cell sarcoma. Arch Pathol Lab Med 108:182, 1984.
336. Kubo T: Clear-cell sarcoma of patellar tendon studied by electron microscopy. Cancer 24:948–953, 1969.
337. Mackenzie DH: Clear cell sarcoma of tendon and aponeuroses with melanin production. J Pathol 114:231–232, 1974.
338. Mechtersheimer G, Tilgen W, Klar E, Möller P: Clear cell sarcoma of tendons and aponeuroses: Case presentation with special reference to immunohistochemical findings. Hum Pathol 20:914–917, 1989.
339. Mii Y, Miyauchi Y, Hohnoki K, et al: Neural crest origin of clear cell sarcoma of tendons and aponeuroses. Ultrastructural and enzyme cytochemical study of human and nude mouse-transplanted tumours. Virchows Arch (A) 415:51–60, 1989.
340. Mukai M, Torikata C, Iri H, et al: Histogenesis of clear cell sarcoma of tendons and aponeuroses. An electron-microscopic, biochemical, enzyme histochemical, and immunohistochemical study. Am J Pathol 114:264–272, 1984.
341. Parker JB, Marcus PB, Martin JH: Spinal melanotic clear cell sarcoma: A light and electron microscopic study. Cancer 46:718–724, 1980.

Spindle Cell Hemangioendothelioma

342. Weiss SW, Enzinger FM: Spindle cell hemangioendothelioma. A low-grade angiosarcoma resembling a cavernous hemangioma and Kaposi's sarcoma. Am J Surg Pathol 10:521–530, 1986.
343. Battocchio S, Facchetti F, Brisigotti M: Spindle cell haemangioendothelioma: Further evidence against its proposed neoplastic nature. Histopathology 22:296–298, 1993.
344. Ding J, Hashimoto H, Imayama S, et al: Spindle cell haemangioendothelioma: Probably a benign vascular lesion not a low-grade angiosarcoma. A clinicopathological, ultrastructural and immunohistochemical study. Virchows Arch (A) 420:77–85, 1992.
345. Fletcher CDM, Beham A, Schmid C: Spindle cell haemangioendothelioma: A clinicopathological and immunohistochemical study indicative of a non-neoplastic lesion. Histopathology 18:291–301, 1991.
346. Imayama S, Murakamai Y, Hashimoto H, Hori Y: Spindle cell hemangioendothelioma exhibits the ultrastructural features of reactive vascular proliferation rather than of angiosarcoma. Am J Clin Pathol 97:279–287, 1992.
347. Lawson JP, Scott G: Case report 602: Spindle cell hemangioendothelioma (SCH) and enchondromatosis (a form of Maffucci syndrome) in a patient with acute myelocytic leukemia (AML). Skeletal Radiol 19:158–162, 1990.
348. Lessard M, Barnhill RL: Spindle cell hemangioendothelioma of the skin. J Am Acad Dermatol 18:393–395, 1988.
349. Scott GA, Rosai J: Spindle cell hemangioendothelioma. Report of seven additional cases of a recently described vascular neoplasm. Am J Dermatopathol 10:281–288, 1988.
350. Zoltie N, Roberts PF: Spindle cell haemangioendothelioma in association with epithelioid haemangioendothelioma. Histopathology 15:544–546, 1989.
351. Tsang WYW, Chan JKC, Fletcher CDM: Recently characterized vascular tumours of skin and soft tissues. Histopathology 19:489–501, 1991.

Angiomatoid Malignant Fibrous Histiocytoma

352. Enzinger FM: Angiomatoid malignant fibrous histiocytoma. A distinct fibrohistiocytic tumor of children and young adults simulating a vascular neoplasm. Cancer 44:2147–2157, 1979.
353. Costa MJ, Weiss SW: Angiomatoid malignant fibrous histiocytoma. A follow-up study of 108 cases with evaluation of possible histologic predictors of outcome. Am J Surg Pathol 14:1126–1132, 1990.
354. Fletcher CDM: Angiomatoid "malignant fibrous histiocytoma": An immunohistochemical study indicative of myoid differentiation. Hum Pathol 22:563–568, 1991.
355. Kanter MH, Duane GB: Angiomatoid malignant fibrous histiocytoma. Cytology of fine needle aspiration and its differential diagnosis. Arch Pathol Lab Med 109:564–566, 1985.
356. Kay S: Angiomatoid malignant fibrous histiocytoma. Report of two cases with ultrastructural observations of one case. Arch Pathol Lab Med 109:934–937, 1985.
357. Leu HJ, Makek M: Angiomatoid malignant fibrous histiocytoma. Case report and electron microscopic findings. Virchows Arch (Pathol Anat) 395:99–107, 1982.
358. Pettinato G, Manivel JC, DeRosa G, et al: Angiomatoid malignant fibrous histiocytoma: Cytologic, immunohistochemical, ultrastructural, and flow cytometric study of 20 cases. Mod Pathol 3:479–487, 1990.
359. Smith MEF, Costa MJ, Weiss SW: Evaluation of CD68 and other histiocytic antigens in angiomatoid malignant fibrous histiocytoma. Am J Surg Pathol 15:757–763, 1991.
360. Sun C-CJ, Toker C, Breitenecker R: An ultrastructural study of angiomatoid fibrous histiocytoma. Cancer 49:2103–2111, 1982.
361. Wegmann W, Heitz PU: Angiomatoid malignant fibrous histiocytoma. Evidence for the histiocytic origin of tumor cells. Virchows Arch (Pathol Anat) 406:59–66, 1985.
362. Fletcher CDM: Angiomatoid fibrous histiocytoma. Am J Surg Pathol 16:426–427, 1992.
363. Leu HJ, Makek M: Angiomatoid malignant fibrous histiocytoma. Arch Pathol Lab Med 110:466–467, 1986.

Plexiform Fibrohistiocytic Tumor

364. Enzinger FM, Zhang R: Plexiform fibrohistiocytic tumor presenting in children and young adults. An analysis of 65 cases. Am J Surg Pathol 12:818–826, 1988.
365. Hollowood K, Holley MP, Fletcher CDM: Plexiform fibrohistiocytic tumour: Clinicopathological, immunohistochemical and ultrastructural analysis in favour of a myofibroblastic lesion. Histopathology 19:503–513, 1991.

Giant Cell Fibroblastoma

366. Abdul-Karim FW, Evans HL, Silva EG: Giant cell fibroblastoma: A report of three cases. Am J Clin Pathol 83:165–170, 1985.
367. Shmookler BM, Enzinger FM: Giant cell fibroblastoma: A peculiar childhood tumor. Lab Invest 46:76A, 1982.
368. Shmookler BM, Enzinger FM: Giant cell fibroblastoma. Anat Pathol 8:1–4, 1984.
369. Alguacil-Garcia A: Giant cell fibroblastoma recurring as dermatofibrosarcoma protuberans. Am J Surg Pathol 15:798–801, 1991.
370. Allen PW, Zwi J: Giant cell fibroblastoma transforming into dermatofibrosarcoma protuberans. Am J Surg Pathol 16:1127–1128, 1992.
371. Barr RJ, Young EM, Liao S-Y: Giant cell fibroblastoma: An immunohistochemical study. J Cutan Pathol 13:301–307, 1986.
372. Chou P, Gonzalez-Crussi F, Mangkornkanok M: Giant cell fibroblastoma. Cancer 63:756–762, 1989.
373. Coyne J, Kaftan SM, Craig RDP: Dermatofibrosarcoma protuberans recurring as a giant cell fibroblastoma. Histopathology 21:184–187, 1992.
374. Dymock RB, Allen PW, Stirling JW, et al: Giant cell fibroblastoma. A distinctive, recurrent tumor of childhood. Am J Surg Pathol 11:263–271, 1987.
375. Fletcher CDM: Giant cell fibroblastoma of soft tissue: A clinicopathological and immunohistochemical study. Histopathology 13:499–508, 1988.
376. Hirose T, Sasaki M, Shintaku M, et al: Giant cell fibroblastoma: A case report. Acta Pathol Jpn 40:540–544, 1990.
377. Kanai Y, Mukai M, Sugiura H, et al: Giant cell fibroblastoma. A case report and immunohistochemical comparison with ten cases of dermatofibrosarcoma protuberans. Acta Pathol Jpn 41:552–560, 1991.
378. Mills AE: Giant cell fibroblastoma. Am J Surg Pathol 12:648–650, 1988.
379. Pinto A, Hwang W-S, Wong AL, Seagram CGF: Giant cell fibroblastoma in childhood immunohistochemical and ultrastructural study. Mod Pathol 5:639–642, 1992.
380. Rosen LB, Amazon K, Weitzner J, Resnick L: Giant cell fibroblastoma. A report of a case and review of the literature. Am J Dermatopathol 11:242–247, 1989.
381. Shmookler BM, Enzinger FM, Weiss SW: Giant cell fibroblastoma. A juvenile form of dermatofibrosarcoma protuberans. Cancer 64:2154–2161, 1989.
382. Chung EB: Pitfalls in diagnosing benign soft tissue tumors in infancy and childhood. Pathol Annu 20:323–386, 1985.
383. Marrogi AJ, Swanson PE, Kyriakos M, Wick MR: Rudimentary meningocele of the skin. Clinicopathologic features and differential diagnosis. J Cutan Pathol 18:178–188, 1991.
384. Kamino H, Lee JY-Y, Berke A: Pleomorphic fibroma of the skin: A benign neoplasm with cytologic atypia. A clinicopathologic study of eight cases. Am J Surg Pathol 13:107–113, 1989.
385. Layfield LJ, Fain JS: Pleomorphic fibroma of skin. A case report and immunohistochemical study. Arch Pathol Lab Med 115:1046–1049, 1991.
386. Beham A, Fletcher CDM: Atypical "pseudosarcomatous" variant of cutaneous benign fibrous histiocytoma: Report of eight cases. Histopathology 17:167–169, 1990.
387. Fukamizu H, Oku T, Inoue K, et al: Atypical ("pseudosarcomatous") cutaneous histiocytoma. J Cutan Pathol 10:327–333, 1983.
388. Leyva WH, Santa Cruz DJ: Atypical cutaneous fibrous histiocytoma. Am J Dermatopathol 8:467–471, 1986.
389. Tamada S, Ackerman AB: Dermatofibroma with monster cells. Am J Dermatopathol 9:380–387, 1987.
390. Beham A, Fletcher CDM: Dermatofibrosarcoma protuberans with areas resembling giant cell fibroblastoma: Report of two cases. Histopathology 17:165–167, 1990.

391. Connelly JH, Evans HL: Dermatofibrosarcoma protuberans. A clinicopathologic review with emphasis on fibrosarcomatous areas. Am J Surg Pathol 16:921–925, 1992.

Postoperative Spindle Cell Nodule and Inflammatory Pseudosarcoma

392. Proppe KH, Scully RE, Rosai J: Postoperative spindle cell nodules of genitourinary tract resembling sarcomas. A report of eight cases. Am J Surg Pathol 8:101–108, 1984.
393. Clement PB: Postoperative spindle-cell nodule of the endometrium. Arch Pathol Lab Med 112:566–568, 1988.
394. Huang W-L, Ro JY, Grignon DJ, et al: Postoperative spindle cell nodule of the prostate and bladder. J Urol 143:824–826, 1990.
395. Hughes DF, Biggart JD, Hayes D: Pseudosarcomatous lesions of the urinary bladder. Histopathology 19:67–71, 1991.
396. Kay S, Schneider V: Reactive spindle cell nodule of the endocervix simulating uterine sarcoma. Int J Gynecol Pathol 4:255–257, 1985.
397. Wick MR, Brown BA, Young RH, Mills SE: Spindle-cell proliferations of the urinary tract. An immunohistochemical study. Am J Surg Pathol 12:379–389, 1988.
398. Young RH: Pseudoneoplastic lesions of the urinary bladder. Pathol Annu (Part 1) 23:67–104, 1988.
399. Roth JA: Reactive pseudosarcomatous response in urinary bladder. Urology 16:635–637, 1980.
400. Ro JY, Ayala AG, Ordóñez NG, et al: Pseudosarcomatous fibromyxoid tumor of the urinary bladder. Am J Clin Pathol 86:583–590, 1986.
401. Sahin AA, Ro JY, El-Naggar AK, et al: Pseudosarcomatous fibromyxoid tumor of the prostate. A case report with immunohistochemical, electron microscopic, and DNA flow cytometric analysis. Am J Clin Pathol 96:253–258, 1981.
402. Goussot JF, Coindre JM, Merlio JP, de Mascarel A: An adult atypical fibromyxoid tumor of the urinary bladder. Tumori 75:79–81, 1989.
403. Hafiz MA, Toker C, Sutula M: An atypical fibromyxoid tumor of the prostate. Cancer 54:2500–2504, 1984.
404. Coyne JD, Wilson G, Sandhu D, Young RH: Inflammatory pseudotumour of the urinary bladder. Histopathology 18:261–264, 1991.
405. Dietrick DD, Kabalin JN, Daniels GF Jr, et al: Inflammatory pseudotumor of the bladder. J Urol 148:141–144, 1992.
406. Jones EC, Clement PB, Young RH: Inflammatory pseudotumor of the urinary bladder. A clinicopathological, immunohistochemical, ultrastructural, and flow cytometric study of 13 cases. Am J Surg Pathol 17:264–274, 1993.
407. Nochomovitz LE, Orenstein JM: Inflammatory pseudotumor of the urinary bladder—possible relationship to nodular fasciitis. Two case reports, cytologic observations, and ultrastructural observations. Am J Surg Pathol 9:366–373, 1985.
408. Young RH, Scully RE: Pseudosarcomatous lesions of the urinary bladder, prostate gland, and urethra. A report of three cases and review of the literature. Arch Pathol Lab Med 111:354–358, 1987.
409. Albores-Saavedra J, Manivel JC, Essenfeld H, et al: Pseudosarcomatous myofibroblastic proliferations in the urinary bladder of children. Cancer 66:1234–1241, 1990.
410. Hollowood K, Fletcher CDM: Pseudosarcomatous myofibroblastic proliferations of the spermatic cord (''proliferative funiculitis''). Histologic and immunohistochemical analysis of a distinctive entity. Am J Surg Pathol 16:448–454, 1992.
411. Forrest JB, King GS, Pittman GR: An atypical myofibroblastic tumor of the bladder resembling a sarcoma. J Okla State Med Assoc 81:222–224, 1988.
412. Bégin LR, Frail D, Brzezinski A: Myofibroblastoma of the tunica testis: Evolving phase of so-called fibrous pseudotumor? Hum Pathol 21:866–868, 1990.
413. Gugliada K, Nardi PM, Borenstein MS, Torno RB: Inflammatory pseudosarcoma (pseudotumor) of the bladder. Radiology 179:66–68, 1991.
414. Yamashina M, Honma T, Uchijima Y: Myofibroblastic pseudotumor mimicking epididymal sarcoma. A clinicopathologic study of three cases. Pathol Res Pract 188:1054–1059, 1992.
415. Lamovec J, Zidar A, Tršinar B, Jančar J: Sclerosing inflammatory pseudotumor of the urinary bladder in a child. Am J Surg Pathol 16:1233–1238, 1992.
416. Stark GL, Feddersen R, Lowe BA, et al: Inflammatory pseudotumor (pseudosarcoma) of the bladder. J Urol 141:610–612, 1989.
417. Allen PW: Nodular fasciitis. Pathology 4:9–26, 1972.
418. Bernstein KE, Lattes R: Nodular (pseudosarcomatous) fasciitis, a nonrecurrent lesion: Clinicopathologic study of 134 cases. Cancer 49:1668–1678, 1982.
419. Meister P, Bückmann F-W, Konrad E: Nodular fasciitis (analysis of 100 cases and review of the literature). Pathol Res Pract 162:133–165, 1978.
420. Montgomery EA, Meis JM: Nodular fasciitis. Its morphologic spectrum and immunohistochemical profile. Am J Surg Pathol 15:942–948, 1991.
421. Das S, Upton JD, Amar AD: Nodular fasciitis of the bladder. J Urol 140:1532–1533, 1988.
422. Meis JM, Enzinger FM: Inflammatory fibrosarcoma of the mesentery and retroperitoneum. A tumor closely simulating inflammatory pseudotumor. Am J Surg Pathol 15:1146–1156, 1991.
423. Roth JA: Letter to the editor. Am J Clin Pathol 98:271, 1992.

Extraskeletal Myxoid Chondrosarcoma

424. Amir D, Amir G, Mogle P, Pogrund H: Extraskeletal soft-tissue chondrosarcoma. Case report and review of the literature. Clin Orthop 198:219–223, 1985.

425. Angervall L, Enerbäck L, Knutson H: Chondrosarcoma of soft tissue origin. Cancer 32:507–513, 1973.
426. Casadei R, Ricci M, Ruggieri P, et al: Chondrosarcoma of the soft tissues. Two different sub-groups. J Bone Joint Surg (Br) 73:162–168, 1991.
427. Dardick I, Lgacé R, Carlier MT, Jung RC: Chordoid sarcoma (extraskeletal myxoid chondrosarcoma). A light and electron microscope study. Virchows Arch (A) 399:61–78, 1983.
428. DeBlois G, Wang S, Kay S: Microtubular aggregates within rough endoplasmic reticulum: An unusual ultrastructural feature of extraskeletal myxoid chondrosarcoma. Hum Pathol 17:469–475, 1986.
429. Enzinger FM, Shiraki M: Extraskeletal myxoid chondrosarcoma. An analysis of 34 cases. Hum Pathol 3:421–435, 1972.
430. Fletcher CDM, McKee PH: Immunohistochemistry and histogenesis of extraskeletal myxoid chondrosarcoma. J Pathol 147:67–68, 1985.
431. Fletcher CDM, Powell G, McKee PH: Extraskeletal myxoid chondrosarcoma: A histochemical and immunohistochemical study. Histopathology 10:489–499, 1986.
432. Fu Y-S, Kay S: A comparative ultrastructural study of mesenchymal chondrosarcoma and myxoid chondrosarcoma. Cancer 33:1531–1542, 1974.
433. Fukuda T, Ishikawa H, Ohnishi Y, et al: Extraskeletal myxoid chondrosarcoma arising from the retroperitoneum. Am J Clin Pathol 85:514–519, 1986.
434. Goldenberg RR, Cohen P, Steinlauf P: Chondrosarcoma of the extraskeletal soft tissues. A report of seven cases and review of the literature. J Bone Joint Surg (Am) 49:1487–1507, 1967.
435. Hachitanda Y, Tsuneyoshi M, Daimaru Y, et al: Extraskeletal myxoid chondrosarcoma in young children. Cancer 61:2521–2526, 1988.
436. Insabato L, Terracciano LM, Boscaino A, et al: Extraskeletal myxoid chondrosarcoma with intranuclear vacuoles and microtubular aggregates in the rough endoplasmic reticulum. Report of a case with fine needle aspiration and electron microscopy. Acta Cytol 34:858–862, 1990.
437. Jacobs GH, Berson SD, Skikne MI, et al: Chordoid sarcoma of the hand. A case report. S Afr Med J 61:630–633, 1982.
438. Kindblom L-G, Angervall L: Myxoid chondrosarcoma of the synovial tissue. A clinicopathologic, histochemical, and ultrastructural analysis. Cancer 52:1886–1895, 1983.
439. Mackenzie DH: The myxoid tumors of somatic soft tissues. Am J Surg Pathol 5:443–458, 1981.
440. Mackenzie DH: The unsuspected soft tissue chondrosarcoma. Histopathology 7:759–766, 1983.
441. Martin RF, Melnick PJ, Warner NE, et al: Chordoid sarcoma. J Clin Pathol 59:623–635, 1973.
442. Mehio AR, Ferenczy A: Extraskeletal myxoid chondrosarcoma with ''chordoid'' features (chordoid sarcoma). Am J Clin Pathol 70:700–705, 1978.
443. Robertson DI, Hogg GR: Chordoid sarcoma. Ultrastructural evidence supporting a synovial origin. Cancer 45:520–527, 1980.
444. Saleh G, Evans HL, Ro JY, Ayala AG: Extraskeletal myxoid chondrosarcoma. A clinicopathologic study of ten patients with long-term follow-up. Cancer 70:2827–2830, 1992.
445. Smith MT, Farinacci CJ, Carpenter HA, Bannayan GA: Extraskeletal myxoid chondrosarcoma. A clinicopathological study. Cancer 37:821–827, 1976.
446. Stout AP, Verner EW: Chondrosarcoma of the extraskeletal soft tissues. Cancer 6:581–590, 1953.
447. Suzuki T, Kaneko H, Kojima K, et al: Extraskeletal myxoid chondrosarcoma characterized by microtubular aggregates in the rough endoplasmic reticulum and tubulin immunoreactivity. J Pathol 156:51–57, 1988.
448. Tseleni-Balafouta S, Arvanitis D, Kakaviatos N, Paraskevakou H: Primary myxoid chondrosarcoma of the thyroid gland. Arch Pathol Lab Med 112:94–96, 1988.
449. Tsuneyoshi M, Enjoji M, Iwasaki H, Shinohara N: Extraskeletal myxoid chondrosarcoma. A clinicopathologic and electron microscopic study. Acta Pathol Jpn 31:439–447, 1981.
450. Turc-Carel C, Cin PD, Rao U, et al: Recurrent breakpoints at 9q31 and 22q12.2 in extraskeletal myxoid chondrosarcoma. Cancer Genet Cytogenet 30:145–150, 1988.
451. Weiss SW: Ultrastructure of the so-called ''chordoid sarcoma.'' Evidence supporting cartilaginous differentiation. Cancer 37:300–306, 1976.
452. Wick MR, Burgess JH, Manivel JC: A reassessment of ''chordoid sarcoma.'' Ultrastructural and immunohistochemical comparison with chordoma and skeletal myxoid chondrosarcoma. Mod Pathol 1:433–443, 1988.
453. Bridge JA, Sanger WG, Neff JR: Translocations involving chromosomes 2 and 13 in benign and malignant cartilaginous neoplasms. Cancer Genet Cytogenet 38:83–88, 1989.
454. Cameron CHS, Kenny BD, Clements WBD, Toner PG: Unusual extraskeletal myxoid chondrosarcoma. Ultrastruct Pathol 16:17–23, 1992.
455. Quagliuolo V, Azzarelli A, Cerasoli S, Audisio RA: Unusual types of chondrosarcoma: Chondrosarcoma arising in soft tissue and in non-skeletal cartilage. Eur J Surg Oncol 14:691–695, 1988.
456. Allen PW: Myxoid tumors of soft tissue. Pathol Annu (Part 1) 15:133–192, 1980.
457. Vuzevski VD, van der Heul RO: Comparative ultrastructure of soft-tissue myxoid tumors. Ultrastruct Pathol 12:87–105, 1988.
458. Chung EB, Enzinger FM: Chondroma of soft parts. Cancer 41:1414–1424, 1978.

Myxoid Dermatofibrosarcoma Protuberans

459. Frierson HF, Cooper PH: Myxoid variant of dermatofibrosarcoma protuberans. Am J Surg Pathol 7:445–450, 1983.

460. Burkhardt BR, Soule EH, Winkelmann RK, Ivins JC: Dermatofibrosarcoma protuberans. Study of fifty-six cases. Am J Surg 111:638–644, 1966.

461. Eisen RN, Tallini G: Metastatic dermatofibrosarcoma protuberans with fibrosarcomatous change in the absence of local recurrence. A case report of simultaneous occurrence with a malignant giant cell tumor of soft parts. Cancer 72:462–468, 1993.

462. Fletcher CDM, Evans BJ, Macartney JC, et al: Dermatofibrosarcoma protuberans: A clinicopathological and immunohistochemical study with a review of the literature. Histopathology 9:921–938, 1985.

463. Fletcher CDM, McKee PH: Sarcomas—a clinicopathological guide with particular reference to cutaneous manifestation. I. Dermatofibrosarcoma protuberans, malignant fibrous histiocytoma and the epithelioid sarcoma of Enzinger. Clin Exp Dermatol 9:451–465, 1984.

464. Lopes JM, Paiva ME: Dermatofibrosarcoma protuberans. A histological and ultrastructural study of 11 cases with emphasis on the study of recurrences and histogenesis. Pathol Res Pract 187:806–813, 1991.

465. McPeak CJ, Cruz T, Nicastri AD: Dermatofibrosarcoma protuberans: An analysis of 86 cases—five with metastasis. Ann Surg 166:803–816, 1967.

466. Taylor HB, Helwig EB: Dermatofibrosarcoma protuberans. A study of 115 cases. Cancer 15:717–725, 1962.

467. duBoulay CEH: Demonstration of alpha-1-antitrypsin and alpha-1-antichymotrypsin in fibrous histiocytomas using the immunoperoxidase technique. Am J Surg Pathol 6:559–564, 1982.

468. Kanai Y, Mukai M, Sugiura H, et al: Giant cell fibroblastoma. A case report and immunohistochemical comparison with ten cases of dermatofibrosarcoma protuberans. Acta Pathol Jpn 41:552–560, 1991.

469. Kindblom L-G, Jacobsen GK, Jacobsen M: Immunohistochemical investigations of tumors of supposed fibroblastic-histiocytic origin. Hum Pathol 13:834–840, 1982.

470. Ma CK, Zarbo RJ, Gown AM: Immunohistochemical characterization of atypical fibroxanthoma and dermatofibrosarcoma protuberans. Am J Clin Pathol 97:478–483, 1992.

471. Miettinen M: Antibody specific to muscle actins in the diagnosis and classification of soft tissue tumors. Am J Pathol 130:205–215, 1988.

472. Fletcher CDM, Theaker JM, Flanagan A, Krausz T: Pigmented dermatofibrosarcoma protuberans (Bednar tumour): Melanocytic colonization or neuroectodermal differentiation? A clinicopathological and immunohistochemical study. Histopathology 13:631–643, 1988.

473. Aiba S, Tabata N, Ishii H, et al: Dermatofibrosarcoma protuberans is a unique fibrohistiocytic tumour expressing CD34. Br J Dermatol 127:79–84, 1992.

473a. Zelger B, Sidoroff A, Stanzl J, et al: Deep penetrating dermatofibroma versus dermatofibrosarcoma protuberans. A clinicopathologic comparison. Am J Surg Pathol 18:677–686, 1994.

473b. Leong AS-Y, Lim MHT: Immunohistochemical characteristics of dermatofibrosarcoma protuberans. Appl Immunohistochem 2:42–47, 1994.

473c. Brathwaite C, Suster S: Dermatofibrosarcoma protuberans. A critical reappraisal of the role of immunohistochemical stains for diagnosis. Appl Immunohistochem 2:36–41, 1994.

474. Alguacil-Garcia A, Unni KK, Goellner JR: Histogenesis of dermatofibrosarcoma protuberans. An ultrastructural study. Am J Clin Pathol 69:427–434, 1978.

475. Dupree WB, Langloss JM, Weiss SW: Pigmented dermatofibrosarcoma protuberans (Bednar tumor). A pathologic, ultrastructural, and immunohistochemical study. Am J Surg Pathol 9:630–639, 1985.

476. Escalona-Zapata J, Fernandez EA, Escuin FL: The fibroblastic nature of dermatofibrosarcoma protuberans. Tissue culture and ultrastructural study. Virchows Arch (Pathol Anat) 391:165–175, 1981.

477. Hashimoto K, Brownstein MH, Jakobiec FA: Dermatofibrosarcoma protuberans. A tumor with perineural and endoneural cell features. Arch Dermatol 110:874–885, 1974.

478. Ozzello L, Hamels J: The histiocytic nature of dermatofibrosarcoma protuberans. Tissue culture and electron microscopic study. Am J Clin Pathol 65:136–148, 1976.

479. Zina AM, Bundino S: Dermatofibrosarcoma protuberans. An ultrastructural study of five cases. J Cutan Pathol 6:265–271, 1979.

480. Erlandson RA, Woodruff JM: Peripheral nerve sheath tumors: An electron microscopic study of 43 cases. Cancer 49:273–287, 1982.

481. Sarode VR, Joshi K, Ravichandran P, Das R: Myxoid variant of primary cutaneous malignant melanoma. Histopathology 20:186–187, 1992.

482. Urso C, Giannotti B, Bondi R: Myxoid melanoma of skin. Arch Pathol Lab Med 114:527–528, 1990.

Nerve Sheath Myxoma

483. Harkin JC, Reed RJ: Tumors of the peripheral nervous system. Atlas of Tumor Pathology, second series, fascicle 3. Washington, DC, Armed Forces Institute of Pathology, 1969.

484. MacDonald DM, Wilson-Jones E: Pacinian neurofibroma. Histopathology 1:247–255, 1977.

485. King DT, Barr RJ: Bizarre cutaneous neurofibromas. J Cutan Pathol 7:21–31, 1980.

486. Aronson PJ, Fretzin DF, Potter BS: Neurothekeoma of Gallager and Helwig (dermal nerve sheath myxoma variant): Report of a case with electron microscopic and immunohistochemical studies. J Cutan Pathol 12:506–519, 1985.

487. Gallager RL, Helwig EB: Neurothekeoma—a benign cutaneous tumor of neural origin. Am J Clin Pathol 74:759–764, 1980.

488. Henmi A, Sato H, Wataya T, et al: Neurothekeoma. Report of a case with immunohistochemical and ultrastructural studies. Acta Pathol Jpn 36:1911–1919, 1986.

489. Kao GF, Penneys NS: Immunohistochemical findings of 34 neurothekeomas (benign peripheral nerve sheath tumor). J Cutan Pathol 17:304, 1990.

490. Paulus W, Jellinger K, Perneczky G: Intraspinal neurothekeoma (nerve sheath myxoma). A report of two cases. Am J Clin Pathol 95:511–516, 1991.

491. Angervall L, Kindblom L-G, Haglid K: Dermal nerve sheath myxoma. A light and electron microscopic, histochemical and immunohistochemical study. Cancer 53:1752–1759, 1984.

492. Fletcher CDM, Chan JK-C, McKee PH: Dermal nerve sheath myxoma: A study of three cases. Histopathology 10:135–145, 1986.

493. Webb JN: The histogenesis of nerve sheath myxoma: Report of a case with electron microscopy. J Pathol 127:35–37, 1979.

494. Allen PW: Myxoid tumors of soft tissues. Pathol Annu 15(Pt 1):133–192, 1980.

495. Holden CA, Wilson-Jones E, MacDonald DM: Cutaneous lobular neuromyxoma. Br J Dermatol 106:211–215, 1982.

496. Reed RJ, Harkin JC: Tumors of the peripheral nervous system. Atlas of Tumor Pathology, second series, fascicle 3, supplement. Washington, DC, Armed Forces Institute of Pathology, 1983.

497. Barnhill RL, Mihm MC Jr: Cellular neurothekeoma. A distinctive variant of neurothekeoma mimicking nevomelanocytic tumors. Am J Surg Pathol 14:113–120, 1990.

498. Calonje E, Wilson-Jones E, Smith NP, Fletcher CDM: Cellular ''neurothekeoma'': An epithelioid variant of pilar leiomyoma? Morphological and immunohistochemical analysis of a series. Histopathology 20:397–404, 1992.

499. Jones TJ, Hammerton W, Shrank AB, Nicholls PE: Cellular neurothekeoma—the Shropshire experience. J Pathol 163:161A, 1991.

500. Rosati LA, Fratamico FCM, Eusebi V: Cellular neurothekeoma. Appl Pathol 4:186–191, 1986.

501. Blumberg AK, Kay S, Adelaar RS: Nerve sheath myxoma of digital nerve. Cancer 63:1215–1218, 1989.

502. Erlandson RA: The enigmatic perineurial cell and its participation in tumors and in tumorlike entities. Ultrastruct Pathol 15:335–351, 1991.

503. Mackenzie DH: The myxoid tumors of somatic soft tissues. Am J Surg Pathol 5:443–458, 1981.

504. Pulitzer DR, Reed RJ: Nerve-sheath myxoma (perineurial myxoma). Am J Dermatopathol 7:409–421, 1985.

505. Wee A, Tan CEL, Raju GC: Nerve sheath myxoma of the breast. A light and electron microscopic, histochemical and immunohistochemical study. Virchows Arch (A) 416:163–167, 1989.

506. Barnhill RL, Dickersin GR, Nickeleit V, et al: Studies on the cellular origin of neurothekeoma: Clinical, light microscopic, immunohistochemical, and ultrastructural observations. J Am Acad Dermatol 25:80–88, 1991.

507. Goldstein J, Lifshitz T: Myxoma of the nerve sheath. Report of three cases, observations by light and electron microscopy and histochemical analysis. Am J Dermatopathol 7:423–429, 1985.

508. Mason MR, Gnepp DR, Herbold DR: Nerve sheath myxoma (neurothekeoma): A case involving the lip. Oral Surg Oral Med Oral Pathol 62:185–186, 1986.

509. Mincer HH, Spears KD: Nerve sheath myxoma in the tongue. Oral Surg 37:428–431, 1974.

510. Sist TC Jr, Greene GW Jr: Benign nerve sheath myxoma: Light and electron microscopic features of two cases. Oral Surg 47:441–444, 1979.

511. Yamamoto H, Kawana T: Oral nerve sheath myxoma. Report of a case with findings of ultrastructural and immunohistochemical studies. Acta Pathol Jpn 38:121–127, 1988.

512. Barnhill RL, Mihm MC Jr, Magro CM: Plexiform spindle cell naevus: A distinctive variant of plexiform melanocytic naevus. Histopathology 18:243–247, 1991.

513. Epstein J, Urmacher C: A cutaneous neoplasm with neural differentiation. Am J Dermatopathol 6:591–593, 1984.

514. Argenyi ZB, LeBoit PE, Santa Cruz D, et al: Nerve sheath myxoma (neurothekeoma) of the skin: Light microscopic and immunohistochemical reappraisal of the cellular variant. J Cutan Pathol 20:294–303, 1993.

515. Ariza A, Bilbao JM, Rosai J: Immunohistochemical detection of epithelial membrane antigen in normal perineurial cells and perineurioma. Am J Surg Pathol 12:678–683, 1988.

516. Theaker JM, Fletcher CDM: Epithelial membrane antigen expression by the perineurial cell: Further studies of peripheral nerve lesions. Histopathology 14:581–592, 1989.

517. Theaker JM, Gatter KC, Puddle J: Epithelial membrane antigen expression by the perineurium of peripheral nerve and in peripheral nerve tumours. Histopathology 13:171–179, 1988.

518. Theaker JM, Gillett MB, Fleming KA, Gatter KC: Epithelial membrane antigen expression by meningiomas, and the perineurium of peripheral nerve. Arch Pathol Lab Med 111:409, 1988.

519. Dover JS, From L, Lewis A: Palisaded encapsulated neuromas. A clinicopathologic study. Arch Dermatol 125:386–389, 1989.

520. Fletcher CDM: Solitary circumscribed neuroma of the skin (so-called palisaded, encapsulated neuroma). A clinicopathologic and immunohistochemical study. Am J Surg Pathol 13:574–580, 1989.

521. Reed RJ, Fine RM, Meltzer HD: Palisaded, encapsulated neuromas of the skin. Arch Dermatol 106:865–870, 1972.

522. Tsang WYW, Chan JKC, Chow LTC, Tse CCH: Perineurioma: An uncommon soft tissue neoplasm distinct from localized hypertrophic neuropathy and neurofibroma. Am J Surg Pathol 16:756–763, 1992.
523. Fletcher CDM, Theaker JM: Digital pacinian neuroma: A distinctive hyperplastic lesion. Histopathology 15:249–256, 1989.

Aggressive Angiomyxoma

524. Steeper TA, Rosai J: Aggressive angiomyxoma of the female pelvis and perineum. Report of nine cases of a distinctive type of gynecologic soft-tissue neoplasm. Am J Surg Pathol 7:463–475, 1983.
525. Bégin LR, Clement PB, Kirk ME, et al: Aggressive angiomyxoma of pelvic soft parts: A clinicopathologic study of nine cases. Hum Pathol 16:621–628, 1985.
526. Tsang WYW, Chan JKC, Lee KC, et al: Aggressive angiomyxoma. A report of four cases occurring in men. Am J Surg Pathol 16:1059–1065, 1992.
527. Destian S, Ritchie WGM: Aggressive angiomyxoma: CT appearance. Am J Gastroenterol 81:711–713, 1986.
528. Hilgers RD, Pai R, Bartow SA, et al: Aggressive angiomyxoma of the vulva. Obstet Gynecol 68:60S–62S, 1986.
529. Llauger J, Pérez C, Coscojuela P, et al: Aggressive angiomyxoma of pelvic soft tissue: CT appearance. Urol Radiol 12:25–26, 1990.
530. Mandai K, Moriwaki S, Motoi M: Aggressive angiomyxoma of the vulva. Report of a case. Acta Pathol Jpn 40:927–934, 1990.
531. Manivel C, Steeper T, Swanson P, Wick M: Aggressive angiomyxoma of the pelvis. An immunoperoxidase study. Lab Invest 56:46A, 1987.
532. Sementa AR, Gambini C, Borgiani L, Comes P: Aggressive angiomyxoma of the pelvis and perineum. Report of a case with immunohistochemical and electron microscopic study. Pathologica 81:463–469, 1989.
533. Sutton GP, Rogers RE, Roth LM, Ehrlich CE: Aggressive angiomyxoma first diagnosed as levator hernia. Am J Obstet Gynecol 161:73–75, 1989.
534. Woods SDS, Essex WB, Hughes ESR, et al: Aggressive angiomyxoma of the female pelvis. Aust NZ J Surg 57:687–688, 1987.
535. Allen PW, Dymock RB, MacCormac LB: Superficial angiomyxomas with and without epithelial components. Report of 30 tumors in 28 patients. Am J Surg Pathol 12:519–530, 1988.

536. Fletcher CDM, Tsang WYW, Fisher C, et al: Angiomyofibroblastoma of the vulva. A benign neoplasm distinct from aggressive angiomyxoma. Am J Surg Pathol 16:373–382, 1992.

Myxoid Leiomyosarcoma

537. Chen KTK, Hafez GR, Gilbert EF: Myxoid variant of epithelioid smooth muscle tumor. Am J Clin Pathol 74:350–353, 1980.
538. King ME, Dickersin GR, Scully RE: Myxoid leiomyosarcoma of the uterus. A report of six cases. Am J Surg Pathol 6:589–598, 1982.
539. Mills SE, Bova GS, Wick MR, Young RH: Leiomyosarcoma of the urinary bladder. A clinicopathologic and immunohistochemical study of 15 cases. Am J Surg Pathol 13:480–489, 1989.
540. Plous RH, Gordon RE, Geller SA: Retrovesical myxoid leiomyosarcoma. Arch Pathol Lab Med 110:1194–1196, 1986.
541. Salm R, Evans DJ: Myxoid leiomyosarcoma. Histopathology 9:159–169, 1985.
542. Young RH, Proppe KH, Dickersin GR, Scully RE: Myxoid leiomyosarcoma of the urinary bladder. Arch Pathol Lab Med 111:359–362, 1987.

Ossifying Fibromyxoid Tumor

543. Akai M, Azuma H, Ohno T, et al: Case report 685. Ossifying fibromyxoid tumor of the soft parts of the upper arm. Skeletal Radiol 20:608–612, 1991.
544. Donner LR: Ossifying fibromyxoid tumor of soft parts: Evidence supporting Schwann cell origin. Hum Pathol 23:200–202, 1992.
545. Enzinger FM, Weiss SW, Liang CY: Ossifying fibromyxoid tumor of soft parts. A clinicopathological analysis of 59 cases. Am J Surg Pathol 13:817–827, 1989.
546. Miettinen M: Ossifying fibromyxoid tumor of soft parts. Additional observations of a distinctive soft tissue tumor. Am J Clin Pathol 95:32–39, 1991.
547. Schofield JB, Krausz T, Stamp GWH, et al: Ossifying fibromyxoid tumour of soft parts: Immunohistochemical and ultrastructural analysis. Histopathology 22:101–111, 1993.
548. Yoshida H, Minamizaki T, Yumoto T, et al: Ossifying fibromyxoid tumor of soft parts. Acta Pathol Jpn 41:480–486, 1991.
549. Guarner J, Dominguez-Malagón HR, Meneses-García A: Ossifying fibromyxoid tumor. Am J Surg Pathol 14:1167–1169, 1990.

CHAPTER 18

Dermatopathology

Philip E. LeBoit, M.D.

This chapter focuses on a few conditions that are particularly problematic in the practice of surgical pathology or are often misdiagnosed by pathologists.

URTICARIAL HYPERSENSITIVITY REACTIONS

Urticarial hypersensitivity reactions produce pink, smooth-surfaced itchy papules. They are sometimes referred to as **urticarial allergic reactions,** or even less informatively as **dermal hypersensitivity reactions,** but few of them are produced by an allergic (type I) immune response. The prototype of an urticarial hypersensitivity reaction is **urticaria,** or **hives.**

CLINICOPATHOLOGIC FEATURES. Urticaria is transient pruritic papules that last less than 48 hours and can be produced by a variety of stimuli. In **acute urticaria,** hives occur shortly after exposure to an offending substance, which is usually easily identified as the trigger. Some patients with acute urticaria develop angioedema, or diffuse swelling of the skin, usually affecting the face but sometimes affecting the larynx and potentially causing asphyxiation. In **chronic urticaria,** the cause is often remote.

Urticarial drug eruptions feature erythematous, often pruritic smooth-surfaced papules, plaques, or nodules. In contrast with urticaria, the lesions are not evanescent and often last for days to weeks. Urticarial drug eruptions are among the most common reactions to drugs.

Urticarial reactions to arthropod assaults produce welts that may fade over days to weeks but on occasion persist for months. The term **arthropod assault** embraces reactions to both stings and bites, whether by insects or arachnids.

An intriguing urticarial hypersensitivity reaction occurs as a complication of pregnancy, and is known as **pruritic urticarial papules and plaques of pregnancy (PUPPP).** PUPPP usually has its onset in the third trimester, and as a rule wanes with parturition. Its lesions are on the abdomen, often following the courses of striae.

In biopsy specimens of acute urticaria, there are usually sparse infiltrates of mononuclear cells around venules of the superficial and deep plexus, along with a few eosinophils and mast cells. Edema of the reticular dermis is evident as increased spaces between collagen bundles. Neutrophils range from few to many. The latter event is referred to as **"neutrophilic urticaria,"** as often occurs in patients whose hives are caused by a physical stimulus such as light, heat, or water.[1] In chronic urticaria, dermal edema is also present, but infiltrates tend to be denser and to contain more eosinophils (Fig. 18–1). Rare patients have dense infiltrates of neutrophils and eosinophils. Patients with so-called **dense infiltrate urticaria** are more likely to have detectable circulating immune complexes.[2]

Changes identical to those of chronic urticaria are commonly found in urticarial drug eruptions. In contrast with urticaria, in which the epidermis is always spared, inflammatory cells can be present in the epidermis in urticarial drug eruptions, accompanied by slight psoriasiform hyperplasia of the epidermis, spongiosis, or vacuolar change at the dermo-epidermal junction. Because the lesions of urticarial drug eruptions are persistent, there can be changes of **lichen simplex chronicus.** In urticaria, lesions fade before persistent rubbing has time to cause these changes.

In urticarial reactions to arthropod assaults, there are dense perivascular and interstitial, superficial and deep infiltrates of lymphocytes, macrophages, eosinophils, and sometimes plasma cells in an inverted wedge-like pattern (Fig. 18–2). The punctum, or point of entry of a stinger or proboscis, can be evident as a small focus of epidermal necrosis. Although the epidermis is sometimes otherwise unaffected, in many cases there is spongiosis adjacent to the punctum, diminishing in intensity laterally. Fibrin thrombi can occlude the lumina of vessels subjacent to the punctum.

Exceptions to this picture can occur in urticarial reactions to the bites and stings of some arthropods. In persistent reactions, lymphoid follicles can be present. In rare cases, infiltrates are entirely lymphocytic. Flea bites feature infiltrates in which neutrophils predominate.

In pruritic urticarial papules and plaques of pregnancy, there are superficial and deep, perivascular and interstitial infiltrates of lymphocytes and eosinophils, accompanied in roughly half of cases by slight diffuse spongiosis.[3]

DIFFERENTIAL DIAGNOSIS. Most clinical dermatologists diagnose urticaria with ease. The main reason that hives are ever biopsied is to rule out **leukocytoclastic vasculitis,** which can present with clinically similar lesions, termed **urticarial vasculitis.** Patients with urticarial vasculitis often have high levels of circulating immune complexes, and some have collagen vascular disease.

The lesions of urticarial vasculitis show leukocytoclastic vasculitis on biopsy. The earliest finding that is specific for diagnosis of leukocytoclastic vasculitis is an infiltrate of neutrophils and nuclear dust around venules (Fig. 18–3). As neutrophils are short-lived, some dust (fragments of nuclei from effete cells) are present wherever there are neutrophils

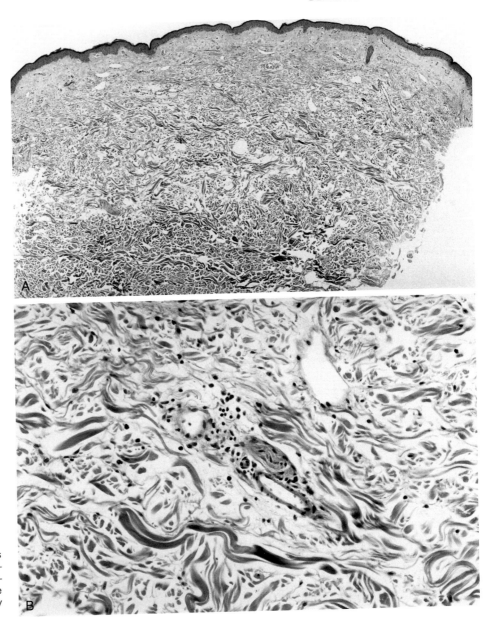

FIGURE 18–1. Urticarial reactions have perivascular interstitial infiltrates that do not involve the epidermis. In urticaria, these infiltrates are often sparse *(A)* and accompanied by edema of the reticular dermis *(B)*.

in any number, and the finding of a few nuclear remnants should not precipitate a diagnosis of vasculitis. Neutrophils predominate in so-called **neutrophilic urticaria.** The mere finding of perivascular neutrophilic infiltrates does not indicate vasculitis. As lesions of urticarial vasculitis evolve, fibrin appears in vessel walls or lumina, or both. Extravasated erythrocytes are scant in the skin-colored or pink papules of urticarial vasculitis, and pathologists should not rely on their presence to make the diagnosis of vasculitis.

Many vesicular and bullous diseases present with urticarial lesions. Sometimes these are transient, but in some patients urticarial lesions predominate over blistering ones. This is particularly common in bullous pemphigoid. **Bullous pemphigoid** is a subepidermal blistering disease that largely affects the elderly. In patients with prolonged urticarial prodromes, severe pruritus may be present while the diagnosis is debated. Many such patients are misdiagnosed as having **erythema multiforme** on clinical grounds, as their lesions are sometimes polycyclic. A biopsy specimen of the urticarial stage of bullous pemphigoid can be misdiagnosed as urticaria, because interstitial eosinophils are common to both conditions. In contrast with urticaria, in which the epidermis is nearly always uninvolved, eosinophils line up along the dermoepidermal junction in the urticarial stage of bullous pemphigoid, and can infiltrate the epidermis, which is often spongiotic (Fig. 18–4). The diagnosis of bullous pemphigoid can be confirmed by direct or indirect immunofluorescence.

ERYTHEMA MULTIFORME

Erythema multiforme is an inflammatory reaction pattern produced by several agents, in which erythematous macules, papules, target-like lesions, and bullae are produced by lymphocytic destruction of basilar keratinocytes. Mild cases affect only the skin (**erythema multiforme minor**). Severe widespread erythema multiforme, or **erythema multiforme major,** is termed the Stevens-Johnson syndrome when it

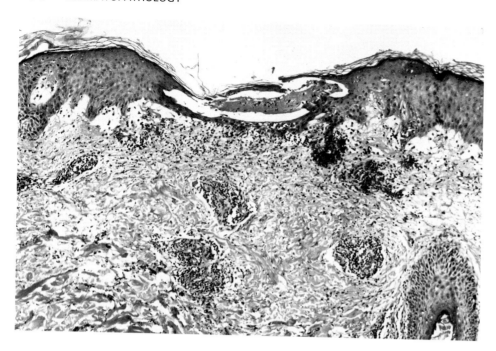

FIGURE 18–2. Urticarial reactions to arthropod assaults show, in addition to dermal infiltrates similar to those of urticaria, spongiotic vesiculation near the site of the bite or sting. Inflammatory changes diminish away from the central punctum.

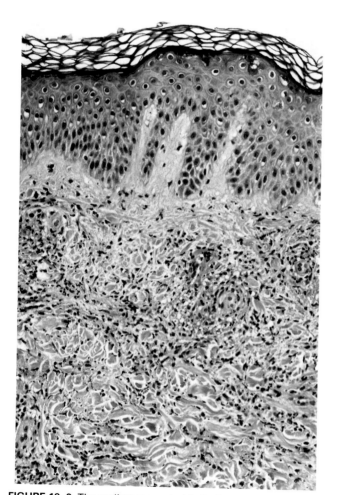

FIGURE 18–3. The earliest recognizable findings of leukocytoclastic vasculitis are infiltrates of neutrophils accompanied by abundant nuclear dust. This change occurs prior to the accumulation of fibrin in vessel walls.

affects mucous membranes and is accompanied by fever and severe systemic symptoms; an even more noxious variant affects the entire integument and is known as **toxic epidermal necrolysis.**

CLINICOPATHOLOGIC FEATURES. The erythematous macules, patches, papules, and blisters of erythema multiforme minor are often symmetrically distributed and favor the skin of the extremities, and in particular tend to occur on the palms. The classic "iris" or "target" lesions are round and have a raised red periphery and a grayish center. In erythema multiforme major, large irregularly shaped areas of the skin are red and tend to blister or slough. Patients with toxic epidermal necrolysis can be denuded of their epidermis by gentle rubbing.

Erythema multiforme minor has long been linked to infection by the herpes simplex virus, because outbreaks often follow symptomatic genital or oral herpes. Viral antigens have been detected in the lesional epidermis of erythema multiforme, as has herpetic genome using *in situ* hybridization and the polymerase chain reaction.[4] Erythema multiforme also occurs in patients with other infections, as a reaction to drugs, and with no obvious cause. The lesions of erythema multiforme usually wane within weeks. Many cases of **"chronic erythema multiforme"** are actually other conditions such as bullous pemphigoid or urticarial hypersensitivity reactions.

Erythema multiforme is the prototypical acute cytotoxic interface dermatitis.[5] In an **interface dermatitis,** the dermoepidermal junction is obscured by inflammatory cells. In erythema multiforme, lymphocytes attack basilar keratinocytes of the epidermis and follicular epithelium, causing vacuolar change and necrosis (Fig. 18–5). In contrast with other interface reactions in which keratinization is affected (e.g., lichen planus), differentiation of keratinocytes is not perturbed. Early on, there are superficial perivascular infiltrates of lymphocytes in addition to a sprinkling of them along the dermoepidermal junction. Only exceptionally is the deep plexus involved or are there more than a very few eosinophils.[4] Later, necrotic keratinocytes form small whorls within the epidermis, as they

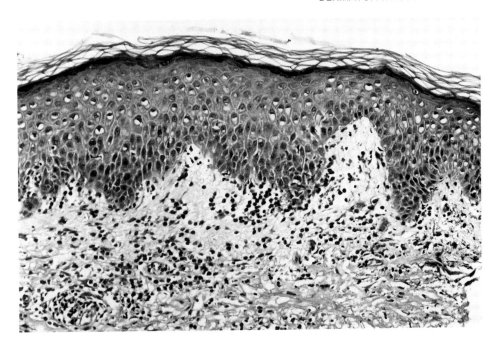

FIGURE 18–4. The urticarial stage of bullous pemphigoid is recognizable because eosinophils accumulate near the dermoepidermal junction, seen here along with edema of papillary dermis.

are transepidermally eliminated. Uncommonly, ballooning (intracellular edema) of keratinocytes results in reticular degeneration of the epidermis.

Blisters of erythema multiforme usually form by the confluence of vacuoles along the dermoepidermal junction and are subepidermal when fully developed (Fig. 18–6).[6] Intraepidermal vesicles can be present early, alongside subepidermal ones. The keratinocytes that form the roof of subepidermal blisters can be viable or partially to entirely necrotic. Necrosis of blister roofs results in the gray centers of some iris lesions.

DIFFERENTIAL DIAGNOSIS. In patients who have received transplanted tissues, or in immunosuppressed patients who have received blood transfusions, **acute cutaneous graft-**

versus-host disease is the principal differential diagnosis. Graft-versus-host disease is caused by cytotoxic damage to the epithelium of the recipient by donor lymphocytes. Amelioration of graft-versus-host disease may require an increase in immunosuppressive therapy.

Both acute cutaneous graft-versus-host disease and erythema multiforme share the same basic histopathologic pattern—vacuolar interface dermatitis with sparse infiltrates of lymphocytes and few to many necrotic keratinocytes. Indeed, the findings early in the course of graft-versus-host disease can be indistinguishable from those of erythema multiforme. In fully formed lesions of acute graft-versus-host disease, there are several changes not seen in erythema multiforme,

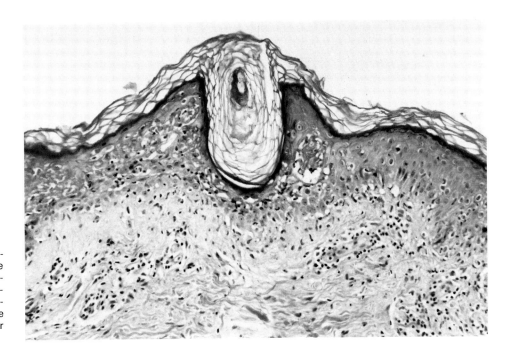

FIGURE 18–5. Erythema multiforme is the prototype of an acute cytotoxic interface dermatitis. Although vacuolar change and necrotic keratinocytes blur the dermoepidermal junction, the basketweave configuration of the cornified layer is unaffected.

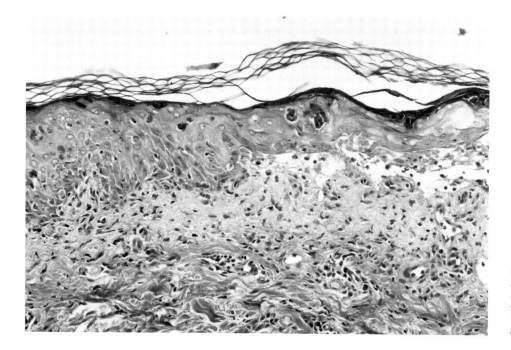

FIGURE 18-6. Vesicles and bullae can form in erythema multiforme, owing to coalescence of vacuoles to form clefts beneath the epidermis. Note the clusters of necrotic keratinocytes above the cleft at the right.

including squamatization of the basal layer and hyperkeratosis, that are not seen in erythema multiforme (Fig. 18–7).[5]

Pityriasis lichenoides et varioliformis acuta, or Mucha-Habermann disease, presents with crops of hemorrhagic papules that crust and then involute spontaneously. On occasion, there can be papulovesicles that elicit a differential diagnosis of erythema multiforme, and such cases can be difficult to resolve because both conditions are interface dermatitides in which lymphocytes predominate (Fig. 18–8). Whorls of necrotic keratinocytes and ballooning of keratinocyte cytoplasms with reticular alteration of the epidermis can occur in both conditions. Whereas Mucha-Habermann disease rou-

tinely involves the deep vascular plexus, erythema multiforme rarely does so. Parakeratosis accounts for the scaly quality of the papules of Mucha-Habermann disease, whereas the lesions of erythema multiforme are smooth until desquamation occurs in their healing phases. A few extravasated erythrocytes can occur early in erythema multiforme, but they are abundant in Mucha-Habermann disease. An authentic **lymphocytic vasculitis** with fibrin in the walls and lumina of venules occurs in approximately 10% of specimens of Mucha-Habermann disease but almost never is present in erythema multiforme. If the differential diagnosis cannot be resolved by light microscopy, polymerase chain reaction to detect herpes simplex viral

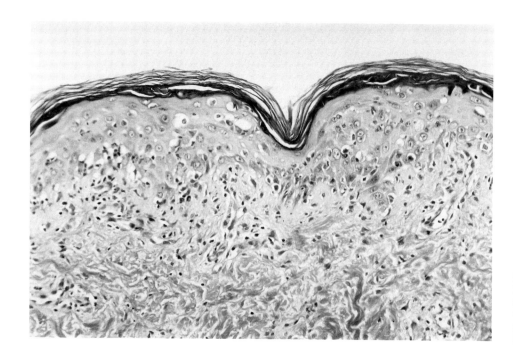

FIGURE 18-7. In acute graft-versus-host disease, basal keratinocytes are squamatized, and hyper- or parakeratosis can occur, features that are uncommon in erythema multiforme.

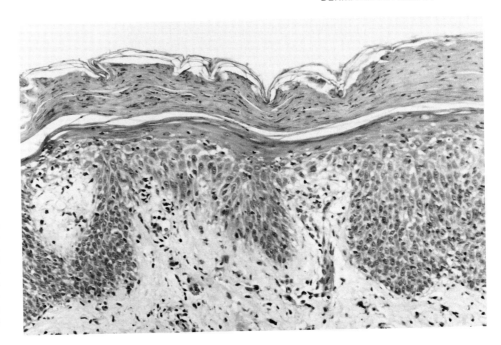

FIGURE 18–8. Mucha-Habermann disease has similar epidermal findings to those of erythema multiforme, but in addition can show psoriasiform epidermal hyperplasia and parakeratosis that sometimes contains neutrophils. Additionally, there can be infiltrates around the deep vascular plexus and fibrin in the walls of venules.

DNA may be useful. Herpetic genomes are evident in the majority of specimens of erythema multiforme minor but are not found in Mucha-Habermann disease.

Staphylococcal scalded skin syndrome was at one time also called toxic epidermal necrolysis and confused with the widespread form of erythema multiforme.[7] Staphylococcal scalded skin syndrome is mediated by a toxin produced by staphylococci infected with a certain phage. It affects infants who lack the ability to metabolize the toxin because of hepatic immaturity and adults with compromised hepatic function.

The distinction between toxic epidermal necrolysis and staphylococcal scalded skin syndrome is one of the few in dermatopathology that a pathologist may be called on to make on frozen section. The treatment and prognosis of these conditions make their distinction important—patients with toxic epidermal necrolysis often need to be admitted to burn units and have a grave prognosis, whereas eradication of staphylococcal infection can lead to a rapid restitution of barrier function in the scalded skin syndrome, as the plane of cleavage is through the granular layer (Fig. 18–9).

UNUSUAL PRESENTATIONS OF PSORIASIS

Psoriasis is a chronic scaling dermatitis that is characterized, in its usual forms, by excessive proliferation of keratinocytes coupled with infiltration of the superficial epidermis by neutrophils. Although the histopathology of fully formed plaques of psoriasis is not a diagnostic dilemma, the disease is so common that its stranger guises are often misinterpreted by pathologists.

CLINICOPATHOLOGIC FEATURES. Both clinicians and pathologists are trained to recognize fully developed plaques of psoriasis. Plaques are symmetrically distributed over extensor surfaces, especially those of the elbows and knees, and are

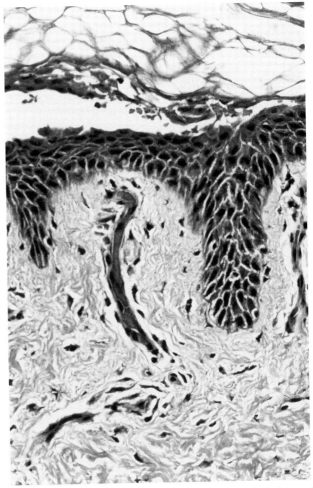

FIGURE 18–9. An acantholytic cleft runs through or just beneath the granular layer in a blister of staphylococcal scalded skin syndrome.

deep red and sharply marginated. Small pustules and micaceous scale are often present.

Guttate psoriasis is apt to be suspected by dermatologists on clinical grounds, but biopsy is often performed to confirm the diagnosis. The term *guttate* derives from the Latin *guttata,* meaning drop-like. Guttate psoriasis often follows an acute upper respiratory illness.

Biopsy specimens of guttate psoriasis do not show the characteristic epidermal hyperplasia with rounded rete ridges of even length and thinning of suprapapillary plates that enable dermatology and pathology residents to recognize sections of plaque stage psoriasis with facility. Instead, there is slight hyperplasia of a pallid epidermis that has rounded rete ridges, and a hint of spongiosis can be detected (Fig. 18–10). Specific clues to the diagnosis of guttate psoriasis are edematous dermal papillae that contain dilated, spiraled capillaries and small mounds of parakeratosis that house neutrophils.[8] Sometimes level sections are necessary to show these findings.

Pustular psoriasis often affects the palms and soles and can be disabling. Large whitish pustules are present in a background of diffuse erythema. Unlike plaques of psoriasis, the epidermis may be only slightly hyperplastic (Fig. 18–11).

Nail biopsies may be done to determine whether a patient has psoriasis, another inflammatory process such as lichen planus, or dermatophytosis. Psoriasis causes pitting of the nails as well as other dystrophic changes. The pits are themselves the product of mounds of parakeratosis that contain neutrophils at their apices.

DIFFERENTIAL DIAGNOSIS. The most difficult differential diagnosis of guttate psoriasis is **pityriasis lichenoides, or Mucha-Habermann disease.** Both conditions are marked by scaly papules. Whereas the infiltrates in plaques of psoriasis are by and large perivascular, those of guttate psoriasis can be prominently interstitial, and sometimes approach a band-like distribution. Both conditions feature mounds of parakeratosis that contain neutrophils. Although necrotic keratinocytes are not generally considered a feature of psoriasis, they can be scattered in the rete ridges of guttate lesions, and

they are found in numbers at the dermoepidermal junction in Mucha-Habermann disease. Erythrocytes can be extravasated into the dermal papillae in both conditions, although this happens more consistently in Mucha-Habermann disease. Level sections are often useful in resolving this difficult differential diagnosis. In Mucha-Habermann disease, vacuolar change and necrotic keratinocytes are consistently found at the dermoepidermal junction throughout a given lesion, whereas such changes are present in minute foci in guttate psoriasis. Even in early guttate lesions of psoriasis, the dermal papillae contain spiraling, ectatic capillaries with capacious lumina. Vascular ectasia can be present in Mucha-Habermann disease but is not a hallmark in the way that it is in psoriasis.

Dermatophytosis or candidiasis can easily be misdiagnosed as psoriasis. Dermatophytosis can simulate every change seen in psoriasis, from vascular dilatation and tortuosity to mounds of parakeratosis surmounted by neutrophils. Unless the clinical presentation is obviously that of psoriasis, a periodic acid-Schiff (PAS)–stained section should be examined when either a superficial or superficial and deep infiltrate accompanies psoriasis-like epidermal changes, and especially when neutrophils and parakeratosis are also present. A hint that a dermatophyte rather than psoriasis may be at fault is layering of two forms of cornified material over the specimen surface, known as the sandwich sign. The combinations include all permutations of compact and basket-weave orthokeratosis, lamellar hyperkeratosis, or parakeratosis.

The differential diagnosis of pustular psoriasis includes other conditions that cause intraepidermal pustules. Pustules that involve the superficial spinous layer and feature neutrophils interlaced between attenuated keratinocytes or that have spongiform pustules occur in candidiasis and dermatophytosis, conditions that can be excluded by staining with periodic acid-Schiff. **Gonococcemia** can cause pustules on the palms or soles but features superficial vessels whose lumina are occluded by thrombi. So-called **pustular bacterid of Andrews** is a condition in which sterile pustules on the volar

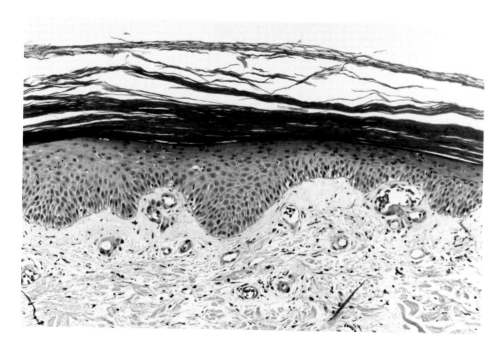

FIGURE 18–10. Guttate psoriasis is often misdiagnosed as "chronic non-specific dermatitis" or as spongiotic or eczematous dermatitis because pathologists are familiar only with the features of fully developed plaques of that disease. Slight epidermal hyperplasia with uneven rete ridges, slight diffuse spongiosis, edematous dermal papillae that contain prominently dilated capillaries, and parakeratosis with neutrophils are the hallmarks of guttate psoriasis. Note that the cornified layer is "dry," i.e., nearly devoid of serum, reflecting the mild degree of spongiosis in guttate psoriasis.

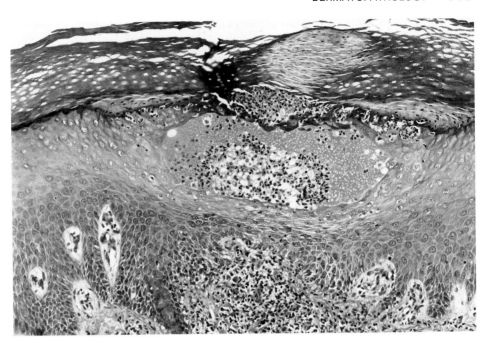

FIGURE 18–11. Pustular psoriasis is often misinterpreted because it lacks many of the features seen in plaques of psoriasis. Clues to the diagnosis are an intraepidermal pustule on acral skin with spongiform pustules adjacent to it, often with little epidermal hyperplasia.

skin of acral surfaces are accompanied by sterile pustules in bone and elsewhere, presumably as a reaction to a bacterial infection. Whether this is an authentic disease or not is unknown.

CHRONIC FIBROSING FORMS OF LEUKOCYTOCLASTIC VASCULITIS

Leukocytoclastic vasculitis usually causes purpuric patches or plaques that resolve in weeks. There are two conditions that begin with leukocytoclastic vasculitis, eventuate in fibrosis, and cause persistent plaques whose clinical diagnosis may be unsuspected and so come to the attention of a surgical pathologist. One condition is misnomerically termed **granuloma faciale,** the other is called **erythema elevatum diutinum.** Granuloma faciale is usually limited to the skin of the face but can also occur at other sites; erythema elevatum diutinum causes a symmetric nodular eruption over extensor surfaces.

CLINICOPATHOLOGIC FEATURES. Patients with granuloma faciale have one or several plaques on the skin of the face that are slightly raised, firm, and tan or yellow. Follicular orifices are patulous. Because the density of follicles is not as high in extrafacial skin, lesions outside the face may not show this feature. Lesions of granuloma faciale are often suspected to be carcinoma by clinicians, and excision is therefore sometimes performed. The lesions have a tendency to recur after attempted surgical extirpation and to be resistant to many medical therapies as well.

Biopsy specimens of granuloma faciale, if taken early enough in the course of the condition, show foci of neutrophilic vasculitis involving venules, as well as dense, diffuse infiltrates that contain many eosinophils and plasma cells (Fig. 18–12). Over time, fibrosis supervenes and can have a concentric pattern surrounding venules or a storiform pattern.[9]

Erythema elevatum diutinum begins with hemorrhagic macules that evolve into plaques, which either resolve or become fibrotic nodules. Early lesions show leukocytoclastic vasculitis; fully developed ones feature dense diffuse neutrophilic infiltrates (Fig. 18–13) that induce fibrosis (Fig. 18–14).[10] Late nodular lesions are sometimes confused with those of **bacillary angiomatosis.** Erythema elevatum diutinum seems to be more prevalent in patients with human immunodeficiency virus (HIV) infection, compounding this problem.[11] There are more vessels in bacillary angiomatosis than in erythema elevatum diutinum, and neutrophils are clumped around aggregations of bacteria. In contrast, neutrophils in erythema elevatum diutinum surround venules. Appropriate silver stains, such as Warthin-Starry, Dieterle, or Steiner, detect bacilli in erythema elevatum diutinum.

DIFFERENTIAL DIAGNOSIS. Granuloma faciale can be difficult to recognize when its vasculitic aspects are obscured by fibrosis and mixed cellular infiltrates of eosinophils and plasma cells. Concentric fibrosis around vessels is a useful clue to the diagnosis. **Dermatophytic folliculitis** sometimes has dense infiltrates of eosinophils and fibrin in venular walls. Level sections are sometimes necessary to detect hyphae in or around hair shafts.

Early papules or plaques of erythema elevatum diutinum resemble other forms of **leukocytoclastic vasculitis** pathologically. In addition to neutrophils and their debris in and around the walls of vessels, there is fibrin in vessel walls, a few extravasated erythrocytes are nearly always present, and there can be increased numbers of small vessels. As plaques eventuate, alternative diagnoses shift to diffuse neutrophilic infiltrates such as **Sweet's syndrome, rheumatoid neutrophilic dermatitis,** and **pyoderma gangrenosum.** In plaques of erythema elevatum diutinum, there are fibrosis and foci of active vasculitis, unlike in these other conditions. As fibrosis becomes more pronounced, nodules develop that resemble the **polypoid variant of dermatofibroma,** in which neutrophils are not apparent.

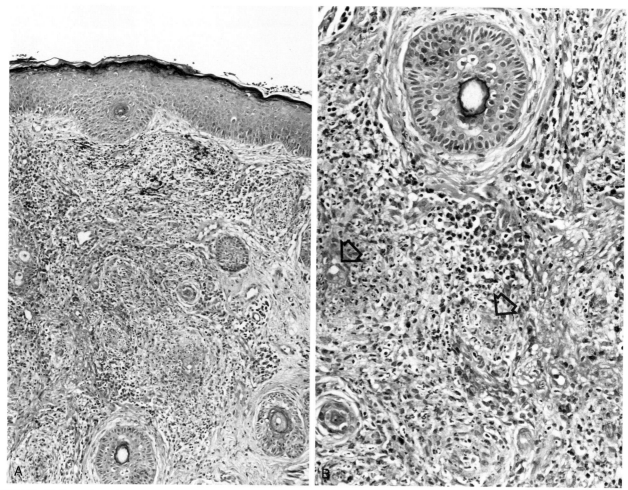

FIGURE 18–12. Granuloma faciale is a chronic fibrosing form of leukocytoclastic vasculitis in which dense mixed infiltrates of inflammatory cells accumulate *(A)*. Neutrophils encircle venules that have fibrin in their walls *(arrows)*, with eosinophils and plasma cells in the background *(B)*. Note that the condition is not truly granulomatous.

PALISADED NEUTROPHILIC AND GRANULOMATOUS DERMATITIS IN PATIENTS WITH SYSTEMIC DISEASE

Palisaded neutrophilic and granulomatous dermatitis is a condition that occurs in patients with collagen vascular, lymphoproliferative, and other systemic diseases. Its histopathologic findings in mature lesions resemble those seen in **rheumatoid nodules,** but the dermis rather than subcutis is involved. Synonyms include **rheumatoid papules, Churg-Strauss granuloma, cutaneous extravascular necrotizing granuloma,** and **interstitial granulomatous dermatitis with arthritis.**[12–14]

CLINICOPATHOLOGIC FEATURES. The most frequent presentation of palisaded neutrophilic and granulomatous dermatitis is as a symmetric, papular eruption over the elbows, knees, and fingers. Many of the papules crust or become umbilicated. Unusual forms include linear cords (misrepresented in the literature as **linear rheumatoid nodules**) and ulcerating plaques, termed **superficial ulcerating rheumatoid necrobiosis.**

Neutrophils predominate early on. Broad collars of fibrin separate small vessels from large zones in which degenerating collagen is mixed with basophilic nuclear dust (Fig. 18–15).[12]

Macrophages palisade around thick bundles of degenerated collagen, basophilic debris, and neutrophils in mature lesions (Fig. 18–16). Later, fibrosis supervenes, neutrophils are few, and palisaded granulomas are less prominent.

DIFFERENTIAL DIAGNOSIS. Early papules differ from those of conventional **leukocytoclastic vasculitis.** There are fewer extravasated erythrocytes, and the palisaded pattern produced by the broad acellular zones of fibrin and lakes of basophilic debris is not present in common leukocytoclastic vasculitis. Fully developed lesions can be mistaken for **granuloma annulare** microscopically. Whereas bundles of collagen in the centers of palisaded foci in granuloma annulare are thin, those in the centers of palisaded neutrophilic and granulomatous dermatitis are thick. Intact neutrophils are scarce in granuloma annulare, but can be abundant in palisaded neutrophilic and granulomatous dermatitis. The basophilia of the centers of granulomatous foci in granuloma annnulare is pale and is due to mucin, whereas that in palisaded neutrophilic and granulomatous dermatitis is deep blue and produced by DNA from effete neutrophils. Late fibrotic lesions can imitate **necrobiosis lipoidica,** with which they share sclerosis, superficial and deep perivascular infiltrates, and palisaded granulomas. Plasma cells are present in necrobiosis lipoidica but are not found often in palisaded neutrophilic and granulomatous der-

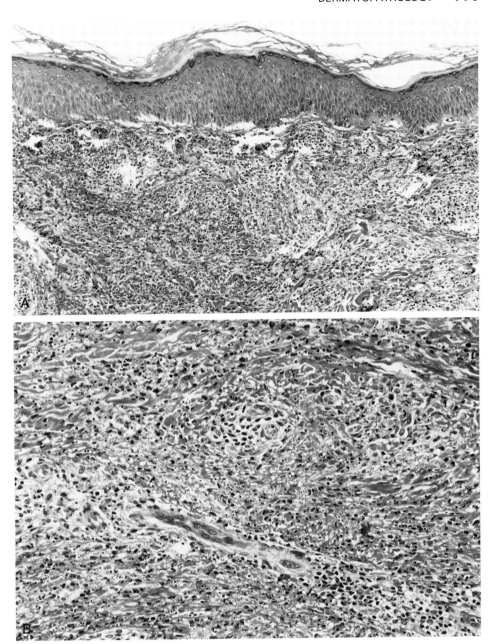

FIGURE 18–13. Dense diffuse neutrophilic infiltrates typify fully developed plaques of erythema elevatum diutinum *(A)*. There is abundant neutrophilic nuclear dust, strewn about in a background of fibrosis *(B)*.

matitis. The tiers of inflammatory cells described in necrobiosis lipoidica are not a feature of these late lesions either.

UNUSUAL VARIANTS OF BASAL CELL CARCINOMA

Basal cell carcinoma is a low-grade carcinoma that differentiates toward the germinative cells of hair follicles. Follicular germs arise in the first trimester of embryonic life as a result of induction by specialized mesenchymal cells that condense to form follicular papillae. Follicular germs are crescentic downgrowths of the epidermis that show peripheral palisading, cells with scant cytoplasm, ovoid nuclei, and inconspicuous nucleoli. The cells of basal cell carcinoma share these features.

CLINICOPATHOLOGIC FEATURES. Basal cell carcinomas are most frequently found on the sun-exposed skin of white patients. A histopathologic classification of basal cell carcinoma that correlates patterns of basal cell carcinoma with behavior recognizes nodular, infiltrative, micronodular, superficial, and morpheic types. **Nodular and superficial basal cell carcinomas** tend to be well-circumscribed, and these types are amenable to simple excision; the other types are less circumscribed and can persist if simple excision of only the clinically apparent lesion is performed.

Basal cell carcinoma often contains keratinizing cells. When numerous, such terms as **keratotic** or **metatypical basal cell carcinoma** have been applied, although some authors reserve the latter for neoplasms in which some of the nests are largely composed of spindled cells that lack peripheral palisading. The centers of nests of nodular or infiltrating basal cell carcinomas can contain squamous keratinocytes. This is especially true in lesions that have been traumatized or biopsied prior to excision. When squamous keratinocytes are confined to the centers of such nests, even if keratinous

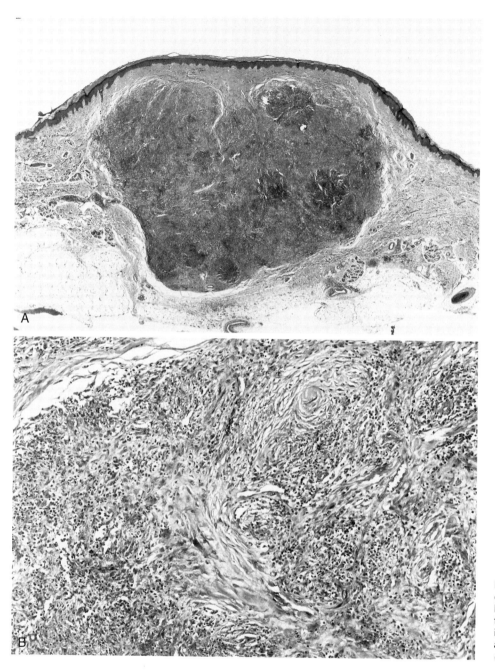

FIGURE 18–14. A nodular lesion of erythema elevatum diutinum *(A)*. Evidence of the vasculitic origins of this fibrosing process can be found in the neutrophilic foci that pepper a background of storiform fibrosis *(B)*.

cystic areas are present, the diagnosis of basal cell carcinoma is easy. However, when entire nests are composed of squamous keratinocytes, the issue arises as to whether the lesion is better termed **basosquamous carcinoma.** My practice is to designate such lesions as invasive carcinoma with areas of basal cell and squamous cell carcinoma, as the imprecise usage of basosquamous and metatypical basal cell carcinoma has confused pathologists and clinicians. Explicit recognition that a component of squamous cell carcinoma is present alerts the clinician that there may be potential for metastasis.

An indolent variant with a unique pattern of growth is the **infundibulocystic type of basal cell carcinoma.**[15] This variant is frequently seen incidentally in the clinically normal skin of patients with the **basal cell nevus syndrome** and was once designated "**nevoid follicular basal cell carcinoma.**"

The clinical lesions tend to be small dome-shaped papules on the skin of the face. Histopathologic examination shows a well-circumscribed neoplasm limited to the superficial dermis, composed of radiating cords of basaloid cells that end in bulbous structures punctuated by small cornifying cysts (Fig. 18–17). The cells of the infundibulocystic type of basal cell carcinoma have monomorphous nuclei and a low mitotic rate.

Several variants of nodular basal cell carcinoma are composed of unusual types of cells. **Granular cell basal cell carcinoma** features nests of polygonal cells with small nuclei and cytoplasm packed with small eosinophilic granules (Fig. 18–18).[16] Granular cells can predominate in all or only some of the nests of a basal cell carcinoma. In the former case, confusion with the common granular cell tumor (a schwannoma) is possible. Granular cell basal cell carcinoma differs

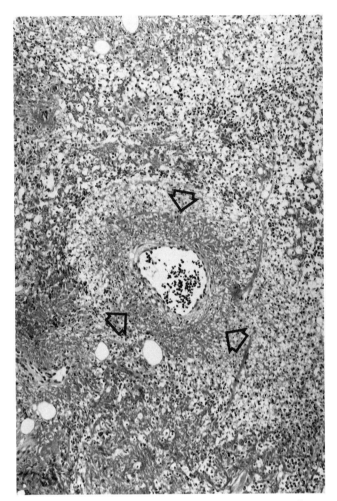

FIGURE 18–15. Palisaded neutrophilic and granulomatous dermatitis of collagen vascular disease can be identified in its early phase by broad collars of fibrin *(arrows)* around venules, peripheral to which is a deeply basophilic background formed by lysed neutrophils.

from **granular cell schwannoma** in that it is composed of discrete nests, rather than sheets of cells, and the fibromyxoid stroma typical of basal cell carcinoma is present.

Basal cell carcinoma with clear cells can pose diagnostic problems if the clear-cell change affects most of the nodules of a specimen.[17, 18] The nests of clear cells do not show peripheral palisading, and their nuclei, like those of granular cell basal cell carcinoma, can be tiny (Fig. 18–19). In some cases, the nodules are surrounded by thickened basement membranes, which may be evidence of trichilemmal differentiation.

Basal cell carcinoma with matrical differentiation is another rare variant that shows a nodular growth pattern. Differentiation toward hair matrix is exemplified by crowded cells with even scantier cytoplasm than is usual in basal cell carcinoma and by the formation of shadow cells (Fig. 18–20). The cells of basal cell carcinoma with matrical differentiation have high mitotic rates, just as their counterparts in the hair bulb do. In basal cell carcinoma with matrical differentiation, some lobules feature mostly matrical and shadow cells, some are admixed with conventional basal cell carcinoma, and others consist entirely of ordinary nodular basal cell carcinoma.

Ducts that resemble those of sweat glands are seen in **nodular, infiltrating, and morpheic patterns of basal cell carci-**

noma as small round spaces with cuticular linings (Fig. 18–21).[19] The cuticles can be highlighted by staining with digested periodic acid-Schiff or by immunoperoxidase staining for carcinoembryonic antigen. These ducts are not merely entrapped eccrine ducts, as they can be widely dispersed throughout large carcinomas. Although an eccrine origin has been posited, they could also represent apocrine differentiation by the pluripotential cells of basal cell carcinoma. Apocrine glands derive from hair follicles, whereas eccrine glands and ducts sprout from the epidermis. Although the secretory portions of apocrine and eccrine glands are easily differentiated, their ducts are indistinguishable. Although ductular differentiation does not change the behavior of a basal cell carcinoma, pathologists should be familiar with this variant so as not to misdiagnose it as an **adnexal carcinoma.**

DIFFERENTIAL DIAGNOSIS. Basal cell carcinoma with areas of overt squamous cell carcinoma can resemble poorly differentiated **squamous cell carcinoma.** This distinction is not critical because the management of these entities is similar. The component of basal cell should show peripheral palisading, fibromyxoid stroma, and clefts that separate neoplastic epithelium from that of stroma.

The infundibulocystic type of basal cell carcinoma is often misdiagnosed as **trichoepithelioma,** because both neoplasms are well-circumscribed collections of cytologically bland basaloid cells, with low mitotic rates, small keratinizing cysts, and "organoid" growth patterns. Infundibulocystic basal cell carcinoma features clefts between the basaloid cells and their stroma, unlike trichoepithelioma, in which clefts are present between collagen bundles. The stroma of trichoepithelioma is more cellular and collagenous. Brownstein described a lesion that he termed **basaloid follicular hamartoma,** which seems indistinguishable from infundibulocystic basal cell carcinoma in many respects.[20]

The granular cell variant of basal cell carcinoma is easily confused with the far more common **schwannian granular cell tumor.** Granular cell basal cell carcinoma is composed of discrete nodules, each surrounded by fibromyxoid stroma, unlike granular cell tumors, which feature sheets of cells with aggregations that are devoid of stroma. Although peripheral palisading may not be evident in nests of basal cell carcinoma with granular cells, clefts are often present between rounded nests of granular cells and their stroma. If there is any doubt, immunoperoxidase staining can be useful. Granular cell basal cell carcinomas stain with broad-spectrum anti-keratin reagents, whereas conventional granular cell tumor does not. Granular cells occur in a wide range of cutaneous neoplasms and do not signify a specific lineage.[21]

Clear-cell basal cell carcinoma can be mistaken for the clear-cell types of **hidradenoma** and squamous cell carcinoma, **tricholemmoma,** and **metastatic renal cell carcinoma.** The nests of clear-cell squamous cell carcinoma often are attached to an epidermis showing changes of carcinoma *in situ.* Unlike the rounded nests of clear-cell basal cell carcinoma, those of clear-cell squamous cell carcinoma tend to be jagged and to contain many dyskeratotic cells. Thickened basement membranes surround the nests of some clear-cell basal cell carcinomas but are not a feature of clear-cell squamous cell carcinoma. Tricholemmomas are benign follicular neoplasms that differentiate toward the outer root sheath, as may clear-cell basal cell carcinoma. Both neoplasms can feature clear cells surrounded by thickened basement membranes.

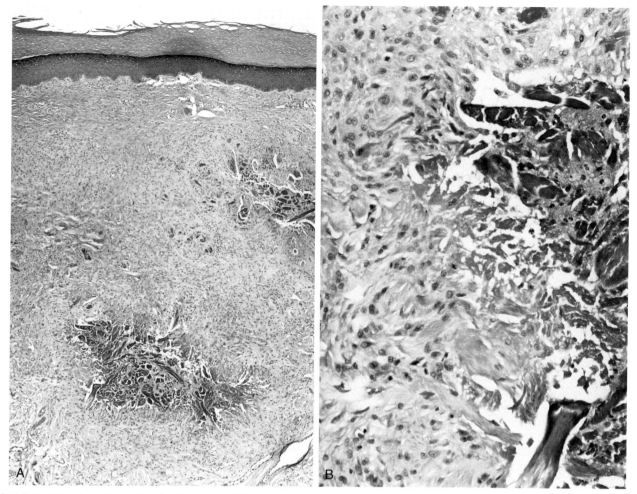

FIGURE 18–16. Later lesions of palisaded neutrophilic and granulomatous dermatitis show palisaded granulomatous foci with broad bundles of altered collagen in their centers *(A)*, between which there are intact neutrophils as well as fragmented ones *(B)*. Intact neutrophils are only rarely present in the centers of the palisaded granulomatous foci of granuloma annulare.

Tricholemmomas are small, vertically oriented with respect to the skin surface, and consist of a single nodule or a few lobules that are attached to the epidermis. The peripheral cells of trichilemmoma have smaller nuclei than those in the rest of the lobule, whereas those of clear-cell basal cell carcinoma have nuclei of approximately the same size as those in the remainder of the nodule. The thickening of the basement membrane in trichilemmoma is usually slight; that seen in clear-cell basal cell carcinoma can be more marked, and the thickness around a single nest can vary greatly.

Basal cell carcinoma with clear cells can be mistaken for clear-cell hidradenoma because both feature lobules of clear cells with monomorphous nuclei. The silhouette of clear-cell hidradenoma is typical of a benign adnexal neoplasm, i.e., the lesion is often taller than it is broad, has smooth borders, and is roughly symmetric. The reverse is the case with clear-cell basal cell carcinoma. The masses of cells in clear-cell hidradenoma are larger, and that lesion often shows a solid-cystic pattern not evident in clear-cell basal cell carcinoma. Ductular differentiation is always present in clear-cell hidradenoma, whereas it has not yet been described in clear-cell basal cell carcinoma.

Renal cell carcinoma can metastasize to the skin, resulting in lobules of clear cells with increased numbers of mitotic figures present just beneath the epidermis. Some metastases of renal cell carcinoma have highly vascular stroma, a feature not evident in clear-cell basal cell carcinoma. Mucinous stroma and clefts separating epithelium from stroma are not generally present in cutaneous metastases of renal cell carcinoma.

Basal cell carcinoma with matrical differentiation can easily be confused with **pilomatricoma** and **matrical carcinoma.**[22] Pilomatricoma, early in its evolution, is rounded and cystic in configuration, with a periphery of matrical cells and a central mass of shadow cells. Basal cell carcinoma with matrical differentiation is always multinodular. If a pilomatricoma ruptures, a multinodular pattern can result, with granulation tissue–like stroma rather than fibromyxoid stroma. Basal cell carcinoma with matrical differentiation is also multinodular, but there are at least some nests typical of nodular basal cell carcinoma, and even those nests that have matrical cells are invested by fibromyxoid stroma.

Basal cell carcinoma with ductular differentiation can simulate several types of adnexal carcinoma. Infiltrating basal cell carcinoma can resemble **microcystic adnexal carcinoma.** These carcinomas share an infiltrative pattern, small cornifying cysts, and ductular spaces lined by eosinophilic cuticles. Carcinoembryonic antigen can be detected by immunoperoxidase staining in the ductular spaces of both neoplasms. Some descriptions of microcystic adnexal carcinoma have impre-

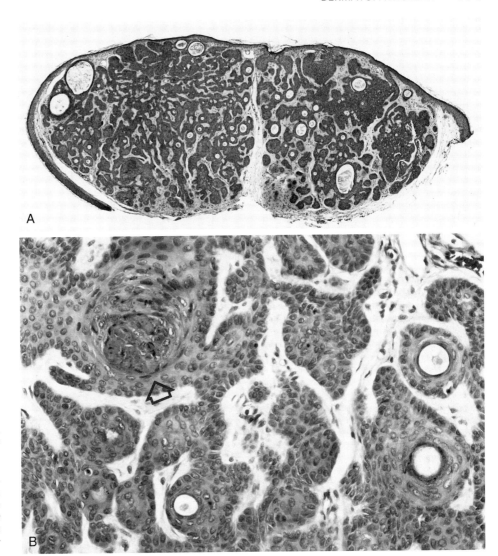

FIGURE 18–17. The infundibulocystic, or nevoid follicular, form of basal cell carcinoma is often well circumscribed and features small cornifying cysts, leading to misinterpretation as trichoepithelioma *(A)*. Unlike trichoepithelioma, there are foci of necrosis *en masse (arrow),* and clefts are present between the epithelium of the neoplasm and its stroma *(B)*.

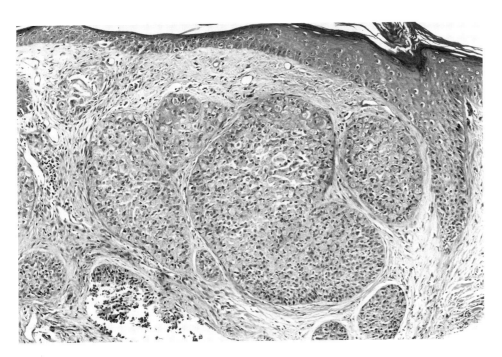

FIGURE 18–18. Basal cell carcinoma with granular cells usually has a nodular growth pattern. Unlike benign granular cell tumors of presumed schwannian origin, small aggregations of granular cells do not occur.

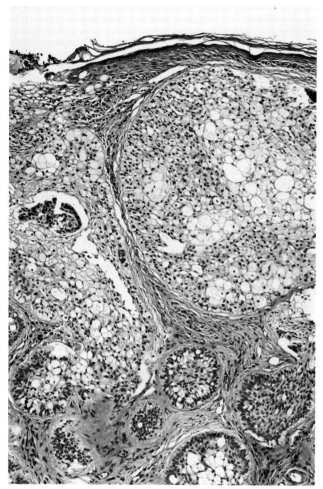

FIGURE 18–19. This example of the clear-cell variant of basal cell carcinoma features some nests with only clear cells and other nests that have a mixture of clear cells and more conventional basaloid cells. As in basal cell carcinoma with granular cells, peripheral palisading is present only in areas in which cells with altered cytoplasm are absent.

cisely claimed that it can be composed of basaloid cells. In fact, the presence of peripheral palisading or aggregations of basaloid cells should call the diagnosis of microcystic adnexal carcinoma into question.

MICROCYSTIC ADNEXAL CARCINOMA

Microcystic adnexal carcinoma is a low-grade carcinoma that features an infiltrative growth pattern, sclerotic stroma, and differentiation toward follicular structures, sweat ducts, or both.

CLINICOPATHOLOGIC FEATURES. Most microcystic adnexal carcinomas occur on the skin of the head and neck as skin-colored indurated plaques. They grow slowly and become bound down to underlying structures, but seldom ulcerate. Occasionally the skin of the trunk or axilla is involved.

Microcystic adnexal carcinomas grow slowly, can be locally destructive, and often invade perineurally. Although a death has been reported from direct extension of a microcystic adnexal carcinoma of the skin of the face, metastases do

not occur. Because of its infiltrative nature, persistence after surgery often occurs.

Excisional specimens of microcystic adnexal carcinoma show a poorly circumscribed neoplasm composed of round or ovoid nests of epithelial cells in the superficial dermis and smaller ovoid nests or strands of cells in the deep dermis and subcutis (Fig. 18–22). There can be connections between nests and the epidermis or follicular epithelium. The nests are composed of cuboidal cells with pale cytoplasm (Fig. 18–23). Atypia is subtle, and mitoses are rare.

The centers of nests of cells in microcystic adnexal carcinoma often contain small cysts with concentrically laminated keratin.[23] Some aggregations have round ductular spaces lined by eosinophilic cuticles in their centers. Squamous whorls are rounded concentric arrays of keratinocytes seen in bulbous aggregations of cells in microcystic adnexal carcinomas. Although most squamous whorls are solid, some have small cysts in their centers, and others contain ducts (Fig. 18–24).

Microcystic adnexal carcinomas on the skin of the trunk almost always lack cysts but contain ductules.[24] Perineural invasion can be present in both facial and truncal lesions.

Exceptional features in microcystic adnexal carcinoma are clusters of sebocytes (Fig. 18–25), areas of clear cells, sometimes with minute, brightly eosinophilic trichohyalin globules, and foci of shadow cells.[25]

The stroma of microcystic adnexal carcinoma is sclerotic. Infiltrates of lymphocytes are generally sparse, but eosinophils are often evident when clear cells are plentiful.

Mounting evidence suggests divergent differentiation in microcystic adnexal carcinomas. Keratinous cysts react with an antibody to pilar keratin, AE13. Sebocytes and clear cells with trichohyalin granules also indicate follicular differentiation. The ductular spaces could be either apocrine or eccrine in nature.

DIFFERENTIAL DIAGNOSIS. The differential diagnosis of microcystic adnexal carcinoma is important because this neoplasm is so frequently mistaken for a benign adnexal neoplasm or for another form of carcinoma. Lesions are most frequently situated on the skin of the face, where clinicians are apt to perform small punch rather than excisional biopsies for cosmetic reasons.

Desmoplastic trichoepithelioma is often found on the face, and its clinical appearance can be similar to that of microcystic adnexal carcinoma.[26] Like microcystic adnexal carcinoma, it features nests or strands of epithelial cells, keratinizing cysts, and sclerotic stroma (Fig. 18–26). Several features differentiate these two sclerosing epithelial neoplasms.[27] Desmoplastic trichoepitheliomas involve the superficial dermis, whereas microcystic adnexal carcinoma, even when lesions first come to clinical attention, often extends into the deep dermis and subcutis. Desmoplastic trichoepitheliomas have smooth borders and are symmetric in configuration. Microcystic adnexal carcinomas have irregular borders and are asymmetric. The strands of desmoplastic trichoepithelioma consist of basaloid cells, as it differentiates toward follicular germ. The cells of microcystic adnexal carcinoma have more abundant, pale cytoplasm and are not palisaded as are those in the largest aggregations of desmoplastic trichoepithelioma. Rudimentary follicular papillae (so-called **papillary mesenchymal bodies**) are sometimes found in desmoplastic trichoepitheliomas, as they are in ordinary trichoepitheliomas, but are absent in microcystic adnexal carcinoma. The nuclei in desmoplastic

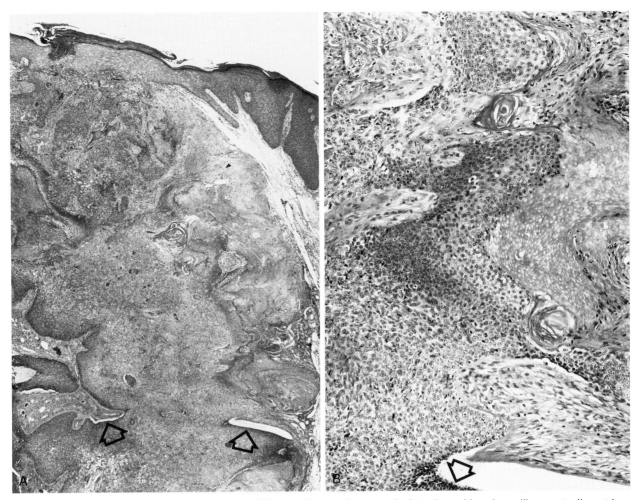

FIGURE 18–20. Basal cell carcinoma with matrical differentiation is often attached to the epidermis, unlike most pilomatricomas. *A,* Broad masses of matrical keratinocytes are present on the left side of the photomicrograph, with a zone of shadow cells on the right. *B,* At higher magnification, the matrical cells can be seen to undergo abrupt keratinization to shadow cells. Note also rims of palisaded basaloid cells adjacent to epithelial-stroma clefts in both photomicrographs, as can be seen in other forms of basal cell carcinoma *(arrows).*

trichoepithelioma are smaller and rounder than those of microcystic adnexal carcinoma. In roughly 10% of specimens of desmoplastic trichoepitheliomas, there are clusters of melanocytic nevus cells, whereas these are not found in microcystic adnexal carcinoma.

Syringomas are sometimes confused histopathologically with microcystic adnexal carcinoma. Syringomas are small skin-colored papules that are often found on infraorbital skin. Unlike microcystic adnexal carcinoma, syringomas are never seen on the upper lip. Dermatologists familiar with the appearances of these conditions are unlikely to confuse them, but microscopically both neoplasms can show small tadpole-shaped aggregations of cells with pale cytoplasm, small cornifying cysts, and small round ductular spaces. Unlike microcystic adnexal carcinoma, syringomas are small, confined to the superficial dermis, and well-circumscribed and do not show perineural invasion. Their distinction in minute specimens can be problematic. Larger aggregations of cells and slight nuclear irregularities in microcystic adnexal carcinoma can be helpful.

Papillary eccrine adenoma is a benign neoplasm found most often as a single lesion on the skin of the arms of black patients. It also has ductular differentiation and sclerotic

stroma. Excisions demonstrate a rounded or ovoid configuration with smooth borders. Within densely sclerotic stroma infiltrated by lymphocytes are rounded nests of cuboidal epithelial cells that form small papillations that project into irregularly shaped lumina. Small foci of necrosis can be present.[28]

In a partial biopsy, papillary eccrine adenoma and a microcystic adnexal carcinoma with ductular differentiation can be difficult to tell apart. The aggregations of microcystic adnexal carcinoma vary in size and configuration more than those of papillary eccrine adenoma. Clinical information can be key— papillary eccrine adenoma is rarely found on the face, and microcystic adnexal carcinoma is unlikely to occur on the extremities. Microcystic adnexal carcinomas are plaques that are often bound down to adjacent structures, whereas papillary eccrine adenomas are freely movable nodules.

Several sclerosing carcinomas can be difficult to distinguish from microcystic adnexal carcinoma. Chief among these are **morpheic basal cell carcinoma,** both with and without eccrine ductal differentiation, eccrine ductular carcinoma, and **adenosquamous carcinoma** of the skin.

Morpheic basal cell carcinoma also presents as an indurated plaque, often on the face or scalp. Although many pathologists

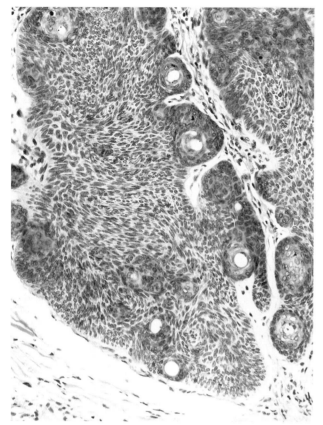

FIGURE 18–21. Small round ductules lined by cuticles can occur in basal cell carcinoma and signify sweat duct differentiation. The exact nature of that differentiation, i.e., eccrine or apocrine, is uncertain.

diagnose morpheic basal cell carcinoma if there is fibrotic stroma or jaggedly shaped nests of neoplastic cells, I reserve the term for lesions that have thin strands of basaloid cells set in collagenous stroma, often parallel to the surface of the skin, and use the term **infiltrating basal cell carcinoma** for the more common variant whose nests have spiky contours. Whereas infiltrating basal cell carcinoma does not resemble microcystic adnexal carcinoma, the morpheic variant can. Distinction is not critical in that both neoplasms require treatment by complete excision, often by micrographic surgery. Both morpheic basal cell carcinoma and microcystic adnexal carcinoma can show perineural invasion, which can result in loss of control of the neoplasm.

Morpheic basal cell carcinoma is composed of basaloid cells, i.e., cells with scant cytoplasm, whose nuclei are closely apposed. The nuclei of morpheic basal cell carcinoma are often diffusely hyperchromatic. In contrast, microcystic adnexal carcinomas have cells with moderate amounts of cytoplasm and have vesicular nuclei. Strands of morpheic basal cell carcinoma are delineated from adjacent fibromyxoid stroma by clefts that contain mucin, whereas no such clefts surround the aggregations of cells in microcystic adnexal carcinoma. In many morpheic basal cell carcinomas, there are a few larger aggregations typical of infiltrating or nodular basal cell carcinoma, whereas larger nests in microcystic adnexal carcinoma can show squamous whorls, cornifying cysts, or ductal differentiation.

Basal cell carcinomas of all histologic types can show ductal differentiation, in which small round lumina bounded by eosinophilic cuticles punctuate aggregations of basaloid cells.[19] Many pathologists are unfamiliar with ductular differentiation in basal cell carcinoma and misinterpret it as another adnexal neoplasm, particularly microcystic adnexal carcinoma.

Eccrine ductular carcinoma resembles the form of microcystic adnexal carcinoma found on the trunk in which keratinizing cysts are few or absent. Elongated tubules occur in both conditions. The chief distinguishing feature is the greater degree of nuclear atypicality seen in eccrine ductular carcinoma. Mitotic figures are rare in microcystic adnexal carcinoma, but can be found in eccrine ductular carcinoma. The distinction between these two adnexal carcinomas is important in that eccrine ductular carcinomas can metastasize, whereas microcystic adnexal carcinomas do not.

Adenosquamous carcinoma of the skin, like microcystic adnexal carcinoma, features poorly circumscribed aggregations of cells that can form both cornifying cysts and ducts, invades along nerves, and can be difficult to excise completely.[29, 30] As many as 50% of cases end fatally, and aggressive therapy early in the course of the disease is critical. Adenosquamous carcinoma is composed of groups of polygonal cells with abundant cytoplasm and focal keratinization (Fig. 18–27). Calcification can occur within glandular spaces. The ductular spaces of adenosquamous carcinoma of the skin can be lined by cells that contain mucin.

DERMATOFIBROSARCOMA PROTUBERANS

Dermatofibrosarcoma protuberans is a low-grade sarcoma of the dermis and superficial subcutis that is composed of spindled cells that have some features of fibroblasts. Perineural fibroblastic differentiation has been proposed on the basis of light and electron microscopic findings.

CLINICOPATHOLOGIC FEATURES. Dermatofibrosarcoma protuberans (DFSP) usually begins as an indurated plaque on the trunk or limbs of males from adolescence to middle age. Plaques of DFSP are often red-purple. Some plaques are depressed beneath the surface of the surrounding skin. If allowed to persist, the nodules from which DFSP derives its name can arise; these are generally deeper in hue. Nodules in which mucin is abundant appear blue.

Slow but relentless growth and recurrence with incomplete excision are characteristic of DFSP. Only rarely does metastasis occur, but infiltration of local tissues makes complete surgical excision desirable. Because the borders of DFSP can be ill defined, wide surgical excision or excision with frozen section guidance followed by removal of a buffer of uninvolved tissue are often used treatments. It is important to make the diagnosis of DFSP the first time that the neoplasm is biopsied, because recurrent lesions are more difficult to treat.

Plaques of DFSP are difficult for the surgical pathologist to recognize, because its cells are cytologically bland, the neoplastic cells can be sparse, and without a nodular component, it may not be suspected clinically. Plaques of DFSP appear to arise in the deep reticular dermis and subcutis as proliferations of spindled cells that form wavy fascicles that

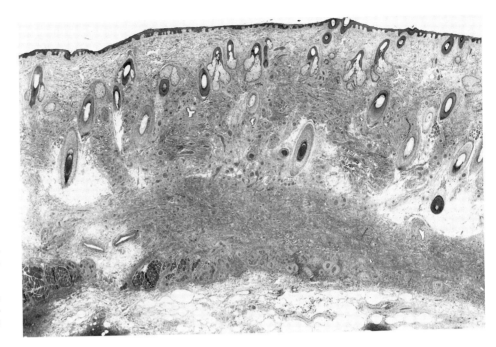

FIGURE 18-22. At scanning magnification, microcystic adnexal carcinoma is deeply infiltrative and associated with a sclerotic stroma. Unfortunately, pathologists are seldom afforded the luxury of a specimen in which these features can be seen.

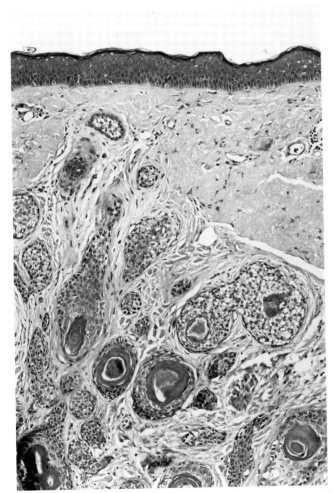

FIGURE 18-23. Nests of cells with clear cytoplasm and small monomorphous nuclei often occur in microcystic adnexal carcinoma.

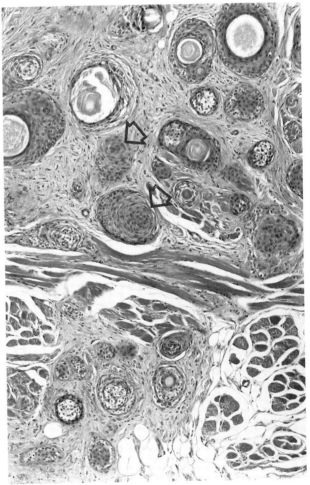

FIGURE 18-24. Small cornifying cysts (signifying infundibular differentiation) and squamous whorls (arrows) can be seen in this example of microcystic adnexal differentiation.

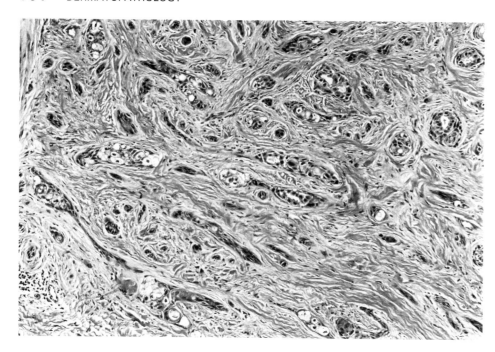

FIGURE 18–25. Slender strands of basaloid cells and sebocytes are present in this microcystic adnexal carcinoma. Microcystic adnexal carcinomas can differentiate toward many portions of the pilo-sebaceous-apocrine unit.

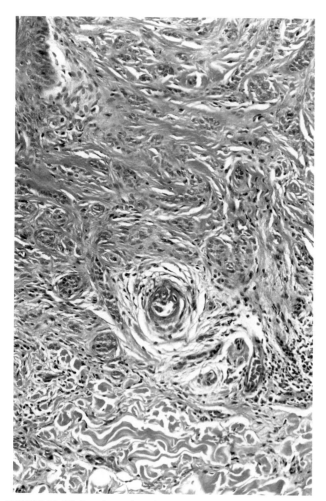

FIGURE 18–26. Another sclerosing adnexal neoplasm, desmoplastic trichoepithelioma, is composed of slender strands of cells with small round nuclei and scant cytoplasm, surrounded by rims of collagen.

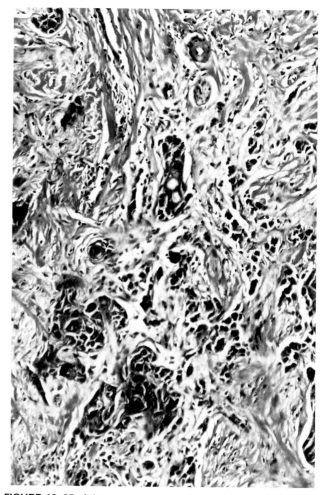

FIGURE 18–27. Adenosquamous carcinoma of the skin is analogous to mucoepidermoid carcinoma as found at other sites. There are keratinizing cells with atypical nuclei and foci of gland formation.

parallel the surface of the epidermis (Fig. 18–28). The papillary and superficial reticular dermis are generally spared. There is often a small or moderate amount of dermal mucin. The dermis can be thinned by plaques of DFSP. Whether this atrophy is due to the neoplasm or indicates an underlying malformation of the dermis is uncertain. The fascicles of spindled cells commonly entrap lipocytes, resulting in a lace-like pattern. When combined with dermal atrophy, the impression on scanning magnification is that adipocytes are situated abnormally superficially. The spindled cells themselves, whether in the dermis or subcutis have sparse finely tapered cytoplasm, and oval to markedly elongated nuclei. The epidermis overlying plaques of DFSP can show slight elongation of its rete ridges.[31]

Nodules of DFSP are easily recognized by surgical pathologists. The spindled cells in nodules have a storiform pattern in which the cells appear to radiate from small acellular areas.

Mitotic figures are more common in nodules than in plaques and range up to 5 per 10 high-power fields (HPF). Some nodules of DFSP contain a population of dendritic melanocytes and are known as pigmented DFSP or Bednar's tumor.

Large nodules of DFSP can harbor areas with a herringbone pattern characteristic of fibrosarcoma.[32] The cells in these zones have higher mitotic rates. Recognition of **fibrosarcoma** arising in DFSP is important, because this transformation is associated with a higher risk of metastasis.

The cells of DFSP have a relatively primitive mesenchymal immunophenotype, containing vimentin, lysozyme, and alpha-1-antichymotrypsin. The **human progenitor cell antigen,** or **CD34,** has been identified in DFSP.[33, 34] Its expression is stronger in the cells of plaques than in those of nodules.

DIFFERENTIAL DIAGNOSIS. The most important entity to be differentiated from DFSP is the common **dermatofibroma,** sometimes referred to by pathologists but never by clinicians

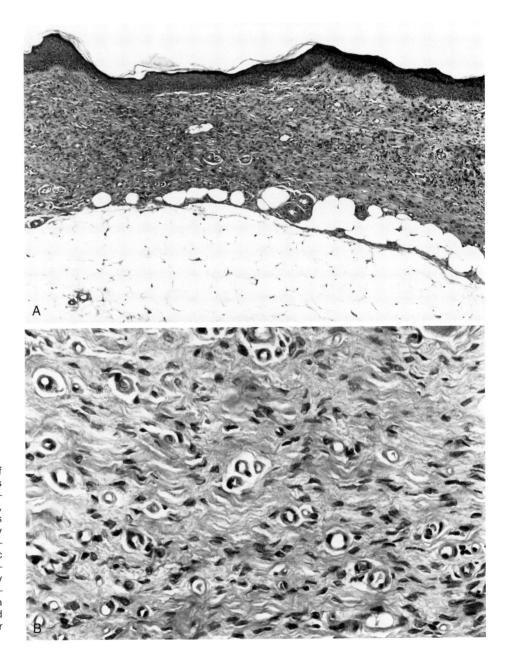

FIGURE 18–28. The plaque stage of dermatofibrosarcoma protuberans features spindled cells aligned parallel to the surface of the epidermis, often entrapping lipocytes. In this example, the dermis is actually thinned by the proliferation, a finding that correlates with an atrophic clinical appearance (A). The spindled cells are seldom strikingly atypical, and a punch biopsy specimen containing areas such as seen in B could easily be misinterpreted as representing a neurofibroma or dermatofibroma.

as **benign cutaneous fibrous histiocytoma.** Dermatofibromas usually are small, dome-shaped brown papules that dermatologists can easily diagnose clinically. Uncommonly, dermatofibromas affect the deep dermis and subcutis and have a multinodular appearance that simulates DFSP. Both dermatofibroma and DFSP are composed of spindled cells with areas of storiform patterns.

Several determinations useful in the differential diagnosis of dermatofibroma and DFSP can be made at scanning magnification. The center of gravity of dermatofibroma is in the mid-dermis, with the exception of the rare multinodular form. In dermatofibroma, spindled cells can extend into septa of the subcutaneous fat, thickening them in a wedge-shaped fashion; DFSP involves the subcutaneous fat differently, with long trabecula of spindled cells that parallel the skin surface, entrapping lipocytes.[31] In dermatofibroma, only a few lipocytes are surrounded by spindled cells. The epidermis overlying most dermatofibromas is hyperplastic, hyperpigmented, and hyperkeratotic. Often, the elongated retia have flat bases. The epidermis above plaques of DFSP is unaffected or shows slight elongation or slight basilar hyperpigmentation. The spindled cells of DFSP, both in plaques and nodules, are monomorphous; those of dermatofibroma can be heterogeneous, with large plump and slender spindled cells in the same microscopic fields. Giant cells are rare in DFSP, whereas hemosiderin-laden giant cells are common in cellular, hemorrhagic lesions of dermatofibroma. Thickened collagen bundles (collagen balls) are often found at the periphery of dermatofibroma but not at that of DFSP.

Many surgical pathologists are under the misapprehension that mitotic figures do not occur or are only rarely found in dermatofibroma, and if present, signify DFSP. Mitoses are common in cellular dermatofibromas and are especially frequent adjacent to areas of necrosis.

Immunohistochemistry can help in the differential diagnosis between dermatofibroma and DFSP. Most dermatofibromas contain a large proportion of cells that stain for Factor XIIIa. Factor XIIIa polymerizes fibrin in coagulation. It is found in macrophages and in a normal cell of the dermis called the **dermal dendrocyte.** Most dermal dendrocytes are inconspicuous in hematoxylin and eosin (H&E)–stained sections and are discounted as fibroblasts. Many believe that dermatofibromas are proliferations of dermal dendrocytes or dermal dendrocytomas. When stained for Factor XIIIa, there are many reactive cells in dermatofibroma, especially at the edges of lesions. In DFSP, there are only scattered dendritic cells, and the majority of spindled cells do not stain (Fig. 18–29).[35]

Dermatofibromas do not stain for CD34, which intensely marks most of the spindled cells of plaques of dermatofibrosarcoma and labels those of nodules less strongly (Fig. 18–30). In addition to differentiating dermatofibroma from DFSP, CD34 is also useful in determining the extent of involvement by recurrent DFSP, when the neoplastic cells are juxtaposed with the fibroblasts of scar tissue, which do not express CD34.

Punch biopsies from sparsely cellular or myxoid areas of DFSP are easily misdiagnosed as a neurofibroma. Both sparsely cellular plaques of DFSP and neurofibroma feature cytologically bland spindled cells with thin bundles of collagen, mucin replete with mast cells, and poor peripheral circumscription. The spindled cells of neurofibroma are more

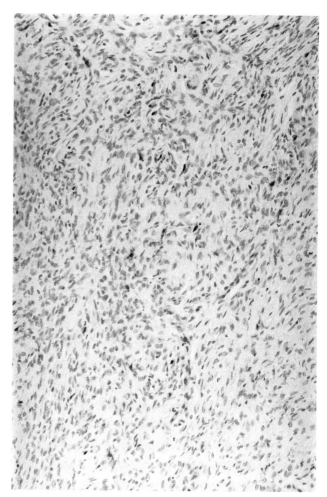

FIGURE 18–29. Factor XIIIa is expressed by only scattered dendritic cells in this immunoperoxidase-stained example of dermatofibrosarcoma protuberans. In contrast, the cells of most dermatofibromas show strong expression of this antigen, especially at the periphery of the lesion.

distinctly S-shaped. Narrow wavy fascicles of spindled cells delineated by clefts are present in neurofibroma and not in DFSP. Staining for S-100 protein can be used to buttress the diagnosis of neurofibroma.

Fibrosarcoma arises in deep soft tissues and only rarely involves the skin. A situation with potential for confusion can occur when a biopsy is taken from a nodule of DFSP with fibrosarcomatous features.[32] The pathologist should sign out such a specimen descriptively, providing the information that such areas can arise within nodules of DFSP and that a larger specimen should be obtained before definitive therapy is carried out.

Large, **multinodular fibrous histiocytomas** can be mistaken for dermatofibrosarcoma protuberans because of their clinical appearance and the unfamiliarity of pathologists with this entity.[36, 37] These lesions can recur after incomplete excision but do not behave aggressively.

Dermatomyofibroma is a recently described entity that may be a form of **fibromatosis** rather than a neoplasm.[38] It features slender spindle cells in fascicles parallel to the epidermal surface, as does dermatofibrosarcoma protuberans. It is more sparsely cellular than DFSP and does not show a

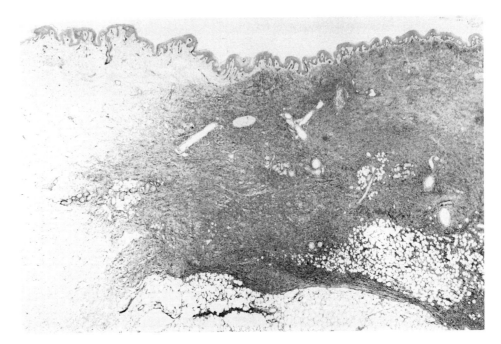

FIGURE 18–30. A dermatofibrosarcoma protuberans stained by immunoperoxidase for CD34. Only a few scattered cells in dermatofibroma express CD34, making this a useful reagent in the differential diagnosis of the two conditions. CD34 also highlights small residual foci of dermatofibrosarcoma protuberans in re-excision specimens, whereas the cells of scars do not express CD34.

lace-like pattern of subcutaneous involvement, and its fascicles lack a wavy pattern.

KAPOSI'S SARCOMA

Kaposi's sarcoma is a proliferation of endothelial cells that often is multicentric and evolves from sparsely cellular patches to densely cellular plaques and nodules. Although its differentiation toward endothelium is no longer under debate, its nature is. Although Kaposi's sarcoma is found in patients infected by the human immunodeficiency virus (HIV), it is not equally prevalent in all risk groups, being far more common in homosexual men than in other infected persons. Epidemiologic evidence suggests that it is caused by a second infectious agent, and some claim that its mode of growth is more in keeping with a reactive hyperplasia than a true neoplasm. This discussion focuses on the patch stage of Kaposi's sarcoma, as its recognition poses a difficult task for surgical pathologists.

CLINICOPATHOLOGIC FEATURES. The earliest lesions of Kaposi's are pink or red macules or patches. Some tiny lesions come to attention only because of the high level of awareness of the disease among homosexual men. Similar macules or patches, were they to have occurred in elderly men of Mediterranean descent (the most common hosts of Kaposi's sarcoma prior to the HIV pandemic), would most likely have been ignored.

Later lesions of Kaposi's sarcoma tend to be darker red and to be plaques, nodules, or tumors. Lesions can range from a few to widespread. Whereas the feet and lower legs were particular sites of predilection in elderly men, the lesions of Kaposi's sarcoma in immunosuppressed patients are widely distributed.

Kaposi described the densely packed spindled cells with extravasated erythrocytes that characterize nodular lesions (Fig. 18–31). It seems doubtful that he would have been able to recognize the changes of the patch stage of the disease that was to be named after him.

The histopathologic features seen in patches of Kaposi's sarcoma were well-described only in the late 1970s.[39] Before then, patches were often regarded as atypical hemangiomas or lymphangiomas. The recognition of the early changes of Kaposi's sarcoma became critical in the early 1980s as the diagnosis of **acquired immunodeficiency syndrome (AIDS)** often rested on their recognition, prior to the advent of serologic testing. Currently, the recognition of Kaposi's sarcoma is still important, as there are several effective treatments, and its occurrence can herald the development of clinically evident disease in patients who had hitherto been seropositive but healthy.

The earliest changes in macules and patches of Kaposi's sarcoma are seen at scanning magnification as a subtle increase in the number of cells with spindled or ovoid shapes seen around small blood vessels and adnexal structures in both the superficial and deep dermis, accompanied by sparse superficial and deep perivascular infiltrates of lymphocytes and a few plasma cells (Fig. 18–32). The spindled cells line elongated spaces that do not contain many erythrocytes. The spaces can vary from narrow and slit-like to large and jagged. When capacious, they often surround preexistent structures such as venules or nerves, which can protrude into them, forming the "promontory sign." As patches evolve, spindled cells and their vascular spaces infiltrate between reticular dermal collagen bundles. It is only at this stage that appreciable numbers of erythrocytes are evident in these spaces, and hemosiderin-laden macrophages appear. Eosinophilic globules, small round pink inclusions seen in the cytoplasms of the cells of Kaposi's sarcoma as the product of phagocytosis of erythrocytes, are not evident until plaques are formed by more extensive infiltration of the dermis.

The plaque and tumor stages of Kaposi's sarcoma do not generally pose a diagnostic problem for pathologists. In plaque stage lesions, there still is a tendency for the cells of Kaposi's sarcoma to surround preexistent structures, and indeed there may be fascicles of spindled cells that course along the paths of the vascular plexuses, small nerves, arrector pili muscles,

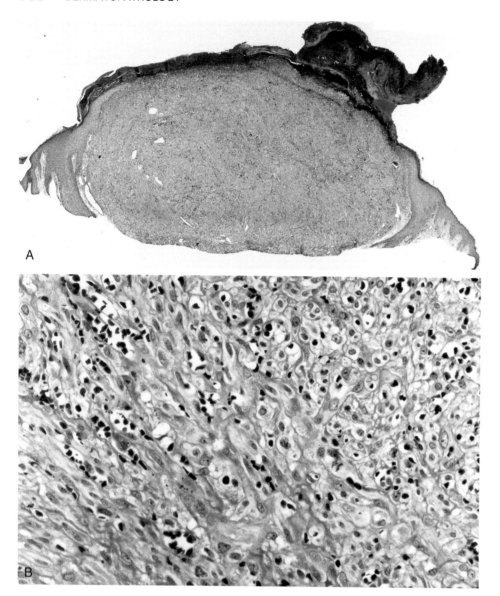

FIGURE 18–31. Kaposi's sarcoma in its classic, nodular form *(A)*. At higher magnification, there is a sieve-like pattern of vascular spaces formed by the spindled cells, some of which contain eosinophilic globules that are the remnants of phagocytized erythrocytes *(B)*.

or eccrine ducts. In nodules of Kaposi's sarcoma, the spindled cells grow to confluence, and unlike the case in earlier lesions, the proliferation is generally well-circumscribed. Slit-like spaces that contain erythrocytes, siderophages, and eosinophilic globules are found in most cases of plaque and nodular stage lesions.[40]

Two detours in this stereotypic evolution of lesions can pose diagnostic problems. These are the so-called angiomatous and pseudogranulomatous types of Kaposi's sarcoma. Both of these types of Kaposi's sarcoma present clinically as papules or nodules.[41] **Angiomatous Kaposi's sarcoma** has well-circumscribed groups of thin-walled, rounded, dilated vessels whose lumina are packed with erythrocytes (Fig. 18–33). Serial sections are sometimes needed to demonstrate areas that are more specific.

The **pseudogranulomatous** type of lesion is composed of small nodules of cells that have abundant pale eosinophilic cytoplasm within which there are small round vascular lumina. Often the groups of cells are in contiguity with adnexal structures. Eosinophilic globules are commonly present.

DIFFERENTIAL DIAGNOSIS. Patches of Kaposi's sarcoma are most often mistaken for two other conditions in which cells

with spindled and ovoid nuclei are dispersed interstitially, namely **dermatofibroma** and **granuloma annulare.** Dermatofibroma is occasionally misdiagnosed clinically as Kaposi's sarcoma, as both lesions can be red-brown or brown papules.[42]

Dermatofibroma can share with Kaposi's sarcoma, in addition to interstitial spindled cells, extravasated erythrocytes and siderophages. Unlike the case in Kaposi's sarcoma, the cells of dermatofibroma do not show a propensity to cluster around preexistent vessels and adnexa. Although both conditions spare the papillary dermis, only dermatofibroma elicits epidermal hyperplasia and hyperpigmentation. Fibrosis is always present in dermatofibroma; it is exceptional in patches of Kaposi's sarcoma. The cells of Kaposi's sarcoma are oval to spindled; dermatofibromas often include a proportion of cells with triangular nuclei. The inflammatory infiltrates of Kaposi's sarcoma include plasma cells, which are not found in dermatofibromas.

In cases in which light microscopy does not resolve this differential diagnosis, immunoperoxidase staining can be useful. Dermatofibromas are composed of a variety of cells, but dermal dendrocytes are among the most frequent and are

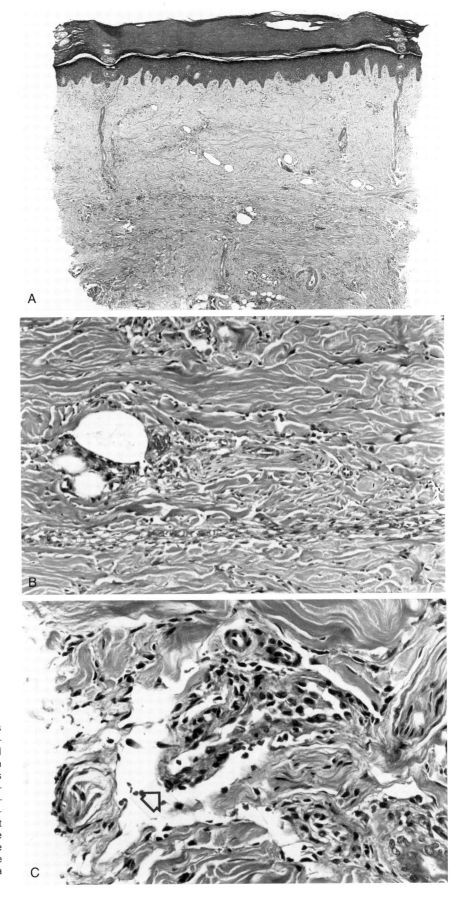

FIGURE 18–32. The patch stage of Kaposi's sarcoma can initially be taken for a superficial and deep perivascular dermatitis, and indeed there are lymphocytes and plasma cells around the vessels of both plexuses *(A)*. However, there are also increased numbers of spindled cells between reticular dermal collagen bundles *(B)* and jagged vascular spaces that surround preexistent structures such as the venule depicted here *(arrow)* jutting into such a space *(C)*. The protrusion of normal structures into the newly formed vessels of Kaposi's sarcoma has been dubbed the "promontory sign."

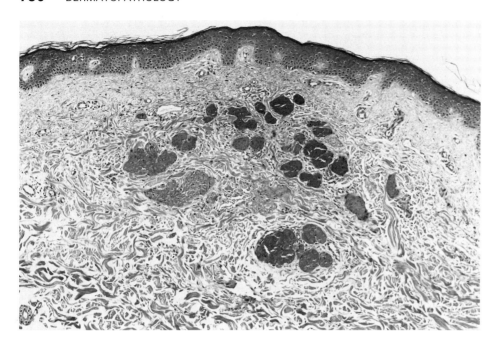

FIGURE 18–33. An angiomatous lesion of Kaposi's sarcoma. This group of thin-walled vessels have lumina packed with erythrocytes. If there is doubt as to the diagnosis, level sections can be cut to unearth such diagnostic findings as eosinophilic globules, spindled cells, and so forth.

particularly dense at the periphery of lesions. Dermal dendrocytes stain with antisera to **Factor XIIIa.**[35] Patches of Kaposi's sarcoma also contain Factor XIIIa–positive cells, albeit more sparsely and in a more diffuse distribution. Whereas the spindled cells of dermatofibroma do not produce a basement membrane, those of Kaposi's sarcoma are found next to vascular spaces lined by **type IV collagen** and **laminin.** Antisera to basement membrane components can be used to outline these spaces in routinely processed material.[43]

The interstitial pattern of **granuloma annulare** can be difficult to distinguish microscopically from early Kaposi's sarcoma. Granuloma annulare is a palisaded granulomatous dermatitis, but early lesions feature lymphocytes around vessels of the superficial and deep plexus, along with macrophages, mast cells, and mucin dispersed interstitially. When the macrophages of this interstitial pattern of granuloma annulare are elongated, they can be confused with the spindled cells of Kaposi's sarcoma.

Several features can be used to distinguish these two conditions. The infiltrates of interstitial granuloma annulare are no denser around adnexa, whereas those of Kaposi's sarcoma begin around follicles, sweat glands, and vessels. Neither extravasated erythrocytes nor hemosiderin is found in granuloma annulare. Plasma cells are a component of the infiltrates of Kaposi's sarcoma but are exceptional in granuloma annulare. In interstitial granuloma annulare, abundant mucin can be detected with a colloidal iron or alcian blue stain; mucin is scant or not increased in Kaposi's sarcoma.

Hemorrhagic dermal scars can simulate macules and patches of Kaposi's sarcoma both clinically and pathologically. Scars contain spindled cells that often parallel the epidermal surface, with similarly oriented collagen fibers that are thinner than the normal bundles of the reticular dermis. The blood vessels in scars are perpendicular or diagonal to the surface. Erythrocytes and siderophages are found in the clefts between collagen bundles in traumatized scars.[42]

Unlike the case in patch stage Kaposi's sarcoma, the changes in dermal scars extend to the dermoepidermal junc-

tion, and the rete ridge pattern of the epidermis is effaced. In patches of Kaposi's sarcoma, the papillary dermis is nearly always spared, and the rete ridge pattern is normal. Although the spindled cells of Kaposi's sarcoma can be parallel to reticular dermal collagen bundles, many spindled cells are clustered around adnexa, whereas the fibroblasts of scars do not show this propensity. The collagen fibers in young scars are thinner than the normal fibers of the reticular dermis; those seen in between the spindled cells of Kaposi's sarcoma are unaffected or very slightly thickened. The demarcation between the changes produced by scarring and the adjacent dermis is sharp, a feature that contrasts with patch stage Kaposi's sarcoma, in which the spindled component diffuses irregularly into the adjacent dermis. Elastic tissue stains demonstrate absent or markedly diminished fibers in scars, with an abrupt margin with the adjacent dermis. The newly formed collagen bundles of scars are less anisotropic than those of the reticular dermis when viewed by polarized light. Immunoperoxidase staining with antisera to type IV collagen or laminin does not demonstrate basement membrane material adjacent to clefts between collagen bundles in scars.

Bacillary angiomatosis, a vasoproliferative reaction to infection with *Bartonella henselae* and *B. quintana,* can be confused with Kaposi's sarcoma both clinically and pathologically.[44] Unlike the case in Kaposi's sarcoma, early lesions of bacillary angiomatosis are minute papules rather than patches, and they evolve into nodules rather than plaques. Even so, clinicians experienced in treating skin disease in immunosuppressed patients often cannot distinguish the two conditions except by biopsy.

Cutaneous lesions of bacillary angiomatosis differ from Kaposi's sarcoma in that there are aggregates of protuberant endothelial cells rather than spindled ones, and infiltrates of neutrophils and neutrophilic nuclear dust rather than plasma cells and lymphocytes (Fig. 18–34).[45] Eosinophilic globules are rare in bacillary angiomatosis, and promontory signs are not found, as lumina are small and round. Purplish clumps of bacilli are often present within the neutrophilic foci, but

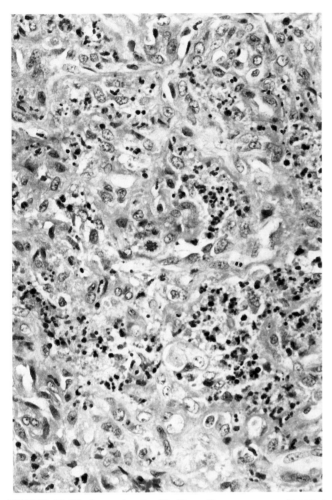

FIGURE 18–34. In contrast with Kaposi's sarcoma, cutaneous lesions of bacillary angiomatosis are composed of polygonal cells with irregular, vesicular nuclei. There are interspersed foci of leukocytoclasis that signify the sites of colonies of organisms. Note the mitotic figure at center, adding to the impression of a vascular neoplasm.

can be difficult to see with poor hematoxylin and eosin stains. The presence of bacilli can be confirmed by Warthin-Starry or similar silver stains, immunoperoxidase staining, or electron microscopy. Distinction between the two conditions is of great clinical importance because bacillary angiomatosis is potentially fatal but easily treated with a variety of antibiotics.[46]

SPITZ'S NEVUS

Spitz's nevus is a benign neoplasm composed of melanocytes with large spindled or ovoid cells. Unlike some variants of blue nevi that also contain large melanocytes, it begins at the dermoepidermal junction and evolves through compound and intradermal stages. Nearly all Spitz's nevi are acquired.

Spitz's nevus is a well-known histopathologic simulant of malignant melanoma, and indeed, the original description by Spitz was of a form of melanoma affecting children.[47] Because the classic features of Spitz's nevus are so well known, this discussion concentrates on its more unusual guises.

CLINICOPATHOLOGIC FEATURES. Spitz's nevi, like other acquired melanocytic neoplasms, begin within the epidermis.

The early Spitz's nevi resemble other melanocytic nevi clinically. **Compound Spitz's nevi** are most often dome-shaped, pink, red, tan, or brown papules. Spitz's nevi in young children can be so deeply erythematous as to resemble hemangiomas. Although most are smooth-surfaced, they are sometimes verrucous. Some exceptional lesions have flat peripheries and a central papule. As compound lesions age and become intradermal, they tend to become tan or skin-colored. Most Spitz's nevi are less than 1.0 cm in diameter, symmetric, and smooth-bordered.

There are several clinical variants of Spitz's nevus that can be mistaken for malignant melanoma. Because many dermatologists have learned that Spitz's nevus is pink or red, the brown or brown-black lesions of the pigmented spindle cell variant are often wrongly assumed to be melanomas.[48] Agminated (grouped) Spitz's nevus presents with several papules within a circumscribed area, sometimes delimited by a *cafe au lait*–colored patch. In eruptive Spitz's nevus, many papules arise within a short period of time. These presentations are alarming, and there have been cases of eruptive Spitz's nevi in which the clinical appearance was similar to that seen in widespread cutaneous metastasis of melanoma.

The concept of a "**malignant Spitz's nevus**" was proposed for cases in which spread to lymph nodes (but not beyond) occurred in patients whose primary lesions were histopathologically similar to Spitz's nevi.[49] The only clinical feature that was distinctive about these neoplasms, which arose mainly in adults, was that their diameter was often more than 1 cm.

The histopathologic appearances of Spitz's nevus are multiform, making its recognition and distinction from **malignant melanoma** one of the major challenges in dermatopathology.

Spitz's nevi begin as proliferations of single melanocytes in the epidermis (Fig. 18–35). They are recognizable even at this embryonic stage by the uniformly large size of their nuclei and by their abundant cytoplasm, which is often separated from that of neighboring keratinocytes by clefts. The cells of an evolving junctional Spitz's nevus tend to be evenly distributed throughout the breadth of a lesion. Often they are spindled and vertically oriented, and many of them are multinucleated. Like their counterparts in compound and intradermal examples, the cytoplasm in most intraepidermal Spitz's nevi is homogeneous.[50] The nuclei are vesicular and can have prominent nucleoli. These are often amphophilic in well-balanced hematoxylin and eosin–stained sections and are seldom brightly eosinophilic.

As an **intraepidermal Spitz's nevus** develops, nests of melanocytes form at the dermoepidermal junction. These nests are often separated by clefts from the adjacent epidermis, and clefts separate the melanocytes within these nests as well. The epidermis above junctional Spitz's nevi becomes progressively hyperplastic and hyperkeratotic, with a thickened granular layer. **Kamino bodies,** which are dull pink agglomerations of necrotic melanocytes and keratinocytes, basement membrane material, and fibronectin, occur in the epidermis in junctional and compound Spitz's nevi.[51] They range in diameter from that of two or three keratinocytes to more than five and have scalloped outlines, surrounded by the crescentic nuclei of degenerating keratinocytes.

Spitz's nevi become compound as nests of melanocytes are incorporated into the papillary dermis, which in turn becomes fibrotic. Superficial compound Spitz's nevi are dome-shaped

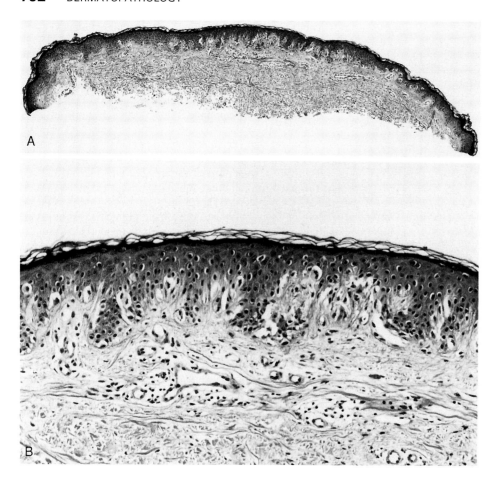

A

B

FIGURE 18–35. An incipient junctional Spitz's nevus. At this early stage, single melanocytes are more common than nested ones *(A)*. The findings seen here differ from those of a simple lentigo or a lentiginous junctional nevus in that many of the melanocytes have spindled shapes and abundant cytoplasm, there are clefts between the cytoplasm of melanocytes and that of neighboring keratinocytes, and some of the melanocytes are multinucleated *(B)*.

(Fig. 18–36). The cytologic features of the dermal cells in such lesions resemble those of their intraepidermal counterparts, although overall cellular and nuclear size tend to diminish with descent. There are perivascular infiltrates of lymphocytes beneath many compound Spitz's nevi, and exceptionally there are dense, band-like infiltrates.

As compound Spitz's nevi progress to involve the reticular dermis, they often become wedge-shaped (Fig. 18–37). Maturation is best assessed in deep Spitz's nevi. Although many pathologists look only for diminished nuclear size, other features should be scrutinized, such as the amount of cytoplasm, the degree of pigmentation of melanocytes, and the sizes of aggregations of melanocytes. Many lesions that have proved to be malignant melanoma were first diagnosed as Spitz's nevi because an overly restrictive definition of maturation was applied.

If left undisturbed, Spitz's nevi eventually become intradermal. Intradermal Spitz's nevi tend to be wedge-shaped, with domed surfaces, but some late compound or intradermal lesions have verrucous surfaces. Desmoplasia is often evident in intradermal Spitz's nevi, and one alternate name for these neoplasms is **"desmoplastic nevus."**[52] Pigmentation is usually absent in intradermal Spitz's nevi, and lymphocytes are scant. Some of the epidermal changes seen above junctional and compound Spitz's nevi may persist in intradermal Spitz's nevi.

One variant of junctional and compound Spitz's nevus that both clinicians and pathologists tend to have difficulty with is the pigmented spindle cell form, sometimes termed **"pigmented spindle cell nevus (of Reed)"** by those who hold that it is not a variant of Spitz's nevus at all, but is instead a separate entity.[48] As mentioned earlier, clinicians may suspect melanoma because they do not know that a Spitz's nevus can be pigmented. Pathologists likewise may be alarmed by intense pigmentation of melanocytes, although pigmentation *per se* is not an informative feature *vis-à-vis* the diagnosis of melanoma.

Some Spitz's nevi have flat peripheries and raised centers (Fig. 18–38), mimicking the **"radial"** and **"vertical"** growth patterns of melanoma. If upward migration of melanocytes is present (as can indeed occur in some Spitz's nevi), many pathologists may be tempted to interpret such a lesion as malignant.

The neoplasms termed **"malignant Spitz's nevus"** have largely been deep, compound lesions that extended into the subcutis (Fig. 18–39). Some have features not seen in conventional Spitz's nevi, such as pigmentation of deep melanocytes, and large nests of melanocytes in the deepest portions of the lesions. Many are ulcerated and larger than 1 cm in diameter.[49]

Agminated Spitz's nevi and **eruptive Spitz's nevi** do not show exceptional histopathologic features in most cases. Spec-

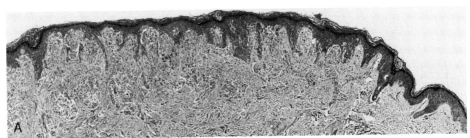

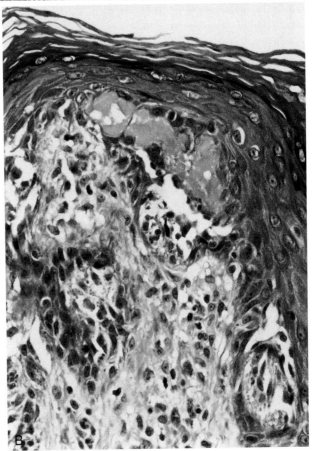

FIGURE 18–36. A compound Spitz's nevus that involves the superficial dermis only. Note the hyperkeratosis and slightly irregular epidermal hyperplasia that stops just beyond the last nest of melanocytes, and also that the neoplasm itself is well circumscribed *(A)*. Kamino bodies *(B)* are found within the epidermis of many Spitz's nevi. They are agglomerations of degenerating keratinocytes, melanocytes, types IV and VII collagen, and fibronectin.

imens that contain several closely set agminated Spitz's nevi can simulate a melanoma in which there are so-called skip areas or one surrounded by satellite lesions. Careful analysis of each of the papules, rather than panic, suffices to make this determination.

DIFFERENTIAL DIAGNOSIS. The differential diagnosis of the intraepidermal stage of Spitz's nevus is **melanoma in situ.** Although in some cases it may be impossible to tell the two conditions apart, intraepidermal Spitz's nevi biopsied at the stage at which single cells still dominate the picture tend to have uniformly larger melanocytes than melanoma *in situ,* which generally has small melanocytes until further in its evolution. Whereas the cells of Spitz's nevi at any stage often have dense-appearing cytoplasm, those of melanoma *in situ* often have abundant pale finely vacuolated cytoplasm. Clefts are nearly always present between the cells of an intraepidermal Spitz's nevus and adjacent melanocytes, but are not obligatory in malignant melanoma *in situ.* As the cells of Spitz's

nevi proliferate and form nests, the diagnosis becomes much easier. Additional features present in junctional Spitz's nevus, such as epidermal hyperplasia, hypergranulosis, and compact hyperkeratosis, are largely absent in malignant melanoma. **Kamino bodies** can be large and numerous in Spitz's nevus. Although they can occur on rare occasion in melanomas, they are often small and few.

As Spitz's nevi become compound, there are additional changes that pathologists can use as aids in their differential diagnosis from malignant melanoma. Symmetry is an attribute of benign nevi in general and Spitz's nevus in particular and not of malignant melanoma. All too many pathologists regard symmetry as referring only to a lesion's silhouette. Although a symmetric outline is a reassuring feature, there are other attributes of symmetry that pathologists should learn to look for. These include the distribution of pigment, the size of nests and the cytologic features of melanocytes at each tier of the dermis, and the distribution of lymphocytes. A lesion

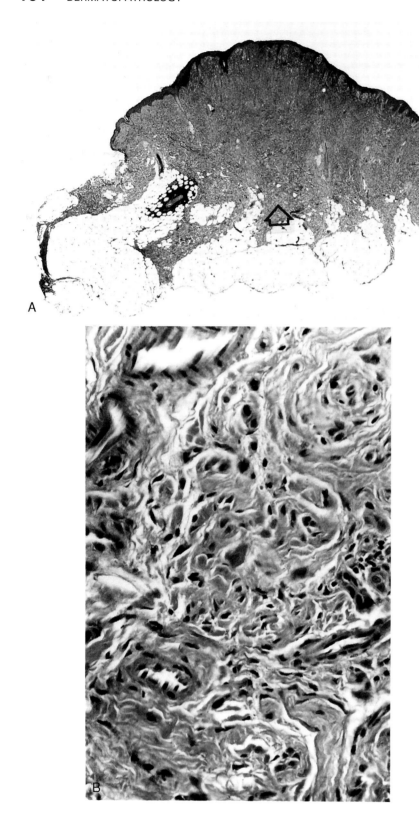

FIGURE 18–37. An intradermal desmoplastic Spitz's nevus. This lesion has the characteristic shape of a wedge with the apex in the deep reticular dermis *(arrow) (A).* Pleomorphic spindled cells lie between thickened collagen bundles *(B).* Unlike the case in desmoplastic melanoma, long fascicles of spindled cells do not occur.

with a perfect wedge shape in which deep pigmentation is present on one side, beneath which there is a dense infiltrate of lymphocytes should be suspected of being a melanoma. "Penumbra" can thus be as important as silhouette.[53]

Intradermal Spitz's nevi elicit a differential diagnosis that includes both **histiocytic proliferations** and **desmoplastic**

malignant melanoma. Reticulohistiocytic granuloma is a condition that presents as solitary skin-colored papules on the skin of the trunk of adults.[54] It can resemble Spitz's nevus clinically and is histopathologically similar in that there is a nodular dermal infiltrate of cells with abundant dense-appearing cytoplasm and vesicular nuclei with prominent cen-

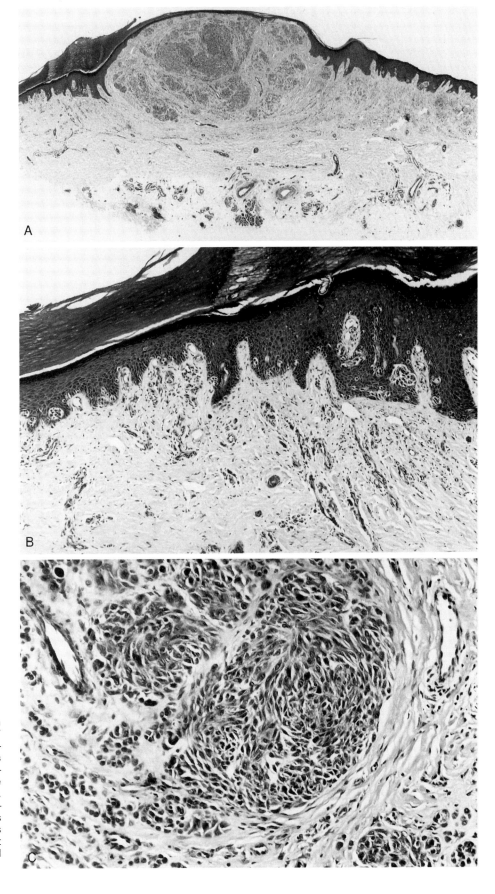

FIGURE 18–38. A Spitz's nevus on acral skin with "radial" and "vertical" growth phases, i.e., a flattish periphery and a nodular center (A). This form can be misdiagnosed as melanoma if one is familiar only with the conventional wedge-shaped type. The periphery has the usual epidermal changes seen overlying a Spitz's nevus (B). The central nodule differs from the changes seen in most Spitz's nevi in that it has a rounded bottom (C).

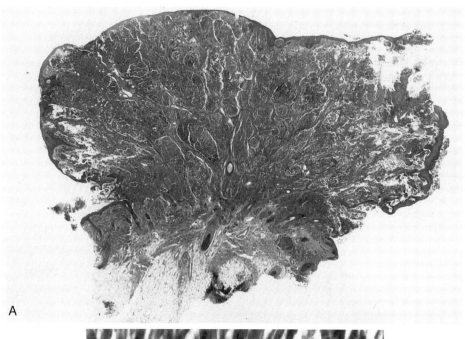

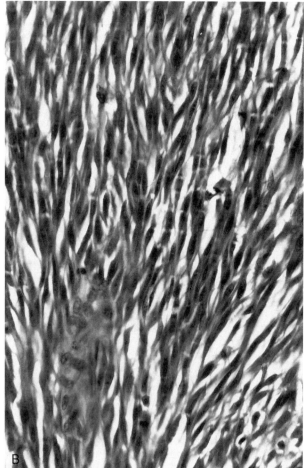

FIGURE 18–39. This so-called malignant Spitz's nevus in a 4-year-old girl metastasized to a local lymph node but not beyond. Its mushroom shape *(A)* is not atypical for a Spitz's nevus in a child, but the dense cellularity of the lesion near its base *(B)* with a high mitotic rate even in the deepest dermal nests is.

tral nucleoli. Papules composed of similar infiltrates occur as disseminated lesions affecting the skin and synovia in the condition known as multicentric reticulohistiocytosis. The hue of the cytoplasm of the cells in reticulohistiocytic granuloma and in multicentric reticulohistiocytosis is distinctive and has been referred to as "muddy rose," and its texture has been likened to ground glass (Fig. 18–40).

Intradermal Spitz's nevus and reticulohistiocytic granuloma can be distinguished by the presence of discrete nests of cells in Spitz's nevus rather than the sheets of cells found in

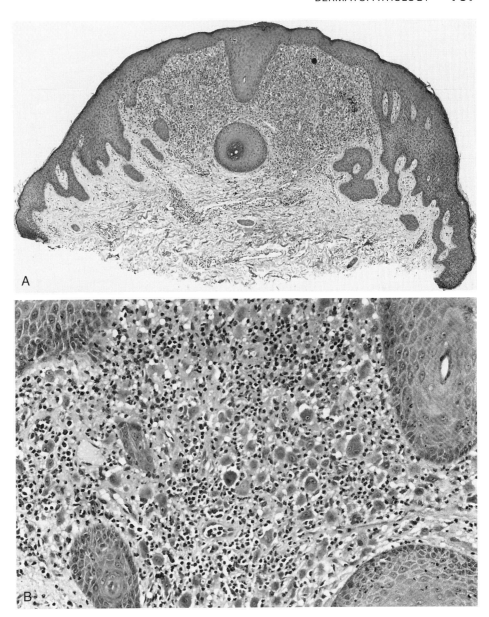

FIGURE 18–40. In solitary reticulohistiocytic granuloma, there are dome-shaped lesions formed by cells with abundant dense cytoplasm and large vesicular nuclei, as there are in Spitz's nevi *(A)*. Unlike in Spitz's nevi, eosinophils and neutrophils are found in the stroma *(B)*.

reticulohistiocytic granuloma. Nests of melanocytes are larger in the superficial portion of even an entirely intradermal Spitz's nevus than in its deeper areas, whereas no such gradient exists in reticulohistiocytic granuloma. Thickened collagen bundles separate aggregations of melanocytes in Spitz's nevus but are not present between the cells of reticulohistiocytic granuloma. In the event that immunoperoxidase stains are performed, it should be kept in mind that S-100 protein is occasionally detected in the cells of reticulohistiocytic granuloma, and that such "histiocytic" markers as alpha-1-antitrypsin and antichymotrypsin, lysozyme, and CD68 can be detected in neoplastic melanocytes.

Intradermal Spitz's nevi are particularly prone to be mistaken for **desmoplastic malignant melanoma** because both feature large melanocytes embedded in sclerotic stroma. There may be no apparent intraepidermal melanoma in as many as one half of desmoplastic melanomas, perhaps because the epidermis over these hard lesions is more apt to be abraded

by trauma, and the re-epithelialized surface may not contain melanocytes. Perineural invasion can occur in both conditions, although its extent is more limited in intradermal Spitz's nevi. The clinical presentation can be helpful in discriminating between these two sclerosing dermal melanocytic neoplasms. Desmoplastic malignant melanoma presents as ill-defined plaques, most often on the skin of the head and neck or trunk of middle-aged or older patients, in contrast with intradermal Spitz's nevi, which are discrete papules.

The arrangement of melanocytes in the dermis is the most useful aid in the histopathologic differential diagnosis between desmoplastic melanoma and intradermal Spitz's nevus.[52] Desmoplastic melanomas are usually poorly circumscribed and asymmetric, whereas intradermal Spitz's nevi usually have a symmetric inverted wedge shape. In intradermal Spitz's nevi, as alluded to earlier, there is an orderly diminution in the size of aggregations of melanocytes with descent into the dermis, whereas in desmoplastic malignant melanoma, aggregations of cells in the depths of a lesion can be larger than those in more superficial portions. Long fascicles of spindled melanocytes are present in desmoplastic malignant melanoma (Fig. 18–41), whereas only short ones are evident in intradermal Spitz's nevus.

Cytologic features are sometimes helpful in this differential diagnosis as well. The nuclei of intradermal Spitz's nevus are usually vesicular and have prominent nucleoli. Some cells contain eosinophilic inclusions, some of which are cross sections of cytoplasmic invaginations. Although the nuclei of melanocytes in desmoplastic melanoma can be bland by conventional cytologic criteria, some can be diffusely hyperchromatic, a finding rare in the cells of Spitz's nevi at any stage of development. Lastly, lymphocytic infiltrates in intradermal Spitz's nevi tend to be sparse and perivascular, whereas those in desmoplastic malignant melanoma are often dense, prominently interstitial, and asymmetrically distributed. Lymphoid follicles are nearly never seen in intradermal Spitz's nevi but occur frequently in the subcutis in desmoplastic melanoma.

MALIGNANT MELANOMA AND OTHER MELANOCYTIC PROLIFERATIONS ARISING IN CONGENITAL MELANOCYTIC NEVI

Congenital melanocytic nevi are malformations of the skin that are thought to result from faulty migration of melanocytes from the neural crest to the basal layer of the epidermis during embryogenesis. These wayward melanocytes are incorporated into the developing dermis and into its adnexa, which they also come to cluster around and within.

CLINICOPATHOLOGIC FEATURES. Congenital melanocytic nevi are arbitrarily classified as small, medium-sized, large, and giant.[55] Large and giant congenital nevi are more apt to show permeation of the deep reticular dermis and the septa of the subcutis by melanocytes. The risk of a melanoma developing in a congenital nevus may be proportionate to the number of melanocytes that constitute the lesion, and thus large congenital nevi give rise to most of the unusual melanocytic proliferations outlined later and to most melanomas that arise in the dermal portion of congenital nevi.

Congenital melanocytic nevi can give rise to several forms of benign melanocytic proliferation that can be mistaken for malignant melanoma, in addition to spawning authentic melanomas. **Simulants of malignant melanoma** arising in congenital nevi include lesions that show pagetoid spread of melanocytes within the epidermis,[56] superficial dermal nodules of large round or ovoid melanocytes with a high mitotic rate, and deep dermal nodules of small round melanocytes that resemble neuroblastoma.[57]

Benign intraepidermal melanocytic proliferations with **pagetoid patterns** were first noted in congenital nevi biopsied shortly after birth (Fig. 18–42). Similar changes have been noted by others in nevi from infants and even young children. The reason that such lesions are biopsied in the first place is that the area of pagetoid intraepidermal growth causes a circumscribed change in pigmentation within a large or medium-sized nevus. The melanocytes that are scattered in pagetoid array in these lesions have relatively monomorphous

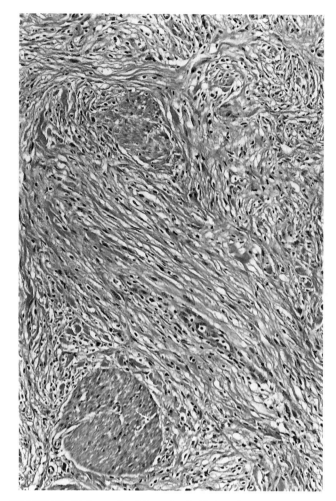

FIGURE 18–41. Long fascicles of spindled melanocytes occur in desmoplastic melanoma but not in Spitz's nevus.

nuclei and abundant pale cytoplasm. Lymphocytes are few, and pale-appearing melanocytes similar to those seen within the epidermis are present in the superficial dermis as small clusters. These cells merge with underlying elements more typical of the dermal component of a congenital nevus.

Proliferative nodules in the superficial portions of large or giant congenital nevi are evident clinically as papules (Fig. 18–43). Biopsy shows largely dermal sheets of melanocytes with slightly more abundant cytoplasm and somewhat more open nuclear chromatin patterns than is evident in the remainder of the nevus. Mitotic figures are also relatively increased in number but are morphologically normal. Lymphocytes are absent, and necrosis is not seen. At the base of these nodules, the melanocytes that constitute them blend with underlying smaller cells.

Other dermal nodules in the deep portions of large or giant congenital nevi have cells with pleomorphic, vesicular nuclei, abundant cytoplasm, and sometimes central foci of necrosis. It is difficult to offer prognostic information on such lesions, but when the mitotic rate is low, these lesions should not be reflexively diagnosed as melanoma (Fig. 18–44).

Large nodules termed proliferative **neurochristic hamartoma** can also occur in large congenital nevi and are usually evident at birth (Fig. 18–45). Polypoid, exophytic, and deeper

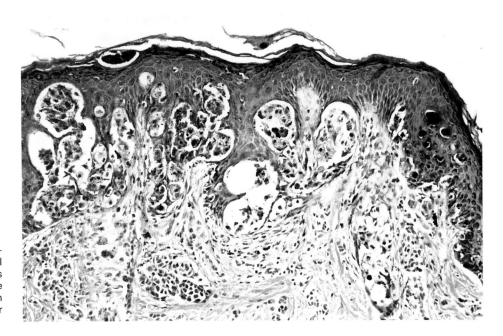

FIGURE 18–42. Pagetoid melanocytic proliferation in a congenital nevus can be misinterpreted as melanoma *in situ.* The large pale cells in the epidermis of this lesion gradually merged with smaller ones deeper in the dermis.

dermal nodular forms have been described.[58, 59] Schwannian differentiation of cytologically bland spindled cells is the preponderant finding, but cartilage, myeloid elements, and striated muscle all can occur in these pluripotential malformations.[57]

Deep dermal nodules of small round cells that resemble those of neuroblastoma but are biologically benign present as large rounded masses within truncal garment–sized nevi. Their cells are monomorphous with minute nucleoli and dispersed chromatin. As maturation occurs, spindled cells begin to predominate.

DIFFERENTIAL DIAGNOSIS. Pagetoid melanocytic proliferations in large congenital nevi in neonates, infants, and young children can be distinguished from melanoma arising in congenital nevi by the absence of lymphocytes and presence of melanocytes with monomorphous nuclei that diminish in size with descent into the dermis. Unlike **superficial spreading melanomas** with pagetoid melanocytes, there is no clear separation between the intraepidermal cells and those in the dermis around appendages.

Proliferative nodules of melanocytes arising in congenital nevi can be distinguished from nodules of malignant melanoma arising in the dermal component of congenital nevi by the absence of marked nuclear atypia, the presence of maturation in the deep portion of the nodule, and the absence of lymphocytes within or beneath the proliferation.

Dermal proliferations of small round cells resembling neuroblastoma and authentic melanomas composed of small round cells capable of metastasis can be difficult to distinguish. Metastatic disease has been documented in infants with congenital nevi in which there were proliferations of small round cells with a high mitotic rate and hyperchromatic nuclei. Until more precise criteria are worked out, cytologic features and mitotic rate are probably the best discriminant features.

Congenital neurochristic hamartomas, because of their composite nature, are difficult to confuse with other melanocytic proliferations arising in congenital nevi.

THE PATCH STAGE OF MYCOSIS FUNGOIDES

Mycosis fungoides is a form of cutaneous T-cell lymphoma that begins as a low-grade malignancy whose cells can grow only within the epidermis but that can eventuate in high-grade lymphoma with the capacity to spread to lymph nodes and viscera. The vast majority of cases have a mature helper T-cell phenotype. The earliest lesions of mycosis fungoides are macules and patches. Plaques and tumors eventuate in an unknown proportion of patients. As plaques and tumors develop, the cells of mycosis fungoides lose their epidermotropic properties and acquire the capacity to proliferate in dermal and extracutaneous environments.

CLINICOPATHOLOGIC FEATURES. Patches of mycosis fungoides are erythematous, slightly scaly, and sometimes wrinkled areas of skin that favor the buttocks, torso, and breasts. They tend to have diffuse margins. Some patches have areas of atrophy, mottled pigmentation, and telangiectasia known as poikiloderma vasculare atrophicans. Patches of mycosis fungoides can persist for many years without change.

The recognition of early patch stage mycosis fungoides is indeed difficult, but can be performed with reasonable accuracy if attention is paid to its characteristic features. It should be emphasized that at the current time there is no overriding advantage, in terms of prognosis, to making a heroic diagnosis of mycosis fungoides based on two or three lymphocytes that are in the wrong place at the wrong time. There are no convincing studies that show that the course of mycosis fungoides is affected by delays of a few months in treatment, but many of the modalities that are employed, such as topical chemotherapy, electron beam radiation, and systemic chemotherapy, have significant morbidity or potential side effects. Because some cases of patch stage mycosis fungoides are "obvious" to clinicians, pathologists are often pressured to make unequivocal diagnoses of that disease based on inadequate material.

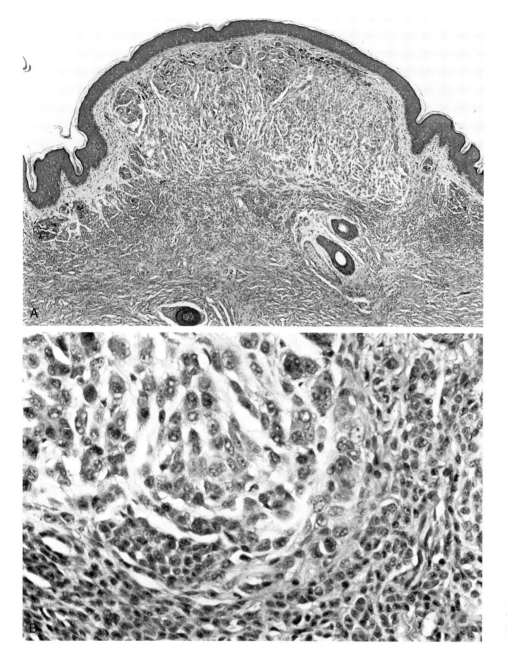

FIGURE 18–43. A papule formed by a proliferative focus in a large congenital nevus *(A)*. There is an abrupt transition between melanocytes with large vesicular nuclei and those with smaller, round nuclei at bottom *(B)*.

The very earliest recognizable changes in mycosis fungoides consist of a sparse infiltrate of small lymphocytes, often without discernible nuclear atypia, around vessels of the superficial plexus, within the papillary dermis, and lodged in the interstices between keratinocytes in the lower half of the epidermis.[60] These findings occur in a background without which a specific inference of mycosis fungoides cannot be made, namely fibrosis of the papillary dermis and slight, psoriasiform hyperplasia of the epidermis. The papillary dermis over most of the skin surface has thin, delicate bundles of collagen. In mycosis fungoides, they are replaced by coarse bundles that are haphazardly or horizontally arranged. The psoriasiform hyperplasia of mycosis fungoides is distinctive. Rete ridges are thin and only slightly elongated.

In early patches of mycosis fungoides, lymphocytes are usually scattered singly within the epidermis or in collections of two or three cells. A distinctive pattern that they can assume has been termed "pearls on a string" and consists of cells linearly arranged on the epidermal side of the basement membrane, without cytopathic effects such as vacuolar change or necrosis of keratinocytes, as would be evident in an interface dermatitis (Fig. 18–46).[61] Early patches of mycosis fungoides are almost wholly composed of lymphocytes. Eosinophils and plasma cells are generally found only in late patches and tumors of mycosis fungoides, respectively.

In late patches of mycosis fungoides, the diagnosis is far easier, because atypia of lymphocytes is the rule rather than the exception, collections of lymphocytes termed Pautrier's microabscesses appear, and the infiltrates within the papillary dermis tend to become band-like.

Poikilodermatous patches of mycosis fungoides feature many findings associated with regression of neoplasms in the

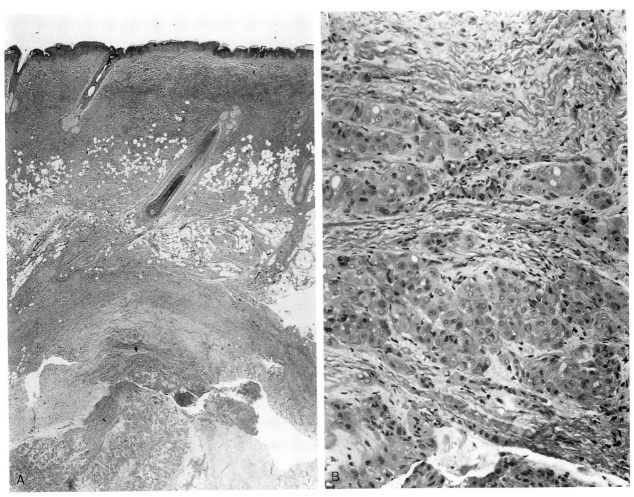

FIGURE 18-44. A nodule has arisen in the subcutaneous portion of this large congenital nevus *(A)*. Large vesicular nuclei are present in the cells of this nodule, which also have small vacuoles in their cytoplasm *(B)*. The cells expressed S-100 protein and HMB-45 but also stained with commercial anti-keratin sera. Unusual nodular proliferations arising in congenital nevi in children, such as this one, should not be assumed to represent melanoma.

skin, such as a diminished rete ridge pattern, marked thickening and fibrosis of the papillary dermis, telangiectases, and melanophages. Sometimes these changes are all that are seen, and a specific diagnosis of mycosis fungoides cannot be made. If a biopsy specimen is of sufficient size, there are often diagnostic findings such as clusters of lymphocytes in the epidermis or lymphocytes aligned along the epidermal side of the junctional zone.

DIFFERENTIAL DIAGNOSIS. Foremost in the differential diagnosis of early patch stage mycosis fungoides are the conditions known to clinicians as **eczematous dermatitis** and known to pathologists and dermatopathologists as the **spongiotic dermatitides.** There are perhaps two dozen inflammatory skin diseases that have spongiotic dermatitis as their principal histopathology. Of these, the ones most commonly confused clinically with mycosis fungoides are **chronic cases of allergic contact dermatitis, chronic nummular dermatitis,** and **small plaque parapsoriasis.**

Allergic contact dermatitis is readily diagnosed by dermatologists when a history of contact exposure is clear-cut or when the pattern of the eruption (i.e., linear, sharply marginated, or geometric) suggests exposure to an exogenous compound. In acute allergic contact dermatitis, there are often vesicles, which practically never are found in mycosis fun-

goides. However, contact dermatitis develops in some patients because they are exposed to minute dosages of contactants over long periods, and despite patch testing, may defy diagnosis.

Nummular dermatitis is a condition whose coin-shaped lesions with scaling, weeping, or crusted surfaces are usually diagnosed clinically. Some long-standing lesions of nummular dermatitis are less obviously eczematous and may be confused with those of mycosis fungoides.

Small plaque parapsoriasis is a condition in which persistent, pink, tan, or yellow, almost imperceptibly raised and slightly scaling lesions occur on the skin of the trunk. Elongated forms are termed **digitate dermatosis.** Although the benignity of this condition has been assumed, some consider it to be an indolent form of patch stage mycosis fungoides.[62]

Spongiotic dermatitis evolves through acute, subacute, and chronic stages. It is the chronic stage that can be mistaken histopathologically for mycosis fungoides. Chronic spongiotic dermatitis, like patch stage mycosis fungoides, features superficial perivascular lymphocytic infiltrates, spongiosis, and compact or lamellar hyperkeratosis. Sometimes areas of the papillary dermis become fibrotic, heightening the resemblance. Important differential findings include the following:

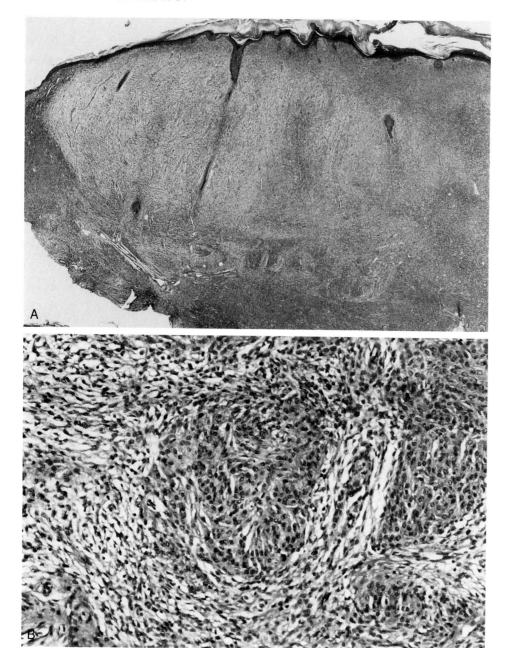

FIGURE 18-45. Proliferative neurochristic hamartoma arising in a large congenital nevus *(A)*. There are small spindled cells and, centrally, round ones forming rosette-like arrangements *(B)*. Unusual forms of mesenchymal differentiation can occur in such areas.

1. Although spongiosis occurs in both conditions, in mycosis fungoides there are disproportionately numerous lymphocytes compared with the degree of spongiosis.

2. Lymphocytes in patch stage mycosis fungoides are commonly arranged linearly above the dermoepidermal junction but not in chronic spongiotic dermatitides.

3. Mounds of parakeratosis that contain serum are commonly found in spongiotic dermatitis but are unusual in mycosis fungoides; indeed, if they are present, indisputable cytologic atypia of lymphocytic nuclei should be present for an outright diagnosis of mycosis fungoides to be rendered. Similar caveats apply for the presence of spongiotic microvesiculation and papillary dermal edema.

4. The infiltrates of allergic contact and nummular dermatitis almost frequently contain eosinophils; only late patches of mycosis fungoides do.

5. Collections of mononuclear cells occur in both conditions, but those due to spongiosis are often heterogeneous in composition and have vase- or flask-like shapes because hydrostatic pressure causes them to rupture laterally as they ascend to the cornified layer.[63]

6. Lymphocytes in acute allergic contact or nummular dermatitis can ascend into the superficial spinous layer but are seen beneath a basket-weave cornified layer in that setting; in mycosis fungoides, they can ascend similarly, but the overlying cornified layer is compact or lamellated.[64]

Adjunctive techniques, such as immunohistochemistry, flow cytometry, and nuclear contour index determination, are of limited benefit in resolving this difficult differential diagnosis. Whereas densely infiltrated specimens can be subjected to

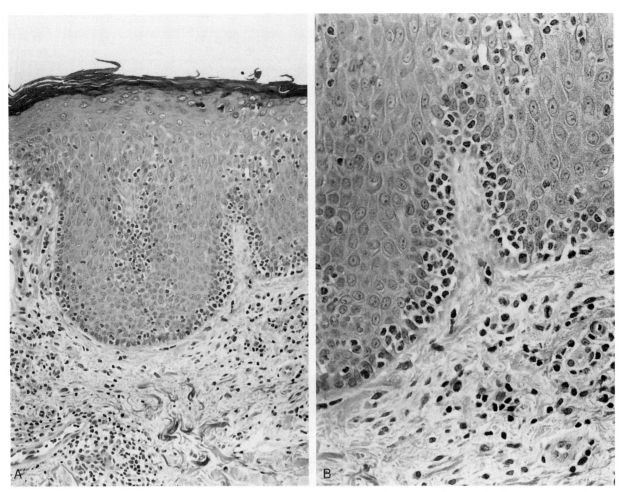

FIGURE 18–46. The patch stage of mycosis fungoides has many histopathologic patterns, but psoriasiform epidermal hyperplasia overlying patchy band-like infiltrates within a fibrotic papillary dermis is one of the more common ones *(A)*. Lymphocytes lie on the epidermal side of the basement membrane, without discernible cytopathic effect, i.e., there is little in the way of vacuolar change and there are few necrotic keratinocytes. This arrangement has been called "pearls on a strand" *(B)*.

T-cell receptor gene rearrangement studies, sparsely infiltrated patches cannot at this time be reliably assessed for clonality. The "gold standard" for the diagnosis of patch stage mycosis fungoides remains light microscopy correlated with clinical information.[61]

References

1. Winkelmann RK, Reizner GT: Diffuse dermal neutrophilia in urticaria. Hum Pathol 19:389–393, 1988.
2. Monroe EW, Schulz CI, Maize JC, Jordon RE: Vasculitis in chronic urticaria: An immunopathological study. J Invest Dermatol 76:528–533, 1981.
3. Lawley TJ, Hertz KC, Wade TR, et al: Pruritic urticarial papules and plaques of pregnancy. JAMA 241:1696–1699, 1979.
4. Patterson JW, Parsons JM, Blaylock WK, Mills AS: Eosinophils in erythema multiforme. Arch Pathol Lab Med 113:36–39, 1989.
5. LeBoit PE: Interface dermatitis. How specific are its histopathologic features? [editorial]. Arch Dermatol 129:1324–1328, 1993.
6. Ackerman AB, Penneys NS, Clark WH: Erythema multiforme exudativum: A distinctive pathological process. Br J Dermatol 84:544–566, 1971.
7. Lyell A: Toxic epidermal necrolysis (the scalded skin syndrome): A reappraisal. Br J Dermatol 100:69–86, 1979.
8. Ragaz A, Ackerman AB: Evolution, maturation and regression of lesions of psoriasis. Am J Dermatopathol 1:199–214, 1979.
9. Perdace FJ, Perry HO: Granuloma faciale: A clinical and histopathologic review. Arch Dermatol 94:387–395, 1966.
10. LeBoit PE, Yen TSB, Wintroub B: The evolution of lesions in erythema elevatum diutinum. Am J Dermatopathol 8:392–402, 1986.
11. LeBoit PE, Cockerell CJ: Nodular lesions of erythema elevatum diutinum in patients infected with the human immunodeficiency virus. J Am Acad Dermatol 28:919–922, 1993.
12. Chu P, Conelly KC, LeBoit, PE: The histopathologic spectrum of palisaded neutrophilic and granulomatous dermatitis in patients with connective tissue disease. Arch Dermatol. 130:1278–1283, 1994.
13. Finan MC, Winkelmann RK: The cutaneous extravascular necrotizing granuloma (Churg-Strauss syndrome). Report and analysis of 30 cases. Medicine 62:142–158, 1983.
14. Smith ML, Jorizzo JL, Semble E, et al: Rheumatoid papules: Lesions showing features of vasculitis and palisading granuloma. J Am Acad Dermatol 20:348–352, 1989.
15. Walsh N, Ackerman AB: Infundibulocystic basal cell carcinoma: A newly described variant. Mod Pathol 3:599–608, 1990.
16. Mrak RE, Baker GF: Granular cell basal cell carcinoma. J Cutan Pathol 14:37–42, 1987.
17. Barnadas MA, Freeman RG: Clear cell basal cell epithelioma: Light and electron microscopic study of an unusual variant. J Cutan Pathol 15:1–7, 1988.
18. Barr RJ, Alpern KS, Santa Cruz DJ, Fretzin DF: Clear cell basal cell carcinoma: An unusual degenerative variant. J Cutan Pathol 20:308–316, 1993.
19. Heenan PJ, Bogle MS: Eccrine differentiation in basal cell carcinoma. J Invest Dermatol 100:295S–299S, 1993.
20. Brownstein MH: Basaloid follicular hamartoma: Solitary and multiple types. J Am Acad Dermatol 27:237–240, 1992.
21. LeBoit PE, Barr RJ, Burall S, et al: Primitive polypoid granular-cell tumor and other cutaneous granular-cell neoplasms of apparent nonneural origin. Am J Surg Pathol 15:48–58, 1991.
22. Manivel C, Wick MR, Mukai K: Pilomatrix carcinoma: An immunohistochemical comparison with benign pilomatrixoma and other benign cutaneous neoplasms of pilar origin. J Cutan Pathol 13:22–29, 1986.
23. Goldstein DJ, Barr RJ, Santa Cruz DJ: Microcystic adnexal carcinoma: A distinct clinicopathological entity. Cancer 50:556–572, 1982.

24. Cooper PH: Sclerosing eccrine carcinoma of sweat ducts (microcystic adnexal carcinoma). Arch Dermatol 122:261–264, 1986.
25. LeBoit PE, Sexton M: Microcystic adnexal carcinoma of the skin. A reappraisal of the differentiation and differential diagnosis of an underrecognized neoplasm. J Am Acad Dermatol 29:609–618, 1993.
26. Brownstein MH, Shapiro L: Desmoplastic trichoepithelioma. Cancer 40:2979–2986, 1977.
27. Takei Y, Fukushiro S, Ackerman AB: Criteria for histologic differentiation of desmoplastic trichoepithelioma (sclerosing epithelial hamartoma) from morphea-like basal cell carcinoma. Am J Dermatopathol 7:207–221, 1985.
28. Sexton M, Maize JC: Papillary eccrine adenoma. A light microscopic and immuno-histochemical study. J Am Acad Dermatol 18:1114–1120, 1988.
29. Weidner N, Foucar E: Adenosquamous carcinoma of the skin. Arch Dermatol 121:775–779, 1985.
30. Banks ER, Cooper PH: Adenosquamous carcinoma of the skin: A report of 10 cases. J Cutan Pathol 18:227–234, 1990.
31. Kamino H: Dermatofibroma extending into the subcutaneous tissue. Differential diagnosis from dermatofibrosarcoma protuberans. Am J Surg Pathol 14:1156–1164, 1990.
32. Wrotonowski U, Cooper PH, Shmookler BM: Fibrosarcomatous change in derma-tofibrosarcoma protuberans. Am J Surg Pathol 12:287–293, 1988.
33. Aiba S, Tabata N, Ishii H, et al: Dermatofibrosarcoma protuberans is a unique fibrohistiocytic tumour expressing CD34. Br J Dermatol 127:79–84, 1992.
34. Kutzner H: Expression of the human progenitor cell antigen CD34 (HPCA-1) distinguishes dermatofibrosarcoma protuberans from fibrous histiocytoma in formalin-fixed paraffin-embedded tissue. J Am Acad Dermatol 28:613–617, 1993.
35. Altman DA, Nickoloff BJ, Fivenson DP: Differential expression of factor XIIIa and CD34 in cutaneous mesenchymal tumors. J Cutan Pathol 20:154–158, 1993.
36. Franquemont DW, Cooper PH, Shmookler BM, Wick MR: Benign fibrous histiocy-toma of the skin with potential for local recurrence: A tumor to be distinguished from dermatofibroma. Mod Pathol 3:158–162, 1990.
37. Fletcher CDM: Benign fibrous histiocytoma of subcutaneous and deep soft tissue: A clinicopathologic analysis of 21 cases. Am J Surg Pathol 14:801–809, 1990.
38. Kamino H, Reddy VB, Gero M, Alba Greco M: Dermatomyofibroma: A benign cutaneous, plaque-like proliferation of fibroblasts and myofibroblasts in young adults. J Cutan Pathol 19:85–93, 1992.
39. Gottlieb GJ, Ackerman AB: Subtle clues to diagnosis in dermatopathology: The patch stage of Kaposi's sarcoma. Am J Dermatopathol 1:165–172, 1979.
40. Kao GF, Johnson FB, Sulica VI: The nature of hyaline (eosinophilic) globules and vascular slits of Kaposi's sarcoma. Am J Dermatopathol 12:256–267, 1990.
41. Gottlieb GJ, Ackerman AB: Kaposi's Sarcoma: A Text and Atlas. Philadelphia, Lea & Febiger, 1988.
42. Blumenfeld W, Egbert BM, Sagebiel RW: Differential diagnosis of Kaposi's sar-coma. Arch Pathol Lab Med 109:123–127, 1984.
43. Penneys NS, Bernstein H, Leonardi C: Confirmation of early Kaposi's sarcoma by polyclonal antibody to type IV collagen. J Am Acad Dermatol 19:447–450, 1988.
44. Koehler JE, Quinn FD, Berger TG, et al: Isolation of Rochalimaea species from cutaneous and osseous lesions of bacillary angiomatosis. N Engl J Med 327:1625–1631, 1992.
45. LeBoit PE, Berger TG, Egbert BM, et al: Bacillary angiomatosis. The histopathology and differential diagnosis of a pseudoneoplastic infection in patients with human immunodeficiency virus disease. Am J Surg Pathol 13:909–920, 1989.
46. LeBoit PE, Berger TG, Egbert BM, et al: Epithelioid haemangioma-like vascular proliferation in AIDS: Manifestation of cat scratch disease bacillus infection? Lancet 1:960–963, 1988.
47. Spitz S: Melanomas of childhood. Am J Pathol 24:591–609, 1948.
48. Barnhill RL, Barnhill MA, Berwick M, Mihm MC: The histologic spectrum of pigmented spindle cell nevus. Hum Pathol 22:52–58, 1991.
49. Smith KJ, Barrett TL, Skelton HGI: Spindle cell and epithelioid cell nevi with atypia and metastasis (malignant Spitz nevus). Am J Surg Pathol 13:931–939, 1989.
50. Panaigo-Pereira C, Maize JC, Ackerman AB: Nevus of large spindle and/or epitheli-oid cells (Spitz's nevus). Arch Dermatol 114:1811–1823, 1978.
51. Kamino H, Flotte TJ, Mischeloff E: Eosinophilic globules in Spitz's nevi. New findings and a diagnostic sign. Am J Dermatopathol 1:319–324, 1979.
52. Barr RJ, Morales RV, Graham JH: Desmoplastic nevus. A distinct histologic variant of mixed spindle cell and epithelioid cell nevus. Cancer 46:557–564, 1980.
53. White WL: Sophie's choice, Rorschach's choice. Am J Dermatopathol 12:630–633, 1990.
54. Purvis WE, Helwig EB: Reticulohistiocytic granuloma (''reticulohistiocytoma'') of the skin. Am J Clin Pathol 24:1005–1015, 1954.
55. Kopf AW, Bart RS, Henessey P: Congenital nevocytic nevi and melanocytic and malignant melanomas. J Am Acad Dermatol 1:123–130, 1979.
56. Silvers DN, Helwig EB: Melanocytic nevi in neonates. J Am Acad Dermatol 4:166–175, 1981.
57. Hendrickson MR, Ross JC: Neoplasms arising in congenital giant nevi. Morphologic study of seven cases and a review of the literature. Am J Surg Pathol 5:109–135, 1981.
58. Clark WH, Elder DE, Guerry, D: Dysplastic nevi and malignant melanoma. In Farmer ER, Hood AF (eds): Pathology of the Skin. Norwalk, CT, Appleton and Lange, 1988, pp 731–735.
59. Manciani M-L, Clark WH, Hayes FA, Herlyn M: Malignant melanoma simulants arising in congenital nevi do not show experimental evidence for a malignant phenotype. Am J Pathol 136:817–829, 1990.
60. Sanchez J, Ackerman AB: The patch stage of mycosis fungoides: Criteria for histologic diagnosis. Am J Dermatopathol 1:5–26, 1979.
61. Nickoloff BJ: Light-microscopic assessment of 100 patients with patch/plaque-stage mycosis fungoides. Am J Dermatopathol 10:469–477, 1988.
62. King-Ismael D, Ackerman AB: Guttate parapsoriasis/digitate dermatosis (small plaque parapsoriasis) is mycosis fungoides. Am J Dermatopathol 14:518–530, 1992.
63. LeBoit PE, Epstein BA: A vase-like shape characterizes the epidermal-mononuclear cell collections seen in spongiotic dermatitis. Am J Dermatopathol 12:612–616, 1990.
64. LeBoit PE: Cutaneous lymphomas and their histopathologic imitators. Semin Der-matol 5:322–333, 1986.

CHAPTER 19

Lymph Node

Lawrence M. Weiss, M.D., Karen L. Chang, M.D., and Daniel A. Arber, M.D.

One of the most important factors in the accurate assessment of diagnostic lymph node biopsies is the proper preparation of the specimen. Preferably, lymph node biopsies should be received fresh, immersed in saline (and not on a dry towel or sponge), and processed immediately by the pathology laboratory. We have found that the choice of fixative is much less important than attention to thin trimming of the specimen and proper fixation. We find neutral buffered formalin to be a perfectly acceptable fixative and prefer it in cases in which Hodgkin's disease is in the differential diagnosis. If a second fixative is to be used, we prefer B5 fixative, because it allows superior preservation of antigens, but other metal-based fixatives are also adequate. The majority of diagnostic lymph node biopsies can be resolved by the light microscopic appearance, and the majority of the remainder of cases can be resolved by a combination of histopathology and paraffin section immunohistochemistry. Some suggested paraffin section immunohistochemical panels are outlined in Table 19–1. In a minority of cases, studies that can be performed only on frozen tissue or cell suspensions are necessary for the diagnosis. We prefer the former, because one may easily snap-freeze a small piece of tissue, and retrieve it later if additional studies are necessary. Studies that can be performed on frozen tissue include a wider variety of monoclonal antibodies than can be applied to paraffin tissues and molecular studies such as analysis of the lymphocyte antigen receptor genes. It is often useful to send a small sterile piece of tissue for microbiologic studies. Cytogenetics also requires sterile tissue and may be helpful in some cases.

When confronted with a diagnostically difficult lymph node biopsy, one should concentrate on making distinctions that are clinically relevant. Some suggested algorithms are given in Tables 19–2, 19–3, and 19–4. Subclassification of Hodgkin's disease is of little clinical relevance today once the nodular, lymphocyte predominance subtype is separated from cases of classic Hodgkin's disease. Similarly, subclassification of non-Hodgkin's lymphoma, after a few important clinicopathologic entities are separated from one another, is also less important (see Table 19–3). When possible, however, cases of non-Hodgkin's lymphoma should be classified according to a standard system such as the Working Formulation or an updated modification shown in Table 19–4.[1] The clinical importance of the immunologic differentiation of B-cell lymphoma versus T-cell lymphoma is still debated among experts in the field and is not a crucial distinction for the large majority of clinicians. In some cases, a definitive diagnosis cannot be established, even after consultation with expert hematopathologists and the performance of all relevant special studies. In these cases, one must acknowledge the uncertainty rather than committing to one diagnosis and hoping for the best. Clinicians may select a treatment regimen that is relatively effective against both Hodgkin's disease and non-Hodgkin's lymphoma if distinction between the two is not possible. Expressed uncertainty can also facilitate rebiopsy if clinically indicated, either immediately or at a later time.

FROZEN SECTION

It is possible to render frozen section diagnoses on lymph node biopsies. The diagnosis may be obvious, such as with a gland-forming metastatic adenocarcinoma or a pigmented metastatic malignant melanoma. However, even in lymphoid lesions, a diagnosis may be possible. We recommend that only a small piece of the tissue be used for the frozen section examination. If necessary, this tissue may be retained frozen for possible future studies. In the rapid evaluation of lymphoid lesions, we urge the performance of scrape preparations or, less preferably, touch imprints in conjunction with the frozen section. Scrape preparations or touch imprints offer superior cytologic detail, whereas the frozen sections provide information concerning the architectural appearance. Regardless of whether or not a diagnosis may be rendered, we always try to determine whether diagnostic tissue has been obtained. When clinical circumstances warrant a rapid diagnosis, we attempt to offer as much of a diagnosis as required to answer the clinical question but do not attempt subtle subclassifications. For example, we believe that a rapid diagnosis of Hodgkin's disease is possible, but subclassification is best deferred until paraffin sections are available (Fig. 19–1).

MALIGNANT LYMPHOMA VERSUS OTHER NEOPLASM

One of the most common problems in surgical pathology is the **undifferentiated malignant neoplasm** involving a lymph node. While in the not-so-distant past, the pathologist often guessed that the tumor was probably a poorly differentiated carcinoma or threw up his or her hands in defeat, the accurate diagnosis of these cases is now well within the capabilities of every surgical pathologist who has access to paraffin immunohistochemistry. With immunohistochemistry, we now recognize a greater spectrum of architectural features of

Table 19–1. **Suggested Panels for Paraffin Section Immunohistochemistry**

Undifferentiated neoplasm	CD45/45RB, keratin, S-100, CD30, (CD20, CD43)
Hodgkin's vs. non-Hodgkin's	CD45/45RB, CD30, CD15, CD20, CD43
Non-Hodgkin's, general	CD45/45RB, CD30, CD20, CD43
Nodular lymphocyte predominance	CD45/45RB, CD20, CD43, CD15
Follicular lymphoma	CD20, CD43, BCL-2
T-cell lymphoma	CD45/45RB, CD30, CD20, CD43, CD45RO
Acute leukemia	CD45/45RB, CD43, CD15, CD68, CD34, myeloperoxidase
Diffuse B-cell lymphoma	CD20, CD43, (CD45RA)
Large-cell lymphoma	CD20, CD45RO, CD43, CD30, epithelial membrane antigen

Parentheses signify optional antibody or antibodies to be ordered with initial screening panel.

Table 19–2. **Practical Approach to Lymph Node Diagnosis**

Is it malignant, benign, or indeterminate?
 I. Malignant
  A. Definitely Hodgkin's
   1. Rye classification
   2. Special variant?
  B. Definitely non-Hodgkin's
   1. Simple classification
   2. Working formulation
   3. Special variant?
  C. Hodgkin's vs. non-Hodgkin's
   1. Consultant?
   2. Rebiopsy?
 II. Benign
  A. Specific pattern?
  B. Specific diagnosis?
 III. Indeterminate
  A. Consultant?
  B. Rebiopsy? Process tissue differently?

Table 19–3. **Simple Classification of Non-Hodgkin's Lymphomas**

1. Low to intermediate grade
  a. Small lymphocytic neoplasms, including mantle cell
  b. Follicular
2. Intermediate to high grade
  a. Diffuse, mixed small- and large-cell
  b. Diffuse, large-cell, including immunoblastic
3. High grade
  a. Lymphoblastic lymphoma
  b. Small, non-cleaved cell lymphoma.

Table 19–4. **Working Formulation for Non-Hodgkin's Lymphomas, with Modifications**

Low grade
Small lymphocytic
  Plasmacytoid
Follicular, predominantly small cleaved cell
Follicular, mixed small cleaved and large-cell
Intermediate grade
Mantle cell lymphoma
Diffuse, predominantly small cleaved cell type (rare)
Diffuse, mixed small cleaved and large-cell type
  Epithelioid cell component
  Polymorphous immunocytoma
Diffuse, predominantly large-cell type
High grade
Large-cell, immunoblastic
  Plasmacytoid
  Clear-cell
  Polymorphous
  Epithelioid cell (rare)
  Anaplastic large cell
Lymphoblastic
Small non-cleaved cell
  Burkitt
  Non-Burkitt

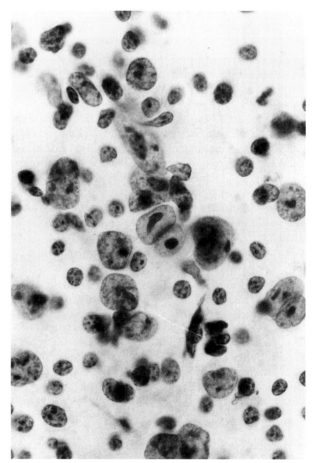

FIGURE 19–1. Hodgkin's disease seen on scrape preparation. Numerous Hodgkin's cells are seen, including a so-called diagnostic Reed-Sternberg cell.

lymphoma than had been appreciated in the past. Cases of malignant lymphoma may show nesting (in-between bands of sclerosis) (Fig. 19–2), a prominent or exclusively sinusoidal architecture (particularly in anaplastic large-cell lymphoma), and even spindling (also in anaplastic large-cell lymphoma). The most helpful features for the diagnosis of lymphoma are the cytologic characteristics of the neoplastic cells. In cases of lymphoma, the neoplastic cells often possess multiple nucleoli and vesicular nuclei that vary in appearance from cell to cell. Although carcinomas may also have vesicular nuclei, the nuclei are usually more monomorphic from cell to cell and often contain only a single nucleolus. In malignant melanoma, the nuclei are usually vesicular with a prominent nucleolus, and often one can identify pseudoinclusions of the cytoplasm in the nucleus if one searches diligently. Hodgkin's disease, particularly the syncytial variant of nodular sclerosing, may also present as an undifferentiated tumor in a lymph node. Morphologic clues that might suggest Hodgkin's disease would include subtotal involvement of the node, admixed inflammatory cells, particularly eosinophils, and areas of necrosis directly adjacent to the neoplastic cells.

We recommend the performance of a panel of antibodies in any case for which there is a question as to the type of tumor present, particularly because the clinical implications

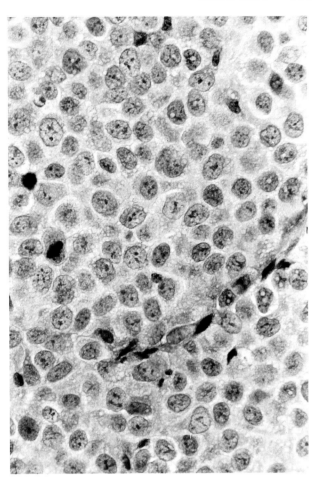

FIGURE 19–3. Malignant melanoma. The histologic features are completely unrevealing—this case lacked features that might suggest the correct diagnosis: melanin pigment, cytoplasmic pseudonuclear inclusions, or prominent eosinophilic nucleoli. Immunostudies performed in this case revealed strong vimentin, S-100, and HMB45 positivity along with keratin and CD45/45RB negativity, providing strong support for the diagnosis of malignant melanoma.

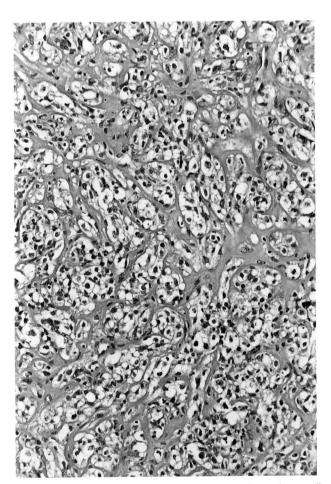

FIGURE 19–2. Sclerosing large-cell lymphoma from the mediastinum with compartmentalization. This appearance may closely mimic carcinoma, neuroendocrine tumor, or other non-lymphomatous neoplasms.

are so great (Fig. 19–3). Although we tailor our panels to the individual case, a CD45/45RB (leukocyte common antigen), keratin, and S-100 stain would constitute an adequate screening panel for most cases. Cases negative with these stains could be investigated further with CD30 (for anaplastic large-cell lymphoma and Hodgkin's disease), CD15 (for Hodgkin's disease and myeloid leukemia, with the caveat that some carcinomas may be CD15-positive), CD43 (for myeloid leukemia and CD45/45RB-negative T-cell lymphoma) and CD20 (for CD45/45RB-negative B-cell lymphoma), and vimentin (for sarcoma and rare S-100–negative malignant melanoma).

If a positive keratin stain is obtained, carcinoma is the most likely diagnosis. In the head and neck, an occult nasopharyngeal primary should be considered; studies for Epstein-Barr virus genomes might prove confirmatory. In an axillary lymph node from a woman, breast carcinoma should be the foremost consideration; however, estrogen receptor immunocytochemical assays and breast-specific monoclonal antibodies are usually negative in the most poorly differentiated breast carcinomas. If embryonal carcinoma is in the differential diagnosis, a CD30 or placental alkaline phosphatase stain may be useful,

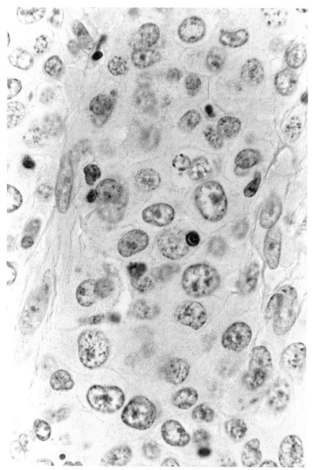

FIGURE 19–4. Immunoblastic lymphoma with keratin staining. Scattered cells show paranuclear dot-like staining for keratin. This case was CD45/45RB-negative, further complicating the diagnosis. Molecular studies revealed clonal immunoglobulin heavy chain gene rearrangements, confirming the diagnosis of lymphoma.

because these antibodies may be positive in this neoplasm. Monoclonal antibody studies for prostate-specific antigen and prostatic acid phosphatase should be performed in older men with carcinomas of unknown origin. One must also keep in mind that a pattern of dot-like cytoplasmic positivity for keratin may be seen in multiple myeloma, highly plasmacytic lymphomas, and rare cases of anaplastic large-cell lymphoma that may also be CD45/45RB-negative (Fig. 19–4). Stains for immunoglobulin light and heavy chains, epithelial membrane antigen, and CD30 may be useful in evaluating these possibilities.

SMALL LYMPHOCYTIC PROLIFERATIONS

There has been a large amount of attention given to small lymphocytic proliferations in the recent hematopathology literature. For the purposes of this discussion, we include lymph node involvement by chronic lymphocytic leukemia, small lymphocytic lymphoma, small lymphocytic lymphoma with plasmacytoid differentiation, mantle cell lymphoma, and monocytoid B-cell lymphoma in this category. By far, the most important distinction to make is the differentiation of a

reactive from a neoplastic proliferation, and fortunately, this is usually easy in lymph node biopsies, although it is often much more difficult in extranodal sites.

Small lymphocytic lymphoma and lymph node involvement by **chronic lymphocytic leukemia** are cytologically indistinguishable from one another; the distinction is based on the absence or presence, respectively, of an absolute lymphocytosis in the peripheral blood or on the extent of marrow involvement. In virtually all cases of these two diseases, complete architectural effacement of the lymph node by a diffuse proliferation of small lymphocytes is seen.[2, 3] Capsular transgression is typical and is often massive in degree. Residual germinal centers may be present in approximately 10% of cases, with obliteration of the mantle zone generally present in those cases. Sinuses are generally not patent but may be seen in approximately 10% of cases. In approximately one half of cases, paler regions that have been termed pseudofollicular proliferation centers are present. These areas tend to be ill-defined and do not possess the mantle zones seen in true germinal centers.

The proliferating cell in small lymphocytic lymphoma and lymph node involvement by chronic lymphocytic leukemia is a small, round lymphocyte, usually morphologically indistinguishable from normal resting lymphocytes (Fig. 19–5). Occasionally, the small cells have minor degrees of chromatin abnormalities, but they are homogeneous from one cell to

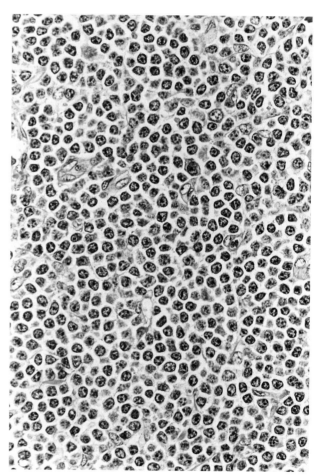

FIGURE 19–5. Small lymphocytic lymphoma. A population of small, round lymphocytes is seen.

another. The mitotic rate is almost always low, consistent with a low-grade lymphoma. These cells are a prominent feature within the pseudofollicular proliferation centers but may also be found scattered among the small lymphocytes in the diffuse areas. These larger cells usually have a round nuclear contour and often contain one or sometimes several prominent nucleoli.

The architectural effacement, along with the monotony of the cellular infiltrate, usually distinguishes lymph node involvement by chronic lymphocytic leukemia or small lymphocytic lymphoma from a reactive process. In doubtful cases, paraffin section immunophenotyping studies can be of great use. The vast majority, if not all cases, of lymph node involvement by chronic lymphocytic leukemia or small lymphocytic lymphoma are B-lineage neoplasms. Therefore, the demonstration of an extensive B-lineage infiltrate outside of the germinal centers is strong evidence for a B-cell lymphoma. Furthermore, a majority of these cases show co-expression of CD43 and CD20.[4] In frozen sections, light chain restriction and aberrant expression of CD5 are almost always present.[5]

A more difficult differential diagnosis is the distinction between lymph node involvement of chronic lymphocytic leukemia or small lymphocytic lymphoma and transformation to a high-grade lymphoma.[3, 6] This transformation, termed **Richter's syndrome,** portends a poor prognosis and occurs in approximately 10% of patients with chronic lymphocytic leukemia and possibly a smaller percentage of patients with small lymphocytic lymphoma. In these cases, the small cell–to–large cell ratio becomes reversed, so that large cells, often with prominent nucleoli, represent the dominant histologic finding, with only a minority of small lymphocytes still present. However, scattered large cells may be commonly found in small lymphocytic lymphoma, and their presence, in the absence of formation of sheets of these cells, does not constitute sufficient evidence for a diagnosis of transformation (Fig. 19–6). Occasionally, the Richter's transformation takes on the appearance of intermediate-sized cells, termed paraimmunoblasts or prolymphocytes by some; the prognosis in these cases appears to be better than that seen with large-cell transformation.[7]

In **small lymphocytic lymphoma with plasmacytoid differentiation,** diffuse effacement is present, and pseudofollicular proliferation centers are usually absent. The proliferating cells of this low-grade lymphoma may be a mixture of small lymphocytes, plasmacytoid lymphocytes, and plasma cells (lymphoplasmacytic variant) or a homogeneous population of plasmacytoid lymphocytes (lymphoplasmacytoid variant) (Fig. 19–7). Intranuclear immunoglobulin inclusions **(Dutcher bodies)** and cytoplasmic immunoglobulin inclusions **(Russell bodies)** may be present and are a helpful clue to the plasmacytic nature of the cells. Scattered epithelioid histiocytes and mast cells may also be present.

In occasional cases, varying numbers of larger lymphoid cells with plasmacytoid features, including plasmacytoid immunoblasts, may be present. When equal numbers of these cells are present, we prefer to classify the lymphoma as intermediate grade (diffuse, mixed small- and large-cell lymphoma, with plasmacytoid features) in the Working Formulation.

Small lymphocytic lymphoma with plasmacytoid features at times may be difficult to distinguish from reactive plasmacytic proliferations. In addition to the paraffin section immunohistochemical studies mentioned earlier for small lymphocytic lymphoma, staining for immunoglobulin light chains in the paraffin sections is usually helpful, owing to the plasmacytic nature of the proliferation. Demonstration of light chain restriction is diagnostic of malignant lymphoma in this setting.

Mantle cell lymphoma is a recently coined term for a malignant lymphoma that has been known under many different names, including germinoma, centrocytic lymphoma, mantle zone lymphoma, intermediate lymphocytic lymphoma, and intermediately differentiated lymphocytic lymphoma.[8] Although the data are sparse, many hematopathologists regard this lymphoma as an intermediate-grade lymphoma, particularly when the proliferation is diffuse, based on some studies that show a median survival of less than 5 years.[8–10] However, similar to low-grade lymphomas, a plateau in the survival curve is not seen, and there is a continuing relapse rate over time. This lymphoma may show either a mantle zone architectural pattern (mantle zone lymphoma) or a diffuse pattern (intermediate lymphocytic lymphoma).[8–10] In the mantle zone pattern, the neoplastic proliferation forms a concentric cuff around residual non-neoplastic germinal centers. Although a mantle zone pattern is not diagnostic for this lymphoma type,[11] the majority of cases of lymphoma with this architectural

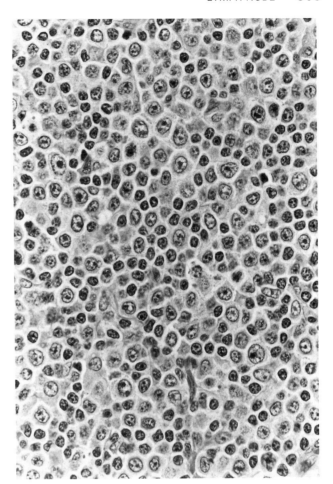

FIGURE 19–6. Small lymphocytic lymphoma with scattered large cells. The number of large cells in this case is not sufficient for a diagnosis of Richter's transformation.

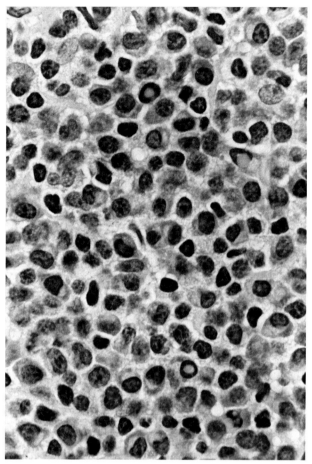

FIGURE 19–7. Small lymphocytic lymphoma with plasmacytoid differentiation. Some cells are small, round lymphocytes, while other cells have abundant eccentrically placed cytoplasm with a paranuclear hof. Note cells with intranuclear inclusions (Dutcher bodies) and cytoplasmic inclusions (Russell bodies).

feature represent mantle cell lymphoma. In the diffuse pattern, diffuse architectural effacement is seen, without pseudofollicular proliferation centers. Cases with a diffuse pattern may have a somewhat worse prognosis than those with a mantle zone pattern.

Cytologically, mantle cell lymphoma is composed of a mixture of small, round lymphocytes and small lymphoid cells with slightly irregular nuclear outlines (Fig. 19–8). The irregularities and chromatin density are less than those seen in the cells of follicular, small cleaved cell lymphoma. In contrast with small lymphocytic lymphoma, admixed large lymphoid cells are not seen in mantle cell lymphoma. In paraffin section immunohistochemistry, the neoplastic cells express the B-lineage marker CD20 and often co-express CD43. In frozen sections, aberrant expression of CD5 is often seen. Molecular studies often demonstrate bcl-1 rearrangements that correlate with a t(11;14)(q13;q32) found in cytogenetic studies.[12]

It is clinically important to distinguish mantle cell lymphoma from follicular lymphoma. In mantle cell lymphoma with a mantle zone pattern, a nodular pattern may be seen on low-power examination, but non-neoplastic germinal centers are almost always present in the center of the nodules, in contrast with the follicles of follicular lymphoma, which con-

tain cytologically malignant cells. Although follicular, small cleaved cell lymphoma may have extensive diffuse areas that can simulate mantle cell lymphoma, there are almost invariably some identifiable neoplastic follicles present to identify the case as follicular lymphoma. It is likely that the majority of the cases classified as **diffuse, small cleaved cell lymphoma** in the Working Formulation study actually represent mantle cell lymphoma.

Monocytoid B-cell (or marginal zone or parafollicular) **lymphoma** represents the neoplastic counterpart of the reactive monocytoid B-cells that are found in a large variety of reactive proliferations such as toxoplasmosis.[13] Architecturally, these lymphomas may show diffuse effacement or may show partial involvement. The lymph node sinuses are almost always involved, and the neoplasm also commonly forms cuffs around non-neoplastic germinal centers. On occasion, the neoplastic cells show invasion of the follicles, a pattern that may mimic follicular lymphoma. Cytologically, the neoplastic cells closely resemble the cells of **hairy cell leukemia.** The nuclei are relatively bland but usually possess slightly irregular nuclear membranes, contain small and inconspicuous nucleoli, and are approximately the same size as, or slightly larger than, the nuclei of small lymphocytes (Fig. 19–9). The most distinctive feature is the presence of relatively abundant clear to pale staining cytoplasm, with distinctive borders

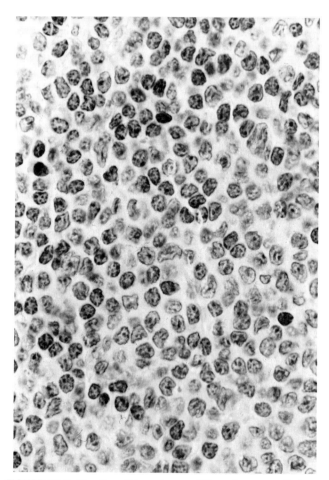

FIGURE 19–8. Mantle cell lymphoma. Although some cells have round nuclear contours, many cells have slightly irregular nuclear contours with irregularities in the chromatin distribution.

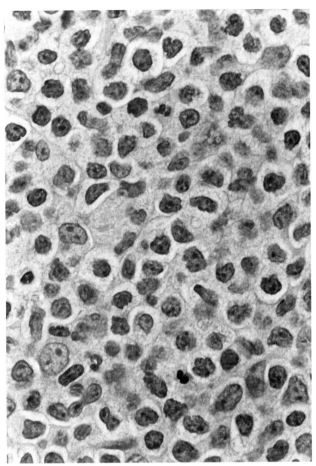

FIGURE 19–9. Monocytoid B-cell lymphoma. The cells have abundant pale cytoplasm. Note admixed neutrophils. The nuclei are slightly more atypical than non-neoplastic monocytoid B cells.

FOLLICULAR LYMPHOMA

Follicular lymphoma represents approximately one third of malignant lymphomas in the United States and a greater percentage of lymphomas in adults. In the assessment of follicular lymphoma versus **follicular hyperplasia,** knowledge of the age of the patient is of critical importance. Follicular lymphomas are rare before the age of 35 years, whereas follicular hyperplasia is very common in the younger ages; therefore, a diagnosis of follicular lymphoma should be made only in the face of overwhelming evidence in this younger age group. However, both follicular lymphoma and reactive hyperplasia commonly occur in the older age group. There are numerous histologic criteria to distinguish follicular lymphoma from follicular hyperplasia, including both architectural and cytologic features, easy to delineate in principle but not always easy to apply in practice.[16] There is no one pathognomonic feature of either a neoplastic or reactive follicle; one must rely on a constellation of findings, weighing each one differently in different cases, depending on its prominence. The architectural criteria are usually the most useful. At low-power magnification, the follicles in follicular lymphoma are usually present back-to-back throughout the lymph node, relatively even in size and shape, and with little intervening interfollicular lymphocytes (Fig. 19–10). The more irregular the follicles are in size and shape, and the further apart

between each cell. Neutrophils and plasma cells are often scattered among the neoplastic infiltrate and are helpful clues to the recognition of this lymphoma. In paraffin sections, the cells express CD20, indicative of a B-cell lineage. In frozen sections, a mature B-lineage phenotype is seen. In contrast with hairy cells, the neoplastic cells of monocytoid B-cell lymphoma are CD25-negative.

Monocytoid B-cell lymphoma is often present as a component of a composite lymphoma.[14] It has been described in direct association with other low-grade lymphomas, such as small lymphocytic lymphoma, often with plasmacytic differentiation, mantle cell lymphoma, and follicular lymphoma. Another feature of monocytoid B-cell lymphoma is its potential to transform to a large-cell lymphoma, either in the same biopsy or at a subsequent time.[15] When sheets of large cells are present even in focal areas, one should consider that transformation has occurred, with an adverse effect on survival.

The most important consideration in the diagnosis of monocytoid B-cell lymphoma is its distinction from a reactive monocytoid B-cell proliferation.[14] Usually, a reactive monocytoid B-cell population is seen focally within a lymph node and is almost always confined to the sinuses. Cytologically, there is a higher mitotic rate, a greater degree of nuclear atypia, and a higher number of admixed large lymphoid cells in lymphoma as compared with a reactive proliferation.

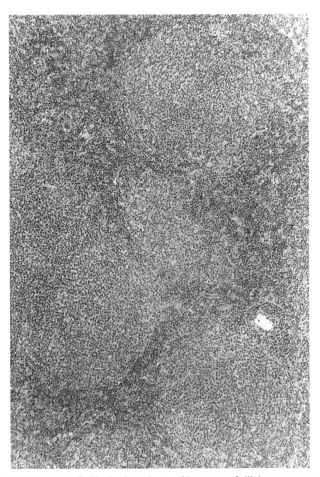

FIGURE 19–10. Follicular lymphoma. Numerous follicles are seen, with little intervening interfollicular space.

they are spaced, the more likely that the lymph node biopsy is benign. Areas of capsular invasion or transgression by follicles, particularly with follicles present in the perinodal adipose tissue, are also useful in establishing a diagnosis of follicular lymphoma, but these features are not often seen. Mantle zones may be present or absent in follicular lymphoma; when absent, follicular lymphoma should be favored, although mantle zones may also be absent in some cases of follicular hyperplasia, most notably in patients with human immunodeficiency virus (HIV) infection.

On high-power magnification, a monomorphous population of small, atypical (''cleaved'') cells in the centers of the follicles is virtually diagnostic of follicular lymphoma (Fig. 19–11). However, often a mixture of small and large cells is present (follicular, mixed small cleaved and follicular, large-cell lymphoma) (Fig. 19–12), and occasionally a predominance of large cells is found (large cleaved and non-cleaved). These latter two patterns are less useful to distinguish between a benign and malignant diagnosis, because reactive hyperplasia usually shows a mixture of cell types and occasionally may contain a predominance of large cells (Fig. 19–13). Tingible body macrophages are generally absent in the follicles of follicular, small cleaved cell lymphoma but may be present in follicular, mixed cell and follicular, large-cell lymphoma. The absence of mitotic figures may favor a diagnosis of follicular lymphoma, but both lymphoma and hyperplasia may contain an abundance of mitotic activity. One very helpful feature in establishing a diagnosis of follicular lymphoma is the presence of small, cleaved cells in the diffuse areas outside of the follicles. This is even more useful when the small, cleaved cells are associated with sclerosis. In occasional cases of follicular lymphoma, foci of sheets of large cells, often associated with sclerosis, may be present.

One major difficulty in the diagnosis of follicular lymphoma occurs in cases of partial involvement of the lymph node by

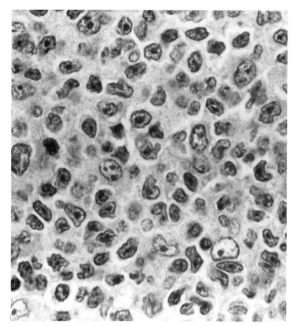

FIGURE 19–12. Follicular, mixed small cleaved and large-cell type. The cellular population is a mixture of small, irregular lymphocytes and occasional larger forms.

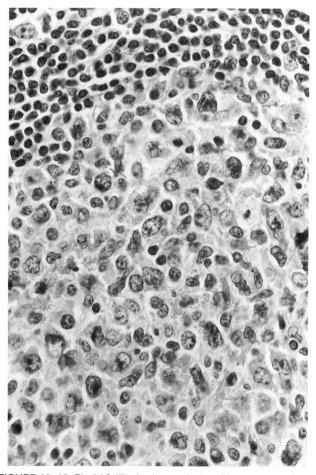

FIGURE 19–13. Florid follicular hyperplasia with monomorphous population of large cells. Note the well-defined mantle zone at the edge.

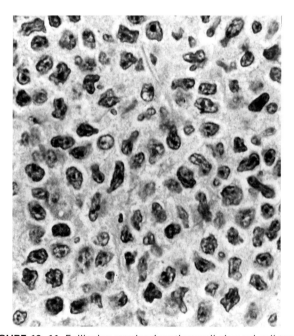

FIGURE 19–11. Follicular, predominantly small cleaved cell type. The predominant cell type is a small lymphocyte with markedly contorted nuclear outlines.

lymphoma. This is particularly common when the sampled lymph nodes are not greatly enlarged. In these cases, many follicles may show reactive features, whereas only focal areas demonstrate the histologic findings indicative of lymphoma. Assessment of all follicles in a specimen is necessary to avoid missing the diagnosis in these cases.

Ancillary studies may be necessary to distinguish follicular lymphomas from reactive hyperplasia in rare cases. In paraffin sections, the staining of a majority of follicular cells by antibodies to bcl-2 protein is diagnostic of lymphoma,[17] although the absence of staining is not diagnostic of hyperplasia, because lack of reactivity may be found in some follicular lymphomas, particularly the large-cell subtype. Application of CD20 to identify sheets of interfollicular B cells present in follicular lymphoma, but generally not in reactive hyperplasia, may also be of use. When frozen sections or cell suspensions are available, determination of the status of the light chains is usually definitive. Follicular lymphomas show light chain restriction or aberrant loss of immunoglobulin expression in the B cells of the follicles.[5] Conversely, in follicular hyperplasia, a mixture of kappa- and lambda-bearing cells is found. Molecular hybridization studies demonstrate clonal rearrangement of the immunoglobulin heavy and light chain genes in virtually all cases of lymphoma, and rearrangement of the bcl-2 gene is found in 60% to 90% of cases.[18] Cytogenetic studies reveal a t(14;18) in 60% to 90% of cases of follicular lymphoma.[19]

Follicular lymphoma is subclassified into three categories based on the relative proportions of small and large cells. **Follicular, predominantly small cleaved cell** and **mixed small cleaved and large-cell** are low-grade lymphomas in the Working Formulation, whereas **follicular, predominantly large-cell** is an intermediate-grade lymphoma.[1] The cutoff between the three groups is arbitrary. In the Working Formulation study, the categories of predominantly small cleaved cell and predominantly large cell are used when the number of small and large cells predominate, respectively, whereas the category of mixed small cleaved and large cell is used when there is no clear preponderance of one cell type over the other. Other studies have attempted a more quantitative approach. For example, Mann and Berard designated cases with 0 to 5 large non-cleaved cells per high-power field as predominantly small cleaved cell, cases with 6 to 15 large non-cleaved cells per high-power field as mixed, and cases with more than 15 large non-cleaved cells as predominantly large cell.[20] However, this classification introduces another subjective element, i.e., discriminating individual cells as cleaved or non-cleaved cell type. Because no method has been shown to have a high degree of reproducibility, we follow the guidelines set forth in the Working Formulation, as they are easy to follow, with the understanding that some decisions may be arbitrary.

DIFFUSE MIXED AND LARGE-CELL LYMPHOMA

Diffuse mixed small- and large-cell lymphoma and the large-cell lymphomas, including large-cell immunoblastic, represent the most heterogeneous subtypes of the non-Hodgkin's lymphomas, including a wide variety of both B- and T-cell lymphomas. The distinction of diffuse mixed small- and large-cell from diffuse large-cell lymphoma in the Work-

ing Formulation is an arbitrary one, based on a highly subjective assessment of the relative number of large cells present. Fortunately, diffuse mixed small- and large-cell lymphoma and diffuse large-cell lymphoma are intermediate-grade neoplasms in the Working Formulation. The recognition of large-cell immunoblastic lymphoma as different from other large-cell lymphomas may also be of lesser importance because the treatment protocols are often similar or identical and the two subtypes may not have a greatly different clinical course or prognosis. Similarly, the clinical importance of the distinction of B- versus T-lineage large-cell lymphoma is a controversial one, and apparently not of critical importance, if any.

These comments notwithstanding, it is still useful for the surgical pathologist to at least attempt to subdivide the diffuse mixed and large-cell lymphoma into specific clinicopathologic entities, if possible. The majority of diffuse mixed and large-cell lymphomas represent B neoplasms, often of follicular center cell type. Evidence of a relationship to follicular lymphoma may be found in the clinical history or with the identification of focal areas of neoplastic follicle formation. The demonstration of a t(14;18) translocation by molecular studies or cytogenetics might also imply indirect proof of a relationship to follicular lymphoma. The presence of sclerosis may also suggest that the lymphoma is follicular center cell–derived. The large-cell lymphomas of follicular center cell origin have traditionally been subdivided into large cleaved cell or non-cleaved cell types.[1] Some investigators have used the identification of these cell types as additional evidence in favor of a follicular cell origin. Large cleaved cells have an irregular cell membrane, possess minimal cytoplasm, and have inconspicuous nucleoli. Non-cleaved cells have a rounded nuclear contour, possess a narrow rim of cytoplasm that may be amphophilic or basophilic, and contain one or more prominent nucleoli, typically situated at their nuclear membrane. We find the definitive identification of large cleaved and non-cleaved cells to be highly subjective and non-reproducible. Therefore, we do not find it helpful toward the recognition of follicular center cell origin nor do we use it for subclassification purposes.

Another B-cell lymphoma that may be classified as diffuse mixed cell type is a variant of lymphoplasmacytoid lymphoma termed polymorphous in the Kiel classification.[21] However, it is poorly described or omitted altogether in most American classifications. It is very similar to small lymphocytic lymphoma with plasmacytoid features but also contains a variable number of plasmacytoid immunoblasts (Fig. 19–14). The number of immunoblasts is fewer than one finds in plasmacytoid immunoblastic lymphoma. Thus, there is a spectrum of lymphomas with plasmacytic features, ranging from small lymphocytic lymphoma with plasmacytoid features to diffuse mixed cell type with plasmacytoid features to large-cell immunoblastic, plasmacytoid type, depending on the frequency of plasmacytoid immunoblasts.

T cell–rich B-cell lymphoma and **histiocyte-rich B-cell lymphoma** are two recently described malignant lymphomas that morphologically correspond to the category of diffuse mixed cell type lymphoma (Figs. 19–15 and 19–16).[22, 23] However, in these two new entities, immunologic studies demonstrate that the large-cell component is neoplastic and B lineage, whereas the small-cell component represents a reactive T-cell infiltrate or histiocytic infiltrate, respectively. Many hematopathologists currently regard these neoplasms as diffuse large-

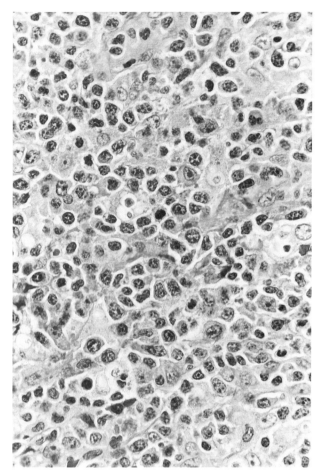

FIGURE 19–14. Diffuse, mixed cell lymphoma with plasmacytoid features (polymorphous immunocytoma of Kiel classification). Note the presence of scattered immunoblasts.

cell lymphomas even though strict morphologic assessment would lead to these lymphomas being diagnosed as diffuse, mixed cell type. Both of these lymphomas may be confused with peripheral T-cell lymphoma if one does not specifically determine the phenotype of the large-cell component. The differential diagnosis of these lymphomas with lymphocyte-predominance Hodgkin's disease is discussed below in the section on the latter entity.

Peripheral T-cell lymphomas are always diffuse lymphomas but are otherwise morphologically heterogeneous, ranging from the Working Formulation categories of diffuse mixed small- and large-cell through diffuse, large-cell to large-cell immunoblastic (Fig. 19–17).[24] Approximately one fourth of cases of diffuse mixed and large-cell lymphomas represent peripheral T-cell lymphomas. Histologic features that might suggest a T-cell rather than a B-cell lineage include selective involvement of the paracortical regions (T-zone lymphoma); a spectrum of cellular atypia; an admixture of eosinophils, plasma cells, and histiocytes (including epithelioid histiocytes); and increased vascularity, particularly in postcapillary venules. Nonetheless, one cannot rely solely on morphologic assessment for the identification of peripheral T-cell lymphoma, because numerous T-cell lymphomas mimic B-cell lymphomas, and vice versa. Immunohistochemistry is necessary for definitive diagnosis; fortunately, this is now possible

in paraffin-fixed tissue in a majority of cases. Positivity for CD45RO and negativity for CD20 constitute strong evidence for a T-cell lymphoma. In addition, CD43 positivity and CD20 negativity also constitute evidence for a T-cell lymphoma once other neoplasms that may also express CD43 (such as acute leukemia or plasmacytoma) have been excluded. In contrast, expression of CD20 or co-expression of CD20 and CD43 or CD45RO is evidence for a B-cell rather than a T-cell lymphoma. Similar to the situation in paraffin sections, when frozen tissue is available for study, the demonstration of one or more pan-T cell markers along with the absence of B-lineage markers is strong evidence that a lymphoid neoplasm is a T- rather than B-lineage lymphoma. Frozen section studies have the added advantage of possibly detecting aberrant absence of one or more pan-T cell antigens, a finding in a majority of cases of peripheral T-cell lymphoma and an important way to exclude a reactive T-cell process.[24]

Within the category of peripheral T-cell lymphoma, there are several entities that affect lymph nodes. The most important clinicopathologic entity to recognize is **human T-cell leukemia/lymphoma,** a neoplasm caused by **HTLV-1** infection.[25] The patients are mostly adults and are usually from

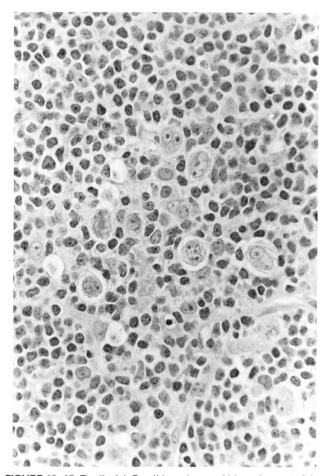

FIGURE 19–15. T cell–rich B-cell lymphoma. Although most of the lymphocytes were found to be T cells, the large atypical cells stained with CD20 (B-lineage marker). The B cells were shown to have monoclonal light chain restriction and were negative for the Hodgkin's disease–associated markers CD15 and CD30. Notice the cell resembling a so-called diagnostic Reed-Sternberg cell—the presence of such cells is not pathognomonic of Hodgkin's disease.

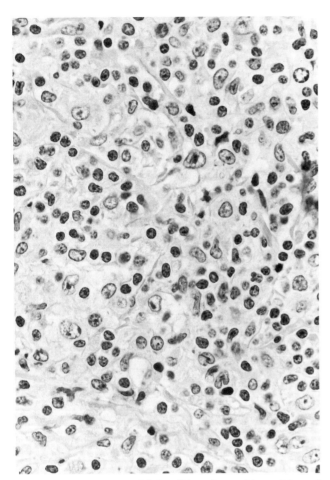

FIGURE 19-16. Histiocyte-rich B-cell lymphoma. Most of the cells in this diffuse lymphoma are small lymphocytes that marked as T cells and histiocytes. Only rare large cells are present; these cells typed as B lineage.

one of the endemic areas of HTLV-1 infection, including the southernmost islands of Japan, areas of the Caribbean, the southeastern United States (affecting mainly blacks), and equatorial Africa. Clinically, the patients invariably have stage IV disease and often have hypercalcemia. The histologic appearance may be indistinguishable from other peripheral T-cell lymphomas, although the neoplastic cells are often highly pleomorphic. A key to the diagnosis is the identification of highly pleomorphic hyperlobated T cells in the peripheral blood, a finding almost always present at some time during the clinical course.

Another variant of peripheral T-cell lymphoma is T-cell lymphoma with high content of epithelioid histiocytes, also known as **Lennert's lymphoma.**[26] In this subtype, the lymph node architecture is effaced by a proliferation of epithelioid histiocytes, present as single cells and in small clusters, but without the formation of well-formed epithelioid granulomas (Fig. 19-18). The key to the diagnosis of this lymphoma is the presence of a population of atypical small, medium-sized, and large lymphoid cells scattered among the histiocytes. This population, which may be subtle to detect, represents the neoplastic element and marks as T-lineage in the large majority of cases. Sarcoidosis should not be confused with this lymphoma, because well-formed granulomas are not seen. Granulomatous infections may be considered in the differen-

tial diagnosis, but they usually have well-formed granulomas and often contain giant cells (an infrequent finding in lymphoma with high content of epithelioid histiocytes) and often contain areas of necrosis adjacent to the histiocytes. If necrosis occurs in this lymphoma, it is seen in areas of atypical cells, and not in the areas of histiocytes. Rarely, small lymphocytic lymphoma with plasmacytoid features may contain large numbers of epithelioid cells.[27] Assessment of immunoglobulin light chains in paraffin sections in cases of doubt avoids confusion with this entity; a polyclonal population of plasma cells is found in T-cell lymphoma with high content of epithelioid histiocytes.

Angioimmunoblastic lymphadenopathy (AILD) is an entity that currently has a highly controversial relationship to peripheral T-cell lymphoma.[28] AILD generally affects elderly people, who usually present with generalized lymphadenopathy, splenomegaly, anemia, a skin rash, and a polyclonal hypergammaglobulinemia. Histologically, the lymph node architecture is usually diffusely effaced, although the subcapsular sinuses may be patent. The vascularity is markedly increased, with numerous small, arborizing vessels (Fig. 19-19). The infiltrate is generally cell-poor and composed of a mixed population of small, regular lymphocytes, plasma cells, histiocytes (including epithelioid histiocytes), immunoblasts, and frequently, eosinophils. Germinal centers are

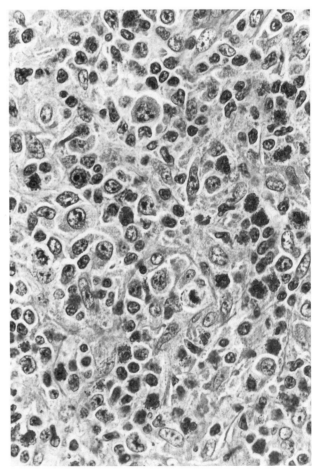

FIGURE 19-17. Peripheral T-cell lymphoma. A spectrum of atypia is present. Contrast this with Figure 19-30, which shows mixed cellularity Hodgkin's disease.

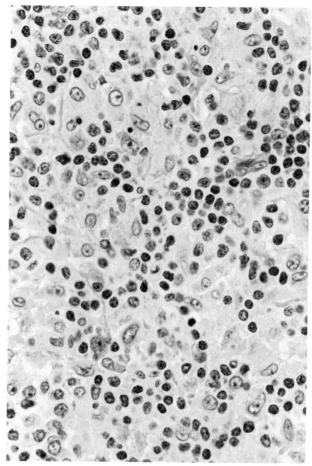

FIGURE 19–18. Malignant lymphoma with high content of epithelioid histiocytes (Lennert's lymphoma). A diffuse admixture of small lymphocytes and epithelioid histiocytes is present. The neoplastic T-cell infiltrate, a population of intermediate-sized cells with nuclear atypia, is very subtle in this case.

either absent or appear ''burnt out.'' Occasionally, there is deposition of an interstitial amorphous, eosinophilic material. An unusual finding in some cases is the presence of large numbers of epithelioid histiocytes, which may lead to confusion with T-cell lymphoma with high content of epithelioid histiocytes. Immunophenotypically, AILD is a proliferation of T cells with scattered polyclonal B immunoblasts and plasma cells.[29] Frozen section immunophenotyping reveals normal T-cell antigen expression without aberrant absence of pan-T cell antigens.

AILD-like lymphoma is a neoplasm very closely related, if not identical, to AILD. Transformation to AILD-like lymphoma is said to have occurred histologically when small clusters to sheets of medium-sized to large lymphoid cells with clear cytoplasm or immunoblastic nuclear features are present in a lymph node biopsy that otherwise shows the histologic features of AILD (Figs. 19–20 and 19–21).[30] Usually, these foci are present around blood vessels. Immunophenotypically, the atypical cells are T lineage and may or may not show absence of pan-T cell antigens.[30] Molecular studies demonstrate clonal rearrangements of the T-cell receptor genes in virtually all these cases, but such findings are not of diagnostic significance in the differential diagnosis with AILD because many cases of AILD also may show clonal rearrange-

ments.[31] These findings, along with similarities in cytogenetic abnormalities between AILD and AILD-like T-cell lymphoma, have led some hematopathologists to suggest that there is no logical reason to separate AILD and AILD-like lymphoma. Nonetheless, most hematopathologists, including the authors, still prefer to attempt to distinguish between these two entities, based on the criteria enumerated here.

Occasional cases of AILD may also terminate in immunoblastic lymphomas of B lineage, possibly arising out of the immunoregulatory abnormalities of this T-cell lymphoproliferative disorder and possibly mediated by Epstein-Barr virus.[31] In these cases, the malignant lymphoma is easy to diagnose and usually shows the morphologic appearance characteristic of a plasmacytic immunoblastic lymphoma. Only the history of a previous biopsy of AILD enables one to know with confidence that it arose in the setting of AILD, because the histologic features of AILD are usually no longer present.

Large-cell immunoblastic lymphoma is a category of the Working Formulation that is much more heterogeneous than the other categories of high-grade malignant lymphomas and does not represent a single clinicopathologic entity. As defined in the Working Formulation, large-cell immunoblastic lymphoma encompasses plasmacytoid, clear-cell, and polymorphous types.[1] In addition, many hematopathologists now include the recently delineated entity of anaplastic large-cell lymphoma in the category of large-cell immunoblastic lymphoma.

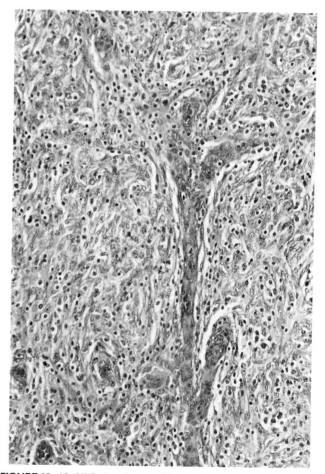

FIGURE 19–19. AILD. A cell-poor diffuse effacement of architecture is present. Note the arborizing vessels.

In **plasmacytoid immunoblastic lymphoma,** diffuse effacement of architecture is usually present, but cases of focal involvement may show selective localization to the sinuses, a pattern that may closely simulate a metastatic neoplasm. The mitotic rate is often very high, and a starry-sky appearance may be often seen, at least focally. The cellular proliferation is relatively homogeneous, with few "host" cells. The neoplastic cells of plasmacytoid immunoblastic lymphoma are large (Fig. 19–22). The nuclei are large with a vesicular chromatin pattern and generally one large, centrally located, basophilic nucleolus. The cytoplasm is abundant, basophilic, intensely pyroninophilic, and eccentrically located. The vast majority of cases are of B lineage; however, rare cases of T-lineage neoplasms with morphologic features of plasmacytoid immunoblastic lymphoma have been described.[24]

The histologic features of plasmacytoid immunoblastic lymphoma may be identical to involvement by anaplastic plasmacytoma or multiple myeloma. The clinical history is of crucial importance, but immunologic studies may also be of use in the distinction. The cells of anaplastic plasmacytoma or multiple myeloma are much more likely to produce IgG or IgA immunoglobulin heavy chain, whereas plasmacytoid immunoblastic lymphoma is much more likely to express IgM. In addition, anaplastic plasmacytoma/multiple myeloma is much more likely to be CD45/45RB-, CD19-, or CD20-negative and CD38- and epithelial membrane antigen–positive than plasmacytoid immunoblastic lymphoma.[32]

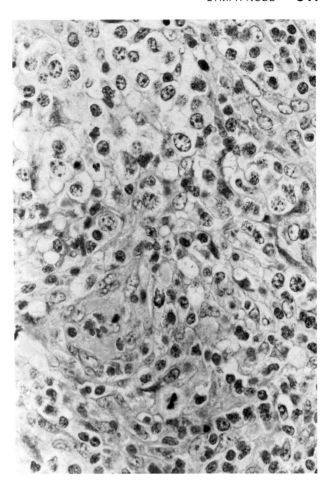

FIGURE 19–21. AILD-like lymphoma (same case as Fig. 19–20). Aggregates of atypical cells with abundant pale cytoplasm are present.

Plasmacytoid immunoblastic lymphoma also may be difficult to distinguish from the non-Burkitt's type of small, non-cleaved cell lymphoma. Compared with the latter entity, the cells of plasmacytoid immunoblastic lymphoma are larger, with a larger nucleus, a larger central nucleolus, and more abundant cytoplasm. Despite these listed differences, there may be transitional cases that defy easy classification into one category or another. This may be particularly true with high-grade lymphomas that develop in HIV-infected patients, a population in which both types of lymphoma are unusually prevalent.

The **clear-cell type of immunoblastic lymphoma** is a somewhat controversial entity. Diffuse effacement of architecture is seen. The characteristic cells of this lymphoma are large, as a result of the presence of abundant, optically clear to pale cytoplasm possessing little pyroninophilia. The nuclei are large and generally have a fine chromatin pattern, with one or more generally small but distinct nucleoli. It was originally thought that this morphologic appearance was specific for a variant of peripheral T-cell lymphoma. However, it is now evident that B-lineage large-cell lymphomas may be composed of cells with abundant clear cytoplasm; these cases may be particularly common in the mediastinum. Therefore, in practice, we usually regard large-cell lymphomas with abundant clear cytoplasm as intermediate-grade lymphomas, despite their position in the Working Formulation.

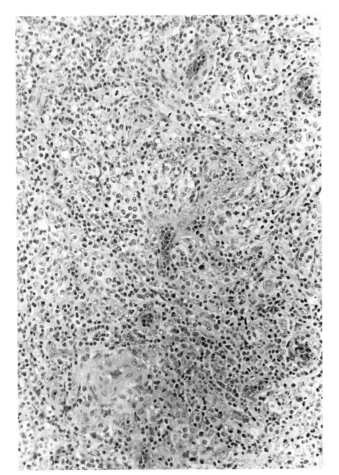

FIGURE 19–20. AILD-like lymphoma. Although the overall pattern is reminiscent of AILD, the cellularity is increased.

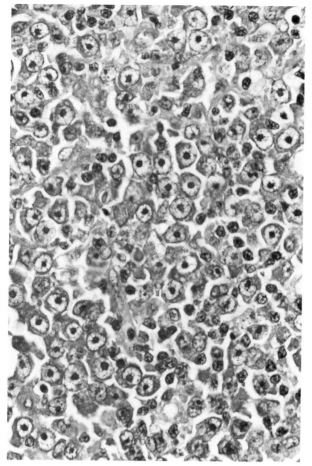

FIGURE 19–22. Plasmacytoid immunoblastic lymphoma. There is a homogeneous population of large cells with large nuclei containing a large central nucleolus and abundant cytoplasm.

The **polymorphous variant of immunoblastic lymphoma** characteristically shows diffuse effacement of lymph node architecture by a mixed population of atypical cells with a wide range of cell size. Many of the large cells are highly pleomorphic, and may have multilobated or multinucleated forms, including Reed-Sternberg–like simulants. Plasma cells, eosinophils, and epithelioid cells are often present; when the latter are a prominent finding and found throughout the infiltrate, this neoplasm may be regarded as a form of malignant lymphoma with high content of epithelioid histiocytes (Lennert's lymphoma). The majority of these lymphomas represent peripheral T-cell lymphomas, although occasional B-cell lymphomas may have these histologic features.

The differential diagnosis of this subtype of immunoblastic lymphoma would include diffuse, mixed small- and large-cell lymphoma and diffuse, large-cell lymphoma of T lineage. These lymphomas form a continuum with no natural divisions separating them. We prefer a diagnosis of polymorphous immunoblastic lymphoma when the large-cell component is the dominant feature and when these cells show a significant degree of cytologic pleomorphism. A more important differential is the distinction of polymorphous immunoblastic lymphoma from Hodgkin's disease, particularly the lymphocyte depletion subtype. In fact, many of the cases previously regarded as lymphocyte depletion Hodgkin's disease are now

recognized to probably represent polymorphous immunoblastic lymphoma.[33] Morphologic features helpful in this distinction include the large number of atypical cells and their pleomorphism in polymorphous immunoblastic lymphoma and the presence of diffuse fibrosis, often enveloping single cells, in lymphocyte depletion Hodgkin's disease. Immunohistochemical studies may be crucial in this setting. The presence of CD45/45RB positivity combined with CD43, CD45RO, or CD20 positivity would favor non-Hodgkin's lymphoma, whereas negativity for these markers along with CD15 positivity would constitute strong evidence for a diagnosis of Hodgkin's disease.

Anaplastic large-cell lymphoma was first described in 1985 on the basis of the expression of the CD30 antigen in this neoplasm.[34] It is now recognized that anaplastic large-cell lymphoma represents a clinicopathologic entity with distinctive histologic characteristics. Clinically, it occurs in two settings: a primary form, which occurs *de novo,* and a secondary form, which occurs subsequent to another type of lymphoma. The primary form shows a male predominance and a bimodal age distribution with peaks at around 25 and 70 years of age. Affected lymph nodes may show architectural effacement, but more commonly show incomplete involvement. Sinusoidal infiltration is very common (Fig. 19–23), and nodules or sheets of tumor within the paracortical regions

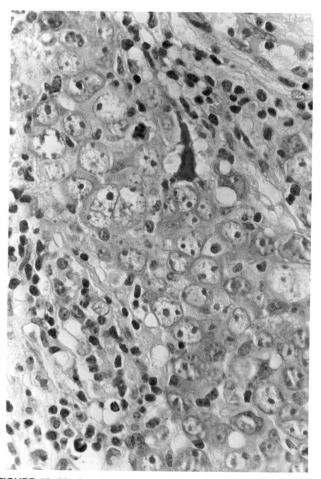

FIGURE 19–23. Anaplastic large-cell lymphoma. Extremely anaplastic lymphoid cells (confirmed by immunostains) are present in a distended sinus.

are also often found. Fibrosis, including both delicate interstitial fibrosis enveloping single cells or small groups of cells and coarse fibrosis dividing the lymphoid parenchyma into nodules, may be seen. Scattered admixed small lymphocytes, histiocytes, neutrophils, and plasma cells are commonly seen, but widespread eosinophilic infiltration is an uncommon feature. Occasional cases may have a high content of reactive histiocytes.

Cytologically, the neoplastic cells are invariably large. The nuclei are large and may be round, ovoid, reniform, highly irregular, multilobulated, or multinucleated.[35] "Jellyfish-like," "donut-like," and Reed-Sternberg–like nuclei all have been described in this neoplasm. The chromatin is often coarsely clumped, interspersed as with areas of clearing. Nucleoli may be multiple or single and are generally prominent, especially when single. Mitotic figures, including atypical forms, are usually readily defined. The cytoplasm is abundant and often eccentrically placed. It may be pale or basophilic and often contains a pale paranuclear hof. The cell membranes are often distinct and may abut one cell on another. In rare cases, the cytoplasm may be spindled and therefore simulate a sarcoma.

Anaplastic large-cell lymphoma is most commonly confused with a metastatic malignant neoplasm, including both carcinoma and malignant melanoma. The most important thing a pathologist can do to diagnose anaplastic large-cell lymphoma is to remember the entity in the differential diagnosis of a malignant neoplasm with a sinusoidal distribution; the greatest pitfall is to diagnose these cases as metastatic undifferentiated malignancy and to not even consider the possibility of the diagnosis. The lymphoid character of the chromatin pattern and the cell-to-cell nuclear variation might suggest the diagnosis of lymphoma. When any doubt exists, a battery of paraffin immunohistochemical studies should resolve the case, including stains for CD45/45RB, CD30, CD43, CD20, keratin, epithelial membrane antigen, and S-100 protein. Inclusion of CD30 in the panel is critical, because a significant minority of these cases may be CD45/45RB-negative. Virtually all cases of anaplastic large-cell lymphoma are CD30-positive, although CD30 positivity may also be seen in occasional cases of non-Hodgkin's lymphoma lacking the morphologic features of this lymphoma. The majority of cases also are positive for epithelial membrane antigen. Therefore, one must seriously consider the diagnosis of anaplastic large-cell lymphoma before regarding a keratin-negative, epithelial membrane antigen–positive neoplasm to be carcinoma. In addition, the majority of cases of anaplastic large-cell lymphoma express the T lineage–associated marker CD45RO, a minority of cases express the B-lineage marker CD20, and rare cases are negative for T- and B-lineage markers (null cell lineage). T-cell receptor or immunoglobulin gene rearrangements are found in a majority of, but not all, cases.[36, 37] Finally, a specific translocation involving 5q35 is found in a substantial number of cases.[38]

Anaplastic large-cell lymphoma may also be confused with Hodgkin's disease. Hodgkin's disease rarely involves sinuses unless there is involvement adjacent to them; selective involvement of the sinuses is exceedingly rare. Extensive infiltration by eosinophils is common in Hodgkin's disease but rare in anaplastic large-cell lymphoma, in which extensive infiltration by plasma cells is not uncommon. The presence of highly bizarre cells such as donut-like cells would favor

anaplastic large-cell lymphoma. In cases in which the diagnosis is uncertain, a battery of immunohistochemical studies, including CD45/45RB, CD30, epithelial membrane antigen, CD20, CD43, and CD15, should allow resolution. Although CD30 is positive in both anaplastic large-cell lymphoma and Hodgkin's disease, anaplastic large-cell lymphoma is usually positive for CD45/45RB, epithelial membrane antigen, and CD20 or CD43, whereas Hodgkin's disease is generally negative for these markers; Hodgkin's disease is generally positive for CD15, and anaplastic large-cell lymphoma is usually negative for this marker.

The entity of malignant histiocytosis or true histiocytic lymphoma should be considered in the differential diagnosis of anaplastic large-cell lymphoma. Malignant histiocytosis as initially defined in the literature was a clinicopathologic entity characterized by malignant cells with morphologic features suggestive of histiocytes present in a sinusoidal distribution.[39, 40] The largest series of malignant histiocytosis were reported before the advent of modern immunohistochemistry. When these cases are studied by the technologies of today, they are almost invariably found to be of lymphoid lineage, with the majority representing CD30-positive neoplasms, best reclassified as anaplastic large-cell lymphoma.[41, 42] The diagnosis of malignant histiocytosis or true histiocytic lymphoma is best made only with the support of comprehensive frozen section immunophenotype and immunogenotypic studies.

LYMPHOBLASTIC LYMPHOMA

Most high-grade malignant lymphomas can be recognized by the monotony of the cellular proliferation and by the high mitotic rate. It is especially important to recognize **lymphoblastic lymphoma** because it constitutes a specific clinicopathologic entity that may require a unique treatment regimen.[43] Lymphoblastic lymphoma most often occurs in childhood and adolescence, although it has been described in all age groups.[44] There is a mediastinal presentation in approximately 50% of cases. Lymphoblastic lymphoma exhibits diffuse effacement of nodal architecture, often with extensive pericapsular involvement. The neoplasm is often recognizable at low magnification by a homogeneous blue appearance, imparted by the high nucleocytoplasmic ratio. A starry-sky pattern may be focally present. At high magnification, the cells of lymphoblastic lymphoma are medium in size and possess nuclei with very fine chromatin and nucleoli that are either indiscernible or inconspicuous (Fig. 19–24). The nuclear outlines may be round ("non-convoluted" type) or highly irregular ("convoluted" type). The mitotic rate is generally high, although variation may occur from case to case. Cytoplasm is very scant in amount. There is usually little or no accompanying lymphoid infiltrate. When present in fibrous tissues and within the adventitia of blood vessels, a single cell file pattern of infiltration may be seen, reminiscent of the pattern of infiltration characteristic of lobular carcinoma of the breast.

In paraffin sections, leukocyte common antigen (CD45/45RB) positivity is seen in approximately 80% to 90% of cases.[45] Because this is one of the lower rates of positivity seen in the malignant lymphomas, the diagnosis of lymphoblastic lymphoma should be kept in mind when one encounters a neoplasm that appears to be lymphoid yet does not express

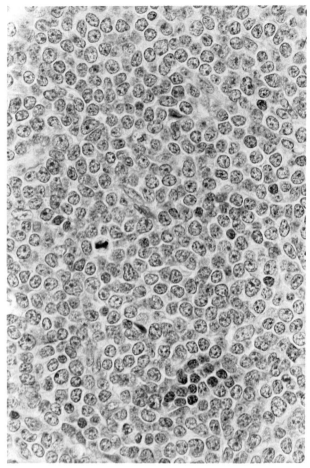

FIGURE 19–24. Lymphoblastic lymphoma. A monomorphous proliferation of medium-sized cells with a fine chromatin pattern and indiscernible cytoplasm is seen. Note the mitotic figure.

leukocyte common antigen. Terminal deoxynucleotidyl transferase (Tdt) can now be detected by paraffin immunohistochemistry in most cases of lymphoblastic lymphoma. Approximately 80% to 90% of cases of lymphoblastic lymphoma are of T lineage,[46] and the majority of these cases are positive for the paraffin T-lineage markers CD45RO and CD43, although CD43 is also expressed in myeloid leukemias. If frozen tissue is available, the T-cell lymphoblastic lymphomas express T-lineage markers, often showing an immature phenotype, e.g., expressing CD1, and either co-expressing CD4 and CD8 or lacking expression of both.[46] Approximately 10% to 20% of cases of lymphoblastic lymphoma express B-lineage markers. Although most of these cases lack immunoglobulin expression (''pre-B''), rare cases expressing immunoglobulin heavy and light chains have been described.[47]

Morphologically and immunologically, lymphoblastic lymphoma is indistinguishable from acute lymphoblastic leukemia. The differentiation is based on peripheral blood and bone marrow findings. Some investigators regard cases with circulating blasts as acute lymphoblastic leukemia,[43] whereas others use the percentage of involved marrow, most often 25%, as the distinguishing feature.[48] Clinically, a much more important neoplasm to distinguish from lymphoblastic lymphoma is acute non-lymphocytic leukemia. The low magnification appearance in the lymph node of both neoplasms may

be identical. Cytologically, there is usually greater cell-to-cell variation in acute non-lymphocytic leukemia, and a greater amount of cytoplasm may be present. The presence of identifiable myeloid precursors, including myelocytes, may raise suspicion of acute non-lymphocytic leukemia, but eosinophils may be found in both neoplasms. In questionable cases, the performance of cytochemical or immunohistochemical studies, e.g., chloroacetate esterase or myeloperoxidase, CD15, and CD68, may resolve the issue. In addition, examination of the bone marrow may be extremely useful.

In suboptimal histologic preparations, lymphoblastic lymphoma may be mistaken for small lymphocytic neoplasms, such as small lymphocytic lymphoma or mantle cell lymphoma. Attention to the high mitotic rate should prevent confusion between the low-grade and high-grade neoplasms. A blastic variant of mantle cell lymphoma has been described that can closely simulate a lymphoblastic neoplasm.[9] The clinical history may be critical in making the distinction, but morphologically, the former neoplasm often retains a focal mantle zone architecture and is more likely to have admixed epithelioid histiocytes. Immunologically, these cases are invariably of B lineage, with immunoglobulin expression, and show anomalous expression of CD5 in frozen sections.

SMALL, NON-CLEAVED CELL LYMPHOMA

It is important to recognize small, non-cleaved cell lymphoma, because this also may represent a distinct entity requiring specific treatment different from other non-Hodgkin's lymphomas. Similar to lymphoblastic lymphoma, small, non-cleaved cell lymphoma is another high-grade lymphoma that is common in childhood; it also commonly occurs in adults, especially in HIV-infected patients. At low magnification, a diffuse effacement of architecture is generally seen, although selective colonization of germinal centers may be present. The mitotic rate is invariably high, and a starry-sky pattern is characteristic (Fig. 19–25). The neoplastic cells possess medium-sized vesicular chromatin, with one to several prominent basophilic nuclei. The cells possess a moderate amount of highly pyroninophilic cytoplasm that is generally eccentric and squares off with the cytoplasm of adjacent cells. Other than scattered tingible-body macrophages, reactive cells are generally not present.

Small, non-cleaved cell lymphoma has been separated into two subtypes based on the cytologic characteristics of the neoplastic cells. In the Burkitt's type, there is great homogeneity from one cell to another (see Fig. 19–25), whereas in the non-Burkitt's type, there is a much greater variability in nuclear size. In addition, non-Burkitt's cells have a greater nuclear irregularity and less prominent nuclear membranes (Fig. 19–26). The nucleoli of non-Burkitt's cells are generally fewer in number (and often single) and larger than in Burkitt's cells. Although there are clinical features such as age and presentation that differ between the two subtypes, subclassification between the two is often difficult, particularly in less than optimal preparations, and decision-making in current clinical protocols generally does not depend on the separation.

Small, non-cleaved cell lymphoma may be difficult to distinguish from lymphoblastic lymphoma at times. Although both lymphomas may show a starry-sky pattern on low magni-

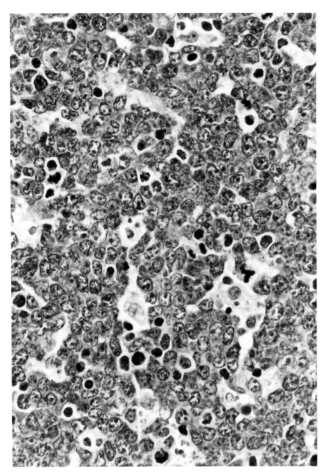

FIGURE 19–25. Small non-cleaved cell lymphoma, Burkitt type. A starry-sky pattern is present.

this characteristic is often difficult to apply in practice. Small, non-cleaved cell lymphoma is much more likely to be composed of a more uniform population of neoplastic cells than the large-cell lymphomas, without much variation from one neoplastic cell to another. In addition, small, non-cleaved cell lymphoma is more likely to be composed almost exclusively of neoplastic cells, whereas the large-cell lymphomas generally have a greater admixture of non-neoplastic elements. In addition, the mitotic rate in small, non-cleaved cell lymphoma is generally higher than in the large-cell lymphomas. Finally, the cells of small, non-cleaved cell lymphoma generally have more nucleoli than those of large-cell lymphomas.

CLASSIC HODGKIN'S DISEASE

For many years, Hodgkin's disease has been classified into the categories of nodular sclerosing, mixed cellularity, lymphocyte predominance (a contraction of lymphocytic and/ or histiocytic [L&H], nodular and diffuse), and lymphocyte depletion (a contraction of diffuse fibrosis and reticular) subtypes. In recent years, it has become evident that L&H lymphocyte predominance may represent a disease entity separate from the remainder of Hodgkin's disease categories, which we will refer to as classic Hodgkin's disease. This section

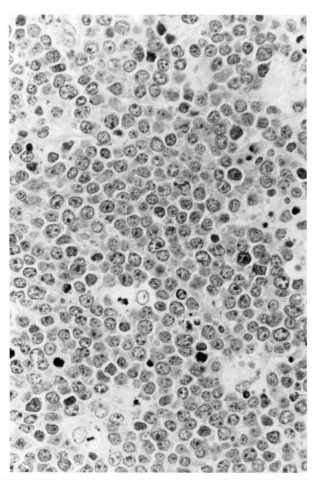

FIGURE 19–26. Small non-cleaved cell lymphoma, non-Burkitt type. A more heterogeneous population of cells is seen than in the Burkitt type.

fication, this is more commonly seen in small, non-cleaved cell lymphoma, especially as a global and not just focal phenomenon. Similarly, both lymphomas may contain a large number of mitoses; however, the mitotic rate in small, non-cleaved cell lymphoma is generally higher than in lymphoblastic lymphoma, with mitoses present throughout the tumor. Lymphoblastic lymphoma may simulate follicular lymphoma through the expansion of connective tissue planes by tumor, but small, non-cleaved cell lymphoma may actually colonize germinal centers. Cytologically, the cells of small non-cleaved cell lymphoma have a greater amount of cytoplasm, which can be demonstrated to be intensely pyroninophilic. The nuclei in small, non-cleaved cell lymphoma are round, whereas they may be round or irregular in lymphoblastic lymphoma. Nucleoli are absent or inconspicuous in lymphoblastic lymphoma, whereas they are generally prominent in small, non-cleaved cell lymphoma. Finally, the neoplastic cells of small, non-cleaved cell lymphoma are of B-cell lineage, and the majority of cases of lymphoblastic lymphoma are of T-cell lineage.

Another difficult problem in differential diagnosis may be the distinction of small, non-cleaved cell lymphoma from diffuse, large-cell lymphoma and large-cell immunoblastic lymphoma. Although the names might suggest that size would be the primary criterion separating small, non-cleaved cell lymphoma from the other two lymphomas, the evaluation of

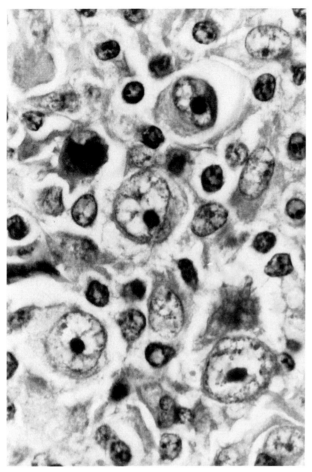

FIGURE 19–27. Hodgkin's disease. Four viable Hodgkin's cells and one "mummified" cell are seen in this field.

The cytoplasm of Hodgkin's cells is generally abundant and acidophilic, amphophilic, or slightly basophilic without a paranuclear hof. At times, particularly in recurrences and at autopsy, Hodgkin's cells may show bizarre nuclear features, making them virtually unrecognizable without a clinical history or performance of special studies;[49, 50] these cells have been termed pleomorphic Hodgkin's cells. In other cases, degenerated Hodgkin's cells are identifiable by a pyknotic nucleus surrounded by contracted eosinophilic cytoplasm; such cells have been called mummified cells. Sometimes, especially in cases of nodular sclerosing Hodgkin's disease fixed in formalin, the cytoplasm of Hodgkin's cells contracts; these cells are commonly referred to as lacunar cells (Fig. 19–28). In lacunar cells, the nucleus tends to be multilobated and often lacks the prominent nucleoli characteristic of most Hodgkin's cells.

Hodgkin's cells of classic Hodgkin's disease possess a characteristic immunophenotype. In paraffin sections, Hodgkin's cells most commonly do not react with CD45/45RB (leukocyte common antigen), CD20, CD43, and CD45RO, but the cells do stain with CD15 and CD30 (Fig. 19–29).[51] However, numerous exceptions occur with all antigens; therefore, reliance on the results of a panel of stains rather than results of a single antibody study is critical. In frozen sections, Hodgkin's cells may be CD45/45RB-positive and may also express a variety of B- and T-lineage antigens.[52] Paraffin section immunohistochemistry is generally sufficient to estab-

discusses classic Hodgkin's disease, and the next section covers L&H lymphocyte predominance.

The diagnosis of classic Hodgkin's disease in most cases is a relatively easy one. Nonetheless, this neoplasm can assume so many variations in its histologic appearance that at times it may mimic a reactive condition, non-Hodgkin's lymphoma, or a non-hematolymphoid neoplasm. The key to the diagnosis of Hodgkin's disease is recognition of the neoplastic element, which we refer to as Hodgkin's cells. These cells are large and contain a large nucleus that may be uninucleated, bi- or multilobated, or bi- or multinucleated (Fig. 19–27). The nuclear membrane is thick, and the chromatin pattern is relatively vesicular, with some coarse chromatin toward the periphery of the nucleus. Each nuclear lobe generally contains a prominent, central eosinophilic nucleolus. Bi- or multilobated and bi- or multinucleated cells with these features have been termed diagnostic Reed-Sternberg (or Sternberg-Reed) cells and are required by many hematopathologists to establish the diagnosis of Hodgkin's disease. However, we do not require their identification for the diagnosis of Hodgkin's disease, although their recognition may be helpful toward establishing the diagnosis. Overemphasis of their importance in establishing the diagnosis of Hodgkin's disease may also lead to the overdiagnosis of Hodgkin's disease when diseases mimicking Hodgkin's disease contain cells morphologically indistinguishable from Hodgkin's cells.

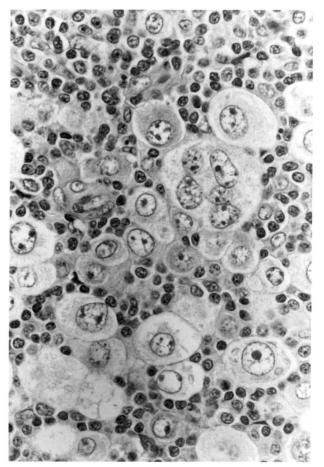

FIGURE 19–28. Nodular sclerosis Hodgkin's disease. Lacunar variants of Hodgkin's cells are demonstrated.

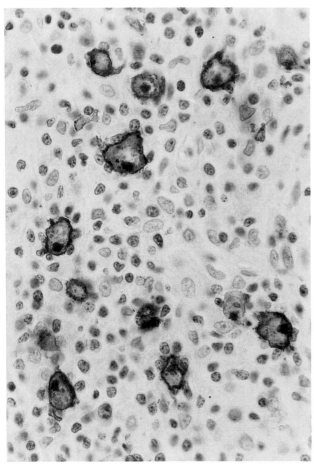

FIGURE 19–29. Hodgkin's disease, immunoperoxidase with CD15 (Leu-M1). A characteristic membrane, cytoplasmic, and paranuclear pattern of staining is seen in the Hodgkin's cells.

lish or rule out a diagnosis of Hodgkin's disease; we often prefer these studies to frozen section immunohistochemistry, because the latter may yield results that are difficult to interpret. Gene rearrangement studies may be of some use in distinguishing Hodgkin's disease from non-Hodgkin's lymphoma if a large clonal population is identified, but the identification of faint rearranged bands or the absence of rearranged bands should be viewed with caution, as faint rearranged bands may be found in some cases of Hodgkin's disease, and some cases of non-Hodgkin's lymphoma may lack detectable clonal antigen receptor gene rearrangements.[53, 54]

The histologic identification of Hodgkin's cells, and therefore of Hodgkin's disease, is facilitated by recognizing the background infiltrate in which Hodgkin's cells are often found (Fig. 19–30). This infiltrate consists of varying numbers of small lymphocytes, eosinophils, plasma cells, histiocytes (including epithelioid histiocytes), neutrophils, and fibroblasts in widely varying proportions. Typically, Hodgkin's cells represent less than 1% of the infiltrate, but may form sheets of cells in rare cases.

Although advances in treatment have rendered subclassification of Hodgkin's disease relatively unimportant for clinical purposes, many hematopathologists still advise subclassification on initial biopsy specimens for purposes of differential diagnosis. The diagnosis of nodular sclerosis generally requires identification of broad collagen bands that often separate the lymphoid parenchyma into nodules. The presence of even focal areas of broad collagen formation warrants classification of a case as nodular sclerosis. The diagnosis of lymphocyte depletion requires recognition of one of the two subtypes, diffuse fibrosis or reticular. In diffuse fibrosis, there is a cell-poor appearance with disorderly reticulum fibrosis that tends to envelop individual cells. In reticular lymphocyte depletion, numerous, often pleomorphic Hodgkin's cells are present. In lymphocyte predominance, only rare Hodgkin's cells are identified. This subtype is discussed in more detail in the section on L&H lymphocyte predominance. All other cases are classified as mixed cellularity, although many hematopathologists recognize an unclassified category, when subclassification cannot be adquately performed.

The diagnosis of most cases of **nodular sclerosis** is straightforward; however, occasional difficulties exist. The primary problem in the diagnosis of nodular sclerosis is recognition of the **syncytial variant** (Fig. 19–31).[55] In this morphologic variant, usually found in the mediastinum, sheets of Reed-Sternberg cells are found, often adjacent to or surrounding an area of necrosis. In some cases, the individual cells clearly have the morphologic features of lacunar cells, but in other cases, the cells are indistinguishable from the neoplastic cells of large-cell or immunoblastic lymphoma, including anaplastic large-cell lymphoma. In addition, the sheets of cells may

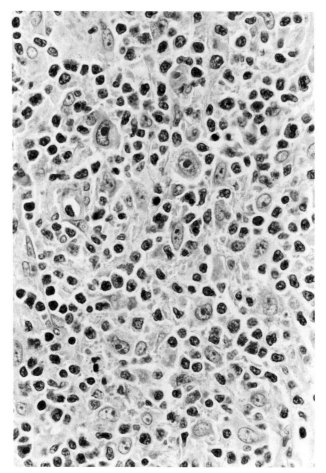

FIGURE 19–30. Mixed cellularity Hodgkin's disease. Four Hodgkin's cells are seen in their typical background. Note the absence of transitional forms.

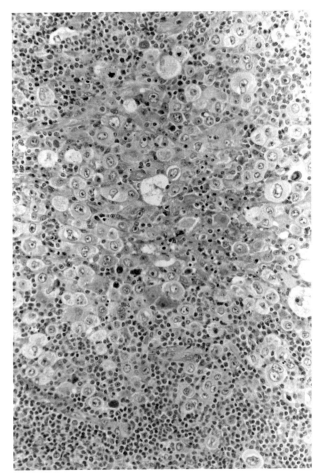

FIGURE 19–31. Nodular sclerosis Hodgkin's disease, syncytial variant. A cohesive sheet of lacunar variants is present.

show cellular cohesion and therefore closely mimic poorly differentiated carcinoma or malignant melanoma. Helpful clues suggesting the diagnosis of Hodgkin's disease include admixed eosinophils, broad bands of fibrosis, and the presence of necrosis directly adjacent to the neoplastic cells. Paraffin section immunohistochemistry is often necessary to establish a definitive diagnosis. The presence of foci of necrosis may raise consideration for necrotizing granulomatous lymphadenitis. Attention to the cytologic features of the cells directly adjacent to the areas of necrosis reveals at least some Hodgkin's cells that can be distinguished from the epithelioid histiocytes of necrotizing granulomas.

Mixed cellularity Hodgkin's disease may be confused with non-Hodgkin's lymphoma. The presence of a high mitotic rate, extension of the infiltrate beyond the lymph node capsule, the absence of eosinophils, and the presence of a spectrum of atypia in small and large cells should alert one to the possibility of a peripheral T-cell lymphoma and prompt performance of immunohistochemical studies.[56, 57] T cell–rich B-cell lymphoma may also be extremely difficult to distinguish from Hodgkin's disease.[22] The histologic distinction between the two often hinges on assessment of the cytologic characteristics of the atypical cells; again, performance of immunohistochemical studies may be essential.

Mixed cellularity Hodgkin's disease may also be difficult to distinguish from reactive immunoblastic proliferations of

the paracortex. In most reactive immunoblastic proliferations, the architecture of the lymph node is retained, although sometimes only focally. The cortex may show florid reactive follicular hyperplasia, and the sinuses may be expanded. The paracortical region often has a mottled appearance owing to the presence of a relatively even distribution of immunoblasts, in contrast with the uneven distribution of Hodgkin's cells typically seen in Hodgkin's disease. In addition, the background infiltrate of reactive immunoblastic proliferations usually contains a maturation sequence of small lymphocytes to plasmacytoid lymphocytes to plasma cells to plasmacytoid immunoblasts (Fig. 19–32).

Interfollicular Hodgkin's disease may be particularly difficult to distinguish from a reactive immunoblastic proliferation. In this rare variant, Hodgkin's cells are found in the interfollicular regions of the lymph node, between retained follicles that are often hyperplastic.[58] Although some cases have more typical areas of Hodgkin's disease elsewhere in the lymph node, the key to its recognition in the remainder of the cases lies in the identification of Hodgkin's cells in the characteristic background, regardless of the overall architectural pattern of the lymph node. Immunohistochemical studies are usually warranted if this variant is suspected and areas more typical of Hodgkin's disease cannot be found.

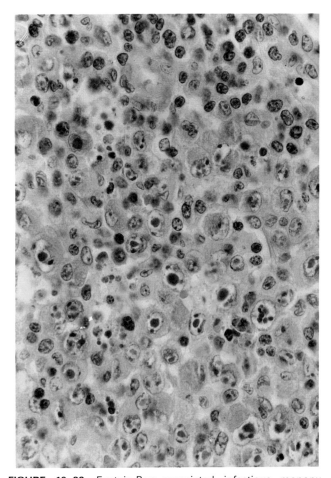

FIGURE 19–32. Epstein-Barr–associated infectious mononucleosis. Although some single cells could easily be mistaken for Hodgkin's cells, the cells show a spectrum of plasmacytoid differentiation.

The **reticular variant of lymphocyte depletion Hodgkin's disease** may be difficult to distinguish from immunoblastic lymphoma, including anaplastic large-cell lymphoma. As discussed earlier, many of the cases that had been diagnosed as the reticular subtype of lymphocyte depletion in the past can now be recognized as pleomorphic variants of non-Hodgkin's lymphoma, with the performance of ancillary studies. The presence of preferential involvement of the sinuses would favor the diagnosis of non-Hodgkin's lymphoma. In addition, the presence of extremely large numbers of Hodgkin's cells (even including, paradoxically, numerous binuclear forms) should also raise suspicion of an immunoblastic lymphoma mimicking Hodgkin's disease. In addition, examination of the bone marrow may be of use, if the typical fibrosing foci of Hodgkin's disease are found. However, in view of the close simulation of morphologic features, it would seem prudent to perform immunohistochemical studies in any case in which a diagnosis of the reticular variant of lymphocyte depletion is considered.

The **diffuse fibrosis subtype of lymphocyte depletion** and **fibroblastic variants of nodular sclerosing** may be confused with a wide variety of neoplasms (Fig. 19–33), including sarcomas such as the inflammatory variant of malignant fibrous histiocytoma. Attention to the clinicopathologic setting and recognition of the fibroblastic component as reactive as opposed to neoplastic should avoid confusion with sarcoma.

L&H LYMPHOCYTE PREDOMINANCE

Participants at the Rye Conference of 1966 combined Lukes and Collins' nodular L&H Hodgkin's disease and diffuse L&H Hodgkin's disease into a new category of **lymphocyte**

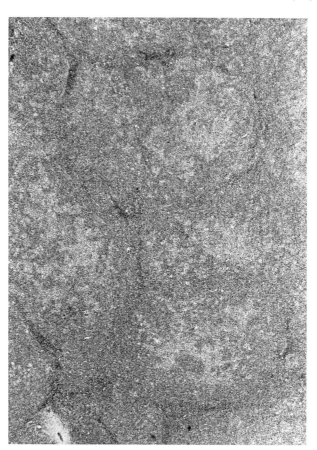

FIGURE 19–34. Nodular L&H lymphocyte predominance Hodgkin's disease. A nodular pattern is seen at low magnification. However, the nodules are larger than generally found in follicular lymphoma.

predominance.[59] In recent years, however, it has become clear that the nodular L&H lymphocyte predominance subtype represents a unique clinicopathologic entity with a clinical course, histology, immunophenotype, and association with non-Hodgkin's lymphoma, all distinct from classic Hodgkin's disease.[60–62] Therefore, the current trend is to separate it from other types of Hodgkin's disease. In nodular L&H lymphocyte predominance, large nodules are present, generally larger but less discrete than the nodules of follicular lymphoma (Fig. 19–34). Within the nodules, and sometimes around the nodules, L&H cells can be identified. L&H cells are large, with large and often multilobated nuclei (Fig. 19–35). The chromatin pattern is generally vesicular, and nucleoli are often evident, although these are smaller than those found in the Reed-Sternberg variants of classic Hodgkin's disease. L&H cells have also been termed ''popcorn'' cells or ''elephant-feet'' cells because of their often polyploid or irregular appearance. These cells mark as B-lineage cells, with CD45 (leukocyte common antigen) and CD20 (B lineage) positivity and lack of staining for CD15 (a marker of Hodgkin's cells of classic Hodgkin's disease) (Fig. 19–36). Often, L&H cells are also positive for epithelial membrane antigen. The other cells in the nodules are small, round lymphocytes that mark as mature B-lineage cells. The internodular cells are mainly T cells, often co-expressing CD57 (Leu-7).[63]

Progressive transformation of germinal centers is a variant of reactive follicular hyperplasia in which the centers of

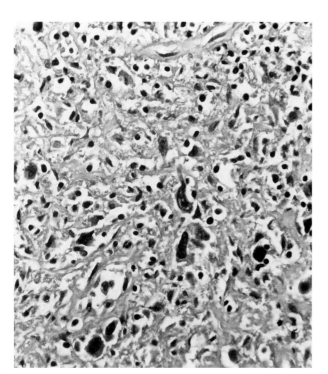

FIGURE 19–33. Nodular sclerosing Hodgkin's disease, fibroblastic variant. Hodgkin's cells are embedded in a background of a fibroblastic proliferation.

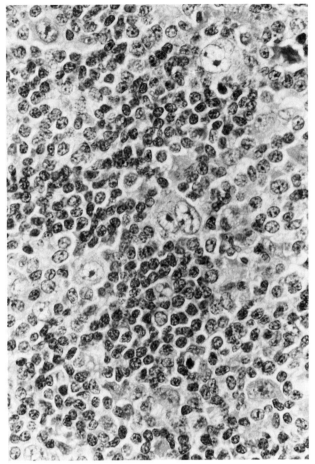

FIGURE 19–35. Nodular L&H lymphocyte predominance Hodgkin's disease. Several L&H ("popcorn") cells are seen. Note the fine nuclear membrane, vesicular chromatin pattern, and the lack of huge nucleoli (although nucleoli are still easily discernible).

one or more follicles become expanded by a proliferation of small lymphocytes, eventually excluding the usual germinal center cells (Fig. 19–37). It is seen most frequently in young males presenting with an asymptomatic solitary enlarged lymph node and is usually unassociated with concomitant or subsequent Hodgkin's disease.[64, 65] Nodular L&H lymphocyte predominance may have a similar low-magnification appearance as progressive transformation; however, in the former, it is common for areas of architectural effacement to be present, with adjacent areas of either normal follicles, hyperplastic follicles, or progressive transformation of germinal centers. The defining difference between nodular L&H lymphocyte predominance and progressive transformation of germinal centers is the presence of the characteristic L&H cells in the former disorder, i.e., a case having histologic features of progressive transformation, yet containing L&H cells, represents nodular L&H lymphocyte predominance.

Nodular L&H lymphocyte predominance may also be difficult to distinguish from classic Hodgkin's disease. The cellular phase of nodular sclerosis may closely mimic nodular L&H lymphocyte predominance. Rarely, sclerosis may be found in the latter, mimicking typical cases of nodular sclerosis. In such borderline cases, immunophenotyping studies are often necessary. As discussed earlier, L&H cells are generally CD45- and CD20-positive and CD15-negative, whereas other

Reed-Sternberg variants are generally CD45- and CD20-negative and CD15-positive.

Rare cases of nodular L&H lymphocyte predominance may be associated with, or transform to, large-cell non-Hodgkin's lymphoma.[62, 66] The key to the diagnosis of non-Hodgkin's lymphoma in such a setting is the presence of sheets of atypical cells in the internodular areas (Fig. 19–38). Borderline cases may occur; in such cases, it is probably wise to err on the side of caution, because the large-cell lymphomas that arise in this setting have had a less aggressive clinical outcome.

Diffuse lymphocyte predominance Hodgkin's disease is another entity currently under re-examination among hematopathologists.[67, 68] We and others suspect that it actually represents two separate diseases that have been confused in the past. Many cases probably represent classic Hodgkin's disease in which Reed-Sternberg cells and variants are difficult to identify. These cases have been called mixed cellularity with lymphocyte predominance by German hematopathologists. Other cases probably represent cases of L&H lymphocyte predominance in which nodularity is absent, minimal, or has been lost over time. We use immunophenotyping studies to separate cases that we encounter in our practice; if the atypical cells are CD45-positive, CD20-positive, and CD15-negative, we would classify a case as L&H lymphocyte predominance, and if the atypical cells are CD45-negative, CD20-negative,

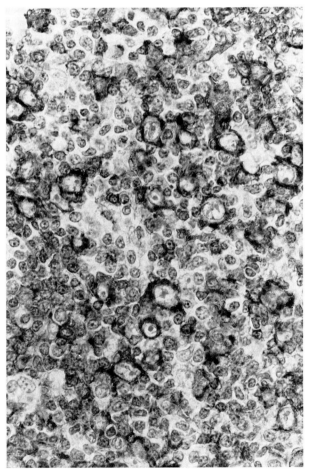

FIGURE 19–36. Nodular L&H lymphocyte predominance Hodgkin's disease; CD20 (L26) stain. The L&H cells are strongly positive for CD20.

and CD15-positive, we would classify a case as classic Hodgkin's disease.

Cases of the diffuse variant of L&H lymphocyte predominance may easily be confused with histiocyte-rich B-cell lymphoma.[23] Epithelioid histiocytes are more common in L&H lymphocyte predominance, whereas the histiocytes in histiocyte-rich B-cell lymphoma are generally non-epithelioid in character. In addition, the presence of even vague nodularity would favor L&H lymphocyte predominance.

Cases of the diffuse variant of L&H lymphocyte predominance may also be confused with T cell–rich B-cell lymphoma.[22] The complete absence of nodularity and the clustering of tumor cells into small aggregates should raise concern for the latter neoplasm. A key feature to examine is the cytologic appearance of the large cells, in an attempt to distinguish L&H cells from the vesicular nuclei more typical of large-cell lymphoma. The large cells of both entities possess a B-lineage phenotype and may express epithelial membrane antigen, but CD57-expressing small lymphocytes, often ringing the L&H cells, are more common in lymphocyte predominance than in T cell–rich B-cell lymphoma.[69] Gene rearrangement studies may be of use, because most cases of T cell–rich B-cell lymphoma reported in the literature have had detectable immunoglobulin gene rearrangements.

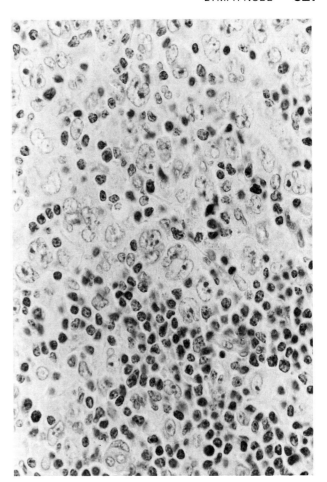

FIGURE 19–38. Large-cell lymphoma arising in nodular L&H lymphocyte predominance Hodgkin's disease. Confluent masses of L&H cells are present.

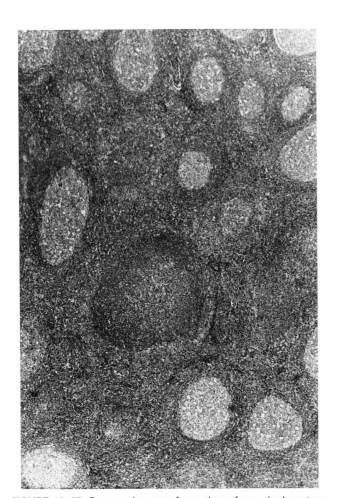

FIGURE 19–37. Progressive transformation of germinal centers. A single progressively transformed germinal center is present, in contrast with the majority of follicles present in this field, which show more typical reactive features.

HISTIOCYTIC PROLIFERATIONS

Sinus histiocytosis with massive lymphadenopathy (Rosai-Dorfman disease) is a rare disorder, but one that should be easily recognized.[70] Involved lymph nodes are enlarged, and the capsule is often fibrotic. At low magnification, there is marked dilatation of the sinuses by distinctive histiocytic-appearing cells (Fig. 19–39). These cells have an intermediate-sized nucleus with a vesicular chromatin pattern and one to several relatively prominent nucleoli (Fig. 19–40). The cytoplasm is very abundant and often contains phagocytosed lymphocytes (lymphophagocytosis or emperipolesis) or other cells, including plasma cells, neutrophils, and red blood cells. Plasma cells are often abundant in the medullary cords. Once the entity is considered, there is usually little diagnostic confusion. In cases of confusion with benign sinus hyperplasia, confirmation of sinus histiocytosis with massive lymphadenopathy may be obtained by demonstrating S-100 positivity in the histiocytic-appearing cells.

In **Langerhans' cell histiocytosis** (histiocytosis X), involved lymph nodes also contain distended sinuses.[71] In this disease, however, the sinus infiltrate is quite different than that seen in sinus histiocytosis with massive lymphadenopathy and consists of a mixed infiltrate of Langerhans' cells, eosinophils, reactive uninucleated and multinucleated histiocytes,

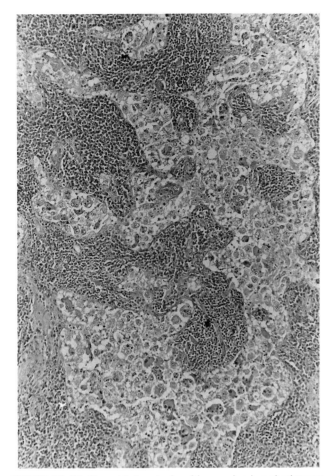

FIGURE 19–39. Sinus histiocytosis with massive lymphadenopathy. A sinusoidal pattern is present.

neutrophils, and small lymphocytes. In some cases, the infiltrate may extend from the sinuses to the adjacent paracortex. The key to the diagnosis is the definitive recognition of the Langerhans' cells as the primary proliferating element in the sinuses. These cells have a characteristic nucleus with a folded, indented, or lobulated nuclear outline, a bland chromatin pattern, and inconspicuous nucleoli (Fig. 19–41). The cytoplasm is generally eosinophilic and moderate in amount. Rare cases may show malignant cytologic features; although some recognize an entity of malignant Langerhans' cell histiocytosis, most hematopathologists believe that the presence of nuclear atypia does not correlate well with subsequent clinical course in most cases.[72] In difficult cases, support for a Langerhans' cell lineage may be obtained in paraffin sections with the demonstration of S-100 in the Langerhans' cells, in frozen sections with the demonstration of CD1 in the cells, or by electron microscopy with the demonstration of Birbeck granules in the cells.

Dermatopathic lymphadenitis, further discussed under the reactive lymphadenopathies, is also characterized by a proliferation of morphologically similar dendritic cells. However, it is usually easily distinguished from Langerhans' cell histiocytosis, because Langerhans' cell histiocytosis primarily affects the sinuses with only secondary involvement of the paracortical regions, and dermatopathic lymphadenitis leads primarily to expansion of the paracortical regions without dendritic cells present in the sinuses.

Rarely, a small focus of Langerhans' cell histiocytosis may be found adjacent to a malignant lymphoma, occurring in either non-Hodgkin's lymphoma or Hodgkin's disease.[73, 74] A sinusoidal localization is not seen in this circumstance. In the majority of such cases, the finding is incidental and without clinical significance, although spread to another site has been reported in at least one patient.

Another rare finding in lymph nodes is prominent sinusoidal dilatation due to massive hemophagocytosis by histiocytes. This phenomenon may be found in several circumstances, including **infection-associated hemophagocytic syndrome, familial hemophagocytic lymphohistiocytosis,** and **secondary hemophagocytic syndrome** associated with malignant lymphoma.[75–79] The histologic appearance of the sinuses is similar in all three conditions. The proliferating histiocytes are cytologically benign and have abundant cytoplasm that contains numerous red blood cells and often other cellular elements, including neutrophils, platelets, lymphocytes, and cellular debris. In both infection-associated hemophagocytic syndrome and familial hemophagocytic lymphohistiocytosis, the remainder of the lymph node usually has a cell-depleted appearance. In secondary hemophagocytic syndrome associated with malignant lymphoma, the malignant lymphoma is most often T lineage, and the lymphoma either may be inti-

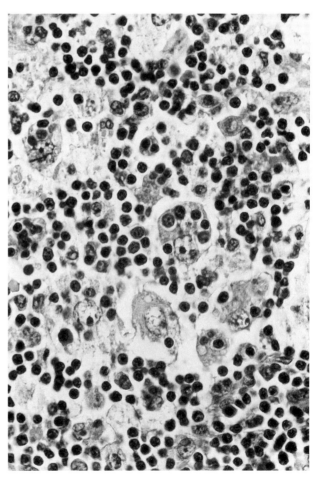

FIGURE 19–40. Sinus histiocytosis with massive lymphadenopathy. The proliferating cells have nuclei with a vesicular chromatin pattern and a distinct nucleolus. The abundant cytoplasm often shows lymphophagocytosis.

mately associated with the phagocytizing histiocytes[77] (Fig. 19–42) or may be found at another site in the body entirely.[78]

As discussed earlier, the diagnosis of malignant histiocytosis or true histiocytic lymphoma is possible only after exhaustive immunophenotypic studies, because the large majority of sinusoidal hematolymphoid neoplasms represent neoplasms of lymphoid derivation, most often large-cell anaplastic lymphoma (Fig. 19–43). One rare setting in which histiocytic malignancies may truly occur is the syndrome of malignant histiocytosis that is associated with a mediastinal germ cell tumor, most commonly a malignant teratoma, with or without yolk sac tumor differentiation.[80]

REACTIVE LYMPHADENOPATHY

In the large majority of cases of reactive lymphadenopathy, a specific diagnosis cannot be given based solely on the histologic features. Generally, we give a description based on the predominant pattern, such as reactive follicular hyperplasia, mixed reactive follicular and paracortical hyperplasia, or reactive paracortical hyperplasia, or based on an important histologic finding, such as the presence of granulomas, necrosis, or vasculitis.

The differential diagnosis between follicular lymphoma and reactive follicular hyperplasia has already been discussed.

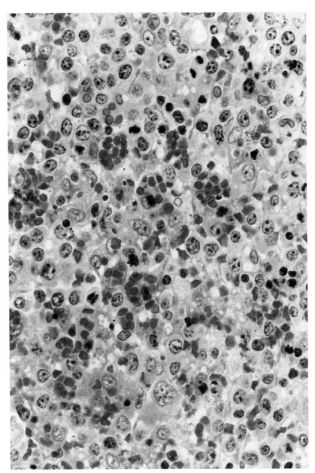

FIGURE 19–42. Malignant lymphoma with benign hemophagocytosis. The histiocyte nuclei are almost obscured by the large amount of hemophagocytosis. The cytologically atypical cells, however, do not exhibit hemophagocytosis.

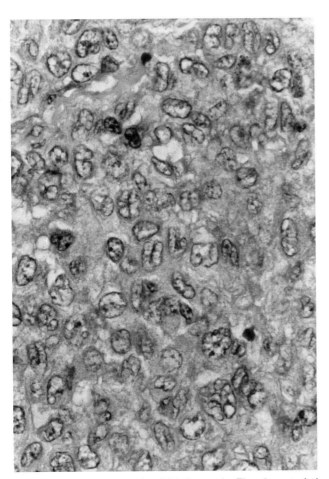

FIGURE 19–41. Langerhans' cell histiocytosis. The characteristic nuclear grooves and folds of the proliferating Langerhans' cells are seen in this field.

Reactive follicular hyperplasia is almost always a nonspecific finding in which a specific cause cannot be assigned; however, there sometimes are clues that might suggest further studies. For example, the presence of numerous plasma cells and plasmacytoid immunoblasts in the paracortical regions along with neutrophils in the sinuses might suggest a collagen vascular disease such as rheumatoid arthritis or Sjögren's syndrome.[81, 82] Similar findings may be found in secondary syphilis, although there is usually a greater degree of fibrosis and the presence of occasional small granulomas and even spirochetes, which sometimes may be demonstrated with a silver-impregnated stain.[83]

The presence of florid reactive follicular hyperplasia in a patient with risk factors for acquired immunodeficiency syndrome (AIDS) should raise consideration of **HIV-related lymphadenopathy.**[84–86] In these cases, one often sees large, highly irregular follicles, often referred to as geographic follicles. The germinal centers may have poorly defined mantle zones or may show follicle lysis, where small lymphocytes are present in the centers of the follicles and are associated with hemorrhage and fragmentation of the follicle into clusters of germinal center cells. Other areas of the lymph node may show atrophic, hypocellular germinal centers ("follicular involution"), with an expanded but lymphocyte-depleted paracortical region. Late in the course of disease, the lymph

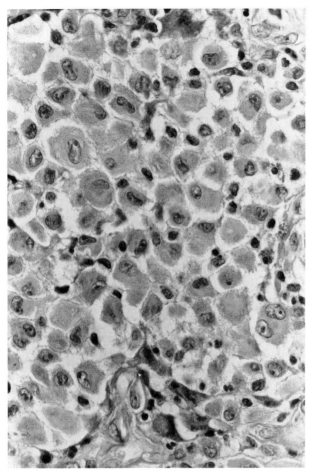

FIGURE 19–43. Peripheral T-cell lymphoma mimicking true histiocytic lymphoma. Despite the histiocytic appearance of the cells, this case lacked histiocytic markers and exhibited monoclonal rearrangements of the beta-T cell receptor gene.

nodes may show absence of germinal centers and marked lymphocyte depletion (''lymphocyte depletion'').

Castleman's disease (angiofollicular lymph node hyperplasia) is in the differential diagnosis of non-specific lymph node hyperplasia.[87] One key to the diagnosis of Castleman's disease is the large size of the excised lymphoid tissue as well as the characteristic capsular fibrosis. In the **unifocal hyaline-vascular variant,** which accounts for approximately 90% of cases, the follicles are usually small and usually contain small vessels with prominent endothelial cells (Fig. 19–44). The mantle zones are usually expanded and contain small lymphocytes in an ''onion-skinning'' pattern around the germinal centers. In addition to its intense vascularity, the interfollicular region often contains scattered plasma cells and plasmacytoid immunoblasts. The hyaline-vascular variant of Castleman's disease may be confused with the follicular involution stage of HIV adenopathy owing to the similar-appearing germinal centers. Attention to clinical information is important, but histologic differences also exist. The interfollicular region in HIV-associated lymphadenopathy tends to have a more polymorphous appearance with greater numbers of plasma cells and lacks the intense vascularity in the interfollicular regions found in Castleman's disease; in addition, fibrosis is more marked in Castleman's disease.

The expanded mantle zones in Castleman's disease must also be distinguished from mantle cell lymphoma. In Castleman's disease, the mantle zone lymphocytes are composed of small, round lymphocytes, different from the cytologically atypical small lymphocytes characteristic of mantle cell lymphoma. Frozen section immunologic studies may be necessary in difficult cases.

In the much rarer **plasma cell type** of Castleman's disease, the germinal centers are indistinguishable from those seen in non-specific reactive follicular hyperplasia. Patients usually have systemic symptoms and numerous abnormal laboratory studies. The characteristic histologic finding is the presence of numerous plasma cells present in the interfollicular areas. The plasma cell variant of Castleman's disease may exist as a unifocal disease similar to the hyaline-vascular variant or may manifest as a multicentric disease.[88] The differential diagnosis for both the unifocal or multicentric plasma cell type of Castleman's disease includes autoimmune disease, HIV-related lymphadenopathy, and lymph nodes involved or adjacent to other neoplasms, particularly Kaposi's sarcoma. Because the histopathologic findings may be indistinguishable among all the above conditions, it is important to obtain complete clinical information and to carefully examine all of the sections for small foci of neoplasm.

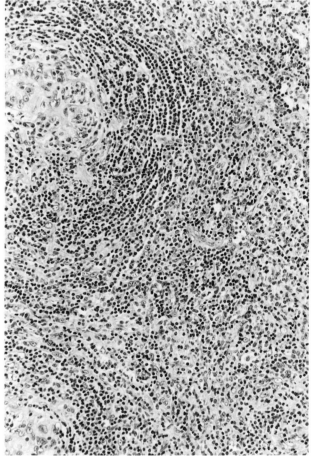

FIGURE 19–44. Castleman's disease, hyaline-vascular type. Note the small but highly vascular germinal center, the well-defined mantle zone with onion-skinning, and the highly vascular expanded interfollicular region.

Toxoplasmic lymphadenopathy typically presents with a florid reactive follicular hyperplasia.[89] In addition, small clusters of epithelioid histiocytes are found in the interfollicular regions that impinge on the germinal centers. Completing the diagnostic triad is infiltration of sinuses with reactive monocytoid B cells. The presence of these three histologic findings is highly specific for toxoplasmosis and should prompt confirmation by serologic studies. Rarely, other lymphadenopathies may show this triad, including HIV-associated lymphadenopathy.[40] The presence of necrosis, even focal, well-formed granulomas, or multinucleated giant cells is highly unusual for toxoplasmosis and should suggest consideration of other diagnoses.

Viral (including Epstein-Barr virus–associated acute infectious mononucleosis) **and postvaccinial lymphadenitis** show similar histologic findings.[90, 91] There is either a mixed reactive follicular and paracortical hyperplasia or a loss of follicles with diffuse effacement of architecture. One often finds a mixed cellular proliferation, including small lymphocytes, plasma cells, plasmacytoid immunoblasts, and histiocytes in the paracortical areas and in the areas of diffuse effacement. Similar histologic findings, sometimes with the addition of numerous eosinophils, may be found in **drug-induced lymphadenopathy.**[92] This polymorphous proliferation usually imparts a mottled appearance and may be confused with interfollicular or mixed cellularity Hodgkin's disease, particularly when eosinophils are present. In Hodgkin's disease, although plasma cells, eosinophils, and histiocytes may be present, there is less of a range of lymphoid cells present; the cells are either small lymphoid cells or Reed-Sternberg variants and diagnostic Reed-Sternberg cells, without plasmacytoid immunoblasts, plasmacytoid lymphocytes, or other transitional lymphoid cells. Occasionally, areas of sheets of immunoblasts, sometimes associated with necrosis, may be found in cases of paracortical or diffuse immunoblastic hyperplasia (Fig. 19–45). These latter areas may easily be confused with non-Hodgkin's lymphomas preferentially involving the paracortical regions, such as is commonly seen in peripheral T-cell lymphoma. Although peripheral T-cell lymphoma also shows a polymorphous infiltrate, the lymphoid proliferation shows a greater range of cytologic atypia, with small atypical lymphocytes, medium-sized atypical lymphocytes, and pleomorphic large lymphoid cells than in hyperplasia.

Immunologic or molecular studies may be very useful in distinguishing the reactive paracortical hyperplasia or effacement due to viral, postvaccinial, or drug-induced lymphadenitis from non-Hodgkin's lymphoma or Hodgkin's disease. In reactive paracortical hyperplasia, most of the immunoblasts mark as B cells, but many of the other cells are of T lineage. In non-Hodgkin's lymphoma of T-cell phenotype, both small and large malignant lymphoid cells mark as T lineage, with only rare B-lineage cells present. In Hodgkin's disease, the atypical cells are generally CD15-positive; however, one must keep in mind that CD15 positivity has been reported in cytomegalovirus-infected cells.[93] In addition, one must remember that CD30 may be expressed on activated reactive lymphoid cells in addition to Reed-Sternberg cells. *In situ* hybridization studies for Epstein-Barr virus may be helpful in distinguishing Epstein-Barr virus–associated acute infectious mononucleosis from other conditions, with the demonstration of large numbers of Epstein-Barr viral genomes in both small and large lymphoid cells.[94] Caution must be exercised, because

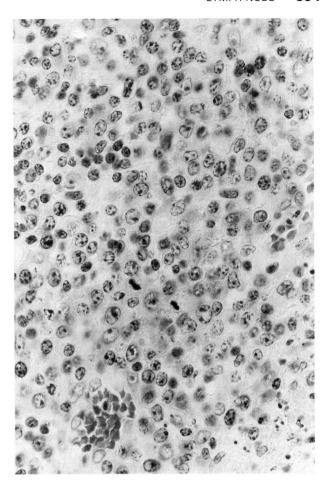

FIGURE 19–45. Herpes lymphadenitis. A diffuse proliferation of immunoblasts is present, closely mimicking a large-cell lymphoma. Other areas of the biopsy showed necrosis and cells with typical herpetic inclusions.

Epstein-Barr virus genomes may be present in the Reed-Sternberg cells in approximately 40% to 50% of cases of Hodgkin's disease. However, in Hodgkin's disease, the virus is present in small numbers and is essentially limited to the Reed-Sternberg cells and variants, with only rare small lymphocytes positive for the virus.

In **dermatopathic lymphadenitis,** there is a diffuse paracortical hyperplasia, with or without reactive follicular hyperplasia.[95] The paracortical regions appear pale and mottled owing to the presence of a mixed population of dendritic cells (both interdigitating reticulum cells and Langerhans' cells), histiocytes, immunoblasts, eosinophils, plasma cells, and varying numbers of small lymphoid cells and immunoblasts showing varying degrees of cytologic atypia (Fig. 19–46). Melanin pigment is usually evident but may be difficult to discern. As discussed earlier, dermatopathic lymphadenitis can be differentiated from Langerhans' cell histiocytosis by its involvement of the paracortical, rather than sinus, regions of the lymph node.

Distinguishing dermatopathic lymphadenitis from lymph node involvement by mycosis fungoides is a much more difficult task. Patients with **mycosis fungoides** often have lymph nodes with dermatopathic changes with or without concomitant mycosis fungoides.[96] In addition, patients with dermatopathic lymphadenitis often have extensive skin lesions for

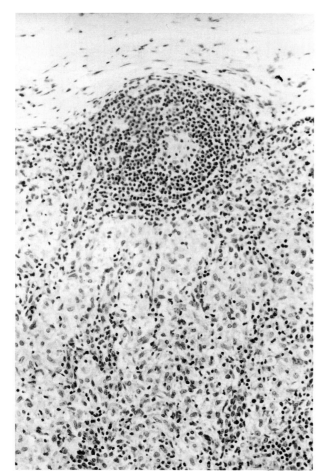

FIGURE 19–46. Dermatopathic lymphadenopathy. The pallor in the interfollicular regions is due to a proliferation of macrophages, interdigitating reticulum cells, and Langerhans' cells.

which mycosis fungoides is considered part of the differential diagnosis. Because single, scattered, and even clusters of atypical lymphocytes may be seen in the dermatopathic lymph nodes of patients with non–mycosis fungoides skin disease, these histologic features are insufficient for a diagnosis of mycosis fungoides. Definite histologic involvement by mycosis fungoides can be established only when architectural effacement by atypical cells is present; even immunologic studies have only a limited role in the differential diagnosis.[97] However, determination of the status of the beta-T cell receptor gene by molecular methods can be very useful in this setting; unfortunately, this procedure generally requires frozen tissue.[98]

Granulomas may be seen in a variety of disorders, including infectious and non-infectious diseases. Sarcoidosis most often manifests as multiple non-caseating granulomas, but the granulomas may occasionally have central areas of fibrinoid necrosis. Infectious agents should be excluded by appropriate special stains and cultures; however, special stains are usually of little use when necrosis is absent. It is also important to consider malignant neoplasms in the differential diagnosis. Involvement of the lymph node by Hodgkin's disease may be obscured by multiple granulomas; in addition, patients with Hodgkin's disease, non-Hodgkin's lymphoma, and other malignant neoplasms may have non-caseating granulomas at uninvolved sites.[99]

The differential diagnosis of caseating granulomas should include mycobacteria and fungi. When necrotizing granulomas are present with central stellate microabscesses, bacterial diseases such as **cat-scratch disease, lymphogranuloma venereum,** and **Yersinial infections** should be considered. Although the organism of cat-scratch disease is said to be identified with a Warthin-Starry stain,[100] we have not been often helped by this stain in cases we considered highly likely to be cat-scratch disease.

Histiocytic necrotizing lymphadenitis (Kikuchi-Fujimoto disease) is a benign, generally self-limited disorder that was first reported in 1972. Histologically, one sees widespread areas of necrosis with abundant karyorrhectic debris and extensive fibrin deposition, usually involving the paracortex.[101] In areas of cellular preservation, sheets of macrophages and large lymphoid cells with single cell necrosis are found (Fig. 19–47). These large cells may closely simulate large-cell lymphoma.[102]

There are several keys to the diagnosis of histiocytic necrotizing lymphadenitis. The first clue is the clinical history, which is usually that of isolated cervical lymphadenopathy occurring in a young woman. However, any age group or lymph node site can be affected, and 20% of cases occur in men. The second clue is the character of the necrosis. In the necrosis that occurs in malignant lymphoma, one generally

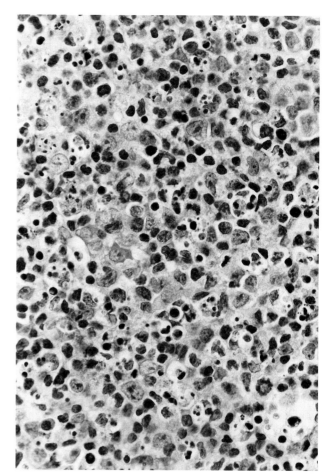

FIGURE 19–47. Histiocytic necrotizing lymphadenitis (Kikuchi-Fujimoto disease). This area mimics a large-cell lymphoma. One clue to the correct diagnosis is the presence of abundant single cell necrosis with karyorrhectic debris.

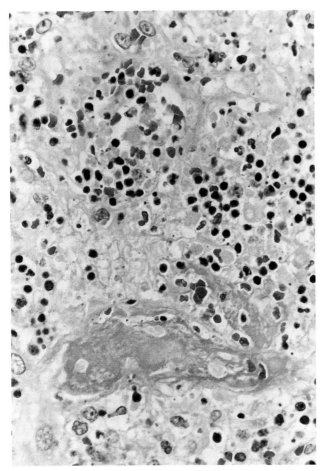

FIGURE 19–48. Kawasaki's disease. This lymph node biopsy shows numerous small vessels with thrombi, in addition to extensive necrosis.

the usual number of plasma cells and, rarely, the deposition of nuclear debris on the walls of vessels or hematoxyphilic bodies. Because of the close morphologic similarities between the two diseases, it may be prudent to obtain serologic studies to rule out systemic lupus erythematosus in all cases in which histiocytic necrotizing lymphadenitis is being seriously considered. **Kawasaki's disease** may also be confused with histiocytic necrotizing lymphadenitis because of the extensive necrosis that may also be present in this condition.[104] Features that distinguish it from necrotizing histiocytic lymphadenitis are the presence of numerous fibrin thrombi in small vessels and the presence of neutrophils (Fig. 19–48).

There are two types of complete lymph node necrosis: liquefactive and infarction.[105] **Liquefactive necrosis** consists of karyorrhectic debris and fragments of neutrophils that completely replace and obliterate the normal lymph node architecture. It is most often infectious in etiology and usually bacterial. Occasionally, there are clues to the specific agent involved, such as when viral inclusions can be identified (Fig. 19–49). In lymph node **infarction,** the areas of necrosis are strongly eosinophilic, consisting of ghosts of cells, indicating ischemia. Granulation tissue is often present at the edge, surrounded by acute and chronic inflammation, and venous thrombosis is seen in some cases. Although vessel disease is a cause of lymph node infarction, a more important association to rule out is that of malignant lymphoma. In one study, 13

sees the ghosts of necrotic cells. Although karyorrhectic debris is abundant in histiocytic necrotizing lymphadenitis, one does not see the ghosts of intact cells. When abundant karyorrhectic debris occurs in the malignant lymphoma, it is virtually always associated with the monomorphic high-grade lymphomas, neoplasms that are usually easy to distinguish from histiocytic necrotizing lymphadenitis. Third, in the cellular areas of histiocytic necrotizing lymphadenitis, although histiocytes and atypical lymphoid cells are present, intact neutrophils are almost invariably absent, and plasma cells usually are not numerous. Fourth, adjacent areas of relatively uninvolved nodal tissue generally show clear-cut reactive changes, including a reactive paracortical immunoblastic proliferation and often highly reactive follicular hyperplasia. Finally, immunophenotyping studies may be useful. The large cells in histiocytic necrotizing lymphadenitis are macrophages and T lymphocytes, usually suppressor cells, whereas the majority of malignant lymphomas are of B-cell phenotype. Phenotyping studies may be useful even in cases with very extensive necrosis, because the antigenic determinants are frequently retained longer than the morphologic appearance of the necrotic cells.

Histiocytic necrotizing lymphadenitis may be confused with a number of other benign conditions. The histologic changes of **systemic lupus erythematosus** may be identical to those of histiocytic necrotizing lymphadenitis.[103] Clues to the recognition of lupus include the presence of more than

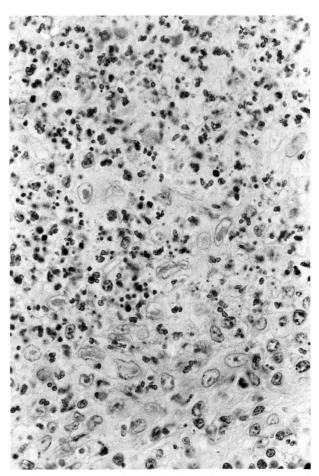

FIGURE 19–49. Herpes lymphadenitis with extensive necrosis. Numerous herpetic inclusions are present.

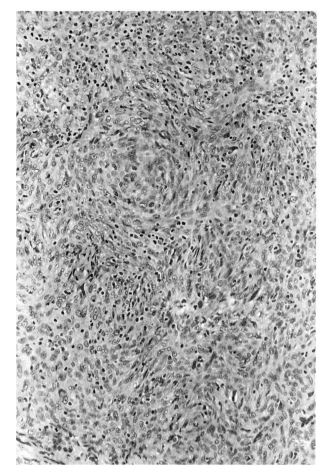

FIGURE 19–50. Dendritic reticulum cell sarcoma. Note the storiform pattern at low magnification.

of 16 patients with infarcted lymph node biopsies subsequently were shown to have malignant lymphoma, usually of large-cell type, on rebiopsy.[106] Occasionally, immunostains performed on completely infarcted areas show retention of immunogenicity and reveal sheets of B-lineage cells, a feature strongly suggestive of malignant lymphoma.[107]

DENDRITIC AND MISCELLANEOUS NON-LYMPHOID PROLIFERATIONS

Dendritic reticulum cell sarcoma and **interdigitating reticulum cell sarcoma** are rare sarcomas showing differentiation toward normal dendritic and interdigitating reticulum cells, respectively.[108] The morphologic features are similar, with a proliferation of ovoid to spindled cells, forming fascicles, nests, whorls, and sometimes a storiform pattern (Fig. 19–50). The neoplastic cells usually possess a bland nucleus and an inconspicuous nucleolus; pseudonuclear inclusions may be found in some cases (Fig. 19–51). One key feature that is often present is an admixture of small lymphocytes scattered as single cells about the tumor or in discrete collections, particularly in perivascular areas.

A suspicion of a diagnosis of reticulum cell sarcoma may be supported by paraffin section immunohistochemical studies. The neoplastic cells of dendritic reticulum cell sarcoma

are usually negative or equivocal for CD45 and negative or positive for S-100 protein, and the cells stain with monoclonal antibodies specific for dendritic reticulum cells, such as R4/23. The neoplastic cells of interdigitating sarcoma are usually positive for CD45RB, S-100, and CD68. The definitive diagnosis of the reticulum cell sarcomas can be established only after exhaustive frozen section immunohistochemical studies document the appropriate dendritic or interdigitating reticulum cell phenotype.

The differential diagnosis of reticulum cell sarcoma includes any lesion that may show spindling of the proliferating cells. This includes malignancies such as rare primary or metastatic sarcoma, metastatic spindle cell carcinoma or melanoma, and rare cases of malignant lymphoma, most commonly CD30-positive lymphomas, which may exhibit spindling.[109] Immunohistochemical studies are extremely useful in cases in which there is a significant level of doubt.

Hemorrhagic spindle cell tumor with amianthoid fibers (palisaded myofibroblastoma) is a rare, benign spindle cell lesion that most commonly occurs in the inguinal region, although it may even more rarely occur in other sites as well.[110, 111] The individual cells possess nuclei with a bland chromatin pattern and low mitotic rate and a spindled cytoplasm that may possess fuchsinophilic globules. As the names used for this tumor imply, additional characteristic features include the presence of variable degrees of hemorrhage, hemo-

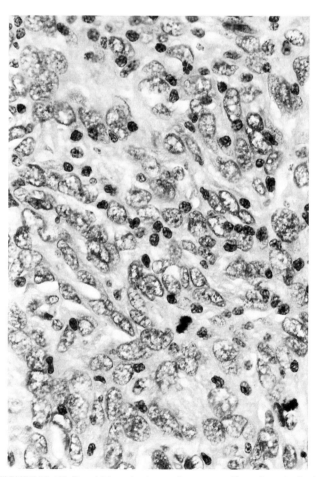

FIGURE 19–51. Dendritic reticulum cell sarcoma. Note the spindled proliferation, with admixed reactive lymphocytes.

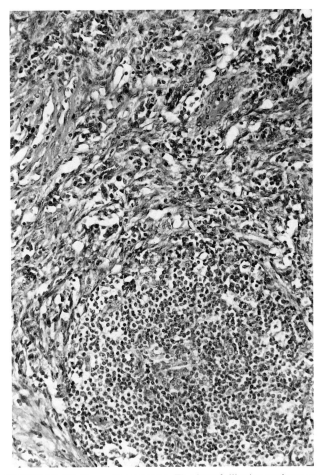

FIGURE 19–52. Kaposi's sarcoma. The interfollicular regions are completely replaced by tumor.

siderin deposits, and granulation tissue; the presence of amianthoid fibers; stellate areas of a peculiar form of collagen deposition; and palisading of nuclei reminiscent of a benign schwannoma. However, paraffin section immunohistochemistry should easily differentiate this lesion from a schwannoma, because the cells are positive for muscle-specific actin (including the globules) and myosin but negative for S-100 protein.

Kaposi's sarcoma may occur in a lymph node in several clinicopathologic settings, including a primary lymphadenopathic form found in endemic (African) regions.[112] More commonly, it occurs as a site of metastatic disease secondary to skin or mucosal involvement in patients with AIDS or immunosuppression due to organ transplantation or malignancies. In advanced lesions, the lymph node shows effacement by a spindled proliferation identical to Kaposi's sarcoma seen in other sites. However, early involvement may be quite subtle and may show preferential involvement of the capsule or subcapsular sinuses, with variable extension into the paracortical regions (Fig. 19–52). Attention should be drawn to areas with ectatic vessels or increased vascular proliferation; nonetheless, a definitive diagnosis is best deferred unless the classic spindle cell areas with PAS-positive hyaline globules are identified.

Kaposi's sarcoma can be distinguished from intranodal hemorrhagic spindle cell tumor with amianthoid fibers by

the more atypical nuclear features and the presence of PAS-positive hyaline globules in the former. In cases of doubt, demonstration of the vascular marker CD34 on the neoplastic cells of Kaposi's sarcoma may be sought.[113] **Vascular transformation of lymph node sinuses,** a relatively common nodal reaction, may also be confused with Kaposi's sarcoma. Vascular transformation of lymph node sinuses is confined to the sinuses, without extension to the capsule or paracortical regions, and does not form a discrete mass.[114] Vascular channels are always present in vascular transformation (although sometimes subtly), and sheets of spindled cells are never found. In addition, cytologic atypia is always lacking in vascular transformation, and hyaline globules are almost always absent.

Kaposi's sarcoma must also be distinguished from benign **inflammatory pseudotumor** of lymph nodes.[115, 116] This disease predominantly affects young adults, presenting with prominent lymphadenopathy, and often having B symptoms. Histologically, there is a proliferation of spindled cells representing fibroblasts and histiocytes, along with scattered inflammatory cells, associated with fibrosis (Fig. 19–53). Cellular atypia is completely lacking. There is usually preferential involvement of the lymph node capsule and trabeculae.

On rare occasions, Kaposi's sarcoma involving the lymph node may be mistaken for **Castleman's disease.** This is

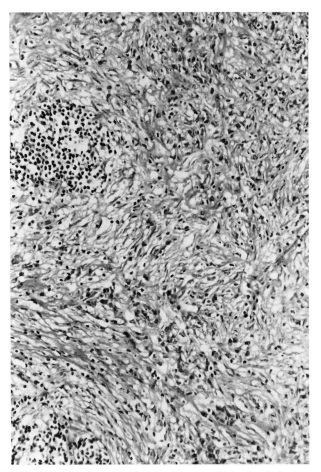

FIGURE 19–53. Inflammatory pseudotumor. A bland spindled proliferation is present, with extensive fibrosis and scattered inflammatory cells.

because the lymphoid tissue adjacent to a focus of Kaposi's sarcoma may show a peculiar hypervascular follicular hyperplasia reminiscent of the follicles of Castleman's disease (Fig. 19–54).[117] If overemphasis is given to this histologic feature, the neoplastic vascular proliferation of Kaposi's sarcoma may be easily mistaken for the hypervascular interfollicular areas of Castleman's disease; attention to the clinicopathologic setting may avoid this pitfall. Rarely, cases of hyaline-vascular Castleman's disease may be complicated by a vascular neoplasm distinct from Kaposi's sarcoma.[118]

The lymph node may also be the site of numerous other rare vascular proliferations, including capillary hemangioma (nodal angiomatosis), epithelioid hemangioma (angiolymphoid hyperplasia with eosinophilia), hemangioendothelioma (including epithelioid, spindle and epithelioid, and polymorphous variants), lymphangioma, and venolymphatic angiodysplasia.[119] In **epithelioid hemangioma,** well-formed epithelioid endothelium-lined vascular channels are present, with frequent admixture of small lymphocytes and eosinophils. This lesion is distinguished from **Kimura's disease** by the lack of the endothelial proliferation in the latter. **Epithelioid hemangioendothelioma** in the lymph node is identical in appearance to the same lesions more commonly found in soft tissue and is more likely to be confused with metastatic carcinoma than

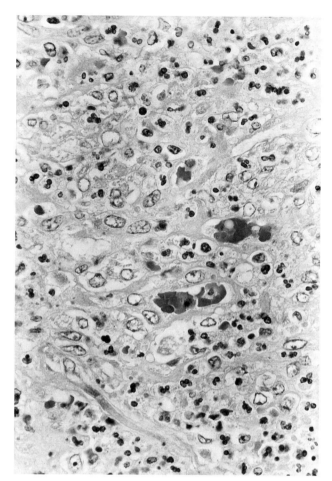

FIGURE 19–55. Bacillary angiomatosis. There is marked vascular proliferation with scattered but numerous neutrophils.

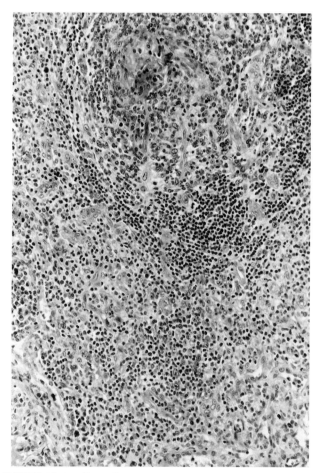

FIGURE 19–54. Kaposi's sarcoma, resembling Castleman's disease. The germinal center is virtually identical to that seen in Castleman's disease, but a malignant vascular proliferation is present in the interfollicular region (lower corners of the photomicrograph).

epithelioid hemangioma. **Spindle and epithelioid hemangioendothelioma** is similar to epithelioid hemangioendothelioma but has a more prominent spindle cell component. **Polymorphous hemangioendothelioma** is variable in appearance and has areas of solid cellular proliferations, areas of primitive vascular differentiation, and areas of an angiomatous component with a lining of plump endothelial cells.

Bacillary angiomatosis represents the most important differential diagnosis of these benign or borderline malignant vascular tumors. This disease is a bacterial infection caused by a *Rickettsia*-like organism and occurs almost always in patients with profound immunodeficiency, such as seen with AIDS. The lymph node shows a disorganized proliferation of vessels lined by plump endothelial cells with scattered neutrophils (Fig. 19–55).[120] The key to the histologic diagnosis is the recognition of the presence of abundant amorphous or granular interstitial substance, which should prompt performance of a Warthin-Starry stain; this will reveal the material to represent numerous short rods. Although the bacillus is identical in appearance to the causative agent of cat-scratch disease, the abundance of organisms, the histologic appearance, and the clinical setting should provide easy distinction between these two diseases.

In addition to purely vascular lesions, mixed vascular and smooth muscle proliferations may occur in lymph node, including lymphangiomyomatosis, angiomyomatous hamartoma, and angiomyolipoma.[119, 121, 122] Finally, pure smooth muscle proliferations may occur, including intranodal leiomyoma, leiomyomatosis, and a reactive smooth muscle proliferation in the lymph node hilum.[123-125]

A variety of glandular inclusions may occur in the lymph node. These include benign inclusions, endometriosis (including decidual changes) and endosalpingiosis, salivary gland inclusions, thyroid inclusions, breast epithelial inclusions, as well as even rarer occurring inclusions from a variety of sites.[126] In general, the key to their recognition is the lack of cytologic atypia. However, some carcinomas metastatic to lymph nodes are notorious for being cytologically bland, e.g., metastatic papillary carcinoma of the thyroid. In all cases, attention to the clinical setting is important, and possible evaluation of potential primary sites may be indicated in some circumstances.

Nevus cells, including blue nevus cells, may also occur as ''rests'' in a lymph node.[127, 128] Keys to the recognition of nevus rests are their cytologic identity to the nevus cells of benign nevocellular or blue nevi of the skin and their predominant location within the capsule rather than the sinuses of the lymph node, although extension into the sinuses from the capsule may occur.

References

1. The Non-Hodgkin's Lymphoma Pathologic Classification Project: National Cancer Institute sponsored study of classifications of non-Hodgkin's lymphomas. Summary and description of a working formulation for clinical usage. Cancer 49:2112–2135, 1982.
2. Ben-Ezra J, Burke JS, Swartz WG, et al: Small lymphocytic lymphoma: A clinicopathologic analysis of 268 cases. Blood 73:579–583, 1989.
3. Dick FR, Maca RD: The lymph node in chronic lymphocytic leukemia. Cancer 41:283–292, 1978.
4. Ngan B-Y, Picker LJ, Medeiros LJ, et al: Immunophenotypic diagnosis of non-Hodgkin's lymphoma in paraffin sections: Co-expression of L60 (Leu22) and L26 antigens correlates with malignant histologic findings. Am J Clin Pathol 91:579–583, 1989.
5. Picker LJ, Weiss LM, Medeiros LJ, et al: Immunophenotypic criteria for the diagnosis of non-Hodgkin's lymphoma. Am J Pathol 128:181–201, 1987.
6. Haraousseau JL, Flandrin G, Tricot G, et al: Malignant lymphoma supervening in chronic lymphocytic leukemia and related disorders—Richter's syndrome: A study of 25 cases. Cancer 48:1302–1308, 1981.
7. Pugh WC, Manning JT, Butler JJ: Paraimmunoblastic variant of small lymphocytic lymphoma/leukemia. Am J Surg Pathol 12:907–917, 1988.
8. Banks PM, Chan J, Cleary ML, et al: Mantle cell lymphoma. A proposal for unification of morphologic, immunologic, and molecular data. Am J Surg Pathol 16:637–640, 1992.
9. Lardelli P, Bookman MA, Sundeen J, et al: Lymphocytic lymphoma of intermediate differentiation. Morphologic and immunophenotypic spectrum and clinical correlations. Am J Surg Pathol 14:752–763, 1992.
10. Perry DA, Bast MA, Armitage JO, et al: Diffuse intermediate lymphocytic lymphoma: A clinicopathologic study with comparison to small lymphocytic lymphoma and diffuse small cleaved cell lymphoma. Cancer 66:1995–2000, 1990.
11. Harris NL, Bhan AK: Mantle-zone lymphoma. A pattern produced by lymphomas of more than one cell type. Am J Surg Pathol 9:872–882, 1985.
12. Williams ME, Westermann CD, Swerdlow SH: Genotypic characterization of centrocytic lymphoma: Frequent rearrangement of the chromosome 11 bcl-1 locus. Blood 76:1387–1391, 1990.
13. Sheibani K, Sohn CC, Burke JS, et al: Monocytoid B-cell lymphoma: A novel B-cell neoplasm. Am J Pathol 124:310–318, 1986.
14. Nathwani BN, Mohrmann RL, Brynes RK, et al: Monocytoid B-cell lymphomas: An assessment of diagnostic criteria and a perspective on histogenesis. Hum Pathol 23:1061–1071, 1992.
15. Traweek ST, Sheibani K, Winberg CD, et al: Monocytoid B-cell lymphoma: Its evolution and relationship to other B-cell neoplasms. Blood 73:573–578, 1989.
16. Nathwani BN, Winberg CD, Diamond LW, et al: Morphologic criteria for the differentiation of follicular lymphoma from florid reactive follicular hyperplasia. Cancer 48:1794–1806, 1981.
17. Pezzella F, Tse AGD, Cordell JL, et al: Expression of the bcl-2 oncogene protein is not specific for the 14;18 chromosomal translocation. Am J Pathol 137:225–232, 1990.
18. Weiss LM, Warnke RA, Sklar J, et al: Molecular analysis of the t(14;18) chromosomal translocation in malignant lymphomas. N Engl J Med 317:1185–1189, 1987.
19. Yunis JJ, Oken MM, Kaplan ME, et al: Distinctive chromosomal abnormalities in histologic subtypes of non-Hodgkin's lymphoma. N Engl J Med 307:1231–1236, 1982.
20. Mann RB, Berard CW: Criteria for the cytologic subclassification of follicular lymphomas: A proposed alternative method. Hematol Oncol 1:187–192, 1982.
21. Lennert K: Histopathology of Non-Hodgkin's Lymphomas (Based on the Kiel Classification). 2nd ed. Berlin, Springer-Verlag, 1981, pp 45–53.
22. Macon WR, Williams ME, Greer JP, et al: T-cell-rich B-cell lymphomas. A clinicopathologic study of 19 cases. Am J Surg Pathol 16:351–363, 1991.
23. Delabie J, Vandenberghe E, Kennes C, et al: Histiocyte-rich B-cell lymphoma. A distinct clinicopathologic entity possibly related to lymphocyte predominant Hodgkin's disease, paragranuloma subtype. Am J Surg Pathol 16:37–48, 1992.
24. Weiss LM, Crabtree GS, Rouse RV, et al: Morphologic and immunologic characterization of 50 peripheral T cell lymphomas. Am J Pathol 118:316–324, 1985.
25. Jaffe ES, Blattner WA, Blayney DW, et al: The pathologic spectrum of adult T-cell leukemia/lymphoma in the United States. Human T-cell leukemia/lymphoma virus-associated lymphoid malignancies. Am J Surg Pathol 8:263–275, 1984.
26. Patsouris E, Nöel H, Lennert K: Histological and immunohistological findings in lymphoepithelioid cell lymphoma (Lennert's lymphoma). Am J Surg Pathol 12:341–350, 1988.
27. Patsouris E, Nöel H, Lennert K: Lymphoplasmacytic/lymphoplasmacytoid immunocytoma with a high content of epithelioid cells. Histologic and immunohistochemical findings. Am J Surg Pathol 14:660–670, 1990.
28. Frizzera G, Moran EM, Rappaport H: Angio-immunoblastic lymphadenopathy with dysproteinaemia. Lancet 1:1070–1073, 1974.
29. Weiss LM, Strickler JG, Dorfman RF, et al: Clonal T-cell populations in angioimmunoblastic lymphadenopathy and angioimmunoblastic lymphadenopathy-like T cell lymphoma. Am J Pathol 122:392–397, 1986.
30. Nathwani BN, Rappaport H, Moran EM, et al: Malignant lymphoma arising in angioimmunoblastic lymphadenopathy. Cancer 41:578–606, 1978.
31. Abruzzo LV, Schmidt K, Weiss LM, et al: B-cell lymphoma arising in angioimmunoblastic lymphadenopathy: A case with oligoclonal gene rearrangements associated with Epstein-Barr virus. Blood 82:241–246, 1993.
32. Strickler JG, Audeh MW, Copenhaver C, et al: Immunophenotypic differences between plasmacytoma/multiple myeloma and immunoblastic lymphoma. Cancer 61:1782–1786, 1988.
33. Kant JA, Hubbard SM, Longo DL, et al: The pathologic and clinical heterogeneity of lymphocyte-depleted Hodgkin's disease. J Clin Oncol 4:284–294, 1986.
34. Stein H, Mason DY, Gerdes J, et al: The expression of the Hodgkin's disease associated antigen Ki-1 in reactive and neoplastic lymphoid tissue: Evidence that Reed-Sternberg cells and histiocytic malignancies are derived from activated lymphoid cells. Blood 66:848–858, 1985.
35. Chan JKC, Ng CS, Hui PK, et al: Anaplastic large cell Ki-1 lymphoma. Delineation of two morphological types. Histopathology 15:11–34, 1989.
36. Weiss LM, Picker LJ, Copenhaver CM, et al: Large cell hematolymphoid neoplasms of uncertain lineage. Hum Pathol 19:967–973, 1988.
37. O'Connor NTJ, Stein H, Gatter KC, et al: Genotypic analysis of large cell lymphomas which express Ki-1 antigen. Histopathology 11:733–740, 1987.
38. Bitter MA, Franklin WA, Larson RA, et al: Morphology in Ki-1 (CD30)-positive non-Hodgkin's lymphoma is correlated with clinical features and the presence of a unique chromosomal abnormality, t(2;5)(p23;q35). Am J Surg Pathol 14:305–316, 1990.
39. Byrne GE, Rappaport H: Malignant histiocytosis. In Akazaki K, Rappaport H, Berard CW, et al (eds): Malignant Disease of the Hematopoietic System. (Gann monograph on cancer research 15). Tokyo, University of Tokyo Press, 1973, pp 145–162.
40. Warnke RA, Kim H, Dorfman RF: Malignant histiocytosis (''histiocytic medullary reticulosis''). I. Clinicopathologic study of 29 cases. Cancer 34:215–230, 1975.
41. Weiss LM, Trela MJ, Cleary ML, et al: Frequent immunoglobulin and T-cell receptor gene rearrangements in ''histiocytic'' neoplasms. Am J Pathol 121:369–373, 1985.
42. Wilson MS, Weiss LM, Gatter KC, et al: Malignant histiocytosis. A reassessment of cases previously reported in 1975 based on paraffin section immunophenotyping studies. Cancer 66:530–536, 1990.
43. Coleman CN, Picozzi VJ, Cox RS, et al: Treatment of lymphoblastic lymphoma in adults. J Clin Oncol 4:1628–1637, 1986.
44. Nathwani BN, Diamond LW, Winberg CD, et al: Lymphoblastic lymphoma: A clinicopathologic study of 95 patients. Cancer 48:2347–2357, 1981.
45. Warnke RA, Gatter KC, Falini B, et al: Diagnosis of human lymphoma with monoclonal antileukocyte antibodies. N Engl J Med 309:1275–1281, 1983.
46. Weiss LM, Bindl JM, Picozzi VJ, et al: Lymphoblastic lymphoma: An immunophenotype study of 26 cases with comparison to T cell acute lymphoblastic leukemia. Blood 67:474–478, 1986.
47. Stroup R, Sheibani K, Misset J-L, et al: Surface immunoglobulin-positive lymphoblastic lymphoma. A report of three cases. Cancer 65:2559–2563, 1990.
48. Murphy SB: Current concepts in cancer. Childhood non-Hodgkin's lymphoma. N Engl J Med 299:1446–1448, 1978.
49. Colby TV, Hoppe RT, Warnke RA: Hodgkin's disease at autopsy: 1972–1977. Cancer 47:1852–1862, 1981.
50. Dolginow D, Colby TV: Recurrent Hodgkin's disease in treated sites. Cancer 48:1124–1126, 1981.
51. Chittal SM, Caverivere P, Schwarting R, et al: Monoclonal antibodies in the diagnosis of Hodgkin's disease. The search for a rational panel. Am J Surg Pathol 12:9–21, 1988.
52. Schmid C, Pan L, Diss T, et al: Expression of B-cell antigens by Hodgkin's and Reed-Sternberg cells in Hodgkin's disease. Am J Pathol 139:475–483, 1991.

53. Weiss LM, Strickler JG, Hu E, et al: Immunoglobulin gene rearrangements in Hodgkin's disease. Hum Pathol 17:1009–1017, 1986.

54. Weiss LM, Picker LJ, Grogan TM, et al: Absence of clonal beta and gamma T-cell receptor gene rearrangements in a subset of peripheral T-cell lymphomas. Am J Pathol 130:436–442, 1988.

55. Strickler JG, Michie SA, Warnke RA, et al: The "syncytial variant" of nodular sclerosing Hodgkin's disease. Am J Surg Pathol 10:470–477, 1986.

56. Osborne BM, Uthman MO, Butler JJ, et al: Differentiation of T-cell lymphoma from Hodgkin's disease: Mitotic rate and S-phase analysis. Am J Clin Pathol 93:227–232, 1990.

57. Butler JJ: The histologic diagnosis of Hodgkin's disease. Semin Diagn Pathol 9:252–256, 1992.

58. Doggett RS, Colby TV, Dorfman RF: Interfollicular Hodgkin's disease. Am J Surg Pathol 7:145–149, 1983.

59. Lukes RJ, Craver LF, Hall TC, et al: Report of the nomenclature committee. Cancer Res 26:1311, 1966.

60. Regula DP, Hoppe RT, Weiss LM: Nodular and diffuse types of lymphocyte predominance Hodgkin's disease. N Engl J Med 318:214–219, 1988.

61. Pinkus GS, Said JW: Hodgkin's disease, lymphocyte predominance type, nodular—further evidence for a B cell derivation. L&H variants of Reed-Sternberg cells express L26, a pan B cell marker. Am J Pathol 133:211–217, 1988.

62. Hansmann ML, Stein H, Fellbaum C, et al: Nodular paragranuloma can transform into high-grade malignant lymphoma of B type. Hum Pathol 20:1169–1175, 1989.

63. Timens W, Visser L, Poppema S: Nodular lymphocyte predominance type of Hodgkin's disease is a germinal center lymphoma. Lab Invest 54:457–461, 1986.

64. Osborne BM, Butler JJ: Clinical implications of progressive transformation of germinal centers. Am J Surg Pathol 8:725–733, 1984.

65. Ferry JA, Zukerberg LR, Harris NL: Florid progressive transformation of germinal centers. A syndrome affecting young men, without early progression to nodular lymphocyte predominance Hodgkin's disease. Am J Surg Pathol 16:252–258, 1992.

66. Sundeen JT, Cossman J, Jaffe ES: Lymphocyte predominant Hodgkin's disease nodular subtype with coexistent "large cell lymphoma." Histological progression or composite malignancy. Am J Surg Pathol 12:599–606, 1988.

67. Hansmann M-L, Stein H, Dallenbach F, et al: Diffuse lymphocyte-predominant Hodgkin's disease (diffuse paragranuloma). A variant of the B-cell-derived nodular type. Am J Pathol 138:29–36, 1991.

68. Nicholas DS, Harris S, Wright DH: Lymphocyte predominance Hodgkin's disease—an immunohistochemical study. Histopathology 16:157–165, 1990.

69. Kamel OW, Gelb A, Shibuya RB, Warnke RA: Leu 7 (CD57) reactivity distinguishes nodular lymphocyte predominance Hodgkin's disease from nodular sclerosing Hodgkin's disease, T-cell-rich B-cell lymphoma and follicular lymphoma. Am J Pathol 142:541–546, 1992.

70. Foucar E, Rosai J, Dorfman RF: Sinus histiocytosis with massive lymphadenopathy (Rosai-Dorfman disease). Review of the entity. Semin Diagn Pathol 7:19–73, 1990.

71. Williams JW, Dorfman RF: Lymphadenopathy as the initial manifestation of histiocytosis X. Am J Surg Pathol 3:405–421, 1979.

72. Risdall RJ, Dehner LP, Duray P, et al: Histiocytosis X (Langerhans' cell histiocytosis). Prognostic role of histopathology. Arch Pathol Lab Med 107:59–63, 1983.

73. Burns BF, Colby TV, Dorfman RF: Langerhans' cell granulomatosis (histiocytosis X) associated with malignant lymphomas. Am J Surg Pathol 7:529–535, 1983.

74. Neumann MP, Frizzera G: The coexistence of Langerhans' cell granulomatosis and malignant lymphoma may take different forms: Report of seven cases with a review of the literature. Hum Pathol 17:1060–1065, 1986.

75. Risdall RJ, McKenna RW, Nesbit ME, et al: Virus-associated hemophagocytic syndrome. A benign histiocytic proliferation distinct from malignant histiocytosis. Cancer 44:993–1002, 1979.

76. Falini B, Piler S, De Solas I, et al: Peripheral T-cell lymphoma associated with hemophagocytic syndrome. Blood 75:434–444, 1990.

77. Soffer D, Okon E, Rosen N, et al: Familial hemophagocytic lymphohistiocytosis in Israel. II. Pathologic findings. Cancer 54:2423–2431, 1984.

78. Wieczorek R, Greco A, McCarthy K, et al: Familial erythrophagocytic lymphohistiocytosis: Immunophenotypic, immunohistochemical and ultrastructural demonstration of the relation to sinus histiocytes. Hum Pathol 17:55–63, 1986.

79. Jaffe ES, Costa J, Fauci AS, et al: Malignant lymphoma and erythrophagocytosis simulating malignant histiocytosis. Am J Med 75:741–749, 1983.

80. DeMent SH: Association between mediastinal germ cell tumors and hematologic malignancies: An update. Hum Pathol 21:699–703, 1990.

81. Kondratowicz GM, Symmons DP, Bacon PA, et al: Rheumatoid lymphadenopathy: A morphological and immunohistochemical study. J Clin Pathol 43:106–113, 1990.

82. Talal N, Schnitzer B: Lymphadenopathy and Sjogren's syndrome. Clin Rheum Dis 3:421–432, 1977.

83. Hartsock RJ, Halling LW, King FM: Luetic lymphadenitis: A clinical and histologic study of 20 cases. Am J Clin Pathol 53:304–314, 1970.

84. Burns BF, Wood GS, Dorfman RF: The varied histopathology of lymphadenopathy in the homosexual male. Am J Surg Pathol 9:287–297, 1985.

85. Turner RR, Levine AM, Gill PS, et al: Progressive histopathologic abnormalities in the persistent generalized lymphadenopathy syndrome. Am J Surg Pathol 11:625–632, 1987.

86. Chadburn A, Metroka C, Mouradian J: Progressive lymph node histology and its prognostic value in patients with acquired immunodeficiency syndrome and AIDS-related complex. Hum Pathol 20:579–587, 1989.

87. Keller AR, Hochholzer L, Castleman B: Hyaline-vascular and plasma-cell types of giant lymph node hyperplasia of the mediastinum and other locations. Cancer 29:670–683, 1972.

88. Frizzera G, Banks PM, Massarelli G, et al: A systemic lymphoproliferative disorder with morphologic features of Castleman's disease: Pathological findings in 15 patients. Am J Surg Pathol 7:211–231, 1983.

89. Dorfman RF, Remington JS: Value of lymph node biopsy in the diagnosis of acute acquired toxoplasmosis. N Engl J Med 289:878–881, 1973.

90. Childs CC, Parham DM, Berard CW: Infectious mononucleosis. The spectrum of morphologic changes simulating lymphoma nodes and tonsils. Am J Surg Pathol 11:122–132, 1987.

91. Hartsock RJ: Postvaccinial lymphadenitis. Hyperplasia of lymphoid tissue that simulates malignant lymphomas. Cancer 21:632–649, 1968.

92. Saltzstein SL, Ackerman LV: Lymphadenopathy induced by anticonvulsant drugs clinically and pathologically mimicking malignant lymphomas. Cancer 12:164–182, 1959.

93. Rushin JM, Riordan GP, Heaton RB, et al: Cytomegalovirus-infected cells express Leu-M1 antigen. A potential source of diagnostic error. Am J Pathol 136:989–995, 1990.

94. Shin SS, Berry GJ, Weiss LM: Infectious mononucleosis. Diagnosis by in situ hybridization in two cases with atypical features. Am J Surg Pathol 15:625–631, 1991.

95. Burke JS, Colby TV: Dermatopathic lymphadenopathy. Comparison of cases associated and unassociated with mycosis fungoides. Am J Surg Pathol 5:343–352, 1981.

96. Colby TV, Burke JS, Hoppe RT: Lymph node biopsy in mycosis fungoides. Cancer 47:351–359, 1981.

97. Weiss LM, Warnke RA, Wood GS: Immunophenotypic differences between dermatopathic lymphadenopathy and lymph node involvement in mycosis fungoides. Am J Pathol 120:179–185, 1985.

98. Weiss LM, Hu E, Wood GS, et al: Clonal rearrangements of the T-cell receptor gene in mycosis fungoides and dermatopathic lymphadenopathy. N Engl J Med 313:539–544, 1985.

99. Kadin ME, Donaldson SS, Dorfman RF: Isolated granulomas in Hodgkin's disease. N Engl J Med 284:859–861, 1970.

100. Miller-Catchpole R, Variakojis D, Vardiman JW, et al: Cat scratch disease: Identification of bacteria in seven cases of lymphadenitis. Am J Surg Pathol 5:343–352, 1986.

101. Dorfman RF, Berry GJ: Kikuchi's histiocytic necrotizing lymphadenitis: An analysis of 108 cases with emphasis on differential diagnosis. Semin Diagn Pathol 5:329–345, 1990.

102. Chamulak GA, Brynes RK, Nathwani BN: Kikuchi-Fujimoto disease mimicking malignant lymphoma. Am J Surg Pathol 14:514–523, 1990.

103. Fox RA, Rosahn PD: The lymph nodes in disseminated lupus erythematosus. Am J Pathol 19:73–79, 1943.

104. Giesker DW, Pastuszak WT, Forouhar FA, et al: Lymph node biopsy for early diagnosis in Kawasaki disease. Am J Surg Pathol 6:493–501, 1982.

105. Strickler JG, Warnke RA, Weiss LM: Necrosis in lymph nodes. Pathol Annu 22(2):253–282, 1987.

106. Cleary KR, Osborne BM, Butler JJ: Lymph-node infarction foreshadowing malignant lymphoma. Am J Surg Pathol 6:435–442, 1982.

107. Norton AJ, Ramsay AD, Isaacson PG: Antigen preservation in infarcted lymphoid tissues. A novel approach to the infarcted lymph node using monoclonal antibodies effective in routinely processed tissues. Am J Surg Pathol 12:759–767, 1988.

108. Weiss LM, Berry GJ, Dorfman RF, et al: Spindle cell neoplasms of lymph nodes of possible reticulum cell lineage. True reticulum cell sarcoma. Am J Surg Pathol 14:405–414, 1990.

109. Chan JKC, Buchanan R, Fletcher CDM: Sarcomatoid variant of anaplastic large cell Ki-1 lymphoma: Report of a case. Am J Surg Pathol 14:983–988, 1991.

110. Suster S, Rosai J: Intranodal hemorrhagic spindle cell tumor with "amianthoid" fibers. Report of six cases of a distinctive mesenchymal neoplasm of the inguinal region that simulates Kaposi's sarcoma. Am J Surg Pathol 13:347–357, 1989.

111. Weiss SW, Gnepp DR, Bratthauer GL: Palisaded myofibroblastoma. A benign mesenchymal tumor of lymph node. Am J Surg Pathol 13:341–346, 1989.

112. Dorfman RF: Kaposi's sarcoma, with special reference to its manifestations in infants and children and to the concepts of Arthur Purdy Stout. Am J Surg Pathol 10(suppl 1):68–77, 1984.

113. Traweek ST, Kandalaft PL, Mehta P, et al: The human hematopoietic progenitor cell antigen (CD34) in vascular neoplasia. Am J Clin Pathol 96:25–31, 1991.

114. Chan JKC, Warnke RA, Dorfman RF: Vascular transformation of sinuses in lymph nodes: A study of its morphological spectrum and distinction from Kaposi's sarcoma. Am J Surg Pathol 15:732–743, 1991.

115. Perrone T, de Wolf-Peeters C, Frizzera G: Inflammatory pseudotumor of lymph nodes, a distinctive pattern of nodal reaction. Am J Surg Pathol 12:351–361, 1988.

116. Davis RE, Warnke RA, Dorfman RF: Inflammatory pseudotumor of lymph nodes: Additional observations and evidence for an inflammatory etiology. Am J Surg Pathol 14:744–756, 1991.

117. Harris NL: Hypervascular follicular hyperplasia and Kaposi's sarcoma in patients at risk for AIDS [letter]. N Engl J Med 310:412, 1984.

118. Gerald W, Kostianovsky M, Rosai J: Development of vascular neoplasia in Castleman's disease: Report of seven cases. Am J Surg Pathol 14:603–614, 1990.
119. Chan JKC, Frizzera G, Fletcher CDM, et al: Primary vascular tumors of lymph nodes other than Kaposi's sarcoma: Analysis of 39 cases and delineation of two new entities. Am J Surg Pathol 16:335–350, 1992.
120. Chan JKC, Lewin KJ, Lombard CM, et al: The histopathology of bacillary angiomatosis of lymph nodes. Am J Surg Pathol 14:430–437, 1991.
121. Brecher ME, Gill WB, Straus FH: Angiomyolipoma with regional lymph node involvement and long-term follow-up study. Hum Pathol 17:962–963, 1986.
122. Cornog JL, Enterline HT: Lymphangiomyoma, a benign lesion of chyliferous lymphatics synonymous with lymphangiopericytoma. Cancer 19:1909–1930, 1966.
123. Horie A, Ishii I, Matsumoto M, et al: Leiomyomatosis in the pelvic lymph node and peritoneum. Acta Pathol Jpn 34:813–819, 1984.
124. Starasoler L, Vuitch F, Albores-Saavedra J: Intranodal leiomyoma, another distinctive primary spindle cell neoplasm of lymph node. Am J Clin Pathol 95:858–862, 1991.
125. Channer JL, Davies JD: Smooth muscle proliferation in the hilum of superficial lymph nodes. Virchows Arch (A) 406:261–270, 1985.
126. Kempson RL: Consultation case. Am J Surg Pathol 2:321–325, 1978.
127. Ridolfi RL, Posen PP, Thaler H: Nevus cell aggregates associated with lymph nodes: Estimated frequency and clinical significance. Cancer 39:164–171, 1977.
128. Epstein JI, Erlandson RA, Rosen PP: Nodal blue nevi, a study of three cases. Am J Surg Pathol 8:907–915, 1984.

CHAPTER 20

Bone Marrow

Diane C. Farhi, M.D.

Disorders of the bone marrow present some unusual problems from the standpoint of surgical pathology. The pathologist not only is confronted with the familiar diagnostic categories of hyperplasia, dysplasia, malignancy, infarct, and fibrosis but must also evaluate perturbations of continuous cell development in the most rapidly dividing tissue of the body. This outstanding feature of the bone marrow produces frequent problems in the diagnosis of myeloproliferative disorders, acute leukemia, and drug reactions and, less often, diagnostic difficulties with uncommon entities such as transient erythroblastopenia of infancy and hematopoietic rebound after chemotherapy.

The sections that follow take up diagnostic problems encountered on a daily basis in the diagnosis of bone marrow samples. As for any other tissue, an organized approach to marrow evaluation is favored, consisting of evaluation of each of the three hematopoietic cell lines (erythroid, granulocytic, and megakaryocytic), non-hematopoietic cells residing or proliferating in the marrow (lymphocytes, plasma cells, histiocytes, mast cells), and supporting stromal cells (fat cells, fibroblasts, osteocytes). An attempt has been made to present problems pertinent to each of these areas and to focus primarily on surgical pathology aspects, with assistance from other types of specimens and techniques. The topics that follow are not intended to provide encyclopedic coverage of bone marrow disorders but rather to assist the surgical pathologist in resolving some of the most critical problems in diagnosis of marrow diseases.

COMMON LESIONS THAT SHARE FEATURES WITH OTHER LESIONS
(With Which They May Be Confused and From Which They Should Be Clearly Distinguished)

Erythroid Hyperplasia

Erythroid hyperplasia is recognized in our laboratory when the myeloid : erythroid (M : E) ratio drops below the normal range of 2.5 : 1 to 3.5 : 1 in a marrow that is of at least normal cellularity for the patient's age. The M : E ratio is calculated from the marrow aspirate differential count or is estimated from microscopic examination of the clot or core biopsy section. An indication of the degree of erythroid hyperplasia should be provided to clinicians and used as a means of comparing sequential biopsies from the same patient. For convenience and ease of reproducibility, we use the term *mild erythroid hyperplasia* when the M : E ratio is less than normal but still greater than 1 : 1, *moderate* when the M : E ratio is about 1 : 1, and *marked* when the M : E ratio is less than 1 : 1 (usually 1 : 1.5 to 1 : 3 or less).

CLINICOPATHOLOGIC FEATURES. The usual setting for erythroid hyperplasia is peripheral red cell loss or destruction through hemorrhage or hemolytic anemia, or ineffective erythropoiesis due to red cell membrane defects, abnormal hemoglobin, or nutrient deficiency. Complete blood count values should be checked for the presence of anemia and other associated abnormal findings. A good clinical history and supporting laboratory data are essential in understanding the pathologic findings and making sure that subtle abnormalities are not overlooked, such as circulating fragmented red cells or hemoglobin C crystals.

DIFFERENTIAL DIAGNOSIS. Erythroid hyperplasia may mimic **chronic lymphocytic leukemia** in both smears and sections, particularly if the material is not optimally prepared (Figs. 20–1 and 20–2). The round, dark nucleus and scant, incompletely hemoglobinized cytoplasm of the polychromatophilic normoblast may be mistaken for a lymphocyte. When the number of normoblasts becomes more than 20%, and in particular when it exceeds 50%, the resemblance to a sea of small lymphocytes becomes clear. Laboratory data and clinical history are not always helpful, as both disorders may be accompanied by anemia and even autoimmune hemolysis. The best way of distinguishing the two is through careful attention to nuclear detail. The normoblast nucleus is quite round, with evenly distributed clumps of chromatin and clear areas of parachromatin, and is centrally located in the cell. The lymphocyte nucleus is irregular, ovoid to elongated, with smudged chromatin and indistinct areas of parachromatin, and is eccentrically located in the cell.

Once normoblasts are identified as such, and not as lymphocytes, a further problem arises in distinguishing reactive or secondary erythroid hyperplasia from **polycythemia vera,** an intrinsic, clonal marrow proliferation. Polycythemia vera is one of the myeloproliferative disorders, and its clinical and laboratory features and criteria for diagnosis have been amply reviewed elsewhere.[1, 2] In practice, findings helpful in separating it from reactive erythroid hyperplasia include (1) peripheral neutrophilia with immature granulocytes ("left shift") and basophilia; (2) absence of anemia and presence of an increased hematocrit; (3) peripheral thrombocytosis with giant or abnormal platelets; (4) increased, and specifically atypical, megakaryocytes, and (5) increased marrow reticulin, a finding which is uncommon but suggestive if present.

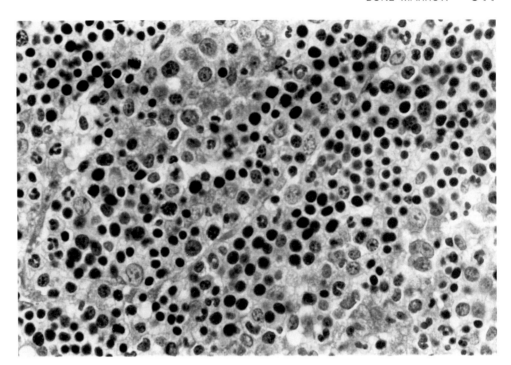

FIGURE 20-1. Bone marrow biopsy, erythroid hyperplasia. Prominent colonies of normoblasts occupy more than half the marrow (myeloid : erythroid ratio less than 1 : 1). These homogeneous round cells may be mistaken for lymphocytes.

Granulocytic Hyperplasia

Like erythroid hyperplasia, granulocytic hyperplasia has not been precisely defined. In our laboratory, the term is used when the M : E ratio exceeds 3 : 1 in a marrow that is at least adequately cellular for the patient's age. The qualifier "mild" is used when the M : E ratio is approximately 4 : 1, "moderate" for an M : E ratio of approximately 5 : 1, and "marked" for an M : E ratio of approximately 8 : 1 or more. Without the presence of atypical or dysplastic changes, the term *granulocytic hyperplasia* is used for reactive disorders of the marrow usually characterized by an increase in all stages of granulocytic maturation.

CLINICOPATHOLOGIC CORRELATION. Granulocytic hyperplasia is seen most often as a consequence of systemic inflammation or infection. It also occurs in association with malignancies, especially solid tumors and **Hodgkin's disease.** The peripheral blood typically shows an absolute increase in neutrophils, with circulating immature forms, and sometimes an increase in eosinophils and basophils as well.

DIFFERENTIAL DIAGNOSIS. The most significant disorder from which granulocytic hyperplasia must be distinguished

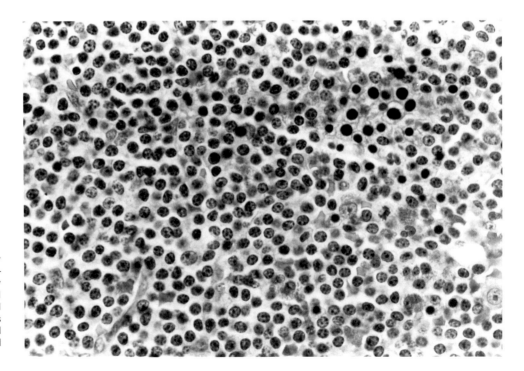

FIGURE 20-2. Bone marrow biopsy, chronic lymphocytic leukemia. The marrow is nearly entirely occupied by small round lymphocytes; a residual island of red cell precursors (normoblasts) is distinguished by very dark, perfectly round nuclei.

is **chronic myelogenous (or granulocytic) leukemia** (CML) (Fig. 20–3). Granulocytic hyperplasia is a reactive, self-limited process linked to an underlying inflammation or malignancy, whereas CML is an intrinsic, clonal marrow disease. Occasionally the two are confused because both are characterized by peripheral neutrophilia with a left shift and both show increased marrow cellularity with a predominance of neutrophils and neutrophil precursors. The distinctive clinical and pathologic findings in CML are well known.[3, 4] Briefly, the pathologic features helpful in identifying CML as opposed to reactive granulocytic hyperplasia include (1) marked peripheral neutrophilia (usually more than $50,000/\mu l$ and typically more than $150,000/\mu l$) with prominent left shift and basophilia; (2) thrombocytosis with giant, abnormal platelets; (3) prominent increase in marrow cellularity usually exceeding 90%; (4) extreme increase in M : E ratio, to 10 : 1 or greater; (5) increased, specifically atypical, megakaryocytes, usually consisting of small, hypolobate forms; (6) increased reticulin fibers, visible with silver stains or in hematoxylin and eosin–stained sections as faint linear strands producing single-filing of myeloid cells; (7) reduction of the **leukocyte alkaline phosphatase** score, usually to 10 or less; and (8) the *sine qua non* of CML, the demonstration of the 9;22 translocation (**Philadelphia chromosome**) by cytogenetic or molecular methods.[5, 6] Molecular analysis should be undertaken in all karyotypically negative cases suspicious for CML in order to confirm the diagnosis.[7]

Two other disorders deserve mention in this context, as they present differential diagnostic problems. Marrow biopsies are occasionally performed for suspected CML when patients have peripheral **neutrophilia due to corticosteroid administration.** Such patients have an absolute increase in circulating neutrophils without a left shift or other abnormalities and typically do not have an increased M : E ratio in the marrow, because the neutrophilia is caused by demargination of neutrophils from vessel walls rather than by increased marrow production.

A second problem occasionally arises with marrow eosinophilia, in trying to separate reactive **eosinophilic hyperplasia** from **hypereosinophilic syndrome.** The former is far more common and is usually seen with a peripheral eosinophilia constituting approximately 5% to 15% of circulating white cells. Reactive eosinophilia is a component of granulocytic hyperplasia in some patients with **carcinoma, lymphoma,** and **Hodgkin's disease,** in patients with parasitic infections (e.g., **visceral larva migrans**), or, rarely, after **tryptophan ingestion.**[8–10] We recently saw such a case in a child with retinoblastoma in which eosinophils constituted more than 20% of the cells in the aspirate differential. In contrast, hypereosinophilic syndrome is a rare, systemic disorder in which peripheral eosinophilia is marked, unassociated with an underlying disorder such as a solid tumor, and is relatively refractory to treatment.[11, 12]

Megaloblastic Change

Megaloblastic change has been well described in numerous standard texts of hematology and may be recognized in smears and in sections of the bone marrow.[13] The classic setting is one of **folate or vitamin B$_{12}$ deficiency.** All dividing cells undergo profound alterations in the synthesis of nucleic acids, manifest as an increased size of the nucleus and a distinctive fine stippling of the chromatin becoming coarser with maturation.[14] These changes are seen most often in the bone marrow, as it is frequently biopsied and is filled with dividing cells. Of the hematopoietic cell lines, the erythroid line demonstrates the changes most clearly, although they are visible in all three. At each stage of erythroid maturation, the nucleus is larger than normal and the chromatin more open, with small clumps becoming larger and darker with maturation. This appearance has led to the term **nuclear:cytoplasmic asynchrony** to reflect the presence of a larger-than-normal nucleus in relatively normal cytoplasm; however, this term does not do justice to

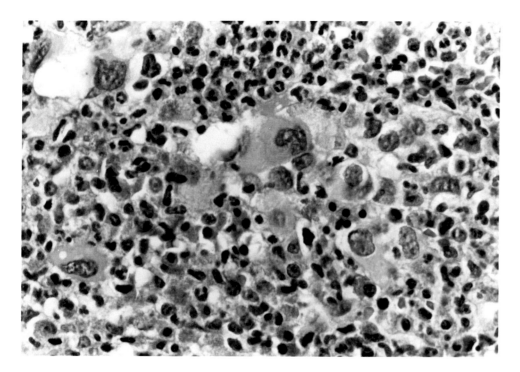

FIGURE 20–3. Bone marrow biopsy, chronic myelogenous leukemia. The marrow is filled with granulocytes and their precursors (myeloid : erythroid ratio more than 5 : 1). Increased numbers of atypical megakaryocytes help distinguish this order from reactive granulocytic hyperplasia.

the nuclear abnormalities, which are present at every stage of cellular development.

CLINICOPATHOLOGIC CORRELATION. The best examples of megaloblastic change are seen in marrow specimens from patients with severe folate or vitamin B_{12} deficiency. In practice, however, mild to moderate degrees of megaloblastosis are much more frequently seen in specimens from patients treated with **chemotherapeutic agents.** Similar, if not indistinguishable, changes may also be seen in patients with the **acquired immunodeficiency syndrome** (AIDS) and **dysmyelopoietic syndromes.** The term **megaloblastoid change** is sometimes used for these findings when not associated with folate or vitamin B_{12} deficiency, but this terminology is morphologically vague and dependent on aspects of the clinical history and/or laboratory data that may be unavailable.

DIFFERENTIAL DIAGNOSIS. Megaloblastic change should be distinguished from dysmyelopoiesis, with which it shares many features.[15] In fact, megaloblastic change is best regarded as an initial stage in dysmyelopoiesis, especially when it is seen only in erythroid precursors. Low-grade dysmyelopoietic syndromes, such as **refractory anemia,** often show megaloblastic change in normoblasts with only subtle additional morphologic abnormalities suggestive of dysplasia. Deletion of the long arm of **chromosome 5 (5q⁻ syndrome)** is also characterized by megaloblastic change in normoblasts.[16] In these and other cases, the distinction between megaloblastic change induced by nutritional deficiencies and that associated with primary marrow disorders may be aided by clinical history and laboratory data, including cytogenetic studies for evidence of a clonal disorder. Megaloblastic change may be mistaken for **acute leukemia,** a classic pitfall in the interpretation of core biopsy sections[17] (Fig. 20–4). This error in diagnosis is most likely to be made when the megaloblastic change is marked, as in florid folate or vitamin B_{12} deficiency, and the sections are examined without evaluation of aspirate smears or touch preparations. Marked megaloblastic change usually occurs with prominent erythroid hyperplasia.

Together, these alterations in the normal marrow produce an increase in cellularity, perceived as a monotonous sea of large, round nuclei surrounded by scant cytoplasm. The resemblance to acute leukemia is strengthened by the occurrence of numerous mitoses in megaloblastosis; however, the mitotic figures seen in florid megaloblastic change are rather unusual, showing very distinct chromosomes spread apart in well-defined metaphase. Differentiation of megaloblastic change from acute leukemia is accomplished by examination of cytologic specimens, including peripheral blood and marrow aspirate smears and touch preparations of the biopsy.

Plasma Cell Hyperplasia

Plasma cells constitute 1% or less of the cell population in the normal adult bone marrow. Reliable data on the percentage of plasma cells in the pediatric marrow are not available, but they appear to constitute an even lower percentage than in adult marrows. An increase in plasma cells becomes appreciable at low to medium power in the aspirate smear when the percentage rises to 2%. Reactive plasma cell hyperplasia ranges from a plasma cell percentage of 2% to an upper limit of usually 10%, although in exceptional cases it may reach as high as 50%.

CLINICOPATHOLOGIC CORRELATION. Plasma cell hyperplasia may accompany a known systemic inflammation, such as infection by **mycobacteria, fungi, viruses** (including the **human immunodeficiency virus** [HIV] and **Epstein-Barr virus**), and other organisms; autoimmune diseases, such as **systemic lupus erythematosus** and **rheumatoid arthritis;** and other disorders, such as **sarcoidosis.**[18] An increase in plasma cells is also seen in a variety of disorders without an identifiable inflammatory component. These include **iron** and **folate deficiency, ethanol** abuse, and **Hodgkin's disease.** In the case of Hodgkin's disease, marrow involvement by the malignancy need not be present in order for plasma cell hyper-

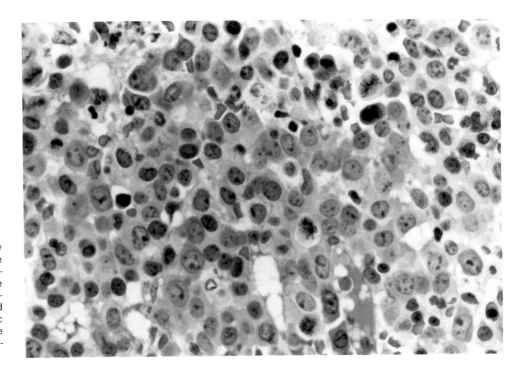

FIGURE 20–4. Bone marrow biopsy, megaloblastic change secondary to pernicious anemia. The marrow presents the appearance of a uniform, monomorphous infiltrate of round cells resembling leukemic blasts; numerous mitoses are seen, typical of marked megaloblastosis.

plasia to occur. In many cases, plasma cell hyperplasia is accompanied by eosinophilic hyperplasia. In others, it occurs in conjunction with **granulomas** and **lymphoid aggregates**. Plasma cell hyperplasia is occasionally overlooked when overshadowed by more striking pathology, such as **acute myeloid leukemia**; in these cases, it likely represents a host response to the tumor.[19]

DIFFERENTIAL DIAGNOSIS. Plasma cell hyperplasia may be difficult to differentiate from increases in other cell types, such as **osteoblasts**, or from **marrow involvement by metastatic carcinoma**. Osteoblasts occur in clusters, as well as singly, and show several features that serve to distinguish them from plasma cells, including a ''shuttlecock'' shape with the nucleus situated at one end of the cell, finely divided chromatin resembling that of a histiocyte, and a large indistinct Golgi zone located away from the nucleus. Carcinoma cells usually occur in clusters and rarely show the basophilia or prominent Golgi zone typical of plasma cells.

The most important diagnostic problem, and one that occurs frequently, is the distinction between reactive plasma cell hyperplasia and **multiple myeloma** or other monoclonal plasma cell proliferations (Fig. 20–5). Four factors may be used to resolve this problem: number (percentage) of plasma cells in the marrow, plasma cell morphology, supporting clinical and laboratory data, and the demonstration of clonality. The number of plasma cells in the marrow is best evaluated as a percentage of cells in the aspirate smear, especially when the percentage is low, as increased plasma cells in the core biopsy are often not appreciable until they constitute 5% or more of the population. Although percentage of plasma cells has been considered a criterion for the diagnosis of multiple myeloma, it is not an absolute one. It should be kept in mind that myeloma may involve the marrow in a patchy or minimal degree and that on rare occasions the bone marrow biopsy may not reveal the disease owing to sampling artifact. Conversely,

reactive hyperplasia may occasionally produce percentages of plasma cells as high as 50%. Thus, differentiation of reactive from malignant disorders of plasma cells is unreliable based on numbers alone.

The next factor, plasma cell morphology, is far more helpful in this differential diagnosis. Care should be taken in every case of plasma cell hyperplasia to note whether the cells are morphologically normal. The most frequent abnormalities seen in neoplastic plasma cells are the appearance of a large, central, single nucleolus and enlargement of both the nucleus and the cytoplasm. Although myeloma may sometimes be manifested as a proliferation of very bizarre cells, in other cases the morphologic changes may be quite subtle. This is particularly true of **light chain disease**, which may appear as a lymphoplasmacytic population with very subtle morphologic derangement.[20, 21] The third factor, supporting clinical and laboratory data, is paramount in establishing a diagnosis of a monoclonal disorder. In fact, it is prudent to regard all diagnoses of plasma cell dyscrasias as clinicopathologic disorders requiring data beyond percentages and morphology. The addition of clinical data derived from skeletal imaging, serum protein analysis, and serum and urine immunoglobulin quantitation and characterization is invaluable in arriving at the correct diagnosis.

With sufficient related clinical and laboratory data, further studies directed at clonality of the marrow plasma cells may not be necessary. Should uncertainty remain, it is practical to perform a limited battery of immunostains of sections of the clot or core biopsy to ascertain the presence of light chain restriction. Stains for kappa and lambda usually suffice, although stains for heavy chains may be desirable for confirmation of the phenotype or evaluation for heavy chain disease.[22] **Gene rearrangement analysis** may reveal B-cell clonality but is not uniformly positive in cases of multiple myeloma.[23]

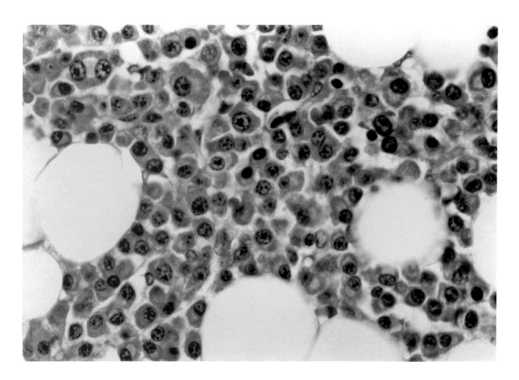

FIGURE 20–5. Bone marrow biopsy, multiple myeloma. Hematopoietic cells are replaced by abnormal plasma cells, showing enlarged nuclei with prominent single nucleoli.

Benign Lymphoid Aggregates

Benign lymphoid aggregates are usually well-circumscribed nodules of small, round lymphocytes occurring in the intertrabecular marrow space (Fig. 20–6). Occasional larger lymphocytes, or more commonly histiocytes, may be admixed; when the histiocytes become numerous, the collections of cells may be termed **lymphohistiocytic aggregates**. **Germinal centers** may be present. Benign lymphoid aggregates are often rimmed by a modest population of eosinophils and/or plasma cells. Cytologically, the lymphocytes are small, with condensed chromatin, and have absent or inconspicuous nucleoli. The nuclear outline is often described as round, but careful examination shows that it is usually ovoid and slightly irregular.

CLINICOPATHOLOGIC CORRELATION. Benign lymphoid aggregates with or without germinal centers occur more frequently in women and in the elderly.[24] They appear to be found with greater frequency in patients with autoimmune disorders, but in the majority of cases no underlying systemic disease can be identified.[25] They are probably best regarded as an expected finding in the older population, of little or no clinical significance.

DIFFERENTIAL DIAGNOSIS. Although benign lymphoid aggregates are not worrisome findings in themselves, their importance lies in distinguishing them from marrow involvement by **malignant lymphoma**[26–30] (Figs. 20–7 and 20–8). Much has been written concerning this difficult distinction, especially because benign lymphoid aggregates carry no clinical implications, but malignant lymphoma in the marrow may warrant a significant change in the staging and clinical management of the patient.

Benign lymphoid aggregates may be separated from low-grade malignant lymphomas, such as lymphoma of small lymphocytic, intermediate, or predominantly small cleaved cell types, primarily on the basis of three morphologic features: degree of involvement, architecture (location and shape), and cytology. In aspirate clot or core biopsy sections showing 30% or more involvement by lymphoid aggregates or infiltrates, the diagnosis of lymphoma is usually evident. The percentage of marrow lymphocytes does not often reach this level in benign adult marrow specimens. Clinical correlation and reliance on architectural and cytologic findings are useful in resolving this differential diagnosis.

Architectural patterns are very helpful, particularly when the aggregates are paratrabecular. This location is highly suggestive of involvement by lymphoma with a small cleaved cell component, although rarely benign lymphoid aggregates may occur in this area. Malignant lymphoma tends to form elongated aggregates that spread out along the trabecula, rather than the round, well-defined nodules typical of benign aggregates. It should be kept in mind that the appearance of a malignant, small cleaved cell infiltrate in the bone marrow is not necessarily an accurate reflection of the cellular composition of the lymphoma as present in lymph nodes but only indicates the presence of small cleaved cells in the lymphoma. This is one of the reasons that lymphoma in the marrow should be diagnosed simply as ''malignant lymphoma'' rather than attaching a specific subtype to the diagnosis.

The second feature of architecture, shape of the aggregate, has been well described for benign aggregates. These are usually quite round, densely cellular, and well-circumscribed, typically showing a small, central blood vessel and a suggestion of peripheral rimming or ''onion-skinning'' by small lymphocytes. Malignant infiltrates are often larger, of irregular shape, without apparent vessels or lymphocyte rimming; however, a very difficult problem arises when trying to use these criteria to separate benign intertrabecular aggregates from intertrabecular involvement by intermediate cell lymphoma. This differential is at times almost impossible to resolve unless

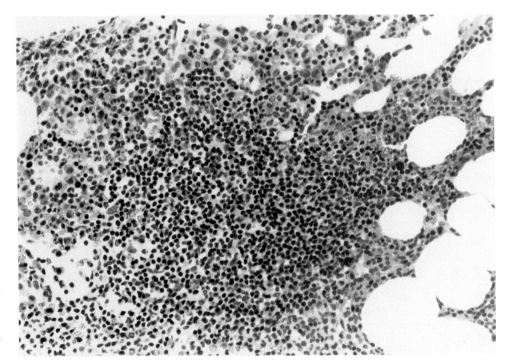

FIGURE 20–6. Bone marrow biopsy, benign lymphoid aggregate. A circumscribed intertrabecular nodule displaces the normal hematopoietic cells and is composed predominantly of small round lymphocytes.

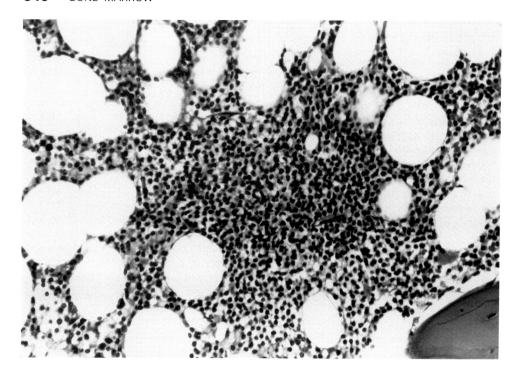

FIGURE 20–7. Bone marrow biopsy, malignant lymphoma, intermediate cell type. A small intertrabecular, circumscribed aggregate is present, composed of small lymphocytes with condensed chromatin. Although the nuclei may be slightly irregular, this feature does not always serve to render a definitive morphologic diagnosis; in such cases, flow cytometry is a very useful adjunct procedure.

the marrow shows widespread lesions or monoclonality can be demonstrated by flow cytometry on the aspirated specimen.

The final morphologic feature, cytology, is less helpful than the preceding. The appearance of a normal lymphocyte in fixed sections of the bone marrow is a slightly irregular, not entirely round, nucleus with scant, inapparent cytoplasm. This description is consistent with the cells of small lymphocytic lymphoma, mantle cell lymphoma, and even some cases of small cleaved cell lymphoma involving the marrow; therefore, cytologic criteria alone may not help resolve the issue. If the cells in a questionable infiltrate are prominently cleaved,

however, and if supporting evidence (such as paratrabecular location) is present, the diagnosis of malignant lymphoma becomes clearer.

Serous Fat Atrophy

Serous fat atrophy, or **gelatinous transformation of the bone marrow**, is the accumulation of pale eosinophilic acellular material among the fat cells (Fig. 20–9). This material usually has a smooth, featureless appearance but occasionally

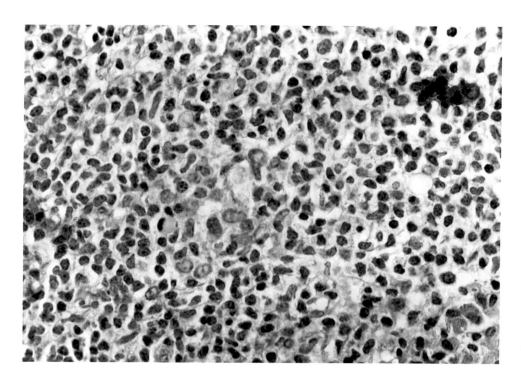

FIGURE 20–8. Bone marrow biopsy, malignant lymphoma. At higher power, the lymphoid cells are significantly more irregular than benign lymphocytes or the cells of chronic lymphocytic leukemia.

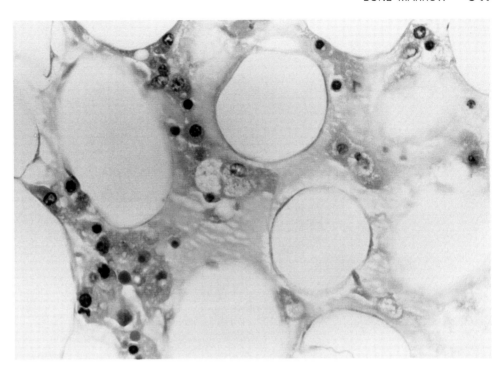

FIGURE 20-9. Bone marrow biopsy, serous fat atrophy secondary to anorexia nervosa. Hematopoietic cells have nearly disappeared, replaced by slightly granular to smooth, featureless extracellular material with properties of an acidic mucopolysaccharide.

shows faint granularity. Staining characteristics show it to be a hyaluronic acid mucopolysaccharide.[31] Its occurrence among fat cells and its resemblance to deposits of serum or plasma proteins have led to the term *serous fat atrophy,* but this is a descriptive term rather than an expression of a known pathophysiologic mechanism.

CLINICOPATHOLOGIC CORRELATION. Serous fat atrophy is most often seen in the context of severe **marrow damage** caused by chemotherapy or, rarely, other toxins or radiation. It is sometimes seen early in the course of **aplastic anemia**, when it probably indicates recent or ongoing marrow damage. In each of these situations, massive hematopoietic cell injury and loss are present. The eosinophilic material may represent accumulated cell membranes and proteins. **Starvation, cachexia, and anorexia** also produce serous fat atrophy of the marrow; in these settings, the changes in marrow fat are likely of the same origin as the fatty changes seen throughout the body and may truly represent atrophy or depletion of fat cells.[32-35] **Hypothyroidism** without malnutrition has been described as producing virtually identical histologic findings.[36]

DIFFERENTIAL DIAGNOSIS. Serous fat atrophy carries implications concerning the presence of marrow damage, and thus should be distinguished from **fibrosis, fibrin deposition, amyloid,** and **foamy histiocytes.** Both fibrosis and foamy histiocytes are cellular processes in which the nuclei, if not always the cytoplasm, are visible. The eosinophilic material seen in fibrosis is collagen and appears fibrillar; that seen with foamy histiocytes is cytoplasm and appears faintly granular or striated, depending on the cause of the histiocytosis (reactive or due to storage disease). Reactive foamy histiocytes are another indication of marrow cell death and may be expected to occur in conjunction with serous fat atrophy after intensive chemotherapy. The cells are readily identified in aspirate smears. Amyloid has a glassy, more deeply eosinophilic appearance, produces positive staining reactions with Congo red and other dyes, and does not occur in a setting of marrow

damage or starvation. Fibrin deposition is seen at the edges of clot and core biopsy sections and is the inevitable result of the trauma of the aspiration and biopsy procedure. It has a very fine, tangled, fibrillar appearance reflective of the natural cross-linking of the fibrin molecule.

Mast Cell Hyperplasia

Mast cells are a normal component of the bone marrow; however, they have not been accurately quantified. As a result, no clear criteria exist defining mast cell hyperplasia. A rough estimate of the expected number of mast cells visible in a normal marrow aspirate is approximately zero to two mast cells per spicule. They are so infrequent under normal circumstances that they are not appreciable in routine hematoxylin and eosin–stained sections of the bone marrow. Hyperplasia of mast cells usually first becomes apparent on examination of the aspirate smear under low or medium power. The characteristic polygonal or elongated outline of a very darkly staining, deep purple mast cell appears as part of a numerous population of cells in the heart of the spicule. Nuclear and cytoplasmic features are indistinct, as this is a very thick part of the smear. In mast cell hyperplasia, the number of mast cells in the center of the spicule may be about six to ten, although occasionally as many as 20 or more mast cells may cluster in and around one spicule (Fig. 20–10). As the number of mast cells increases, they begin to spread out into the surrounding hematopoietic cells, where they appear as distinctive dark purple, prominently granulated cells. Each spicule in a marrow preparation shows similar findings, indicating that mast cell hyperplasia occurs throughout the marrow.

CLINICOPATHOLOGIC CORRELATION. Mast cell hyperplasia occurs most often in the setting of mild marrow damage, due to **toxins, alcohol,** or **radiation,** and in the presence of marrow infiltration by myeloid disorders or low-grade lymphoma, such

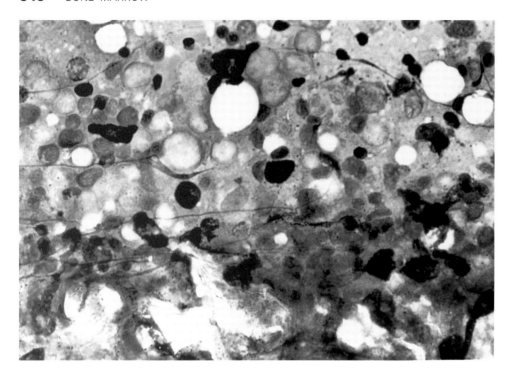

FIGURE 20–10. Bone marrow aspirate, mast cell hyperplasia. Dark, polygonal to ovoid mast cells cluster in the heart of the aspirate spicule and spread out into the thinner areas at the spicule's edge. They are by comparison relatively inapparent in sections even when hyperplastic.

as **malignant lymphoma** of small lymphocytic, mantle cell, or cleaved cell type or **hairy cell leukemia**.[37, 38] When mast cells are noticeably increased, an effort should be made to uncover one of these underlying disorders. In some cases, the appearance of mast cell hyperplasia is the first clue to subtle involvement of the marrow by malignant lymphoma.

DIFFERENTIAL DIAGNOSIS. Mast cell hyperplasia should be distinguished from basophilia and from marrow involvement by systemic mastocytosis. In separating mast cell hyperplasia from basophilia, the single most useful morphologic criterion is the shape of the nucleus. Mast cells have round to ovoid nuclei; basophils have indistinctly but definitely lobated nuclei. The intensity of granule staining may make evaluation of nuclear morphology difficult; in this case, examination of cells at the edge of the spicular center, where cellular morphology is clearer, may help. Other features aiding in the distinction include cytoplasmic outline (mast cells are ovoid, triangular, or spindled; basophils are round) and staining characteristics (mast cell granules and nucleus are blue-purple or violet; basophil nuclei are red-purple).

Mast cell hyperplasia may become so marked as to raise a question of **systemic mastocytosis,** a primary, uncontrolled proliferation of mast cells[39] (Fig. 20–11). Cytologically, mast cells are similar in both reactive and neoplastic proliferations. Systemic mastocytosis, unlike reactive mast cell hyperplasia, is associated with specific clinical signs and symptoms, presents as a diffuse infiltrative lesion of the marrow, and is not found in the setting of an underlying disorder, such as marrow damage or malignant lymphoma. **Marrow fibrosis** may be quite prominent in systemic mastocytosis but is inconspicuous in most cases of mast cell hyperplasia. Circulating mast cells occur in **mast cell leukemia** but are not seen in mast cell hyperplasia.

Aplastic Anemia

Aplastic anemia is the loss of all three hematopoietic cell lines, producing a profoundly hypocellular marrow and peripheral blood pancytopenia.[40-44] Criteria for the required degrees of pancytopenia and hypocellularity have been proposed by the International Aplastic Anemia Study Group and include an absolute granulocyte count of less than $0.5\% \times 10^9$/L, platelets less than 20×10^9/L, and reticulocytes less than 1% of red cells after correction for the hematocrit. The morphologic bone marrow diagnosis associated with aplastic anemia is marked trilineal hypoplasia.[45]

CLINICOPATHOLOGIC CORRELATION. Marrow specimens from patients with aplastic anemia typically arrive with a clinical history of fatigue and lightheadedness due to anemia, ecchymoses and petechiae due to thrombocytopenia, and/or fever and infection due to granulocytopenia. Patients may be of either sex and of any age. A history of exposure to toxins (such as benzene, paint, or organic solvents), radiation, viruses (especially hepatitis), or autoimmune disorder is present in approximately 50% of patients, but this history may not be uncovered until after the diagnosis is made.

DIFFERENTIAL DIAGNOSIS. Occasionally marked trilineal hypoplasia must be distinguished from the normal variants of marrow cellularity seen in elderly patients and from sampling artifact. Marrow cellularity steadily decreases throughout life, receding from the most distal parts of the skeleton into the axial skeleton. The posterior iliac crest is chosen as a biopsy site in most patients because it offers ease of accessibility and access to hematopoietically active marrow in both young and older individuals. After the age of 70, however, hematopoiesis may recede even further into the axial skeleton, leaving the pelvic girdle nearly devoid of dividing marrow cells. This disappearance of functional marrow is familiar to pathologists examining histologic sections of resected femoral heads from elderly patients. It is important to compare marrow cellularity with peripheral blood counts, particularly in material from older individuals, to avoid the erroneous impression of hypocellularity. Sampling artifact producing the appearance of true hypocellularity occurs not only on a regular basis in the elderly but also at times in specimens from patients who have under-

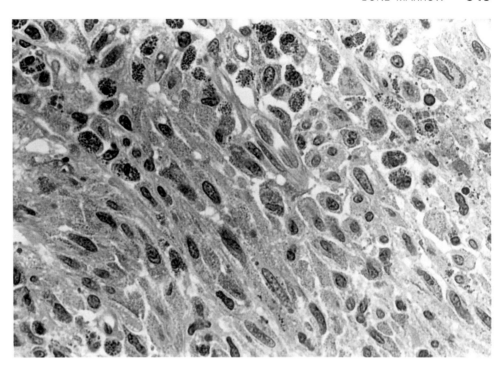

FIGURE 20–11. Bone marrow biopsy, systemic mastocytosis. Mast cells have proliferated as a sheet of ovoid to elongated cells with a prominent fibrotic background.

gone **pelvic irradiation**. These may include patients with a history of Hodgkin's disease or bowel and genitourinary malignancies. Again, comparison of the marrow findings with peripheral blood counts and attention to the clinical background usually serve to avert a diagnosis of aplastic anemia.

Acute Lymphoblastic Leukemia

Acute lymphoblastic leukemia (ALL) is a marrow-based neoplastic proliferation of lymphoblasts.[46] The cells may bear either early T-cell or early B-cell markers; ALL of mature B-cell phenotype (L3 or Burkitt's-type morphology) is not discussed in this section.

CLINICOPATHOLOGIC CORRELATION. ALL may occur at any age, but is most common in the young (children between 1 and 5 years of age) and the elderly. The clinical history usually reveals signs and symptoms consistent with the recent onset of bone marrow failure, similar to those seen in aplastic anemia.

DIFFERENTIAL DIAGNOSIS. Recognition of increased blasts is generally not difficult given good cytologic preparations, such as smears or touch preparations of the core biopsy. The latter are particularly useful when an aspirate cannot be obtained (dry tap). Diagnostic problems arise in the following areas: the distinction between ALL and **acute myeloid leukemia** or **acute leukemia of mixed lymphoid-myeloid phenotype;** the separation of ALL from marrow involvement by **malignant lymphoma;** the differentiation of recurrent or residual ALL from **regenerating primitive hematopoietic precursors;** and potential confusion of ALL with other **small round-cell tumors of childhood**.

The distinction between ALL and acute myeloid or mixed leukemia is important in arriving at an accurate prognosis and providing appropriate therapy; thus, considerable effort is expended in immunologic and other studies aimed at delineating the phenotype and genotype of the malignant cells. In brief, cytochemical studies help confirm myeloid origin but

do not identify lymphoid origin. Flow cytometry identifies both myeloid and lymphoid phenotypes, as well as mixtures of both lymphoid and myeloid blasts on one hand and blast populations bearing a mixed lymphoid-myeloid phenotype on the other.[47] **Gene rearrangement studies** confirm clonality in lymphoblast populations but may also reveal immunoglobulin rearrangements in myeloblasts.[48] These studies may serve to resolve problems in classifying acute leukemia, especially when the morphology is compatible with either a pleomorphic ALL (FAB L2) or an undifferentiated or minimally differentiated AML (FAB M0 or M1). It may also be difficult to distinguish ALL from **acute basophilic leukemia,** because the granules in the latter may be inconspicuous or taken for the findings in granular ALL.[49, 50]

Separation of ALL from marrow involvement by lymphoma presents a problem when the type of **lymphoma** is either **lymphoblastic** or large cell. Lymphoblastic lymphoma commonly affects the marrow at diagnosis or during the clinical course.[51] This disorder is usually of early T-cell and rarely of early or pre-B cell phenotype.[52–54] As the cells themselves are virtually indistinguishable from those of ALL, the distinction has come to rest on the percentage of blasts in the marrow. Currently, if 25% or more of the marrow population is composed of lymphoblasts at presentation, the disease is termed ALL, whether or not a mediastinal mass is noted. If the percentage is less than 25% and a mass is present, the diagnosis of lymphoblastic lymphoma is made. The malignant cells of large-cell lymphoma may resemble blasts, especially in smears and touch preparations, but examination of the clot or core biopsy sections usually reveals mass lesions similar to metastases rather than the uniform percolation of cells throughout the marrow typical of acute leukemia. **Flow cytometry** and analysis for **terminal deoxynucleotidyl transferase** (TdT) also help distinguish lymphoma from ALL.

Mention should be made of the phenomenon of **regenerating** early **hematopoietic** or lymphoid **cells** seen in marrow samples after intensive chemotherapy or marrow transplantation.[55, 56] Such cells have most often been reported to bear B-cell markers, including intracytoplasmic μ (mu) heavy chain. The appearance of this reactive cell population after treatment for ALL may easily be mistaken for failure to eradicate the malignant lymphoblasts.

Lastly, ALL may be difficult to separate on morphologic grounds from other neoplasms of small, essentially round cells. Helpful clues to the presence of a non-hematopoietic neoplasm include the findings of cohesiveness among cells in smears, architectural organizations into nodules or epithelial structures in sections, absence of hematolymphoid markers by flow cytometry, and immunostains characteristic of epithelial or neuroendocrine cells. These points are further addressed later.

Acute Promyelocytic Leukemia

Acute promyelocytic leukemia (APL) has been well described as a proliferation of heavily granulated myeloid precursors, regarded as abnormal promyelocytes. A micro-granular variant with minute granules, too small to be resolved with routine staining and light microscopy, has also been described.[57, 58] A characteristic, although not invariable, feature is the presence of large neoplastic cells filled with abundant Auer rods. The translocation of part of chromosome 17 to chromosome 15, or **t(15;17),** is such a constant finding in this subtype of acute myeloid leukemia (AML) that it has become a virtual *sine qua non* for the diagnosis.[59]

CLINICOPATHOLOGIC CORRELATION. Patients with APL have, in addition to the usual presenting signs and symptoms of acute leukemia, a marked propensity to develop **disseminated intravascular coagulation** (DIC). The presence of DIC at the time of diagnosis is not restricted to the APL subtype of acute myeloid leukemia, but the association is so strong that APL should be considered in patients with acute leukemia and DIC.

DIFFERENTIAL DIAGNOSIS. Other types of AML and even regenerating normal promyelocytes may at times be mistaken for APL. In considering other types of AML, those most likely to be confused with APL are prominently granulated variants of AML with maturation (FAB M2) and acute basophilic leukemia. Neither shows blasts containing abundant **Auer rods,** and neither is characterized by the 15;17 translocation. **Acute basophilic leukemia** is composed of blasts and maturing basophils with fewer but larger and more basophilic granules; electron microscopy confirms the basophilic rather than neutrophilic nature of the granules. In addition to positive reactions with the usual cytochemical stains, basophil granules stain with toluidine blue.

Proliferating myeloid precursors may also produce a resemblance to APL, particularly in the marrow of a patient recently treated for APL. The percentage of **promyelocytes** (and usually accompanying myelocytes) is high in marrow specimens rebounding from intensive chemotherapy or from drug-induced neutropenia. This wave of synchronously regenerating cells may appear as a relatively monomorphous population of myeloid precursors similar to APL. The resemblance to APL may be heightened by the unusually prominent neutrophil granulation induced by the administration of **granulocyte-** and **granulocyte-monocyte colony stimulating factor** (G-CSF, GM-CSF).[60] In such cases, the clinical setting and

absence of t(15;17) are sufficient to exclude the possibility of APL.

Myeloproliferative Disorders

Myeloproliferative disorders (MPD) are clonal proliferations of hematopoietic cells characterized by involvement of all three cell lines and persistence of maturation, at least until the terminal phase.[61] In most cases, an increase in one cell line predominates, although this is not invariable. Thus, an increase primarily in red cell precursors is termed **polycythemia vera** (Fig. 20–12), in white cell precursors is termed **chronic granulocytic** or **chronic myelogenous leukemia** (CML), and in megakaryocytes is termed **essential** (or primary) **thrombocythemia.** The fourth myeloproliferative disorder, **myelofibrosis with myeloid metaplasia,** shares features of the other three but has as a prominent component the presence of increased marrow reticulin fibers. All four disorders are closely related morphologically and may show similar terminal phases, including blast crisis and profound marrow fibrosis.

CLINICOPATHOLOGIC CORRELATION. Myeloproliferative disorders typically affect middle-aged to older adults, although chronic myelogenous leukemia occurs in a younger age group extending to children as young as 5 years of age. Patients either are asymptomatic or present with signs and symptoms of marrow failure (anemia, granulocytopenia, thrombocytopenia) or coagulation abnormalities (hemorrhage, thrombosis) referable to the production of abnormal platelets. Symptoms accompanying splenomegaly occur as the spleen becomes progressively enlarged; splenic infarct may complicate the clinical findings.

DIFFERENTIAL DIAGNOSIS. Approached from a surgical pathology standpoint, the myeloproliferative disorders are more similar than different. The clot and core biopsy sections reveal a hypercellular marrow in most cases, with adequate maturation of hematopoietic cells and an increase in megakaryocytes. The M : E ratio is usually elevated, except in polycythemia vera, the only myeloproliferative disorder in which red cell production predominates. Reticulin fibers with resulting **myelofibrosis** are increased compared with normal specimens. The problems in differential diagnosis fall into three categories: differentiating MPD from reactive conditions, subclassifying cases of MPD, and separating MPD from myelodysplastic syndromes.

The distinction between a myeloproliferative disorder and a reactive process is not always easily made. Both are characterized by **neutrophilia** and an increase in circulating immature granulocytes (left shift); however, in addition, MPD shows basophilia, thrombocytosis, and giant platelets in most cases. Marked degrees of neutrophilia, more than 50,000 white cells per microliter, are more consistent with MPD. The marrow in MPD is more likely to show increased reticulin and a proliferation of morphologically atypical megakaryocytes. The clinical history may include an underlying inflammatory process suggestive of reactive leukocytosis, or may point instead to a chronic abnormality in the peripheral blood typical of MPD. Splenomegaly is a finding in favor of MPD. The **leukocyte alkaline phosphatase** score, if very low, suggests CML. Demonstration of the **Philadelphia chromosome,** or 9;22 translocation, by conventional cytogenetic analysis or

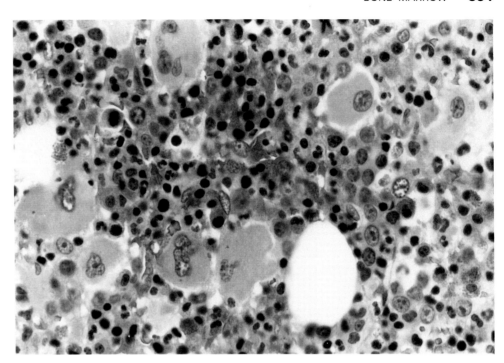

FIGURE 20-12. Bone marrow biopsy, polycythemia vera. The marrow is occupied by abundant red cell precursors (normoblasts) and increased, atypical megakaryocytes.

molecular techniques is virtually required for the diagnosis of CML, although other subtypes of MPD may rarely show this translocation as well. Cytogenetic studies, aside from revealing a 9;22 translocation, may be very helpful in identifying a clonal process; however, the absence of a demonstrable clonal abnormality does not exclude MPD.

The second problem, resolution of the subtype of MPD, usually requires clinical and laboratory data in addition to the morphologic changes seen in the marrow sections. Occasional cases cannot be accurately subtyped and may be classified only as MPD rather than as a specific entity.

Thirdly, the separation of MPD from **myelodysplastic syndromes** (MDS) is sometimes difficult. Dysplasia of hematopoietic precursors is not considered a hallmark of MPD, whereas it is a required finding in MDS. Nevertheless, megakaryocytes are clearly abnormal in most cases of MPD, and even neutrophils may show subtle changes. Thus, the distinction between these two sets of marrow disorders is not always clear-cut. The criteria proposed by the French-American-British Cooperative Group are useful in establishing the diagnosis of MDS.[62] In rare cases, the differential diagnosis of MPD or MDS cannot be resolved and becomes clearer only on subsequent marrow examinations.

ATYPICAL PRESENTATIONS IN THE BONE MARROW OF COMMON LESIONS

Lymphocytosis

Lymphocytes constitute a significant component of the marrow population in children, averaging approximately 20% to 30% of the cells in specimens from patients younger than 2 years of age (Fig. 20–13). The percentage declines in adult life to about 5% to 10%, although normal ranges occasionally

reach 20%. Lymphocytosis of the marrow may be regarded as a percentage of lymphocytes substantially in excess of these values.

CLINICOPATHOLOGIC CORRELATION. Patients with benign, **reactive lymphocytosis** in the marrow may or may not show peripheral lymphocytosis. Often no definite underlying disorder is uncovered. Occasionally such patients have concurrent viral or other infections, a chronic inflammatory process, a solid tumor, or history of recent chemotherapy.

DIFFERENTIAL DIAGNOSIS. In other organs, an increase in reactive lymphocytes is taken as a morphologic sign of chronic inflammation. In the bone marrow, chronic inflammation is not recognized as a primary disorder; rather, an increase in lymphocytes is usually interpreted as part of a systemic reaction to chronic inflammation. In this context, marrow lymphocytosis is often accompanied by reactive **plasmacytosis** and sometimes by **eosinophilia** or **mastocytosis.**

Marrow lymphocytosis must be distinguished from the normal complement of lymphocytes, especially in children, and from involvement of the marrow by low-grade **malignant lymphoma** or **acute lymphoblastic leukemia.** The cells of malignant lymphoma are not always clearly different from normal lymphocytes as seen in aspirate smears, particularly if the lymphoma is of small lymphocytic or intermediate-cell type. Hairy cells and lymphoma cells of the small cleaved type show more well-defined abnormalities, which have been amply described elsewhere. Sections of the clot and/or core biopsy are very helpful in evaluating a marrow sample with increased lymphocytes. **Flow cytometry** and **gene rearrangement analysis** may establish polyclonality versus monoclonality in difficult cases.

Infarcts

Infarcts of the bone marrow are necrotic areas of either native hematopoietic cells or malignant infiltrates (Figs.

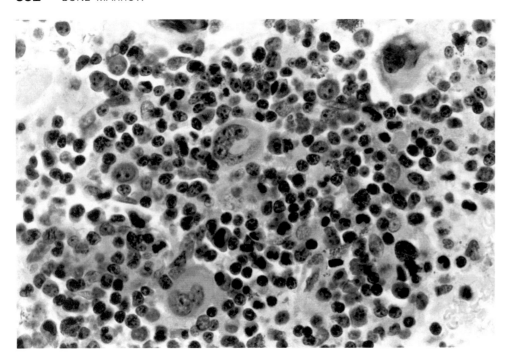

FIGURE 20–13. Bone marrow biopsy, lymphocytosis. Lymphocytes constitute approximately 50% of marrow cells in this child recovering from transient erythroblastopenia of childhood. Other viral or autoimmune disorders may produce a similar appearance, resembling a lymphoproliferative disorder.

20–14 and 20–15). The bony trabeculae may be necrotic as well but are usually viable. Cell ghosts or outlines may persist in necrotic areas, providing a clue to the presence of a preexisting **metastasis** or **acute leukemia** as opposed to the expected heterogeneity of normal or reactive marrow cells.

CLINICOPATHOLOGIC CORRELATION. Infarcts of the marrow may be heralded by bone pain, often multifocal, or may be asymptomatic. They occur in a variety of settings, including **sickling diseases** (hemoglobins S-S, S-C, and S-D), **sepsis** (viral and bacterial infections), **metastatic tumor,** and **acute leukemia.**[63–69] The mechanism by which necrosis occurs is probably variable, mediated by red cell sludging in the case of the sickling disorders, vascular compromise or production of tumor necrosis factor in the case of malignant tumors, and the production of toxins by microorganisms.

DIFFERENTIAL DIAGNOSIS. Infarcts are difficult to recognize in aspirate smears, where they appear as necrotic cells in a background of hazy, acellular material. In sections, they must be distinguished from the effects of **over-decalcification,** which may produce a similar eosinophilic appearance without clear nuclear detail. Infarcts should be separated from accumulations of **fibrin** or **fibrosis,** which may also appear relatively hypocellular or acellular. These distinctions are important, because the presence of an infarct carries great implications

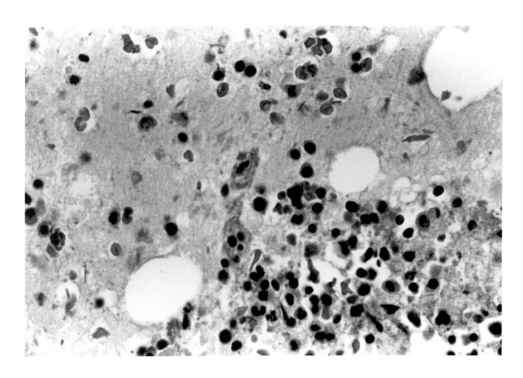

FIGURE 20–14. Bone marrow biopsy, necrosis secondary to hemoglobin S-C disease. Viable areas composed primarily of normoblasts are surrounded by an amorphous residue of necrotic cells, in which occasional sickled cells are visible.

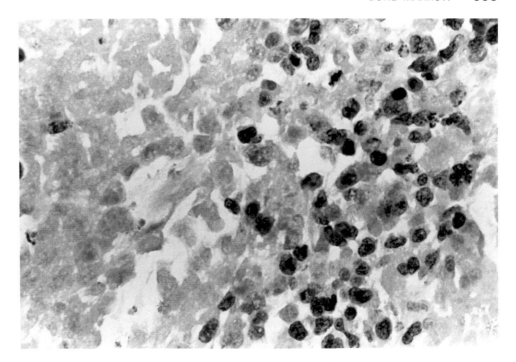

FIGURE 20–15. Bone marrow biopsy, necrosis secondary to malignant lymphoma. A cluster of intact lymphoma cells is seen in conjunction with the ghosts of similar but necrotic tumor cells. Immunohistochemistry and flow cytometry are useful in elucidating the nature of the underlying malignancy in this setting.

regarding the possibility of a serious underlying disorder. Every effort should be made to ascertain the nature of the primary disease, including careful study of viable areas with appropriate investigation of malignant lesions, if found. Thorough investigation often requires multiple sections and selective immunostaining of well-preserved, viable areas of malignant cells.

Fibrosis

Fibrosis takes two forms in the bone marrow: the proliferation of **reticulin** fibers as seen in the myeloproliferative disorders, and the production of dense, eosinophilic **collagen** more typical of fibrosis in other tissues. Reticulin is normally found in the marrow as linear strands of faintly-staining material forming part of the supporting stroma around bony trabeculae and blood vessels. The strands are brought out by silver stains. Increased reticulin is manifest as a proliferation of strands among hematopoietic cells, often constraining the cells into linear configurations. Fibrosis caused by the accumulation of dense collagen resembles that seen in other organs.

CLINICOPATHOLOGIC CORRELATION. Increased reticulin production is a finding typical of the **myeloproliferative disorders;** in fact, one of these disorders, myelofibrosis with myeloid metaplasia, is named for the marked increase in marrow reticulin. The marrow is not often the site of dense collagen formation; in these cases, evidence for marrow injury should be sought, such as prior biopsy or radiation effect. This type of fibrosis is also characteristic of certain types of **metastatic carcinoma** (see later discussion).

DIFFERENTIAL DIAGNOSIS. Fibrosis must be distinguished from other conditions creating the appearance of hypocellular, eosinophilic material, such as fibrin, amyloid, necrotic tissue, and metastatic carcinoma with a desmoplastic reaction (e.g., **carcinoma of the breast** and **prostate**). Furthermore, dense collagen fibrosis may be part of the background of **Hodgkin's**

disease. A thorough examination of the fibrotic area may reveal patches of cellularity composed of lymphocytes, plasma cells, eosinophils, and diagnostic or variant Reed-Sternberg cells (Fig. 20–16). Mention should also be made of an uncommon entity called **fibrohistiocytic lesion with eosinophilia,** a focal abnormality of the marrow in which fibroblasts, histiocytes, eosinophils, and mast cells proliferate. This lesion is of unknown etiology and should not be confused with Hodgkin's disease, although it may accompany it.

Metastatic Carcinoma

The bone marrow is a frequent site of metastasis, in which lesions appear much as they do in other organs and lymph nodes, with the addition of bony changes.

CLINICOPATHOLOGIC CORRELATION. Marrow metastases are usually uncovered in the course of aspirations and biopsies performed for staging purposes. Such patients have a known history of a primary tumor. In other cases, metastases are discovered during the course of a work-up for fever of unknown origin or suspected mass lesion. Primary sites commonly include breast, lung, and prostate; however, nearly any primary carcinoma may find its way into the bone marrow.[70, 71]

DIFFERENTIAL DIAGNOSIS. The recognition of a metastasis is usually not difficult, except in the case of a markedly fibrotic and/or osteoblastic lesion. These may be mistaken for marrow fibrosis or a primary bone lesion. These stromal reactions are most likely to accompany metastases from **breast** and **prostate carcinoma.** In these cases, the malignant cells may be compressed into elongated, barely visible nuclei with inapparent cytoplasm, surrounded by collagen and new bone formation. It is helpful in such situations to maintain a high index of suspicion and pursue identification of the malignant cells with appropriate immunostains for epithelial mark-

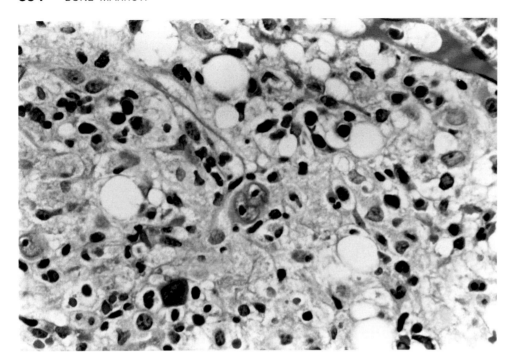

FIGURE 20–16. Bone marrow biopsy, Hodgkin's disease. Patchy fibrotic areas with a hematolymphoid cell population may be mistaken for marrow fibrosis or a fibrohistiocytic lesion with eosinophilia. Close examination of such areas in Hodgkin's disease may reveal diagnostic Reed-Sternberg cells (as shown) or variants, serving to distinguish this malignancy from other causes of marrow fibrosis.

ers.[72–75] Deeper cuts into the tissue may also reveal more typical adenocarcinoma morphology.

Metastatic Small Round-cell Tumors

The group of tumors designated as small round-cell malignancies includes **Ewing's sarcoma, neuroblastoma,** related **neuroendocrine tumors,** and **lymphoma and leukemia.**

CLINICOPATHOLOGIC CORRELATION. Small round-cell tumors are typically childhood malignancies, although on occasion they may occur in adults. They are discovered in the bone marrow in the course of staging for a known primary tumor or in an attempt to document the diagnosis of malignancy when a mass is relatively inaccessible.

DIFFERENTIAL DIAGNOSIS. Much has been written concerning the cellular origins of small round-cell tumors and the difficulties attendant in making these diagnoses.[76] This section focuses on two aspects of the problem: identification of tumor cells in aspirates and core biopsies, and separation of non-hematopoietic malignancies from leukemia and lymphoma.

Small round-cell tumor cells in bone marrow aspirates appear as both single cells and tumor clusters or groups of cohesive cells (Fig. 20–17). They differ from the expected population of hematopoietic cells in having no specific features of maturation, such as primary or secondary granules, nuclear lobation, or cytoplasmic hemoglobinization. Single cells may resemble blasts, as they show a high nucleocytoplasmic ratio, but they are usually slightly larger and have coarser nuclear chromatin and indistinct nucleoli. With diligent searching, clusters of cohesive cells are virtually always found and may show nuclear molding, a very helpful criterion for a non-hematopoietic malignancy. In the appropriate setting, such as metastatic neuroblastoma, pseudorosette formation may be identified. In clot and core biopsy sections, small round-cell tumors appear as cohesive masses of small, dark,

relatively featureless cells with a high nucleocytoplasmic ratio. In neuroblastoma, pseudorosettes may be seen. Some tumors may be accompanied by fibrosis, but this is not a constant feature. Indeed, these tumors have instead a propensity to blend almost imperceptibly with surrounding hematopoietic tissue, making the recognition of small metastases very difficult. In the case of a very small suspected metastasis, it is helpful to compare the histologic sections with the aspirate smears, because the majority of metastases involve both and the tumor may be seen more clearly in one or the other.

The separation of hematolymphoid from other malignancies is crucial, because their clinical management is quite different. They may be distinguished through cytologic and histologic characteristics, as described previously, and by techniques aimed at determining the cell of origin. These include immunostaining, **flow cytometry,** and genetic studies such as conventional cytogenetic analysis, **gene rearrangement,** and oncogene analysis. In the majority of cases, staining for a basic battery of cell markers, including leukocyte common antigen and non-hematopoietic markers, should be sufficient if the cytologic and histologic features are not clear.

OTHER UNCOMMON LESIONS OF THE BONE MARROW

Artifacts

The most troublesome artifact in marrow evaluation is probably the frequent occurrence of **naked nuclei** in aspirate smears. These are overlooked when the problem is hematopoietic maturation or the diagnosis of a benign disorder, but when one is scrutinizing the smear for the presence of a malignancy, naked nuclei suddenly become prominent. This is particularly true when the differential diagnosis includes the small round-cell tumors. Naked nuclei, like these tumor

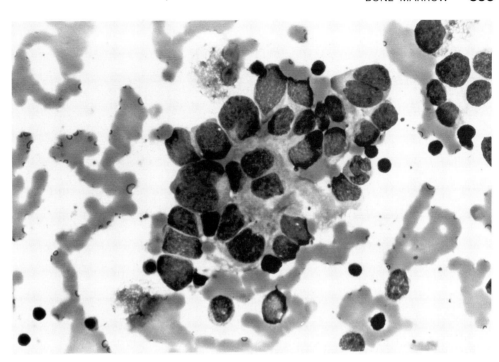

FIGURE 20–17. Bone marrow aspirate, metastatic neuroblastoma. A cluster of darkly-staining cells with a high nucleocytoplasmic ratio is seen, resembling leukemia or lymphoma but showing cohesiveness and nuclear molding.

cells, appear as dark, relatively featureless cells occurring in clusters; however, they do not show clearly identifiable cytoplasm or a cytoplasmic membrane. The chromatin is smudgy. The clustering is only apparent and is created by numerous naked nuclei in close proximity; true nuclear molding is not seen. The cells producing this effect are usually normoblasts or lymphocytes; thus, this phenomenon is most common in a background of erythroid hyperplasia or abundant lymphocytes. Because the latter is the rule in marrow specimens from young children, great care must be taken in avoiding overinterpretation of naked nuclei in this age group. The safest rule is never to derive diagnostic information from damaged cells or naked nuclei.

A second artifact that may cause difficulties is the presence of **fibrin.** This stringy, amorphous material may be mistaken for **amyloid, fibrous tissue,** colonies of **actinomycetes,** and even **granulomas.** As with naked nuclei, care must be taken to identify definite cytoplasmic and nuclear features to make the diagnosis of fibrosis or granulomas. Both amyloid and fibrin are eosinophilic extracellular materials (Figs. 20–18 and 20–19).[77] They differ in location and staining characteristics. Fibrin typically occurs at the periphery of a core biopsy section or in the interstices of marrow particles in a clot section, whereas amyloid occurs within the hematopoietic tissue or around marrow vessels. Fibrin has a finely fibrillar structure and is rather pale-staining; amyloid has a dense, glassy quality, is deeply eosinophilic, and stains positively with the usual stains for amyloid.

Bone Disorders

The bony trabeculae may at times be overlooked in the routine examination of the core biopsy. The diagnosis of bony disorders is not usually the primary reason for marrow biopsy, unless the procedure is performed specifically for the evaluation of **osteopetrosis** or **metabolic bone disease.** However,

osteoporosis and **osteomalacia** may be seen in many specimens and should be recognized as a secondary diagnosis.

Osteoporosis is found in specimens from the elderly and those who may be inactive as a result of chronic disease.[78] It is seen as a marked thinning of bony trabeculae, with slender, attenuated profiles of bone and round to oval cross sections of trabeculae instead of the usual elongated club shapes. The round cross sections seem to be floating in the hematopoietic tissue, much as alveolar wall cross sections appear in emphysematous lung tissue. Osteomalacia is found in specimens from patients with renal insufficiency (Fig. 20–20) and nutritional disorders; the latter may be one reason for the finding of this bony change in patients with hematolymphoid malignancies.[79] In addition, T- and B-cell malignancies may be associated with hypercalcemia mediated by the production of factors stimulating bone resorption. The effect on bone morphology as seen in routine bone marrow biopsy specimens is not well defined but likely includes both osteoporosis and osteomalacia. Morphologically, osteomalacia is characterized by increased osteoclastic (and often osteoblastic) activity, Howship's lacunae, widening of the osteoid seams, and peritrabecular fibrosis. Rarely are all three well-developed; this is most likely to occur in cases of hyperparathyroidism or the secondary hyperparathyroidism accompanying renal failure.

Paget's disease of bone has been known to occur in iliac crest biopsies but is an extremely rare finding.[80] The prominent cement lines and mosaic appearance of this bony disorder may be observed even in small specimens, such as core biopsies.

Hemophagocytosis

Hemophagocytosis is included in this section as a reminder that it is a normal component of the bone marrow. Thus, a specific diagnosis of hemophagocytosis should represent a significant increase over the expected number of histiocytes

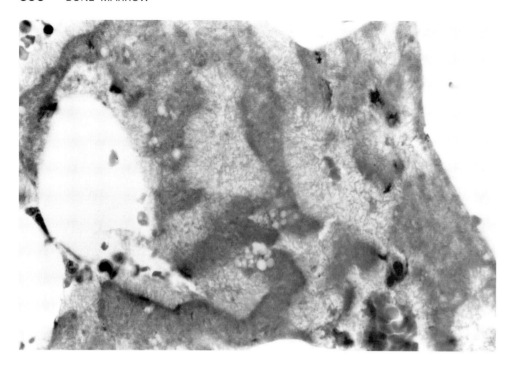

FIGURE 20–18. Bone marrow clot, fibrin. Clouds of faintly fibrillar material show an almost architectural pattern of cords and clusters resembling bacterial colonies, necrotic tissue, or amyloid.

containing ingested marrow elements. In order to appreciate the background level of hemophagocytosis in the marrow, one may make use of smears or sections. Histiocytes with cytoplasmic remnants of normoblasts are best seen individually in smears, where they tend to occur close to the center of the spicule. They are difficult to visualize in routinely stained sections but are brought out by the Prussian blue stain for iron. This stain serves to highlight the histiocytes, which may then be examined for the presence of recognizable normoblast nuclei. If only phagocytized normoblasts are identified, the process is termed **erythrophagocytosis;** if more than

the erythroid cell line is seen as ingested material, the term **hemophagocytosis** is used.

Excessive or abnormal hemophagocytosis, or erythrophagocytosis, is seen in the setting of marrow damage, as after chemotherapy, and in the course of marrow involvement by infection and malignancy.[81, 82] As a dominant finding, it provides the basis for the diagnosis of the **familial erythrophagocytic lymphohistiocytic syndrome** and the related, if not identical, **virus-** or other **microorganism-associated hemophagocytic syndrome.**[83] In these disorders, evidence of phagocytosis of more than one cell line should be present.

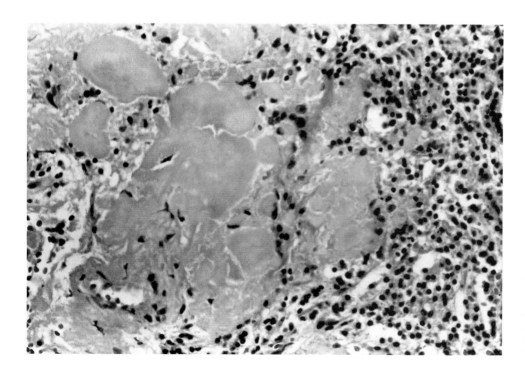

FIGURE 20–19. Bone marrow biopsy, amyloidosis secondary to multiple myeloma. Nodular masses of extracellular material resemble non-specific debris, fibrin, or fibrosis; the adjacent cellular infiltrate is composed of atypical plasma cells, providing a clue to the correct diagnosis.

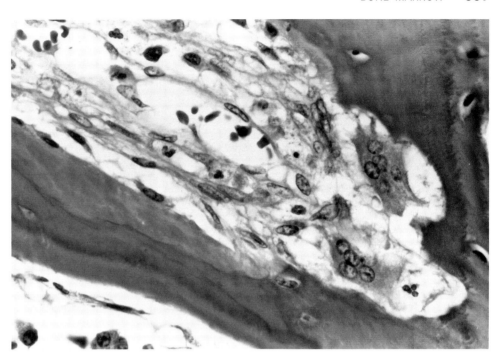

FIGURE 20–20. Bone marrow biopsy, osteomalacia secondary to chronic renal failure (renal osteodystrophy). The bony trabeculae are irregular, showing marked widening of the osteoid seams, peritrabecular fibrosis, and increased osteoclastic activity with prominent Howship's lacunae.

Erythrophagocytosis may occur in cell types other than the histiocyte, such as malignant T cells and plasma cells, but this phenomenon is not further discussed here.

Transient Erythroblastopenia of Childhood

This disorder is included because of the importance in distinguishing transient erythroblastopenia of childhood (TEC) from **congenital hypoplastic anemia** (CHA, or **Diamond-Blackfan anemia**).[84, 85] TEC and CHA are both characterized by a profound reduction in erythroid precursors, but they have many clinical, laboratory, and prognostic differences. TEC is a benign, self-limited disorder with a seasonal incidence suggestive of viral transmission, although no etiologic agent has yet been implicated. It occurs in children approximately 2 to 4 years of age. Normoblasts are virtually absent, but there are no other morphologic or maturational abnormalities. Red cell precursors return, and the hematocrit rises within about 1 to 2 months; therapy is generally unnecessary and ineffective. CHA is a congenital near-absence of red cell precursors presenting in the first few months of life and may be likened to a myelodysplastic syndrome or aplastic anemia in its persistence of a stem cell defect. Normoblasts are almost absent in the marrow, but additional dysplastic changes may be seen, unlike in TEC. In trying to distinguish the two from a pathologic standpoint, it may be useful to obtain additional laboratory information. CHA patients have evidence of persistence or reactivation of fetal patterns of hematopoiesis, such as production of **fetal hemoglobin,** of **i antigen** rather than **I antigen** on red blood cells, and fetal levels of red blood cell enzymes; these are lacking in TEC patients.

Both TEC and CHA should be separated from the effects of **parvovirus B19 infection** in children.[86] Parvovirus produces marked destruction of normoblasts, especially in patients undergoing chemotherapy for acute leukemia or malignant lymphoma or those with hemolytic red cell disorders, such as the sickling hemoglobinopathies. The occurrence of highly distinctive **giant pronormoblasts** is virtually diagnostic of parvovirus-induced red cell injury.

Rebound of Hematopoietic Precursors After Chemotherapy

Early hematopoietic cells constitute a very small percentage of the normal bone marrow, but increase severalfold in the **marrow recovering from chemotherapy** or other causes of cytopenia.[55, 56, 87] From a normal level of less than 1% of the marrow population, these cells may increase to 5% to 10% of the marrow cells; in exceptional cases, the percentage may even exceed that required for the diagnosis of acute leukemia, or 30%. This phenomenon may be more common with the administration of **cytokine therapy.** It may thus become difficult to distinguish such an increase in immature cells from the malignant population the chemotherapy was intended to eliminate. The terminology for these cells is still somewhat problematic; they probably correspond to cells described as **hematogones,** but in other cases they may simply be termed blasts or immature hematopoietic progenitor or precursor cells.

Flow cytometry is currently the best method for identifying this population, which bears CD34 and few other hematopoietic markers. Cell surface marker analysis is also a reliable way to establish that such a cell population is not identical to the targeted malignant blast population. Chromosomal abnormalities may also separate malignant from normal cells. Morphologically, regenerating precursors may resemble the patient's malignant cells, particularly if the leukemic cells have few distinguishing features, such as granules. Too few viable cells may be obtained from recently treated marrow specimens to permit flow cytometric or cytogenetic analysis. In these cases the possibility of regenerating cells must be kept in mind to prevent an unwarranted diagnosis of persistent or recurrent **acute leukemia.**

References

1. Ellis JT, Peterson P: The bone marrow in polycythemia vera. Pathol Annu 13:383–403, 1979.
2. Ellis JT, Peterson P, Geller SA, et al: Studies of the bone marrow in polycythemia vera and the evolution of myelofibrosis and second hematologic malignancies. Semin Hematol 23:144–155, 1986.
3. Kantarjian HM, Talpaz M, Gutterman JU: Chronic myelogenous leukemia—past, present, and future. Hematol Pathol 2:91–120, 1988.
4. Thiele J, Thienel C, Zankovich R, et al: Prognostic features at diagnosis of chronic myeloid leukaemia with special emphasis on histological parameters. Med Oncol Tumor Pharmacother 5:49–60, 1988.
5. Nowell PC, Hungerford DA: A minute chromosome in human chronic granulocytic leukemia. Science 132:1497–1498, 1960.
6. Rowley JD: A new consistent chromosomal abnormality in chronic myelogenous leukaemia identified by quinacrine fluorescence and Giemsa staining. Nature 243:290–293, 1973.
7. Ganesan TS, Rassool F, Gui AP, et al: Rearrangement of the bcr gene in Philadelphia chromosome-negative chronic myeloid leukemia. Blood 68:957–960, 1986.
8. Stefanini M, Claustro JC, Motos RA, et al: Blood and bone marrow eosinophilia in malignant tumors. Cancer 68:543–548, 1992.
9. Kim CJ, Park SH, Chi JG: Idiopathic hypereosinophilic syndrome terminating as disseminated T-cell lymphoma. Cancer 67:1064–1069, 1991.
10. Talpos DC, Carstens SA, Silverman J, et al: Perimyositis with perineuritis and myofiber type grouping in the eosinophilia myalgia syndrome associated with tryptophan ingestion. Am J Surg Pathol 15:222–226, 1991.
11. Fauci AS, Harley JB, Roberts WC, et al: The idiopathic hypereosinophilic syndrome. Ann Intern Med 97:78–92, 1982.
12. Chusid MJ, Dale DC, West BC, et al: The hypereosinophilic syndrome. Medicine 54:1–27, 1975.
13. Krause JR: The bone marrow in nutritional deficiencies. Hematol Oncol Clin North Am 2:557–566, 1988.
14. Perry J, Chanarin I, Deacon R, et al: Methylation of DNA in megaloblastic anaemia. J Clin Pathol 43:211–212, 1990.
15. Bennett JM, Catovsky D, Daniel MT, et al: Proposals for the classification of the myelodysplastic syndromes. Br J Haematol 51:189–199, 1982.
16. Mahmood T, Robinson WA, Hamstra RD, Wallner SF: Macrocytic anemia, thrombocytosis and nonlobulated megakaryocytes. The 5q⁻ syndrome, a distinct entity. Am J Med 66:946–950, 1979.
17. Dokal IS, Cox TM, Galton DAG: Vitamin B-12 and folate deficiency presenting as leukaemia. Br Med J 330:1263–1264, 1990.
18. Rosenthal NS, Farhi DC: Bone marrow findings in connective tissue disease. Am J Clin Pathol 92:650–653, 1989.
19. Rosenthal NS, Farhi DC, Fox RM, et al: Marrow cellularity as a predictor of adequate cell yield for transplantation. Am J Clin Pathol 101:81–84, 1994.
20. Buxbaum JN, Chuba JV, Hellman GC, et al: Monoclonal immunoglobulin deposition disease: Light chain and light and heavy chain deposition diseases and their relation to light chain amyloidosis: Clinical features, immunopathology, and molecular analysis. Ann Intern Med 1121:455–464, 1990.
21. Sun NCJ, Fishkin BG, Nies KM, et al: Lymphoplasmacytic myeloma: An immunological, immunohistochemical and electron microscopic study. Cancer 43:2268–2278, 1979.
22. Hitzman JL, Li C-Y, Kyle A: Immunoperoxidase staining of bone marrow sections. Cancer 48:2438–2446, 1981.
23. Humphries JE, Dressman HK, Williams ME: Immunoglobulin gene rearrangement in multiple myeloma: Limitations of Southern blot analysis. Hum Pathol 22:966–971, 1991.
24. Maeda K, Hyun BH, Rebuck JW: Lymphoid follicles in bone marrow aspirates. Am J Clin Pathol 67:41–48, 1977.
25. Farhi DC: Germinal centers in the bone marrow. Hematol Pathol 3:133–136, 1989.
26. Navone R, Valpreda M, Pich A: Lymphoid nodules and nodular lymphoid hyperplasia in bone marrow biopsies. Acta Haematol 74:19–22, 1985.
27. Bartl R, Frisch B, Burkhardt R, et al: Lymphoproliferations in the bone marrow: Identification and evolution; classification and staging. J Clin Pathol 37:233–254, 1984.
28. Mennemeyer RP, Kjeldsberg CR: Isolated lymphoid hyperplasia of the bone marrow simulating malignant lymphoma. Am J Clin Pathol 65:45–48, 1976.
29. Rywlin AM, Ortega RS, Dominguez CJ: Lymphoid nodules of bone marrow: Normal and abnormal. Blood 43:389–400, 1974.
30. Faulkner-Jones BE, Howie AJ, Boughton BJ, et al: Lymphoid aggregates in bone marrow: Study of eventual outcome. J Clin Pathol 41:768–775, 1988.
31. Cornbleet PJ, Moir RC, Wolf PL: A histochemical study of bone marrow hypoplasia in anorexia nervosa. Virchows Arch A Pathol Anat Histopathol 374:239–247, 1977.
32. Tavassoli M, Eastlund DT, Yam LT, et al: Gelatinous transformation of bone marrow in prolonged self-induced starvation. Scand J Haematol 16:311–319, 1976.
33. Smith RRL, Spivak JL: Marrow cell necrosis in anorexia nervosa and involuntary starvation. Br J Haematol 60:525–530, 1985.
34. Mant MJ, Faragher BS: The haematology of anorexia nervosa. Br J Haematol 23:737–749, 1972.
35. Lampert F, Lau B: Bone marrow hypoplasia in anorexia nervosa. Eur J Pediatr 124:65–71, 1976.
36. Savage RA, Sipple C: Marrow myxedema: Gelatinous transformation of marrow ground substance in a patient with severe hypothyroidism. Arch Pathol Lab Med 111:375–377, 1987.
37. Travis WD, Li C-Y, Yam LT, et al: Significance of systemic mast cell disease with associated hematologic disorders. Cancer 62:965–972, 1988.
38. Travis WD, Li C-Y, Bergstralh EJ: Solid and hematologic malignancies in 60 patients with systemic mast cell disease. Arch Pathol Lab Med 113:365–368, 1989.
39. Horny HP, Parwaresch MR, Lennert K: Bone marrow findings in systemic mastocytosis. Hum Pathol 16:808–814, 1985.
40. Camitta BM, Storb R, Thomas ED: Aplastic anemia: Pathogenesis, diagnosis, treatment and prognosis. N Engl J Med 306:645–652, 1982.
41. Nissen C: The pathophysiology of aplastic anemia. Semin Hematol 28:313–318, 1991.
42. Alter BP, Potter NU, Li FP: Classification and aetiology of the plastic anaemias. Clin Haematol 7:431–444, 1978.
43. Williams DM, Lynch RE, Cartwright GE: Prognostic factors in aplastic anaemia. Clin Haematol 7:467–474, 1978.
44. Frickhofen N, Kaltwasser JP, Schrezenmeier H, et al: Treatment of aplastic anemia with antilymphocyte globulin and methylprednisolone with or without cyclosporine. N Engl J Med 342:1297–1304, 1991.
45. dePlanque MM, VanKrieken JHJM, Kluin-Nelemans HC, et al: Bone marrow histopathology of patients with severe aplastic anaemia before treatment and at follow-up. Br J Haematol 72:439–444, 1989.
46. Bleyer WA: Acute lymphoblastic leukemia in children. Cancer 65:689–695, 1990.
47. Wiersma SR, Ortega J, Sobel E, et al: Clinical importance of myeloid-antigen expression in acute lymphoblastic leukemia of childhood. N Engl J Med 324:800–808, 1991.
48. Farhi DC, Luckey CN: Prospective gene rearrangement studies and multiparameter analysis of acute myeloid leukemia. Am J Clin Pathol 95:702–708, 1991.
49. Wick MR, Li C-Y, Pierre RV: Acute nonlymphocytic leukemia with basophilic differentiation. Blood 60:38–45, 1982.
50. Stein P, Peiper S, Butler D, et al: Granular acute lymphoblastic leukemia. Am J Clin Pathol 79:426–430, 1983.
51. Steinherz PG, Siegel SE, Bleyer WA, et al: Lymphomatous presentation of childhood acute lymphoblastic leukemia. Cancer 68:751–758, 1991.
52. Quintanilla-Martinez L, Zukerberg LR, Harris NL: Prethymic adult lymphoblastic lymphoma: A clinicopathologic and immunohistochemical analysis. Am J Surg Pathol 16:1075–1084, 1992.
53. Sander CA, Jaffe ES, Gebhardt FC, et al: Mediastinal lymphoblastic lymphoma with an immature B-cell immunophenotype. Am J Surg Pathol 16:300–305, 1992.
54. Stroup R, Sheibani K, Misset JL, et al: Surface immunoglobulin-positive lymphoblastic lymphoma. Cancer 65:2559–2563, 1990.
55. Kobayashi SD, Seki K, Suwa N, et al: The transient appearance of small blastoid cells in the marrow after bone marrow transplantation. Am J Clin Pathol 96:191–195, 1991.
56. Caldwell CW, Poje E, Helikson MA: B-cell precursors in normal pediatric bone marrow. Am J Clin Pathol 95:816–823, 1991.
57. Bennett JM, Catovsky D, Daniel MT, et al: A variant form of hypergranular promyelocytic leukaemia (M3). Br J Haematol 44:169–170, 1980.
58. McKenna RW, Parkin J, Bloomfield CD, et al: Acute promyelocytic leukaemia: A study of 39 cases with identification of a hyperbasophilic microgranular variant. Br J Haematol 50:201–214, 1982.
59. Weil SC, Rosner GL, Reid MS, et al: Translocation and rearrangement of myeloperoxidase gene in acute promyelocytic leukemia. Science 240:790–792, 1988.
60. Ryder JW, Lazarus HM, Farhi DC: Bone marrow and blood findings after marrow transplantation and rhGM-CSF therapy. Am J Clin Pathol 97:631–637, 1992.
61. Wolf BC, Neiman RS: The bone marrow in myeloproliferative and dysmyelopoietic syndromes. Hematol Oncol Clin North Am 2:669–694, 1988.
62. Bennett JM, Catovsky D, Daniel MT, et al: Proposals for the classification of the myelodysplastic syndromes. Br J Haematol 51:189–199, 1982.
63. Murphy RG, Greenberg ML: Osteonecrosis in pediatric patients with acute lymphoblastic leukemia. Cancer 65:1717–1721, 1990.
64. Pardoll DM, Rodeheffer RJ, Smith RRL, et al: Aplastic crisis due to extensive bone marrow necrosis in sickle cell disease. Arch Intern Med 142:2223–2225, 1982.
65. Laso FJ, Gonzalez-Diaz M, Paz JI, et al: Bone marrow necrosis associated with tumor emboli and disseminated intravascular coagulation. Arch Intern Med 143:2220, 1983.
66. Hicks CB, Redmond J III: Adult hemolytic-uremic syndrome and bone marrow necrosis. West J Med 141:680–681, 1984.
67. Pui C-H, Stass S, Green A: Bone marrow necrosis in children with malignant disease. Cancer 56:1522–1525, 1985.
68. Mehta K, Pawel BR, Gadol C: Bone marrow necrosis in leukemic-phase follicular lymphoma. Arch Pathol Lab Med 115:89–92, 1991.
69. Conrad ME, Studdard H, Anderson LJ: Case report: Aplastic crisis in sickle cell disorders: Bone marrow necrosis and human parvovirus infection. Am J Med Sci 295:212–215, 1988.
70. Ceci G, Franciosi V, Nizzoli R, et al: The value of bone marrow biopsy in breast cancer at time of diagnosis: A prospective study. Cancer 61:96–98, 1988.
71. Garrett TJ, Gee TS, Lieberman PH, et al: The role of bone marrow aspiration and biopsy in detecting marrow involvement by nonhematologic malignancies. Cancer 38:2401–2403, 1976.

72. Kubic VL, Brunning RD: Immunohistochemical evaluation of neoplasms in bone marrow biopsies using monoclonal antibodies reactive in paraffin-embedded tissue. Mod Pathol 2:618–629, 1989.

73. Berger U, Bettelheim R, Mansi JL, et al: The relationship between micrometastases in the bone marrow, histopathologic features of the primary tumor in breast cancer and prognosis. Am J Clin Pathol 90:1–6, 1988.

74. Cote RJ, Rosen PP, Hakes TB, et al: Monoclonal antibodies detect occult breast carcinoma metastases in the bone marrow of patients with early stage disease. Am J Surg Pathol 12:333–340, 1988.

75. Beiske K, Myklebust AT, Aamdal S, et al: Detection of bone marrow metastases in small cell lung cancer patients. Am J Pathol 141:531–538, 1992.

76. Triche TJ, Askin RB, Kissane JM: Neuroblastoma, Ewing's sarcoma, and the differential diagnosis of small-, round-, blue-cell tumors. In Finegold M (ed): Pathology of Neoplasia in Children and Adolescents. (Vol 18 in the Major Problems in Pathology Series.) Philadelphia, WB Saunders, 1986.

77. Wu SS-H, Bady K, Anderson JJ, et al: The predictive value of bone marrow morphologic characteristics and immunostaining in primary (AL) amyloidosis. Am J Clin Pathol 96:95–99, 1991.

78. Raisz LG: Local and systemic factors in the pathogenesis of osteoporosis. N Engl J Med 318:818–828, 1988.

79. Nuovo MA, Dorfman HD, Sun C-CJ, et al: Tumor-induced osteomalacia and rickets. Am J Surg Pathol 13:588–599, 1989.

80. Wittels B: Surgical Pathology of Bone Marrow—Core Biopsy Diagnosis. (Vol 17 in the Major Problems in Pathology Series.) Philadelphia, WB Saunders, 1985.

81. Gonzalez CL, Medeiros LJ, Braziel RM, et al: T-cell lymphoma involving subcutaneous tissue: A clinicopathologic entity commonly associated with hemophagocytic syndrome. Am J Surg 15:17–27, 1991.

82. Ooe K: Pathogenesis and clinical significance of hemophagocytic syndrome: Hypothesis. Ped Pathol 12:309–312, 1992.

83. Favara BE: Hemophagocytic lymphohistiocytosis: A hemophagocytic syndrome. Semin Diagn Pathol 9:63–74, 1992.

84. Glader BE: Diagnosis and management of red cell aplasia in children. Hematol Oncol Clin North Am 1:431–447, 1987.

85. Hays T, Lane PA, Shafer F: Transient erythroblastopenia of childhood. Am J Dis Child 143:605–607, 1989.

86. Wodzinski MA, Lilleyman JS: Transient erythroblastopenia of childhood due to human parvovirus B19 infection. Br J Haematol 73:127–128, 1989.

87. Foot ABM, Potter MN, Ropner JE, et al: Transient erythroblastopenia of childhood with CD10, TdT, and cytoplasmic μ lymphocyte positivity in bone marrow. J Clin Pathol 43:857–859, 1990.

CHAPTER 21

The Spleen

Barbara C. Wolf, M.D., and Diane C. Farhi, M.D.

Pathologic processes involving the spleen are often a source of confusion for the surgical pathologist, because it is rare for pathologists to have the opportunity to study spleens whose morphologic features have not been altered by previous therapy or postmortem autolysis. Optimal evaluation of the histopathologic changes in the spleen requires that careful attention be paid to details of fixation and tissue processing. The periodic acid-Schiff (PAS) stain is often helpful, because it highlights the architectural framework and because it may assist in the recognition of the lineage of hematopoietic cells present. Romanowsky-stained touch imprints of the cut surface of the spleen can aid in its evaluation, particularly in identifying platelet sequestration or erythrophagocytosis or when cytochemical stains are needed. Additionally, in some cases, the diagnosis of lymphoproliferative disorders and the subtyping of leukemic processes in the spleen may require ancillary techniques such as immunohistochemistry, flow cytometric analysis, or molecular diagnostic studies.

It is also important to realize that the study of disorders involving the spleen often requires an understanding of the overall clinical picture. It may be necessary to know the status of the patient's peripheral blood and whether or not other lymphoid organs or the bone marrow are involved with the disease process.

THE NORMAL SPLEEN

Pathologic processes affecting the spleen can be best understood in light of its normal structure and function.[1] The spleen is composed of two anatomic and functional compartments. The white pulp accounts for the bulk of the lymphoid tissue and is responsible for its immunologic function. The white pulp is intimately associated with the splenic arterial circulation, which is surrounded by a cuff of lymphocytes termed the periarterial lymphoid sheath (PALS), which is an admixture of B and T cells.[2-5] Lymphoid follicles occur periodically, usually at arterial branches. The germinal center and its surrounding mantle zone are predominantly B-cell areas, encased by the paler outer marginal zone that is an extension of the PALS.[6]

The red pulp of the spleen is composed of vascular sinuses and the cords of Billroth, which contain numerous macrophages with long dendritic processes.[7, 8] The splenic sinuses are lined by endothelial cells that are not joined by tight junctions. This unique structure provides a discontinuous barrier for passage of cells from the cords of Billroth into the sinuses, allowing the spleen to act as a filter of the peripheral blood, trapping senescent or defective circulating cells, which are then destroyed by the cordal macrophages.[9-15]

COMMON LESIONS THAT SHARE FEATURES WITH OTHER LESIONS (With Which They May Be Confused and From Which They Should Be Clearly Distinguished) (Table 21-1)

Benign Lesions of the White Pulp

Immunologic Reactions

Disorders of the splenic white pulp produce a grossly nodular pattern. Non-neoplastic proliferations of splenic lymphoid tissue may on occasion be so exuberant as to mimic lymphoproliferative disorders.[1] The evolving activated immune response, characterized by reactive **follicular hyperplasia of the malpighian corpuscles,** and often accompanied by a **plasmacytosis** around small arterioles, is usually easy to recognize. This is the typical reaction pattern of the spleen to blood-borne antigens, particularly bacterial, and is a normal finding in children and young adults as a result of their frequent exposure to new antigens. The white pulp shows tripartite follicles, usually with well-formed mantle and marginal zones (Fig. 21-1). The germinal centers themselves contain transformed lymphocytes, often with many mitotic figures, and tingible body macrophages.

In contrast, the pattern of white pulp response to viral infections may be more difficult to recognize histologically. This so-called early activated immune reaction, or **immunoblastic hyperplasia,** usually results in only mild expansion of the white pulp, and therefore the spleen may appear unremarkable grossly. On microscopic examination, particularly at low power, the white pulp may appear immunologically unstimulated, because the follicles lack germinal centers and distinct mantle zones. However, high-power examination reveals evidence of immunologic activation. There is a proliferation of transformed lymphocytes and immunoblasts, which occasionally may also infiltrate the vascular structures, resulting in splenic rupture.[16, 17] This pattern is also characteristic of hypersensitivity reactions and graft rejection.[18, 19]

Occasionally, the proliferation of immunoblasts in the early activated immune reaction may be so prominent as to mimic splenic involvement by malignant lymphoma. However, it should be remembered that the vast majority of **large-cell lymphomas** would be expected to produce tumor masses rather than a miliary pattern of expansion of the white pulp nodules. The presence of a mixed cell population in the white pulp should also aid in the recognition of a benign lesion. Alternatively, in some cases binucleated immunoblasts may suggest Reed-Sternberg cells, mimicking **Hodgkin's disease,** although it is also unusual for Hodgkin's disease to produce a miliary pattern of white pulp involvement.[20–22]

The early activated pattern of the splenic immune response is also seen in chronic autoimmune disorders when the patients have been treated with corticosteroid therapy.[23–27] Steroids suppress germinal center formation, although the phagocytic function of the red pulp remains intact.[28] Therefore, in cases of **immune thrombocytopenic purpura** and **autoimmune hemolytic anemia,** touch imprints can be essential in making the diagnosis, because phagocytosis is often more easily demonstrable than in tissue sections.

Granulomatous Disorders

Granulomatous disorders involving the spleen include lipogranulomas, infectious granulomas, and sarcoidal-type granulomas.[29] **Lipogranulomas,** lipid droplets in the white pulp usually without giant cell response, are common incidental findings.[30, 31] Similarly, **infectious granulomas** usually cause little difficulty in diagnosis.[32, 33]

Sarcoidal-type granulomas may be found in the spleen of patients with a variety of disorders associated with aberrant immune function.[29, 34] These granulomas are found in the white pulp in intimate association with the arterial circulation. Histologically, these are non-caseating granulomas composed of epithelioid histiocytes with occasional giant cells. Such granulomas are commonly found in the spleen in sarcoidosis.[35] Histologically identical granulomas were described in the spleens of patients with Hodgkin's disease by Kadin et al.[36] and may also be found in the liver, lymph nodes, and bone marrow. They are usually seen in patients whose spleen is not involved with Hodgkin's disease itself, although occasionally there may be concomitant granulomas and Hodgkin's disease.[37] These granulomas do not imply splenic involvement, nor do they alter the stage of disease or treatment modality.[29, 34]

Sarcoidal-type granulomas may occasionally be seen in the spleens of patients with non-Hodgkin's lymphomas, although this is a less frequent finding.[34] They may also be found in association with non-malignant diseases, including severe combined immunodeficiency and selective IgA deficiency.[1] The common thread among disorders associated with these granulomas appears to be **immunodeficiency,** most probably impaired T-cell function. The morphology is the same regardless of the underlying disease. If such granulomas are found unexpectedly in a spleen removed for other purposes, the pathologist must first rule out an infectious cause. The differential diagnosis then depends on clinical correlation.

Dysproteinemias

The term *dysproteinemias* refers to a group of benign and malignant disorders characterized by aberrant immunoglobulin production.[1] This immunoglobulin may be either monoclonal or polyclonal but occurs in the absence of a recognizable antigenic stimulus and is not self-limited. These disorders tend to involve both the white pulp and the red pulp. Evidence of immunoglobulin production is often seen, including the presence of plasmacytoid lymphocytes and cells with intranuclear inclusions of immunoglobulin, so-called Dutcher bodies. There may also be Mott cells, containing numerous intracytoplasmic globules, as well as Russell bodies, which are cytoplasmic or extracellular aggregates of immunoglobulin. Although characteristic of systemic amyloidosis, amyloid may also be seen in association with other dysproteinemias[38] (Fig. 21–2).

The autoimmune disorders, associated with the autoantibody production, were discussed previously. The dysproteinemias associated with polyclonal hypergammaglobulinemia include **immunoblastic lymphadenopathy** and **Castleman's disease.** These rare conditions are discussed in a later section. The dysproteinemias associated with monoclonal gammopathies include systemic **amyloidosis,** the **heavy chain diseases, plasma cell leukemia,** and **Waldenstrom's macroglobulinemia.** Because these disorders share morphologic features, their diagnosis often cannot be made on examination of the spleen alone, but may require bone marrow biopsy as well as serum and/or urine immunoelectrophoresis.[39–43]

Cold agglutinin disease, associated with an IgM paraprotein, may also have a monoclonal lymphoplasmacytic infiltrate in the spleen, which in some cases may herald an underlying B-cell lymphoma, in spite of its non-neoplastic morphologic appearance.

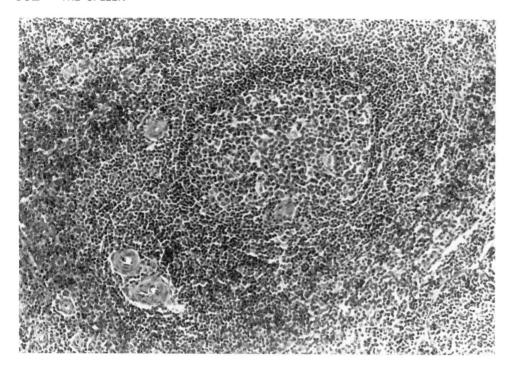

FIGURE 21–1. Spleen, follicular hyperplasia. Eccentric to a splenic arteriole, a well-formed germinal center is surrounded by a mantle zone of small dark lymphocytes and an indistinct marginal zone of pale-staining lymphocytes.

Benign Lesions of the Red Pulp

The majority of pathologic processes involving the red pulp produce a diffuse enlargement of the spleen with obliteration of the white pulp markings, in contrast with the grossly nodular pattern that is apparent with many disorders of the white pulp.[1] Splenomegaly of any cause may result in **hypersplenism.** Expansion of the red pulp results in prolonged exposure of the formed elements of the blood to the acidotic, hypoxic environment of the cords of Billroth, where they are susceptible to destruction and phagocytosis by the cordal macrophages.[44, 45] Hypersplenism is the most frequent indication for therapeutic splenectomy. In contrast, **hyposplenism,** which refers to the decreased or absent function of the spleen, is rarely of clinical significance. Exceptions to this occur in children and immunosuppressed adults, in whom the absence of the spleen may predispose to overwhelming sepsis.[46–49]

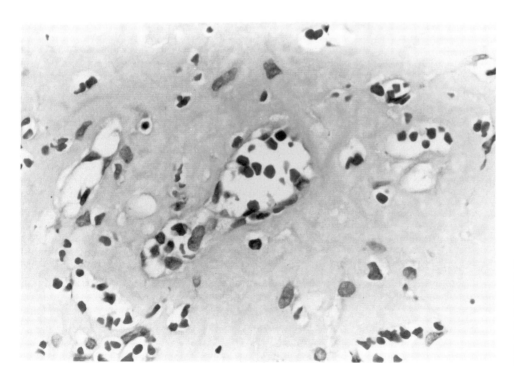

FIGURE 21–2. Spleen, amyloidosis secondary to plasma cell dyscrasia. The splenic cords are nearly replaced and the vascular sinuses compressed by the massive extracellular accumulation of amyloid. The underlying plasma cell dyscrasia is not apparent morphologically.

Non-neoplastic Disorders of Circulating Blood Cells

Hypersplenism either may be related to disorders of the spleen itself, in which the expansion of the red pulp results in trapping of normal circulating blood cells, or may be secondary to abnormalities in the blood cells themselves, rendering them more susceptible to trapping in the spleen as it performs its normal filtration function.[50, 51] Congenital forms of hypersplenism include **hereditary spherocytosis** (Fig. 21–3) and **elliptocytosis, sickle cell disease,** and some of the **hemoglobinopathies.**[52-56] Abnormal erythrocytes lack the plasticity necessary to squeeze through the potential apertures between the vascular sinus lining cells to return to the venous circulation. Acquired disorders of circulating blood cells include the **immune cytopenias,**[55-60] in which antibody-coated cells are trapped in the red pulp of the spleen. Erythrocytes containing parasites such as **malarial organisms** are also trapped.[61, 62] In histologic sections, the red pulp cords appear congested.

Disorders of Cordal Macrophages

Disorders of cordal macrophages can result in prominent splenomegaly, with the gross appearance similar to that of other red pulp diseases. The storage diseases, particularly the lipid storage diseases, result in a proliferation of cordal macrophages leading to hypersplenism. In particular, the adult form of **Gaucher's disease, Niemann-Pick disease,** and **ceroid histiocytosis** may result in cytopenias, although these are usually mild. Gaucher's cells can usually be recognized in routine sections by the "wrinkled tissue paper" appearance of their cytoplasm[63-65] (Fig. 21–4). The macrophages in ceroid histiocytosis may closely mimic those of Niemann-Pick disease, in which the cells appear foamy owing to numerous small cytoplasmic vacuoles.[63, 66] Ceroid is a product of lipid oxidation and polymerization. Ceroid-containing histiocytes

appear somewhat dirty brown in hematoxylin and eosin–stained sections.[66-68] They are PAS-positive, acid fast, and stain with the Prussian blue for iron. The tissue Giemsa stain reveals an intense dark staining of the cytoplasm, similar to that seen in Romanowsky-stained bone marrow smears, resulting in the term **"sea blue histiocytes."** The so-called syndrome of the sea blue histiocyte is characterized by prominent splenomegaly.[67-69] When associated with thrombocytopenia and oculocutaneous albinism, the term **Hermansky-Pudlak syndrome** has been adopted.[70] However, ceroid-containing histiocytes are non-specific and may be seen in a variety of unrelated disorders.

The **infection-associated hemophagocytic syndromes,**[71, 72] as well as the **familial hemophagocytic disorders,**[73, 74] are characterized by splenomegaly with cytopenias. The infection-associated forms occur primarily in children and in immunosuppressed adults and are usually associated with herpes or adenovirus infection,[71] although cases have been reported in association with bacterial, fungal, and parasitic infections.[72] The red pulp of the spleen, as well as other lymphoreticular organs, shows a proliferation of benign-appearing cordal macrophages with prominent phagocytosis of erythrocytes, platelets, and granulocytes. This must be distinguished from the so-called malignant histiocytosis, in which the red pulp of the spleen is infiltrated by bizarre tumor cells, associated with erythrophagocytosis by benign-appearing macrophages.[75-77] This is a poorly understood disorder, many cases of which are probably not actually proliferations of neoplastic macrophages. Some cases probably represent examples of infection-associated hemophagocytic syndromes, and others are actually non-Hodgkin's lymphomas.

The differentiated histiocytoses were formerly termed **Langerhans cell histiocytosis or histiocytosis X.**[78, 79] The cell of origin is the Langerhans cell, which has a histiocyte-like appearance, often with abundant amphophilic or eosinophilic

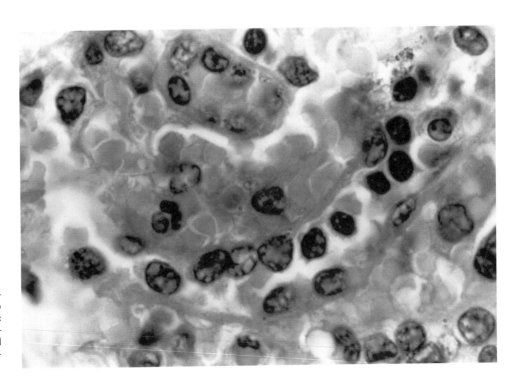

FIGURE 21–3. Spleen, hereditary spherocytosis. Adjacent to a vascular sinus, the splenic cord is packed with phagocytized red blood cells. Red blood cell morphology does not appear abnormal.

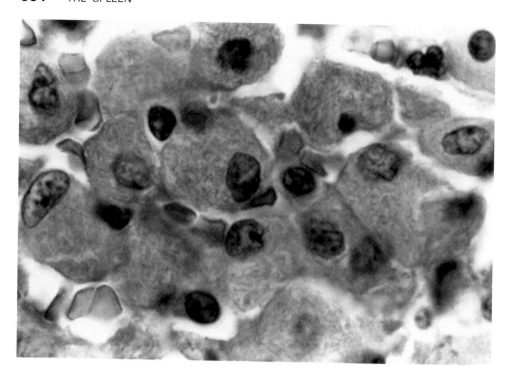

FIGURE 21–4. Spleen, Gaucher's disease. The enlarged histiocytes show regular, ovoid nuclei and abundant finely granular to vaguely striated ("wrinkled tissue paper") cytoplasm.

cytoplasm and characteristic nuclear grooves. Splenomegaly is typical of the disseminated form of differentiated histiocytosis, or **Letterer-Siwe disease.**[80, 81] This is a disorder of childhood with an ominous prognosis, although most investigators believe the differentiated histiocytoses to be reactive rather than neoplastic.

Non-hematopoietic Lesions

Splenic hamartomas are benign lesions that are usually incidental findings, although occasionally they may result in hypersplenism as a result of trapping of circulating hematopoietic cells.[82, 83] Grossly they present as well-circumscribed mass lesions. Microscopically they resemble the normal splenic red pulp, with slit-like vascular spaces that may mimic a hemangioma.

Hemangiomas are the most common benign tumors of the spleen.[84, 85] Although they are also most often incidental findings, occasionally cytopenias may result from sequestration of hematopoietic cells. The gross appearance is usually that of a well-circumscribed blue-red nodule, occasionally with areas of infarction (Fig. 21–5). The cavernous hemangioma is the most common and must be distinguished from angiosarcoma by the lack of cytologic atypia. The capillary hemangioma may resemble a splenic hamartoma. Hemangiomas may also resemble the early stages of **splenic peliosis,** in which small cysts result from dilatation of the red pulp sinuses. Peliosis of the spleen is usually associated with **peliosis hepatis,** and most cases have been reported in patients treated with either anabolic steroids or oral contraceptives.[86–88] In its advanced stages, there are grossly visible blood-filled spaces in the red pulp with varying degrees of organization. They tend to have a perifollicular location and are usually lined by attenuated sinus lining cells.

A newly described benign splenic vascular lesion, termed **littoral cell angioma,** may be more difficult to distinguish

from a malignant vascular tumor.[89] This lesion is composed of anastomosing vascular channels, lined by tall endothelial cells that may demonstrate phagocytosis. There may be papillary projections, similar to those seen in angiosarcomas, although there is little atypia. Immunohistologic studies have shown both endothelial and histiocytic differentiation.

Splenic cysts are usually asymptomatic, although splenectomy is occasionally performed for diagnostic purposes because of the presence of a mass lesion.[85] The most common cyst is the so-called **false cyst,** which lacks epithelial lining and is presumed to be traumatic in origin. **Epidermoid cysts** are usually unilocular and have a trabeculated lining, which is most often stratified squamous epithelium[90–92] (Fig. 21–6).

Malignant Lesions of the White Pulp

Non-Hodgkin's Lymphomas

The morphologic features of the spleen in non-Hodgkin's lymphomas have been well characterized for tumors of B-cell lineage. The majority of lymphomas involving the spleen are part of a disseminated systemic process. Primary lymphomas of the spleen are uncommon. The B-cell lymphomas most often produce white pulp involvement, with a nodular appearance on gross examination. However, red pulp involvement may occur in any malignant lymphoma with leukemic dissemination. The diagnosis of low-grade B-cell lymphomas in the spleen may sometimes be difficult and may rest on examination of other organs or on immunologic or molecular studies. **Small lymphocytic lymphoma,** with morphologic features in lymphoid organs identical to those of chronic lymphocytic leukemia, in its early stages produces uniform expansion of the white pulp nodules, which may resemble the immunologically unstimulated.[93–95] However, high-power microscopic examination usually reveals admixed prolympho-

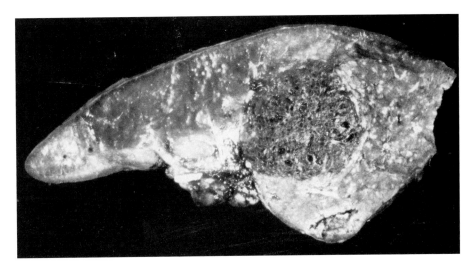

FIGURE 21–5. Spleen, cavernous hemangioma. A well-circumscribed nodule is seen surrounded by unremarkable red and white pulp. The large vascular spaces are readily apparent and typical of a cavernous hemangioma.

cytes. Additionally, even in the early stages, there is often subtle involvement of the red pulp. It is helpful to examine the splenic hilar lymph nodes. Knowledge of bone marrow and/or peripheral blood involvement also assists in the diagnosis. Later in the course of small lymphocytic lymphoma, red pulp involvement predominates, resulting in obliteration of white pulp markings.

Splenic involvement in **small cleaved cell and mixed small- and large-cell lymphomas** usually produces irregular expansion of all of the malpighian corpuscles, with a grossly visible miliary pattern.[96] Microscopic determination of involvement by small cleaved cell lymphoma is usually not difficult, owing to the monomorphous population of small cleaved lymphocytes.[93] The recognition of mixed small- and large-cell lymphoma may be more difficult, because it may mimic a reactive process. However, the cell population is bimorphic, rather than showing a range of transformed lym-

phocytes with tingible body macrophages as is seen in reactive germinal centers, and the red pulp plasmacytosis typically seen in the evolving immune reaction is absent.

Intermediate-cell lymphoma, which may present with prominent splenomegaly and hypersplenism, also shows a miliary pattern of involvement of the white pulp[96, 97] (Figs. 21–7 and 21–8). The tumor cells tend to proliferate in wide mantle zones around benign, often atrophic or hyalinized germinal centers. The tumor cells are somewhat irregular, and there may be admixed small round and cleaved lymphocytes.[98] The residual benign germinal centers may make it difficult to distinguish the tumor nodules from reactive follicles. The recognition of red pulp involvement, as well as documentation of involvement of lymph nodes or bone marrow, aids in the diagnosis of this disorder. In some cases, however, the diagnosis of malignancy requires ancillary studies. Similarly, the newly described entity termed **marginal zone lymphoma**

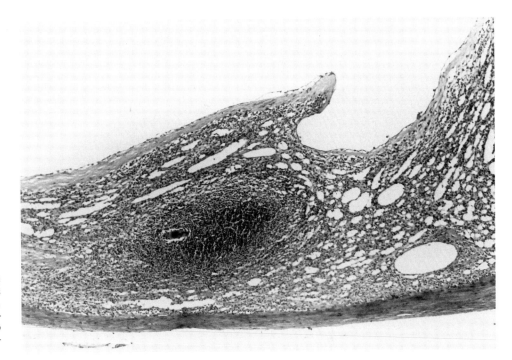

FIGURE 21–6. Spleen, splenic cyst. The cyst wall *(top)* is smooth and lined by epithelium. The cyst is surrounded by unremarkable red and white pulp and the splenic capsule *(bottom).*

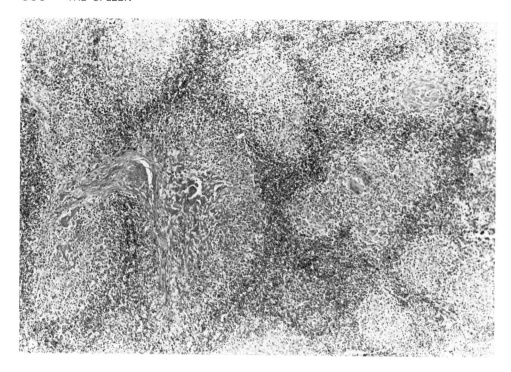

FIGURE 21-7. Spleen, intermediate-cell lymphoma. Uniform enlargement of the white pulp is seen in a miliary pattern.

may present with prominent splenomegaly.[99] The tumor cells, medium-sized lymphocytes, proliferate around the lymphoid follicles, which they may also infiltrate. The morphologic pattern and immunophenotypic characteristics of this low-grade B-cell lymphoma suggest origin from the marginal zone lymphocytes.

Large-cell lymphomas of B-cell lineage usually produce solitary or multiple tumor masses, often without a discernible relationship to the white pulp (Fig. 21–9). On gross examination, the differential diagnosis includes Hodgkin's disease

and metastatic carcinoma. Rarely, large-cell lymphomas may present as primary splenic tumors and with diffuse involvement.[100]

The morphology of the spleen in **T-cell lymphoproliferative disorders** is less well characterized. Anecdotal evidence indicates that most lymphomas of mature T-cell phenotype involve the red pulp in a pattern mimicking the leukemic disorders[101–107] (Fig. 21–10). The tumor may be associated with a striking erythrophagocytosis by benign cordal macrophages. Several immunophenotypic studies have indicated

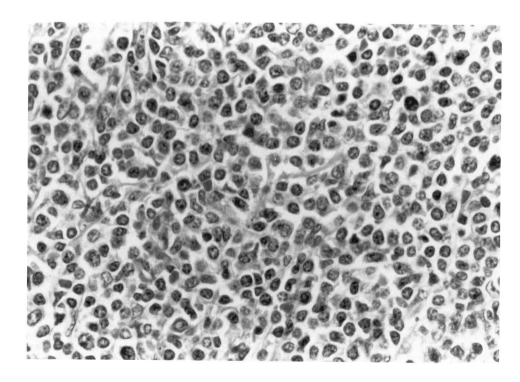

FIGURE 21-8. Spleen, intermediate-cell lymphoma. The white pulp surrounding the splenic arteriole is filled with small, slightly irregular lymphocytes admixed with small round and with small cleaved lymphocytes.

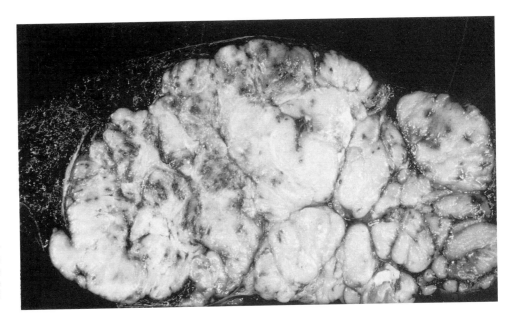

FIGURE 21–9. Spleen, primary large-cell lymphoma. Massive involvement by pale gray-white tumor replaces much of the parenchyma. A rim of spared splenic tissue is seen *(left).*

that some cases originally reported as **malignant histiocytosis** were actually lymphomas, usually of a mature T-cell phenotype.

Other types of T-cell lymphomas may have characteristic patterns in the spleen. Early splenic involvement in the disseminated stages of the cutaneous T-cell lymphomas may produce a striking expansion of the PALS.[94, 104, 105] Diffuse red pulp involvement usually supervenes in the later course of the disease. **Lymphoblastic lymphoma** tends to involve the white pulp, particularly in areas adjacent to the PALS.[93]

Hodgkin's Disease

The diagnosis of Hodgkin's disease in the spleen rarely presents a problem to the surgical pathologist, because the majority of patients already carry the diagnosis. The spleen is involved in more than one third of patients undergoing staging laparotomy.[106] Nodular sclerosis and mixed cellularity are the subtypes most commonly involving the spleen. Splenic involvement in the lymphocyte predominant subtype is rare.[17] Lymphocyte depletion is an uncommon subtype that usually does involve the spleen.[108, 109]

The gross appearance of Hodgkin's disease is usually that of single or multiple masses, therefore mimicking the appearance of large-cell lymphomas or metastatic tumors (Fig. 21–11). Occasionally splenic involvement may be very subtle, with only 1- to 2-mm nodules in the white pulp.[110–113] The gross examination of the spleen in Hodgkin's disease must be very meticulous. The importance of documenting the splenic involvement is that it indicates that the liver and bone marrow

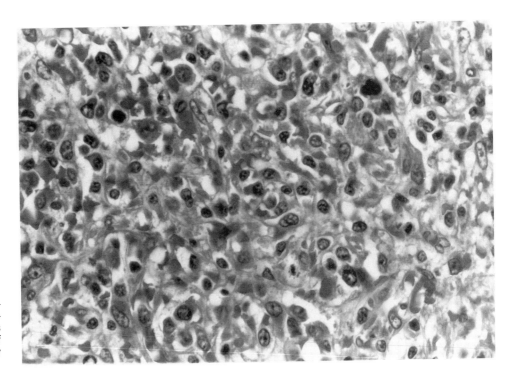

FIGURE 21–10. Spleen, peripheral T-cell lymphoma. The normal splenic architecture is obscured by an admixture of small and large, occasionally hyperchromatic, lymphocytes.

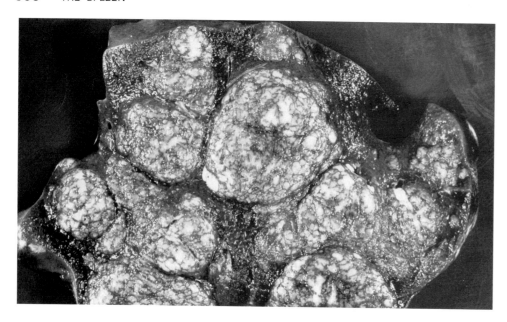

FIGURE 21–11. Spleen, Hodgkin's disease. Multiple firm, gray-white nodules enlarge and distort the spleen, sparing intervening parenchyma.

are also at risk, because these organs are almost never involved if the spleen is not. Additionally, the documentation of splenic involvement may alter the treatment modality.

Microscopic examination of the spleen in the early stages of Hodgkin's disease may also be subtle. Early involvement is usually in the marginal zones of the white pulp and the PALS. The criteria for diagnosis of Hodgkin's disease in the spleen, as well as other non-lymphoid organs, in a patient with a previous biopsy-proven diagnosis are not as stringent as those in a patient without a prior diagnosis.[114] In a previously diagnosed patient, the documentation of splenic disease requires the identification of one of the Reed-Sternberg variants, such as the lacunar cell or mononuclear variant, in an appropriate cellular population. Diagnostic Reed-Sternberg cells need not be found. If the patient does not have a prior nodal diagnosis, the identification of a diagnostic Reed-Sternberg cell is mandatory. It may be difficult to subtype Hodgkin's disease on examination of the spleen, unless the identification of characteristic cells of one subtype is made.[111]

Dysproteinemias

Hepatosplenomegaly may be a feature of **Waldenstrom's macroglobulinemia,** which, like **plasma cell leukemia** and **multiple myeloma,** tends to affect the red pulp more severely than the white.[115, 116] In macroglobulinemia, lymphocytes, plasma cells, and plasmacytoid lymphocytes, sometimes associated with immunoblasts, may infiltrate the red pulp, simulating involvement by acute leukemia. Clinically significant involvement of the spleen in multiple myeloma and plasma cell leukemia is uncommon and usually occurs as a terminal manifestation.[117, 118]

Malignant Lesions of the Red Pulp

Leukemias

The gross appearance of spleens involved in leukemic processes is that of red pulp disease, with a diffuse, homogeneous

cut surface.[119] The degree of splenomegaly varies with the type of leukemia and with the duration of the disease. In general, the chronic leukemias present a much more striking splenomegaly than do the acute forms. Microscopically, early involvement may be difficult to detect, because there may just be subtle infiltration of the red pulp. Eventually, the white pulp is obliterated. It is often very difficult to determine the subtype of the leukemia on examination of histologic sections. If a patient does not have a previous diagnosis, cytochemical studies can be performed on touch preparations, or flow cytometric analysis on fresh tissue.

Several leukemic disorders do produce characteristic morphologic changes in the spleen. The appearance of **chronic lymphocytic leukemia (CLL)** is histologically identical to that seen in small lymphocytic lymphoma. Early involvement in B-cell CLL produces a miliary expansion of the white pulp, before the red pulp involvement predominates.[93–95] Splenic involvement in **T-cell CLL,** or **leukemia of large granular lymphocytes,** may result in massive splenomegaly associated with neutropenia and a minimal bone marrow lymphocytosis.[120] The lymphocytes have more abundant cytoplasm, and azurophilic granules may be discernible.

Chronic myeloid leukemia also produces massive splenomegaly. Histologic examination reveals immature granulocytes at varying stages of maturation, often accompanied by megakaryocytes and clusters of normoblasts. The recognition of eosinophilic myelocytes in histologic sections may assist in the diagnosis. Sudden enlargement of the spleen in chronic myeloid leukemia may herald the transition to accelerated phase, or blast crisis.[121, 122] The spleen is the most common site of extramedullary origin of blast crisis. In blast transformation, the spleen usually shows a homogeneous cut surface. Occasionally, however, there may be grossly visible nodules that represent clusters of proliferating blasts. Chronic monocytic leukemia is a rare disorder that may present with prominent splenomegaly and infiltration of the red pulp by mature-appearing monocytes that may demonstrate phagocytosis of other blood elements.[123]

Hairy cell leukemia also produces characteristic morphologic findings in the spleen.[124, 125] Massive splenomegaly,

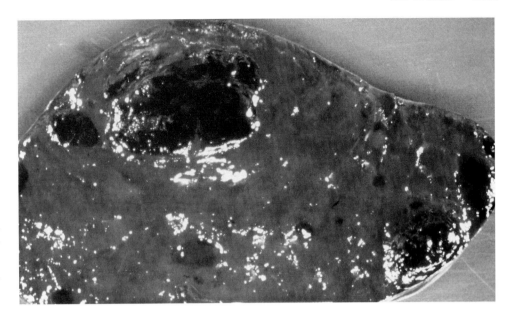

FIGURE 21–12. Spleen, hairy cell leukemia. The red pulp has a smooth, homogeneous appearance owing to a leukemic pattern of infiltration; the white pulp is inapparent. The uniform cut surface of the spleen is interrupted by cyst-like blood-filled venous lakes.

cytopenias, inconspicuous lymphadenopathy, and subtle peripheral blood involvement are typical presenting features. The spleen has a deep red cut surface as a result of sequestration of blood (Fig. 21–12). The hairy cells have round to oval or bean-shaped nuclei and copious pale cytoplasm. The cytologic features may be best seen on touch preparations. A characterisic finding is the presence of pseudosinuses.[126] These venous lakes lack ring fibers and are lined by hairy cells. They may produce grossly visible nodules that resemble a hemangioma (Fig. 21–13).

Prominent splenomegaly with cytopenias is also often a presenting feature of **prolymphocytic leukemia,** in which the white blood cell count tends to be extraordinarily high.[127, 128]

The tumor cells have vesicular nuclei, often with prominent central nucleoli and abundant cytoplasm. The majority of cases have shown B-cell lineage. Although red pulp involvement is the typical pattern of infiltration, rarely there may be nodular involvement of the white pulp, resembling involvement by a lymphoma. A newly described entity termed **splenic lymphoma with circulating villous lymphocytes** [129–131] and the disorders described as **hairy cell leukemia variants**[132] have clinical, morphologic, and immunophenotypic features linking them to both prolymphocytic leukemia and hairy cell leukemia. Splenic lymphoma with villous lymphocytes is a B-cell disorder characterized by splenomegaly, often a monoclonal serum paraprotein, and peripheral blood involvement

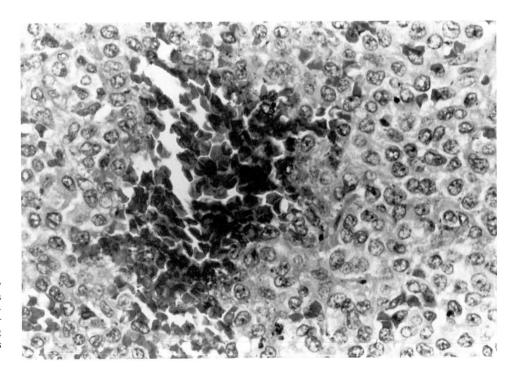

FIGURE 21–13. Spleen, hairy cell leukemia. The red pulp is diffusely infiltrated by pale-staining cells with ovoid or indented nuclei and abundant cytoplasm. A small pseudosinus or blood lake is present.

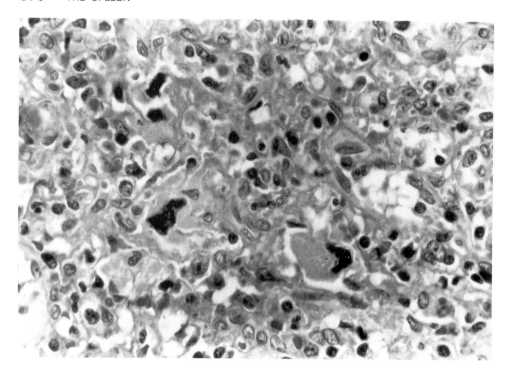

FIGURE 21-14. Spleen, agnogenic myeloid metaplasia. The vascular sinuses are patent, but the cords are widened by a diverse population of hematopoietic cells, including dysplastic megakaryocytes.

by lymphoid cells with irregular cytoplasmic outlines. Histologic examination of the spleen in these cases has shown variable degrees of involvement of the red and white pulp, associated with lymphoplasmacytic differentiation.

Myeloproliferative Disorders

Extramedullary hematopoiesis, or **myeloid metaplasia,** may occur in the spleen in a variety of disorders. The pathogenesis of the myeloid metaplasia appears to be related to medullary fibrosis, resulting in alteration of the bone marrow vascular sinus structures, allowing hematopoietic precursors access to the circulation. **Leukoerythroblastosis** leads to so-called splenic extramedullary hematopoiesis as the spleen performs its normal filtration function, trapping circulating immature hematopoietic cells. Any process that is associated with bone marrow fibrosis, including infections and metastic carcinoma in the bone marrow, may therefore lead to splenic extramedullary hematopoiesis. Evaluation of the spleen in these disorders therefore requires an understanding of the overall clinical picture.

Extramedullary hematopoiesis is characteristic of **agnogenic myeloid metaplasia** and the spent phase of **polycythemia vera,** in which the accumulation of hematopoietic precursors may lead to massive splenomegaly and hypersplenism.[133-136] The red pulp shows the presence of trilinear hematopoietic precursors (Fig. 21-14). Normoblasts and megakaryocytes are usually easy to recognize on morphologic grounds. The recognition of immature granulocytes may necessitate immunohistochemical or cytochemical studies. In contrast, the erythrocytic phase of polycythemia vera, in which the bone marrow shows no reticulin fibrosis and leukoerythroblastosis is absent, is associated with only modest splenomegaly. The spleen in uncomplicated polycythemia vera shows only a striking congestion of the red pulp.[137] Similarly, **essential thrombocythemia** is usually not associated with

splenic extramedullary hematopoiesis.[138-140] The cords appear somewhat "dirty" as a result of the accumulation of platelets. Touch imprints demonstrate platelet phagocytosis. In the late stages of essential thrombocythemia, autoinfarction of the spleen may occur owing to platelet pooling, resulting in an atrophic spleen with **Gamna-Gandy bodies,** similar to that seen in late stages of sickle cell disease. Leukemic transformation similar to that seen in the accelerated phase of chronic myeloid leukemia may supervene in any of the chronic myeloproliferative disorders.

UNCOMMON LESIONS OF THE SPLEEN (Table 21-2)

Lesions of the White Pulp

Dysproteinemias

The dysproteinemias associated with polyclonal hypergammaglobulinemia include **angioimmunoblastic lymphadenopathy** and **Castleman's disease,** although the latter may rarely be associated with a monoclonal gammopathy. Splenic

Table 21-2. Uncommon Lesions of the Spleen

I. Lesions of the White Pulp
  A. Dysproteinemias
    1. Immunoblastic lymphadenopathy
    2. Castleman's disease
  B. Systemic mastocytosis
II. Lesions of the Red Pulp
  A. Inflammatory pseudotumor
  B. Non-hematopoietic malignancies
    1. Angiosarcoma
  C. Metastatic carcinoma

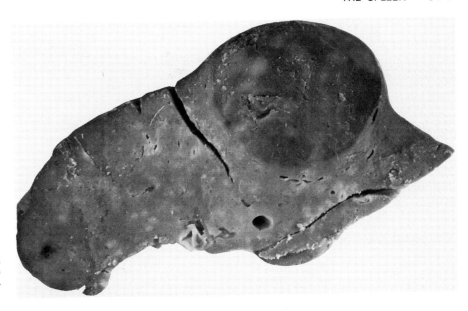

FIGURE 21–15. Spleen, pseudotumor. A bulging nodule resembling red pulp shows compression of surrounding normal splenic parenchyma.

involvement is rare in these disorders. In many cases, the morphologic features in the spleen are subtle and non-specific.

Angioimmunoblastic lymphadenopathy with dysproteinemia (AILD), or immunoblastic lymphadenopathy (IBL), was originally believed to be a hyperimmune B-cell proliferation associated with a defect in immunoregulatory T cells.[141-143] It now appears, however, that this disorder may represent a T-cell proliferation, with clonal rearrangement of the T-cell receptor genes, and many such cases are now considered to be lymphomas of T-cell origin. The majority of descriptions of splenic morphology of AILD/IBL have come from autopsy series, although in occasional cases splenectomy is performed in patients with severe immune hemolytic anemia.[141, 142] In some reported cases, the spleens have shown non-specific follicular hyperplasia. Other spleens show a polymorphous proliferation of lymphoid cells in the white pulp similar to that seen in lymph nodes, with lymphoid cells at all stages of transformation and occasional plasma cells. The red pulp may also be infiltrated by similar cells. The vascular proliferation seen in involved lymph nodes does not appear to be seen in the spleen. In patients who have received chemotherapy, the spleen often shows lymphoid depletion and fibrosis.

Although **Castleman's disease, or angiofollicular lymph node hyperplasia,** was originally described as having two distinct subtypes, it is now believed that the clinical and morphologic features of these subtypes in many cases overlap.[144, 145] Occasional cases of multicentric Castleman's disease

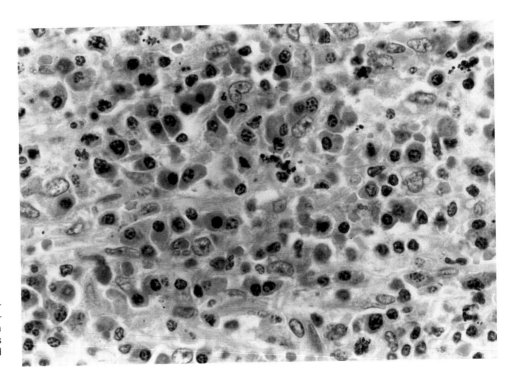

FIGURE 21–16. Spleen, pseudotumor. The normal splenic architecture is absent, replaced by a proliferation of plasma cells admixed with histiocytes and lymphocytes.

involving the spleen have been reported.[144, 146, 147] The majority have shown features of the plasma cell variant, which is the usual histology of lymph nodes in the disseminated disease, with large reactive follicles in the white pulp and a striking perifollicular plasma cell infiltrate. Other examples have shown foci reminiscent of the hyaline vascular pattern, usually seen in lymph nodes in localized cases, in which atrophic follicles are surrounded by a concentric proliferation of small lymphocytes and in which hyalinized vessels are often seen entering the follicles. The spleens in some cases of systemic Castleman's disease have shown features of both subtypes, indicating that a distinction between the two may be arbitrary.[147]

Systemic Mastocytosis

Splenic involvement in systemic mast cell disease may occasionally lead to clinically apparent splenomegaly.[148] Early involvement may show a marginal zone of distribution, with the characteristic mast cells having oval or bean-shaped nuclei and abundant gray cytoplasm rimming the white pulp nodules.[148] Other cases may show diffuse red pulp involvement.[149, 150] There may also be a variable degree of fibrosis and eosinophilia.

Lesions of the Red Pulp

Inflammatory Pseudotumor

Inflammatory pseudotumor of the spleen is an uncommon lesion that may mimic a malignancy both grossly and microscopically.[151–154] The lesion tends to be poorly circumscribed and infiltrates surrounding structures (Fig. 21–15). Microscopically, there is an admixture of spindle cells and a pleocytotic inflammatory infiltrate that may contain numerous plasma cells and histiocytes (Fig. 21–16).

Non-hematopoietic Malignancies

Primary sarcomas of the spleen are extremely rare, although there have been recent reports of splenic **Kaposi's sarcoma**[155] and **primary malignant fibrous histiocytoma**.[156] Most sarcomas of the spleen are of vascular origin.[157, 158] The histologic appearance of **splenic angiosarcomas** is widely variable. The lesions range from those with well-formed vascular channels, mild atypia, and a low mitotic rate, which previously have been termed hemangioendotheliomas, to frankly malignant tumors with solid areas and papillary growths. Because there may be a wide range of differentiation within a given tumor, it is difficult to predict clinical behavior on the basis of histologic findings, and therefore these tumors should all be considered angiosarcomas. They usually present as poorly delimited nodular masses, although occasionally angiosarcomas may involve the spleen diffusely. Extensive sampling of these lesions is essential to identify the more obviously sarcomatous regions.

Metastatic Carcinoma

Metastatic carcinoma to the spleen is uncommon and usually occurs only in patients with disseminated disease.[159, 160] The most common primary sites are breast, lung, and melanoma. Metastatic carcinoma to the spleen usually produces single or multiple tumor masses.

References

1. Wolf BC, Neiman RS: Disorders of the Spleen. Philadelphia, WB Saunders, 1989.
2. Christensen BE, Jonsson V, Matre R, Tonder O: Traffic of T and B lymphocytes in the normal spleen. Scand J Haematol 20:246–257, 1978.
3. Millikin PD: The nodular white pulp of the human spleen. Arch Pathol 87:247–258, 1969.
4. Weiss L: The structure of the normal spleen. Semin Hematol 2:205–227, 1965.
5. Weiss L, Tavassoli M: Anatomical hazards to the passage of erythrocytes through the spleen. Semin Hematol 7:372–380, 1970.
6. Millikin PD: Anatomy of germinal centers in human lymphoid tissue. Arch Pathol 83:499–503, 1966.
7. Bishop MB, Lansing LS: The spleen: A correlative overview of normal and pathologic anatomy. Hum Pathol 13:334–342, 1982.
8. Rappaport H: The pathologic anatomy of the splenic red pulp. In Lennert K, Harms D (eds): Die Milz. Berlin, Springer-Verlag, 1970, p 25.
9. Burke JS, Simon GT: Electron microscopy of the spleen. I. Anatomy and microcirculation. Am J Pathol 58:127–156, 1970.
10. Chen LT, Weiss L: Electron microscopy of the red pulp of the human spleen. Am J Anat 134:425–457, 1972.
11. Hirasaw Y, Tokuhiro H: Electron microscopic studies on the normal human spleen: Especially on the red pulp and the reticulo-endothelial cells. Blood 35:201–212, 1970.
12. King JT, Puchtler H, Sweat F: Ring fibers in human spleens. Arch Pathol 85:237–244, 1968.
13. Weiss L: A scanning electron microscopic study of the spleen. Blood 43:665–691, 1974.
14. Crosby WH: Normal functions of the spleen relative to red blood cells. A review. Blood 14:399–408, 1959.
15. Crosby WH: Splenic remodeling of red cell surfaces. Blood 50:643–665, 1977.
16. Rawsthorne GB, Cole TP, Kyle RJ: Spontaneous rupture of the spleen in infectious mononucleosis. Br J Surg 57:396–398, 1970.
17. Smith EB, Custer RP: Rupture of the spleen in infectious mononucleosis. A clinicopathologic report of seven cases. Blood 1:317–398, 1946.
18. Gowing NFC: Infectious mononucleosis: Histopathologic aspects. Pathol Annu 1:1–20, 1975.
19. Lukes JJ, Cox FH: Clinical and morphologic findings in thirty fatal cases of infectious mononucleosis. Am J Pathol 34:586, 1958.
20. Gordon HW, McMahon NJ, Rosen RB: Reed-Sternberg cells in a patient with infectious mononucleosis. Lab Invest 22:498, 1970.
21. Lukes RJ, Tindle BH, Parker JW: Reed-Sternberg-like cells in infectious mononucleosis. Lancet 2:1003–1004, 1969.
22. Tindle BH, Parker JW, Lukes RJ: ''Reed-Sternberg cells'' in infectious mononucleosis. Am J Clin Pathol 58:607–617, 1972.
23. Gugliotta L, Isacchi G, Guarini A, et al: Chronic idiopathic thrombocytopenic purpura (ITP): Site of platelet sequestration and results of splenectomy. A study of 197 patients. Scand J Haematol 26:407–412, 1981.
24. Karpatkin S: Autoimmune thrombocytopenic purpura. J Am Soc Hematol 56:329–343, 1980.
25. McMillan R: Chronic idiopathic thrombocytopenic purpura. N Engl J Med 304:1135–1147, 1981.
26. Tavassoli M, McMillan R: Structure of the spleen in idiopathic thrombocytopenic purpura. Am J Clin Pathol 64:180–191, 1975.
27. Rappaport H, Crosby WH: Autoimmune hemolytic anemia. II. Morphologic observations and clinicopathologic correlations. Am J Pathol 33:429–449, 1957.
28. Hassan NMR, Neiman RS: The pathology of the spleen in steroid-treated immune thrombocytopenic purpura. Am J Clin Pathol 84:433–438, 1985.
29. Collins RD, Neiman RS: Granulomatous diseases of the spleen. In Ioachim HL (ed): Pathology of Granulomas. New York, Raven Press, 1983, p 189.
30. Warner NE, Friedman NB: Lipogranulomatous pseudosarcoid. Arch Intern Med 45:662–673, 1956.
31. Wiland OK, Smith EB: Lipid globules in the lymphoid follicles of the spleen. Arch Pathol 64:623–628, 1957.
32. Klemperer P: The pathologic anatomy of splenomegaly. Am J Clin Pathol 6:99–158, 1936.
33. Kuo T, Rosai J: Granulomatous inflammation in splenectomy specimens: Clinicopathologic study of 20 cases. Arch Pathol 98:261–268, 1974.
34. Neiman RS: Incidence and importance of splenic sarcoid-like granulomas. Arch Pathol Lab Med 101:518–521, 1977.
35. Kay S: Sarcoidosis of the spleens report of four cases with a twenty-three year follow-up in one case. Am J Pathol 26:427–443, 1950.
36. Kadin ME, Donaldson SS, Dorfman RF: Isolated granulomas in Hodgkin's disease. N Engl J Med 283:859–861, 1970.
37. Sacks EL, Donaldson SS, Gordon J, Dorfman RF: Epithelioid granulomas associated with Hodgkin's disease: Clinical correlations in 55 previously untreated patients. Cancer 41:562–567, 1978.
38. MacPherson AIS, Richmon J, Stuart AE: The Spleen. Springfield, IL, Charles C Thomas, 1973, pp 98–101.
39. Franklin EC: Mu chain disease. Arch Intern Med 135:71–72, 1975.

40. Jonsson V, Videbaek A, Axelsen NH, Harboe N: Mu chain disease in a case of chronic lymphocytic leukemia and malignant histiocytoma. I. Clinical aspects. Scand J Haematol 16:209–217, 1976.
41. Frangione B, Franklin EC: Heavy chain diseases: Clinical features and molecular significance of the disordered immunoglobulin structure. Semin Hematol 10:53–64, 1973.
42. Kyle RA, Greipp PR, Banks PM: The diverse picture of gamma heavy-chain diseases. Report of seven cases and review of the literature. Mayo Clin Proc 56:439–451, 1981.
43. Seligmann M, Mihaesco E, Preud'homme JL, et al: Heavy chain disease: Current findings and concepts. Immunol Rev 48:145–167, 1979.
44. Dameshek W: Hypersplenism. Bull N Acad Med 31:113–131, 1955.
45. Crosby WH: Hypersplenism. Ann Rev Med 13:127–146, 1962.
46. Ellis EF, Smith RT: The role of the spleen in immunity with special reference to the post-splenectomy problem in infants. Pediatrics 37:111–119, 1966.
47. Kitchens CS: The syndrome of post-splenectomy fulminant sepsis: Case report and review of the literature. Am J Med Sci 274:303–310, 1977.
48. Smith CH, Erlandson M, Schulman I, et al: Hazard of severe infection in splenectomized infants and children. Am J Med 23:390–404, 1957.
49. Van Wyck DB: Overwhelming post-splenectomy infection (OPSI): The clinical syndrome. Lymphology 16:107–114, 1983.
50. LaCelle PL: Alteration of membrane deformability in hemolytic anemias. Semin Hematol 7:355–371, 1970.
51. Motulsky AG, Casserd F, Giblett ER, et al: Anemia and the spleen. N Engl J Med 259:1164–1169, 1958.
52. Bowdler AJ: The spleen and haemolytic disorders. Clin Haematol 4:231–246, 1975.
53. Jacobs HS: The defective red blood cell in hereditary spherocytosis. Ann Rev Med 20:41–46, 1969.
54. Jacob HS: Hereditary spherocytosis: A disease of the red cell membrane. Semin Hematol 2:139–164, 1965.
55. Weed RI: Hereditary spherocytosis: A review. Arch Intern Med 135:1316–1323, 1975.
56. Finch CA: Pathophysiologic aspects of sickle cell anemia. Am J Med 53:1–6, 1972.
57. Allgood JW, Chaplin H: Idiopathic acquired autoimmune hemolytic anemia: A review of forty-seven cases treated from 1955 through 1965. Am J Med 43:254–273, 1967.
58. Bowdler AJ: The role of the spleen and splenectomy in autoimmune hemolytic disease. Semin Hematol 13:335–348, 1976.
59. Laszlo J, Jones R, Silberman HR, Banks PM: Splenectomy for Felty's syndrome. Clinicopathologic study of 27 patients. Arch Intern Med 138:597–602, 1978.
60. Wiseman BK, Doan CA: Primary splenic neutropenia: Newly recognized entity closely related to congenital hemolytic icterus and essential thrombocytopenic purpura. Ann Intern Med 16:1097–1117, 1942.
61. Schnitzer B, Soderman TM, Mead MC, et al: An ultrastructural study of the red pulp of the spleen in malaria. Blood 41:207–218, 1973.
62. Wyler DJ: Splenic functions in malaria. Lymphology 16:121–127, 1983.
63. Groopman JE, Golde DW: The histiocytic disorders: A pathophysiologic analysis. Ann Intern Med 94:95–107, 1981.
64. Lee RE, Peters SP, Glew RH: Gaucher's disease: Clinical, morphologic and pathogenetic considerations. Pathol Annu 2:309–339, 1977.
65. Peters SP, Lee RE, Glew RH: Gaucher's disease, a review. Medicine 56:425–441, 1977.
66. Long RG, Lake BD, Pettie JE, et al: Adult Niemann-Pick disease. Its relationship to the syndrome of the sea-blue histiocyte. Am J Med 62:627–635, 1977.
67. Silverstein MN, Ellefson RD: The syndrome of the sea-blue histiocyte. Semin Hematol 9:299–307, 1972.
68. Silverstein MN, Ellefson RD, Ahern EJ: The syndrome of the sea-blue histiocyte. N Engl J Med 282:1–4, 1970.
69. Sawitsky A, Rosner F, Chodsky S: The sea-blue histiocyte syndrome, a review: Genetic and biochemical studies. Semin Hematol 9:285–297, 1972.
70. Schinella RA, Greco MA, Garay SM, et al: Hermansky-Pudlak syndrome: A clinicopathologic study. Hum Pathol 16:366–376, 1985.
71. Risdall RJ, McKenna RW, Nesbit ME, et al: Virus-associated hemophagocytic syndrome. A benign histiocytic proliferation distinct from malignant histiocytosis. Cancer 44:993–1002, 1979.
72. Risdall RJ, Brunning RD, Hernandez JI, Gordon DH. Bacteria-associated hemophagocytic syndrome. Cancer 54:2968–2972, 1984.
73. Perry MC, Harrison EG Jr, Burgert EO, Gilchrist GS: Familial erythrophagocytic lymphohistiocytosis: Report of two cases and clinicopathologic review. Cancer 38:209–218, 1976.
74. Fullerton P, Ekert H, Hosking C, Tauro GP: Hemophagocytic reticulosis: A case report with investigations of immune and white cell function. Cancer 36:441–445, 1975.
75. Lampert IA, Catovsky D, Bergier N: Malignant histiocytosis: A clinicopathologic study of 12 cases. Br J Haematol 40:65–77, 1978.
76. Warnke RA, Kim H, Dorfman RF: Malignant histiocytosis (histiocytic medullary reticulosis): I. Clinical pathologic study of 29 cases. Cancer 35:215–230, 1975.
77. Vardiman JW, Byrne GE, Rappaport H: Malignant histiocytosis with massive splenomegaly in asymptomatic patients. Cancer 36:419–427, 1975.
78. Callihan TR: The surgical pathology of the differentiated histioses. In Jaffe ES (ed): Surgical Pathology of the Lymph Nodes and Related Organs. Philadelphia, WB Saunders, 1985, p 357.
79. Enriquez P, Dahlin DC, Hayles AB, et al: Histiocytosis X: A clinical study. Mayo Clin Proc 99:42–48, 1967.
80. Lipton EL: Hematolytic and pancytopenic syndrome associated with Letterer-Siwe disease. Pediatrics 14:533–541, 1954.
81. Nezelof C, Frileux-Harbert F, Cronier-Sachot J: Disseminated histiocytosis X. Analysis of prognostic factors based on a retrospective study of 50 cases. Cancer 44:1824–1838, 1979.
82. Falk S, Stutte HJ: Hamartomas of the spleen: A study of 20 biopsy cases. Histopathology 14:603–612, 1989.
83. Silverman ML, LiVolsi VA: Splenic hamartoma. Am J Clin Pathol 70:224–229, 1978.
84. Butler JJ: Pathology of the spleen in benign and malignant conditions. Histopathology 7:453–474, 1983.
85. Garvin DF, King FM: Cysts and non-lymphomatous tumors of the spleen. Pathol Annu 16(pt I):61–80, 1981.
86. Garcia RL, Khan MK, Berlin RB: Peliosis of the spleen with rupture. Hum Pathol 13:177–179, 1982.
87. Lacson A, Berman LD, Neimas RS: Peliosis of the spleen. Am J Clin Pathol 71:586–590, 1979.
88. Tada T, Wakabayashi T, Kishimoto H: Peliosis of the spleen. Am J Clin Pathol 79:708–713, 1983.
89. Falk S, Stutte HJ, Frizzera G: Littoral cell angioma: A novel splenic vascular lesion demonstrating histiocytic differentiation. Am J Surg Pathol 15:1023–1033, 1991.
90. Blank E, Campbell JR: Epidermoid cysts of the spleen. Pediatrics 51:75–84, 1973.
91. Robbins FG, Yellin AE, Lingua RW, et al: Splenic epidermoid cysts. Ann Surg 187:231–235, 1968.
92. Sirinek KR, Evans WE: Nonparasitic splenic cysts. Case report of epidermoid cysts with review of the literature. Am J Surg 126:8–13, 1973.
93. Burke JS: Surgical pathology of the spleen: An approach to the differential diagnosis of splenic lymphomas and leukemias. Part I. Diseases of the white pulp. Am J Surg Pathol 5:551–563, 1981.
94. Burke JS: The diagnosis of lymphoma and lymphoid proliferations in the spleen. In Jaffe ES (ed): Surgical Pathology of the Lymph Nodes and Related Organs. Philadelphia, WB Saunders, 1985, p 249.
95. Evans HL, Butler JJ, Youness EL: Malignant lymphoma, small lymphocytic type: A clinicopathologic study of 84 cases with suggested criteria for intermediate lymphocytic lymphoma. Cancer 41:1440–1455, 1978.
96. Mann RB: Follicular lymphoma and lymphocytic lymphoma of intermediate differentiation. In Jaffe ES (ed): Surgical Pathology of the Lymph Nodes and Related Organs. Philadelphia, WB Saunders, 1985, p 165.
97. Narang S, Wolf BC, Neiman RS: Malignant lymphoma presenting with prominent splenomegaly. A clinicopathologic study with special reference to intermediate cell lymphoma. Cancer 55:1948–1957, 1985.
98. Weisenburger DD, Linder J, Daley DT, Armitage JO: Intermediate lymphocytic lymphoma: An immunohistologic study with comparison to other lymphocytic lymphomas. Hum Pathol 18:781–790, 1987.
99. Schmid C, Kirkham N, Dii T, Isaacson PG: Splenic marginal zone cell lymphoma. Am J Surg Pathol 16:455–466, 1992.
100. Harris NL, Aisenberg AC, Meyer JE, et al: Diffuse large cell (histiocytic) lymphoma of the spleen. Clinical and pathologic characteristics of ten cases. Cancer 54:2460–2467, 1984.
101. Brouet J-C, Flandrin G, Sasportes M, et al: Chronic lymphocytic leukemia of T-cell origin: Immunological and clinical evaluation in eleven patients. Lancet 2:890–893, 1975.
102. Pandolfi F, De Rossi G, Semenzato G, et al: Immunologic evaluation of T chronic lymphocytic leukemia cells: Correlation among phenotype, functional activities and morphology. Blood 59:688–695, 1982.
103. Uchiyama T, Yodoi J, Sagawa K, et al: Adult T-cell leukemia: Clinical and hematologic features of 16 cases. Blood 50:481–492, 1977.
104. Rappaport H, Thomas LB: Mycosis fungoides: The pathology of extracutaneous involvement. Cancer 34:1198–1229, 1974.
105. Variakojis D, Rosas-Uribe A, Rappaport H: Mycosis fungoides: Pathologic findings in staging laparotomies. Cancer 33:1589–1600, 1974.
106. Kadin ME, Glatstein E, Dorfman RF: Clinicopathologic studies of 117 untreated patients subjected to laparotomy for the staging of Hodgkin's disease. Cancer 27:1277–1295, 1971.
107. Trudel M, Krikorian J, Neiman RS: Lymphocyte predominance Hodgkin's disease: Clinical and morphologic heterogeneity. Cancer 59:99–106, 1987.
108. Neiman RS, Rosen PJ, Lukes RJ: Lymphocyte-depletion Hodgkin's disease: A clinicopathologic entity. N Engl J Med 288:751–755, 1973.
109. Zellers RA, Thibodeau SN, Banks PM: Primary splenic lymphocyte-depletion Hodgkin's disease. Am J Clin Pathol 94:453–457, 1990.
110. Diebold J, Temmin J: Etude anatomo-pathologique des prelevements effectues au cours de 250 laparotomies exploratrices pour maladie de Hodgkin. Ann Pathol 25:341, 1980.
111. Farrer-Brown G, Bennett MH, Harrison CV, et al: The diagnosis of Hodgkin's disease in surgically excised spleens. J Clin Pathol 25:294–300, 1972.
112. Neiman RS: Current problems in the histopathologic diagnosis and classification of Hodgkin's disease. Pathol Annu 2:289–328, 1978.
113. Desser PK, Moran EM, Eultmann JE: Staging of Hodgkin's disease and lymphoma. Med Clin North Am 57:479–498, 1973.
114. Lukes RJ: Criteria for involvement of lymph nodes, bone marrow, spleen and liver in Hodgkin's disease. Cancer Res 31:1755–1767, 1971.

115. Cohen RJ, Bohannon RA, Wallerstein RO: Waldenstrom's macroglobulinemia. A study of ten cases. Am J Med 41:274–284, 1966.

116. Dutcher TF: The histopathology of macroglobulinemia of Waldenstrom. J Natl Cancer Inst 22:887–917, 1959.

117. Rappaport H: Tumors of the hematopoietic system. In Atlas of Tumor Pathology, section III, fascicle 8. Washington, DC, Armed Forces Institute of Pathology, 1966, p 207.

118. Shaw MT, Twele TW, Nordquist RE: Plasma cell leukemia: Detailed studies and response to therapy. Cancer 33:813–819, 1974.

119. Burke JS: Surgical pathology of the spleen: An approach to the differential diagnosis of splenic lymphomas and leukemias. Part II. Diseases of the red pulp. Am J Surg Pathol 5:681–694, 1981.

120. Pandolfi F, Loughran TP Jr, Starkebaum G, et al: Clinical course and prognosis of the lymphoproliferative disease of granular lymphocytes: A multi-center study. Cancer 65:341–348, 1990.

121. Baccarani M, Zaccarai A, Santucci AM, et al: A simultaneous study of bone marrow, spleen and liver in chronic myeloid leukemia: Evidence for differences in cell compositions and karyotypes. Ser Haematol 8:81–112, 1975.

122. Brandt L: Comparative study of bone marrow and extramedullary haematopoietic tissue in chronic myeloid leukaemia. Ser Haematol 8:75–80, 1975.

123. Bearman RM, Kjeldsberg CR, Pangalsi GA, Rappaport H: Chronic monocytic leukemia in adults. Cancer 48:2239–2255, 1981.

124. Burke JS, MacKay B, Rappaport H: Hairy cell leukemia (leukemic reticuloendotheliosis), II. Ultrastructure of the spleen. Cancer 34:2267–2272, 1976.

125. Katayama I, Finkel HE: Leukemic reticuloendotheliosis: A clinicopathologic study with review of the literature. Am J Med 57:115–126, 1974.

126. Nanba K, Soban EJ, Bowling MC, et al: Splenic pseudosinuses and hepatic angiomatous lesions: Distinctive features of hairy cell leukemia. Am J Clin Pathol 67:415–426, 1977.

127. Bearman RM, Pangalis GA, Rappaport H: Prolymphocytic leukemia: Clinical, histopathological and cytochemical observations. Cancer 42:2360–2372, 1978.

128. Galton DAG, Goldman JM, Wiltshaw E, et al: Prolymphocytic leukemia. Br J Haematol 24:7–23, 1974.

129. Melo JV, Hedge U, Parreira A, et al: Splenic B cell lymphoma with circulating villous lymphocytes: Differential diagnosis of B cell leukaemias with large spleens. J Clin Pathol 40:642–651, 1987.

130. Mulligan SP, Matutes E, Dearden C, et al: Splenic lymphoma with villous lymphocytes: Natural history and response to therapy in 50 cases. Br J Haematol 78:206–209, 1991.

131. Rousselet M-C, Gardembas-Pain M, Renier G, et al: Splenic lymphoma with circulating villous lymphocytes: A report of a case with immunologic and ultrastructural studies. Hematopathology 97:1, 147–152, 1992.

132. Catovsky D, O'Brien M, Melo JV, et al: Hairy cell leukemia (HCL) variant: An intermediate disease between HCL and B prolymphocytic leukemia. Semin Oncol 11:362–369, 1984.

133. Glew RH, Haese WH, McIntyre PA: Myeloid metaplasia with myelofibrosis: The clinical spectrum of extramedullary hematopoiesis and tumor formation. Johns Hopkins Med J 132:253–270, 1973.

134. Laszlo J: Myeloproliferative disorders (MPD): Myelofibrosis, myelosclerosis, extramedullary hematopoiesis, undifferentiated MPD and hemorrhagic thrombocythemia. Semin Hematol 12:409–432, 1975.

135. Ward HP, Block MH: The natural history of agnogenic myeloid metaplasia (AMM) and a critical evaluation of its relationship to the myeloproliferative syndrome. Medicine 50:357–420, 1971.

136. Wolf BC, Neiman RS: Myelofibrosis with myeloid metaplasia: Pathophysiologic implications of the correlation between bone marrow changes and progression of splenomegaly. Blood 65:803–809, 1985.

137. Wolf BC, Banks PM, Mann RB, Neiman RS: Splenic hematopoiesis in polycythemia vera: A morphologic and histologic study. Am J Clin Pathol 89:69–75, 1988.

138. Hardisty RM, Wolff HH: Haemorrhagic thrombocythaemia: A clinical and laboratory study. Br J Haematol 1:390–405, 1955.

139. Marsh GW, Lewis SM, Szur L: The use of Cr-labelled heat-damaged red cells to study splenic function. II. Splenic atrophy and thrombocythaemia. Br J Haematol 12:167–171, 1966.

140. Ozur FL, Truax WE, Miesch DC, Levin WC: Primary hemorrhagic thrombocythemia. Am J Med 28:807–823, 1960.

141. Frizzera G, Morgan EM, Rappaport H: Angio-immunoblastic lymphadenopathy: Diagnosis and clinical course. Am J Med 59:803–818, 1975.

142. Lukes RJ, Tindle BH: Immunoblastic lymphadenopathy: A hyperimmune entity resembling Hodgkin's disease. N Engl J Med 292:1–8, 1975.

143. Neiman RS, Dervan P, Haudenschild C, et al: Angioimmunoblastic lymphadenopathy: An ultrastructural and immunologic study with review of the literature. Cancer 41:507–518, 1978.

144. Frizzera G, Massarelli G, Banks PM, Rosai J: A systemic lymphoproliferative disorder with morphologic features of Castleman's disease. Am J Surg Pathol 7:211–231, 1983.

145. Frizzera G: Castleman's disease: More questions than answers. Hum Pathol 16:202–205, 1985.

146. Gaba AR, Stein RS, Sweet DL, Variakojis D: Multicentric giant lymph node hyperplasia. Am J Clin Pathol 69:86–90, 1978.

147. Weisenburger DD: Multicentric angiofollicular lymph node hyperplasia: Pathology of the spleen. Am J Surg Pathol 12:176–181, 1988.

148. Travis WD, Li CY: Pathology of the lymph node and spleen in systemic mast cell disease. Mod Pathol 1:4–14, 1988.

149. Webb TA, Li CY, Yam LT: Systemic mast cell disease: A clinical and pathologic study of 26 cases. Cancer 49:927–938, 1982.

150. Brunning RD, McKenna RW, Rosai J, et al: Systemic mastocytosis. Extracutaneous manifestations. Am J Surg Pathol 7:425–438, 1983.

151. Cotelingham JD, Jaffe ES: Inflammatory pseudotumor of the spleen. Am J Surg Pathol 8:375–380, 1984.

152. Dalal BI, Greenberg H, Quinonez GE, Gough JC: Inflammatory pseudotumor of the spleen: Morphological, radiological, immunophenotypic, and ultrastructural features. Arch Pathol Lab Med 115:1062–1064, 1991.

153. Monforte-Munoz H, Ro JY, Manning JT, et al: Inflammatory pseudotumor of the spleen: Report of two cases with a review of the literature. Hematopathology 96:491–495, 1991.

154. Sheahan DK, Wolf BC, Neiman RS: Inflammatory pseudotumor of the spleen: A clinicopathologic study of three cases. Hum Pathol 19:1024–1029, 1988.

155. Sarode VR, Datta BN, Savitri K, et al: Kaposi's sarcoma of spleen with unusual clinical and histologic features. Arch Pathol Lab Med 115:1042–1044, 1991.

156. Sieber SC, Lopez V, Rosai J, Buckley PJ: Primary tumor of the spleen with morphologic features of malignant fibrous histiocytoma: Immunohistochemical evidence for a macrophage origin. Am J Surg Pathol 14:1061–1070, 1990.

157. Chen KTK, Bolles JC, Gilbert EF: Angiosarcoma of the spleen: Report of two cases and review of the literature. Arch Pathol Lab Med 103:122–124, 1979.

158. Smith VC, Eisenberg BL, McDonald EC: Primary splenic angiosarcoma: Case report and literature review. Cancer 55:1625–1627, 1985.

159. Cummings OW, Mazur MT: Breast carcinoma diffusely metastatic to the spleen: A report of two cases presenting as idiopathic thrombocytopenia purpura. Am J Clin Pathol 97:484–489, 1992.

160. Marymont JH Jr, Gross S: Patterns of metastatic cancer in the spleen. Am J Clin Pathol 40:58–66, 1963.

CHAPTER 22

The Central Nervous System

Samuel Hensley, M.D., and James G. Smirniotopoulos, M.D.

LOW-GRADE ASTROCYTOMA (Versus Reactive Gliosis, Cerebral Infarction, Inflammatory Demyelinating Pseudotumor, Cystic Meningioma, Oligodendroglioma, and Progressive Multifocal Leukoencephalopathy)

Astrocytomas are one of the most common primary neuroglial neoplasms but can be confused with a host of neuropathologic entities. A familiarity with the diagnostic criteria for low-grade astrocytoma and each of the other entities should allow the surgical pathologist to arrive at the correct diagnosis.

Low-grade Diffuse Fibrillary Astrocytoma

Neoplastic transformation of astrocytes results in an array of tumors the clinical and histologic diversity of which is much greater than in other types of intracranial neoplasms. This discussion centers on the low-grade diffuse astrocytomas derived from fibrillary astrocytes. Although these neoplasms exhibit limited biologic aggressiveness, with time, dedifferentiation or anaplastic transformation is likely.

CLINICOPATHOLOGIC FEATURES. Low-grade fibrillary astrocytomas of the cerebral hemispheres occur primarily in young and middle-aged adults, with a peak incidence in the fourth decade. There is a slight male predilection. These tumors can arise in any white matter site but are most common in the cerebral hemispheres. Their frequency is directly proportional to the volume of white matter in a given area of brain.

Clinically these slowly growing neoplasms typically present with seizure activity, signs of increased intracranial pressure, sensory or motor deficits, or altered cognition. Headaches are also occasionally reported.

The prognosis for these patients has steadily improved in recent years, partly as a result of megavoltage radiotherapy, oral corticosteroids, improved surgical techniques and anesthesia, and more effective anticonvulsant drugs.[1] This improved survival may also be related to earlier diagnosis in the era of computed tomography (CT) and magnetic resonance imaging (MRI) scans.[1] The current median survival is the range of 5 to 7 years. Interestingly, most deaths occur only after dedifferentiation to an anaplastic astrocytoma or glioblastoma.[1, 2]

Although the precise criteria and number of tiers have varied, grading systems have been recognized as providing prognostically useful information for many years. The grading scheme proposed by Kernohan and Sayre[3] has been largely replaced or modified by further studies.[4–7]

An in-depth study of the grading of diffuse fibrillary astrocytomas is beyond the scope of this discussion. Yet, because of its helpfulness in understanding the clinical course of these tumors, grading is summarized generally in this discussion. A three-tier system, as originally proposed by Ringertz,[8] has been in use, which separates diffuse astrocytomas into well-differentiated or low-grade astrocytoma, anaplastic astrocytoma, and glioblastoma.[4, 6]

Well-differentiated astrocytomas are characterized by low cellularity, mild nuclear atypia, infrequent or absent mitotic figures, and a lack of capillary endothelial proliferation and necrosis.

Anaplastic astrocytomas demonstrate increased cellularity, variable nuclear pleomorphism, and hyperchromasia (anaplasia), along with scattered mitotic figures. Infiltration of the surrounding neuropil with the production of perivascular, subpial, and perineuronal cell aggregates has also been associated with anaplastic astrocytomas.[5]

Glioblastoma is differentiated from anaplastic astrocytoma by the presence of foci of necrosis.[4, 6]

The inherent difficulty encountered in grading neoplasms is that it is an arbitrary division of a continuous spectrum of histologic changes into distinct, separate categories. Borderline cases of intermediate malignancy may be encountered that do not fit well in a particular grade and have an unpredictable clinical course.

Other modalities have been studied with the hope that prognostication can be further refined. Two of the most promising areas involve measuring cell proliferation indices and cytogenetic analysis.

The rate of cell proliferation can be accurately measured by injecting bromodeoxyuridine (BUdR), a thymidine analogue, before surgery. BUdR is taken up by cells in S phase, and the proliferating cells can subsequently be identified by immunoperoxidase staining using an anti-BUdR monoclonal antibody available commercially. The percentage of positive cells is then expressed as the labeling index. These indices have correlated closely with histologic grading and survival.[9–12] Similar measurements can be performed with an indirect immunoperoxidase technique using a monoclonal antibody Ki-67, which reacts with nuclear proteins expressed in the G, S, G_2, and M phases of the cell cycle.[13] It seems likely that such measuring of the proliferating cell pool will complement histologic grading in the future.[14]

Although experience is limited, cytogenetic analysis also shows promise of complementing histologic grading by providing independent prognostic information. In a recent report, survival time was significantly longer for patients whose tumors had normal or non-clonal karyotypes than for those whose tumors had clonal abnormalities, irrespective of tumor grade.[15]

In surgical biopsies, the overall gross features of these low-grade astrocytomas are rarely helpful because most specimens tend to be small. The rare pure low-grade astrocytoma examined by autopsy has a smooth white or gray cut surface with occasional small cysts. The tumor is poorly demarcated and can obsure the normally distinct gray-white junction.

Microscopically, low-grade diffuse fibrillary astrocytomas exhibit a delicate background of neuroglial fibers formed by multiple cell processes of neoplastic astrocytes. There is often only a mild increase in the background cellularity, with the tumor cells dispersed in an uneven fashion (Fig. 22–1). The nuclei are usually hyperchromatic and slightly larger than in normal astrocytes, exhibit mild nuclear irregularities, and range in contour from round to oval (Fig. 22–2). The amount of cytoplasm is variable. Some cells may contain abundant eosinophilic cytoplasm. In other cells, the quantity of cytoplasm is minimal, and their nuclei appear to be simply embedded in the background neuropil. Calcifications are occasionally found in association with small capillaries.

Smear preparations with or without frozen section may be very helpful. Although the uneven spread of cells within the

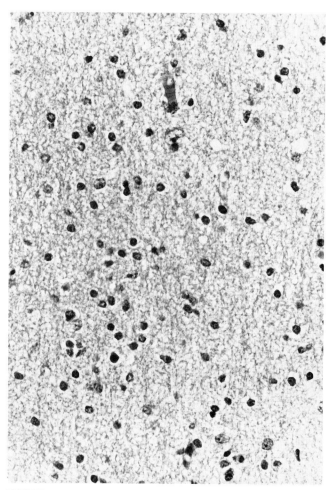

FIGURE 22–2. Astrocytoma. The minimally enlarged nuclei exhibit slight nuclear membrane irregularity and hyperchromasia in low-grade astrocytomas. (H&E ×300)

neuropil cannot be assessed using this technique, cytologic detail is excellent and may be an invaluable aid in diagnosing astrocytomas.

Immunoperoxidase stain for glial fibrillary acidic protein (GFAP) is usually strongly positive in well-differentiated astrocytomas. S-100, a less specific marker, is also generally positive. Staining for cytokeratin (CK) and epithelial membrane antigen (EMA) is rarely positive.[16, 17]

Astrocytomas composed predominantly of large, plump astrocytes with abundant eosinophilic cytoplasm with one or more eccentric nuclei have been termed **gemistocytic astrocytomas.**[5] This otherwise low-grade variant of diffuse astrocytoma shows a propensity for anaplastic transformation. This impression is further supported by a report that concluded that the presence of at least 20% gemistocytes in a glial neoplasm is a poor prognostic sign, and it was proposed that gemistocytic astrocytomas be classified as anaplastic astrocytomas for treatment purposes.[18]

DIFFERENTIAL DIAGNOSIS. Although various entities can simulate astrocytomas, most are discussed and contrasted with well-differentiated astrocytoma in following sections.

At this point it should be noted that gliosis, a reactive proliferation secondary to many forms of parenchymal damage, shares some features with astrocytoma and, especially in small biopsies, many cause considerable diagnostic difficulty.

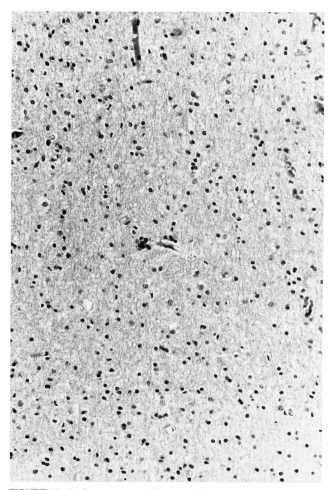

FIGURE 22–1. Astrocytoma. The neoplastic astrocytes, in small ill-defined clusters, are responsible for the overall mild increase in cellularity of the white matter. (H&E ×150)

Within the white matter of the cerebral hemispheres, reactive gliosis is generally marked by sheets of reactive astrocytes that are usually evenly spaced through the neuropil (Fig. 22–3) as compared with the non-random cell clusters of low-grade astrocytoma. Intermingled with these cells may be other astrocytes with abundant eosinophilic cytoplasm and discrete cell processes. In addition to these hypertrophic astrocytes, there is frequently a mixed population of cells, including macrophages and/or lymphocytes. There is usually only a mild increase in cellularity. The nuclear changes of mild atypia and enlargement may closely resemble the changes seen in well-differentiated fibrillary astrocytoma. The presence of hemosiderin suggests a reactive glial proliferation to some unidentified but often non-neoplastic process.

A common feature of low-grade astrocytoma that is rarely seen in reactive gliosis is the presence of microcystic degeneration, sometimes leading to grossly apparent cysts. The deposition of calcium also occurs more frequently in astrocytomas. Mitotic figures are infrequently identified but, if present, are strong presumptive evidence of neoplasia in this setting. Macrophages, just mentioned in association with reactive gliosis, are not generally associated with astrocytomas.

The presence of subpial, subependymal, perivascular, or

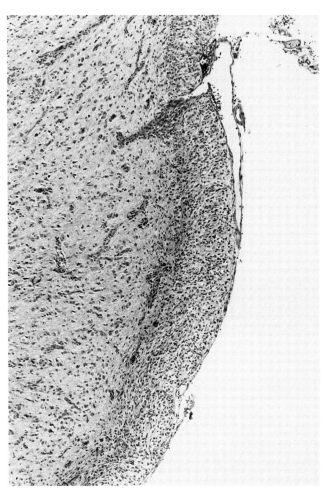

FIGURE 22–4. Astrocytoma. Subpial, perivascular, and perineuronal accumulation of neoplastic cells is typical of an infiltrating glioma. (H&E ×75)

perineuronal aggregates of cells is also a strong indicator of astrocytoma and, as noted earlier, is a finding that has been associated with dedifferentiation[5] in low-grade fibrillary astrocytomas (Fig. 22–4).

Cerebral Infarction

All forms of anoxia produce similar patterns of brain injury that vary histologically over time. Lesions at stages in which sheets of macrophages and reactive capillaries dominate can be particularly confusing, especially on frozen section. Most commonly, the localized lesion that can resemble low-grade astrocytoma occurs secondary to vascular occlusion. Because the therapy and prognosis for these two conditions are so different, the importance of accurate diagnosis is evident.

CLINICOPATHOLOGIC FEATURES. Although cerebral infarcts most commonly present with a sudden focal neurologic deficit that reaches its maximum effect in minutes or hours, some infarcts, especially of thrombotic origin, may present with vague symptoms evolving over a course of days. In this latter situation, the clinical history may be inconclusive and suggest the possibility of a cerebral neoplasm.

Microscopically, infarcts proceed through a series of stages over time. By 6 to 8 hours after ischemic insult, the brain

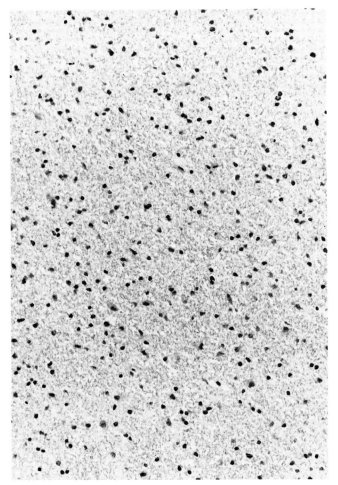

FIGURE 22–3. Reactive Gliosis. Reactive gliosis generally shows a more even, homogeneous distribution of cells with low overall cellularity; however, overlapping features result in diagnostic difficulty. (H&E ×200)

tissue exhibits edema along with swelling of capillary endothelial cells. There is perinuclear clearing in oligodendrocytes, and ischemic neurons assume a characteristic appearance with pyknotic nuclei and contracted hypereosinophilic cytoplasm. At this stage, neutrophils may be prominent. Infarcts at this early stage are rarely biopsied. The less common slowly progressive infarcts are occasionally biopsied, usually at 1 to 3 weeks, by which time the CT scan suggests a neoplasm, and the microscopic features have changed considerably.

Within 48 hours, the tissue necrosis is apparent histologically, and an influx of macrophages begins to phagocytize the necrotic debris. In the following days, the neurons disappear, and the macrophage infiltration imparts a startling cellularity to the process[19] (Fig. 22–5).

These macrophages, which may show a tendency to aggregate around blood vessels, typically contain round nuclei with evenly dispersed chromatin. The cell borders are sharp, and the cytoplasm is variably vacuolated (Fig. 22–6). Immunohistochemically, there is no staining for GFAP. HAM-56, a macrophage-specific marker, has demonstrated both sensitivity and specificity for these infarct-associated macrophages.[20]

Residual astrocytes typically undergo reactive changes and contain abundant eosinophilic cytoplasm and prominent cell processes. The border zone may also contain reactive irregular

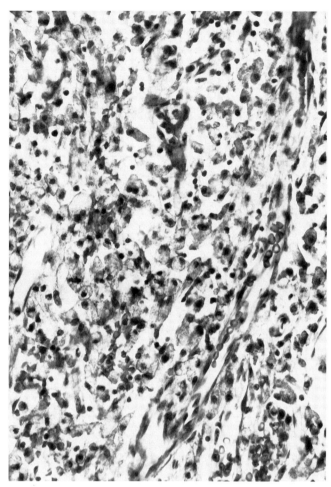

FIGURE 22–6. Cerebral Infarction. The macrophages, which account for the increased cellularity, are recognized by their sharp cytoplasmic borders, vacuolated cytoplasm, and small round nuclei. (H&E ×300)

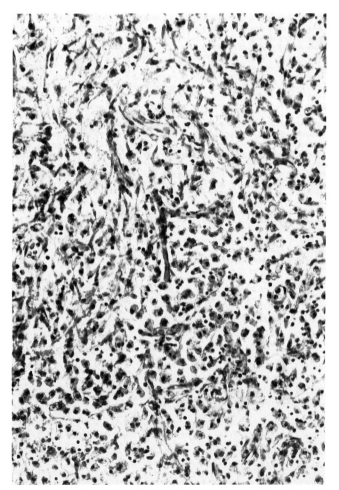

FIGURE 22–5. Cerebral Infarction. The vascular proliferation and increased cellularity can simulate a neoplastic process. (H&E ×200)

capillaries. Although these capillaries generally lack the florid capillary endothelial hyperplasia typical of high-grade astrocytoma, their presence along with marked parenchymal cellularity has been confused with both low- and high-grade astrocytoma, especially on frozen section.

DIFFERENTIAL DIAGNOSIS. The differential diagnosis that arises when a 2- to 4-week-old infarct is biopsied includes **low-grade astrocytoma, high-grade astrocytoma,** and **demyelinating pseudotumor.**

Consideration of low-grade astrocytoma is suggested by the presence of proliferative vascular changes and an increased cellularity secondary to an infiltrate of bland-appearing cells. The ability to make the correct diagnosis is dependent on recognizing that these cells are macrophages. An extremely helpful diagnositic aid at the time of frozen section is a smear preparation. In this technique, a small tissue fragment is placed on a slide, smeared to a thin sheet, and rapidly fixed. Macrophages are identified by such cytologic features as bland nuclei and sharp cell borders, described previously, whereas neoplastic astrocytes typically show slight nuclear irregularity and delicate cytoplasmic processes.

On permanent sections, this distinction may be difficult, especially in cases with superimposed freeze artifact or suboptimal fixation. Immunoperoxidase staining for HAM-56, a macrophage marker discussed previously, may be definitive. HAM-56 has demonstrated cross-reactivity with endothelial but not glial cells.[20]

Identification of the cells as macrophages should alert the surgical pathologist to the possibility of a reactive process, because macrophages are uncommon in astrocytomas.

The same approach applies to excluding a high-grade astrocytoma, which may have been considered because of the high cellularity, necrosis, and reactive vascular changes seen in cerebral infarcts. The lack of cytologic anaplasia quickly excludes this diagnostic possibility.

Inflammatory demyelinating pseudotumors also contain sheets of macrophages; however, unlike cerebral infarcts, necrosis is absent and silver stains demonstrate relatively well preserved axons.

Inflammatory Demyelinating Pseudotumor (IDP)

This process has been increasingly recognized in recent years as a focal cerebral lesion with radiographic features closely simulating a primary or metastatic neoplasm. The changes are secondary to diffuse demyelination in a circumscribed area with associated edema and mass effect. Less frequently the process may begin with multiple areas of involvement occurring simultaneously.[21, 22] In this case, the differential diagnosis is more likely to center on an infectious process rather than a neoplasm.

CLINICOPATHOLOGIC FEATURES. The age of onset is extremely variable, extending from 8 to 77 years in the largest available series.[22] The clinical symptoms at presentation are also quite varied, depending on the area of involvement. Presenting symptoms include aphasia, ataxia, headache, muscle weakness, seizures, and difficulties with cognition. Single or multiple foci of demyelination may be present initially in the deep white matter of the cerebral hemispheres, with occasional extension across the corpus callosum. Dramatic clinical improvement often follows steroid therapy, with partial or complete resolution of the abnormal areas on CT scans. No predilection has been noted for involvement of periventricular areas, optic nerve, or brain stem, sites commonly involved in classic multiple sclerosis.

The etiology of this process is obscure, and the diversity of the theories developed to explain it account for the lack of a generally agreed upon terminology for this process. Several authors have considered these lesions to be multiple sclerosis plaques that have attained sufficient size to mimic a neoplastic process.[23-25] That this phenomenon can occur during the course of **multiple sclerosis (MS)**[26] or as a presenting sign is well recognized. The course of MS is classically marked by exacerbations and remissions. If each exacerbation is followed by neuroradiologic studies, occasional especially large plaques with mass effect are identified. The prognosis and clinical course of these patients are probably similar to typical MS. If a past history of MS is available, the difficulty in reaching the correct diagnosis is greatly diminished, because the possibility of a demyelinating process is already under consideration.

Some studies,[22] however, indicate that most of these lesions represent a single event and that long-term follow-up does not show the typical MS course. It has been suggested that these areas of demyelination represent a variant of postinfectious-postvaccination encephalitis (PPE),[27] similar to cases seen after swine flu vaccination.[28] Although PPE usually consists of microscopic perivenous foci of inflammation and demyelination, large areas of demyelination have been reported in this condition.[29, 30] The prognosis of most patients is good, with an initial response to steroids and subsequent total recovery or stable deficits without the relentless progressive course of typical MS. Unfortunately, it is not possible to determine at initial presentation which patients will go on to develop MS. In lieu of an agreed upon nomenclature based on etiology or clinical parameters, we favor the use of the term **inflammatory demyelinating pseudotumor (IDP)** for this process, although another proposed term is "large focal tumor-like demyelinating lesions."[22]

When there is no prior history of MS and the lesion is a single large mass, there may be marked difficulty in establishing this diagnosis, especially for the pathologist. Furthermore, there is often a strong presumptive diagnosis of neoplasia based on the neurosurgeon's impressions and the radiologic findings. As will be discussed in detail, the cellularity of the biopsy may lead to a frozen section diagnosis of low-grade astrocytoma, or after multiple biopsies, the frozen section diagnosis is finally deferred. The process so closely simulates a neoplasm clinically that even if permanent sections are interpreted correctly, the surgeon may contemplate re-biopsy to obtain tissue "diagnostic" of neoplasia.

Histologically, a moderate increase in cellularity is produced by sheets of macrophages with vacuolated cytoplasm and well-defined cell borders (Fig. 22–7). The macrophage nuclei are small and darkly staining. Hypertrophic astrocytes with abundant eosinophilic cytoplasm are present but less prominent. Occasional small blood vessels are surrounded by cuffs of lymphocytes. If sampled, the border with adjacent brain is distinct, and silver stains show relative preservation of axons within the areas of demyelination. No necrosis is apparent.

DIFFERENTIAL DIAGNOSIS. The mistaken diagnosis of **low-grade astrocytoma** can be avoided by recognizing that the cellularity of the biopsies is accounted for mainly by sheets of macrophages with distinct cell borders and bland round nuclei. This distinction may be difficult, especially in cases with superimposed freeze artifact or suboptimal fixation. Immunoperoxidase staining for HAM-56, a macrophage marker, may be definitive. HAM-56 has demonstrated cross-reactivity with endothelial but not glial cells.[20] The clear demarcation from adjacent brain is also helpful if this marginal zone has been biopsied. Although scans may suggest a high-grade primary or metastatic tumor, the lack of cellular anaplasia precludes these diagnoses.

A subacute **cerebral infarct** contains abundant macrophages and may be considered as a diagnostic possibility. The presence of areas of necrosis and associated axon destruction are typical of infarction and are not found in IDP. In addition, cerebral infarcts are generally delimited by a vascular distribution pattern on scans, whereas IDP typically is not and often crosses the midline to involve both cerebral hemispheres.

Cystic Changes with Intracranial Meningiomas

Although the great majority of meningiomas are solid neoplasms, a small percentage show prominent tumoral cyst for-

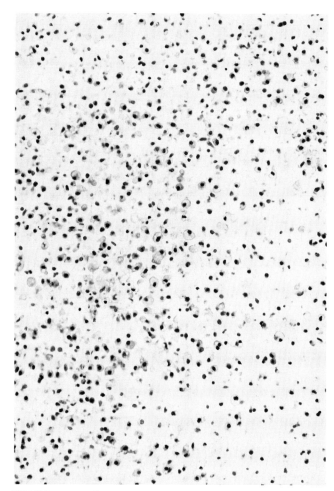

FIGURE 22–7. **Inflammatory Demyelinating Pseudotumor.** As in cerebral infarction, sheets of macrophages account for the increased cellularity. (H&E ×150)

mation. Large peritumoral cysts have also been described in the surrounding compressed brain parenchyma. Because this finding is so uncommon in meningiomas, the correct diagnosis may not be suspected before surgery. In fact, a low- or high-grade glioma may be the favored preoperative diagnosis given the presence of cystic changes and the well-known ability of gliomas to infiltrate the meninges, closely mimicking a meningioma.

CLINICOPATHOLOGIC FEATURES. Grossly cystic meningiomas account for only 1.7% to 4.6% of intracranial meningiomas.[31, 32] They do not differ from meningiomas lacking cystic change with regard to age, site, sex predilection, or prognosis. The majority occur over the cerebral convexities or in a parasagittal location.

Cystic change can occur within the meningioma or in the adjacent neural parenchyma. Four types of cystic meningiomas have been described, depending on the location of the cyst: (1) centrally located intratumoral cyst; (2) peripherally located intratumoral cyst; (3) peritumoral cyst in adjacent parenchyma; and (4) peritumoral cyst between tumor and the adjacent parenchyma.[33, 34] Intratumoral cysts may result from microcystic degeneration, ischemic necrosis, or hemorrhage.[31]

Grossly, meningiomas often appear bosselated with multiple protruding nodules. Attachment to the dura is a general

finding. The consistency varies from soft and spongy to firm and gritty. The presence of cysts grossly is very unusual, and when present, these cysts can range in size from barely visible to large, smooth-walled cysts that occupy a major portion of the tumor.

Microscopically, these neoplasms typically have the features of common meningioma variants (meningothelial, transitional, fibroblastic, and so on). Microcysts filled with a protein-rich fluid are usually present, and these microcysts can in turn become confluent, producing grossly apparent cysts (Figs. 22–8 and 22–9). Hemosiderin deposition from prior hemorrhage is prominent in some tumors. Some reported examples of this tumor[35] are particularly difficult to diagnose because they lack certain characteristic histologic features of meningiomas such as margination of nuclear chromatin, whorl formation, and islets of syncytial cells. Because the tumor cells are artifactually separated, they appear to have cytoplasmic processes, a feature mimicking low-grade astrocytomas.

Compressed brain tissue adjacent to a meningioma may become edematous with subsequent secondary cystic degeneration. The result can be reactive gliosis and fibroblastic reaction.[36]

Meningothelial meningiomas most clearly exhibit the classic ultrastructural features of meningiomas, including the intricate interdigitation of cell membranes joined by desmosomes

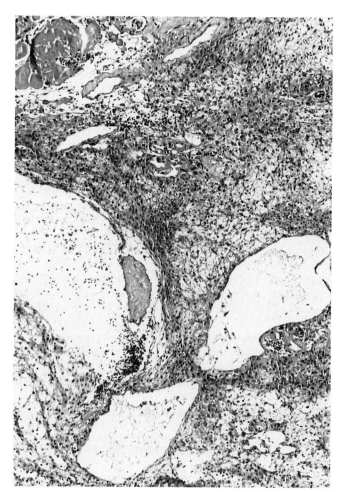

FIGURE 22–8. **Cystic Meningioma.** Irregular cysts filled with proteinaceous fluid result in grossly cystic meningiomas. (H&E ×75)

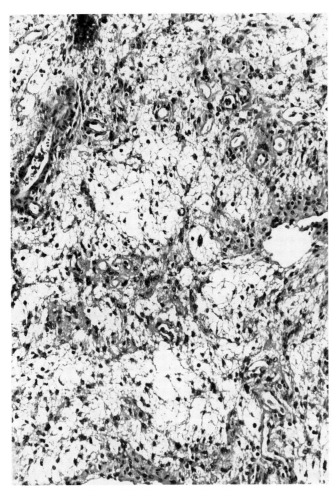

FIGURE 22–9. Cystic Meningiomas. Cyst formation frequently begins in foci of microcystic degeneration. Separation of meningothelial cells can result in cytoplasmic distortions that simulate astrocytic cell processes. (H&E ×150)

and other intercellular junctions. The concentric arrangement of neoplastic cells around blood vessels is also typical. Microvilli, indicative of epithelial differentiation, are sometimes numerous, especially in the secretory variant.[37] Intracytoplasmic tonofilaments are associated with the desmosomes. Fibroblastic variants may exhibit these features to a limited extent.

DIFFERENTIAL DIAGNOSIS. This differential diagnosis can be difficult on hematoxylin and eosin (H&E)–stained sections, especially at frozen section or in small biopsies. On frozen or permanent sections, the first and most important factor is simple awareness of this diagnostic possibility. If the tumor location is common for meningiomas and dural attachment is demonstrated, one should not exclude the possibility of meningioma in favor of **low-grade astrocytoma** simply because of tumoral cyst formation. At the time of frozen section, a cytologic smear preparation may be helpful.[38]

If typical features of meningioma, including whorl and psammoma bodies, are present, a diagnosis can be made with reasonable certainty.

If, as in some previously mentioned reports,[34, 35] these features are lacking, then adequate tissue should be obtained and immunohistochemical stains for GFAP and EMA performed. The presence of distinct membrane staining by EMA is characteristic of meningiomas and helps exclude astocytoma from

further consideration. GFAP stains the cell processes in astrocytoma but not in meningiomas. These immunoperoxidase stains are thus very helpful in this differential diagnosis.

Electron microscopy, although rarely required, can also be helpful. The typical ultrastructural features of meningiomas, although obscured by large amounts of fluid, may be present focally. The presence of desmosomes and intracytoplasmic filaments would help establish the diagnosis of cystic meningioma.[39]

Microcystic meningiomas may also be confused with **hemangioblastomas** with meningeal/dural attachment. The meningiomas, however, usually contain thick-walled vessels and often lack cytoplasmic lipid in spite of their vacuolated appearance. Again, EMA immunoperoxidase staining helps confirm the meningothelial derivation of this neoplasm. **Meningeal hemangiopericytomas** may also undergo cystic degeneration.

Oligodendroglioma

Oligodendrogliomas are composed of neoplastic oligodendrocytes, the neoplastic counterpart of cells that function in the formation and maintenance of myelin. The histologic appearance in the most common variant of this neoplasm is so distinctive as to be one of the easiest diagnoses for neophyte pathologists. The difficulty arises from the fact that this tumor can exhibit a wide spectrum of histologic variations. For the purposes of our limited discussion here, we are concerned with variations that can create diagnostic difficulties with low-grade astrocytoma. Some variants can mimic high-grade astrocytoma, and this topic is discussed in the appropriate section.

CLINICOPATHOLOGIC FEATURES. Oligodendrogliomas account for approximately 4% to 5% of intracranial gliomas[40] and occur with a 2 : 1 male preponderance.[41] This is usually a tumor of adulthood; however, childhood examples are not rare. Peak incidence occurs in the fifth and sixth decades.

Most oligodendrogliomas occur in the cerebral hemispheres, particularly in the frontal and temporal lobes, although, as is the case with astrocytomas, no white matter site is exempt.

Grossly, these tumors are well-demarcated and have a gray-tan to pink cut surface. Hemorrhages are not uncommon and change the otherwise relatively homogeneous appearance. Cystic changes are occasionally encountered.

The most common histologic variant of this neoplasm consists of sheets of cells that are segregated in lobules by arching capillary vessels. The tumor cell nuclei are small, round, and surrounded by a zone of perinuclear clearing (Fig. 22–10). This gives a "honeycomb" or "fried egg" appearance. The cells may be closely packed with no glial fibers present or dispersed within a neuropil background.

Capillary endothelial proliferation is occasionally seen without other atypical features such as pleomorphism, increased cellularity, or necrosis. Calcifications are common and may be found in the neoplasm or adjacent brain parenchyma. An immunoperoxidase marker specific for oligodendrogliomas has not been identified.[42]

A potentially confusing factor in the microscopic evaluation and diagnosis of oligodendrogliomas is the high percentage (more than 50%) of tumors with admixed reactive astrocytes. This problem is further complicated by the admixture of neo-

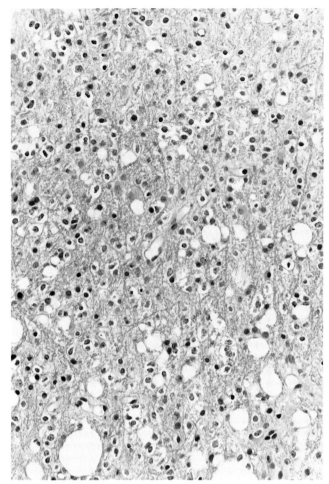

FIGURE 22–10. Oligodendroglioma. Neoplastic oligodendroglia are typically recognized by the uniform round nuclei and prominent perinuclear halos. (H&E ×200)

plastic astrocytes in many examples. These features have given rise to terms such as *mixed glioma* and *oligoastrocytoma*. Although these entities clearly exist, we believe such terms should be reserved for tumors with distinct areas of each tumor type. In particular, the habit of labeling any oligodendroglioma with scattered, often reactive, astrocytes as a mixed glioma is particularly to be avoided.

It has been noted more frequently in recent years, especially since the advent of immunoperoxidase stains, that cells intermediate between neoplastic astrocytes and oligodendrocytes are present in some tumors.[43] These cells are rounded and more discrete than fibrillary or gemistocytic astrocytes owing to lack of the delicate radiating astrocytic cell processes. The cytoplasm, however, contains abundant intermediate filaments that stain strongly for GFAP, a feature not usually associated with benign or neoplastic oligodendrocytes (Fig. 22–11). These cells have been designated as **gliofibrillary oligodendrocytes (GFOCs).**[43] Discrete foci of gemistocytic astrocytes identified by their long cell processes may also be present in oligodendrogliomas. The ability to differentiate gemistocytic astrocytes from GFOCs is of more than academic interest as stressed by a recent large study.[44] In this study, there was no reported prognostic significance for GFOCs, but a 50%

decrease in survival was noted when gemistocytic astrocytes were present.

The prognosis of oligodendrogliomas and its relationship to histologic features has been controversial in recent years. Before 1983, oligodendrogliomas were viewed as unpredictable, and grading schemes were considered of little value. Subsequently, a large retrospective review of cases from the Armed Forces Institute of Pathology[45] supported the contention that histologic grading can be effective in estimating prognosis. These findings were independently supported by further study.[46, 47] More recently, a large study based on the Mayo Clinic experience[48] found that tumor grade was the single factor most strongly associated with survival.

These studies have conflicted concerning the number of tiers in the grading system and exact criteria for each grade. The grouping of several microscopic features is common to most attempts. These features, which include increased cellularity, pleomorphism, mitotic figures, necrosis, and vascular proliferation, allow the separation of oligodendrogliomas into separate groups with distinct prognostic differences.

DIFFERENTIAL DIAGNOSIS. The differential diagnosis of **low-grade astrocytoma** and oligodendroglioma may not be difficult if the process is adequately sampled and characteristic features of either of these entities are clearly recognizable.

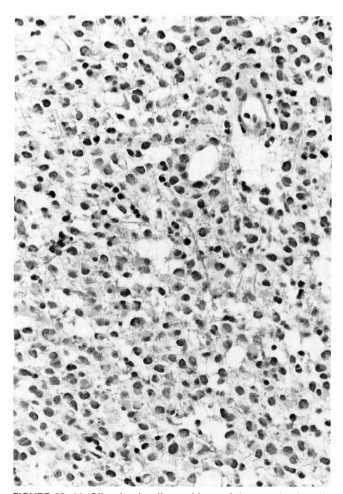

FIGURE 22–11. Oligodendroglioma. Many of the neoplastic cells contain abundant glassy eosinophilic cytoplasm while lacking cell processes typical of astrocytic differentiation. These are termed gliofibrillary oligodendrocytes. (H&E ×240)

However, in certain settings, the correct diagnosis may not be immediately apparent. Frozen sections can be especially challenging. Because the typical perinuclear halos, so distinctive for oligodendroglioma, are artifacts of fixation and therefore absent in frozen sections, a valuable diagnostic aid is missing. The delicate arching capillaries are very helpful if present. Otherwise it may be necessary to depend more heavily on cytologic smear preparations. The cytology of oligodendrogliomas consists of a cellular smear composed of fairly monotonous cells with small round nuclei and scanty or absent cytoplasm.

Because the surgical approach to low-grade oligodendrogliomas is similar to that for astrocytomas, we generally render a frozen section diagnosis of low-grade glioma and, after reminding the neurosurgeon of the importance of adequate sampling, await permanent sections before rendering a final more specific diagnosis.

On permanent sections, the microscopic features discussed previously usually allow a definitive diagnosis. If arching capillaries and perinuclear halos are not prominent, two additional features may be helpful. Oligodendrogliomas widely infiltrate the cortex and produce a prominent pattern of neuronal satellitosis. Although astrocytomas can also show neuronal satellitosis, the pattern in some oligodendrogliomas is particularly striking. Also, the typical small rounded nuclei of the neoplastic oligodendrocytes contrast with those of the low-grade neoplastic astrocytes, which are more oval to angulated.

Finally, provided the previous discussion of infrequent GFAP positivity in oligodendrogliomas is kept in mind, this immunoperoxidase stain may be very helpful in establishing the correct diagnosis. Negative staining strongly supports a diagnosis of oligodendroglioma. Should the GFAP stain be positive and if numerous delicate cell processes are highlighted, this would support the diagnosis of low-grade astrocytoma.

Progressive Multifocal Leukoencephalopathy

Progressive multifocal leukoencephalopathy (PML) is a viral disease affecting the brain predominantly in immunocompromised hosts. Prior to the recent acquired immunodeficiency syndrome (AIDS) epidemic, PML was a rare disorder seen in terminal cancer patients, in individuals treated with immunosuppressive drugs, and in chronic disorders such as tuberculosis.[49] With the increased incidence of AIDS, PML is now seen much more frequently. The condition is due to infection by a **polyoma-type virus,** designated as the JC virus. Infrequently a second polyoma virus (SV40) has been recovered and appears to be an etiologic agent.

CLINICOPATHOLOGIC FEATURES. PML occurs over a wide age range and affects both sexes. Recently with the inclusion of AIDS patients, a male predominance has been seen because most symptomatic HIV-positive individuals to date have been male. PML has a reported incidence of as high as 3.8% in AIDS.[50]

Because the disease begins as multiple small foci of demyelination scattered through the central nervous system, a variety of symptoms would be expected.[51] The symptom complex includes cognitive dysfunction, blindness, motor and sensory alteration, and brain stem dysfunction. Infrequently a confluent area of demyelination occurs with associated mass effect, resulting in clinical consideration of a neoplastic process.

The disease may be rapidly progressive, with death occurring within a few months. Most deaths occur by 1 year after diagnosis, although long survivals and spontaneous remissions have been described.[52, 53]

An autopsy examination of the gross brain shows a typical appearance consisting of multiple variably sized areas of necrosis in the deep white matter and along the gray-white junction. These foci may be discrete or confluent.

Microscopically, multiple foci of demyelination are present in an asymmetric distribution that is unrelated to blood vessels or vascular supply (Fig. 22–12). The surrounding oligodendrocytes, which are responsible for myelin sheath formation, show degeneration and nuclear changes typical of viral infection. These nuclear changes range from non-specific dense clumped chromatin to diffuse homogenization of chromatin (ground-glass change) (Fig. 22–13) to discrete eosinophilic nuclear inclusions with a surrounding halo.

Surrounding astrocytes exhibit variable pleomorphism, with occasional bizarre giant forms identified. These atypical astrocytes exhibit abortive infection. They contain viral nucleic acids but only occasionally express early or late viral

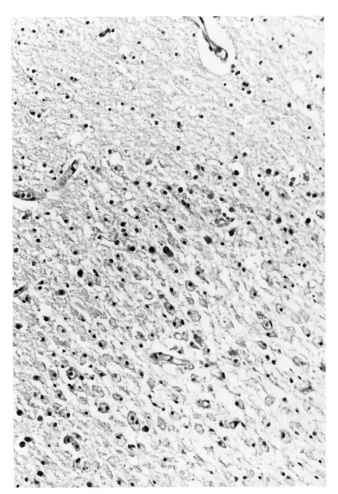

FIGURE 22–12. PML. Foci of demyelination contain scattered macrophages and are surrounded by cells with hyperchromatic nuclei. (H&E ×150)

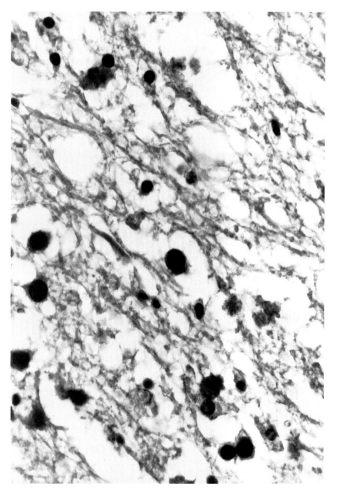

FIGURE 22–13. PML. The virus-infected oligodendrocytes seen at the periphery of the demyelination in PML most frequently exhibited nuclear hyperchromasia or ground-glass homogenization of the nuclear chromatin. (H&E ×600)

proteins.[54] With time, the foci of demyelination degenerate, and foamy macrophages infiltrate the area. A scant lymphoid infiltrate is usually present. Occasionally an intense inflammatory reaction composed primarily of lymphocytes and plasma cells has been noted in both HIV-positive and HIV-negative patients with PML. Speculation as to a possible co-infection with other opportunistic organisms was considered in one study, but no other infectious process could be identified.[50] Consequently, a heavy inflammatory reaction may be an infrequently observed part of the histomorphologic spectrum of PML.

Immunoperoxidase stains and DNA *in situ* hybridization probes have been used to confirm infection. In addition, detection of JC virus in cerebrospinal fluid in a high percentage of symptomatic patients by polymerase chain reaction (PCR) amplification has been demonstrated.[55, 56] Ultrastructurally, the viral particles appear as 30 to 40-nm spheres and filaments measuring 20 to 34 nm in diameter. Crystalline arrays of virus have also been encountered.

DIFFERENTIAL DIAGNOSIS. The primary consideration in the differential diagnosis is the distinction of PML from astrocytoma. This becomes a problem most frequently when neuroradiologic studies show a single lesion with mass effect as opposed to the usual finding of multiple hypodense areas.

If enough of the lesion is sampled, the presence of viral inclusions within oligodendrocytes, demyelination, and atypical astrocytes allow for a correct diagnosis of PML. If only a small tissue sample such as a stereotactic biopsy from the center of the mass is available, there may be only atypical astrocytes and macrophages. Viral inclusions may be lacking, and the degeneration of axons obscures the demyelination. In this setting, the presence of numerous macrophages, an uncommon feature in astrocytomas, should suggest demyelination and the possibility of PML. Immunostains or DNA hybridization may identify cells infected with the JC (polyoma) virus and are helpful.

In larger tissue samples, confusion could arise with **demyelinating pseudotumor** or other causes of demyelination. The presence of viral inclusions in oligodendrocytes and atypical astrocytes are, however, confined to PML.

Neuroradiologic Correlations in Low-grade Astrocytoma Differential Diagnosis

Neuropathologists and neuroradiologists frequently collaborate, an arrangement that often results in improved diagnostic accuracy. Although frequently not yielding a specific diagnosis, the CT and MRI scans should be regarded as complementary techniques that provide helpful diagnostic insights. An experienced neuropathologist is careful to correlate histologic features with neuroradiologic studies before arriving at a final diagnosis.

The histologic grade of an adult **cerebral astrocytoma** can often be predicted quite accurately based on its imaging appearances on CT and MR.[57–60] Adult supratentorial fibrillary low-grade astrocytomas (LGA) are usually homogeneous solid masses and only rarely show contrast enhancement (Fig. 22–14).[57–60] Because they are infiltrating lesions, they often have remarkably little mass effect, especially when compared with the overall size of abnormality. The lesion is seen as a decreased density on CT and altered signal intensity on MRI (decreased on T1-weighted images and increased on T2-weighted images). Low-grade astrocytomas may produce very subtle changes in density and mass effect and may be missed entirely. Unfortunately, these imaging features allow LGA to be confused with other common entities such as cerebral infarction, other types of glioma (e.g., oligodendroglioma), demyelinating disease, and PML (Figs. 22–15 and 22–16). However, there are some important differential features that can be used to separate these other possibilities.

Cerebral infarction typically presents with an acute onset of symptoms. On both CT and MRI, the gray matter is almost invariably involved (>90%), whereas in neoplasms the gray matter is the major site of involvement in less than 2% of cases.[61] In contrast, peritumoral ''vasogenic'' edema, commonly associated with many types of neoplasms, usually tracks along the short and long association fiber tracts of the white matter and does not affect the gray matter.[61–63] The involvement of the gray matter in an infarct is seen as swelling of the gyri with effacement of the sulci. Infarcts can usually be linked to a particular vascular territory and therefore have an angular geometric shape, either a triangle or a trapezoid, with its base on the cortex. Infarcts, like LGA, also have decreased density on CT and increased water signal on MRI

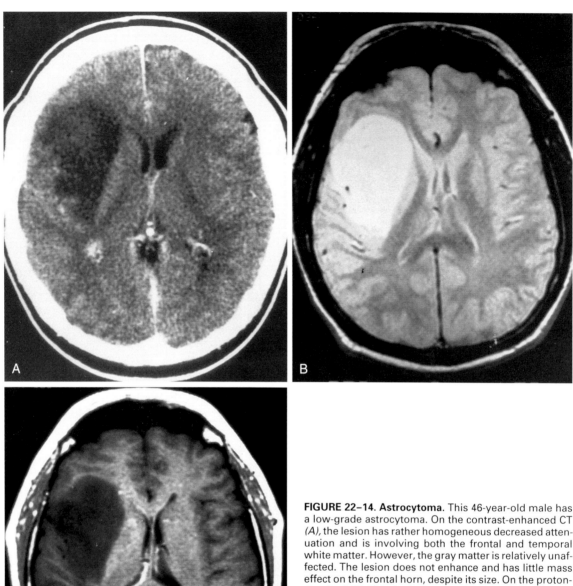

FIGURE 22–14. Astrocytoma. This 46-year-old male has a low-grade astrocytoma. On the contrast-enhanced CT *(A)*, the lesion has rather homogeneous decreased attenuation and is involving both the frontal and temporal white matter. However, the gray matter is relatively unaffected. The lesion does not enhance and has little mass effect on the frontal horn, despite its size. On the proton-density MRI *(B)*, the lesion has increased signal compared with both cerebrospinal fluid and brain. The T1-weighted MRI after Gd-DTPA *(C)*, like the CT, does not show any evidence of enhancement because the blood-brain barrier is intact. In LGA, because vasogenic edema is unlikely when the blood-brain barrier is intact, the visualized abnormality is usually entirely or at least mostly neoplasm. (Contrast this with glioblastoma multiforme, in which a large part of the abnormality and mass effect comes from vasogenic edema produced by the neoplasm.)

(dark on T1-weighted and bright on T2-weighted) as a result of the edema (both cytotoxic and vasogenic) (see Fig. 22–15). Edema in an infarct follows a predictable time course and is often not visible until the second day after ictus and usually reaches a peak in 3 to 5 days.[64] Thereafter, the amount of edema and the amount of swelling and mass effect become reduced, and the sulci open up as the gyri become atrophic. Serial imaging should demonstrate reduced mass on examinations performed during or after the second week following ictus; however, there are cases in which mass effect persists for 3 weeks or more.[65]

As many as 90% of cerebral infarcts demonstrate contrast enhancement at some time during their clinical course, and this is typically most obvious (in terms of both intensity and incidence) during the second through fourth weeks after ictus.[66] Although CT may appear "normal" early in the course of an infarction, some studies have shown that 80% of patients have a positive CT, with as many as one third of patients showing enhancements, within the first 24 hours after infarction.[67] The enhancement of an infarct is usually dependent on the re-establishment of a blood supply (either through re-opening of an obstruction, collateral flow, or capillary

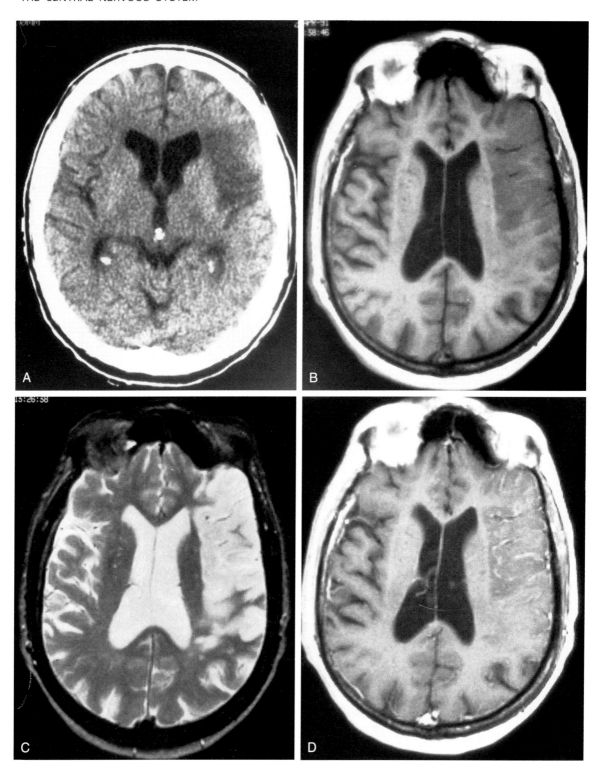

FIGURE 22–15. Infarct. This 68-year-old male has an infarct in the territory of the middle cerebral artery (MCA). In contrast with LGA, there is prominent involvement of the gray matter, with effacement of the sulci. This is seen on the plain CT *(A),* and on both the T1-weighted *(B)* and T2-weighted *(C)* MRI scans. Predominant or significant gray matter involvement is very suggestive of infarction. On the Gd-DTPA–enhanced T1-weighted MRI *(D),* the pattern of enhancement is "gyriform" along the surface of the infarcted cortex. This is also highly suggestive of infarction but can also be seen in other conditions.

ingrowth during the healing phase). Enhancement in an is-chemic or infarcted brain produces a serpentine or "gyriform" pattern typically limited to the superficial gray matter of the cortex, and, less often, there may be enhancement of the deep gray nuclei (see Fig. 22–15). Serial or follow-up imaging

examinations are often recommended for questionable cases. Although the gyriform pattern of enhancement can be useful in differential diagnosis, there is controversy regarding the use of contrast infusions in acute stroke. Some authors feel that iodinated agents may exacerbate an acute infarct.[68]

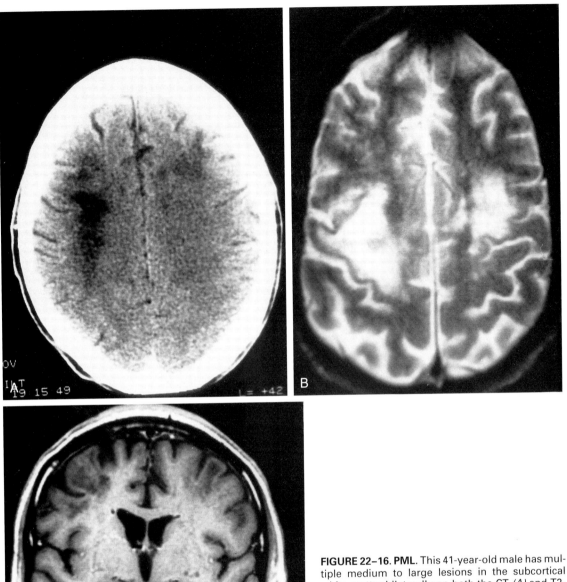

FIGURE 22–16. PML. This 41-year-old male has multiple medium to large lesions in the subcortical white matter bilaterally on both the CT *(A)* and T2-weighted MRI *(B)*. The coronal T1-weighted MRI *(C)* shows how the lesions are predominantly peripheral, occasionally within a gyrus. The lesions do not have either mass effect or enhancement. The presence of involvement in multiple, widely separated, vessel territories and the sparing of the gray matter make infarction (even embolic) unlikely. Although LGA is an infiltrating process, usually there is some mass effect, even though minimal.

Progressive multifocal leukoencephalopathy (PML) typically shows multifocal white matter disease but may present initially with only a single lesion visible on imaging. The lesions of PML, like infarcts and LGA, are usually homogeneous abnormalities, do not enhance, and lack mass effect. These lesions have decreased attenuation of CT and are bright foci on T2-weighted MRI (see Fig. 22–16). There may be large lesions that, unlike an infarct, involve more than one vascular territory, often in both cerebral hemispheres. Serial or follow-up examination shows relatively rapid progression over time (often within weeks), with both enlargement of lesions and development of new foci of disease. Large map-

like lesions form as multiple small foci of demyelination coalesce. Thus, PML can often be identified because of the characteristic "geographic" pattern, in which the lesions extend from the deep centrum semiovale up to the cortical gray matter of the gyri, but the gray matter itself is normal. In AIDS patients, however, PML may actually involve the cortical gray matter and may rarely cross the corpus callosum and/or be complicated by hemorrhage.[69]

It may be difficult to distinguish PML from atypical or aggressive **multiple sclerosis (MS)** on imaging studies. Most cases of typical multiple sclerosis present a pattern of involvement that is quite distinct from PML. In more than 90%

of cases, the majority of acute MS plaques in the cerebral hemispheres appear as small punctate lesions near the lateral edges of the lateral ventricles.[70, 71] MS plaques are usually smaller and more numerous than the lesions of PML. Unlike PML, MS plaques may show acute contrast enhancement, but this is usually self-limited for only approximately 6 to 8 weeks. It must be recalled that this enhancement can be suppressed with steroid treatment. The enhancement in an MS plaque is usually peripheral (ring enhancement) and follows the advancing edge of the inflammation. Large MS plaques may have a round or oval configuration and usually do not extend up to the cortex or subcortical ventricle, but rather cluster about the ventricles. Therefore, MS plaques do not form a geographic margin under the gray matter.

Large solitary foci of demyelination may occasionally exhibit mass effect along with peripheral contrast enhancement on scans, thus closely simulating a glioma.[72] The diagnosis of inflammatory demyelinating pseudotumor should be considered even if involvement of the corpus callosum is documented. These features are more commonly confused with high-grade gliomas, as noted in the section on "ring-enhancing" masses.

Relatively "pure" **oligodendrogliomas,** those composed of more than 75% oligodendrocytes, can present a highly suggestive pattern on imaging studies. These characteristic features include a superficial location, especially in the frontal lobe; several scattered areas of cystic change; infiltration into the cortex (as evidenced by abnormal gray matter enhancement); extensive calcifications, especially areas of infiltrated cortex; and evidence of slow growth by clinical history, or by the presence of a scalloped erosion of the inner table of the calvarium overlying the tumor.[73]

Thirty to ninety percent of oligodendrogliomas have calcifications on CT.[74] These may be detected on plain films in as many as 75% of cases.[75] A characteristic pattern of calcifications seen as a dot-dash or even a continuous curvilinear gyriform pattern of increased attenuation on CT can be seen in the cortex after tumor infiltration. Although routine MRI pulse sequences are often insensitive to small (psammomatous) calcifications, many oligodendrogliomas contain calcium in large "chunks" that can easily be detected without using special scan routines.

HIGH-GRADE ASTROCYTOMA/ GLIOBLASTOMA (Versus Gliosarcoma, Pleomorphic Xanthoastrocytoma, Oligodendroglioma, Cerebral Lymphoma, Metastatic Carcinoma, and Germinoma)

Glioblastomas are one of the most common primary tumors of the central nervous system, especially in older individuals. Because these neoplasms are relatively frequent at any institution with a neurosurgery service, the common manifestations and histologic features are usually readily recognized. Two potential diagnostic pitfalls do exist. Some glioblastomas have unusual microscopic features, of little or no prognostic significance, which can result in an incorrect diagnosis. Conversely there are uncommon entities with very different prognoses, which have features that can lead to an erroneous

diagnosis of glioblastoma with potentially catastrophic consequences. In both cases, it is important to consider the full diagnostic differential to arrive at a correct diagnosis.

Glioblastoma

Glioblastomas are generally regarded as the expression of progressive anaplasia in astrocytomas, mixed oligoastrocytomas, and less frequently oligodendrogliomas. The time course of these changes is variable but probably rather short. Tumors arising in low-grade gliomas have been termed secondary glioblastomas, whereas those with no associated low-grade component are termed primary. Primary glioblastoma may result from rapid overgrowth of a previous small low-grade glioma or could be due to a *de novo* primitive tumor with a proclivity to differentiate along astrocyte or oligodendroglial lines.

CLINICOPATHOLOGIC FEATURES. Glioblastomas occur most frequently in the sixth decade[6] and account for 15% to 20% of all intracranial tumors.[76] A male predilection of approximately 3 : 2 is noted. The tumor arises in the white matter, with frontal and temporal lobes as preferred sites. Involvement of the contralateral cerebral hemisphere by extension across the corpus callosum is not unusual. This discussion deals primarily with the most common cerebral hemisphere variants.

The clinical symptoms in these patients vary greatly depending on tumor location, rate of growth, and time course of a preceding low-grade astrocytoma. Glioblastomas, as may all brain tumors, can produce both generalized symptoms related to tumor size and increased intracranial pressure, as well as focal symptoms based on compression or infiltration of specific brain areas.

Expanding size and increased intracranial pressure are related to tumor bulk, cerebral edema, and degree of cerebrospinal fluid pathway obstruction. Symptoms classically associated with increased intracranial pressure include headache, mental status changes, vomiting, and less commonly generalized seizures. Localizing signs include focal seizures along with various patterns of motor and sensory deficit. Various syndromes are described depending on the primary lobe involved. A more detailed discussion is beyond the scope of this chapter but is of value in understanding clinical symptomatology in brain tumors.[77]

Microscopically, the tumor cells, at least focally, have pink cytoplasm, cell processes, and an associated neuropil background typical of astrocytic differentiation. The tumors are typically diffuse and highly cellular. Individual tumor cells exhibit marked nuclear hyperchromasia and often extreme pleomorphism. Sheets of small undifferentiated-appearing cells may constitute a portion of glioblastomas. Capillary endothelial hyperplasia is usually prominent and may consist of capillaries arranged in glomeruloid formation. In our opinion, and that of others,[4, 6] the *sine qua non* for diagnosis of glioblastoma multiforme as opposed to anaplastic astrocytoma are the irregular areas of necrosis often accompanied by pseudopalisading by adjacent tumor cells seen only in glioblastoma (Fig. 22–17).

At this juncture, two points should be emphasized. First, necrosis with or without the pseudopalisade arrangement carries the same poor prognosis. Second, in small stereotactic biopsies, which are becoming increasingly common, an extremely cellular pleomorphic astrocytoma with vascular proliferation and appropriate neuroradiologic appearance may represent a glioblastoma, although no necrosis is found in the small sample. If frozen sections are performed, the neurosurgeon should be told of the possibility that the samples are inadequate to distinguish between anaplastic astrocytoma and glioblastoma. The neurosurgeon can then decide whether the clinical importance of making this distinction overrides the risk of further biopsies.

Rare distinctive variants of glioblastoma can cause diagnostic difficulties. These include the **lipid-rich epithelioid glioblastoma**, the **giant cell (monstrocellular) glioblastoma**, and glioblastomas with foci of epithelioid appearance.

Lipid-rich Epithelioid Glioblastoma

Malignant gliomas with heavily lipidized cells have been described[78] for some time and the name "lipid-rich epithelioid glioblastoma" has been suggested.[79]

These neoplasms consist of lobules and sheets of cells separated by thin fibrovascular septa (Fig. 22–18). The individual tumor cells contain abundant clear to vacuolated cytoplasm. The epithelioid appearance is enhanced by the presence of sheets of cells with distinct cell membranes and lack of cell processes (Fig. 22–19). Some areas more typical of astrocytoma, or glioblastoma may be present, but typically the

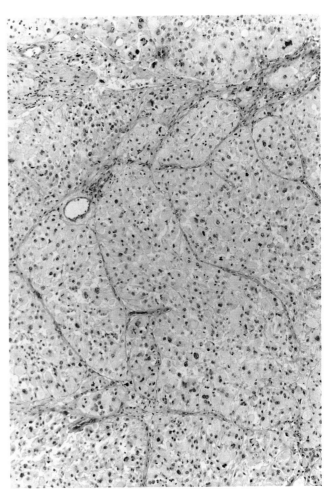

FIGURE 22–18. Lipid-rich Epithelioid Glioblastoma. Sheets of tumor cells are divided into variably sized lobules by a delicate fibrovascular septum. (H&E ×75)

majority of cells of these tumors are heavily lipidized. Mitotic figures and areas of necrosis are generally present.

Distinguishing this tumor from metastatic clear-cell carcinoma (kidney, adrenal, and other organs) is difficult with routine stains because the prominent intracellular lipid accumulation obscures glial features such as abundant eosinophilic cytoplasm and cell processes. Periodic acid-Schiff (PAS) stain with and without diastase demonstrates a high content of glycogen in metastatic renal cell carcinoma, whereas lipid-rich glioblastoma is glycogen poor.

Immunoperoxidase stains are helpful but must be interpreted with caution. Because both cytokeratin (CK) and epithelial membrane antigens (EMA) have been reported in astrocytomas,[16, 17] their presence is not diagnostic of metastatic carcinoma.

GFAP has been considered a very specific marker for astrocytoma but rarely has been described in carcinomas.[80, 81] The diagnosis of lipid-rich epithelioid glioblastoma can be made confidently when areas of more typical high-grade astrocytoma are present and when the immunoperoxidase stains are strongly GFAP-positive with weak to negative staining for CK and EMA.

Occasionally when staining results are equivocal and sampling is limited, it is reasonable to suggest non-invasive imaging of the kidneys.[79]

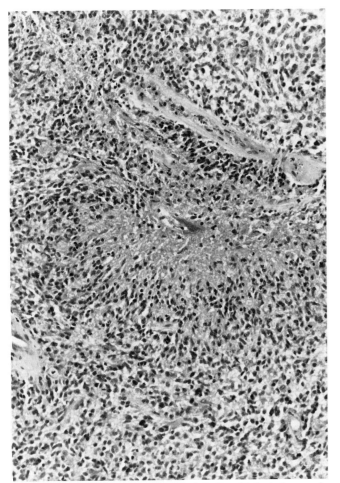

FIGURE 22–17. Glioblastoma. High cellularity with foci of necrosis and vascular proliferation are typical. (H&E ×150)

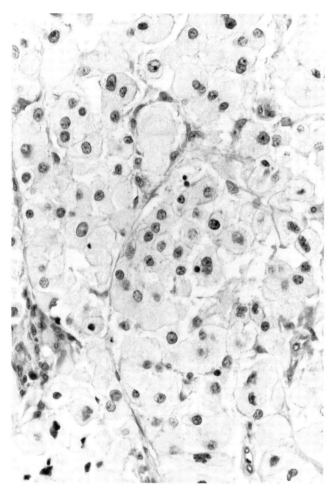

FIGURE 22–19. Lipid-rich Epithelioid Glioblastoma. The tumor cell cytoplasm is vacuolated, and cell processes are lacking. The distinct cytoplasmic borders contribute to the epithelioid appearance. (H&E ×300)

Immunoperoxidase stains are helpful in eliminating **balloon cell melanomas** and sarcomas with xanthomatous change from the differential list. Melanomas usually stain for HMB-45 (melanoma-specific antigen) and are negative for GFAP and CK. Sarcomas are usually negative for both GFAP and cytokeratin.

There have been no reports of positive staining for GFAP in adrenal cortical carcinoma, a helpful feature to exclude a metastasis from the adrenal gland.

Giant Cell (Monstrocellular) Glioblastoma

A particular variant of glioblastoma, designated as giant cell (monstrocellular) glioblastoma, has been described that is composed predominantly of very large, bizarre, often multinucleated cells with eosinophilic cytoplasm and pleomorphic nuclei (Figs. 22–20 and 22–21). These neoplasms grossly appear well-defined, and the temporal lobe has been the preferred site in some series.[82] These tumors generally show only scanty vascular proliferation but large foci of reticulin deposition. Areas of necrosis may be present, but the typical palisading arrangement is often absent. A heavy infiltrate of lymphocytes is present in many examples, and the suggestion has been made that this lymphoid reaction may account for

the overall prolonged survivals compared with the usual glioblastoma.[83] Immunoperoxidase staining is positive for GFAP in many of the cells.

Other explanations have been offered for the somewhat improved survivals noted in some series.[82, 84] Glioma cell cycle studies show slowed proliferation in giant cells.[85, 86] Kinetic analyses have indicated that the rate of tumor growth correlates most closely with the size of the proliferating component. Different degrees of malignancy relate to the size of the growth fraction in a given tumor.[87] The large number of giant cells may be accompanied by a smaller proliferating component, accouting for a somewhat improved prognosis in comparison with more typical glioblastomas.

Also, in spite of microscopic infiltration of the adjacent brain and leptomeninges, the gross circumscription and frequent occurrence in the temporal lobe may allow a more frequent total gross excision. If only a microscopic amount of tumor is left, the time to recurrence would be expected to be increased, resulting in prolonged survival.

Glioblastoma with Epithelial-like Structures

"Adenoid" formations and areas of squamous metaplasia have been described in gliosarcomas and uncomplicated gli-

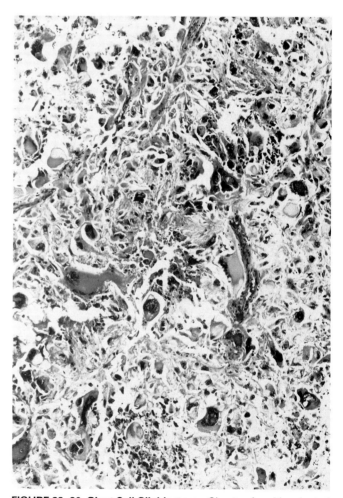

FIGURE 22–20. Giant Cell Glioblastoma. Sheets of multinucleated pleomorphic cells predominate in giant cell glioblastoma. (H&E ×75)

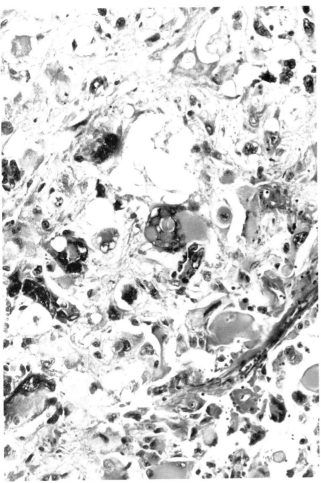

FIGURE 22-21. Giant Cell Glioblastoma. Grotesque multinucleated cells with abundant eosinophilic cytoplasm are present, with minimal capillary endothelial proliferation. (H&E ×150)

oblastomas. The adenoid formations were described in five cases of gliosarcoma[88] and consist of clusters of cuboidal cells forming a cribriform pattern and structures resembling ducts and glands of metastatic adenocarcinoma. Areas of squamous metaplasia with keratinization and pearl formation have also been described.[89]

These epithelial-like areas do not change the prognosis for glioblastomas but may prompt concern that a second malignancy is present elsewhere that has metastasized to the central nervous system. Strong GFAP staining in the adenoid foci and lack of membrane staining for epithelial membrane antigen are helpful findings in eliminating a metastatic adenocarcinoma. Squamous metaplasia may fail to stain with GFAP, whereas cytokeratin and EMA show a typical staining pattern for squamous epithelium. In this case, it may still be possible to avoid a metastatic work-up if one is aware of the possibility of squamous metaplasia in glioblastomas and if the squamous cells are bland and lack the degree of cellular anaplasia usually seen in metastatic squamous cell carcinoma.

Gliosarcoma

Gliosarcomas are neoplasms with a high-grade astrocytoma/glioblastomatous component and sarcomatous

component. This is usually a result of sarcomatous transformation occurring in the mesenchymal component of an otherwise typical glioblastoma. Examples have also been reported in which meningeal sarcomas are associated with a neoplastic change in the surrounding neuroepithelial tissue, resulting in a similar mixed tumor that has been termed a "sarcoglioma."[90] Various types of sarcoma have been described in these tumors,[91, 92] including rhabdomyosarcoma,[93] malignant fibrohistiocytoma,[92] angiosarcoma, fibrosarcoma, and osteochondrosarcomas.[91, 94]

CLINICOPATHOLOGIC FEATURES. The gliosarcoma does not significantly differ from glioblastoma with regard to age at diagnosis, sex, and clinical presentation. Metastases may occur more frequently, but generally the survival is short and this factor is not usually of clinical significance. Gliosarcomas have been estimated to occur in 2% to 8% of glioblastomas.[95, 96]

Two gross findings have been noted[95] that are more typical of gliosarcoma than of glioblastoma: the gliosarcomas are more likely to arise in the temporal lobe, and they were more likely to be grossly circumscribed with occasional meningeal attachment.

Microscopically, the anaplastic astrocytoma/glioblastoma component contains all the histologic features described previously. The sarcomatous component most commonly resembles a fibrosarcoma with parallel rows of elongated fusiform nuclei and eosinophilic cytoplasm forming irregular fascicles. In addition, the sarcoma exhibits frank histologic and cytologic evidence of malignancy, including high cellularity, mitotic figures, nuclear atypia, and in many cases irregular areas of necrosis (Fig. 22-22).

The sarcomatous component is thought to arise in association with the florid vascular hyperplasia that is prominent in high-grade gliomas. These vascular formations are sometimes surrounded by a proliferation of mesenchymal spindled cells (Fig. 22-23). With sarcomatous transformation, these mesenchymal cells proliferate and infiltrate the surrounding high-grade glioma. The cell of origin for the sarcoma is uncertain, and the issue provokes conflicting opinions, with some authors favoring endothelium,[97] perivascular fibroblasts,[98] or histiocyte-mediated sarcomatous proliferations of other mesenchymal cells.[99]

An immunoperoxidase stain for GFAP is helpful in separating the neuroepithelial and mesenchymal components. The neuroepithelial tissue stains strongly GFAP-positive, with no positive staining in the adjacent sarcoma. Although the sarcoma is thought to arise from the hyperplastic vessels, endothelial markers such as Factor VIII–related antigen and *Ulex europaeus* are usually negative, although positive staining has been reported.[97]

DIFFERENTIAL DIAGNOSIS. The distinction between a pure glioblastoma and gliosarcoma may be difficult, especially given the presence of prominent spindling that is sometimes seen in high-grade astrocytomas (anaplastic astrocytoma and glioblastoma multiforme). Such spindled astrocytomatous cells may show marked nuclear elongation with a fascicular growth pattern strongly reminiscent of mesenchymal sarcomas. The presence of GFAP positivity as mentioned previously is very helpful in identifying spindled neoplastic astrocytes. A recent report emphasizes the difficulty that can be encountered in attempting to make this distinction.[100]

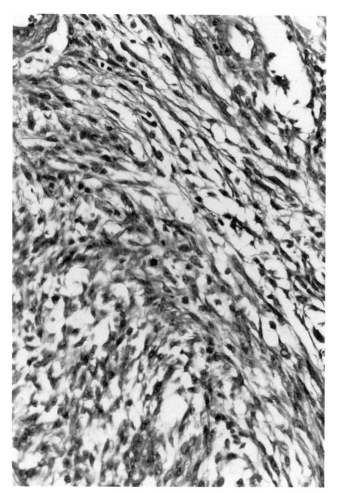

FIGURE 22–22. Gliosarcoma. Fascicles of spindled cells exhibit nuclear atypia and scattered mitotic figures. (H&E ×240)

Because the sarcomatous component may arise late in the course of a glioblastoma, the original biopsy may show only features of glioblastoma, with a later re-excision or autopsy study revealing a superimposed sarcoma. Conversely, if the sarcomatous changes occur early in the time course of the high-grade glioma, the sarcoma may overgrow the original glioma and result in a neoplasm composed predominantly of high-grade sarcoma. If sampling is limited, the gliomatous component may be missed.

A particular problem that may arise at the time of frozen section involves gliosarcomas with a prominent sarcomatous component. Because these neoplasms exhibit better gross circumscription than pure glioblastomas and may have a meningeal attachment, the surgeon's evaluation may favor a meningioma. The presence of fascicles of spindled cells on frozen section could lead to a cursory review and diagnosis of meningioma, with the correct diagnosis determined only with permanent sections. To avoid this pitfall, it is necessary to recognize that the nuclear atypia, cellularity, mitotic figures, and necrosis, if present, favor a sarcoma. At this point, the surgeon can be informed that the frozen section is suggestive of a meningeal sarcoma and that a gliosarcoma cannot be excluded as a diagnostic possibility.

Also pertinent to this overview, it should be noted that sarcomas have been reported to arise in association with oligodendrogliomas.[101, 102]

Pleomorphic Xanthoastrocytoma (PXA)

Pleomorphic xanthoastrocytomas are low-grade astrocytomas with areas of cellular pleomorphism often resulting in the mistaken diagnosis of high-grade glioma. Although this neoplasm has been recognized for some years as a distinct entity,[103] some questions remain concerning the spectrum of histologic changes and their relationship to aggressiveness.

CLINICOPATHOLOGIC FEATURES. PXA, although occurring primarily in children and young adults, has been reported at older ages.[104] No sex preponderance has been noted. The tumor occurs in supratentorial sites, with a predilection for superficial temporal and parietal lobes.

PXA generally has a favorable clinical course, with cures and long symptom-free postoperative survival to be expected.[103, 105–107] Recurrent tumors have been re-excised and usually do not appear to have evolved to an obviously malignant glioma.[103, 107, 108] It is important to realize that a PXA may recur as a glioblastoma at varying intervals after surgery.[109, 110]

Grossly the neoplasms tend to be large, relatively well circumscribed, and partially cystic. A distinct yellow coloration is present when cellular lipid is abundant.

The microscopic appearance is quite distinctive. The central portion of the tumor is cellular and consists of astrocytic cells

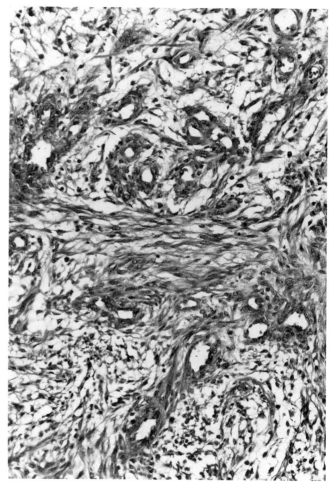

FIGURE 22–23. Gliosarcoma. Sarcomatous transformation appears to begin as a perivascular proliferation of small fascicles of spindled mesenchymal cells. (H&E ×150)

exhibiting various degrees of nuclear atypia and hyperchromasia (Fig. 22–24). The cytoplasm ranges from eosinophilic to vacuolated depending on the cytoplasmic lipid content (Fig. 22–25). In some areas, the cells are surrounded by a reticulin network. Perivascular cuffs of lymphocytes are often present. Necrosis is not a feature of this tumor. Mitotic activity is generally low, with labeling studies using proliferating cell nuclear antigen showing rates similar to those for low-grade astrocytomas.[111] The suggestion has been made that an increased mitotic rate may signal transformation to a high-grade astrocytoma.[112] Focally, neoplastic infiltration of the surrounding neuropil at the periphery of the tumor belies its gross circumscription. As would be expected, the tumor cells stain positively with GFAP. An uncommon feature that has been reported is the presence of a very large number of capillary-sized vessels sometimes associated with fibromatous areas within the tumor. The term *angiomatous variant of PXA* has been suggested for this neoplasm.[113]

Typical PXA associated with neoplastic ganglion cells has been reported.[104, 114, 115] In one example, the PXA and ganglio-gliomatous components were distinct.[114] In the other examples, the ganglion cells were admixed in the PXA.[104, 115]

Electron microscopy is remarkable for the demonstration of a continuous basal lamina surrounding and following the

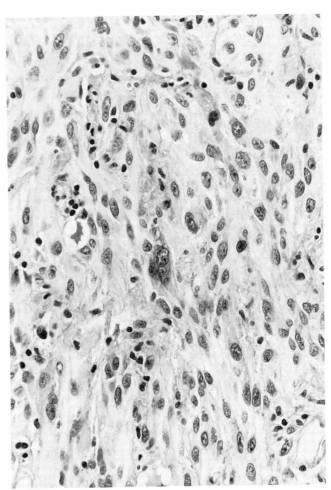

FIGURE 22–25. PXA. Areas more typical of low-grade astrocytoma are characteristically present, especially at the periphery. (H&E ×300)

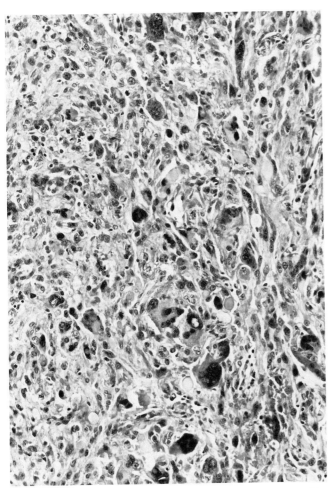

FIGURE 22–24. PXA. Focally, the PXA contains pleomorphic, hyperchromatic, occasionally multinucleated cells with variably vacuolated cytoplasm. (H&E ×150)

plasma membranes of individual neoplastic astrocytes, an ultrastructural feature that accounts for the reticulin deposition noted on histochemical staining. This finding has led to the suggestion that the neoplasm is derived from subpial astrocytes, because they also exhibit basement membranes.[103]

DIFFERENTIAL DIAGNOSIS. The two main pathologic entities that may be confused with PXA are **lipidized glioblastomas** and **meningeal fibrous histiocytomas.**

In differentiating PXA from glioblastoma, it should be noted that the latter has a higher mitotic rate and areas of necrosis are common (see section on Lipid-rich Epithelioid Glioblastoma). Marked vascular hyperplasia is not usually a feature of PXA but accompanies most glioblastomas. The young age and superficial tumor location, most commonly in temporal and parietal lobes, are also helpful in making this distinction.

The separation of PXA from meningeal fibrous histiocytoma/xanthoma can be difficult because of certain morphologic similarities. Some of the first neoplasms reported as PXA[103] were previously reported as fibrous xanthomas of the meninges.[116]

The recognition of PXA as a glial tumor is based on the finding of typical infiltrating astrocytoma at the periphery of many tumors, GFAP positivity of the neoplastic cells, and published reports of late recurrence of some PXAs as small-cell glioblastomas.[110] The first two features are of diagnostic help to the surgical pathologist.

The possibility was recently raised again that PXA is a mesenchymal tumor of the meninges, identical to benign fibrous histiocytomas elsewhere in the body.[117] The presence of positive staining for numerous monocyte-histiocyte markers by immunoperoxidase methods and only focal GFAP staining at the tumor periphery have led some investigators to these conclusions.

Given the fact that histiocyte markers have been described in various gliomas,[118, 119] the presence of these markers in PXA does not in itself seem sufficient reason to doubt the existence of PXA as a distinct glial neoplasm. GFAP positivity considered in concert with the previously described feature of typical low-grade astrocytoma at the periphery supports the glial origin of this tumor. In addition, the previously described electron microscopic findings in PXA of a continuous basal lamina is not typical of fibrous histiocytoma.[110] We find these features to be of value in making the diagnosis of PXA and thus separating it from meningeal fibrous histiocytomas.

Oligodendroglioma

A more detailed discussion of oligodendrogliomas is included in the section on differentiating oligodendrogliomas from low-grade astrocytomas. The features described there are helpful in that perinuclear halos, calcifications, and arching blood vessels are often present at least focally in high-grade variants.

Although some features of low-grade or well-differentiated oligodendroglioma are retained, the high-grade variants show some combination of increased cellularity, nuclear pleomorphism, vascular endothelial hyperplasia, mitotic figures, and scattered foci of necrosis[120] (Figs. 22–26 and 22–27). Several studies have stressed the prognostic significance of grading oligodendrogliomas.

In the absence of residual features typical of oligodendroglioma, it may not be possible to distinguish a high-grade oligodendroglioma from a glioblastoma. The prognostic implications of such a distinction is moot, because clinical behavior of the neoplasms and their therapy are similar.

Primary Cerebral Lymphoma

These neoplasms are by definition clinically isolated to the central nervous system (CNS) but resemble their systemic counterparts. Ocular involvement is also sometimes associated with primary cerebral lymphomas.[121]

CLINICOPATHOLOGIC FEATURES. Primary cerebral lymphomas can occur at virtually all ages. In the past, most of these tumors arose in otherwise healthy patients who were usually elderly. Most presentations were after age 55. More recently, cerebral lymphomas in younger patients have increased in incidence and are associated with compromise of the immune system, as seen in patients with AIDS and with patients having undergone organ transplantation. In addition to this age-related increased incidence of cerebral lymphoma, an unexplained increase has also been noted in the older age group without known immunologic anomalies.[122]

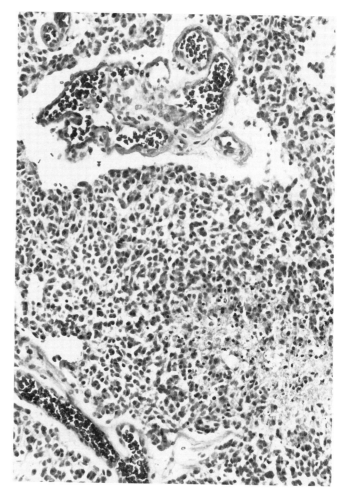

FIGURE 22–26. Oligodendroglioma. Prominent capillary endothelial hyperplasia combined with increased cellularity and necrosis in oligodendroglioma can simulate a glioblastoma. (H&E ×150)

The increased incidence of primary cerebral lymphoma in immunocompromised patients is presumed to be secondary to defects in immune surveillance that allow monoclonal proliferations of malignant lymphoid cells to develop. Regardless of the immune status, Epstein-Barr virus (EBV) has been suggested as an etiologic agent. Although several studies to clarify the role of EBV have been undertaken,[123–129] the results have been conflicting. At this time, it seems reasonable to state that the Epstein-Barr virus genome is present by *in situ* hybridization in a significant number of cerebral lymphomas associated with an immunocompromised status. It seems likely that the virus plays an etiologic role in this setting. The incidence of the viral genome is much lower in immunocompetent patients, and the role of the virus in this group is unclear.

Primary CNS lymphomas may present as a solitary mass or as multiple discrete intraparenchymal or intradural masses. Diffuse meningeal or periventricular lesions have also been described. Infrequently the initial presentation may be intra-ocular (uveitis/vitreitis).[121]

The macroscopic appearance is highly variable, with some nodules appearing grossly distinct, whereas other foci blend imperceptibly with the surrounding parenchyma. Often the cut surface is smooth and white, although a variegated appearance due to hemorrhage and necrosis is not uncommon. Tumors presenting in the meninges and periventricular regions may appear as a poorly defined thickening over the brain surface or along the ventricular lining.

Microscopic examination shows dense cellularity in the center of the mass lesion with a gradual decrease in cellularity as the neoplastic lymphoid cells infiltrate the adjacent parenchyma. The infiltrating border of neoplastic cells extends along perivascular spaces and is present diffusely in the neuropil (Fig. 22–28). Of diagnostic significance, the tumor cells not only extend along perivascular spaces but invade the adjacent vessels in an angiotrophic pattern similar to that of some systemic lymphomas. The vascular wall invasion results in an increase in perivascular reticulin fibers that form irregular concentric rings in which tumor cells appear entrapped (Fig. 22–29).

Primary CNS lymphomas can be composed of the same spectrum of atypical cells seen in nodal lymphomas. However, a nodular form has not been described. Most CNS tumors consist of large cells with smooth to cleaved nuclear membranes. Immunoblastic forms are common, especially in immunocompromised patients. Pure small-cell lymphomas are less frequent.[130]

These neoplasms are predominantly of B-cell lineage as demonstrated by immunoperoxidase stains for B- and T-cell

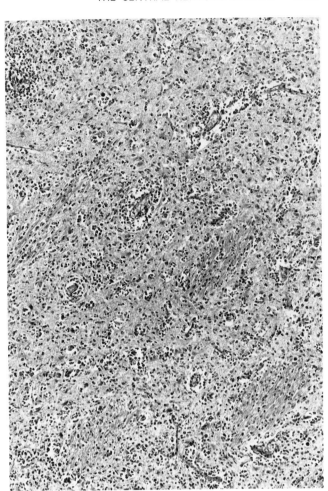

FIGURE 22–28. Cerebral Lymphoma. The infiltration of malignant lymphoid cells through brain parenchyma with associated reactive astrocytic changes can suggest a high-grade glioma at low power. (H&E ×75)

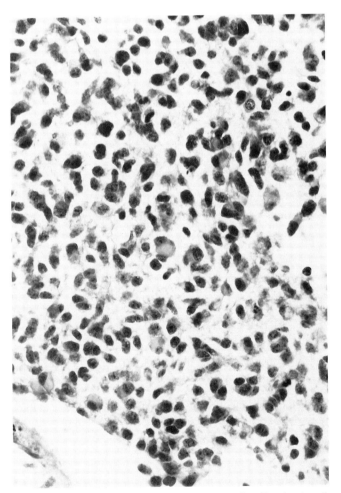

FIGURE 22–27. Oligodendroglioma. High-grade oligodendroglioma exhibits greater nuclear pleomorphism and cellularity than the low-grade variants. (H&E ×400)

markers.[131–133] The B-cell lineage has also been demonstrated by immunoglobulin gene rearrangement studies.[134] Primary CNS T-cell lymphomas have been reported but make up a very small percentage of the overall number.[135–139]

DIFFERENTIAL DIAGNOSIS. With routine H&E staining, an occasional problem arises in differentiating **high-grade astrocytoma** and lymphoma. A peripheral biopsy in particular often shows infiltrating lymphoid cells surrounded by neuropil. Although the tumor cells do not possess distinct glial cytoplasmic processes, the ''neuropil background'' may lead to a hasty diagnosis of high-grade astrocytoma. An especially helpful feature in recognizing lymphoma is its perivascular extension with vascular wall invasion and the formation of concentric bands of perivascular reticulin. Although glioma cells may be oriented around vessels, they are infrequently identified within the vascular walls.

Immunoperoxidase stains are quite helpful in this differential diagnosis. Astrocytic differentiation is generally confirmed by staining for GFAP. Lymphoid cells do not stain with this marker but are positive for leukocyte common antigen (LCA). Further diagnostic specificity is obtained by employing a battery of B- and T-cell markers if the LCA is positive.

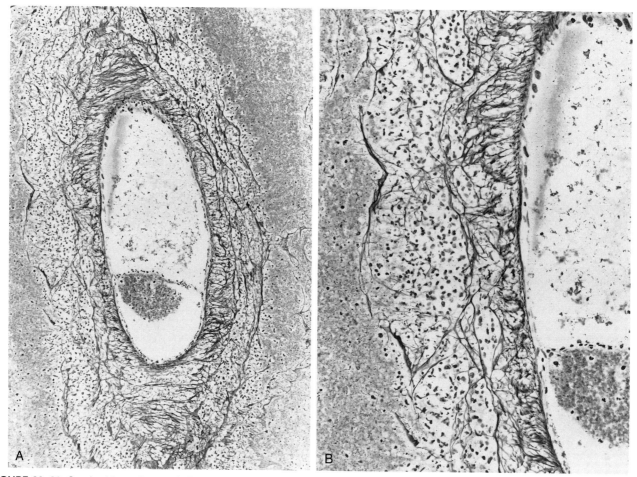

FIGURE 22–29. Cerebral Lymphoma. *A,* The lymphoid cells infiltrate vessel walls with an increased concentric deposition of reticulin. (Retic ×75) *B,* At high magnification, full-thickness permeation of the vessel wall is apparent. (Retic ×150)

Metastatic poorly differentiated carcinomas can resemble lymphomas and consequently cause diagnostic difficulties. Again, however, vascular wall invasion by neoplastic cells and the associated concentric reticulin formation in lymphomas, when present, strongly suggest this to be the correct diagnosis. In addition, metastatic carcinomas generally consist of cohesive sheets or nests of cells with distinct cell borders, and all but the undifferentiated carcinomas may show at least isolated foci of glandular or squamous differentiation. If necessary, an immunoperoxidase battery containing LCA and anti-epithelial antibodies such as cytokeratin and EMA may be employed to reach a definitive diagnosis.

Metastatic Carcinoma

Hematogenous spread of carcinoma to the central nervous system may be encountered in different settings by the surgical pathologist. When a carcinoma has been identified previously in another organ, the brain biopsy may be employed therapeutically to remove an apparent solitary metastasis or employed diagnostically to exclude a second primary malignancy. The setting in which the greatest diagnostic confusion is apt to occur is with a solitary poorly differentiated metastasis from an unknown primary site. The distinction of some poorly differentiated carcinomas from anaplastic glioma is difficult.

CLINICOPATHOLOGIC FEATURES. Although a small peak is noted in childhood resulting from metastases of pediatric solid tumors, the vast majority of metastases occur in later life, during the sixth and seventh decades in particular.

In adults, the relative incidence of primary sites varies among published reports and series depending on the type of medical services and subspecialties available, patient demographics, and whether the studies were based on autopsy or surgical cases.

An estimate of the relative incidence of primary sites resulting in CNS metastases and based on surgical series is lung 25%, breast 20%, skin (melanoma) 10%, kidney 10%, and gastrointestinal tract 5%.[140] A slight male preponderance has been noted in the past because of the high incidence of lung cancer in men. Given the increasing incidence of this disease in females, the number of CNS metastases in these patients can be expected to increase steadily.

The distribution of brain metastases demonstrates a marked preference for the cerebral hemispheres as opposed to the cerebellum or brain stem. Although all areas of the cerebral hemispheres are vulnerable, a greater than expected number based on brain volume occur in the vascular "watershed" zones of the anterior, middle, and posterior cerebral arteries, one assumption being that tumor microemboli pass as far distally as the vessel size permits.[141] An unexplained but noteworthy phenomenon is the increased incidence of cerebellar metastases from tumors of the gastrointestinal tract and pelvis.[141] The increased vascularity of the cerebral cortex seems to explain the frequency of metastatic tumor deposits within the cortex and at the gray-white junction.

The clinical presentations of a CNS metastasis can be sudden, with severe headache and alteration of consciousness usually secondary to an acute hemorrhage. Epileptic seizures may also be the first symptom of metastatic disease. More frequently, the symptoms are slowly progressive and most commonly consist of headache, nausea, vomitting, unilateral motor weakness, and mental changes.[142]

On gross autopsy inspection, metastatic foci tend to be discrete and spherical, with surrounding softness and edema in adjacent brain. The cut surface appearance and consistency are extremely variable and are influenced by tumor necrosis, hemorrhage, and the extent of a fibroblastic reaction.

Microscopically, most metastatic carcinomas are clearly recognized as such and present no diagnostic challenge. The cohensive sheets of tumor may exhibit glandular, squamous, or clear-cell features that may at least suggest a site of origin.

Poorly differentiated carcinomas and amelanotic melanomas often consist of cohesive sheets of cells with distinct cell borders and abundant clear to eosinophilic cytoplasm lacking cell processes. The nuclei are often remarkable for large eosinophilic nucleoli and prominent areas of clear nucleoplasm and clumped chromatin. Broad foci of necrosis are often present, sparing a cuff of tumor cells located around blood vessels. Metastatic carcinoma tends to be well demarcated from the adjacent brain in periphery biopsies.

DIFFERENTIAL DIAGNOSIS. Occasionally poorly differentiated metastatic carcinomas may be difficult to distinguish from **anaplastic astrocytoma** and **glioblastoma,** especially those with epithelioid features.

Several H&E features are helpful in making this distinction. Unlike the previous description of metastatic carcinomas, high-grade astrocytomas usually retain a fibrillarity to the background that is a result of interwoven cell processes. The boundary is indistinct, and the surrounding brain frequently shows features of low-grade astrocytoma. Subpial, subependymal, and perineuronal cell aggregates beyond the gross tumor margin are more typical of high-grade gliomas. In addition, foci of necrosis in glioblastomas are frequently stellate or serpiginous, with pseudopalisading as previously described, a feature lacking in metastatic carcinoma.

A battery of immunoperoxidase stains, including GFAP, HMB-45 (melanoma specific antigen), cytokeratin (CK), EMA, and LCA provide helpful diagnostic clues.

With rare exceptions,[78–80] GFAP is considered a highly specific marker for astrocytomas. Conversely, CK and EMA staining are infrequent and focal in astocytomas, whereas diffuse positive staining, especially with EMA, is typical of metastatic carcinoma.

An intriguing and potentially useful observation that has been reported[143, 144] is that metastatic brain tumors have a significantly higher proliferative potential than high-grade gliomas. This finding can be demonstrated by Ki-67 labeling index or by nucleolar organizer region (NOR) score.[143]

NORs are fragments of DNA containing ribosomal RNA genes, present in the nucleoli of proliferating cells, which have been shown to accurately reflect cellular proliferation. Scoring is based on number of NORs per nucleus as demonstrated by a silver colloid stain on paraffin-embedded tissue.[143]

The results of labeling with Ki-67, a monoclonal antibody to nuclear proteins expressed in proliferating cells, parallel those obained by NOR score.

Both have been shown to be significantly higher in metastatic carcinomas than in high-grade gliomas, indicating a higher proliferative activity in CNS metastases.[143, 144] In addition to providing information on the size of the proliferating cell pool, the results may be helpful in separating high-grade astrocytomas from poorly differentiated metastatic carcinomas.

Amelanotic melanomas can be particularly difficult to differentiate from high-grade astrocytoma on H&E stains. Positive staining for HMB-45 in the absence of a reaction for GFAP or CK supports the diagnosis of melanoma. An LCA is also included to help exclude a cerebral lymphoma, which fails to react with any of the above stains except LCA. The previous discussion about rates of cell proliferation may also be applicable to separating metastatic melanoma from high-grade astrocytomas.

In most cases, a consideration of the histologic features in association with the immunoperoxidase stains and potentially cell proliferation analysis allows a correct diagnosis.

Germinoma

Germinomas are germ cell tumors of the CNS identical to those arising in the gonads (seminoma, dysgerminoma) and other areas. That such tumors are included in the differential diagnosis of high-grade astrocytomas should not be surprising. In our own consultative experience and in that of others, suprasellar germinoma has on occasion been misdiagnosed as a glioblastoma.

CLINICOPATHOLOGIC FEATURES. Germinomas occur most frequently in the pineal gland and the suprasellar region, although non-midline sites have been reported.[145, 146] Pineal germinomas occur three times more frequently in males than in females. In the suprasellar location, the sex incidence is roughly equal.[147, 148] Although pineal tumors are rare, accounting for 0.5% to 1% of intracranial tumors, germinomas occur in this location and account for 50% of pineal tumors.[149]

Grossly, germinomas present with a uniform tan-gray cut surface with vague lobulations and occasional foci of hemorrhage. Small tumors may be encapsulated but most are large ill-defined masses with infiltration of the surrounding brain.

Microscopically, the neoplasm is composed of nests or sheets of cells with variably spaced fibrous septa containing lymphocytes (Fig. 22–30). A granulomatous response is sometimes present in the surrounding brain or within the tumor itself. The tumor cells are large with prominent nuclei. The nuclei are round to oval with distinct nuclear membranes and contain unevenly distributed nuclear chromatin and large central nucleoli. The cytoplasm is eosinophilic to clear, and the cytoplasmic membranes are usually distinct (Fig. 22–31).

Germinomas may be admixed with other germ cell elements, a finding which, if present, makes confusion with glioblastoma even less likely.

DIFFERENTIAL DIAGNOSIS. The only features this uncommon tumor shares with **high-grade astrocytoma/glioblastoma** are that both are cellular and both have a histologic appearance suggesting a high-grade neoplasm.

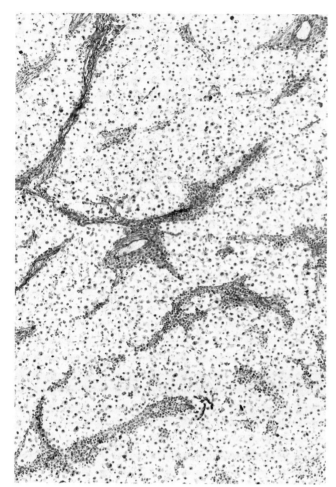

FIGURE 22–30. Germinoma. Cohesive sheets of neoplastic cells in germinomas are divided into lobules by fibrovascular septa with numerous lymphocytes. (H&E ×75)

If both diagnoses are under consideration, immunoperoxidase stains are extremely helpful. Germinomas stain for placental alkaline phosphatase and occasionally for human chorionic gonadotropin.[150] Positive staining for GFAP should not occur. High-grade astrocytomas are GFAP-positive and negative for germ cell markers. This diagnostic distinction is of critical importance in that germinomas are highly radiosensitive and long-term survivals and cures have reported.[151, 152]

Except in the setting of AIDS, **cerebral lymphomas** are rare in the young age group at highest risks for germinomas. On small biopsies, this differential could arise, however, and is usually resolved by an immunoperoxidase stain for LCA, which stains lymphoid cells. However, care must be exercised in interpreting this stain, because germinomas often contain numerous small reactive lymphocytes that are reactive with LCA. The large neoplastic germ cells conversely do not stain with LCA.

Neuroradiologic Correlations in the Differential Diagnosis of Glioblastoma Multiforme

The term **ring enhancement** is used to describe lesions with central regions that do not accumulate contrast on CT, MRI, or radionuclide scanning. Ring lesions can be caused by a variety of processes, including glioblastoma multiforme (GBM) and many other neoplasms in our list of differential diagnoses. Usually the central non-enhancing area is avascular—either necrosis in a malignancy (e.g., GBM or metastasis) or cyst formation in a benign glioma (e.g, pleomorphic xanthoastrocytoma). Occasionally, the enhancement is due to a reactive process surrounding damaged tissue (e.g., hematoma, contusion, infarct, or abscess) or represents a zone of advancing inflammation (e.g., multiple sclerosis [MS], inflammatory demyelinating pseudotumor [IDP], or cerebritis).

Additional features such as location and the morphology of the ring can help narrow the possibilities. A solitary large, deep, white matter, ring-enhancing mass with surrounding vasogenic edema is typical of a GBM. Active MS plaques or IDP can also form large and often solitary lesions with considerable mass effect, peripheral enhancement, and surrounding edema. Careful review of the scans may reveal some differential features. When an aggressive neoplasm becomes necrotic (whether primary or metastatic), the enhancing rim is frequently thick (>2 cm) and is often extremely irregular or "shaggy" along its inner margin (Fig. 22–32).[153] That pattern can be distinguished from the enhancing rim of a MS plaque, which is usually relatively uniform in thickness, thin (<1 cm), and has a smooth inner margin.

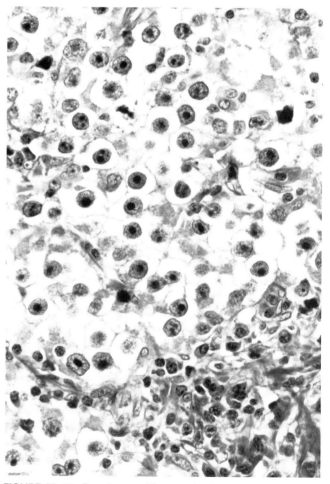

FIGURE 22–31. Germinoma. The neoplastic germ cells are large with distinct cell borders and pale to clear cytoplasm. The nuclei are centrally located, round to oval, and contain one or two eosinophilic nucleoli. (H&E ×400)

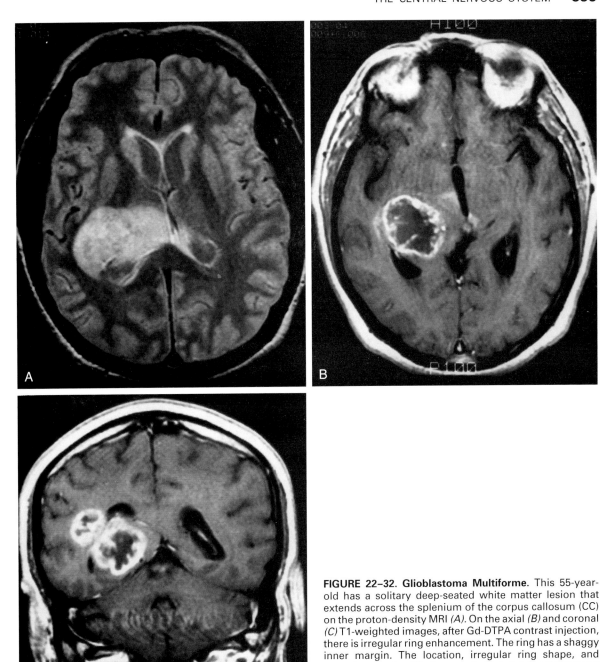

FIGURE 22–32. Glioblastoma Multiforme. This 55-year-old has a solitary deep-seated white matter lesion that extends across the splenium of the corpus callosum (CC) on the proton-density MRI *(A)*. On the axial *(B)* and coronal *(C)* T1-weighted images, after Gd-DTPA contrast injection, there is irregular ring enhancement. The ring has a shaggy inner margin. The location, irregular ring shape, and spread across the CC all suggest a high-grade astrocytoma or GBM.

Although evidence of spread across the corpus callosum can be seen in as many as 75% of GBM, it is not a specific finding and can also be seen in primary cerebral lymphomas, inflammatory demyelinating pseudotumors, and some oligodendrogliomas. However, spread through these dense commissural tracts is distinctly uncommon for metastatic disease.

Pleomorphic xanthoastrocytomas typically are located in the superficial temporal and parietal lobes and frequently contain a central cyst with mural nodule formation on CT scans.

Another entity in the differential of GBM is primary cerebral lymphoma. Although this neoplasm has a range of radiographic appearances, lymphomas often show a homogeneous pattern of contrast enhancement as opposed to the peripheral or ring enhancement around a low-density necrotic center in GBM.

Oligodendrogliomas, as noted previously in the discussion of the neuroradiology of low-grade gliomas, often have a characteristic appearance on scans. They can be disturbingly heterogeneous and may resemble a multiloculated GBM with multiple arcs of "rim enhancement" surrounding nonenhancing regions. In an oligodendroglioma, the nonenhancing areas usually contain mucoid material as opposed to the necrotic tumor of GBM. Infiltration of the cortex with subsequent contrast enhancement and calcifications are features suggestive of oligodendroglioma.

A contrast-enhancing mass in the suprasellar or pineal area in a child or young adult is suggestive of a germinoma. Occasionally, spread along walls of the ventricular system is identified by a band of contrast enhancement.

CAPILLARY HEMANGIOBLASTOMA VERSUS METASTATIC RENAL CELL CARCINOMA

Hemangioblastomas are generally regarded as vascular neoplasms and are relatively uncommon. These benign neoplasms are of particular interest because of their association with a central nervous system phakomatosis (von Hippel-Lindau disease). This association should always be kept in mind, although the majority of hemangioblastomas occur as isolated tumors. In one series, 23% of hemangioblastomas occurred as part of this phakomatosis.[154]

The **von Hippel-Lindau syndrome** is an autosomal dominant inherited disorder that is related to an abnormal gene focus on chromosome 3. The syndrome is a large nosologic entity with multisystem abnormalitities, which may include retinal angiomatosis, solitary or multiple cerebellar or spinal hemangioblastomas, renal cell carcinoma, pheochromocytoma, visceral cysts in multiple organs, and papillary cystadenomas of the epididymis. Other anomalies have also been described with lesser frequency.

Complicating consideration of this phakomatosis is the large number of cases that show only some of these components. Variable manifestations, or formes frustes, are the rule rather than the exception. Of particular interest to our discussion is the association with renal cell carcinomas, which have also been shown to be related, in some cases, to a gene on chromosome 3. Both von Hippel-Lindau syndrome and renal cell carcinoma have been associated with similar deletions of chromosome 3. The deleted area is believed to contain a suppressor gene that inhibits the development of renal cell carcinoma, hemangioblastoma, and other tumors associated with this phakomatosis.[155, 156]

CLINICOPATHOLOGIC FEATURES. Hemangioblastomas are generally said to account for 1% to 2.5% of all intracranial tumors.[154] No age is exempt. However, the majority occur around the third or fourth decade and involve males more frequently than females.[157] The cerebellum is the most common site, with lateral lobes, vermis, and the paramedian regions possibly involved. The spinal cord is the next most likely site, with brain stem involvement reported infrequently.

Another clinical finding is the presence of **polycythemia** in approximately 5% to 30% of patients with hemangioblastomas.[155] This polycythemia usually resolves after surgical resection of the tumor and has been shown to be secondary to production of an **erythropoietin-like substance** that is

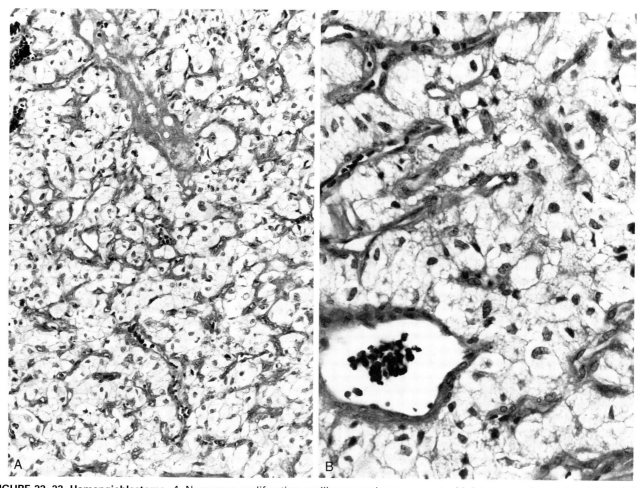

FIGURE 22–33. Hemangioblastoma. A, Numerous proliferating capillary vessels are present with interspersed vacuolated, lipid-laden stromal cells. (H&E ×150) B, Cell borders are less distinct between stromal cells than is usually the case with renal cell carcinoma. (H&E ×300)

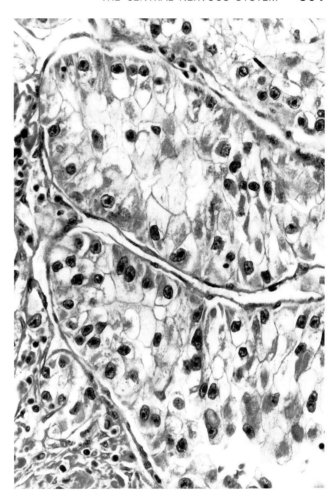

FIGURE 22–34. Renal Cell Carcinoma. The lobules of metastatic renal cell carcinoma contain cells with crisp, distinctive cytoplasmic membranes. (H&E ×300)

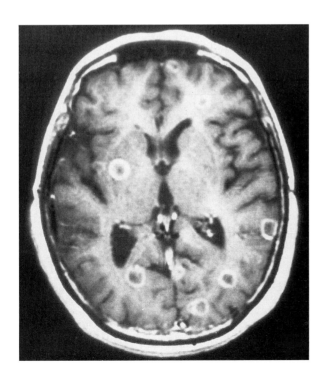

FIGURE 22–35. Metastases. This 70-year-old female has metastatic adenocarcinoma. The T1-weighted MRI after gadolinium demonstrates multiple lesions. Most of them are small and either cortical, subcortical, or in the deep gray matter. All of the lesions show a central region of necrosis that does not enhance.

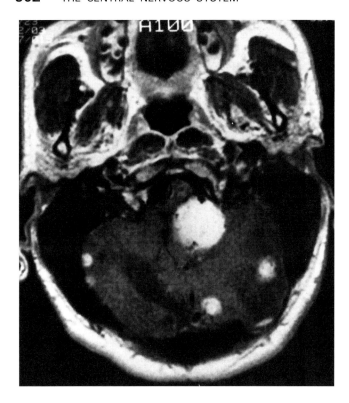

FIGURE 22–36. Hemangioblastoma. In another patient with von Hippel-Lindau disease, there are multiple lesions, seen here as nodular enhancement on the Gd-DTPA T1-weighted MRI. Although this could suggest metastases, at least one of the lesions has an associated cystic region that is not rimmed by enhancement. That suggests fluid accumulation, rather than necrosis, and makes metastasis less likely.

similar to the hormone produced by the kidney. This ectopic hormone product accounts for the finding of foci of erythropoiesis in some hemangioblastomas.[158]

Erythropoietin production has been confirmed by immunohistochemical techniques[159, 160] and by a newly developed radioimmunoassay for human erythropoietin.[155] Erythropoietin messenger RNA has also been found with elevated tumor levels of the hormone and erythrocytosis.[161]

The immunohistochemical studies demonstrate that the cell responsible for hormone secretion is a small cell with finely granular cytoplasm. Ultrastructurally, these cells contain round membrane-bound secretory granules ultrastructurally. The ultrastructural features of these cells are typical of mast cells.

Grossly, these tumors often present as variably sized mural nodules within a cyst cavity. The neoplastic mass, whether

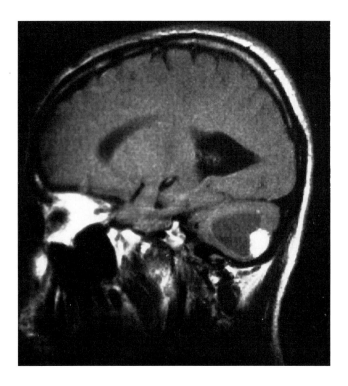

FIGURE 22–37. Hemangioblastoma. Parasagittal gadolinium-enhanced T1-weighted MRI in a 36-year-old male with von Hippel-Lindau (VHL) disease shows the highly suggestive "cyst with mural nodule" morphology. Approximately one third of hemangioblastomas have this morphology, but one third may form a solid nodule and one third may have a complex shape that is partially solid and partially cystic. The absence of complete circumferential ring enhancement is uncommon for both necrotic neoplasms and abscesses.

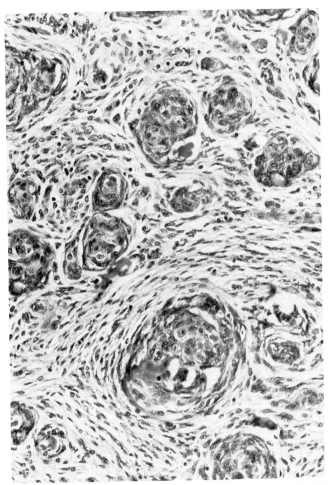

FIGURE 22–38. Meningioma. An admixture of meningothelial whorls and fascicles of spindled cells are typically present. (H&E ×200)

occurring in the cyst wall or as a solid mass, appears well-demarcated and as a firm darkened cut surface. The presence of abundant lipid can give the mass a yellow-tan color.

Microscopically, the tumor is composed of numerous thin-walled capillaries lined by plump to flattened endothelial cells. Interspersed between proliferating vascular channels are variable numbers of stromal cells (Fig. 22–33). Reticulin stains outline the blood vessels and help delineate the intervening stromal cells. The number of stromal cells may be low, but in some examples these cells predominate, and when abundant cytoplasmic lipid droplets are present, the cytoplasm has a foamy vacuolated appearance. Glycogen is also present, as demonstrated by appropriate histochemical stains or electron microscopy.

When large quantities of lipid are absent, it may become difficult to separate the endothelial and stromal cells on H&E stains alone. The stromal cell nuclei can occasionally exhibit significant nuclear irregularity and hyperchromasia and cause unnecessary alarm. Mitotic figures are uncommon. As mentioned earlier, small erythropoietic islands can create confusion unless this diagnosis is kept in mind.

Electron microscopic studies have demonstrated that the neoplasm is composed of endothelial cells, pericytes, stromal cells, and small granular cells. The stromal cells are sur-rounded by electron-dense extracellular material with intermediate junctions between stromal cells. The cytoplasm contains 6-nm microfilaments, which are occasionally condensed into dense bundles. The cytoplasm also contains vacuoles, lipid droplets, mitochondria, and infrequent Golgi structures.[162] These features are typical of the stromal cells; however, a single diagnostic feature is lacking.

The prognosis is generally good for this benign tumor, although as many as 25% do recur. In one study,[157] certain clinical and pathologic features influenced the likelihood of tumor recurrence. Hemangioblastomas occurring with the associated phakomatosis had a large rate of recurrence. Male sex and young age at presentation (younger than 30 years) correlated positively with tumor recurrences. Grossly and microscopically, the tumors most likely to recur were small (approximately 3 cm) and solid to partially cystic with a large component of eosinophilic as opposed to lipid-laden stromal cells.

DIFFERENTIAL DIAGNOSIS. The differential diagnosis between a hemangioblastoma and metastatic renal cell carcinoma may be difficult in certain clinical settings. Consider for example a middle-aged patient who presents with cerebellar and spinal cord masses. Either before biopsy or shortly afterward a large renal mass is identified on CT scan. The clinicians are immediately concerned as to whether the CNS neoplasms represent foci of ''benign'' hemangioblastoma or metastatic renal cell carcinoma.

Renal cell carcinomas have been reported to frequently metastasize to brain and do share some histologic features with hemangioblastoma.[141] Both tumors are highly vascular and contain tumor cells with clear to vacuolated cytoplasm. In addition, both neoplasms may exhibit erythropoietin production with associated polycythemia.

However, there are features that help with this differential diagnostic problem. Firstly, the clear cells of renal cell carcinoma generally show very distinct cell borders in keeping with their epithelial nature. In hemangioblastomas, the lipidized stromal cells may aggregate, but such distinct-appearing cell membranes are uncommon (Fig. 22–34). The presence of numerous muscular arteries is also more typical of a metastatic renal cell carcinoma. It has been stated that renal cell carcinoma cells contain more glycogen than the stromal cells of hemangioblastoma. This may be true, but the overlap is such that, in our experience, the PAS stain is often not definitive. Of particular help is an immunoperoxidase stain for EMA, which does stain renal tumor cells but not the stromal cells of hemangioblastoma.[163, 164]

Electron microscopy can be helpful in assessing whether the tumor has epithelial features of adenocarcinoma. Ultrastructurally, renal cell carcinomas are characterized by abundant intracytoplasmic glycogen and lipid. The cell membranes are joined by junctional complexes, and microvilli are often prominent.

One diagnostic pitfall that can be avoided by good communication between pathologist and neurosurgeon is the mistaken diagnosis of astrocytoma. This is particularly true in the instance in which a cyst is present with a mural nodule. If the cyst wall is biopsied first for frozen sections and the pathologist is only informed of a ''cerebellar mass,'' the presence of intense gliosis and Rosenthal's fibers may strongly suggest a pilocytic astrocytoma. Again this mistake can be

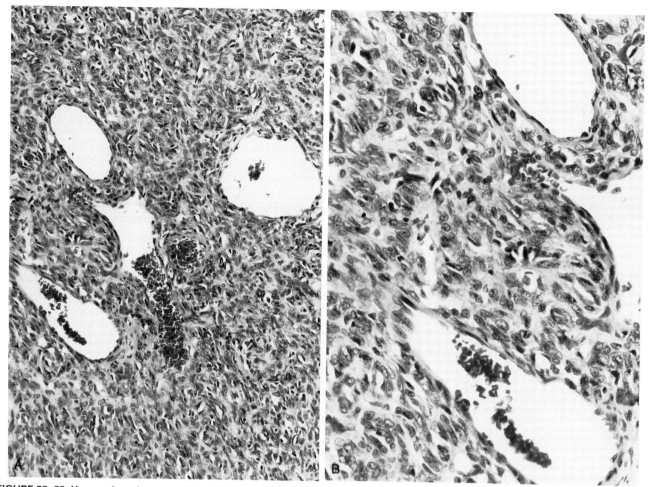

FIGURE 22–39. Hemangiopericytoma. *A,* Irregular blood vessels, lined by a single layer of endothelium, are surrounded by haphazardly arranged spindled neoplastic cells. (H&E ×150) *B,* The tumor cells are spindled to oval with mild nuclear pleomorphism and ill-defined cytoplasm. (H&E ×300)

avoided if the patient's age is considered, the CT scans reviewed, and the area of biopsy discussed with the surgeon.

An additional diagnostic problem may occur when the tumor is sampled but frozen section artifacts are present that distort the microscopic appearance. It is often difficult to distinguish stromal from endothelial cells, and given the nuclear pleomorphism discussed earlier in some hemangioblastomas, a diagnosis of metastatic tumor or high-grade glioma may also be considered.

If hemangioblastoma is considered in the differential diagnosis, a fat stain on frozen section material demonstrates the fat globules so typical of hemangioblastoma. Because, with the exception of renal cell carcinoma mentioned earlier, such globules are infrequent in metastatic tumors and usually absent in high-grade gliomas, their presence may be helpful in resolving the differential diagnosis. It has also been noted[159] that hemangioblastomas contain a variable number of mast cells, which can be highlighted by metachromatic stains on frozen sections.

NEURORADIOLOGIC CORRELATION. Metastatic disease to the brain parenchyma is usually hematogenously disseminated and presents with multiple lesions located near the cortical gray-white junction. In most cases the distribution of brain metastases favors the cerebral hemispheres, paralleling the distribution of cerebral blood flow (Fig. 22–35).

Intra-axillary, primary cerebellar neoplasms in the adult include **hemangioblastoma (HB)** and **high-grade gliomas (GBM).** Hemangioblastomas represent approximately 1.5% of all primary intracranial neoplasms [165, 166] and approximately 5% of all posterior fossa neoplasms.[75] Solitary lesions of the cerebellum, without any associated supratentorial masses, should first be considered as primary neoplasms, although metastatic disease to the cerebellum may occur as solitary or multiple masses, without any supratentorial lesions.[167] Melanoma and lung and breast cancer have a low incidence of solitary metastasis (24%, 28%, and 31%, respectively), whereas other primary sources have a higher rate of single nodules (urinary tract 44%, GI tract 47%).[142] It has been suggested that the cerebellum receives a disproportionately larger number of metastases (per unit volume) from certain primary sites (e.g., lung 22%, breast 29%, and especially GI 41%) but is host for a disproportionately lower rate from other sources (e.g., urinary tract 7%) as compared with the cerebrum.[142] A solitary cerebellar metastasis from a renal cell carcinoma (RCC) is less likely than a hemangioblastoma; and multiple lesions, only in the cerebellum, are much more likely to be HB in von Hippel-Lindau disease, and not metastatic RCC—even if the patient has a known renal cell carcinoma (Fig. 22–36). Overall, a patient with RCC has a metastasis to the brain parenchyma (only one fifth of which is cerebellum)

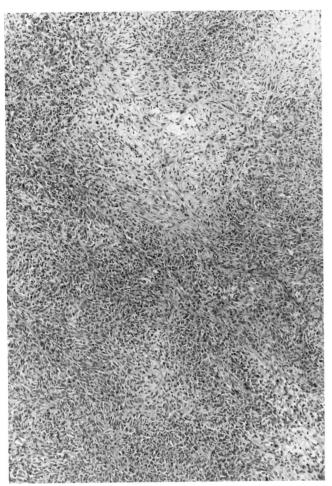

FIGURE 22–40. Hemangiopericytoma. Irregular areas of reduced tumor cellularity are often striking on low-power inspection. (H&E ×75)

in 2% to 17% of cases, and asymptomatic metastases are found in less than 4% of patients with known RCC.[142, 168–170]

Hemangioblastomas may form a classic cystic mass, with the neoplastic tissue limited to a mural nodule, in about one third of cases. HB may also form solid masses (one third) or partially cystic masses with complex architecture (one third) (Figs. 22–36 and 22–37). When HB is cystic or partially cystic, imaging may be characteristic. The cyst portion of an HB may be exophytic to the neoplasm. As such, it may not be lined by tumor, but rather has a wall composed of non-neoplastic tissue. Therefore, the wall does not enhance when contrast MRI or CT scans are performed. The presence of a cystic cerebellar lesion, without a complete circle of enhancement, is strongly suggestive of a hemangioblastoma in an adult (>30 years). It is important to remember that in patients with von Hippel-Lindau disease, the hemangioblastomas may present in the late teens and early twenties. Multiple lesions, which can vary from solid to cystic, can be confused with metastases.

MENINGIOMA VERSUS HEMANGIOPERICYTOMA
(Angioblastic Meningioma)

Meningiomas are tumors that arise from the superficial meninges and from areas lined by pia and arachnoid cells.

Most of these tumors arise from the arachnoid cells, especially those associated with arachnoid villi within dural veins and sinuses.

The hemangiopericytoma is a controversial neoplasm in that some observers feel that it is a distinct entity, unrelated to other meningiomas.[171–176] Others argue that there are overlapping features that suggest a kinship between classic meningiomas and meningeal tumors with an hemangiopericytic growth pattern.[177, 178]

Although we believe that these neoplasms are separate, unrelated entities that share the common feature of arising in the meninges, the argument is primarily of academic interest. The matter of prime importance is that tumors with a hemangiopericytic pattern have histologic and biologic characteristics of malignancy. For therapeutic and prognostic reasons, the recognition of this tumor as distinct from classic meningiomas is thus essential.

CLINICOPATHOLOGIC FEATURES. Symptomatic meningiomas have a broad age range, with most occurring between ages 40 and 60, with a median around 46 years.[179] Infrequently this neoplasm occurs in childhood[180] or with advanced age. Of interest, there is a strong female predilection of 1.5:1 to 3:1 with intracranial meningiomas. Spinal meningiomas exhibit a female preponderance of 4:1 to 5:1.[179, 181] Recurrences have been noted in 6% to 22% of cases without reference to completeness of excision or other parameters.

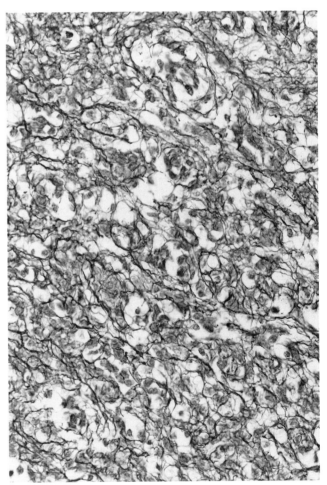

FIGURE 22–41. Hemangiopericytoma. Reticulin stains show a dense meshwork of reticulin fibers surrounding the blood vessels and individual tumor cells. (Retic ×300)

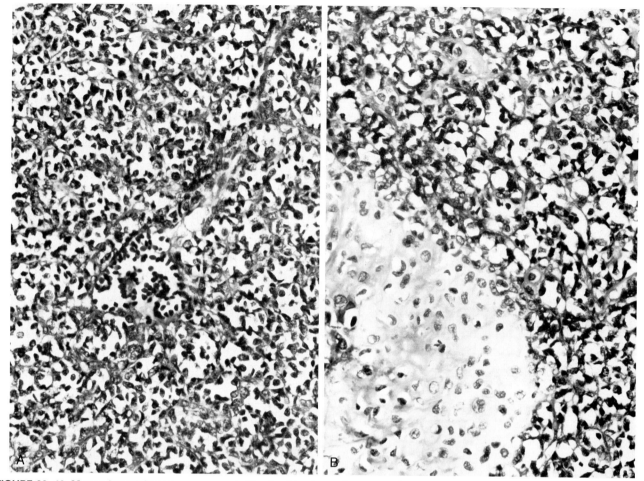

FIGURE 22–42. Mesenchymal Chondrosarcoma. *A,* Sheets of haphazardly arranged undifferentiated tumor cells and dilated vessels in meningeal mesenchymal chondrosarcomas can closely resemble hemangiopericytoma. (H&E ×300) *B,* When abrupt islands of well-differentiated cartilage are present, the diagnosis of mesenchymal chondrosarcoma is simplified. (H&E ×300)

Extraneural metastasis is rare (approximately 0.1%) and is seen mostly with malignant variants.[182]

Conversely, hemangiopericytomas have a somewhat earlier median age of occurrence (40 years) and a slight but distinct male preponderance of 1.25 : 1.[179, 183, 184] Recurrences are frequent, with one large review article showing an overall recurrence rate of approximately 60%.[184] Another long-term follow-up series demonstrated recurrence rates at 1, 5, and 10 years after surgery of 15%, 65%, and 76%, respectively.[183] An average rate of extraneural metastasis is 20%.[184] Lung and bone are the most frequent metastatic sites.

Both meningiomas and hemangiopericytomas arise throughout the central nervous system, with the cortical convexity and parasagittal areas being favored sites.

Grossly, hemangiopericytomas are lobulated soft, highly vascular neoplasms without prominent cystic changes that often show dural attachment. Meningiomas are typically firm but have similar sites of origin, focal dural attachment, and infrequently a cystic cut surface. No gross finding is pathognomonic for either entity.

Microscopically, the appearances are quite different. Meningiomas are best known for cellular whorls with associated laminated calcifications (psammoma bodies). Spindled cells are also sometimes present that resemble fibroblasts and are arranged in interlacing bundles (Fig. 22–38). The number of variations on this common theme is large and is well covered in one monograph.[185] Immunoperoxidase stains are frequently positive for vimentin, epithelial membrane antigen, and less frequently for S-100 protein.[175] The biologic behavior of meningiomas is not always predictable. Various histologic features have been found that are associated with tumor aggressiveness, including foci of necrosis, high mitotic rate, nuclear pleomorphism, increased cellularity, and invasion of adjacent brain.[186, 187] A papillary growth pattern is also associated with aggressive biologic potential.[188, 189] Less frequently reported features thought to be associated with recurrence include hypervascularity, hemosiderin deposition, and growth of tumor cells in sheets with prominent nucleoli.[181] One study suggests that intraoperative infusion of bromodeoxyuridine (BUdR) can be used to label cells in DNA synthesis (S phase). Early results indicate that this labeling index (LI) is predictive of recurrence risk.[187] Labeled cells are identified by immunohistochemical methods. In another study, the recurrence rates correlated well with the LI. If this finding is supported by further study, a proliferation index may be used as a sensitive gauge for the probability of tumor recurrence.[187, 190]

Hemangiopericytomas are highly cellular and are composed of tightly packed cells interspersed between thin-walled,

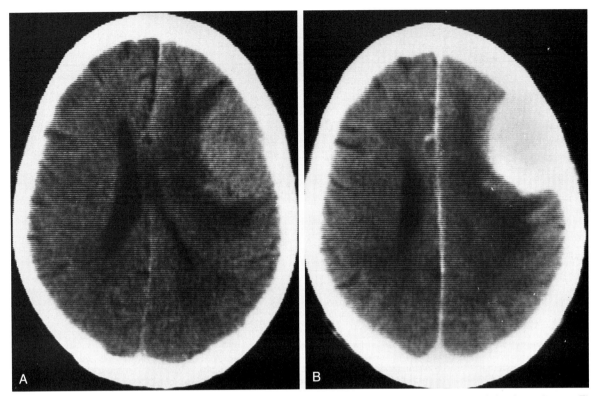

FIGURE 22–43. Meningioma. A typical meningioma is a unilobular hemispherical mass with a broad-based dural attachment. The lesion is usually hyperdense compared with brain on the precontrast image *(A)*, and the adjacent calvarium may show hyperostosis. After contrast infusion *(B)*, enhancement is typically dense and homogeneous.

endothelium-lined vessels of variable size. Some large anastomotic vessels have been described as having a "staghorn" arrangement. The neoplastic cells possess small oval to spindled nuclei with indistinct cytoplasm (Fig. 22–39). Interlacing bundles or fascicles of spindled cells are not a feature of this tumor. Irregular foci of reduced cellularity are often seen and are helpful in recognizing hemangiopericytomas (Fig. 22–40). Reticulin staining reveals a dense meshwork that surrounds individual tumor cells (Fig. 22–41). Immunoperoxidase stains for Factor VIII and *Ulex europaeus* show positive staining of endothelial cells lining the vessels but not the actual neoplastic cells. These cells, presumably derived from pericytes, stain positively for actin and vimentin but negative for desmin and EMA.

Two large studies conflict on the importance of tumor histology in predicting the length of survival.[183, 184] Both, however, concur that histologic features do not influence the rate of recurrence.

DIFFERENTIAL DIAGNOSIS. The pattern of hemangiopericytomas is distinctive, and a diagnosis can usually be made with confidence on H&E stains. If confirmation is needed, the reticulin preparation is quite helpful. The individual neoplastic cells in hemangiopericytomas are surrounded by a reticulin network, whereas meningiomas are reticulin-poor with broad areas exhibiting negative staining. Immunoperoxidase stains for EMA are positive in meningiomas and negative in hemangiopericytomas.[175]

The recognition of hemangiopericytomas has assumed even greater importance with reports[183, 184] showing a longer period to first recurrence and prolonged survival if the tumor is

recognized and radiation therapy is administered after the first surgery.

Another malignant tumor should be considered in the differential diagnosis of hemangiopericytoma. **Mesenchymal chondrosarcoma** may show a hemangiopericytomatous pattern focally and has been described arising in the meninges.[191] The

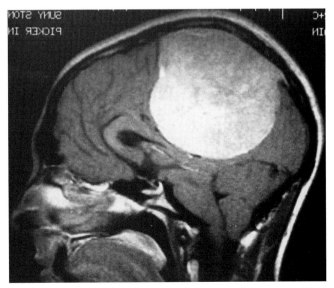

FIGURE 22–44. Meningioma. This T1-weighted MRI after Gd-DTPA enhancement shows the characteristics of a typical meningioma: homogeneous enhancement, a unilobular mass with a broad-based dural attachment, and a dural "tail sign."

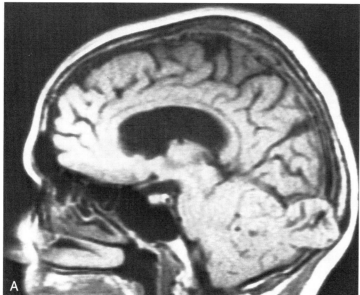
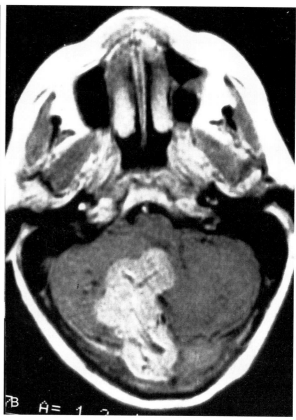

FIGURE 22–45. Hemangiopericytoma. On the precontrast *(A)* and post-contrast *(B)* T1-weighted MRI, the hemangiopericytoma is lobulated, has a narrow base of dural attachment with a "mushroom" shape, and has eroded through the calvarium. There are multiple curvilinear signal voids (dark lines within the tumor) from large vessels within the tumor. As solitary features, these findings can be seen in typical meningiomas. However, when taken together, they suggest hemangiopericytoma.

presence of cartilage islands and areas of decreased reticulin deposition are useful criteria to establish a diagnosis of mesenchymal chondrosarcoma (Fig. 22–42).

NEURORADIOLOGIC CORRELATION. The meningioma typically presents as a dural-based lesion. The mass may grow as an *en plaque* thickening or "carpeting" along the inner table of the calvarium. This pattern is seen most often in the skull base, along the floor and lateral margins of the anterior fossa. Much more commonly, the meningioma grows as a globose mass, roughly hemispherical, with a broad base against the dura, which may be the falx or tentorium, or most frequently the dura lining the calvarium (Fig. 22–43). The angle formed between the tumor and the dura is usually obtuse. The edge of the meningioma may show the "tail sign," in which a tapered bit of tissue extends away from the mass, apparently creeping along the dural surface (Fig. 22–44). Meningiomas are usually homogeneous masses, without cavitation (cyst or necrosis). On precontrast CT, they are hyperdense compared with the brain, yet without calcium or hemorrhage (see Fig. 22–43). On MRI, they may be isointense to gray matter but can be recognized by varying the pulse sequence (scan parameters) to change their signal. Even when isointense, they may be identified because of their location (broad-based on the dura) and as extra-axial by the pattern of brain displacement ("cortical buckling") (see Fig. 22–44). On both CT and MRI, meningiomas usually show homogeneous enhancement (see Fig. 22–43).

Hemangiopericytomas (HPC) may mimic meningiomas on imaging. However, they often show certain suggestive features (Fig. 22–45). Unlike meningiomas, HPC often forms a highly lobulated mass rather than a smooth hemispheric shape and may have a narrow base, forming an acute margin with the dura. HPC can have large internal signal voids (SV) on MRI, indicating a massive amount of tumor neovascularity. Hemangiopericytoma is more likely to be associated with bone destruction rather than the hyperostosis seen in 15% to 25% of meningiomas.

References

1. Vertosick FT, Selker RG, Arena VC: Survival of patients with well-differentiated astrocytomas diagnosed in the era of computed tomography. Neurosurgery 28:496–501, 1991.
2. Muller W, Afra D, Schroder R: Supratentorial recurrences of gliomas: Morphologic studies with relation to time intervals in gliomas. Acta Neurochir (Wien) 37:75–91, 1977.
3. Kernohan JW, Sayre GP: Tumors of the Central Nervous System. Washington, DC, Armed Forces Institute of Pathology, 1952.
4. Nelson JS, Tsukada Y, Schoenfeld D, et al: Necrosis as a prognostic criterion in malignant supratentorial, astrocytic tumors. Cancer 52:550–554, 1983.
5. Zulch KJ: Histological Typing of Tumors of the Central Nervous System. Geneva, World Health Organization, 1979.
6. Burger PC, Vogel FS, Green SB: Glioblastoma and anaplastic astrocytomas: Pathologic criteria and prognostic implications. Cancer 56:1106–1111, 1985.
7. Daumas-Duport C, Scheithauer B, O'Fallon J, et al: Grading of astrocytoma: A simple and reproducible grading method. Cancer 62:2152–2165, 1988.
8. Ringertz N: Grading of gliomas. APMIS 27:51–64, 1950.
9. Hoshino T, Rodriguez LA, Cho KG, et al: Prognostic implications of the proliferative potential of low-grade astrocytoma. J Neurosurg 69:839–842, 1988.
10. Nishizaki T, Orita T, Furutani Y, et al: Flow-cytometric DNA analysis and immunohistochemical measurement of Ki-67 and BUdR labeling indices in human brain tumors. J Neurosurg 70:379–384, 1989.
11. Fujimaki T, Matsutani M, Nakamura O, et al: Correlation between bromodeoxyuridine-labeling indices and patient prognosis in cerebral astrocytic tumors of adults. Cancer 67:1629–1634, 1991.
12. Labrousse F, Daumas-Duport C, Batorski L, et al: Histological grading and bromodeoxyuridine labeling index of astrocytomas. J Neurosurg 75:202–205, 1991.
13. Raghavan R, Steart PV, Weller RO: Cell proliferation patterns in the diagnosis of astrocytomas, anaplastic astrocytomas and glioblastoma multiforme: A Ki-67 study. Neuropathol Appl Neurobiol 16:123–133, 1990.

14. Revesz T, Alsanjar N, Darling JL, et al: Proliferating cell nuclear antigen (PCNA): Expression in samples of human astrocytic gliomas. Neuropath Appl Neurobiol 19:152–158, 1993.

15. Kimmel DW, O'Fallon JR, Scheithauer BW: Prognostic value of cytogenetic analysis in human cerebral astrocytomas. Ann Neurol 31:534–542, 1992.

16. Ng H-K, Lo STH: Cytokeratin immunoreactivity in gliomas. Histopathology 14:359–368, 1989.

17. Hitchcock E, Morris CS: Cross reactivity of anti-epithelial membrane antigen monoclonal for reactive and neoplastic glial cells. J Neurooncol 4:345–352, 1987.

18. Krouwer HGJ, Davis RL, Silver P, et al: Gemistocytic astrocytomas. J Neurosurg 74:399–406, 1991.

19. Burger PC, Vogel FS: Cerebrovascular disease. Am J Pathol 92:257–313, 1978.

20. Hulette CM, Downey BT, Burger PC: Macrophage markers in diagnostic neuropathology. Am J Surg Pathol 16(5):493–499, 1992.

21. Ishihara O, Yamaguchi Y, Matsuishi T, et al: Multiple ring enhancement in a case of acute reversible demyelinating disease of childhood suggestive of acute multiple sclerosis. Brain Dev 6:401–406, 1984.

22. Kepes J: Large focal tumor-like demyelinating lesions of the brain. Intermediate entity between multiple sclerosis and acute disseminated encephalomyelitis? A study of 31 cases. Ann Neurol 33:18–27, 1993.

23. Hunter SB, Ballinger WE, Rubin JJ: Multiple sclerosis mimicking brain tumor. Arch Pathol Lab Med 111:464–468, 1987.

24. Van der Velden M, Bots GTAM, Endtz LJ: Cranial CT in multiple sclerosis showing a mass effect. Surg Neurol 12:307–310, 1979.

25. Sagar HJ, Warlow CP, Shelson PWE, et al: Multiple sclerosis with clinical and radiological features of cerebral tumor. J Neurol Neurosurg Psychiatry 45:802–808, 1982.

26. Rieth KG, Di Chiro G, Cromwell LD, et al: Primary demyelinating disease simulating glioma of the corpus callosum. J Neurosurg 55:620–624, 1981.

27. Poser CM: Neurological complications of swine influenza vaccination. Acta Neurol Scand 66:413–431, 1982.

28. de la Monte SM, Ropper AH, Dickersin GR, et al: Relapsing central and peripheral demyelinating diseases. Unusual pathologic features. Arch Neurol 43:626–629, 1986.

29. Walker RWH, Gawler J: Serial cerebral CT abnormalities in relapsing acute disseminated encephalomyelitis. J Neurol Neurosurg Psychiatry 52:1100–1102, 1989.

30. Donovan MK, Lenn NJ: Postinfectious encephalomyelitis with localized basal ganglia involvement. Pediatr Neurol 5:311–313, 1989.

31. Fortuna A, Ferrante L, Acqui M, et al: Cystic meningiomas: Report of two cases. Acta Neurochir (Wien) 90:23–30, 1988.

32. Parisi G, Tropea R, Giuffrida S, et al: Cystic meningiomas: Report of seven cases. J Neurosurg 64:35–38, 1986.

33. Nauta HJW, Tucker WS, Horsey WJ, et al: Xanthochromic cysts associated with meningioma. J Neurol Neurosurg Psychiatry 42:529–535, 1979.

34. Odake G: Cystic meningioma: Report of three patients. Neurosurgery 30:935–940, 1992.

35. Henry JM, Schwartz FT, Sartawi MA, et al: Cystic meningiomas simulating astrocytomas. J Neurosurg 40:647–650, 1974.

36. Rengachary S, Batnitzky S, Kepes JJ, et al: Cystic lesions associated with intracranial meningiomas. Neurosurgery 4:107–114, 1979.

37. Alguacil-Garcia A, Pettigrew NM, Sima AAF: Secretory meningioma. A distinct subtype of meningioma. Am J Surg Pathol 10:102–111, 1986.

38. Kobayashi S: Meningioma, neurilemmoma and astrocytoma specimens obtained with squash method for cytodiagnosis. A cytologic immunochemical study. Acta Cytol 37:913–922, 1993.

39. Kepes JJ: Electron microscopy of meningiomas. In Meningiomas—The Biology, Pathology and Differential Diagnosis. New York, Raven Press, 1982, pp 150–182.

40. Russell DS, Rubinstein LJ: Pathology of Tumors of the Nervous System. Baltimore, Williams & Wilkins, 1989, pp 172–173.

41. Mork SJ, Lindegaard KF, Halvorsen TB, et al: Oligodendroglioma: Incidence and biologic behavior in a defined population. J Neurosurg 63:881, 1985.

42. Nakagawa Y, Perentes E, Rubinstein LJ: Immunohistochemical characterizaton of oligodendrogliomas: An analysis of multiple markers. Acta Neuropathol (Berl) 72:15–22, 1986.

43. Herpers MJHM, Budka H: Glial fibrillary acidic protein (GFAP) in oligodendroglial tumors: Gliofibrillary oligodendroglioma and transitional oligoastrocytoma as subtypes of oligodendroglioma. Acta Neuropathol (Berl) 64:265–272, 1984.

44. Kros JM, Van Eden CG, Stefanko SZ, et al: Prognostic implications of glial fibrillary acidic protein containing cell types in oligodendrogliomas. Cancer 66:1204–1212, 1990.

45. Smith MT, Ludwig CL, Godfrey AD, et al: Grading of oligodendrogliomas. Cancer 52:2107–2114, 1983.

46. Kros JM, Troost D, Van Eden CG, et al: Oligodendroglioma—A comparison of two grading systems. Cancer 61:2251–2259, 1988.

47. Burger PC, Rawlings CE, Cox EB, et al: Clinicopathologic correlations in the oligodendroglioma. Cancer 59:1345–1352, 1987.

48. Shaw EG, Scheithauer BW, O'Fallon JR, et al: Oligodendrogliomas: The Mayo Clinic experience. J Neurosurg 76:428–434, 1992.

49. Greenlee JE: Progressive multifocal leukoencephalopathy. Curr Clin Top Infect Dis 10:140–156, 1989.

50. Hair LS, Nuovo G, Powers JM, et al: Progressive multifocal leukoencephalopathy in patients with human immunodeficiency virus. Hum Pathol 23:663–667, 1992.

51. von Einsiedel RW, Fife TD, Aksamit AJ, et al: Progressive multifocal leukoencephalopathy in AIDS: A clinicopathologic study and review of literature. J Neurol 240:391–406, 1993.

52. Hedley-Whyte ET, Smith BP, Tyler HR, et al: Multifocal leukoencephalopathy with remission and five year survival. J Neuropathol Exp Neurol 25:107–116, 1966.

53. Padgett BL, Walker DL: Virologic and serologic studies of progressive multifocal leukoencephalopathy. In Sever JL, Madden DL (eds): Polyomaviruses and Human Neurological Diseases. New York, Alan R. Liss, 1983, pp 107–117.

54. Greenlee JE, Stroop WG: JC virus nucleic acids in the atypical astrocytes of progressive multifocal leukoencephalopathy. Neurology 38:118, 1988.

55. Moret H, Guichard M, Matherson S, et al: Virological diagnosis of progressive multifocal leukoencephalopathy: Detection of JC virus DNA in cerebrospinal fluid and brain tissue of AIDS patients. J Clin Microbiol 31:3310–3313, 1993.

56. Gibson PE, Knowles WA, Hand JF, et al: Detection of JC virus in the cerebrospinal fluid of patients with progressive multifocal leukoencephalopathy. J Med Virol 39:278–281, 1993.

57. Dean BL, Drayer BP, Bird RD, et al: Gliomas: Classification with MR imaging. Radiology 174:411–415, 1990.

58. Butler AR, Horii SC, Kricheff II, et al: Computed tomography in astrocytomas. Radiology 129:433–439, 1978.

59. Kelley PJ, Daumas-Suport C, Kisper DB, et al: Imaging-based stereotaxic serial biopsies in untreated intracranial glial neoplasms. J Neurosurg 66:865–874, 1987.

60. Earnest F, Kelly PJ, Scheithauer BW, et al: Cerebral astrocytomas: Histological correlation of MR and CT enhancement with stereotactic biopsy. Radiology 166:823–827, 1988.

61. Monajati A, Heggeness L: Patterns of edema in tumors vs. infarcts: Visualization of white matter pathways. AJNR 3:251–255, 1982.

62. Fishman RA: Brain edema. N Engl J Med 293:706–711, 1975.

63. Cowley AR: Influence of fiber tracts on the CT appearance of cerebral edema: Anatomic-pathologic correlation. AJNR 4:915–925, 1983.

64. O'Brian MD: Ischemic cerebral edema. A review. Stroke 10:623–627, 1979.

65. Campbell JK, Houser OW, Stevens JC, et al: Computed tomography and radionuclide imaging in the evaluation of ischemic stroke. Radiology 126:695–702, 1978.

66. Caille JM, Guibert F, Bidabe AM, et al: Enhancement of cerebral infarcts with CT. Computerized Tomography 4:73–77, 1980.

67. Wall SD, Brant-Zawadski M, Jeffrey RB, et al: High frequency CT findings within 24 hours after cerebral infarction. AJNR 2:553–557, 1981.

68. Kendall BE, Pullicino P: Intravascular contrast injection in ischemic lesions. II. Effect on prognosis. Neuroradiology 19:241–243, 1980.

69. Mark AS, Atlas SW: Progressive multifocal leukoencephalopathy in patients with AIDS: Appearance on MR images. Radiology 173:517–520, 1989.

70. Runge VM, Price AC, Kirshner HS, et al: The evaluation of multiple sclerosis by magnetic resonance imaging. Radiographics 6:203–212, 1986.

71. Uhlenbrock D, Seidel D, Gehlen W, et al: MR imaging in multiple sclerosis: Comparison with clinical, CSF, and visual evoked potential findings. AJNR 9:59–67, 1988.

72. Mastrostefano R, Occhipinti E, Bigotti G, et al: Multiple sclerosis plaque simulating cerebral tumor: Case report and review of the literature. Neurosurgery 21:244–246, 1987.

73. Lee Y, Van Tassel P: Intracranial oligodendrogliomas: Imaging findings in 35 untreated cases. AJR 152:361–369, 1989.

74. Vonofakos D, Marcu H, Hacker H: Oligodendrogliomas: CT patterns with emphasis on features indicating malignancy. J Comput Assist Tomogr 3:783–788, 1979.

75. Martin F, Lemmen LJ: Calcification in intracranial neoplasms. Am J Pathol 28:1107–1131, 1952.

76. Russell DS, Rubinstein LJ: Glioblastoma multiforme. In Pathology of Tumors of the Nervous System, 5th ed. Baltimore, Williams & Wilkins, 1989, p 219.

77. Rosenberg RN: Intracranial neoplasms. In The Clinical Neurosciences, Vol 1. New York, Churchill Livingstone, 1983, pp 246–250.

78. Kepes JJ, Rubinstein LJ: Malignant gliomas with heavily lipidized (foamy) tumor cells: A report of three cases with immunoperoxidase study. Cancer 47:2451–2459, 1981.

79. Rosenblum MK, Erlandson RA, Budzilovich GN: The lipid-rich epithelioid glioblastoma. Am J Surg Pathol 15(10):925–934, 1991.

80. Budka H: Non-glial specificities of immunocytochemistry for the glial fibrillary acidic protein (GFAP): Triple expression of GFAP, vimentin and cytokeratins in papillary meningioma and metastasizing renal carcinoma. Acta Neuropathol (Berl) 72:43–54, 1986.

81. Cosgrove M, Fitzgibbons PL, Sherrod A, et al: Intermediate filament expression in astrocytic neoplasms. Am J Surg Pathol 13:141–145, 1989.

82. Margetts JC, Kalyan-Raman UP: Giant-celled glioblastoma of brain. A clinicopathological and radiological study of ten cases (including immunohistochemistry and ultrastructure). Cancer 63:524–531, 1989.

83. Palma L, Celli P, Maleci L, et al: Malignant monstrocellular brain tumours. A study of 42 surgically treated cases. Acta Neurochir (Wien) 97:17–25, 1989.

84. Burger PC, Vollmer RT: Histologic factors of prognostic significance in glioblastoma multiforme. Cancer 46:1179–1186, 1980.

85. Gluszcz A, Alwasials J, Papierz W, et al: Morphologic observations of dysplastic gliomas heterotransplanted to experimental animals. Acta Neuropathol (Berl) 31:21–28, 1975.

86. Hoshino T, Wilson CS, Ellis WG: Gemistocytic astrocytes in gliomas. An autoradiographic study. J Neuropathol Exp Neurol 34:263–281, 1975.

87. Hoshino T, Wilson CB: Cell kinetic analyses of human malignant brain tumors (gliomas). Cancer 44:956, 1979.

88. Kepes JJ, Fulling KH, Garcia JH: The clinical significance of "adenoid" formations of neoplastic astrocytes, imitating metastatic carcinoma, in gliosarcomas. A review of five cases. Clin Neuropathol 1:139–150, 1982.

89. Mork SJ, Rubinstein LJ, Kepes JJ, et al: Patterns of epithelial metaplasia in malignant gliomas. II. Squamous differentiation of epithelial-like formations in gliosarcomas and glioblastomas. J Neuropathol Exp Neurol 47:101–118, 1988.

90. Lalitha VS, Rubinstein LJ: Reactive glioma in intracranial sarcoma: A form of mixed sarcoma and glioma ("sarcoglioma"). Cancer 43:246–257, 1979.

91. Banerjee AK, Sharma BS, Kak VK, et al: Gliosarcoma with cartilage formation. Cancer 63:518–523, 1989.

92. Ng H-K, Poon WS: Gliosarcoma of the posterior fossa with features of a malignant fibrous histiocytoma. Cancer 65:1161–1166, 1990.

93. Barnard RO, Bradford R, Scott T: Gliomyosarcoma. Acta Neuropathol (Berl) 69:23–27, 1986.

94. Sarimiento J, Ferrer K, Pons L, et al: Cerebral osteochondrosarcoma-glioblastoma multiforme. Acta Neurochir (Wien) 50:335–341, 1979.

95. Morantz RA, Feigin I, Ransohoff J: Clinical and pathological study of 24 cases of gliosarcoma. J Neurosurg 45:398–408, 1976.

96. Meis JM, Ho KL, Nelson JS: Gliosarcoma: A histologic and immunohistochemical reaffirmation. Mod Pathol 3:19–24, 1990.

97. Slowik F, Jellinger K, Gaszó L, Fischer J: Gliosarcomas: Histological, immunohistochemical, ultrastructural, and tissue culture studies. Acta Neuropathol (Berl) 67:201–210, 1985.

98. Grant JW, Steart PV, Aguzzi A, et al: Gliosarcoma: An immunohistochemical study. Acta Neuropathol 79:305–309, 1989.

99. Kochi N, Budka H: Contribution of histiocytic cells to sarcomatous development of the gliosarcoma. Acta Neuropathol (Berl) 73:124–130, 1987.

100. Jones H, Steart PV, Weller RO: Spindle-cell glioblastoma or gliosarcoma? Neuropathol Appl Neurobiol 17:177–187, 1991.

101. Feigin I, Ransohoff J, Lieberman A: Sarcoma arising in oligodendroglioma of the brain. J Neuropathol Exp Neurol 35:679–684, 1976.

102. Pasquier B, Couderc P, Pasquier D, et al: Sarcoma arising in oligodendroglioma of the brain. Cancer 42:2753–2758, 1978.

103. Kepes JJ, Rubinstein LJ, Eng LF: Pleomorphic xanthoastrocytoma: A distinctive meningocerebral glioma of young subjects with relatively favorable prognosis. Cancer 44:1839–1852, 1979.

104. Kros JM, Vecht CJ, Stefanko SZ: The pleomorphic xanthoastrocytoma and its differential diagnosis: A study of five cases. Hum Pathol 22:1128–1135, 1991.

105. Gomez JG, Garcia JH, Colon LE: A variant of cerebral glioma called pleomorphic xanthoastrocytoma: Case report. Neurosurgery 16:703–706, 1985.

106. Kepes JJ: Pleomorphic xanthoastrocytoma: The birth of a diagnosis and a concept. Brain Pathol 3:269–274, 1993.

107. Heyerdahl Strom E, Skullerud K: Pleomorphic xanthoastrocytoma: Report of five cases. Clin Neuropathol 2:188–191, 1983.

108. Jones M, Drut R, Raglia G: Pleomorphic xanthoastrocytoma: A report of two cases. Pediatr Pathol 1:459–467, 1983.

109. Weldon-Linne CM, Victor TA, Groothuis DR, et al: Pleomorphic xanthoastrocytoma. Ultrastructural and immunohistochemical study of a case with rapidly fatal outcome following surgery. Cancer 52:2055–2063, 1983.

110. Kepes JJ, Rubinstein LJ, Ansbacher L, et al: Histopathological features of recurrent pleomorphic xanthoastrocytomas: Further corroboration of the glial nature of this neoplasm. A study of three cases. Acta Neuropathol 78:585–593, 1989.

111. Allegranza A, Girlando S, Arrigoni GL, et al: Proliferating cell nuclear antigen expression in central nervous system neoplasms. Virchows Arch A Pathol Anat Histopathol 419:417–423, 1991.

112. MaCaulay RJB, Jay V, Hoffman HK, et al: Increased mitotic activity as a negative prognostic indicator in pleomorphic xanthoastrocytoma. J Neurosurg 79:761–768, 1993.

113. Sugita Y, Kepes JJ, Shigemori M, et al: Pleomorphic xanthoastrocytoma with desmoplastic reaction: Angiomatous variant. Report of two cases. Clin Neurol 9:271–278, 1990.

114. Furuta A, Takahashi H, Ikuta F, et al: Temporal lobe tumor demonstrating ganglioglioma and pleomorphic xanthoastrocytoma components. J Neurosurg 77:143–147, 1992.

115. Lindboe CF, Cappelen J, Kepes JJ: Pleomorphic xanthoastrocytoma as a component of a cerebellar ganglioglioma: Case report. Neurosurgery 31:353–355, 1992.

116. Kepes JJ, Kepes M, Slowik F: Fibrous xanthomas and xanthosarcomas of the meninges and the brain. Acta Neuropathol (Berl) 23:187–199, 1973.

117. Paulus W, Peiffer J: Does the pleomorphic xanthoastrocytoma exist? Problems in the application of immunological techniques to the classification of brain tumors. Acta Neuropathol 76:245–252, 1988.

118. Ng H-K, Lo STH: Immunostaining for alpha-1-antichymotrypsin and alpha-1-antitrypsin in gliomas. Histopathology 13:79–87, 1988.

119. Zuccarello M, Sawaya R, Ray MB: Immunohistochemical demonstration of alpha-1-proteinase inhibitor in brain tumors. Cancer 60:804–809, 1987.

120. Burger PC, Rawlings CE, Cox EB: Clinicopathologic correlations in the oligodendroglioma. Cancer 59:1345–1352, 1987.

121. Hochberg FH, Miller DC: Primary central nervous system lymphoma. J Neurosurg 68:835–853, 1988.

122. Eby NL, Grufferman S, Flannelly CM: Increasing incidence of primary brain lymphoma in the US. Cancer 62:2461–2465, 1988.

123. Nakhleh RE, Manivel JC, Copenhaver CM: In-situ hybridization for the detection of Epstein-Barr virus in central nervous system lymphomas. Cancer 67:444–448, 1991.

124. Bashir R, Luka J, Cheloha K, et al: Expression of Epstein-Barr virus proteins in primary CNS lymphoma in AIDS patients. Neurology 43:2358–2362, 1993.

125. Paulus W, Jellinger K, Hallas C, et al: Human herpesvirus-6 and Epstein-Barr virus genome in primary cerebral lymphomas. Neurology 43:1591–1593, 1993.

126. Murphy JK, Young LS, Bevan IS, et al: Demonstration of Epstein-Barr virus in primary brain lymphoma by in situ DNA hybridization in paraffin wax embedded tissue. J Clin Pathol 43:220–223, 1990.

127. Bashir RM, Hochberg FH, Harris NL, et al: Variable expression of Epstein-Barr virus genome as demonstrated by in-situ hybridization in central nervous system lymphomas in immunocompromised patients. Mod Pathol 3:429–434, 1990.

128. List AF, Greer JP, Cousar JP: Primary brain lymphoma in the immunocompetent host: Relation to Epstein-Barr virus. Mod Pathol 3:609–612, 1990.

129. Bignon YJ, Clavelou P, Ramos F: Detection of Epstein-Barr virus sequences in primary brain lymphoma without immunodeficiency. Neurology 41:1152–1153, 1991.

130. Bonnin JM, Garcia JH: Primary malignant non-Hodgkin's lymphoma of the central nervous system. Path Annu 22:353–375, 1987.

131. Kumanishi T, Washiyama K, Saito T: Primary malignant lymphoma of the brain: An immunohistochemical study of eight cases using a panel of monoclonal and heterologous antibodies. Acta Neuropathol (Berl) 71:190–196, 1986.

132. Murphy JK, O'Brien CJ, Ironside J: Morphologic and immunophenotypic characterization of primary brain lymphomas using paraffin-embedded tissue. Histopathology 15:449–460, 1989.

133. Nakhleh RE, Manivel JC, Hurd D: Central nervous system lymphomas. Arch Pathol Lab Med 113:1050–1056, 1989.

134. Kumanishi T, Washiyama K, Nishiyama A: Primary malignant lymphoma of the brain: Demonstration of immunoglobulin gene rearrangements in four cases by the Southern blot hybridization technique. Acta Neuropathol 79:23–26, 1989.

135. Grant JW, von Deimling A: Primary T-cell lymphoma of the central nervous system. Arch Pathol Lab Med 114:24–27, 1990.

136. Kanavaros P, Mikol J, Nemeth J, et al: Primary T-cell lymphoma of the central nervous system. Res Pract 189:93–98, 1993.

137. Inoue M, Kawaguchi T, Yokoyama H, et al: Primary T-cell lymphoma with myelopathy associated HTLV-1. Neurosurgery 27:148–151, 1990.

138. Mineura K, Sawataishi J, Sasajima T, et al: Primary central nervous system involvement of the so-called "peripheral T-cell lymphoma." Report of a case and review of the literature. J Neurooncol 16:235–242, 1993.

139. Bednar MM, Sallerni A, Flanagan ME: Primary central nervous system T-cell lymphoma. J Neurosurg 74:668–672, 1991.

140. Burger PC, Scheithauer BW, Vogel FS: Metastatic neoplasms. In Burger PC, Scheithauer BW, Vogel FS: Surgical Pathology of the Nervous System and Its Coverings, 3rd ed. New York, Churchill Livingstone, 1991, p 405.

141. Delattre JY, Krol G, Thaler HT, et al: Distribution of brain metastases. Arch Neurol 45:741–744, 1988.

142. Takakura K, Sano K, Hirano A, et al: Metastatic tumors of the central nervous system. New York, Igaku-Shoin, 1982, p 19.

143. Hara A, Hirayama H, Sakai N, et al: Nucleolar organizer region score and Ki-67 labelling index in high-grade gliomas and metastatic brain tumors. Acta Neurochir (Wien) 109:37–41, 1991.

144. Burger PC, Shibata T, Kleihues P: The use of monoclonal antibody Ki-67 in the identification of proliferating cells: Application to surgical pathology. Am J Surg Pathol 10:611–617, 1986.

145. Rueda-Pedraza ME, Heigetz SA, Sesterhenn IA, et al: Primary intracranial germ cell tumors in the first two decades of life: A clinical, light-microscopic, and immunohistochemical analysis of 54 cases. Perspect Pediatr Pathol 10:160–207, 1987.

146. Kobayashi T, Kageyama N, Kida Y, et al: Unilateral germinomas involving the basal ganglia and thalamus. J Neurosurg 55:55–62, 1981.

147. Legido A, Packer RJ, Sutton LN, et al: Suprasellar germinomas in childhood: A reappraisal. Cancer 63:340–344, 1989.

148. Takeuchi J, Handa H, Nagata I: Suprasellar germinoma. J Neurosurg 49:41–48, 1978.

149. Russell DS, Rubinstein LJ: Germinoma. In Russell DS, Rubinstein LJ: Pathology of Tumors of the Nervous System, 5th ed. Baltimore, Williams & Wilkins, 1989, p 669.

150. Scheithauer BW: Neuropathology of pineal region tumors. Clin Neurosurg 32:351–383, 1985.

151. Edwards MSB, Hudgins RJ, Wilson CB, et al: Pineal region tumors in children. J Neurosurg 68:689–697, 1988.

152. Rich TA, Cassady JR, Strand RD, et al: Radiation therapy for pineal and suprasellar germ cell tumors. Cancer 55:932–940, 1985.

153. Hesselink JR, Press GA: MR contrast enhancement of intracranial lesions with Gd-DTPA. Radiol Clin North Am 26:873–887, 1988.

154. Neumann HP, Eggert HR, Weigel K, et al: Hemangioblastomas of the central nervous system. A 10-year study with special reference to von Hippel-Lindau syndrome. J Neurosurg 70:24–30, 1989.

155. Horton JC, Harsh GR, Fisher JW, et al: Von Hippel-Lindau disease and erythrocytosis: Radioimmunoassay of erythropoietin in cyst fluid from a brainstem hemangioblastoma. Neurology 41:753–754, 1991.

156. Seizinger BR, Rouleau GA, Ozelius LJ, et al: Von Hippel-Lindau disease maps to the region of chromosome 3 associated with renal cell carcinoma. Nature 332:268–269, 1989.

157. de la Monte SM, Horowitz SA: Hemangioblastomas: Clinical and histopathological factors correlated with recurrence. Neurosurgery 25:695–698, 1989.

158. Kamitani H, Masuzawa H, Sato J, et al: Erythropoietin in haemangioblastoma: Immunohistochemical and electron microscopy studies. Acta Neurochir (Wien) 85:56–62, 1987.

159. Bohling T, Haltia M, Rosenlof K: Erythropoietin in capillary hemangioblastoma: An immunohistochemical study. Acta Neuropathol (Berl) 74:324–328, 1987.

160. Trimble M, Caro J, Talalla A, et al: Secondary erythrocytosis due to a cerebellar hemangioblastoma: Demonstration of erythropoietin mRNA in the tumor. Blood 78:599–601, 1991.

161. Kamitani H, Masuzawa H, Sato J, et al: Capillary hemangioblastoma: Histogenesis of stromal cells. Acta Neuropathol (Berl) 73:370–378, 1987.

162. Hufnagel TJ, Kim JH, True LD, et al: Immunohistochemistry of capillary hemangioblastoma. Immunoperoxidase-labeled antibody staining resolves the differential diagnosis with metastatic renal cell carcinoma, but does not explain the histogenesis of the capillary hemangioblastoma. Am J Surg Pathol 13(3):207–216, 1989.

163. Andrew SM, Gradwell E: Immunoperoxidase labelled antibody staining in differential diagnosis of central nervous system haemangioblastomas and central nervous system metastases of renal carcinomas. J Clin Pathol 39:917–919, 1986.

164. Martin F, Lemmen LJ: Calcification in intracranial neoplasms. Am J Pathol 28:1107–1131, 1952.

165. Green JR, Waggener JD, Kriegsfeld BA: Classification and incidence of neoplasms of the central nervous system. In Thompson RA, Green JR (eds): Advances in Neurology, Vol 15. New York, Raven Press, 1976, pp 51–55.

166. Baker JL, Houser OQ, Campbell JK: National Cancer Institute Study: Evaluation of computed tomography in the diagnosis of intracranial neoplasms. I. Overall results. Radiology 36:91–96, 1980.

167. Carmel PW, Mawad M: CT scanning of the posterior fossa. Clin Neurosurg 29:51–102, 1982.

168. Richards P, McKissock W: Intracranial metastasis. Br Med J 1:15–18, 1963.

169. Potts DG, Abbott GF, von Sneidern JV: National Cancer Institute Study: Evaluation of computed tomography in the diagnosis of intracranial neoplasms. III. Metastatic tumors. Radiology 136:657–664, 1980.

170. Marshall ME, Pearson T, Simpson W, et al: Low incidence of asymptomatic brain metastases in patients with renal cell carcinoma. Urology 36:300–302, 1990.

171. Kruse F Jr: Hemangiopericytoma of the meninges (angioblastic meningioma of Cushing and Eisenhardt). Clinicopathologic aspects and follow-up studies in 8 cases. Neurology (NY) 11:771–777, 1961.

172. Popoff NA, Malinin TI, Rosomoff HC: Fine structure of intracranial hemangiopericytoma and angiomatous meningioma. Cancer 34:1187–1197, 1974.

173. Pena CE: Intracranial hemangiopericytoma. Ultrastructural evidence of its leiomyoblastic differentiation. Acta Neuropathol (Berl) 33:279–284, 1975.

174. Goellner JR, Laws ER, Soule EH, et al: Hemangiopericytoma of the meninges. Mayo Clinic experience. Am J Clin Pathol 70:375–380, 1978.

175. Winek RR, Scheithauer BW, Wick MR: Meningioma, meningeal hemangiopericytoma (angioblastic meningioma), peripheral hemangiopericytoma, and acoustic schwannoma. A comparative immunohistochemical study. Am J Surg Pathol 13(4):251–261, 1989.

176. Burger PC, Scheithauer BW, Vogel FS: Surgical Pathology of the Nervous System and Its Coverings, 3rd ed. New York, Churchill Livingstone, 1991, p 107.

177. Russell DS, Rubinstein LJ: Pathology of Tumors of the Nervous System. Baltimore, Williams & Wilkins, 1989, pp 477–478.

178. Horten BD, Urich H, Rubinstein LJ, et al: The angioblastic meningioma: A reappraisal of a nosological problem. J Neurol Sci 31:387–410, 1977.

179. Schroder R, Firsching R, Kochanek S: Hemangiopericytoma of meninges. Zentralbl Neurochir 47:191–199, 1986.

180. Germano IM, Edwards MSB, Davis RL, et al: Intracranial meningiomas of the first two decades of life. J Neurosurg 80:447–453, 1994.

181. de la Monte S, Flickinger J, Linggood RM: Histopathologic features predicting recurrence of meningiomas following subtotal resection. Am J Surg Pathol 10(2):836–843, 1986.

182. Kepes JJ: Metastases of meningiomas. In Meningiomas—The Biology, Pathology, and Differential Diagnosis. New York, Raven Press, 1982, pp 190–199.

183. Guthrie BL, Ebersode MJ, Scheithauer BW, et al: Meningeal hemangiopericytoma: Histopathological features, treatment and long-term follow-up of 44 cases. Neurosurgery 25:514–522, 1989.

184. Mena H, Ribas JL, Pezeshkpour LH: Hemangiopericytoma of the central nervous system: A review of 94 cases. Hum Pathol 22:84–91, 1991.

185. Kepes JJ: Light microscopic features of meningiomas. In Meningiomas—Biology, Pathology, and Differential Diagnosis. New York, Raven Press, 1982, pp 64–149.

186. Mahmood A, Caccamo DV, Tomecek FJ, et al: Atypical and malignant meningiomas: A clinicopathologic review. Neurosurg 33:955–963, 1993.

187. Shibuya M, Hoshino T, Ito S, et al: Meningiomas: Clinical implications of a high proliferative potential determined by bromodeoxyuridine labeling. Neurosurgery 30:494–498, 1992.

188. Ludwin SK, Rubinstein LJ, Russell DS: Papillary meningioma: A malignant variant of meningioma. Cancer 36:1363–1373, 1975.

189. Pasquier B, Gasnier F, Pasquier D: Papillary meningioma: Clinicopathologic study of seven cases and review of the literature. Cancer 58:299–305, 1986.

190. Salmon I, Kiss R, Levivier M, et al: Characterization of nuclear DNA content, proliferation index, and nuclear size in a series of 181 meningiomas, including benign primary, recurrent, and malignant tumors. Am J Surg Pathol 17(3):239–247, 1993.

191. Parker JR, Zarabi MC, Parker JC Jr: Intracerebral mesenchymal chondrosarcoma. Ann Clin Lab Sci 19:401–407, 1989.

CHAPTER 23

Triviomas

Noel Weidner, M.D., and Ronald L. Goldman, M.D.

. . . nor is there any better way to advance the proper practice of medicine than to give our minds to the discovery of the usual law of nature, by careful investigation of cases of rarer forms of disease.

WILLIAM HARVEY, 1657

Loosely defined, a **"trivioma"** may be stated to represent an anatomic finding, usually microscopic, that, for varying reasons, is rare and often insignificant. In addition to "trivioma," creative synonyms coined by surgical pathologists are **"nebuloma," "incidentaloma,"** and **"rarey."** Those that defy explanation have been considered **"ignoromas"** by some. It should be noted, however, that these "lesions" are of import for three reasons: (1) they may be confused with entities of more portentous clinical significance; (2) they may, through a discussion of their pathogenesis and differential diagnosis, serve as an important teaching model; and (3) they may be pathogenetically related to lesions that are of clinical significance, and, as a corollary, it should be noted that such clinically significant lesions have been described in the literature either before or after initial recognition of the trivioma.

We initially attempted to include every conceivable candidate for trivioma. Although computerized aid is available to cope with the worldwide information explosion, such an all-inclusive attempt is impractical for a variety of reasons. Thus, this collection is admittedly arbitrary, not only in that references have been selected largely from major English-language publications, but primarily because its source is from the authors' own personal and referral material. The following selected examples will prove illustrative.

LIESEGANG RINGS

The literature, still relatively scant, now contains several studies devoted to peculiar eosinophilic ring-like bodies that are rather striking but essentially inconsequential structures. They are usually observed in cysts containing hemorrhagic or proteinaceous material, or within necroinflammatory tissue, and are the result of alternating diffusion and precipitation in colloidal solutions that are supersaturated *in vitro* or *in vivo*.[1, 2] The rings and the phenomenon that induces them are named after R. E. Liesegang, a German biochemist who produced them *in vitro*.[1] This fact demonstrates that a trivial physical-chemical phenomenon can find its trivial pathologic analogue, even if it takes almost a century to do so.

Liesegang rings have been observed in renal and perirenal hemorrhagic cysts (and, in some cases, in cytologic preparations of the cyst fluid),[2–4] and we have recently encountered such a case (Fig. 23–1). They have also been described in various inflammatory and necrotic processes in the kidney, synovium, conjunctiva and eyelid, solitary bone cyst, pleura, pericardium, omentum, breast, epididymis, fallopian tube, ovarian and extraovarian endometriosis, and nasal sinus.[2, 5–9] Liesegang rings vary greatly in size, measuring from 7 to 800 μm, and shape. They are round or oval, occasionally irregular, uniformly eosinophilic, and vary from hyaline to faintly laminated, with centers that are hollow or contain granular or amorphous material; radial striations are sometimes present.[3] The one apparent practical point is that Liesegang rings have been mistaken for parasites, particularly one or another stage of the giant kidney worm *Dioctophyma renale*.[10, 11]

Surgical pathologists have undoubtedly encountered Liesegang rings many times and in diverse lesions but have paid little or no attention to them, an example of the modified dictum of Goethe, to wit: "We recognize only what we see, we see only what we know."

HETEROTOPIC GLIAL TISSUE IN THE UTERUS

Heterotopic glial tissue is best known for its occurrence in the craniofacial region, either in the form of pure glial tissue in the nose or as a dominant component within brain heterotopia in the nasal-oropharyngeal area; such deposits are deemed to be based on developmental aberrations.[12–16] Of importance, heterotopic glial tissue in the craniofacial region can be associated with considerable fibrosis, which can obscure the diagnosis.

Vastly different in their pathogenesis are the even rarer examples of ectopic glial tissue in the uterus,[17–20] which are thought in virtually all instances to be a result of persistent localized and circumscribed growth of implanted fetal remnants after instrumentation associated with a spontaneous or elective abortion—a unique form of a fetal heterograft. Only approximately 40 cases have been recorded, most representing variably sized polypoid masses of the cervix, associated with metrorrhagia or postcoital bleeding in multiparous women, months to years after an abortion. Occasionally, similar symptoms may be present, unassociated with a grossly discernible lesion. The heterotopia, usually cervical, may be associated with similar deposits in the endometrium, or the latter may rarely occur without cervical involvement. The glia has been devoid of neurons, which are thought to degenerate, the glia

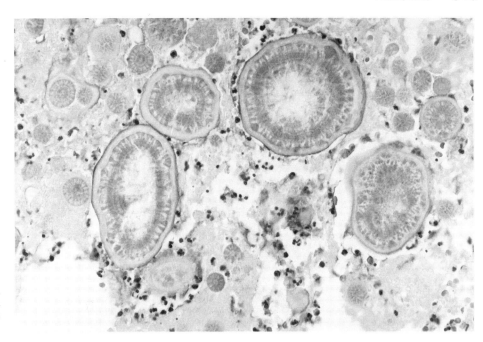

FIGURE 23-1. Liesegang rings in perirenal cyst. Note characteristic polymorphism. The prominent radial striations are an inconstant feature.

remaining because it may survive with a minimal blood supply[21] and persist because of its weak antigenicity.[18, 19] Rarely, the glia may be associated with bone, cartilage, choroid plexus, adipose tissue, and keratinizing squamous epithelium, thought to represent remnants of the fetal head, the most incompletely evacuated part during abortion.[18, 19] Only rarely have patients been asymptomatic, the heterotopia occurring as an incidental finding in uterine curettings. We have seen several such cases (Fig. 23-2), suggesting the possibility that the glial component may go unrecognized or unreported. A minority of the examples have had a negative history of sexual intercourse, but obviously, concealed pregnancies cannot be totally excluded.[18] Thus, the case of Young et al.[21] is of particular interest in that the patient was said to give a reliably negative coital history. However, as the authors point out, their case exhibited a pattern of deep infiltration, more compatible with a low-grade fibrillary astrocytoma, either possibly arising on the basis of metaplasia (neometaplasia) of mullerian origin or possibly being of teratoid origin. In the latter regard, it is pertinent to note the case of Shepherd et al.,[22] who described ectopic glia in the subcutis of the chest wall in a 2-year-old girl. Such a location similarly raises the possibility of unilateral teratoid differentiation in association with an aberration in germ cell migration.

Although glial tissue in the uterus represents a unique type of ectopy, heterotopias, in general, are due to developmental error, metaplasia, benign metastasis, or the rare emergence of a dominant (monophyletic) solitary tissue in a putative extragonadal teratoma. It should be noted that other peculiar heterotopias[23, 24] are difficult if not impossible to understand using standard pathogenetic explanations. Indeed, Kurman and Prabha[24] quote G.W. Nicholson in his account of the theories of origin in endometriosis: ''It can do us nothing but good to examine these theories and point at their shortcomings, and to humble ourselves and confess our ignorance of the true explanation.''

THECAL METAPLASIA OF THE ADRENAL

Reed and Patrick[25] and Wong and Warner[26] were among the first to report thecal metaplasia of the adrenal gland. Others have subsequently confirmed these observations.[27-29] The diagnosis is made when one finds a focus of basophilic spindle cells in the adrenal cortex, usually attached to the capsule, that closely resembles ovarian theca or more cellular variants of thecomas (Fig. 23-3).[29] Nearly all cases of thecal metaplasia of the adrenal have been found incidentally in postmenopausal women, although rare cases occur in men.[29] It has been estimated that 2.5% to 4% of adrenals from postmenopausal women may contain such tissue, if carefully sampled. The lesions are often multiple and bilateral, and as many as 10 foci have been reported in a single patient. The thecal tissues are thought to arise by metaplasia of undifferentiated but embryologically competent mesenchymal cells under the influence of certain endocrine stimuli occurring late in life. Gonadal failure appears to be important, and one 77-year-old man with thecal metaplasia also had acquired bilateral testicular atrophy. Capsular-based blastema cells, having the dual capacities for forming adrenal cortex and gonadal stroma, are retained in the adrenals as well as in the gonads in postnatal life. This occurs because the adrenals and the gonads develop in close proximity to one another during embryogenesis. Of additional interest, **granulosa–theca cell tumor, virilizing Leydig cell adenoma, and intracortical Leydig cells within an aldosterone-secreting adenoma** have been reported to occur rarely in the adrenals of women.[29a, 29b, 29c]

BENIGN PERINEURAL INVASION AND NERVE-EPITHELIAL INTERMINGLING

Until relatively recently, surgical pathologists had equated the presence of epithelial structures within the perineural space

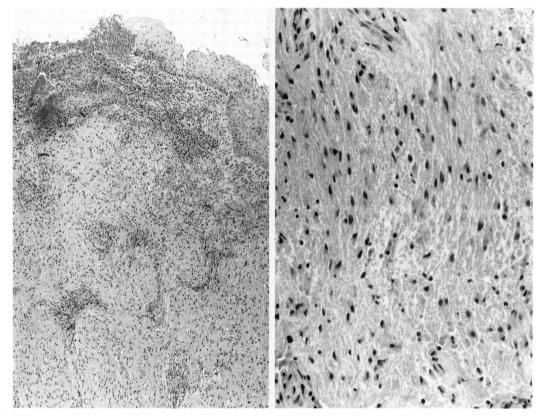

FIGURE 23–2. Uterine curettings contain, as an "incidental finding," bundles of glial tissue in a cervical segment.

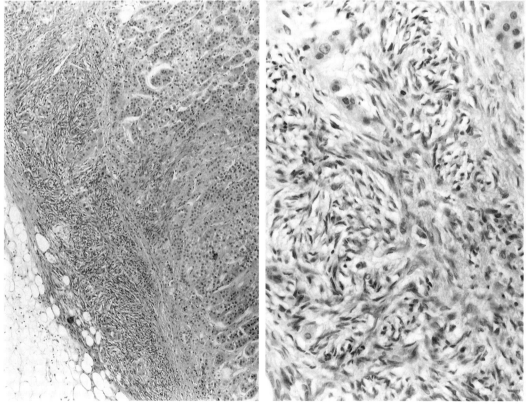

FIGURE 23–3. Adrenal with capsular and subcapsular thecal metaplasia. Entrapped cortical cells are evident.

or within nerves with carcinomatous invasion of these structures. The view that this intimate association does not always have such a sinister connotation has been established by reports that have described the presence of histologically benign epithelial neural infiltration in several organs, almost invariably in association with some type of underlying local hyperplastic lesion, usually composed of both exuberant epithelial and stromal proliferation[30-43] (Fig. 23–4). The mechanism by which benign epithelial tissue assumes the capacity to seemingly invade nerves and perineural spaces remains unknown. The usual presence, in these circumstances, of a proliferative, but similarly benign, process suggests the possibility that mechanical forces may produce displacement along tissue planes that offer paths of least resistance.[33] However, such structural intermingling has also been described in apparently normal prostatic,[36, 44] pancreatic,[37] and parotid tissue,[45] so that a mechanism involving hyperplasia of neighboring tissues in adult life may not be the only one involved. It has been suggested that all of these types of neural interactions represent an acquired[44-46] or congenital[47, 48] intermingling mediated by localized release of nerve growth factor. It should be noted that in addition to neural invasion, associated invasion of veins[38, 49, 50] and arteries[49, 50] has been documented in some instances, suggesting an intrinsic aggressive potential on the part of the epithelial conformations, implying a possible nexus between these two pathogenetic alternatives.

Neural invasion (nerve-epithelial intermingling) is not synonymous with malignancy, and it must be appreciated that histologically benign epithelial structures can be encountered in both a perineural and an intraneural location.

UNUSUALLY SITUATED PARAGANGLIA

Extra-adrenal paragangliomas, whether they are of sympathetic or parasympathetic derivation, chromaffin or non-chromaffin, and functional or non-functional, have been described in a wide variety of locations,[51-56] although the majority are located in the head, neck, and retroperitoneum. Despite this geographic ubiquity, congeneric normal paraganglionic tissue has been largely absent. It has been suggested that this inconspicuousness is attributable to the scant number and minute size of normal paraganglionic tissue[57] (Fig. 23–5). Other reasons are that they may be easily overlooked in the course of examination of histopathologic material, or that their true nature is unrecognized or, conversely that they may be overdiagnosed as primary or metastatic carcinoma. In addition to well-known sites, normal paraganglionic tissue has been described in the gallbladder,[57, 58] subcapsular splenic parenchyma,[57] mesosigmoid,[59] and prostate.[60-62] In these locations, sometimes the paraganglionic tissue has been described first, followed by reports of a paraganglioma in the organ in point, and sometimes the converse has been true.[63]

Of practical import is the misinterpretation of this "triviomatous tissue" as representing either metastatic or primary carcinoma. MacKinon and Mickels noted four cases, two clear-cell renal carcinomas and two testicular teratomas with clear-cell foci, in which groups of clear cells in sympathetic ganglia, removed as part of a retroperitoneal resection, caused difficulty and transitory misinterpretation as metastatic clear-cell carcinoma.[64] However, perhaps the most difficult differen-

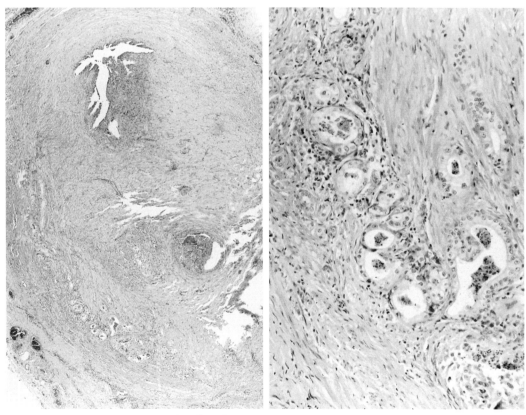

FIGURE 23–4. Vasitis nodosa. Detailed view shows benign tubules with pseudoinfiltrative pattern.

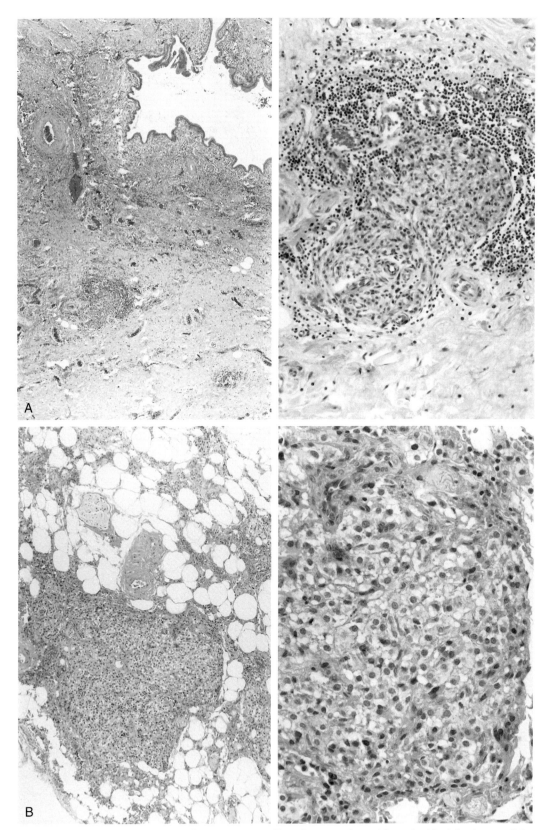

FIGURE 23–5. *A,* Gallbladder with characteristic discrete paraganglion. Cases such as this make ideal ''unknowns'' for pedantic and pedagogic purposes. *B,* Retroperitoneal paraganglion. Such structures should not be confused with metastatic carcinoma.

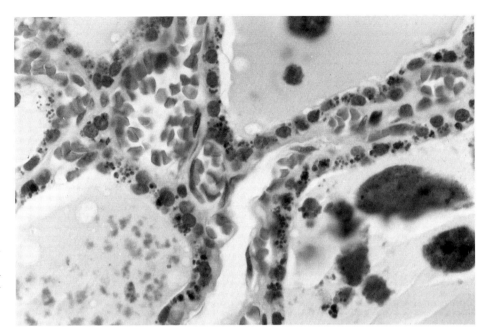

FIGURE 23–6. The black thyroid. Minocycline-induced pigment in follicular epithelium and colloid. Such deposition results in gross black discoloration but is of no functional significance. Thyroidectomy was performed for a thyroid adenoma, which was not blackened.

tial diagnosis involves distinction of prostatic paraganglia, either suburethral or subcapsular, from small acinar-solid primary adenocarcinoma of the prostate. The development of immunohistochemical techniques facilitates such differentiation, the paraganglial tissue exhibiting an affinity for neuroendocrine markers and an absence of epithelial and prostatic epithelial markers.[60] In order to recognize this differential diagnosis, one must first be aware of prostatic paraganglionic tissue and also keep in the back of his or her mind the fact that rare prostatic paraganglial and various types of neuroendocrine neoplasms[65–67] may exhibit a somewhat similar immunohistochemical profile, although such neoplasms are of sufficient morphologic dissimilarity to cause little trouble in their interpretation.[68]

THE BLACK THYROID

Finding a black thyroid gland has been associated in most cases with **chronic minocycline use,** but occasional idiopathic cases occur that are not associated with minocycline use.[69–73] Besides thyroid pigmentation, chronic minocycline administration can be associated with increased skin pigmentation, black bones, and blue-black discoloration of the substantia nigra or atherosclerotic plaques.[72] Thyroid function is normal (unless another lesion is present), and light microscopy of the black thyroid shows numerous brown granules within the cytoplasm of the otherwise normal thyroid epithelium. Also, brown deposits may be found in the colloid (Fig. 23–6). The nature of the pigment or, more likely, pigments is unclear, but it has been variably considered neuromelanin, lipofuscin, and/or a minocycline oxidation product.[72] In any event, the pigment(s) appears to be a naturally occurring degenerative product gradually accumulating in normal but "aging" thyroid epithelium. The marked accumulation seen with minocycline administration appears to be an exaggeration of this normally occurring process. Of interest, thyroid adenomas arising within a background of black thyroid are often pigment

free. Finally, before making a diagnosis of black thyroid, other causes of thyroid pigmentation must be excluded, such as **hemochromatosis** and **ochronosis**.

References

1. Liesegang RE: Uber einige Eigenschaften von Gallerton. Naturw Wochschr 11:353–362, 1896.
2. Tuur SM, Nelson AM, Gibson DW, et al: Liesegang rings in tissue. How to distinguish Liesegang rings from the giant kidney worm, *Dioctophyma renale.* Am J Surg Pathol 11:598–605, 1987.
3. Sneige N, Dekmezian RH, Silva EG, et al: Pseudoparasitic Liesegang structures in perirenal hemorrhagic cysts. Am J Clin Pathol 89:148–153, 1988.
4. Katz LB, Ehya H: Liesegang rings in renal cyst fluid. Diagn Cytopathol 6:197–200, 1990.
5. Sneige N, Batsakis JG, Hawkins RA, Doble HP II: Pseudoparasitic (Liesegang) bodies in paranasal sinus. J Laryngol Otol 102:730–732, 1988.
6. Kragel PJ, Williams J, Garvin D, Goral AB: Solitary bone cyst of the radius containing Liesegang's rings. Am J Clin Pathol 92:831–833, 1989.
7. Clement PB, Young RH, Scully RE: Liesegang rings in the female genital tract. A report of three cases. Int J Gynecol Pathol 8:271–276, 1989.
8. Boss JH, Misslevitch I: Liesegang rings in tissue [letter]. Am J Surg Pathol 13:524–525, 1989.
9. Schwartz DA, Bellin HJ: Liesegang rings developing within intraperitoneal endometriotic implants. A case report. J Reprod Med 36:403–406, 1991.
10. Fernando SSE: The giant kidney worm (*Dioctophyma renale*) infection in man in Australia. Am J Surg Pathol 7:281–284, 1983.
11. Sun T, Turnbull A, Lieberman PH, Sternberg SS: Giant kidney worm (*Dioctophyma renale*) mimicking retroperitoneal neoplasm. Am J Surg Pathol 10:508–512, 1986.
12. Knox R, Pratt M, Garvin AJ, White B: Heterotopic lingual brain in the newborn. Arch Otolaryngol Head Neck Surg 115:630–632, 1989.
13. Momose F, Hashimoto K, Shioda S: Heterotopic brain tissue in the oropharynx. Report of a case. Oral Surg Oral Med Oral Pathol 68:682–685, 1989.
14. Garcia MG, Avila CG, Arranz JSL, Garcia JG: Heterotopic brain tissue in the oral cavity. Oral Surg Oral Med Oral Pathol 66:218–222, 1988.
15. Bossen EH, Hudson WR: Oligodendroglioma arising in heterotopic brain tissue of the soft palate and nasopharynx. Am J Surg Pathol 11:571–574, 1987.
16. Wilkins RB, Hofmann RJ, Byrd WA, Font R: Heterotopic brain tissue in the orbit. Arch Ophthalmol 105:390–392, 1987.
17. Brown LJR, Wells M: Heterotopic adipose and glial tissue in the endometrium with staining for glial fibrillary acidic protein. Case report. Br J Obstet Gynaecol 93:637–639, 1986.
18. Luevano-Flores E, Sotelo J, Tena-Suck M: Glial polyp (glioma) of the uterine cervix. Report of a case with demonstration of glial fibrillary acidic protein. Gynecol Oncol 21:385–390, 1985.
19. Gronroos M, Meurman L, Kahra K: Proliferating glia and other heterotopic tissues in the uterus. Fetal homografts? Obstet Gynecol 61:261–266, 1983.
20. Nelson LM, Callicott JH Jr: Pregnancy after gliosis uteri (endometrii). JAMA 248:2311–2313, 1982.

21. Young RH, Kleinman GM, Scully RE: Glioma of the uterus. Report of a case with comments on histogenesis. Am J Surg Pathol 5:695–699, 1981.

22. Shepherd NA, Coates PJ, Brown AA: Soft tissue gliomatosis—heterotopic glial tissue in the subcutis. A case report. Histopathology 11:655–660, 1987.

23. Takahashi T, Ishikura H, Kato H, et al: Ectopic thyroid follicles in the submucosa of the duodenum. Virchows Archiv A 418:547–550, 1991.

24. Kurman RJ, Prabha C: Thyroid and parathyroid glands in the vaginal wall. Report of a case. Am J Clin Pathol 59:503–507, 1973.

25. Reed RJ, Patrick JT. Nodular hyperplasia of the adrenal cortical blastema. Bull Tulane Univ Med Fac 26:151–157, 1967.

26. Wong TW, Warner NE: Ovarian thecal metaplasia in the adrenal gland. Arch Pathol 92:319–328, 1971.

27. Fidler WJ: Ovarian thecal metaplasia in adrenal glands. Am J Clin Pathol 67:318–323, 1977.

28. Carney JA: Unusual tumefactive spindle-cell lesions in the adrenal glands. Hum Pathol 18:980–985, 1987.

29. Romberger CH, Wong TW. Thecal metaplasia in the adrenal gland of a man with acquired bilateral testicular atrophy. Arch Pathol Lab Med 113:1071–1075, 1989.

29a. Orsell RC, Bassler TJ: Theca granulosa cell tumor arising in adrenal. Cancer 31:474–477, 1973.

29b. Pollack WJ, McConnell CF, Hilton C, Lavine RL: Virilizing Leydig cell adenoma of adrenal gland. Am J Surg Pathol 10:816–822, 1986.

29c. Lack EE, Nauta RJ: Intracortical Leydig cells in a patient with an aldosterone-secreting adrenal cortical adenoma. J Urol Pathol 1:411–418, 1994.

30. Taylor HB, Norris HJ: Epithelial invasion of nerves in benign diseases of the breast. Cancer 20:2245–2249, 1967.

31. Davies JD: Neural invasion in benign mammary dysplasia. J Pathol 109:225–231, 1973.

32. Gould VE, Rogers DR, Sommers SC: Epithelial-nerve intermingling in benign breast lesions. Arch Pathol 99:596–598, 1975.

33. Goldman RL, Azzopardi JG: Benign neural invasion in vasitis nodosa. Histopathology 6:309–315, 1982.

34. Balogh K, Travis WD: The frequency of perineurial ductules in vasitis nodosa. Am J Clin Pathol 82:710–713, 1984.

35. Kiser GC, Fuchs EF, Kessler S: The significance of vasitis nodosa. J Urol 136:42–44, 1986.

36. Carstens PHB: Perineural glands in normal and hyperplastic prostates. J Urol 123:686–688, 1980.

37. Goldman RL: Benign neural invasion in chronic pancreatitis. J Clin Gastroenterol 6:41–44, 1984.

38. Cooper PH, Wolfe JT III: Perioral keratoacanthomas with extensive perineural invasion and intravenous growth. Arch Dermatol 124:1397–1401, 1988.

39. Wagner RF Jr, Cottel WI, Smoller BR, Kwan T: Perineural invasion associated with recurrent sporadic multiple self-healing squamous carcinomas [letter]. Arch Dermatol 123:1275–1276, 1987.

40. Stern JB, Stout DA: Trichofolliculoma showing perineural invasion. Trichofolliculo-carcinoma? Arch Dermatol 115:1003–1004, 1979.

41. Stern JB, Haupt HM: Reexcision perineural invasion. Not a sign of malignancy. Am J Surg Pathol 14:183–185, 1990.

42. Roth LM: Endometriosis with perineural invasion. Am J Clin Pathol 59:807–809, 1973.

43. Costa J: Benign epithelial inclusions in pancreatic nerves [letter]. Am J Clin Pathol 67:306–307, 1977.

44. Cramer SF: Benign glandular inclusion in prostatic nerve. Am J Clin Pathol 75:854–855, 1981.

45. Cramer SF, Heggeness LM: Benign glandular inclusions in parotid nerve. Am J Clin Pathol 90:220–222, 1988.

46. DeSchryver-Kecskameti K, Balogh K, Neet KE: Nerve growth factor and the concept of neural-epithelial interactions: Immunohistochemical observations in two cases of vasitis nodosa and six cases of prostatic adenocarcinoma. Arch Pathol Lab Med 111:833–835, 1987.

47. Behr MM, Gould AR, George DI Jr: Intraneural epithelial islands associated with a periapical cyst. Oral Surg Oral Med Oral Pathol 57:58–62, 1984.

48. Perrone T: Vessel-nerve intermingling in benign infantile hemangioendothelioma [letter]. Hum Pathol 16:198, 1985.

49. Balogh K, Travis WD: Benign vascular invasion in vasitis nodosa. Am J Clin Pathol 83:426–430, 1985.

50. Azzopardi JG: Problems in Breast Pathology. Philadelphia, WB Saunders, 1979, pp 172–174.

51. Badalament RA, Kenworthy P, Pelligrini A, Drago JR: Paraganglioma of urethra. Urology 38:76–78, 1991.

52. Bacchi CE, Schmidt RA, Brandao M, et al: Paraganglioma of the spermatic cord. Report of a case with immunohistochemical and ultrastructural studies. Arch Pathol Lab Med 114:899–901, 1990.

53. Hitanant S, Sriumpi S, Na-sangkla S, et al: Paraganglioma of the common hepatic duct. Am J Gastroenterol 79:485–488, 1984.

54. Young RW, Thrasher TV: Nonchromaffin paraganglioma of the uterus. A case report. Arch Pathol Lab Med 106:608–609, 1982.

55. Freschi M, Sassi I: Paraganglioma della colecisti. Pathologica 82:459–463, 1990.

56. Miller TA, Weber TR, Appleman HD: Paraganglioma of the gallbladder. Arch Surg 105:637–639, 1972.

57. Kuo TT, Anderson CB, Rosai J: Normal paraganglia in human gallbladder. Arch Pathol 97:46–47, 1974.

58. McDonald EC: Nonneoplastic paraganglionic tissue in the gallbladder wall. J Tenn Med Assoc 83:225–226, 1990.

59. Freedman SR, Goldman RL: Normal paraganglion in the mesosigmoid. Hum Pathol 12:1037–1038, 1981.

60. Rode J, Bentley A, Parkinson C: Paraganglial cells of urinary bladder and prostate. Potential diagnostic problem. J Clin Pathol 43:13–16, 1990.

61. Blessing MH, Lehman HD, Dahl M: Sog Glomera in Bereich der Prostata. Urologe (A) 22:270–273, 1983.

62. Freedman SR, Goldman RL: Normal paraganglia in the human prostate. J Urol 113:874–875, 1975.

63. Goldman RL: Unusually situated paragangliomas [letter]. Am J Surg Pathol 1:279, 1977.

64. MacKinon J, Mickels J: Paraganglion cells mimicking clear cell carcinoma. Histopathology 3:459–465, 1979.

65. Voges GE, Wipperman F, Duber C, Hohenfellner R: Pheochromocytoma in the pediatric age group. The prostate—an unusual location. J Urol 144:1219–1221, 1990.

66. diSant'Agnese PA: Neuroendocrine differentiation and prostatic carcinoma. The concept ''comes of age.'' Arch Pathol Lab Med 112:1097–1099, 1988.

67. diSant'Agnese PA: Neuroendocrine differentiation in human prostatic carcinoma. Hum Pathol 23:287–296, 1992.

68. Ostrowski ML, Wheeler TM: Paraganglia of the prostate: Location, frequency, and differentiation from prostatic adenocarcinoma. Am J Surg Pathol 18:412–420, 1994.

69. Gordon G, Sparano BM, Kramer AW, et al: Thyroid gland pigmentation and minocycline therapy. Am J Pathol 117:98–109, 1984.

70. Alexander CB, Herrera GA, Jaffe K, Yu H: Black thyroid: Clinical manifestations, ultrastructural findings, and possible mechanisms. Hum Pathol 16:72–78, 1985.

71. Ohaki Y, Misugi K, Hasegawa H: ''Black thyroid'' associated with minocycline therapy. A report of an autopsy case and review of the literature. Acta Pathol Jpn 36:1367–1375, 1986.

72. Landas SK, Schelper RL, Tio FO, et al: Black thyroid syndrome: Exaggeration of a normal process. Am J Clin Pathol 85:411–418, 1986.

73. Rumbak MJ, Pitcock JA, Palmieri GMA, Robertson JT: Black bones following long-term minocycline treatment. Arch Pathol Lab Med 115:939–941, 1991.

Index

Note: Page numbers in *italics* refer to illustrations; page numbers followed by t refer to tables.

A

Abortive rosette(s), in malignant peripheral neuroectodermal tumor, 683–684, *686*

Abortus, hydropic, 559, *560–561*, 562t

Acidophilic rhabdomyoblast(s), vs. epithelioid sarcoma, *698*

Acinar cell carcinoma, pancreatic, 275–276, *275–276*
  vs. pancreatic endocrine tumors, 272

Acinar cell cystadenocarcinoma, pancreatic, 276

Acinic cell carcinoma, 45–47, *46*
  papillary-cystic, vs. intestinal-type adenocarcinoma of head and neck, 80–81
  pulmonary, 108–110, *110*

ACIS (adenocarcinoma in situ), cervical, 549, 550, *550–551*

Acoustic neuroma(s), vs. adenomatous tumors of middle ear, 86

Acquired immunodeficiency syndrome (AIDS), cystic lymphoid hyperplasia in, vs. benign lymphoepithelial cysts, 84
  enteropathy in, 213–214, *214*
  liver disease in, 296–298
  lymphadenopathy in, 829–830
  with progressive multifocal leukoencephalopathy, 883–884, *883–884*

Acral lentiginous melanoma, vulvar, 537

Actinomycosis, colonic, 228–229

Acute lymphoblastic leukemia (ALL), 849–850

Acute promyelocytic leukemia (APL), 850

Addison's disease, and autoimmune oophoritis, 458

Adenocanthoma(s), colonic, 245
  esophageal, *181*, 181–182

Adenocarcinoma, adrenal, vs. adenomatoid adrenal tumors, 404
  basal cell, of salivary glands, 28, *28*
  cervical, 549–555. See also *Cervical adenocarcinoma.*
  endometrial. See also *Endometrial adenocarcinoma.*
  enteric-type, sinonasal, 80–81, *82*
  fetal, 102–103, *102–103*
  hepatic, vs. hepatocellular tumors, 300–301
  in small intestine, 214
  intestinal-type, nasopharyngeal, 80–81, *82*
  low-grade, polymorphous, of salivary glands, 47, *48–49*
  melanotic, anorectal, 245

Adenocarcinoma (*Continued*)
  microacinar, of prostate, vs. adenomatous hyperplasia, 347, *348–349*
    vs. sclerosing adenosis, 346–347, *346–347*
  mucinous, colonic, 243, *244*
    vs. appendiceal mucocele, 233
    vs. colitis cystica profunda, 225
  of appendix, *250*, 250–251
  of bladder, clear-cell, vs. nephrogenic adenoma, 337–338, *339*
    vs. cystitis cystica, 334–337, *336–338*
  of gallbladder, 309–310
    vs. xanthogranulomatous cholecystitis, 308
  pulmonary, vs. adenoid cystic carcinoma, 106–107
    vs. mesothelioma, 4t
  vaginal, vs. clear-cell carcinoma, 542
  vs. gestational choriocarcinoma, 585

Adenofibroma(s), clear-cell, ovarian, 439
  mullerian, stromal and epithelial components of, 514t
  ovarian, vs. clear-cell ovarian carcinoma, 441, *441–442*
  papillary, cervical, vs. villoglandular cervical adenocarcinoma, 554
  pulmonary, *135*, 137
  uterine, vs. adenosarcoma, 508, *509*, 511t

Adenoid cystic carcinoma, esophageal, 180–181
  of breast, vs. collagenous spherulosis, 640, *641*
  of prostate, vs. basal cell adenoma/hyperplasia, 350, *353*
  of salivary glands, 28–29, *29–30*
    vs. polymorphous low-grade adenocarcinoma, 47
  pulmonary, 106–107, *106–107*
  vs. thymoma, 144, *147*

Adenoid formation(s), in glioblastoma, 890–891

Adenoid pattern, thymoma with, *144*

Adenoma(s), adrenal, vs. adrenal cortical carcinoma, 383t–384t, 383–384
    vs. incidental cortical nodules, 377
  adrenal cortical, 377–379, *378–379*
    vs. myelolipoma, 400
  alveolar, *133*, 133–134
  canalicular, vs. basal cell tumors of salivary glands, 29, *31*

Adenoma(s) (*Continued*)
  colonic, flat, *235*, 235–236
    goblet cell–rich, vs. hyperplastic-adenomatous colonic polyps, 240
    serrated, *241*
    vs. dysplastic idiopathic inflammatory bowel disease, 241
    with invasive carcinoma, 241–243, *243*
  ductal, of breast, vs. sclerosing papillary proliferations, 633–634, *634*
  eccrine, papillary, vs. microcystic adnexal carcinoma, 781
  esophageal, 177
  follicular, of thyroid, with follicular papillary carcinoma, 72, *72*
  gastric, 197–198, *199*
  hepatocellular, 302t, 303–304
  lactating, vs. lobular carcinoma in situ, 649, *650*
  Leydig cell, adrenal, 400
  mucinous, vs. appendiceal mucocele, 233, *234*
  mucous gland, pulmonary, *134–135*, 136–137
  nephrogenic, of bladder, vs. clear-cell adenocarcinoma, 337–338, *338*
  of breast, pleomorphic, 659, *661*
    tubular, vs. pseudoangiomatous hyperplasia of mammary stroma, 639, *639*
  of nipple ducts, vs. salivary/sweat gland–like breast tumors, 660
  of parathyroid, 174
  of salivary glands, monomorphic, 25–31, *25–32*
    pleomorphic, 25–31, *26–32*
    vs. basal cell tumors of salivary glands, 29, *30*
    vs. epithelial-myoepithelial carcinoma, 49
    vs. polymorphous low-grade adenocarcinoma, 47
  pancreatic, glycogen-rich, *263*, 263–264
  renal cortical, 321–324, *323–324*
  syringomatous, of nipple, 659, *661*

Adenomatoid odontogenic tumor(s), vs. ameloblastoma, 14

Adenomatoid tumor(s), adrenal, 403–404, *404*
  endometrial, 469, *473*
  myometrial, 522, *523*
  of fallopian tubes, vs. carcinoma, 518

Adenomatous hyperplasia, of prostate, vs. microacinar adenocarcinoma, 347, *348–349*

Adenomatous polyposis, familial, 235

919

G

ISBN 0-7216-6464-4

90038

9 780721 664644